SAUNDERS

Comprehensive
Review for
NCLEX-RN

SAUNDERS
Comprehensive
Review for
NCLEX-RN

Linda Anne Silvestri, MSN, RN

Assistant Professor of Nursing
Clinical Coordinator, Nursing Program
Salve Regina University
Newport, Rhode Island

President
Professional Nursing Seminars, Inc.
Charlestown, Rhode Island

W.B. Saunders Company
A *Harcourt Health Sciences Company*
Philadelphia   London   New York   St. Louis   Sydney   Toronto

W.B. SAUNDERS COMPANY
A *Harcourt Health Sciences Company*

The Curtis Center
Independence Square West
Philadelphia, Pennsylvania 19106

Library of Congress Cataloging-in-Publication Data

Saunders comprehensive review for NCLEX-RN / Linda Anne Silvestri.

p.   cm.

ISBN 0–7216–7795–9

1. Nursing—Examinations, questions, etc.   I. Title.
  [DNLM: 1. Nursing Care examination questions.   2. Nursing Process
  examination questions.   WY 18.2 S587s 1999]

RT55.S484 1999   610.73′076—dc21

DNLM/DLC   98–3399

SAUNDERS COMPREHENSIVE REVIEW FOR NCLEX-RN   ISBN 0–7216–7795–9

Printed in the United States of America.

Last digit is the print number: 9   8   7   6   5   4

To my parents,

To my mother, Frances Mary, and in loving memory of my father, Arnold Lawrence, who taught me to always love, care, and be the best that I could be.

NOTICE

Nursing is an ever-changing field. Standard safety precautions must be followed, but as new research and clinical experience broaden our knowledge, changes in treatment and drug therapy become necessary or appropriate. Readers are advised to check the product information currently provided by the manufacturer of each drug to be administered to verify the recommended dose, the method and duration of administration, and the contraindications. It is the responsibility of the treating physician, relying on experience and knowledge of the patient, to determine dosages and the best treatment for the patient. Neither the publisher nor the editor assumes any responsibility for any injury and/or damage to persons or property.

THE PUBLISHER

About the Author

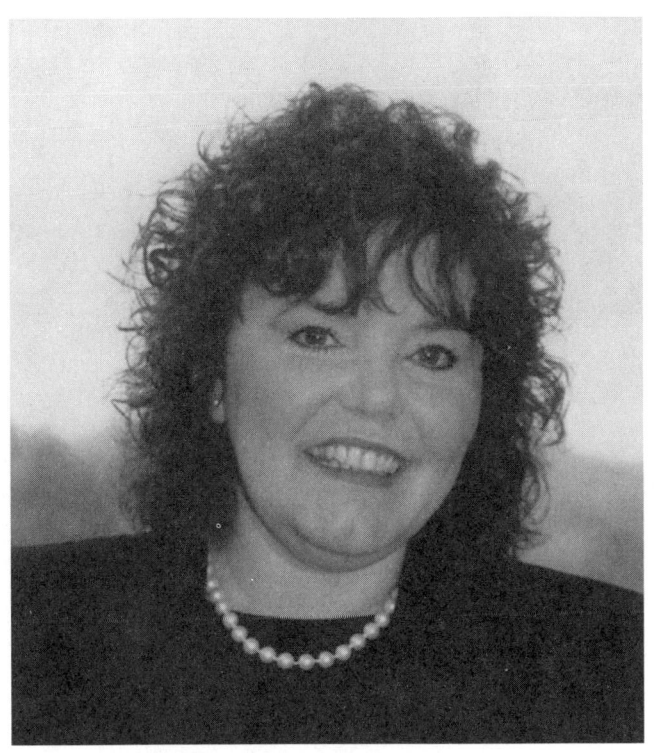

Linda Anne Silvestri received her diploma in nursing at Cooley Dickinson Hospital School of Nursing in Northampton, Massachusetts. Afterwards, she worked at Baystate Medical Center in the trauma center and in the pediatric and acute care units. She later received her BSN from American International College in Springfield, Massachusetts.

A native of Springfield, Massachusetts, Linda began her teaching career as an instructor of medical-surgical nursing and leadership-management nursing at Baystate Medical Center School of Nursing in 1981. In 1985, she earned her MSN from Anna Maria College, Paxton, Massachusetts, with a dual major in Nursing Management and Patient Education.

Linda moved to Rhode Island in 1989 and began teaching advanced medical-surgical nursing and psychiatric nursing to RN and LPN students at the Community College of Rhode Island. While teaching at the Community College of Rhode Island, a group of students approached Linda, asking her to help them prepare for the NCLEX. Based on her past experience as an NCLEX item writer, she developed a comprehensive review course and hired faculty from the University of Rhode Island, Community College of Rhode Island, and Rhode Island College to teach specific clinical areas for the courses.

In 1991, Linda established Professional Nursing Seminars, Inc., dedicated to conducting NCLEX-RN review courses and assisting nursing graduates to achieve their goals of becoming Registered Nurses. The next year, her company began conducting NCLEX-PN review courses. During 1994, she was courted by Salve Regina University in Newport, Rhode Island, to conduct review courses for their program. Later that same year, Salve Regina University invited her to work as an Assistant Professor and Clinical Coordinator of the Nursing Program, where she teaches in the areas of acute care, community and family health, and NCLEX review. She is currently matriculated at the University of Rhode Island in the PhD in Nursing Program.

Today, Linda Silvestri's company conducts NCLEX review courses throughout New England. She is the successful author of numerous NCLEX-RN and NCLEX-PN review products, including *Saunders Comprehensive Review for NCLEX-RN, Saunders Q&A Review for NCLEX-RN, Saunders Computerized AssessTest for NCLEX-RN,* and *Saunders Instructor's Resource Package for NCLEX-RN.*

Contributors

Marion G. Anema, PhD, RN
Dean, Nursing Program, Professor of Nursing, Tennessee State University, Nashville, Tennessee

Marianne P. Barba, MS, RN
Associate Professor of Nursing, Salve Regina University, Newport, Rhode Island

Carole A. Baxter, EdD, RN
Vice President for Academic Affairs, Lancaster Institute for Health Education, Lancaster, Pennsylvania

Eloise M. Brotzman, MSEd, MSN, RN
Nursing Instructor, St. Luke's School of Nursing, Bethlehem, Pennsylvania

Reitha Cabaniss, MSN, RN
Nursing Faculty, Bevill State Community College, Sumiton, Alabama

Darlene Nebel Cantu, MSN, RNC
Assistant Director, School of Professional Nursing, Baptist Health System, San Antonio, Texas

Shannon Irene Chase, RN
Student, Department of Nursing, Salve Regina University, Newport, Rhode Island

Jane Anne Claffy, MSN, RNC
Nursing Instructor, Saint Vincent Hospital School of Nursing, New York, New York

Alice D. Coomes, MSN, RN
Assistant Professor of Nursing, Kentucky Wesleyan College, Owensboro, Kentucky

Gloria Coschigano, MSN, RN, CS
Assistant Professor of Nursing, Westchester Community College, Valhalla, New York

Jean W. Davis, MS, RN, CS
Assistant Professor of Nursing, Barry University School of Nursing, Miami Shores, Florida

Jean DeCoffe, MSN, RN
Assistant Professor of Nursing, Salve Regina University, Newport, Rhode Island

Carole A. Devine, MSN, RN
Associate Professor of Nursing, Community College of Rhode Island, Newport, Rhode Island

Kerry H. Fater, PhD, RN, CS
Associate Professor of Nursing, University of Massachusetts-Dartmouth, North Dartmouth, Massachusetts

Ginette G. Ferszt, MSN, RN, CS
Nursing Faculty, University of Rhode Island, College of Nursing, Kingston, Rhode Island

Cathy Fortenbaugh, MSN, RN, AOCN, CNS, C
Nurse Educator, Helene Fuld School of Nursing, Trenton, New Jersey

Jane H. Freeman, EDD, RN
Associate Professor of Nursing, Jacksonville State University, Jacksonville, Alabama

Rita S. Glazebrook, PhD, RNC
Associate Professor of Nursing, St. Olaf College, Northfield, Minnesota

Joyce Hammer, MSN, RN
Lecturer of Nursing, Wayne State University, Detroit, Michigan

Jacqueline Lynne Harris, MN, SC, RN, ONC
Assistant Professor, Harding University, Searcy, Arkansas

Mary Ann Hogan, MSN, RN
Medical-Surgical Level Coordinator, Baystate Medical Center School of Nursing, Springfield, Massachusetts

Mary Kathleen Jackson, BSN, RN
Instructor of Nursing, Southeastern Community College, Whiteville, North Carolina

Gail M. Johnson, EdD, MSN, RN
Nursing Faculty, Helene Fuld School of Nursing, Trenton, New Jesey

Katherine Theresa Jorgensen, MSN, RN
Assistant Professor of Nursing, University of South Dakota, Vermillion, South Dakota

Teresa Leonard, MSN, RN, CCRN, RN
Assistant Professor of Nursing, University of North Alabama, Florence, Alabama

Carol O. Long, PhD, RN

Assistant Professor of Nursing, Arizona State University, Tempe, Arizona

Marilyn Lusk, MSN, MS, RN

Nursing Faculty, Mohave Community College, Kingman, Arizona

Elisa Mangosing Lemmon, MSN, RN, C

Program Coordinator, Riverside School of Professional Nursing, Newport News, Virginia

Linda Ann Martin, MSN, RN, CS

Faculty Coordinator, St. Francis Medical Center School of Nursing, Trenton, New Jersey

Dorothy Mae Mathers, MSN, RN

Assistant Professor of Nursing, Pennsylvania College of Technology, Williamsport, Pennsylvania

Jo Ann Barnes Mullaney, PhD, RN, CS

Professor of Nursing/RRN Coordinator, Salve Regina University, Newport, Rhode Island

Betsy Nield, MS, RNC

Professor of Nursing, Community College of Rhode Island, Warwick, Rhode Island

Patricia A. Parsons, MSN, RN

Director of Nursing, Riverland Community College, Austin, Minnesota

Elizabeth Phillip, MSN, RN

Nursing Faculty, St. Luke's School of Nursing, Bethlehem, Pennsylvania

Ethel Pruden, MSN, RN

Assistant Professor of Nursing, Armstrong Atlantic State University, Savannah, Georgia

Marion Sawyier, MSN, RN

Faculty at Albuquerque Technical-Vocational Institute, Albuquerque, New Mexico

Nancy Schlapman, PhD, RN

Coordinator of the Baccalaureate Nursing Program, Indiana University, Kokomo, Indiana

Jane Schlickau, MN, RN, ARNP/CNS

Associate Professor of Nursing, Southwestern College, Winfield, Kansas

Shellie Simons, MS, RN

Chairperson, Division of Nursing, Roxbury Community College, Boston, Massachusetts

Marian I. Stewart, MSN, RN

Associate Professor of Nursing, Level II Coordinator, Motlow State Community College, Tullahoma, Tennessee

Lynn Tesh, MSN, RN

Departmental Chair, Health Occupations and Human Services, Randolph Community College, Asheboro, North Carolina

Laurent W. Valliere, BS

Vice President, Professional Nursing Seminars, Inc., Charlestown, Rhode Island; Area Manager, Training Services, Henkels & McCoy, Inc., Blue Bell, Pennsylvania

Cheryl J. Vitacco-Grab, MSN, RNC

Instructor of Nursing, Lancaster Institute for Health Education, Lancaster, Pennsylvania

Loretta A. Wack, MSN, CRRN, FNP, CPNP

Associate Professor of Nursing, Nursing Program Coordinator, Blue Ridge Community College, Weyers Cave, Virginia

Reviewer List

Betty Nash Blevins, MSN, RN, CCRN, CS
Bluefield State College, Bluefield, West Virginia

Clara Willard Boyle, EdD, RN
Salem State College, Salem, Massachusetts

Bonita Eileen Broyles, EdD, BSN, RN
Piedmont Community College, Roxboro, North Carolina

Mary L. Centa, BA, RN, CNOR
Coordinator, Surgical Technology and Perioperative Nursing, Community College of Denver, Denver, Colorado

Captain Marla J. DeJong, MS, RN, CCRN, CEN
Wilford Hall Medical Center, Lackland Air Force Base, Texas

Lenora D. Follett, MS, RN
Assistant Professor, Department of Nursing, Pacific Union College, Angwin, California

Diane M. Ford, MS, RN, CCRN
Andrews University, Berrien Springs, Michigan

Mary Jo Gay, MSN, RN
Missouri Western State College, St. Joseph, Missouri

Susan V. Gille, PhD, RN, CS, NP-C, FNP
Missouri Western State College, St. Joseph, Missouri

Beth Hammer, MSN, RN, ANP
Zablocki Veterans Affairs Medical Center, Milwaukee, Wisconsin

Ann Putnam Johnson, EdD, RN, CS
Western Carolina University, Cullowhee, North Carolina

Brenda P. Johnson, MSN, RN
Assistant Professor, Southeast Missouri State University, Cape Girardeau, Missouri

Joyce L. Kee, MS, RN
Associate Professor Emerita, College of Nursing, University of Delaware, Newark, Delaware

Denise LeBlanc, BSCN, RN, ENC(c)
Professor, School of Health Sciences, Humber College, Toronto, Ontario

Marquita Lindsey, BSN, RNC
Caddo-Kiowa Vocational Technical School, Ft. Cobb, Oklahoma

Gene Livingston, BS, MEd, RN
Texarkana College, Texarkana, Texas

Mary Jo Melby, BS, RN
Great Plains Area Vo-Tech School, Lawton, Oklahoma

Dorothy M. Obester, PhD, RN
St. Francis College, Loretto, Pennsylvania

Beth Perdue, MSN, RN
Former Instructor, El Centro College, Dallas, Texas

Conchita Quimbo-Rader, MA, RN
Chilton Memorial Hospital, Pompton Plains, New Jersey

Mary E. Sampel, MSN, RN
Saint Louis University, St. Louis, Missouri

Janice G. Sample, MNSc, CNRN, RN
Texarkana College, Texarkana, Texas

Susan T. Sanders, MSN, RN, CNAA
Motlow State Community College, Tullahoma, Tennessee

Karen G. Tarnow, PhD, RN
School of Nursing, University of Kansas, Kansas City, Kansas

David Tilton, BSN, RN
Harrison Hospital, Bremerton, Washington

Linda G. Waite, MN, RN, CCRN
Clinical Nurse Specialist, Kaiser Permanente Medical Center, San Rafael, California

Janice S. Williams, MSN, RN, CS
Department of Nursing, Presentation College, Aberdeen, South Dakota

Marion Yavorka, MSN, RN
School of Nursing, Mercy Hospital, Pittsburgh, Pennsylvania

Student Reviewer List

Melissa D. Ball
Salve Regina University, Newport, Rhode Island

Keri A. Bourassa
Salve Regina University, Newport, Rhode Island

Judith A. Brown
Regis University, Denver, Colorado

Lori Chieka
Salve Regina University, Newport, Rhode Island

Patrick J. Driscoll
Widener University, Springfield, Pennsylvania

Melinda A. Figueiredo
Salve Regina University, Newport, Rhode Island

Michelle Hertz
Salve Regina University, Newport, Rhode Island

MaryAnn Hickey
Salve Regina University, Newport, Rhode Island

Karla Marie Klassen
The College of St. Catherine, St. Paul, Minnesota

Amanda Mandel
Salve Regina University, Newport, Rhode Island

Erica Anne Markey
Salve Regina University, Newport, Rhode Island

Amy E. Munson
Beebe Medical Center, Lewes, Delaware

Delores L. Rogers
Winston-Salem State University, Winston-Salem, North Carolina

Pamela Rosen
University of Rochester, Rochester, New York

Denise J. Servoss
Salve Regina University, Newport, Rhode Island

Nannette Tyson
Georgia Southwestern State University, Americus, Georgia

Tresa K. Vinyard
Southeast Missouri State University, Cape Girardeau, Missouri

Cindy Wilkins
Nebraska Methodist College of Nursing and Allied Health, Omaha, Nebraska

Ashley Williams
Union University, Jackson, Tennessee

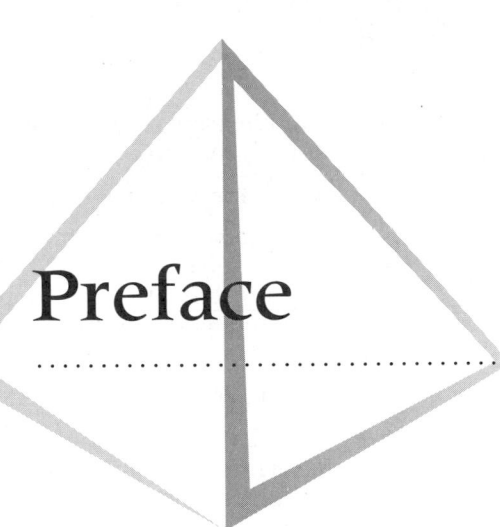

Preface

"To know that even one life has breathed easier because you have lived, this is to have succeeded."

RALPH WALDO EMERSON

Welcome to *Saunders Pyramid to Success!*

The *Saunders Comprehensive Review for NCLEX-RN* is one of a series of products designed to assist you in achieving your goal of becoming a registered nurse. The *Saunders Comprehensive Review for NCLEX-RN* will provide you with a comprehensive review of all of the nursing content areas specifically related to the new 1998 CAT NCLEX-RN test plan implemented by the National Council of State Boards of Nursing.

ORGANIZATION

The *Saunders Comprehensive Review for NCLEX-RN* contains 21 units and 75 chapters. The chapters are designed to identify specific components of nursing content. Each chapter contains practice questions reflective of the chapter content and of the 1998 CAT NCLEX-RN test plan.

The new test plan identifies a framework based on Client Needs. These Client Needs categories include Safe, Effective Care Environment; Health Promotion and Maintenance; Psychosocial Integrity; and Physiological Integrity. All of the chapters address all components of the test plan framework. However, Units I through IV include content that specifically addresses the Client Needs category, Safe, Effective Care Environment. Units V through VIII and Unit XX provide a focus on Health Promotion and Maintenance. Units IX through XVIII emphasize Physiological Integrity, and Unit XIX focuses on Psychosocial Integrity.

UNIT I: NCLEX-RN PREPARATION

Chapter 1 addresses all of the information about the 1998 CAT NCLEX-RN test plan and the testing procedures related to the examination. This chapter answers all of those questions that you may have regarding the testing procedures.

Chapter 2 discusses the issue of NCLEX-RN preparation from a nonacademic view and provides an emphasis on a holistic approach for your individual test preparation. This chapter identifies the components of a structured study plan and pattern, anxiety reduction techniques, and personal focus issues.

Nursing students want to hear what other students have to say about their experiences with NCLEX-RN. Students seek that view of what it is really like to take an NCLEX-RN examination. Chapter 3 is written by a nursing student who recently took the NCLEX-RN examination. The chapter addresses the issue of what the examination is all about and includes the student's "story of success."

Test Taking Strategies is an important component of success in taking such an important examination. Chapter 4, *Test Taking Strategies,* includes all of those important strategies that will assist in teaching you how to read a question, how not to read into a question, and how to use the process of elimination and various other strategies to select the correct response from the options presented.

UNIT II: ISSUES IN NURSING

Unit II addresses relevant nursing issues reflective of the components of the CAT NCLEX-RN test plan. Chapter 5, *Cultural Diversity,* identifies cultures and the related factors that promote maintenance of cultural identity when caring for culturally diverse clients. Chapter 6, *Ethical and Legal Issues,* provides a review of the ethical and legal considerations important to the practice of nursing and relevant to the components of the test plan. Chapter 7, *Leadership and Management Issues,* identifies issues pertinent to the practice of nursing.

UNIT III: NURSING SCIENCES

The chapters in this unit specifically address areas that students have identified as areas of concern requiring review. Chapter 8, *Fluids and Electrolytes,* and Chapter 9, *Acid-Base Balance,* highlight the key components of physiology, then introduce the necessary nursing assessments and nursing interventions required in caring for a client with an acid-base imbalance. Chapter 10, *Laboratory Values,* identifies common laboratory studies, normal values, and significant information related to the specific laboratory test.

Chapter 11, *Nutrition,* addresses the various food groups and important nutritional components of specific diet therapy. This chapter will assist in your review of the selection of the correct food or the foods to avoid with certain physiological conditions, as these type of questions are certainly addressed in the CAT NCLEX-RN test plan. Chapter 12, *Total Parenteral Nutrition (TPN),* Chapter 13, *Intravenous Therapy,* and Chapter 14, *Administration of Blood Products,* stress all of the key components of nursing care for a client. These chapters focus on the nurse's role in the administration of these therapies and in monitoring for complications.

UNIT IV: FUNDAMENTAL SKILLS

Chapter 15, *Providing a Safe Environment,* addresses nursing care specific to client safety and the measures that promote environmental safety. Chapter 16, *Administering Medication and Intravenous Solutions,* includes the important components related to conversions tables and calculations of medication dosages, intravenous (IV) solutions and flow rates, IV medications, and unit doses such as heparin and insulin. Chapter 17, *Basic Life Support,* has been included to assist you in reviewing the steps in cardiopulmonary resuscitation and the Heimlich maneuver and to refresh your memory on the priorities to be addressed in emergency situations. Chapter 18, *Perioperative Nursing Care,* addresses the key components related to caring for the client requiring surgery. Chapter 19, *Positioning Clients,* identifies safe client positions specific to various surgical and diagnostic procedures, and Chapter 20, *Care of a Client with a Tube,* addresses the various types of tubes, such as chest, gastrointestinal, or renal tubes, that have always been very confusing to students, particularly in terms of their purpose and the nursing care involved.

UNITS V THROUGH VIII: GROWTH AND DEVELOPMENT AND MATERNITY AND PEDIATRIC NURSING

Unit V, *Growth and Development Across the Life Span,* addresses the common theories of growth and development utilized in the profession of nursing. Unit VI, *Maternity Nursing,* includes chapters that address maternity issues, the care of the newborn, and maternity and newborn medications. Unit VII, *Pediatric Nursing,* and Unit VIII, *Pediatric Medications and Calculations,* focus on the components of pediatric care and the specifics related to administering medication to the child.

UNITS IX THROUGH XVIII: ADULT HEALTH

Units IX through XVIII address the components of Adult Health and are divided based on specific body systems, including the integumentary, endocrine, gastrointestinal, respiratory, cardiovascular, renal, eye and ear, neurological, and musculoskeletal system, and oncology nursing. These chapters incorporate all of the Client Needs components of the CAT NCLEX-RN test plan with a particular emphasis on Physiological Integrity. Each unit includes a pharmacology chapter that provides a comprehensive review of the medications specific to that body system.

UNIT XIV: MENTAL HEALTH NURSING

This unit primarily addresses the Psychosocial Integrity of the Client Needs component of the test plan. Specific mental health disorders are addressed. This unit includes a chapter that provides a comprehensive review of the psychiatric medications.

UNIT XX: THE GERONTOLOGICAL CLIENT

Unit XX focuses on the variations to caring for the gerontological client. This unit reviews the age-related factors and differences that the nurse needs to consider when caring for an elderly client.

UNIT XXI: COMPREHENSIVE TEST QUESTIONS

Unit XXI contains a comprehensive examination and contains practice questions related to all of the content areas addressed in this book. It consists of 300 questions representative of the percentages identified in the NCLEX-RN test plan.

SPECIAL FEATURES OF THE BOOK

PYRAMID TERMS

Each content area begins with *Pyramid Terms,* the definitions of important related terms signficant to the content contained in the chapter. Additionally, these *Pyramid Terms* are in bold type throughout the content section.

PYRAMID TO SUCCESS

The *Pyramid to Success,* a unit or chapter introduction, provides you with an overview of the chapter, guidance and direction regarding the focus of review in the particular content area, and its relative importance to the 1998 CAT NCLEX-RN test plan. Specific nursing content areas, as specified in the test plan, are identified. The *Pyramid to Success* reviews the Nursing Process and the Client Needs as they pertain to the content in that unit or chapter.

Nursing Process. The steps of the Nursing Process provide a systematic and organized method of providing care to clients. Although the 1998 CAT NCLEX-RN test plan addresses Nursing Process as an integrated concept or process in the test plan, each chapter or unit introduction provides a general nursing care plan specific to the content area. This has been incorporated to provide you with the highlights of care related to Nursing Process that you need to keep in mind as you are moving through the content area of the chapter.

Client Needs. The Client Needs are identified at the beginning of each unit or chapter. The Client Needs section identifies the significant content of the unit or chapter that is representative of the CAT NCLEX-RN test plan. These points are the specific components to keep in mind as you review the chapter outline.

PYRAMID POINTS

Pyramid Points ◆ are the bullets that are placed at specific content areas throughout the chapters. The *Pyramid Points* provide you with immediate recognition of content that is important in preparation for CAT NCLEX-RN. These bullets identify areas of content that typically appear on CAT NCLEX-RN.

PRACTICE QUESTIONS

While preparing for NCLEX-RN, it is crucial for students to practice questions. This book contains 2700 practice questions. The accompanying software includes all the questions from the book, plus an additional 600 questions for a total of 3300 test questions. Each of the 75 chapters is followed by practice questions in the NCLEX format.

The answer sections for the practice questions include the correct answer and the *Rationale* for the correct and incorrect answers. The structure of the answer section is unique and provides the following information for every question:

The rationale provides you with the significant information regarding both correct and incorrect options.

Test-Taking Strategy. The test taking strategy provides you with the logical path in selecting the correct option and assists you in selecting an answer to a question you must guess. Specific suggestions for review are identified in the test-taking strategy.

Question Categories. Each question is identified based on the categories used by the CAT NCLEX-RN test plan. Additional content categories are provided with each question to assist you in identifying areas in need of review. The categories identified with each practice question includes Level of Cognitive Ability, Phase of Nursing Process, Client Needs, and the specific nursing Content Area. All categories are identified by their full names, so that you do not need to memorize codes or abbreviations.

Reference Source. The reference source and page number is provided so you can easily find that information that you need to review in your undergraduate nursing textbooks.

PHARMACOLOGY AND MEDICATION CALCULATIONS REVIEW

Students consistently verbalize that pharmacology is an area in which they need assistance. CAT NCLEX-RN 1998 is incorporating pharmacology in the examination to a greater extent than in the past. Therefore, these chapters have been included for your review and practice. This book includes 12 pharmacology chapters, a medication and intravenous (IV) calculation chapter, and a pediatric medication calculation chapter. Each of these chapters is followed by a practice test using the same question format as described above. This book contains over 400 pharmacology questions.

NCLEX-RN REVIEW SOFTWARE

Packaged in the back of this book you will find a CD-ROM containing NCLEX-RN review software.

This software contains 3300 questions, 2700 from the book and 600 additional questions. This Windows and Macintosh compatible program offers three testing modes for review:

Quiz—10 randomly chosen questions on a specific content area. Results are provided after you answer all 10 questions.

Study—10 randomly chosen questions on a specific content area. The answer, comprehensive rationale, and test-taking strategy appear after answering each question. Results are provided after you answer all 10 questions.

Examination—100 randomly chosen questions from the entire pool of 3300 questions. Results are given and review is provided after you answer all 100 questions.

The software allows you to customize your review and determine your areas of strength and weakness. It also provides you with a wealth of practice test questions while at the same time simulating the NCLEX-RN experience on the computer.

HOW TO USE THIS BOOK

Saunders Comprehensive Review for NCLEX-RN is especially designed to help you with your successful journey to the peak of the *Saunders Pyramid to Success,* becoming a registered nurse. As you begin your journey through this book, you will be introduced to all of the important points regarding the CAT NCLEX-RN examination, the process of testing and the unique and special tips regarding how to prepare yourself for this important examination.

You should begin your process through the *Saunders Pyramid to Success* by reading all of Unit I in this book and becoming familiar with the important points regarding the CAT NCLEX-RN examination. Read the chapter from the nursing graduate who recently passed NCLEX-RN and heed what this graduate has to say about the examination. The test-taking strategy chapter will provide you with those important strategies that will guide you in selecting the correct option, or assist you in selecting an answer to a question you must guess. Read this chapter and practice these strategies as you proceed through your journey with this book. Continue your journey by reading each of the chapters and content areas. Review the Pyramid Terms, the Nursing Process, and specific components of the nursing process that are general to the content area, and identify the Client Needs specific to the test plan in that area. Read each of the content areas focusing on the Pyramid Points that identify those areas most likely to be tested on the CAT NCLEX-RN.

As you read each chapter, identify your strengths and those areas in need of further review. Highlight these areas and test your strength and ability by taking all of the practice tests provided at the end of the chapters. Be sure to read all of the rationales and test-taking strategies. The rationale provides you with significant information regarding both the correct and incorrect options. The test-taking strategy offers you the logical path to selecting the correct option. The strategy also identifies content areas that you need to review if you had difficulty answering the question. Use the reference source listed so you can easily find the information you need to review.

After reviewing all the chapters in the book, turn to Unit XXI, the Comprehensive Test. Take the examination and then review each question, answer, and rationale. Identify any areas requiring further review, then take the time to review those areas again.

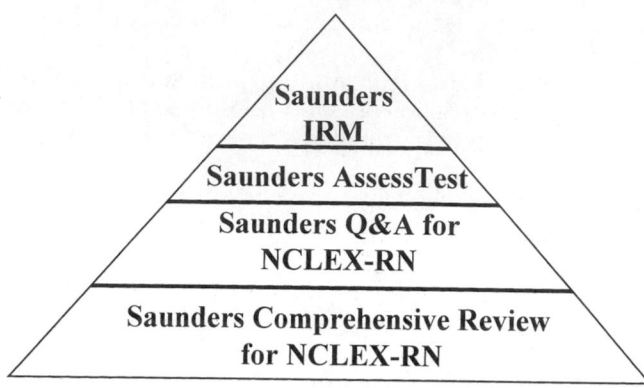

After using this book to review specific content areas, continue on your journey through the *Saunders*

Pyramid to Success with the companion book, *Saunders Q&A Review for NCLEX-RN*, for additional practice questions. The companion book and its accompanying software offer you 3450 practice questions on specific areas outlined by the 1998 CAT NCLEX-RN test plan. With practice questions uniquely focused on steps of the nursing process and categories of client needs, you can assess your level of competence on these types of questions. To determine your readiness for CAT NCLEX-RN, you will use the next step in the *Saunders Pyramid to Success*, the *Saunders Computerized AssessTest for NCLEX-RN*, which is a unique software program containing 1200 NCLEX-RN style questions. The software provides detailed analysis similar to standardized nursing examinations. The final component of the *Saunders Pyramid to Success* is the *Saunders Instructor's Resource Package for NCLEX-RN*. This manual and CD-ROM accompany the Saunders program of NCLEX-RN review products. Be sure to ask your nursing program director and nursing faculty about the CD-ROM and its use for a review course or a self-paced review in your school's computer laboratory.

Good luck with your journey through the *Saunders Pyramid to Success*. I wish you continued success throughout your new career as a Registered Nurse!

Linda Anne Silvestri, MSN, RN

To All Future Registered Nurses,

Congratulations to you!
You should be very proud and pleased with yourself on your most recent well-deserved accomplishment of completing your nursing program to become a registered nurse. I know that you have worked very hard to become successful and that you have proved to yourself that indeed you can achieve your goals.

In my opinion, you are about to enter the most wonderful and rewarding profession that exists. Your willingness, desire, and ability to assist those who need nursing care will bring great satisfaction to your life.

In the profession of nursing, your learning will be a lifelong process. This aspect of the profession makes it stimulating and dynamic. Your learning process will continue to expand and grow as the profession continues to evolve. Your next very important endeavor will be the learning process involved to achieve success in your examination to become a registered nurse.

I am excited and pleased to be able to provide you with the *Saunders Pyramid to Success* products that will prepare you for your next important professional goal, becoming a registered nurse. I want to thank all of my former nursing students that I have assisted in preparing for NCLEX-RN for their willingness to offer ideas regarding their needs in preparing for licensure. Student ideas have certainly added a special uniqueness to all of the products available in *Saunders Pyramid to Success*.

Saunders Pyramid to Success products provide you with everything that you need to prepare for NCLEX-RN. These products include material that is required for NCLEX-RN preparation for all nursing students regardless of educational background, specific strengths, areas in need of improvement, or clinical experience during the nursing program.

So, let's get started and begin our journey through the *Pyramid to Success* and welcome to the wonderful profession of nursing!

Sincerely,

Linda Anne Silvestri MSN, RN

Linda Anne Silvestri, MSN, RN

Acknowledgments

Sincere appreciation and warmest thanks are extended to the many individuals who in their own way have contributed to the publication of this book.

First, I want to thank all of my nursing students at the Community College of Rhode Island in Warwick, who approached me in 1991 and persuaded me to assist them in preparing to take the NCLEX-RN examination. Their enthusiasm and inspiration led to the commencement of my professional endeavors in conducting NCLEX-RN review courses for nursing students. I also thank the numerous nursing students who have attended my review courses for their willingness to share their needs and ideas. Their input has certainly added a special uniqueness to this publication. I wish to acknowledge all of the nursing faculty who taught in my NCLEX-RN review courses. Their commitment, dedication, and expertise has certainly assisted the nursing students in achieving success with the NCLEX-RN. Additionally, I want to acknowledge Laurent W. Valliere for his contribution to this publication, for teaching in my NCLEX-RN review courses, and for his commitment and dedication in assisting my nursing students to prepare for NCLEX-RN from a nonacademic point of view.

I would also like to acknowledge Patricia Mieg, Senior Educational Representative, who encouraged me to submit my ideas and initial work to the W. B. Saunders Company and for initiating my meeting with Maura Connor.

I sincerely acknowledge and thank Maura Connor, Senior Acquisitions Editor, for the opportunity to provide this unique and exciting comprehensive review book to all nursing students. Her commitment to facilitating nursing students in achieving success complemented my professional expectations for this publication. I thank Maura for her expert professional guidance, extraordinary support, and for her patience as I prepared this publication. Her caring and warm personality along with her energy, enthusiasm, and professional direction have certainly led me to success in the creation of this publication.

I want to acknowledge all of the staff at the W. B. Saunders Company for their tremendous assistance throughout the preparation and production of this publication. A special thank you to all of them. I would like to thank Victoria Legnini, Editorial Assistant, for her help throughout this project. Her expert organizational skills maintained order for all of the work that I submitted for manuscript production. I also thank all of the special people in the production department at W. B. Saunders Company: Jeff Gunning, Production Manager, David Saracco, Software Production Manager, Agnes Byrne, Project Supervisor, and Wynette Kommer, Copy Editor. I also had the fortunate opportunity to work with Andrea Stingelin, Director of Marketing, and Cindy Fortunato, Marketing Manager, whose support and special creativity assisted with this publication.

I want to acknowledge my parents who opened my door of opportunity in education. I thank my mother, Frances Mary, for all of her love, support, and assistance as I continuously worked to achieve my professional goals. I thank my father, Arnold Lawrence, who always provided insightful words of encouragement. My memories of his love and support will always remain in my heart.

I also thank my sister, Dianne Elodia, my brother, Lawrence Peter, and my niece, Gina Marie, who were continuously supportive, giving, and helpful during my research and preparation of this publication.

A very special thank you to Sarah Miller for her continuous support and dedication to my work and for her assistance each and every moment as I prepared my work for publication.

I want to acknowledge all of the contributors who provided many of the practice questions contained in this publication and to the many faculty and student reviewers for their thoughts and ideas. A special thank you to Dr. Jo Ann Mullaney from Salve Regina University in Newport, Rhode Island, for her numerous and expert contributions to this publication and to Shannon Chase, RN, for providing a chapter to this publication regarding her experiences with NCLEX-RN. I sincerely thank Mary Ann Hogan, MSN, RN who has always encouraged and supported me through my professional endeavors. Her numerous contributions to this publication is a reflection of her dedication to the profession of nursing and to nursing students.

I also need to thank Salve Regina University for the opportunity to educate nursing students in the baccalaureate nursing program and for its support during my research and writing of this publication. I would like to especially acknowledge Dr. Eileen Donnelly, Chairperson of the Department of Nursing at Salve Regina University, for her continuous support, academic mentoring, and astute vision regarding the future of the profession of nursing.

I wish to acknowledge the University of Rhode Island, College of Nursing, for providing me with the opportunity for professional growth in my nursing education, particularly Dr. Donna Schwartz Barcott and Dr. Suzie Kim, my academic advisors in the doctoral program at the university.

I wish to acknowledge the Community College of Rhode Island who provided me the opportunity to educate nursing students in the Associate Degree of Nursing Program, and a special thank you to Patricia Miller, MSN, RN, and Michelina McClellan, MS, RN, from Baystate Medical Center, School of Nursing, Springfield, Massachusetts, who were my very first mentors in nursing education.

Lastly, a very special thank you to all my nursing students—past, present, and future. Your love and dedication to the profession of nursing and your commitment to provide health care will bring never ending rewards!

Linda Anne Silvestri, MSN, RN

Contents

UNIT I

NCLEX-RN
Preparation

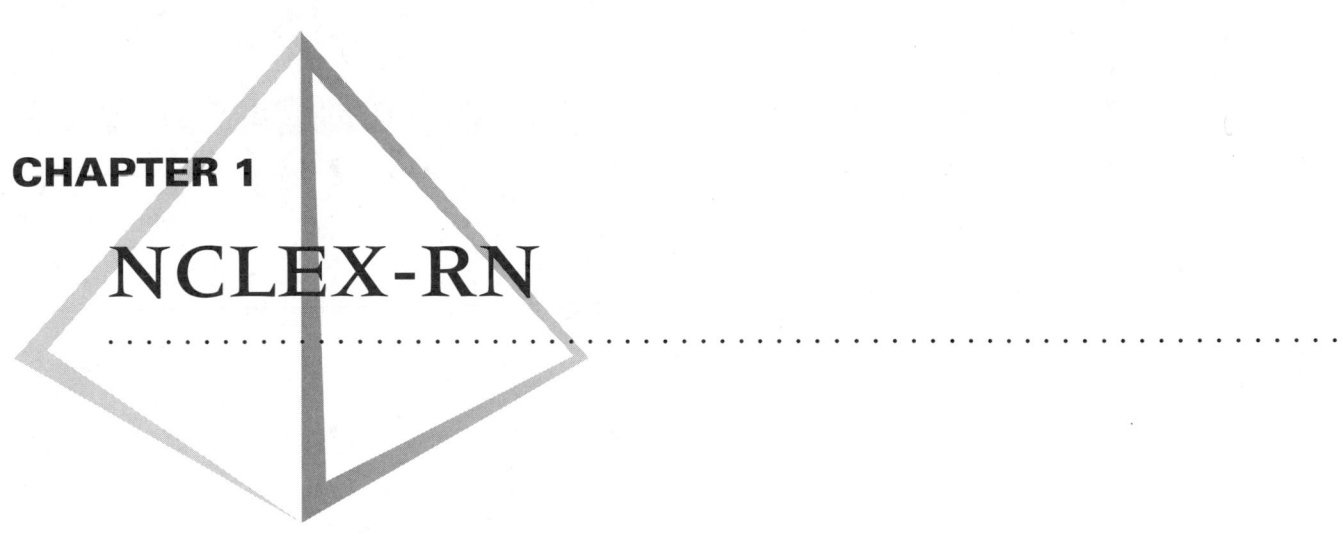

CHAPTER 1
NCLEX-RN

THE PYRAMID TO SUCCESS

Welcome to the Pyramid to Success!

Saunders Comprehensive Review for NCLEX-RN is specially designed to help you begin your successful journey to the peak of the Pyramid, becoming a Registered Nurse! As you begin your journey, you will be introduced to all the important points regarding the NCLEX-RN examination, the process of testing, and the unique and special tips regarding how to prepare yourself for this very important examination. You will read what a nursing graduate who recently passed NCLEX-RN has to say about the examination. All those important Test-Taking Strategies are detailed. These details will guide you in selecting the correct option or assist you in selecting an answer to a question you must guess at.

Each of the content areas in this book begins with the Pyramid to Success. The Pyramid to Success addresses specific points related to NCLEX-RN, including the Pyramid Terms, the Nursing Process, and Client Needs. Pyramid Terms are key words that are defined and are boldfaced throughout each chapter to attract you toward those significant NCLEX points. The Nursing Process is outlined as a guide and includes the significant areas to address in a particular content area. The Client Needs area lists the related content that is a component of the NCLEX-RN.

Throughout each chapter, you will find the Pyramid Points that identify those areas most likely to be tested on NCLEX-RN. Read each content chapter and identify your strengths and those areas in need of further review. Test your strengths and abilities by taking all the practice tests provided in this book. Be sure to read all the rationales and the test-taking strategies. The rationale provides you with significant information regarding both the correct and incorrect options. The test-taking strategy provides you with the logical path to selecting the correct option. The test-taking strategy also identifies the content area to review, if required. The reference source and page number are provided so that you can easily find the information that you need to review. Each question is coded based on the Cognitive Level of Ability, the Phase of Nursing

Process, the Client Needs category, and the nursing content area.

Following the completion of your comprehensive review in this book, continue on your journey though the Pyramid to Success with the companion book, *Saunders Q & A for NCLEX-RN*, which provides you with over 3400 practice questions based on the NCLEX-RN test plan. Then, you are ready for the Saunders AssessTest, a computer disk program that contains 1200 NCLEX-RN-style questions to help you determine your readiness for NCLEX-RN.

Let's begin our journey through The Pyramid to Success!

THE EXAMINATION PROCESS

An important step in the Pyramid to Success is to become as familiar as possible with the examination process. A significant amount of anxiety can occur in candidates facing the challenge of this examination. Knowing what the examination is all about, and knowing what you will encounter during the process of testing will assist in alleviating fear and anxiety. The information contained in this chapter addresses the procedures related to the development of the NCLEX-RN Test Plan, the components of the Test Plan, and the answers to the questions most commonly asked by nursing students and graduates preparing to take the NCLEX-RN. The information related to the development of the NCLEX-RN Test Plan, the components of the Test Plan, and the testing procedures were adapted from the *Test Plan for the National Council Licensure Examination for Registered Nurses*, National Council of State Boards of Nursing, Chicago, 1997, and *The NCLEX Process*, National Council of State Boards of Nursing, Chicago, 1995.

DEVELOPMENT OF THE TEST PLAN

As an initial step in the test development process, the National Council of State Boards of Nursing considers the legal scope of nursing practice as governed by state laws and regulations, including the Nurse Practice Act. The National Council uses these laws to define the areas on NCLEX-RN that will assess the competence of candidates for nurse licensure.

The National Council of State Boards of Nursing also conducts a Job Analysis study to determine the framework for the Test Plan for NCLEX-RN. Since nursing practice continues to change, this study is conducted every 3 years. The results of this study, most recently conducted in 1996, provided the structure for the new Test Plan implemented in April of 1998.

JOB ANALYSIS STUDY

The participants of this study are selected by a stratified random sampling process. They include newly licensed registered nurses from all types of basic education programs. The participants are given a list of nursing activities and are asked how often they performed these activities in practice: this is called the frequency rating. The participants are also asked whether they could sometimes, or never, omit performing a nursing activity without having a major impact on the client's well-being. This is called the criticality rating. The participant is then asked to indicate the setting in which he or she performed the specific nursing activities. The analysis of the data obtained from this study is used in developing the framework for NCLEX-RN.

THE TEST PLAN

The content of NCLEX-RN reflects the activities that a minimally competent, newly registered nurse must be able to perform in order to provide clients with safe and effective nursing care. The questions are written to address the Levels of Cognitive Ability, Client Needs, and Integrated Concepts and Processes as identified in the Test Plan.

LEVELS OF COGNITIVE ABILITY

The NCLEX-RN examination includes questions at the cognitive levels of knowledge, comprehension, application, and analysis. Most of the questions are written at the application and analysis levels because the practice of nursing requires the application of knowledge, skills, and abilities. This means that the test taker will be required to analyze and/or apply the facts provided in the test question (Box 1–1).

CLIENT NEEDS

In the new Test Plan implemented in April 1998, the National Council of State Boards of Nursing has identified a test plan framework based on *Client Needs*. This framework was selected based on the analysis of the findings in the Job Analysis study, and because Client Needs provides a structure for defining nursing actions and competencies across all settings for all clients. The National Council of State Boards of Nursing identifies four major categories of Client Needs. These categories are further divided into subcategories, and the percentage of test questions in each subcategory is identified (Table 1–1).

BOX 1–1. Level of Cognitive Ability

The nurse is caring for a client with a T5 spinal cord injury. The client complains of a severe headache and is feeling anxious. The nurse notes the client is sweating and is bradycardic and hypertensive. Which of the following interventions is most appropriate initially?

1 Check for bladder distention
2 Notify the physician
3 Medicate the client with an analgesic
4 Discuss the client's feelings of anxiety

Answer: 1

Rationale: This question requires the test taker to analyze the data provided in order to determine the most appropriate nursing action. The test taker needs to know the signs and symptoms of autonomic dysreflexia and the potential causes, such as a full bladder or bowel. The analysis of the data provided in the question will direct the test taker to the correct option.

Level of Cognitive Ability: **Analysis**

Reference
Hartshorn, J., Sole, M.L., Lamborn, M. (1997). *Introduction to critical care nursing* (2nd ed.). Philadelphia: W.B. Saunders. p. 305.

SAFE, EFFECTIVE CARE ENVIRONMENT

The Safe, Effective Care Environment category includes two subcategories: Management of Care, and Safety and Infection Control. Management of Care (7%–13%) addresses content that tests the knowledge, skills, and ability required to provide integrated, cost-effective care to clients by coordinating, supervising, and/or collaborating with members of the multidisciplinary health care team. Safety and Infection Control (5%–11%) addresses content that tests the knowledge, skills, and ability required to protect clients and health care personnel from environmental hazards (Box 1–2).

TABLE 1–1. Client Needs and the Percentage of Test Questions

Safe, Effective Care Environment	
Management of Care	7%–13%
Safety and Infection Control	5%–11%
Health Promotion and Maintenance	
Growth and Development Through the Life Span	7%–13%
Prevention and Early Detection of Disease	5%–11%
Psychosocial Integrity	
Coping and Adaptation	5%–11%
Psychosocial Adaptation	5%–11%
Physiological Integrity	
Basic Care and Comfort	7%–13%
Pharmacological and Parenteral Therapies	5%–11%
Reduction of Risk Potential	12%–18%
Physiological Adaptation	12%–18%

BOX 1-2. Safe, Effective Care Environment

MANAGEMENT OF CARE

The charge nurse in an Intensive Care Unit observes a client who is agitated and incoherent. The nurse suspects that the client is experiencing a reaction to medication. In planning a safe environment for this client, the most appropriate intervention is to:

1 Request that the physician order restraints and sedation
2 Ask the family to stay with the client
3 Have a nurse observe the client
4 Utilize a multidisciplinary approach to plan care

Answer: 4

Rationale: This question addresses the subcategory of Management of Care, in the Client Needs category of Safe, Effective Care Environment. The nurse has the responsibility to provide safe and effective care. Options 1, 2, and 3 rely on other individuals to care for the client. Option 4 addresses an integrated, multidisciplinary health care team approach.

Reference
Gillies, D. (1994). *Nursing management: A systems approach.* Philadelphia: W.B. Saunders. pp. 114–115.

SAFETY AND INFECTION CONTROL

Which of the following nursing actions will decrease the risk for developing an infection in clients receiving total parenteral nutrition (TPN)?

1 Assessing vital signs at 4-hour intervals
2 Instructing the client to perform a Valsalva maneuver during intravenous tubing changes
3 Administering acetaminophen (Tylenol) before changing the central line dressing
4 Using aseptic technique in handling the total parenteral nutrition solution and tubing

Answer: 4

Rationale: This question addresses the subcategory of Safety and Infection Control, in the Client Needs category of Safe, Effective Care Environment. It addresses content related to Surgical Asepsis. Clients receiving total parenteral nutrition are at high risk for developing an infection. Concentrated glucose solutions are excellent media for bacterial growth. Using aseptic technique in handling all equipment and solutions is paramount to prevention. Option 1 will detect signs of an infection but is not associated with prevention. Options 2 and 3 do not relate to infection. Aseptic technique is critical to prevent infection!

Reference
Black, J., & Matassarin-Jacobs, E. (1997). *Medical-surgical nursing: Clinical management for continuity of care* (5th ed.). Philadelphia: W.B. Saunders. pp. 1754–1756.

HEALTH PROMOTION AND MAINTENANCE

The Health Promotion and Maintenance category includes two subcategories: Growth and Development Through the Life Span, and Prevention and Early Detection of Disease. Growth and Development Through the Life Span (7%–13%) addresses content that tests the knowledge, skills, and ability required to assist the client and significant others through the normal, expected stages of growth and development from conception through advanced old age. Prevention and Early Detection of Disease (5%–11%) addresses content that tests the knowledge, skills, and ability required to manage and provide care for clients in need of prevention and early detection of health problems (Box 1–3).

PSYCHOSOCIAL INTEGRITY

The Psychosocial Integrity category includes two subcategories: Coping and Adaptation and Psychosocial Adaptation. Coping and Adaptation (5%–11%) addresses content that tests the knowledge, skills, and ability required to promote the client's ability to cope, adapt, and/or problem solve situations related to illnesses or stressful events. Psychosocial Adaptation (5%–11%) addresses content that tests the knowledge, skills, and ability required to manage and provide care for clients with acute or chronic mental illnesses (Box 1–4).

PHYSIOLOGICAL INTEGRITY

The Physiological Integrity category includes four subcategories: Basic Care and Comfort, Pharmacological and Parenteral Therapies, Reduction of Risk Potential, and Physiological Adaptation. Basic Care and Comfort (7%–13%) addresses content that tests the knowledge, skills, and ability required to provide comfort and assistance in the performance of activities of daily living. Pharmacological and Parenteral Therapies (5%–11%) addresses content that tests the knowledge, skills, and ability required to manage and provide care related to the administration of medications and parenteral therapies. Reduction of Risk Potential (12%–18%) addresses content that tests the knowledge, skills, and ability required to reduce the likelihood that clients will develop complications or health problems related to existing conditions, treatments, or procedures. Physiological Adaptation (12%–18%) addresses content that tests the knowledge, skills, and ability required to manage and provide care to clients with acute, chronic, or life-threatening physical health conditions (Box 1–5).

INTEGRATED CONCEPTS AND PROCESSES OF THE TEST PLAN

The National Council of State Boards of Nursing has identified seven concepts and processes that are fundamental to the practice of nursing (Table 1-2). These concepts and processes are a component of

---

BOX 1–3. Health Promotion and Maintenance

GROWTH AND DEVELOPMENT THROUGH THE LIFE SPAN

Which of the following activities would best promote health and maintenance among older adults?
1 Gardening every day for an hour
2 Cycling three times a week for 20 minutes
3 Sculpting once a week for 40 minutes
4 Walking three to five times a week for 30 minutes

Answer: 4

Rationale: This question addresses the subcategory of Growth and Development Through the Life Span, in the Client Needs category of Health Promotion and Maintenance. Exercise and activity are essential for health promotion and maintenance in the older adult and to achieve an optimal level of functioning. One of the best exercises for an older adult is walking, progressing to 30-minute sessions three to five times each week. Swimming and dancing are also beneficial.

Reference
Black, J., & Matassarin-Jacobs, E. (1997). *Medical-surgical nursing: Clinical management for continuity of care* (5th ed.). Philadelphia: W.B. Saunders. p. 85.

PREVENTION AND EARLY DETECTION OF DISEASE

Which of the following client statements indicates an understanding of the measures that can be taken to prevent thrombophlebitis?
1 "I am taking oral contraceptives to avoid pregnancy, which can cause venous stasis."
2 "I avoid sitting or standing in one position for prolonged periods."
3 "I'm glad I don't need to wear those ugly stockings anymore."
4 "I have decreased my fluid consumption to 1 glass of water a day."

Answer: 2

Rationale: This question addresses the subcategory of Prevention and Early Detection of Disease, in the Client Needs category of Health Promotion and Maintenance. Avoidance of sitting or standing for a prolonged period of time is one of the measures for the prevention of venous stasis and thrombophlebitis. Active and passive range of motion exercises, early ambulation, and postoperative deep breathing are additional preventive measures. Taking oral contraceptives may cause hypercoagulability in some individuals. Compression stockings are used to promote venous return, maintain normal coagulability, and prevent injury to the endothelial wall. Adequate hydration is maintained to prevent hypercoagulability.

Reference
Luckmann, J. (1997). *Saunders manual of nursing care.* Philadelphia: W.B. Saunders. p. 1019.

---

the Test Plan and are incorporated throughout the categories of Client Needs.

ITEM WRITERS

NCLEX-RN item writers are selected by the National Council of State Boards of Nursing following an extensive application process. The item writers are registered nurses who are clinical experts and experienced in writing test items. Most of the item writers are nursing educators; however, clinical nurse specialists are also selected to participate in this process. These item writers voluntarily submit an application to become an item writer and must meet specific established criteria designated by the National Council in order to be accepted as a participant in the process.

CAT NCLEX-RN

The term NCLEX-RN stands for National Council Licensure Examination for Registered Nurses. CAT NCLEX-RN is a computer-administered, multiple choice examination that the nursing graduate must take and pass in order to practice as a registered nurse. This examination measures the test candidate's knowledge, skills, and abilities required to perform

safely and competently as a newly licensed, entry-level registered nurse.

COMPUTER ADAPTIVE TESTING (CAT)

The acronym CAT stands for Computer Adaptive Testing. CAT provides a uniqueness to the examination that the candidate will take, as the examination adapts to each test taker's skill level. The CAT is an examination that is assembled interactively as the candidate answers the questions. All the test questions are stored in a large test bank and are categorized based on the Test Plan structure and the level of difficulty of the question. With the CAT method of testing, an examination is created and tailored to test the candidate's knowledge and abilities while fulfilling

---

TABLE 1–2. Integrated Concepts and Processes of the Test Plan

Nursing process	Documentation
Caring	Self-care
Communication	Teaching/learning
Cultural awareness	

BOX 1–4. Psychosocial Integrity

COPING AND ADAPTATION

The hospice nurse visits a client dying of ovarian cancer. During the visit, the client says, "If I can just live long enough to attend my daughter's graduation, I'll be ready to die." Which phase of coping is this client experiencing?

1 Isolation
2 Bargaining
3 Depression
4 Acceptance

Answer: 2

Rationale: This question addresses the subcategory of Coping and Adaptation in the Client Needs category of Psychosocial Integrity. Bargaining is the phase of coping in which the dying person tries to negotiate, as in this case, making deals with God or fate. Read the client statement in the case and determine the coping mechanism that the client is expressing verbally.

Reference
Carson, V., & Arnold, E. (1996). *Mental health nursing: The nurse-patient journey.* Philadelphia: W.B. Saunders. pp. 130–131.

PSYCHOSOCIAL ADAPTATION

The visiting nurse observes that the elderly male client is confined to his room by his daughter-in-law. When the nurse suggests he walk to the den and join the family, he says, "I'm in everyone's way; my son needs for me to stay here." The most important action for the nurse to take is to:

1 Suggest to the client and daughter-in-law that they consider a nursing home for the client
2 Suggest appropriate resources to the client and daughter-in-law, such as respite care and senior citizens
3 Say nothing as it is best for the nurse to remain neutral and wait to be asked for help
4 Say to the son, "Confining your father to his room is inhuman"

Answer: 2

Rationale: This question addresses the subcategory of Psychosocial Adaptation in the Client Needs category of Psychosocial Integrity. Assisting clients and families to become knowledgeable about available community support systems is a role and responsibility of the nurse. The suggestion to commit the client to a nursing home is premature. Observing that the client has begun to be confined to his room makes it necessary for the nurse to intervene legally and ethically, so option 3 is not appropriate and is passive in terms of advocacy. Option 4 is incorrect and judgmental. Caregiver stress and burnout are thought to account for much of the abuse of elderly people.

Reference
Carson, V., & Arnold, E. (1996). *Mental health nursing: The nurse-patient journey.* Philadelphia: W.B. Saunders. pp. 1068–1073.

Test Plan requirements. The candidate will not waste time answering questions that are far above or below her or his competency level.

When you answer a question on CAT NCLEX-RN, the computer will calculate a competency skill estimate based on the answer that you selected. If you selected a correct answer to a question, the computer scans the test bank and selects a more difficult question. If you selected an incorrect answer, the computer scans the test bank and selects an easier question. This process continues until the test plan requirements are met and a reliable pass or fail decision is made.

THE PROCESS OF REGISTRATION

The initial step in the registration process is that candidates apply to the State Board of Nursing in the state in which they intend to obtain licensure. (The address and telephone numbers of Boards of Nursing in all states and territories of the United States are provided at the end of this chapter.) You need to obtain information from the Board of Nursing regarding the specific registration process, as the process may vary from state to state. It is very important that you follow the registration instructions and complete the registration forms precisely and accurately. Registration forms not properly completed, or not accompanied by the proper fees in the required method of payment, will be returned to you and will delay testing. The initial fee for the application process may vary from state to state. Each Board of Nursing will set its initial license fee according to its own needs. The registration forms will identify the registration and testing service fees. When the Board of Nursing receives the completed registration form, based on the criteria established by the Board, your eligibility is determined, and the Board authorizes your admission to the examination.

Once your eligibility to test has been determined by the Board of Nursing in the jurisdiction in which licensure is requested, the valid NCLEX registration is processed and an Authorization to Test form will be sent to you. You cannot make an appointment until the Board of Nursing declares eligibility and you receive an Authorization to Test form. The Authorization to Test form will provide a candidate identification number and an authorization number, and these numbers will be needed to make an appointment with the testing center.

SPECIAL TESTING CIRCUMSTANCES

A candidate who is requesting special accommodations should contact the Board of Nursing prior to submitting a registration form. The Board of Nursing will provide you with the procedures for the request. Testing accommodations for candidates with disabili-

BOX 1–5. Physiological Integrity

BASIC CARE AND COMFORT

The client has slight weakness in the right leg. Based on this assessment, the nurse determines that the client would benefit most from the use of a:

1 Walker
2 Wooden crutch
3 Lofstrand crutch
4 Straight leg cane

Answer: 4

Rationale: This question addresses the subcategory of Basic Care and Comfort in the Client Needs category of Physiological Integrity. A straight leg cane is useful for the client with slight weakness in one leg. A walker is beneficial to the client with greater or bilateral weakness, or who is at risk for falls. Wooden crutches are often used by clients with a leg cast. Lofstrand crutches aid clients who need crutches but have limited arm strength.

Reference
Lammon, C., Foote, A., Leli, P., et al. (1995). *Clinical nursing skills.* Philadelphia: W.B. Saunders. pp. 238–239.

PHARMACOLOGICAL AND PARENTERAL THERAPIES

The nurse is caring for a client with a diagnosis of chronic angina pectoris. The client is receiving sotalol (Betapace), 80 mg PO daily. Which of the following would indicate that the client is experiencing a side effect related to the medication?

1 Difficulty in swallowing
2 Diaphoresis
3 Dry mouth
4 Bradycardia

Answer: 4

Rationale: This question addresses the subcategory of Pharmacological and Parenteral Therapies in the Client Needs category of Physiological Integrity. Sotalol (Betapace) is a betaadrenergic blocking agent. Side effects include bradycardia, palpitations, difficulty in breathing, irregular heart beat, signs of congestive heart failure (CHF), cold hands and feet. Gastrointestinal disturbances, anxiety and nervousness, and unusual tiredness and weakness can also occur.

Reference
Hodgson, B., & Kizior, R. (1998). *Saunders nursing drug handbook 1998.* Philadelphia: W.B. Saunders. p. 940.

REDUCTION OF RISK POTENTIAL

The client with acute myocardial infarction receives therapy with al-teplase recombinant (tPA). The nurse assesses for complications of this treatment. Which assessment data would the nurse document as indicating a possible complication?

1 Epistaxis
2 Vomiting
3 ST segment elevation on ECG
4 Absent pedal pulses

Answer: 1

Rationale: This question addresses the subcategory of Reduction of Risk Potential in the Client Needs category of Physiological Integrity. Bleeding is a major side effect of tPA therapy. The bleeding can be superficial or internal and can be spontaneous. The other options do not correlate with the side effects of tPA therapy. Resolution of ST segment elevation is one of the expected results of tPA therapy.

Reference
Hodgson, B., & Kizior, R. (1998). *Saunders nursing drug handbook 1998.* Philadelphia: W.B. Saunders. p. 1098.

PHYSIOLOGICAL ADAPTATION

The nurse reviews the blood gas results of a client with Guillain-Barré syndrome. The nurse analyzes the results and determines that the client is experiencing respiratory acidosis. Which of the following validates the nurse's findings?

1 pH 7.40, P_{CO_2} 52 mmHg
2 pH 7.35, P_{CO_2} 40 mmHg
3 pH 7.25, P_{CO_2} 50 mmHg
4 pH 7.50, P_{CO_2} 30 mmHg

Answer: 3

Rationale: This question addresses the subcategory of Physiological Adaptation in the Client Needs category of Physiological Integrity. The normal pH is 7.35 to 7.45. The normal P_{CO_2} is 35 to 45 mmHg. In respiratory acidosis, the pH is down and the P_{CO_2} is up. Remember that in a respiratory imbalance you will find an opposite response between the pH and the P_{CO_2}. Also remember that the pH is down in an acidotic condition. Options 1 and 4 reflect an elevated pH, which indicates an alkalotic condition. Option 2 reflects a normal blood gas result. Option 3 is the only option that reflects an acidotic condition.

Reference
Black, J., & Matassarin-Jacobs, E. (1997). *Medical-surgical nursing: Clinical management for continuity of care* (5th ed.). Philadelphia: W.B. Saunders. p. 334.

ties must be authorized by the Board of Nursing. Following Board of Nursing approval, the National Council of State Boards reviews the requested accommodations to assure that the proposed modification does not affect the psychometric properties of NCLEX or cause a security risk.

MAKING AN APPOINTMENT TO TEST

The CAT NCLEX-RN examination is administered on a year-round basis. You will be provided with a list of testing centers and their telephone numbers. Note the expiration date on the Authorization to Test form. You must schedule and make an appointment prior to this expiration date. You may take the test at any approved testing center and do not have to test in the same jurisdiction in which you are seeking licensure. An eligible candidate taking NCLEX for the first time will be offered an appointment date within 30 days of the telephone call to the testing center. Repeat candidates will be offered an appointment date within 45 days of the telephone call to the testing center. A confirmation notice will not be sent to you, therefore it is important to note the date and time of the appointment. When you call the test center, it is also important to verify the address and the directions to the testing center.

CANCELING OR RESCHEDULING AN APPOINTMENT

If for any reason you need to cancel your appointment to test, remember that three business days' (Monday through Saturday) notice is required. The original appointment must be canceled before a new appointment can be scheduled.

LATE ARRIVALS TO THE TEST CENTER

It is important that you arrive at the testing center 30 minutes before the test is scheduled. Candidates arriving late for the scheduled testing appointment may be required to forfeit the NCLEX appointment. If it is necessary for the appointment to be forfeited, candidates will need to re-register for the examination and pay an additional fee. The Board of Nursing will be notified that the candidate will not test.

A few days prior to your scheduled date of testing, take the time to drive to the testing center to determine its exact location, the length of time required to arrive to that destination, and any potential obstacles that might delay you, such as road construction, traffic, or parking sites.

THE TESTING CENTER

The test center is designed to ensure complete security of the testing process. Strict candidate identification requirements have been established. To be admitted to the testing center, it is imperative that you bring the Authorization to Test form, along with two forms of identification. Both forms of identification must be signed by you, and one must contain your photograph. The name on the photograph identification must bear the same name as stated on the Authorization to Test form. Examples of acceptable forms of identification will be included in the information received with the Authorization to Test form. You will be required to sign in and out on the test center log form. Each candidate will be thumbprinted and photographed at the test center, and the photograph will accompany the NCLEX results to confirm the candidate's identity. Personal belongings are not allowed in the testing room. Secure storage will be provided for the candidate; however, storage space is small so you must plan accordingly. In addition, the testing center will not assume responsibility for your personal belongings. The testing waiting areas are generally small, therefore friends or family members who accompany you are not permitted to wait in the testing center while you are taking the NCLEX-RN.

Once you have completed the admission process and a brief orientation, the proctor will escort you to the assigned computer. You will be seated at an individual table, with an appropriate work space that includes computer equipment, appropriate lighting, scratch paper, and a pencil. Unauthorized scratch paper may not be brought into or removed from the testing room. Eating, drinking, and smoking are not allowed in the testing room. A video camera is located in the testing room, and full sound and motion videotaping of all test sessions occurs.

Keep your two forms of identification with you at all times. You cannot leave the testing room without the permission of the proctor. If you leave the testing room for any reason, you will be required to show two forms of identification to be readmitted. You must follow the directions given by the test center staff and must remain in your seat during the test, except when authorized to leave. If you feel that you have a problem with the computer, need more scratch paper, or need the proctor for any reason, you must raise your hand to notify the proctor.

THE COMPUTER

You do not need any computer experience to take a CAT NCLEX-RN examination. Only two computer keys are needed to take the CAT examination, the space bar and the enter key. The space bar key will allow you to scroll the options, and the enter key will allow you to highlight and select an answer. The enter key must be struck twice to record the answer choice and to proceed to the next question. A key board tutorial is provided and administered to all test takers prior to the start of the examination. In addition, a proctor is present to assist in explaining the use of the computer to assure your full understanding of how to proceed.

CAT NCLEX-RN TEST QUESTIONS

The examination is composed of individual, or "stand alone," test questions. This means that there is no case situation to accompany the question. With this type of question, you can expect that the question

---

BOX 1–6.   Appearance of an Individual Test Item on the Computer Screen

The most appropriate method for feeding the infant with cleft lip or palate is:	•1 With the head in an upright position 2 With the infant in a lying position 3 With the infant in a side-lying position 4 With the infant prone

The client is admitted with a diagnosis of myasthenia gravis. Pyridostigmine (Mestinon) is prescribed for the client. An adverse effect of this medication is:

1 Muscle cramps
2 Mouth ulcers
3 Depression
4 Unexplained weight gain

---

will appear on the lefthand side of the screen with the four responses on the righthand side of the screen or the question appears across the top of the screen with the four responses below (Box 1–6).

You must answer the test question presented on the computer screen or the test will not move on. This means that you will not be able to skip questions, go back and review questions, or go back and change answers. Students preparing for CAT NCLEX-RN become anxious and frustrated because questions cannot be skipped and returned to at a later time during the examination process. Remember, in a CAT examination, once an answer is recorded, all subsequent answers administered depend, to an extent, on the response selected for that question. Skipping and returning to earlier questions is not compatible with the logical methodology of a computerized adaptive test. Additionally, it is important to recall the number of times you may have changed a correct answer to an incorrect one on a pencil and paper nursing examination during your nursing education. The inability to skip questions or go back to change previous answers will not disadvantage you. Actually, you will not fall into that "trap" of changing a correct answer to an incorrect one with CAT. There is no penalty for guessing on CAT NCLEX-RN. Remember, the answer to the question will be right there in front of you. If you need to guess, utilize your nursing knowledge to its fullest extent, as well as all the test-taking strategies provided to you in Chapter 4 of this book.

TESTING TIME

The maximum testing time will be 5 hours, including the short keyboard tutorial and any rest breaks. There is no minimum amount of examination time. A mandatory 10-minute break will be taken after 2 testing hours, and an optional 10-minute break can be taken at the end of 3.5 hours of testing time. The computer screen will notify you of the time for these breaks. You must leave the testing room during breaks. You may leave the room for additional unscheduled breaks, but no additional testing time will be allowed.

LENGTH OF THE EXAMINATION

The minimum number of questions that you may need to answer in order to meet adequate testing in each area of the test plan is 75. Sixty of these questions will be real (scored) questions, and 15 of these questions will be try-out (unscored) questions. The maximum number of questions you may need to answer will be 265. Again, of these 265 questions, 15 will be try-out (unscored) questions. The try-out questions are not identified as such. In other words, you do not know which questions are the unscored questions.

COMPLETING THE EXAMINATION

Once the test is completed, you will complete a brief computer-delivered questionnaire about your testing experience. After this questionnaire is completed, the test proctor will collect all scratch paper, sign you out, and permit you to leave.

PROCESSING RESULTS

Upon completion of the examination, results are transmitted electronically to the data center at the Testing Service. Your results are transmitted to the Board of Nursing in the state in which you applied for licensure. A paper copy of the results is mailed to the Board of Nursing within 48 hours after the examination is completed. The Board of Nursing will mail the results to you. You should not telephone the Testing Center, the National Council, or the State Board of Nursing for results. Results will not be given to candidates over the telephone.

INTERSTATE ENDORSEMENT

Since the CAT NCLEX-RN is a national examination, you can apply to take the examination in any state. Once licensure is received, the registered nurse can apply for Interstate Endorsement. The procedures and requirements for Interstate Endorsement may vary from state to state, and these procedures can be obtained from the State Board of Nursing in the state in which endorsement is sought.

STATE BOARDS OF NURSING

Alabama Board of Nursing
P.O. Box 303900
Montgomery, AL 36130-3900
(205) 242-4060

Alaska Board of Nursing
3601 C. St., Suite 722
Anchorage, AK 99503
(907) 561-2878

American Samoa Health Services Regulatory Board
LBJ Tropical Medical Center
Pago Pago, American Samoa 96799
(684) 633-1222

Arizona State Board of Nursing
1651 E. Morton, Suite 150
Phoenix, AZ 85020
(602) 255-5092

Arkansas State Board of Nursing
1123 South University, Suite 800
Little Rock, AR 72204
(501) 686-2700

California Board of Registered Nursing
P.O. Box 944210
Sacramento, CA 94244-2100
(213) 897-3590

Colorado State Board of Nursing
1560 Broadway, Suite 670
Denver, CO 82002
(303) 894-2435

Connecticut Department of Public Health
Division of Medical Quality Assurance
P.O. Box 260490
Hartford, CT 06126-0490
(860) 509-7603

Delaware Board of Nursing
Cannon Bldg., P.O. Box 1401
Dover, DE 19901
(302) 739-4522

District of Columbia Board of Nursing
614 H. St. NW
Washington, DC 20013
(202) 727-7856

Florida State Board of Nursing
111 E. Coastline Dr. East
Jacksonville, FL 32202
(904) 798-4858

Georgia Board of Nursing
166 Pryor St., S.W.
Atlanta, GA 30334
(404) 656-3943

Guam Board of Nurse Examiners
P.O. Box 2816
Agana, Guam 96910
(671) 734-7295

Hawaii Board of Nursing
Box 3469
Honolulu, HI 99503
(808) 586-2695

Idaho State Board of Nursing
P.O. Box 83720
Boise, ID 83720-0061
(208) 334-3110

Illinois Department of Professional Regulations
320 W. Washington St.
Springfield, IL 62786
(217) 785-9465

Indiana State Board of Nursing
402 W. Washington St.
Indianapolis, IN 46204
(317) 233-4405

Iowa Board of Nursing
1223 E. Court Ave.
Des Moines, IA 50319
(515) 281-4828

Kansas State Board of Nursing
900 S.W. Jackson St., Suite 551S
Topeka, KS 66612-1256
(913) 296-3782

Kentucky Board of Nursing
312 Whittington Pky., Ste. 300
Louisville, KY 40222-5172
(502) 329-7000

Louisiana State Board of Nursing
150 Baronne St., Suite 912
New Orleans, LA 70112
(504) 568-5464

Maine State Board of Nursing
35 Anthony Ave.
State House Station 158
Augusta, ME 04333-0158
(207) 264-5275

Maryland Board of Nursing
4140 Patterson Ave.
Baltimore, MD 21215-2254
(301) 764-5124

Massachusetts Board of Registration in Nursing
100 Cambridge St., Rm. 150
Boston, MA 02202
(617) 727-3060

Michigan Board of Nursing
P.O. Box 30018, 611 West Ottawa
Lansing, MI 48909
(517) 373-1600

Minnesota Board of Nursing
2700 University Ave., W. 108
St. Paul, MN 55114
(612) 643-2565

Mississippi Institution of Higher Learning
3825 Ridgewood Rd.
Jackson, MS 39211
(601) 982-6448

Missouri State Board of Nursing
3605 Missouri Blvd.
Jefferson City, MO 65102
(314) 751-0080

Montana State Board of Nursing
Arcade Bldg., 111 Jackson
Helena, MT 59620-0513
(406) 444-2071

Nebraska Bureau of Examining Bd.
P.O. Box 95007
Lincoln, NE 68509
(402) 471-2115

Nevada State Board of Nursing
4335 S. Industrial Rd., #430
Las Vegas, NV 89103
(702) 739-1575

New Hampshire State Board of Nursing
Division of Public Health, 6 Hazen Dr.
Concord, NH 03301
(603) 271-2323

New Jersey Board of Nursing
P.O. Box 45010
Newark, NJ 07101
(201) 504-6493

New Mexico Board of Nursing
4206 Louisiana N.E., Suite A
Albuquerque, NM 87109
(505) 841-8340

New York State Board of Nursing
The Cultural Center, Room 3023
Albany, NY 12230
(518) 486-2967

North Carolina Board of Nursing
P.O. Box 2129
Raleigh, NC 27602
(919) 782-3211

North Dakota Board of Nursing
919 S. 7th St., Suite 504
Bismarck, ND 58504-5881
(701) 224-2974

Ohio Board of Nursing
77 S. High St., 17th Floor
Columbus, OH 43266-0316
(614) 466-9800

Oklahoma Board of Nursing
2915 N. Classen Blvd., Suite 524
Oklahoma City, OK 73106
(405) 525-2076

Oregon State Board of Nursing
800 N.E. Oregon St., #25
Portland, OR 97232
(503) 731-4745

Pennsylvania State Board of Nursing
P.O. Box 2649
Harrisburg, PA 17105
(717) 783-7142

Counsel of Higher Education of Puerto Rico
P.O. Box 23305, UPR Station
Rio Piedras, PR 00931-3305
(809) 758-3350, Ext. 2305

Rhode Island Board of Nursing Education
and Nurse Registration
3 Capital Hill
Providence, RI 02908-5097
(401) 277-2827

State Board of Nursing for South Carolina
220 Executive Center Dr., Suite 220
Columbia, SC 29210
(803) 731-1648

South Dakota Board of Nursing
3307 South Lincoln
Sioux Falls, SD 57105
(605) 335-4973

Tennessee Board of Nursing
283 Plus Park Blvd.
Nashville, TN 37217
(615) 367-6232

Texas Board of Nurse Examiners
9101 Burnett Rd., Suite 105
Austin, TX 78752
(512) 835-8660

Utah State Board of Nursing
160 E. 300 South, Box 45805
Salt Lake City, UT 84145
(801) 530-6736

Vermont Board of Nursing
Licensing and Registration Div.
109 State Street
Montpelier, VT 05602
(802) 828-2396

Virgin Islands Board of Nursing Licensure
P.O. Box 4247
Charlotte Amalie, VI 00803
(809) 776-7397

Virginia State Board of Nursing
6606 W. Broad Street, 4th Fl.
Richmond, VA 23230-1717
(804) 662-9909

Washington State Nursing Care
Quality Assurance Commission
1300 Quincy, Box 47864
Olympia, WA 98504-7864
(206) 753-3726

West Virginia Board of Examiners for
Registered Nurses
101 Dee Drive
Charleston, WV 25311-1620
(304) 558-3596

Wisconsin Department of Regulation & Licensing
P.O. Box 8935
Madison, WI 53708-8935
(608) 267-2357

State of Wyoming Board of Nursing
2301 Central Ave., Barret Bldg.
Cheyenne, WY 82002
(307) 777-7601

BIBLIOGRAPHY

Black, J., & Matassarin-Jacobs, E. (1997). *Medical-surgical nursing: Clinical management for continuity of care* (5th ed.). Philadelphia, W.B. Saunders

Carson, V., & Arnold, E. (1996). *Mental health nursing: The nurse-patient journey.* Philadelphia: W.B. Saunders.

Gillies, D. (1994). *Nursing management: A systems approach.* Philadelphia: W.B. Saunders.

Hartshorn, J., Sole, M.L. & Lamborn, M. (1997). *Introduction to critical care nursing,* (2nd ed). Philadelphia, W.B. Saunders.

Hodgson, B., & Kizior, R. (1998). *Saunders nursing drug handbook 1998.* Philadelphia: W.B. Saunders.

Lammon, C.B., Foote, A.W., Leli, P.G., et al. (1995). *Clinical nursing skills.* Philadelphia: W.B. Saunders.

Luckmann, J. (1997). *Saunders manual of nursing care.* Philadelphia: W.B. Saunders.

National Council of State Boards of Nursing. (1995). *The NCLEX process.* Chicago: Author.

National Council of State Boards of Nursing. (1997). *Plan for the National Council licensure examination for registered nurses.* Chicago: Author.

National League for Nursing. (1995). *State-Approved Schools of Nursing R.N.* New York: Author.

CHAPTER 2

Pathways to Success

Laurent W. Valliere, B.S.

THE FOUNDATION

The foundation of Pathways to Success begins with a positive attitude and developing short- and long-term goals. Both a positive attitude and a list of goals will lead you toward achievement and success. Without these components, the Pathway to Success leads to nowhere and has no end point. You will expend energy and valuable time and will experience exhaustion without any accomplishment. Therefore, it is imperative that you take the time to develop that positive attitude and to establish your short- and long-term goals.

Where do you start? To begin this process, find a comfortable position, close your eyes, inhale, hold your breath to a count of 4, exhale slowly, and relax. Repeat this breathing exercise several times until you begin to feel relaxed and free from anxiety. Allow your mind to become void of all chatter. Now, you are in control and your mind can see for miles. Your highway of life has a multitude of destinations that you may travel. It is now time for you to select the order of your journey.

THE LIST

It is time to create "The List." The List is your set of goals. At this time, you may or may not have a scheduled date for taking NCLEX-RN. Begin by developing the goals you wish to accomplish today, tomorrow, and into the future. Allow yourself the opportunity to list all that is flowing from your uninhibited thought process. Write your goals on a piece of paper. When the List is complete, it is time to bank it away for 2 or 3 days. After 2 or 3 days, retrieve and review the List and begin the process of planning for preparing for the licensing examination.

THE PLAN

Now that you have the List in order, let us begin by looking at your goals that relate to the studying for the licensing examination.

The first task is to decide what study pattern works best for you. Take the time to review what has worked most successfully for you in the past. These questions must be addressed in order to establish the correct plan for study. Ask yourself:

Do I work better <u>alone</u> or in a group study environment?

If I work best in a group, does the group consist of one, two, or more study partners?

Who are these study partners?

How long should my study sessions last?

Does the time of day that I study make a difference for me?

Do I retain more if I study in the morning?

How does my work schedule affect my study pattern?

How do I balance my family obligations with my need to study?

Do I have a comfortable study area at home or do I need to find an environment that is conducive to my study needs?

"The Plan" must include how you will manage your study needs with the demands of your family and friends. Take time to think about how you will balance your everyday commitments with your plan for study. Your family and friends are key players in your life and are going to become a part of your Pyramid to Success. After you have established your study needs, communicate your needs, and the importance of your study plan in achieving your goal of becoming a Registered Nurse, to your family and friends.

A difficult part of the Plan may include how you will deal with those family and friends who choose not to participate in your Pyramid to Success. What if the individual or individuals choose not to be part of the Pyramid? Then you are faced with a decision. You must weigh all the factors carefully. You must keep your goals in mind, and remember that your need for positive momentum is critical. Your decision may not be an easy one, but must be one that will help you ensure that your goal of becoming a Registered Nurse is achieved. Remember, a positive momentum and goal achievement needs to be shared by all who support you.

The Plan must include a schedule. Establish a realistic schedule that includes your daily, weekly, and future goals, and adhere to it. This consistency will provide advantages to you and to those supporting you. A daily schedule allows you to plan your topic areas more carefully. Adherence to the Plan helps you develop a rhythm that can only enhance your retention and positive momentum. Those supporting you will share this rhythm and will be able to schedule their activities and life better because you are consistent with your study schedule. You are moving forward and you are in Control!

POSITIVE PAMPERING

Positive momentum can be maintained only if you are properly balanced. This means that you must continue to care for yourself. Proper exercise, diet, and positive mental stimulation are critical to achieving your goal of becoming a Registered Nurse. Just as you have developed a schedule for study, you should have a schedule that includes some fun and some form of physical activity. It is your choice: aerobics, running, weight lifting, bowling, or whatever makes you feel good about yourself. Time spent away from the hard study schedule and devoted to some form of fun and physical exercise pays its rewards 100-fold. You will feel alive and more energetic with a schedule that includes these activities.

Establish good eating habits. Stay away from fatty foods as they will slow you down. Eat lighter meals and more frequently. Include complex carbohydrates in your diet for energy and be careful not to include too much caffeine in your daily diet. Feel good about yourself, as you are in control. Take the time to pamper yourself with activities that make you feel even better about who you are. Make dinner reservations at your favorite restaurant with someone who is special and is supporting your goal to become a Registered Nurse. Take walks in a place that has a particular tranquility that enables you to reflect on the positive momentum you have maintained. Whatever it is, wherever it takes you, allow yourself the time to do some Positive Pampering.

FINAL PREPARATION

You have established the foundation of your Pyramid. You are moving forward and you are in control. When you receive your date and time for the NCLEX-RN, you may immediately think, "I am not ready!"

Stop! Reflect on all you have achieved. Think about your goal achievement and the organization of the positive life momentum with which you have surrounded yourself. Think about all those individuals who love and support your effort to be a Registered Nurse. Believe that the challenge that waits you is one you have successfully prepared for and will lead you to your goal, becoming a Registered Nurse!

Take a deep breath and organize the remaining days so that they support your educational and personal needs. Support your positive momentum with a visual technique. Write your name in large letters and write the letters R.N. after it. Post one or more of these visual reinforcements in areas that you frequent. This form of motivational technique works for many individuals preparing for this examination.

Through all that you have accomplished to this point, it is imperative that you not fall into the trap of expecting too much of yourself. The idea of perfection must not drive you to a point that causes your positive momentum to hesitate. You must believe in who you are, as you are, and stay focused on your goal. Allow yourself the opportunity to continue to carry out your plan in a manner that is most conducive to who you are, not someone else. The day and time are at hand. Write down the date and time and underneath write the word "YES." Post this next to your name plus R.N.

You must ensure that you have command over how to get to the testing center. A test run is a must. Time the drive and allow for road construction or whatever may occur to slow the traffic down. On the test run, once you arrive at the test facility you may want to walk into it. Walk in and become familiar with the lobby and the surroundings. This may help alleviate some of the peripheral nervousness associated with entering an unknown building. Remember, you must do whatever it takes to keep yourself in control. If familiarizing yourself with the facility will help you maintain positive momentum, by all means, be sure to do so! Who is in control? You are!

It is time to check your study plan and make the necessary adjustments now that a firm date and time are set. Adjust your review so that it flows to your needs and so that your study plan ends 2 days before the examination. Remember that the mind is like a muscle. If it is overworked, it has no strength or stamina. Your strategy is to rest the body and the mind on the day before the examination. Your strategy is to stay in control and allow yourself the opportunity to be absolutely fresh and attentive the day of the examination. This will help you control the nervousness that is natural, achieve the clear thought processes required, and be confident that you have done all that is necessary to prepare and conquer this challenge. Plan the day before your examination just as you have planned your study schedule. This day is to be one of pleasure. Treat yourself to what you enjoy the most.

Relax! You have prepared yourself well for the challenge of tomorrow. Allow yourself a good night's sleep and wake up the day of the examination knowing you are absolutely ready to succeed. Look at your name with R.N. after it and the word, "YES"! Wake up believing in yourself and that all you have accomplished is about to propel you to the professional level of Registered Nurse. Allow yourself plenty of time, eat a nutritious breakfast, and groom yourself for success. You are ready to meet the challenges of the day and overcome any obstacle that may face you. Today will soon be history and tomorrow will bring you the envelope on which you read your name with the words, Registered Nurse, after it.

Be proud and confident of your achievements. You have worked hard to achieve your goal of becoming a Registered Nurse. If you believe in yourself and your goals, no one person or obstacle can move you off the pathway that leads to success, to the peak of the Pyramid!

Congratulations, and I wish you the very best in your career as a Registered Nurse!

CHAPTER 3

The NCLEX-RN Examination: From a Student's Perspective

Shannon Chase, R.N.

The time for me to take my boards was approaching. Many overwhelming questions flew through my mind. How was I going to study? Where do I start? What do I do? And, of course, the most important question was "Will I pass?"

Since I had entered nursing school, I had been preparing for NCLEX. Each class I took was to enhance my knowledge in the subject of nursing and to prepare me for NCLEX. Therefore, I felt that the best place to begin was with a nursing review book.

The nursing review book contained both review and practice questions and answers. As I reviewed and answered the practice questions, my strengths and weaknesses and areas where I needed to focus became evident and clear to me.

After reading through the review book, I focused on my weakest areas by going back to my class notes and textbooks to review nursing content area that I was unsure of. I made sure that I understood what I was studying. Anything I was unclear on, I looked up for further explanation. My primary focus for preparation was using the review book, and I moved back to my textbooks only when I was unfamiliar with an area of nursing content.

During my final semester of college, I attended a seminar that provided a review of nursing content and provided some great test-taking strategies. I found that using these test-taking strategies really helped me in looking at a question clearly and determining what is really being asked in the stem of the question. I also spent time answering computer-based questions. This was also an important component of preparation. Practicing computer questions gave me a sense of what the NCLEX would be like, gave me exposure to important nursing content areas, and provided the opportunity to develop my test-taking skills further.

Understanding test-taking strategies and developing sound test-taking skills are very important. Test-taking strategies help you avoid reading into the question, and, when all else fails, it is important to use these strategies to make an educated guess!

It is important to establish some type of routine or schedule for studying. NCLEX isn't something that you can cram for. Each day I reviewed nursing content for 1 to 2 hours. I paced myself with my study plan and didn't allow myself to become overwhelmed. I made time to spend with family and friends, maintained a summer job, and studied.

Support and a positive environment are critical. I was very fortunate because everyone in my life was very supportive. When my friends would call and ask what I was doing, they usually received the same answer, "Studying." My friends were supportive and allowed me to achieve my daily study goals without pressuring me. I would do my bit of studying for the day, and then go out and have some fun! Fun time is very important for balance in life and success.

The entire time I was preparing for NCLEX, I tried to keep a regular sleep pattern and eat healthy. Sleep is important, and if I didn't get enough I would have fallen asleep studying. I consistently ate a well-balanced diet and that helped me feel good, not only physically, but also mentally. Eating properly also helped my studying. Remember, you need to feed your body and your brain!

After scheduling my appointment for NCLEX, the reality set in. I would be taking NCLEX soon. I was instantly nervous, but took a slow deep breath and told myself, "You have plenty of time to prepare, and you are in control." I calmed myself down and relaxed. I knew it was important to take things one step at a time and not to become overwhelmed. I remained focused on my goal of daily study and my goal of passing NCLEX. I made a promise to myself that the night before the examination would be a relaxing one. I made plans to go out with some friends and informed them that I needed to be in early. Until that night arrived, though, I knew I needed to continue studying. Through clinical work and classes, I had learned many things. Now, the time was approaching to put this knowledge to the test. By reviewing, the material I had already learned was reinforced, and anything I had missed along the way was now learned.

The day of my examination was quickly approaching. I kept my promise to myself. The day before the examination, I did not allow myself to open a single nursing book. I spent the day at work and the evening with my friends. I treated the day like any other day and did not question what tomorrow would be like. Knowing that I had to arrive early in the morning, I made sure to be home and in bed at a reasonable hour.

When I awoke the day of the examination, the reality of the day set in. There was no more time to study, and if I didn't know it by now, I probably never would. I jumped into the shower and continuously told myself "You are in control." My mother was great! She made me a healthy breakfast and I was on my way. I remembered that I had been told not to eat fatty foods because they make you sluggish and tired. Today, I needed to be wide awake!

My mother accompanied me to the testing center. While I was there taking the test, she planned to do some shopping and catch up on her reading. It was nice to have someone to talk to on the long drive to the testing center, and it kept my mind off the examination. A bit of advice; be sure to allow extra time to get to the testing center. You don't want to be late and you certainly don't need the additional anxiety that "running late" will produce. In fact, it is a great idea to do a "test drive" to the testing center a week before your scheduled time.

At about 8:25 A.M. I entered the testing center. My appointment was for 9:00 A.M., but I was told to arrive 30 minutes early. Several people were already there. I instantly wondered, "Are they all here for NCLEX?" Quickly I learned that I was the only one taking the nursing examination. Everyone at the testing center was friendly and wished me well. Before entering the testing room, I was thumbprinted and my picture was taken. I was given scratch paper, pencils, and earplugs and told to bring my two forms of identification into the testing room. The proctor explained everything, including the mandatory break that must be taken after 2 hours of testing. The proctor told me to read all the directions for the test, which would be on the computer.

I entered the testing room, sat down at the computer, and began. I read the directions, answered the sample questions, and then began answering the test questions. When I reached 50 questions, I couldn't help but wonder how many questions I had left. I read every question carefully, looking for key words such as except, initially, and best. I had trained my mind so well that those important key words stood out clearly. At around 70 questions, I remembered thinking that I could have as few as 5 questions left to answer. Then it happened! I answered question number 75 and my computer shut down. The computer screen read that I had completed the examination.

After that, I answered some questions requested for a survey and questions about the testing experience. After completing these, I raised my hand and was dismissed. I was done! The test was over!

I gathered my belongings from the locker where I had left them, signed out, and left. When I got to the car, my mother was there. All she said was "So, how did it go?" I answered, "It went." I knew I had done my best and knew that I had to wait to find out how well I did. No matter what the outcome would be, I knew that I had done all that I could do to prepare and that I needed to move on with my life.

The worst part of the process was not the examination but the waiting period following it. In my state, results are sent out in 7 to 10 business days. Beginning on the seventh business day, I began to get very anxious. No results came. The days passed, and on what would have been the tenth business day, the envelope with my results arrived. I was so nervous opening it. When I was finally able to open the envelope, all I saw were the words "has passed." I began bouncing all over the house!

Looking back on the experience, I can describe it as stressful but rewarding. I need to say that in addition to my study patterns and what I studied, the thing that helped me the most in preparing was a person, and that was Linda Silvestri. Linda had been my academic advisor since my freshman year in nursing school and has always been supportive. Through her NCLEX review classes, I learned what to focus on specifically. Without her, I don't know where I would be today. Through her guidance, the support of my family and friends, especially my mother, and my dedication, I am now a registered nurse!

My experience with NCLEX is something I will never forget. My advice to anyone who reads this is that when preparing for boards, don't try to cram, establish a daily schedule, and stay focused and in control. Spread your studying out over a period of time and do a little every day. Also, make the most of your nursing classes and clinical experiences. Every little thing that you learn will be with you when you sit down before that computer to take NCLEX. It was a difficult examination, and I would never tell anyone differently, but with determination and dedication, your dream will come true!

Best of luck to all future RNs!

CHAPTER 4
Test-Taking Strategies

....

I. The Pyramid to Success (Box 4–1)

II. The Components of the Question

A. Strategy 1
  1. Identify the components of the question
  2. Identify the "CASE SITUATION" from the "STEM" (see C below)
  3. Read all the options carefully and thoroughly
B. The Case Situation
  1. The case situation gives you the information about a clinical health problem and the information you need to consider in answering the question
  2. It is extremely important to read all the information and every word in the case situation
C. The Stem
  1. The stem usually comes after the case situation and asks you something about it
  2. The stem asks you to solve a problem and select an answer
  ✗3. Read the stem very carefully and specifically identify exactly what the question is asking
D. The Options
  1. The options are all of the answers and you must select one
  2. Read all the options very carefully and then reread the stem of the question before selecting the answer

---

BOX 4–1. The Pyramid to Success

Read the questions and options thoroughly and carefully!
Ask yourself, "What is the question really asking me?"
Be alert to key words and true and false stems!
Eliminate the incorrect options!
Use all your nursing knowledge, your clinical experiences, and your test-taking skills to answer the question!

---

  3. Use the process of elimination and eliminate the incorrect options
  4. Once you have eliminated the incorrect options, read the stem again and identify specifically what the question is asking before selecting your answer

III. The Critical Elements of the Question

A. Strategy 2
  1. Identify the critical elements of the case situation and the stem of the question
  2. The critical elements are the key words or phrases in the case situation and the stem of the question
B. Key Words or Phrases
  1. The key words or phrases focus your attention on critical ideas in the case, in the stem, and in the options
  2. Some of the key words or phrases you should look for and focus your attention on include
    a. Early or late
    b. Immediately
    c. Most likely or least likely
    d. Initial
    e. First
    f. Best
    g. Most appropriate
    h. On the day of
    i. After several days
  3. The key words will make a difference in your selection of an answer (Box 4–2)

IV. The Client of the Question

A. Strategy 3
  1. Identify the client of the question
  2. The client is the person who is the focus of the question
B. The Client
  1. It is important to remember that the client of

BOX 4–2. Key Words in the Question

Which of the following is an EARLY sign of shock?

Which of the following is a LATE sign of shock?

ON THE DAY OF surgery, following a transurethral resection of the prostate (TURP), the nurse notes that the client's urine is bright red in color. Which of the following nursing actions is appropriate?

AFTER SEVERAL DAYS, following a transurethral resection of the prostate (TURP), the nurse notes that the client's urine is bright red in color. Which of the following nursing actions is appropriate?

Noting the key words or phrases in each of these situations will assist in directing you to select the correct option.

The EARLY signs of shock are quite different from the LATE signs of shock!

Bright red urine might be expected ON THE DAY OF surgery following a transurethral resection of the prostate (TURP) but would not be expected AFTER SEVERAL DAYS!

True {
   a. Most
   b. Best
   c. Best judgment
   d. Initial
   e. First
   f. Chief
   g. Immediate
}

C. False Response Stem
   1. False response stems use key words that ask you to select an answer which is NOT true regarding the situation and question
   2. False response stems may utilize the following key words or phrases

False {
   a. Except
   b. Least likely
   c. Need for further education
   d. Lowest priority
   e. Incorrect
   f. Unsafe
}

the question may not necessarily be the person with the health problem
   2. In the test question, the client may be a relative, friend, spouse, significant other, or even another nurse
 ★ 3. Identify the client of the question and select an answer that relates to and most directly addresses that client

V. The Issue of the Question

A. Strategy 4
   1. Identify the issue of the question
   2. The issue of the question is the specific subject content that the question is asking about
B. The Issue
   1. Identifying the issue of the question will assist in eliminating the incorrect options and direct you to selecting the correct response
   2. The issue of the question can include
      a. A medication
      b. A side effect or toxic effect of a medication
      c. A procedure
      d. A complication
      e. A specific nursing action

VI. The Type of Stem in the Question

A. Strategy 5
   1. Identify the type of stem in the question
   2. The stem can be either a true response stem or a false response stem
 ★ B. True Response Stem
   1. True response stems use key words that ask you to select an answer which is true regarding the situation and the question
   2. True response stems may utilize the following key words or phrases

VII. Eliminating the Incorrect Options

A. Strategy 6
   1. Using the process of elimination, eliminate the incorrect options before selecting an answer
   2. Be alert to the key words or phrases and to the true and the false response stems
B. Distracters
   1. Distracters are options that are made to look like correct answers but, in fact, are not
   2. They are intended to "distract" you from answering questions correctly
   3. There are three "distracters" and one correct answer
   4. Use the process of elimination and eliminate the incorrect options
   5. Be alert to the key words and to the true and the false response stems
   6. Once you have eliminated the incorrect options, read the stem again and identify specifically what the question is asking before selecting your answer

VIII. Questions That Require Prioritizing

A. Strategy 7
   1. Identify the key words in the question that indicate the need for you to prioritize
   2. Key words include the following
      a. Initial
      b. Essential
      c. Vital
      d. Immediate
      e. Highest
      f. Best
      g. Most
B. Strategy 8
   1. Utilize MASLOW'S HIERARCHY OF NEEDS THEORY to prioritize

2. Physiological needs come FIRST, so select an answer that addresses physiological needs
3. When a physiological need is not addressed in the question, safety needs receive priority, and in this situation select an answer that addresses safety

C. Strategy 9
1. Utilize the ABCs when selecting an answer
2. Remember the order of priority of AIRWAY, BREATHING, AND CIRCULATION!

D. Strategy 10
1. Use the nursing process to prioritize
2. Remember that assessment is the first step in the nursing process
3. When you are asked to select your first or initial nursing action, use and follow the steps of the nursing process to select your response
4. If an answer contains the concept of assessment or collection of client data, select that answer

IX. The Nursing Process (Box 4–3)

A. Assessment
1. Assessment questions address the process of gathering subjective and objective data relative to the client, confirming that data, and communicating and documenting the data
2. Remember that assessment is the first step in the nursing process
3. When you are asked a question regarding your initial or first nursing action, select the option that addresses an assessment action
4. If an assessment action is not one of the options, follow the steps of the nursing process as your guide to select your initial or first action
5. When answering questions that focus on assessment, look for key words in the options that reflect assessment
6. Key words or phrases that reflect assessment
   a. Observe
   b. Monitor
   c. Check
   d. Obtain information
   e. Find out
   f. Determine
   g. Assess
   h. Ascertain

B. Analysis
1. Analysis questions are the most difficult as they require understanding of the principles of physiological responses
2. Analysis questions will require interpretation of the data based on assessment
3. Analysis questions address formulation of nursing diagnoses and the communication and documentation of the results of the process of analysis
4. These questions will require critical thinking and determining the rationale for therapeutic interventions related to the specific issue addressed in the question
5. Avoid reading into the question

C. Planning
1. Planning questions will require prioritizing nursing diagnoses, determining goals and outcome criteria for goals of care, developing the plan of care, and communicating and documenting the plan of care
2. Remember that this is a nursing examination, and the answer to the question involves something that is included in the nursing care plan, rather than the medical plan

D. Implementation
1. This examination is about NURSING, so focus on the nursing action rather than on the medical action, unless the question is asking you what prescribed action is anticipated
2. Implementation questions address the process of organizing and managing care, counseling and teaching, providing care to achieve established goals, supervising and coordinating care, and communicating and documenting nursing interventions
3. On NCLEX-RN, the only client that you need to be concerned about is the client in the question you are answering
4. When you are answering a question, remember that this client is your only assigned client
5. Answer the question as if the situation were textbook and ideal, and the nurse had all the time and resources needed and readily available at the client's bedside

E. Evaluation
1. Evaluation questions focus on comparing the actual outcomes of care with the expected outcomes
2. These questions address evaluating the client's ability to implement self-care, evaluating health care team members' ability to implement care, and the process of communicating and documenting evaluation findings
3. These questions focus on how the nurse should monitor or make a judgment concerning a client's response to therapy or to a nursing action

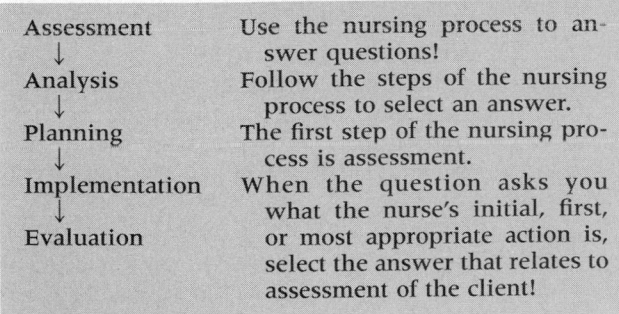

BOX 4–3. Steps of the Nursing Process

Assessment ↓	Use the nursing process to answer questions!
Analysis ↓	Follow the steps of the nursing process to select an answer.
Planning ↓	The first step of the nursing process is assessment.
Implementation ↓	When the question asks you what the nurse's initial, first, or most appropriate action is, select the answer that relates to assessment of the client!
Evaluation	

4. In an evaluation question, be alert to false response stems as they are frequently used in evaluation-type questions

5. The question may ask for the client's statement that indicates INACCURATE information regarding the issue in the question

X. Client Needs

A. Safe, Effective Care Environment
 1. These questions address the provision that the nurse meets client needs for a safe and effective care environment by providing and directing nursing care that promotes achievement of coordinated care, environmental safety, and safe and effective treatments and procedures
 2. Be alert to safety needs addressed in a question!
 3. Remember the importance of handwashing, siderails, and call bells!

B. Physiological Integrity
 1. These questions address the provision that the nurse meets the physiological integrity needs of clients with acute and chronic conditions and clients at risk for the development of complications from treatments or management modalities
 2. The nurse provides and directs care to promote physiological adaptation, reduction of risk potential, and provision of basic care
 3. Be careful not to read into the question
 4. These questions will require you to think critically and determine the rationale for the correct response
 5. Remember that physiological needs are a priority and are addressed first!
 6. Remember to utilize the ABCs when selecting an answer addressing physiological integrity
 7. Remember the order of priority of AIRWAY, BREATHING, AND CIRCULATION!

C. Psychosocial Integrity
 1. These questions address the provision that the nurse meets the psychosocial needs of the client in stress and crisis-related situations throughout the life span by promoting psychosocial adaptation and coping, and adaptation abilities in the client
 2. Communication Questions
    a. Identify the use of therapeutic communication tools
    b. When answering communication questions, utilization of communication tools indicates a CORRECT answer
    c. When answering communication questions, utilization of communication blocks indicates an INCORRECT answer (Box 4–4)

D. Health Promotion and Maintenance
 1. These questions address the provision that the nurse meets client needs for health promotion and maintenance throughout the life span by providing and directing care to clients and significant others
 2. It involves promoting growth and development throughout the life span, promoting self-care and providing support systems, and the prevention and early treatment of disease
 3. Utilize the teaching/learning theory if the question addresses client education, remembering that client motivation and client readiness to learn is the FIRST priority
 4. Be alert to those true and false response stems with questions that address health promotion and maintenance

XI. Pyramid Points (Box 4–5)

A. Unfamiliar Content
 1. Answer questions utilizing your nursing knowledge, clinical experience, and test-taking skills
 2. If the content of the question is unfamiliar and you are unable to answer questions using your nursing knowledge, look for a global response, similar distracters, or similar words in the question and in the options

B. The Global Response *cover-all*
 1. When more than one option appears to be correct, look for a global response
 2. A global response is one that is a general statement and may include the ideas of other options within it

C. Similar Distracters
 1. If you don't know the answer, try looking for similar distracters
 2. Remember that there is only ONE answer
 3. If two options say the same thing or include

BOX 4–4. Communication Tools and Blocks

TOOLS	BLOCKS
Being silent	Giving advice
Offering self	Showing approval/ disapproval
Showing empathy	Using cliché and false reassurance
Focusing	Requesting an explanation, "Why?"
Restatement	Devaluing client feelings
Validation/ clarification	Being defensive
Giving information	Focusing on inappropriate issues
Dealing with the here and now	Placing the client's issues on "hold"

Always focus on the client's feelings FIRST! If an answer reflects the client's feelings, select that answer!

BOX 4–5. Pyramid Points

- If the question asks for an immediate action or response, all answers may be correct; therefore, base your selection on priorities.
- Reword a difficult question but, if you do so, be careful not to change the intent of the question.
- Look for the most common or typical response.
- Relate the situation to something that you are familiar with and try to visualize the client as you go through the case situation and the question.
- Look for answers that focus on the client as a worthy human being or are directed toward feelings.
- With medication calculations, talk yourself through each step and be sure the answer makes sense.
- If there are words in the stem that are unfamiliar, try to figure out the meaning in terms of the context of the sentence, or break down the word using your medical terminology skills.
- If one option includes qualifiers such as GENERALLY, USUALLY, or TENDS TO and other options do not, select that option.

- Absolute terminology, such as ALWAYS, NEVER, ALL, EVERY, NONE, and MUST, tends to make a statement false.
- Unusual or highly technical language typically indicates that the option is not correct.
- Remember that lengthy questions are not always the most difficult.
- Answer all questions as if the situation were ideal and the nurse had all the time and resources needed.
- Remember, the only client you need to be concerned about is the one in the question you are answering.
- Pace yourself and concentrate and focus on one item at a time.
- Do not become frustrated!
- Be patient with yourself!

SMILE!
BELIEF!
CONFIDENCE!
CONTROL!
SUCCESS!

the same idea, then NEITHER OF THESE OPTIONS can be the answer
4. The answer has to be the option that is different
D. Similar Words
1. If you do not know the answer, look for a similar word or phrase used in the stem or the case situation and in one of the options
2. If you find a word, feeling, or behavior that is used in the stem or the case situation and is

repeated in one of the options, that option MAY be the correct answer (Box 4–5)

BIBLIOGRAPHY

Leahy, J., & Kizilay, P. (1998). *Foundations of nursing practice: A nursing process approach.* Philadelphia; W. B. Saunders.

National Council of State Boards of Nursing (1997). *Plan for the National Council licensure examination for registered nurses.* Chicago: Author.

Varcarolis, E. (1998). *Foundations of psychiatric-mental health nursing* (3rd ed.). Philadelphia: W. B. Saunders.

UNIT II

Issues in Nursing

CHAPTER 5

Cultural Diversity

PYRAMID TERMS

Acculturation—Process of learning norms, beliefs, and behavioral expectations of a group.

Belief—Something accepted as true and accepted by an ethnocultural group.

Cultural Assimilation—Occurs when individuals from a minority group are absorbed by the dominant culture and take on the characteristics of the dominant culture.

Cultural Competence—Having the knowledge, understanding, and skills regarding a diverse culture that allow one to provide acceptable care.

Cultural Diversity—The differences among people that result from ethnic, racial, and cultural variables.

Cultural Imposition—The tendency to impose one's own beliefs, values, and patterns of behavior on individuals from another culture.

Culture—Refers to the structures of knowledge, beliefs, behaviors, ideas, attitudes, values, habits, customs, languages, symbols, rituals, ceremonies, and practices that are unique to a particular group of people.

Dominant Culture—The group whose values prevail within a society.

Ethnic—A group of people who have had different experiences from those of the dominant culture by status, background, residence, religion, education, or other factors that functionally unify the group.

Ethnicity—A cultural group's perception of themselves, or the group identity. This self-perception influences how the group members are perceived by others.

Ethnocentrism—An assumption of cultural superiority, and an inability to accept another culture's ways.

Minority Group—An ethnic, racial, or religious group that constitutes less than a numerical majority of the population.

Oppression—Is based on cultural biases and stems from values, beliefs, traditions, and cultural expectations. Occurs when the rules, modes, and ideals of one group are imposed on another group.

Race—Refers to a grouping of people based on biological similarities. Members of a racial group have similar physical characteristics, such as blood group, facial features, and color of skin, hair, and eyes.

Racism—Discrimination directed toward individuals who are misperceived to be inferior due to biological differences. A form of oppression.

Stereotyping—An expectation that all people within the same racial, ethnic, or cultural group act alike and share the same beliefs and attitudes.

Subculture—A group of people with characteristic patterns of behavior that distinguish the group from the larger culture or society.

Values—Principles and standards that have meaning and worth to an individual, family, group, or community.

◆ THE PYRAMID TO SUCCESS

Often, nurses are caring for clients who come from different **ethnic,** cultural, and religious backgrounds from their own. Awareness of and sensitivity to the unique health and illness **beliefs** and practices are essential in the delivery of safe and effective care. Acknowledgment and acceptance of cultural differences with a nonjudgmental attitude are essential in providing culturally sensitive care. The **belief** underlying the NCLEX-RN Test Plan is that people are unique individuals and define their own systems of daily living, which reflects their **values,** motives, and lifestyles. Cultural Awareness is a concept and process that is fundamental to the practice of nursing and is integrated throughout the categories of Client Needs, the framework for NCLEX-RN.

NURSING PROCESS

ASSESSMENT

Ethnic heritage
Native language
Religious practices
Food preferences
Health care beliefs

Family role and function
Family patterns of health care
Social networks and supports
Educational experiences

ANALYSIS: Focus on developing a list of actual and potential nursing diagnoses based on data collected from the process of Assessment. Identify client and family interpretation of the problem and the possible effective measures when developing the actual or potential nursing diagnoses.

PLANNING

Develop the plan of care based on the unique characteristics of the individual. Include the client, family, and community in the plan of care as appropriate. Consult with client and family regarding the plan of care.

IMPLEMENTATION

Utilize data gathered during assessment to adjust interventions, in order to meet the unique needs of the client. Incorporate interventions that are compatible with the client's cultural heritage, educational level, and language. Provide care using a nonjudgmental approach. Respect client and family needs based on their cultural practices and preferences.

EVALUATION

Determine compatibility of plan with client and family in meeting needs based on cultural practices and preferences. Adjust plan of care as appropriate based on meeting expectations and needs.

◆ CLIENT NEEDS

SAFE, EFFECTIVE CARE ENVIRONMENT

Cultural awareness
Caring
Communication
Advocacy
Client rights
Confidentiality
Ethical and legal responsibilities
Consultations and referrals

HEALTH PROMOTION AND MAINTENANCE

Cultural awareness
Caring
Communication
Family planning and family systems
Health and wellness
Lifestyle choices

PSYCHOSOCIAL INTEGRITY

Cultural awareness
Caring
Communication
Coping mechanisms
Religious and spiritual influences on health
Support systems

PHYSIOLOGICAL INTEGRITY

Cultural awareness
Caring
Communication
Nutritional preferences (Box 5–1)
Comfort practices
Practices or restrictions related to procedures and treatments

---

BOX 5–1. Dietary Practices and Preferences

African-Americans
Fried foods
Pork, greens, rice
Some pregnant African-Americans engage in pica

Asian-Americans
Soy sauce
Raw fish
Rice

European-Americans
Carbohydrates (potatoes)
Red meat

Hispanic-Americans
Beans
Fried foods
Spicy foods
Chili
Carbonated beverages

Native Americans
Blue cornmeal
Fish
Game
Fruits and berries
Navajos prefer meat and blue cornmeal and tend to avoid consumption of milk

---

I. African-Americans

A. Communication
   1. Languages include English or Black English
   2. Head nodding does not necessarily mean agreement

3. Direct eye contact is often viewed as being rude
4. Nonverbal communication is very important
5. It is considered to be intrusive to ask personal questions of someone on initial contact or meeting

B. Space
   1. Close personal space is important
   2. Touching another's hair is sometimes viewed as offensive

C. Social Roles
   1. Large, extended family networks are important
   2. Women serve as both breadwinners and care-takers
   3. Religion is usually Protestant (Baptist) (see Box 5–2)
   4. Strong church affiliation with community is important
   5. Social organizations are strong within communities

D. Health and Illness
   1. Harmony with nature
   2. No separation of body, mind, and spirit
   3. Illness is a disharmonious state that may be caused by demons or spirits
   4. Illness can be prevented by nutritious meals, rest, and cleanliness

E. Health Risks
   1. Lactose intolerance
   2. Keloid formation
   3. Sickle cell anemia
   4. Hypertension
   5. Cancer (especially stomach and esophageal)
   6. Coronary heart disease

F. Implementation
   1. Avoid **stereotyping**
   2. Do not label Black English as an unacceptable form of language
   3. Clarify meaning of client's verbal and nonverbal behavior
   4. Be flexible and avoid rigidity in scheduling care
   5. Encourage involvement with family
   6. A folk healer or herbalist may be consulted before the individual seeks medical treatment

---

BOX 5–2. Religions and Dietary Practices

Seventh Day Adventist (Church of God)
Alcohol, coffee, and tea prohibited.
Some groups prohibit meat.

Baptist
Alcohol prohibited.
Discourage consumption of coffee and tea.

Buddhism
Alcohol and drug use discouraged.
Some sects are vegetarian.

Roman Catholicism
Fasting on Ash Wednesday and Good Friday.
Optional fasting during Lent season.
During Lent, discourage meat on Friday.
Children and the ill are exempt from fasting.

Church of Jesus Christ of Latter-Day Saints (Mormon)
Alcohol, coffee, and tea prohibited.
Limited consumption of meat.
First Sunday of the month is time for fasting.

Hinduism
Beef and veal prohibited.
Many individuals are vegetarians.
Limited consumption of meat.
Fasting occurs on specific days of the week according to which God the person worships.
Children are not allowed to participate in fasting.
Fasting rituals vary from complete abstinence to consumption of only one meal per day.

Islam
Pork prohibited.
Any meat product not ritually slaughtered is prohibited.
Avoidance of alcohol and drugs.
During Ramadan (9th month of Mohammedan year), fasting occurs during daytime.

Jehovah's Witness
Prohibition of any foods to which blood has been added.
Can consume animal flesh that has been drained.

Judaism
Dietary kosher laws must be adhered to by Orthodox believers.
Meats allowed include animals that are vegetable eaters, cloven-hoofed animals, and animals that are ritually slaughtered.
Fish that have scales and fins are allowed.
Any combination of meat and milk is prohibited.
During Yom Kippur, 24-hour fasting.
Pregnant women and those who are seriously ill are exempt from fasting.
During Passover week, only unleavened bread is eaten.

Pentecostal (Assembly of God)
Alcohol is prohibited.
Avoid consumption of anything to which blood has been added.
Some individuals avoid pork.

Russian Orthodox
Abstention from meat and dairy products on Wednesdays, Fridays, and during Lent.
During Lent, all animal products, including dairy products, are forbidden.
Fasting during Advent.
Exceptions from fasting include illness and pregnancy.

II. Asian-Americans

A. Communication
   1. Languages include Chinese, Japanese, Korean, Vietnamese, English
   2. Silence is valued
   3. Eye contact is considered rude
   4. Criticism or disagreement is not expressed verbally
   5. The word "no" is interpreted as disrespect for others
B. Space
   1. Social distance is important
   2. Usually do not touch others during conversation
   3. Touch is unacceptable with members of opposite sex
   4. The head is considered to be sacred, therefore touching someone on the head is disrespectful
C. Social Roles
   1. Immediate and extended family loyalty and honor are valued
   2. Family unit is very structured and hierarchical
   3. Men have the power and authority, and the women are expected to be obedient
   4. Education is viewed as important
   5. Religions include Taoism (Buddhism), Islam, Christianity (see Box 5–2)
D. Health and Illness
   1. Health is a state of physical and spiritual harmony with nature and a balance between positive and negative energy forces (yin and yang)
   2. A healthy body is viewed as a gift from ancestors
   3. Illness is viewed as an imbalance between yin and yang
   4. Illness is attributed to prolonged sitting or lying, or to overexertion
E. Health Risks
   1. Lactose intolerance
   2. Hypertension
   3. Cancer (stomach and liver)
F. Implementation
   1. Avoid physical closeness and excessive touch and only touch the client's head when necessary, informing the client before doing so
   2. Limit eye contact
   3. Avoid gesturing with hands
   4. Clarify responses to questions
   5. Be flexible and avoid rigidity in scheduling care
   6. Encourage involvement with family
   7. A traditional healer may be consulted before the individual seeks out medical treatment

III. European-Americans

A. Communication
   1. Languages include national languages, English
   2. Silence can be used to show respect or disrespect for another, depending on situation
   3. Eye contact is viewed as indicating trustworthiness

B. Space
   1. Aloof and tend to avoid close physical contact
   2. Handshakes are used for formal greetings
C. Social Roles
   1. The nuclear family is the basic unit; the extended family is important
   2. The man is the dominant figure
   3. Religion includes Judeo-Christian (see Box 5–2)
   4. Community social organizations are important
D. Health and Illness
   1. Health is usually viewed as an absence of disease or illness
   2. Have a tendency to be stoical when expressing physical concerns
E. Health Risks
   1. Heart disease
   2. Thalassemia
   3. Breast cancer
   4. Diabetes
F. Implementation
   1. Monitor and assess client's body language
   2. Respect client's personal space
   3. Home remedies may be the first method of treatment used

IV. Hispanic-Americans

A. Communication
   1. Languages include Spanish or Portuguese with various dialects
   2. Tend to be verbally expressive, yet confidentiality is important
   3. Eye behavior is significant; for example, the "evil eye" can be given to a child if a person looks at and admires a child without touching the child
   4. Avoiding eye contact indicates respect and attentiveness
   5. Direct confrontation is disrespectful, and the expression of negative feeling is impolite
   6. Dramatic body language, such as gestures or facial expressions, is used to express emotion or pain
B. Space
   1. Comfortable with close proximity to others
   2. Very tactile and use embraces and handshakes
   3. Value the physical presence of others
   4. Politeness and modesty are essential
C. Social Roles
   1. The nuclear family is the basic unit; the extended family is highly regarded
   2. Needs of the family take precedence over individual family member's needs
   3. Man is the decision maker and breadwinner, and the woman is the caretaker and homemaker
   4. Religion includes Catholicism (see Box 5–2)
D. Health and Illness
   1. Health may be a reward from God or a result of good luck

2. Health results from a state of balance between "hot and cold" forces and "wet and dry" forces
3. Illness occurs as a result of God's punishment for sins

E. Health Risks
   1. Lactose intolerance
   2. Diabetes
   3. Parasites?

F. Implementation
   1. Communicate with male head of family
   2. Protect privacy
   3. Offer to call priest or other clergy because of the significance of religious practices related to illnesses
   4. Always touch a child when examining
   5. Be flexible and avoid rigidity in scheduling care

V. Native Americans

A. Communication
   1. Languages include English, Navajo, and other tribal languages
   2. Silence indicates respect for the speaker
   3. Speak in a low tone of voice and expect others to be attentive
   4. Eye contact is avoided because it is a sign of disrespect
   5. Body language is important

B. Space
   1. Personal space is very important
   2. Will lightly touch another person's hand during greetings
   3. Massage is used for the newborn infant to promote bonding between infant and mother
   4. Touching a dead body is prohibited

C. Social Roles
   1. Very family oriented
   2. Basic family unit is the extended family and often includes people from several households
   3. In some tribes, grandparents are viewed as family leaders
   4. Elders are honored
   5. Children are taught to respect traditions
   6. The father does all the work outside the home, and the mother assumes responsibility for domestic duties
   7. Sacred myths and legends provide spiritual guidance
   8. Religion and healing practices are integrated
   9. Community social organizations are important

D. Health and Illness
   1. Health is a state of harmony between the person, the family, and the environment
   2. Illness is caused by supernatural forces and disequilibrium between person and environment

E. Health Risks
   1. Tuberculosis
   2. Diabetes
   3. Heart disease
   4. Arthritis
   5. American Eskimos are susceptible to glaucoma?

F. Implementation
   1. Clarify communication
   2. Understand that the client may be attentive even when eye contact is absent
   3. Be attentive to own use of body language
   4. Obtain input from extended family members
   5. Encourage client to personalize space in which health care is delivered—for example, to bring personal items or objects to the hospital
   6. In the home, assess for the availability of running water, and modify infection control and hygiene practices as necessary

PRACTICE QUESTIONS

1. The nurse is conducting an admission assessment of an African-American client scheduled for a hernia repair. Which of the following assessment data are of least priority during the initial assessment?
   1 Cardiovascular assessment data
   2 Neurological assessment data
   3 Respiratory assessment data
   ④ Psychosocial assessment data

2. The nurse is caring for an African-American client. The nurse enters the room and, following a greeting and introduction to the client, the nurse begins to describe the angiogram procedure scheduled for the following day. The client turns away from the nurse. Which of the following nursing actions is most appropriate?
   ① Continue with the explanation
   2 Ask the client if he or she can hear the nurse
   3 Walk around to the client so that the nurse faces the client
   4 Leave the room and return later to continue with the explanation

3. The nurse caring for an African-American client is reviewing the plan of care. The client frequently nods the head during the review. The nurse interprets this behavior as:
   1 The client agrees with the plan
   ② The client may not necessarily agree with the plan
   3 The client would like to hear more about the plan
   4 The client is very anxious

4. The nursing instructor is providing a session on cultural beliefs related to health and illness. Following the session, the instructor asks the nursing student to describe the beliefs of an African-American in regard to illness. Which of the following would be the most appropriate response?
   1 Illness is due to an imbalance between yin and yang
   2 Illness is punishment for sins
   ③ Illness is a disharmonious state that may be caused by demons and spirits
   4 Illness is due to lack of exercise

5. The nurse is planning to instruct the African-American client about nutrition. When developing the plan, the nurse is aware that a common dietary practice of the African Americans is to:
   1. Eat fried foods
   2. Eat rice as the basis for all meals
   3. Eat red meat
   4. Eat raw fish

6. The nurse caring for an Asian-American client plans care considering the client's view of illness. Which of the following most appropriately describes the Asian-American's view of illness?
   1. Illness is caused by supernatural forces
   2. Illness is punishment for sins
   3. Illness is a disharmonious state that may be caused by demons and spirits
   4. Illness is due to an imbalance between yin and yang

7. The nurse develops a plan of care for an Asian-American client. Which of the following would not be a component of the plan of care?
   1. Avoid physical closeness
   2. Limit eye contact
   3. Avoid hand gestures
   4. Provide light touch to the head for comfort

8. The nurse consults with a nutritionist regarding the dietary preferences of an Asian-American client. Which of the following foods would most appropriately be included in the dietary plan?
   1. Red meat
   2. Rice
   3. Fried foods
   4. Fruits

9. The European-American client maintains eye contact with the nurse during a conversation regarding the preoperative teaching plan. The nurse interprets this nonverbal communication as:
   1. Rudeness
   2. Arrogance
   3. Indicating uneasiness
   4. Indicating trustworthiness

10. The nurse develops a plan of care for a European-American client. The nurse considers the practices and preferences of the culture when planning the care. Which of the following practices and preferences are not a characteristic of this ethnic group?
    1. Community social organizations are important
    2. Health is often viewed as an absence of disease or illness

3. Appear stoic when expressing physical concerns
4. The woman is the dominant figure

11. The nurse calls the dietary department to obtain a dinner meal for a European-American client who was admitted to the hospital at 4:00 P.M. The physician prescribed a diet "as tolerated." Considering the practices and preferences of the European-American, which of the following foods would the nurse request for the meal?
    1. Red meat and potatoes
    2. Blue cornmeal
    3. Kosher foods
    4. Rice

12. A Hispanic-American mother brings her child to the clinic for an examination. Which of the following would be most important during the assessment of the child?
    1. Avoiding eye contact
    2. Touching the child during the examination
    3. Avoiding speaking to the child
    4. Using body language only

13. The nurse is caring for a Hispanic-American client admitted with a diagnosis of diabetic ketoacidosis. Several family members are present. Which of the following behaviors, if displayed by the family members, would the nurse interpret as characteristic of this cultural group?
    1. Dramatic body language
    2. Consistently expressing negative feelings
    3. Maintaining consistent eye contact
    4. Consistently confronting the nurse directly

14. The nurse develops a plan of care for the Native American client, considering the practices and preferences of the culture. Which of the following practices and preferences are not a characteristic of this ethnic group?
    1. Religion and healing practices
    2. Touching the body of a dead family member
    3. Avoidance of eye contact
    4. Use of healing practices

15. The nurse caring for an Orthodox Jewish client plans a diet that adheres to the practices of Judaism. Which of the following is not a practice of Judaism?
    1. Eating fish with scales and fins is allowed
    2. Meat is allowed if ritually slaughtered
    3. Only unleavened bread is eaten during Passover week
    4. Meat and milk can be eaten together

ANSWERS

1. **4**

Rationale: The psychosocial assessment is the lowest priority during the initial admission assessment. In the African-American culture, it is considered to be intrusive to ask personal questions on the initial contact or meeting. Additionally, cardiovascular, neurological, and respiratory assessments include physiological assessments, which would be the priority assessments.

Test-Taking Strategy: Knowledge regarding the characteristics of the African-American culture will assist in answering the question. Use Maslow's Hierarchy of Needs Theory to answer the question. Note that the question asks for the least priority. Options 1, 2, and 3 address physiological needs. Option 4 addresses the psychosocial need and is the correct answer to the question.

Level of Cognitive Ability: Application
Phase of Nursing Process: Assessment
Client Needs: Physiological Integrity
Content Area: Fundamental Skills

Reference
Swanson, J., & Nies, M. (1997). *Community health nursing: Promoting the health of aggregates* (2nd ed.). Philadelphia: W. B. Saunders. p. 488.

2. **1**

Rationale: In the African-American culture, direct eye contact is often viewed as being rude. If the client turns away from the nurse during a conversation, the best action is to continue with the conversation. Walking around to the client so that the nurse faces the client is in direct conflict with the cultural practice. Asking the client if she or he can hear the nurse or leaving the room and returning later to continue with the explanation may be viewed as a rude gesture by the client.

Test-Taking Strategy: Understanding the characteristics of this cultural group will assist in answering the question. Utilize the process of elimination. Eliminate options 2 and 4 first, as these are nontherapeutic actions. From the remaining two options, option 1 is the most therapeutic. If you had difficulty with this question, take time now to review the communication practices of this cultural group!

Level of Cognitive Ability: Application
Phase of Nursing Process: Implementation
Client Needs: Psychosocial Integrity
Content Area: Fundamental Skills

Reference
Swanson, J., & Nies, M. (1997). *Community health nursing: Promoting the health of aggregates* (2nd ed.). Philadelphia: W. B. Saunders. p. 488.

3. **2**

Rationale: In the African-American culture, head nodding does not necessarily mean that the client is in agreement with what is being presented. The nurse needs to be alert to nonverbal communication. It is important for the nurse to validate the client's nonverbal communication.

Test-Taking Strategy: Understanding the characteristics of this cultural group will assist in answering the question.

Take time now to review the importance and meaning of nonverbal communication if you had difficulty with this question!

Level of Cognitive Ability: Analysis
Phase of Nursing Process: Analysis
Client Needs: Psychosocial Integrity
Content Area: Fundamental Skills

Reference
Swanson, J., & Nies, M. (1997). *Community health nursing: Promoting the health of aggregates* (2nd ed.). Philadelphia: W. B. Saunders. p. 488.

4. **3**

Rationale: In the African-American culture, illness is viewed as a disharmonious state that may be caused by demons and spirits. The goal of treatment, from the traditional African perspective, is to remove the harmful spirit from the body of the ill person. Asian-Americans believe that illness is due to an imbalance between yin and yang and due to prolonged sitting or lying, or to overexertion.

Test-Taking Strategy: Knowledge regarding the beliefs related to health and illness of the various cultures would assist in answering the question. From this point, use the process of elimination in determining the correct option. If you had difficulty with the question, take time now to review these various beliefs!

Level of Cognitive Ability: Analysis
Phase of Nursing Process: Evaluation
Client Needs: Psychosocial Integrity
Content Area: Fundamental Skills

Reference
Swanson, J., & Nies, M. (1997). *Community health nursing: Promoting the health of aggregates* (2nd ed.). Philadelphia: W.B. Saunders. p. 489.

5. **1**

Rationale: African-American food preferences include pork, greens, rice, and fried foods. Asian-Americans eat raw fish, rice, and soy sauce. Hispanic-Americans prefer beans, fried foods, spicy foods, chili, and carbonated beverages. European-Americans prefer carbohydrates and red meat.

Test-Taking Strategy: Knowledge of the food practices and preferences related to the various cultures is required to answer the question. Knowledge that African-Americans are at risk for hypertension and coronary artery disease may assist in directing you to option 1. If you had difficulty with this question, take time now to review the food preferences associated with the African-American culture!

Level of Cognitive Ability: Analysis
Phase of Nursing Process: Planning
Client Needs: Physiological Integrity
Content Area: Fundamental Skills

Reference
Leahy, J., & Kizilay, P. (1998). *Foundations of nursing practice: A nursing process approach.* Philadelphia: W. B. Saunders. p. 1105.

6. **4**

Rationale: Asian-Americans believe that illness is due to an imbalance between yin and yang and due to prolonged sitting or lying, or to overexertion. In the African-American culture, illness is viewed as a disharmonious state that may be caused by demons and spirits. Native Americans believe that illness is caused by supernatural forces.

Test-Taking Strategy: Knowledge of the beliefs related to health and illness of the various cultures would assist in answering the question. From this point, utilize the process of elimination in determining the correct option. If you had difficulty with the question, take time now to review these various beliefs!

Level of Cognitive Ability: Analysis
Phase of Nursing Process: Analysis
Client Needs: Psychosocial Integrity
Content Area: Fundamental Skills

Reference
Luckmann, J. (1997). *Saunders manual of nursing care.* Philadelphia: W.B. Saunders. p. 41.

7. 4

Rationale: Avoiding physical closeness, limiting eye contact, avoiding hand gestures, and clarifying responses to questions are all a component of the plan of care for an Asian-American client. In the Asian-American culture, the head is considered to be sacred, therefore touching someone on the head is disrespectful. Touch the client's head only when necessary, and inform the client before doing so.

Test-Taking Strategy: Utilize knowledge regarding the characteristics of the Asian-Americans and the process of elimination to answer the question. Note that options 1, 2, and 3 are similar in that they all address a lack of physical contact. Option 4 is the different option. If you had difficulty with this question, take time now to review the beliefs associated with this culture!

Level of Cognitive Ability: Application
Phase of Nursing Process: Planning
Client Needs: Psychosocial Integrity
Content Area: Fundamental Skills

Reference
Luckmann, J. (1997). *Saunders manual of nursing care.* Philadelphia: W.B. Saunders. p. 474.

8. 2

Rationale: Asian-American food preferences include raw fish, rice, and soy sauce. African-American food preferences include pork, greens, rice, and fried foods. Hispanic-Americans prefer beans, fried foods, spicy foods, chili, and carbonated beverages. European-Americans prefer carbohydrates and red meat.

Test-Taking Strategy: Knowledge of the food practices and preferences related to the various cultures is required to answer the question. Correlate rice with Asian-Americans. This may assist when answering other questions similar to this one. If you had difficulty with this question, take time now to review the food preferences associated with the Asian-American culture!

Level of Cognitive Ability: Analysis
Phase of Nursing Process: Planning
Client Needs: Physiological Integrity
Content Area: Fundamental Skills

Reference
Leahy, J., & Kizilay, P. (1998). *Foundations of nursing practice: A nursing process approach.* Philadelphia: W. B. Saunders. p. 1106.

9. 4

Rationale: In the European-American culture, eye contact is viewed as indicating trustworthiness. It is a nursing responsibility, however, to monitor the client's body language and respect the client's personal space when implementing care.

Test-Taking Strategy: Utilize knowledge regarding the verbal and nonverbal communication practices associated with the European-American culture to answer the question. Use the process of elimination, noting that options 1, 2, and 3 are similar in that they indicate a negative response. Option 4 is the only option indicating positiveness. If you had difficulty with this question, take time now to review the communication practices of the European-American culture!

Level of Cognitive Ability: Analysis
Phase of Nursing Process: Analysis
Client Needs: Psychosocial Integrity
Content Area: Fundamental Skills

Reference
Purnell, L., & Paulanka, B. (1998). *Transcultural healthcare: A culturally competent approach.* Philadelphia: F. A. Davis. p. 357.

10. 4

Rationale: In the European-American culture, the man is the dominant figure. Community social organizations are important in this culture. Health is often viewed as an absence of disease or illness. European-Americans tend to be aloof and avoid physical contact and appear stoic when expressing physical concerns.

Test-Taking Strategy: Utilize knowledge of the practices and beliefs associated with the European-American culture to answer the question. If you had difficulty with this question, take time now to review the practices and beliefs of the European-American culture!

Level of Cognitive Ability: Analysis
Phase of Nursing Process: Analysis
Client Needs: Psychosocial Integrity
Content Area: Fundamental Skills

Reference
Purnell, L., & Paulanka, B. (1998). *Transcultural healthcare: A culturally competent approach.* Philadelphia: F. A. Davis. p. 358.

11. 1

Rationale: Food preferences of European-Americans include carbohydrates as potatoes and red meat. Native American preferences include blue cornmeal, fish, game, fruits, and berries. Asian-Americans prefer rice and raw fish. Dietary kosher laws are adhered to by members of the Jewish community.

Test-Taking Strategy: Knowledge of the food preferences of cultural groups will assist in answering the question. Utilize the process of elimination, remembering that kosher foods are important to the Jewish population, blue cornmeal to Native Americans, and rice to Asian-Americans. Take time now to review food preferences of the various cultures if you had difficulty with this question!

Level of Cognitive Ability: Analysis
Phase of Nursing Process: Planning
Client Needs: Physiological Integrity
Content Area: Fundamental Skills

Reference
Purnell, L., & Paulanka, B. (1998). *Transcultural healthcare: A culturally competent approach.* Philadelphia: F. A. Davis. p. 363.

12. **2**

Rationale: In the Hispanic-American culture, eye behavior is significant. The "evil eye" can be given to a child if a person looks at and admires a child without touching the child. Therefore, touching the child during the examination is very important. Although avoiding eye contact indicates respect and attentiveness, this is not the most important intervention during the assessment of a child. Avoiding speaking to the child and using body language only are not therapeutic interventions.

Test-Taking Strategy: Utilize the process of elimination. Eliminate options 3 and 4 first as they are basically similar. From the remaining two options, select the intervention that is most therapeutic, that being touch. If you had difficulty with this question, take time now to review the characteristics associated with Hispanic-Americans!

Level of Cognitive Ability: Application
Phase of Nursing Process: Implementation
Client Needs: Psychosocial Integrity
Content Area: Fundamental Skills

Reference
Purnell, L., & Paulanka, B. (1998). *Transcultural healthcare: A culturally competent approach.* Philadelphia: F. A. Davis. p. 400.

13. **1**

Rationale: Characteristics of the Hispanic-American culture include the use of dramatic body language, such as gestures or facial expressions, to express emotion or pain. Their belief is that direct confrontation is disrespectful, and the expression of negative feelings is impolite. Additionally, in this culture, avoiding direct eye contact indicates respect and attentiveness.

Test-Taking Strategy: Knowledge of the beliefs and traditions of this culture is required to answer this question. From this knowledge, use the process of elimination to answer the question. If you had difficulty with this question, take time now to review the beliefs of the Hispanic-American culture!

Level of Cognitive Ability: Analysis
Phase of Nursing Process: Analysis
Client Needs: Psychosocial Integrity
Content Area: Fundamental Skills

Reference
Purnell, L., & Paulanka, B. (1998). *Transcultural healthcare: A culturally competent approach.* Philadelphia: F. A. Davis. p. 400.

14. **2**

Rationale: In the Native American culture, touching a dead body is prohibited. The use of religion and healing practices is integrated into health care and illness practices. Eye contact is avoided because it is a sign of disrespect.

Test-Taking Strategy: Utilize the process of elimination based on knowledge of the beliefs of this cultural group. Eliminate options 1 and 4 first because they are similar. Remembering that eye contact is a sign of disrespect will direct you to the correct option, option 2. If you had difficulty with this question, take time now to review the traditional beliefs of the Native American!

Level of Cognitive Ability: Analysis
Phase of Nursing Process: Analysis
Client Needs: Psychosocial Integrity
Content Area: Fundamental Skills

Reference
Leahy, J., & Kizilay, P. (1998). *Foundations of nursing practice: A nursing process approach.* Philadelphia: W.B. Saunders. p. 1109.

15. **4**

Rationale: Dietary kosher laws must be adhered to by Orthodox believers. Meats allowed include animals that are vegetable eaters, cloven-hoofed animals, and animals that are ritually slaughtered. Fish that have scales and fins are allowed; however, any combination of meat and milk is prohibited. During Passover week, only unleavened bread is eaten.

Test-Taking Strategy: Read the question carefully, noting the word "not" in the stem of the question. Knowledge regarding the dietary practices in Judaism is required to answer the question. If you had difficulty with the question, take time now to review the dietary practices of this cultural group!

Level of Cognitive Ability: Analysis
Phase of Nursing Process: Analysis
Client Needs: Psychosocial Integrity
Content Area: Fundamental Skills

Reference
Purnell, L., & Paulanka, B. (1998). *Transcultural healthcare: A culturally competent approach.* Philadelphia: F. A. Davis. pp. 380–381.

REFERENCES

Black, J., & Matassarin-Jacobs, E. (1997). *Medical surgical nursing: Clinical management for continuity of care* (5th ed.). Philadelphia: W.B. Saunders.

DeLaune, S., & Ladner, P. (1998). *Fundamentals of nursing standards and practice.* Albany, NY: Delmar.

Ignatavicius, D., Workman, M., & Mishler, M. (1995). *Medical surgical nursing: A nursing process approach* (2nd ed.). Philadelphia: W.B. Saunders.

Leahy, J., & Kizilay, P. (1998). *Foundations of nursing practice: A nursing process approach.* Philadelphia: W.B. Saunders.

Luckmann, J. (1997). *Saunders manual of nursing care.* Philadelphia: W.B. Saunders.

Purnell, L., & Paulanka, B. (1998). *Transcultural healthcare: A culturally competent approach.* Philadelphia: F. A. Davis.

Swanson, J., & Nies, M. (1997). *Community health nursing: Promoting the health of aggregates* (2nd ed.). Philadelphia: W.B. Saunders.

CHAPTER 6

Ethical and Legal Issues

PYRAMID TERMS

Advance Directive—Written document, recognized by state law, that provides directions concerning the provision of care when a person is unable to make his or her own treatment choices.

Advocacy—Acting on behalf of the client, protecting the clients' rights to make their own decisions.

Consent—Voluntary act by which a person agrees to allow someone else to do something.

Ethics—Concerns the distinction between right and wrong on the basis of a body of knowledge, not just on the basis of opinions.

Informed Consent—The client understands the reason for the proposed intervention, with its benefits and risks, and agrees to the treatment by signing a consent form.

Law—A system composed of general rules governing conduct, and the procedures for resolving disputes when rules are not followed.

Malpractice—Failure to meet the standards of acceptable care, which results in harm to another person.

Negligence—Failure to provide care that a reasonable person would ordinarily use in a similar circumstance.

Patient's Bill of Rights—Includes the rights and responsibilities of clients receiving care.

Values—Beliefs and attitudes that may influence behavior and the process of decision making.

PYRAMID TO SUCCESS

Across all settings in the practice of nursing, nurses are frequently confronted with **ethical** and legal issues related to client care. It is the responsibility of the professional nurse to be aware of the **ethical** principles, **laws,** and guidelines related to providing safe and quality care to clients. In the Pyramid to Success, focus on **ethical** practices; the Nurse Practice Act; Client Rights, particularly confidentiality; and **informed consent, advocacy,** documentation, **advance directives,** death and dying, and organ donation.

NURSING PROCESS

ASSESSMENT

Client values
Cultural and religious beliefs
Client rights
Standards of Care
Ethical and legal responsibilities

ANALYSIS: Determine actual and potential nursing diagnoses based on ethical and legal considerations related to the client treatment plan

PLANNING	IMPLEMENTATION	EVALUATION
Develop the plan of care based on the ethical and legal considerations related to the client. Include the client and family in the plan of care as appropriate. Consult with client and family in planning care.	Identify own value system. Function within the guidelines of the Nurse Practice Act, Standards of Care, Code of Ethics, and agency policies and procedures and legal system. Identify cultural and religious preferences of the client. Develop a caring and nonjudgmental relationship with client. Provide care functioning as a client advocate and protect client rights. Respect client and family needs based on their value system.	Determine compatibility of plan with client and family in meeting needs based on their value system and legal responsibilities. Client rights are upheld.

◆ CLIENT NEEDS

SAFE, EFFECTIVE CARE ENVIRONMENT

Advance directives
Advocacy
Client rights
Confidentiality
Ethical practice
Incident reports
Informed consent
Legal responsibilities
Organ donation

HEALTH PROMOTION AND MAINTENANCE

Developmental stages and transitions
Family systems
Lifestyle choices

PSYCHOSOCIAL INTEGRITY

Grief and loss
Support systems
Chemical dependency
Abuse/neglect

PHYSIOLOGICAL INTEGRITY

Basic care and comfort
Alterations in body systems
Potential complications of tests and procedures

I. Ethics and Values

A. **Ethics:** The branch of philosophy that concerns the distinction between right and wrong on the basis of a body of knowledge, not just on the basis of opinions
B. Morality: Behavior in accordance with customs or tradition, usually reflecting personal or religious beliefs
C. Teleology
   1. Ethical theory that states that the value of a situation is determined by its consequences
   2. Principle of Utility states that the act must result in the greatest amount of good for the greatest number of people involved in a situation
D. Deontology: Ethical theory that considers the intrinsic significance of the act itself as the criterion for determination of good

E. Ethical principles: Codes that direct or govern our actions (Box 6–1)
F. **Values:** Beliefs and attitudes that may influence behavior and the process of decision making
G. Values clarification: Process of analyzing one's own values to better understand what is truly important
H. Ethical Codes
   1. Provide broad principles for determining and evaluating client care
   2. Are not legally binding, but in most states, the Board of Nursing has authority to reprimand nurses for unprofessional conduct that results from violation of an ethical code
   3. Specific ethical codes
      a. The Code for Nurses developed by the International Council of Nurses
      b. American Nurses Association (ANA) Code of **Ethics**
I. Ethical dilemma
   1. Occurs when there is a conflict between two or more ethical principles

BOX 6–1. Ethical Principles	
Autonomy	Respect for an individual's right to self determination
Nonmaleficence	The obligation to do or cause no harm to another
Beneficence	The duty to do good to others and to maintain a balance between benefits and harms. Paternalism is an undesirable outcome of beneficence, in which the health care provider decides what is best for the client and attempts to encourage the client to act against his or her own choices
Justice	The equitable distribution of potential benefits and tasks
Veracity	The obligation to tell the truth
Fidelity	The duty to do what one has promised

2. There is no correct decision
3. The nurse must make a choice between two alternatives that are equally unsatisfactory
4. Ethical reasoning is the process of thinking through what one ought to do in an orderly and systematic manner to provide justification of actions based on principles

J. **Advocate**
1. A person who speaks up for or acts on the behalf of a client, protects the client's right to make her or his own decisions, and upholds the principle of fidelity
2. Represents the client's viewpoint to others
3. Avoids letting personal **values** influence **advocacy** for the client
4. Supports client decision even when it conflicts with own preferences or choices

K. **Ethics** committees
1. Multidisciplinary approach to facilitate dialogue regarding ethical dilemmas
2. Develop and establish policies and procedures for the prevention and resolution of dilemmas

II. Regulation of Nursing Practice

A. Nurse Practice Act
1. A series of statutes enacted by each state legislature to regulate the practice of nursing in that state
2. Nursing practice acts set educational requirements for the nurse, distinguish between nursing and medical practice, and define the scope of nursing practice
3. Additional issues covered by the nurse practice acts include licensure requirement for protection of the public, grounds for disciplinary action, rights of the nurse licensee if a disciplinary action is taken, and related topics
4. All nurses are responsible for knowing the provisions of the act of the state or province in which they work

B. Standards of care
1. Guidelines by which the nurse should practice
2. Guidelines for determining whether nurses performed duties in an appropriate manner
3. If nurses do not perform duties within accepted standards of care, they place themselves in jeopardy of legal action
4. If nurses are named as defendants in a **malpractice** lawsuit and it is shown that neither the accepted standards of care outlined by the state or province nursing practice act nor the policies of the employing institution were followed, the nurses' legal liability is clear

C. Employee guidelines
1. Respondent superior: Employer will be held liable for any negligent acts of an employee if the alleged negligent act occurred during the employment relationship and was within the scope of the employee's responsibilities

2. Contracts
   a. Nurses are responsible for carrying out the terms of a contractual agreement with the employee agency and the client
   b. The nurse employee relationship is governed by established employee handbooks and client care policies and procedures that create obligations, rights, and duties between those parties

3. Institutional policies
   a. Written policies and procedures of the employing institution that detail how nurses are to perform their duties
   b. Policies and procedures are usually quite specific and are located in manuals in most health care facilities
   c. Although policies are not **laws,** courts generally rule against nurses who violate policies
   d. If the nurse practices nursing in accordance with the client care policies and procedures established by the employer, functions within the job responsibility, and provides care consistent with the care in a nonnegligent manner, the potential for liability is minimized

D. Hospital staffing
1. Nurses should not walk out when staffing is inadequate because charges of abandonment can be made
2. Nurses in short staffing situations are obligated to make a report to nursing administration

E. Floating
1. An acceptable legal practice used by hospitals to solve their understaffing problems
2. Legally, a nurse cannot refuse to float unless a union contract guarantees that nurses can work only in a specified area or the nurse can prove lack of knowledge for the performance of assigned tasks
3. Nurses in a floating situation must not assume responsibility beyond their level of experience or qualification
4. Nurses who float should inform the supervisor of any lack of experience in caring for the type of clients on the new nursing unit
5. The nurse should request and be given orientation to the new unit

F. Disciplinary action
1. Boards of nursing may deny, revoke, or suspend any license to practice as a registered nurse in accordance with their statutory authority
2. Causes for disciplinary action
   a. Unprofessional conduct
   b. Conduct that could adversely affect the health and welfare of the public

c. Breach in client confidentiality
d. Failure to use sufficient knowledge, skills, or nursing judgment
e. Physically or verbally abusing a client
f. Assuming duties without sufficient preparation
g. Knowingly delegating to unlicensed personnel nursing care that places the client at risk for injury
h. Failure to accurately maintain a record for each client
i. Falsifying a client's record
j. Leaving a nursing assignment without properly notifying appropriate personnel

III. Legal Liability

A. **Laws**
1. Nurses are governed by civil and criminal **law** in roles as providers of services, employees of institutions, and private citizens
2. A nurse has a personal and legal obligation to provide a standard of client care expected of a reasonably competent professional nurse
3. Professional nurses are held responsible (liable) for harm resulting from their negligent acts, or their failure to act

B. Types of **laws** (Box 6–2)

C. **Negligence** and **malpractice**
1. Conduct that falls below the standard of care
2. Can include acts of commission as well as acts of omission
3. If a nurse gives care that does not meet appropriate standards, he or she may be held liable for **negligence**

BOX 6–2. Types of Laws	
Contract Law	Concerned with enforcement of agreements among private individuals
Civil Law	Concerned with relationships among people and the protection of a person's rights Violation may cause harm to an individual or property, but no grave threat to society exists
Criminal Law	Concerned with relationships between individuals and governments and with acts that threaten society and its order A crime is an offense against society that violates a law and is defined as a misdemeanor (less serious nature) or felony (serious nature)
Tort Law	Civil wrong, other than a breach in contract, in which the law allows an injured person to seek damage from a person who caused the injury

4. **Malpractice** is **negligence** on the part of a nurse
5. **Malpractice** is determined if the nurse owed a duty to the client and did not carry out the duty, and the client was injured because the nurse failed to perform the duty
6. Proof of liability
   a. Duty: At the time of injury, a duty existed between the plaintiff and defendant
   b. Breach of duty: The defendant breached duty of care to the plaintiff
   c. Causation: The breach of the duty was the legal cause of injury to the client
   d. Injury: The plaintiff experienced injury or damages or both and can be compensated by **law**

D. Professional liability insurance
1. Nurses need their own liability insurance for protection against **malpractice** lawsuits
2. Having one's own insurance provides the nurse protection as an individual and allows the nurse to have an attorney present who has only the nurse's interests in mind

E. Good Samaritan **laws**
1. Passed by a state legislature
2. Encourage health care professionals to assist in emergency situations without fear of being sued for the care provided
3. These **laws** limit liability and offer legal immunity for people helping in an emergency providing they give reasonable care
4. Immunity from suit applies only when all the conditions of the state **law** are met, such as the health care provider receives no compensation for the care provided and the care given is not intentionally negligent

F. Controlled substances
1. Adhere to facility policies and procedures concerning administration of controlled substances, which is governed by federal and state **laws**
2. Controlled substances must be kept securely locked, and only authorized personnel should have access to them

IV. Legal Risk Areas

A. Assault
1. Occurs when a person puts another person in fear of a harmful or an offensive contact
2. The victim fears and believes harm will result as a result of the threat

B. Battery: An intentional touching of another's body without the other's **consent**

C. Invasion of privacy: Includes violating confidentiality, intruding on private client or family matters, and sharing client information with unauthorized persons

D. False imprisonment
1. Occurs when a client is not allowed to leave

a health care facility when there is no legal justification to detain the client

2. Occurs when restraining devices are used without an appropriate clinical need

3. A client can sign an "Against Medical Advice" form when the client refuses care and is competent to make decisions

4. Document circumstances in the medical record to avoid allegations by the client that cannot be defended

E. Defamation: Occurs when information is communicated to a third party that causes damage to someone's reputation, either in writing (libel) or verbally (slander)

F. Fraud: Results from a deliberate deception intended to produce unlawful gains

V. Client Rights

A. Patient's Bill of Rights
1. Increases health care providers' awareness of the need to treat clients in an ethical and legal manner and encourages protection of rights
2. Key elements of a client's rights with which nurses should be familiar include **informed consent** and confidentiality

B. Confidentiality
1. A special relationship exists between two persons in which information discussed will not be shared with a third party who is not directly involved in the client's care
2. Nurses are bound to protect client confidentiality by most nurse practice acts, by ethical principles and standards, and by institutional and agency policies and procedures
3. Treatment records cannot be released to any third party without the client's written **consent** and only after agency policies and procedures are followed
4. Information release may be mandatory when ordered by a court, or when state statutes require reporting child abuse, communicable diseases, or other associated incidents

C. **Informed consent**
1. **Consent** is the client's approval to have his or her body touched by a specific individual
2. Legally, the client must be mentally competent to give **consent** for procedures
3. Prior to granting a **consent,** the client must be fully informed regarding treatment, tests, surgery, and so on, and must understand both the intended outcome and the potentially harmful results
4. **Consent** must be obtained by the physician, surgeon, or other medical practitioner performing the treatment or procedure
5. In most states, when a nurse is involved in the **informed consent** process, the nurse is only witnessing the signature of the client on the **informed consent** form

6. If a client is determined by a court to be unable to make decisions and is declared incompetent or under a legal disability, a personal guardian is appointed by the court to make decisions

7. An **informed consent** can be waived for urgent medical and surgical intervention as long as institutional policy so indicates

8. Parental or guardian **consent** should be obtained before treatment is initiated on a minor except in an emergency, in situations where the **consent** of the minor is sufficient such as treatment of a sexually transmitted disease, or if a court order or other legal authorization has been obtained

9. Minors who are married or emancipated from parents and those seeking treatment for sexually transmitted diseases can sign an informed **consent** form

10. A client has the right to refuse information and waive the **informed consent** and undergo treatment, but this decision must be documented in the medical record

VI. Legal Safeguards

A. Risk management
1. A planned method to identify, analyze, and evaluate risks followed by a plan for reducing the frequency of accidents and injuries
2. Programs are based on a systematic reporting system of incidents or unusual occurrences

B. Incident reports
1. A tool used as a means of identifying and improving client care
2. Follow specific documentation guidelines
3. Fill out completely, accurately, and factually
4. The report form should not be copied or placed in the client's record
5. No reference should be made to the report form in the client record
6. Not a substitute for a complete entry in the client's record regarding the incident

C. Physician's orders
1. The nurse is obligated to carry out physician's orders except when the nurse believes the order is inappropriate
2. A nurse carrying out an inaccurate order may be legally responsible for any harm suffered by the client
3. Clarify an unclear or inappropriate order with the physician
4. If no resolution occurs regarding the order in question, contact the nurse manager or supervisor
5. See Box 6–3 concerning telephone orders

D. Documentation
1. Legally required by accrediting agencies, state licensing **laws,** and state nurse and medical practice acts

---

BOX 6–3. Telephone Orders

- Date and time the entry
- Repeat the order to the physician and record the order given
- Sign the order beginning with t.o. (telephone order), write physician's name, and sign the order
- If another nurse witnessed the order, that signature follows
- The physician needs to countersign the order within a time frame according to agency policy

---

2. Follow agency guidelines and procedures (Box 6–4)

E. Client/family teaching
  1. Provide complete instructions in a language client can understand
  2. Document client and family teaching, what was taught, evaluation of understanding, who was present during the teaching
  3. Inform client of what would happen if information shared during teaching is not followed

VII. Legal Documents for Decision Making

A. Wills
  1. Some agencies have specific policies that

BOX 6–4. Documentation Guidelines

NARRATIVE

- Use a black pen
- Date and time entries
- Provide objective, factual, and complete documentation
- Document care, medications, treatments, and procedures as soon as possible after completed
- Document client responses to interventions
- Document consent for or refusal of treatments
- Document calls made to other health care providers
- Do not document for others or change documentation for other individuals
- Sign and title each entry
- Use quotes as appropriate for subjective data
- Use correct spelling, grammar, and punctuation
- Avoid unacceptable abbreviations
- Avoid judgmental or evaluative statements, such as "uncooperative client"
- Do not leave blank spaces on documentation forms
- Follow agency policies when an error is made (draw one line through the error, initial, and date)
- Follow agency guidelines regarding late entries

COMPUTERIZED

- Use only the user ID code, name, or password
- Never lend access ID to another
- Maintain privacy and confidentiality of documented information printed from the computer

---

prohibit the nurse from signing as witness to this legal document for a client
  2. If a nurse witnesses a legal document, the nurse must document the event and the factual circumstances surrounding the signing in the medical record
  3. Documentation should include who was present, any significant comments by the client, and the nurse's observations of the client's conduct during the process

B. **Advance directive**
  1. Written document recognized by state **law** that provides directions concerning the provision of care when a person is unable to make his or her own treatment choices
  2. Must be made part of the medical record
  3. The physician must be notified of its presence so orders can be written consistent with the client's wishes

C. Living will: Document prepared by a competent adult that provides direction regarding medical care in the event of a person's incapacitation or otherwise becoming unable to make decisions personally

D. Durable power of attorney
  1. Also called health care proxy
  2. An authorization that enables any competent individual to name someone to exercise decision-making authority under specific circumstances on the individual's behalf

VIII. Death and Dying

A. Right of informed refusal: A competent adult has the right to refuse treatment, even life-sustaining treatment

B. Do not resuscitate (DNR) orders
  1. A written order must be present and must be reviewed on a regular basis
  2. Specific agency guidelines must be followed regarding when and under what circumstances an oral DNR order is acceptable
  3. The client or legal representative must provide **informed consent** for the DNR status
  4. Both DNR and CPR (cardiopulmonary resuscitation) must be clearly defined so that other treatment not refused by the client will be continued

C. Organ transplant: The option to accept an organ transplant can be refused

D. Organ donation
  1. Any person 18 years of age or older may become an organ donor by written **consent**
  2. Informed choice to donate an organ can take place with the use of a written document signed by the client prior to death, a will, donor card, or **advance directive**
  3. A family member or legal guardian may authorize donation of the decedent's organs in the absence of appropriate documentation

4. All 50 states have adopted the Uniform Anatomical Gift Act for cadaveric organ donation
E. Autopsy
   1. Medical examination of the body after death for the purpose of determining the cause of death
   2. Required by state **law** in certain circumstances, such as a sudden death or a death that occurs under suspicious circumstances
   3. If no oral or written instructions were given by the decedent, state **law** determines who has the authority to **consent** to any autopsy requested on a voluntary basis
   4. Documentation regarding **consent** must be present before the body can be released for autopsy
F. Assisted suicide
   1. Legal support exists for a client to refuse life-sustaining procedures and for health care providers to honor the client's voluntary and informed decision by withdrawing or withholding treatment
   2. Taking an active role in assisting a client to die is a criminal offense in many states

◆ **IX. Reporting Responsibilities**

A. Requirements: Nurses are required to report certain communicable diseases or criminal activities such as abuse, gunshot or stab wounds, assaults, homicides, and suicides to the appropriate authorities
◆ B. The impaired nurse
   1. If a nurse suspects that a coworker is abusing chemicals, the nurse must report the individual to nursing administration in a confidential manner with the goal of treatment being the priority issue
   2. Nursing administration then notifies the board of nursing regarding the nurse's behavior
C. Occupational Safety and Health Administration (OSHA)
   1. Requires that an employer provide a safe workplace for employees according to regulations
   2. Employees can confidentially report working conditions that violate regulations
   3. An employee who does not report unsafe working conditions can be retaliated against by the employer
D. Sexual harassment
   1. Prohibited by state and federal **laws**
   2. Includes unwelcome conduct of a sexual nature
   3. Follow agency policies and procedures to handle reporting a concern or complaint

PRACTICE QUESTIONS

1. The nurse enters the client's room and finds the client lying on the floor. Following assessment of the client, the nurse calls the nursing supervisor and the physician to inform them of the occurrence. The nursing supervisor instructs the nurse to complete an incident report. The nurse understands that incident reports allow the analysis of adverse client events by:
   1 Evaluating quality care and the potential risks for injury to the client
   2 Determining the effectiveness of nursing interventions
   3 Providing a method of reporting injuries to local, state, and federal agencies
   4 Providing clients with necessary stabilizing treatments

2. The nurse observes that the client received pain medication 1 hour ago from another nurse, but that the client still has severe pain. The nurse has previously observed this same occurrence. The nurse practice act requires the observing nurse to do which of the following?
   1 Talk with the nurse who gave the medication
   2 Report the information to a supervisor
   3 Call the impaired nurse organization
   4 Report the information to the police

3. A client has died and a family member is asked about the funeral arrangements. The family member refuses to discuss the issue. The nurse's most appropriate action is to:
   1 Provide information needed for decision making
   2 Assess risk of harm to self and refer family member to mental health professional
   3 Demonstrate acceptance of family member's feelings
   4 Remain with family member without discussing funeral arrangements

4. A client arrives in the emergency room and is assessed by the nurse. The client is staggering, confused, and verbally abusive. The client complains of a headache from drinking alcohol and is asking for medication. The nurse explains to the client that the physician will need to perform an assessment prior to the administration of medication. When the client becomes verbally abusive, the nurse obtains leather restraints and threatens to place the client in the restraints. With which of the following can the client legally charge the nurse as a result of the nursing action?
   1 Assault
   2 Battery
   3 Negligence
   4 Invasion of privacy

5. A nurse lawyer provides an education session to the nursing staff regarding client rights. A staff nurse asks the lawyer to describe an example that might relate to invasion of client privacy. Which of the following indicates a violation of this right?

1 Taking photographs of the client without consent
2 Telling the client that he or she cannot leave the hospital
3 Threatening to place the client in restraints
4 Performing a surgical procedure without consent

6. The nurse calls the physician of a client scheduled for a cardiac catheterization because the client has numerous questions regarding the procedure and has requested to speak to the physician. The physician is very upset and arrives at the unit to visit the client after prompting by the nurse. The nurse is outside the client's room and hears the physician tell the client in a derogatory manner that the nurse "doesn't know anything." Which legal tort has the physician violated?
   1 Libel
   2 Slander
   3 Assault
   4 Negligence

7. The nurse calls the physician regarding a new medication order because the dosage prescribed is higher than the recommended dosage. The nurse is unable to locate the physician and the medication is due to be administered. Which of the following actions would the nurse take?
   1 Hold the medication until the physician can be contacted
   2 Administer the dose prescribed
   3 Administer the recommended dose until the physician can be located
   4 Contact the nursing supervisor

8. The nurse enters a client's room and finds the client sitting on the floor. The nurse performs a thorough assessment and assists the client back to bed. The nurse completes an incident report and notifies the physician of the incident. Which of the following is the next appropriate nursing action regarding the incident?
   1 Make a copy of the incident report for the physician
   2 Place the incident report in the client's chart
   3 Document a complete entry in the client's record concerning the incident
   4 Document in the client's record that an incident report has been completed

9. A nursing graduate is employed as a staff nurse in a local hospital. During orientation the new graduate asks the nurse educator about the need to obtain professional liability insurance. The most appropriate response by the nurse educator is:
   1 "The hospital's liability insurance will cover your actions."
   2 "It is very expensive and not necessary."
   3 "Nurses are encouraged to have their own malpractice insurance."

4 "The majority of suits are filed against physicians and the hospital."

10. A nurse witnesses an automobile accident and provides care to the open wound of a young child at the scene of the accident. The family is extremely grateful and insists that the nurse accept monetary compensation for the care provided to the child. Because of the family insistence, the nurse accepts the compensation to avoid offending the family. The child develops an infection and sepsis and is hospitalized. The family files suit against the nurse who provided care to the child at the scene of the accident. Which of the following is accurate regarding the nurse's immunity from this suit?
    1 The Good Samaritan Law will protect the nurse
    2 The Good Samaritan Law will protect the nurse if the care given at the scene was not negligent
    3 The Good Samaritan Law will not provide immunity from suit if the nurse accepted compensation for the care provided
    4 The Good Samaritan Law protects lay persons and not professional health care providers

11. A client brought to the emergency department after a serious accident is unconscious and bleeding profusely. Surgery is required immediately in order to save the client's life. In regard to informed consent for the surgical procedure, which of the following is the best action?
    1 Try calling the client's spouse to obtain telephone consent prior to the surgical procedure
    2 Transport the client to the operating room immediately as required by the physician without obtaining an informed consent
    3 Ask the friend who accompanied the client to the emergency department to sign the consent form
    4 Call the nursing supervisor to initiate a court order for the surgical procedure

12. The registered nurse arrives at work and is told to report (float) to the intensive care unit for the day because the ICU is understaffed and needs additional nurses to care for the clients. The nurse has never worked in the ICU. Which of the following is the most appropriate nursing action?
    1 Refuse to float to the ICU
    2 Call the hospital lawyer
    3 Call the nursing supervisor
    4 Report to the ICU and identify tasks that can be safely performed

13. The home health care nurse arrives at the client's home for the scheduled home visit. The client's lawyer is present and the client is preparing a living will. The living will requires that the client's signature be witnessed, and the client asks

the nurse to witness the signature. Which of the following is the most appropriate nursing action?
1   Sign the living will as a witness to signature only
2   Sign the will, clearly identifying credentials and employment agency
3   Decline to sign the will
④   Call the home health care office and speak to the supervisor prior to signing the will

14. An elderly woman is brought to the emergency department. On physical assessment, the nurse notes old and new ecchymotic areas on both arms and buttocks. The nurse asks the client how the bruises were sustained. The client, although reluctant, tells the nurse in confidence that her daughter frequently hits her if she gets in the way. Which of the following is the most appropriate nursing response?
1   "I promise I will not tell anyone but let's see what we can do about this."
②   "I have a legal obligation to report this type of abuse."
3   "Let's talk about ways that will prevent your daughter from hitting you."
4   "This should not be happening, and if it happens again you must call the emergency department."

15. A client tells the home health care nurse of the decision to refuse external cardiac massage. Which of the following is the most appropriate nursing action?
1   Notify the physician of the client's request
②   Document the client's request in the home health nursing care plan
3   Conduct a client conference with the home health care staff to share the client's request
4   Discuss the client's request with the family

16. A client is brought to the emergency room by the ambulance team following collapse at home. Cardiopulmonary resuscitation is attempted but is unsuccessful. The wife of the client tells the nurse that the client is an organ donor and that the eyes are to be donated. Which of the following is the most appropriate nursing action?
1   Elevate the head of the bed of the deceased and place dry sterile dressings over the eyes
2   Call the National Donor Association to confirm that the client is a donor
③   Close the deceased client's eyes and place wet saline gauze pads and an ice pack on the eyes
4   Ask the wife to obtain the legal documents regarding organ donation from the lawyer

17. A client asks the nurse how to become an organ donor. Which of the following would not be a component of the nurse's response?
1   Donor must be 18 years or older
2   The donation is done by written consent
3   Your family is responsible for making that decision at the time of death
④   Clients have the right to donate their own organs for transplantation

18. The nurse recognizes that which of the following interventions is unlikely to facilitate effective communication between the dying client and his or her family?
1   The nurse encourages the client and family to identify and discuss feelings openly
②   The nurse makes decisions for the client and family in order to relieve them of unnecessary demands
3   The nurse assists the client and family in carrying out spiritually meaningful practices
4   The nurse maintains a calm attitude and one of acceptance when the family or client expresses anger

19. The client had a colon resection. A Levin tube was in place when a regular diet was brought to the client's room. The client did not want to eat solid food and asked that the physician be called. The nurse persisted in the belief that the solid food was the correct diet. The client ate two meals and subsequently had additional surgery due to complications. The determination of negligence in this situation is based on:
1   A duty existed and it was breached
②   Not calling the physician
3   The dietary department sending the wrong food
4   The nurse's beliefs

20. A 39-year-old man learned today that his 36-year-old wife has an incurable cancer and is expected to live not more than a few weeks. The nurse identifies which of these responses by the husband as indicative of effective individual coping:
1   He states that he will not allow his wife to come home to die
2   He immediately arranges for their three teenaged children to live with relatives in another state
③   He expresses his anger at God and the physicians for allowing this to happen
4   He refuses to visit his wife in the hospital or to discuss her illness

ANSWERS

1. 1

Rationale: Proper documentation of unusual occurrences, incidents, and accidents, and the nursing actions taken as a result of the occurrence are internal to the institution or agency and allow the nurse and administration to review the quality of care and determine any potential risks present.

Test-Taking Strategy: Use the process of elimination to determine the purpose of incident reports. Eliminate option 2 because incident reports are not routinely filled out for interventions. Eliminate option 3 because incident reports are not used to report occurrences to other agencies. Medical records are used for this purpose. Option 4 is unrelated to the purpose of an incident report. If you had difficulty with this question, take time now to review the purpose of incident reports!

Level of Cognitive Ability: Analysis
Phase of Nursing Process: Analysis
Client Needs: Safe, Effective Care Environment
Content Area: Fundamental Skills

Reference
Black, J., & Matassarin-Jacobs, E. (1997). *Medical surgical nursing: Clinical management for continuity of care* (5th ed.). Philadelphia: W. B. Saunders. p. 130.

2. 2

Rationale: Nurse practice acts require reporting the suspicion of impaired nurses. The board of nursing has jurisdiction over the practice of nursing and may develop plans for treatment and supervision. This suspicion needs to be reported to the nursing supervisor, who will then report to the board of nursing.

Test-Taking Strategy: Use the principles of prioritizing when answering this question. By reporting the information, the nurse alerts the institution to the potential problem and sets the stage for further investigation and appropriate action.

Level of Cognitive Ability: Analysis
Phase of Nursing Process: Implementation
Client Needs: Safe, Effective Care Environment
Content Area: Fundamental Skills

Reference
Brent, N. (1997). *Nurses and the law.* Philadelphia: W. B. Saunders p. 347.

3. 4

Rationale: The family member is exhibiting the first stage of grief—denial. Option 1 may be an appropriate intervention for the bargaining stage. Option 2 may be an appropriate intervention for the depression stage. Option 3 is an appropriate intervention for the acceptance or reorganization and restitution stage.

Test-Taking Strategy: The stem asks for the "most" appropriate action. Utilize the therapeutic communication techniques, and you should easily be directed to option 4. Remember to address client and family feelings first. Review the grieving process and therapeutic communication techniques now, if you had difficulty with this question!

Level of Cognitive Ability: Application
Phase of Nursing Process: Implementation
Client Needs: Psychosocial Integrity
Content Area: Fundamental Skills

Reference
Leahy, J., & Kizilay, P. (1998). *Foundations of nursing practice: A nursing process approach.* Philadelphia: W. B. Saunders. p. 226.

4. 1

Rationale: An assault occurs when a person puts another person in fear of a harmful or offensive contact. For this intentional tort to be actionable, the victim must be aware of the threat of harmful or offensive contact. Battery is the actual contact with one's body. Negligence involves actions below the standards of care. Invasion of privacy occurs when the individual's private affairs are unreasonably intruded into.

Test-Taking Strategy: Note the key word "threatens" in the question. This key word should easily direct you to option 1. If you had difficulty with this question, take time now to review the descriptions associated with the terms in each option!

Level of Cognitive Ability: Analysis
Phase of Nursing Process: Analysis
Client Needs: Safe, Effective Care Environment
Content Area: Fundamental Skills

Reference
Leahy, J., & Kizilay, P. (1998). *Foundations of nursing practice: A nursing process approach.* Philadelphia: W. B. Saunders. p. 66.

5. 1

Rationale: Invasion of privacy takes place when an individual's private affairs are unreasonably intruded into. Telling the client that she or he cannot leave the hospital constitutes false imprisonment. Threatening to place a client in restraints constitutes assault. Performing a surgical procedure without consent is an example of battery.

Test-Taking Strategy: The key phrase is "invasion of client privacy." This key phrase should easily direct you to option 1. If you had difficulty with this question, take time now to review those situations that include invasion of privacy!

Level of Cognitive Ability: Analysis
Phase of Nursing Process: Analysis
Client Needs: Safe, Effective Care Environment
Content Area: Fundamental Skills

Reference
Leahy, J., & Kizilay, P. (1998). *Foundations of nursing practice: A nursing process approach.* Philadelphia: W. B. Saunders. p. 67.

6. 2

Rationale: Defamation takes place when something untrue is said (slander) or written (libel) about a person, resulting in injury to that person's good name and reputation. An assault occurs when a person puts another person in fear of a harmful or an offensive contact. Negligence involves the actions of professionals that fall below the standard of care for a specific professional group.

Test-Taking Strategy: You should easily eliminate options 3 and 4 first. Recalling that slander constitutes verbal defamation will easily direct you to option 2. If you had difficulty with this question, review the torts identified in each option!

Level of Cognitive Ability: Analysis
Phase of Nursing Process: Analysis
Client Needs: Safe, Effective Care Environment
Content Area: Fundamental Skills

Reference
Leahy, J., & Kizilay, P. (1998). *Foundations of nursing practice: A nursing process approach.* Philadelphia: W. B. Saunders. p. 68.

7. 4

Rationale: If the physician writes an order that requires clarification, it is the nurse's responsibility to contact the physician for clarification. If there is no resolution regarding the order because the physician cannot be located, or because the order remains as it was written after talking with the physician, the nurse should then contact the nurse manager or supervisor for further clarification as to what the next step should be. Under no circumstances should the nurse proceed to carry out the order until clarification is obtained.

Test-Taking Strategy: Eliminate options 2 and 3 first because they are similar and unsafe actions. Holding the medication can result in client injury. The nurse needs to take action. Option 4 clearly identifies the required action in this situation. Review nursing responsibilities related to physician's orders now, if you had difficulty with this question!

Level of Cognitive Ability: Application
Phase of Nursing Process: Implementation
Client Needs: Safe, Effective Care Environment
Content Area: Fundamental Skills

Reference
Leahy, J., & Kizilay, P. (1998). *Foundations of nursing practice: A nursing process approach.* Philadelphia: W. B. Saunders. p. 70.

8. 3

Rationale: The incident report is confidential and privileged information and should not be copied, placed in the chart, or have any reference made to it in the client's record. The incident report is not a substitute for a complete entry in the client's record concerning the incident.

Test-Taking Strategy: Eliminate options 2 and 4 first because they are similar. Recalling that incident reports should not be copied will direct you to option 3. Review nursing responsibilities related to incident reports now, if you had difficulty with this question!

Level of Cognitive Ability: Application
Phase of Nursing Process: Implementation
Client Needs: Safe, Effective Care Environment
Content Area: Fundamental Skills

Reference
Leahy, J., & Kizilay, P. (1998). *Foundations of nursing practice: A nursing process approach.* Philadelphia: W. B. Saunders. p. 72.

9. 3

Rationale: Nurses need their own liability insurance for protection against malpractice law suits. Nurses erroneously assume that they are protected by an agency's professional liability policies. Usually when a nurse is sued, the employer is also sued for the nurse's actions or inactions. Even though this is the norm, nurses are encouraged to have their own malpractice insurance.

Test-Taking Strategy: Note that the issue of the question relates to "obtaining professional liability insurance." This issue should easily direct you to option 3. Review liability related to malpractice insurance now, if you had difficulty with this question!

Level of Cognitive Ability: Analysis
Phase of Nursing Process: Implementation
Client Needs: Safe, Effective Care Environment
Content Area: Fundamental Skills

Reference
Leahy, J., & Kizilay, P. (1998). *Foundations of nursing practice.* Philadelphia: W. B. Saunders. p. 72.

10. 3

Rationale: A Good Samaritan law is passed by a state legislature to encourage nurses and other health care providers to provide care to a person when an accident, emergency, or injury occurs, without fear of being sued for the care provided. Called immunity from suit, this protection usually applies only if all the conditions of the law are met, such as that the health care provider received no compensation for the care provided, and the care given is not willfully and wantonly negligent.

Test-Taking Strategy: If you read the question carefully, you will note the key phrase "accept monetary compensation." This will easily direct you to option 3. Additionally, options 1, 2, and 4 are similar. Review the Good Samaritan law now, if you had difficulty with this question!

Level of Cognitive Ability: Analysis
Phase of Nursing Process: Analysis
Client Needs: Safe, Effective Care Environment
Content Area: Fundamental Skills

Reference
Leahy, J., & Kizilay, P. (1998). *Foundations of nursing practice: A nursing process approach.* Philadelphia: W. B. Saunders. p. 73.

11. 2

Rationale: Generally the informed consent of an adult client is not needed in only two instances. One instance is when an emergency is present and delaying treatment for the purpose of obtaining informed consent would result in injury or death to the client. The second instance is when the client waives the right to give informed consent.

Test-Taking Strategy: Option 3 can be easily eliminated first. Note the key phrase "surgery is required immediately." Options 1 and 4 would delay treatment and should be eliminated. Review the issues surrounding informed consent now, if you had difficulty with this question!

Level of Cognitive Ability: Application
Phase of Nursing Process: Implementation
Client Needs: Safe, Effective Care Environment
Content Area: Fundamental Skills

Reference
Leahy, J., & Kizilay, P. (1998). *Foundations of nursing practice: A nursing process approach.* Philadelphia: W. B. Saunders. pp. 74–75.

12. 4

Rationale: Floating is an acceptable legal practice used by hospitals to solve their understaffing problems. Legally, a nurse cannot refuse to float unless a union contract guarantees that nurses can work only in a specified area or the nurse can prove the lack of knowledge for the performance of assigned tasks. When encountering this situation, nurses should set priorities and identify potential areas of harm to the client.

Test-Taking Strategy: Note the key phrase "most appropriate." This may indicate that more than one option may be correct. Options 1 and 2 can be eliminated first. From the remaining options, it is premature to call the nursing supervisor. Option 4 is most appropriate. Review nursing responsibilities related to "floating" now, if you had difficulty with this question!

Level of Cognitive Ability: Application
Phase of Nursing Process: Implementation
Client Needs: Safe, Effective Care Environment
Content Area: Fundamental Skills

Reference
Brent, N. (1997). *Nurses and the law.* Philadelphia: W. B. Saunders. p. 391.

13. **3**

Rationale: Living wills are required to be in writing and signed by the client. The client's signature either must be witnessed by specified individuals or notarized. Many states prohibit any employee, including a nurse of a facility where the client is receiving care, from being a witness.

Test-Taking Strategy: Note the key phrase "most appropriate." This may indicate that more than one option may be correct. Options 1 and 2 are similar and should be eliminated first. From the remaining options, option 3 is most appropriate. Review legal implications associated with wills now, if you had difficulty with this question!

Level of Cognitive Ability: Application
Phase of Nursing Process: Implementation
Client Needs: Safe, Effective Care Environment
Content Area: Fundamental Skills

Reference
Brent, N. (1997). *Nurses and the law.* Philadelphia: W. B. Saunders. p. 251.

14. **2**

Rationale: Confidential issues are not to be discussed with nonmedical personnel or the person's family or friends without the person's permission. Clients should be assured that information is kept confidential, unless it places the nurse under a legal obligation. The nurse must report situations related to child or elder abuse, gunshot wounds, and certain infectious diseases.

Test-Taking Strategy: Option 4 can be eliminated first because this action does not protect the client from injury. Options 1 and 3 are similar and should be eliminated. Review the nursing responsibilities related to reporting obligations now, if you had difficulty with this question!

Level of Cognitive Ability: Application
Phase of Nursing Process: Implementation
Client Needs: Safe, Effective Care Environment
Content Area: Fundamental Skills

Reference
Luckmann, J. (1997). *Saunders manual of nursing care.* Philadelphia: W. B. Saunders. p. 84.

15. **1**

Rationale: External cardiac massage is one type of treatment that a client can refuse. The most appropriate nursing action is to notify the physician because a written Do Not Resuscitate (DNR) order from the physician must be present. The DNR order must be reviewed or renewed on a regular basis per agency policy.

Test-Taking Strategy: The key phrase "most appropriate" may indicate that more than one option may be correct.

Prioritize the options. Although options 2, 3, and 4 may be appropriate, remember that first a physician's written order is necessary. Review DNR procedures now, if you had difficulty with this question!

Level of Cognitive Ability: Application
Phase of Nursing Process: Implementation
Client Needs: Safe, Effective Care Environment
Content Area: Fundamental Skills

Reference
Leahy, J., & Kizilay, P. (1998). *Foundations of nursing practice: A nursing process approach.* Philadelphia: W. B. Saunders. p. 76.

16. **3**

Rationale: When a corneal donor dies, the eyes are closed and gauze pads wet with saline are placed over them with a small ice pack. Within 2 to 4 hours the eyes are enucleated. The cornea is usually transplanted within 24 to 48 hours. The head of the bed should also be elevated.

Test-Taking Strategy: Note that the key issue relates to donation of the eyes. This should assist in directing you to eliminating options 2 and 4. From the remaining options, knowledge regarding care of the eyes of the deceased who is a donor is required. This knowledge should direct you to option 3. Review this procedure now, if you had difficulty with the question!

Level of Cognitive Ability: Application
Phase of Nursing Process: Implementation
Client Needs: Safe, Effective Care Environment
Content Area: Fundamental Skills

Reference
Monahan, F., & Neighbors, M. (1998). *Medical-surgical nursing: Foundations for clinical practice* (2nd ed.). Philadelphia: W. B. Saunders. p. 1954.

17. **3**

Rationale: The client has the right to donate her or his own organs for transplantation. Any person 18 years of age or older may become an organ donor by written consent. In the absence of appropriate documentation, a family member or legal guardian may authorize donation of the decedent's organs.

Test-Taking Strategy: Note the key word "not" in the stem of the question. Using the process of elimination and the issues related to client rights will easily direct you to option 3. If you had difficulty with this question, take time now to review the procedure for organ donation!

Level of Cognitive Ability: Application
Phase of Nursing Process: Implementation
Client Needs: Safe, Effective Care Environment
Content Area: Fundamental Skills

References
Leahy, J., & Kizilay, P. (1998). *Foundations of nursing practice: A nursing process approach.* Philadelphia: W. B. Saunders. p. 76.

18. **2**

Rationale: Maintaining effective and open communication among family members affected by death and grief is of the greatest importance. The nurse looks for ways to maintain and enhance communication, as well as preserving the family's sense of self-direction and control. Option 1 describes encouraging discussion of feelings and is likely to enhance communication. Option 3 is also an effective intervention, because spiritual practices give meaning to life and have an impact on how people react to crisis. Option 4 is also an effective technique, as the client and family need to know that someone will be there who is supportive and nonjudgmental. Option 2 describes the nurse removing autonomy and decision making from the client and family, who are already experiencing feelings of loss of control in that they cannot change the process of dying. This is an ineffective intervention that can further impair communication.

Test-Taking Strategy: Read the stem carefully, and note the key words "unlikely" and "facilitate." This question is asking you to identify the negative response, so it is important to read each possible answer carefully before deciding which to choose. Understanding that people in crisis usually feel helpless and unable to control their circumstances can assist in identifying option 2 as a response that further removes control.

Level of Cognitive Ability: Analysis
Phase of Nursing Process: Analysis
Client Needs: Psychosocial Integrity
Content Area: Fundamental Skills

Reference
Carson, V., & Arnold, E. (1996). *Mental health nursing: The nurse-patient journey.* Philadelphia: W. B. Saunders. p. 680.

19. **1**

Rationale: For negligence to be proved, there must be a duty, then a breach of duty; the breach of duty must cause the injury, and damages or injury must be experienced. Options 2, 3, and 4 do not fall under the criteria for negligence. Option 1 is the only response that fits the criteria of negligence.

Test-Taking Strategy: Options 2, 3, and 4 do not directly support the issue of negligence because it would be difficult to determine that these elements caused injury. The focus relates to what the nurse is responsible for. Option 1 is a broad, general response to the question. Review the legal elements of nursing practice and criteria for negligence now, if you had difficulty with this question!

Level of Cognitive Ability: Analysis
Phase of Nursing Process: Analysis
Client Needs: Safe, Effective Care Environment
Content Area: Fundamental Skills

Reference
Brent, N. (1997). *Nurses and the law.* Philadelphia: W. B. Saunders. pp. 42, 51–52.

20. **3**

Rationale: The expression of anger is known to be a normal response to impending loss, and the anger may be directed toward the self, the dying person, God or other spiritual being, or the caregivers. Options 1 and 2 indicate possibly rash and unilateral decisions made by the husband, without taking into consideration anyone else's feelings. There is strong evidence of denial in option 4, as he refuses to see or discuss his wife. The only "normal" or expected response by the husband is 3.

Test-Taking Strategy: In the stem, note the key phrase "effective individual coping." Knowledge of the stages of grief associated with loss is essential in answering this question. Each of the four possible options seems negative unless carefully considered within the framework of responses to grief and loss. Look for the option that uses the same terminology as the stages of death and dying. Anger stands out as the only concept that matches the expected stages of coping with grief and loss.

Level of Cognitive Ability: Analysis
Phase of the Nursing Process: Analysis
Client Needs: Psychosocial Integrity
Content Area: Fundamental Skills

Reference
Carson, V., & Arnold, E. (1996). *Mental health nursing: The nurse-patient journey.* Philadelphia: W. B. Saunders. p. 670.

BIBLIOGRAPHY

Black, J., & Matassarin-Jacobs, E. (1997). *Medical surgical nursing: Clinical management for continuity of care* (5th ed.). Philadelphia: W. B. Saunders.
Brent, N. (1997). *Nurses and the law.* Philadelphia: W. B. Saunders.
Carson, V., & Arnold, E. (1996). *Mental health nursing: The nurse-patient journey.* Philadelphia: W. B. Saunders.

Leahy, J., & Kizilay, P. (1998). *Foundations of nursing practice: A nursing process approach.* Philadelphia: W. B. Saunders.
Luckmann, J. (1997). *Saunders manual of nursing care.* Philadelphia: W. B. Saunders.
Monahan, F., & Neighbors, M. (1998). *Medical-surgical nursing: Foundations for clinical practice* (2nd ed.). Philadelphia: W. B. Saunders.

CHAPTER 7

Leadership and Management Issues

PYRAMID TERMS

Authority—Legitimate power or official right to act

Accountability—A moral concept that involves acceptance by the professional nurse of the consequences of a decision or action

Case Management—Represents an interdisciplinary health care delivery system designed to promote appropriate use of hospital personnel and material resources to maximize hospital revenues while providing for optimal outcome of care

Change—A dynamic process that leads to an alteration in behavior

Critical Paths—Provide effective clinical management systems for monitoring care and for reducing or controlling the length of hospital stay

Delegation—Process of transferring a selected nursing task in a situation to an individual who is competent to perform that specific task

Empowerment—An interpersonal process of enabling others to do for themselves

Leadership—The interpersonal process that involves motivating and guiding others to achieve goals

Management—The accomplishment of tasks either by one's self or by directing others

Power—Ability to do or act that results in the achievement of desired results

Responsibility—The duty to act

Variances—Actual deviations or detours from the critical paths

◆ PYRAMID TO SUCCESS

The professional nurse is both a leader and a manager. As described in the NCLEX-RN Test Plan, the professional nurse needs to provide integrated, cost effective care to clients by coordinating, supervising, and/or collaborating with members of the multidisciplinary health care team. Pyramid points focus on concepts of **leadership** and **management, case management,** resource **management,** the **change** process, and the process of **delegation.**

NURSING PROCESS

ASSESSMENT

Health care setting
Multidisciplinary health care team
Support systems
Resources
Risk potential

ANALYSIS: Determine organizational structure and functioning of health care setting

---

PLANNING	IMPLEMENTATION	EVALUATION
Develop management plan and leadership style based on organizational goals. Plan client care to provide continuity.	Identify organizational mission and goals. Manage the health care environment congruent with the organizational mission and goals. Function within the guidelines of the Nurse Practice Act, Standards of Care, Code of Ethics, and agency policies and procedures and legal system. Plan client care assignments appropriately, considering continuity of care. Provide care functioning as a client advocate. Initiate the change process as appropriate to assure continuous quality improvement.	Care to the client is congruent with organizational mission and goals. Continuous quality improvement in client care occurs.

◆ CLIENT NEEDS

SAFE, EFFECTIVE CARE ENVIRONMENT

Case management
Concepts of management
Continuous quality improvement
Delegation and supervision
Consultation and referrals
Resource management

HEALTH PROMOTION AND MAINTENANCE

Family systems
Disease prevention
Health and wellness
Health screening
Health promotion programs

PSYCHOSOCIAL INTEGRITY

Support systems
Therapeutic milieu

PHYSIOLOGICAL INTEGRITY

Basic care and comfort
Reduction of risk potential

I. Health Care Delivery Systems

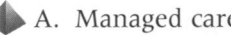A. Managed care
   1. Designed to control the cost of health services and promote a continuum of care through the development and use of integrated services
   2. Emphasizes the promotion of health, client education and responsible self-care, early identification of disease, and the use of health care resources
   3. The practice of prospectively paying predetermined amounts of money to selected providers to maintain the health of a defined population
   4. To control health care costs, employers limit employee choices to less costly managed programs or encourage employees to elect managed care options
   5. Managed care organizations, through contractual agreements, enter into a variety of relationships with providers to meet the needs of members
   6. Less costly to provide this type of care than that associated with acute care and hospitalization
   7. Physicians receive a specific monetary amount per member per month to provide care irrespective of services rendered, which provides the incentive to keep the client healthy
   8. Requires that physicians authorize specialty care and limit use of hospital-based services to promote efficient cost effective care and appropriate use of resources
B. Health maintenance organizations (HMOs)
   1. Offer comprehensive coverage for hospital and physician services in exchange for a fixed, prepaid fee
   2. Both an insurance company and a health care delivery system
   3. Costs and premiums are low for employer and beneficiary
C. Preferred provider organizations
   1. Represent an arrangement between employers and insurance companies that provides member services from a selected group of providers
   2. The choice of physicians is comprehensive, and members can elect to see any participating physician without prior authorization
D. Exclusive provider organization
   1. Parallels preferred provider organization except that beneficiaries are limited to those providers who are participating physicians for any required health care service
   2. Employee premiums are the lowest in the managed care arena
E. **Case management**
   1. Represents an interdisciplinary health care delivery system designed to promote appropriate use of hospital personnel and material resources to maximize hospital

revenues while providing for optimal outcome of care

2. Provides a care process that assists hospitals and health care providers to standardize the appropriate use of resources

3. Manages client care by managing the client care environment

F. **Critical paths**

1. Developed based on appropriate standards of care

2. Provide effective clinical **management** systems for monitoring care and for reducing or controlling the length of hospital stay

3. Developed through the collaborative efforts of physicians, nurses, pharmacists, and other interdisciplinary caregivers, with the goal of improving the quality and outcomes of care

4. The goal of **critical paths** is to anticipate and recognize negative **variance** early so that appropriate action can be taken and better client outcomes can result

5. **Variances**

a. Actual deviations or detours from the **critical paths**

b. Positive **variance** occurs when the client achieves maximum benefit and is discharged earlier than anticipated on his or her **critical path**

c. Negative **variance** occurs when untoward events prevent a timely discharge, and the length of stay is longer than planned for a client on a specific **critical path**

d. **Variance** analysis occurs continually as the case manager and other caregivers monitor client outcomes against the **critical path**

e. Accurate monitoring of **critical paths** with **variance** analysis can estimate the financial impact of client care

f. If the **variance** is predictable, negotiation with insurers for an additional length of stay can maximize client care revenues

G. Levels of prevention

1. Primary prevention: Relates to health promotion activities and specific protection for disease or illness

2. Secondary prevention: Focuses on the early diagnosis and prompt treatment of disease

3. Tertiary prevention: Represented by rehabilitative services

H. Health care settings

1. Hospital care

2. Home care

3. Hospice care

4. Long-term care

5. Surgical centers

6. Ambulatory care

7. Public health departments

II. Formal Organizations

A. Mission statement: Communicates in broad terms the reason for existence, the geographical area

the organization serves, and attitudes and beliefs within which the organization functions

B. Goals and objectives: Measurable activities specific to the development of designated services and programs of an organization

C. Organizational chart: Depicts and communicates how activities are arranged, how **authority** relationships are defined, and how communication channels are established

D. Procedures and protocols

1. Guides in defining appropriate courses of actions

2. Procedure defines a task

3. Protocol signifies the definition of a clinical process

E. Centralization: When decisions are made by a limited number of individuals at the top of the organization, or by managers of a department or unit, and thereafter communicated to the employees

F. Decentralization: **Authority** is distributed throughout the organization to allow for increased **responsibility** and **delegation** in decision making

III. Nursing Delivery Systems

A. Functional nursing

1. Involves a task approach to client care, with major tasks being delegated by the charge nurse to individual members of the team

2. Goals are concerned with work productivity at the lowest possible cost

3. Tasks are generally assigned to the lowest-skilled paid workers who are available to do the work

B. Team nursing

1. The team is generally led by a registered nurse who is responsible for assessing, diagnosing, planning, and evaluating each client's plan of care

2. Each staff member works fully within the realm of his or her educational and clinical expertise

3. Each staff member is accountable for client care and outcomes of care delivered in accordance with the licensing and practice scope as determined by hospital policy and state law

4. Characterized by a large degree of respect and maturity of team members and a high degree of communication and collaboration between members

C. Primary nursing

1. Focuses on client outcomes as opposed to nursing tasks

2. Concerned with keeping the nurse at the bedside, actively involved in client care, while planning goal-directed, individualized client care

BOX 7–1. Managerial Functions

Planning	Determining objectives and identifying methods that lead to achievement of those objectives
Organizing	Using resources (human and material) to achieve predetermined outcomes
Directing	Guiding and motivating others to meet the expected outcomes
Controlling	Using performance standards as criteria for measuring success, and taking corrective action
Decision making	Identifying a problem and deciding which alternative(s) can best achieve the objectives

IV. Professional Responsibilities

◆ A. **Accountability**
  1. The process that mandates that individuals are answerable for their actions and have an obligation (or duty) to act
  2. Assuming only the responsibilities that are within one's scope of practice
  3. Not assuming **responsibility** for activities in which competency has not been achieved
  4. Involves admitting mistakes rather than blaming others, and evaluating the outcomes of one's own actions
  5. Includes a **responsibility** to the client to be competent, to render nursing services in accordance with standards of nursing practice, and to adhere to the professional ethic code

◆ B. **Leadership**
  1. The interpersonal process that involves motivating and guiding others to achieve goals
  2. A method of modeling accountable behavior to others

◆ C. **Management:** The accomplishment of tasks either by one's self or by directing others

  D. Managerial Functions (Box 7–1)

◆ E. **Leadership** styles
  1. Autocratic
     a. Leader-focused
     b. Leader maintains strong control, makes the decisions, and solves all problems
     c. Leader dominates the group
     d. Leader commands rather than makes suggestions or seeks input
  2. Democratic
     a. Also called participative **leadership**
     b. Based on the belief that every group member should have input into development of goals and problem solving
     c. Leader acts primarily as a facilitator and a resource person
     d. Leader is concerned for each member of the group
     e. More participative and much less

authoritarian than the autocratic **leadership** style
  3. Laissez-faire
     a. Leader assumes a passive, nondirective, and inactive approach
     b. **Leadership** responsibilities are either assumed by the members of the group or completely relinquished
     c. All decision making is left to the group, with the leader giving little if any guidance, support, or feedback
     d. Behavior by the group may be permissible due to the leader's lack of limit setting and stated expectations
  4. Situational
     a. Utilizing a combination of styles based on current circumstances and events
     b. **Leadership** styles are assumed according to the needs of the group and tasks to be achieved

  F. **Leadership** qualities
  1. Communication
     a. Listens actively to others
     b. Communicates in an assertive manner, speaks directly and honestly to others
     c. Differentiates aggressive, passive, and assertive behavior to communicate appropriately in a given situation (Box 7–2)
  2. Credibility
     a. Enhances a nurse's **accountability**
     b. Individuals who perform well are those who can influence others
  3. Critical thinking
     a. An individual with an open-minded, questioning attitude
     b. The ineffective leader is one who falls into routine ways of thinking without even being aware of what is happening
  4. Initiating action
     a. Initiates measures to solve problems
     b. Puts ideas into action and demonstrates flexibility
     c. If an approach is ineffective, the leader is not hesitant to try another approach

BOX 7–2. Types of Behavior

AGGRESSIVE BEHAVIOR

Occurs when an individual meets one's own needs regardless of the impact on others

PASSIVE BEHAVIOR

Giving up one's own rights and not having one's own needs met

ASSERTIVE BEHAVIOR

Occurs when an individual seeks to meet one's own needs while respecting the rights of others

5. Risk taking
    a. Involves taking actions to solve problems
    b. Risk-taking activities are goal directed
6. Persuasiveness and influence
    a. Motivates and inspires others to achieve goals
    b. Understands how to use **power** effectively and does not dominate but rather motivates others
    c. Persuasiveness can create enthusiasm, encourage collaboration, and increase cohesiveness among team members

V. Delegation

A. Process of transferring a selected nursing task in a situation to an individual who is competent to perform that specific task
B. A tool for nurse leaders that encourages team members to develop skills
C. Professional nurses will be delegating tasks to unlicensed assistive personnel (UAP) and to licensed personnel
D. The Nurse Practice Act defines which aspects of care can be delegated and which must be performed by the registered nurse
E. Even though a task may be delegated to someone, the nurse who delegates maintains **accountability** for the overall nursing care of the client
F. Only the task, not the ultimate **accountability,** may be delegated to another
G. Guidelines
    1. Determine which tasks can be delegated and to whom
    2. Match the task to the delegate based on the Nurse Practice Act and appropriate position descriptions
    3. Communicate a feeling of confidence to the delegate and provide feedback promptly after the task is performed
    4. Maintain continuity of care as much as possible when assigning client care

VI. Power

A. Ability to do or act and results in the achievement of desired results
B. Powerful people are able to modify behavior and influence others to **change,** even when others are resistant to **change**
C. Effective nurse leaders use **power** to improve the delivery of care and to enhance the profession
D. **Power** that is effective is **power** that is shared
E. Types of **power** (Box 7–3)

VII. Empowerment

A. An interpersonal process of enabling others to do for themselves
B. Occurs when individuals are better able to influence what happens to them

BOX 7–3. Types of Power	
Reward	Ability to provide incentives
Coercive	Ability to punish
Referent	Based on attraction; others wanting to associate with one
Expert	Based on having an expert knowledge base and skill level
Legitimate	Based on a position in society
Personal	Derives from a high degree of self-confidence
Informational	Occurs when one person provides explanations about why another should behave in a certain way

C. Involves open communication, mutual goal setting, and decision making
D. Nurses can **empower** clients through advocacy

VIII. The **Change** Process

A. A dynamic process that leads to an alteration in behavior
B. Types of **change**
    1. Planned **change:** A deliberate effort to improve a situation
    2. Unplanned **change**
        a. **Change** that just happens
        b. It is unpredictable and may be imposed by others or by uncontrollable natural events
C. Resistance to **change**
    1. Resistance occurs when the individual rejects proposed new ideas without critically thinking about the proposal
    2. **Change** requires energy
    3. There is no guarantee that the **change** activity will lead to positive outcomes (Box 7–4)

BOX 7–4. Reasons for Resisting Change
CONFORMITY
Going along with others to avoid conflict
DISSIMILAR BELIEFS AND VALUES
Differences that can impede positive **change**
HABIT
Routine, set behaviors are often hard to **change**
SECONDARY GAINS
Benefits or pay-off is present and so desirable that there is no incentive to **change**
THREATS TO SATISFY BASIC NEEDS
Change may be perceived as a threat to self-esteem, security, or survival
FEAR
Fear of failure and fear of the unknown

D. Overcoming barriers
 1. Create a flexible and adaptable environment
 2. **Change** should be planned and goal-directed by people
 3. Include all involved in the plan for **change**
 4. Focus on the benefits of the **change** in relation to improvement of client care
 5. Evaluate the process on an ongoing basis, keeping everyone informed of the progress
 6. Provide positive feedback to all involved
 7. **Change** takes time, therefore commitment is necessary

PRACTICE QUESTIONS

1. The clinical nurse manager provides an inservice educational session to the staff nurses. The topic of this discussion is case management. Which of the following is not a characteristic of case management and would not be included in the discussion?
 1 Represents a primary health prevention focus managed by a single case manager
 2 Manages client care by managing the client care environment
 3 Designed to promote appropriate use of hospital personnel and material resources
 4 Maximizes hospital revenues while providing for optimal outcome of client care

2. The nurse is reviewing the critical paths of the clients on the nursing unit. In performing a variance analysis, which of the following would indicate the need for further action and analysis?
 1 A client's family attending a diabetic teaching session
 2 Canceling physical therapy sessions on the weekend
 3 Normal vital signs and absence of wound infection in a postoperative client
 4 A client demonstrating accurate medication administration following teaching

3. A new nursing graduate is attending an agency orientation regarding the nursing model of practice implemented in the facility. The nurse is told that the nursing model is a team nursing approach. Which of the following is a characteristic of this type of nursing model of practice?
 1 A task approach method is used to provide care to clients
 2 A single RN is responsible for providing nursing care to a group of clients
 3 Managed care concepts and tools are used in providing client care
 4 Nursing personnel are led by an RN leader in providing care to a group of clients

4. The nurse manager attends a conference, and the topic of discussion is leadership styles. The nurse is seeking a leadership style that will best empower staff toward excellence. Which leadership style would the nurse select to achieve this goal?
 1 Autocratic
 2 Situational
 3 Democratic
 4 Laissez-faire

5. The nurse manager has implemented a change in the method of the nursing delivery system from functional to team nursing. A nursing assistant is resistant to the change and is not taking an active part in facilitating the process of change. Which of the following would be the best approach in dealing with the nursing assistant?
 1 Ignore the resistance
 2 Exert coercion with the nursing assistant
 3 Provide a positive reward system for the nursing assistant
 4 Confront the nursing assistant to encourage verbalization of feelings regarding the change

6. A community health nurse is working with food services in a rural school setting. A goal for the school dietary program is to avoid nutritional deficiencies and enhance children's nutritional status through healthy dietary practices. In implementing interventions by levels of prevention, which of the following would be a primary prevention intervention that the nurse could use?
 1 Case finding in the school to identify dietary practices
 2 School screening programs for early detection of children with poor eating habits
 3 Providing educational programs, literature, and posters to promote awareness of healthy eating
 4 Conduct a community-wide dietary screening activity to detect community dietary trends

7. A community health nurse working in a school setting was concerned because parents were not participating in health activities designed to promote child safety. In this situation, the most appropriate first action would be to:
 1 Perform a thorough assessment of district census data
 2 Perform an analysis of health problems related to child safety
 3 Develop a focused child safety program
 4 Find a new method of marketing the child safety programs

8. The nurse is a member of a community task force on violence. The task force recognizes that it has insufficient data to make decisions about specific interventions. Using the nursing process, the first activity that the nurse would suggest to the task force is to:
 1 Call other communities similar in size to determine what they do
 2 Develop a general educational program related to violence

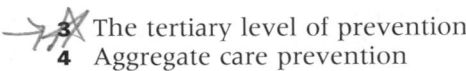

3 Conduct a community survey to assess community perceptions regarding violence

4 Develop a pamphlet on violence to be distributed to the community

9. A community health nurse is working with disaster relief following a tornado. The nurse's goal with the overall community is to prevent as much injury and death as possible from the uncontrollable event. Finding safe housing for survivors, providing support to families, organizing counseling, and securing physical care when needed are all examples of which type of prevention?
   1 The primary level of prevention
   2 The secondary level of prevention

3 The tertiary level of prevention
4 Aggregate care prevention

10. The registered nurse is planning the client assignments. Which of the following is the least appropriate assignment for the nursing assistant?
   1 Assist a 12-year-old boy with Down's syndrome, profoundly developmentally disabled, to eat lunch
   2 Obtain a temperature on a 29-year-old woman receiving the final 30 minutes of a whole blood transfusion
   3 Accompany a 51-year-old man, being discharged to home following a bowel resection 8 days ago, to his transportation
   4 Collect a urine specimen from a 70-year-old woman admitted 3 days ago

ANSWERS

1. 1

Rationale: Case management represents an interdisciplinary health care delivery system to promote appropriate use of hospital personnel and material resources to maximize hospital revenues while providing for optimal outcome of care.

Test-Taking Strategy: Knowledge regarding the characteristics of case management is necessary to answer this question. Use the process of elimination in selecting the correct option. Note the key word "not" in the stem of the question. Also, note the key word "single" in the correct option to this question. Review the characteristics of case management now, if you had difficulty with this question!

Level of Cognitive Ability: Analysis
Phase of Nursing Process: Analysis
Client Needs: Safe, Effective Care Environment
Content Area: Fundamental Skills

Reference
Rocchiccioli, J., & Tilbury, M. (1998). *Clinical leadership in nursing.* Philadelphia: W. B. Saunders. pp. 38–39.

2. 2

Rationale: Variances are actual deviations or detours from the critical paths. Variances can be either positive or negative, avoidable or unavoidable, and can be caused by a variety of things. Positive variance occurs when the client achieves maximum benefit and is discharged earlier than anticipated. Negative variance occurs when untoward events prevent a timely discharge. Variance analysis occurs continually in order to anticipate and recognize negative variance early so that appropriate action can be taken.

Test-Taking Strategy: Use the process of elimination in identifying the negative variance. Options 1, 3, and 4 identify positive outcomes. Option 2 identifies a negative outcome. Review the purpose of variance analysis now, if you had difficulty with this question!

Level of Cognitive Ability: Analysis
Phase of Nursing Process: Analysis
Client Needs: Safe, Effective Care Environment
Content Area: Fundamental Skills

Reference
Rocchiccioli, J., & Tilbury, M. (1998). *Clinical leadership in nursing.* Philadelphia: W. B. Saunders. p. 42.

3. 4

Rationale: In team nursing, nursing personnel are led by an RN leader in providing care to a group of clients. Option 1 identifies functional nursing. Option 2 identifies primary nursing. Option 3 identifies a component of case management.

Test-Taking Strategy: Note that the issue of the question relates to team nursing. Keep this issue in mind and use the process of elimination. Option 4 is the only option that identifies the concept of a team approach. Review the various types of nursing delivery systems now, if you had difficulty with this question!

Level of Cognitive Ability: Analysis
Phase of Nursing Process: Analysis
Client Needs: Safe, Effective Care Environment
Content Area: Fundamental Skills

Reference
Rocchiccioli, J., & Tilbury, M. (1998). *Clinical leadership in nursing.* Philadelphia: W. B. Saunders. p. 30.

4. 3

Rationale: Democratic styles best empower staff toward excellence because this style of leadership allows nurses an opportunity to grow professionally. The autocratic style is task oriented and directive. Situational leadership style utilizes a style depending on the situation and events. Laissez-faire allows staff to work without assistance, direction, or supervision.

Test-Taking Strategy: Note the key phrase "empower staff toward excellence." Knowledge of the characteristics of the various leadership styles and this key phrase will assist in directing you to option 3. If you had difficulty with this question, take time now to review the various leadership styles!

Level of Cognitive Ability: Analysis
Phase of Nursing Process: Planning
Client Needs: Safe, Effective Care Environment
Content Area: Fundamental Skills

Reference
Rocchiccioli, J., & Tilbury, M. (1998). *Clinical leadership in nursing.* Philadelphia: W. B. Saunders. pp. 103–104.

5. **4**

Rationale: Confrontation is an important strategy to meet resistance head-on. Face-to-face meetings to confront the issue at hand will allow verbalization of feelings, identification of problems and issues, and development of strategies to solve the problem. Option 1 will not address the problem. Option 2 may produce additional resistance. Option 3 may provide a temporary solution to the resistance but will not specifically address the concern.

Test-Taking Strategy: Options 1 and 2 can be easily eliminated first. From the remaining options, select option 4 over option 3 because this option specifically addresses the issue and would provide problem-solving measures. If you had difficulty with this question, take time now to review the strategies associated with dealing with resistance to change!

Level of Cognitive Ability: Application
Phase of Nursing Process: Implementation
Client Needs: Safe, Effective Care Environment
Content Area: Fundamental Skills

Reference
Rocchiccioli, J., & Tilbury, M. (1998). *Clinical leadership in nursing.* Philadelphia: W. B. Saunders. pp. 188–192.

6. **3**

Rationale: Primary prevention interventions are those measures that keep illness, injury, or potential problems from occurring, therefore option 3 is correct. Option 1 is a tertiary prevention measure; options 2 and 4 are secondary prevention measures that seek to detect existing health problems or trends.

Test-Taking Strategy: Note the issue of the question "primary prevention intervention." Knowledge that primary prevention interventions are those measures that keep illness from occurring will direct you to option 3. If you had difficulty with this question, take time now to review the levels of prevention!

Level of Cognitive Ability: Application
Phase of Nursing Process: Implementation
Client Needs: Health Promotion and Maintenance
Content Area: Fundamental Skills

Reference
Leahy, J., & Kizilay, P. (1998). *Foundations of nursing practice: A nursing process approach.* Philadelphia: W. B. Saunders. pp. 83–84.

7. **1**

Rationale: In this situation, the best action is to determine the appropriateness of the planned health activities. The first step is to assess. This would then be followed by option 2, analysis, and then by options 3 and 4, implementation.

Test-Taking Strategy: Use the steps of the nursing process to answer the question. Option 1 addresses the process of assessment, the first step of the nursing process!

Level of Cognitive Ability: Application
Phase of Nursing Process: Implementation
Client Needs: Health Promotion and Maintenance
Content Area: Fundamental Skills

Reference
Swanson, J., & Nies, M. (1997). *Community health nursing: Promoting the health of aggregates* (2nd ed.). Philadelphia: W. B. Saunders. p. 110.

8. **3**

Rationale: An assessment activity is always the first step in the nursing process. Options 2 and 4 are implementation measures. Option 1 is a part of analysis of a variety of assessment data. Option 3 addresses assessment of the community that is the issue of the question!

Test-Taking Strategy: Use the steps of the nursing process to answer the question. Options 2 and 4 can be eliminated first because they are not indicative of the first step of the nursing process. Options 1 and 3 relate to assessment. Select option 3 over option 1 because it directly relates to the community of concern.

Level of Cognitive Ability: Application
Phase of Nursing Process: Implementation
Client Needs: Health Promotion and Maintenance
Content Area: Fundamental Skills

Reference
Swanson, J., & Nies, M. (1997). *Community health nursing: Promoting the health of aggregates* (2nd ed.). Philadelphia: W. B. Saunders. p. 110.

9. **3**

Rationale: Tertiary prevention involves the reduction of the amount and degree of disability, injury, and damage following a crisis. Primary prevention means keeping the crisis from ever occurring, and secondary prevention focuses on reducing the intensity and duration of a crisis. There is no known aggregate care prevention level.

Test-Taking Strategy: Identify the scenario in the question. Focus on this scenario and utilize knowledge regarding the various levels of prevention to answer the question. If you had difficulty with this question, take time now to review the levels of prevention!

Level of Cognitive Ability: Analysis
Phase of Nursing Process: Analysis
Client Needs: Safe, Effective Care Environment
Content Area: Fundamental Skills

Reference
Leahy, J., & Kizilay, P. (1998). *Foundations of nursing practice: A nursing process approach.* Philadelphia: W. B. Saunders. pp. 83–84.

10. **1**

Rationale: The nurse must determine the most appropriate assignment based on the skills of the staff member and the needs of the client. In this case, the least appropriate assignment for a nursing assistant would be assisting with feeding a profoundly developmentally disabled child. The child is likely to have difficulty in eating, and therefore a higher potential for complications such as choking and aspiration. The remaining three options include nothing to indicate that these tasks carry any unforeseen risk (the blood transfusion is nearly complete; the client is being discharged to home postoperatively; and a urine sample is needed).

Test-Taking Strategy: Note the key phrase "least appropriate" in the stem of the question. Use the process of elimination. Consider the ABCs, and recall the principles of delegation and supervision of the work of others in answering the question. Work that is delegated to others must be done consistent with the individual's level of expertise and licensure or lack of licensure. Review the principles of delegation now, if you had difficulty with this question!

Level of Cognitive Ability: Application
Phase of Nursing Process: Implementation
Client Needs: Safe, Effective Care Environment
Content Area: Fundamental Skills

Reference
Rocchiccioli, J., & Tilbury, M. (1998). *Clinical leadership in nursing.* Philadelphia: W. B. Saunders. p. 140.

BIBLIOGRAPHY

Leahy, J., & Kizilay, P. (1998). *Foundations of nursing practice: A nursing process approach.* Philadelphia: W. B. Saunders.

Luckmann, J. (1997). *Saunders manual of nursing care.* Philadelphia: W. B. Saunders.

Monahan, F., & Neighbors, M. (1998). *Medical-surgical nursing: Foundations for clinical practice* (2nd ed.). Philadelphia: W. B. Saunders.

Rocchiccioli, J., & Tilbury, M. (1998). *Clinical leadership in nursing.* Philadelphia: W. B. Saunders.

Swanson, J., & Nies, M. (1997). *Community health nursing: Promoting the health of aggregates* (2nd ed.). Philadelphia: W. B. Saunders.

UNIT III

Nursing Sciences

CHAPTER 8

Fluids and Electrolytes

. . . .

PYRAMID TERMS

Fluid Volume Deficit—Dehydration in which water and electrolytes are lost in the same proportion. The goal of treatment is to restore fluid volume, replace electrolytes as needed, and eliminate the cause of the fluid volume deficit.

Fluid Volume Excess—An actual excess of total body fluid or a relative fluid excess in one or more fluid compartments. Also called overhydration or fluid overload. The goal of treatment is to restore fluid balance, correct electrolyte imbalances if present, and eliminate or control the underlying cause of the overload.

Homeostasis—The tendency of biological systems to maintain relatively constant conditions in the internal environment while continuously interacting with and adjusting to changes originating within or outside the system.

Hypercalcemia—A high serum calcium level that exceeds 11 mg/dL or 5.5 mEq/L.

Hypocalcemia—A low serum calcium level below 4.5 mEq/L or below 9 mg/dL.

Hyperkalemia—A high serum potassium level greater than 5.1 mEq/L.

Hypokalemia—A low serum potassium level below 3.5 mEq/L, or potassium deficit. Potassium deficit is the most common electrolyte imbalance and is potentially life threatening.

Hypermagnesemia—An increased magnesium serum level of 2.3 mEq/L or 2.6 mg/dL. *(greater than)*

Hypomagnesemia—A decreased serum magnesium level of less than 1.5 mEq/L or 1.8 mg/dL.

Hypernatremia—A condition in which the serum sodium concentration is greater than 145 mEq/L.

Hyponatremia—A sodium deficit in which there is too little sodium in the serum, less than 135 mEq/L.

Hyperphosphatemia—A serum phosphate level greater than 4.5 mg/dL or 2.6 mEq/L.

Hypophosphatemia—A serum phosphate level below 3.0 mg/dL or below 1.8 mEq/L.

Third-Space Losses—A fluid shift from the intravascular space into another part of the body where the fluid is not functional.

PYRAMID TO SUCCESS

Pyramid points focus primarily on the assessment of a fluid and electrolyte imbalance, implementation, and evaluating the expected outcomes. Fluid and electrolytes constitute a content area that is complex and sometimes difficult to understand. It is important to understand cell functions and properties and the concepts related to body fluids as outlined in this chapter. Review this content. Pyramid points focus on the common fluid and electrolyte disturbances. Focus on the pyramid points related to the causes, assessment, and related treatments (Box 8-1).

BOX 8-1. Pyramid to Success

Identify clients at risk
Causes of the excess or deficit
Clinical manifestations
Respiratory alterations
ECG changes
Neurological changes
Normal laboratory values
Treatment measures

NURSING PROCESS

ASSESSMENT

Vital signs
Determine clients at risk for fluid or electrolyte imbalance

Signs and symptoms noted in the client
Laboratory results
Health maintenance patterns

ANALYSIS:	**Fluid volume excess**	Alteration in elimination	Altered tissue perfusion
	Fluid volume deficit	Impaired gas exchange	Altered thought processes
	Ineffective breathing pattern	Potential for injury	Altered health maintenance

PLANNING

The client tolerates measures initiated to maintain normal fluid and electrolyte balance. The client remains free of complications associated with the fluid and electrolyte imbalance. The client describes appropriate health care measures to prevent fluid and electrolyte imbalance.

IMPLEMENTATION

Identify clients at risk for a fluid or electrolyte imbalance. Monitor vital signs. Monitor cardiovascular, respiratory, and neurological status. Monitor for signs and symptoms indicative of a fluid or electrolyte imbalance. Monitor laboratory results. Initiate measures as prescribed to treat the imbalance. Monitor for complications associated with the imbalance or interventions. Monitor for and document the outcomes of interventions. Instruct client in the appropriate measures to prevent alterations in fluid and electrolyte balance.

EVALUATION

Fluid and electrolyte values are within normal limits. The client demonstrates compliance with the prescribed treatment plan.

CLIENT NEEDS

SAFE, EFFECTIVE CARE ENVIRONMENT

Asepsis and preventing infection in the client and health care personnel when obtaining laboratory studies and when administering IVs

Protection and safety of the client when an imbalance exists, particularly when changes in respiratory, cardiac, or neurological status occur, or when the client is at risk for complications such as seizures, respiratory depression, or dysrhythmias.

HEALTH PROMOTION AND MAINTENANCE

Education related to medication and diet management

Instruct the client and family about the potential risk for a fluid and electrolyte imbalance

Instruct the client and family on the signs and symptoms associated with an imbalance, measures to prevent the imbalance, and actions to take if signs and symptoms occur.

PSYCHOSOCIAL INTEGRITY

Reassure the client experiencing symptoms related to a fluid and electrolyte imbalance

Provide support and continuously inform the client of the purpose for prescribed interventions.

PHYSIOLOGICAL INTEGRITY

Identify clients at risk for a fluid or electrolyte imbalance

Monitor laboratory values

Monitor for complications related to the imbalance

Manage emergencies

Identify the expected and unexpected responses to treatment, and document accordingly.

I. Concepts of Fluid and Electrolyte Balance

A. Electrolytes
   1. Description: When a substance is dissolved in solution and some of its molecules split or dissociate into electrically charged atoms or ions (Box 8–2)
   2. Measurement
      a. To measure volume of fluids, the metric system is used to measure liters (L) or milliliters (mL)
      b. The unit of measure that expresses the

BOX 8–2. Cell Properties

Atom—The smallest part of an element that still has the properties of the element. Composed of particles known as the proton (positive charge), neutron (neutral), and electron (negative charge).

Protons and neutrons are in the nucleus of the atom; therefore, the nucleus is positively charged.

Electrons carry a negative charge and revolve around the nucleus. As long as the number of electrons is the same as the number of protons, there is no net charge on the atom, that is, it is neither positive nor negative. Atoms may gain, lose, or share electrons and then no longer are neutral.

Molecule—When two or more atoms combine to form a substance.

Ion—When an atom carries an electrical charge because it has either gained or lost electrons. Some ions carry a negative electrical charge, and some carry a positive charge.

Cation—When an ion carries a positive charge and it has given away or lost electrons. The result is fewer electrons than protons, and the result is a positive charge.

Anion—An ion that has gained electrons and therefore carries a negative charge. When an ion has gained or taken on electrons, it assumes a negative charge and the result is a negatively charged ion.

combining activity of an electrolyte is the milliequivalent (mEq)

  c. One milliequivalent of any cation will always react chemically with one milliequivalent of an anion

  d. Milliequivalents provide information about the number of anions or cations available to combine with other cations or anions

B. Body Fluid Compartments

  1. Description

    a. Fluid in each of the body compartments contain electrolytes

    b. Each compartment has a particular composition of electrolytes, which differs from that of other compartments

    c. To function normally, body cells must have fluids and electrolytes

    d. The electrolytes must be in the right compartments in the right amounts

    e. A specific kind and amount of certain electrolytes must be available for normal cell function

    f. Whenever an electrolyte moves out of a cell, another electrolyte moves in to take its place

    g. The number of cations and anions must be the same for **homeostasis** to exist

    h. Compartments are separated by semipermeable membranes

  2. Intracellular compartments

    a. Refers to all fluid inside the cells

    b. Most of the body fluids are inside the cells

  3. Extracellular compartment: Refers to all fluid outside the cells

  4. Intravascular compartment: Fluid that is within blood vessels

  5. Interstitial fluids: Fluid between the cells and blood vessels

C. Body Fluid

  1. Description

    a. Provides transportation of nutrients to the cells and carries waste products from the cells

    b. Total body fluid amounts to about 60% of body weight

    c. A loss of 10% of body fluid in the adult is serious

    d. A loss of 20% of the body fluid content in the adult is fatal

  2. Constituents of body fluids

    a. Body fluids consist of water and dissolved substances

    b. The largest single fluid constituent of the body is water

    c. Some substances such as glucose, urea, and creatinine do not dissociate in solution, that is, they do not separate from their complex form into simpler substances when they are in solutions

    d. Other substances do dissociate; for example, when sodium chloride (NaCl) is in a solution, it dissociates or separates into two parts or elements

D. Body Fluid Transport

  1. Diffusion

    a. The movement of particles in all directions through a solution

    b. The process by which a solute may spread through a solution or solvent

    c. Solute is the substance that is dissolved

    d. Solvent is the solution in which the solute is dissolved

    e. Diffusion of a solute will spread the molecules from an area of high concentration to an area of lower concentration

    f. A permeable membrane will allow substances to pass through it without restriction

    g. A selectively permeable membrane will allow some solutes to pass through without restriction but will prevent other solutes from passing freely

    h. Diffusion occurs within fluid compartments and from one compartment to another if the barrier between the compartments is permeable to the diffusing substances

  2. Osmosis

    a. Osmotic pressure is the force that draws the water from a less concentrated solution through a selectively permeable membrane into a more concentrated solution

    b. If a membrane is permeable to water but not to all the solutes present, it is a selective or semipermeable membrane

    c. When the solvent or water moves across the membrane, it is called osmosis

    d. Osmosis is the diffusion of solvent across a membrane in response to a concentration gradient usually from a solution of lesser to one of greater solute concentration

    e. When there is a more concentrated solution on one side of a selectively permeable membrane and a less concentrated solution on the other side, a pull called osmotic pressure draws the water through the membrane to the more concentrated side or the side with more solute

  3. Filtration

    a. Filtration is the movement of solutes and solvents by hydrostatic pressure

    b. Hydrostatic pressure is the force exerted by the weight of a solution

    c. The movement is from an area of greater pressure to an area of lesser pressure

  4. Osmolality

    a. Refers to the number of osmotically active particles per kilogram of water

b. In the body, osmotic pressure is measured in milliosmols

c. The normal osmolality of plasma is 280 to 294 mOsm/kg

5. Hydrostatic pressure

a. The force of the fluid pressing outward against some surface

b. When there is a difference in the hydrostatic pressure on two sides of a membrane, water and diffusible solutes move out of the solution that has the higher hydrostatic pressure by the process of filtration

c. At the arterial end of the capillary, the hydrostatic pressure is greater than the osmotic pressure; therefore, fluids and diffusible solutes move out of the capillary

d. At the venous end, the osmotic pressure or pull is greater than the hydrostatic pressure, and fluids and some solutes move into the capillary

e. The excess fluid and solutes remaining in the interstitial spaces are returned to the intravascular compartment by the lymph channels

E. Movement of Body Fluid

1. Description

a. Cell membranes separate the interstitial fluid from the intravascular fluid

b. These barriers are selectively permeable, that is, the cell membrane and the capillary wall will allow water and some solutes free passage through them

c. The solute is the substance that is dissolved

d. Several forces affect the movement of water and solutes through the walls of cells and capillaries

e. The greater the number of particles in the concentrated solution, the more pull there will be to move the water through the membrane

f. Fluids and electrolytes must be kept in balance for health; when they remain out of balance, death can occur

g. If the body loses more electrolytes than fluids, as can happen in diarrhea, then the extracellular fluid will contain less electrolytes or less solutes than the intracellular fluid

2. Isotonic solutions (Table 8–1)

a. When the solutions on both sides of a selectively permeable membrane have established equilibrium or are equal in concentration, they are then isotonic

b. An example of an isotonic solution is 0.9% sodium chloride, which is referred to as isotonic saline solution or normal saline solution

c. This means that it is isotonic to human

Table 8–1. Tonicity of Intravenous Fluids

Solution	Tonicity
0.45% saline (½ NS) *Distilled H₂O*	Hypotonic
0.9% saline (NS)	Isotonic
5% dextrose in water (5% D/W)	Isotonic
5% dextrose in 0.225% saline (5% D/¼ NS)	Isotonic
Lactated Ringer's solution (RL)	Isotonic
5% dextrose in lactated Ringer's solution	Hypertonic
5% dextrose in 0.45% saline (5% D/½ NS)	Hypertonic
5% dextrose in 0.9% saline (5% D/NS)	Hypertonic
10% dextrose in water (10% D/W)	Hypertonic

cells and thus there will be very little osmosis

d. Other solutions that are isotonic are 5% dextrose, 5% dextrose in 0.225% saline, and lactated Ringer's solution

3. Hypotonic solutions (Table 8–1)

a. When a solution contains a lower concentration of salt than other solutions, it is hypotonic

b. A hypotonic solution has less salt or more water than an isotonic solution

c. 0.45% saline is a hypotonic solution

d. Distilled water is an example of a hypotonic solution since it does not have solutes in it

e. Since distilled water is hypotonic to the cells, osmosis would continue in an attempt to bring about balance or equality

4. Hypertonic solutions (Table 8–1)

a. A solution that has a higher concentration of solutes than another solution is a hypertonic solution

b. Hypertonic solutions include 10% dextrose in water, 5% dextrose in 0.9% saline, 5% dextrose in 0.45% saline, 5% dextrose in lactated Ringer's solution

5. Osmotic pressure

a. The force that draws the solvent from a solution with more solvent activity through a selectively permeable membrane to a solution with less solvent activity

b. The amount of osmotic pressure is determined by the relative number of particles of solute on the side of greater concentration

c. When the solutions on each side of a selectively permeable membrane are equal in concentration, they are isotonic

d. A hypotonic solution has less solute than an isotonic solution, whereas a hypertonic solution contains more solute

e. If the selectively permeable membrane will allow the solvent to pass through but will not allow the solute through freely, the solvent will move to the side of greater solute concentration

6. Active transport
   a. If an ion is to move through a membrane from an area of low concentration to an area of high concentration, an active transport system is necessary
   b. An active transport system moves molecules or ions uphill against concentration and osmotic pressure
   c. The energy for active transport is supplied by metabolic processes in the cell
   d. Substances that are actively transported through the cell membrane include ions of sodium, potassium, calcium, iron, and hydrogen, some of the sugars, and the amino acids

F. Body Fluid Excretion
   1. Description
      a. Fluids leave the body by several routes, including the skin, lungs, gastrointestinal (GI) tract, and kidneys
      b. The kidneys excrete the largest quantity of fluid
      c. As long as all organs are functioning normally, the body is able to maintain balance in its fluid content
   2. Skin
      a. Water is lost through the skin by diffusion in the amounts of 300 to 400 mL per day
      b. Water is also lost through the skin by perspiration
      c. The amount of water lost by perspiration will vary depending on the temperature of the environment and of the body
      d. Average amount of water lost by perspiration is 100 mL per day
   3. Lungs
      a. Water is lost from the lungs through expired air that is saturated with water vapor
      b. The amount of water lost from the lungs will vary with the rate and depth of respiration
      c. The average amount of water lost from the lungs is 300 to 400 mL per day
      d. Water lost from the lungs and the skin by diffusion is called insensible loss because the individual is unaware of losing that water
   4. GI tract
      a. Large quantities of water are secreted into the GI tract, but almost all of this fluid is reabsorbed
      b. A very large volume of electrolyte-containing liquids moves into the GI tract and then returns again into the extracellular fluid
      c. The average amount of water lost in the feces is 200 mL per day, equal to the amount of water gained through the oxidation of foods
      d. Severe diarrhea will result in the loss of large quantities of fluids and electrolytes

5. Kidneys
   a. Play a major role in regulating fluid and electrolyte balance
   b. Normal kidneys can adjust the amount of water and electrolytes leaving the body
   c. The quantity of fluid excreted by the kidneys is determined by the amount of water ingested and the amount of waste and solutes excreted
   d. The usual quantity of urine output is approximately 1400 mL per day; however, this will vary greatly depending on fluid intake, amount of perspiration, and other factors (Box 8–3)

G. Body Fluid Replacement
   1. Description: Water enters the body through three sources: oral liquids, water in foods, and water formed by oxidation of foods
   2. Amounts
      a. The average total amount of water taken into the body from all three sources is 2400 mL per day
      b. About 10 mL of water is released by the metabolism of each 100 calories of fat, carbohydrates, or proteins
   3. Electrolytes
      a. Electrolytes are present in both foods and liquids
      b. With a normal diet, an excess of essential electrolytes is taken in and the unused electrolytes are excreted

H. Maintaining Fluid and Electrolyte Balance
   1. Description
      a. **Homeostasis** is a term that indicates the relative stability of the internal environment
      b. Concentration and composition of body fluids must be nearly constant
      c. In the client, when one of the substances, either fluids or electrolytes, is deficient, it must be replaced either normally by the intake of food and water or by therapy such as IVs and/or medications
      d. When the client has an excess of fluid or electrolytes, therapy is directed toward assisting the body to eliminate the excess
   2. Kidneys: Play a major role in controlling all types of balance in fluid and electrolytes
   3. Adrenal glands: Through the secretion of aldosterone, the adrenal glands also aid in controlling extracellular fluid volume by regulating the amount of sodium reabsorbed by the kidneys

---

BOX 8–3. Daily Body Fluid Excretion

Skin by diffusion = 350 mL
Skin by perspiration = 100 mL
Lungs = 350 mL
Feces = 200 mL
Kidneys = 1400 mL

4. Antidiuretic hormone (ADH): ADH from the pituitary gland regulates the osmotic pressure of extracellular fluid by regulating the amount of water reabsorbed by the kidney

II. Fluid Volume Deficit

A. Description
   1. Dehydration in which water and electrolytes are lost in the same proportion
   2. The goal of treatment is to restore fluid volume, replace electrolytes as needed, and eliminate the cause of the **fluid volume deficit**

B. Causes
   1. Vomiting
   2. Diarrhea
   3. Increased respirations
   4. Use of diuretics and increased urine output
   5. Insufficient IV fluid replacement
   6. GI suctioning
   7. Draining fistulas
   8. Ileostomy or colostomy drainage

C. Assessment
   1. Increased respirations
   2. Increased heart rate
   3. Decreased central venous pressure (CVP)
   4. Weight loss
   5. Poor skin turgor
   6. Dry mucous membranes
   7. Decrease in urine volume
   8. Urine is dark in color and odorous
   9. Increased specific gravity of the urine
   10. Increased hematocrit
   11. Altered level of consciousness
   12. Confusion

D. Implementation
   1. Assess vital signs
   2. Assess neck and hand vein filling
   3. Assess mucous membranes and skin turgor
   4. Monitor hematocrit and electrolyte values
   5. Replace fluids by PO or IV (lactated Ringer's solution, 0.9% normal saline) as prescribed
   6. Administer medications as prescribed
   7. Monitor weight daily
   8. Monitor I&O (intake and output)
   9. Test urine for specific gravity
   10. Monitor bowel sounds

III. Fluid Volume Excess

A. Description
   1. An actual excess of total body fluid or a relative fluid excess in one or more fluid compartments
   2. Also called overhydration or fluid overload
   3. The goal of treatment is to restore fluid balance, correct electrolyte balances if present, and eliminate or control the underlying cause of the overload

B. Causes
   1. Excessive administration of oral or IV fluids
   2. The use of hypotonic fluids to replace isotonic fluid losses
   3. Decreased kidney function
   4. Congestive heart failure
   5. Cirrhosis
   6. SIADH (syndrome of inappropriate antidiuretic hormone)
   7. Cushing's syndrome
   8. Excessive irrigation of body cavities or organs
   9. Excessive ingestion of table salt

C. Assessment
   1. Cough
   2. Dyspnea
   3. Rales
   4. Tachypnea
   5. Tachycardia
   6. Increased blood pressure and bounding pulse
   7. Elevated central venous pressure
   8. Neck and hand vein distention
   9. Pitting edema
   10. Weight gain
   11. Decreased hematocrit
   12. Flushed skin
   13. Headache
   14. Altered level of consciousness
   15. Confusion

D. Implementation
   1. Assess vital signs
   2. Position client in semi-Fowler's position
   3. Administer diuretics as prescribed
   4. Restrict fluids as prescribed
   5. Monitor I&O
   6. Monitor weight daily
   7. Assess for edema
   8. Provide a low sodium diet as prescribed
   9. Monitor laboratory values

IV. Hypokalemia

A. Description
   1. A low serum potassium level below 3.5 mEq/L, or potassium deficit (Box 8–4)
   2. Potassium deficit is the most common

BOX 8–4. Potassium (K)	
Normal Value 3.5 mEq/L to 5.1 mEq/L	
Potassium-Containing Foods	
Apricots	Chocolate
Avocados	Beef
Bananas	Pork
Cantaloupes	Veal
Figs	Carrots
Peaches	Potatoes
Prunes	Spinach
Raisins	Tomatoes

electrolyte imbalance and is potentially life threatening

B. Causes
  1. Decreased intake of potassium
  2. Excessive urinary loss
  3. Use of nonpotassium-sparing diuretics
  4. Chronic use of corticosteroids
  5. Vomiting
  6. Gastric suction
  7. Diarrhea
  8. Laxative abuse
  9. Colitis
  10. Excessive perspiration
  11. Malnutrition
  12. Rapid weight loss diets
  13. Acute alcoholism
  14. Cushing's syndrome
  15. Burns or massive trauma
  16. Uncontrolled diabetes
  17. Alkalosis

C. Assessment
  1. Muscle cramping, weakness, and paralysis
  2. Fatigue
  3. Weak and slow pulse
  4. Dyspnea
  5. Tetany and loss of deep tendon reflexes
  6. Mental changes, such as depression or hallucinations
  7. Dysrhythmias
  8. ECG shows peaked P waves, flat T waves, depressed ST segment, and U waves
  9. Respiratory arrest

D. Implementation
  1. Assess vital signs
  2. Assess neuromuscular activity
  3. Monitor I&O
  4. Assess renal function before administering potassium
  5. Administer potassium supplements as prescribed orally or IV
  6. Oral potassium chloride has an unpleasant taste and should be taken with juice or other desired liquid
  7. Oral potassium preparations can cause GI irritation and should not be taken on an empty stomach
  8. If the client complains of abdominal pain, distention, nausea, vomiting, diarrhea, or GI bleeding, the oral potassium may need to be discontinued
  9. When potassium is added to an IV solution, shake the bag and invert it to ensure that the potassium is evenly distributed
  10. Never give an IV bolus injection of potassium; dilute before administering
  11. A client receiving more than 10 mEq potassium per hour should be placed on a cardiac monitor, and the infusion should be controlled by an infusion device
  12. Monitor for cardiac changes during the administration of potassium
  13. Monitor electrolyte values

  14. Monitor IV site; if phlebitis or infiltration occurs, the IV should be stopped immediately and restarted at another site
  15. Instruct client not to use salt substitutes containing potassium unless prescribed by the physician

V. Hyperkalemia

A. Description: A high serum potassium level greater than 5.1 mEq/L
B. Causes
  1. Renal failure
  2. Cell damage
  3. Addison's disease
  4. Metabolic acidosis
  5. Excessive oral or parenteral administration of potassium
  6. Excessive use of potassium-based salt substitutes
  7. Transfusion of stored blood with red blood cell (RBC) release of potassium

C. Assessment
  1. CNS stimulation
  2. Listlessness, muscle weakness, flaccid paralysis
  3. Abdominal cramps
  4. Dysrhythmias
  5. ECG shows wide, flat P wave, widened QRS complex, prolonged PR interval, depressed ST segment, and narrow, peaked T waves

D. Implementation
  1. Monitor vital signs
  2. Monitor for pulse or ECG changes, particularly bradycardia
  3. Emergency treatment includes rapid IV administration of 250 mL of 10% to 20% dextrose with 10 to 20 units of regular insulin to move excess potassium into the cells
  4. Administer sodium polystyrene sulfonate (Kayexalate) orally or by enema, which absorbs the potassium into the GI tract
  5. Monitor for calcium and magnesium loss when using Kayexalate
  6. Monitor kidney function
  7. Give fluids to increase urinary output as prescribed
  8. Prepare for peritoneal dialysis or hemodialysis as prescribed
  9. When blood transfusions are prescribed for a client with a potassium imbalance, the client should receive fresh blood if possible because transfusions of stored blood may elevate the potassium level as the breakdown of older blood cells releases potassium
  10. Teach clients to avoid foods high in potassium
  11. Instruct client to avoid the use of salt substitutes or other potassium-containing substances

VI. Hyponatremia

A. Description: A sodium deficit in which there is too little sodium in the serum, less than 135 mEq/L (Box 8–5)

B. Causes
1. GI, renal, and **third-space losses**
2. Drinking excess water
3. Increased perspiration
4. Skin loss through draining skin lesions
5. Lack of sodium intake
6. Potent diuretics
7. GI suction
8. Irrigation of GI tube with plain water
9. Central nervous system (CNS) trauma
10. Adrenal insufficiency
11. SIADH
12. Cancer, such as oat cell of the lungs or leukemia

C. Assessment
1. Postural blood pressure changes
2. Rapid, thready pulse and tachycardia
3. Muscle twitching
4. Lethargy, muscular weakness
5. Poor skin turgor
6. Flat hand and neck veins
7. Cold, clammy skin
8. Oliguria as the deficit worsens
9. Cramps, vomiting
10. Headache
11. Apprehension
12. Mental confusion
13. Seizures
14. Increased RBC count

D. Implementation
1. Assess vital signs
2. Measure I&O
3. Monitor weight
4. Assess skin turgor and mucous membranes
5. Avoid tap water enemas
6. Use normal saline rather than sterile water for irrigation
7. Administer sodium replacement by IV as prescribed
8. Encourage foods high in sodium
9. Encourage juices and bouillon
10. If the client is taking lithium, monitor lithium level, as **hyponatremia** can cause diminished lithium excretion, resulting in toxicity

VII. Hypernatremia

A. Description: A condition in which the serum sodium concentration is greater than 145 mEq/L

B. Causes
1. Decreased water intake or excessive loss of water
2. Watery diarrhea
3. Enteral nutrition and total parenteral nutrition (TPN) deplete the cells of water
4. The administration of sodium chloride by IV without water replacement

---

BOX 8–5. Sodium (Na)

Normal Value
135–145 mEq/L

Sodium-Containing Foods

Common table salt	Corn flakes
Bacon	Processed oat cereals
Corned beef	Crackers
Canned crab	Green olives
Frankfurters	Pickles
Lunch meat	Pretzels
Bouillon cubes	Processed salad dressings
Cheese	Soy sauce
Bread stuffing mixes	Ketchup

---

5. Excessive administration of sodium bicarbonate
6. Use of corticosteroids
7. Cushing's syndrome
8. Impaired renal function

C. Assessment
1. Changes in personality
2. Agitation
3. Decreased level of consciousness
4. Confusion
5. Seizures
6. Twitching
7. Irregular muscle contractions
8. Skeletal muscle weakness
9. Oliguria
10. Edema
11. Tachycardia
12. Dry, sticky mucous membranes
13. Elevated temperature
14. Flushed skin
15. Thirst

D. Implementation
1. Monitor vital signs
2. Monitor I&O
3. Monitor electrolyte values
4. Increase water intake orally or by IV with salt-free solutions
5. Provide water between meals or feedings
6. Encourage client to drink 8 to 10 glasses of water daily
7. Provide additional water to clients receiving tube feedings

VIII. Hypocalcemia

A. Description: A severe calcium deficit below 4.5 mEq/L or below 9 mg/dL (Box 8–6)

B. Causes
1. Inadequate dietary intake of calcium
2. Decreased albumin level
3. Increased intake of dietary protein
4. Long-term immobilization and bone demineralization
5. Excessive GI losses from diarrhea or wound draining
6. Acute pancreatitis

BOX 8–6. Calcium (Ca)

Normal Value

4.5 mEq/L to 5.5 mEq/L, or 9 to 11 mg/dL

Sources

Dairy products	Kale
Milk	Mustard greens
Creamed soups	Rhubarb
Oysters	Spinach
Sardines	Turnip greens
Almonds	Antacids containing
Macaroni	calcium salts
Molasses	

7. Generalized peritonitis
8. Massive infection
9. Burns
10. Diuretic phase of renal failure
11. Excessive administration of blood
12. Parathyroidectomy
13. Inadequate vitamin D consumption
14. **Hyperphosphatemia** ↑
15. Calcium-excreting drugs, such as diuretics, caffeine, anticonvulsants, heparin, laxatives, nicotine

C. Assessment
1. Increased neuromuscular excitability
2. Tingling, numbness, hyperactive reflexes
3. Muscle cramps
4. Tetany
5. Positive Trousseau's or Chvostek's sign
6. Seizures
7. Insomnia
8. Memory impairment
9. Irritability
10. Anxiety
11. Depression
12. Cardiac dysrhythmias
13. ECG shows prolongation of QT interval

D. Implementation
1. Monitor vital signs
2. Monitor for the presence of Chvostek's and Trousseau's signs
3. Provide a quiet environment and avoid overstimulation
4. Initiate seizure precautions
5. Administer calcium orally or IV
6. Administer vitamin D to aid in the absorption of calcium from the intestinal tract
7. Administer calcium supplements 1 to 2 hours after meals to maximize intestinal absorption
8. Keep 10% calcium gluconate on hand for acute calcium deficit
9. Monitor calcium levels closely after thyroid surgery
10. Instruct client taking calcium-excreting drugs to have serum calcium levels checked periodically
11. Teach proper use of antacids or laxatives

12. Instruct client to consume foods high in calcium
13. If **hyperphosphatemia** is present, restrict dietary intake of phosphorus

IX. Hypercalcemia ↑

A. Description: A serum calcium level that exceeds 11 mg/dL or 5.5 mEq/L

B. Causes
1. Increased bone reabsorption or destruction
2. Excessive administration of vitamin D
3. Excessive intake of calcium supplements
4. Excessive ingestion of milk, antacids, and products containing calcium
5. Use of thiazide diuretics
6. Neoplasms
7. Paget's disease
8. Thyroid toxicosis
9. Multiple fractures
10. Adrenal insufficiency
11. Use of lithium
12. Albumin changes
13. Hyperparathyroidism
14. Multiple myeloma
15. Renal disease

C. Assessment
1. Hypotonicity of muscles
2. Lethargy, muscle weakness
3. Deep bone pain
4. Pathological fractures
5. Confusion
6. Thirst
7. Abdominal pain
8. Nausea, vomiting, weight loss
9. Constipation
10. Dysrhythmias
11. ECG shows shortened QT interval
12. Flank pain
13. Renal calculi

D. Implementation
1. Monitor vital signs
2. Monitor for dysrhythmias
3. Restrict dietary calcium
4. Increase mobility
5. Assist with passive range of motion exercises when ambulation is not possible
6. Move clients carefully
7. Monitor for the development of pathological fractures
8. Strain urine to check for urinary stones
9. Monitor for severe flank or abdominal pain
10. Monitor level of consciousness
11. Monitor for confusion and neurological changes
12. Avoid large doses of vitamin D supplements
13. Avoid administering calcium-containing IV fluids such as lactated Ringer's
14. Administer saline and sodium sulfate to induce diuresis
15. Administer IV or oral phosphate
16. Administer calcitonin (Calcimar) as prescribed

17. Administer fluids during diuretic therapy
18. Avoid the use of thiazide diuretics

X. Hypomagnesemia

A. Description: A decreased serum magnesium level of less than 1.5 mEq/L or 1.8 mg/dL (Box 8–7)
B. Causes
   1. Decreased magnesium intake
   2. Excessive loss of calcium and potassium
   3. Vomiting
   4. Diarrhea
   5. Nasogastric (NG) suction
   6. GI losses
   7. Intestinal malabsorption
   8. Intestinal fistulas
   9. Increased renal excretion
   10. Prolonged diuretic therapy
   11. Excessive use of aminoglycosides
   12. Rapid administration of citrated blood
   13. Renal disease
   14. Chronic alcoholism
   15. Diabetic ketoacidosis
   16. Burns
   17. Pancreatitis
C. Assessment
   1. Neurological irritability
   2. Tremors
   3. Tetany
   4. Positive Chvostek's and Trousseau's signs
   5. Seizures
   6. Acute confusion
   7. Weakness
   8. Muscular excitability
   9. Ataxia
   10. Dysrhythmias
   11. ECG shows broadening of T waves, shortening of ST segment, prolonged QT interval, and widened QRS complex
   12. In severe deficiency, inverted T waves and prominent U waves
   13. Laryngeal stridor, coma, or sudden death if severe
D. Implementation
   1. Monitor vital signs
   2. Monitor for dysrhythmias
   3. Monitor for neuromuscular changes
   4. Monitor I&O
   5. Initiate seizure precautions
   6. Administer oral or IV magnesium
   7. Monitor calcium and potassium levels and administer calcium and potassium as prescribed if levels are low
   8. Monitor serum magnesium levels every 12 to 24 hours when client is receiving magnesium by IV
   9. Monitor for reduced deep tendon reflexes suggesting **hypermagnesemia** during administration of magnesium
   10. Instruct client to eat foods high in magnesium, calcium, and potassium

XI. Hypermagnesemia

A. Description: An increased magnesium serum level of 2.3 mEq/L or 2.6 mg/dL
B. Causes
   1. Advanced renal failure
   2. Excessive use of laxatives containing magnesium
   3. Overuse of antacids
   4. Extracellular **fluid volume deficit**
   5. Treatment of severe toxemia of pregnancy with magnesium
   6. Untreated acute diabetic ketoacidosis
   7. Hemodialysis with hard water or dialysate too high in magnesium
   8. Adrenal insufficiency
   9. Pheochromocytoma
C. Assessment
   1. Neurological depression
   2. Drowsiness
   3. Lethargy
   4. Bradycardia
   5. Dysrhythmias
   6. ECG shows peaked T waves, prolonged PR and QT intervals, widened QRS complexes
   7. Respiratory depression
   8. Paralysis of respiratory center
   9. Paralysis of voluntary muscles
   10. Severe hypotension along with nausea and vomiting
   11. Muscle weakness
   12. Areflexia
   13. Loss of deep tendon reflexes
   14. Coma
D. Implementation
   1. Monitor vital signs
   2. Monitor for respiratory depression
   3. Monitor for hypotension, bradycardia, and dysrhythmias
   4. Monitor neurological and muscular activity
   5. Monitor level of consciousness
   6. Remove the source of the excess magnesium
   7. Increase renal excretion by forcing fluids or administering diuretics
   8. Administer 10% calcium gluconate as prescribed if serum levels are over 7 mEq/L to aid in reversing CNS depression

BOX 8–7. Magnesium (Mg)

Normal Value
1.5 to 2.3 mEq/L, or 1.8 to 2.6 mg/dL

Sources

Unprocessed cereal grains	Dairy products
	Dried fruit
Nuts	Meat
Chocolate	Fish
Legumes	Drinking water that has not
Green, leafy vegetables	been processed through a water softener

9. Mechanical ventilation in severe magnesium excess
10. Pacemaker for bradycardia
11. Dialysis with magnesium-free dialysate if renal function is impaired
12. Instruct clients regarding avoiding the use of laxatives and antacids containing magnesium

XII. Hypophosphatemia

A. Description: A serum phosphate level below 3.0 mg/dL or below 1.8 mEq/L (Box 8–8)
B. Causes
1. Decreased nutritional intake
2. Poor absorption from the bowel due to a lack of vitamin D
3. Intake of carbonate antacids
4. Malabsorption syndrome
5. Increased renal excretion due to hyperparathyroidism or renal insufficiency
6. Diabetic ketoacidosis
7. Steatorrhea
8. A poor nutritional state, as in alcoholism
9. Fever
10. Long-term TPN
11. Burns
12. Hepatic disease
C. Assessment
1. Anorexia
2. Dysphasia
3. Weakness
4. Malaise, lethargy
5. Skeletal pain and aches
6. Bone pain
7. Pathological fractures
8. Pulmonary insufficiency
9. Tachypnea
10. Shallow respirations
11. Confusion, stupor, delirium
12. Seizures
13. Hematological changes
D. Implementation
1. Monitor respiratory status
2. Move client carefully
3. Administer potassium phosphate
4. Assess renal system before administering phosphorus
5. Monitor calcium, phosphorus, sodium, and chloride levels
6. Administer vitamin D
7. Monitor for decreased neuromuscular activity
8. Monitor for calcium excess and kidney stones
9. Monitor for hematological changes
10. Monitor clients receiving TPN for electrolyte imbalances
11. Instruct client regarding the use of antacids

XIII. Hyperphosphatemia

A. Description: A serum phosphate level greater than 4.5 mg/dL or 1.8 mEq/L

BOX 8–8. Phosphorus

Normal Value
3.0 to 4.5 mg/dL, or 1.8 to 2.6 mEq/L

Sources

Almonds	Cocoa
Peanuts	Chocolate
Walnuts	Cheese
Barley	Eggs
Bran	Milk
Oatmeal	Beef
Wheat and rye	Liver
Dried beans and peas	Pork
Legumes	Poultry
Lentils	Fish
Pumpkin	Sardines
Squash	Soft drinks

B. Causes
1. Excessive dietary intake of phosphorus
2. Overuse of phosphate-containing laxatives or enemas
3. Hypoparathyroidism
4. Vitamin D intoxication
5. Renal failure
6. Adrenal insufficiency
7. Excessive bone growth in infants and children
8. Metabolic and hormonal imbalances
9. Tissue damage
C. Assessment
1. Neurological excitability
2. Hyperreflexia, tetany
3. Positive Chvostek's or Trousseau's sign
4. Seizures
5. Conjunctivitis
6. Pruritus
7. Renal deposits leading to renal failure
D. Implementation
1. Increase fecal excretion of phosphorus by binding phosphorus from food in the GI tract (aluminum hydroxide gel)
2. Prepare for dialysis if prescribed
3. Administer calcium if **hypocalcemia** exists

Table 8–2. Electrocardiographic Changes in Electrolyte Imbalances

Hypokalemia	*Hyperkalemia*
Peaked P waves	Wide, flat P wave
Flat T waves	Widened QRS complex
Depressed ST segment	Prolonged PR interval
U waves	Depressed ST segment
	Narrow, peaked T waves
Hypocalcemia	*Hypercalcemia*
Prolongation of QT interval	Shortened QT interval
Hypomagnesemia	*Hypermagnesemia*
Broadening of T waves	Peaked T waves
Shortening of ST segment	Prolonged PR and QT intervals
Prolonged QT interval	Widened QRS complexes
Widened QRS	

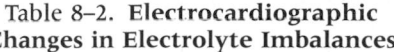

4. Monitor for neuromuscular irritability
5. Monitor for hyperreflexia, tetany, and seizures
6. Monitor for signs of **hypocalcemia**
7. Monitor for Trousseau's and Chvostek's signs
8. Instruct clients to avoid phosphate-containing medications, including laxatives and enemas
9. Instruct clients to decrease their intake of foods high in phosphorus
10. Instruct clients how to take phosphate-binding medications, emphasizing that these should be taken with meals or immediately after meals

PRACTICE QUESTIONS

1. Normal saline 0.9% 1000 mL IV solution is prescribed for the client. The IV is to run at 100 mL per hour. The nurse understands that which of the following is not a characteristic of this type of solution?
   1 Is isotonic with the plasma and other body fluids
   2 Is hypotonic with the plasma and other body fluids
   3 Does not affect the plasma osmolarity
   4 Is the same solution as sodium chloride 0.9%

2. The nurse hears the attending physician asking the intern to prescribe a hypotonic IV solution for the client. Which of the following IV solutions would the nurse expect the intern to prescribe?
   1 0.45% saline (½ NS)
   2 5% dextrose in water (5% D/W)
   3 10% dextrose in water (10% D/W)
   4 5% dextrose in 0.9% saline (5% D/NS)

3. Lactated Ringer's solution (RL) is prescribed for the postoperative client. A nursing student is caring for the client. The nursing instructor asks the student about the tonicity of the prescribed IV solution. Which of the following is correct regarding the tonicity of the solution?
   1 Isotonic
   2 Normotonic
   3 Hypotonic
   4 Hypertonic

4. The nurse is reading the physician's progress notes in the client's record and reads that the physician has documented "insensible fluid loss of approximately 800 mL daily." The nurse understands that this type of fluid loss can occur through:
   1 The GI tract
   2 Urinary output
   3 Wound drainage
   4 The skin

5. Which of the following clients is least likely at risk for the development of third spacing?
   1 The client with cirrhosis
   2 The client with diabetes mellitus
   3 The client with sepsis
   4 The client with renal failure

6. The nurse is caring for a client with a fluid volume deficit. Which of the following clients is at risk for fluid volume deficit?
   1 A client with a colostomy
   2 A client with cirrhosis
   3 A client with congestive heart failure
   4 A client with decreased kidney function

7. The nurse is caring for a client who has been taking diuretics on a long-term basis. A fluid volume deficit is suspected. Which of the following assessment findings would be noted in the client with this condition?
   1 Rales
   2 Increased blood pressure
   3 Decreased hematocrit
   4 Decreased central venous pressure (CVP)

8. The nurse is caring for a client with a fluid volume excess. Which of the following clients is at risk for fluid volume excess?
   1 The client with renal failure
   2 The client with an ileostomy
   3 The client on diuretics
   4 The client on GI suctioning

9. The nurse is caring for a client with cirrhosis. On assessment, the nurse notes that the client is dyspneic, and rales are heard on auscultation. The nurse suspects fluid volume excess. What additional signs would the nurse expect to note in this client if a fluid volume excess is present?
   1 A decreased central venous pressure
   2 A weak and thready pulse
   3 An increase in blood pressure
   4 An increased urine output

10. The clinic nurse performs an assessment on a client with a history of congestive heart failure. The client has been taking diuretics on a long-term basis. The nurse reviews the medication record, knowing that which of the following medications, if prescribed for this client, would place the client at risk for hypokalemia?
    1 Spironolactone (Aldactone)
    2 Bumetanide (Bumex)
    3 Triamterene (Dyrenium)
    4 Amiloride HCl (Midamor)

11. The nurse is caring for a client with a potassium deficit. Which of the following clients is at risk for a potassium deficit?
    1 The client on NG suction
    2 The client with renal disease
    3 The client with Addison's disease
    4 The client in metabolic acidosis

Hyponatremia

12. The nurse analyzes the electrolyte results and notes that the potassium level is 3.2 mEq/L. Which of the following would the nurse note on the ECG as a result of the laboratory value?
    1 Elevated T waves
    2 Absent P waves
    3 Elevated ST segment
    → **4** U waves

13. The nurse prepares to administer potassium IV as prescribed for a client with hypokalemia. Which of the following would not be a part of the nurse's plan regarding the preparation and administration of the potassium?
    1 Prepare the medication for bolus administration
    2 Obtain a controlled IV infusion pump
    3 Dilute in appropriate amount of normal saline
    4 Monitor urine output during administration

14. The nurse instructs a client at risk for hypokalemia about the foods high in potassium that should be included in the daily diet. Which of the following foods is the least likely source of potassium?
    1 Spinach
    2 Carrots
    3 Apricots
    4 Apple

15. The nurse analyzes the electrolyte values and notes a potassium level of 5.5 mEq/L. Which of the following clients is at risk for the development of a potassium value at this level?
    → **1** The client who sustained a traumatic burn *hyper*
    2 The client with Cushing's syndrome *hypo*
    3 The client with colitis *hypo*
    4 The client who has been overusing laxatives *hypo*

16. The nurse analyzes the electrolyte results and notes that the potassium level is 5.4 mEq/L. Which of the following would the nurse note on the ECG as a result of the laboratory value?
    → **1** Narrow, peaked T waves
    2 Prominent U wave
    3 ST segment elevation
    4 Peaked P wave

17. The nurse prepares to administer sodium polystyrene sulfonate (Kayexalate) to the client. Prior to administering the medication, the nurse reviews the action of the medication and understands that it:
    1 Releases bicarbonate in exchange for primarily sodium ions
    2 Releases sodium ions in exchange for primarily bicarbonate ions
    → **3** Releases sodium ions in exchange for primarily potassium ions
    4 Releases potassium ions in exchange for primarily sodium ions

18. The nurse analyzes the electrolyte values and notes a sodium level of 130 mEq/L. Which of the following clients is at risk for the development of a sodium value at this level?
    → **1** The client with SIADH *hypo*
    2 The client with an inadequate daily water intake *hyper*
    3 The client with watery diarrhea *hyper*
    4 The client with renal disease *hyper*

19. The nurse is caring for a client with leukemia. On assessment, the nurse notes that the client has poor skin turgor and has flat neck and hand veins. The nurse suspects hyponatremia. What additional signs would the nurse expect to note in this client if hyponatremia is present?
    1 Dry, sticky mucous membranes *hyper*
    → **2** Postural blood pressure changes
    3 Intense thirst *hyper*
    4 Slow, bounding pulse ——

20. The nurse is caring for a client with an NG tube. NG tube irrigations are prescribed to be performed once every shift. The serum electrolyte results indicate a potassium level of 4.5 mEq/L and a sodium level of 132 mEq/L. Based on these laboratory findings, which solution is the most appropriate to use for the NG irrigation?
    1 Tap water
    2 Distilled water
    3 Sterile water
    4 Normal saline

21. The clinic nurse analyzes the serum sodium level and notes that the client's level is 150 mEq/L. The nurse reports the serum sodium level to the physician, and the physician prescribes dietary instructions based on the sodium level. Which of the following foods will the nurse instruct the client to avoid?
    1 Spinach
    2 Squash
    3 Processed oat cereals
    4 Molasses

22. The nurse analyzes the serum calcium level and notes that the client's level is 4.0 mEq/L. Which of the following conditions most likely caused this serum calcium level?
    → **1** Prolonged bed rest
    2 Excessive administration of vitamin D
    3 Renal disease
    4 Multiple myeloma

23. The nurse is assessing a client with a suspected diagnosis of hypocalcemia. Which of the following assessment signs would not be an indication of this diagnosis?
    → **1** Hypotonicity of the muscles *hyper*
    2 Tingling sensations *hypo*
    3 Hyperactive reflexes *hypo*
    4 Positive Trousseau's sign *hypo*

24. The nurse caring for a client with hypocalcemia would expect to note which of the following changes on the ECG?
    1. Absent P waves
    2. Elevated T waves
    3. Depressed ST segment
    4. Prolonged QT interval *hypo*

    (hyper = shortened)

25. The nurse is caring for a client with Paget's disease. The serum calcium level is 6.2 mEq/L. Which of the following medications would the nurse anticipate to be prescribed for the client?
    1. Calcium gluconate *Tx for hypo*
    2. Calcium chloride *Tx for hypo*
    3. Calcitonin (Calcimar) *hyper*
    4. Large doses of vitamin D *Avoid*

26. The nurse caring for a client with pancreatitis analyzes the laboratory results. The nurse notes a magnesium level of 1.0 mEq/L. Which of the following ECG changes would the nurse expect to note based on the magnesium level?
    1. Peaked T waves
    2. Shortened ST segment
    3. Absent P waves
    4. Prolonged PR interval

27. The nurse is caring for a client with pheochromocytoma. The laboratory results reveal a magnesium level of 6.0 mEq/L. Which of the following assessment signs would the nurse most likely expect to note in the client based on this magnesium level?

    1. Tetany
    2. Muscular excitability
    3. Tremors
    4. Loss of deep tendon reflexes

28. The nurse analyzes the serum phosphate level and notes that the client's level is 1.0 mEq/L. Which of the following conditions most likely caused this serum phosphate level?
    1. Alcoholism
    2. Hypoparathyroidism
    3. Renal failure
    4. Acromegaly

29. The nurse is instructing a client how to decrease the intake of phosphorus in the diet. Which of the following foods contain the least amount of phosphorus?
    1. Oranges
    2. Eggs
    3. Beans
    4. Almonds

30. The nurse is caring for a client with renal failure. The serum phosphorus level is reported as 7.0 mg/dL. Which of the following medications would the nurse expect to be prescribed for the client?
    1. Calcium gluconate
    2. Calcium chloride
    3. Aluminum hydroxide gel (Amphogel)
    4. Calcitonin (Calcimar)

ANSWERS

1. **2**

Rationale: Sodium chloride 0.9% is the same solution as normal saline 0.9%. This solution is isotonic, and isotonic solutions are frequently used for IV infusion because they do not affect the plasma osmolarity. A fluid into which cells can be placed without affecting the cell size is described as being isotonic with the cells.

Test-Taking Strategy: Utilize the process of elimination and knowledge regarding the concepts related to body fluids. If you knew that normal saline was the same as sodium chloride, you could eliminate option 4. Note the word "normal" saline. This should provide you with the key that options 1 and 3 are incorrect options for this question as stated. Remember, "normal" is isotonic and would not affect plasma osmolarity!

Level of Cognitive Ability: Analysis
Phase of Nursing Process: Analysis
Client Needs: Physiological Integrity
Content Area: Fundamental Skills

Reference
Lee, C., Barrett, C., & Ignatavicius, D. (1996). *Fluids and electrolytes: A practical approach* (4th ed.). Philadelphia: F. A. Davis. p. 6.

2. **1**

Rationale: 5% dextrose in water (5% D/W) is an isotonic solution. 10% dextrose in water (10% D/W) and 5% dextrose in 0.9% saline (5% D/NS) are hypertonic solutions. 0.45% saline (½ NS) is hypotonic and is probably the only hypotonic solution used in clinical situations. Distilled water is another example of a hypotonic solution. Hypotonic solutions contain a lower concentration of salt or more water than an isotonic solution.

Test-Taking Strategy: Note the similarities in options 2, 3, and 4. All these solutions contain dextrose. Option 1 is different from the others. Select the option that is different! If you had difficulty with this question, take time now to review the tonicity of the various IV solutions!

Level of Cognitive Ability: Analysis
Phase of Nursing Process: Planning
Client Needs: Physiological Integrity
Content Area: Fundamental Skills

References
Lee, C., Barrett C., & Ignatavicius, D. (1996). *Fluids and electrolytes: A practical approach* (4th ed.). Philadelphia: F. A. Davis. p. 207.
Ignatavicius, D., Workman, M., & Mishler, M. (1995). *Medical-surgical nursing: A nursing process approach* (2nd ed.). Philadelphia: W. B. Saunders. p. 272.

3. **1**

Rationale: Lactated Ringer's solution (RL) is an isotonic solution. Other isotonic solutions include 5% dextrose in water (5% D/W), 0.9% saline (NS), and 5% dextrose in 0.225% saline (5% D/¼ NS). 0.45% saline (½ NS) is hypotonic. 10% dextrose in water (10% D/W) and 5% dextrose in 0.9% saline (5% D/NS) and 5% dextrose in 0.45% saline (5% D/½ NS) are hypertonic solutions.

Test-Taking Strategy: Knowledge regarding the tonicity of the various IV solutions is required to answer the question. If you had difficulty with this question, take time now to review this content!

Level of Cognitive Ability: Analysis
Phase of Nursing Process: Analysis
Client Needs: Safe, Effective Care Environment
Content Area: Fundamental Skills

References
Lee, C., Barrett, C., & Ignatavicius, D. (1996). *Fluids and electrolytes: A practical approach* (4th ed.). Philadelphia: F. A. Davis. p. 207.
Ignatavicius, D., Workman, M., & Mishler, M. (1995). *Medical-surgical nursing: A nursing process approach* (2nd ed.). Philadelphia: W. B. Saunders. p. 272.

4. **4**

Rationale: Sensible losses are those of which the person is aware, such as through wound drainage, GI tract losses, and urination. Insensible losses may occur without the person's awareness. Insensible losses occur daily through the skin and the lungs.

Test-Taking Strategy: Utilize the process of elimination, noting the similarity between options 1, 2, and 3. Note that the issue of the question is fluid loss. In options 1, 2, and 3, these types of losses can be measured for accurate output. Fluid loss through the skin cannot be accurately measured, only approximated. If you had difficulty with this question, take time now to review the difference between sensible and insensible fluid loss!

Level of Cognitive Ability: Analysis
Phase of Nursing Process: Analysis
Client Needs: Physiological Integrity
Content Area: Fundamental Skills

Reference
Lee, C., Barrett, C. & Ignatavicius, D. (1996). *Fluids and electrolytes: A practical approach* (4th ed.). Philadelphia: F. A. Davis. pp. 8–9.

5. **2**

Rationale: Fluid that shifts into the interstitial spaces and remains there is referred to as third-space fluid. Common sites for third spacing include the abdomen, pleural cavity, peritoneal cavity, and pericardial sac. Third-space fluid is physiologically useless because it does not circulate to provide nutrients for the cells. Risk factors include clients with liver or kidney disease, major trauma, burns, sepsis, wound healing or major surgery, malignancy, GI malabsorption, malnutrition, and alcoholic or elderly clients.

Test-Taking Strategy: Utilize the process of elimination. Eliminate options 1 and 4 first as it is likely that fluid balance disturbances will occur with these conditions. From the remaining two options, sepsis is the option that is most acute and, therefore, is most similar to options 1 and 4, the incorrect options. Take time now to review the risk factors associated with third spacing if you had difficulty with this question!

Level of Cognitive Ability: Analysis
Phase of Nursing Process: Assessment
Client Needs: Physiological Integrity
Content Area: Fundamental Skills

Reference
Black, J., & Matassarin-Jacobs, E. (1997). *Medical-surgical nursing: Clinical management for continuity of care* (5th ed.). Philadelphia: W. B. Saunders. pp. 289–290.

6. **1**

Rationale: Causes of a fluid volume deficit include vomiting, diarrhea, conditions that cause increased respirations or increased urinary output, insufficient IV fluid replacement, draining fistulas, or an ileostomy or colostomy. A client with cirrhosis, congestive heart failure (CHF), or decreased kidney function is at risk for fluid volume excess.

Test-Taking Strategy: Read the question carefully, noting that it asks for the client at risk for a deficit. Read each option and think about the fluid imbalance that can occur in each. Utilize the process of elimination. The clients presented in options 2, 3, and 4 retain fluid. The only condition that can cause a deficit is that condition noted in option 1. If you had difficulty with this question, take time now to review the causes of fluid volume deficit!

Level of Cognitive Ability: Analysis
Phase of Nursing Process: Assessment
Client Needs: Physiological Integrity
Content Area: Fundamental Skills

Reference
Lee, C., Barrett, C., & Ignatavicius, D. (1996). *Fluids and electrolytes: A practical approach* (4th ed.). Philadelphia: F. A. Davis. pp. 16–24.

7. **4**

Rationale: Assessment signs in a client with a fluid volume deficit include increased respirations and heart rate, decreased CVP, weight loss, poor skin turgor, dry mucous membranes, decreased urine volume, increased specific gravity of the urine, dark-colored and odorous urine, an increased hematocrit, and altered level of consciousness. The normal CVP is between 4 and 11 mm H_2O. A client with dehydration has a low CVP. The assessment signs in options 1, 2, and 3 are seen in a client with fluid volume excess.

Test-Taking Strategy: Knowledge regarding the assessment signs in fluid volume deficit is required to answer the question. Eliminate options 1 and 2 first. Rales are noted in a fluid volume excess, as is an increased BP. Remembering that CVP reflects the pressure under which blood is returned to the superior vena cava and right atrium should direct you to the correct option, option 4. Pressure (volume) would be decreased in a fluid volume deficit. If you had difficulty with this question, take time now to review the assessment signs noted in fluid volume deficit!

Level of Cognitive Ability: Analysis
Phase of Nursing Process: Assessment
Client Needs: Physiological Integrity
Content Area: Fundamental Skills

References
Lee, C., Barrett, C., & Ignatavicius, D. (1996). *Fluids and electrolytes: A practical approach* (4th ed.). Philadelphia: F. A. Davis. p. 23.
Black, J., & Matassarin-Jacobs, E. (1997). *Medical-surgical nursing: Clinical management for continuity of care* (5th ed.). Philadelphia: W. B. Saunders. p. 1233.

8. 1

Rationale: The causes of fluid volume excess include decreased kidney function, CHF, cirrhosis, the use of hypotonic fluids to replace isotonic fluid losses, excessive irrigation of body fluids, and excessive ingestion of table salt. The client with an ileostomy, the client on diuretics, and the client on GI suctioning are at risk for fluid volume deficit.

Test-Taking Strategy: Read the question carefully, noting that it asks for the client at risk for an excess. Read each option and think about the fluid imbalance that can occur in each. Utilize the process of elimination. The clients presented in options 2, 3, and 4 lose fluid. The only condition that can cause an excess is that condition noted in option 1. If you had difficulty with this question, take time now to review the causes of fluid volume excess!

Level of Cognitive Ability: Analysis
Phase of Nursing Process: Assessment
Client Needs: Physiological Integrity
Content Area: Fundamental Skills

References

Lee, C., Barrett, C., & Ignatavicius, D. (1996). *Fluids and electrolytes: A practical approach* (4th ed.). Philadelphia: F. A. Davis. p. 25.
Black, J., & Matassarin-Jacobs, E. (1997). *Medical-surgical nursing: Clinical management for continuity of care* (5th ed.). Philadelphia: W. B. Saunders. p. 285.

9. 3

Rationale: Assessment findings associated with fluid volume excess include cough, dyspnea, rales, tachypnea, tachycardia, an elevated BP and a bounding pulse, an elevated CVP, weight gain, edema, neck and hand vein distention, altered level of consciousness, and a decreased hematocrit.

Test-Taking Strategy: Knowledge regarding the assessment signs in fluid volume excess is required to answer the question. Remember that CVP reflects the pressure under which blood is returned to the superior vena cava and right atrium. Pressure (volume) would be elevated in a fluid volume excess. If you had difficulty with this question, take time now to review the assessment signs noted in fluid volume excess!

Level of Cognitive Ability: Analysis
Phase of Nursing Process: Assessment
Client Needs: Physiological Integrity
Content Area: Fundamental Skills

References

Lee, C., Barrett, C., & Ignatavicius, D. (1996). *Fluids and electrolytes: A practical approach* (4th ed.). Philadelphia: F. A. Davis. p. 25.
Black, J., & Matassarin-Jacobs, E. (1977). *Medical-surgical nursing: Clinical management for continuity of care* (5th ed.). Philadelphia: W. B. Saunders. p. 287.

10. 2

Rationale: Bumetanide (Bumex) is a loop diuretic. The client on this medication would be at risk for hypokalemia. Spironolactone (Aldactone), triamterene (Dyrenium), and amiloride HCl (Midamor) are potassium-sparing diuretics. Other potassium-sparing diuretics include amiloride HCl and hydrochlorothiazide (Moduretic), spironolactone and hydrochlorothiazide (Aldactazide), and triamterene and hydrochlorothiazide (Dyazide, Maxzide).

Test-Taking Strategy: Knowledge regarding the diuretics that are in the classification of potassium sparing is required to answer this question. It is important to know which medications are in this classification. Take time now to learn

these medications if you had difficulty with this question. You are likely to see a question on NCLEX-RN related to this medication classification!

Level of Cognitive Ability: Analysis
Phase of Nursing Process: Assessment
Client Needs: Physiological Integrity
Content Area: Pharmacology

Reference

Hodgson, B., & Kizior, R. (1998). *Saunders nursing drug handbook 1998*. Philadelphia: W. B. Saunders. pp. 41–43, 126–128, 494–496, 942–944, 1021–1022.

11. 1

Rationale: Potassium-rich GI fluids are lost through GI suction, placing the client at risk for hypokalemia. The client with renal disease and Addison's disease and the client in metabolic acidosis are at risk for hyperkalemia.

Test-Taking Strategy: Read the question carefully, noting that it asks for the client at risk for hypokalemia. Read each option and think about the electrolyte loss that can occur in each. Utilize the process of elimination. Option 1 clearly identifies a loss of body fluid. If you had difficulty with this question, take time now to review the causes of hypokalemia!

Level of Cognitive Ability: Analysis
Phase of Nursing Process: Assessment
Client Needs: Physiological Integrity
Content Area: Fundamental Skills

Reference

Lee, C., Barrett, C., & Ignatavicius, D. (1996). *Fluids and electrolytes: A practical approach* (4th ed.). Philadelphia: F. A. Davis. pp. 62, 67.

12. 4

Rationale: A serum potassium level below 3.5 mEq/L is indicative of hypokalemia. Potassium deficit is the most common electrolyte imbalance and is potentially life threatening. ECG changes include peaked P waves, flat T waves, depressed ST segment, and prominent U waves.

Test-Taking Strategy: Knowledge of the normal potassium level is required to answer this question. From the information in the question, you need to determine that this condition is a hypokalemic one. From this point, it is necessary to know the ECG changes that are expected when hypokalemia exists. If you had difficulty with this question, take time now to review the ECG changes that occur in hypokalemia!

Level of Cognitive Ability: Analysis
Phase of Nursing Process: Analysis
Client Needs: Physiological Integrity
Content Area: Fundamental Skills

Reference

Black, J., & Matassarin-Jacobs, E. (1997). *Medical-surgical nursing: Clinical management for continuity of care* (5th ed.). Philadelphia: W. B. Saunders. p. 308.

13. 1

Rationale: Potassium administered IV must always be diluted in IV fluid. The usual concentration of IV potassium is 20 to 40 mEq/L. Potassium is not given IM and is never given by bolus (IV push). Giving potassium by IV push can result in cardiac arrest. Saline dilution is recommended and dextrose is avoided because it increases intracellular potassium shifting. Always agitate IV bags before hanging them. Monitor the IV site carefully because potassium is very irritating to the veins, and the risk of phlebitis exists. Monitor urinary output during administration and contact the physician if the urinary output is less than 30 mL/hr.

Test-Taking Strategy: Knowledge regarding the administration of IV potassium is required to answer the question. By the process of elimination, you should be able to select the correct option. Although some medications can be given by IV bolus, administering potassium in this manner is life threatening. If you had difficulty with this question, take time now to review potassium administration. You are likely to find a question related to this content on NCLEX-RN!

Level of Cognitive Ability: Application
Phase of Nursing Process: Planning
Client Needs: Safe, Effective Care Environment
Content Area: Pharmacology

Reference
Black, J., & Matassarin-Jacobs, E. (1997). *Medical-surgical nursing: Clinical management for continuity of care* (5th ed.). Philadelphia: W. B. Saunders. pp. 306–308.

14. **4**

Rationale: An apple provides approximately 3 mEq of potassium per serving. Spinach and carrots (½ cup cooked) and 4 apricots provide approximately 7 mEq of potassium per serving.

Test-Taking Strategy: Knowledge regarding the potassium content of foods is required to answer this question. Take the time now to learn the foods that are high and low in potassium content. You are likely to find a question related to this content on NCLEX-RN!

Level of Cognitive Ability: Application
Phase of Nursing Process: Implementation
Client Needs: Health Promotion and Maintenance
Content Area: Fundamental Skills

Reference
Black, J., & Matassarin-Jacobs, E. (1997). *Medical-surgical nursing: Clinical management for continuity of care* (5th ed.). Philadelphia: W. B. Saunders. p. 313.

15. **1**

Rationale: A serum potassium level greater than 5.1 mEq/L is indicative of hyperkalemia. Clients who experience cellular shifting of potassium as in the early stages of massive cell destruction, such as in trauma, burns, sepsis, or with metabolic or respiratory acidosis (with the exception of diabetic acidosis), are at risk for hyperkalemia. The client with Cushing's syndrome or colitis and the client who has been overusing laxatives are at risk for hypokalemia.

Test-Taking Strategy: Utilize the process of elimination, eliminating options 3 and 4 first as they are similar, both being reflective of a GI loss. Remembering that cell destruction causes potassium shifts may assist in directing you to the correct option. Remember that Cushing's presents a risk for hypokalemia and Addison's presents a risk for hyperkalemia. If you had difficulty with this question, take time now to review the risk factors associated with hyperkalemia!

Level of Cognitive Ability: Analysis
Phase of Nursing Process: Assessment
Client Needs: Physiological Integrity
Content Area: Fundamental Skills

Reference
Black, J., & Matassarin-Jacobs, E. (1997). *Medical-surgical nursing: Clinical management for continuity of care* (5th ed.). Philadelphia: W. B. Saunders. p. 311.

16. **1**

Rationale: A serum potassium level above 5.4 mEq/L is indicative of hyperkalemia. ECG changes include a wide, flat P wave; prolonged PR interval; widened QRS complex; narrow, peaked T waves; and a depressed ST segment.

Test-Taking Strategy: Knowledge of the normal potassium level is required to answer this question. From the information in the question, you need to determine that this condition is a hyperkalemic one. From this point, it is necessary to know the ECG changes that are expected when hyperkalemia exists. If you had difficulty with this question, take time now to review the ECG changes that occur in hyperkalemia!

Level of Cognitive Ability: Analysis
Phase of Nursing Process: Analysis
Client Needs: Physiological Integrity
Content Area: Fundamental Skills

Reference
Black, J., & Matassarin-Jacobs, E. (1997). *Medical-surgical nursing: Clinical management for continuity of care* (5th ed.). Philadelphia: W. B. Saunders. p. 308.

17. **3**

Rationale: Sodium polystyrene sulfonate is a cation exchange resin used in the treatment of hyperkalemia. The resin either passes through the intestine or is retained in the colon. It releases sodium ions in exchange for primarily potassium ions. The therapeutic effect occurs 2 to 12 hours after oral administration and longer after rectal administration.

Test-Taking Strategy: Knowledge regarding this medication is required to answer the question. Looking closely at the name of the medication (Kayexalate) may provide you with assistance regarding the action of the medication. If you had difficulty with this question, take time now to review the action of this very important medication!

Level of Cognitive Ability: Analysis
Phase of Nursing Process: Analysis
Client Needs: Physiological Integrity
Content Area: Pharmacology

Reference
Hodgson, B., & Kizior, R. (1998). *Saunders nursing drug handbook 1998*. Philadelphia: W. B. Saunders. p. 935.

18. **1**

Rationale: Hyponatremia is evidenced by a serum sodium level of less than 135 mEq/L. Hyponatremia can result secondary to SIADH (syndrome of inappropriate secretion of antidiuretic hormone). The client with an inadequate daily water intake, watery diarrhea, or renal disease is at risk for hypernatremia.

Test-Taking Strategy: Knowledge regarding normal sodium levels and the causes of hyponatremia is required to answer the question. Take time now to review the normal laboratory values and the causes of hyponatremia if you had difficulty with this question!

Level of Cognitive Ability: Analysis
Phase of Nursing Process: Assessment
Client Needs: Physiological Integrity
Content Area: Fundamental Skills

Reference
Black, J., & Matassarin-Jacobs, E. (1997). *Medical-surgical nursing: Clinical management for continuity of care* (5th ed.). Philadelphia: W. B. Saunders. p. 296.

19. **2**

Rationale: Postural blood pressure changes occur in the client with hyponatremia. Dry, sticky mucous membranes and intense thirst are seen in clients with hypernatremia. A slow, bounding pulse is not indicative of hyponatremia. In hyponatremia, a rapid, thready pulse would be noted.

Test-Taking Strategy: Knowledge regarding the signs of hyponatremia is certainly helpful in answering the question. Note the information provided in the question. If the client has poor skin turgor, then the client is unlikely to have dry, sticky mucous membranes. Eliminate option 3 next as it is similar to option 1. A client with dry, sticky mucous membranes is likely to have intense thirst. From this point, you need to rely on your knowledge to assist in selecting the correct option. If you have difficulty with this, take time now to review the assessment signs associated with hyponatremia!

Level of Cognitive Ability: Analysis
Phase of Nursing Process: Assessment
Client Needs: Physiological Integrity
Content Area: Fundamental Skills

Reference
Lee, C., Barrett, C., & Ignatavicius, D. (1996). *Fluids and electrolytes: A practical approach* (4th ed.). Philadelphia: F. A. Davis. p. 78.

20. **4**

Rationale: A potassium level of 4.5 mEq/L is within normal range. A sodium level of 132 mEq/L is low, indicating hyponatremia. In clients with hyponatremia, normal (isotonic) saline should be used rather than sterile water for GI irrigations.

Test-Taking Strategy: Utilize the process of elimination to answer the question. Note that sterile water, distilled water, and tap water are similar. The only option that is different is option 4. Select the option that is different. If you had difficulty with this question, take time now to review the care of the client experiencing hyponatremia!

Level of Cognitive Ability: Application
Phase of Nursing Process: Implementation
Client Needs: Safe, Effective Care Environment
Content Area: Fundamental Skills

Reference
Lee, C., Barrett, C., & Ignatavicius, D. (1996). *Fluids and electrolytes: A practical approach* (4th ed.). Philadelphia: F. A. Davis. p. 80.

21. **3**

Rationale: The normal serum sodium level is 135 to 145 mEq/L. A serum sodium level of 150 mEq/L is indicative of hypernatremia. Based on this finding, the nurse would instruct the client to avoid foods high in sodium. Spinach and molasses are good food sources of calcium. Squash is high in phosphorus.

Test-Taking Strategy: Knowledge regarding the normal serum sodium level is required to answer this question. After determining that the client has hypernatremia, determining the food to avoid is the issue. Utilize the process of elimination. Eliminate options 1 and 2 first because these are basically very healthy foods. From the remaining two options, note the word "processed" in option 3. Processed foods tend to be higher in sodium content. This is the food to avoid. Take time now to review foods high in sodium content if you had difficulty with this question!

Level of Cognitive Ability: Application
Phase of Nursing Process: Planning
Client Needs: Health Promotion and Maintenance
Content Area: Fundamental Skills

Reference
Mahan, L., & Escott-Stump, S. (1996). *Krause's food, nutrition and diet therapy* (9th ed.). Philadelphia: W. B. Saunders. p. 742.

22. **1**

Rationale: The normal serum calcium level is 4.5 mEq/L to 5.5 mEq/L or 9 to 11 mg/dL. A client with a serum calcium level of 4.0 mEq/L is experiencing hypocalcemia. The excessive administration of vitamin D, renal disease, and multiple myeloma are causative factors associated with hypercalcemia. Although immobilization can initially cause hypercalcemia, the long-term effect of prolonged bed rest is hypocalcemia.

Test-Taking Strategy: Knowledge regarding the normal serum calcium level will assist in determining that the client is experiencing hypocalcemia. If you had difficulty with this question, take time now to review the causative factors associated with hypocalcemia!

Level of Cognitive Ability: Analysis
Phase of Nursing Process: Assessment
Client Needs: Physiological Integrity
Content Area: Fundamental Skills

Reference
Lee, C., Barrett, C., & Ignatavicius, D. (1996). *Fluids and electrolytes: A practical approach* (4th ed.). Philadelphia: F. A. Davis. pp. 98–99.

23. **1**

Rationale: Hypotonicity of the muscles is seen in hypercalcemia. Signs of hypocalcemia include tingling sensations, hyperactive reflexes, and a positive Trousseau's or Chvostek's sign. Additional signs of hypocalcemia include increased neuromuscular excitability, muscle cramps, tetany, seizures, insomnia, irritability, memory impairment, and anxiety.

Test-Taking Strategy: Utilize the process of elimination, noting that options 2, 3, and 4 are similar in that they all reflect a hyperactivity of the neuromuscular system. The option that is different is option 1, and the stem of the question asks for the assessment sign that would not be an indication of the diagnosis presented in the question. Take time now to review the assessment signs noted in hypocalcemia if you had difficulty with this question!

Level of Cognitive Ability: Analysis
Phase of Nursing Process: Assessment
Client Needs: Physiological Integrity
Content Area: Fundamental Skills

References
Lee, C., Barrett, C., & Ignatavicius, D. (1996). *Fluids and electrolytes: A practical approach* (4th ed.). Philadelphia: F. A. Davis. p. 100.
Black, J., & Matassarin-Jacobs, E. (1997). *Medical-surgical nursing: Clinical management for continuity of care* (5th ed.). Philadelphia: W. B. Saunders. p. 317.

24. 4

Rationale: ECG changes that occur in a client with hypocalcemia include a prolonged QT interval. In hypercalcemia, a shortened QT interval occurs.

Test-Taking Strategy: Knowledge regarding the ECG changes that occur in calcium imbalances is required to answer this question. Correlate QT interval with calcium imbalances and correlate "prolonged" with hypocalcemia and "shortened" with hypercalcemia. This may help you remember what changes would occur in these conditions. If you had difficulty with this question, take time now to review the ECG changes that occur in these conditions!

Level of Cognitive Ability: Analysis
Phase of Nursing Process: Assessment
Client Needs: Physiological Integrity
Content Area: Fundamental Skills

Reference
Black, J., & Matassarin-Jacobs, E. (1997). *Medical-surgical nursing: Clinical management for continuity of care* (5th ed.). Philadelphia: W. B. Saunders. pp. 317, 320.

25. 3

Rationale: The normal serum calcium level is 4.5 mEq/L to 5.5 mEq/L or 9 to 11 mg/dL. This client is experiencing hypercalcemia. Calcium gluconate and calcium chloride are medications used in the treatment of tetany that occurs from acute hypocalcemia. In hypercalcemia, large doses of vitamin D need to be avoided. Calcitonin (Calcimar), a thyroid hormone, decreases the plasma calcium level by increasing the incorporation of calcium into the bones, thus keeping it out of the serum.

Test-Taking Strategy: Knowledge regarding the normal serum calcium level will assist in determining that the client is experiencing hypercalcemia. With this knowledge, you can easily eliminate options 1 and 2 because you would not administer medication that would add calcium to the body. Remembering that excessive vitamin D is a causative factor of hypercalcemia will assist in eliminating option 4, leaving option 3 as the correct choice. If you had difficulty with this question, take time now to review the treatment for hypercalcemia!

Level of Cognitive Ability: Application
Phase of Nursing Process: Implementation
Client Needs: Physiological Integrity
Content Area: Pharmacology

References
Black, J., & Matassarin-Jacobs, E. (1997). *Medical-surgical nursing: Clinical management for continuity of care* (5th ed.). Philadelphia: W. B. Saunders. p. 321.
Lee, C., Barrett, C., & Ignatavicius, D. (1996). *Fluids and electrolytes: A practical approach* (4th ed.). Philadelphia: F. A. Davis. p. 108.

26. 2

Rationale: The normal magnesium level is 1.5 to 2.3 mEq/L or 1.8 to 2.6 mg/dL. A magnesium level of 1.0 mEq/L indicates hypomagnesemia. Options 1 and 4 would be found on an ECG in a client experiencing hypermagnesemia. Option 2, along with broadening of T waves, prolonged QT interval, and widened QRS, is indicative of hypomagnesemia. An absent P wave is seen in a client with atrial fibrillation.

Test-Taking Strategy: Knowledge regarding the normal serum magnesium levels and ECG changes that occur are required to answer the question. If you had difficulty with

this question, take time now to review the normal magnesium level and the ECG changes that occur in both hypomagnesemia and hypermagnesemia.

Level of Cognitive Ability: Analysis
Phase of Nursing Process: Assessment
Client Needs: Physiological Integrity
Content Area: Fundamental Skills

Reference
Black, J., & Matassarin-Jacobs, E. (1997). *Medical-surgical nursing: Clinical management for continuity of care* (5th ed.). Philadelphia: W. B. Saunders. pp. 323–324.

27. 4

Rationale: The normal magnesium level is 1.5 to 2.3 mEq/L or 1.8 to 2.6 mg/dL. A client with a magnesium level of 6.0 mEq/L is experiencing hypermagnesemia. Assessment signs include neurologic depression, drowsiness and lethargy, loss of deep tendon reflexes, respiratory paralysis, and loss of consciousness. Tetany, muscular excitability, and tremors are seen in a client with hypomagnesemia.

Test-Taking Strategy: Knowledge regarding the normal magnesium level and the associated signs related to an imbalance is helpful in answering the question. Utilize the process of elimination, noting that options 1, 2, and 3 are similar in that they reflect neurological excitability. If you had difficulty with this question, take time now to review the assessment signs found in magnesium imbalances!

Level of Cognitive Ability: Analysis
Phase of Nursing Process: Assessment
Client Needs: Physiological Integrity
Content Area: Fundamental Skills

Reference
Black, J., & Matassarin-Jacobs, E. (1997). *Medical-surgical nursing: Clinical management for continuity of care* (5th ed.). Philadelphia: W. B. Saunders. p. 324.

28. 1

Rationale: The normal serum phosphate level is 3.0 to 4.5 mg/dL. The client in this question is experiencing hypophosphatemia. Causative factors relate to low or decreased nutritional intake and poor absorption from the bowel or malabsorption syndrome. A poor nutritional state is associated with alcoholism. Hypoparathyroidism, renal failure, and acromegaly are causative factors of hyperphosphatemia.

Test-Taking Strategy: Knowledge regarding the normal phosphate level is required to determine the condition that this client is experiencing. From this point, it is necessary to know the causes of hypophosphatemia. If you had difficulty with this question, take time now to review the causative factors associated with hypophosphatemia!

Level of Cognitive Ability: Analysis
Phase of Nursing Process: Assessment
Client Needs: Physiological Integrity
Content Area: Fundamental Skills

Reference
Lee, C., Barrett, C., & Ignatavicius, D. (1996). *Fluids and electrolytes: A practical approach* (4th ed.). Philadelphia: F. A. Davis. pp. 114, 118.

29. 1

Rationale: An orange contains 18 mg of phosphorus. One egg contains 86 mg; beans (½ cup), 137 mg; and almonds (½ cup), 184 mg of phosphorus.

Test-Taking Strategy: Knowledge regarding the foods high in phosphorus is required to answer the question. The question asks for the food that contains the least amount of phosphorus. If you had difficulty with the question, it is important to review the foods that are high in phosphorus!

Level of Cognitive Ability: Application
Phase of Nursing Process: Implementation
Client Needs: Health Promotion and Maintenance
Content Area: Fundamental Skills

Reference
Mahan, L., & Escott-Stump, S. (1996). *Krause's food, nutrition, and diet therapy* (9th ed.). Philadelphia: W. B. Saunders. p. 132.

30. **3**

Rationale: The normal serum phosphorus level is 3.0 to 4.5 mg/dL or 1.8 to 2.6 mEq/L. The client in this question is experiencing hyperphosphatemia. The phosphorus level needs to be lowered. Certain medications can be given to increase fecal excretion of phosphorus by binding phospho-rus to the food in the GI tract. Aluminum hydroxide gel (Amphogel) is one such medication. Calcium gluconate and calcium chloride are medications used in the treatment of tetany that occurs from acute hypocalcemia. Calcitonin (Calcimar), a thyroid hormone, decreases the plasma calcium level by increasing the incorporation of calcium into the bones, thus keeping it out of the serum.

Test-Taking Strategy: Utilize the process of elimination in answering the question. Note the similarity in options 1, 2, and 4. All relate to calcium in some way. Option 3 is the option that is different. If you had difficulty with this question, take time now to review the treatments associated with phosphorus imbalances!

Level of Cognitive Ability: Analysis
Phase of Nursing Process: Planning
Client Needs: Safe, Effective Care Environment
Content Area: Pharmacology

Reference
Lee, C., Barrett, C., & Ignatavicius, D. (1996). *Fluids and electrolytes: A practical approach* (4th ed.). Philadelphia: F. A. Davis. p. 120.

BIBLIOGRAPHY

Black, J., & Matassarin-Jacobs, E. (1997). *Medical-surgical nursing: Clinical management for continuity of care* (5th ed.). Philadelphia: W. B. Saunders.

Hodgson, B., & Kizior, R. (1998). *Saunders nursing drug handbook 1998.* Philadelphia: W. B. Saunders.

Ignatavicius, D., Workman, M., & Mishler, M. (1995). *Medical-surgical nursing: A nursing process approach* (2nd ed.). Philadelphia: W. B. Saunders.

Lee, C., Barrett, C., & Ignatavicius, D. (1996). *Fluids and electrolytes: A practical approach* (4th ed.). Philadelphia: F. A. Davis.

Mahan, L., & Escott-Stump, S. (1996). *Krause's food, nutrition, and diet therapy* (9th ed.). Philadelphia: W. B. Saunders.

CHAPTER 9

Acid-Base Balance

....

PYRAMID TERMS

Allen's Test—Testing for collateral (radial or ulnar) circulation to the hand before performing an arterial puncture in the radial artery.

Respiratory Acidosis—The total concentration of buffer base is lower than normal, with a relative increasing hydrogen ion (H^+) concentration, thus a greater number of H^+ are circulating in the blood than can be absorbed by the buffer system. Caused by primary defects in the function of the lungs or by changes in normal respiratory patterns due to secondary problems. Any condition that causes an obstruction of the airway or depresses respiratory status can cause **respiratory acidosis**

Respiratory Alkalosis—A deficit of carbonic acid (H_2CO_3) or a decrease in hydrogen ion concentration. Results from the accumulation of base or from a loss of acid without a comparable loss of base in the body fluids. Due to conditions that cause overstimulation of the respiratory status.

Metabolic Acidosis—The total concentration of buffer base is lower than normal, with a relative increase in the H^+ concentration. It occurs as a result of losing buffer bases or retaining too many acids without sufficient bases. It occurs in conditions such as renal failure, diabetic ketoacidosis, and production of lactic acid, and from the ingestion of toxins, such as aspirin.

Metabolic Alkalosis—A deficit of or loss of H^+ or acids or an excess of base (bicarbonate). Results from the accumulation of base or from a loss of acid without a comparable loss of base in the body fluids. Caused by conditions resulting in hypovolemia, the loss of gastric fluid, excessive bicarbonate intake, the massive transfusion of whole blood, and hyperaldosteronism.

PYRAMID TO SUCCESS

Acid-base imbalance is a content area that is sometimes viewed as complex to understand. It is important to understand the description of each imbalance and then review the causes of each disorder, correlating the pathophysiology to each cause. From this point, note the assessment signs related to each disorder and the treatment associated with the clinical manifestations (Box 9–1).

BOX 9–1. Pyramid to Success

Identify clients at risk
Causes of the imbalance
Clinical manifestations
Respiratory alterations
Electrolyte values
Treatment measures
Analyzing arterial blood gases
Allen's test

NURSING PROCESS

ASSESSMENT

Pre-existing conditions	Cyanosis
Vital signs	Headache
Respiratory status	Vertigo
Restlessness	Lightheadedness
Mental status changes	Visual disturbances
Nausea	Paresthesias
Vomiting	Tetany
Diarrhea	Convulsions
Fruity-smelling breath due to improper fat metabolism	ECG changes
Diaphoresis	Abnormal electrolyte or blood gas values

ANALYSIS: Ineffective Airway Clearance   Fluid Volume Excess
Ineffective Breathing Patterns   Anxiety
Impaired Gas Exchange   Potential for Injury
Fluid Volume Deficit   Potential for Infection

PLANNING

Client will maintain a patent airway. Client requests breathing assistance when needed. Client is oriented to person, time, and place. Client maintains an adequate fluid balance. Client demonstrates anxiety-reducing techniques. Client remains free from injury. Client remains free of signs and symptoms of infection.

IMPLEMENTATION

Monitor vital signs. Monitor for signs of respiratory distress. Administer oxygen as prescribed. Assist with breathing techniques and breathing aids as prescribed. Educate and encourage appropriate breathing patterns. Use caution when caring for ventilator clients so that the client is not forced to take breaths too deeply or rapidly. Assess level of consciousness (LOC) for central nervous system (CNS) depression. Provide emotional support and reassurance to the client. Monitor electrolyte values. Maintain intake and output (I&O) to assist with fluid replacement. Initiate safety precautions for convulsions and coma. Administer antibiotics for infection as prescribed. Administer medications as prescribed.

EVALUATION

Vital signs are within normal limits. Breathing patterns are effective. Pulmonary function is normal. Blood gas values are within normal range. Client performs breathing techniques appropriately. Client remains oriented. Serum electrolytes and laboratory values are within normal range. Client remains free of infection. Client remains free of injury. Anxiety is reduced. Complications related to acid-base imbalances are prevented.

CLIENT NEEDS

SAFE, EFFECTIVE CARE ENVIRONMENT

Invasive procedures, such as arterial blood gas specimens or treatments, related to the various acid-base imbalances
Asepsis, standard (universal) precautions
Providing safety to the client when implementing various treatments for the acid-base disorders

HEALTH PROMOTION AND MAINTENANCE

Identify those clients at risk for an acid-base disturbance
Instruct the client and family about the prevention, early detection, and treatment measures for health disorders

PSYCHOSOCIAL INTEGRITY

Provide emotional support to the client and to the family
Support systems

PHYSIOLOGICAL INTEGRITY

Identify clients at risk for an acid-base disturbance
Reduce the likelihood that an alteration will occur
Monitor for changes in status and complications
Administer and monitor medications, IV fluids, and other prescribed therapies
Document the expected and unexpected responses to the therapy
Obtain arterial blood gases
Provide wound care when blood is obtained for a blood gas determination
Analyze the results from an arterial blood gas study.

I. Hydrogen Ions, Acids, and Bases

A. Hydrogen Ions (H^+)
  1. Vital to life
  2. Expressed as pH
  3. Circulate in the body in two forms:
     a. Volatile hydrogen of carbonic acid
     b. Nonvolatile form of hydrogen and organic acids
B. Acids
  1. Produced as end products of metabolism
  2. Contain hydrogen ions
  3. Hydrogen ion donors, which means that acids give up H^+ to neutralize or decrease the strength of an acid or to form a weaker base
  4. The strength of an acid is determined by the number of hydrogen ions it contains

5. The number of hydrogen ions in body fluid determines its acidity, alkalinity, or neutrality
6. The lungs excrete 13,000 to 30,000 mEq of volatile hydrogen per day in the form of H_2CO_3 as carbon dioxide (CO_2)
7. The kidneys excrete 50 mEq of nonvolatile acids per day

C. Bases
1. Contain no H^+
2. Hydrogen ion acceptors
3. Accept H^+ from acids to neutralize or decrease the strength of a base or to form a weaker acid

ll. Regulatory Systems for Hydrogen Ion Concentration in the Blood

A. Buffers
1. The fastest-acting regulatory system
2. Provide immediate protection against changes in H^+ concentration in the extracellular fluid
3. Reactors that function only to keep the pH within the narrow limits of stability when too much acid or base is released into the system
4. React immediately with acids or bases to minimize changes in pH
5. Absorb or release H^+ as needed
6. Serve as a transport mechanism that carries excess H^+ to the lungs
7. Once the primary buffer systems react, they are consumed, and this leaves the body less able to withstand further stress until they are replaced

B. Primary Buffer Systems in Extracellular Fluid
1. Hemoglobin (Hgb) system
   a. In the red blood cells (RBCs)
   b. Maintains acid-base balance by a process called chloride shift
   c. Chloride shifts in and out of the cells in response to the level of oxygen (O_2) in the blood
   d. For each chloride ion that leaves an RBC, a bicarbonate ion enters
   e. For each chloride ion that enters an RBC, a bicarbonate ion leaves
2. Plasma proteins system
   a. Functions in conjunction with the liver to vary the amount of H^+ in the chemical structure of protein
   b. Plasma proteins have the ability to attract or release H^+
3. Carbonic acid/bicarbonate system
   a. Maintains a pH of 7.4 with a ratio of 20 parts bicarbonate to 1 part carbonic acid (20:1)
   b. This ratio (20:1) determines H^+ concentration of body fluid
   c. Carbonic acid concentration is controlled by the excretion of CO_2 by the lungs; the

rate and depth of respiration changes in response to changes in CO_2
   d. Bicarbonate concentration is controlled by the kidneys, which selectively retain or secrete bicarbonates in response to the body needs
4. Phosphate buffer system
   a. Present in the cells and body fluids
   b. Especially active in the kidneys
   c. Acts like bicarbonate and clears spare H^+

C. Lungs
1. Body's second defense that interacts with the buffer system to maintain acid-base balance
2. In acidosis, the pH goes down and the respiratory rate and depth go up in an attempt to blow off acids; the carbonic acid created by the neutralizing action of bicarbonate can be carried to the lungs, where it is reduced to CO_2 and water and exhaled, thus H^+ are inactivated and excreted
3. In alkalosis, the pH goes up and the respiratory rate and depth go down; the CO_2 is retained, and the carbonic acid builds to neutralize and decrease the strength of excess bicarbonate
4. The action of the lungs is reversible in controlling an excess or deficit
5. The lungs can hold H^+ until the deficit is corrected or can inactivate H^+, changing them to water molecules to be exhaled as CO_2, thus correcting the excess
6. The process of correcting a deficit or excess takes 10 to 30 seconds to complete
7. The lungs are capable of inactivating only H^+ carried by H_2CO_3; excess H^+ created by other problems must be excreted by the kidneys

D. Kidneys
1. The ultimate correction of acid-base disturbances is dependent on the kidneys, even though the renal excretion of acids and alkali occurs more slowly
2. Compensation requires a few hours to several days; however, it is more thorough and selective than that of other regulators
3. In acidosis, the pH goes down, and excess H^+ are secreted into the tubules and combine with buffers for excretion in the urine
4. In alkalosis, the pH goes up, and bicarbonate ions move into the tubules, combine with sodium, and are excreted in the urine
5. Selective regulation of bicarbonate in the kidneys
   a. The kidneys restore bicarbonate by the release of H^+ and holding bicarbonate ions
   b. Extra H^+ are excreted in the urine in the form of phosphoric acid
   c. The alteration of certain amino acids in the renal tubules results in a diffusion of ammonia into the kidneys, and the

ammonia combines with extra H^+ and is excreted in the urine

E. Potassium
1. Plays an exchange role in maintaining acid-base balance
2. The body changes the potassium (K) level by drawing H^+ into the cell or by pushing them out of the cell
3. The K level changes to compensate for H^+ level changes
4. In acidosis, the body protects itself from the acid state by moving H^+ into the cell; therefore, K moves out to make room for H^+; the K level goes up
5. In alkalosis, the cells release H^+ into the blood in an attempt to increase the acidity of the blood and combat alkalinity; the K moves into the cells and the K level goes down

III. Respiratory Acidosis

A. Description: The total concentration of buffer base is lower than normal, with a relative increasing H^+ concentration; thus, a greater number of H^+ are circulating in the blood than can be absorbed by the buffer system
B. Causes
1. Due to primary defects in the function of the lungs or changes in normal respiratory patterns from secondary problems
2. Remember that any condition that causes an obstruction of the airway or depresses respiratory status can cause **respiratory acidosis**
3. Hypoventilation
   a. Carbon dioxide is retained and the H^+ increase, leading to the acid state
   b. Carbonic acid is retained and the pH goes down
4. Infection
   a. Caused by inflammation and bacterial agents
   b. Aeration decreases owing to the obstruction of airways
5. Medications
   a. Sedatives, narcotics, and anesthetics depress the respiratory center, leading to hypoventilation
   b. An increase in H^+ occurs, leading to CO_2 narcosis
6. Pneumonia
   a. Caused by infection, irritants, and immobility
   b. Obstruction of airway passages leads to inadequate oxygenation due to fluid accumulation
7. Atelectasis: Excessive mucus collection, with the collapse of alveolar sacs caused by mucus plugs, infectious drainage, or anesthetic drugs, results in decreased respirations
8. Brain trauma: Excessive pressure on the

respiratory center or medulla oblongata depresses respirations
9. Emphysema: Loss of elasticity of alveolar sacs restricts air flow in and out, primarily out, leading to an increased CO_2 level
10. Asthma: Spasms due to allergens, irritants, or emotions cause the smooth muscles of the bronchioles to constrict
11. Bronchitis: Inflammation causes airway obstruction
12. Pulmonary edema: Extracellular accumulation of fluid in acute congestive heart failure (CHF) causes disturbances in alveolar diffusion and perfusion
13. Bronchiectasis
    a. Bronchi become dilated due to inflammation
    b. Destructive changes and weakness in the walls of the bronchi occur

C. Assessment
1. In an attempt to compensate, the respiratory rate and depth increase
2. Headache
3. Mental status changes
4. Confusion
5. Drowsiness
6. Restlessness
7. Visual disturbances
8. Diaphoresis
9. Cyanosis as the hypoxia becomes more acute
10. Hyperkalemia
11. Rapid and irregular pulse leading to dysrhythmias and ventricular fibrillation

D. Implementation
1. Maintain patent airway
2. Improve ventilation and aeration based on the clinical manifestations
3. Monitor for signs of respiratory distress
4. Administer oxygen as prescribed
5. Place client in semi-Fowler's position unless contraindicated
6. Encourage and assist the client to turn, cough, and deep breathe
7. Prepare to administer chest physiotherapy and postural drainage as prescribed
8. Encourage hydration to thin secretions unless excess fluid intake is contraindicated
9. Suction client as necessary
10. Reduce restlessness by improving ventilation rather than by the administration of sedatives and narcotics
11. Monitor electrolyte values
12. Avoid the use of tranquilizers, narcotics, and hypnotics because they further depress respirations
13. Administer antibiotics for infection as prescribed

IV. Respiratory Alkalosis

A. Description: A deficit of H_2CO_3 and a decrease in H^+ concentration; results from the accumulation of base or from a loss of acid without a comparable loss of base in the body fluids

B. Causes
 1. Due to conditions that cause overstimulation of the respiratory status
 2. Hyperventilation: Rapid respirations cause the blowing off of CO_2 and this leads to a decrease in H_2CO_3
 3. Hysteria: Often neurogenic in nature and related to a psychoneurosis; however, this condition leads to vigorous breathing and excessive exhaling of CO_2
 4. Overventilation by mechanical ventilators: the administration of O_2 and the depletion of CO_2 can occur from mechanical ventilation; the client may be hyperventilated by mechanical ventilation
 5. Conditions that increase metabolism, such as fever
 6. Pain or brain trauma: Causes overstimulation of the respiratory center in the brain stem, with resultant carbonic acid deficit
 7. Salicylates: Stimulate the respiratory center, causing hyperventilation
 8. Hypoxia: Causes respiratory stimulation, with resultant carbonic acid deficit

C. Assessment
 1. Initially, the hyperventilation and respiratory stimulation will cause abnormal rapid respirations (tachypnea); in an attempt to compensate, respiratory rate and depth then go down
 2. Headache
 3. Mental status changes
 4. Vertigo
 5. Lightheadedness
 6. Paresthesias such as tingling of the fingers and toes
 7. Hypokalemia
 8. Hypocalcemia
 9. Tetany
 10. Convulsions

D. Implementation
 1. Maintain a patent airway
 2. Provide emotional support and reassurance to the client
 3. Encourage appropriate breathing patterns
 4. Assist with breathing techniques and apply breathing aids as prescribed
   a. Voluntary holding of breath
   b. Rebreathe exhaled CO_2
   c. Rebreathing mask as prescribed
   d. Carbon dioxide breaths as prescribed
 5. Provide cautious care with ventilator clients so that the client is not forced to take breaths too deeply or rapidly
 6. Monitor electrolyte values
 7. Administer medications as prescribed
 8. Prepare to administer calcium gluconate for tetany as prescribed

V. Metabolic Acidosis

A. Description: The total concentration of buffer base is lower than normal, with a relative increase in the H^+ concentration; occurs as a result of losing too many bases and holding too many acids without sufficient bases

B. Causes
 1. Diabetes/diabetic ketoacidosis: An insufficient supply of insulin causes increased fat metabolism, leading to an excess accumulation of ketones or other acids; the bicarbonate then ends up being exhausted
 2. Renal insufficiency/failure
   a. Increased waste products of protein metabolism are retained
   b. Excessive acids build up, and bicarbonate is unable to maintain acid-base balance
 3. Insufficient metabolism of carbohydrates
   a. When an insufficient supply of O_2 is available for the proper burning of carbohydrates, glucose, and water, lactic acid increases
   b. The insufficient metabolism of carbohydrates causes lactic acidosis
 4. Excessive ingestion of acetylsalicylic acid (aspirin) causes an increase in the H^+ concentration
 5. Severe diarrhea: Intestinal and pancreatic secretions are normally alkaline, therefore, excessive loss of base leads to acidosis
 6. Malnutrition: Improper metabolism of nutrients causes fat catabolism, leading to an excess build-up of ketones and acids
 7. High fat diet: A high intake of fat causes a much too rapid accumulation of the waste products of fat metabolism, leading to a build-up of ketones and acids

C. Assessment
 1. In an attempt to blow off the extra CO_2 and compensate for the acidosis, hyperpnea with Kussmaul's respirations occurs
 2. Headache
 3. Nausea
 4. Vomiting
 5. Diarrhea
 6. Fruity-smelling breath due to improper fat metabolism
 7. Twitching
 8. Mental dullness
 9. Drowsiness
 10. Stupor
 11. Coma
 12. Convulsions

D. Implementation
 1. Determine the cause of the acidosis
 2. Maintain a patent airway
 3. Assess LOC for CNS depression
 4. Monitor electrolyte values
 5. Maintain intake and output (I&O) and assist with fluid and electrolyte replacement as prescribed

6. Initiate safety precautions for convulsions and coma
7. Prepare to administer IV solutions as prescribed such as isotonic saline, 5% dextrose and ½ normal saline, sodium lactate or bicarbonate to increase the buffer base
8. Monitor the K level very closely; when acidosis is being treated, K will move back into the cell and the blood level will drop

E. Implementation in Diabetes/Diabetic Ketoacidosis
   1. Insulin is given to hasten the movement of serum glucose into the cell, thereby decreasing the concurrent ketosis
   2. When glucose is being properly metabolized, the body will stop converting fats to glucose
   3. Monitor for circulatory collapse due to polyuria, which may result from the hyperglycemic state, as polyuria or diuresis may lead to extracellular volume deficit

F. Implementation in Renal Failure
   1. In renal failure, dialysis may be used to remove protein and waste products, thereby lessening the acidotic state
   2. A diet low in protein and high in calories will lessen the amount of protein waste products due to protein catabolism; this in turn, will lessen the acidosis

VI. Metabolic Alkalosis

A. Description: A deficit of H_2CO_3 and a decrease in hydrogen ion concentration; results from the accumulation of base or from a loss of acid without a comparable loss of base in the body fluids

B. Causes
   1. Results from a malfunction of metabolism leading to an increased amount of available basic solution in the blood and a decrease in available acids in the blood
   2. Ingestion of excess sodium bicarbonate causes an increase in the amount of base in the blood
   3. Excessive vomiting leads to an excessive loss of acids
   4. Gastrointestinal suctioning leads to an excessive loss of acids from the suctioning
   5. Diuretics: The loss of H^+ and chloride causes a compensatory increase in the bicarbonate in the blood
   6. Hyperaldosteronism: Increased renal tubular reabsorption of sodium occurs with the resultant loss of hydrogen ions
   7. Massive transfusion of whole blood: The citrate anticoagulant used for the storage of blood is metabolized to bicarbonate

C. Assessment
   1. In an attempt to compensate, respiratory rate and depth go down to conserve CO_2
   2. Nausea
   3. Vomiting

BOX 9–2. Normal Blood Gas Values

- pH   7.35–7.45
- PCO_2 35–45 mmHg
- HCO_3 22–27 mEq/L
- PO_2 80–100 mmHg

---

4. Diarrhea
5. Numbness and tingling in the extremities
6. Restlessness and twitching in the extremities
7. Hypokalemia
8. Hypocalcemia
9. Sinus tachycardia
10. Dysrhythmias

D. Implementation
   1. Maintain a patent airway
   2. Monitor vital signs
   3. Monitor I&O
   4. Monitor electrolyte values
   5. Monitor for muscle weakness
   6. Institute safety precautions for tetany and convulsions
   7. Prepare to replace K and chloride (Cl) as prescribed
   8. Prepare to administer medications as prescribed to promote the kidney's excretion of bicarbonate
   9. Prepare to administer acidifying solutions such as ammonium chloride and arginine chloride as prescribed

VII. Arterial Blood Gases (Box 9–2)

A. Obtaining an Arterial Blood Gas Specimen
   1. Obtain vital signs
   2. Determine whether the client has an arterial line in place
   3. Perform **Allen's test** to determine the presence of collateral circulation (Box 9–3)
   4. Assess factors that may affect the accuracy of the results, such as changes in the O_2 settings, suctioning within the last 20 minutes, and client activities
   5. Assist with the specimen draw by preparing a heparinized syringe
   6. Provide emotional support to the client
   7. Apply pressure immediately to the puncture site for 5 minutes, and for 10 minutes if the client is taking anticoagulants

---

BOX 9–3. Performing Allen's Test

Ask client to make a tight fist
Apply direct pressure over the client's ulnar and radial arteries
While pressure is applied, ask the client to open the hand
Remove pressure from the ulnar artery and assess the color of the extremity distal to the pressure point

8. Appropriately label the specimen and transport on ice to the laboratory
9. Record the client's temperature and the type of supplemental oxygen that the client is receiving on the laboratory form

B. Respiratory Imbalances
   1. Remember, the respiratory function indicator is the PCO_2
   2. In a respiratory imbalance, you will find an opposite response between the pH and the PCO_2; in other words, the pH will be up with a PCO_2 down, or the pH will be down with an elevated PCO_2
   3. Remember, the pH is down in an acidotic condition and is elevated in an alkalotic condition
   4. Look at the pH and the PCO_2 to determine whether the condition is a respiratory problem
   5. **Respiratory Acidosis**
      a. The pH is down
      b. The PCO_2 is up
   6. **Respiratory Alkalosis**
      a. The pH is up
      b. The PCO_2 is down

C. Metabolic Imbalances
   1. Remember, the metabolic function indicator is the bicarbonate (HCO_3)
   2. In a metabolic imbalance, you will find a corresponding response between the pH and the HCO_3
   3. In other words, the pH will be up and the HCO_3 will be up, or the pH will be down and the HCO_3 will be down
   4. Remember, the pH is down in an acidotic condition and is elevated in an alkalotic condition
   5. Look at the pH and the HCO_3 to determine whether the condition is a metabolic problem
   6. **Metabolic acidosis**
      a. The pH is down
      b. The HCO_3 is down
   7. **Metabolic alkalosis**
      a. The pH is up
      b. The HCO_3 is up

D. Compensation
   1. **Respiratory acidosis** and **Respiratory alkalosis**
      a. When compensation has occurred, the pH will be within normal limits
      b. The blood gas result reflects partial compensation if the HCO_3 is abnormal
      c. The blood gas result reflects an uncompensated condition if the HCO_3 is normal
   2. **Metabolic acidosis** and **Metabolic alkalosis**
      a. When compensation has occurred, the pH will be within normal limits
      b. The blood gas result reflects partial compensation if the PCO_2 is abnormal
      c. The blood gas result reflects an uncompensated condition if the PCO_2 is normal

E. Analyzing Arterial Blood Gas Results (Box 9–4)

BOX 9–4. Analyzing Arterial Blood Gas Results

If you can remember the following pyramid points and steps, you will be able to analyze any blood gas report!

PYRAMID POINTS

In acidosis, the pH is down.
In alkalosis, the pH is up.
The respiratory function indicator is the PCO_2.
The metabolic function indicator is the HCO_3.

PYRAMID STEPS

Look at the blood gas report.

Pyramid Step 1
Look at the pH. Is it up or down? If it is up, it reflects alkalosis. If it is down, it reflects acidosis.

Pyramid Step 2
Look at the PCO_2. Is it up or down? If it reflects an opposite response to the pH, then you know that the condition is a respiratory imbalance. If it does not reflect an opposite response to the pH, then move on to Pyramid Step 3.

Pyramid Step 3
Look at the HCO_3. Does the HCO_3 reflect a corresponding response with the pH? If it does, then the condition is a metabolic imbalance.

Pyramid Step 4
Remember, compensation has occurred if the pH is in a normal range of 7.35–7.45. If the pH is not within normal range, look at the respiratory or metabolic function indicators.

Respiratory Imbalances:
If the condition is a respiratory imbalance, look at the HCO_3 to determine the state of compensation.
If the HCO_3 is normal, then the condition is uncompensated. If the HCO_3 is abnormal, then the condition is partial compensation.

Metabolic Imbalances:
If the condition is a metabolic imbalance, look at the PCO_2 to determine the state of compensation.
If the PCO_2 is normal, then the condition is uncompensated. If the PCO_2 is abnormal, then the condition is partial compensation.

PRACTICE QUESTIONS

1. The client with a diagnosis of chronic obstructive pulmonary disease (COPD) is most likely to experience what type of acid-base imbalance?
   1. Respiratory acidosis
   2. Respiratory alkalosis
   3. Metabolic acidosis
   4. Metabolic alkalosis

2. The nurse reviews the blood gas results of a client with Guillain-Barré syndrome. The nurse analyzes the results and determines that the client is experiencing respiratory acidosis. Which of the following validates the nurse's findings?
   1   pH 7.40, PCO_2 52 mmHg
   2   pH 7.35, PCO_2 40 mmHg
   3   pH 7.25, PCO_2 50 mmHg
   4   pH 7.50, PCO_2 30 mmHg

3. The nurse is caring for a client with adult respiratory distress syndrome (ARDS). Blood gas results indicate a pH of 7.50 and a PCO_2 of 30 mmHg. The nurse has determined that the client is experiencing respiratory alkalosis. Which of the following laboratory values would the nurse expect to note?
   1   Sodium level, 145 mEq/L
   2   Potassium level, 3.2 mEq/L
   3   Magnesium level, 2.0 mEq/L
   4   Phosphorus level, 2.3 mEq/L

4. The nurse is caring for a client with pneumonia. Blood gas results indicate a pH of 7.45, PCO_2 of 30 mmHg, and HCO_3 of 22 mEq/L. The nurse analyzes these results as:
   1   Metabolic acidosis, compensated
   2   Metabolic alkalosis, uncompensated
   3   Respiratory alkalosis, compensated
   4   Respiratory acidosis, uncompensated

5. The client is scheduled for blood to be drawn from the radial artery for an arterial blood gas (ABG) determination. An Allen's test is performed prior to drawing the blood to determine the adequacy of the:
   1   Radial circulation
   2   Ulnar circulation
   3   Femoral circulation
   4   Carotid circulation

6. The nurse is caring for a client with a nasogastric tube that is attached to low suction. The client is at risk for which of the following acid-base disorders?
   1   Respiratory acidosis
   2   Respiratory alkalosis
   3   Metabolic acidosis
   4   Metabolic alkalosis

7. The client with an ileostomy is at risk for developing which of the following acid-base disorders?
   1   Respiratory acidosis
   2   Respiratory alkalosis
   3   Metabolic acidosis
   4   Metabolic alkalosis

8. The nurse is caring for a client with diabetic ketoacidosis and documents that the client is experiencing Kussmaul's respirations. Based on this documentation, which of the following did the nurse observe?
   1   Respirations that are abnormally deep, regular, and increased in rate
   2   Respirations that are regular but abnormally slow
   3   Respirations that are labored and increased in depth and rate
   4   Respirations that cease for several seconds

9. Excessive use of oral antacids containing sodium or calcium HCO_3 can result in which of the following acid-base disturbances?
   1   Respiratory alkalosis
   2   Respiratory acidosis
   3   Metabolic acidosis
   4   Metabolic alkalosis

10. The nurse is caring for a client with renal failure. Blood gas results indicate a pH of 7.30, a PCO_2 of 32 mmHg, and an HCO_3 of 20 mEq/L. The nurse has determined that the client is experiencing metabolic acidosis. Which of the following laboratory values would the nurse expect to note?
    1   Sodium of 145 mEq/L
    2   Magnesium, 2.0 mEq/L
    3   Potassium, 5.2 mEq/L
    4   Phosphorus, 2.3 mEq/L

ANSWERS

1. **1**

Rationale: Respiratory acidosis is most often due to hypoventilation. Chronic respiratory acidosis is most commonly caused by COPD. In end-stage disease, pathological changes lead to airway collapse, air trapping, and disturbance of ventilation-perfusion (V/Q) relationships. Acute respiratory acidosis also occurs in these clients when superimposed respiratory infection or concurrent respiratory disease increases the work of breathing.

Test-Taking Strategy: Knowledge regarding the causes of respiratory acidosis is necessary to answer this question. Remembering that hypoventilation results in respiratory acidosis will direct you toward the correct option. Review the causes of respiratory acidosis now, if you had difficulty with this question!

Level of Cognitive Ability: Analysis
Phase of Nursing Process: Analysis
Client Needs: Physiological Integrity
Content Area: Fundamental Skills

Reference
Black, J., & Matassarin-Jacobs, E. (1997). *Medical-surgical nursing: Clinical management for continuity of care* (5th ed.). Philadelphia: W. B. Saunders. p. 333.

2. **3**

Rationale: The normal pH is 7.35 to 7.45. The normal PCO_2 is 35 to 45 mmHg. In respiratory acidosis, the pH is down and the PCO_2 is up.

Test-Taking Strategy: Remember that in a respiratory imbalance you will find an opposite response between the pH and the PCO_2. Also remember that the pH is down in an acidotic condition. Options 1 and 4 reflect an elevated pH, which indicates an alkalotic condition. Option 2 reflects a normal blood gas result. Option 3 is the only option that reflects an acidotic condition.

Level of Cognitive Ability: Analysis
Phase of Nursing Process: Assessment
Client Needs: Physiological Integrity
Content Area: Fundamental Skills

Reference

Black, J., & Matassarin-Jacobs, E. (1997). *Medical-surgical nursing: Clinical management for continuity of care* (5th ed.). Philadelphia: W. B. Saunders. p. 334.

3. **2**

Rationale: Clinical manifestations of respiratory alkalosis include tachypnea, hyperpnea, weakness, paresthesias, tetany, dizziness, convulsions, coma, hypokalemia, and hypocalcemia.

Test-Taking Strategy: Knowledge regarding the clinical manifestations of respiratory alkalosis, along with normal laboratory values, will assist you in answering the question. By the process of elimination, you can then determine that the only abnormal laboratory value is the K level, option 2.

Level of Cognitive Ability: Analysis
Phase of Nursing Process: Analysis
Client Needs: Physiological Integrity
Content Area: Fundamental Skills

Reference

Black, J., & Matassarin-Jacobs, E. (1997). *Medical-surgical nursing: Clinical management for continuity of care* (5th ed.). Philadelphia: W. B. Saunders. p. 334.

4. **3**

Rationale: The normal pH is 7.35 to 7.54. Compensation occurs when the pH returns to a normal value. In a respiratory condition, an opposite effect will be seen between the pH and the PCO_2. In an alkalotic condition, the pH is up. Clients with pneumonia are at risk for respiratory alkalosis as a result of hypoxemia.

Test-Taking Strategy: Remember that in a respiratory imbalance you will find an opposite response between the pH and the PCO_2 as indicated in the question. Therefore, options 1 and 2 can be eliminated. Also remember that the pH is up in an alkalotic condition and compensation occurs as evidenced by a normal pH. Option 3 reflects a respiratory alkalotic condition and compensation and describes the blood gas values as indicated in the question. Review the steps related to reading blood gas values if you had difficulty with this question!

Level of Cognitive Ability: Analysis
Phase of Nursing Process: Analysis
Client Needs: Physiological Integrity
Content Area: Fundamental Skills

Reference

Black, J., & Matassarin-Jacobs, E. (1997). *Medical-surgical nursing: Clinical management for continuity of care* (5th ed.). Philadelphia: W. B. Saunders. p. 338.

5. **2**

Rationale: Before radial puncture for obtaining an arterial specimen for ABGs, an Allen's test should be performed to determine adequate ulnar circulation. Failure to assess collateral circulation could result in severe ischemic injury to the hand if damage to the radial artery occurs with arterial puncture.

Test-Taking Strategy: Knowledge regarding the purpose and procedure for the Allen's test is required to answer this question. Protection of the client from injury during diagnostic procedures is a priority nursing responsibility. Review the purpose and procedure of the Allen's test now, if you had difficulty with this question!

Level of Cognitive Ability: Analysis
Phase of Nursing Process: Assessment
Client Needs: Physiological Integrity
Content Area: Fundamental Skills

Reference

Black, J., & Matassarin-Jacobs, E. (1997). *Medical-surgical nursing: Clinical management for continuity of care* (5th ed.). Philadelphia: W. B. Saunders, p. 339.

6. **4**

Rationale: Loss of gastric fluid via nasogastric suction or vomiting causes metabolic alkalosis due to the loss of hydrochloric acid (HCl). This results in an alkalotic condition.

Test-Taking Strategy: If you can remember that HCl acid is lost when the client is on nasogastric suction, this will direct you to the option identifying an alkalotic condition. Since the question addresses a situation other than a respiratory one, the acid-base disorder would be a metabolic condition. If you had difficulty with this question, review the causes of metabolic alkalosis now!

Level of Cognitive Ability: Analysis
Phase of Nursing Process: Analysis
Client Needs: Physiological Integrity
Content Area: Fundamental Skills

Reference

Black, J., & Matassarin-Jacobs, E. (1997). *Medical-surgical nursing: Clinical management for continuity of care* (5th ed.). Philadelphia: W. B. Saunders. p. 336.

7. **3**

Rationale: Intestinal secretions high in HCO_3 may be lost through enteric drainage tubes, an ileostomy, or with diarrhea. The decreased HCO_3 level creates the actual base deficit of metabolic acidosis.

Test-Taking Strategy: Remembering that intestinal fluids are primarily alkaline will assist you in selecting the correct option. When excess HCO_3 is lost, acidosis will result. Note that the client in the question has a gastrointestinal disorder. This will direct you toward a metabolic disorder. If you had difficulty with this question, review the causes of metabolic acidosis now!

Level of Cognitive Ability: Analysis
Phase of Nursing Process: Assessment
Client Needs: Physiological Integrity
Content Area: Fundamental Skills

References

Black, J., & Matassarin-Jacobs, E. (1997). *Medical-surgical nursing: Clinical management for continuity of care* (5th ed.). Philadelphia: W. B. Saunders. p. 336.

Ignatavicius, D., Workman, M., & Mishler, M. (1995). *Medical-surgical nursing: A nursing process approach* (2nd ed.). Philadelphia: W. B. Saunders. p. 337.

8. **1**

Rationale: Kussmaul's respirations are abnormally deep, regular, and increased in rate. In bradypnea, respirations are regular but abnormally slow. In hyperpnea, respirations are labored and increased in depth and rate. Apnea is described as respirations that cease for several seconds.

Test-Taking Strategy: Knowledge regarding the descriptions for alterations in breathing pattern is required to answer the question. Kussmaul's respirations occur in diabetic ketoacidosis. Review the characteristics of these types of respirations now, if you had difficulty with this question.

Level of Cognitive Ability: Analysis
Phase of Nursing Process: Assessment
Client Needs: Physiological Integrity
Content Area: Fundamental Skills

Reference

Potter, P., & Perry, A. (1997). *Fundamentals of nursing: Concepts, process and practice* (4th ed.). St. Louis: Mosby–Year Book. p. 624.

9. **4**

Rationale: Increases in base components occur as a result of oral or parenteral ingestion of bicarbonates, carbonates, acetates, citrates, and lactates. Excessive use of oral antacids containing sodium or calcium HCO_3 can cause a metabolic alkalosis.

Test-Taking Strategy: Remembering that antacids contain HCO_3 and that an excess oral intake will increase HCO_3 will assist in directing you to the correct option. Review the causes of metabolic alkalosis now, if you had difficulty with the question!

Level of Cognitive Ability: Analysis
Phase of Nursing Process: Analysis
Client Needs: Physiological Integrity
Content Area: Fundamental Skills

Reference

Black, J., & Matassarin-Jacobs, E. (1997). *Medical-surgical nursing: Clinical management for continuity of care* (5th ed.). Philadelphia: W. B. Saunders. p. 335.

10. **3**

Rationale: Clinical manifestations of metabolic acidosis include hyperventilation, drowsiness, confusion, headache, or coma. Hyperkalemia will occur. The pH will be less than 7.35 and the HCO_3 lower than 22 mEq/L.

Test-Taking Strategy: Knowledge regarding the clinical manifestations of metabolic acidosis along with normal laboratory values will assist you in answering the question. By the process of elimination, you can then determine that the only abnormal laboratory value is the potassium level, option 3.

Level of Cognitive Ability: Analysis
Phase of Nursing Process: Analysis
Client Needs: Physiological Integrity
Content Area: Fundamental Skills

Reference

Black, J., & Matassarin-Jacobs, E. (1997). *Medical-surgical nursing: Clinical management for continuity of care* (5th ed.). Philadelphia: W. B. Saunders. p. 335.

BIBLIOGRAPHY

Black, J. M., & Matassarin-Jacobs, E. (1997). *Medical surgical nursing: Clinical management for continuity of care* (5th ed.). Philadelphia: W. B. Saunders.

Craven, R. F., & Hirnle, C. J. (1996). *Fundamentals of nursing: Human health and function* (2nd ed.). Philadelphia: J. B. Lippincott.

Hodgson, B., & Kizior, R. (1988). *Saunders nursing drug handbook 1998.* Philadelphia: W. B. Saunders.

Ignatavicius, D., Workman, M. L., & Mishler, M. (1995). *Medical surgical nursing: A nursing process approach* (2nd ed., Vol. 1). Philadelphia: W. B. Saunders.

Lee, C., Barrett, C., & Ignatavicius, D. (1996). *Fluid and electrolytes: A practical approach* (4th ed.). Philadelphia: F. A. Davis.

Luckmann, J. (1997). *Saunders manual of nursing care.* Philadelphia: W. B. Saunders.

Potter, P., & Perry, A. (1997). *Fundamentals of nursing: Concepts, process, and practice* (4th ed.). St. Louis: Mosby–Year Book.

Smeltzer, S., & Bare, B. (1996). *Brunner and Suddarth's textbook of medical surgical nursing* (8th ed.). Philadelphia: J. B. Lippincott.

CHAPTER 10

Laboratory Values

PYRAMID TERMS

Capillary Puncture—Preferred for a peripheral blood smear

Venipuncture—Allows procurement of larger quantities of blood for testing; the antecubital veins are the veins of choice because of ease of access

Serum—Blood plasma from which clotting agents have been removed

Plasma—The fluid ground substance; what remains after the cells have been removed from a sample of whole blood

◆ PYRAMID TO SUCCESS

This chapter identifies the normal adult values of the most common laboratory tests. If you are familiar with the normal values, you of course will be able to determine whether an abnormality exists. It is unlikely that a question on NCLEX-RN will simply ask you what a normal value may be. The questions on NCLEX-RN related to laboratory values will require you to identify whether the laboratory value is normal or abnormal, and then you will be required to think critically about the effects of the laboratory value in terms of the client.

Pyramid points focus on awareness of the normal values of the most common laboratory tests, therapeutic levels in **serum** of commonly prescribed medications, and determination of the need to implement specific actions based on the findings. When a question is presented on NCLEX-RN regarding a specific laboratory value, note the disorder presented in the question and the associated body organ that is affected as a result of the disorder. This process will assist you in determining the correct answer.

For example, if the question is asking you about the immune status of a client receiving chemotherapy, assessment of laboratory values will focus on the white blood cell count and the neutrophils. You are required to analyze these results as low and determine the specific client need, which in this case would be the risk for infection. In the client receiving chemotherapy who has a low white blood cell count, your plan centers on the immune system and protecting that client from infection. Implementation focuses on preventive interventions related to infection, perhaps protective isolation measures. Evaluation may focus on maintenance of a normal temperature in the client.

Box 10–1 lists abbreviations found in laboratory values.

BOX 10–1. Pyramid Abbreviations

g/dL—gram per deciliter
µg/dL—microgram per deciliter
mg/dL—milligram per deciliter
mEq/L—milliequivalent per liter
U/L—unit per liter
mm/hr—millimeter per hour
IU/L—International Unit per liter
µg/mL—microgram per milliliter
ng/mL—nanogram per milliliter
µU/mL—microunit per milliliter
mL/kg—milliliter per kilogram

NURSING PROCESS

ASSESSMENT

Specific client preparation required for test
Specific postprocedure measures
Significant laboratory value specific to the client's condition
Significant value as compared with a normal finding
Signs and symptoms in the client based on an abnormal laboratory value

---

ANALYSIS: Interpreting the laboratory value
Comparing the data with the normal values
Identifying significant signs and symptoms
Determining the client's needs or problems
Formulating a nursing diagnosis based on identified needs

PLANNING	IMPLEMENTATION	EVALUATION
Client identifies purpose of test. Client describes laboratory test preparation. Client describes postprocedure measures. Client identifies the need for follow-up testing.	Explain purpose of test to client. Obtain informed consent if required. Inform client of specific test preparation. Initiate standard (universal) or other precautions as necessary. Maintain asepsis. Instruct client in post-test procedures and need for follow-up. Note whether the laboratory value is abnormal. Monitor for signs and symptoms that will occur as a result of the abnormality. Report significant results to the physician. Initiate prescribed interventions based on the laboratory results. Document the effectiveness of interventions and follow-up laboratory studies.	Client prepares for the laboratory study. Client performs postprocedure measures. Client complies with prescribed interventions. Client obtains follow-up testing as required.

◆ CLIENT NEEDS

SAFE, EFFECTIVE CARE ENVIRONMENT

Informed consent for specific procedures
Handling infectious materials
Asepsis
Standard (universal) and other precautions

HEALTH PROMOTION AND MAINTENANCE

Client preparation for laboratory test
Post-test procedures
Signs and symptoms that indicate the need to notify the health care provider
Importance of follow-up laboratory studies
Community resources available for the follow-up

PSYCHOSOCIAL INTEGRITY

Communicate purpose of test to client
Provide psychosocial comfort during testing
Identify support systems
Communicate with the client regarding laboratory results
Describe specific interventions required based on the results

PHYSIOLOGICAL INTEGRITY

Comfort interventions
Normal values of the most common laboratory tests
Significant laboratory values

Therapeutic serum medication levels of commonly prescribed medications
Determination of the need to implement specific actions based on the findings
Monitoring for clinical manifestations associated with the abnormal laboratory value
Monitoring for potential complications related to the test

I. Electrolytes (Table 10–1)

A. **Serum** sodium (Na)
1. Description
   a. Na is a major cation of extracellular fluid
   b. Na maintains osmotic pressures and acid-base balance and transmits nerve impulses
   c. Na is absorbed from the small intestine and excreted in urine in amounts dependent on dietary intake
   d. Minimum daily requirement of Na is 15 mEq

Table 10–1. Normal Adult Electrolyte Values

Sodium	136–145 mEq/L
Potassium	3.5–5.1 mEq/L
Chloride	98–107 mEq/L
Bicarbonate (venous)	22–29 mEq/L

2. Value: 135 to 145 mEq/L
3. Nursing considerations
   a. Do not draw blood during hemodialysis
   b. Drawing blood samples proximal to IV infusion of sodium chloride will falsely elevate results

B. **Serum** potassium (K)
1. Description
   a. K is a major intracellular cation
   b. K regulates cellular water balance, electrical conduction in muscle cells, and acid-base balance
   c. The body obtains K through dietary ingestion, and the kidneys either preserve or excrete K depending upon cellular need
   d. K levels are used to evaluate cardiac dysrhythmias, renal dysfunction, mental confusion, GI distress, and IV replacement therapy
2. Value: 3.5 to 5.1 mEq/L
3. Nursing considerations
   a. Do not draw blood during hemodialysis
   b. Use of a tourniquet and pumping the hand prior to venous sampling can increase the value
   c. Do not draw blood from a site where an IV infusion exists
   d. If the client is receiving K, note on the laboratory form
   e. Clients with elevated WBC counts and platelet counts may have falsely elevated K levels

C. **Serum** chloride
1. Description
   a. Chloride is a hydrochloric acid salt that is the most abundant body anion in the extracellular fluid
   b. Chloride functions in counterbalancing cations such as sodium, and acts as a buffer during oxygen (O_2) and carbon dioxide (CO_2) exchange in red blood cells
   c. Chloride aids in digestion, osmotic pressure, and water balance
2. Value: 98 to 107 mEq/L
3. Nursing considerations
   a. Do not draw blood during hemodialysis
   b. Draw blood from an extremity that does not have saline infusing into it
   c. Do not allow client to clench/unclench hand prior to blood draw
   d. Any condition accompanied by prolonged vomiting, diarrhea, or both will alter levels

II. Coagulation Studies

A. Activated partial thromboplastin time (APTT)
1. Description
   a. Evaluates how well the coagulation sequence is functioning by measuring the amount of time it takes for recalcified, citrated **plasma** to clot after partial thromboplastin is added to it
   b. Screens for deficiencies and inhibitors of all coagulation factors except VII and XIII
   c. Most commonly used to monitor heparin therapy and screen for coagulation disorders
2. Value: 20 to 36 seconds, depending on the type of activator used
3. Nursing considerations
   a. If client is on intermittent heparin therapy, draw sample one hour prior to next scheduled dose
   b. Do not draw samples during hemodialysis
   c. Do not draw samples from an arm in which heparin is infusing
   d. Transport specimen to the laboratory immediately
   e. If the value is prolonged, initiate bleeding precautions

B. Prothrombin time (PT) and International Normalized Ratio (INR)
1. Description
   a. Prothrombin is a vitamin K–dependent glycoprotein produced by the liver that is necessary for firm fibrin clot formation
   b. Each laboratory establishes a normal value or control based on the method used to perform the test (PT)
   c. The PT measures the amount of time it takes for clot formation and is used to monitor the response to warfarin (Coumadin) therapy or to screen for dysfunction involving the extrinsic system resulting from liver disease, vitamin K deficiency, or disseminated intravascular coagulation (DIC)
   d. A PT value within 2 seconds (plus or minus) of the control is considered normal
   e. The INR standardizes the PT ratio and is calculated by raising the observed PT ratio to the power of the International Sensitivity Index specific to the thromboplastin reagent used
2. Values
   a. Normal PT is 9.6 to 11.8 seconds (adult male) and 9.5 to 11.3 seconds (adult female)
   b. INR of 2.0 to 3.0 for standard Coumadin therapy
   c. INR of 3.0 to 4.5 for high-dose Coumadin therapy
3. Nursing considerations
   a. Blood for a baseline PT should be drawn before starting anticoagulation therapy
   b. Do not draw blood during hemodialysis
   c. Note time of collection on the laboratory form
   d. Provide direct pressure to the site for 3 to 5 minutes if a coagulation defect is present
   e. Concurrent therapy with heparin can lengthen PT for up to 5 hours after dosing
   f. Diets high in green leafy vegetables can

increase the absorption of vitamin K, which shortens the PT

    g. A PT greater than 30 seconds places the client at risk for hemorrhage

    h. Oral anticoagulation therapy usually maintains the PT at 1.5 to 2 times the laboratory control value

C. Clotting time
1. Description: Measures the time required for the interaction of all factors involved in the clotting process
2. Value: 8 to 15 minutes
3. Nursing considerations
    a. The client should not receive heparin therapy for 3 hours prior to specimen collection
    b. The test result is prolonged by any anticoagulant therapy, test tube agitation, or higher temperature changes

D. Platelet count
1. Description
    a. Platelets function in hemostatic plug formation, clot retraction, and coagulation factor activation
    b. Platelets are produced by the bone marrow to function in hemostasis
2. Value: 150,000 to 400,000 cells/μL
3. Nursing considerations
    a. Do not draw a specimen during hemodialysis
    b. Monitor the site for bleeding in clients with known thrombocytopenia
    c. High altitudes, chronic cold weather, and exercise increase platelet counts
    d. Bleeding precautions should be instituted in clients with a low platelet count

III. Serum Gastrointestinal Studies

A. Albumin
1. Description
    a. Albumin is the major plasma protein of blood
    b. Albumin maintains oncotic pressure and transports bilirubin, fatty acids, medications, hormones, and other substances that are insoluble in water
2. Value: 3.4 to 5 g/dL
3. Nursing considerations
    a. Draw from an extremity that does not have an IV infusing into it
    b. Instruct client to consume a low-fat diet on the day of the test

B. Alkaline phosphatase
1. Description
    a. Alkaline phosphatase is an enzyme normally found in bone, liver, intestine, and placenta
    b. The level rises during periods of bone growth, liver disease, and bile duct obstruction
2. Value: 4.5 to 13 King-Armstrong units/dL

3. Nursing considerations
    a. The client may be requested to fast 10 to 12 hours prior to the test
    b. Hepatotoxic medications administered within 12 hours prior to specimen collection invalidate the test
    c. Do not draw the specimen during hemodialysis
    d. Transport the specimen to the laboratory immediately

C. Ammonia
1. Description
    a. Ammonia is a waste product from nitrogen breakdown during protein metabolism
    b. Ammonia is metabolized by the liver and excreted by the kidneys as urea
    c. Elevated levels due to hepatic dysfunction may lead to encephalopathy
    d. Not a reliable indicator of hepatic coma
2. Value: 15 to 45 μg/dL
3. Nursing considerations
    a. Instruct the client to fast, except for water, and refrain from smoking for 8 to 10 hours
    b. Do not draw the specimen during hemodialysis
    c. Place the specimen in an ice-water bath
    d. Transport to the laboratory immediately

D. Amylase
1. Description
    a. Amylase is an enzyme produced by the pancreas and salivary glands that aids in the digestion of complex carbohydrates
    b. Amylase is excreted by the kidneys
    c. In acute pancreatitis, amylase starts rising at least 2 hours after the onset, peaks at about 24 hours, and returns to normal in 2 to 3 days after the onset
    d. Normal **serum** amylase may occur in pancreatitis, especially chronic pancreatitis
2. Value: 50 to 180 Somogyi U/dL in the adult, and 20 to 160 Somogyi U/dL in the older adult
3. Nursing considerations
    a. List medications that the client has taken 24 hours prior to the test on the laboratory form
    b. Identify medications that may cause false-positive or false-negative results
    c. Results are invalidated if the specimen was obtained less than 72 hours after cholecystography with radiopaque dyes

E. Bilirubin
1. Description
    a. Bilirubin is produced by the liver, spleen, and bone marrow and is also a by-product of hemoglobin breakdown
    b. Total bilirubin levels can be broken down into direct bilirubin, which is primarily excreted via the intestinal tract, and indirect bilirubin, which circulates primarily in the blood stream
    c. Total bilirubin levels rise with any type of

jaundice, whereas direct and indirect levels rise depending on the etiology of the jaundice

2. Values
   a. Bilirubin, direct: 0 to 0.3 mg/dL
   b. Bilirubin, indirect: 0.1 to 1.0 mg/dL
   c. Bilirubin, total: less than 1.5 mg/dL
3. Nursing considerations
   a. Do not draw the specimen during hemodialysis
   b. Instruct the client to eat a diet low in yellow foods such as carrots, yams, yellow beans, and pumpkin, 3 to 4 days before sampling
   c. Instruct the client to fast for 4 hours before sampling
   d. Note that results will be elevated with the use of alcohol, morphine, theophylline, ascorbic acid, and aspirin
   e. Note that results are invalidated if the client received a radioactive scan within 24 hours prior to the test

F. Cholesterol, total
   1. Description: Cholesterol is present in all body tissues and is a major component of low-density lipoproteins (LDL), brain and nerve cells, cell membranes, and some gallstones
   2. Value: 120 to 200 mg/dL
   3. Nursing considerations
      a. Instruct the client to fast from foods and fluid, except for water, for 12 to 14 hours and from alcohol for 24 hours prior to the test
      b. Instruct the client that the evening meal prior to the test should be free of high-cholesterol foods
      c. Cholesterol levels tend to decrease temporarily with major illness or surgery

G. Lipase
   1. Description
      a. Lipase is a pancreatic enzyme that changes fats and triglycerides into fatty acids and glycerol
      b. In acute pancreatitis, **serum** lipase begins to increase in 2 to 6 hours, peaks at 12 to 30 hours, and remains elevated, but slowly decreases, for 2 to 4 days
   2. Value: 31 to 186 U/L
   3. Nursing considerations
      a. Endoscopic retrograde cholangiopancrea-tography (ERCP) may increase lipase activity
      b. Traumatic **venipuncture** can inhibit lipase activity

II. Lipids, total
   1. Description
      a. Blood lipids consist of cholesterol, triglycerides, and phospholipids
      b. A lipid profile helps determine the risk factors in coronary artery disease
   2. Value: 400 to 800 mg/dL
   3. Nursing considerations

   a. Instruct the client to fast from food and fluids for 12 hours prior to the test
   b. Oral contraceptives may increase the levels of lipids in the **serum**

I. Triglycerides
   1. Description
      a. Triglycerides comprise a major part of very-low-density lipoproteins (VLDL) and a small part of low-density lipoproteins (LDL)
      b. Triglycerides are synthesized in the liver from fatty acids, protein, and glucose and are obtained from the diet
   2. Values
      a. Normal range: 10 to 190 mg/dL
      b. Borderline high: 200 to 400 mg/dL
      c. High: 400 to 1000 mg/dL
      d. Very high: greater than 1000 mg/dL
   3. Nursing considerations
      a. Instruct the client to fast for 12 hours prior to the test
      b. Instruct the client to avoid alcohol and refined carbohydrates for 3 days prior to the test

J. Protein
   1. Description
      a. Reflects the total amount of albumin and globulins in the **serum**
      b. Protein regulates osmotic pressure and is comprised of coagulation factors for hemostasis, enzymes, hormones, tissue growth and repair, and pH buffers
   2. Value: 6.0 to 8.0 g/dL
   3. Nursing considerations
      a. Do not draw blood during hemodialysis
      b. Do not draw in an extremity with an IV infusion
      c. Instruct client to avoid a high-fat diet for 8 hours prior to the test

K. Uric acid
   1. Description
      a. Uric acid is formed as the purines adenine and guanine, and it is continuously metabolized during the formation and degradation of DNA and RNA, and from the metabolism of dietary purines
      b. Elevated amounts deposit in joints and soft tissue and cause gout
      c. Conditions of fast cell turnover, as well as slowed renal excretion of uric acid, may cause uricemia
      d. Elevated amounts of urinary uric acid precipitate into urate stones in the kidneys
   2. Values
      a. Men: 4.5 to 8 ng/dL
      b. Women: 2.5 to 6.2 ng/dL
   3. Nursing considerations
      a. Instruct client to fast for 8 hours prior to the test
      b. Aminophylline, caffeine, and vitamin C may cause falsely elevated results

◆ **IV. Glucose Studies**

A. Fasting blood glucose (FBS)
   1. Description
      a. Glucose is a monosaccharide found in fruits and is formed from the digestion of carbohydrates and the conversion of glycogen by the liver
      b. Glucose is the body's main source of cellular energy and is essential for brain and erythrocyte function
      c. FBS levels are used to help diagnose diabetes mellitus and hypoglycemia (Table 10–2)
   2. Nursing considerations
      a. Instruct client to fast for 8 to 12 hours prior to the test
      b. Instruct a diabetic client to withhold morning insulin or oral hypoglycemic medication until after the blood is drawn

B. Glucose tolerance test (GTT)
   1. Description
      a. Aids in the diagnosis of diabetes mellitus
      b. If the glucose levels peak at higher than normal at 1 and 2 hours after injection or ingestion of glucose and are slower than normal to return to fasting levels, then diabetes mellitus is confirmed
   2. Nursing considerations
      a. Instruct the client to eat a high-carbohydrate (200 to 300 g) diet for 3 days before the test
      b. Instruct the client to avoid alcohol, coffee, and smoking for 36 hours before testing
      c. Instruct the client to fast for 10 to 16 hours prior to the test
      d. Instruct the client to avoid strenuous exercise for 8 hours before and after the test
      e. Instruct the diabetic client to withhold morning insulin or oral hypoglycemic medication
      f. Instruct the client that the test will take 3 to 5 hours and requires intravenous or oral administration of glucose and multiple blood samples

C. Glycosylated hemoglobin
   1. Description
      a. Glycosylated hemoglobin is blood glucose bound to hemoglobin
      b. HbA1c (a glycosylated hemoglobin A) is a reflection of how well blood glucose levels have been controlled for up to the prior 4 months
      c. Hyperglycemia in diabetics is usually a cause of an increase in HbA1c
   2. Values
      a. Values are expressed as a percentage of total hemoglobin
      b. Nondiabetic: 5.5% to 8.5%
      c. Diabetic with good control: 7.5% to 11.4%
      d. Diabetic with moderate control: 11.5% to 15%
      e. Diabetic with poor control: greater than 15%
   3. Nursing consideration: Fasting is not required

V. Renal Function Studies

A. **Serum** creatinine
   1. Description
      a. A very specific indicator of renal function, revealing the balance between creatinine formation and excretion
      b. Increased levels indicate a slowing of the glomerular filtration rate
   2. Value: 0.6 to 1.3 mg/dL
   3. Nursing considerations
      a. Do not draw blood during hemodialysis
      b. Instruct the client to avoid excessive exercise for 8 hours and avoid excessive red meat intake for 24 hours before the test

B. Blood urea nitrogen (BUN)
   1. Description
      a. Urea nitrogen is the nitrogen portion of urea, a substance formed in the liver through an enzymatic protein breakdown process
      b. Urea is normally freely filtered through the renal glomeruli, with a small amount reabsorbed in the tubules and the remainder excreted in the urine
      c. Elevated values may result from prerenal, renal, or postrenal causes
   2. Value: 5 to 20 mg/dL
   3. Nursing considerations
      a. Do not draw blood during hemodialysis
      b. Both creatinine levels and urea nitrogen levels should be analyzed when evaluating renal function

VI. Serum Enzymes

A. Creatine phosphokinase
   1. Description
      a. Creatine phosphokinase is an enzyme found in muscle and brain tissue and reflects tissue catabolism due to cell trauma
      b. The test is performed to detect myocardial or skeletal muscle damage or central nervous system damage

Table 10–2. Normal Adult Glucose Values

Glucose, fasting	70–105 mg/dL
Glucose monitoring (capillary blood)	60–110 mg/dL
Glucose tolerance test, oral	
Baseline fasting	70–105 mg/dL
30 minute fasting	110–170 mg/dL
60 minute fasting	120–170 mg/dL
90 minute fasting	100–140 mg/dL
120 minute fasting	70–120 mg/dL
Glucose, 2 hour postprandial	<140 mg/dL

c. Isoenzymes include CK-BB (brain), CK-MB (heart), and CK-MM (muscles)

d. CK-BB is found mainly in brain tissue, CK-MB is found mainly in cardiac muscle, and CK-MM is found mainly in skeletal muscle

2. Values

a. Creatine phosphokinase-MM: 5 to 70 U/L

b. Creatine phosphokinase-MB: 0 to 7 U/L

c. Creatine phosphokinase-BB: 0.3 U/L

3. Nursing considerations

a. If the test is to evaluate skeletal muscle, instruct the client to avoid strenuous physical activity for 24 hours prior to the test

b. Instruct the client to avoid ingestion of alcohol for 24 hours prior to the test

c. Invasive procedures and IM injections may falsely elevate CK levels

B. Lactate dehydrogenase (LD or LDH)

1. Description

a. The isoenzymes that are particularly affected with acute myocardial infarction are LDH_1 and LDH_2

b. This enzyme begins to elevate approximately 24 hours after myocardial infarction and peaks in 48 to 72 hours; thereafter, it returns to normal, usually within 7 to 14 days (Table 10–3)

c. The presence of an LD flip (when LD_1 is greater than LD_2) is helpful in diagnosing a myocardial infarction

2. Nursing considerations

a. LDH isoenzymes should be interpreted in view of the clinical findings

b. Testing should be repeated on 3 consecutive days

VII. Erythrocyte Studies

A. Erythrocyte sedimentation rate

1. Description

a. The rate at which erythrocytes settle out of anticoagulated blood in 1 hour

b. Not diagnostic of any particular disease but indicates that a disease process is ongoing

2. Value: 0 to 30 mm/hr depending on age

3. Nursing consideration: Fasting is not necessary, but a fatty meal may cause **plasma** alterations

B. Hemoglobin and hematocrit

1. Description

Table 10–3. Normal Adult Lactate Dehydrogenase

Lactate dehydrogenase	70–200 IU/L
Lactate dehydrogenase isoenzymes	
LDH_1	14%–26%
LDH_2	29%–39%
LDH_3	20%–26%
LDH_4	8%–16%
LDH_5	6%–16%

Table 10–4. Normal Adult Hemoglobin and Hematocrit Levels

Hemoglobin	
Male	14–16.5 g/dL
Female	12–15 g/dL
Hematocrit	
Male	42%–52%
Female	35%–47%

a. Hemoglobin is the main component of erythrocytes and serves as the vehicle for the transportation of oxygen and carbon dioxide

b. Hemoglobin determinations are important in determining anemia

c. Hematocrit determines red blood cell mass and is an important measurement in the determination of anemia or polycythemia (Table 10–4)

2. Nursing consideration: Fasting is not required

C. **Serum** iron

1. Description

a. Iron is mostly found in hemoglobin

b. Iron acts as a carrier of oxygen from the lungs to the tissues and indirectly aids in return of carbon dioxide to the lungs

c. Aids in diagnosing anemias and hemolytic disorders

2. Value

a. Male: 65 to 175 μg/dL

b. Female: 50 to 170 μg/dL

3. Nursing considerations

a. Do not draw blood during hemodialysis

b. The level will be increased if the client has ingested iron prior to the test

D. Red blood cell (RBC) count

1. Description

a. RBCs function in hemoglobin transport, which results in delivery of oxygen to the body tissues

b. RBCs are formed by red bone marrow, have a life span of 120 days, and are removed from the blood by the liver, spleen, and bone marrow

c. Aid in diagnosing anemias and blood dyscrasias

d. Evaluate the body's ability to produce red blood cells in sufficient numbers

2. Values

a. Women: 4 to 5.5 million/μL

b. Men: 4.5 to 6.2 million/μL

3. Nursing consideration: Do not draw blood during hemodialysis

VIII. Elements

A. Calcium

1. Description

a. A cation that is absorbed into the bloodstream from dietary sources and functions in bone formation, nerve impulse transmission, and contraction of myocardial and skeletal muscles

    b. Aids in blood clotting by converting prothrombin to thrombin

  2. Value: 8.6 to 10.2 mg/dL or 4.5 to 5.5 mEq/L

  3. Nursing considerations

    a. Do not draw blood during hemodialysis

    b. Instruct the client to eat a diet with normal calcium levels (800 mg/day) for 3 days before the test

    c. Instruct the client that fasting may be required for 8 hours prior to the test

B. Magnesium

  1. Description

    a. Used as an index to determine metabolic activity and renal function

    b. Magnesium is needed in the blood-clotting mechanism, regulates neuromuscular activity, acts as a cofactor that modifies the activity of many enzymes, and has an effect on the metabolism of calcium

  2. Value: 1.5 to 2.3 mEq/L or 1.8 to 2.6 mg/dL

  3. Nursing considerations

    a. Do not draw blood during hemodialysis

    b. Prolonged use of magnesium products will cause falsely increased levels, especially if renal damage is present

    c. Prolonged IV or total parenteral nutrition (TPN) therapy, blood transfusions, or prolonged nasogastric suctioning may cause falsely decreased results

C. Phosphorus

  1. Description

    a. Phosphorus is important in bone formation, energy storage and release, urinary acid base buffering, and carbohydrate metabolism

    b. High concentrations of phosphorus are stored in bone and skeletal muscle

    c. Phosphorus is absorbed from food and excreted by the kidneys

  2. Value: 2.5 to 4.5 mg/dL or 1.8 to 2.6 mEq/L

  3. Nursing considerations

    a. Do not draw blood during hemodialysis

    b. Instruct the client to fast prior to the test

IX. Thyroid Studies

A. Description

  1. Performed if a thyroid disorder is suspected

  2. Helpful to differentiate primary thyroid disease from secondary causes and from abnormalities in thyroxine-binding globulin levels

B. Values

  1. Thyroid-stimulating hormone (thyrotropin; TSH): 0.2 to 5.4 μU/mL

  2. Thyroxine (T_4): 5.0 to 12.0 μg/dL

  3. Thyroxine, free (FT_4): 0.8 to 2.4 ng/dL

  4. Triiodothyronine (T_3): 80 to 230 ng/dL

C. Nursing consideration: Test results are invalid if

the client had undergone a radionuclide scan within 7 days prior to the test

X. White Blood Cells

A. Description

  1. White blood cells function in the body's immune defense system

  2. The WBC count assesses each leukocyte distribution

B. Value: 4500 to 11,000/μL (Table 10–5)

C. Nursing considerations

  1. A "shift to the left" means there is an increased number of immature neutrophils in the peripheral blood

  2. A low total WBC count with a left shift indicates a recovery from bone marrow depression or an infection of such intensity that the demand for neutrophils in the tissue is greater than the capacity of the bone marrow to release them in the circulation

  3. A high total WBC count with a left shift indicates an increased release of neutrophils by the bone marrow in response to an overwhelming infection or inflammation

  4. A "shift to the right" means cells have more than the usual number of nuclear segments; found in liver disease, Down's syndrome, or megaloblastic and pernicious anemia

XI. Hepatitis Tests

A. Description

  1. Tests include radioimmunoassay (RIA) and enzyme-linked immunosorbent assay (ELISA)

  2. Serologic tests for specific hepatitis virus markers assist in defining the specific type of hepatitis

B. Values

  1. The presence of IgM antibody to hepatitis A virus (IgM anti-HAV) and the total antibody to hepatitis A virus (total anti-HAV) identify the disease

  2. Detection of core antigen (HB_cAg), envelope antigen (HB_eAg), and surface antigen (HB_sAg), or their corresponding antibodies, constitutes hepatitis B assessment

  3. Hepatitis C is confirmed by the presence of antibodies to hepatitis C (anti-HCV)

  4. Serologic hepatitis delta virus (HDV) determination is made by detection of the hepatitis D antigen (HDAg) early in the course

Table 10–5. Normal Adult White Blood Cell Differential

Neutrophils	56% or 1800–7800/μL
Bands	3% or 0–700/μL
Eosinophils	2.7% or 0–450/μL
Basophils	0.3% or 0–200/μL
Lymphocytes	34% or 1000–4800/μL
Monocytes	4% or 0–800/μL

Table 10–6. **Normal Adult Values: Urine Tests**

Name of Test	Value
Chloride	110–250 mEq/24 hr
Magnesium	7.3–12.2 mg/dL/day
Potassium	25–125 mEq/24 hr
Protein	40–150 mg/24 hr
Sodium	40–220 mEq/24 hr
Uric acid	250–750 mg/24 hr
pH	4.5–7.8
Specific gravity	1.016 and 1.022

of the infection and by detection of anti-HDV antibody in the later disease stages

5. Hepatitis E virus (HEV) is serologically distinct

C. Nursing consideration: If using RAI technique, the injection of radionuclides within 1 week prior to the test may falsely elevate results

▲ **XII. AIDS Testing**

A. Description
1. Detects human immunodeficiency virus (HIV), types 1 and 2 (HIV-1/2), that causes AIDS
2. Tests used to determine the presence of antibodies to HIV-1 include ELISA, Western blot (WB), and indirect fluorescent antibody (IFA)
3. A single reactive ELISA test by itself cannot be used to diagnose AIDS and should be repeated in duplicate with the same blood sample; if

Table 10–7. **Therapeutic Serum Medication Levels**

Medication	Therapeutic Range
▲ Acetaminophen (Tylenol)	10–20 µg/mL
Amikacin (Amikin)	25–30 µg/mL
Amitriptyline (Elavil)	120–150 ng/mL
▲ Carbamazepine (Tegretol)	5–12 µg/mL
Chloramphenicol (Chloromycetin)	10–20 µg/mL
Desipramine (Norpramin)	150–300 ng/mL
Digitoxin (Crystodigin)	15–25 ng/mL
▲ Digoxin (Lanoxin)	0.5–2.0 ng/mL
Disopyramide (Norpase)	2–5 µg/mL
Ethosuximide (Zarontin)	40–100 µg/mL
▲ Gentamicin (Garamycin)	5–10 µg/mL
Imipramine (Tofranil)	150–300 ng/mL
Lidocaine (Xylocaine)	1.5–5.0 µg/mL
▲ Lithium (Lithobid)	0.5–1.3 mEq/L
▲ Magnesium sulfate	4–7 mg/dL
Nortriptyline (Aventyl)	50–150 ng/mL
Phenobarbital (Luminal)	10–30 µg/mL
▲ Phenytoin (Dilantin)	10–20 µg/mL
Primidone (Mysoline)	5–20 µg/mL
Procainamide (Pronestyl)	4–10 µg/mL
Propranolol (Inderal)	50–100 ng/mL
Quinidine (Quinaglute, Cardioquin)	2–5 µg/mL
Salicylate	100–250 µg/mL
▲ Theophylline (Aminophylline, Theo-Dur)	10–20 µg/mL
Tobramycin (Nebcin)	5–10 µg/mL
Valproic acid (Depakene)	50–100 µg/mL

repeatedly reactive, follow-up tests using WB or IFA should be done
4. A positive WB or IFA is considered confirmatory for HIV
5. A positive ELISA that fails to be confirmed by WB or IFA should not be considered negative and repeat testing should take place in 3 to 6 months

B. Nursing considerations
1. Maintain issues of confidentiality surrounding HIV testing
2. Follow prescribed state regulations and protocols related to reporting positive test results

XIII. Urine Tests

A. See Table 10–6

XIV. Therapeutic Serum Medication Levels

A. See Table 10–7

PRACTICE QUESTIONS

1. The nurse is assigned to a 40-year-old client admitted with chronic pancreatitis. The nurse anticipates a serum amylase level that is most similar to which of the following values?
   1 50 Somogyi U/dL
   2 100 Somogyi U/dL
   3 300 Somogyi U/dL
   4 500 Somogyi U/dL

2. The adult client with hepatic encephalopathy has a serum ammonia level of 95 µg/dL and receives treatment with lactulose syrup. The nurse evaluates that the client had the best and most realistic response if the level changed to which of the following after medication administration?
   1 80 µg/dL
   2 40 µg/dL
   3 20 µg/dL
   4 5 µg/dL

3. The client who has fallen from a ladder and fractured three ribs has arterial blood gas results of pH, 7.38; PaCO$_2$, 38 mmHg; PaO$_2$, 86 mmHg; HCO$_3^-$, 23 mEq/L. The nurse interprets that the client's blood gases indicate which of the following?
   1 Normal results
   2 Metabolic alkalosis
   3 Metabolic acidosis
   4 Respiratory acidosis

4. The adult client has undergone lumbar puncture to obtain cerebrospinal fluid (CSF) for analysis. The nurse assesses for which of the following negative values if the CSF is normal?

1 Protein
2 Glucose
3 White blood cells
4 Red blood cells

5. The client is suspected of having myocardial infarction. The nurse assesses for elevations in which of the following isoenzyme values reported with the creatinine phosphokinase (CPK) level?
   1 MM
   2 MB
   3 BB
   4 MK

6. The adult male client has had laboratory work done as part of a routine physical examination. The nurse interprets that the client may have a mild degree of renal insufficiency if which of the following serum creatinine levels is found?
   1 0.6 mg/dL
   2 1.1 mg/dL
   3 1.9 mg/dL
   4 3.5 mg/dL

7. The client with a history of seizure disorder is compliant with medication therapy and is admitted with seizure activity. Phenytoin (Dilantin) is administered to the client by the IV push route, and subsequently a serum Dilantin level is drawn. The nurse evaluates that the medication therapy has been most effective if the laboratory result is:
   1 3 μg/mL
   2 8 μg/mL
   3 16 μg/mL
   4 24 μg/mL

8. The client who takes theophylline for chronic obstructive pulmonary disease (COPD) is seen in the urgent care center for respiratory distress. Just prior to initiating therapy, a baseline theophylline (aminophylline) level is drawn. Once the client is stabilized, the nurse begins discharge teaching. The nurse would be especially vigilant to include information about complying with medication therapy if the client's baseline result was:
   1 6 μg/mL
   2 11 μg/mL
   3 15 μg/mL
   4 18 μg/mL

9. The nurse checks the laboratory result for a serum digoxin level that was drawn on a client earlier in the day. The result is 2.4 ng/mL. Which of the following is the most important action on the part of the nurse?
   1 Record the normal value on the client's flowsheet
   2 Administer the next dose of the medication as scheduled
   3 Check the client's last pulse rate
   4 Notify the physician

10. The client is receiving a continuous IV infusion of heparin in the treatment of deep vein thrombosis. The client's activated partial thromboplastin time (aPTT) level is 65 seconds. The client's baseline before the initiation of therapy was 30 seconds. The nurse anticipates that which of the following actions is needed?
    1 Shut off the heparin drip
    2 Decrease the rate of the heparin drip
    3 Leave the rate of the heparin drip as is
    4 Increase the rate of the heparin drip

11. The client with atrial fibrillation who is receiving maintenance therapy of warfarin sodium (Coumadin) has a prothrombin time of 30 seconds. The nurse anticipates which of the following orders?
    1 Holding the next dose of warfarin
    2 Administering the next dose of warfarin
    3 Increasing the next dose of warfarin
    4 Adding a dose of heparin

12. The adult client who has had preadmission testing before surgery has had blood drawn for determination of serum electrolytes. The nurse would report which of the following abnormal values to the surgeon's office preoperatively?
    1 Sodium of 148 mEq/L
    2 Potassium of 3.8 mEq/L
    3 Chloride of 101 mEq/L
    4 Bicarbonate of 26 mEq/L

13. The adult client with a critically high potassium level has received sodium polystyrene sulfonate (Kayexalate). The nurse evaluates that the medication was most effective if the client's repeat serum potassium level is:
    1 6.2 mEq/L
    2 5.8 mEq/L
    3 5.4 mEq/L
    4 4.9 mEq/L

14. The client with a history of cardiac disease is due for a morning dose of furosemide (Lasix). The nurse would report which of the following serum potassium levels before administering the dose of furosemide?
    1 3.8 mEq/L
    2 3.2 mEq/L
    3 4.8 mEq/L
    4 4.2 mEq/L

15. The diabetic client has had a fasting blood glucose sample drawn. The nurse would report which of the following results as a critical value?
    1 150 mg/dL
    2 225 mg/dL
    3 290 mg/dL
    4 340 mg/dL

16. The adult client with a history of GI bleeding has a platelet count of 300,000 cells μL. Which of the following actions by the nurse is most appropriate upon reading this report?
    1 Report the abnormally low count
    2 Report the abnormally high count
    3 Place the client on bleeding precautions
    4 Place the normal report in the client's medical record

17. The adult client with hepatic cirrhosis has been taking a diet with optimal amounts of protein, since neither excess nor deficiency of protein has been helpful. The nurse evaluates the client's status as most satisfactory if the total protein level is which of the following values in the normal range?
    1 0.4 g/dL
    2 3.7 g/dL
    3 6.4 g/dL
    4 9.8 g/dL

18. The client is seen in the urgent care center for complaints of chest pain 4 days ago. Since that time, the client has not been feeling well and fatigues easily. The nurse would suspect myocardial infarction at the time of chest pain if which of the following isoenzymes for LDH came back positive?
    1 LDH_1
    2 LDH_3
    3 LDH_4
    4 LDH_5

19. The adult client was diagnosed with acute pancreatitis 9 days ago. The nurse interprets that the client is recovering from this episode if the serum lipase level drops to which of the following values, which is just beneath the upper limit of normal?
    1 20 IU/L
    2 80 IU/L
    3 175 IU/L
    4 350 IU/L

20. The client who suffered a crush injury to the leg has a highly positive urine myoglobin level. The nurse assesses this particular client carefully for signs of:
    1 Cerebrovascular accident
    2 Acute tubular necrosis
    3 Respiratory failure
    4 Myocardial infarction

21. The nurse has an order to test the stool of a client with Hemoccult slides. The nurse would question the order if the client were taking which of the following medications that could cause false-negative results?
    1 Ascorbic acid
    2 Colchicine
    3 Iodine
    4 Acetylsalicylic acid

22. The adult female client has a hemoglobin level of 10.8 g/dL. The nurse interprets that this result is most likely due to which of the following factors in the client's history?
    1 Chronic obstructive pulmonary disease (COPD)
    2 Heart failure
    3 Dehydration
    4 Iron deficiency anemia

23. The adult male client admitted with dehydration has received fluid volume replacement. The nurse evaluates that the client has had adequate fluid resuscitation if the client's repeat hematocrit level has decreased to which of the following values in the normal range?
    1 56%
    2 48%
    3 39%
    4 34%

24. The diabetic client has a glycosylated hemoglobin A_{1c} level of 8%. Based on this test result, the nurse plans to teach the client about the need to:
    1 Avoid infection
    2 Take in adequate fluids
    3 Prevent hyperglycemia
    4 Prevent hypoglycemia

25. The client has been diagnosed as having syndrome of inappropriate antidiuretic hormone (SIADH) secretion following cranial surgery. The nurse interprets that this complication is not resolving if which of the following urine specific gravity measurements is obtained?
    1 1.002
    2 1.016
    3 1.020
    4 1.030

26. The nurse is caring for the client who is immunosuppressed with a diagnosis of cancer. The nurse would consider implementing neutropenic precautions if the client's white blood cell (WBC) count were:
    1 2000/μL
    2 5800/μL
    3 8400/μL
    4 11,500/μL

27. The 22-year-old adult had a cholesterol level determined at a screening sponsored by a local health club. The nurse volunteering at the screening teaches the client that diet and exercise should be used as tools to keep the total cholesterol level under:
    1 150 mg/dL
    2 200 mg/dL
    3 250 mg/dL
    4 300 mg/dL

28. The 78-year-old client has been admitted for urinary tract infection and dehydration. The nurse evaluates that the client has received adequate volume replacement if the blood urea nitrogen (BUN) level drops to:
    1 35 mg/dL
    2 29 mg/dL
    3 15 mg/dL
    4 7 mg/dL

29. The client is at risk for developing disseminated intravascular coagulopathy (DIC). The nurse would become most concerned with which of the following fibrinogen levels?
    1 390 mg/dL

    2 290 mg/dL
    3 190 mg/dL
    4 90 mg/dL

30. The client in renal failure is hospitalized with pneumonia. Because the client's oxygen saturation levels are low, the physician orders arterial blood gases to be drawn. The client's results are pH, 7.32; $PaCO_2$, 44 mmHg; PaO_2, 78 mmHg; and HCO_3^-, 19 mEq/L. The nurse interprets these results to indicate:
    1 Respiratory acidosis
    2 Respiratory alkalosis
    3 Metabolic acidosis
    4 Metabolic alkalosis

ANSWERS

1. **3**

Rationale: The normal serum amylase level is 50 to 180 Somogyi U/dL in the adult, and 20 to 160 Somogyi U/dL in the older adult. With chronic cases of pancreatitis, the rise in serum amylase levels usually does not exceed three times the normal value. In acute pancreatitis, the value may exceed five times the normal value.

Test-Taking Strategy: Familiarity with the normal serum amylase level is needed to answer this question. Note the key word "chronic" in the question. It is also necessary to understand the effects of pancreatitis on this laboratory value. Review these effects now, if you had difficulty with this question!

Level of Cognitive Ability: Analysis
Phase of Nursing Process: Assessment
Client Needs: Physiological Integrity
Content Area: Adult Health/Gastrointestinal

Reference:
Chernecky, C., & Berger, B. (1997). *Laboratory tests and diagnostic procedures* (2nd ed.). Philadelphia: W..B. Saunders. pp. 186–187.

2. **2**

Rationale: The normal serum ammonia level is 15 to 45 μg/dL. In the client with hepatic encephalopathy, the serum level is not likely to drop below normal, nor is it likely to drop into the low-normal range. The most optimal yet realistic change would be to 40 μg/dL, which falls into the high-normal range. A level of 80 μg/dL represents insufficient effect of the medication.

Test-Taking Strategy: Familiarity with the normal serum ammonia level is needed to answer this question. It is also necessary to understand the association between hepatic encephalopathy and this laboratory value. Review this test briefly, and the desirable effects of this medication now, if you had difficulty with this question!

Level of Cognitive Ability: Analysis
Phase of Nursing Process: Evaluation
Client Needs: Physiological Integrity
Content Area: Adult Health/Gastrointestinal

Reference:
Chernecky, C., & Berger, B. (1997). *Laboratory tests and diagnostic procedures* (2nd ed.). Philadelphia: W. B. Saunders. p. 179.

3. **1**

Rationale: The client's results fall in the normal range for pH (7.35 to 7.45), $PaCO_2$ (35 to 45 mmHg), and bicarbonate level (22 to 26 mEq/L). With acidosis, the pH would be less than 7.35; with alkalosis, the pH would be greater than 7.45. Carbon dioxide levels would be high with respiratory acidosis, whereas bicarbonate levels would be low if there were metabolic acidosis.

Test-Taking Strategy: Specific knowledge related to arterial blood gas analysis is needed to answer this question correctly. If needed, review the essentials of this content area at this time!

Level of Cognitive Ability: Analysis
Phase of Nursing Process: Analysis
Client Needs: Physiological Integrity
Content Area: Adult Health/Respiratory

Reference:
Chernecky, C., & Berger, B. (1997). *Laboratory tests and diagnostic procedures* (2nd ed.). Philadelphia: W. B. Saunders. pp. 252–256.

4. **4**

Rationale: The adult with normal cerebrospinal fluid has no red blood cells in the CSF. The client may have small levels of white blood cells (0 to 3 per mm³). Protein (15 to 45 mg/dL) and glucose (40 to 80 mg/dL) are normally present in CSF.

Test-Taking Strategy: To answer this question accurately, it is necessary to understand which of the aforementioned components are present and absent in the cerebrospinal fluid. If needed, take a few moments to review the basics of this procedure and the normal results!

Level of Cognitive Ability: Analysis
Phase of Nursing Process: Assessment
Client Needs: Physiological Integrity
Content Area: Adult Health/Neurological

Reference:
Chernecky, C., & Berger, B. (1997). *Laboratory tests and diagnostic procedures* (2nd ed.). Philadelphia: W. B. Saunders. pp. 346–347.

5. **2**

Rationale: CPK is a cellular enzyme that can be fractionated into three isoenzymes. The MM band reflects CPK from skeletal muscle. The MB band reflects CPK from cardiac muscle. This is the level that elevates with myocardial infarction. The BB band reflects CPK from the brain. There is no MK band.

Test-Taking Strategy: To answer this question correctly, it is necessary to have specific knowledge of the isoenzymes that are produced with elevations in this enzyme. If needed, take a few moments now to review this important laboratory value for detecting myocardial infarction!

Level of Cognitive Ability: Analysis
Phase of Nursing Process: Assessment
Client Needs: Physiological Integrity
Content Area: Adult Health/Cardiovascular

Reference:
Chernecky, C., & Berger, B. (1997). *Laboratory tests and diagnostic procedures* (2nd ed.). Philadelphia: W. B. Saunders. pp. 324–326.

6. **3**

Rationale: The normal serum creatinine level for a man is 0.6 to 1.3 mg/dL. The normal value for women is 0.5 to 1.0 mg/dL. The client with a mild degree of renal insufficiency would have a slightly elevated level, which would be the value of 1.9 mg/dL. Creatinine levels of 3.5 mg/dL may be associated with acute or chronic renal failure.

Test-Taking Strategy: Note that the key word in this question is "mild." This tells you that the correct answer will be an abnormal value, but perhaps not the most abnormal of all the options. Use your knowledge of this common laboratory test to choose correctly. Review the normal value of this laboratory test now, if you had difficulty with this question!

Level of Cognitive Ability: Analysis
Phase of Nursing Process: Analysis
Client Needs: Physiological Integrity
Content Area: Adult Health/Renal

Reference:
Chernecky, C., & Berger, B. (1997). *Laboratory tests and diagnostic procedures* (2nd ed.). Philadelphia: W. B. Saunders. pp. 415–416.

7. **3**

Rationale: The therapeutic range for a serum phenytoin (Dilantin) level is 10 to 20 μg/mL. If the level is below the therapeutic range, the client may continue to experience seizure activity. If the level is too high, the client could experience phenytoin toxicity.

Test-Taking Strategy: To answer this question accurately, specific knowledge is needed about the normal range of results for this laboratory test. If needed, take a few moments to review and learn this material at this time!

Level of Cognitive Ability: Analysis
Phase of Nursing Process: Evaluation
Client Needs: Physiological Integrity
Content Area: Adult Health/Neurological

Reference:
Chernecky, C., & Berger, B. (1997). *Laboratory tests and diagnostic procedures* (2nd ed.). Philadelphia: W. B. Saunders. pp. 805–806.

8. **1**

Rationale: The therapeutic range for a serum theophylline (or aminophylline) level is 10 to 20 μg/mL. If the level is below the therapeutic range, the client may experience frequent exacerbations of the disorder. This client, in particular, needs reinforcement of the importance of continuing to take prescribed medications. If the level is within the therapeutic range, the client is most likely compliant with medication therapy. Compliant clients may also benefit from intermittent reinforcement of the importance of medication compliance.

Test-Taking Strategy: Note that the key words in this question are "especially vigilant." This implies that more than one option may be partially correct, but that one response is clearly better than the others. Familiarity with the therapeutic level of theophylline is needed to select the correct option. Review this therapeutic range now, if you had difficulty with this question!

Level of Cognitive Ability: Analysis
Phase of Nursing Process: Evaluation
Client Needs: Physiological Integrity
Content Area: Adult Health/Respiratory

Reference:
Hodgson, B., & Kizior, R. (1998). *Saunders nursing drug handbook 1998.* Philadelphia: W. B. Saunders. pp. 44–47.

9. **4**

Rationale: The normal therapeutic range for digoxin is 0.5 to 2.0 ng/mL. A value of 2.4 exceeds the therapeutic range, and it could be toxic to the client. The most important action is to notify the physician, who may give further orders about holding further doses of digoxin. Option 1 is incorrect because the value is not normal. The next dose should not be administered automatically. Checking the client's pulse is not incorrect but may have limited value. Depending on the time that has elapsed since the last assessment, it may be more useful to do a current assessment of the client's status.

Test-Taking Strategy: Note that the question contains the key words "most important." This implies that more than one or all of the options may be partially correct. To choose correctly, it is necessary to be familiar with the therapeutic range for this medication. If this question was difficult, take a few moments to review the information on this important and commonly used medication, and measurement of its therapeutic serum level!

Level of Cognitive Ability: Application
Phase of Nursing Process: Implementation
Client Needs: Physiological Integrity
Content Area: Adult Health/Cardiovascular

Reference:
Hodgson, B., & Kizior, R. (1998). *Saunders nursing drug handbook 1998.* Philadelphia: W. B. Saunders. pp. 324–326.

10. **3**

Rationale: The normal aPTT varies between 20 and 36 seconds, depending on the type of activator used in testing. The therapeutic dose of heparin for treatment of deep vein thrombosis is to keep the aPTT between 1.5 and 2.5 times normal. Thus, the client's aPTT is within the therapeutic range, and the dose should remain unchanged.

Test-Taking Strategy: To answer this question accurately, it is necessary to be familiar with both the normal aPTT level and the therapeutic level needed following institution of heparin therapy. If this question was difficult, review this important and frequently encountered content area now. You are likely to find a question related to this concept on NCLEX-RN!

Level of Cognitive Ability: Analysis
Phase of Nursing Process: Planning
Client Needs: Physiological Integrity
Content Area: Adult Health/Cardiovascular

Reference:
Chernecky, C., & Berger, B. (1997). *Laboratory tests and diagnostic procedures* (2nd ed.). Philadelphia: W. B. Saunders. p. 780.

11. **1**

Rationale: The normal PT is 9.6 to 11.8 seconds (adult male) and 9.5 to 11.3 seconds (adult female). A therapeutic PT level is 1.3 to 1.5 times greater than the client's control level. Since the value stated is extremely high (and perhaps near the critical range), the nurse should anticipate that the client would not receive further doses at this time. If the level were too high, then the antidote (vitamin K) could also be administered.

Test-Taking Strategy: To answer this question accurately, it is necessary to be familiar with both the normal PT level and the therapeutic level needed following institution of warfarin therapy. If this question was difficult, review this important and frequently encountered content area now. You are likely to find a question related to this concept on NCLEX-RN!

Level of Cognitive Ability: Analysis
Phase of Nursing Process: Planning
Client Needs: Physiological Integrity
Content Area: Adult Health/Cardiovascular

Reference:
Chernecky, C., & Berger, B. (1997). *Laboratory tests and diagnostic procedures* (2nd ed.). Philadelphia: W. B. Saunders. p. 847.

12. **1**

Rationale: The normal serum electrolyte ranges for adults is as follows: sodium, 136 to 145 mEq/L; potassium, 3.5 to 5.1 mEq/L; chloride, 98 to 107 mEq/L; bicarbonate (venous), 22 to 29 mEq/L. The only abnormal value identified is the serum sodium. The nurse reports any abnormal preoperative laboratory values to the surgeon's office.

Test-Taking Strategy: Familiarity with normal serum electrolyte values is needed to answer this question. If this question was difficult, take the time to memorize these common laboratory values now!

Level of Cognitive Ability: Analysis
Phase of Nursing Process: Implementation
Client Needs: Physiological Integrity
Content Area: Fundamental Skills

Reference:
Chernecky, C., & Berger, B. (1997). *Laboratory tests and diagnostic procedures* (2nd ed.). Philadelphia: W. B. Saunders. p. 470.

13. **4**

Rationale: The normal adult serum potassium level is 3.5 to 5.3 mEq/L. Option 4 is the only option reflecting a value that has dropped down into the normal range.

Test-Taking Strategy: Note the key phrase "critically high." You would expect that this medication is administered to lower the potassium level. Familiarity with normal serum potassium levels is needed to answer this question. If this question was difficult, take the time to memorize this common laboratory value now!

Level of Cognitive Ability: Analysis
Phase of Nursing Process: Evaluation
Client Needs: Physiological Integrity
Content Area: Fundamental Skills

Reference:
Chernecky, C., & Berger, B. (1997). *Laboratory tests and diagnostic procedures* (2nd ed.). Philadelphia: W. B. Saunders. p. 470.

14. **2**

Rationale: The normal adult serum potassium level is 3.5 to 5.3 mEq/L. Option 2 is the only value that falls below the therapeutic range. Administering furosemide to a client with a low potassium level and a cardiac history could precipitate ventricular dysrhythmias in the client.

Test-Taking Strategy: Familiarity with the normal serum potassium level is needed to answer this question. This will assist you in identifying the value that is not within normal range. If this question was difficult, take the time to memorize this common laboratory value now!

Level of Cognitive Ability: Application
Phase of Nursing Process: Implementation
Client Needs: Physiological Integrity
Content Area: Adult Health/Renal

Reference:
Chernecky, C., & Berger, B. (1997). *Laboratory tests and diagnostic procedures* (2nd ed.). Philadelphia: W. B. Saunders. p. 470.

15. **4**

Rationale: The normal fasting blood glucose is 70 to 105 mg/dL in the adult client. A critical level is considered to be one that exceeds 300 mg/dL. This makes option 4 the correct choice.

Test-Taking Strategy: Note the key phrase "critical value." This will assist in directing you to option 4. Familiarity with the normal fasting serum glucose level is needed to answer this question. If this question was difficult, take the time to memorize this common laboratory value now!

Level of Cognitive Ability: Application
Phase of Nursing Process: Implementation
Client Needs: Physiological Integrity
Content Area: Adult Health/Endocrine

Reference
Chernecky, C., & Berger, B. (1997). *Laboratory tests and diagnostic procedures* (2nd ed.). Philadelphia: W. B. Saunders. p. 565.

16. **4**

Rationale: A normal platelet count ranges from 150,000 to 400,000 cells/μL. The nurse should place the report containing the normal laboratory value in the client's medical record.

Test-Taking Strategy: Remember that options that are similar are not likely to be correct. With this in mind, eliminate options 1 and 3 first. To discriminate between the final two options, it is necessary to be familiar with the normal range for this laboratory test. Since this is a common hematological study, the normal range is worth memorizing!

Level of Cognitive Ability: Application
Phase of Nursing Process: Implementation
Client Needs: Physiological Integrity
Content Area: Adult Health/Gastrointestinal

Reference
Chernecky, C., & Berger, B. (1997). *Laboratory tests and diagnostic procedures* (2nd ed.). Philadelphia: W. B. Saunders. p. 815.

17. 3

Rationale: The normal range for total serum protein level in the adult client is 6.0 to 8.0 g/dL, making option 3 the correct choice. The client with cirrhosis often has low total protein levels from inadequate nutrition. Excess protein is not helpful, though, since a function of the liver is to metabolize protein. This may not be done well by the diseased liver.

Test-Taking Strategy: Familiarity with the normal total protein level is needed to answer this question. If needed, take a few moments to review this important laboratory range now!

Level of Cognitive Ability: Analysis
Phase of Nursing Process: Evaluation
Client Needs: Physiological Integrity
Content Area: Adult Health/Gastrointestinal

Reference
Chernecky, C., & Berger, B. (1997). *Laboratory tests and diagnostic procedures* (2nd ed.). Philadelphia: W. B. Saunders. p. 843.

18. 1

Rationale: The isoenzymes that are particularly affected with acute myocardial infarction are LDH_1 and LDH_2. LDH begins to elevate approximately 24 hours after myocardial infarction and peaks in 48 to 72 hours. Thereafter, it returns to normal, usually within 7 to 14 days.

Test-Taking Strategy: Familiarity with the cardiac isoenzymes for LDH is needed to answer this question. If needed, take a few moments to review this important laboratory data now!

Level of Cognitive Ability: Analysis
Phase of Nursing Process: Analysis
Client Needs: Physiological Integrity
Content Area: Adult Health/Cardiovascular

Reference
Luckmann, J. (1997). *Saunders manual of nursing care.* Philadelphia: W. B. Saunders. p. 1047.

19. 3

Rationale: The normal serum lipase level is 31 to 186 IU/L. The client who is recovering from acute pancreatitis usually has elevated lipase levels for approximately 10 days after onset of symptoms. This makes lipase a valuable test in monitoring the client's pancreatic function, since serum amylase levels usually return to normal 3 days after onset of symptoms. Option 3 is the only option that contains a value just under the peak of normal.

Test-Taking Strategy: Familiarity with the serum lipase level is needed to answer this question. If needed, take a few moments to review the range for this laboratory study now!

Level of Cognitive Ability: Analysis
Phase of Nursing Process: Evaluation
Client Needs: Physiological Integrity
Content Area: Adult Health/Gastrointestinal

Reference
Chernecky, C., & Berger, B. (1997). *Laboratory tests and diagnostic procedures* (2nd ed.). Philadelphia: W. B. Saunders. p. 674.

20. 2

Rationale: The normal urine myoglobin level is negative. After extensive muscle destruction or damage, myoglobin is released into the blood stream, where it is cleared from the body by the kidneys. When a large amount of myoglobin is being cleared from the body, there is risk of the renal tubules being clogged with myoglobin, causing acute tubular necrosis. This is one form of acute renal failure.

Test-Taking Strategy: Familiarity with this laboratory study is needed to answer this question. It is also necessary to understand the nature and consequences of crush injury. You might be able to deduce the correct option by noting that the question addresses a urine result. This will assist in directing you to option 2.

Level of Cognitive Ability: Application
Phase of Nursing Process: Assessment
Client Needs: Physiological Integrity
Content Area: Adult Health/Renal

Reference
Chernecky, C., & Berger, B. (1997). *Laboratory tests and diagnostic procedures* (2nd ed.). Philadelphia: W. B. Saunders. p. 745.

21. 1

Rationale: Ascorbic acid can interfere with the result of occult blood testing, causing false-negative findings. Colchicine and iodine can cause false-positive results. Acetylsalicylic acid would either have no effect on results or could cause a positive result, since aspirin is irritating to the stomach lining.

Test-Taking Strategy: Specific knowledge of interfering factors with occult blood testing is needed to answer this question accurately. If this question was difficult, a brief review of this test may be useful!

Level of Cognitive Ability: Application
Phase of Nursing Process: Implementation
Client Needs: Safe, Effective Care Environment
Content Area: Adult Health/Gastrointestinal

Reference
Jaffee, M., & McVan, B. (1997). *Davis's laboratory and diagnostic test handbook.* Philadelphia: F. A. Davis. p. 819.

22. 4

Rationale: The normal hemoglobin level for an adult female client is 12 to 15 g/dL. Iron deficiency anemia can result in lower hemoglobin levels. Heart failure and COPD may increase the hemoglobin level because of the need by the body for more oxygen-carrying capacity. Dehydration may increase the hemoglobin level by hemoconcentration.

Test-Taking Strategy: Evaluate each of the responses in terms of whether it is likely to raise or lower the hemoglobin level. The wording of the question tells you that there is clearly only one correct answer. Review the normal hemoglobin level now, if you had difficulty with this question!

Level of Cognitive Ability: Analysis
Phase of Nursing Process: Analysis
Client Needs: Physiological Integrity
Content Area: Fundamental Skills

Reference
Chernecky, C., & Berger, B. (1997). *Laboratory tests and diagnostic procedures* (2nd ed.). Philadelphia: W. B. Saunders. p. 593.

23. 2

Rationale: The normal hematocrit level for an adult male is 42% to 52%. The client who is dehydrated has an elevated level owing to hemoconcentration. The client's level may be expected to drift back down to within the normal range once fluid volume has been adequately restored. Thus, option 2 is the only correct choice. Option 1 is too high, while options 3 and 4 are low.

Test-Taking Strategy: Familiarity with this laboratory study is needed to answer this question. Since this is a very common laboratory study, it would be useful to have this one committed to memory!

Level of Cognitive Ability: Analysis
Phase of Nursing Process: Evaluation
Client Needs: Physiological Integrity
Content Area: Fundamental Skills

Reference
Chernecky, C., & Berger, B. (1997). *Laboratory tests and diagnostic procedures* (2nd ed.). Philadelphia: W. B. Saunders. p. 591.

24. **3**

Rationale: The normal level for glycosylated hemoglobin A_{1c} is 3.5% to 6.0%. This test measures the amount of glucose that has become permanently bound to the RBCs from circulating glucose. Elevations in blood glucose will cause elevations in the amount of glycosylation. Thus, the test is useful in detecting clients who have periods of hyperglycemia that are undetected in other ways. Elevations indicate continued need for teaching related to prevention of hyperglycemic episodes.

Test-Taking Strategy: Familiarity with this test and its significance is needed to answer this question accurately. Take a few moments to review this increasingly common test now if you have the need. You are likely to find a question related to this laboratory test on NCLEX-RN!

Level of Cognitive Ability: Application
Phase of Nursing Process: Planning
Client Needs: Health Promotion and Maintenance
Content Area: Adult Health/Endocrine

Reference
Chernecky, C., & Berger, B. (1997). *Laboratory tests and diagnostic procedures* (2nd ed.). Philadelphia: W. B. Saunders. p. 576.

25. **4**

Rationale: The possible urine specific gravity measurement ranges from 1.010 to 1.035, with the normal range being between 1.016 and 1.022. Elevations may occur with SIADH, because the kidneys are stimulated to reabsorb water, thus causing unusual concentration of the urine. Option 1 represents a low value, which may be seen with diabetes insipidus. Options 2 and 3 reflect normal values.

Test-Taking Strategy: Familiarity with this test and its significance is needed to answer this question accurately. Take a few moments to review this common urine measurement now if you have the need!

Level of Cognitive Ability: Analysis
Phase of Nursing Process: Evaluation
Client Needs: Physiological Integrity
Content Area: Adult Health/Neurological

Reference
Chernecky, C., & Berger, B. (1997). *Laboratory tests and diagnostic procedures* (2nd ed.). Philadelphia: W. B. Saunders. p. 921.

26. **1**

Rationale: The normal WBC count ranges from 4500 to 11,000/μL. The client who is immunosuppressed has a decrease in the number of circulating WBCs. The nurse implements neutropenic precautions when the client's values fall sufficiently under the low-normal level. The specific value for implementing neutropenic precautions is usually determined by agency policy.

Test-Taking Strategy: Familiarity with this test and its significance is needed to answer this question accurately. Take a few moments to review this common hematological test now if you have the need. You are likely to find a question related to this laboratory test on NCLEX-RN!

Level of Cognitive Ability: Application
Phase of Nursing Process: Planning
Client Needs: Safe, Effective Care Environment
Content Area: Adult Health/Oncology

Reference:
Chernecky, C., & Berger, B. (1997). *Laboratory tests and diagnostic procedures* (2nd ed.). Philadelphia: W. B. Saunders. p. 451.

27. **2**

Rationale: The client should be counseled to keep the total cholesterol level under 200 mg/dL. This will aid in prevention of atherosclerosis, which can lead to a number of cardiovascular disorders later in life.

Test-Taking Strategy: To answer this question accurately, it is necessary to be familiar with this specific laboratory value. Because of the importance of the health problems resulting from atherosclerosis, it would be a helpful value to have memorized!

Level of Cognitive Ability: Application
Phase of Nursing Process: Implementation
Client Needs: Health Promotion and Maintenance
Content Area: Adult Health/Cardiovascular

Reference:
Chernecky, C., & Berger, B. (1997). *Laboratory tests and diagnostic procedures* (2nd ed.). Philadelphia: W. B. Saunders. p. 364.

28. **3**

Rationale: The normal BUN for the older adult is 8 to 21 mg/dL. Thus option 3 is correct. Values such as those in options 1 and 2 reflect continued dehydration. Option 4 reflects a lower than normal value, which may occur with fluid overload, among other conditions.

Test-Taking Strategy: To answer this question accurately, it is necessary to be familiar with this specific laboratory value. Because it is such a common laboratory study, this one would be quite useful to have memorized!

Level of Cognitive Ability: Analysis
Phase of Nursing Process: Evaluation
Client Needs: Physiological Integrity
Content Area: Adult Health/Renal

Reference:
Chernecky, C., & Berger, B. (1997). *Laboratory tests and diagnostic procedures* (2nd ed.). Philadelphia: W. B. Saunders. p. 1003.

29. **4**

Rationale: The normal fibrinogen level is 180 to 340 mg/dL for men and 190 to 420 mg/dL for women. A critical value is one that is less than 100 mg/dL. With DIC, the fibrinogen level drops because fibrinogen is used up in the clotting process. For these reasons, the nurse would become most concerned with the level of 90 mg/dL.

Test-Taking Strategy: Note that the stem contains the key words "most concerned." This tells you that more than one or all of the options may be partially or totally correct. Knowing that DIC causes the value to fall, you would select the value that is the lowest. Review this normal value and manifestations that occur in DIC now, if you had difficulty with this question!

Level of Cognitive Ability: Analysis
Phase of Nursing Process: Assessment
Client Needs: Physiological Integrity
Content Area: Adult Health/Cardiovascular

Reference:
Jaffee, M., & McVan, B. (1997). *Davis's laboratory and diagnostic test handbook.* Philadelphia: F. A. Davis. p. 1369.

30. **3**

Rationale: The normal range for results of ABGs are pH, 7.35 to 7.45; $PaCO_2$, 35 to 45 mmHg; and bicarbonate level, 22 and 26 mEq/L. With acidosis, the pH is less than 7.35; with alkalosis, the pH is greater than 7.45. Carbon dioxide levels would be high with respiratory acidosis, whereas bicarbonate levels would be low if there were metabolic acidosis. Through the process of elimination, then, the client's results indicate metabolic acidosis, which is also compatible with the abnormality expected with renal failure.

Test-Taking Strategy: Specific knowledge related to arterial blood gas analysis is needed to answer this question correctly. If needed, review the essentials of this content area at this time!

Level of Cognitive Ability: Analysis
Phase of Nursing Process: Analysis
Client Needs: Physiological Integrity
Content Area: Adult Health/Renal

Reference:
Chernecky, C., & Berger, B. (1997). *Laboratory tests and diagnostic procedures* (2nd ed.). Philadelphia: W. B. Saunders. pp. 252–256.

BIBLIOGRAPHY

Black, J.M., & Matassarin-Jacobs, E. (1997). *Medical-surgical nursing: Clinical management for continuity of care* (5th ed.). Philadelphia: W. B. Saunders.

Chernecky, C., & Berger, B. (1997). *Laboratory tests and diagnostic procedures* (2nd ed.). Philadelphia: W. B. Saunders.

Hodgson, B., & Kizior, R. (1998). *Saunders nursing drug handbook 1998.* Philadelphia: W. B. Saunders.

Jaffee, M., & McVan, B. (1997). *Davis's laboratory and diagnostic test handbook.* Philadelphia: F. A. Davis.

Leahy, J., & Kizilay, P. (1998). *Foundations of nursing practice: A nursing process approach.* Philadelphia: W. B. Saunders.

Lehne, R. (1998). *Pharmacology for nursing care* (3rd ed.). Philadelphia: W. B. Saunders.

Luckmann, J. (1997). *Saunders manual of nursing care.* Philadelphia: W. B. Saunders.

Monahan, F., & Neighbors, M. (1998). *Medical-surgical nursing: Foundations for clinical practice* (2nd ed.). Philadelphia: W. B. Saunders.

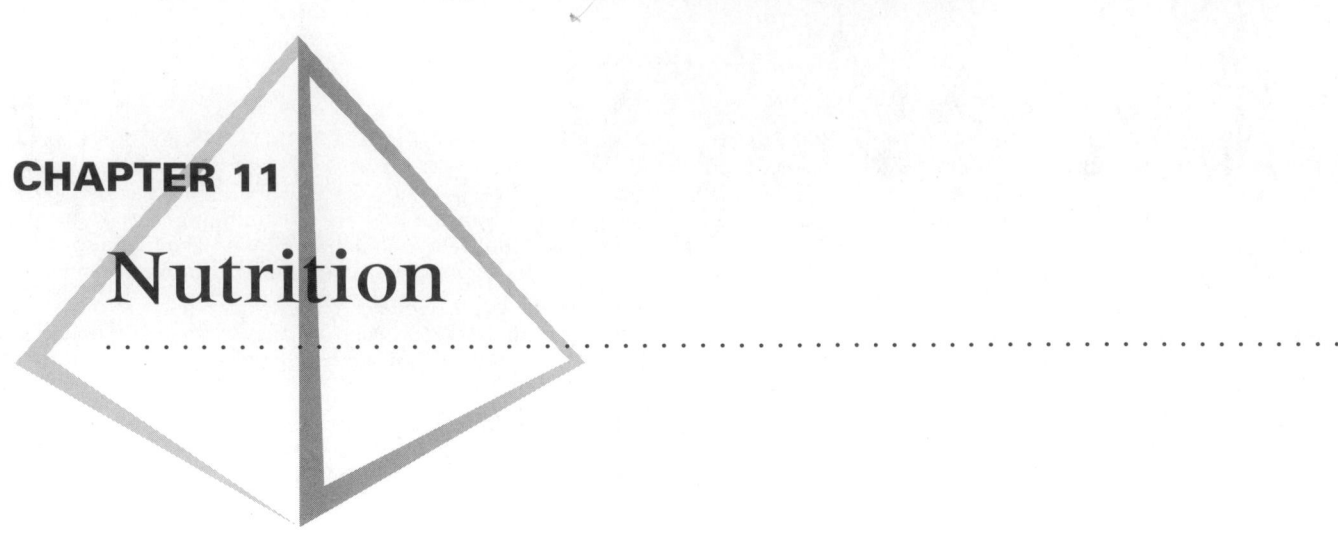

CHAPTER 11

Nutrition

PYRAMID TERMS

Absorption—Passage of digested nutrients through the wall of the stomach or small intestine into the blood or lymph system.

Anorexia—A lack of appetite with no desire to eat.

Digestion—The breakdown of carbohydrates, fats, and proteins into monosaccharides, fatty acids, and amino acids.

Enteral Nutrition—Administering nutrition with liquefied foods into the gastrointestinal (GI) tract via a tube.

Malnutrition—The deficiency of nutrients required to maintain development and maintenance of the human body.

Metabolism—Ongoing chemical process within the body that converts digested nutrients into energy for the functioning of the body cells.

Nutrients—Includes carbohydrates, fats/lipids, proteins, vitamins, minerals, and water and must be supplied in adequate amounts to provide energy, growth, development, and maintenance of the human body.

◆ PYRAMID TO SUCCESS

Nutrition is a basic need that must be met for all clients. Nurses must have the knowledge required to educate and care for healthy clients, as well as clients with nutritional needs or disorders requiring alterations in dietary measures. NCLEX-RN will address the dietary measures required for basic needs and for particular body system alterations. When presented with a question related to nutrition, consider the client diagnosis and the particular requirement or restriction necessary for treatment of the disorder. Pyramid points focus on the common types of therapeutic diets, nutrients contained in food items, and enteral feedings.

NURSING PROCESS

ASSESSMENT

Nutritional history
Age
Meal patterns
Food preferences
Sociocultural or religious considerations
Appetite
Nutritional intake
Height and weight
Elimination schedule
Laboratory data
Physical problems related to eating
Existing disorders

ANALYSIS: Altered Nutrition: Less Than Body Requirements
Altered Nutrition: More Than Body Requirements

PLANNING

Client maintains intake and output balance and consumes proper amounts of foods. Client complies with diet therapy. Client tolerates tube feeding.

IMPLEMENTATION

Perform nutritional assessment, including history, physical examination, and diagnostic data. Incorporate a diet considering nutritional needs, physiological disorders, and sociocultural and religious preferences. Monitor food and fluid intake. Instruct client in prescribed diet. Inform client of the purpose and importance of prescribed diet. Encourage client to select foods. Monitor tube feedings if prescribed and client's ability to tolerate feeding. Monitor laboratory values. Initiate dietary consult as necessary.

EVALUATION

Food and fluid intake and output are balanced. Client describes appropriate diet. Client independently selects own foods. Client tolerates tube feedings. Laboratory values are within normal limits.

◆ **CLIENT NEEDS**

SAFE, EFFECTIVE CARE ENVIRONMENT

Dietary consultation
Standard (universal) and other precautions
Asepsis

HEALTH PROMOTION AND MAINTENANCE

Lifestyle choices
Disease prevention
Health and wellness
Health promotion programs
Physical assessment
Dietary teaching

PSYCHOSOCIAL INTEGRITY

Religious and cultural influences on health
Lifestyle changes

PHYSIOLOGICAL INTEGRITY

Nutrition and oral hydration
Elimination
Enteral feedings
Laboratory values
Fluid and electrolyte imbalances
Alteration in body systems

I. Nutrients

A. Carbohydrates (Table 11–1)
1. The preferred source of energy
2. Includes sugars, starches, and cellulose, and provides 4 cal/g
3. Promotes normal fat **metabolism,** spares protein, and enhances lower GI function
4. Major food sources include milk, grains, fruits, and vegetables

5. Inadequate carbohydrate intake affects **metabolism**
B. Fats (Table 11–2)
1. Provide a concentrated source of energy and a stored form of energy
2. Spare protein, improve satiety and palatability
3. Protect internal organs and maintain body temperature
4. Enhance **absorption** of the fat-soluble vitamins
5. Provide 9 cal/g
6. Inadequate fat intake leads to clinical manifestations of sensitivity to cold, skin lesions, increased risk of infection, and amenorrhea in women
7. Diets high in fat can lead to obesity and increase the risk of cardiac disease and some cancers
C. Proteins (Box 11–1)
1. Made from amino acids, critical to all aspects of growth and development of body tissues, and provide 4 cal/g
2. Build and repair body tissues, regulate fluid balance, maintain acid-base balance, produce antibodies, provide energy, and produce enzymes and hormones

Table 11–1. Carbohydrate Food Sources

Glucose	Fructose	Cellulose	Lactose
Grapes	Honey	Bran	Milk
Oranges	Fruits	Apples	
Dates		Beans	
Corn		Cabbage	
Carrots			

Sucrose	Starch
Granulated table sugar	Wheat
Molasses	Corn
Apricots	Oats
Peaches	Rye
Plums	Barley
Honeydew and cantaloupe	Potatoes and pasta
Peas and corn	Beets, carrots, and peas

BOX 11–1. Protein Food Sources

Meats
Dairy products
Cereal products
Dried beans

Table 11–2. Fat Food Sources

Saturated Fats	Monounsaturated Fats
Beef	Duck and goose
Lunch meats	Eggs
Hard yellow cheeses	Olive and peanut oils
Butter	

Polyunsaturated Fats	Cholesterol
Safflower oil	Animal products
Corn oil	Egg yolks
Sunflower oil	Liver and organ meats

3. Essential amino acids (EAAs) are required in the diet because the body cannot manufacture them
4. High-quality proteins or complete proteins such as eggs, dairy products, meat, fish, and poultry contain adequate amounts of EAAs
5. Foods that do not contain EAAs in sufficient amounts are lower quality or incomplete proteins
6. Inadequate protein can cause protein energy **malnutrition** and severe wasting of fat and muscle tissue

D. Vitamins (Box 11–2)
1. Facilitate **metabolism** of proteins, fats, and carbohydrates; act as a catalyst for metabolic functions; promote life and growth processes; and maintain and regulate body functions
2. Fat-soluble vitamins A, D, E, and K can be stored in the body, so an excess can cause toxicity
3. The B vitamins and vitamin C are water

soluble, are not stored in the body, and can be excreted in the urine
4. Vitamin K acts as a catalyst for facilitating blood-clotting factors, especially prothrombin
5. Vitamin C produces collagen, a vital component in wound healing
6. Vitamin A maintains eyesight and epithelial linings

E. Minerals (Box 11–3)
1. Components of hormones, cells, tissues, and bones

BOX 11–2. Food Sources of Vitamins

WATER-SOLUBLE

Vitamin C (ascorbic acid): Citrus fruits, tomatoes, broccoli, cabbage
Vitamin B_1 (thiamine): Pork, nuts, whole grain cereals, legumes
Vitamin B_2 (riboflavin): Milk, lean meats, fish, grains
Niacin: Meats, poultry, fish, beans, peanuts, grains
Vitamin B_6 (pyridoxine): Yeast, corn, meat, poultry, fish
Vitamin B_{12} (cobalamin): Meat, liver
Folic acid: Green, leafy vegetables; liver, beef, and fish; legumes; grapefruit and oranges

FAT-SOLUBLE

Vitamin A: Liver, egg yolk, whole milk, green and orange vegetables, fruits
Vitamin D: Fortified milk, fish oils, cereals
Vitamin E: Vegetable oils; green, leafy vegetables; cereals; apricots, apples, and peaches
Vitamin K: Green, leafy vegetables; cauliflower, and cabbage

BOX 11–3. Food Sources of Minerals

CALCIUM

Milk and dairy products
Dark green, leafy vegetables
Sardines
Fortified orange juice

CHLORIDE

Salt

MAGNESIUM

Whole-grain products
Nuts and beans
Bananas
Green, leafy vegetables

PHOSPHORUS

Meat and dairy products
Meats
Whole grains
Legumes and nuts

POTASSIUM

Dried fruits
Baked potato
Cantaloupe
Bananas
Spinach
Milk
Steak
Beans

SODIUM

Canned foods
Cheeses
Ham, pork, sausages, lunch meats, frankfurters
Soy sauce
Salt

IRON

Liver, meats
Egg yolk
Dark-green vegetables
Breads and cereals

ZINC

Meats
Eggs
Leafy vegetables
Protein-rich foods

2. Act as catalysts for chemical reactions and enhancers of cell function
3. Almost all foods contain some form of minerals
4. A deficiency of minerals can occur in chronically ill or hospitalized clients

II. Food Guide Pyramid (Fig. 11–1)

A. Groups six broad families of foods with similar kinds of **nutrients** together
B. Levels of the pyramid
   1. Level one (base of the pyramid)
      a. Bread, cereal, rice, and pasta group
      b. Daily recommendation is 6 to 11 servings
   2. Level two
      a. Vegetables and fruit group
      b. Daily recommendation is 3 to 5 servings of vegetables and 2 to 4 servings of fruit
   3. Level three
      a. Includes the milk, yogurt, and cheese group and the meats, poultry, fish, dry beans and peas, eggs, and nuts group
      b. Daily recommendation is 2 to 3 servings for each group
      c. The recommendation for the milk group depends on the various life stages of the individual
   4. Peak of the pyramid
      a. Includes the fats and sweets group
      b. Foods are high in fats, sugar, or alcohol and are to be eaten sparingly because they are kilocalorie-dense, nutrient-sparse foods

III. Therapeutic Diets

A. Clear liquid diet
   1. Indications
      a. Serves a primary function of providing fluids and electrolytes to prevent dehydration
      b. Initial feeding after complete bowel rest
      c. Used to feed a malnourished person or a person who has not had any oral intake for some time
      d. Bowel preparation for surgery or tests
      e. Postsurgical diet
      f. Diarrhea
   2. Nursing considerations
      a. Clear liquid is deficient in energy and most **nutrients**
      b. The body digests and absorbs clear liquids easily
      c. Contributes to little or no residue in the GI tract
      d. Can be unappetizing and boring
      e. Client should not stay on a clear liquid diet for more than a day or two
      f. Consists of foods that are relatively transparent to light, are in liquid form at body temperature, and may be semisolid when cooled
      g. Foods include water, bouillon, clear broth, carbonated beverages, either regular or decaffeinated coffee, fruit drinks or strained fruit juices, gelatin, hard candy, honey, lemonade, popsicles, tea
      h. Client may have salt or sugar
      i. Dairy products are not allowed

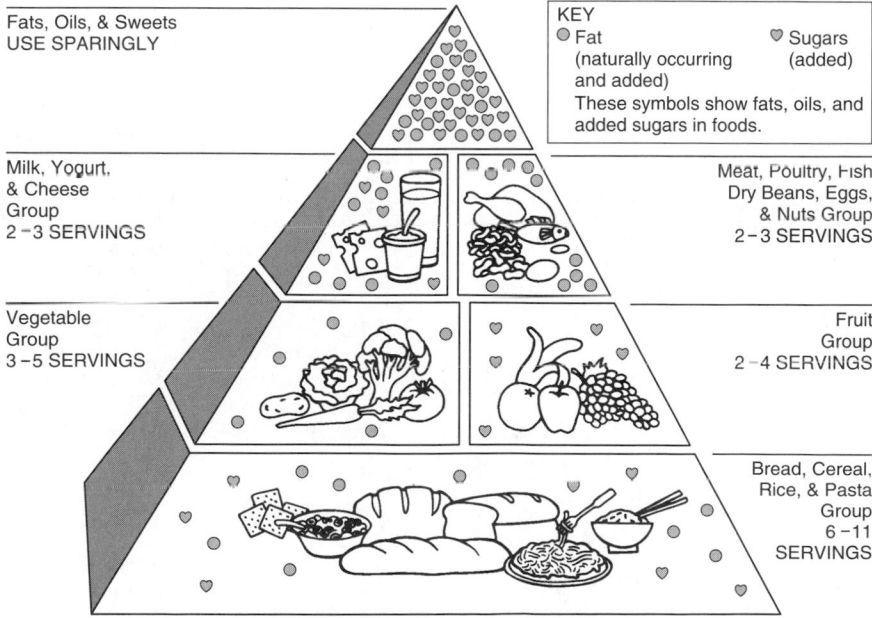

FIGURE 11–1. The food guide pyramid.

B. Full liquid diet
   1. Indication: May be used as a second diet after clear liquids following surgery, or for the client who is unable to chew or swallow
   2. Nursing considerations
      a. Nutritionally deficient in energy and most **nutrients**
      b. Includes both clear and opaque liquid foods and those that liquefy at body temperature
      c. Foods include all clear liquids, butter, margarine, cream, cooked and strained cereals, cream custard, soft cooked or scrambled eggs, plain ice cream, breakfast drinks, milk, mashed potatoes, pudding, sherbet, strained soups, strained vegetable and fruit juices
C. Soft diet
   1. Indications
      a. Used in clients with dental problems, clients with poor-fitting dentures, and clients who have difficulty chewing or swallowing
      b. Used for ulcerations of the mouth or gums, oral surgery, broken jaw, plastic surgery of head or neck, dysphagia, stroke, AIDS
      c. Therapeutic for clients with impaired **digestion** and/or **absorption** due to conditions such as ulcerative colitis and Crohn's disease
   2. Nursing considerations
      a. Clients with mouth sores should be served foods at cooler temperatures
      b. Clients who have difficulty in chewing and swallowing because of a reduced flow of saliva can increase salivary flow by sucking on sour candy or gum
      c. Encourage the client to eat a variety of foods
      d. Provide plenty of fluids with meals to ease chewing and swallowing of foods
      e. Sucking fluids through a straw may be easier than drinking them from cup or glass
      f. All foods and seasonings are permitted
      g. Liquid, chopped, puréed or regular foods with a soft consistency are best tolerated
      h. Avoid foods that contain nuts or seeds as these can become easily trapped in the mouth and cause discomfort
      i. Raw fruits and vegetables, fried foods, and whole grains are avoided
D. Bland diet
   1. Indication: Used for gastritis, ulcers, reflux esophagitis, congestive heart failure (CHF), myocardial infarction
   2. Nursing considerations
      a. Bland foods are less likely to form gas than are regular diets
      b. Eliminate foods that stimulate gastric acid secretions
      c. Eliminate foods that are irritating to the gastric mucosa

d. Foods to be avoided include alcohol; caffeine and caffeine-containing beverages such as cola, cocoa, coffee, and tea; fried foods; pepper and spicy foods
E. Low-residue/low-fiber diet
   1. Indications
      a. Supplies foods that are least likely to form an obstruction when the intestinal tract is narrowed by inflammation or scarring, or when GI motility is slowed
      b. Used for inflammatory bowel disease, ileostomy, colostomy, partial obstructions of the intestinal tract, enteritis, or diarrhea
   2. Nursing considerations
      a. Foods high in carbohydrate are usually low in residue and include white bread, cereals, pasta
      b. Foods to be avoided are raw fruits (except bananas), vegetables, seeds, plant fiber, and whole grains
      c. Dairy products are limited to two servings a day
F. High-fiber diet
   1. Indications
      a. Used in constipation
      b. Used in irritable bowel syndrome and when the primary symptom of irritable bowel syndrome is alternating constipation and diarrhea
      c. Helps regulate blood glucose in clients with diabetes mellitus
      d. Helps control blood cholesterol in clients with heart disease
   2. Nursing considerations
      a. Provides 20 to 25 grams of dietary fiber daily
      b. Adds volume and weight to the stool and speeds the movement of undigested materials through the intestine
      c. Consists of fruits and vegetables

BOX 11–4. Foods High in Fat

- Canned, cured, salted, or smoked meats
- Lunch meats
- Sausage, ham, bacon, and hot dogs
- Organ meats
- Caviar
- Whole milk
- Buttermilk
- Ice cream, half-and-half cream
- Eggnog, nondairy creamer, high-fat cheeses
- Fried foods
- Butter rolls, egg bread, bagels, biscuits, muffins, doughnuts, sweet rolls, pancakes, French toast, cheese and butter crackers, cereal containing coconut oil or nuts
- Potato chips, corn chips, other fried snacks
- Grains prepared with eggs, milk, cream, fat, or vegetable shortening
- Butter, lard, margarine, salad dressings, chocolates, palm oil, cashews, pistachios, macadamia nuts

G. Fat-controlled diet (Box 11–4)
   1. Indications
      a. Indicated for atherosclerosis, diabetes, hyperlipidemia, hypertension, myocardial infarct (MI), nephrotic syndrome, and renal failure
      b. Reduces the risk of heart disease
   2. Nursing consideration: Limit both the total amount of fats as well as amounts of polyunsaturated, monounsaturated, and saturated fats and cholesterol
H. High-calorie diet
   1. Indications: Severe stress, burns, cancer, human immunodeficiency virus (HIV) infection, chronic obstructive pulmonary disease (COPD), respiratory failure
   2. Nursing considerations
      a. High-calorie diets are also high-protein diets because the purpose of the diet is to build or maintain lean body mass
      b. Add fats to foods whenever possible
      c. Add nuts and dried fruits such as raisins to desserts or cereals
      d. Add sugar to food and eat high-calorie desserts
      e. Encourage snacks between meals, such as milkshakes and instant breakfasts
I. Sodium restriction diet (Box 11–5)
   1. Indications: Hypertension, CHF, kidney diseases, cardiac diseases, cirrhosis
   2. Nursing considerations (Box 11–6)

BOX 11–5. Foods High in Sodium

- Highly salted snacks
- Barbecue sauce
- Bouillon cubes
- Catsup
- Celery salt, seeds, or leaves
- Chili sauce
- Garlic salt
- Horseradish
- Meat extracts
- Sauces and tenderizers
- Monosodium glutamate
- Prepared mustard, olives, onion salt, pickles, relishes, saccharin, soy sauce, and other sauces
- Canned foods and commercial foods made with milk, ice cream, sherbet, artichokes, beets, carrots, cabbage, sauerkraut, and spinach
- Maraschino cherries; glazed fruit and dried fruits; grains; kidneys; canned, salted, or smoked meats
- Bacon, lunch meats, hot dogs, corned beef, kosher meats, shellfish, and codfish; regular cheeses; egg substitutes; peanut butter
- Salted butter or margarine, salt pork, commercial salad dressing, and salted nuts
- Baking powder and baking soda
- Pudding mixes
- Molasses
- Instant cocoa mixes
- Candy, cakes, cookies, sweetened gelatin mixes, pastry, puddings, and biscuit mix

---

BOX 11–6. Sodium-Free Spices and Flavorings

Allspice, almond extract, bay leaves, caraway seeds, cinnamon, curry powder, garlic powder or garlic, ginger, lemon extract, maple extract, marjoram, mustard powder, and nutmeg

---

      a. The amount of sodium allowed varies from 250 mg to about 4 g of sodium daily
      b. A no-added-salt diet includes no salt at the table and lightly salting foods during cooking
      c. Foods allowed on a sodium-restricted diet include dried or instant cereals, puffed wheat, puffed rice, and shredded wheat
J. Protein-restriction diet
   1. Indications: Acute renal failure, chronic renal disease, cirrhosis, and hepatic coma
   2. Nursing considerations
      a. Provides enough protein to maintain nutritional status but not enough to allow the build-up of waste products from protein **metabolism** (40 to 60 g of protein daily)
      b. The lower the amount of protein allowed, the more important it becomes that all protein included in the diet be of high quality
      c. An adequate total energy intake is critical for clients on protein-restricted diets because, without adequate energy, protein will be used for energy rather than in protein synthesis
      d. To boost energy intake, clients may use fats and concentrated sweets from margarine, creamed butter, hard candy, jelly, and sugar whenever possible
      e. Special low-protein products such as pastas, bread, cookies, wafers, and gelatin made with wheat starch can improve energy intake and add variety to the diet
      f. Carbohydrates in powdered or liquid forms can also provide additional energy
      g. Vegetables and fruits contain some protein, and for very low protein diets, these foods must be calculated into the diet
      h. Foods are limited from the milk, meat, bread, and starch exchange
K. High-protein diet
   1. Indications: Tissue building, burns, liver disease, and maternity clients
   2. Nursing considerations
      a. High-protein diets correct protein loss or assist with tissue repair by increasing the intake of protein food sources
      b. Increase foods such as meat, fish, fowl, and dairy products
      c. May need protein supplements
L. Low-calcium diet
   1. Indication: To prevent renal calculi (Table 11–3)

Table 11-3. Diets for Renal Calculi

Alkaline Ash Diet

To increase pH
Milk
Fruits except cranberries, plums, and prunes
Rhubarb
Vegetables
Small amounts of beef, halibut, veal, trout, and salami allowed

Acid Ash Diet

To decrease pH
Eggs
Meat
Cranberries, plums, prunes
Fish
Poultry
Oysters

2. Nursing considerations
   a. Decrease the total intake of calcium to prevent further stone formation
   b. Avoid whole grains, milk and dairy products, and green leafy vegetables
M. Low-purine diet
   1. Indication: Used to treat gout
   2. Nursing considerations
      a. Purine is a precursor for uric acid that forms stones and crystals
      b. Avoid glandular meats, gravies, and high meat quantities
N. High-iron diet
   1. Indication: Used in anemia
   2. Nursing considerations
      a. Replace iron deficit from inadequate intake or loss
      b. Include organ meats, meat, egg yolks, whole wheat products, leafy vegetables, dried fruit, legumes
O. Diet for diverticular disease
   1. Foods with seeds need to be avoided as they get trapped in the diverticula and cause irritation
   2. Foods to avoid include whole grain breads and cereals, fruits, vegetables, dried beans, peas, and nuts
   3. Gas-forming foods should be avoided in clients with irritable bowel syndrome (Box 11-7)
P. Fluid restriction (Box 11-8)
   1. Indications: Acute renal failure—oliguric phase, chronic renal disease, cirrhosis, CHF, hepatic coma, MI

BOX 11-7. Gas-Forming Foods

Apples, artichokes, barley, beans, bran, broccoli, Brussels sprouts, cabbage, celery, cherries, coconuts, eggplant, figs, honey, melons, milk, molasses, nuts, onions, radishes, soybeans, wheat, and yeast

BOX 11-8. Measures to Relieve Thirst

Chew gum or suck hard candy
Freeze fluids so they take longer to consume
Add lemon juice to water to make it more refreshing
Gargle with refrigerated mouthwash

2. Nursing considerations
   a. Usually this diet restricts those foods that are composed largely of water
   b. Restrict carbonated beverages, coffee, juices, milk, tea, water, frozen yogurt, gelatin, ice cream, ice milk, Popsicles, sherbet, soup, cream, liquid medications
Q. Carbohydrate-controlled diet
   1. Indications
      a. Helps maintain normal glucose levels in clients with disorders that cause blood glucose levels to rise or fall abnormally, such as diabetes or hypoglycemia
      b. Used for diabetes mellitus, hypoglycemia, lactose intolerance, galactosemia, dumping syndrome, obesity, and overweightness
   2. Nursing considerations
      a. Adjust energy intake from foods so as to provide specific amounts and types of carbohydrates
      b. The exchange list system is most frequently used to plan carbohydrate-controlled diets
R. Miscellaneous diets
   1. See Box 11-9 for foods high in potassium.
   2. See Box 11-10 for foods high in phosphorus.

IV. The Exchange System

A. Starches and breads
   1. One bread is equal to 15 g of carbohydrate, 3 g of protein, trace of fat, and 80 calories
   2. Equal to ¾ cup ready-to-eat cereal, ⅓ cup cooked beans, ½ cup corn
B. Meats
   1. One lean meat is equal to 7 g of protein, 3 g of fat, and 55 calories
   2. One meat exchange is equal to 1 ounce

BOX 11-9. High Potassium Foods

Vegetables, artichokes, asparagus, beets, broccoli, Brussels sprouts, cabbage, dried beans and peas, green beans, kale, mixed vegetables, parsnips, pinto beans, potatoes, pumpkins, spinach, squash, tomato juice, tomatoes, turnip greens, vegetable juice, winter squash, yams. Apricots, avocados, bananas, cantaloupes, dates, figs, grapefruit, honeydew melon, kiwi fruit, nectarines, orange juice, papayas, peaches, pears, pineapples, prune juice, prunes, raisins, rhubarb, strawberries, tangerines. Chocolate, cocoa, meat, milk, molasses, peanuts, walnuts, wheat germ

3. One ounce of lean meat is equal to 1 ounce of chicken meat without skin, 1 ounce of any fish, ¼ cup of canned tuna, 1 ounce low-fat cheese
4. Medium-fat meats
   a. One medium-fat meat is equal to 7 g of protein, 5 g of fat, and about 75 calories
   b. One ounce of medium-fat meat is equal to 1 ounce of lean meat in protein content but has 5 g of fat
   c. Equal to 1 ounce of pork loin, 1 egg, ¼ cup of creamed cottage cheese
5. High-fat meats
   a. One high-fat meat is equal to 7 g of protein, 8 g of fat, and 100 calories
   b. A hotdog counts as 1 high-fat meat exchange plus 1 fat exchange
   c. One ounce of high-fat meat is equal to 1 ounce of lean meat in protein content but includes an extra 1 fat
   d. Equal to 1 ounce of ham, 1 ounce of cheddar cheese, 1 small hotdog
   e. Peanut butter is like a meat in terms of its protein content
   f. One tablespoon of peanut butter is equal to 1 high-fat meat
   g. One tablespoon of peanut butter is equal to 7 g of protein, 8 g of fat, and 100 calories
C. Vegetables
   1. One vegetable is equal to 5 g of carbohydrate, 2 g of protein, and 25 calories
   2. One half cup of carrots is equal to ½ cup of greens, ½ cup of Brussels sprouts, ½ cup of beets
D. Fruits
   1. One fruit is equal to 15 g of carbohydrate and 60 calories
   2. One-half banana is equal to 1 small apple, ½ grapefruit, ½ cup orange juice
E. Milks
   1. One milk is equal to 12 g of carbohydrate, 8 g of protein, trace of fat, and 90 calories
   2. One cup of nonfat milk is equal to 1 cup of nonfat plain yogurt, 1 cup of nonfat buttermilk, or ½ cup evaporated nonfat milk
F. Fats
   1. One fat is equal to 5 g fat and 45 calories
   2. One teaspoon (tsp) of butter is equal to 1 tsp of margarine, 1 tsp of any oils, 1 tablespoon of salad dressing, 1 strip of bacon, 5 large olives, 10 whole peanuts
G. Legumes

BOX 11–10. High Phosphorus Foods

Canned fish, cocoa, chocolate, dried beans and peas, dried fruits, game meats, milk and milk products, nuts, organ meats, peanut butter, whole grains, breads and cereals

---

1. Similar to meats, are rich in protein and iron and are lower in fat than meat
2. Contain starch
3. One cup of legumes is equal to 1 lean meat plus 2 starches
4. One cup of legumes is equal to 30 g of carbohydrates, 13 g of protein, 3 g of fat, and 215 calories

V. Enteral Nutrition

A. Description: Provides liquefied foods into the GI tract via a tube
B. Indications
   1. When the GI tract is functional but oral intake is not feasible
   2. Used for clients with swallowing problems, burns, major trauma, liver failure, or severe **malnutrition**
C. Tubes
   1. Nose to stomach (nasogastric)
   2. Nose to duodenum or jejunum (nasoduodenal/nasojejunal)
   3. Stomach (gastrostomy)
   4. Jejunum (jejunostomy)
D. Administration
   1. Bolus
      a. Resembles normal meal feeding patterns
      b. Approximately 300 to 400 mL of formula is administered over a 30- to 60-minute period every 3 to 6 hours
   2. Continuous
      a. Administered continually for 24 hours
      b. An infusion pump regulates the flow
   3. Cyclical
      a. Administered either in the daytime or nighttime for 8 to 16 hours
      b. An infusion pump regulates the flow
      c. Feedings at night allow for more freedom during the day
E. Administering enteral feedings
   1. Position client in high Fowler's on right side if comatose
   2. Warm feeding to room temperature to prevent diarrhea and cramps
   3. Aspirate all stomach contents (residual), measure the amount, and return the contents to the stomach to prevent electrolyte imbalances
   4. Usually, if the residual is less than 100 to 150 mL, the feeding is administered; if greater than 150 mL, hold the feeding
   5. Assess tube placement by aspirating the gastric contents and measuring the pH (should be 4 or less)
   6. Note that the best method to check placement is by x-ray
   7. Assess bowel sounds; hold the feeding and notify the physician if the bowel sounds are absent
   8. Use a feeding pump for continuous or cyclic feedings

9. Flush tubing with water following feeding to maintain fluid balance and patency of tube
10. For bolus feeding, leave the client in a high Fowler's position for 30 minutes after feeding
11. For a continuous feeding, keep client in a 30-degree Fowler position at all times

F. Prevention of complications
   1. Diarrhea
      a. Use fiber-containing feedings
      b. Administer feeding slowly and at room temperature
   2. Aspiration
      a. Verify tube placement
      b. Do not administer feeding if the residual is greater than 150 mL
      c. Keep head of bed elevated
      d. If aspiration occurs, suction as needed, monitor temperature for aspiration pneumonia, auscultate lung sounds and assess the respiratory rate, and prepare to obtain a chest radiograph
   3. Clogged tube
      a. Use liquid forms of medication, if possible
      b. Flush the tube with water before and after medication administration
      c. Flush the tube with 20 to 50 mL of water before and after bolus feeding
      d. Flush with water every 4 hours for continuous feeding
   4. Vomiting
      a. Administer feedings slowly, and for bolus feedings, make the feeding last for 30 minutes
      b. Measure abdominal girth
      c. Do not allow feeding to run dry
      d. Do not allow air to enter the tubing
      e. Administer feeding at room temperature
      f. Elevate the head of the bed
      g. Administer antiemetics as prescribed
      h. If the client vomits, place in side-lying position

PRACTICE QUESTIONS

1. An alkaline ash diet is prescribed for the client with renal calculi. Which of the following diet menus would be selected for this type of diet?
   1 A spinach salad, milk, and a banana
   2 Pasta with shrimp, tossed salad, and a plum
   3 Turkey, rice, and cranberries
   4 Peanut butter sandwich, salad, and prunes

2. A low sodium diet has been prescribed for the client with hypertension. Following diet teaching, which of the following foods, if selected from the menu by the client, would best indicate an understanding of this diet?
   1 Tomato soup
   2 Baked turkey
   3 Chicken gumbo soup
   4 Boiled shrimp

3. The home health nurse is providing dietary instructions to a client with gout. Which of the following foods would the nurse instruct the client to avoid?
   1 Macaroni products
   2 Cornbread
   3 Scallops
   4 Chocolate

4. A clear liquid diet has been prescribed for the client with gastroenteritis. Which of the following nutritional items would be most appropriate to offer to the client?
   1 Orange juice
   2 Strained soup
   3 Fat-free broth
   4 Soft custard

5. Spironolactone (Aldactone), a diuretic, is prescribed for the client with CHF. Which of the following foods would the nurse instruct the client to avoid?
   1 Bananas
   2 Cranberry juice
   3 Plum
   4 Cheddar cheese

6. The diabetic client has been instructed in the dietary exchange system. The client asks the nurse if bacon is allowed in the diet. Which of the following responses is most appropriate?
   1 "Bacon is much too high in fat."
   2 "Bacon is not allowed."
   3 "One strip of bacon may be eaten if you eliminate one teaspoon of butter."
   4 "Bacon may be eaten if you eliminate one meat item from your diet."

7. The client has been diagnosed with ulcerative colitis. Which of the following diets would the nurse anticipate would be prescribed for the client?
   1 High-residue
   2 Low-residue
   3 High-carbohydrate
   4 Low-fat

8. The client with heart disease is instructed regarding a low-fat diet. The nurse evaluates that the client understands the diet if the client states a food item to avoid is:
   1 Apples
   2 Oranges
   3 Avocado
   4 Cherries

9. The clinic nurse instructs a client to increase the content of riboflavin in the diet. Which of the following food items is especially high in riboflavin?
   1 Milk
   2 Liver

3 Chicken

4 Eggs

10. The substance abuse clinic nurse is providing dietary instructions to clients. A client asks the nurse about the foods that are high in thiamine. Which food is especially rich in this vitamin?
    1 Chicken
    2 Broccoli
    3 Pork
    4 Milk

11. The nurse caring for a client with a neurological disorder is planning care to maintain nutritional status. The nurse is concerned about the client's swallowing ability. Which of the following food items would be avoided in this client's diet?
    1 Cheese casserole
    2 Scrambled eggs
    3 Mashed potatoes
    4 Spinach

12. The nurse is planning a diet for the client with acute renal failure. Which of the following dietary components would be restricted in this client's diet?
    1 Carbohydrates
    2 Fats
    3 Vitamins
    4 Potassium

13. The nurse is preparing a diet plan for the postgastrectomy client with dumping syndrome. Which of the following would not be a component of this teaching plan?
    1 Lie down after eating
    2 Drink liquids with meals
    3 Eat small meals six times daily
    4 Avoid concentrated sweets

14. The nurse is preparing a diet plan for the client who is taking warfarin (Coumadin) daily. Which of the following foods will the nurse instruct the client to exclude from the diet?
    1 Pasta
    2 Broccoli
    3 Oranges
    4 Potatoes

15. A client has been diagnosed with pernicious anemia. In planning care for the client, the nurse anticipates that the client will be treated with:
    1 Thiamine
    2 Iron
    3 Vitamin B$_{12}$
    4 Folic acid

16. An elderly postoperative client has been tolerating a full liquid diet and the nurse plans to advance the diet to solid food as prescribed. Which assessment is most important for the nurse to make prior to advancing the diet to solids?

1 Food preferences

2 Cultural preferences

3 Presence of bowel sounds

4 Ability to chew

17. A burned client is transferred to the nursing unit, and a regular diet has been prescribed. Which dietary items should the nurse encourage the client to eat in order to promote wound healing?
    1 Veal, potatoes, Jell-O, orange juice
    2 Peanut butter and jelly sandwich, cantaloupe, tea
    3 Chicken breast, broccoli, strawberries, milk
    4 Spaghetti with tomato sauce, garlic bread, ginger ale

18. The nurse is caring for a postoperative client. The physician has prescribed a clear liquid diet. In planning to initiate this diet, which of the following would the nurse place at the bedside?
    1 Code cart
    2 A straw
    3 Cardiac monitor
    4 Suction equipment

19. When assisting a client to eat who has had a cerebrovascular accident (CVA), the nurse can best promote independence by which of these actions?
    1 Offer only puréed foods
    2 Sit the client in high Fowler's position
    3 Place the food tray on the unaffected side
    4 Encourage the client to eat with other clients who have had CVAs

20. The nurse has completed diet teaching for a client on a low-sodium diet for hypertension. The nurse evaluates that further teaching is necessary when the client makes which of these statements?
    1 "This diet will help lower my blood pressure."
    2 "The reason I need lower salt intake is to reduce fluid retention."
    3 "This diet is not a replacement for my antihypertensive medications."
    4 "Frozen foods are lowest in sodium."

21. The nurse conducting a weight loss program prepares to monitor a client's weight loss. What method would most accurately assess the effectiveness of weight loss?
    1 Daily weights
    2 Serum protein levels
    3 Calorie counts
    4 Daily intake and output

22. The clinic nurse is monitoring a client with anorexia nervosa. Which statement, if made by a client, would indicate to the nurse that treatment has been effective?
    1 "I no longer have a weight problem."
    2 "I don't want to starve myself anymore."
    3 "I'll eat until I don't feel hungry."
    4 "My friends and I went out to lunch today."

23. The clinic nurse is instructing a pregnant client about nutrition. Which of the following would the nurse include in this client's teaching plan?
    1 The nutritional status of the mother significantly influences fetal growth and development
    2 All mothers are at high risk for nutritional deficiencies
    3 Calcium is not important until the third trimester
    4 Iron supplements are not necessary unless the mother has iron deficiency anemia

24. A client with lung cancer receiving chemotherapy tells the nurse that the food on the meal tray tastes "funny." Which of the following is the most appropriate nursing intervention?
    1 Keep the client NPO
    2 Administer an antiemetic as prescribed
    3 Provide oral hygiene care frequently
    4 Consult with the physician regarding an order for total parenteral nutrition (TPN)

25. A client is on a diet designed to avoid concentrated sugars. The nurse evaluates that the client understands the diet plan if which of these diets is selected by the client?
    1 Strawberry yogurt, lettuce salad, coffee
    2 Chicken salad, tomato, Jell-O, instant iced tea
    3 Peanut butter and jelly sandwich, sherbet, cola
    4 Tuna sandwich, lettuce salad, watermelon, herbal tea

26. A client who has a gastrostomy tube for feeding refuses to participate in the plan of care, will not make eye contact, and does not speak to the family or visitors. The nurse assesses that this client is using which type of coping mechanism?
    1 Self-control
    2 Problem-solving
    3 Accepting responsibility
    4 Distancing

27. A client receiving enteral feedings develops abdominal distension and diarrhea shortly after initiation of the feedings. When reviewing the nursing history for this client, which of these notations warrants the nurse calling the physician?
    1 Prior history of enteral feedings
    2 Difficulty in swallowing
    3 History of hemorrhoids
    4 Lactose intolerance since childhood

28. The nurse is formulating a plan of care for a client receiving enteral feedings. Which nursing diagnosis is of highest priority for this client?
    1 Altered nutrition, less than body requirements
    2 High risk for aspiration
    3 High risk for fluid volume deficit
    4 Diarrhea

29. The nurse is preparing to administer a feeding to the client receiving enteral nutrition through a nasogastric tube. What is the priority nursing action?
    1 Measuring intake and output
    2 Weighing the client
    3 Adding blue food coloring to the formula to aid in diagnosing aspiration
    4 Determining tube placement

30. The nurse has completed discharge teaching with the family of a client who is to have enteral feedings at home. Which method of evaluation should the nurse use to best determine the family's competence in performing the feeding procedure?
    1 Return demonstration of the feeding procedure
    2 Selection of appropriate equipment for the feeding procedure
    3 Written testing on the steps of the feeding procedure
    4 Verbal description of the feeding procedure by each member of the family

ANSWERS

1. **1**

Rationale: In an alkaline ash diet, all fruits are allowed except cranberries, prunes, and plums. Options 2, 3, and 4 represent an acid ash diet.

Test-Taking Strategy: Knowledge regarding the foods included and restricted in an alkaline ash diet is required to eliminate the incorrect options. Remembering that cranberries, prunes, and plums are not allowed in an alkaline ash diet will direct you to the correct option. Review the foods allowed in this diet now, if you had difficulty with this question!

Level of Cognitive Ability: Analysis
Phase of Nursing Process: Implementation
Client Needs: Physiological Integrity
Content Area: Adult Health/Renal

Reference
Mahan, L., & Escott-Stump, S. (1996). *Krause's food, nutrition, & diet therapy* (9th ed.). Philadelphia: W. B. Saunders. p. 780.

2. **2**

Rationale: Regular soup (1 cup) contains 900 mg Na. Fresh shellfish (1 oz) contains 50 mg Na. Poultry (1 oz) contains 25 mg Na.

Test-Taking Strategy: Eliminate options 1 and 3 first because they are similar. Also recall that canned foods are high in sodium. From the remaining two options, select option 2 over option 4, remembering that shellfish is also high in sodium. Review foods high in sodium now, if you had difficulty with this question!

Level of Cognitive Ability: Analysis
Phase of Nursing Process: Evaluation
Client Needs: Health Promotion and Maintenance
Content Area: Adult Health/Cardiovascular

Reference
Mahan, L., & Escott-Stump, S. (1996). *Krause's food, nutrition, & diet therapy* (9th ed.). Philadelphia: W. B. Saunders. p. 744.

3. 3

Rationale: Scallops should be omitted from the diet of a client who has gout because of the high purine content. The food items identified in options 1, 2, and 4 contain a negligible purine content and may be consumed daily by the client with gout.

Test-Taking Strategy: Knowledge regarding high-purine foods is required to answer this question. Review foods high in purine now, if you had difficulty with this question!

Level of Cognitive Ability: Application
Phase of Nursing Process: Implementation
Client Needs: Health Promotion and Maintenance
Content Area: Adult Health/Musculoskeletal

Reference
Mahan, L., & Escott-Stump, S. (1996). *Krause's food, nutrition, & diet therapy* (9th ed.). Philadelphia: W. B. Saunders. p. 895.

4. 3

Rationale: A clear liquid diet consists of foods that are relatively transparent. The food items in options 1, 2, and 4 would be included in a full liquid diet.

Test-Taking Strategy: Remember that a clear liquid diet consists of foods that are relatively transparent. By the process of elimination, you should easily select option 3 because this is the only food item that is transparent. Review food items allowed on a clear liquid and full liquid diet now, if you had difficulty with this question!

Level of Cognitive Ability: Application
Phase of Nursing Process: Implementation
Client Needs: Physiological Integrity
Content Area: Adult Health/Gastrointestinal

Reference
Luckmann, J. (1997). *Saunders manual of nursing care.* Philadelphia: W. B. Saunders. p. 311.

5. 1

Rationale: Aldactone is a potassium (K)-sparing diuretic, and the client should avoid foods high in potassium. A banana contains 451 mg of K. Cranberry juice (1 cup) contains 61 mg of K. A plum contains 48 mg of K, and 1 oz of cheddar cheese contains 28 mg of K.

Test-Taking Strategy: Knowledge that Aldactone is a potassium-sparing diuretic will easily direct you to option 1. If you had difficulty with this question, review this medication and foods high in K now!

Level of Cognitive Ability: Application
Phase of Nursing Process: Implementation
Client Needs: Physiological Integrity
Content Area: Adult Health/Cardiovascular

References
Mahan, L., & Escott-Stump, S. (1996). *Krause's food, nutrition, & diet therapy* (9th ed.). Philadelphia: W. B. Saunders. p. 1016.
Hodgson, B., & Kizior, R. (1998). *Saunders nursing drug handbook 1998.* Philadelphia: W. B. Saunders. pp. 942–944.

6. 3

Rationale: Bacon is a component of the fat group in the exchange system. One tsp of butter is equal to 1 tsp of margarine, 1 tsp of any oil, 1 tablespoon of salad dressing, 1 strip of bacon, 5 large olives, or 10 whole peanuts.

Test-Taking Strategy: Note the key phrase "most appropriate" in the stem of the question. Eliminate options 1 and 2 because they are similar. Select option 3 over option 4 knowing that bacon is an item of the fat group. Review foods in the exchange system now, if you had difficulty with this question!

Level of Cognitive Ability: Application
Phase of Nursing Process: Implementation
Client Needs: Health Promotion and Maintenance
Content Area: Adult Health/Endocrine

Reference
Monahan, F., & Neighbors, M. (1998). *Medical-surgical nursing: Foundations for clinical practice* (2nd ed.). Philadelphia: W. B. Saunders. p. 1233.

7. 2

Rationale: A low-residue (low-fiber) diet places less strain on the intestines because this type of diet is easier to digest. This diet is used for ulcerative colitis, diverticulitis, and irritable bowel syndrome.

Test-Taking Strategy: Note that the diagnosis in the question refers to an inflammation in the colon. With this in mind, you should easily be directed to option 2, the diet that would place the least strain on the intestinal tract. If you had difficulty with this question, take time now to review the diet prescribed for ulcerative colitis!

Level of Cognitive Ability: Analysis
Phase of Nursing Process: Planning
Client Needs: Physiological Integrity
Content Area: Adult Health/Gastrointestinal

Reference
Luckmann, J. (1997). *Saunders manual of nursing care.* Philadelphia: W. B. Saunders. p. 311.

8. 3

Rationale: Fruits and vegetables, except avocado, olives, and coconut, contain minimal amounts of fat.

Test-Taking Strategy: Knowledge regarding the fat content of fruits is required to answer this question. Options 1 and 2 can be easily eliminated. From the remaining two options, remember that avocado is high in fat content. You are likely to find a question related to these food items on NCLEX-RN!

Level of Cognitive Ability: Analysis
Phase of Nursing Process: Evaluation
Client Needs: Health Promotion and Maintenance
Content Area: Adult Health/Cardiovascular

Reference
Luckmann, J. (1997). *Saunders manual of nursing care.* Philadelphia: W. B. Saunders. p. 311.

9. 2

Rationale: Riboflavin is present in a variety of foods of animal and vegetable origin. Good sources are meats, chicken, eggs, and milk. Liver, however, has an especially high riboflavin content.

Test-Taking Strategy: Note the key phrase "especially high" in the stem of the question. This may indicate that more than one option may contain riboflavin. Knowledge regarding food items high in riboflavin is required to answer this question. If you are unfamiliar with these foods, take time now to review!

Level of Cognitive Ability: Application
Phase of Nursing Process: Implementation
Client Needs: Health Promotion and Maintenance
Content Area: Fundamental Skills

Reference
Lehne, R. (1998). *Pharmacology for nursing care* (3rd ed.). Philadelphia: W. B. Saunders. p. 811.

10. 3

Rationale: Thiamine is present in a variety of foods of plant and animal origin. Pork products are especially rich in the vitamin. Other good sources include peanuts, asparagus, and whole grain and enriched cereals.

Test-Taking Strategy: Note the key phrase "especially rich" in the stem of the question. This may indicate that more than one option may contain thiamine. Knowledge regarding food items high in thiamine is required to answer this question. If you are unfamiliar with these foods, take time now to review this important content!

Level of Cognitive Ability: Application
Phase of Nursing Process: Implementation
Client Needs: Health Promotion and Maintenance
Content Area: Adult Health/Gastrointestinal

Reference
Lehne, R. (1998). *Pharmacology for nursing care* (3rd ed.). Philadelphia: W. B. Saunders. p. 811.

11. 4

Rationale: In general, flavorful and very warm or well-chilled foods with texture stimulate the swallow reflex. Moist pastas, casseroles, egg dishes, and potatoes are usually effective. Raw vegetables, chunky vegetables such as diced beets, and stringy vegetables such as spinach, corn and peas are foods commonly excluded from the diet of a client with a poor swallow reflex. Clients should be warned not to wash food down with liquids.

Test-Taking Strategy: Note the key phrases "avoid" and "swallowing ability." Use the process of elimination to select option 4 as the food with the least amount of substance or consistency. If you had difficulty with this question, take time now to review feeding measures for a client with an altered swallow reflex!

Level of Cognitive Ability: Application
Phase of Nursing Process: Implementation
Client Needs: Physiological Integrity
Content Area: Adult Health/Neurological

Reference
Mahan, L., & Escott-Stump, S. (1996). *Krause's food, nutrition, & diet therapy* (9th ed.). Philadelphia: W. B. Saunders. p. 869.

12. 4

Rationale: Most of the excretion of potassium and the control of potassium balance are normal functions of the kidneys. In the client with renal failure, potassium intake must be restricted as much as possible (30 to 50 mEq/day). The primary mechanism of potassium removal during acute renal failure (ARF) is dialysis. Options 1, 2, and 3 are not normally restricted in the client with ARF.

Test-Taking Strategy: Noting the diagnosis of the client in this question will assist in directing you to option 4. Use the process of elimination and eliminate options 1, 2, and 3 because these items would least likely promote a workload on the kidneys. Review the therapeutic diet in the client with ARF now, if you had difficulty with this question!

Level of Cognitive Ability: Analysis
Phase of Nursing Process: Planning
Client Needs: Physiological Integrity
Content Area: Adult Health/Renal

Reference
Mahan, L., & Escott-Stump, S. (1996). *Krause's food, nutrition, & diet therapy* (9th ed.). Philadelphia: W. B. Saunders. pp. 776–777.

13. 2

Rationale: The client with dumping syndrome should be placed on a high-protein, moderate-fat, and high-calorie diet. The client should avoid drinking liquids with meals. Frequent small meals are encouraged, and the client should avoid concentrated sweets.

Test-Taking Strategy: Note the key word "not" in the stem of the question. Use the process of elimination, selecting option 2 as the item that will contribute to the problems associated with dumping syndrome. If you had difficulty with this question, take time now to review the diet associated with this disorder!

Level of Cognitive Ability: Application
Phase of Nursing Process: Planning
Client Needs: Physiological Integrity
Content Area: Adult Health/Gastrointestinal

Reference
Mahan, L., & Escott-Stump, S. (1996). *Krause's food, nutrition, & diet therapy* (9th ed.). Philadelphia: W. B. Saunders. p. 605.

14. 2

Rationale: Anticoagulant medications act to prevent coagulation by antagonizing the action of vitamin K. When a client is taking an anticoagulant, foods high in vitamin K are often omitted from the diet. Vitamin K is found in large amounts in green, leafy vegetables, especially broccoli, cabbage, turnip greens, and lettuce. Pasta, oranges, and potatoes are very low in vitamin K.

Test-Taking Strategy: Knowledge regarding the relationship between Coumadin and vitamin K is required to answer this question. Note the key word "exclude" and select the food item that is highest in vitamin K. If you had difficulty with this question, take time now to review foods high in vitamin K!

Level of Cognitive Ability: Analysis
Phase of Nursing Process: Planning
Client Needs: Physiological Integrity
Content Area: Pharmacology

Reference
Mahan, L., & Escott-Stump, S. (1996). *Krause's food, nutrition, & diet therapy* (9th ed.). Philadelphia: W. B. Saunders. p. 91.

15. 3

Rationale: Pernicious anemia is caused by a deficiency of vitamin B_{12}. Treatment consists of monthly injections of vitamin B_{12}. Thiamine is most often prescribed for the client with alcoholism. Iron is administered for iron deficiency anemia and folic acid for folic acid deficiency.

Test-Taking Strategy: Knowledge regarding the relationship between pernicious anemia and vitamin B_{12} is required to answer this question. If you are unfamiliar with this disorder, take time now to review!

Level of Cognitive Ability: Analysis
Phase of Nursing Process: Planning
Client Needs: Physiological Integrity
Content Area: Adult Health/Gastrointestinal

Reference

Mahan, L., & Escott-Stump, S. (1996). *Krause's food, nutrition, & diet therapy* (9th ed.). Philadelphia: W. B. Saunders. p. 724.

16. 4

Rationale: It may be necessary to modify a client's diet to a soft or mechanically chopped diet if the client has difficulty chewing. Food and cultural preferences should be ascertained on admission. Bowel sounds should have previously been assessed and present before introducing any diet.

Test-Taking Strategy: Note the key word "elderly." Eliminate options 1 and 2 first because they are similar. Eliminate option 3 next because the client has been tolerating a liquid diet, therefore bowel sounds have been present. The issue relates to consistency of food. Option 4 is the only option that addresses a factor affecting food consistency.

Level of Cognitive Ability: Application
Phase of Nursing Process: Assessment
Client Needs: Physiological Integrity
Content Area: Fundamental Skills

Reference

Craven, R., & Hirnle, C. (1996). *Fundamentals of nursing: Human health and function* (2nd ed.). Philadelphia: Lippincott-Raven. p. 1051.

17. 3

Rationale: Protein and vitamin C are necessary for wound healing. Poultry and milk are good sources of protein. Broccoli and strawberries are good sources of vitamin C. Peanut butter is a source of niacin. Gelatin (Jell-O) and jelly have no nutrient value. Spaghetti is a complex carbohydrate.

Test-Taking Strategy: Remember that all components of an option must be correct to make the option correct. Knowledge that protein and vitamin C are necessary for wound healing would assist in selecting the option that contains those nutrients. Eliminate options 1 and 2 first because jelly and Jell-O have no nutrient value related to healing. From the remaining options, select option 3 over option 4 because of the greater nutrient value in these food items. Review foods high in protein and vitamin C now, if you had difficulty with this question!

Level of Cognitive Ability: Analysis
Phase of Nursing Process: Analysis
Client Needs: Physiological Integrity
Content Area: Fundamental Skills

Reference

Mahan, L., & Escott-Stump, S. (1996). *Krause's food, nutrition, & diet therapy* (9th ed.). Philadelphia: W. B. Saunders. p. 674.

18. 4

Rationale: In a postoperative client, a concern related to initiating a diet is aspiration. Suction equipment must be available. A cardiac monitor and a code cart are unnecessary. A straw may help the client sip fluids but is not necessary.

Test-Taking Strategy: Note the key word "postoperative." Use the ABCs—airway, breathing, and circulation—to answer this question. Option 4 will maintain airway clearance. If you had difficulty with this question, take time now to review care to the postoperative client!

Level of Cognitive Ability: Application
Phase of Nursing Process: Planning
Client Needs: Safe, Effective Care Environment
Content Area: Fundamental Skills

Reference

Craven, R., & Hirnle, C. (1996). *Fundamentals of nursing: Human health and function* (2nd ed.). Philadelphia: Lippincott-Raven. pp. 674–675.

19. 3

Rationale: Independence is promoted by allowing the client to have control in a given situation. Placing the client's tray on the unaffected side will facilitate the client's ability to perform the activity of eating. Options 1, 2, and 4 do not offer the client control.

Test-Taking Strategy: Note the key phrase "promote independence." With this issue in mind, by the process of elimination, you should easily be directed to option 3. Review measures related to promoting independence now, if you had difficulty with this question!

Level of Cognitive Ability: Application
Phase of Nursing Process: Implementation
Client Needs: Psychosocial Integrity
Content Area: Adult Health/Neurological

Reference

Monahan, P., & Neighbors, M. (1998). *Medical-surgical nursing: Foundations for clinical practice* (2nd ed.). Philadelphia: W. B. Saunders. p. 813.

20. 4

Rationale: A low-sodium diet is used as an adjunct to antihypertensive medications for treatment of hypertension. Sodium retains fluid, which leads to hypertension secondary to increased fluid volume. Frozen foods use salt as a preservative and should not be encouraged as part of a low-sodium diet.

Test-Taking Strategy: Note the key phrase "further teaching is necessary." Use the process of elimination in selecting the correct option. Eliminate options 1, 2, and 3 because these are accurate statements related to hypertension. If you had difficulty with this question, take time now to review the treatment of hypertension and foods high in sodium!

Level of Cognitive Ability: Analysis
Phase of Nursing Process: Evaluation
Client Needs: Health Promotion and Maintenance
Content Area: Adult Health/Cardiovascular

Reference

Mahan, L., & Escott-Stump, S. (1996). *Krause's food, nutrition, & diet therapy* (9th ed.). Philadelphia: W. B. Saunders. p. 742.

21. 1

Rationale: The most accurate measurement of weight loss is daily weighing of the client at the same time, in the same clothes, and using the same scale. Options 2, 3, and 4 assist in measuring nutrition and hydration status rather than actual loss of pounds.

Test-Taking Strategy: Note the key phrase "most accurate." Also note the similar words in the question and option. If you had difficulty with this question, take time now to review the methods of monitoring weight loss!

Level of Cognitive Ability: Application
Phase of Nursing Process: Assessment
Client Needs: Physiological Integrity
Content Area: Fundamental Skills

Reference
Mahan, L., & Escott-Stump, S. (1996). *Krause's food, nutrition, & diet therapy* (9th ed.). Philadelphia: W. B. Saunders. p. 371.

22. 4

Rationale: In anorexia nervosa, the client tries to establish identity and control by self-imposed starvation. Options 1, 2, and 3 are verbalizations of the client's intentions. Option 4 is a measurable action that can be verified.

Test-Taking Strategy: Note the key phrase "that treatment has been effective." With this in mind, use the process of elimination and select the option that is measurable. Option 4 is the only measurable action.

Level of Cognitive Ability: Analysis
Phase of Nursing Process: Evaluation
Client Needs: Psychosocial Integrity
Content Area: Mental Health

Reference
Carson, V., & Arnold, E. (1996). *Mental health nursing: The nurse-patient journey.* Philadelphia: W. B. Saunders. pp. 916–917.

23. 1

Rationale: Poor nutrition during pregnancy can negatively influence fetal growth and development. Although pregnancy poses some nutritional risk for the mother, not all clients are at high risk. Calcium is critical during the third trimester but must be increased from the onset of pregnancy. Intake of dietary iron is usually insufficient for the majority of pregnant women and iron supplements are routinely encouraged.

Test-Taking Strategy: Eliminate option 2 because of the absolute term "all." Note the absolute term "not" in options 3 and 4. Option 1 is a general statement true for any stage of pregnancy and is the most global statement.

Level of Cognitive Ability: Application
Phase of Nursing Process: Planning
Client Needs: Physiological Integrity
Content Area: Maternity

Reference
Mahan, L., & Escott-Stump, S. (1996). *Krause's food, nutrition, & diet therapy* (9th ed.). Philadelphia: W. B. Saunders. p. 193.

24. 3

Rationale: Chemotherapy may cause distortion of taste. Frequent oral hygiene aids in preserving taste function. Keeping a client NPO increases nutritional risks. Antiemetics are used when nausea and vomiting are a problem. TPN is used when oral intake is not possible.

Test-Taking Strategy: The issue of the question is a change in taste sensation. Eliminate options 1, 2, and 4 because they are unrelated to the issue of the question. Option 3 is the only option that addresses the issue of the question. If you had difficulty with this question, take time now to review interventions related to nutrition in the client receiving chemotherapy!

Level of Cognitive Ability: Application
Phase of Nursing Process: Implementation
Client Needs: Physiological Integrity
Content Area: Adult Health/Oncology

Reference
Mahan, L., & Escott-Stump, S. (1996). *Krause's food, nutrition, & diet therapy* (9th ed.). Philadelphia: W. B. Saunders. p. 818.

25. 4

Rationale: Concentrated sugars are found in fruit yogurt, gelatin desserts, prepared drink mixes, jelly, and sherbet.

Test-Taking Strategy. Use knowledge of foods containing concentrated sugar to answer the question. Note that option 4 is the only option that does not identify a prepared food item. Review foods containing concentrated sugar now, if you had difficulty with this question!

Level of Cognitive Ability: Analysis
Phase of Nursing Process: Evaluation
Client Needs: Health Promotion and Maintenance
Content Area: Fundamental Skills

Reference
Mahan, L., & Escott-Stump, S. (1996). *Krause's food, nutrition, & diet therapy* (9th ed.). Philadelphia: W. B. Saunders. p. 34.

26. 4

Rationale: Self-control is demonstrated by stoicism and hiding feelings. Problem-solving involves making plans and verbalizing what will be done. Accepting responsibility places the responsibility for a situation on one's self. Distancing is an unwillingness or inability to discuss events.

Test-Taking Strategy: Note the key phrases "refuses," "will not," and "does not." These phrases indicate ineffective coping. Option 4, distancing, is indicative of ineffective coping. If you had difficulty with this question, take time now to review coping mechanisms!

Level of Cognitive Ability: Analysis
Phase of Nursing Process: Assessment
Client Needs: Psychosocial Integrity
Content Area: Adult Health/Gastrointestinal

Reference
Luckmann, J. (1997). *Saunders manual of nursing care.* Philadelphia: W. B. Saunders. p. 316.

27. 4

Rationale: A lactose intolerance would require that the client be placed on a lactose-free formula. The physician would need to be notified to change the order. Options 1, 2, and 3 would not warrant notification of the physician.

Test-Taking Strategy: The question addresses a rationale for physician notification. Option 1 indicates that the client has tolerated this treatment before. Option 2 is an indication for enteral feeding. Option 3 is most commonly associated with constipation, not diarrhea. Option 4 warrants notifying the physician to change to a lactose-free formula. If you had difficulty with this question, take time now to review the complications of tube-feeding formulas!

Level of Cognitive Ability: Analysis
Phase of Nursing Process: Implementation
Client Needs: Physiological Integrity
Content Area: Fundamental Skills

Reference
Luckmann, J. (1997). *Saunders manual of nursing care.* Philadelphia: W. B. Saunders. p. 319.

28. **2**

Rationale: Any condition in which GI motility is slowed or esophageal reflux is possible places a client at risk for aspiration. Options 1 and 4 may be appropriate nursing diagnoses but are not of highest priority. Option 3 is not likely to occur in this client.

Test-Taking Strategy: Note the key phrase "highest priority." Use the ABCs—airway, breathing, and circulation. Option 2 addresses airway management. Options 1, 3, and 4 are possible problems but not as high a priority as airway maintenance.

Level of Cognitive Ability: Application
Phase of Nursing Process: Planning
Client Needs: Safe, Effective Care Environment
Content Area: Fundamental Skills

Reference
Luckmann, J. (1997). *Saunders manual of nursing care.* Philadelphia: W. B. Saunders. p. 316.

29. **4**

Rationale: Initiating a tube feeding prior to checking tube placement can lead to serious complications such as aspiration. Options 1 and 2 are part of the total plan of care for a client on enteral feedings. Option 3 is instituted for a client who has been identified as a high risk for aspiration. Option 4 is the priority nursing action.

Test-Taking Strategy: Utilize the ABCs—airway, breathing, and circulation—and the nursing process to answer the question. Option 4 relates to assessment and to the risk of aspiration. If you had difficulty with this question, take time now to review nursing interventions when initiating a tube feeding!

Level of Cognitive Ability: Application
Phase of Nursing Process: Implementation
Client Needs: Physiological Integrity
Content Area: Fundamental Skills

Reference
Luckmann, J. (1997). *Saunders manual of nursing care.* Philadelphia: W. B. Saunders. p. 316.

30. **1**

Rationale: Return demonstration is the most reliable evaluation of procedure performance. Selection of equipment is included in a return demonstration. Written testing is not useful for performance testing of procedures. Verbal description does not allow the nurse to observe the psychomotor skill needed to perform the procedure.

Test-Taking Strategy: Note the similar words in question and option. "Performing" in the question and "demonstration" in the option indicate action. Review teaching/learning principles now, if you had difficulty with this question!

Level of Cognitive Ability: Analysis
Phase of Nursing Process: Evaluation
Client Needs: Health Promotion and Maintenance
Content Area: Fundamental Skills

Reference
Luckmann, J. (1997). *Saunders manual of nursing care.* Philadelphia: W. B. Saunders. p. 316.

BIBLIOGRAPHY

Carson, V., & Arnold, E. (1996). *Mental health nursing: The nurse-patient journey.* Philadelphia: W. B. Saunders.

Craven, R., & Hirnle, C. (1996). *Fundamentals of nursing: Human health and function* (2nd ed.). Philadelphia: Lippincott-Raven.

Dudek, S. (1997). *Nutrition handbook for nursing practice* (3rd ed.). Philadelphia: Lippincott-Raven.

Hodgson, B., & Kizior, R. (1998). *Saunders nursing drug handbook 1998.* Philadelphia: W. B. Saunders.

Leahy, J., & Kizilay, P. (1998). *Foundations of nursing practice: A nursing process approach.* Philadelphia: W. B. Saunders.

Lehne, R. (1998). *Pharmacology for nursing care* (3rd ed.). Philadelphia: W. B. Saunders.

Luckmann, J. (1997). *Saunders manual of nursing care.* Philadelphia: W. B. Saunders.

Mahan, L., & Escott-Stump, S. (1996). *Krause's food, nutrition, & diet therapy* (9th ed.). Philadelphia: W. B. Saunders.

Monahan, F., & Neighbors, M. (1998). *Medical surgical nursing: Foundations for clinical practice* (2nd ed.). Philadelphia: W. B. Saunders.

CHAPTER 12

Total Parenteral Nutrition (TPN)

PYRAMID TERMS

Central Parenteral Nutrition (CPN)—Parenteral nutrition, administered through the subclavian or internal jugular vein, that is used when feeding must last longer than 7 days.

Fat Emulsion—Administered during TPN therapy; provides up to 30% of caloric (energy) needs, provides nonprotein calories, and prevents fatty acid deficiency.

Malnutrition—Poor nourishment resulting from improper diet or from some defect in metabolism that prevents the body from using its food properly.

Peripheral Parenteral Nutrition (PPN)—Parenteral nutrition administered through a peripheral vein; used for short-term therapy (5 to 7 days) and when the client needs only small concentrations of carbohydrates, fats, and proteins

◆ PYRAMID TO SUCCESS

The NCLEX-RN test plan addresses TPN as related content in the Client Needs area of Physiological Integrity and Pharmacological and Parenteral Therapies. Pyramid points focus on the precautions related to the administration of TPN and **fat emulsions,** nursing interventions, and the interventions required in monitoring for complications. Pyramid points also focus on home care instructions for the client receiving TPN at home.

NURSING PROCESS

ASSESSMENT

Vital signs
Signs of infection
IV site
Physician orders
TPN and fat emulsion solutions
Signs of complications
Client teaching

ANALYSIS: Potential for Infection
Potential for Fluid Volume Excess
Potential for Hyperglycemia or Hypoglycemia
Potential for Air Embolism

PLANNING	IMPLEMENTATION	EVALUATION
Client is free of signs and symptoms of infection. Client gains no more than 2 to 3 pounds of weight per week. Client is free of signs and symptoms of hyperglycemia and hypoglycemia. Client exhibits no signs of air embolism.	Monitor temperature. Monitor for signs of infection. Monitor IV site. Monitor intake and output (I&O). Monitor daily weight. Auscultate lung sounds. Monitor glucose levels. Monitor for signs and symptoms of hyperglycemia and hypoglycemia. Initiate measures to prevent the occurrence of air emboli. Monitor for signs of air emboli.	Vital signs remain within normal limits. Lung sounds are clear. Target weight is achieved. Glucose levels remain within normal limits. Client remains free of complications. Client demonstrates care related to the administration of TPN.

CLIENT NEEDS

SAFE, EFFECTIVE CARE ENVIRONMENT

Informed consent
Dietary consultation
Home health care referral
Asepsis
Standard precautions

HEALTH PROMOTION AND MAINTENANCE

Disease prevention
Health and wellness
Client and family teaching
Assessment of complications

PSYCHOSOCIAL INTEGRITY

Role changes
Promoting self-care
Support systems

PHYSIOLOGICAL INTEGRITY

Nutrition
Assistance with care
Rest and sleep
Central venous access device
TPN
Laboratory values
Monitoring for potential complications
Monitoring for expected effects
Documentation

I. Total Parenteral Nutrition (TPN)

A. Description
   1. Supplies necessary nutrients via veins
   2. Supplies carbohydrates in the form of dextrose, fats in special emulsified form, proteins in the form of amino acids, vitamins, minerals, and water
   3. Prevents subcutaneous fat and muscle protein from being catabolized by the body for energy
B. Indications
   1. When the gastrointestinal (GI) tract is severely dysfunctional or nonfunctional
   2. For clients who can take some oral nutrition but not enough to meet the body's needs
   3. Clients with multiple GI surgeries, GI trauma, severe intolerance to enteral feedings, or intestinal obstructions, or when the bowel needs to rest for healing
   4. Clients with AIDS, cancer, or malnutrition
C. Components
   1. Carbohydrates
      a. Mainly in the form of glucose
      b. Range from 5% for **peripheral parenteral nutrition** to 50% to 70% hypertonic solution for **central parenteral nutrition**
      c. Provides 60% to 70% of caloric (energy) needs
   2. Amino acids: Provides 5% to 15% of the total calories
   3. Lipid (**fat emulsions**)
      a. Provides up to 30% of caloric (energy) needs
      b. Provides nonprotein calories and prevents fatty acid deficiency
   4. Vitamins
   5. Minerals
   6. Electrolytes
   7. Insulin may be added to control the blood glucose level because of the high concentration of glucose in the TPN
   8. Heparin may be added to reduce the build-up of a fibrinous clot at the catheter tip
D. Intravenous sites
   1. **Peripheral parenteral nutrition (PPN)**
      a. Administered through a peripheral vein
      b. Used for short periods (5 to 7 days) and when the client needs only small concentrations of carbohydrates, fats, and proteins
      c. Volume is usually limited to 2000 to 3000 mL/day, providing a calorie value of 2000 kcal/day
      d. Used to deliver isotonic or mildly hypertonic solutions
      e. The delivery of highly hypertonic solutions into peripheral veins can cause sclerosis, phlebitis, or swelling
   2. **Central parenteral nutrition (CPN)**
      a. Administered through the subclavian or internal jugular veins

b. Used when feeding must last longer than 7 days

c. Used when the client requires a larger concentration of carbohydrates (greater than 10% dextrose)

d. An inline filter is required to remove crystals from the solution; for standard solutions, a 0.22-micron (m) filter can be used

II. Precautions

A. When a central line is inserted, placement is confirmed by chest radiograph

B. Check TPN with physician order

C. To help prevent infection and solution incompatibility, IV medications and blood are not given through the TPN line

D. TPN is always delivered via an electronic infusion device, preferably a volumetric pump

E. In severely dehydrated clients, the albumin level may drop initially as treatment restores hydration

F. With severely malnourished clients, monitor for "refeeding syndrome" (a rapid drop in potassium, magnesium, and phosphate serum levels)

G. Abnormal liver function values may indicate an intolerance to or an excess in lipid emulsions, or problems with metabolism with glucose and protein

H. Abnormal renal function tests indicate an excess of amino acids

I. When infusion of hypertonic dextrose is stopped, an infusion of 10% dextrose should be instituted and maintained for 1 to 2 hours to prevent hypoglycemia

J. Solutions should be stored under refrigeration and administered within 24 hours (remove from refrigerator 0.5 to 1 hour before use)

K. Preparations that are cloudy or darkened should be discarded

III. Nursing Interventions

A. Monitor weight
   1. Ideal weight gain is 1 pound per week
   2. Rapid weight gain may indicate fluid overload

B. Initiate feeding slowly to avoid cardiac overload

C. Monitor electrolytes

D. Monitor capillary glucose every 6 hours

E. Monitor partial thromboplastin time (PTT) and prothrombin time (PT) for clients receiving anticoagulants

F. Monitor liver and renal function tests

G. Use an IV tubing filter and change IV tubing every 24 hours or according to agency protocol

H. Wean client from TPN

IV. Administering Fat Emulsion

A. This is an isotonic solution and may be administered through a peripheral vein

B. Assess for allergy to eggs, a contraindication for lipid infusion

C. Use vented tubing

D. May be infused in the same vein as dextrose amino acid solutions

E. The Y-connector through which the fat will flow should be placed below any inline filter because particles in the **fat emulsion** are too large to pass through filters

F. Administer slowly for the first 15 to 30 minutes, and monitor for adverse reactions, such as dyspnea, cyanosis, and allergic responses; use a 4- to 6-hour rate for 250 to 500 mL of **fat emulsion** thereafter

G. Observe for separation of emulsion, and do not use if separation occurs

H. Monitor for hyperlipidemia

V. Prevention of Complications (Box 12–1)

A. Infection
   1. Use strict aseptic technique when cleansing the IV site and administering IV fluid
   2. Monitor temperature
   3. Assess site for redness, swelling, tenderness, or drainage
   4. If signs of infection occur at the site, the IV line must be removed and restarted at a different site
   5. In the event of fever, sepsis should be suspected
   6. To assess for sepsis, blood for culture should be drawn, and the tip of the catheter should be cultured for bacteria

B. Hyperglycemia
   1. Monitor IV hourly
   2. Monitor glucose and ketone levels
   3. Never "speed up" parenteral feeding
   4. Administer insulin as prescribed
   5. Monitor for malaise; deep, rapid breathing; excessive urinary output

C. Fluid overload
   1. Monitor I&O
   2. Weigh daily
   3. Monitor for bounding pulse, jugular vein distention, headache, increased blood pressure, and crackles on lung auscultation

D. Air embolism
   1. Tape tubing connections
   2. Instruct client to use the Valsalva maneuver whenever the line is opened
   3. Place client in left side-lying position with

BOX 12–1. Complications of Total Parenteral Nutrition

Infection
Hyperglycemia
Fluid overload
Air embolism

BOX 12–2. Home Care Instructions

- How to administer and maintain TPN fluids
- How to change a sterile dressing
- Weigh daily at the same time in the same clothes
- Stress that a weight gain of more than 0.5 kg (1.1 lb) per day may indicate excessive fluid intake and should be reported
- Check urine for sugar and acetone and report abnormalities immediately
- Check for signs and symptoms of infection, thrombosis, air embolism, and displacement
- For symptoms of thrombosis, the client should report edema of the arm or catheter insertion site, neck pain, and jugular vein distention
- Symptoms of an air embolus should be taught to another person in the client's home and include confusion, pallor, lightheadedness, tachycardia, tachypnea, hypotension, anxiety, and unresponsiveness
- Leaking of fluid from the insertion site or pain or discomfort as the fluids are infused may indicate displacement of the catheter; this must be reported immediately

head lower than feet if air embolism is suspected, and contact the physician

E. Home care instructions (Box 12–2)

PRACTICE QUESTIONS

1. The client has been discharged to home on TPN. With each visit, the home care nurse assesses which of the following parameters most closely in monitoring this therapy?
   1 Temperature and weight
   2 Temperature and blood pressure
   3 Pulse and weight
   4 Pulse and blood pressure

2. The nurse is monitoring the client who may be started on TPN. The nurse interprets that the client is at risk of severe malnutrition if the albumin level drops below which critical cut-off level?
   1 4.5 g/dL
   2 3.5 g/dL
   3 2.5 g/dL
   4 1.5 g/dL

3. The nurse is caring for a group of adult clients on the acute care nursing unit. The nurse interprets that which of the following clients would be the least likely candidate for TPN?
   1 A 66-year-old client with extensive burns
   2 A 42-year-old client who had an open cholecystectomy
   3 A 35-year-old client with persistent nausea and vomiting from chemotherapy
   4 A 27-year-old client with severe exacerbation of regional enteritis (Crohn's disease)

4. The physician has ordered that the client be started on TPN with a solution containing 25% glucose. The client has a peripheral IV line in place. The nurse should plan to do which of the following?
   1 Hang the solution as ordered
   2 Hang the solution but only at half the rate
   3 Dilute the solution with sterile water to half-strength
   4 Question the order

5. The nurse is planning to hang the first bag of TPN solution via the central line of an assigned client. The nurse plans to obtain which of the following most essential pieces of equipment before hanging the solution?
   1 Electronic infusion pump
   2 Blood glucose meter
   3 Urine test strips
   4 Noninvasive blood pressure monitor

6. The home care nurse is monitoring the malnourished client's response to TPN. The client's weight 1 week ago was 114 pounds. The nurse interprets that the client is not gaining weight too rapidly if this morning's weight was:
   1 122 pounds
   2 116 pounds
   3 120 pounds
   4 118 pounds

7. The nurse is assigned to the client receiving TPN who had a blood glucose measurement done at 06:00. The nurse writes on the client's clinical worksheet for the day that the blood glucose level should be checked at which of the following times?
   1 10:00
   2 12:00
   3 16:00
   4 18:00

8. The client is receiving nutrition by means of TPN. The nurse assesses the client for which of the following signs of hyperglycemia?
   1 Nausea, vomiting, and oliguria
   2 Sweating, chills, and abdominal pain
   3 Pallor, weak pulse, and thirst
   4 Weakness, thirst, and increased urine output

9. At 8:00 A.M. the nurse checks the amount of solution left in a TPN infusion bag for an assigned client. It is a 3000-mL bag with 1000 mL remaining. The solution is running at a rate of 100 mL/hour. The bag was hung the previous day at 12:00 noon. The nurse plans to change the infusion bag and tubing today at:
   1 8:00 P.M.
   2 4:00 P.M.
   3 2:00 P.M.
   4 12:00 noon

10. The nurse is changing the central line dressing of the client receiving TPN. The nurse notes that the catheter insertion site appears reddened. The nurse next assesses which of the following items?
    1 Tightness of tubing connections
    2 Client's temperature
    3 Expiration date on the bag
    4 Time of last dressing change

11. The nurse is preparing to hang a fat emulsion. The nurse notes that fat globules are visible at the top of the solution. The nurse takes which of the following actions?
    1 Run the bottle under warm water
    2 Roll the bottle gently
    3 Shake the bottle vigorously
    4 Obtain a different bottle

12. The nurse is assigned to a client receiving TPN. The nurse assesses the client at 8:00 A.M. and checks the solution, which is being administered through an electronic infusion pump. The nurse next returns at which time to check the status of the TPN?
    1 4:00 P.M.
    2 12:00 noon
    3 10:00 A.M.
    4 9:00 A.M.

13. The client is being weaned from TPN and is expected to begin taking solid food today. The ongoing solution rate has been 100 mL/hr. The nurse anticipates that which of the following orders regarding the TPN solution will accompany the diet order?
    1 Discontinue the TPN
    2 Continue current orders for TPN
    3 Decrease TPN rate to 50 mL/hr
    4 Hang 1000 mL 5% dextrose in water

14. The client is receiving TPN with fat emulsion piggybacked into the IV line. The nurse notices during rounds that the fat emulsion has infused too quickly. The nurse immediately assesses the client for which of the following manifestations of fat overload?
    1 Fever and pruritic urticaria
    2 Hypothermia and muscle weakness
    3 Hypertension and decreased urine output
    4 Bradycardia and chest pain

15. The client receiving TPN may begin to take small amounts of clear liquids today. The nurse completes which of the following most important assessments before giving the client anything by mouth?
    1 Client's appetite
    2 Client's weight today
    3 Presence of swallow reflex
    4 Adequate pulse and blood pressure

16. The client has had extensive surgery on the GI tract and has been started on TPN. The client tells the nurse, "I think I'm going crazy . . . I feel like I'm starving and yet that bag is supposed to be feeding me." The best response by the nurse is:
    1 "Don't worry. Many others in your situation say the same thing."
    2 "That is unusual. I wonder if the solution is being mixed correctly?"
    3 "Maybe you should ask your doctor about that; I've never heard of that before."
    4 "That is because the empty stomach sends signals to the brain to stimulate hunger."

17. The nurse is preparing to change the TPN solution bag and tubing. The client's central venous line is located in the right subclavian vein. The nurse asks the client to do which of the following most essential items during the tubing change?
    1 Take a deep breath and hold it
    2 Exhale slowly and evenly
    3 Turn the head to the left
    4 Turn the head to the right

18. The nurse is caring for the restless client who is beginning nutritional therapy with TPN. The nurse should plan to ensure that which of the following is done to prevent the client from injury?
    1 Monitor blood glucose levels every 12 hours
    2 Tape all connections in the TPN system
    3 Monitor temperature once daily
    4 Calculate daily I&O

19. The client with TPN infusing has disconnected the tubing from the central line catheter. The nurse suspects air embolism. The nurse should immediately place the client in which of the following positions?
    1 On the left side with the head higher than the feet
    2 On the left side with the head lower than the feet
    3 On the right side with the head higher than the feet
    4 On the right side with the head lower than the feet

20. The client receiving TPN complains of headache. The nurse notes that the client has an increased blood pressure, bounding pulse, jugular vein distention, and bilateral crackles. The nurse interprets that the client is experiencing which of the following complications of TPN therapy?
    1 Hyperglycemia
    2 Air embolism
    3 Sepsis
    4 Fluid overload

21. The nurse is educating the client about home parenteral nutrition. The nurse identifies which of the following learning needs as most critical to address in the teaching plan, since complications from lack of knowledge in this area are the most common reason for hospital readmission?
    1 Catheter care
    2 Infusion rate
    3 Blood glucose monitoring
    4 Measurement of daily weight

22. The client receiving TPN suddenly spikes a fever. The nurse notifies the physician, who orders that the solution and tubing be changed. The nurse should do which of the following with the discontinued materials?
    1 Return them to the hospital pharmacy
    2 Send them to the laboratory for culture
    3 Save them for return to the manufacturer
    4 Discard them in the unit trash

23. The nurse enters the room of the client receiving TPN and discovers that the electronic infusion pump has been shut off. After checking the line for patency and restarting the infusion, the nurse assesses the client for which of the following signs and symptoms?
    1 Nausea, weakness, headache, thirst, and excessive urination
    2 Sudden temperature elevation, chills, and diaphoresis
    3 Weakness, headache, tingling around the mouth, apprehension, and diaphoresis
    4 Dyspnea, tachycardia, hypotension, and disorientation

24. The nurse is making initial rounds at the beginning of the shift. The TPN bag of an assigned client is empty. Which of the following solutions readily available on the unit should the nurse hang until another TPN solution is mixed and delivered to the nursing unit?
    1 5% dextrose in water
    2 5% dextrose in 0.9% sodium chloride
    3 5% dextrose in Ringer's lactate
    4 10% dextrose in water

25. At the beginning of the shift, the nurse assesses the client receiving TPN with fat emulsion piggybacked to the line. The nurse notes that the fat emulsion tubing has an inline filter. Which of the following actions by the nurse is most appropriate?

    1 Inspect the filter for clogging
    2 Remove the filter
    3 Leave the system alone
    4 Check the line for patency

26. The nurse has an order to hang a fat emulsion for a client with an existing infusion of TPN via a central venous line. Of the following areas, where would be the best place for the nurse to attach the fat emulsion tubing?
    1 Directly into the central line catheter
    2 To a peripheral IV line
    3 To the proximal Y-connector of the TPN tubing
    4 To the distal Y-connector of the TPN tubing

27. The nurse is monitoring the status of the client's fat emulsion infusion. The nurse notes that the infusion is 1 hour behind. Which of the following actions by the nurse is most appropriate?
    1 Adjust the line to run wide open until the solution is back on time
    2 Leave the fat emulsion infusion rate as it is
    3 Adjust the rate to catch up over the next 2 hours
    4 Adjust the rate to catch up over the next hour

28. The nurse has an order to hang a TPN solution containing glucose, amino acids, and vitamins. The nurse should plan to get which of the following most important items from the supply area when preparing the solution for infusion?
    1 A microdrip tubing
    2 A tubing extension set
    3 A new central line dressing kit
    4 An inline filter

29. The client is being weaned from parenteral nutrition to oral feedings. The nurse should use which of the following items as the best indicator of continued nutritional adequacy?
    1 I&O
    2 Calorie count
    3 Serum electrolytes
    4 Trace element levels

30. The client receiving TPN in the home setting has a weight gain of 4 pounds in 1 week. The nurse next assesses the client focusing on which of the following?
    1 Peripheral edema and breath sounds
    2 Headache and thirst
    3 Elevated pulse and blood pressure
    4 Polyuria and skin tenting

ANSWERS

1. 1

Rationale: The client receiving TPN at home should have the temperature monitored as a means of detecting infection, which is a potential complication of this therapy. The infection could also result in sepsis, since the catheter is in a blood vessel. The client's weight is tracked as a measure of the effectiveness of this nutritional therapy. Other vital signs are good parameters to assess, but they do not relate specifically to the effects of TPN.

Test-Taking Strategy: The key words in the question are "TPN" and "most closely." This tells you that more than one or all of the options may be partially or totally correct. Remember also that when there are multiple parts to an option, all the parts must be correct in order for that option to be correct. Use knowledge of purposes and complications of TPN to make a choice. Review these important assessments now, if you had difficulty with this question!

Level of Cognitive Ability: Application
Phase of Nursing Process: Assessment
Client Needs: Health Promotion and Maintenance
Content Area: Fundamental Skills

Reference
Taylor, C., Lillis, C., & LeMone, P. (1997). *Fundamentals of nursing: The art and science of nursing care* (3rd ed.). Philadelphia: Lippincott-Raven. p. 1198.

2. 3

Rationale: The serum albumin level is an excellent indicator of the need for TPN. The client whose albumin level drops below 2.5 g/dL is at severe risk of malnutrition. It is hoped that clients would be started on TPN before the level drops this far. The normal serum albumin level in the adult is 3.3 to 5 g/dL.

Test-Taking Strategy: Familiarity with the normal range for this laboratory test is needed to answer this question correctly. If needed, take a few moments to review this test now!

Level of Cognitive Ability: Analysis
Phase of Nursing Process: Analysis
Client Needs: Physiological Integrity
Content Area: Fundamental Skills

References
Jaffee, M., & McVan, B. (1997). *Davis's laboratory and diagnostic test handbook.* Philadelphia: F. A. Davis. p. 914.
Taylor, C., Lillis, C., & LeMone, P. (1997). *Fundamentals of nursing: The art and science of nursing care* (3rd ed.). Philadelphia: Lippincott-Raven. p. 1193.

3. 2

Rationale: TPN is indicated in clients whose GI tracts are not functional, or who cannot take in a diet enterally for extended periods of time. Examples of these conditions include the clients outlined in options 1, 3, and 4. Other clients are those who have had extensive surgery, have multiple fractures, are septic, or have advanced cancer or AIDS. The client with the open cholecystectomy is not a candidate because this client would resume a diet within 5 days or so.

Test-Taking Strategy: Note that the question contains the key words "TPN" and "least likely." This tells you that the correct option is the client who does not require this type of nutritional support. Use nursing knowledge of these various conditions and baseline knowledge of the purposes of TPN to make your selection.

Level of Cognitive Ability: Analysis
Phase of Nursing Process: Analysis
Client Needs: Physiological Integrity
Content Area: Fundamental Skills

Reference
Taylor, C., Lillis, C., & LeMone, P. (1997). *Fundamentals of nursing: The art and science of nursing care* (3rd ed.). Philadelphia: Lippincott-Raven. pp. 1193, 1196.

4. 4

Rationale: Peripheral vessels are used for solutions containing up to 10% glucose. A TPN solution with 25% glucose is hypertonic. The nurse should question the order in the absence of a central venous access line. Options 2 and 3 are unrealistic and are not legal. The nurse does not independently change a physician order, although one may be questioned with sufficient reason.

Test-Taking Strategy: Note the key phrase "25% glucose." Use knowledge related to TPN and principles related to ethical-legal nursing practice to answer this question. This will allow you to eliminate each of the incorrect options systematically. Review base solutions of TPN now, if you had difficulty with this question!

Level of Cognitive Ability: Application
Phase of Nursing Process: Planning
Client Needs: Safe, Effective Care Environment
Content Area: Fundamental Skills

Reference
Taylor, C., Lillis, C., & LeMone, P. (1997). *Fundamentals of nursing: The art and science of nursing care* (3rd ed.). Philadelphia: Lippincott-Raven. p. 1193.

5. 1

Rationale: The nurse obtains an electronic infusion pump before hanging a TPN solution. Because of the high glucose load, it is necessary to use an infusion pump to ensure that the solution does not infuse too rapidly or fall too far behind. Because the client's blood glucose is monitored every 6 to 8 hours during administration of TPN, a blood glucose meter will also be needed, but this is not the most essential item needed prior to hanging the solution. Urine test strips (to measure glucose) are rarely used today since the advent of blood glucose monitoring. A noninvasive blood pressure cuff is totally unnecessary for this procedure.

Test-Taking Strategy: Note that the question contains the key words "most essential" and "before hanging." This tells you that the correct option is one that is needed to start the infusion. Utilize knowledge of principles of TPN administration to eliminate each of the incorrect options easily. Review these principles now, if you had difficulty with this question!

Level of Cognitive Ability: Application
Phase of Nursing Process: Planning
Client Needs: Safe, Effective Care Environment
Content Area: Fundamental Skills

Reference
Taylor, C., Lillis, C., & LeMone, P. (1997). *Fundamentals of nursing: The art and science of nursing care* (3rd ed.). Philadelphia: Lippincott-Raven. p. 1193.

6. **2**

Rationale: The client receiving TPN should not gain more than 3 pounds per week, with optimal weight gain being 1 to 2 pounds per week. The nurse evaluates client weight as a measure of the effectiveness of TPN. The weight goal for the client on TPN is individual and depends on the client's metabolic needs and baseline weight (whether underweight, overweight, or at optimal weight). The correct answer, option 2, shows a reasonable weight gain of 2 pounds per week.

Test-Taking Strategy: To answer this question accurately, it is necessary to be familiar with the nursing considerations related to TPN therapy and expected outcomes. If this question was difficult, take a few moments to review the essentials of TPN at this time!

Level of Cognitive Ability: Analysis
Phase of Nursing Process: Evaluation
Client Needs: Health Promotion and Maintenance
Content Area: Fundamental Skills

Reference
Taylor, C., Lillis, C., & LeMone, P. (1997). *Fundamentals of nursing: The art and science of nursing care* (3rd ed.). Philadelphia: Lippincott-Raven. p. 1193.

7. **2**

Rationale: The client's blood glucose level should be monitored every 6 hours while receiving TPN. Depending on agency policy, this may be done every 8 hours instead. It is unnecessary to monitor the blood glucose level every 4 hours (option 1). Monitoring every 10 or 12 hours (options 3 and 4) is insufficient.

Test-Taking Strategy: To answer this question accurately, it is necessary to know the parameters for blood glucose monitoring for the client receiving TPN, and also to understand military time. If needed, review these procedures now!

Level of Cognitive Ability: Application
Phase of Nursing Process: Implementation
Client Needs: Physiological Integrity
Content Area: Fundamental Skills

Reference
Taylor, C., Lillis, C., & LeMone, P. (1997). *Fundamentals of nursing: The art and science of nursing care* (3rd ed.). Philadelphia: Lippincott-Raven. p. 1193.

8. **4**

Rationale: The high glucose concentration in TPN places the client at risk for hyperglycemia. Signs of hyperglycemia include polyuria, polydipsia, blurred vision, nausea and vomiting, and abdominal pain. If the client presents with these symptoms, the blood glucose level should be checked immediately.

Test-Taking Strategy: Remember that in order for an option to be correct, all the parts of that option must be correct. Begin to answer this question by eliminating options 2 and 3 as least plausible. Choose option 4 over option 1 because the client has increased urine output rather than decreased urine output with hyperglycemia. Review the signs of hyperglycemia now, if you had difficulty with this question!

Level of Cognitive Ability: Application
Phase of Nursing Process: Assessment
Client Needs: Physiological Integrity
Content Area: Fundamental Skills

Reference
Monahan, F., & Neighbors, M. (1998). *Medical-surgical nursing. Foundations for clinical practice* (2nd ed.). Philadelphia: W. B. Saunders. p. 1246.

9. **4**

Rationale: TPN solution, like IV solutions, should be changed every 24 hours for infection control purposes. Infection control is also aided by use of aseptic technique with bag and tubing changes. Most agencies recommend that tubing be changed every 24 hours along with the bag, although some facilities recommend changing tubing every 48 to 72 hours. Specific agency policies should always be adhered to.

Test-Taking Strategy: To answer this question accurately, it is necessary to know that the infusion bag should be changed every 24 hours. This will help you eliminate all the incorrect options easily. If this question was difficult, take a few moments to review principles related to TPN at this time!

Level of Cognitive Ability: Application
Phase of Nursing Process: Planning
Client Needs: Safe, Effective Care Environment
Content Area: Fundamental Skills

Reference
Taylor, C., Lillis, C., & LeMone, P. (1997). *Fundamentals of nursing: The art and science of nursing care* (3rd ed.). Philadelphia: Lippincott-Raven. p. 1194.

10. **2**

Rationale: Redness at the catheter insertion site is a possible indication of infection, which could lead to sepsis. The nurse would next assess for other signs of infection. Of the choices given, the temperature is the next item to assess for infection. The tightness of connections should be assessed each time the TPN is checked; if loose, it would result in leakage, not skin redness. The expiration date on the bag is a viable alternative, but that also should be checked at the time the solution is hung, and with each shift change.

Test-Taking Strategy: The key word in the question is "next." To answer this question correctly, it is necessary to understand the significance of the information in the stem as it relates to infection. This would guide you to look for another client-related factor that could indicate infection. Note that option 2 is the only option that relates to physiological integrity!

Level of Cognitive Ability: Application
Phase of Nursing Process: Assessment
Client Needs: Physiological Integrity
Content Area: Fundamental Skills

Reference
Taylor, C., Lillis, C., & LeMone, P. (1997). *Fundamentals of nursing: The art and science of nursing care* (3rd ed.). Philadelphia: Lippincott-Raven. p. 1194.

11. **4**

Rationale: The nurse should not hang a fat emulsion that has visible fat globules. Another solution should be obtained and used instead. In a container that has TPN plus fat emulsion in one solution (three-in-one), the solution should not be used if there is a visible "ring."

Test-Taking Strategy: Remember that options that are similar are not likely to be correct. With this in mind, eliminate options 2 and 3 first. Discriminate between the final two options by knowing the significance of seeing fat globules in the solution. You could also reason the correct option by imagining the potential adverse impact of fat globules entering the client's blood stream.

Level of Cognitive Ability: Application
Phase of Nursing Process: Implementation
Client Needs: Safe, Effective Care Environment
Content Area: Fundamental Skills

Reference
Luckmann, J. (1997). *Saunders manual of nursing care.* Philadelphia: W. B. Saunders. p. 317.

12. 4

Rationale: The status of the TPN infusion should be checked hourly. This helps ensure that the system is running properly and minimizes the possibility that the client will become hyperglycemic or hypoglycemic because of problems with the infusion pump.

Test-Taking Strategy: To answer this question accurately, it is necessary to be familiar with the standard time frames for checking IV solutions and TPN solutions, even when infusing by electronic pump devices. If needed, take a few moments to review the key elements of these procedures now!

Level of Cognitive Ability: Application
Phase of Nursing Process: Implementation
Client Needs: Physiological Integrity
Content Area: Fundamental Skills

Reference
Luckmann, J. (1997). *Saunders manual of nursing care.* Philadelphia: W. B. Saunders. p. 318.

13. 3

Rationale: When a client begins taking a diet following a period of receiving parenteral nutrition, the TPN is usually continued at half the rate initially. Clients often have anorexia after being without food for some time, and the digestive tract is also not used to producing the digestive enzymes that will be needed. Maintaining the solution at half rate allows the client to remain adequately nourished during the transition to a normal diet. It also helps prevent sudden hypoglycemia. Even before clients are started on a solid diet, they are given clear liquids followed by full liquids to further ease the transition.

Test-Taking Strategy: To answer this question correctly, it is necessary to be familiar with TPN and the process of weaning. If needed, take a few moments to review the concepts related to weaning at this time!

Level of Cognitive Ability: Analysis
Phase of Nursing Process: Analysis
Client Needs: Physiological Integrity
Content Area: Fundamental Skills

Reference
Luckmann, J. (1997). *Saunders manual of nursing care.* Philadelphia: W. B. Saunders. p. 321.

14. 1

Rationale: Signs and symptoms of fat overload include fever, leukocytosis, hyperlipidemia, pruritic urticaria, and possibly focal seizures. Hepatosplenomegaly may also be present. The nurse assesses for these signs if a fat emulsion solution infuses too rapidly. Parenteral solutions are infused by electronic pumps to help prevent occurrences such as these.

Test-Taking Strategy: To answer this question accurately, it is necessary to be able to recognize signs and symptoms of fat overload. If needed, take a few moments to review these now!

Level of Cognitive Ability: Application
Phase of Nursing Process: Assessment
Client Needs: Physiological Integrity
Content Area: Fundamental Skills

Reference
Luckmann, J. (1997). *Saunders manual of nursing care.* Philadelphia: W. B. Saunders. p. 321.

15. 3

Rationale: The nurse ensures that the client has intact gag and swallow reflexes. Another important assessment is the presence of bowel sounds. Pulse, blood pressure, and weight are ongoing assessments but are not the most important, given the wording of the question. The client may be expected to have a poor appetite after being without oral intake for a period of time.

Test-Taking Strategy: To answer this question accurately, it is necessary to understand basic physical assessment techniques and the process of weaning from TPN. Option 3 is most closely associated with the issue of the question, feeding the client. This will allow you to eliminate each of the incorrect options systematically.

Level of Cognitive Ability: Application
Phase of Nursing Process: Assessment
Client Needs: Physiological Integrity
Content Area: Fundamental Skills

Reference
Luckmann, J. (1997). *Saunders manual of nursing care.* Philadelphia: W. B. Saunders. p. 321.

16. 4

Rationale: The stomach does send signals to the brain when it is empty to stimulate hunger. The client should be told that this is normal. Some clients also experience food cravings for the same reason. Options 1 and 3 will block the communication process. Option 2 will produce fear in the client.

Test-Taking Strategy: Begin to answer this question by eliminating option 2 first. This response frightens the client and lessens trust in the health care team. Next eliminate options 1 and 3. These statements block communication and do not respond to the client's concerns. Option 4 is the only response that acknowledges the client's concern and addresses it.

Level of Cognitive Ability: Application
Phase of Nursing Process: Implementation
Client Needs: Psychosocial Integrity
Content Area: Fundamental Skills

Reference
Leahy, J., & Kizilay, P. (1998). *Foundations of nursing practice: A nursing process approach.* Philadelphia: W. B. Saunders. p. 784.

17. 1

Rationale: The client should be asked to perform the Valsalva maneuver during tubing changes. This helps avoid air embolism during tubing changes. This is commonly achieved by asking the client to take a deep breath and hold it. If the line is on the right, it may be helpful to have the client turn the head to the left. This allows more room for the nurse to work. However, it is not the most essential action. The other responses are incorrect.

Test-Taking Strategy: Note that the question contains the key words "most essential." This tells you that more than one or all of the responses may be partially or totally correct. Use priority setting to choose correctly. Review the procedure for TPN bag and tubing change now, if you had difficulty with this question!

Level of Cognitive Ability: Application
Phase of Nursing Process: Planning
Client Needs: Safe, Effective Care Environment
Content Area: Fundamental Skills

Reference
Leahy, J., & Kizilay, P. (1998). *Foundations of nursing practice: A nursing process approach.* Philadelphia: W. B. Saunders. p. 785.

18. **2**

Rationale: The nurse should plan to tape all connections in the tubing. This will help prevent the restless client from pulling them apart accidentally. The nurse should also monitor I&O, but this does not specifically relate to a risk for injury as presented in the stem. Client temperature and blood glucose levels should be monitored every 8 hours and every 6 to 8 hours, respectively. This will help detect signs of infection and hyperglycemia early. Options 1 and 3 are also incorrect because the time frames are too infrequent.

Test-Taking Strategy: Note that the question has the key words "restless," "ensure," "prevent," and "injury." These multiple cues guide you to look for the most critical action needed to maintain safety in the client who is restless. Use nursing knowledge to prioritize your answer.

Level of Cognitive Ability: Application
Phase of Nursing Process: Planning
Client Needs: Safe, Effective Care Environment
Content Area: Fundamental Skills

Reference
Leahy, J., & Kizilay, P. (1998). *Foundations of nursing practice: A nursing process approach.* Philadelphia: W. B. Saunders. p. 785.

19. **2**

Rationale: When air embolism is suspected, the client should be placed in a left side-lying position. The head should be lower than the feet. This position is utilized to try to minimize the effect of the air traveling as a bolus to the lungs by trapping it in the right side of the heart.

Test-Taking Strategy: Specific knowledge of client positioning to manage this dangerous complication is needed to answer this question accurately. Take a few moments to review this material if this question was difficult!

Level of Cognitive Ability: Application
Phase of Nursing Process: Implementation
Client Needs: Physiological Integrity
Content Area: Fundamental Skills

Reference
Leahy, J., & Kizilay, P. (1998). *Foundations of nursing practice: A nursing process approach.* Philadelphia: W. B. Saunders. p. 785.

20. **4**

Rationale: The client's signs and symptoms are consistent with fluid overload. The increased intravascular volume increases the blood pressure, while the pulse rate increases

as the heart tries to pump the extra fluid volume. The volume also causes neck vein distention and shifting of fluid into the alveoli, resulting in lung crackles.

Test-Taking Strategy: To answer this question accurately, it is necessary to be familiar with the various complications of TPN and their manifestations. If needed, take a few moments to review the signs and symptoms of these complications now!

Level of Cognitive Ability: Analysis
Phase of Nursing Process: Analysis
Client Needs: Physiological Integrity
Content Area: Fundamental Skills

Reference
Leahy, J., & Kizilay, P. (1998). *Foundations of nursing practice: A nursing process approach.* Philadelphia: W. B. Saunders. p. 785.

21. **1**

Rationale: The nurse places highest priority in teaching the client proper techniques in catheter care. Catheter infection is the most common reason why clients on home TPN are readmitted to the hospital. The client should also know the infusion rate, as well as the importance of monitoring weight and blood glucose.

Test-Taking Strategy: Note that the question contains the key phrases "most critical" and "most common reason." This tells you that more than one option is partially or totally correct. It is necessary to use nursing knowledge related to TPN to prioritize the answer. Proper catheter care will reduce the risk of infection. Review home care measures now, if you had difficulty with this question!

Level of Cognitive Ability: Application
Phase of Nursing Process: Planning
Client Needs: Health Promotion and Maintenance
Content Area: Fundamental Skills

Reference
Leahy, J., & Kizilay, P. (1998). *Foundations of nursing practice: A nursing process approach.* Philadelphia: W. B. Saunders. p. 785.

22. **2**

Rationale: When the client spikes a sudden temperature, or when a low-grade temperature is noted and persists, the solution and tubing should be changed and the discontinued materials should be cultured for infectious organisms. The other responses are incorrect.

Test-Taking Strategy: To answer this question accurately, it is necessary to correlate the elevated temperature with infection of the IV line. This would allow you to eliminate each of the incorrect options systematically. Identifying the issue of the question, infection, should direct you to option 2.

Level of Cognitive Ability: Application
Phase of Nursing Process: Implementation
Client Needs: Safe, Effective Care Environment
Content Area: Fundamental Skills

Reference
Monahan, F., & Neighbors, M. (1998). *Medical-surgical nursing: Foundations for clinical practice* (2nd ed.). Philadelphia: W. B. Saunders. p. 987.

23. **3**

Rationale: If the pump that is infusing TPN becomes shut off for a period of time, the nurse assesses the client for signs and symptoms of hypoglycemia. These include weakness, headache, tingling around the mouth or in extremities, apprehension, diaphoresis, thirst, and hunger. The other signs and symptoms described are hyperglycemia (option 1), infection (option 2), and air embolism (option 4).

Test-Taking Strategy: To answer this question correctly, it is necessary to be able to anticipate the complications that the client receiving TPN may experience. It is also necessary to be familiar with their associated signs and symptoms. This knowledge will allow you to eliminate each of the incorrect options systematically. Review the complications associated with TPN now, if you had difficulty with this question!

Level of Cognitive Ability: Application
Phase of Nursing Process: Assessment
Client Needs: Physiological Integrity
Content Area: Fundamental Skills

Reference

Monahan, F., & Neighbors, M. (1998). *Medical-surgical nursing: Foundations for clinical practice* (2nd ed.). Philadelphia: W. B. Saunders. pp. 987–988.

24. **4**

Rationale: The solution containing the highest amount of glucose should be hung until the new TPN becomes available. Since TPN solutions contain high glucose concentrations (either 25% glucose with central TPN or 10% glucose with peripheral TPN), the 10% glucose solution is the best of the choices presented. The selection of solution should be one that minimizes the risk of hypoglycemia.

Test-Taking Strategy: To answer this question correctly, it is necessary to understand that this particular client is at risk for hypoglycemia. With this in mind, you would then select the solution that minimizes this risk to the client. Remember also that options that are similar are not likely to be correct. Each of the incorrect options representing solutions commonly stocked on the nursing unit contain only 5% dextrose.

Level of Cognitive Ability: Application
Phase of Nursing Process: Implementation
Client Needs: Physiological Integrity
Content Area: Fundamental Skills

Reference

Monahan, F., & Neighbors, M. (1998). *Medical-surgical nursing: Foundations for clinical practice* (2nd ed.). Philadelphia: W. B. Saunders. p. 989.

25. **2**

Rationale: The most appropriate action by the nurse is to remove the filter. This is because the filter could disrupt the emulsion or occlude.

Test-Taking Strategy: To answer this question accurately, it is necessary to know that an inline filter should not be used with fat emulsions. There is no other answer that is correct. If needed, take a few moments to review the key concepts related to fat emulsion therapy!

Level of Cognitive Ability: Application
Phase of Nursing Process: Implementation
Client Needs: Safe, Effective Care Environment
Content Area: Fundamental Skills

Reference

Monahan, F., & Neighbors, M. (1998). *Medical-surgical nursing: Foundations for clinical practice* (2nd ed.). Philadelphia: W. B. Saunders. p. 990.

26. **3**

Rationale: The nurse should piggyback the fat emulsion to the proximal Y-connector of the TPN line. The two solutions are compatible and should be joined at the Y-connector most proximal to the client's central line. This allows the fat emulsion to infuse into a large-diameter catheter. If necessary, fat emulsion may be hung via a peripheral line since the solution is isotonic.

Test-Taking Strategy: Note that the question contains the key word "best." This means that more than one or all of the options may be partially or totally correct. Use the information provided in the stem plus your knowledge of fat emulsion and TPN therapy to prioritize your answer. Review the procedure for the administration of fat emulsions now, if you had difficulty with this question!

Level of Cognitive Ability: Application
Phase of Nursing Process: Implementation
Client Needs: Safe, Effective Care Environment
Content Area: Fundamental Skills

Reference

Monahan, F., & Neighbors, M. (1998). *Medical-surgical nursing: Foundations for clinical practice* (2nd ed.). Philadelphia: W. B. Saunders. p. 990.

27. **2**

Rationale: The nurse should not increase the rate of a fat emulsion to make up the difference if the infusion falls behind. Doing so could place the client at risk for fat overload. The same principle applies to TPN; increasing the rate suddenly in that case could cause hyperglycemia and fluid overload.

Test-Taking Strategy: Note that the question contains the key words "most appropriate." Remember also that options that are similar are not likely to be correct. This guides you to eliminate options 3 and 4 first. Choose option 2 over option 1 using knowledge of fat emulsion infusion therapy and principles related to client safety. Review these safety principles now, if you had difficulty with this question!

Level of Cognitive Ability: Application
Phase of Nursing Process: Implementation
Client Needs: Safe, Effective Care Environment
Content Area: Fundamental Skills

References

Luckmann, J. (1997). *Saunders manual of nursing care.* Philadelphia: W. B. Saunders. p. 320.
Monahan, F., & Neighbors, M. (1998). *Medical-surgical nursing: Foundations for clinical practice* (2nd ed.). Philadelphia: W. B. Saunders. p. 990.

28. **4**

Rationale: TPN that does not have fat emulsion added should have an inline filter added to trap any microorganism, air, or crystals in the solution. Fat emulsions are not recommended to be infused through filters because the small pores clog the filter and thus the tubing. Macrodrip, not microdrip, tubing should be used. It is not necessary to change the dressing purely because a bag is being hung. Extension sets are used only as needed, depending on insertion site and client mobility.

Test-Taking Strategy: Note that the question contains the key words "most important." This tells you that more than one or all of the options may be partially or totally correct.

Begin to answer this question by eliminating options 1 and 3 first. Choose option 4 over option 2 because it should be used on all clients.

Level of Cognitive Ability: Application
Phase of Nursing Process: Planning
Client Needs: Safe, Effective Care Environment
Content Area: Fundamental Skills

Reference
Lehne, R. (1998). *Pharmacology for nursing care* (3rd ed.).

29. **2**

Rationale: The best indicator of whether the client is taking in adequate oral nourishment following TPN is a calorie count. This gives an idea of the total calories consumed and the distribution of the diet in terms of protein, fat, and carbohydrate. I&O is useful as a measure of fluid balance, and the laboratory studies identified give an indication of electrolyte balance.

Test-Taking Strategy: Note that the stem of the question contains the key words "best indicator." This tells you that more than one or all of the options may be partially or totally correct. Use nursing knowledge related to nutrition to prioritize your answer.

Level of Cognitive Ability: Application
Phase of Nursing Process: Evaluation
Client Needs: Health Promotion and Maintenance
Content Area: Fundamental Skills

Reference
Luckmann, J. (1997). *Saunders manual of nursing care.* Philadelphia: W. B. Saunders. p. 321.

30. **1**

Rationale: The client who has a weight gain of 3 pounds per week while receiving TPN is likely to have fluid retention. Optimal weight gain on TPN is 1 to 2 pounds per week. All the other responses are incorrect.

Test-Taking Strategy: To answer this question accurately, it is necessary to understand the anticipated benefits and complications related to TPN. Knowledge of physical assessment parameters related to this area is also useful. If needed, take a few minutes to review the key aspects of TPN at this time!

Level of Cognitive Ability: Application
Phase of Nursing Process: Assessment
Client Needs: Physiological Integrity
Content Area: Fundamental Skills

Reference
Pinnell, N. (1996). *Nursing pharmacology.* Philadelphia: W. B. Saunders. p. 1034.

BIBLIOGRAPHY

Jaffee, M., & McVan, B. (1997). *Davis's laboratory and diagnostic test handbook.* Philadelphia: F. A. Davis.

Leahy, J., & Kizilay, P. (1998). *Foundations of nursing practice: A nursing process approach.* Philadelphia: W. B. Saunders.

Lehne, R. (1998). *Pharmacology for nursing care* (3rd ed.). Philadelphia: W. B. Saunders.

Luckmann, J. (1997). *Saunders manual of nursing care.* Philadelphia. W. B. Saunders.

Mahan, L., & Escott-Stump, S. (1996). *Krause's food, nutrition, & diet therapy* (9th ed.). Philadelphia: W. B. Saunders.

Monahan, F., & Neighbors, M. (1998). *Medical-surgical nursing: Foundations for clinical practice* (2nd ed.). Philadelphia: W. B. Saunders.

Pinnell, N. (1996). *Nursing pharmacology.* Philadelphia: W. B. Saunders. p. 1034.

Taylor, C., Lillis, C., & LeMone, P. (1997). *Fundamentals of nursing: The art and science of nursing care* (3rd ed.). Philadelphia: Lippincott-Raven.

CHAPTER 13

Intravenous Therapy

PYRAMID TERMS

Isotonic—Solutions that have the same osmolality as body fluids.

Hypotonic—Solutions that are more dilute or have a lower osmolality than body fluids.

Hypertonic—Solutions that are more concentrated or have a higher osmolality than body fluids.

Phlebitis—An inflammation of the vein that can occur from either mechanical or chemical (medication) trauma or a local infection.

Infiltration—Seepage of the intravenous (IV) fluid out of the vein into the surrounding interstitial spaces.

Air Embolism—The bolus of air that enters the vein through an inadequately primed IV line, from a loose connection, or during tubing change or removal of the IV.

Speed Shock—Occurs when the IV infusion is administered too rapidly, resulting in fluid volume overload.

◆ PYRAMID TO SUCCESS

Professional nurses are responsible for managing and providing care to clients receiving IV therapy. Pyramid points focus on the safe measures required to initiate and maintain an IV, monitoring for complications related to the IV, and the initiation of measures required when an IV complication occurs. The focus is on the signs and symptoms of infiltration, phlebitis, circulatory overload, and air embolism, and the treatment measures associated with each.

NURSING PROCESS

ASSESSMENT

Physician's order related to IV therapy
IV administration techniques
Hydration status, electrolyte balance, acid-base balance
Health history and existing conditions
Vital signs
Weight and intake and output (I&O)
Cardiovascular assessment
Integumentary assessment
Gastrointestinal (GI) assessment
Renal assessment

ANALYSIS: Fluid Volume Deficit
Fluid Volume Excess
Potential for Complications

PLANNING	IMPLEMENTATION	EVALUATION
Client maintains adequate I&O and hydration status. Client is free of signs and symptoms of complications related to IV therapy. Client or family identifies care measures related to the IV.	Assess physician's order related to IV therapy. Assess health history and existing conditions in client. Perform IV administration techniques according to agency policy. Monitor IV frequently. Monitor vital signs, weight, and I&O. Monitor electrolytes and hydration status. Monitor for complications related to IV therapy. Teach client or family about care of the IV. Initiate home care support services as necessary.	Fluid balance and electrolyte balance is established. Client tolerates IV therapy without complications. Client or family demonstrates appropriate care of IV.

◆ CLIENT NEEDS

SAFE, EFFECTIVE CARE ENVIRONMENT

Informed consent for central venous catheters
Consultation to surgeon if necessary
Error prevention in administering IVs
Handling hazardous or infectious materials
Asepsis
Standard (universal) precautions

HEALTH PROMOTION AND MAINTENANCE

Health and wellness
Lifestyle choices related to home care of IV
Teaching client and family regarding care of IV

PSYCHOSOCIAL INTEGRITY

Assessment of coping mechanisms
Support systems in the home for caring for IV

PHYSIOLOGICAL INTEGRITY

Intravenous therapy
Parenteral therapies
Expected effects of IV therapy
Monitoring laboratory values for fluid and electrolyte imbalances
Monitoring for complications of IV therapy

I. Intravenous Therapy

A. Purpose and uses
   1. Used to sustain clients who are unable to take substances orally
   2. Replaces water, electrolytes, and nutrients more rapidly than oral administration
   3. Provides immediate access to the vascular system for the rapid delivery of specific solutions without the time required for GI tract absorption
   4. Provides a vascular route for the administration of medication or blood components
B. Types of solutions (Table 13–1)
   1. **Isotonic**
      a. Solutions with the same osmolality as body fluids
      b. Do not enter the cells because there is no osmotic force to shift the fluids
      c. Increase extracellular fluid (ECF) volume

   2. **Hypotonic**
      a. Solutions that are more dilute or have a lower osmolality than body fluids
      b. Dilute extracellular fluid and cause movement of water into cells by osmosis
      c. These solutions should be administered slowly to prevent cellular edema
   3. **Hypertonic**
      a. Solutions that are more concentrated or have a higher osmolality than body fluids
      b. Concentrate ECF and cause movement of water from cells into the ECF by osmosis
   4. Crystalloids
      a. Solutions that contain electrolytes
      b. May be used for fluid volume replacement
   5. Colloids
      a. Also called plasma expanders
      b. Pull fluid from the interstitial compartment into the vascular compartment
      c. Used to increase the vascular volume rapidly, such as in hemorrhage or severe hypovolemia

II. Intravenous Devices

A. IV cannulas
   1. Steel needles or butterfly set
      a. A wing-tip needle with a metal cannula, plastic or rubber wings, and a plastic catheter or hub
      b. The needle is 0.5 to 1.5 mm in length with needle gauge sizes from 16 to 26
      c. Used when the infusion time will be short
      d. **Infiltration** is more common with these devices
      e. The butterfly infusion set may commonly be used in children and elderly people, whose veins are likely to be small or fragile
   2. Plastic cannulas
      a. May be either an over-the-needle device or an in-needle catheter
      b. Over-the-needle consists of a plastic catheter mounted over a needle; after venipuncture, the catheter is guided off the needle and into the vein
      c. Over-the-needle is preferred for rapid

Table 13–1. **Types of Intravenous Solutions**

Solution	Tonicity
0.45% saline (½ NS)	Hypotonic
0.9% saline (NS)	Isotonic
0.225% saline (¼ NS)	Hypotonic
0.33% saline (⅓ NS)	Hypotonic
3% saline (3% NS)	Hypertonic
5% saline (5% NS)	Hypertonic
5% dextrose in water (D5W)	Isotonic before administration; hypotonic effect in the body after sugar enters cells
10% dextrose in water (D10W)	Hypertonic before administration; hypotonic effect in the body after sugar enters cells
5% dextrose in 0.9% saline (5% D/NS)	Hypertonic
5% dextrose in 0.45% saline (5% D/½ NS)	Hypertonic before administration; hypotonic effect in the body after sugar enters cells
5% dextrose in 0.225% saline (5% D/¼ NS)	Isotonic before administration; hypotonic effect in the body after sugar enters cells
Lactated Ringer's (RL) solution	Isotonic
5% dextrose in lactated Ringer's solution	Hypertonic
Dextran	Colloid
Albumin	Colloid

infusion and is more comfortable for the client

d. After venipuncture, the in-needle catheter is guided through the needle into the vein, and the needle is removed from the catheter

e. The in-needle catheter can cause catheter embolism if the tip of the cannula breaks

f. The in-needle and over-the-needle catheters are primarily used for short term therapy

B. IV gauges
1. The smaller the gauge number, the larger the outside diameter of the cannula
2. The size used depends on the solution to be administered and the diameter of the available vein
3. Larger gauges allow a higher fluid rate than smaller ones and allow the administration of higher concentrations of solutions
4. For rapid emergency fluid administration, blood products, or anesthetics, use a large gauge, such as a 14-, 16-, 18-, or 19-gauge needle
5. For peripheral fat infusions, use a 20- or 21-gauge
6. For standard IV fluid and clear liquid medications, use a 22- or 24-gauge
7. If the client has very small veins, use a 24- to 25-gauge

C. IV containers
1. Container may be glass or plastic
2. Squeeze the plastic bag to ensure intactness and assess glass bottle for any cracks before hanging
3. Do not write on the plastic IV bag with a marking pen because it may be absorbed into the solution
4. Use a label and a ballpoint pen for marking the bag, placing the label onto the bag

D. Vented and nonvented tubing
1. A vent allows air to enter the IV container as the fluid leaves

2. A vented adapter can be used to add a vent to a nonvented IV tubing system
3. Use nonvented tubing for flexible containers
4. Use a vented tubing for glass or rigid plastic containers to allow air to enter and displace the fluid as it leaves; fluid will not flow from a rigid IV container unless it is vented

E. Drip chambers
1. Microdrip chamber
   a. Normally this has a short vertical metal piece where the drop forms
   b. Delivers between 50 and 60 drops per millimeter
   c. Read the tubing package to determine how many drops per milliliter are delivered (drop factor)
   d. Used if fluid will be infused at a slow rate (less than 50 mL per hour)
   e. Used if the solution contains potent medication that needs to be titrated, such as in a critical care setting or in pediatrics
2. Macrodrip chamber
   a. Drop factor varies from 8 to 20 drops per millimeter
   b. Used if the solution is thick or is to infuse rapidly
   c. Read the tubing package to determine how many drops per milliliter are delivered (drop factor)

F. Filters
1. Provide protection by preventing particles from entering the client's veins
2. Used in IV lines to trap small particles such as undissolved antibiotics or salt, or medications that have precipitated in solution
3. Assess the agency policy regarding the use of filters
4. Use a 0.22-micron filter for most solutions, a 1.2-micron filter for solutions containing lipids or albumin, and a special filter for blood components
5. Change filters every 24 to 72 hours (depending on agency policy) to prevent bacterial growth

G. Tubing
   1. Add extension tubing for children, clients who are restless, or clients who have special mobility needs
   2. Use shorter secondary tubing for piggyback solutions, connecting them to the injection sites nearest the drip chamber
   3. Use special tubing for medication that absorbs into plastic
H. Needleless systems
   1. Include recessed needles, plastic cannulas, or one-way valves, and decrease the exposure to contaminated needles
   2. Do not administer total parenteral nutrition (TPN) or blood products through a one-way valve
I. Intermittent infusion sets
   1. Used when intravascular accessibility is desired for intermittent administration of medications by either IV push or IV piggyback
   2. An IV lock is attached for intermittent infusion devices
   3. Patency is maintained with periodic flushing with normal saline solution
   4. When administering medication, flush with 1 to 2 mL (depending on agency policy) of **isotonic** saline to confirm placement of the cannula; administer the prescribed medication, then flush the cannula again with 1 to 2 mL (depending on agency policy) of **isotonic** saline to maintain patency

III. Selection of a Peripheral Venous Site

A. Veins in the hand, forearm, and antecubital fossa are suitable sites
B. Veins in the lower extremities are not suitable due to the risk of thrombus formation and possible pooling of medication in areas of decreased venous return (Box 13–1)
C. Veins in the scalp and feet may be suitable sites for infants
D. The most frequently used sites are the veins of the forearm, because the bones of the forearm act as a natural support and splint
E. Assess the veins of both arms very closely before selecting a site
F. Start the IV infusion distally to provide the option of proceeding up the extremity if the vein is ruptured or **infiltration** occurs; if **infiltration** occurs from the antecubital vein, the lower veins usually cannot be used for further puncture sites

---

BOX 13–1. Peripheral Intravenous Sites to Avoid

- Edematous extremity
- An arm that is weak, traumatized, or paralyzed
- The arm on the same side as a mastectomy
- An arm that has an arteriovenous fistula or shunt for dialysis

---

G. Determine the client's dominant side and select the opposite side for a venipuncture site
H. Bending the elbow on the arm with an IV may easily obstruct the flow of solution, causing **infiltration** that could lead to thrombophlebitis
I. Avoid checking the blood pressure on the arm receiving the IV infusion
J. Do not place restraints over the venipuncture site
K. Use an armboard when the venipuncture site is located in an area of flexion

IV. Adding Medication to an IV

A. Assess for compatibility of medication and solution
B. When adding medication to the bag, mix the bag end-to-end several times before hanging it to disperse the medication
C. Ensure that medication can be mixed into soft plastic, as some medications absorb into the soft plastic and should only be mixed in glass

V. Administering IV Solutions

A. The IV solution should be checked against the physician's orders for the type, amount, percent of solution, and rate of flow
B. Assess the health status and medical disorders present in the client
C. Assess situations that contraindicate particular IV solutions
D. Wash hands thoroughly before inserting an IV and before working with an IV
E. Use sterile technique when inserting an IV and when changing the dressing over the IV site
F. When inserting an IV, clean the skin with an antimicrobial solution with an inner to outer circular motion
G. Prime the tubing to remove air from the system
H. Change the venipuncture site every 48 to 72 hours, depending on agency policy
I. Change the IV dressing every 72 hours, when the dressing is wet or contaminated, or as specified by agency policy
J. Change the IV tubing every 24 to 72 hours, depending on agency policy
K. Label the tubing, dressing, and solution bags clearly, including the date and time when changed
L. Do not let an IV bag or bottle hang for more than 24 hours
M. Do not allow the IV tubing to touch the floor
N. Before adding medications or solutions, swab access ports with 70% alcohol, another equally effective solution, or as specified by the agency policy

VI. IV Precautions

A. An IV can cause initial pain and discomfort on insertion for the client
B. An IV provides a route of entry for microorganisms into the body

C. Medications enter the blood immediately, and any adverse reactions or allergic responses can occur immediately

D. Fluid overload or electrolyte imbalances can occur from an excessive or too rapid infusion of fluids

E. Incompatibilities between certain solutions and medications can occur

F. Clients with renal and liver diseases, elderly clients, and very young persons cannot tolerate an excessive fluid volume, and the risk of fluid overload exists with these clients

G. A client with congestive heart failure is usually not given a saline solution because this type of fluid encourages the retention of water and would therefore exacerbate heart failure by increasing the fluid overload

H. A diabetic client typically does not receive dextrose (sugar) solutions

VII. Complications (Table 13–2)

A. Infection
   1. Description
      a. The entry of microorganisms into the body through the venipuncture site
      b. Venipuncture interrupts the integrity of the skin, the first line of defense against infection

Table 13–2. Signs of Complications of Intravenous Therapy

Complication	Signs
Phlebitis	Heat, redness, tenderness at site
	Not swollen or hard
	IV infusion sluggish
Thrombophlebitis	Hard and cordlike vein
	Heat, redness, tenderness at site
	IV infusion sluggish
Infiltration	Edema, pain, and coolness at site
	May or may not have a blood return
Catheter embolism	Decrease in blood pressure (BP)
	Pain along vein
	Weak, rapid pulse
	Cyanosis of nailbeds
	Loss of consciousness
Fluid overload	Increased BP
	Distended jugular veins
	Rapid breathing
	Dyspnea
	Moist cough and crackles
Speed shock	Flushed face
	Severe headache
	Chest pain
	Irregular pulse
	Decreased BP
	Loss of consciousness
	Cardiac arrest can occur
Air embolus	Tachycardia
	Dyspnea
	Cyanosis
	Hypotension
	Decreased level of consciousness

c. The longer the therapy continues, the greater the risk of infection

2. At-risk clients
   a. Immunocompromised clients from diseases such as cancer or acquired immunodeficiency syndrome (AIDS)
   b. Clients receiving treatments, such as chemotherapy, that have altered or lowered the WBC count
   c. Elderly client, because aging alters the effectiveness of the immune system

3. Prevention and implementation
   a. Assess client for predisposition or risk for infection
   b. Maintain strict asepsis when caring for the IV site
   c. Monitor vital signs, particularly temperature
   d. Monitor WBC counts
   e. Perform frequent assessment and monitor for local inflammation at the IV site
   f. Check fluid containers for cracks, leaks, or cloudiness or other evidence of contamination
   g. Change tubing and site dressing every 24 to 72 hours according to agency policy
   h. Use antimicrobial ointment at the IV site
   i. Label the IV site, bag or bottle, and tubing with the date and time to ensure that it is changed on time according to agency policy
   j. Ensure that the IV solution is not hanging for more than 24 hours
   k. Monitor for systemic infection, which will include malaise, headache, chills, fever, nausea, vomiting, backache, tachycardia
   l. If infection occurs, discontinue the IV, place a sterile cover on the venipuncture device for possible culture, and notify the physician
   m. Prepare to obtain blood cultures as prescribed if infection occurs
   n. Restart an IV in the opposite arm to differentiate sepsis from local infection at the IV site
   o. Document the assessment of the finding related to infection

B. Tissue damage
   1. Description
      a. Tissues most commonly damaged include the skin, veins, and subcutaneous tissue
      b. Tissue damage can be uncomfortable and can cause permanent negative effects
   2. Prevention and implementation
      a. Use a careful and gentle approach when applying a tourniquet
      b. Avoid tapping the skin over the vein when starting an IV
      c. Monitor for ecchymosis when penetrating the skin with the cannula
      d. Assess for any allergies to tape or dressing adhesives

e. Notify the physician if tissue damage is suspected

f. Document the assessment of the tissue damage and its effects

C. **Phlebitis** and thrombophlebitis

1. Description

a. An inflammation of the vein that can occur from either mechanical or chemical (medication) trauma or a local infection

b. Phlebitis can cause the development of a clot (thrombophlebitis)

2. Prevention and implementation

a. Use an IV cannula smaller than the vein and avoid very small veins when administering irritating solutions

b. Avoid using the lower extremities as an access area for the IV

c. Avoid venipuncture over an area of flexion

d. Anchor the cannula and a loop of tubing securely with tape

e. Use an armboard or a splint if the client is restless or active

f. Change the venipuncture site every 48 to 72 hours, depending on agency policy

g. If **phlebitis** occurs, remove the IV device immediately and restart it in the opposite extremity

h. Notify the physician if **phlebitis** is suspected, and apply warm, moist compresses as prescribed

i. If thrombophlebitis occurs, never irrigate the IV catheter; remove the IV, notify the physician, and restart in the opposite extremity

j. Document the assessment of the **phlebitis** or thrombophlebitis and its effects

D. Infiltration

1. Description

a. A form of tissue damage that is also called extravasation

b. Seepage of the IV fluid out of the vein into the surrounding interstitial spaces

c. Occurs when an access device has become dislodged or perforates the wall of the vein, or when vein back pressure occurs due to a clot or venospasm

2. Prevention and implementation

a. Avoid venipuncture over an area of flexion

b. Anchor the cannula and a loop of tubing securely with tape

c. Use an armboard or splint if the client is restless or active

d. Assess the IV site for pain, edema, or coolness, comparing it with the opposite extremity

e. Monitor the IV rate for a decrease or a halt in flow

f. Evaluate the IV site for **infiltration** by occluding the vein proximal to the IV site; if the IV fluid continues to flow, the cannula is probably outside the vein (infiltrated); if the IV flow stops after occluding the vein, the IV device is still in the vein

g. Lower the IV fluid container below the IV site and monitor for the appearance of blood in the IV tubing; if blood appears, the IV device is in the vein

h. If **infiltration** has occurred, the IV device is removed immediately

i. Do not to rub an infiltrated area, which can cause the development of a hematoma

j. If **infiltration** has occurred, elevate the extremity and apply compresses (warm or cool, depending on the solution and the physician's order) over the affected area

k. Document the assessment of the **infiltration,** its effects, and the action taken

E. Catheter embolism

1. Description: The tip of the catheter breaks off during IV insertion or removal, resulting in the possibility of an embolus

2. Prevention and implementation

a. Remove the catheter carefully

b. Inspect the catheter when removed

c. If the catheter tip has broken off, place a tourniquet high on the limb of the IV site, notify the physician immediately, prepare to obtain an x-ray, and prepare the client for surgery to remove pieces if prescribed

F. Circulatory overload

1. Description: Results from the administration of fluids too rapidly or in a client at risk for fluid overload

2. Prevention and implementation

a. Identify clients at risk for circulatory overload

b. Calculate and monitor the drip rate frequently

c. Use an infusion controller device and frequently check the drip rate or pump setting, particularly in clients at risk for overload

d. Add a time strip to the IV bag or bottle

e. If circulatory overload occurs, elevate the head of the bed, keep the client warm, assess for edema, decrease the drip rate to a minimum at a keep vein open (KVO) rate, notify the physician

f. Document the assessment and actions taken

G. **Speed shock**

1. Description: The IV infusion is administered too rapidly, resulting in fluid volume overload

2. Prevention and implementation

a. Calculate and monitor the drip rate frequently

b. Use an infusion controller device and frequently check the drip rate or pump setting

c. Add a time strip to the IV bag or bottle

d. If **speed shock** occurs, stop the infusion, notify the physician, and monitor VS (vital signs)

H. Electrolyte overload
   1. Description: An electrolyte imbalance caused by too rapid, excessive, or inappropriate IV solution
   2. Prevention and implementation
      a. Assess laboratory value reports
      b. Verify the correct solution
      c. Calculate and monitor the drip rate
      d. Use an infusion controller device and frequently check the drip rate or pump setting
      e. Add a time strip to the IV bag or bottle
      f. Place a colored sticker on the bag or bottle if a medication has been added to the IV solution
I. Hematoma
   1. Description: The collection of blood in the tissues following an unsuccessful venipuncture or after the venipuncture site is discontinued
   2. Prevention and implementation
      a. When starting an IV, avoid piercing the posterior wall of the vein
      b. Do not apply a tourniquet to an extremity immediately following an unsuccessful venipuncture
      c. When discontinuing an IV, apply pressure to the site for at least 1 minute and elevate the extremity; apply pressure longer for clients with a bleeding disorder on anticoagulants
      d. Monitor for hard and painful lumps at the site
      e. If a hematoma develops, elevate the extremity and apply pressure and ice as prescribed
J. **Air embolism**
   1. Description: A bolus of air enters the vein through an inadequately primed IV line, from a loose connection, or during tubing change or removal of the IV
   2. Prevention and implementation
      a. Prime tubing with fluid before use and monitor for any air bubbles in the tubing
      b. Secure all connections
      c. Replace the IV fluid before the bag or bottle is dry
      d. If an air embolus is suspected, clamp the tubing, turn the client on the left side with the head of the bed lowered to trap the air in the right atrium, and notify the physician
      e. A possible "mill wheel murmur," a continuous loud, turning sound over the precordium due to air in the right ventricle, may be heard

VIII. Central Venous Catheters

A. Description
   1. Placed in large central veins, such as the superior vena cava
   2. Used to deliver hyperosmolar solutions, to measure central venous pressure, to infuse TPN or multiple IV infusions or medications
   3. Catheter position is determined by x-ray following insertion
   4. May have a single, double, or triple lumen
   5. May be inserted peripherally and threaded through the basilic or cephalic vein into the superior vena cava, centrally through the internal jugular or subclavian veins, or surgically tunneled through subcutaneous tissue into the cephalic vein
   6. With multilumen catheters, more than one medication can be administered at the same time without incompatibility problems, and there is only one insertion site for care
   7. For central line insertion, tubing change, and line removal, place client in the Trendelenburg position if not contraindicated and instruct the client to perform the Valsalva maneuver to increase pressure in central veins while the system is open
B. Tunneled central venous catheters
   1. A more permanent type of catheter, such as the Hickman or Broviac, used for long-term IV therapy
   2. May be single or multilumen
   3. Inserted in the operating room, and the catheter is threaded into the lower part of the vena cava at the entrance of the right atrium
   4. The catheter will be fitted with an intermittent infusion devise to allow access as needed and to keep the system closed and intact
   5. Patency is maintained with a heparin flush per agency policy
   6. Groshong's catheters require only normal saline instillation for patency
C. Vascular access ports
   1. Surgically implanted under the skin; used for long-term administration of repeated IV therapy
   2. Require palpation and injection through the skin into the self-sealing port for access with a noncoring needle such as a Huber-point needle
   3. Patency is maintained by periodic flushing with a diluted heparin solution per agency policy
D. Peripherally inserted central catheter (PICC) line
   1. Used for long-term IV therapy, frequently in the home
   2. The basilic vein is usually used, but the median cubital and cephalic veins in the antecubital area can also be used
   3. Threaded so that the catheter tip may terminate in either the axillary or subclavian vein or superior vena cava
   4. A small amount of bleeding may occur at the time of insertion and continue for 24 hours, but bleeding thereafter is not expected
   5. **Phlebitis** is a common complication
   6. Insertion is below the heart level; therefore, **air embolism** is not common

PRACTICE QUESTIONS

1. The nurse has just added potassium chloride, 20 mEq, to an IV bag of 1000 ml 5% dextrose in water. The nurse should next:
   1 Rotate the bag gently
   2 Place the time tape on the IV
   3 Attach the tubing to the client
   4 Check the solution again for particles

2. The nurse is preparing to administer an antibiotic by intermittent IV infusion, piggybacked to a mainline IV. The nurse should plan to administer the antibiotic by:
   1 Disconnecting the main solution and plugging in the antibiotic
   2 Hanging the antibiotic solution higher than the mainline IV
   3 Hanging the antibiotic solution lower than the mainline IV
   4 Hanging the antibiotic solution level with the mainline IV

3. The client with a heparin lock has an order to receive 1000 mL 5% dextrose in 0.45% sodium chloride. After gathering the appropriate equipment, the nurse takes which of the following actions first before spiking the IV bag with the tubing?
   1 Uncaps the spike portion of the tubing
   2 Uncaps the distal end of the tubing
   3 Closes the roller clamp on the IV tubing
   4 Opens the roller clamp on the IV tubing

4. The nurse is inserting an IV line into a client's vein. The nurse interprets that the catheter is correctly placed when the nurse first notes which of the following?
   1 The vein is distended under the needle
   2 The client does not complain of discomfort
   3 The catheter advances easily
   4 There is blood return in the backflash chamber of the catheter

5. The nurse has an order to infuse 1000 mL of 5% dextrose in lactated Ringer's at 80 mL/hr. The nurse time-tapes the bag with a start time of 07:00. After making hourly marks on the time-tape, the nurse notes that the completion time for the bag is:
   1 17:00
   2 17:30
   3 19:30
   4 21:00

6. The nurse is explaining the advantages of a peripherally inserted central catheter (PICC) to a client scheduled to have one inserted. Which of the following would not be included by the nurse in an explanation of the advantages of this type of catheter?

1 It is cost effective
2 It is the ideal catheter for short-term use
3 There is less pain and discomfort
4 This type of catheter is very reliable

7. The nurse has given instructions to the client being discharged to home with a PICC. The nurse evaluates that the client does not fully understand the information given if the client states he will:
   1 Have a repair kit available in the home for use if needed
   2 Wear a Medic-Alert tag or bracelet
   3 Keep activity level to a minimum while this catheter is in place
   4 Keep the insertion site protected when in the shower or bath

8. The nurse is assessing the IV dressing of a client with a peripheral IV infusion running. The date on the dressing is 3/20 (March 20). The nurse calculates that the dressing should be changed on which of the following dates?
   1 3/21
   2 3/23
   3 3/25
   4 3/27

9. The nurse is doing a routine assessment of a client's peripheral IV site. The nurse notes that the site is cool, pale, and swollen. The IV has stopped running. The nurse interprets that which of the following has probably occurred?
   1 Infiltration
   2 Phlebitis
   3 Thrombosis
   4 Infection

10. The nurse assesses that the client has developed phlebitis at the site of a current IV infusion. Which of the following actions are contraindicated by the nurse?
    1 Discontinue the IV catheter at that site
    2 Notify the physician
    3 Apply warm, moist packs to the site
    4 Start a new line in a proximal portion of the same vein

11. The nurse is orienting a new RN to the nursing unit. The nurse would intervene if the newcomer did which of the following while changing the hospital gown of a client with a peripheral IV line being used for fluid replacement?
    1 Used a hospital gown with snaps at the sleeves
    2 Put the bag and tubing through the sleeve, followed by the client's arm
    3 Disconnected the IV tubing from the angio-catheter
    4 Removed the tubing temporarily from an infusion pump after closing the roller clamp

12. The nurse is making a worksheet for assessments to be made during the shift on assigned clients. The nurse writes on the plan to check the IV of an assigned client receiving fluid replacement therapy every:
    1 4 hours
    2 3 hours
    3 2 hours
    4 1 hour

13. The client had a 1000-mL bag of 5% dextrose in 0.9% sodium chloride hung at 07:00. The nurse making rounds at 08:00 finds the client complaining of a pounding headache and is dyspneic, with chills, apprehension, and an increased pulse rate. The IV bag has 300 mL remaining. The first action of the nurse is to:
    1 Shut off the infusion
    2 Discontinue the angiocatheter
    3 Sit the client up in bed
    4 Call the physician

14. The nurse is assessing the insertion site of a peripheral IV catheter. The nurse notes the site to be reddened, warm, painful, and slightly edematous in the area of the vein that is proximal to the IV catheter. The nurse interprets that this is most likely due to:
    1 Infiltration of the IV line
    2 Phlebitis of the vein
    3 Hypersensitivity to the IV solution
    4 An allergic reaction to the IV catheter material

15. The nurse has an order to convert an existing IV to a heparin lock. After priming the device, the nurse makes the switch from the IV to the lock while doing which of the following with the non-dominant hand?
    1 Holding pressure on the vein distal to the insertion site
    2 Stabilizing the hub of the angiocatheter
    3 Closing the roller on the IV tubing
    4 Pinching the IV tubing near the insertion site

16. The nurse must teach the client scheduled for discharge about the management of home IV infusion therapy. The nurse begins the process by first teaching the client principles related to:
    1 Proper handwashing technique
    2 The handling of equipment
    3 Where to obtain supplies
    4 How to report signs of infection

17. The nurse has a written order to discontinue an IV line. The nurse removes the catheter by withdrawing the catheter while applying pressure to the site with a(n):
    1 Alcohol swab
    2 Betadine swab
    3 Band-Aid
    4 Sterile 2×2 gauze

18. The nurse has an order to infuse a 50-mL solution containing 150 mg of ranitidine (Zantac) by IV piggyback over 30 minutes BID. The administration set has a drop factor of 10 gtt/mL. The nurse would regulate the roller clamp on the infusion set to deliver how many drops per minute?
    1 9
    2 17
    3 30
    4 50

19. The nurse is preparing to insert an IV angiocatheter in the client's inner forearm. Before cannulating the vein, the nurse cleanses the entry site using which of the following motions?
    1 Scrubbing from wrist toward elbow
    2 Scrubbing from elbow toward wrist
    3 Using a circular motion from the center outward
    4 Using a circular motion inward toward the center

20. The client requiring IV insertion has difficult veins to find. The nurse plans to avoid doing which of the following to help distend the vein?
    1 Placing a cool compress over the site for 10 to 15 minutes
    2 Placing a warm compress over the site for 10 to 15 minutes
    3 Lowering the arm below heart level
    4 Lightly tapping over the vein after applying a tourniquet

21. The nurse has just inserted an IV line on a client. Which of the following actions does the nurse complete last after cannulating the vein?
    1 Attaching the primed IV tubing
    2 Observing for signs of infiltration
    3 Beginning the flow of IV fluid
    4 Releasing the tourniquet

22. The nurse has an order to administer diazepam (Valium), 5 mg, IV push through an IV line of 1000 mL 5% dextrose in 0.45% sodium chloride with 40 mEq potassium chloride added. Which of the following should the nurse plan to do first to carry out this order?
    1 Draw up the medication in a 3-mL syringe
    2 Check the compatibility of diazepam with the IV solution
    3 Check the client's identification bracelet
    4 Pinch off the IV tubing above the injection port

23. The nurse is about to administer an IV push medication through a heparin lock. The nurse should do which of the following with the non-dominant hand while piercing the heparin lock port with the dominant one?
    1 Apply pressure over the catheter insertion site
    2 Hold a watch that has a second hand
    3 Stabilize the port of the heparin lock
    4 Wipe with an alcohol swab

24. The nurse is caring for a client who has just had insertion of a central venous catheter done at the bedside. The nurse would check the results of which of the following before beginning an IV infusion ordered to run at 125 mL/hr?
    1 Portable chest radiograph
    2 Lung scan
    3 Serum electrolytes
    4 Serum osmolality

25. The client is hypovolemic and plasma expanders are not available. The nurse anticipates that which of the following solutions available on the unit will be ordered?
    1 5% dextrose in 0.45% sodium chloride
    2 5% dextrose in water
    3 0.9% sodium chloride
    4 0.45% sodium chloride

26. The nurse has taught an RN orientee about care of a multilumen central venous catheter. The nurse evaluates that the orientee has understood the information presented if the orientee states to discard and replace the injection cap on a lumen:
    1 At the change of each shift
    2 Whenever blood is drawn from the lumen
    3 After administration of each medication
    4 Once a week

27. The nurse must temporarily remove the IV line from an electronic infusion pump while it is still attached to the client's IV catheter. The nurse makes sure to take which of the following most essential actions?

    1 Ensure that the pump is unplugged
    2 Check the amount of solution that has infused
    3 Close the roller clamp on the IV tubing
    4 Assess the insertion site while in the client's room

28. The client is scheduled to be discharged to home with continuous IV infusion therapy. The nurse questions the issue regarding whether the client is a good candidate for this type of therapy after first noting that the client:
    1 Is medically stable
    2 Has a telephone
    3 Has a working refrigerator
    4 Lives alone

29. The nurse primes the IV tubing, and then uncaps the distal end of the tubing to attach a needleless device. Before attachment, however, the tubing drops and hits the top of the medication cart. The nurse should plan to do which of the following?
    1 Attach a new needleless device
    2 Change the IV tubing
    3 Wipe the tubing port with Betadine
    4 Scrub the needleless device with an alcohol swab

30. The nurse is completing a time tape for a 1000-mL IV bag that is scheduled to infuse over 8 hours. The nurse has just placed the 11:00 marking at the 500 mL level. The nurse would place the mark for 12:00 at which of the following levels on the time tape?
    1 425 mL
    2 400 mL
    3 375 mL
    4 350 mL

ANSWERS

1. **1**

Rationale: After adding a medication to a bag of IV solution, the nurse should agitate or rotate the bag gently to mix the medication evenly in the solution. Then the nurse should attach the label stating which medication was added. The nurse can then place a time tape if this has not been done. The IV solution should have been checked for particulate matter before adding the medication to the solution.

Test-Taking Strategy: Note that the question contains the key word "next." This denotes a particular time sequence. Visualize and think through the steps of adding medication to an IV bag, and make your choice accordingly. Review the procedure for adding potassium to an IV bag now, if you had difficulty with this question!

Level of Cognitive Ability: Application
Phase of Nursing Process: Implementation
Client Needs: Safe, Effective Care Environment
Content Area: Fundamental Skills

Reference
Leahy, J., & Kizilay, P. (1998). *Foundations of nursing practice: A nursing process approach.* Philadelphia: W. B. Saunders. p. 488.

2. **2**

Rationale: For an intermittent IV infusion that is piggy-backed to the mainline IV, the intermittent infusion (in this case, the antibiotic) is placed higher than the mainline solution. This allows gravity to assist in infusing the medication. Once the intermittent infusion is complete, the mainline IV will resume at the drip rate set for the secondary infusion. For this reason, it is also important to remember to check the infusion frequently and reset the main drip rate correctly once the secondary infusion is complete.

Test-Taking Strategy: This question tests a fundamental principle related to intravenous therapy. Think about the principles related to gravity when answering this question. If this question was difficult, take a few moments to review the key aspects of this procedure at this time!

Level of Cognitive Ability: Application
Phase of Nursing Process: Planning
Client Needs: Safe, Effective Care Environment
Content Area: Fundamental Skills

Reference
Leahy, J., & Kizilay, P. (1998). *Foundations of nursing practice: A nursing process approach.* Philadelphia: W. B. Saunders. p. 813.

3. 3

Rationale: The nurse should first clamp the tubing to prevent the solution from running freely through the tubing once it is attached to the IV bag. The nurse should next uncap the proximal (spike) portion of the tubing. Then, the roller clamp is opened slowly and the fluid is allowed to flow through the tubing in a controlled fashion to prevent air from remaining in parts of the tubing. Finally, the distal end of the tubing is uncapped and attached to the needle or needleless device, which is then attached to the client's heparin lock. An alternative method is to uncap the distal end of the tubing and attach the tubing directly to the hub of the client's IV line.

Test-Taking Strategy: This question tests a specific procedure related to IV therapy. Attempt to visualize this process in order to answer the question correctly. If this question was difficult, take a few moments to review the key aspects of this procedure at this time!

Level of Cognitive Ability: Application
Phase of Nursing Process: Implementation
Client Needs: Safe, Effective Care Environment
Content Area: Fundamental Skills

Reference
Leahy, J., & Kizilay, P. (1998). *Foundations of nursing practice: A nursing process approach.* Philadelphia: W. B. Saunders. pp. 489–490.

4. 4

Rationale: The IV catheter has been successfully placed in the lumen of the vein when there is blood backflash in the IV catheter. The vein should have been distended from the tourniquet before the vein is cannulated. Client discomfort varies with the client, the site, and the nurse's insertion technique and is not a reliable measure of catheter placement. The nurse should not advance the catheter until placement in the vein is already verified by blood return.

Test-Taking Strategy: Specific knowledge of the steps of starting an intravenous catheter is needed to answer this question accurately. Note the key phrase "correctly placed." Use the process of elimination to answer the question. This key phrase will assist in directing you to the correct option. If needed, take a few moments to review the theory basics of this procedure now!

Level of Cognitive Ability: Analysis
Phase of Nursing Process: Analysis
Client Needs: Physiological Integrity
Content Area: Fundamental Skills

Reference
Leahy, J., & Kizilay, P. (1998). *Foundations of nursing practice: A nursing process approach.* Philadelphia: W. B. Saunders. p. 817.

5. 3

Rationale: At a rate of 80 mL per hour, the 1000-mL bag will be finished infusing in 12.5 hours. This brings the end time to 19:30, using military time.

Test-Taking Strategy: To answer this question accurately, it is necessary to be familiar with the key points related to time-taping an IV and also to be familiar with military time. This question is a fundamental and important question related to the client with an IV line. If this question was difficult, review either or both of these areas!

Level of Cognitive Ability: Application
Phase of Nursing Process: Implementation
Client Needs: Safe, Effective Care Environment
Content Area: Fundamental Skills

Reference
Taylor, C., Lillis, C., & LeMone, P. (1997). *Fundamentals of nursing: The art and science of nursing care* (3rd ed.). Philadelphia: Lippincott-Raven. pp. 1414–1415.

6. 2

Rationale: This type of catheter is intended for clients needing long-term catheter placement. It is cost effective, because the catheter does not need routine replacement, as do peripheral IV catheters. The catheter is more comfortable for the client, because the discomfort of catheter changes is avoided. The catheter is also very reliable. It is less likely to infiltrate and can be used for administration of a number of different type of medications.

Test-Taking Strategy: The key words in this question are "not" and "advantages." This tells you that the correct answer will be an incorrect statement about this type of catheter. Use general nursing knowledge about the purposes of this catheter to choose correctly. The key phrase "short-term" will assist in directing you to option 2. Review the characteristics of a PICC catheter now, if you had difficulty with this question!

Level of Cognitive Ability: Application
Phase of Nursing Process: Planning
Client Needs: Physiological Integrity
Content Area: Fundamental Skills

Reference
Leahy, J., & Kizilay, P. (1998). *Foundations of nursing practice: A nursing process approach.* Philadelphia: W. B. Saunders. p. 813.

7. 3

Rationale: The client should be taught that there are only minor activity restrictions with this catheter. The client should protect the site during bathing and should carry a Medic-Alert identification. The client should have a repair kit in the home for PRN use, since it is a long-term catheter.

Test-Taking Strategy: Note that the key words in the question are "does not fully understand." This tells you that the correct answer will be an option that is an incorrect statement. Use knowledge of basic care of PICC lines to make your choice. If needed, do a brief review of this increasingly commonly used catheter!

Level of Cognitive Ability: Analysis
Phase of Nursing Process: Evaluation
Client Needs: Health Promotion and Maintenance
Content Area: Fundamental Skills

Reference
Leahy, J., & Kizilay, P. (1998). *Foundations of nursing practice: A nursing process approach.* Philadelphia: W. B. Saunders. p. 814.

8. 2

Rationale: The IV site should be changed every 48 to 72 hours, which is every 2 to 3 days. With an insertion date of 3/20, the due date for change, depending on agency policy, would be either 3/22 or 3/23. It would be unnecessary, uncomfortable, and not cost effective to change the site on a daily basis. Changing the site every 5 to 7 days (options 3 and 4) would place the client at higher risk of infection or other catheter complications.

Test-Taking Strategy: To answer this question accurately, it is necessary to be familiar with the standard accepted guidelines for IV site maintenance. If this question was difficult, take a few moments to review these key concepts at this time!

Level of Cognitive Ability: Application
Phase of Nursing Process: Planning
Client Needs: Physiological Integrity
Content Area: Fundamental Skills

Reference

Leahy, J., & Kizilay, P. (1998). *Foundations of nursing practice: A nursing process approach.* Philadelphia: W. B. Saunders. p. 814.

9. **1**

Rationale: An infiltrated IV is one that has dislodged from the vein and is lying in subcutaneous tissue. The pallor, coolness, and swelling are the result of IV fluid being deposited in the subcutaneous tissue. When the pressure in the tissues exceeds the pressure in the tubing, the flow of the IV solution will stop. The corrective action is to remove the catheter and start a new line. The other three options are likely to be accompanied by warmth at the site, not coolness.

Test-Taking Strategy: To answer this question accurately, it is necessary to be familiar with the signs and symptoms that accompany complications of IV therapy. If this question was difficult, take a few moments to review the signs of infiltration now!

Level of Cognitive Ability: Analysis
Phase of Nursing Process: Analysis
Client Needs: Physiological Integrity
Content Area: Fundamental Skills

Reference

Leahy, J., & Kizilay, P. (1998). *Foundations of nursing practice: A nursing process approach.* Philadelphia: W. B. Saunders. p. 822.

10. **4**

Rationale: The nurse should discontinue the IV at the phlebitic site and apply warm, moist compresses to the area to speed resolution of the inflammation. Since phlebitis has occurred, the nurse also notifies the physician about the IV complication. The nurse should restart the IV in a different vein than the one with the phlebitis.

Test-Taking Strategy: The key word in this question is "contraindicated." This tells you that the correct answer is an incorrect nursing action. Use knowledge of basic principles related to the handling of IV complications to make your selection. Review nursing interventions related to phlebitis now, if you had difficulty with this question!

Level of Cognitive Ability: Application
Phase of Nursing Process: Implementation
Client Needs: Physiological Integrity
Content Area: Fundamental Skills

Reference

Leahy, J., & Kizilay, P. (1998). *Foundations of nursing practice: A nursing process approach.* Philadelphia: W. B. Saunders. p. 822.

11. **3**

Rationale: The tubing should not be removed from the IV catheter. With each break in the system, there is an increased chance of introducing bacteria into the system, leading to infection. This is poor aseptic technique. Each of the other methods described is acceptable.

Test-Taking Strategy: Note the key words "intervene" in the question and "disconnected" in the correct option. Use knowledge of basic principles related to intravenous therapy and asepsis to answer this question. Review these principles now, if you had difficulty with this question!

Level of Cognitive Ability: Application
Phase of Nursing Process: Implementation
Client Needs: Safe, Effective Care Environment
Content Area: Fundamental Skills

Reference

Leahy, J., & Kizilay, P. (1998). *Foundations of nursing practice: A nursing process approach.* Philadelphia: W. B. Saunders. p. 818.

12. **4**

Rationale: Safe nursing practice includes monitoring an IV infusion at least once per hour in an adult client. The IV may be checked even more frequently depending on whether medication is also being infused.

Test-Taking Strategy: To answer this question accurately, it is necessary to be familiar with the specific time frames indicated in this nursing procedure. If this question was difficult, take a few moments now to review the essentials of safe IV administration!

Level of Cognitive Ability: Application
Phase of Nursing Process: Planning
Client Needs: Physiological Integrity
Content Area: Fundamental Skills

Reference

Leahy, J., & Kizilay, P. (1998). *Foundations of nursing practice: A nursing process approach.* Philadelphia: W. B. Saunders. p. 819.

13. **1**

Rationale: The client's symptoms are compatible with speed shock. This may be verified by noting that 700 mL has infused in the course of a single hour. The "first" action of the nurse is to shut off the infusion. Other actions may follow in rapid sequence. The nurse may elevate the head of the bed to aid the client's breathing. The physician is also notified immediately. The angiocatheter does not need to be removed. It may continue to be needed once the crisis is over.

Test-Taking Strategy: To answer this question accurately, it is necessary to be able to recognize signs of speed shock and know the appropriate interventions. Note that the question contains the key words "first action." This tells you that more than one or all of the options are likely to be correct actions. It is necessary for you to be able to discriminate which of them is most crucial in terms of sequence. Review nursing actions related to this complication now, if you had difficulty with this question!

Level of Cognitive Ability: Analysis
Phase of Nursing Process: Implementation
Client Needs: Physiological Integrity
Content Area: Fundamental Skills

Reference

Taylor, C., Lillis, C., & LeMone, P. (1997). *Fundamentals of nursing: The art and science of nursing care* (3rd ed.). Philadelphia: Lippincott-Raven. p. 1422.

14. **2**

Rationale: Phlebitis at an IV site can be distinguished by client discomfort at the site, as well as by redness, warmth, and swelling proximal to the catheter. The line should be discontinued, and a new line should be inserted at a different site. The remaining options are incorrect.

Test-Taking Strategy: Remember that options that are similar are not likely to be correct. In this case, options 3 and 4 are similar and are therefore discarded. Choose option 2 over option 1 by knowing the signs and symptoms of common IV complications. Review these signs and symptoms now, if you had difficulty with this question!

Level of Cognitive Ability: Analysis
Phase of Nursing Process: Analysis
Client Needs: Physiological Integrity
Content Area: Fundamental Skills

Reference
Leahy, J., & Kizilay, P. (1998). *Foundations of nursing practice: A nursing process approach.* Philadelphia: W. B. Saunders. p. 822.

15. **2**

Rationale: The nondominant hand is used to stabilize the angiocatheter, ensuring that it does not become dislodged or pulled out during the changeover. Holding pressure on the vein distal to the IV site accomplishes nothing. The IV roller clamp should be closed before the nurse attempts to switch the line over to the heparin lock. The line should be shut off and not pinched prior to the change.

Test-Taking Strategy: Remember that options that are similar are not likely to be correct. Thus, begin to answer this question by eliminating options 3 and 4 first. Choose option 2 over option 1, using critical thinking skills to determine what each of them would accomplish. You could also choose correctly by knowing this basic nursing procedure!

Level of Cognitive Ability: Application
Phase of Nursing Process: Implementation
Client Needs: Safe, Effective Care Environment
Content Area: Fundamental Skills

Reference
Taylor, C., Lillis, C., & LeMone, P. (1997). *Fundamentals of nursing: The art and science of nursing care* (3rd ed.). Philadelphia: Lippincott-Raven. p. 1424.

16. **1**

Rationale: There are many components to a teaching plan for the client being discharged to home with ongoing IV therapy. The teaching should begin with an emphasis on proper handwashing technique. This is essential for prevention of infection. The client or family member may then learn how to handle and utilize the equipment, change the dressing, and assess for signs of infection. The client must learn where to obtain necessary supplies, if applicable; some home infusion companies deliver supplies to the client's home. Finally, the client or family member should know to report signs of infection promptly.

Test-Taking Strategy: The key word in the question is "first." This tells you that more than one option may be a correct action, but that one of them is of greater priority, or should be completed before the others. Use knowledge of basic medical asepsis to choose correctly. Remember that handwashing is always the first step!

Level of Cognitive Ability: Application
Phase of Nursing Process: Implementation
Client Needs: Health Promotion and Maintenance
Content Area: Fundamental Skills

Reference
Leahy, J., & Kizilay, P. (1998). *Foundations of nursing practice: A nursing process approach.* Philadelphia: W. B. Saunders. p. 823.

17. **4**

Rationale: A dry, sterile dressing such as a sterile 2×2 is used to apply pressure to the site while the angiocatheter is discontinued. This material is absorbent, sterile, and nonirritating to the site. A Betadine swab or alcohol swab would irritate the opened puncture site and would not stop the blood flow. A Band-Aid may be used to cover the site once hemostasis has occurred.

Test-Taking Strategy: Visualize this procedure and think about each of the items identified in the options to answer the question. Familiarity with this basic nursing procedure is needed to answer this question correctly. If needed, take a few minutes to review this procedure at this time!

Level of Cognitive Ability: Application
Phase of Nursing Process: Implementation
Client Needs: Safe, Effective Care Environment
Content Area: Fundamental Skills

Reference
Luckmann, J. (1997). *Saunders manual of nursing care.* Philadelphia. W. B. Saunders. p. 256.

18. **2**

Rationale: The formula for calculating IV drip rates is:

$$\text{gtt/min} = \frac{\text{volume (mL)} \times \text{drop factor (gtt/mL)}}{\text{time (in min)}}$$
$$= \frac{50 \text{ mL} \times 10 \text{ gtt/mL}}{30 \text{ min}}$$
$$= \frac{500}{30}$$
$$= 16.66 \text{ or } 17 \text{ gtt/min}$$

Test-Taking Strategy: To calculate the answer to this question correctly, you must be familiar with the standard formula for calculating IV flow rates. If you answered incorrectly, take a few moments to relearn this formula now!

Level of Cognitive Ability: Application
Phase of Nursing Process: Implementation
Client Needs: Physiological Integrity
Content Area: Fundamental Skills

Reference
Leahy, J., & Kizilay, P. (1998). *Foundations of nursing practice: A nursing process approach.* Philadelphia: W. B. Saunders. p. 813.

19. **3**

Rationale: The nurse cleans the skin using a circular motion from inward to outward. This is the standard accepted aseptic technique to carry microorganisms away from the insertion site. It is the same technique used in cleansing any area using surgical asepsis.

Test-Taking Strategy: To answer this question, it is necessary only to be familiar with principles of asepsis. Knowledge of these principles allows you to choose correctly even without specific knowledge of IV insertion techniques. Review the basic principles of asepsis now, if you had difficulty with this question!

Level of Cognitive Ability: Application
Phase of Nursing Process: Implementation
Client Needs: Safe, Effective Care Environment
Content Area: Fundamental Skills

Reference
Leahy, J., & Kizilay, P. (1998). *Foundations of nursing practice: A nursing process approach.* Philadelphia: W. B. Saunders. p. 816.

20. 1

Rationale: The nurse would avoid placing a cool compress over the site. Cold causes vasoconstriction while warmth causes vasodilatation. It is also helpful to have the client lower the arm below heart level before applying the tourniquet to let gravity aid in venous distention. Lightly tapping over the vein also helps distend it and makes it visible from the surface.

Test-Taking Strategy: Use principles of gravity and blood flow and knowledge of applications of heat and cold to answer this question. Since the question contains the key word "avoid," you would look for the option that is an incorrect nursing action. Review the principles related to initiating an IV now, if you had difficulty answering this question!

Level of Cognitive Ability: Application
Phase of Nursing Process: Planning
Client Needs: Physiological Integrity
Content Area: Fundamental Skills

Reference
Luckmann, J. (1997). *Saunders manual of nursing care.* Philadelphia. W. B. Saunders. p. 251.

21. 2

Rationale: After cannulating the vein, the nurse attaches the primed IV tubing to the angiocatheter. The nurse then releases the tourniquet and starts the flow of IV solution. Finally, the nurse observes the site, looking for signs of infiltration.

Test-Taking Strategy: Familiarity with the procedure for beginning an IV line is needed to answer this question. You could also deduce the correct answer by utilizing concepts related to general IV therapy and blood flow. Attempt to visualize this procedure in answering the question. Review this procedure now, if you had difficulty with this question!

Level of Cognitive Ability: Application
Phase of Nursing Process: Implementation
Client Needs: Safe, Effective Care Environment
Content Area: Fundamental Skills

Reference
Taylor, C., Lillis, C., & LeMone, P. (1997). *Fundamentals of nursing: The art and science of nursing care* (3rd ed.). Philadelphia: Lippincott-Raven. p. 1407.

22. 2

Rationale: The nurse should first check the compatibility of the medication with the ingredients in the IV solution. (In this case, diazepam does not have Y-site compatibility with potassium chloride.) This allows the nurse to determine whether to disconnect the IV at the site and flush the line (which requires additional flush solution to be drawn up), or to get an order to get a second line started (depending on the particular client need). The nurse then draws up the medication, checks the ID bracelet to verify client identity, pinches off the tubing above the Y-site, and injects the medication slowly through the port nearest the IV insertion site.

Test-Taking Strategy: Use basic principles related to administration of medications to answer this question. Note that the stem of the question contains the key word "first." This tells you that you will need to think through the process to determine the sequence of activities. Determining medication compatibility is the first step!

Level of Cognitive Ability: Application
Phase of Nursing Process: Planning
Client Needs: Physiological Integrity
Content Area: Fundamental Skills

Reference
Luckmann, J. (1997). *Saunders manual of nursing care.* Philadelphia. W. B. Saunders. p. 255.

23. 3

Rationale: The nurse uses the nondominant hand to stabilize the port of the heparin lock, which prevents the catheter from moving in the vein and possibly infiltrating. The port should be wiped with an alcohol swab before the port is pierced, not at the same time of piercing. The nurse needs a watch or clock with a second hand to time medication injection, but this does not have to be held in the nondominant hand. There is no reason to apply pressure over the catheter insertion site. This added pressure would cause resistance and make the medication harder to inject.

Test-Taking Strategy: Familiarity with this medication administration procedure is needed to answer this question correctly. Visualize the options presented in the stem to help you make your choice. If needed, review this basic procedure now!

Level of Cognitive Ability: Application
Phase of Nursing Process: Implementation
Client Needs: Safe, Effective Care Environment
Content Area: Fundamental Skills

Reference
Luckmann, J. (1997). *Saunders manual of nursing care.* Philadelphia. W. B. Saunders p. 257.

24. 1

Rationale: Before beginning administration of large volumes of IV solution, the nurse should assess whether the results of the chest radiograph reveal that the catheter is in the proper place. This is necessary to prevent infusion of IV fluid into pulmonary or subcutaneous tissues. The other options are incorrect.

Test-Taking Strategy: Note the key phrase "central venous catheter done at the bedside." To answer this question correctly, it is necessary to know potential complications associated with insertion of central venous lines, and how to detect them. If this question was difficult, briefly review the principles of care for this catheter following insertion!

Level of Cognitive Ability: Application
Phase of Nursing Process: Assessment
Client Needs: Safe, Effective Care Environment
Content Area: Fundamental Skills

Reference
Leahy, J., & Kizilay, P. (1998). *Foundations of nursing practice: A nursing process approach.* Philadelphia: W. B. Saunders. p. 813.

25. 1

Rationale: Five percent dextrose in 0.45% sodium chloride is a hypertonic solution. An advantage of hypertonic solutions is that they may be used to treat hypovolemia when plasma expanders are not readily available. Options 2 and 3 are isotonic solutions. Option 4 is a hypotonic solution.

Test-Taking Strategy: Familiarity with concepts related to fluid and electrolyte balance and fluid shifts is needed to answer this question. If this question was difficult, review the nature and purposes of hypertonic, isotonic, and hypotonic IV solutions!

Level of Cognitive Ability: Analysis
Phase of Nursing Process: Analysis
Client Needs: Physiological Integrity
Content Area: Fundamental Skills

Reference

Leahy, J., & Kizilay, P. (1998). *Foundations of nursing practice: A nursing process approach.* Philadelphia: W. B. Saunders. p. 811.

26. **2**

Rationale: The injection cap should be discarded and a new one applied once it has been removed from the actual lumen. It is removed whenever bloodwork is drawn from the port. This is done to reduce systemic infection, which has been shown to be caused by contaminated caps. In addition, each agency has a policy that guides the frequency of routine cap changes (often every 48 hours).

Test-Taking Strategy: To answer this question correctly, it is necessary to understand the uses of the ports on a central venous catheter, and to know the basic principles involved in controlling infection with them. If you are not familiar with this material, take a few moments at this time to review these catheters and their care!

Level of Cognitive Ability: Analysis
Phase of Nursing Process: Evaluation
Client Needs: Safe, Effective Care Environment
Content Area: Fundamental Skills

Reference

Taylor, C., Lillis, C., & LeMone, P. (1997). *Fundamentals of nursing: The art and science of nursing care* (3rd ed.). Philadelphia: Lippincott-Raven. p. 1404.

27. **3**

Rationale: When the tubing is removed from an electronic infusion pump, it is most essential that the roller clamp on the IV tubing has been shut. Otherwise, the client will receive a bolus of fluid from tubing that is wide open. The client could then suffer fluid overload or drug toxicity, depending on the solution hanging. It is also good nursing practice to check the volume infused and to assess the IV site while in the room. There is no reason to unplug the machine.

Test-Taking Strategy: Note that the key words in the question are "most essential." This means that more than one option is likely to be correct, and that you must prioritize your answer. Use Maslow's hierarchy of needs, specifically safety needs, to choose correctly!

Level of Cognitive Ability: Application
Phase of Nursing Process: Implementation
Client Needs: Physiological Integrity
Content Area: Fundamental Skills

Reference

Luckmann, J. (1997). *Saunders manual of nursing care.* Philadelphia. W. B. Saunders. p. 248

28. **4**

Rationale: One of the common criteria for continuous IV infusion therapy in the home setting is having a part-time or full-time caregiver to assist the client with the therapy. The client should also be medically stable. Finally, the client should have a refrigerator for storage of infusion supplies, and access to a telephone.

Test-Taking Strategy: Note that the key words are "good candidate" and "questions." This leads you to look for an option that is not satisfactory or helpful to the client. Prioritize and use the process of elimination to make your choice.

Level of Cognitive Ability: Analysis
Phase of Nursing Process: Analysis
Client Needs: Health Promotion and Maintenance
Content Area: Fundamental Skills

Reference

Luckmann, J. (1997). *Saunders manual of nursing care.* Philadelphia. W. B. Saunders. p. 260.

29. **2**

Rationale: The nurse should change the IV tubing. The tubing has become contaminated and could result in systemic infection to the client. Wiping the port with Betadine is insufficient and would be contraindicated regardless, since the catheter will be attached directly to an angiocatheter in the client's vein. The needleless device has not been contaminated and does not need replacement. Cleansing would not be indicated either.

Test-Taking Strategy: Use knowledge of basic infection control measures and IV therapy concepts to answer this question. There is clearly only one correct choice. Review aseptic technique now, if you had difficulty with this question!

Level of Cognitive Ability: Application
Phase of Nursing Process: Planning
Client Needs: Safe, Effective Care Environment
Content Area: Fundamental Skills

Reference

Leahy, J., & Kizilay, P. (1998). *Foundations of nursing practice: A nursing process approach.* Philadelphia: W. B. Saunders. p. 813.

30. **3**

Rationale: If the IV is scheduled to run over 8 hours, then the hourly rate is 125 mL per hour. Using 500 mL as the reference point, the next hourly marking would be at 375 mL, which is 125 mL less than 500. The rates that would accompany the markings in options 1, 2, and 3 are 75 mL, 100 mL, and 150 mL per hour, respectively.

Test-Taking Strategy: Use basic principles related to pharmacology mathematics and IV administration to answer this question. If this question was difficult, take time to review this essential material!

Level of Cognitive Ability: Application
Phase of Nursing Process: Implementation
Client Needs: Safe, Effective Care Environment
Content Area: Fundamental Skills

Reference

Leahy, J., & Kizilay, P. (1998). *Foundations of nursing practice: A nursing process approach.* Philadelphia: W. B. Saunders. p. 818.

BIBLIOGRAPHY

Leahy, J., & Kizilay, P. (1998). *Foundations of nursing practice: A nursing process approach.* Philadelphia: W. B. Saunders.

Lehne, R. (1998). *Pharmacology for nursing care* (3rd ed.). Philadelphia: W. B. Saunders.

Luckmann, J. (1997). *Saunders manual of nursing care.* Philadelphia. W. B. Saunders.

Mahan, L., & Escott-Stump, S. (1996). *Krause's food, nutrition, & diet therapy* (9th ed.). Philadelphia: W. B. Saunders.

Monahan, F., & Neighbors, M. (1998). *Medical-surgical nursing: Foundations for clinical practice* (2nd ed.). Philadelphia: W. B. Saunders.

Taylor, C., Lillis, C., & LeMone, P. (1997). *Fundamentals of nursing: The art and science of nursing care* (3rd ed.). Philadelphia: Lippincott-Raven.

CHAPTER 14

Administration of Blood Products

....

PYRAMID TERMS

ABO—ABO represents a type of antigen system. The ABO type of the donor should be compatible with the recipient's. Type A can match with types A or O; type B can match with types B or O; type O can match only with type O; type AB can match with A, B, or O.

Autologous Donation—A donation of the client's own blood before a scheduled procedure.

Blood Salvage—An autologous donation that involves suctioning blood from body cavities, joint spaces, or other closed body sites during a procedure.

Crossmatching—The testing of the donor's blood and the recipient's blood for compatibility.

Compatibility—Determined by two different types of antigen systems, the ABO system antigens and the Rh antigen, present on the membrane surface of the red blood cells (RBCs).

Circulatory Overload—A complication resulting from the infusion of blood at a rate too rapid for size, cardiac status, or clinical condition of the recipient.

Designated Donor—A designated donation occurs when recipients pick their own donors.

Disease Transmission—Diseases can be transmitted through blood transfusions, the most common being hepatitis C. The incidence of transmission of human immunodeficiency virus (HIV) is rare since routine donor testing was implemented in 1985.

Fresh-Frozen Plasma—Administered to increase the level of clotting factors in clients with such a deficiency.

Iron Overload—A delayed transfusion complication; it can occur in clients receiving over 100 units of blood over a period of time.

Platelets—Administered to clients with low platelet counts and to thrombocytopenic clients who are actively bleeding or scheduled for an invasive procedure.

RBCs (Red Blood Cells)—Used to replace erythrocytes lost as a result of trauma or surgical interventions, or in clients with bone marrow suppression.

Rh—Represents a type of antigen system. Rh-negative blood can be given to an Rh-negative or Rh-positive recipient.

Septicemia—The presence of infective agents or their toxins in the blood stream. Septicemia is a serious disease and must be treated promptly, otherwise the infection leads to circulatory collapse, profound shock, and death.

Transfusion Reaction—A hemolytic transfusion reaction is caused by blood type or Rh incompatibility. An allergic transfusion reaction is most often seen in clients with a history of allergy. A febrile transfusion reaction most commonly occurs in clients with antibodies directed against the transfused white blood cells (WBCs). A bacterial transfusion reaction is seen after transfusion of contaminated blood products.

Whole Blood—Composed of RBCs, plasma, and plasma proteins; it is administered in conditions of acute and massive blood loss.

◆ PYRAMID TO SUCCESS

Pyramid points focus on the safe administration of blood components, managing and providing care related to the procedure for administering blood components, and monitoring for complications. Focus is on the safe procedure related to administering blood and on the signs and symptoms of **transfusion reaction**. Pyramid points also focus on the immediate interventions if a **transfusion reaction** occurs, and evaluation and documentation of expected and unexpected effects of the therapy.

NURSING PROCESS

ASSESSMENT

Physician's order for the type of blood component and volume

Determine rate of infusion by physician order or, if not specified, by agency policy

Informed consent

Client's vital signs (VS); renal, circulatory, and respiratory status; and ability to tolerate fluids

Temperature for elevation

Determine whether the client has ever experienced any previous reactions to blood transfusions

---

ANALYSIS: Risk for infection Risk for transfusion reaction

Risk for fluid volume excess

PLANNING

Client will remain free of infection. Client will maintain fluid balance. Client will remain free of injury.

IMPLEMENTATION (see also Box 14–1)

Always maintain body fluid precautions. If the temperature is elevated, notify the physician before beginning the transfusion. A fever may be a cause for delaying the transfusion in addition to masking a possible symptom of an acute transfusion reaction. Insert an IV flushed with NS (normal saline) and maintain at a KVO (keep vein open) rate. A central catheter is an acceptable venous access option for blood transfusions. A 19- to 20-gauge or larger needle will be needed to achieve a maximum flow rate of blood products and prevent damage to RBCs; if a smaller-gauge needle must be used, RBCs may be diluted with 0.9% NS. Blood products should be infused through administration sets designed specifically for blood; use a Y-tubing or straight tubing blood administration set that contains a filter designed to trap fibrin clots and other debris that accumulates during blood storage. Premedicate the client with acetaminophen (Tylenol) or diphenhydramine hydrochloride (Benadryl) as prescribed if the client has a history of adverse reactions. If prescribed, oral medications should be administered 30 minutes before the transfusion is started, and IV medications may be given immediately before the transfusion is started. Begin the transfusion slowly under close supervision. During the transfusion, monitor the client for signs and symptoms of transfusion reaction. The first 10 to 15 minutes of the transfusion are the most critical and the nurse must stay with client. If a major ABO incompatibility exists or a severe allergic reaction occurs, it is usually evident within the first 50 mL of the transfusion. If no reaction is noted within the first 15 minutes, the flow can be increased to the prescribed rate. The recommended rate of infusion varies with the blood component being transfused and the client's condition. Generally infusion is as quick as the client's condition allows. Components containing few RBCs and platelets may be infused rapidly, but caution should be taken to avoid circulatory overload. Vital signs and lung sounds should be taken before the transfusion and again after the first 15 minutes and every hour until 1 hour after the transfusion has been discontinued. Instruct the client to report anything unusual immediately. If a reaction occurs, stop the transfusion, change the IV tubing down to the IV site, keep the IV line open with NS, notify the physician and blood bank, and return the blood bag and tubing to the blood bank. If a reaction occurs, do not leave the client alone, and monitor for any life-threatening symptoms. If a reaction occurs, obtain appropriate laboratory samples, according to agency policies, such as blood and urine samples (free hemoglobin indicates that RBCs were hemolyzed). Document the client's tolerance to the administration of the blood product. Monitor the appropriate laboratory values and document the effectiveness of treatment related to the specific type of blood product.

EVALUATION

Vital signs remain within normal limits. Fluid balance is maintained. Client will remain free of injury. Laboratory values return to within normal range.

CLIENT NEEDS

SAFE EFFECTIVE CARE ENVIRONMENT

Informed consent
Continuity of care and close supervision during transfusion
Handling hazardous and infectious material
Asepsis
Standard (universal) precautions

HEALTH PROMOTION AND MAINTENANCE

Lifestyle choices related to blood administration
Teaching the client about the signs of a transfusion reaction

PSYCHOSOCIAL INTEGRITY

Communication regarding the procedure for blood administration
Religious and cultural considerations related to blood administration

PHYSIOLOGICAL INTEGRITY

Safe administration of blood
Venous access devices for blood administration
Monitoring for complications related to blood administration
Monitoring laboratory values
Monitoring for expected effects
Complete documentation

I. Types of Blood Components

A. **RBCs**
   1. Used to replace erythrocytes
   2. Packed **RBCs** are usually supplied in 250-mL unit bags; however, they can be supplied in 250- to 350- or 350- to 400-mL bags; always check the unit for the volume of the blood component
   3. The normal erythrocyte count in men is 4.6 to 6.2 million/mm³ and in women, 4.2 to 5.4 million/mm³
   4. Each unit increases hemoglobin by 1 g/dL and hematocrit by 2% to 3%; the change in laboratory values takes 4 to 6 hours to appear
   5. Evaluation of an effective response is based on the resolution of the symptoms of anemia and an increase of the erythrocyte count
B. **Whole Blood**
   1. Rarely used; treatment with a specific blood component is usually prescribed
   2. Used to resolve hypovolemic shock due to hemorrhage
   3. Contains **RBCs**, plasma, and plasma proteins, and each unit normally contains 500 mL; always check the bag for the volume of the blood component
   4. Evaluation of an effective response is based on the resolution of the symptoms of hypovolemia
C. **Platelets**
   1. **Platelets** are used to treat thrombocytopenia and **platelet** dysfunctions
   2. **Crossmatching** is not required but is usually done (**platelet** concentrates contain few **RBCs**)

> ### BOX 14–1. Precautions Related to Blood Administration
>
> - A large volume of refrigerated blood infused rapidly through a central catheter into the ventricle of the heart can cause cardiac dysrhythmias
> - No solution other than NS should be added to blood components
> - Medications are never added to blood transfusions
> - To avoid the risk of **septicemia**, infusions (1 unit) should not exceed 4 hours
> - The blood administration set should be changed every 4 to 6 hours or according to institution policy to reduce the risk of **septicemia**
> - Blood will be released from the blood bank only to personnel as specified by agency policy
> - The name and identification (ID) number of the intended recipient must be provided to the blood bank, and a documented permanent record of this information is maintained
> - Blood should be transported from the blood bank to only one client at a time to prevent blood delivery to the wrong client
> - The most critical phase of the transfusion is confirming product compatibility and verifying client identify
> - Two RNs need to check the physician's order, the client's identity, and the ID band and number verifying that it is identical to the blood component tag
> - At the bedside, ask the client to state her or his name, and compare it with the name on the ID bracelet
> - The blood bag tag, label, and requisition form are assessed to ensure that ABO and Rh types are compatible
> - The blood bag label is checked to ensure that the correct components have been issued; if there are any inconsistencies or questions, notify the blood bank immediately
> - Always check the bag for the date of expiration; components expire at midnight on the day marked on the bag unless otherwise specified
> - Inspect the blood bag for leaks, abnormal color, clots, excessive air, and bubbles
> - Blood must be administered within 30 minutes as this is the maximal allowable time out of monitored storage
> - Blood bank regulations state that refrigerated components may not be returned to blood banks if they have been warmed to more than 10°C
> - NEVER refrigerate blood in refrigerators other than those used in blood banks; if the blood is not administered within 30 minutes, return it to the blood bank

   3. The volume in a unit of **platelets** may vary from 50 to 70 mL per unit to 200 to 400 mL per unit; always check the bag for the volume of the blood component
   4. **Platelets** are administered immediately upon receipt from the blood bank and are given rapidly, usually over 15 to 30 minutes
   5. The normal **platelet** count is 150,000 to 350,000/mm³; each unit will increase the platelet count by 5000 to 10,000/mm³

6. Evaluation of an effective response is based on improvement in the **platelet** count, and **platelet** counts are normally evaluated 1 hour and 18 to 24 hours after the transfusion

D. **Fresh-Frozen Plasma**
1. **Fresh-frozen plasma** may be used to provide clotting factors or volume expansion; it contains no platelets
2. It is infused within 6 hours of thawing while clotting factors are still viable and is infused as rapidly as possible
3. **Rh** and **ABO** compatibility are required for the transfusion of plasma products
4. A unit normally contains 200 to 250 mL; always check the bag for the volume of the blood component
5. Normal prothrombin time (PT) is 9.6 to 11.8 sec (adult male) and 9.5 to 11.3 sec (adult female), and the normal partial thromboplastin time (PTT) is 20 to 36 sec, depending on the type of activator used
6. Evaluation of an effective response is assessed by monitoring coagulation studies, particularly the PT and PTT, and resolution of hypovolemia

II. Types of Blood Donations

A. **Autologous**
1. A donation of the client's own blood before a scheduled procedure; it reduces the risk of disease transmission and potential transfusion complications
2. Not an option for a client with leukemia or bacteremia
3. A donation can be made every 3 days if the hemoglobin remains at or above 11 g/dL
4. Donations should begin within 5 weeks of the transfusion date and end at least 3 days before the date of transfusion

B. **Blood Salvage**
1. An **autologous donation** that involves suctioning blood from body cavities, joint spaces, or other closed body sites
2. Blood may need to be "washed," a special process that removes tissue debris before reinfusion

C. **Designated Donation**
1. Occurs when recipients designate their own compatible donors
2. It does not reduce the risk of contracting infections transmitted by the blood; however, recipients feel more comfortable identifying their donors

III. Compatibility

A. Client blood samples are drawn and labeled at the bedside when drawn; the client is asked to state his or her name, which is compared with the name on the identification bracelet
B. The recipient's **ABO** and **Rh** types are identified
C. An antibody screen is done to determine the presence of antibodies other than anti-A and anti-B
D. **Crossmatch testing** is done in which donor **RBCs** are combined with recipient's serum and Coombs' serum; **crossmatch** is compatible if no **RBC** agglutination has occurred
E. In an emergency, O-negative **RBCs** and AB plasma can be safely administered to most clients without serologic testing

IV. Infusion Controllers and Pumps

A. Infusion controllers and pumps may be used to administer blood products if designed to function with opaque solutions; however, the negative pressure exerted by the cassette of the machine can cause **RBC** hemolysis
B. Always consult manufacturer guidelines for the controller or pump
C. Special manual pressure cuffs may be used to increase the flow rate but should not exceed 300 mmHg
D. Standard sphygmomanometer cuffs are not to be used to increase flow rate because they do not exert uniform pressure against all parts of the bag

V. Blood Warmers

A. Blood warmers may be used to prevent hypothermia and decrease reactions
B. Special warmers have been designed specifically for this purpose, and only devices specifically tested and approved for this use can be used
C. Do not warm blood products in a microwave or in hot water

VI. Complications
A. **Transfusion Reactions**
1. Signs of an immediate **transfusion reaction**
   a. Chills and diaphoresis
   b. Rapid, thready pulse
   c. Pallor and cyanosis
   d. Muscle aches, back pain, or chest pain
   e. Headache
   f. Apprehension
   g. Tingling and numbness
   h. Dyspnea, cough, wheezing, or rales
   i. Nausea, vomiting, abdominal cramping, and diarrhea
   j. Rashes, hives, itching, and swelling
2. Signs of **transfusion reaction** in an unconscious client
   a. Weak pulse
   b. Fever
   c. Tachycardia or bradycardia
   d. Hypotension
   e. Visible hemoglobinuria
   f. Oliguria or anuria
3. Delayed **transfusion reactions**
   a. Reactions can occur days to years after a transfusion
   b. Signs include fever, mild jaundice, and decreased hematocrit

B. **Circulatory Overload**
  1. Description: Caused by infusion of blood at a rate too rapid for the client to tolerate
  2. Assessment
     a. Cough, dyspnea, chest pain, rales, and pulmonary edema
     b. Headache
     c. Hypertension
     d. Tachycardia and a rapid, bounding pulse
     e. Distended neck veins
  3. Implementation
     a. Slow the rate of infusion
     b. Place the client in an upright position, with the feet in a dependent position
     c. Administer oxygen, diuretics, and morphine as prescribed
     d. Phlebotomy may also be a method of prescribed treatment
C. **Septicemia**
  1. Description: Occurs with the transfusion of blood contaminated with microorganisms
  2. Assessment
     a. Rapid onset of chills and high fever
     b. Vomiting
     c. Diarrhea
     d. Hypotension
     e. Shock
  3. Implementation
     a. Obtain blood cultures and cultures of the blood bag
     b. Administer IV fluids, antibiotics, vasopressors, and steroids as prescribed
D. **Iron Overload**
  1. Description: Can occur in clients receiving over 100 units of blood over a period of time
  2. Assessment
     a. Vomiting
     b. Diarrhea
     c. Hypotension
     d. Altered hematological values
  3. Implementation
     a. Deferoxamine (Desferal), administered IV or subcutaneously, removes accumulated iron via the kidneys
     b. Urine turns red as iron is excreted following administration of Desferal; treatment is discontinued when serum ion levels return to normal
E. **Disease Transmission**
  1. The most common disease transmission is hepatitis C, manifested by anorexia, nausea, vomiting, dark urine, and jaundice; it usually occurs within 4 to 6 weeks of the transfusion
  2. The incidence of transmission of HIV is rare since routine donor testing was implemented in 1985
F. Hypocalcemia and citrate intoxication
  1. Citrate in transfused blood binds with calcium and is excreted
  2. Assess serum calcium pre- and post-transfusion

G. Hyperkalemia
  1. Stored blood liberates potassium through hemolysis
  2. The older the blood, the greater the risk of hyperkalemia
  3. Assess the date on the blood as well as the serum potassium pre- and post-transfusion

PRACTICE QUESTIONS

1. The client has an order to receive 2 units of packed RBCs. The nurse begins to assess the client's knowledge of the procedure by asking which of the following initial questions?
   1 "Have you ever had a transfusion before?"
   2 "Have you ever gone into anaphylactic shock from transfusion in the past?"
   3 "Can you tell me everything the doctor told you about why you need the transfusion?"
   4 "Does the idea of receiving blood frighten you in any way?"

2. The nurse is preparing to transfuse a unit of packed RBCs for an assigned client. The nurse teaches the client that it is most important to report which of the following signs immediately?
   1 Mild discomfort at the catheter site
   2 Chills, itching, or rash
   3 Unusual sleepiness or fatigue
   4 Headache, nausea, or vomiting

3. The client has an order to receive a unit of packed RBCs. The nurse chooses which of the following solutions to keep the line open after inserting an IV angiocatheter for the blood product infusion?
   1 5% dextrose in 0.9% sodium chloride
   2 5% dextrose in water
   3 0.9% sodium chloride
   4 Lactated Ringer's solution

4. The nurse must insert an IV line to use for blood transfusion for an assigned client. The nurse selects an angiocatheter that has a minimum size of which of the following to ensure that the catheter has a large enough bore for this procedure?
   1 24-gauge
   2 22-gauge
   3 19-gauge
   4 16-gauge

5. The nurse is preparing to infuse a unit of blood to an assigned client. The nurse asks which of the following members of the health care team available on the nursing unit to assist in checking the unit of blood?
   1 Pharmacist
   2 Phlebotomist
   3 Nursing assistant
   4 Registered nurse

6. The nurse who is about to begin a blood transfusion knows that blood cells start to deteriorate after a certain period of time. The nurse checks

which of the following items carefully before beginning the transfusion to assure this has not happened?

1 Blood identification number
2 Expiration date
3 Blood group and type
4 Presence of clots

7. The nurse is beginning to transfuse a client with a unit of blood. Just prior to starting the infusion, it is most important for the nurse to assess:
   1 Skin color
   2 Oxygen saturation
   3 Vital signs
   4 Latest hematocrit

8. The nurse has completed checking a unit of blood for an assigned client with another nurse. The nurse plans to remain in this client's room and asks the second nurse to monitor other assigned clients for how long?
   1 5 minutes
   2 15 minutes
   3 30 minutes
   4 60 minutes

9. The client in hemorrhagic shock requires rapid transfusion with multiple units of blood. The nurse uses which of the following devices to prevent cardiac dysrhythmias during the transfusions?
   1 Blood-warming device
   2 Electronic infusion device
   3 Noninvasive blood pressure monitor
   4 Continuous cardiac monitor

10. The client receiving a blood transfusion rings the call bell for the nurse. Upon entering the room, the nurse notes that the client is flushed and dyspneic and is complaining of generalized itching. The nurse interprets that the client is experiencing:
    1 Fluid overload
    2 Bacteremia
    3 Hypovolemic shock
    4 Transfusion reaction

11. The client is suspected of having a transfusion reaction. After stopping the blood transfusion, the nurse immediately takes which of the following actions as the most prudent pending further orders?
    1 Discontinue the IV line
    2 Convert the line to a heparin lock
    3 Keep normal saline running to keep vein open
    4 Change the solution to 5% dextrose in water

12. The client who was receiving a blood transfusion has experienced a transfusion reaction. The nurse should plan to send the blood bag to which of the following areas after discontinuing the unit from the client?
    1 Risk management department
    2 Laboratory

3 Pharmacy
4 Blood bank

13. The nurse is preparing to begin a blood transfusion on an assigned client. Which of the following missing items would be most important for the nurse to retrieve or obtain in order to proceed with client identification?
    1 Identification bracelet
    2 Social security number
    3 Client address
    4 Medical record number

14. The nurse is preparing a unit of packed RBCs for transfusion. Before attaching the unit of blood and priming the tubing, the nurse assures that the tubing has which of the following?
    1 A slide clamp
    2 An inline filter
    3 A microdrip chamber
    4 An air vent

15. A client is told by the physician that a blood transfusion is needed, and that a blood sample must be drawn first for blood typing and cross-match. After the physician leaves, the client asks the nurse, "What exactly is a blood type, anyway?" The nurse should incorporate which of the following statements in a response?
    1 The blood type represents an antibody that normally circulates in the blood plasma
    2 The blood type represents an antigen that normally circulates in the blood plasma
    3 The blood type represents an antigen found on the surface of the red blood cells
    4 The blood type represents an antibody found on the surface of the red blood cells

16. The Rh-negative client has given birth to an Rh-positive baby. The nurse prepares to administer which of the following medications as per agency protocol?
    1 Flunisolide (Rhinalar)
    2 Methotrexate (Rheumatrex)
    3 Rheaban
    4 RhoGAM

17. The client requiring upcoming surgery is extremely anxious about the need for possible blood transfusion during or after surgery. The nurse advises the client to do which of the following as the most effective way to eliminate this risk?
    1 Take iron supplements before surgery to boost hemoglobin levels
    2 Request that any donated blood be screened twice by the blood bank
    3 Ask a friend or family member to donate blood ahead of time
    4 Donate autologous blood prior to the surgery

18. The nurse assesses the client's temperature prior to beginning a blood transfusion. The temperature is 100.6°F orally. The nurse interprets that

which of the following actions would be most appropriate?

1 Begin the transfusion as ordered
2 Hold the blood and call the physician
3 Begin the transfusion after administering an antihistamine
4 Hold the blood until the client receives 600 mg of acetaminophen (Tylenol)

19. The client with hypovolemic shock requires plasma expansion. The nurse interprets that this client would benefit most from replacement of which of the following blood products?

1 Albumin
2 Platelets
3 Cryoprecipitate
4 Gamma globulin

20. The nurse is orienting a newly licensed nurse to the clinical nursing unit. They are co-assigned to a client due to be transfused with a unit of packed RBCs. The experienced nurse instructs the orientee that the unit of blood must be hung within how many minutes after obtaining it from the blood bank?

1 15
2 30
3 45
4 60

21. The client is receiving the second unit of packed red blood cells (PRBCs), which have been preserved with citrate phosphate-dextrose-adenine (CPDA-1). The client begins to complain of circumoral tingling and tingling in the fingers. The nurse takes which of the following corrective actions?

1 Slows the rate of transfusion
2 Stops the blood
3 Speeds up the flow rate of the blood
4 Adds more saline to the blood

22. A client with a low hemoglobin level and hematocrit is scheduled to receive a blood transfusion. When giving a health history, this client tells the nurse about having previously experienced a transfusion reaction characterized only by fever. The nurse relays this information to the physician and the blood bank, anticipating that the client will need to receive:

1 Granulocytes
2 Leukocyte-poor RBCs
3 Platelets
4 Fresh-frozen plasma

23. The nurse has finished infusing a unit of granulocytes to an assigned client. The nurse notes the results of which follow-up laboratory study to evaluate the effectiveness of this therapy?

1 Hemoglobin
2 Hematocrit
3 WBC count
4 Platelet count

24. The nurse is checking a unit of blood with another nurse prior to initiating a transfusion. The nurse notes that the blood type, Rh, expiration date, and unit number on the bag match the requisition. There is a discrepancy, however, in the client's name. Which of the following actions should the nurse plan to take next?

1 Hang the unit of blood since the blood information matches
2 Cross out the incorrect name and write in the correct one
3 Notify the physician that the client will not receive any blood
4 Call the blood bank about the discrepancy

25. The nurse is beginning to transfuse a client with a unit of blood. After priming the line and attaching the unit of blood, the nurse begins the transfusion at which of the following drip rates?

1 20 gtt/min
2 40 gtt/min
3 60 gtt/min
4 80 gtt/min

26. Within an hour after beginning to transfuse a unit of packed RBCs to an assigned client, the nurse finds the client to be restless, with complaints of chills and back pain. The nurse notes that there is dark-colored urine in the Foley catheter drainage bag. The nurse interprets that the client is most likely experiencing which of the following reactions?

1 Delayed hemolytic
2 Acute hemolytic
3 Hyperkalemic
4 Allergic

27. The client ordered to receive a transfusion has experienced a rash with pruritus during previous transfusions. The nurse anticipates that which of the following medications will be ordered as pretreatment for this client before beginning the transfusion?

1 Acetaminophen (Tylenol)
2 Ibuprofen (Motrin)
3 Diphenhydramine (Benadryl)
4 Allopurinol (Zyloprim)

28. The client receiving a blood transfusion begins to exhibit flushing, stridor, and a drop in blood pressure. The nurse initially obtains which of the following medications from the emergency cart to have ready for use as ordered?

1 Aminophylline
2 Lidocaine
3 Norepinephrine
4 Epinephrine

29. The nurse has transfused a unit of packed RBCs, which has a 250-mL bag of 0.9% sodium chloride (normal saline) attached. The follow-up IV order is to hang a 1000-mL bag of 5% dextrose in water. Which of the following steps would the

nurse take in the process of discontinuing the completed transfusion?
1 Aspirate the IV line before connecting the IV solution tubing
2 Disconnect the tubing while there is blood in the line and attach the IV solution tubing
3 Infuse the rest of the normal saline before changing from the blood tubing to the IV tubing
4 Flush the blood tubing with normal saline before changing to the IV tubing

30. The client has received a transfusion of platelets. The nurse evaluates that the client is benefiting most from this therapy if the client exhibits which of the following?
1 Decline of temperature to normal
2 Decrease in oozing from puncture sites and gums
3 Increased hemoglobin level
4 Increased hematocrit level

ANSWERS

1. **1**

Rationale: Asking the client about personal experiences with transfusion therapy provides a good starting point for client teaching about this procedure. Options 2 and 4 are not helpful because they may frighten the client. Option 3 is incorrect because it could make the client ill at ease, particularly if the client does not feel totally at ease with the information presented.

Test-Taking Strategy: The key words in the question are "client's knowledge" and "initial." This tells you that the correct answer is the best starting point for discussion about the transfusion therapy. Options 2 through 4 all have emotionally laden trigger words, including "anaphylactic shock," "everything," and "frighten," respectively, which make them incorrect. This is an example of a question when a response that is closed-ended is the best "initial" communication.

Level of Cognitive Ability: Application
Phase of Nursing Process: Assessment
Client Needs: Physiological Integrity
Content Area: Fundamental Skills

Reference
Luckmann, J. (1997). *Saunders manual of nursing care*. Philadelphia: W. B. Saunders. p. 1163.

2. **2**

Rationale: The client is taught to report chills, itching, or rash immediately. These could possibly be signs of transfusion reaction and would require the nurse to stop the transfusion. Mild discomfort at the catheter site may be indicative of a problem or could result from the size of the IV catheter required to infuse the blood product. Sleepiness, fatigue, headache, nausea, or vomiting are unrelated to transfusion reaction.

Test-Taking Strategy: Note that the key words in the question are "most important" and "immediately." This tells you that more than one or all of the options may be partially or totally correct. Knowing that a transfusion reaction is of most concern to the nurse, you must prioritize your answer to select the option that characterizes this problem. Review the signs of a transfusion reaction now, if you had difficulty with this question!

Level of Cognitive Ability: Application
Phase of Nursing Process: Implementation
Client Needs: Physiological Integrity
Content Area: Fundamental Skills

Reference
Luckmann, J. (1997). *Saunders manual of nursing care*. Philadelphia: W. B. Saunders. p. 1164.

3. **3**

Rationale: Sodium chloride (normal saline, NS) 0.9% is an isotonic solution that is standardly used both to precede and follow infusion of blood products. Dextrose is not used because it could result in clumping and subsequent hemolysis of red blood cells. Lactated Ringer's is not the solution of choice with this procedure.

Test-Taking Strategy: Familiarity with blood administration methods is needed to answer this question accurately. Remember that NS is the solution that is compatible with red blood cells. If this question was difficult, take a few moments to review this key area at this time.

Level of Cognitive Ability: Application
Phase of Nursing Process: Planning
Client Needs: Physiological Integrity
Content Area: Fundamental Skills

Reference
Luckmann, J. (1997). *Saunders manual of nursing care*. Philadelphia: W. B. Saunders. p. 1163.

4. **3**

Rationale: The IV catheter should have a minimum size of 18 or 19 gauge to be used for transfusion. This assures that the bore of the catheter is large enough to prevent damage to the blood cells.

Test-Taking Strategy: Specific knowledge of blood administration methods and techniques is needed to answer this question accurately. If this question was difficult, take a few moments to review this key area at this time!

Level of Cognitive Ability: Application
Phase of Nursing Process: Planning
Client Needs: Physiological Integrity
Content Area: Fundamental Skills

Reference
Taylor, C., Lillis, C., & LeMone, P. (1997). *Fundamentals of nursing: The art and science of nursing care* (3rd ed.). Philadelphia: Lippincott-Raven. p. 1425.

5. **4**

Rationale: The nurse asks a second registered nurse to check the unit of blood, according to agency policy. This minimizes the risk of error in checking information on the blood bag, and thereby minimizes risk of harm or injury to the client. The other responses are incorrect.

Test-Taking Strategy: Specific knowledge of blood administration methods and techniques is needed to answer this question accurately. If this question was difficult, take a few moments to review this key area at this time!

Level of Cognitive Ability: Application
Phase of Nursing Process: Implementation
Client Needs: Safe, Effective Care Environment
Content Area: Fundamental Skills

Reference

Luckmann, J. (1997). *Saunders manual of nursing care*. Philadelphia: W. B. Saunders. p. 1163.

6. **2**

Rationale: The nurse notes the expiration date on the unit of blood to assure that the blood is fresh. Blood cells begin to degenerate over time, so safe storage is limited to 35 days. Careful notation of the expiration date by the nurse is an essential part of the verification process that is done before hanging a unit of blood. Also noted are the blood identification (unit) number, blood group and type, and client's name. The nurse does also inspect the unit of blood for clots and returns the unit to the blood bank if any are found.

Test-Taking Strategy: The key word in this question is "deteriorates." To answer this question correctly, you must know which part of the pretransfusion verification procedure relates to the "freshness" of the unit of blood. A review of each of the options should allow you to eliminate each of the incorrect options systematically. Review the procedure for checking blood now, if you had difficulty with this question!

Level of Cognitive Ability: Application
Phase of Nursing Process: Implementation
Client Needs: Physiological Integrity
Content Area: Fundamental Skills

Reference

Taylor, C., Lillis, C., & LeMone, P. (1997). *Fundamentals of nursing: The art and science of nursing care* (3rd ed.). Philadelphia: Lippincott-Raven. p. 1426.

7. **3**

Rationale: A change in vital signs may indicate that a transfusion reaction is occurring. This is why the nurse assesses vital signs prior to the procedure, every 15 minutes for the first half hour, and every half hour thereafter.

Test-Taking Strategy: The key words in the question are "just prior" and "most important." This tells you that more than one of the options may be partially or totally correct. Use knowledge of blood transfusions and client assessment to prioritize your answer. Additionally, vital signs is the most global response!

Level of Cognitive Ability: Application
Phase of Nursing Process: Assessment
Client Needs: Physiological Integrity
Content Area: Fundamental Skills

Reference

Black, J., & Matassarin-Jacobs, E. (1997). *Medical-surgical nursing: Clinical management for continuity of care* (5th ed.). Philadelphia: W. B. Saunders. p. 1527.

8. **2**

Rationale: The nurse must remain with the client for the first 15 minutes of a transfusion, which is the most frequent period during which a transfusion reaction may occur. This enables the nurse to quickly detect a reaction and intervene quickly.

Test-Taking Strategy: Specific knowledge related to blood transfusion procedure is needed to answer this question accurately. Remember, the client needs to be directly monitored for the first 15 minutes of the transfusion. If needed, take a few moments now to review this procedure and its key elements!

Level of Cognitive Ability: Application
Phase of Nursing Process: Planning
Client Needs: Physiological Integrity
Content Area: Fundamental Skills

Reference

Black, J., & Matassarin-Jacobs, E. (1997). *Medical-surgical nursing: Clinical management for continuity of care* (5th ed.). Philadelphia: W. B. Saunders. p. 1527.

9. **1**

Rationale: Rapid transfusion of blood that is cold places the client at risk for cardiac dysrhythmias. To prevent this occurrence, the nurse warms the blood as indicated, using a blood-warming device. Electronic infusion devices are not helpful in this case, since the infusion must be rapid, and infusion devices are generally used to control the flow rate. In addition, not all infusion devices are made to handle blood or blood products. Blood pressure and cardiac monitoring equipment are useful in client assessment but do not prevent complications from occurring. Rather they are useful in early detection.

Test-Taking Strategy: Note that the key words in this question are "rapid" and "prevent." This tells you that the correct answer is one that will minimize the risk of cardiac dysrhythmias. Knowledge related to complications of transfusion therapy and hemorrhagic shock enables you to use critical thinking skills to choose correctly.

Level of Cognitive Ability: Application
Phase of Nursing Process: Implementation
Client Needs: Physiological Integrity
Content Area: Fundamental Skills

Reference

Black, J., & Matassarin-Jacobs, E. (1997). *Medical-surgical nursing: Clinical management for continuity of care* (5th ed.). Philadelphia: W. B. Saunders. pp. 1526–1527.

10. **4**

Rationale: The signs and symptoms exhibited by the client are consistent with transfusion reaction. With fluid overload, the client would be expected to have crackles in addition to dyspnea. With bacteremia, the client should have fever, which is not part of the clinical picture presented. There is no correlation between the signs mentioned and hypovolemic shock. The signs are indicative of allergic reaction, which is one type of blood transfusion reaction.

Test-Taking Strategy: To answer this question correctly, it is necessary to be able to recognize and accurately interpret signs of transfusion reaction. If needed, review the complications of blood administration and this key content area related to transfusion therapy at this time!

Level of Cognitive Ability: Analysis
Phase of Nursing Process: Analysis
Client Needs: Physiological Integrity
Content Area: Fundamental Skills

Reference

Black, J., & Matassarin-Jacobs, E. (1997). *Medical-surgical nursing: Clinical management for continuity of care* (5th ed.). Philadelphia: W. B. Saunders. p. 1528.

11. **3**

Rationale: If a transfusion reaction is suspected, the nurse stops the transfusion and allows normal saline to infuse pending further physician orders. This maintains a patent IV access line and aids in maintaining the client's intravascular volume. The nurse would not discontinue the IV line, because then there would be no IV access route. Normal saline is the solution of choice over solutions containing dextrose because saline does not cause RBCs to clump.

Test-Taking Strategy: Note that the question contains the key words "most prudent" and "pending further orders." This tells you that the correct answer is one that is done while waiting for definitive physician's orders. Begin to answer this question by eliminating options 1 and 4 as totally incorrect. Choose option 3 over option 2 knowing that normal saline is used when administering a unit of blood, or by knowing that it is more prudent to support the client with IV fluid to maintain intravascular volume.

Level of Cognitive Ability: Application
Phase of Nursing Process: Implementation
Client Needs: Physiological Integrity
Content Area: Fundamental Skills

Reference

Taylor, C., Lillis, C., & LeMone, P. (1997). *Fundamentals of nursing: The art and science of nursing care* (3rd ed.). Philadelphia: Lippincott-Raven. pp. 1427,1429.

12. **4**

Rationale: The nurse returns the blood transfusion bag containing any remaining blood to the blood bank. This allows the blood bank to complete any follow-up testing procedures needed once a transfusion reaction has been documented.

Test-Taking Strategy: Specific knowledge related to routine transfusion-related procedures is needed to answer this question accurately. Knowing that blood is issued from the blood bank may help you eliminate each of the incorrect options fairly easily. If needed, take a few moments to review this content area now!

Level of Cognitive Ability: Application
Phase of Nursing Process: Planning
Client Needs: Safe, Effective Care Environment
Content Area: Fundamental Skills

Reference

Black, J., & Matassarin-Jacobs, E. (1997). *Medical-surgical nursing: Clinical management for continuity of care* (5th ed.). Philadelphia: W. B. Saunders. p. 1529.

13. **1**

Rationale: The identification bracelet that is placed on the client at admission is the most important item for proper client identification before hanging a unit of blood. The ID bracelet contains the client's name, age, physician name, room number, and a hospital and/or medical record identification number. It contains the same information that is present on the client's addressograph card, which is stamped on all client requisitions. The social security number and address are irrelevant for the procedure described. The medical record number would most likely be present on the client ID bracelet, which is the better answer.

Test-Taking Strategy: Note that the question contains the key words "most important." This tells you that more than one or all of the options may be partially or totally correct. Begin to answer the question by eliminating options 2 and 3 first as incorrect. Choose option 1 over option 4 because it is the most global answer.

Level of Cognitive Ability: Application
Phase of Nursing Process: Implementation
Client Needs: Safe, Effective Care Environment
Content Area: Fundamental Skills

Reference

Black, J., & Matassarin-Jacobs, E. (1997). *Medical-surgical nursing: Clinical management for continuity of care* (5th ed.). Philadelphia: W. B. Saunders. p. 1525.

14. **2**

Rationale: The tubing used for blood administration has an inline filter. This helps assure that any particles larger than the size of the filter are caught in the filter and are not infused into the client. The tubing should have a roller clamp rather than a slide clamp for greater accuracy and control. The tubing should be macrodrip, not microdrip, to allow blood to flow freely through the drip chamber. An air vent is unnecessary, since the blood bag is not made of glass.

Test-Taking Strategy: The wording of the question tells you that there is clearly only one correct answer to the question. Read each option carefully and visualize the process of blood administration. Review concepts related to tubing used for blood administration now, if you had difficulty with this question!

Level of Cognitive Ability: Application
Phase of Nursing Process: Implementation
Client Needs: Safe, Effective Care Environment
Content Area: Fundamental Skills

Reference

Black, J., & Matassarin-Jacobs, E. (1997). *Medical-surgical nursing: Clinical management for continuity of care* (5th ed.). Philadelphia: W. B. Saunders. p. 1525.

15. **3**

Rationale: The major blood types are A, B, AB, and O. The blood type indicates an antigen that is found on the surface of the RBCs. Antigens can stimulate the production of antibodies. These antibodies are actually formed only when that specific antigen has gained entry into the body. For example, a person with type B blood has "B" antigen on the RBCs, and has agglutinins to cause clumping of "A" antigens.

Test-Taking Strategy: Specific knowledge related to the meaning of blood groups is needed to answer this question. If needed, take a few moments to review these basic concepts now!

Level of Cognitive Ability: Analysis
Phase of Nursing Process: Analysis
Client Needs: Physiological Integrity
Content Area: Fundamental Skills

Reference
Black, J., & Matassarin-Jacobs, E. (1997). *Medical-surgical nursing: Clinical management for continuity of care* (5th ed.). Philadelphia: W. B. Saunders. p. 1525.

16. 4

Rationale: RhoGAM (Rh₀ D immune globulin) is administered to prevent the client from developing a permanent active immunity to an Rh antigen. Rheaban is an antidiarrheal agent. Flunisolide (Rhinalar) is a nasal inhalation glucocorticoid. Methotrexate (Rheumatrex) is an antimetabolite used in the treatment of various cancers and to treat rheumatoid arthritis that does not respond to conventional therapy.

Test-Taking Strategy: To answer this question accurately, it is necessary to be familiar with RhoGAM and its intended purpose. If needed, take a few minutes to review this medication and those identified in the options at this time!

Level of Cognitive Ability: Application
Phase of Nursing Process: Planning
Client Needs: Health Promotion and Maintenance
Content Area: Fundamental Skills

References
Deglin, J., & Vallerand, A. (1997). *Davis's drug guide for nurses* (5th ed.). Philadelphia: F. A. Davis. pp. 116,537,771,1051.
Taylor, C., Lillis, C., & LeMone, P. (1997). *Fundamentals of nursing: The art and science of nursing care* (3rd ed.). Philadelphia: Lippincott-Raven. p. 1428.

17. 4

Rationale: Donating autologous blood to be reinfused as needed during or after surgery eliminates the risk of crossinfection from contaminated blood. The next most effective way is to ask a family member to donate blood prior to surgery. Blood banks do not provide extra screening on request. Preoperative iron supplements are helpful for iron deficiency anemia but are not most helpful in replacing blood lost during the surgery.

Test-Taking Strategy: Note that the question contains the key words "most effective." This tells you that more than one or all of the options may be partially or totally correct. Note the key word "autologous" in the correct option. Utilize knowledge related to disease transmission and blood donation procedures to answer this question!

Level of Cognitive Ability: Application
Phase of Nursing Process: Implementation
Client Needs: Physiological Integrity
Content Area: Fundamental Skills

Reference
Taylor, C., Lillis, C., & LeMone, P. (1997). *Fundamentals of nursing: The art and science of nursing care* (3rd ed.). Philadelphia: Lippincott-Raven. p. 1428.

18. 2

Rationale: If the client has a temperature equal to or greater than 100°F, the unit of blood should be held until the physician is notified and has the opportunity to give further orders. The other responses are incorrect.

Test-Taking Strategy: Familiarity with basic procedures related to blood administration is needed to answer this question correctly. Eliminate options 1 and 3 as they are similar. Select option 2 over option 4 remembering that the physician needs to be notified prior to initiating blood, if the temperature is elevated. If needed, take a few moments to review this content at this time!

Level of Cognitive Ability: Analysis
Phase of Nursing Process: Analysis
Client Needs: Physiological Integrity
Content Area: Fundamental Skills

Reference
Taylor, C., Lillis, C., & LeMone, P. (1997). *Fundamentals of nursing: The art and science of nursing care* (3rd ed.). Philadelphia: Lippincott-Raven. p. 1428.

19. 1

Rationale: Albumin may be used as a plasma expander. Platelets are used when the client's platelet count is low. Cryoprecipitate is useful in treating bleeding from hemophilia or disseminated intravascular coagulopathy because it is rich in clotting factors. Gamma globulin is used in the treatment of gamma globulin deficiencies.

Test-Taking Strategy: Specific knowledge of the benefits and uses of various blood products is needed to answer this question. The key phrase is "requires plasma expansion." If needed, take a few moments to review the various blood component therapies at this time!

Level of Cognitive Ability: Analysis
Phase of Nursing Process: Analysis
Client Needs: Physiological Integrity
Content Area: Fundamental Skills

Reference
Black, J., & Matassarin-Jacobs, E. (1997). *Medical-surgical nursing: Clinical management for continuity of care* (5th ed.). Philadelphia: W. B. Saunders. p. 278.

20. 2

Rationale: Blood must be hung within 30 minutes after obtaining it from the blood bank. After that time, the blood temperature will be in excess of 50°F and could be unsafe for use.

Test-Taking Strategy: Familiarity with basic procedures related to blood administration is needed to answer this question correctly. If needed, take a few moments to review this important content at this time!

Level of Cognitive Ability: Application
Phase of Nursing Process: Implementation
Client Needs: Physiological Integrity
Content Area: Fundamental Skills

Reference
Black J., & Matassaren-Jacobs, E. (1997). *Medical-Surgical Nursing: Clinical management for continuity of care* (5th ed.) Philadelphia: W. B. Saunders p. 1525.

21. 1

Rationale: The citrate preservative found in many units of PRBCs may bind onto calcium in the client's blood stream, effectively lowering the serum calcium level. The client then exhibits signs and symptoms of hypocalcemia. These include tingling around the mouth and in the fingers, muscle cramps, and hyperreflexia and nervousness. They can also progress in extreme cases to convulsions, hypotension, and cardiac arrest. This is referred to as citrate toxicity. The appropriate nursing action is to slow the infusion rate of the blood.

Test-Taking Strategy: Options 3 and 4 can be easily eliminated. To select accurately from the remaining two options, it is necessary to understand the effects of the citrate preservative on the electrolyte balance in the body, specifically the calcium level. If needed, take a few moments to review this type of reaction and the nursing management indicated!

Level of Cognitive Ability: Application
Phase of Nursing Process: Implementation
Client Needs: Physiological Integrity
Content Area: Fundamental Skills

Reference

Leahy, J., & Kizilay, P. (1998). *Foundations of nursing practice: A nursing process approach.* Philadelphia: W. B. Saunders. pp. 825–826.

22. **2**

Rationale: The client who has a low hemoglobin level and hematocrit requires replacement of RBCs. Febrile reactions without hemolysis usually occur in clients who have had transfusions in the past. The client develops antibodies in response to exposure to antigens of the surface of infused granulocytes, lymphocytes, or platelets. This reaction may be prevented or minimized by administering leukocyte-poor RBCs.

Test-Taking Strategy: The key phrases in this question are "low hemoglobin level and hematocrit" and "characterized only by fever." This tells you that the client has a limited reaction to transfusions in the past. It also indicates that the client needs transfusion of a blood product containing RBCs. Using either line of reasoning may help you eliminate each of the incorrect options systematically!

Level of Cognitive Ability: Analysis
Phase of Nursing Process: Analysis
Client Needs: Physiological Integrity
Content Area: Fundamental Skills

Reference

Leahy, J., & Kizilay, P. (1998). *Foundations of nursing practice: A nursing process approach.* Philadelphia: W. B. Saunders. pp. 823–824.

23. **3**

Rationale: The client who has neutropenia may receive a transfusion of granulocytes, or white blood cells. These are often clients with severe infections who are unresponsive to antibiotic therapy. The nurse notes the results of follow-up WBC counts to evaluate the effectiveness of therapy. The nurse continues to monitor the client for signs and symptoms of infection.

Test-Taking Strategy: A basic understanding of the different types of cells available for transfusion is needed to answer this question correctly. Recalling that granulocytes are a component of WBCs will assist in directing you to option 3. If needed, take a few moments to review the key points related to types of blood products at this time!

Level of Cognitive Ability: Analysis
Phase of Nursing Process: Evaluation
Client Needs: Physiological Integrity
Content Area: Fundamental Skills

Reference

Leahy, J., & Kizilay, P. (1998). *Foundations of nursing practice: A nursing process approach.* Philadelphia: W. B. Saunders. p. 824.

24. **4**

Rationale: The nurse should plan to call the blood bank to notify them of the discrepancy. The unit should not be hung, and information on the requisition or bag should not be altered in any way. The nurse may choose to call the physician, but the nature of that communication would be to report a delay in the transfusion due to the problem, not to report that there would be no transfusion.

Test-Taking Strategy: The key words in the question are "discrepancy" and "next." This tells you that the question is seeking a response that indicates the behavior of the nurse after analyzing this clinical problem. Knowledge of basic transfusion-related procedures should help you eliminate each of the incorrect options systematically.

Level of Cognitive Ability: Application
Phase of Nursing Process: Planning
Client Needs: Safe, Effective Care Environment
Content Area: Fundamental Skills

Reference

Leahy, J., & Kizilay, P. (1998). *Foundations of nursing practice: A nursing process approach.* Philadelphia: W. B. Saunders. p. 828.

25. **1**

Rationale: The nurse begins the transfusion at a rate of 20 drops per minute. Blood tubing typically has a drop factor of 10 drops per mL. A drip rate of 20 drops per minute indicates that only 2 mL infuses each minute. After 15 minutes, the nurse adjusts the transfusion rate upward as long as the client is tolerating the procedure without adverse changes in condition.

Test-Taking Strategy: Familiarity with basic procedures related to blood administration is needed to answer this question correctly. Remembering that the first 15 minutes is the most critical time, your best selection is the slowest rate of infusion. If needed, take a few moments to review this content at this time!

Level of Cognitive Ability: Application
Phase of Nursing Process: Implementation
Client Needs: Physiological Integrity
Content Area: Fundamental Skills

Reference

Leahy, J., & Kizilay, P. (1998). *Foundations of nursing practice: A nursing process approach.* Philadelphia: W. B. Saunders. p. 829.

26. **2**

Rationale: The client is experiencing an acute hemolytic reaction to the transfusion. The nurse in this instance would immediately stop the infusion and notify the physician. A delayed hemolytic reaction typically occurs from 2 to 14 days after transfusion. A hyperkalemic reaction occurs when blood is transfused that has been stored for too long, resulting in RBC hemolysis. The client experiencing a hyperkalemic type of reaction would exhibit nausea, muscle weakness or paresthesias, apprehension, bradycardia, ECG changes, and possibly cardiac arrest. An allergic reaction is characterized by flushing, nausea and vomiting, respiratory stridor, hypotension, and other signs of anaphylaxis.

Test-Taking Strategy: To answer this question accurately, it is necessary to be able to recognize the symptoms of various common transfusion reactions. If needed, take a few moments to review the key differences among them at this time. You are likely to find a question related to transfusion reactions on NCLEX-RN!

Level of Cognitive Ability: Analysis
Phase of Nursing Process: Analysis
Client Needs: Physiological Integrity
Content Area: Fundamental Skills

Reference

Leahy, J., & Kizilay, P. (1998). *Foundations of nursing practice: A nursing process approach.* Philadelphia: W. B. Saunders. pp. 825–826.

27. 3

Rationale: An urticaria reaction is characterized by a rash accompanied by pruritus. This type of transfusion reaction is prevented by pretreating the client with an antihistamine, such as diphenhydramine. Acetaminophen is an analgesic and motrin is a nonsteroidal antinflammatory drug. Allopurinol is an antigout medication.

Test-Taking Strategy: To answer this question accurately, it is necessary to be familiar with this particular type of reaction and the type of medication that may be utilized in its prevention. Use the process of elimination, recalling the classifications of the medications noted in each option. If needed, take a few moments to review the key elements of blood transfusion reactions and their management at this time!

Level of Cognitive Ability: Analysis
Phase of Nursing Process: Analysis
Client Needs: Physiological Integrity
Content Area: Pharmacology

Reference

Hodgson, B., & Kizior, R. (1998). *Saunders nursing drug handbook 1998.* Philadelphia: W. B. Saunders. pp. 331–333.
Leahy, J., & Kizilay, P. (1998). *Foundations of nursing practice: A nursing process approach.* Philadelphia: W. B. Saunders. pp. 825–826.

28. 4

Rationale: The symptoms exhibited by the client are compatible with an allergic reaction to the transfusion. Other common symptoms of allergic reaction are nausea and vomiting, diarrhea, and loss of consciousness. The nurse prepares to administer epinephrine and steroid medications as ordered. Norepinephrine is a sympathetic agonist used to treat hypotension, but it is not indicated in allergic reaction. Lidocaine is an antidysrhythmic medication. Aminophylline is a bronchodilator, which could possibly be prescribed if needed to treat bronchospasm.

Test-Taking Strategy: Note the key word in the stem of the question, which is "initially." This tells you that more than one or all of the options may be partially or totally correct. However, only one of the options is the first action of the nurse. In this case, you would eliminate options 2 and 3 first. You would choose option 4 over option 1 because it is the first-line agent used in management of severe allergic (anaphylactic) reaction.

Level of Cognitive Ability: Application
Phase of Nursing Process: Implementation
Client Needs: Physiological Integrity
Content Area: Pharmacology

Reference

Leahy, J., & Kizilay, P. (1998). *Foundations of nursing practice: A nursing process approach.* Philadelphia: W. B. Saunders. pp. 825–826.

29. 4

Rationale: When a unit of blood has finished infusing, the line is cleared of blood with approximately 10 to 20 mL of normal saline before hanging the next IV. This assures that the IV solution containing dextrose will not come in contact with the blood, which could cause RBC hemolysis.

Test-Taking Strategy: Familiarity with basic procedures related to blood administration is needed to answer this question correctly. Visualize the procedure as you select the correct option, remembering that NS is the only solution to be used with blood administration. If needed, take a few moments to review this content at this time!

Level of Cognitive Ability: Application
Phase of Nursing Process: Implementation
Client Needs: Physiological Integrity
Content Area: Fundamental Skills

Reference

Leahy, J., & Kizilay, P. (1998). *Foundations of nursing practice: A nursing process approach.* Philadelphia: W. B. Saunders. p. 830.

30. 2

Rationale: Platelets are necessary for proper blood clotting. The client with insufficient platelets may exhibit frank bleeding, or oozing of blood from puncture sites, wounds, and mucous membranes. A temperature would decline to normal following infusion of granulocytes if those cells were then instrumental in fighting infection in the body. An increased hemoglobin level and hematocrit would be seen when the client has received transfusion of red blood cells.

Test-Taking Strategy: To answer this question accurately, it is necessary to understand the potential uses and benefits of various types of blood product transfusions. If this question was difficult, review the key types of blood products available for transfusion. Remember, also, that options that are similar are not likely to be correct. With this in mind, you may immediately eliminate options 3 and 4 as incorrect.

Level of Cognitive Ability: Analysis
Phase of Nursing Process: Evaluation
Client Needs: Physiological Integrity
Content Area: Fundamental Skills

Reference

Leahy, J., & Kizilay, P. (1998). *Foundations of nursing practice: A nursing process approach.* Philadelphia: W. B. Saunders. p. 824.

BIBLIOGRAPHY

Black, J., & Matassarin-Jacobs, E. (1997). *Medical-surgical nursing: Clinical management for continuity of care* (5th ed.). Philadelphia: W. B. Saunders.
Deglin, J., & Vallerand, A. (1997). *Davis's drug guide for nurses* (5th ed.). Philadelphia: F. A. Davis.
Hodgson, B., & Kizior, R. (1998). *Saunders nursing drug handbook 1998.* Philadelphia: W. B. Saunders.
Ignatavicius, D., Workman, M., & Mishler, M. (1995). *Medical-surgical nursing: A nursing process approach* (2nd ed.). Philadelphia: W. B. Saunders.
Lammon, C., Foote, A., Leli, P., et al. (1995). *Clinical nursing skills.* Philadelphia: W. B. Saunders.

Leahy, J., & Kizilay, P. (1998). *Foundations of nursing practice: A nursing process approach*. Philadelphia: W. B. Saunders.

Lehne, R. (1998). *Pharmacology for nursing care* (3rd ed.). Philadelphia: W. B. Saunders.

Luckmann, J. (1997). *Saunders manual of nursing care*. Philadelphia: W. B. Saunders.

Monahan, F., & Neighbors, M. (1998). *Medical-surgical nursing: Foundations for clinical practice* (2nd ed.). Philadelphia: W. B. Saunders.

Taylor, C., Lillis, C., & LeMone, P. (1997). *Fundamentals of nursing: The art and science of nursing care* (3rd ed.). Philadelphia: Lippincott-Raven.

Fundamental Skills

CHAPTER 15

Providing a Safe Environment

....

PYRAMID TERMS

Nosocomial Infections—Infections acquired in the hospital or other health care facility that were not present or incubating at the time of the client's admission; also referred to as hospital-acquired infections.

Physical Restraints—Restriction of client movement through the application of a device.

Chemical Restraints—Medications given to inhibit a specific behavior or movement.

Poison—Any substance that impairs health and can destroy life when ingested, inhaled, or otherwise absorbed by the body.

Standard Precautions—Guidelines used by all health care providers with all clients to reduce the risk of infection for clients and caregivers.

Transmission-Based Precautions—Guidelines that are used in addition to Standard Precautions and are to be used for specific syndromes that are highly suspicious for infections until a diagnosis is confirmed.

PYRAMID TO SUCCESS

Safety and Infection Control is a subcategory of the Client Needs component, Safe, Effective Care Environment, of the test plan for NCLEX-RN. Pyramid points focus on maintaining environmental safety, preventing accidents, the use of **restraints**, and priority nursing actions in the event of an emergency or a disaster. Pyramid points also focus on **Standard and Transmission-Based Precautions** and the measures required to handle hazardous and infectious materials.

NURSING PROCESS

ASSESSMENT

Age
Lifestyle, cultural and religious practices
Sensory and perceptual alterations
Mental status
Health history
Presence of infections
Risk factors related to injury or infection

Laboratory values
History of falls
Knowledge level
Ability to communicate
Mobility
Nutrition and elimination patterns
Home safety

ANALYSIS:	Risk for injury.	Risk for infection.

PLANNING	IMPLEMENTATION	EVALUATION
Client will identify factors that increase the potential for injury. Client will identify internal and external factors that increase the risk of injury. Client will implement safety measures that decrease the risk of injury.	Assess actual and potential risk for injury. Assess effects of medication on the client. Implement environmental precautions. Use infection control practices. Comply with agency's environmental and safety guidelines. Use equipment according to the manufacturer's guidelines and agency's policies. Implement emergency measures during fires or disasters. Document assessment findings, risk potential, and measures implemented to provide safety. Initiate client education regarding the identification of hazards and health promotion practices. Collaborate with other health care members to assure client safety	Client remains free of preventable injuries. Client remains free of nosocomial infections. Client complies with health safety measures.

CLIENT NEEDS

SAFE, EFFECTIVE CARE ENVIRONMENT

Maintaining precautions to prevent accidents
Disaster planning
Standard and Transmission-Based Precautions
Handling hazardous and infectious materials
Guidelines regarding the use of restraints

HEALTH PROMOTION AND MAINTENANCE

Home safety assessment
Assisting clients and families to identify environmental hazards in the home
Client and family education regarding accident prevention
Client and family education to prevent the spread of infection
Client and family education regarding measures to be implemented in an emergency

PSYCHOSOCIAL INTEGRITY

Cultural and religious lifestyles
Sensory/perceptual alterations
Support systems

PHYSIOLOGICAL INTEGRITY

Providing comfort and assistance to client
Assisting the client with activities of daily living (ADLs)
Use of assistive devices to prevent injury
Managing and providing care to clients with infectious diseases
Priority nursing actions in an emergency

I. Environmental Safety

A. Fire Safety (Box 15–1)
    1. Keep open spaces free of clutter
    2. Clearly mark fire exits
    3. Know the location of all fire alarms, exits, and extinguishers (Table 15–1; Box 15–2)
    4. Know the telephone number for reporting fires
    5. Know the agency's fire drill and evacuation plan
    6. Never use the elevator in the event of a fire
    7. Turn off oxygen and appliances in the vicinity of the fire
    8. In the event of a fire, if the client is on life support, maintain the client's respiratory status manually with an Ambu-bag until the client is moved away from the threat of the fire
    9. In the event of a fire, ambulatory clients can be directed to walk by themselves to a safe area, and in some cases may be able to assist in moving clients in wheelchairs
    10. Bedridden clients are generally moved from the scene of a fire by a stretcher, their bed, or a wheelchair
    11. If a client must be carried from the area of a fire, appropriate transfer techniques need to be used
    12. If fire department personnel are at the scene of the fire, they can help evacuate clients
B. Electrical Safety
    1. Electrical equipment must be maintained in good working order and should be grounded
    2. Use a three-pronged electrical cord
    3. In a three-pronged electrical cord, the longer prong of the cord is the ground; the other two prongs carry the power to the piece of electrical equipment
    4. Any electrical equipment that the client brings into the health care facility must be inspected for safety prior to use
    5. Check electrical cords and outlets for exposed, frayed, and damaged wires
    6. Avoid overloading any circuit
    7. Read warning labels on all equipment; never operate unfamiliar equipment
    8. Use safety extension cords only when absolutely necessary and tape to the ground with electrical tape
    9. Never run electrical wiring under carpets
    10. Never pull a plug using the cord; always grasp the plug itself
    11. Never use electrical appliances near sinks, bathtubs, or other water sources
    12. Always disconnect a plug from the outlet before cleaning equipment or appliances
    13. If a client receives an electrical shock, turn off the electricity before touching the client
C. Radiation Safety
    1. Know the health care agency protocols and guidelines
    2. Label potentially radioactive material
    3. To reduce exposure to radiation
        a. The time spent near the source should be limited
        b. The distance from the source should be as great as possible
        c. A shielding device such as a lead apron should be used
    4. Monitor radiation exposure with a film badge
    5. Place client with a radiation implant in a private room

---

BOX 15–1. Priority Actions in the Event of a Fire

Remember the mnemonic **RACE** to set priorities in the event of a fire:

R—Rescue: Remove all clients from the vicinity of a fire

A—Alarm: Activate the fire alarm; report a fire before attempting to extinguish it

C—Confine: Close doors and windows when a fire is detected

E—Extinguish: Extinguish the fire, using the appropriate fire extinguisher

Table 15–1. Fire Extinguishers

Type	Class of Fires
Type A: Water	Wood, draperies, upholstery, paper, and rubbish
Types B and C: Carbon dioxide or dry chemical	Flammable liquids or gases, grease, and electrical
Types A, B, or C: Multipurpose, dry chemical	Any fire

6. Never touch dislodged implants
7. Wear gloves when handling body discharges

D. Disposal of Infectious Wastes
1. Handle all infectious materials as a hazard
2. Dispose of waste in designated areas only, using proper containers for disposal
3. Ensure that infectious material is properly labeled
4. Needles should not be recapped, bent, or broken
5. Dispose of all sharps immediately after use in closed, puncture-resistant disposal containers that are leakproof and labeled or color coded

E. Falls
1. See Box 15–3 for measures to prevent falls.

F. Restraints
1. Protective devices used to limit the physical activity of a client or to immobilize a client or an extremity
2. **Physical Restraints**: Restrict client movement through the application of a device
3. **Chemical Restraints**: Medications given to inhibit a specific behavior or movement
4. Implementation
   a. When **restraints** are necessary, the physician's orders should state the type of restraint and specific client behaviors for which **restraints** are to be used, and identify a limited time frame for use (Box 15–4)
   b. Physicians' orders for **restraints** should be renewed within a specific time frame according to the agency's policy
   c. **Restraints** are not to be ordered PRN
   d. The reason for the **restraints** should be given to the client and the family, and their permission should be sought

BOX 15–2. Using a Fire Extinguisher

Remember the mnemonic PASS to use a fire extinguisher:

P—Pull the pin
A—Aim at the base of the fire
S—Squeeze the handles
S—Sweep the fire from side to side

BOX 15–3. Measures to Prevent Falls

Assess client's risk for falling
Assign clients at risk for falling to rooms near the nurses' station
Alert all personnel to the client's risk for falling
Orient client to physical surroundings
Instruct client to seek assistance when getting up
Explain use of call bell system
Keep bed in the low position with side rails up if required
Lock all beds, wheelchairs, and stretchers
Keep personal items within reach
Eliminate clutter and obstacles in client's room
Provide adequate lighting
Reduce bathroom hazards
Maintain client's toileting schedule throughout the day

   e. **Restraints** should not interfere with any treatments or affect the client's health problem
   f. Use a clove hitch knot so that the restraint can be changed and released easily
   g. Assure that there is enough slack on the straps to assure some movement of the body part
   h. Secure the restraint to the bed frame, not to side rails
   i. Assess skin integrity and neurovascular and circulatory status every 30 minutes
   j. Release the **restraints** at least every 2 hours to permit muscle exercise and promote circulation
   k. Continually assess the need for **restraints**
5. Alternatives to **restraints**
   a. Orient client and family to surroundings
   b. Explain all procedures and treatments to client and family
   c. Encourage family and friends to stay with the client and utilize sitters for clients who need supervision
   d. Assign confused and disoriented clients to rooms near the nurses' station

BOX 15–4. Documentation Points with Use of a Restraint

Reason for restraint
Method of restraint
Date and time of application of restraint
Duration of use of the restraint and client's response
Release from restraint with periodic exercise and circulatory, neurovascular, and skin assessment
Assessment of continued need for restraint
Evaluation of the client response

e. Provide appropriate visual and auditory stimuli to client, such as clocks, radio
f. Place familiar items near the client's bedside, such as family pictures
g. Maintain toileting routines
h. Eliminate bothersome treatments, such as tube feedings, as soon as possible
i. Evaluate all medications that the client is receiving
j. Use relaxation techniques with the client
k. Institute exercise and ambulation schedules as client's condition allows

G. **Poisons**
1. Any substance that impairs health and can destroy life when ingested, inhaled, or otherwise absorbed by the body
2. Specific antidotes or treatments are available for only some types of **poisons**
3. The capacity of body tissue to recover from the **poison** determines the reversibility of the effect
4. **Poison** can impair the respiratory, circulatory, central nervous, hepatic, gastrointestinal (GI) and renal systems of the body
5. The toddler, preschooler, and young school-aged child must be protected from accidental **poisoning**
6. In older adults, diminished eyesight and impaired memory may result in accidental ingestion of poisonous substances or an overdose of prescribed medications
7. The Poison Control Center phone number should be visible on the telephone in homes with small children; in all cases of expected **poisoning**, the number should be called immediately
8. Implementation
a. Remove any obvious materials from the mouth, eyes, or body area immediately
b. Identify the type and amount of substance ingested
c. Call the Poison Control Center before attempting an intervention
d. If victim vomits or vomiting is induced, save vomitus if requested to do so and deliver it to the Poison Control Center
e. If instructed by the Poison Control Center to take the person to the emergency department, call an ambulance
f. Vomiting is never induced following ingestion of lye, household cleaners, grease, or petroleum products
g. Vomiting is never induced in an unconscious victim

II. Disasters

A. Know the agency's disaster plan
B. Internal disasters are those in which the agency is in danger
C. External disasters occur in the community, and many victims will be brought to the health care facility for care
D. When the health care agency is notified of a disaster, specific plans as specified in the agency policy must be carried out

III. Nosocomial Infections

A. Description
1. Also referred to as hospital-acquired infections
2. Infections acquired in the hospital or other health care facility that were not present or incubating at the time of the client's admission
3. Illness impairs the body's normal defense mechanism
4. The hospital environment provides exposure to a variety of virulent organisms that the client has not been exposed to in the past; therefore, the client has not developed resistance to these organisms
5. Infections can be transmitted by health care personnel who fail to practice proper handwashing procedures or fail to change gloves between client contacts
B. Drug-resistant **nosocomial infections**
1. Vancomycin-resistant enterococci (VRE)
2. Methicillin-resistant *Staphylococcus aureus* (MRSA)
3. Multidrug-resistant (MDR) tuberculosis (TB)

IV. Standard Precautions

A. Description
1. Combines the major features of Universal Precautions (UP) and Body Substance Isolation (BSI)
2. Must be practiced with all clients
3. Promotes handwashing and the use of gloves, masks, eye protection, and gowns when appropriate for client contact
B. Precautions
1. Blood
2. All body fluids, secretions and excretions, and contaminated items regardless of whether or not they contain visible blood
3. Nonintact skin
4. Mucous membranes
C. Implementation
1. Handle all blood and body fluids from all clients as if they are contaminated
2. Gloves should be removed and hands washed between client care
3. Masks, eye protection, or face shields are worn if client care activities may generate splashes or sprays of blood or body fluid
4. Gowns are worn if soiling of clothing is likely from blood or body fluid
5. Wash hands after removing a gown
6. Client care equipment is properly cleaned and reprocessed, and single-use items are discarded

7. Contaminated linen is placed in leakproof bags and handled to prevent skin and mucous membrane exposure
8. Needles are disposed of uncapped, or a mechanical device for recapping is used if necessary
9. All sharp instruments and needles are discarded in a puncture-resistant container
10. Clean up spills of blood or body fluids with a solution of bleach and water (diluted 1:10) or agency-approved disinfectant

V. Transmission-Based Precautions

A. Airborne Precautions
 1. Diseases
  a. Measles
  b. Chickenpox (varicella)
  c. Disseminated varicella zoster (shingles)
  d. Pulmonary or laryngeal TB
 2. Barrier protection
  a. Private room for client
  b. Negative air-flow pressure in room of 6 to 12 exchanges per hour
  c. Discharge of air outdoors or high-efficiency particulate air (HEPA) filtration system if air is recirculated
  d. Keep room door closed
  e. Wear an N95 respirator when entering the room of a client with known or suspected infectious TB or clients with measles and varicella, if not immune to these diseases
B. Droplet Precautions
 1. Diseases
  a. Diphtheria (pharyngeal)
  b. Rubella
  c. Streptococcal pharyngitis
  d. Mycoplasma or meningococcal pneumonia
  e. Scarlet fever in infants and younger children
  f. Pertussis
  g. Mumps
 2. Barrier Protection
  a. Private room for client
  b. A mask is required when within 3 feet of the client
  c. Place a mask on the client during transport
C. Contact Precautions
 1. Diseases
  a. Respiratory syncytial virus (RSV)
  b. *Shigella* and other enteric pathogens
  c. Major wound infections
  d. Herpes simplex
  e. Scabies
  f. Disseminated varicella zoster (shingles)
  g. Colonization or infection with multidrug-resistant organism
 2. Barrier protection
  a. Private room for client
  b. Wear gloves and a gown when in contact with client

PRACTICE QUESTIONS

1. The nurse enters a client's room and finds that the wastebasket is on fire. The nurse immediately assists the client out of the room. The next nursing action would be to:
 1 Confine the fire by closing the room door
 2 Activate the fire alarm
 3 Call for help
 4 Extinguish the fire

2. A nurse enters the nursing lounge and discovers that a chair is on fire. The nurse activates the alarm, closes the lounge door, and obtains the fire extinguisher to extinguish the fire. The nurse pulls the pin on the fire extinguisher. The next appropriate action would be to:
 1 Squeeze the handle on the extinguisher
 2 Aim at the base of the fire
 3 Sweep the fire from side to side with the extinguisher
 4 Sweep the fire from top to bottom with the extinguisher

3. The home care nurse performs a home safety assessment and discovers that a client is using a space heater to heat the apartment. Which of the following instructions would the nurse provide to the client regarding the use of the space heater?
 1 A space heater should not be used in an apartment
 2 The space heater needs to be placed at least 3 feet from anything that can burn
 3 The space heater should be placed in the hallway at night
 4 The space heater should be kept at low setting at all times

4. The nurse is preparing to initiate an IV containing a high dose of potassium to a client and plans to use an IV pump. The nurse brings the pump to the bedside and prepares to plug the pump cord into the wall. There is no available receptacle in the wall socket. Which of the following is the most appropriate nursing action?
 1 Use an extension cord from the nurse's lounge for the pump plug
 2 Initiate the IV without the use of a pump
 3 Plug in the pump cord in the available plug above the room sink
 4 Contact the electrical maintenance department for assistance

5. The nurse obtains an order from the physician to restrain the client using a jacket restraint. The nurse instructs the nursing assistant to apply the restraint to the client. Which of the following observations, if made by the nurse, would indicate inappropriate application of the restraint?
 1 A clove hitch knot in the restraint strap
 2 Restraint straps are safely secured to the side rails

3 The jacket restraint is secure and two fingers can easily slide between the restraint and the client's skin

4 The jacket restraint strap does not tighten when force is applied against it

6. The nurse is giving a report to the nursing assistant who will be caring for a client with hand restraints. The nurse instructs the nursing assistant to assess the skin integrity of the restrained hands:
   1 Every 30 minutes
   2 Every 2 hours
   3 Every 3 hours
   4 Every 4 hours

7. The nurse is planning care for a client with an internal radiation implant. Which of the following is not an appropriate component of this plan of care?
   1 Placing the client in a semiprivate room at the end of the hallway
   2 Wearing gloves when emptying the client's bedpan
   3 Keeping all linens in the room until the implant is removed
   4 Wearing a lead apron when providing direct care to the client

8. A mother calls the home care nurse and tells the nurse that her 3-year-old child has just ingested liquid furniture polish. The home care nurse would direct the mother to immediately:
   1 Administer ipecac to induce vomiting
   2 Bring the child to the emergency room
   3 Call an ambulance
   4 Call the Poison Control Center

9. The emergency room nurse receives a telephone call and is informed that a tornado hit a local residential area and numerous casualties have occurred. The victims will be brought to the emergency room. The initial nursing action would be which of the following?
   1 Prepare the triage rooms
   2 Obtain additional supplies from the central supply department
   3 Activate the agency disaster plan
   4 Obtain additional nursing staff to assist in treating the casualties

10. The nurse is caring for a client with a nosocomial infection caused by methicillin-resistant *S. aureus* (MRSA). Contact precautions are initiated. The nurse prepares to provide colostomy care to the client. Which of the following protective items will be required to perform this procedure?
    1 Gloves, gown, and goggles
    2 Gloves and goggles
    3 Gloves, gown, and shoe protectors
    4 Gloves and a gown

ANSWERS

1. **2**

Rationale: The order of priority in the event of a fire is to rescue the clients in immediate danger. The next step is to activate the fire alarm. The fire is then confined by closing all doors, and lastly, the fire is extinguished.

Test-Taking Strategy: Remember the mnemonic RACE to prioritize in the event of a fire. R—Rescue clients in immediate danger; A—Alarm, sound the alarm; C—Confine the fire by closing all doors; E—Extinguish or evacuate. If you had difficulty with this question, take time now to review fire safety!

Level of Cognitive Ability: Application
Phase of Nursing Process: Implementation
Client Needs: Safe, Effective Care Environment
Content Area: Fundamental Skills
Reference
Leahy, J., & Kizilay, P. (1998). *Foundations of nursing practice: A nursing process approach.* Philadelphia: W. B. Saunders. p. 393.

2. **2**

Rationale: A fire can be extinguished by smothering it with a blanket or by the use of a fire extinguisher. To use the extinguisher, the pin is pulled first. The extinguisher should then be aimed at the base of the fire. The handle of the extinguisher is then squeezed and the fire is extinguished by sweeping from side to side to coat the area evenly.

Test-Taking Strategy: Remember the mnemonic PASS to prioritize in the use of a fire extinguisher. PASS—Pull the pin; A—Aim at the base of the fire; S—Squeeze the handle; S—Sweep from side to side to coat the area evenly. If you had difficulty with this question, take time now to review the appropriate use of a fire extinguisher!

Level of Cognitive Ability: Application
Phase of Nursing Process: Implementation
Client Needs: Safe, Effective Care Environment
Content Area: Fundamental Skills

Reference
Leahy, J., & Kizilay, P. (1998). *Foundations of nursing practice. A nursing process approach*. Philadelphia: W. B. Saunders. pp. 392–393.

3. **2**

Rationale: Space heaters need to be used appropriately as they present a great risk of fire. A space heater needs to be placed at least 3 feet from anything that can burn. Placing a heater in a hallway does not guarantee that it will be 3 feet from anything that can burn. A low setting does not reduce the risk of fire. A space heater can be used in an apartment if there is ample space and safety precautions are followed.

Test-Taking Strategy: Use the process of elimination, keeping in mind the issue related to fire safety. Note that option 2 is the only option that specifically defines a safety measure related to the use of a space heater. Review fire safety prevention measures in the home now, if you had difficulty with this question!

Level of Cognitive Ability: Application
Phase of Nursing Process: Implementation
Client Needs: Safe, Effective Care Environment
Content Area: Fundamental Skills

Reference
Leahy, J., & Kizilay, P. (1998). *Foundations of nursing practice: A nursing process approach*. Philadelphia: W. B. Saunders. p. 392.

4. **4**

Rationale: The nurse needs to utilize hospital resources for assistance. A regular extension cord should not be used because it poses the risk of fire. The use of electrical appliances near a sink also presents a hazard. An IV that contains a high dose of potassium should be administered by the use of a pump.

Test-Taking Strategy: Note the key phrase "high dose" in the question. This will assist in easily eliminating option 2. Recalling safety issues related to electrical hazards will assist in eliminating options 1 and 3. If you had difficulty with this question, take time to review electrical safety!

Level of Cognitive Ability: Application
Phase of Nursing Process: Implementation
Client Needs: Safe, Effective Care Environment
Content Area: Fundamental Skills

Reference
Leahy, J., & Kizilay, P. (1998). *Foundations of nursing practice: A nursing process approach*. Philadelphia: W. B. Saunders p. 389.

5. **2**

Rationale: A clove hitch knot should be used for applying a restraint because it does not tighten when force is applied against it and allows quick and easy removal of the restraint in case of an emergency. The restraint strap is secured to the bed frame and never to the side rail to avoid accidental injury in the event that the side rail is released. The jacket restraint should be secure, and one to two fingers should easily slide between the restraint and the client's skin.

Test-Taking Strategy: Note the key word "inappropriate" in the stem of the question. This indicates that you are looking for a response that identifies an inaccurate measure related to the application of restraints. The phrase "secured to the side rails" in option 2 should direct your attention as an inappropriate action. Review guidelines related to the application of restraints now, if you had difficulty with this question!

Level of Cognitive Ability: Analysis
Phase of Nursing Process: Evaluation
Client Needs: Safe, Effective Care Environment
Content Area: Fundamental Skills

Reference
Leahy, J., & Kizilay, P. (1998). *Foundations of nursing practice: A nursing process approach*. Philadelphia: W. B. Saunders. pp 399–400.

6. **1**

Rationale: The nurse should instruct the nursing assistant to assess restraints and skin integrity every 30 minutes. Additionally, restraints need to be released at least every 2 hours to permit muscle exercise and promote circulation. Agency guidelines regarding the use of restraints should always be followed.

Test-Taking Strategy: Knowledge regarding the use of restraints is required to answer this question. In this situation, it is best to select the option that identifies the most frequent time frame. You are likely to find a question related to restraints on NCLEX-RN!

Level of Cognitive Ability: Application
Phase of Nursing Process: Implementation
Client Needs: Physiological Integrity
Content Area: Fundamental Skills

Reference
Lammon, C., Foote, A., & Leli P., et al. (1995). *Clinical nursing skills*. Philadelphia: W. B. Saunders, p. 292.

7. **1**

Rationale: A private room with a private bath is essential if a client has an internal radiation implant. This is necessary to prevent accidental exposure of radiation to other clients. Options 2, 3, and 4 are accurate interventions for a client with a radiation implant.

Test-Taking Strategy: Note the key phrase "not an appropriate." Option 2 can be eliminated first because this is a component of standard precautions for all clients. Options 3 and 4 can be eliminated next because they directly relate to radiation safety. Review radiation safety principles now, if you had difficulty with this question!

Level of Cognitive Ability: Application
Phase of Nursing Process: Planning
Client Needs: Safe, Effective Care Environment
Content Area: Fundamental Skills

Reference
Craven, R., & Hirnle, C. (1996). *Fundamentals of nursing: Human health and function* (2nd ed.). Philadelphia: Lippincott-Raven. pp. 703–704.

8. **4**

Rationale: If a poisoning occurs, the Poison Control Center should be contacted immediately. Vomiting should not be induced if the victim is unconscious or if the substance ingested was a strong corrosive or petroleum product. Bringing the child to the emergency room and calling an ambulance would not be the initial actions as this would delay treatment. The Poison Control Center may advise the mother to bring the child to the emergency department, and if this is the case, the mother should call an ambulance.

Test-Taking Strategy: Note the key word "immediately" in the stem of the question. Eliminate options 2 and 3 because these options will delay treatment. Recalling that vomiting should not be induced if a corrosive substance was ingested will assist in eliminating option 1. Review poison control measures now, if you had difficulty with this question!

Level of Cognitive Ability: Application
Phase of Nursing Process: Implementation
Client Needs: Physiological Integrity
Content Area: Child Health

Reference
Craven, R., & Hirnle, C. (1996). *Fundamentals of nursing: Human health and function* (2nd ed.). Philadelphia: Lippincott-Raven. p. 711.

9. **3**

Rationale: In an external disaster, many people will be brought to the emergency room for treatment. Although options 1, 2, and 4 may be components of preparing for the casualties, the initial nursing action must be to activate the disaster plan.

Test-Taking Strategy: Note the key word "initial" in the stem of the question. Use the process of elimination in determining the priority action. Note that option 3 is the global response. Review procedures related to management of a disaster now, if you had difficulty with this question!

Level of Cognitive Ability: Application
Phase of Nursing Process: Implementation
Client Needs: Safe, Effective Care Environment
Content Area: Fundamental Skills

Reference
Craven, R., & Hirnle, C. (1996). *Fundamentals of nursing: Human health and function* (2nd ed.). Philadelphia: Lippincott-Raven. p. 710.

10. **1**

Rationale: Goggles are worn to protect the mucous membranes of the eye during interventions that may produce splashes of blood, body fluids, secretions, and excretions. In addition, contact precautions require the use of gloves, and a gown should be worn if direct client contact is anticipated. Shoe protectors are not necessary.

Test-Taking Strategy: Note the key phrases "contact precautions" and "colostomy." Use the process of elimination in determining the necessary items required to care for this client. If you had difficulty with this question, take time now to review transmission-based precautions!

Level of Cognitive Ability: Application
Phase of Nursing Process: Implementation
Client Needs: Safe, Effective Care Environment
Content Area: Fundamental Skills

Reference
Leahy, J., & Kizilay, P. (1998). *Foundations of nursing practice: A nursing process approach.* Philadelphia: W. B. Saunders. pp 1237–1238.

BIBLIOGRAPHY

Black, J., & Matassarin-Jacobs, E. (1997). *Medical-surgical nursing; Clinical management for continuity of care* (5th ed.). Philadelphia: W. B. Saunders.

Craven, R., & Hirnle, C. (1996). *Fundamentals of nursing: Human health and function* (2nd ed.). Philadelphia: Lippincott-Raven.

DeLaune, S., & Ladner, P. (1998). *Fundamentals of nursing: Standards and practice.* Albany, NY: Delmar.

Hodgson, B., & Kizior, R. (1998). *Saunders nursing drug handbook 1998.* Philadelphia: W. B. Saunders.

Lammon, C., Foote, A., Leli, P., et al. (1995). *Clinical nursing skills.* Philadelphia: W. B. Saunders.

Leahy, J., & Kizilay, P. (1998). *Foundations of nursing practice: A nursing process approach.* Philadelphia: W. B. Saunders.

Luckmann, J. (1997). *Saunders manual of nursing care.* Philadelphia: W. B. Saunders.

Monahan, F., & Neighbors, M. (1998). *Medical-surgical nursing: Foundations for clinical practice* (2nd ed.). Philadelphia: W. B. Saunders.

CHAPTER 16

Administering Medication and Intravenous Solutions

....

PYRAMID TERMS

Conversion—Conversion is the first step in the calculation of a medication problem.

Generic Name—The generic name is the official accepted name of a drug.

Milliequivalent—Milliequivalent, abbreviated mEq, is an expression of the number of grams of a medication contained in 1 mL of a normal solution.

Parenteral—Parenteral always means injection route. Injections are administered by intravenous (IV), intramuscular (IM), and subcutaneous (SQ, SC) methods. Percentage solutions express the number of grams of the medication per 100 mL of solution.

Reconstitution—Powders must be dissolved with a sterile diluent before use, and usually sterile water or normal saline is used. The dissolving procedure is called reconstitution.

Ratio Solutions—Ratio solutions express the number of grams of the medication per total milliliters of solution.

Trade Name—The trade name, also called brand name or proprietary name, is followed by the sign ® meaning that the name is a registered trademark.

Unit—Unit, abbreviated as U or u, measures a medication in terms of its action, not its physical weight.

◆ PYRAMID TO SUCCESS

When a medication or intravenous calculation question is presented, the nurse should always use the appropriate formula to calculate the problem. Short-cuts should not be used when calculating these problems. The problem and answer should be labeled with the correct measurement. Be careful with decimal points. It is important to place the decimal points in the correct places or the answer will be incorrect. When calculating the problem, the nurse evaluates whether the answer is within reason and makes sense. In the clinical setting, the nurse should always seek assistance if unsure of the accuracy in calculating.

On CAT NCLEX-RN, it is important to check the calculation before selecting the answer to the question. REMEMBER, on CAT NCLEX-RN, the correct answer will be on the screen. Following the formula, placing the decimal points in the correct places, and checking the accuracy of the calculation will ensure selection of the correct answer!

PRACTICE MAKES PERFECT!

NURSING PROCESS

ASSESSMENT

Medication order
Five rights: right medication, right dose, right client, right route, and right time
Client's history of allergies
Client's current condition and the purpose for the medication or intravenous solution
Client's understanding of the purpose of the medication
Need for conversion when preparing a dose of medication

ANALYSIS:	Potential for Injury	Risk for Fluid Volume Excess
	Risk for Infection	Knowledge Deficit

PLANNING	IMPLEMENTATION	EVALUATION
Client will remain free of injury. Client will remain free of infection. Client will maintain fluid balance. Client will verbalize purpose of medication or intravenous solution. Client will respond appropriately to the medication.	Assess medication order. Ask client about a history of allergies. Assess client's current condition. Assess vital signs. Monitor client for signs of infection. Monitor client for signs of fluid overload. Assess the five rights: right medication, right dose, right client, right route, and right time. Assess the need for conversion when calculating the correct dose of medication. Prepare and administer medication or intravenous solution once correct dosage is determined. Determine client's understanding regarding the prescribed medication. Determine client's understanding of the purpose of the medication. Teach client about medication. Document the administration of the prescribed therapy and client's response to the therapy.	Correct dosage is determined and administered to client. Client's vital signs remain within normal limits. Client does not develop an infection, fluid overload, or adverse medication reaction. Client responds appropriately to the medication or intravenous solution. Effectiveness of the medication is achieved. Client verbalizes purpose of prescribed therapy.

CLIENT NEEDS

SAFE, EFFECTIVE CARE ENVIRONMENT

Client rights
Medication calculations
Intravenous fluid and medication calculations
Error prevention
Handling hazardous and infectious materials
Asepsis
Standard precautions

HEALTH PROMOTION AND MAINTENANCE

Physical assessment of client
Client teaching regarding prescribed medication(s) or IV therapy
Disease prevention

PSYCHOSOCIAL INTEGRITY

Utilization of support systems
Communication
Caring and providing emotional comfort
Cultural awareness
Use of coping mechanisms

PHYSIOLOGICAL INTEGRITY

Administration of medications and IV therapy
Expected effects of pharmacological therapy
Actions, side effects, and untoward effects of medications and IV therapy
Unexpected responses to therapy
Alterations in body systems
Laboratory values
Monitoring hemodynamics
Fluid and electrolyte imbalances

I. Drug Measurement Systems

A. Metric system
 1. The basic units of metric measures are meter, liter, and gram (Table 16–1)
  a. Meter measures length
  b. Liter measures volume
  c. Gram measures weight
B. Apothecary and Household Systems (Table 16–2)

 1. The apothecary and household systems are the oldest of the medication measurement systems
 2. The four apothecary measures sometimes used are the grain, minim, dram, and ounce
  a. Grain measures weight
  b. Minim, dram, and ounce measure volume
 3. The three household measures commonly used are the tablespoon, teaspoon, and drop
C. Additional Common Drug Measures
 1. **Milliequivalent**
  a. Abbreviated mEq
  b. Is an expression of the number of grams of a medication contained in 1 mL of a normal solution
  c. Example: Potassium
 2. **Unit**
  a. Abbreviated as U or u; measures a medication in terms of its action, not its physical weight
  b. Examples: Penicillin, heparin, insulin

II. Conversions

A. Conversion Between Metrics Units (Box 16–1)
 1. The metric system is a decimal system; therefore, conversions between the units in this system can be done either by dividing or

Table 16–1. Metric System

Abbreviations	Equivalents
meter—m	1 mg = 1000 μg or 0.001 g
liter—L	1 gm = 1000 mg
gram—g, gm, Gm	1 mL = 0.001 L or 1 mL
milligram—mg, mgm	1 kg = 1000 g
microgram—μg, mcg	1 μg = 0.000001 g
kilogram—kg, Kg	1 mL = 1 cc or 0.001 L
milliliter—mL	1 kg = 2.2 lb
cubic centimeter—cc	1 L = 1000 mL

Table 16–2. **Apothecary and Household Systems**

Abbreviations	Equivalents
grain—gr	gr 1 = 60 mg
dram—dr	gr 5 = 300 mg
ounce—oz	gr 15 = 1000 mg or 1 g
minim—min, M, or m	gr 1/150 = 0.4 mg
quart—qt	1 oz = 30 mL
pint—pt	1 dr = 4 mL
drop—gtt	1 T = 15 mL or 3 tsp
tablespoon—T or tbs	1 t or tsp = 5 mL
teaspoon—t or tsp	1 min = 1 gtt
pound—lb	15 min = 1 mL
	60 min = 1 dr
	8 dr = 1 oz
	1 qt = 1000 mL or 1 L
	1 qt = 2 pt or 32 oz
	1 pt = 16 oz
	16 oz = 1 lb
	2.2 lb = 1 kg

BOX 16–2. Calculating Equivalents Between Two Systems

Calculating equivalents between two systems may be done using the method of ratio and proportion!

PROBLEM:

The physician orders nitroglycerin, gr 1/150. The medication label reads 0.4 mg per tablet. How many tablets will you administer to the client?

gr 1 : 60 mg = gr 1/150 : X mg
60 × 1/150 = X
X = 0.4 mg (1 tablet)

---

multiplying by 1000 or by moving the decimal point three places to the right or three places to the left

2. In the metric system, to convert larger to smaller multiply by 1000 or move the decimal 3 places to the right
3. In the metric system, to convert smaller to larger divide by 1000 or move the decimal 3 places to the left

B. Conversion Between Apothecary, Household, and Metric Systems
   1. Conversions between the metric, apothecary, and household measures are equivalent, not equal, measures
   2. Conversion to equivalent measures between systems is necessary when a medication order is written in one system but the medication label is stated in another
   3. Medications are not always ordered and prepared in the same system of measurement; it is therefore necessary to convert units from one system to another

---

BOX 16–1. Conversion Between Metric Units

1. PROBLEM:

Convert 2 grams to milligrams.

Solution:

Change a larger unit to a smaller unit.
2.000 grams = 2000 mg (moving decimal 3 places to right)

2. PROBLEM:

Convert 250 mL to liters.

Solution:

Change a smaller unit to a larger unit.
250 mL = 0.250 L or 0.25 L (moving decimal 3 places to left)

---

4. Conversion is the first step in the calculation of dosages
5. Calculating equivalents between two systems may be done using the method of ratio and proportion (Box 16–2)

III. Celsius and Fahrenheit Temperature (Table 16–3)

A. To convert Fahrenheit to Celsius, subtract 32 and divide the result by 1.8
B. To convert Celsius to Fahrenheit, multiply by 1.8 and add 32

IV. Medication Labels

A. A medication label will contain both the **generic** and **trade name** of the medication
B. The **generic name** is the official accepted name of a medication; the **generic name** is not capitalized
C. The trade name, also called brand name or proprietary name, is followed by the sign ®, meaning the name is registered; trade names are capitalized or written with the first letter capitalized
D. Each medication has only one official name but may have several trade names, each for the exclusive use of the company that manufactures the medication

E. Always check expiration dates on medication labels

V. Medication Orders (Box 16–3)

A. In a medication order, the name of the medication is written first, followed by the dosage, route, and frequency

---

Table 16–3. **Celsius and Fahrenheit Temperature**

Fahrenheit to Celsius
To convert Fahrenheit to Celsius, subtract 32 and divide result by 1.8
Formula: $C = (F - 32) \div 1.8$

Celsius to Fahrenheit
To convert Celsius to Fahrenheit, multiply by 1.8 and add 32
Formula: $F = 1.8 C + 32$

BOX 16–3. Medication Orders

Name of client
Date and time when order written
Name of medication to be given
Dosage of medication
Route
Time and frequency of administration
Signature of person writing the order

B. If there are any questions or inconsistencies with the written order, the person who wrote the order must be contacted immediately, and the order must be verified

VI. Oral Medications

A. Scored tablets contain an indented mark to make possible breakage for partial dosages; when necessary, scored tablets (those marked for division) can be divided in halves or quarters
B. Enteric-coated tablets and sustained-released capsules delay absorption until the medication reaches the small intestine; these medications should not be crushed
C. Capsules contain a powdered or oily medication in a gelatin cover
D. Oral liquids are supplied in solution form and contain a specific amount of medication in a given amount of solution, as stated on the label
E. The Medicine Cup
    1. Has a capacity of 30 mL or 1 ounce
    2. Is used for oral liquids
    3. Is calibrated to measure teaspoons, tablespoons, and drams
    4. To pour accurately, hold the medication cup at eye level, then line up the measure that is needed and pour
F. Volumes of less than 5 mL are measured using a syringe with the needle removed
G. A calibrated dropper is used when giving medicine to children and when adding small amounts of liquid to water or juice; calibrations are in milliliters, cubic centimeters, drops, or minims

VII. Parenteral Medications

A. **Parenteral** always means injection route, and **parenteral** medications are administered by intravenous (IV), intramuscular (IM), or subcutaneous (SC) routes.
B. **Parenteral** medications are packaged in single-use ampules, single and multiple-use rubber-stoppered vials, and premeasured syringes and cartridges
C. The nurse should not administer more than 3 mL per IM or SC injection site, as volumes larger than 3 mL are difficult for a single injection site to absorb
D. Always question excessively large or small volumes of medication

E. The standard 3-mL (cc) syringe is used to measure most injectable medications; it is calibrated in tenths (0.1) of a mL (Fig. 16–1)
F. The calibrations on a syringe are read from the top black ring on the syringe, not the raised middle section and not the bottom ring
G. Injection Cartridges
    1. Tubex and Carpuject are trade names of two widely used injection cartridges
    2. These cartridges slip into plastic injectors that provide a plunger for injection of the medication
    3. The cartridge is prefilled with sterile medication and is labeled with the medication name and dosage
    4. The cartridges contain a volume of 2.5 mL and are calibrated in tenths
    5. The cartridges are routinely overfilled with 0.1 to 0.2 mL of medication to allow for manipulation of the syringe to expel air from the needle prior to injection
    6. The cartridges are designed to provide sufficient capacity to allow for the addition of a second medication when combined dosages are prescribed
    7. The prefilled syringe is to be used once and discarded; if the nurse is to give less than a full single dose provided, the nurse needs to discard the extra amount before injecting the client
H. Standard medication doses are to be rounded to the nearest tenth (0.1) of a mL or cc and measured on the mL scale; for example, 1.25 mL is rounded to 1.3 mL
I. When volumes larger than 3 mL are required, a 5-, 6-, 10-, or 12-mL syringe may be used; these syringes are calibrated in fifths (Fig. 16–2)
J. Syringes larger than 12 mL are calibrated in full mL measures
K. Tuberculin Syringe (Fig. 16–3)
    1. Holds a total capacity of 1 mL or cc and is used to measure small or critical amounts of medications such as allergen extract, vaccine, or a child's medication
    2. It is calibrated in hundredths (0.01) of a mL, with each one tenth (0.1) marked on the metric scale
L. Insulin Syringe (Fig. 16–4)
    1. The standard U-100 insulin syringe is used to measure U-100 insulin only; it is calibrated for a total of 100 units, or 1 mL (cc)
    2. The Lo-Dose U-100 insulin syringe is used for measuring small amounts of U-100 insulin; it is calibrated for a total of 50 units, or 0.5 mL (cc)
    3. Insulin should not be measured in any other type of syringe
    4. When the insulin order states to combine Regular and NPH Insulin, remember "R.N." Draw "R"egular insulin first, and then draw the "N"PH insulin

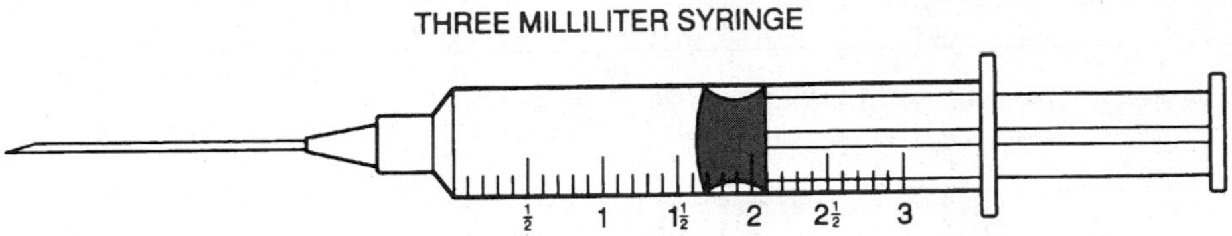

THREE MILLILITER SYRINGE

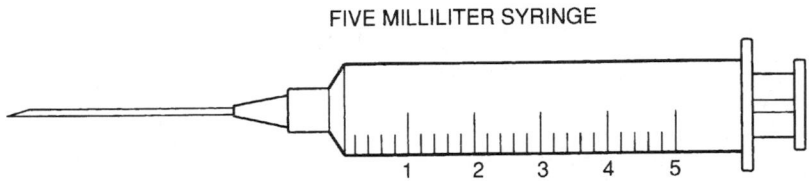

FIGURE 16–1. Three milliliter syringe. (From Kee, J., & Marshall, S. [1996]. *Clinical calculations: With applications to general and specialty areas* [3rd ed.]. Philadelphia: W. B. Saunders.)

FIVE MILLILITER SYRINGE

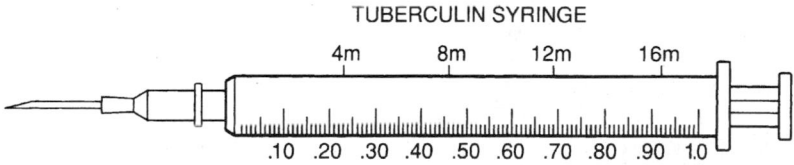

FIGURE 16–2. Five milliliter syringe. (From Kee, J., & Marshall, S. [1996]. *Clinical calculations: With applications to general and specialty areas* [3rd ed.]. Philadelphia: W. B. Saunders.)

TUBERCULIN SYRINGE

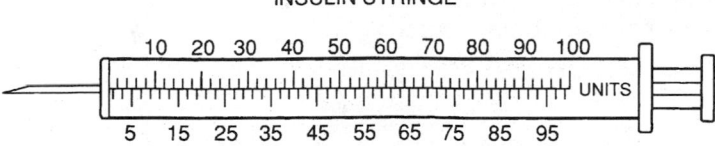

FIGURE 16–3. Tuberculin syringe. (From Kee, J., & Marshall, S. [1996]. *Clinical calculations: With applications to general and specialty areas* [3rd ed.]. Philadelphia: W. B. Saunders.)

INSULIN SYRINGE

FIGURE 16–4. Insulin syringe. (From Kee, J., & Marshall, S. [1996]. *Clinical calculations: With applications to general and specialty areas* [3rd ed.]. Philadelphia: W. B. Saunders.)

In reconstituting the medication, locate the instructions on the label or in the vial package insert and read and follow the directions carefully.

Instructions will state the volume of diluent to be used and the resulting volume of the reconstituted medication.

Often the powdered medication adds volume to the solution in addition to the amount of diluent added.

When you reconstitute a multiple-dose vial, label the medication vial with the date and time of preparation, your initials, and the date of expiration.

It is also important to label the strength per volume.

The total volume of the prepared solution will always exceed the volume of the diluent you add.

VIII. Injectable Medications in Powder Form

A. Some medications become unstable when stored in solution form and are therefore packaged in powder form
B. Powders must be dissolved with a sterile diluent before use, and usually sterile water or normal saline is used. The dissolving procedure is called **reconstitution** (Box 16–4)

IX. Calculating the Correct Dosage (Table 16–4)

A. When calculating oral medications, check the calculation and question an order if the amount is for more than three tablets
B. When calculating parenteral medications, check the calculation and question an order if the amount to be given is too large a dose
C. Regardless of the source of the error, if the nurse gives an incorrect dose, the nurse is legally responsible for the action
D. Be sure that all measures are in the same system, and all units are in the same size, converting when necessary; carefully consider what is the reasonable amount of the medication that should be administered
E. Round standard injection doses to tenths and measure in a 3-mL syringe
F. Round small, critical, or children's doses to hundredths and measure in the 1-mL tuberculin syringe

Table 16–4. Formula for Calculating a Medication Dosage

$$\frac{D \text{ (Desired)}}{A \text{ (Available)}} \times Q \text{ (Quantity)} = X$$

D (Desired) = The dosage that the physician ordered
A (Available) = The dosage strength as stated on the medication label
Q (Quantity) = The volume that the dosage strength is available in, such as tablets, capsules, or mL

X. Calculating Dosages Expressed as Ratio or Percent

A. **Percentage Solutions**
   1. Express the number of grams of the medication per 100 mL of solution
   2. Example: Calcium gluconate 10% = 10 g of pure medication per 100 mL of solution
B. **Ratio Solutions**
   1. Express the number of grams of the medication per total milliliters of solution
   2. Example: Epinephrine 1:1000 = 1 g pure medication per 1000 mL solution

XI. Intravenous Flow Rates

A. Monitor IVs every 30 minutes for adults and every 15 minutes for children
B. If the IV is running behind schedule, collaborate with the physician to determine the client's ability to tolerate an increased flow rate, particularly those clients with cardiac, pulmonary, renal, and neurological conditions
C. The nurse should never arbitrarily speed up an IV to catch up if the IV is running behind schedule
D. Whenever an IV rate is increased, the nurse should assess the client for increased heart rate, increased respirations, or increased lung congestion, which could indicate fluid overload
E. IV fluids are most frequently ordered on the basis of milliliters per hour to be administered
F. The volume ordered is administered by adjusting the rate at which the IV infuses, which is counted in drops (gtt) per minute
G. Most flow rate calculations involve changing milliliters per hour into drops per minute
H. IV Tubing
   1. Calibrated in drops per milliliter, and this calibration is needed for calculating flow rates
   2. A standard or macrodrip set is used for routine adult IV administrations, depending on the manufacturer and type of tubing; it will require 10, 15, or 20 gtt to equal 1 mL
   3. A mini- or microdrip set is used when more exact measurements are needed, in intensive care units and in pediatric units
   4. In a mini- or microdrip set, 60 gtt is equal to 1 mL
   5. The calibration, in gtt per mL, is written on the IV tubing package

XII. Calculations

A. See Table 16–5

XIII. Electronic IV Flow Rate Regulators

A. Controller
   1. Works on the same principle of gravity as a regular IV drip, with the rate of flow being maintained by rapid compression and

BOX 16–5. Infusions Ordered by Unit Dosage per Hour

Calculation of these problems requires a two-step process:

1. Determine the amount of medication in 1 mL.
2. Determine the infusion rate or mL per hour.

PROBLEM:

Continuous heparin by IV drip, 1000 units per hour
Available: IV bag of 500 mL D5W with 25,000 units of heparin
How many milliliters per hour are required to give the correct dose?

Solution:

STEP 1. Calculate the **units** per mL.

$$\frac{\text{Known amount of medication in solution}}{\text{Total volume of diluent}} =$$
$$\text{Amount of medication per mL}$$

$$\frac{25,000 \text{ units}}{500 \text{ mL}} = 50 \text{ units per 1 mL}$$

STEP 2. Calculate mL per hour

$$\frac{\text{Dose per hour desired}}{\text{Concentration per mL}} =$$
$$\text{Infusion rate or mL per hour}$$

$$\frac{1000 \text{ units}}{50 \text{ units}} = 20 \text{ mL per hour}$$

PROBLEM:

Continuous Regular Insulin by IV at 10 units per hour
Available: IV bag of 100 mL NS with 50 units regular insulin
How many mL per hour are required to give the correct dose?

Solution:

STEP 1:

$$\frac{\text{Known amount of medication in solution}}{\text{Total volume of diluent}} =$$
$$\text{Amount of medication per mL}$$

$$\frac{50 \text{ units}}{100 \text{ mL}} = 0.5 \text{ unit per mL}$$

$$1 \text{ mL} = 0.5 \text{ unit}$$

STEP 2:

$$\frac{\text{Dose per hour desired}}{\text{Concentration per mL}} =$$
$$\text{Infusion rate or mL per hour}$$

$$\frac{10 \text{ units}}{0.5 \text{ unit}} = 20 \text{ mL per hour}$$

Table 16–5. Formulas for Intravenous Calculations

Flow Rates

$$\frac{\text{Total volume} \times \text{gtt factor}}{\text{Time in minutes}} = \text{gtt per min}$$

Infusion Time

$$\frac{\text{Total volume to infuse}}{\text{mL per hour being infused}} = \text{Infusion time}$$

3. Because controllers work by gravity, the height of the solution bag is critical and must be maintained at a minimum of 36 inches above the controller
4. The nurse should continue to assess the amount of IV solution in the IV container and monitor the controller to ensure proper functioning of the machine

B. Pump
1. A pump is different from a controller in that it physically pumps fluid against resistance
2. Gravity is not a factor in the use of a pump, and the height of the IV solution bag is not a critical factor
3. The flow rate on a pump is set in milliliters per hour
4. The nurse should continue to assess the amount of IV solution in the IV container and monitor the pump to ensure proper functioning of the machine

XIV. Calculating Infusions Ordered by Unit Dosage per Hour (Box 16–5)

A. The most common medications that will be ordered by **unit** dosage per hour and to run by continuous infusion are heparin and Regular Insulin

B. Calculation of these problems requires a two-step process:
1. Determine the amount of medication in 1 mL
2. Determine the infusion rate or milliliters per hour

Medication and Intravenous Calculations

. . . .

PRACTICE QUESTIONS

1. The physician orders 1000 mL of 0.9% NS to run over 12 hours. The drop factor is 15 drops per 1 mL. What is the flow rate in drops per minute?
   1 15 drops per minute
   2 17 drops per minute
   3 21 drops per minute
   4 23 drops per minute

2. The physician orders an IV dose of 400,000 units

decompression of the IV tubing by the machine
2. The desired flow rate is set on the controller in milliliters per hour

of penicillin G benzathine (Bicillin). The label on the 10-mL ampule sent from the pharmacy reads penicillin G benzathine (Bicillin), 300,000 units per mL. How much medication will you prepare to administer the correct dose?

1 1.3 mL
2 13 mL
3 1.5 mL
4 10 mL

3. The physician's order reads potassium chloride (KCl), 30 mEq, to be added to 1000 mL NS and to be administered over a 10-hour period. The label on the medication bottle reads 40 mEq (KCl) per 20 mL. How many milliliters of potassium chloride (KCl) are needed to administer the correct dose of medication?

1 10 mL
2 15 mL
3 20 mL
4 50 mL

4. The physician orders 3000 mL of D5W to run over a 24-hour period. The drop factor is 10 drops per 1 mL. What is the flow rate in drops per minute?

1 15 drops per minute
2 17 drops per minute
3 21 drops per minute
4 24 drops per minute

5. The physician's order reads clindamycin phosphate (Cleocin Phosphate), 0.3 g in 50 mL NS to be administered IV over 30 minutes. The medication label reads clindamycin phosphate (Cleocin Phosphate), 900 mg in 6 mL. How many milliliters of the medication are needed to administer the correct dose?

1 1 mL
2 2 mL
3 3 mL
4 5 mL

6. The physician's order reads phenytoin (Dilantin), 0.2 g PO BID. The medication label states 100-mg capsules. How many capsule(s) will you prepare to administer one dose?

1 1 capsule
2 2 capsules
3 3 capsules
4 4 capsules

7. The physician orders 1000 mL of ½% NS to run over 8 hours. The drop factor is 15 drops per 1 mL. What is the flow rate in drops per minute?

1 20 drops per minute
2 22 drops per minute
3 28 drops per minute
4 31 drops per minute

8. The physician orders 2000 mL of D5½% NS to run over 24 hours. The drop factor is 15 drops per 1 mL. What is the flow rate in drops per minute?

1 15 drops per minute
2 17 drops per minute
3 21 drops per minute
4 28 drops per minute

9. The physician orders heparin sodium (Liquaemin), 1300 units per hour by continuous IV infusion. The pharmacy prepares the medication and delivers an IV bag labeled heparin (Liquaemin), 20,000 units per 250 mL D5W. An infusion pump must be used to administer the medication. How many milliliters per hour are required to deliver the correct dose?

1 12 mL
2 16 mL
3 20 mL
4 22 mL

10. The physician's order reads cyanocobalamin (vitamin B_{12}) 1000 µg IM. The medication label reads cyanocobalamin (vitamin B_{12}), 0.5 mg per mL. How many milliliters will you administer to the client?

1 0.5 mL
2 1 mL
3 2 mL
4 3 mL

11. The physician orders 3000 mL of D5W to be administered over a 24-hour period. How many milliliters per hour are to be administered?

1 50 mL per hour
2 75 mL per hour
3 100 mL per hour
4 125 mL per hour

12. Gentamicin sulfate (Garamycin), 80 mg in 100 mL NS, is to be administered in one half hour. The drop factor is 10 drops per mL. What is the flow rate in drops per minute?

1 43 drops
2 33 drops
3 23 drops
4 18 drops

13. The physician's order reads levothyroxine (Synthroid), 150 µg PO daily. The medication label reads Synthroid, 0.1 mg per tablet. How many tablet(s) will you administer to the client?

1 1 tablet
2 1.5 tablets
3 2 tablets
4 2.5 tablets

14. Cefuroxime axetil (Ceftin), 1 g in 50 mL NS, is to be administered over 30 minutes. The drop factor is 15 drops per mL. What is the flow rate in drops per minute?

1 15 drops
2 25 drops
3 20 drops
4 22 drops

15. The physician orders 1000 mL D5W to run at 125 mL per hour. How many hours will 1 liter run?
    1 8 hours
    2 10 hours
    3 12 hours
    4 15 hours

16. The physician orders 500 mL of 0.9% NS to run over 5 hours. The drop factor is 10 drops per 1 mL. What is the flow rate in drops per minute?
    1 15 drops
    2 17 drops
    3 20 drops
    4 22 drops

17. The physician orders 1 unit of packed red blood cells to run over 4 hours. The unit of blood contains 250 mL. The drop factor is 10 drops per 1 mL. What is the flow rate in drops per minute?
    1 15 drops
    2 17 drops
    3 10 drops
    4 20 drops

18. The physician orders 3000 mL of 0.9% NS to run over 24 hours. The drop factor is 15 drops per 1 mL. What is the flow rate in drops per minute?
    1 17 drops per minute
    2 20 drops per minute
    3 24 drops per minute
    4 31 drops per minute

19. The physician's order reads quinidine gluconate (Quinaglute), 0.3 g PO BID. The medication label reads quinidine gluconate (Quinaglute), 150-mg tablets. How many tablet(s) will you prepare to administer one dose?
    1 0.5 tablet
    2 1 tablet
    3 2 tablets
    4 3 tablets

20. The physician orders tetracycline hydrochloride (Achromycin), 0.5 g PO QID. The label on the bottle of medication reads tetracycline hydrochloride (Achromycin), 250-mg tablets. How many tablet(s) will you give to administer the correct dose?
    1 0.5 tablet
    2 1 tablet
    3 2 tablets
    4 3 tablets

21. The physician's order reads triazolam (Halcion), 125 μg PO at HS daily. The medication bottle is labeled triazolam (Halcion), 0.125-mg tablets. How many tablet(s) will you administer to the client?
    1 1 tablet
    2 1.5 tablets
    3 2 tablets
    4 2.5 tablets

22. The physician orders heparin sodium (Liquaemin), 800 units per hour by continuous IV infusion. The pharmacy prepares the medication and delivers an IV bag labeled heparin, 20,000 units per 250 mL D5W. An infusion pump must be used to administer the medication. How many milliliters per hour are required to deliver the correct dose?
    1 10 mL per hour
    2 17 mL per hour
    3 20 drops per minute
    4 22 drops per minute

23. The physician's order reads atenolol (Tenormin), 0.025 g PO QD. The medication bottle reads atenolol (Lopressor), 50-mg tablets. How many tablet(s) will you administer to the client?
    1 0.5 tablet
    2 1 tablet
    3 2 tablets
    4 3 tablets

24. The physician's order reads hydromorphone hydrochloride (Dilaudid), 3 mg IM q4h PRN. The medication label reads hydromorphone hydrochloride (Dilaudid), 4 mg per 1 mL. Which of the following represents the accurate dose to be administered to the client?
    1 1.5 mg
    2 4 mg
    3 0.8 mL
    4 1.3 mL

25. The physician orders heparin sodium (Liquaemin), 1200 units per hour by continuous IV infusion. The pharmacy prepares the medication and delivers an IV bag that is labeled heparin, 25,000 units per 500 mL D5W. An infusion pump must be used to administer the medication. How many mL per hour are required to deliver the correct dose?
    1 12 mL per hour
    2 16 mL per hour
    3 22 mL per hour
    4 24 mL per hour

26. The physician orders heparin sodium (Liquaemin), 5000 units SC q12h. The vial reads heparin, 10,000 units per mL. How many mL will you administer to the client?
    1 0.5 mL
    2 0.1 mL
    3 1.0 mL
    4 2.0 mL

27. The physician's order states heparin sodium (Liquaemin), 750 units per hour by continuous IV infusion. The concentration of the heparin is 12,500 units in 250 mL of D5W. You note that the infusion pump is set at 15 mL per hour. Which of the following nursing actions will you

implement regarding the rate set on the infusion pump?
1 Decrease the flow rate to 10 mL per hour
2 Decrease the flow rate to 8 mL per hour
3 Increase the flow rate to 18 mL per hour
4 Leave the flow rate at 15 mL per hour

28. The physician orders Regular Insulin, 8 units per hour by continuous IV infusion. The pharmacy prepares the medication and delivers an IV bag labeled 100 units of Regular Insulin in 100 mL NS. An infusion pump must be used to administer the medication. How many milliliters per hour are required to deliver the correct dose?
1 1 mL per hour
2 4 mL per hour
3 8 mL per hour
4 10 mL per hour

29. The physician's order reads digoxin (Lanoxin), 0.25 mg PO daily. The medication label reads digoxin (Lanoxin), 0.125 mg per tablet. How many tablet(s) will you administer to the client?
1 0.5 tablet
2 1 tablet
3 1.5 tablets
4 2 tablets

30. The physician's order reads meperidine hydrochloride (Demerol), 80 mg IM PRN. The medication label reads meperidine hydrochloride (Demerol), 100 mg per mL. Which of the following represents the accurate dose to be administered to the client?
1 1.25 mL
2 100 mL
3 0.8 mL
4 1 mL

31. The physician orders heparin sodium (Liquaemin), 650 units SC q12h. The medication vial reads heparin sodium (Liquaemin), 1000 units per mL. The nurse prepares to administer the morning dose. Which of the following represents the accurate dose to be administered to the client?
1 1.5 mL
2 0.7 mL
3 1.3 mL
4 1.0 mL

32. The physician orders heparin sodium (Liquaemin), 900 units per hour by continuous IV infusion. The pharmacy prepares the medication and delivers an IV bag labeled heparin, 25,000 units per 500 mL D5W. An infusion pump must be used to administer the medication. How many milliliters per hour are required to deliver the correct dose?
1 12 mL per hour
2 16 mL per hour

3 18 mL per hour
4 20 mL per hour

33. The physician orders trimethobenzamide hydrochloride (Tigan), 250 mg IM PRN. The medication label reads trimethobenzamide hydrochloride (Tigan), 200 mg per 2 mL. How much medication will the nurse prepare to administer the correct dose?
1 0.4 mL
2 1.0 mL
3 1.25 mL
4 2.5 mL

34. The physician orders Regular Insulin, 10 units per hour by continuous IV infusion. The pharmacy prepares the medication and then delivers an IV bag labeled 50 units of Regular Insulin in 100 mL NS. An infusion pump must be used to administer the medication. How many milliliters per hour are required to deliver the correct dose?
1 5 mL per hour
2 10 mL per hour
3 15 mL per hour
4 20 mL per hour

35. The physician orders meperidine hydrochloride (Demerol), 35 mg IM stat. The medication label states meperidine hydrochloride (Demerol), 50 mg per mL. How many milliliters will you prepare to administer to the client?
1 0.5 mL
2 0.6 mL
3 0.7 mL
4 1.0 mL

36. The physician orders prochlorperazine (Compazine), 25 mg q4h IM PRN. The medication label states prochlorperazine (Compazine), 10 mg per mL. How many milliliters will you prepare to administer to the client?
1 0.5 mL
2 2.0 mL
3 2.5 mL
4 2.9 mL

37. The physician orders potassium chloride elixir (KCl), 20 mEq PO BID. The medication label states potassium chloride (KCl), 30 mEq per 15 mL. The nurse prepares to administer the morning dose. How many milliliters will the nurse administer to the client?
1 10 mL
2 15 mL
3 32 mL
4 40 mL

38. The physician orders atropine sulfate, 0.4 mg IM stat. The medication label states atropine sulfate, 0.3 mg per 0.5 mL. Which of the following represents the accurate dose to administer to the client?

1 0.1 mL
2 0.4 mL
3 0.5 mL
4 0.7 mL

39. The physician orders levodopa (Dopar), 1 g PO BID. The medication label states 500-mg tablets. How many tablet(s) will the nurse administer at the evening dose?
    1 2 tablets
    2 3 tablets
    3 4 tablets
    4 5 tablets

40. The physician orders zidovudine (AZT), 0.2 g PO q4h. The medication label states zidovudine (AZT), 100-mg tablets. How many tablet(s) will you prepare to administer for one dose?
    1 0.5 tablet
    2 1 tablet
    3 1.5 tablets
    4 2 tablets

41. The physician orders pentobarbital (Nembutal), 0.15 g PO HS. The medication label reads pentobarbital (Nembutal), 50-mg capsules. How many capsule(s) will you administer to the client?
    1 1 capsule
    2 2 capsules
    3 3 capsules
    4 4 capsules

42. The physician orders atropine sulfate, gr 1/300 to be administered. The medication label states atropine sulfate, 0.5 mg per 0.5 mL. How many milliliters will you administer to the client?
    1 0.1 mL
    2 0.2 mL
    3 1 mL
    4 2 mL

43. The home care nurse makes a home visit to the client. The client tells the nurse that the physician's instructions state to take ibuprofen (Advil), 0.4 g for mild pain. The medication bottle states ibuprofen (Advil), 200-mg tablets. How many tablet(s) will the nurse instruct the client to take?
    1 0.5 tablet
    2 1 tablet
    3 2 tablets
    4 1.5 tablets

44. The physician's order states to administer aspirin (acetylsalicylic acid), 650 mg PO for a temperature above 38° Celsius. The medication bottle states aspirin (acetylsalicylic acid), gr 5 per tablet. The nurse takes the client's temperature and notes that it is 101° Fahrenheit. Which of the following actions will the nurse take?
    1 Do not administer the aspirin (acetylsalicylic acid) at this time
    2 Check the client's temperature in 30 minutes

3 Administer 2 tablets
4 Administer 3 tablets

45. The physician orders codeine sulfate, gr ½ PO q4h PRN. The medication bottle reads codeine sulfate, 15-mg tablets. How many tablet(s) will the nurse administer to the client?
    1 0.5 tablet
    2 1 tablet
    3 1.5 tablets
    4 2 tablets

46. The physician's order reads kanamycin sulfate (Kantrex), 300 mg IM. The directions on the medication bottle read: Add 2.7 mL sterile water for injection to make 1 g per 3 mL. After reconstitution, how many milliliters will you prepare to administer the correct dose?
    1 0.3 mL
    2 0.9 mL
    3 1.2 mL
    4 1.5 mL

47. The physician's order reads morphine sulfate, gr ⅛ IM stat. The medication ampule states morphine sulfate, 10 mg per mL. How many milliliters will the nurse prepare to administer the correct dose?
    1 0.5 mL
    2 0.75 mL
    3 0.85 mL
    4 1.5 mL

48. The physician orders brompheniramine maleate (Dimetane), 6 mg PO BID. The medication label reads brompheniramine maleate (Dimetane), 4-mg tablets. How many tablet(s) will you prepare to administer one dose?
    1 1 tablet
    2 1.5 tablets
    3 2 tablets
    4 2.5 tablets

49. The physician orders phenobarbital sodium (Luminal), 25 mg PO q6h. The medication label reads phenobarbital sodium (Luminal), 10 mg per 4 mL. How many milliliters will you prepare to administer one dose?
    1 4 mL
    2 10 mL
    3 15 mL
    4 25 mL

50. The physician orders furosemide (Lasix), 40 mg PO daily. The medication label reads furosemide (Lasix), 20 mg per tablet. How many tablet(s) will you prepare to administer one dose?
    1 1 tablet
    2 2 tablets
    3 3 tablets
    4 4 tablets

ANSWERS

1. **3**—20.8, or 21 drops per minute

Formula:

$$\frac{\text{Total volume in mL} \times \text{drop factor}}{\text{Time in minutes}} =$$

$$\text{Flow rate in drops per minute}$$

$$\frac{1000 \text{ mL} \times 15 \text{ drops}}{720 \text{ minutes}} = \frac{15,000}{720}$$

$$= 20.8, \text{ or } 21 \text{ drops per minute}$$

2. **1**—1.3 mL

Formula:

$$\frac{\text{Desired}}{\text{Available}} \times \text{mL} = \text{mL per dose}$$

$$\frac{400,000 \text{ units}}{300,000 \text{ units}} \times 1 \text{ mL} = \text{mL per dose}$$

$$\frac{400,000}{300,000} = 1.3 \text{ mL}$$

3. **2**—15 mL

Formula:

$$\frac{\text{Desired}}{\text{Available}} \times \text{mL} = \text{mL per dose}$$

$$\frac{30 \text{ mEq}}{40 \text{ mEq}} \times 20 \text{ mL} = 15 \text{ mL}$$

4. **3**—20.8, or 21 drops per minute

Formula:

$$\frac{\text{Total volume in mL} \times \text{drop factor}}{\text{Time in minutes}} =$$

$$\text{Flow rate in drops per minute}$$

$$\frac{3000 \text{ mL} \times 10 \text{ drops}}{1440 \text{ minutes}} = \frac{30,000}{1440}$$

$$= 20.8, \text{ or } 21 \text{ drops per minute}$$

5. **2**—2 mL

Formula:

$$\frac{\text{Desired}}{\text{Available}} \times \text{mL} = \text{mL per dose}$$

$$\frac{0.3 \text{ g}}{900 \text{ mg}} \times 6 \text{ mL}$$

Convert 0.3 g to mg:
In the metric system, to convert larger to smaller multiply by 1000, or move the decimal 3 places to the right.

0.3 g = 300 mg

$$\frac{300 \text{ mg}}{900 \text{ mg}} \times 6 \text{ mL} = \frac{1800}{900} = 2 \text{ mL}$$

6. **2**—2 capsules

$$\frac{\text{Desired}}{\text{Available}} \times \text{Capsules} = \text{Capsules per dose}$$

$$\frac{0.2 \text{g}}{100 \text{ mg}} \times 1 \text{ capsule}$$

Formula:

Convert 0.2 g to mg:
In the metric system, to convert larger to smaller multiply by 1000 or move the decimal 3 places to the right.

0.2 g = 200 mg

$$\frac{200 \text{ mg}}{100 \text{ mg}} \times 1 \text{ capsule} = 2 \text{ capsules}$$

7. **4**—31.2, or 31 drops per minute

Formula:

$$\frac{\text{Total volume in mL} \times \text{drop factor}}{\text{Time in minutes}} =$$

$$\text{Flow rate in drops per minute}$$

$$\frac{1000 \text{ mL} \times 15 \text{ drops}}{480 \text{ minutes}} = \frac{15,000}{480} = 31.2, \text{ or } 31 \text{ drops per minute}$$

8. **3**—20.8, or 21 drops per minute

Formula:

$$\frac{\text{Total volume in mL} \times \text{drop factor}}{\text{Time in minutes}} =$$

$$\text{Flow rate in drops per minute}$$

$$\frac{2000 \text{ mL} \times 15 \text{ drops}}{1440 \text{ minutes}} = \frac{30,000}{1440} = 20.8, \text{ or } 21 \text{ drops per minute}$$

9. **2**—16.25, or 16 mL per hour
Calculation of this problem requires a two-step process. First, you need to determine the amount of heparin in 1 mL. The next step is to determine the infusion rate, or milliliters per hour.

Step 1:

Formula:

$$\frac{\text{Known amount of medication}}{\text{Total volume of diluent}} = \text{Amount of medication per mL}$$

$$\frac{20,000 \text{ units}}{250 \text{ mL}} = 80 \text{ units per mL}$$

1 mL = 80 units

Step 2:

Formula:

$$\frac{\text{Dose per hour desired}}{\text{Concentration per mL}} = \text{Infusion rate or mL per hour}$$

$$\frac{1300 \text{ Units}}{80 \text{ Units per mL}} = 16.25, \text{ or } 16 \text{ mL per hour}$$

10. **3**—2 mL

Formula:

$$\frac{\text{Desired}}{\text{Available}} \times \text{mL} = \text{mL per dose}$$

$$\frac{1000 \text{ μg}}{0.5 \text{ mg}} \times 1 \text{ mL} = \text{mL per dose}$$

Convert 1000 μg to mg:
In the metric system, to convert smaller to larger divide by 1000 or move the decimal 3 places to the left.

1000 μg = 1.0 mg

$$\frac{1.0 \text{ mg}}{0.5 \text{ mg}} \times 1 \text{ mL} = \frac{1.0}{0.5} = 2 \text{ mL}$$

11. **4**—125 mL per hour

Formula:

$$\frac{\text{Total volume in mL}}{\text{Number of hours}} = \text{Amount of mL per hour}$$

$$\frac{3000 \text{ mL}}{24 \text{ hours}} = 125 \text{ mL per hour}$$

12. **2**—33 drops per minute

Formula:

$$\frac{\text{Total volume in mL} \times \text{drop factor}}{\text{Time in minutes}} =$$

$$\text{Flow rate in drops per minute}$$

$$\frac{100 \text{ mL} \times 10 \text{ drops}}{30 \text{ minutes}} = \frac{1000}{30} = 33.3, \text{ or } 33 \text{ drops per minute}$$

13. **2**—1.5 tablets

Formula:

$$\frac{\text{Desired}}{\text{Available}} \times \text{Tablets} = \text{Per dose}$$

$$\frac{150 \text{ μg}}{0.1 \text{ mg}} \times 1 \text{ tablet} = \text{tablet(s) per dose}$$

Convert 150 μg to mg:
In the metric system, to convert smaller to larger divide by 1000 or move the decimal 3 places to the left.

150 μg = 0.15 mg

$$\frac{0.15 \text{ mg}}{0.1 \text{ mg}} \times 1 \text{ tablet} = \frac{0.15}{0.1} = 1.5 \text{ tablets}$$

14. **2**—25 drops per minute

Formula:

$$\frac{\text{Total volume in mL} \times \text{drop factor}}{\text{Time in minutes}} =$$

$$\text{Flow rate in drops per minute}$$

$$\frac{50 \text{ mL} \times 15 \text{ drops}}{30 \text{ minutes}} = \frac{750}{30} = 25 \text{ drops per minute}$$

15. **1**—8 hours

Formula:

$$\frac{\text{Total volume in mL}}{\text{mL per hour}} = \text{Infusion time in hours}$$

1 liter = 1000 mL

$$\frac{1000 \text{ mL}}{125 \text{ mL}} = 8 \text{ hours}$$

16. **2**—16.6, or 17 drops per minute

Formula:

$$\frac{\text{Total volume in mL} \times \text{drop factor}}{\text{Time in minutes}} =$$

$$\text{Flow rate in drops per minute}$$

$$\frac{500 \text{ mL} \times 10 \text{ drops}}{300 \text{ minutes}} = \frac{5000}{300} = 16.6, \text{ or } 17 \text{ drops per minute}$$

17. **3**—10.4, or 10 drops per minute

Formula:

$$\frac{\text{Total volume in mL} \times \text{drop factor}}{\text{Time in minutes}} =$$

$$\text{Flow rate in drops per minute}$$

$$\frac{250 \text{ mL} \times 10 \text{ drops}}{240 \text{ minutes}} = \frac{2500}{240} = 10.4, \text{ or } 10 \text{ drops per minute}$$

18. **4**—31.2, or 31 drops per minute

Formula:

$$\frac{\text{Total volume in mL} \times \text{drop factor}}{\text{Time in minutes}} =$$

$$\text{Flow rate in drops per minute}$$

$$\frac{3000 \text{ mL} \times 15 \text{ drops}}{1400 \text{ minutes}} = \frac{45,000}{1440}$$

$$= 31.2, \text{ or } 31 \text{ drops per minute}$$

19. **3**—2 tablets

Formula:

$$\frac{\text{Desired}}{\text{Available}} \times \text{Tablet} = \text{Number of tablets per dose}$$

$$\frac{0.3 \text{ g}}{150 \text{ mg}} \times 1 \text{ tablet} = \text{number of tablets per dose}$$

Convert 0.3 g to mg:
In the metric system, to convert larger to smaller multiply by 1000 or move the decimal 3 places to the right.

0.3 g = 300 mg

$$\frac{300 \text{ mg}}{150 \text{ mg}} \times 1 \text{ tablet} = \frac{300 \text{ mg}}{150 \text{ mg}} = 2 \text{ tablets}$$

20. **3**—2 tablets

Formula:

$$\frac{\text{Desired}}{\text{Available}} \times \text{Tablet} = \text{Number of tablets per dose}$$

$$\frac{0.5 \text{ g}}{250 \text{ mg}} \times 1 \text{ tablet} = \text{number of tablets per dose}$$

Convert 0.5 g to mg:
In the metric system, to convert larger to smaller multiply by 1000 or move the decimal 3 places to the right.

0.5 g = 500 mg

$$\frac{500 \text{ mg}}{250 \text{ mg}} \times 1 \text{ tablet} = \frac{500 \text{ mg}}{250 \text{ mg}} = 2 \text{ tablets}$$

21. **1**—1 tablet

Formula:

$$\frac{\text{Desired}}{\text{Available}} \times \text{Tablet} = \text{Number of tablets per dose}$$

$$\frac{125 \text{ μg}}{0.125 \text{mg}} \times 1 \text{ tablet} = \text{tablet(s) per dose}$$

Convert 125 μg to mg:
In the metric system, to convert smaller to larger divide by 1000 or move the decimal 3 places to the left.

125 μg = 0.125 mg

$$\frac{0.125 \text{ mg}}{0.125 \text{ mg}} \times 1 \text{ tablet} = \frac{0.125}{0.125} = 1 \text{ tablet}$$

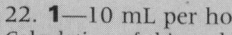

22. **1**—10 mL per hour

Calculation of this problem requires a two-step process. First, you need to determine the amount of heparin in 1 mL. The next step is to determine the infusion rate, or mL per hour.

Step 1:

Formula:

$$\frac{\text{Known amount of medication}}{\text{Total volume of diluent}} = \text{Amount of medication per mL}$$

$$\frac{20{,}000 \text{ units}}{250 \text{ mL}} = 80 \text{ units per mL}$$

1 mL = 80 units

Step 2:

Formula:

$$\frac{\text{Dose per hour desired}}{\text{Concentration per mL}} = \text{Infusion rate or mL per hour}$$

$$\frac{800 \text{ units}}{80 \text{ units per mL}} = 10 \text{ mL per hour}$$

23. **1**—0.5 tablet

Formula:

$$\frac{\text{Desired}}{\text{Available}} \times \text{Tablet} = \text{Number of tablets per dose}$$

$$\frac{0.025 \text{ g}}{50 \text{ mg}} \times 1 \text{ tablet} = \text{Number of tablets per dose}$$

Convert 0.025 g to mg:

In the metric system, to convert larger to smaller multiply by 1000 or move the decimal 3 places to the right.

0.025 g = 25.0 mg

$$\frac{25 \text{ mg}}{50 \text{ mg}} \times 1 \text{ tablet} = \frac{25 \text{ mg}}{50 \text{ mg}} = 0.5 \text{ tablet}$$

24. **3**—0.8 mL

Formula:

$$\frac{\text{Desired}}{\text{Available}} \times \text{mL} = \text{mL per dose}$$

$$\frac{3 \text{ mg}}{4 \text{ mg}} \times 1 \text{ mL}$$

$$\frac{3}{4} = 0.75 \text{ or } 0.8 \text{ mL}$$

25. **4**—24 mL per hour

Calculation of this problem requires a two-step process. First, you need to determine the amount of heparin in 1 mL. The next step is to determine the infusion rate, or mL per hour.

Step 1:

Formula:

$$\frac{\text{Known amount of medication}}{\text{Total volume of diluent}} = \text{Amount of medication per mL}$$

$$\frac{25{,}000 \text{ Units}}{500 \text{ mL}} = 50 \text{ units per mL}$$

1 mL = 50 units

Step 2:

Formula:

$$\frac{\text{Dose per hour desired}}{\text{concentration per mL}} = \text{Infusion rate, or mL per hour}$$

$$\frac{1200 \text{ units}}{50 \text{ units per mL}} = 24 \text{ mL per hour}$$

26. **1**—0.5 mL

Formula:

$$\frac{\text{Desired}}{\text{Available}} \times \text{mL} = \text{mL per dose}$$

$$\frac{5000 \text{ Units}}{10{,}000 \text{ Units}} \times 1 \text{ mL} = \frac{5000}{10{,}000} = 0.5 \text{ mL}$$

27. **4**—Leave the flow rate at 15 mL per hour, as this is the correct dose

Calculation of this problem requires a two-step process. First, you need to determine the amount of heparin in 1 mL. The next step is to determine the infusion rate, or mL per hour.

Step 1:

Formula:

$$\frac{\text{Known amount of medication}}{\text{Total volume of diluent}} = \text{Amount of medication per mL}$$

$$\frac{12{,}500 \text{ units}}{250 \text{ mL}} = \text{units per mL}$$

1 mL = 50 units

Step 2:

Formula:

$$\frac{\text{Dose per hour desired}}{\text{Concentration per mL}} = \text{Infusion rate, or mL per hour}$$

$$\frac{750 \text{ units}}{50 \text{ units per mL}} = 15 \text{ mL per hour}$$

28. **3**—8 mL per hour

Calculation of this problem requires a two-step process. First, you need to determine the amount of Regular Insulin in 1 mL. The next step is to determine the infusion rate, or mL per hour.

Step 1:

Formula:

$$\frac{\text{Known amount of medication}}{\text{Total volume of diluent}} = \text{Amount of medication per mL}$$

$$\frac{100 \text{ units}}{100 \text{ mL}} = 1 \text{ unit per mL}$$

1 mL = 1 unit

Step 2:

Formula:

$$\frac{\text{Dose per hour desired}}{\text{Concentration per mL}} = \text{Infusion rate, or mL per hour}$$

$$\frac{8 \text{ units}}{1 \text{ unit per mL}} = 8 \text{ mL per hour}$$

29. **4**—2 tablets

Formula:

$$\frac{\text{Desired}}{\text{Available}} \times \text{Tablet} = \text{Number of tablets per dose}$$

$$\frac{0.25 \text{ mg}}{0.125 \text{ mg}} \times 1 \text{ tablet} = \frac{0.25}{0.125} = 2 \text{ tablets}$$

30. **3**—0.8 mL

Formula:

$$\frac{\text{Desired}}{\text{Available}} \times \text{mL} = \text{mL per dose}$$

$$\frac{80 \text{ mg}}{100 \text{ mg}} \times 1 \text{ mL}$$

$$\frac{80}{100} = 0.8 \text{ mL}$$

31. **2**—0.7 mL

Formula:

$$\frac{\text{Desired}}{\text{Available}} \times \text{mL} = \text{mL per dose}$$

$$\frac{650 \text{ Units}}{1000 \text{ Units}} \times 1 \text{ mL}$$

$$\frac{650}{1000} = 0.65 \text{ mL, or } 0.7 \text{ mL}$$

32. **3**—18 mL per hour

Calculation of this problem requires a two-step process. First, you need to determine the amount of heparin in 1 mL. The next step is to determine the infusion rate, or milliliters per hour.

Step 1:

Formula:

$$\frac{\text{Known amount of medication}}{\text{Total volume of diluent}} = \text{Amount of medication per mL}$$

$$\frac{25,000 \text{ units}}{500 \text{ mL}} = \text{units per mL}$$

1 mL = 50 units

Step 2:

Formula:

$$\frac{\text{Dose per hour desired}}{\text{Concentration per mL}} = \text{Infusion rate, or mL per hour}$$

$$\frac{900 \text{ units}}{50 \text{ units per mL}} = 18 \text{ mL per hour}$$

33. **4**—2.5 mL

Formula:

$$\frac{\text{Desired}}{\text{Available}} \times \text{mL} = \text{mL per dose}$$

$$\frac{250 \text{ mg}}{200 \text{ mg}} \times 2 \text{ mL}$$

$$\frac{500}{200} = 2.5 \text{ mL}$$

34. **4**—20 mL per hour

Calculation of this problem requires a two-step process. First, you need to determine the amount of Regular Insulin in 1 mL. The next step is to determine the infusion rate, or milliliters per hour.

Step 1:

Formula:

$$\frac{\text{Known amount of medication}}{\text{Total volume of diluent}} = \text{Amount of medication per mL}$$

$$\frac{50 \text{ units}}{100 \text{ mL}} = 0.5 \text{ unit per mL}$$

1 mL = 0.5 unit

Step 2:

Formula:

$$\frac{\text{Dose per hour desired}}{\text{Concentration per mL}} = \text{Infusion rate, or mL per hour}$$

$$\frac{10 \text{ units}}{0.5 \text{ unit per mL}} = 20 \text{ mL per hour}$$

35. **3**—0.7 mL

Formula:

$$\frac{\text{Desired}}{\text{Available}} \times \text{mL} = \text{mL per dose}$$

$$\frac{35 \text{ mg}}{50 \text{ mg}} \times 1 \text{ mL}$$

$$\frac{35}{50} = 0.7 \text{ mL}$$

36. **3**—2.5 mL

Formula:

$$\frac{\text{Desired}}{\text{Available}} \times \text{mL} = \text{mL per dose}$$

$$\frac{25 \text{ mg}}{10 \text{ mg}} \times 1 \text{ mL}$$

$$\frac{25}{10} = 2.5 \text{ mL}$$

37. **1**—10 mL

Formula:

$$\frac{\text{Desired}}{\text{Available}} \times \text{mL} = \text{mL per dose}$$

$$\frac{20 \text{ mEq}}{30 \text{ mEq}} \times 15 \text{ mL}$$

$$\frac{300}{30} = 10 \text{ mL}$$

38. **4**—0.7 mL

Formula:

$$\frac{\text{Desired}}{\text{Available}} \times \text{mL} = \text{mL per dose}$$

$$\frac{0.4 \text{ mg}}{0.3 \text{ mg}} \times 0.5 \text{ mL}$$

$$\frac{0.4}{0.3} \times 0.5 = 0.66, \text{ or } 0.7 \text{ mL}$$

39. **1**—2 tablets

Formula:

$$\frac{\text{Desired}}{\text{Available}} \times \text{Tablet} = \text{Number of tablets per dose}$$

$$\frac{1 \text{ g}}{500 \text{ mg}} \times 1 \text{ tablet} = \text{number of tablets per dose}$$

Convert 1 g to mg:

In the metric system, to convert larger to smaller multiply by 1000 or move the decimal 3 places to the right.

1 g = 1000 mg

$$\frac{1000 \text{ mg}}{500 \text{ mg}} \times 1 \text{ tablet} = \frac{1000 \text{ mg}}{500 \text{ mg}} = 2 \text{ tablets}$$

40. **4**—2 tablets

Formula:

$$\frac{\text{Desired}}{\text{Available}} \times \text{Tablet} = \text{Number of tablets per dose}$$

$$\frac{0.2 \text{ g}}{100 \text{ mg}} \times 1 \text{ tablet} = \text{number of tablets per dose}$$

Convert 0.2 g to mg:
In the metric system, to convert larger to smaller multiply by 1000 or move the decimal 3 places to the right.

0.2 g = 200 mg

$$\frac{200 \text{ mg}}{100 \text{ mg}} \times 1 \text{ tablet} = \frac{200 \text{ mg}}{100 \text{ mg}} = 2 \text{ tablets}$$

41. **3**—3 capsules

Formula:

$$\frac{\text{Desired}}{\text{Available}} \times \text{Capsule} = \text{Number of capsules per dose}$$

$$\frac{0.15 \text{ g}}{50 \text{ mg}} \times 1 \text{ capsule} = \text{number of capsules per dose}$$

Convert 0.15 g to mg:
In the metric system, to convert larger to smaller multiply by 1000 or move the decimal 3 places to the right.

0.15 g = 150 mg

$$\frac{150 \text{ mg}}{50 \text{ mg}} \times 1 \text{ capsule} = \frac{150 \text{ mg}}{50 \text{ mg}} = 3 \text{ capsules}$$

42. **2**—0.2 mL

Formula:

$$\frac{\text{Desired}}{\text{Available}} \times \text{mL} = \text{Number of mL per dose}$$

$$\frac{\text{gr } ^1/_{300}}{0.5 \text{ mg}} \times 0.5 \text{ mL} = \text{mL per dose}$$

Convert gr $^1/_{300}$ to mg:

60 mg : gr 1 :: X mg : gr $^1/_{300}$

$$1X = {}^1/_{300} \times 60/1$$

$$X = 60/300 = {}^1/_5 \text{ mg, or } 0.2 \text{ mg}$$

$$\frac{0.2 \text{ mg}}{0.5 \text{ mg}} \times 0.5 \text{ mL} = \frac{0.1 \text{ mg}}{0.5 \text{ mg}} = 0.2 \text{ mL}$$

43. **3**—2 tablets

Formula:

$$\frac{\text{Desired}}{\text{Available}} \times \text{Tablet} = \text{Number of tablets per dose}$$

$$\frac{0.4 \text{ g}}{200 \text{ mg}} \times 1 \text{ tablet} = \text{number of tablets per dose}$$

Convert 0.4 g to mg:
In the metric system, to convert larger to smaller multiply by 1000 or move the decimal 3 places to the right.

0.4 g = 400 mg

$$\frac{400 \text{ mg}}{200 \text{ mg}} \times 1 \text{ tablet} = \frac{400 \text{ mg}}{200 \text{ mg}} = 2 \text{ tablets}$$

44. **3**—Administer 2 tablets
Calculation of this problem requires more than one step. First, convert Fahrenheit to Celsius and then calculate the dose to be administered.

Step 1:
Convert Fahrenheit to Celsius

Formula:
To convert Fahrenheit to Celsius, subtract 32 and divide result by 1.8

$$C = (F - 32) \div 1.8$$
$$C = (101 - 32) \div 1.8$$
$$C = (69) \div 1.8$$
$$C = 38.3$$

Step 2:

Formula:

$$\frac{\text{Desired}}{\text{Available}} \times \text{Tablet} = \text{Number of tablets per dose}$$

$$\frac{650 \text{ mg}}{\text{gr } 5} \times 1 \text{ tablet} = \text{tablets per dose}$$

Convert mg to gr:

gr 1 : 60 mg :: X gr : 650 mg

$$60X = 650$$
$$X = \text{gr } 10.8$$

$$\frac{\text{gr } 10.8}{\text{gr } 5} \times 1 \text{ tablet} = \frac{10.8}{5} = 2.16, \text{ or } 2 \text{ tablets}$$

45. **4**—2 tablets

Formula:

$$\frac{\text{Desired}}{\text{Available}} \times \text{Tablet} = \text{Number of tablets per dose}$$

$$\frac{\text{gr } ^1/_2}{15 \text{ mg}} \times \text{Tablet} = \text{tablets per dose}$$

Convert gr $^1/_2$ to mg:

60 mg : gr 1 :: x mg : gr $^1/_2$

$$1X = {}^1/_2 \times 60/1$$
$$X = 60/2 = 30 \text{ mg}$$

$$\frac{30 \text{ mg}}{15 \text{ mg}} \times 1 \text{ tablet} = \frac{30}{15} = 2 \text{ tablets}$$

46. **2**—0.9 mL

Formula:

$$\frac{\text{Desired}}{\text{Available}} \times \text{mL} = \text{mL per dose}$$

$$\frac{300 \text{ mg}}{1 \text{g}} \times 3 \text{ mL} = \text{mL per dose}$$

Convert 300 mg to g:
In the metric system, to convert smaller to larger divide by 1000 or move the decimal 3 places to the left.

300 mg = 0.3 g

$$\frac{0.3 \text{ g}}{1 \text{ g}} \times 3 \text{ mL} = \frac{0.9}{1} = 0.9 \text{ mL}$$

47. **2**—0.75 mL

Formula:

$$\frac{\text{Desired}}{\text{Available}} \times \text{mL} = \text{mL per dose}$$

$$\frac{\text{gr } ^1/_8}{10 \text{ mg}} \times 1 \text{ mL} = \text{mL per dose}$$

Convert gr ⅛ to mg:

60 mg : gr 1 :: X mg : gr ⅛

$$1X = \frac{1}{8} \times 60/1$$

$$X = 60/8 = 7.5 \text{ mg}$$

$$\frac{7.5 \text{ mg}}{10 \text{ mg}} \times 1 \text{ mL} = \frac{7.5}{10} = 0.75 \text{ mL}$$

48. **2**—1.5 tablets

Formula:

$$\frac{\text{Desired}}{\text{Available}} \times \text{Tablet} = \text{Number of tablets per dose}$$

$$\frac{6 \text{ mg}}{4 \text{ mg}} \times 1 \text{ tablet} = \frac{6}{4} = 1.5 \text{ tablets}$$

49. **2**—10 mL

Formula:

$$\frac{\text{Desired}}{\text{Available}} \times \text{mL} = \text{mL per dose}$$

$$\frac{25 \text{ mg}}{10 \text{ mg}} \times 4 \text{ mL} = \frac{100}{10} = 10 \text{ mL}$$

50. **2**—2 Tablets

Formula:

$$\frac{\text{Desired}}{\text{Available}} \times \text{Tablet(s)} = \text{Tablet(s) per dose}$$

$$\frac{40 \text{ mg}}{20 \text{ mg}} \times 1 \text{ tablet} = \frac{40}{20} = 2 \text{ tablets}$$

BIBLIOGRAPHY

Brown, M., & Mulholland, J. (1996). *Drug calculations, process, and problems for clinical practice* (5th ed.). St. Louis: Mosby–Year Book.

Curren, A., & Munday, L. (1996). *Math for meds: Dosages and solutions.* San Diego, CA: Wallcur.

Hodgson, B., & Kizior, R. (1998). *Saunders nurse's drug handbook 1998.* Philadelphia: W. B. Saunders.

Kee, J., & Hayes, E. (1997). *Pharmacology: A nursing process approach* (2nd ed.). Philadelphia: W. B. Saunders.

Kee, J., & Marshall, S. (1996). *Clinical calculations: With applications to general and specialty areas* (3rd ed.). Philadelphia: W. B. Saunders.

Kuhn, M. (1998). *Pharmaco-therapeutics: A nursing process approach* (4th ed.). F. A. Davis.

Leahy, J., & Kizilay, P. (1998). *Foundations of nursing practice: A nursing process approach.* Philadelphia: W. B. Saunders.

Lehne, R. (1998). *Pharmacology for nursing care* (3rd ed.). Philadelphia: W. B. Saunders.

Skidmore, L. (1997). *Mosby's drug guide for nurses* (2nd ed.). St. Louis: C. V. Mosby.

CHAPTER 17

Basic Life Support

....

PYRAMID TERMS

Automated External Defibrillator (AED)—Converts ventricular fibrillation into a perfusing rhythm and allows for early defibrillation by first responders.

Basic Life Support (BLS)—Providing oxygen to the brain, heart, and other vital organs until help arrives.

Cardiopulmonary Resuscitation (CPR)—An interchangeable term for Basic Life Support.

Head Tilt–Chin Lift—Preferred method to open the victim's airway.

Heimlich Maneuver—Method of rescue to remove foreign objects from a choking victim.

Jaw Thrust Maneuver—Method used to open a victim's airway if a neck injury is suspected.

PYRAMID TO SUCCESS

The Pyramid to Success focuses on the emergency measures related to performing **Basic Life Support**. Focus on the points related to the breaths and compression ratio with one-man and two-man adult **CPR** and **CPR** in the infant and child. Pyramid points focus on airway management in **CPR** and in performing the **Heimlich maneuver**. Focus on the correct hand placements for cardiac compressions and the differences between the adult, child, and infant. Remember prior to initiating **CPR**, determining unresponsiveness is the initial action. Remember the ABCs: airway, breathing, and circulation, when performing **CPR**.

NURSING PROCESS

ASSESSMENT

Responsiveness or consciousness	Breathing
Airway	Circulation

ANALYSIS: Ineffective airway clearance
Ineffective breathing pattern
Impaired gas exchange

PLANNING	IMPLEMENTATION	EVALUATION
Client maintains a patent airway. Client demonstrates an effective breathing pattern. Client maintains adequate gas exchange.	Assess airway, breathing, and circulation. Maintain open airway. Provide ventilations to victim as necessary. Perform chest compressions as necessary. Perform Heimlich maneuver if necessary. Evaluate response to interventions continuously.	Airway is patent. Breathing patterns are normal. Adequate circulation is maintained.

CLIENT NEEDS

SAFE, EFFECTIVE CARE ENVIRONMENT

Advanced directives regarding client's documented requests
Advocacy regarding client's wishes
Client rights
Ethical and legal responsibilities
Standard (universal) precautions

HEALTH PROMOTION AND MAINTENANCE

Health promotion programs
Teaching significant other to perform basic life support (BLS)

PSYCHOSOCIAL INTEGRITY

Religious, spiritual, and cultural influences
Communication and emotional support to significant other

PHYSIOLOGICAL INTEGRITY

Alterations in cardiopulmonary system
Handling medical emergencies
Use of special equipment
Administration of emergency medications and IVs
Documentation of response to BLS

I. Basic Life Support (BLS) (Box 17–1)

A. Providing oxygen to the brain, heart, and other vital organs until help arrives
B. Also known as cardiopulmonary resuscitation (CPR)

II. Adult BLS

A. Description: An adult can be defined as an individual 8 years of age or older
B. Airway
 1. Remember that assessment is the first step of the nursing process
 2. The first thing you would do in assessing a victim of sudden illness or accident is to assess unconsciousness or unresponsiveness
 3. Assess the victim for 5 to 10 seconds
 4. Gently shake the victim's shoulders and ask "Are you OK?" In shaking the victim, be alert to the potential for a head or neck injury
 5. Call for help: "Help! Help!"
 6. If the victim is unresponsive, activate the emergency medical system (EMS)
 7. Place the victim in a supine position on a firm, flat surface and kneel near the shoulders of the victim
 8. Open the airway
 9. The **head-tilt–chin-lift** is the preferred method for opening the airway; if there is a neck injury, the **jaw thrust maneuver** is used to open the airway
 10. Look for any foreign material, liquids, or solids in the victim's mouth; wipe out any foreign material with a hooked index or middle finger
C. Breathing
 1. Assess breathing
 2. Maintain an open airway and place your ear over the victim's nose and mouth
 3. Look for the chest to rise and fall, listen for air moving in and out of the lungs, and feel for the flow of air

---

BOX 17–1. The ABCs of Basic Life Support (BLS)

A—Airway
B—Breathing
C—Circulation

Each step of the ABCs of BLS begins with assessment!

---

 4. Breathing Victim
  a. Place the victim on his or her side in the recovery position if no cervical trauma is suspected
  b. Roll the victim onto the side as a unit (without twisting) to help maintain an open airway
  c. If trauma or injury is suspected, the victim should not be moved
 5. Nonbreathing Victim
  a. Pinch the nostrils closed, give two full ventilations (breaths) of 1.5 to 2 seconds per breath
  b. In the adult, give 10 to 12 ventilations per minute or one every 5 to 6 seconds
  c. If you are unsuccessful in giving the breath or ventilation, reposition the victim's head and try again
  d. Improper chin and head position is the most common cause of difficulty in ventilating the victim
  e. If you are still unsuccessful, check the victim's mouth for a foreign body or for loose dentures (remove dentures only if they interfere with the mouth seal)
  f. Clear the airway and try to ventilate again
  g. Be alert to gastric distention when giving ventilations
D. Circulation
 1. Assess circulation; always check for the absence of a pulse before beginning chest compressions on the victim
 2. Maintain an open airway and palpate for a carotid pulse for 5 to 10 seconds
 3. If there is a pulse, give 10 to 12 ventilations a minute, or one every 5 to 6 seconds
 4. Recheck the pulse after 1 minute; if there is no pulse, start chest compressions on the victim
E. Chest Compressions
 1. Hand placement
  a. Correct placement of the hands for chest compressions is crucial
  b. Always recheck the landmarks for chest compressions; hand placement is on the lower half of the sternum
  c. With the hand closest to the victim's feet, locate the lower margin of the rib cage
  d. Move your fingertips along the margin to the notch where the ribs meet the sternum
  e. Place the middle finger on the notch and the index finger next to the middle finger
  f. Place the heel of the opposite hand next to the index finger and place the other hand on top
 2. Complications of chest compressions
  a. Laceration of internal organs such as the liver, spleen, stomach
  b. Punctured lungs

c. Fractured ribs or sternum

d. Gastric distention

III. Adult One-Man BLS

A. The ratio is 15:2; that is, 15 chest compressions to 2 ventilations

B. The rate of compressions is 80 to 100 a minute at a depth of 1.5 to 2 inches

C. Perform four complete cycles, then reassess the victim

D. Check the carotid pulse after the first four cycles of **CPR** and every few minutes thereafter; if no pulse is felt, continue **CPR**

IV. Adult Two-Man BLS

A. One person is at the victim's side performing chest compressions; one person is at the victim's head, maintaining an open airway, monitoring the carotid pulse, and doing the rescue breathing

B. The adult ratio for two-man **BLS** is 5 to 1 or 5 compressions at a rate of 80 to 100 per minute, and 1 ventilation at 1.5 to 2 seconds per breath

C. When the second rescuer arrives at the scene, he or she must identify himself or herself and tell the first rescuer that he or she knows two-man **CPR**

D. The second rescuer then activates EMS if this hasn't been done, and then returns to the scene to help

E. The second rescuer can perform one-man **CPR** if the first rescuer is fatigued; or, the first rescuer finishes 15 compressions, gives 2 ventilations, moves to the head, opens the airway, and checks the carotid pulse

F. If there is no pulse, the first rescuer announces "No pulse, continue **CPR**"

G. The second rescuer locates the landmark for chest compressions

H. The two rescuers begin **CPR** at a ratio of 5 compressions to 1 ventilation

I. At the end of 1 minute, the ventilator checks for a pulse and checks for breathing; if none, the ventilator says, "No pulse, continue **CPR**"

J. When the compressor becomes tired, the compressor may call for a switch in position, stating "Switch (change), 2, 3, 4, 5"

K. The ventilator gives a breath and moves to the chest and locates the correct hand placement or landmark for chest compressions

L. The compressor moves to the head and checks for a carotid pulse; if no pulse, the rescuer states "No pulse, continue **CPR**"

V. Pediatric BLS

A. Description

1. A child can be defined as an individual between the ages of 1 and 8 years of age

2. An infant can be defined as an individual under 1 year old

B. Airway

1. Assess unresponsiveness

2. Gently shake the victim; be alert to the potential for a head or neck injury

3. Call out for help

4. Position the victim

5. Open the airway using the **head-tilt–chin-lift** or the **jaw thrust** if a neck injury is suspected

6. With infants, place the head in a sniffing or neutral position

7. With a child, tilt the head back slightly farther than you would if the victim were an infant

C. Breathing

1. Assess for breathing

2. Maintain an open airway and place your ear over the victim's nose and mouth

3. Look for the chest to rise and fall, listen for air moving in and out of the lungs, and feel for the flow of air on your cheek

4. Breathing victim: Keep the airway open

5. Nonbreathing victim

a. Give two ventilations at 1 to 1.5 seconds per breath

b. If unsuccessful, reposition the victim's head

c. If still unsuccessful, check for a foreign body in the victim's mouth

d. With the infant, provide ventilations by mouth to mouth and nose

e. With the larger child, provide ventilations by mouth to mouth

f. With the infant and child, give 20 ventilations per minute or 1 every 3 seconds

g. Provide 1 minute of rescue breathing, then activate EMS

D. Circulation

1. Assess circulation

2. If the victim is older than 1 year, assess circulation via the carotid pulse

3. If the victim is younger than 1 year, assess circulation via the brachial pulse

4. The ratio is 5 compressions to 1 ventilation

5. Reassess the victim after 20 cycles (approximately 1 minute), and activate EMS if not already done

6. Continue to reassess every few minutes

7. Infant chest compressions

a. The imaginary line between the nipples is located over the breast bone (sternum)

b. The index finger of the hand farthest from the infant's head is placed just under the intermammary line where it intersects the sternum

c. The area of compression is one fingerwidth below this intersection, at the location of the middle and ring fingers

d. Using 2 to 3 fingers, the breast bone is compressed 0.5 to 1 inch at 100 times a minute

8. Chest compressions for a child
   a. The location for hand placement is the same as for an adult
   b. Depress the chest 1 to 1.5 inches at 100 times a minute with the heel of one hand

VI. The Choking Victim and Heimlich Maneuver

A. Conscious Adult
   1. Ask the victim, "Are you choking?"
   2. The victim won't be able to speak or cough if choking
   3. If the victim's airway is partially obstructed, you will hear a crowing sound; encourage the victim to cough
   4. Relieve the obstruction by the **Heimlich maneuver** (Box 17–2)
   5. Perform the **Heimlich maneuver** until the object is dislodged or the victim becomes unconscious
B. Unconscious Adult
   1. Assess consciousness by gently shaking the victim and place the victim in a supine position
   2. Call for help; activate EMS
   3. Open the airway
   4. Assess breathing
   5. Attempt ventilation
   6. Reposition the head if unsuccessful; reattempt ventilation
   7. Relieve the obstruction by the **Heimlich maneuver** with five thrusts, then fingersweep the mouth
   8. To perform the **Heimlich maneuver**, kneel astride the thighs, place the heel of one hand on top of the other between the umbilicus and xiphoid process and give five thrusts in and up with the heel of the bottom hand
   9. To open the airway, grasp the tongue and lower jaw between your thumb and fingers, lift the jaw, and insert the index finger in a hooking motion to relieve the obstruction
   10. Reattempt ventilation
   11. Repeat the sequence of breaths, five abdominal thrusts, and fingersweep until successful

---

BOX 17–2. Heimlich Maneuver

Stand behind the victim
   Place arms around the victim's waist
   Make a fist
   Place the thumb side of the fist just above the umbilicus (belly button) and well below the xiphoid process
   Perform five quick in and up thrusts (between the umbilicus and xiphoid process)
   Use chest thrusts for the markedly obese or for advanced pregnancy victim

---

12. Be sure to assess the victim's pulse and respirations
13. Perform **CPR** if required

C. Choking Child or Infant
   1. Choking is suspected in infants and children experiencing acute respiratory distress associated with coughing, gagging, or stridor (high-pitched noisy breathing)
   2. Allow the victim to continue to cough if the cough is forceful
   3. If the cough is ineffective or the victim develops increased respiratory difficulty accompanied by a high-pitched noise while inhaling, help is needed
   4. Conscious child
      a. Assess for obstruction by asking the child, "Are you choking?"
      b. Relieve the obstruction by the **Heimlich maneuver** until the obstruction is dislodged or the victim becomes unconscious
   5. Unconscious child
      a. Assess unconsciousness
      b. Call for help
      c. Activate the EMS
      d. Open the airway by the **head-tilt–chin-lift**
      e. Check for breathing
      f. Attempt ventilation
      g. If unsuccessful, reposition the head; reattempt ventilation
      h. Relieve the obstruction using the **Heimlich maneuver**, giving five thrusts and fingersweep the mouth only if the object is seen
      i. Reattempt ventilation
      j. Repeat the sequence
      k. Assess pulse and respirations
      l. Perform **CPR** if required
   6. Conscious infant
      a. Assess for obstruction and note breathing problems
      b. Relieve the obstruction by five back blows and five chest thrusts in the infant
      c. Straddle infant over your arm, place the infant's head lower than the trunk, and support the head firmly, holding the jaw
      d. Give five back blows with the heel of your hand between the shoulder blades
      e. Turn the infant; place the head lower than the trunk
      f. Give five chest thrusts at the same location as for chest compressions
      g. Check for the object and remove if seen
      h. Blind fingersweeps are avoided in infants and small children since the object may be pushed back farther into the airway, causing further obstruction
      i. Continue until the object is removed or the victim becomes unconscious
   7. Unconscious infant
      a. Assess consciousness by gentle taps

b. Call for help; activate the EMS
c. Open the airway by the **head-tilt–chin-lift**
d. Check for breathing
e. Attempt ventilation
f. Reposition the head if unsuccessful; reattempt ventilation
g. Relieve the obstruction by five back blows and five chest thrusts
h. Fingersweep the mouth only if the object is seen
i. Reattempt ventilation
j. Repeat the sequence
k. Perform **CPR** if required (Box 17–3)

VII. Automated External Defibrillator (AED)

A. Description
   1. Used to convert ventricular fibrillation into a perfusing rhythm
   2. Differentiates nonventricular fibrillation rhythms and allows for early defibrillation by first responders
B. Implementation
   1. Attach **AED** leads to the victim
   2. Turn on the **AED** and push the button to activate the analyzer
   3. Follow instructions given for the **AED**, usually to "assess," "stand back," "shock," and "reassess"
   4. Evaluate for return of the pulse, and if pulseless, repeat defibrillation as directed up to three times, then perform **CPR**

PRACTICE QUESTIONS

1. The client is brought into the emergency room in ventricular fibrillation (VF). The advanced cardiac life support (ACLS) nurse prepares to defibrillate by placing conductive gel pads on which part of the chest?
   1 On the upper and lower half of the sternum
   2 On the upper right chest below the clavicle and to the left of the nipple in the midaxillary line
   3 On the right shoulder and in the back of the left shoulder
   4 Parallel between the umbilicus and the right nipple

2. The nurse on the day shift walks into a client's room and finds the client unresponsive. The client is not breathing and does not have a pulse. The nurse immediately calls out for help. The next nursing action is which of the following?
   1 Ventilate with a mouth-to-mask device
   2 Start chest compressions
   3 Give the client oxygen
   4 Open the airway

3. The nurse is performing CPR on an adult client. The correct hand placement that the nurse uses for chest compressions is which of the following?
   1 Placing the hands on the lower third of the sternum
   2 Placing the hands on the upper half of the sternum
   3 Placing the hands on the upper third of the sternum
   4 Placing the hands on the lower half of the sternum

4. A nurse witnesses a neighbor's husband sustain a fall from the roof of the house. The nurse rushes to the victim and determines the need to open the airway. Which method is most appropriate to open the airway in this victim?
   1 Head tilt–chin lift
   2 Neutral or sniffing position
   3 Modified head tilt–chin lift
   4 Jaw thrust maneuver

5. The nurse is preparing to do the Heimlich maneuver on a 3-year-old conscious child. The correct hand placement to perform this maneuver is which of the following?
   1 Between the umbilicus and the groin
   2 Between the groin and the abdomen
   3 Between the umbilicus and the xiphoid process
   4 Between the lower abdomen and the chest

6. The nurse is performing CPR on a 7-year-old child. How many breaths per minute will the nurse deliver to the child?
   1 12 breaths per minute
   2 16 breaths per minute
   3 18 breaths per minute
   4 20 breaths per minute

7. When performing CPR on an infant, the rate of compression should be:
   1 At least 60 times per minute
   2 At least 80 times per minute
   3 At least 100 times per minute
   4 At least 160 times per minute

8. A nursing instructor teaches a group of students about BLS. The instructor asks a student to identify the most appropriate location to assess the pulse of an infant. Which of the following, if stated by the student, would indicate that the

---

BOX 17–3. Pyramid Points

Do not interrupt CPR for more than 5 seconds!
STOP CPR ONLY IF:
   Pulse and respiration return
   Emergency Medical System arrives
   The rescuer becomes exhausted
   A physician declares the victim dead

student understands the appropriate assessment procedure?

1 Brachial
2 Carotid
3 Popliteal
4 Radial

9. The nurse is teaching CPR to a group of community members. The nurse asks a member of the group to describe the reason that blind fingersweeps are avoided in infants. Which of the following responses is accurate?

1 The object may be forced back farther into the throat
2 The mouth is too small to see the object
3 The object may have been swallowed
4 The infant may bite down on the finger

10. The nurse is performing CPR on an adult client. When one performs chest compressions, the sternum should be depressed:

1 $1/2$ to $3/4$ inch
2 $3/4$ to 1 inch
3 $21/2$ to 3 inches
4 $11/2$ to 2 inches

ANSWERS

1. **2**

Rationale: The ACLS nurse would place one gel pad on the upper right chest below the clavicle and the other to the left of the nipple with the center in the midaxillary line. The nurse would then place the electrode paddles over the pads, apply firm pressure, and charge the defibrillator to an initial energy of 200 joules. The nurse then ensures that oxygen has been turned away from the client. The nurse loudly and clearly commands all personnel to clear contact with the client and the bed and ensures their compliance before delivering the shock.

Test-Taking Strategy: Consider the anatomical location of the heart to answer the question. This will easily assist in eliminating options 1, 3, and 4. If you had difficulty with this question, take time now to review the correct placement of pads for defibrillation!

Level of Cognitive Ability: Application
Phase of Nursing Process: Planning
Client Needs: Safe, Effective Care Environment
Content Area: Adult Health/Cardiovascular

Reference
Ignatavicius, D., Workman, M., & Mishler, M. (1995). *Medical-surgical nursing: A nursing process approach* (2nd ed.). Philadelphia: W. B. Saunders. pp. 878–879.

2. **4**

Rationale: The next nursing action is to open the airway. Ventilation cannot be initiated unless the airway is opened. Chest compressions are started after the airway is opened and ventilation is initiated. Oxygen may be helpful at some point, but the airway is opened first.

Test-Taking Strategy: Visualize the steps of BLS to answer the question. Recalling the ABCs—airway, breathing, and circulation—will assist in directing you to option 4. Review the steps of BLS now, if you had difficulty with this question!

Level of Cognitive Ability: Application
Phase of Nursing Process: Implementation
Client Needs: Physiological Integrity
Content Area: Adult Health/Cardiovascular

Reference
Ignatavicius, D., Workman, M., & Mishler, M. (1995). *Medical-surgical nursing: A nursing process approach* (2nd ed.). Philadelphia: W. B. Saunders. p. 874.

3. **4**

Rationale: If a pulse is not present, chest compressions will need to be initiated. Determine proper hand placement for chest compressions by locating the notch where the rib margin meets the sternum, and place the middle finger on this notch and the index finger next to it. Then, place the heel of the opposite hand on the lower half of the sternum close to the index finger. Remove the first hand and place it on top of the hand on the sternum and begin chest compressions. This location is the lower half of the sternum.

Test-Taking Strategy: Consider the anatomical location of the heart to answer this question. Eliminate options 2 and 3 first because this location would be ineffective. The lower half of the sternum is the most effective location for chest compressions. If you had difficulty with this question, take time now to review landmarks for chest compressions!

Level of Cognitive Ability: Application
Phase of Nursing Process: Implementation
Client Needs: Physiological Integrity
Content Area: Adult Health/Cardiovascular

Reference
Ignatavicius, D., Workman, M., & Mishler, M. (1995). *Medical-surgical nursing: A nursing process approach* (2nd ed.). Philadelphia: W. B. Saunders. p. 877.

4. **4**

Rationale: If a neck injury is suspected, the jaw thrust maneuver is used to open the airway. The head tilt–chin lift produces hyperextension of the neck and could cause complications if a neck injury is present. The neutral or sniffing position is used to open the airway in an infant. There is no such position as a modified head tilt–chin lift.

Test-Taking Strategy: Eliminate option 2 first since this position is utilized in an infant. Eliminate options 1 and 3 next because they are similarly stated. Knowledge of BLS will direct you toward option 4. If you had difficulty with this question, review the appropriate methods to open an airway!

Level of Cognitive Ability: Application
Phase of Nursing Process: Planning
Client Needs: Physiological Integrity
Content Area: Adult Health/Neurological

Reference
Leahy, J., & Kizilay, P. (1998). *Foundations of nursing practice: A nursing process approach.* Philadelphia: W. B. Saunders. p. 971.

5. 3

Rationale: To perform the Heimlich maneuver, the rescuer stands behind the victim and places the arms directly under the victim's axillae and around the victim. The thumb side of one fist is placed against the victim's abdomen in the midline, slightly above the navel and well below the tip of the xiphoid process. The fist is grasped with the other hand and a series of upward thrusts are delivered. Care must be taken not to touch the xiphoid process or the lower margins of the rib cage because force applied to these structures may damage internal organs.

Test-Taking Strategy: Eliminate options 1 and 2 first because they are similar. To select between the remaining options, consider the anatomical location and the effect of the maneuver in dislodging an obstruction. If you had difficulty with this question, take time now to review the correct hand placement for the Heimlich maneuver!

Level of Cognitive Ability: Application
Phase of Nursing Process: Planning
Client Needs: Physiological Integrity
Content Area: Child Health

Reference
Ashwill, J., & Droske, S. (1997). *Nursing care of children: Principles and practice.* Philadelphia: W. B. Saunders. p. 325.

6. 4

Rationale: In a child between the ages of 1 and 8 years, 20 breaths per minute are delivered. Initially, the nurse would give the child two breaths at 1 to 1.5 seconds per breath.

Test-Taking Strategy: Knowledge regarding the BLS maneuvers in a child is required to answer this question. You are likely to find a question related to this content on NCLEX-RN. If you had difficulty with this question, take time now to review BLS in a child!

Level of Cognitive Ability: Application
Phase of Nursing Process: Implementation
Client Needs: Physiological Integrity
Content Area: Child Health

Reference
Ashwill, J., & Droske, S. (1997). *Nursing care of children: Principles and practice.* Philadelphia: W. B. Saunders. p. 326.

7. 3

Rationale: In an infant, the rate of chest compressions is at least 100 per minute.

Test-Taking Strategy: Consider the normal heart rate of an infant to answer this question. You can easily eliminate options 1 and 2 because of the low rates identified in the options. Eliminate option 4 because this rate would be much too rapid for an infant. If you had difficulty with this question, take time now to review BLS for an infant!

Level of Cognitive Ability: Application
Phase of Nursing Process: Implementation
Client Needs: Physiological Integrity
Content Area: Child Health

Reference
Ashwill, J., & Droske, S. (1997). *Nursing care of children: Principles and practice.* Philadelphia: W. B. Saunders. p. 326.

8. 1

Rationale: When assessing a pulse in an infant (under 1 year of age), the pulse should be checked at the brachial artery. The infant's relatively short, fat neck makes palpation of the carotid artery difficult.

Test-Taking Strategy: Knowledge regarding circulatory assessment in an infant is required to answer this question. Options 3 and 4 can be easily eliminated. Consider the body structure of an infant to assist in directing you to option 1. Review cardiac assessment and BLS in an infant now, if you had difficulty with this question!

Level of Cognitive Ability: Analysis
Phase of Nursing Process: Evaluation
Client Needs: Physiological Integrity
Content Area: Child Health

Reference
Ashwill, J., & Droske, S. (1997). *Nursing care of children: Principles and practice.* Philadelphia: W. B. Saunders. p. 323.

9. 1

Rationale: Blind fingersweeps are not recommended for infants and children because of the risk of forcing the object farther down into the airway. Options 2, 3, and 4 are not directly related to the issue of the question.

Test-Taking Strategy: Utilize the ABCs—airway, breathing, and circulation—to answer this question. Option 1 addresses the concern of airway patency. If you had difficulty with this question, take time now to review obstructed airway management of an infant or child!

Level of Cognitive Ability: Analysis
Phase of Nursing Process: Evaluation
Client Needs: Physiological Integrity
Content Area: Child Health

Reference
Ashwill, J., & Droske, S. (1997). *Nursing care of children: Principles and practice.* Philadelphia: W. B. Saunders. p. 323.

10. 4

Rationale: When performing CPR on an adult client, the sternum should be depressed 1.5 to 2 inches.

Test-Taking Strategy: Knowledge regarding the procedure for performing chest compressions on an adult client is required to answer the question. Note the key word "adult" in the question. Consider the normal body structure of an adult to assist in answering the question. If you had difficulty with this question, take time now to review adult BLS!

Level of Cognitive Ability: Application
Phase of Nursing Process: Implementation
Client Needs: Physiological Integrity
Content Area: Adult Health/Cardiovascular

Reference
Ignatavicius, D., Workman, M., & Mishler, M. (1995). *Medical-surgical nursing: A nursing process approach* (2nd ed.). Philadelphia: W. B. Saunders. p. 877.

BIBLIOGRAPHY

Ashwill, J., & Droske, S. (1997). *Nursing care of children: Principles and practice.* Philadelphia: W. B. Saunders.

Black, J., & Matassarin-Jacobs, E. (1997). *Medical-surgical nursing; Clinical management for continuity of care* (5th ed.). Philadelphia: W. B. Saunders.

Ignatavicius, D., Workman, M., & Mishler, M. (1995). *Medical-surgical nursing: A nursing process approach* (2nd ed.). Philadelphia: W. B. Saunders.

Leahy, J., & Kizilay, P. (1998). *Foundations of nursing practice: A nursing process approach.* Philadelphia: W. B. Saunders.

Luckmann, J. (1997). *Saunders manual of nursing care.* Philadelphia: W. B. Saunders.

Monahan, F., & Neighbors, M. (1998). *Medical-surgical nursing: Foundations for clinical practice* (2nd ed.). Philadelphia: W. B. Saunders.

CHAPTER 18

Perioperative Nursing Care

PYRAMID TERMS

Atelectasis—A collapsed or airless state of the lung that may be the result of airway obstruction due to accumulated secretions or failure of the client to deep breathe. It is the most common postoperative complication and usually occurs 1 to 2 days postoperatively.

Extended Postoperative Stage—The period of at least 1 to 4 days postoperatively.

Immediate Postoperative Stage—The period of 1 to 4 hours after surgery.

Intermediate Postoperative Stage—The period of 4 to 24 hours after surgery.

Wound Dehiscence—An opening of the wound edges.

Wound Evisceration—Protrusion of internal organs through an opening in wound edges.

PYRAMID TO SUCCESS

Pyramid points focus on teaching client and family or significant other in the preoperative stage, preparing the client for the operative procedure, assuring that prescribed preoperative procedures have been performed, and that the results of the procedures are within the expected range and are documented. In the postoperative stage, pyramid points focus on monitoring for surgical complications and on the implementation of initial nursing measures if a complication arises. Pyramid points also focus on preparing the client for discharge, teaching related to the prescribed treatments, and the mobilization of home care support services as needed.

NURSING PROCESS

ASSESSMENT

Major complaint
Pre-existing conditions that increase the risk of surgery
Allergies
Client's present lifestyle related to diet, exercise, substance abuse, and support systems
Vital signs
Breath sounds
Level of consciousness, alertness, and orientation
Circulatory status and capillary refill
Nutritional status
Nausea or vomiting
Obesity, malnutrition, or dietary deficiency
Presence of conditions that may produce nutritional deficiencies
Urinary output
Bowel sounds
Muscular weakness
Laboratory results
Anxiety levels, fears, and emotional issues
Financial concerns

ANALYSIS: Ineffective Airway Clearance

PLANNING	IMPLEMENTATION	EVALUATION
The client maintains an effective airway. The client demonstrates the use of coughing and deep breathing exercises and the use of an incentive spirometer.	Monitor vital signs. Monitor lung sounds and signs of breathing distress. Assist with repositioning. Instruct on proper coughing and breathing techniques. Encourage client to demonstrate techniques and use of incentive spirometer. Assist client with splinting incision. Encourage ambulation.	Vital signs remain within normal limits. The client coughs and deep breathes and uses assistive devices.

ANALYSIS: Pain

PLANNING	IMPLEMENTATION	EVALUATION
The client requests pain medication. The client demonstrates and uses relaxation and noninvasive techniques to control anxiety and postoperative pain.	Assess pain level using a 1 to 10 pain scale. Administer pain medication as prescribed, noting time and effect of last dosage of medication. Utilize noninvasive pain control techniques. Document the effectiveness of pain control measures.	The client achieves pain control.

ANALYSIS: Alteration in Nutrition

PLANNING	IMPLEMENTATION	EVALUATION
The client tolerates intake as prescribed.	Monitor I&O. Monitor for signs of dehydration. Maintain IV fluids as prescribed. Assess for nausea and vomiting. Administer antiemetics as prescribed. Monitor electrolyte values. Offer ice chips as prescribed. Resume diet with clear liquids, advancing diet as prescribed. Document I&O and client's ability to tolerate food and fluids.	Fluid and electrolyte status remains normal. Weight remains normal.

ANALYSIS: Potential for Infection

PLANNING	IMPLEMENTATION	EVALUATION
The surgical wound remains clean and dry.	Maintain aseptic techniques. Monitor for signs and symptoms of infection. Assess the wound area, drains, and dressings frequently for signs of infection. Administer prophylactic antibiotics as prescribed.	The client is free of infection.

ANALYSIS: Potential for Alteration in Elimination

PLANNING	IMPLEMENTATION	EVALUATION
The client maintains an adequate urinary output. The client resumes normal bowel patterns.	Assess bladder for distention. Monitor for urinary output. Monitor for bowel sounds. Encourage ambulation. Monitor for bowel movement and return of normal bowel patterns.	Normal urinary and bowel patterns return.

ANALYSIS: Anxiety and Fear

PLANNING	IMPLEMENTATION	EVALUATION
The client expresses feelings related to surgery.	Allow the client to talk about concerns and fears related to surgery. Teach the client relaxation techniques to deal with preoperative anxiety and postoperative pain. Describe any alterations in body appearance or function, or lifestyle changes that may occur. Assist the client to adapt to any changes resulting from the surgery. Arrange for a visit from someone who has undergone the same surgical procedure. Assist the client to set realistic goals regarding any lifestyle changes.	The client expresses a positive outlook for the impending surgery. The client sets goals and makes decisions regarding care.

ANALYSIS: Knowledge Deficit

PLANNING	IMPLEMENTATION	EVALUATION
The client verbalizes understanding of the events that will occur before, during, and following surgery. The client verbalizes the prescribed treatment plan for discharge. The client expresses feelings of personal control regarding rehabilitation.	Initiate preoperative teaching regarding the events of surgery. Instruct client and family in the prescribed discharge plan. Develop a rehabilitation program that maximizes client control and involvement. Include family members in the discussion regarding the rehabilitation process. Refer the client to appropriate support groups.	The client describes the rehabilitation process. The client utilizes support groups. The client participates actively in the rehabilitation process.

CLIENT NEEDS

SAFE, EFFECTIVE CARE ENVIRONMENT

Advance directives
Client rights
Informed consent for the surgical procedure
Informing the client of the surgical process
Providing safety to the medicated client
Surgical asepsis
Standard (Universal) Precautions
Monitoring for surgical infection

HEALTH PROMOTION AND MAINTENANCE

Expected body image changes
Client and family teaching related to the prescribed discharge plan
Health and wellness to prevent complications
Promoting lifestyle choices
Appropriate referral to support services

PSYCHOSOCIAL INTEGRITY

Assessment of psychosocial concerns
Promoting an environment that will allow the client to express concerns
Unexpected body image changes
Assisting the client to develop coping methods
Support systems

PHYSIOLOGICAL INTEGRITY

Safe administration of preoperative and postoperative medications

Safe administration of IV fluids and blood products as prescribed

Providing respiratory therapy

Providing basic care and comfort

Monitoring for surgical complications

Monitoring for wound infection

Monitoring for unexpected responses to treatments and procedures

Initiating nursing interventions when surgical complications arise

Perioperative Nursing Care

. . . .

I. Preoperative Care

A. Obtaining Informed Consent
  1. The surgeon is responsible for obtaining the consent for surgery
  2. No sedation should be administered to the client before signing the consent
  3. Minors may need a parent or legal guardian to sign the consent form
  4. Older clients may need a legal guardian to sign the consent form
  5. The nurse may witness the client signing the operative permit, but the nurse must be sure that the client has understood the surgeon's explanation of the surgery
  6. The nurse needs to document the witnessing of the signing of the operative permit, after the client acknowledges understanding the procedure

B. Nutrition
  1. Assess the physician's orders regarding the NPO status prior to surgery
  2. Solid foods and liquids are withheld for 6 to 8 hours prior to general anesthesia and for 3 hours before surgery with local anesthesia, to avoid aspiration
  3. Prepare to initiate an IV and administer IV fluids as prescribed
  4. Prepare to administer total parenteral nutrition (TPN) to clients who are malnourished, have protein or metabolic deficiencies, or cannot ingest foods

C. Elimination
  1. If the client is to have intestinal or abdominal surgery, an enema or laxative or both may be prescribed the night before surgery
  2. The client should void immediately before surgery
  3. Prepare to insert a Foley catheter if prescribed
  4. If a Foley catheter is in place, it should be emptied immediately before surgery and the amount and quality of urine output documented

D. Surgical Site
  1. Prepare to clean the surgical site with a mild antiseptic soap the night before surgery, as prescribed
  2. Prepare to shave the operative site as prescribed
  3. Hair should be shaved only if it will interfere with the surgical procedure and only if prescribed
  4. Shaving of hair, if prescribed, should be done in the direction of hair growth with a sharp razor, and caution should be used to prevent cuts or epidermal damage

E. Preoperative Client Teaching (Boxes 18–1 and 18–2)
  1. Inform the client about what to expect postoperatively
  2. Inform the client to notify the nurse if any pain is experienced postoperatively and that pain medication will be prescribed to be given as the client requests
  3. Teach noninvasive pain relief measures, such as relaxation, distraction techniques, and guided imagery
  4. Instruct the client to use the noninvasive pain relief techniques before the pain occurs and as soon as the pain is noticed
  5. Demonstrate the use of a client-controlled analgesia pump if its use is prescribed
  6. Inform the client not to hestiate to request pain medication when needed
  7. Inform the client that requesting a narcotic after surgery will not make the client a drug addict
  8. The client should be instructed not to smoke for at least 12 hours before surgery
  9. Instruct the client in deep breathing and coughing techniques, the use of incentive spirometry, and the importance of performing the techniques postoperatively to prevent the development of pneumonia and **atelectasis**
  10. Instruct client in leg and foot exercises to prevent venous stasis of blood and to facilitate venous blood return
  11. Instruct client how to splint an incision and to turn and reposition
  12. Inform the client of any invasive devices that may be needed following surgery, such as a nasogastric tube, drain, Foley catheter, epidural catheter, intravenous or subclavian lines
  13. Inform the client not to pull on any of the invasive devices, as they will be removed as soon as possible

F. Psychosocial Preparation
  1. Be alert to the client's anxiety level
  2. Answer any questions or concerns the client may have regarding surgery
  3. Allow time for privacy for the client to prepare for surgery psychologically
  4. Provide support and assistance as needed

G. Preoperative Checklist
  1. Assure that the client has an identification bracelet on
  2. Assess for allergy

BOX 18-1. Client Teaching

LEG AND HIP EXERCISES

Instruct the client to press the back of the knees against the bed, and then to relax knees.

This contracts and relaxes the thigh and calf muscles to prevent thrombus formation.

Instruct the client to rotate each foot in a circle at least ten times an hour.

Have the client flex the knee and thigh, straighten the leg up in the air, and hold for 5 seconds before lowering, performing the exercise ten times per day.

COUGHING AND DEEP-BREATHING EXERCISES

Instruct the client that a sitting position gives the best lung expansion for coughing and deep-breathing exercises.

Instruct the client to breathe deeply three times, inhaling through the nostrils and exhaling through the mouth.

Instruct the client that the third breath should be held for 3 seconds, then the client should forcefully cough out three times.

The client should perform this exercise every 2 hours.

SPLINTING INCISION

If the surgical incision is abdominal or thoracic, instruct client to place a pillow, or one hand with the other hand on top, over the incisional area.

During deep breathing and coughing, the client presses gently against the incisional area to splint or support it.

INCENTIVE SPIROMETRY

Instruct client to assume a sitting position.

Instruct client that lips need to cover the mouthpiece completely.

Instruct client to inhale slowly and maintain a constant flow through the unit.

When maximal inspiration is reached, client should hold the breath for 2 to 3 seconds and then exhale slowly.

Instruct client that the number of breaths should not exceed 12 breaths per minute.

BOX 18-2. Medications That Can Affect the Surgical Client

ANTIBIOTICS

Potentiate the action of anesthetic agents.

If taken for 2 weeks before surgery, aminoglycosides such as gentamicin (Garamycin), tobramycin (Nebcin), and neomycin (Mycifradin) may cause mild respiratory depression from depressed neuromuscular transmission.

ANTIDYSRHYTHMICS

Reduce cardiac contractility and impair cardiac conduction during anesthesia.

ANTICOAGULANTS

Alter normal clotting factors and increase the risk of hemorrhaging.

Aspirin (acetylsalicylic acid [ASA]) and ibuprofen (Motrin, Advil) are commonly used medications that can alter clotting mechanisms.

They should be discontinued at least 48 hours before surgery.

ANTICONVULSANTS

Long-term use of certain anticonvulsants can alter the metabolism of anesthetic agents.

ANTIHYPERTENSIVES

Can interact with anesthetic agents and cause bradycardia, hypotension, and impaired circulation.

CORTICOSTEROIDS

Cause adrenal atrophy and reduce the body's ability to withstand stress.

Before and during surgery, dosages may be temporarily increased.

INSULIN

The need for insulin after surgery in a diabetic may be reduced, because the client's nutritional intake is decreased.

Stress response and IV administration of glucose solutions can increase insulin dosage requirements after surgery.

DIURETICS

Potentiate electrolyte imbalances after surgery.

ANTIDEPRESSANTS

May lower the blood pressure during anesthesia.

ANTICHOLINERGICS

Medications with anticholinergic effects increase the potential for confusion.

3. Review the preoperative checklist to be sure that each item is addressed before the client is transported to surgery
4. Assure that consent forms were signed for the operative procedure, for any blood transfusions, for disposal of a limb, or for surgical sterilization procedures
5. Assure that a history and physical examination were completed and documented in the client's record
6. Assure that consultations prescribed were completed and documented in the client's record
7. Assure that the prescribed laboratory results are documented in the client's record
8. Assure that ECG and chest radiograph reports are noted in the client's record
9. Assure that blood type and screen or type and cross-match is noted in the client's record
10. Document that the client has voided prior to surgery

11. Remove jewelry, makeup, dentures, hairpins, nail polish, glasses, and any prosthesis
12. Document that valuables were given to the client's family members or locked in the hospital safe
13. Document that the prescribed preoperative medication was given
14. Monitor and document the client's vital signs
15. Document the last time the client ate or drank

H. Preoperative Medications
   1. Prepare to administer preoperative medications as prescribed or on call to the operating room immediately before the surgery
   2. Instruct the client that he or she will feel drowsy after the medications are given
   3. After administering the preoperative medications, keep the client in bed with the side rails up
   4. Place the call bell next to the client, instruct the client not to get out of bed and to call for assistance if needed

I. Arrival in the Operating Room
   1. When the client arrives in the operating room, the operating room nurse will verify the identification bracelet with the client's verbal response and will review the client's chart
   2. The operating room nurse will confirm the operative procedure and site to be operated on
   3. The client's chart will be checked for completeness
   4. The client's chart will be reviewed for consent forms, history and physical examination, and allergic reaction information
   5. Physician's orders will be reviewed and verified that they were carried out
   6. The IV line may be initiated at this time if prescribed
   7. The anesthesia team will administer the prescribed anesthesia

II. Postoperative Care

A. Immediate Stage
   1. Description: The period of 1 to 4 hours after surgery
   2. Respiratory system
      a. Monitor vital signs
      b. Monitor airway patency and adequate ventilation, since prolonged mechanical ventilation during anesthesia may affect postoperative lung function
      c. Remember that extubated clients who are lethargic may not be able to maintain an airway
      d. Monitor for secretions and remove them by suctioning, if the client is unable to clear the airway by coughing

   e. Observe chest movement for symmetry and the use of accessory muscles
   f. Monitor oxygen administration if prescribed
   g. Monitor pulse oximetry
   h. Encourage coughing and deep breathing exercises as soon as possible
   i. Auscultate lungs, noting rate, depth, and quality of respirations: the respiratory rate should be greater than 10 and less than 30
   j. Assess breath sounds, noting any stridor, wheezing, or crowing, which can indicate partial obstruction, bronchospasm, or laryngospasm
   k. Assess breath sounds, noting any crackles or rhonchi, which may indicate pulmonary edema
   l. Monitor client for signs of **atelectasis**, pneumonia, and pulmonary embolism
3. Cardiovascular system
   a. Assess the client's color
   b. Observe capillary refill, mucous membranes, and sclera
   c. Assess peripheral pulses and for peripheral edema
   d. Monitor for bleeding
   e. Assess pulse for rate and rhythm
   f. A bounding pulse may indicate hypertension, fluid overload, or excitement
   g. Monitor for signs of hypertension and hypotension
   h. Monitor for cardiac dysrhythmias
   i. Assess for Homan's sign, particularly in clients in lithotomy position during surgery, as these clients may be predisposed to developing deep vein thrombosis
4. Musculoskeletal system
   a. Assess the client for moving extremities
   b. Assess physician's orders regarding client positioning or restrictions
   c. Unless contraindicated, place client in a low Fowler's position after surgery to increase the size of the thorax
   d. Avoid positioning the client in a supine position until pharyngeal reflexes have returned
   e. If the client is comatose or semicomatose, position on the side and keep an oral airway in place
5. Neurological system
   a. Assess level of consciousness
   b. Closely monitor the client who may be drowsy or unconscious
   c. Frequent periodic attempts to awaken the client should continue until the client awakens
   d. Orient client to environment
   e. Speak in a soft tone and filter out extraneous noises in the environment

f. Maintain body temperature and prevent heat loss by providing the client with warm blankets and raising the room temperature as necessary

6. Temperature control
   a. Monitor temperature
   b. Monitor for signs of hypothermia that may result from anesthesia, a cool operating room, and exposure of the skin and internal organs during surgery
   c. Apply warm blankets and continue oxygen as prescribed if client is shivering

7. Integumentary system
   a. Assess surgical site, drains, and wound dressings
   b. Monitor for and document any drainage or bleeding from the surgical site
   c. Assess skin for redness, abrasions, or breakdown that may have resulted from surgical positioning

8. Fluid and electrolyte balance
   a. Monitor IV administration as prescribed
   b. Accurately record I&O
   c. Monitor for signs of hypocalcemia, hyperglycemia, and metabolic and respiratory acidosis and alkalosis

9. Gastrointestinal system
   a. Monitor for nausea and vomiting
   b. Maintain patency of nasogastric tube if present
   c. Monitor for abdominal distention
   d. Monitor for return of bowel sounds

10. Renal system
    a. Assess bladder for distention
    b. Monitor color, quantity, and quality of urine output if a Foley catheter is present
    c. Expect client to void 6 to 8 hours following the surgical procedure, depending on the type of anesthesia administered

11. Pain management
    a. Assess for pain
    b. Assess the type of anesthetic used and preoperative medication that the client received, and note whether the client received any pain medications in the postanesthesia period
    c. Inquire about the type and location of pain
    d. Ask the client to rate the degree of pain on a scale of 1 to 10, with 10 being the most severe
    e. Monitor such objective data as facial expressions, body gestures, pulse rate, blood pressure, and respirations
    f. Inquire about the effectiveness of the last pain medication
    g. Administer pain medication as prescribed
    h. If a narcotic has been prescribed, during the initial administration assess the client every 30 minutes for respiratory rate and pain relief

   i. Utilize noninvasive measures to relieve postoperative pain, including distraction, comfort measures, positioning, back rubs, and providing a quiet and restful environment
   j. Document effectiveness of pain medication

B. Intermediate Stage
   1. Description: The period of 4 to 24 hours after surgery
   2. Respiratory system
      a. Monitor vital signs
      b. Continue assessments as during the immediate stage
      c. Monitor patency of airway, verifying that the lungs are clear on auscultation
      d. Encourage coughing and deep breathing
   3. Cardiovascular system
      a. Monitor circulatory status, such as peripheral pulses, capillary refill, and the absence of edema, numbness, and tingling
      b. Encourage the use of antiembolism stockings, if prescribed, to promote venous return, strengthen muscle tone, and prevent pooling of secretions in the lungs
   4. Musculoskeletal system
      a. Assess for movement in all extremities and encourage ambulation
      b. Before ambulation, instruct the client to sit at the edge of the bed with the feet supported
      c. If client is unable to get out of bed, turn client every 1 to 2 hours
   5. Neurological system
      a. Assess level of consciousness
      b. Maintain orientation to the environment
   6. Integumentary system
      a. Assess surgical site and drains
      b. Monitor temperature and wound for signs of infection
      c. Maintain a dry and intact dressing
      d. Reinforce wound with a sterile dressing if necessary, and notify the physician if bleeding occurs from the site
      e. Change dressings as prescribed, noting the amount of bleeding or drainage, odor, and intactness of sutures or staples
      f. Use an abdominal binder for obese and debilitated individuals to prevent rupture of the incision
      g. Drains should be patent, and there should be minimal bleeding or drainage
      h. Prepare to assist with the removal of drains as prescribed by the physician when the drainage amount becomes insignificant
   7. Gastrointestinal system
      a. Monitor I&O
      b. Monitor for nausea and vomiting
      c. Turn the unconscious client to a side-lying position if vomiting occurs, and

have suctioning equipment available and ready to use

d. Administer frequent mouth care

e. Maintain the NPO status until the gag reflex returns and peristalsis returns

f. Continue IV fluids as prescribed until the client can tolerate fluids

g. When oral fluids are permitted, start with ice chips and water

h. Ensure that the client advances to clear liquids and then to a regular diet as tolerated

i. Assess for bowel sounds in all four quadrants

j. Monitor the client for gas pains and encourage ambulation

8. Renal system

a. Monitor urinary output (should be greater than 30 mL per hour)

b. If the client does not have a Foley catheter, client is expected to void within 6 to 8 hours postoperatively, and assure that the amount is at least 200 mL

9. Pain management

a. Assess for pain

b. Inquire about the type and location of pain

c. Ask the client to rate the degree of pain on a scale of 1 to 10, with 10 being the most severe

d. Monitor such objective data as facial expressions, body gestures, pulse rate, blood pressure, and respirations

e. Inquire about the effectiveness of the last pain medication

f. Administer pain medication as prescribed

g. Utilize noninvasive measures to relieve postoperative pain, including distraction, comfort measures, positioning, back rubs, and providing a quiet and restful environment

h. Document effectiveness of pain medication

C. Extended Stage

1. Description: The period of at least 1 to 4 days postoperatively

2. Implementation

a. Continue to assess and observe the client's body systems during this stage

b. Monitor for signs of infection, such as redness, swelling and tenderness at the surgical site, fever, and leukocytosis

c. Encourage active range of motion exercises every 2 hours

d. Continue to encourage ambulation, which will promote peristalsis and the passage of fluid and flatus

e. Increase ambulation every day to increase muscle strength

f. Encourage the client to perform as many activities of daily living as possible

g. Instruct client to eat foods that are high in protein and vitamin C content to promote wound healing

III. Pneumonia and Atelectasis (Box 18–3)

A. Description

1. Pneumonia, an inflammation of the alveoli caused by an infectious process, may develop 3 to 5 days postoperatively because of infection, aspiration, or immobility

2. **Atelectasis**, a collapse of the alveoli with retained mucus secretions, is the most common postoperative complication and usually occurs 1 to 2 days postoperatively

B. Assessment

1. Assess for factors that may increase the risk of pneumonia and **atelectasis**

2. Dyspnea

3. Increased respiratory rate

4. Crackles over involved lung area

5. Cyanosis

6. Elevated temperature

7. Weakness

8. Productive cough

9. Chest pain

C. Implementation

1. Assess lung and breath sounds

2. Reposition the client every 1 to 2 hours

3. Encourage the client to use the incentive spirometer, cough, and deep breathe

4. Provide postural drainage

5. Suction to clear secretions if client is unable to cough

6. Encourage fluid intake

7. Encourage early ambulation

IV. Hypoxia

A. Description: An inadequate concentration of oxygen in arterial blood

B. Assessment

1. Restlessness

2. Dyspnea

3. Hypertension

4. Tachycardia

5. Diaphoresis

6. Cyanosis

C. Implementation

1. Monitor for signs of hypoxia

2. Monitor for depressed respirations

3. Monitor lung sounds

BOX 18–3. Postoperative Complications

Pneumonia and atelectasis	Urinary retention
Hypoxia	Constipation
Pulmonary embolism	Paralytic ileus
Hemorrhage	Wound infection
Shock	Wound dehiscence
Thrombophlebitis	Wound evisceration

4. Encourage coughing and deep breathing and use of incentive spirometry
5. Turn and reposition client
6. Monitor pulse oximetry
7. Eliminate cause of hypoxia
8. Administer oxygen as prescribed

V. Pulmonary Embolism

A. Description: An embolus blocking the pulmonary artery and disrupting blood flow to one or more lobes of the lung
B. Assessment
  1. Dyspnea
  2. Sudden sharp chest or upper abdominal pain
  3. Cyanosis
  4. Tachycardia
  5. A drop in blood pressure
C. Implementation
  1. Monitor vital signs
  2. Notify the physician immediately

VI. Hemorrhage

A. Description: The loss of a large amount of blood externally or internally in a short period of time
B. Assessment
  1. Hypotension
  2. Weak and rapid pulse
  3. Cool, clammy skin
  4. Rapid breathing
  5. Restlessness
  6. Reduced urine output
C. Implementation
  1. Provide pressure to the site of bleeding
  2. Notify physician immediately
  3. Administer oxygen as prescribed
  4. Administer IV and blood replacement as prescribed
  5. Prepare client for surgical procedure if necessary

◆ VII. Shock

A. Description: Loss of circulatory fluid volume that is usually caused by hemorrhage
B. Assessment
  1. Hypotension
  2. Weak and rapid pulse
  3. Cool, clammy skin
  4. Rapid breathing
  5. Restlessness
  6. Disorientation
  7. Slow capillary refill
  8. Reduced urine output
C. Implementation
  1. If shock develops, elevate the legs
  2. If the client had spinal anesthesia, do not elevate the legs any higher than placing them on a pillow, otherwise diaphragm muscles could be impaired
  3. Determine and treat cause of shock

4. Monitor level of consciousness
5. Monitor vital signs for increased pulse or decreased blood pressure
6. Monitor I&O
7. Measure urine and specific gravity
8. Assess color, temperature, turgor, and moisture of skin and mucous membranes
9. Administer fluids, blood, and colloid solutions as prescribed

VIII. Thrombophlebitis

A. Description
  1. Inflammation of a vein, often accompanied by clot formation
  2. Veins in legs are most commonly affected
B. Assessment
  1. Vein inflammation
  2. Aching or cramping pain
  3. Vein feels hard and cordlike and is tender to touch
  4. Elevated temperature
  5. Positive Homan's sign
C. Implementation
  1. Monitor legs for swelling, inflammation, cyanosis, pain, tenderness, and venous distention
  2. Elevate the extremity 30 degrees without allowing any pressure on the popliteal area
  3. Encourage coughing and deep breathing
  4. Encourage the use of antiembolism stockings as prescribed
  5. Remove antiembolism stockings twice a day to wash and inspect the legs
  6. Utilize intermittent pneumatic compression stockings as prescribed
  7. Perform passive range of motion every 2 hours if the client is on bed rest
  8. Encourage early ambulation as prescribed
  9. Do not allow the client to dangle the legs
  10. Instruct the client not to sit in one position for an extended period of time
  11. Administer heparin or warfarin (Coumadin) as prescribed

IX. Urinary Retention

A. Description
  1. Involuntary accumulation of urine in the bladder from loss of muscle tone
  2. Due to the effects of anesthetics and narcotic analgesics
  3. Appears 6 to 8 hours after surgery
B. Assessment
  1. Inability to void
  2. Restlessness
  3. Distended bladder
  4. Hypertension
  5. Lower abdominal pain
  6. Diaphoresis
  7. On percussion, the bladder sounds like a drum

C. Implementation
  1. Assess for distended bladder
  2. Monitor for voiding
  3. Monitor for hypertension
  4. Encourage ambulation when prescribed
  5. Encourage fluid intake unless contraindicated
  6. Assist the client to void by helping to stand
  7. Provide privacy
  8. Pour warm water over the perineum
  9. Allow the client to hear running water
  10. Catheterize the client as prescribed after all noninvasive techniques have been attempted

X. Constipation

A. Description
  1. Infrequent passage of stool
  2. When the client resumes a solid diet postoperatively, failure to pass stool within 48 hours is a cause for concern
B. Assessment
  1. Abdominal distention
  2. Absence of bowel movements
  3. Anorexia, headache, and nausea
C. Implementation
  1. Assess bowel sounds
  2. Encourage fluid intake up to 3000 mL per day unless contraindicated
  3. Encourage early ambulation
  4. Encourage consumption of fiber and roughage
  5. Administer stool softeners and laxatives as prescribed
  6. Provide privacy and adequate time for bowel elimination

XI. Ileus

A. Description
  1. Failure of appropriate forward movement of bowel contents
  2. May occur as a result of anesthetic medications or manipulation of the bowel during the surgical procedure
B. Assessment
  1. Nausea and vomiting postoperatively
  2. Abdominal distention
  3. Absence of bowel sounds, bowel movement, or flatus
C. Implementation
  1. Monitor bowel sounds
  2. Maintain NPO status until bowel sounds return
  3. Maintain patency of NG tube
  4. Encourage ambulation
  5. Administer IV fluids or TPN as prescribed
  6. Administer medications as prescribed to increase GI motility and secretions

XII. Wound Infection

A. Description
  1. Caused by poor aseptic technique or a contaminated wound before surgical exploration
  2. Usually occurs 3 to 6 days after surgery
  3. Purulent material may exit from the drains or separated wound edges
B. Assessment
  1. Fever and chills
  2. Warm, tender, painful, and inflamed incision site
  3. Edematous skin at incision and tight skin sutures
  4. Elevated white blood cell count
C. Implementation
  1. Monitor temperature
  2. Monitor incision site for approximation of suture line, edema, or bleeding, and signs of infection
  3. Maintain patency of drains
  4. Monitor drains and assess drainage amount, color, and consistency
  5. Keep drain and tubes away from incision line and maintain asepsis
  6. Change dressing as prescribed
  7. Administer antibiotics as prescribed

XIII. Wound Dehiscence

A. Description
  1. Separation of the abdominal wound edges at the suture line
  2. Usually occurs 6 to 8 days after surgery
B. Assessment
  1. Increased drainage
  2. Opened wound edges
  3. Appearance of underlying tissues through the wound
C. Implementation
  1. Notify the physician immediately
  2. Cover the wound with a sterile normal saline dressing
  3. Place the client in low Fowler's position with knees bent to prevent abdominal tension
  4. Prevent wound infection
  5. Administer antiemetics as prescribed to prevent vomiting and further strain on incision
  6. Instruct the client to splint incision when coughing

XIV. Wound Evisceration

A. Description
  1. Protrusion of the internal organs through an opening in wound edges
  2. Most common among obese clients, clients who had abdominal surgery, or those who have poor wound-healing ability
  3. Usually occurs 6 to 8 days after surgery
  4. Wound evisceration is an emergency

BOX 18–4. Postoperative Discharge Teaching

- Assess the client's readiness to learn, educational level, and desire to change or modify lifestyle
- Assess the need for resources needed for home care
- Demonstrate care of the incision and how to change the dressing
- Instruct the client to cover the incision with plastic if showering is allowed
- Be sure the client is provided with a 48-hour supply of dressings for home use
- Instruct the client on the importance of returning to the physician's office for a check-up
- Instruct the client that sutures are usually removed in the physician's office 7 to 10 days after surgery
- Inform the client that staples are removed 7 to 14 days after surgery and that the skin may become slightly reddened when they are ready to be removed
- Steri-Strips may be applied to provide extra support after the sutures are removed
- Instruct the client on the use of medications, their purpose, doses, administration, and side effects
- Instruct the client on diet
- Instruct client to drink 6 to 8 glasses of liquid a day
- Instruct the client on activity levels
- Instruct the client to resume normal activities gradually
- Instruct the client to avoid lifting for 6 weeks if a major surgical procedure was performed
- Instruct the client with an abdominal incision not to lift anything weighing 10 pounds or more and not to engage in any activities that involve pushing or pulling
- Clients usually can return to work in 6 to 8 weeks as prescribed by the physician
- Instruct the client on the signs and symptoms of complications and when to call a physician

B. Assessment
   1. Discharge of serosanguineous fluid from a previously dry wound
   2. The appearance of loops of bowel or other abdominal contents through the wound
   3. The client may report feeling a popping sensation after coughing or turning
C. Implementation
   1. Notify the physician immediately
   2. Cover the wound with a sterile normal saline dressing
   3. Place the client in low Fowler's position with knees bent to prevent abdominal tension
   4. Prevent wound infection
   5. Administer antiemetics as prescribed to prevent vomiting and further strain on incision
   6. Instruct the client to splint incision when coughing

XV. Ambulatory Surgery

A. Criteria for Client Discharge
   1. Is alert and oriented
   2. Has voided
   3. Has no respiratory distress
   4. Is able to ambulate, swallow, and cough
   5. Has minimal pain
   6. Is not vomiting
   7. Has minimal, if any, bleeding from incision site
   8. A responsible adult is available to drive the client home
   9. The surgeon has signed a release form
B. Discharge Teaching (Box 18–4)
   1. Should be performed prior to the date of the scheduled procedure
   2. Provide written instructions to the client and family regarding the specifics of care
   3. Instruct the client and family of postoperative complications that can occur
   4. Provide appropriate resources for home care support
   5. Instruct the client not to drive for 24 hours if general anesthesia was used
   6. Inform client to call the surgeon, ambulatory center, or emergency department if postoperative problems occur
   7. Instruct the client to keep follow-up appointments with surgeon

PRACTICE QUESTIONS

1. Before a client has surgery, diagnostic tests such as a complete blood count, serum electrolyte analysis, coagulation studies, and serum creatinine are performed to screen for pre-existing abnormalities. Which of these laboratory results would indicate to the nurse that the surgery may be postponed?
   1 Sodium (Na^+), 140 mEq/L
   2 Hemoglobin (Hgb), 9.2 g/dL
   3 Platelets, 200,000/mm³
   4 Serum creatinine, 0.9 mg/100 mL

2. The nurse should include which of the following activities in the nursing care plan for the client on the day of surgery?
   1 Remove colored nail polish from the nails
   2 Report immediately any increase in blood pressure or pulse
   3 Verify that the client has not eaten for the last 24 hours
   4 Avoid oral hygiene and rinsing with mouthwash

3. Emergency surgery is scheduled for a client with a bowel obstruction. The nurse is unable to obtain informed consent from the client because the client has been receiving narcotic analgesics and is very sedated. Which of the following is the most appropriate action?

1 Perform the surgery without an informed consent

2 Call the family and tell them that they must come to the hospital immediately to sign the informed consent

3 Obtain a telephone consent from the family member, assuring that the oral consent is witnessed by two persons

4 Have the client sign the consent form because this is an emergency situation

4. Most clients have some fear of surgery. The extent to which a client fears surgery depends on several factors, including past experiences with surgery and preconceptions about surgery. To alleviate the client's fears and misconceptions about surgery, the nurse should first:

1 Provide explanations about procedures involved in the planned surgery.

2 Explain all nursing care and possible discomfort that may result.

3 Tell the client that preoperative fear is normal.

4 Ask the client to discuss information known about planned surgery.

5. In an evaluation of the preoperative teaching of the use of the incentive spirometer, which of the following statements indicates that the client does not clearly understand the procedure?

1 "My lips should cover the mouthpiece completely."

2 "I should inhale slowly to maintain a constant flow through the unit."

3 "After maximum inspiration, I should hold my breath for 2 to 3 seconds, then exhale slowly."

4 "I can use the incentive spirometer in any position to achieve optimal lung expansion."

6. The nurse performs a preoperative assessment on a client who is scheduled for surgery in 1 week in the ambulatory care surgical center. On assessment, the nurse notes that the client has a history of arthritis and has been taking aspirin (acetylsalicylic acid [ASA]). Which of the following information is most appropriate to provide to the client regarding the aspirin?

1 Continue to take the aspirin as prescribed

2 Decrease the dose of the aspirin to half of what is normally taken

3 Discontinue the aspirin immediately

4 Discontinue the aspirin 48 hours before the scheduled surgery

7. An older person requires less anesthetic medication to produce anesthesia. Additionally, it takes longer for an older person to eliminate the anesthetic agents from the body. Which of the following statements best explains the reason for the reduction of anesthetic medication dosage in the older person?

1 The increase of fatty tissue allows anesthetic agents, which have an affinity for fatty tissue, to concentrate in body fat

2 The decrease in liver size increases the rate at which the liver can inactivate many anesthetics

3 The decrease in plasma proteins causes less of the anesthetic agents to remain free or unbound

4 An increase in the function of kidney cells increases the excretion of waste products and anesthetics

8. The nurse preparing a client for surgery reviews the client's medication record. The client is to be NPO after midnight. Which of the following medications, if noted on the client's record, would the nurse question?

1 Cyclobenzaprine (Flexeril)

2 Fentanyl (Duragesic)

3 Allopurinol (Zyloprim)

4 Prednisone (Deltasone)

9. When applying the safety strap across the client's legs on the operating table, the nurse should avoid pressure on the popliteal nerve. Which of the following nursing actions would be most appropriate to avoid this pressure?

1 Apply the safety strap 2 inches above the knees

2 Apply the safety strap 2 inches below the knees

3 Apply the safety strap 6 inches above the knees

4 Apply the safety strap over the ankles

10. During a surgical procedure, the nurse is responsible for the maintenance of the health of the client by preventing the extremities from dangling over the sides of the table. If the extremities are allowed to dangle over the edge of the table, this action may cause:

1 An increase in pulse rate

2 Nerve and muscle damage

3 A drop in blood pressure

4 The extremities to get tired

11. On admission to the postanesthesia room, the nurse obtains the client's vital signs. The blood pressure is 100/60 mmHg, pulse is 90, and respiration rate is 20. Which of the following nursing actions should be performed first?

1 Cover the client with a warm blanket

2 Shake gently to arouse

3 Recheck the vital signs in 5 minutes

4 Call the surgeon immediately

12. On the arrival of the client to the surgical unit after surgery, the nurse should first:

1 Check the dressing to assess for bleeding

2 Check tubes or drains for patency

3 Assess the patency of the airway

4 Assess the vital signs to compare with preoperative measurements

13. Through the prevention of postoperative complications, the nurse promotes rapid convalescence. Which of the following would be most indicative of a potential postoperative complication that requires further observation?
    1 Urinary output of 20 mL/hour
    2 Temperature of 37.6°C (99.6°F)
    3 Serous drainage on the surgical dressing
    4 Blood pressure of 100/70 mmHg

14. Postoperatively, the client should be assessed frequently for secretions in the lungs. The nurse understands the importance of respiratory assessment since accumulated secretions can lead to:
    1 Pulmonary edema
    2 Pneumonia
    3 Fluid imbalance
    4 Carbon dioxide retention

15. A tube or drain may be inserted in a client's body near the wound after surgery if it is anticipated that fluid may collect. Which of the following nursing actions would be inappropriate in the care of a tube or drain?
    1 Maintain aseptic technique when emptying
    2 Observe for bright red, bloody drainage
    3 Check drain/tube for patency
    4 Secure by curling or folding and taping firmly to body

16. The goal of respiratory care for the postoperative client is to maintain pulmonary ventilation that is adequate to prevent hypoxemia and hypercapnia. The pulse oximeter is a noninvasive method for continuous monitoring of the client. Which of the following is an expected measurement determined by the pulse oximeter?
    1 Oxygen saturation, 95% to 100%
    2 Blood pressure, 120/80 to 130/80 mmHg
    3 Respiration rate, 18 to 22 breaths per minute
    4 Temperature, 36.7° to 37.2°C (98.0° to 99.0°F)

17. The nurse assesses the client's surgical incision for signs of infection. Which of the following would not be indicative of a potential infection?
    1 The presence of serous drainage
    2 Warm, red, tender skin around the incision
    3 Chills and fever
    4 The presence of purulent drainage

18. When assessing a client's surgical incision, the nurse notes an increase in the amount of drainage, a separation of the incision line, and the appearance of underlying tissue. Which of the following is the most appropriate initial action?
    1 Clean the wound, using aseptic technique, and apply a sterile, dry dressing
    2 Apply a sterile dressing soaked with normal saline to the wound
    3 Leave the incision open to the air to assist in drying the drainage
    4 Cover the wound with a Betadine-soaked dressing

19. The nurse monitors the postoperative client for signs of complications. Which of the following would indicate a sign of a potential complication?
    1 Faint bowel sounds heard in all four quadrants
    2 A negative Homan's sign
    3 A blood pressure of 120/70 with a pulse of 90
    4 Increasing restlessness

20. Discharge planning and teaching should begin at the time of the client's admission to the hospital. Which of the following instructions would be least appropriate to include in the postoperative discharge plan of care?
    1 Wound care
    2 Activity restrictions
    3 Personal hygiene
    4 Turn and deep breathe

ANSWERS

1. **2**

Rationale: Routine screening tests include a complete blood count, serum electrolyte analysis, coagulation studies, and serum creatinine tests. The complete blood count includes the hemoglobin analysis. All these values are within normal range except hemoglobin. If a client has a low hemoglobin level, the surgery will be postponed.

Test-Taking Strategy: Knowledge of the normal values for serum sodium, hemoglobin, platelets, and creatinine is required to answer this question. If you know the normal values for these tests, use the process of elimination to determine the correct option. Take time now to review these laboratory values, if you had difficulty answering this question!

Level of Cognitive Ability: Analysis
Phase of Nursing Process: Analysis
Client Needs: Physiological Integrity
Content Area: Fundamental Skills

Reference
Potter, P., & Perry, A. (1997). *Fundamentals of nursing: Concepts, process, and practice* (4th ed.). St. Louis: Mosby–Year Book. pp. 1389, 1390.

2. **1**

Rationale: Nail polish should be removed from the nails for the pulse oximeter to check oxygen saturation. Some increase in blood pressure and pulse is common because of anxiety. The client usually has a restriction of food and fluids for 8 hours prior to surgery instead of 24 hours. Oral hygiene is allowed, but the client should not swallow any water.

Test-Taking Strategy: All these interventions relate to nursing care that promotes safety during surgery. Utilize the principles associated with prioritization when answering this question. Remember the ABCs of Airway, Breathing, and Circulation. Monitoring the oxygen saturation level through the nails would assess airway, breathing, and circulation. Note the word "any" in option 2. Absolute terminology tends to make a statement false. Options 3 and 4 include incorrect information. Review general preoperative care now, if you had difficulty with this question!

Level of Cognitive Ability: Application
Phase of Nursing Process: Planning
Client Needs: Safe, Effective Care Environment
Content Area: Fundamental Skills

Reference

Leahy, J., & Kizilay, P. (1998). *Foundations of nursing practice: A nursing process approach.* Philadelphia: W. B. Saunders. p. 1183.

3. **3**

Rationale: Every effort must be made to obtain permission from a responsible family member to perform surgery if the client is unable to sign the consent form. A telephone consent must be witnessed by two persons who hear the family member's oral consent. The two witnesses then sign the consent with the name of the family member, noting that an oral consent was obtained. In emergencies, the client may be unable to sign and family members may not be available. In this type of a situation, the physician is legally permitted to perform surgery without consent. Consent is not informed if it is obtained from a client who is confused, unconscious, mentally incompetent, or under the influence of sedatives.

Test-Taking Strategy: Knowledge regarding the implications related to informed consent is required to answer this question. Note the key phrase "most appropriate" in the question. Eliminate options 1 and 4 first. From the remaining two options, select option 3 because it is legally acceptable to obtain a telephone permission from a family member if it is witnessed by two persons. Take time now to review the implications surrounding informed consent, if you had difficulty with this question. You are likely to see a question related to informed consent on NCLEX-RN!

Level of Cognitive Ability: Application
Phase of Nursing Process: Implementation
Client Needs: Safe, Effective Care Environment
Content Area: Fundamental Skills

Reference

Potter, P., & Perry, A. (1997). *Fundamentals of nursing: Concepts, process, and practice* (4th ed.). St. Louis: Mosby–Year Book. p. 1393.

4. **4**

Rationale: Explanations should begin with the information that the client knows. By providing the client with explanations of care and procedures, the nurse can assist the client in handling fears for a smooth preoperative experience. Clients who are calm and emotionally prepared for surgery withstand anesthesia better and experience fewer postoperative complications.

Test-Taking Strategy: All these interventions relate to the psychosocial aspects of preoperative preparation. Remember always to focus on the client's feelings and knowledge first, such as option 4. Additionally, option 4 is the only option that addresses assessment, the first step of the nursing process!

Level of Cognitive Ability: Application
Phase of Nursing Process: Implementation
Client Needs: Psychosocial Integrity
Content Area: Fundamental Skills

Reference

Black, J., & Matassarin-Jacobs, E. (1997). *Medical-surgical nursing: Clinical management for continuity of care* (5th ed.). Philadelphia: W. B. Saunders. pp. 458–459.

5. **4**

Rationale: For optimal lung expansion with an incentive spirometer, the client should assume the semi-Fowler's or high Fowler's position. The mouthpiece should be covered completely while the client inhales slowly with a constant flow through the unit. The breath should be held for 2 to 3 seconds before exhaling slowly.

Test-Taking Strategy: Knowledge of the procedure for using the incentive spirometer is required to answer the question. Options 1, 2, and 3 are correct steps in the procedure for the incentive spirometer. Option 4 is incorrect. For optimal lung expansion, the head should be elevated to decrease the pressure of the internal organs on the diaphragm and to increase the expansion of the diaphragm. If you had difficulty with this question, take time now to review the correct procedure related to the use of an incentive spirometer!

Level of Cognitive Ability: Analysis
Phase of Nursing Process: Evaluation
Client Needs: Health Promotion and Maintenance
Content Area: Fundamental Skills

Reference

Leahy, J., & Kizilay, P. (1998). *Foundations of nursing practice: A nursing process approach.* Philadelphia: W. B. Saunders. p. 868.

6. **4**

Rationale: Anticoagulants alter normal clotting factors and increase the risk of hemorrhage. Aspirin has properties that can alter the clotting mechanism and should be discontinued at least 48 hours before surgery.

Test-Taking Strategy: Knowledge regarding the medications that affect the surgical client is required to answer this question. Note the key phrase "most appropriate" in the question. Option 3 can be eliminated first because the surgery is 1 week away. Option 2 should be eliminated because it addresses adjusting dosages. Remember that aspirin has properties that can alter normal clotting factors. Knowledge regarding the risk for hemorrhage following surgery would assist in directing you to option 4. If you had difficulty with this question, take time now to review medications that affect the client preparing for surgery!

Level of Cognitive Ability: Analysis
Phase of Nursing Process: Implementation
Client Needs: Safe, Effective Care Environment
Content Area: Pharmacology

Reference

Potter, P., & Perry, A. (1997). *Fundamentals of nursing: Concepts, process, and practice* (4th ed.). St. Louis: Mosby–Year Book. p. 1384.

7. 1

Rationale: An older person needs less anesthetic medication to produce anesthesia, and it takes longer for the older person to eliminate anesthetic agents. One reason for the reduction of dosage is that the percentage of fatty tissue increases as people age. Anesthetic agents that have an affinity for fatty tissue concentrate in body fat and the brain. Another reason is that older clients may have low plasma proteins, particularly when malnourished. With decreased plasma proteins, more of the anesthetic agent remains free or unbound, which results in a more potent action. Reduction in liver size decreases the rate at which the liver can inactivate many anesthetic agents. The decreased functioning of kidney cells reduces excretion of waste products and anesthetic agents.

Test-Taking Strategy: Knowledge of the action of anesthetic agents and their effects on the body of an older person is required to answer this question. Read each option carefully. Through the process of elimination, you should select option 1 as the best explanation for a reduction of anesthetic agents for the older person. If you had difficulty with this question, take time now to review the effects of medications on the older person!

Level of Cognitive Ability: Analysis
Phase of Nursing Process: Analysis
Client Needs: Physiological Integrity
Content Area: Fundamental Skills

Reference
Smeltzer, S., & Bare, B. (1996). *Brunner and Suddarth's textbook of medical-surgical nursing* (8th ed.). Philadelphia: Lippincott-Raven. p. 377.

8. 4

Rationale: Prednisone (Deltasone) is a glucocorticoid. When stress is severe, glucocorticoids are essential to support life. Before and during surgery, dosages may be temporarily increased. Cyclobenzaprine (Flexeril) is a skeletal muscle relaxant. Fentanyl (Duragesic) is an opioid analgesic. Allopurinol (Zyloprim) is an antigout medication.

Test-Taking Strategy: Knowledge regarding medications that may have special implications for the surgical client is required to answer this question. Glucocorticoids are extremely important medications to be familiar with. You are likely to find a question related to this content on NCLEX-RN. Take time now to review glucocorticoids if you had difficulty with this question!

Level of Cognitive Ability: Analysis
Phase of Nursing Process: Analysis
Client Needs: Physiological Integrity
Content Area: Pharmacology

References
Potter, P., & Perry, A. (1997). *Fundamentals of nursing: Concepts, process, and practice* (4th ed.). St. Louis: Mosby–Year Book. p. 1384.
Hodgson, B., & Kizior, R. (1998). *Saunders nursing drug handbook 1998.* Philadelphia: W. B. Saunders. pp. 24, 269, 405.

9. 1

Rationale: The safety strap is applied to prevent the client from falling off the surgery table. The strap should be applied 2 inches above the knees to avoid pressure on the popliteal nerve.

Test-Taking Strategy: Knowledge regarding the anatomy related to the location of the popliteal nerve is helpful to answer this question. Use the process of elimination and identify the key phrase in the question. The phrase "most appropriate" indicates that one answer is correct. Through the process of elimination, determine that option 1 is the only correct statement. Options 2, 3, and 4 contain the incorrect position for the safety strap. Take time now to review the anatomical location of the popliteal nerve if you had difficulty with this question!

Level of Cognitive Ability: Application
Phase of Nursing Process: Implementation
Client Needs: Physiological Integrity
Content Area: Fundamental Skills

Reference
Leahy, J., & Kizilay, P. (1998). *Foundations of nursing practice: A nursing process approach.* Philadelphia: W. B. Saunders. p. 1199.

10. 2

Rationale: Whatever the client's position is on the operating table, the nurse is responsible for the safety of the client. The client's extremities should not be allowed to dangle over the sides of the table because this may impair circulation or cause nerve and muscle damage.

Test-Taking Strategy: Note the key word in the question that will assist in selecting the correct option. The word "cause" indicates an effect or one correct answer. Through the process of elimination, determine that option 2 is correct. The client is anesthetized, therefore the sense of position or tiredness is absent. The vital signs would not be affected significantly either, therefore options 1, 3, and 4 are not correct.

Level of Cognitive Ability: Analysis
Phase of Nursing Process: Evaluation
Client Needs: Physiological Integrity
Content Area: Fundamental Skills

References
Black, J., & Matassarin-Jacobs, E. (1997). *Medical-surgical nursing: Clinical management for continuity of care* (5th ed.). Philadelphia: W. B. Saunders. p. 477.
Polaski, A., & Tatro, S. (1996). *Luckmann's core principles and practices of medical-surgical nursing.* Philadelphia: W. B. Saunders. p. 102.

11. 3

Rationale: On admission to the postanesthesia unit, the nurse assesses airway patency, vital signs, and level of consciousness immediately. A drop in blood pressure slightly below a client's preoperative baseline reading is common after surgery. Warm blankets are applied to maintain the client's body temperature. Level of consciousness can be assessed by the evaluation of the client's response to light touch and verbal stimuli.

Test-Taking Strategy: The principles of prioritizing should be used to answer this question. The ABCs, Airway, Breathing, and Circulation, should be utilized also. The assessment of vital signs in option 3 takes priority over warming the client in option 1 and arousing the client in option 2. The vital signs are within normal limits following a surgical procedure, therefore the surgeon does not need to be notified immediately. Review postoperative assessment now if you had difficulty with this question!

Level of Cognitive Ability: Application
Phase of Nursing Process: Implementation
Client Needs: Physiological Integrity
Content Area: Fundamental Skills

Reference

Black, J., & Matassarin-Jacobs, E. (1997). *Medical-surgical nursing: Clinical management for continuity of care* (5th ed.). Philadelphia: W. B. Saunders. pp. 481–483.

12. **3**

Rationale: The nurse must assess the surgical client immediately on returning to the clinical unit. The patency of the airway and respiratory function are always evaluated first. The nurse then performs an assessment of the cardiovascular function, the condition of the surgical site, and function of the central nervous system. If the airway is not patent, immediate measures must be taken for the survival of the client.

Test-Taking Strategy: Use the principles of prioritization when answering this question. Remember your ABCs: Airway, Breathing, and Circulation. Airway patency is the first action to be taken, therefore option 3 is correct. Options 1, 2, and 4 are all nursing actions that should be performed after a patent airway has been established.

Level of Cognitive Ability: Application
Phase of Nursing Process: Assessment
Client Needs: Physiological Integrity
Content Area: Fundamental Skills

Reference

Smeltzer, S., & Bare, B. (1996). *Brunner and Suddarth's textbook of medical-surgical nursing* (8th ed.). Philadelphia: Lippincott Raven. pp. 394, 396.

13. **1**

Rationale: Urine output is maintained at a minimum of at least 30 mL/hour for an adult. An output of less than 30 mL for each of 2 consecutive hours should be reported to the physician. A temperature above 37.7°C (100°F) or below 36.1°C (97°F) and a falling systolic blood pressure under 90 mmHg are usually considered reportable at once. The client's preoperative or baseline blood pressure is used to make informed postoperative comparisons. Moderate or light serous drainage from the surgical site is considered normal.

Test-Taking Strategy: Knowledge of the normal ranges for temperature, blood pressure, urinary output, and wound drainage is necessary to determine the correct answer. Through the process of elimination, you can determine that the urinary output is the only observation that is not within the normal range. Option 1 is the correct response. Take time now to review normal postoperative assessment findings, if you had difficulty with this question!

Level of Cognitive Ability: Analysis
Phase of Nursing Process: Assessment
Client Needs: Physiological Integrity
Content Area: Fundamental Skills

Reference

Black, J., & Matassarin-Jacobs, E. (1997). *Medical-surgical nursing: Clinical management for continuity of care* (5th ed.). Philadelphia: W. B. Saunders. p. 484.

14. **2**

Rationale: The most common postoperative respiratory problems are atelectasis, pneumonia, and pulmonary emboli. Pneumonia is the inflammation of lung tissue that causes productive cough, dyspnea, and crackles. Pulmonary edema usually results from left-sided heart failure and can be caused by drugs, fluid overload, and smoke inhalation. Carbon dioxide retention results from inability to exhale carbon dioxide in conditions such as chronic obstructive pulmonary disease. Fluid imbalance can be a deficit or excess related to fluid loss or overload.

Test-Taking Strategy: Knowledge of postoperative respiratory complications is necessary to answer this question. Through a process of elimination, you will determine that the usual complication postoperatively is pneumonia, option 2. Options 1, 3, and 4 occur with other respiratory problems, such as chronic obstructive pulmonary disease. Take time now to review the common postoperative complications if you had difficulty with this question!

Level of Cognitive Ability: Application
Phase of Nursing Process: Assessment
Client Needs: Physiological Integrity
Content Area: Fundamental Skills

References

Black, J., & Matassarin-Jacobs, E. (1997). *Medical-surgical nursing: Clinical management for continuity of care* (5th ed.). Philadelphia: W. B. Saunders. p. 1169.
Polaski, A., & Tatro, S. (1996). *Luckmann's core principles and practices of medical-surgical nursing*. Philadelphia: W. B. Saunders. pp. 109–110.

15. **4**

Rationale: Aseptic technique must be used when emptying the drainage container or changing the dressing, to avoid contamination of the wound. Usually the drainage from the wound is pale, red, and watery. Active bleeding will be bright red in color. The tube/drain should be checked for patency to provide an exit for the fluid/blood to promote healing. Ensure that drainage flows freely and that there are no kinks in the tubes/drains. Curling/folding the tube/drain prevents the flow of the drainage.

Test-Taking Strategy: Knowledge of the care of tubes/drains is necessary to answer this question. Read the question carefully, noting the word "inappropriate." Through a process of elimination, you will determine that the nursing action in option 4 is inappropriate. Options 1, 2, and 3 are appropriate nursing actions in the care of tubes and drains. If you had difficulty with this question, take time now to review nursing care for the client with a surgical drain!

Level of Cognitive Ability: Application
Phase of Nursing Process: Implementation
Client Needs: Physiological Integrity
Content Area: Fundamental Skills

References

Polaski, A., & Tatro, S. (1996). *Luckmann's core principles and practices of medical-surgical nursing*. Philadelphia: W. B. Saunders. p. 105.
Potter, P., & Perry, A. (1997). *Fundamentals of nursing: Concepts, process, and practice* (4th ed.). St. Louis: Mosby–Year Book. pp. 1436–1437.

16. **1**

Rationale: Pulse oximetry is a noninvasive method of continuously monitoring the oxygen saturation of hemoglobin (SaO_2). The pulse oximeter does not measure arterial blood gases, but it is an effective tool to monitor the client for subtle or sudden changes in oxygen saturation. It does not measure temperature, blood pressure, or respiratory rate.

Test-Taking Strategy: Knowledge of the purpose of the pulse oximeter is necessary to answer this question. Through the process of elimination, you can determine that the correct answer is option 1. Options 2, 3, and 4 can be eliminated since these responses do not measure oxygen saturation. If you had difficulty with this question, take time now to review the purpose and expected results of pulse oximetry!

Level of Cognitive Ability: Analysis
Phase of Nursing Process: Evaluation
Client Needs: Physiological Integrity
Content Area: Fundamental Skills

Reference
Black, J., & Matassarin-Jacobs, E. (1997). *Medical-surgical nursing: Clinical management for continuity of care* (5th ed.). Philadelphia: W. B. Saunders. pp. 1051–1055.

17. **1**

Rationale: Wound infection is an invasion of deep or superficial wound tissues by pathogenic microorganisms. Signs and symptoms include warm, red, and tender skin around the incision. The client may have fever and chills. Purulent material may exit from drains or from separated wound edges. The infection may be caused by poor aseptic technique and a contaminated wound before surgical exploration. It appears 3 to 6 days after surgery.

Test-Taking Strategy: Knowledge regarding the signs and symptoms of wound infection is required to answer this question. Use the process of elimination in selecting the correct option. Read the question carefully, noting that the question is asking for the sign that does not indicate infection. Options 2, 3, and 4 indicate signs of infection. Serous drainage is sometimes normally noted at a surgical incision. Remember, however, that an increased flow of serosanguineous fluid from a surgical incision may be a sign of dehiscence.

Level of Cognitive Ability: Analysis
Phase of Nursing Process: Assessment
Client Needs: Physiological Integrity
Content Area: Fundamental Skills

Reference
Potter, P., & Perry, A. (1997). *Fundamentals of nursing: Concepts, process, and practice* (4th ed.). St. Louis: Mosby–Year Book. p. 1422.

18. **2**

Rationale: Wound dehiscence is the separation of wound edges at the suture line. Signs and symptoms include increased drainage and the appearance of underlying tissues. It usually occurs 6 to 8 days after surgery. The client should be instructed to remain quiet and to avoid coughing or straining. The client should be positioned to prevent further stress on the wound. Sterile dressings such as ABD pads soaked with sterile normal saline should be used to cover the wound. The physician needs to be notified.

Test-Taking Strategy: Knowledge regarding care to the wound when dehiscence occurs is required to answer this question. Use the process of elimination. Eliminate option 3 first as this action would only expose the open wound and underlying tissues to infection. Eliminate options 1 and 4 next. A dry dressing and a dressing soaked with Betadine will irritate the exposed body tissues. Take time now to review emergency care when dehiscence or evisceration occurs, if you had difficulty with this question!

Level of Cognitive Ability: Application
Phase of Nursing Process: Implementation
Client Needs: Physiological Integrity
Content Area: Fundamental Skills

References
Potter, P., & Perry, A. (1997). *Fundamentals of nursing: Concepts, process, and practice* (4th ed.). St. Louis: Mosby–Year Book. p. 1422.

19. **4**

Rationale: Increasing restlessness noted in a client is a sign that requires continuous and close monitoring, as it could indicate a potential complication, such as shock. Faint bowel sounds heard in all four quadrants is a normal occurrence. A negative Homan's sign is also normal. A positive Homan's sign, however, may indicate thrombophlebitis. A blood pressure of 120/70 with a pulse of 90 is a relatively normal sign.

Test-Taking Strategy: Use the process of elimination in answering the question. Eliminate options 1, 2, and 3, as these are normal, expected findings. If you had difficulty with this question, take time now to review the normal, expected postoperative findings and the signs and symptoms of postoperative complications!

Level of Cognitive Ability: Analysis
Phase of Nursing Process: Assessment
Client Needs: Physiological Integrity
Content Area: Fundamental Skills

References
Potter, P., & Perry, A. (1997). *Fundamentals of nursing: Concepts, process, and practice* (4th ed.). St. Louis: Mosby–Year Book. pp. 1421–1422.

20. **4**

Rationale: The type of planning and instruction required varies with each individual and type of surgery. Specific instructions that the client needs to receive prior to discharge should include wound care, activity restrictions, dietary instructions, postoperative medication instructions, personal hygiene, and follow-up appointments. Turning and deep breathing are taught in the preoperative period.

Test-Taking Strategy: Use the strategy of selecting the response that is different. Options 1, 2, and 3 refer to information that needs to be taught postoperatively. Option 4 refers to information that should be taught preoperatively. In this question, the correct answer is the response that is different. Take time now to review the client education points related to discharge teaching, both preoperatively and postoperatively, if you had difficulty with this question!

Level of Cognitive Ability: Application
Phase of Nursing Process: Planning
Client Needs: Health Promotion and Maintenance
Content Area: Fundamental Skills

Reference
Polaski, A., & Tatro, S. (1996). *Luckmann's core principles and practices of medical-surgical nursing.* Philadelphia: W. B. Saunders. p. 114.

BIBLIOGRAPHY

Black, J., & Matassarin-Jacobs, E. (1997). *Medical-surgical nursing: Clinical management for continuity of care* (5th ed.). Philadelphia: W. B. Saunders.

Hodgson, B., & Kizior, R. (1998). *Saunders nursing drug handbook 1998*. Philadelphia: W. B. Saunders.

Lammon, C., Foote, A., Leli, P., et al. (1995). *Clinical nursing skills*. Philadelphia: W. B. Saunders.

Leahy, J., and Kizilay, P. (1998). *Foundations of nursing practice: A nursing process approach*. Philadelphia: W. B. Saunders.

Lehne, R. (1998). *Pharmacology for nursing care* (3rd ed.). Philadelphia: W. B. Saunders.

Luckmann, J. (1997). *Saunders manual of nursing care*. Philadelphia: W. B. Saunders.

O'Toole, M. (ed.). (1997). *Miller-Keane encyclopedia & dictionary of medicine, nursing, & allied health* (6th ed.). Philadelphia: W. B. Saunders.

Phipps, W., Cassmeyer, V., Sands, J., & Lehman, M. (1995). *Medical-surgical nursing: Concepts and clinical practice* (5th ed.). St. Louis: Mosby–Year Book.

Polaski, A., & Tatro, S. (1996). *Luckmann's core principles and practices of medical-surgical nursing*. Philadelphia: W. B. Saunders.

Potter, P., & Perry, A. (1997). *Fundamentals of nursing: Concepts, process, and practice* (4th ed.). St. Louis: Mosby–Year Book.

Smeltzer, S., & Bare, B. (1996). *Brunner and Suddarth's textbook of medical-surgical nursing* (8th ed.). Philadelphia: Lippincott-Raven.

CHAPTER 19

Positioning Clients

··

PYRAMID TERMS

Fowler's Position—The client is supine and the head of the bed is elevated to 45°.

Low Fowler's Position (Semi-Fowler's)—The client is supine and the head of the bed is elevated to 30°.

High Fowler's Position—The client is supine and the head of bed is elevated to 90°.

Lateral (Side-Lying) Position—The client is lying on the side, and the head and shoulders are aligned with the hips and the spine and are parallel to the edge of the mattress. The head, neck, and upper arm are supported by a pillow. The lower shoulder is pulled forward slightly and, along with the elbow, flexed at 90°. The legs are flexed or extended. A pillow is placed to support the back.

Lithotomy Position—The client is lying on the back with the hips and knees flexed at right angles and the feet in stirrups.

Prone Position—The client is lying on the abdomen, with head turned to the side. The shoulders are abducted and rotated 90°, with arms flexed at the elbows and palms facing downward along the side of the head. The legs are extended and slightly separated. The feet should extend over the bottom of the mattress, with the ankles at a 90° angle, or be supported at a 90° angle with sandbags.

Supine (Dorsal Recumbent) Position—The client is lying on the back. The head and shoulders are usually slightly elevated with a small pillow. The arms and legs are extended, and the legs are slightly abducted.

Sims' Position (Semiprone)—The client is lying on the side with the body turned prone at 45°. The spine is parallel with the mattress, and shoulders and hips are aligned. The face is supported by a small pillow. The lower arm is behind the body, with the shoulder retracted and hyperextended, and the elbow is slightly flexed. The lower leg is extended, with the upper leg flexed at the hip and knee to a 45 to 90° angle. The ankles are supported at 90°.

PYRAMID TO SUCCESS

Nursing responsibility includes positioning clients in a safe and appropriate manner to provide safety and comfort. Knowledge regarding the client position required for a certain procedure or condition is expected (Fig. 19–1). It is the nurse's responsibility to reduce the likelihood and prevent the development of complications related to an existing condition, prescribed treatment, or medical and surgical procedure. It is imperative that the nurse review the physician's orders following treatments and procedures to assess for orders regarding positioning and mobility.

NURSING PROCESS

ASSESSMENT

Determine current client condition and prescribed treatments or procedures
Identify the general and specific protective measures for the prescribed procedure or treatment
Assess the status and need for informed consent
Monitor the client's condition

ANALYSIS:	Risk for injury Alteration in comfort Risk for infection	Altered protection Risk for impaired skin integrity Impaired physical mobility

PLANNING	IMPLEMENTATION	EVALUATION
Client will remain free from injury. Client will verbalize comfort control measures. Client will be free of infection. Protective function of the client's skin will be maintained. Client will demonstrate a gradual return to previous level of mobility.	Determine status and need for informed consent and notify the physician if informed consent has not been obtained for a specific procedure requiring one. Assess vital signs. Monitor client condition as determined by specific condition and restrictions. Maintain safety measures as necessary. Place side rails up and place client's call bell within reach. Turn and reposition client as indicated based on restrictions related to condition. Initiate measures to provide comfort. Notify physician if an elevation in temperature occurs. Monitor skin for redness and signs of breakdown. Provide adequate rest, hydration, and intake as determined by condition. Observe dressings and insertion sites for bleeding or signs of infection. Document status of client condition.	Client remains free of injury. Vital signs remain within normal limits. Interventions employed to provide comfort are effective. Insertion sites on the skin remain free of infection. Skin integrity remains intact. Prescribed level of activity is maintained.

CLIENT NEEDS

SAFE, EFFECTIVE CARE ENVIRONMENT

Informed consent
Appropriate positioning
Environmental and personal safety
Protective measures
Medical and surgical asepsis

HEALTH PROMOTION AND MAINTENANCE

Physical assessment
Instructions regarding the need for prescribed therapies

PSYCHOSOCIAL INTEGRITY

Providing comfort and support to the client
Assisting the client to utilize coping mechanisms
Keeping the family informed of client progress

PHYSIOLOGICAL INTEGRITY

Use of assistive devices
Immobility
Comfort measures for rest and sleep
Providing nutrition and oral intake
Providing personal hygiene as needed
Preventing complications

I. Providing Safety and Comfort

A. Integumentary System
  1. Autograft
     a. Following surgery, site is immobilized for 3 to 7 days
     b. Immobilization provides the time needed for the graft to adhere and attach to the wound bed
  2. Burns of the face and head
     a. Elevate the head of the bed to prevent or reduce facial and head edema
     b. This position will prevent edema surrounding the head and tracheal area
  3. Circumferential burns of the extremities
     a. Elevate the extremities above the level of the heart
     b. This position will prevent or reduce dependent edema
  4. Skin graft
     a. Elevate and immobilize the graft site
     b. Avoid weight-bearing
     c. This position will prevent movement and shearing of the graft and disruption of tissue
B. Reproductive System
  1. Mastectomy
     a. Position client with the head of the bed elevated at least 30° **(semi-Fowler's)**, with the affected arm elevated on a pillow to promote lymphatic fluid return after the removal of axillary lymph nodes
     b. Turn client only to back and unaffected side
  2. Perineal and vaginal procedures: place client in **lithotomy** position
C. Endocrine System
  1. Hypophysectomy
     a. Elevate the head of the bed
     b. This position will prevent increased intracranial pressure
  2. Thyroidectomy
     a. Place in **semi-Fowler's** position to reduce swelling and edema in the neck area
     b. Sandbags or pillows may be used to support the client's head or neck
D. Gastrointestinal System
  1. Hemorrhoidectomy
     a. Assist client to a **lateral (side-lying)** position

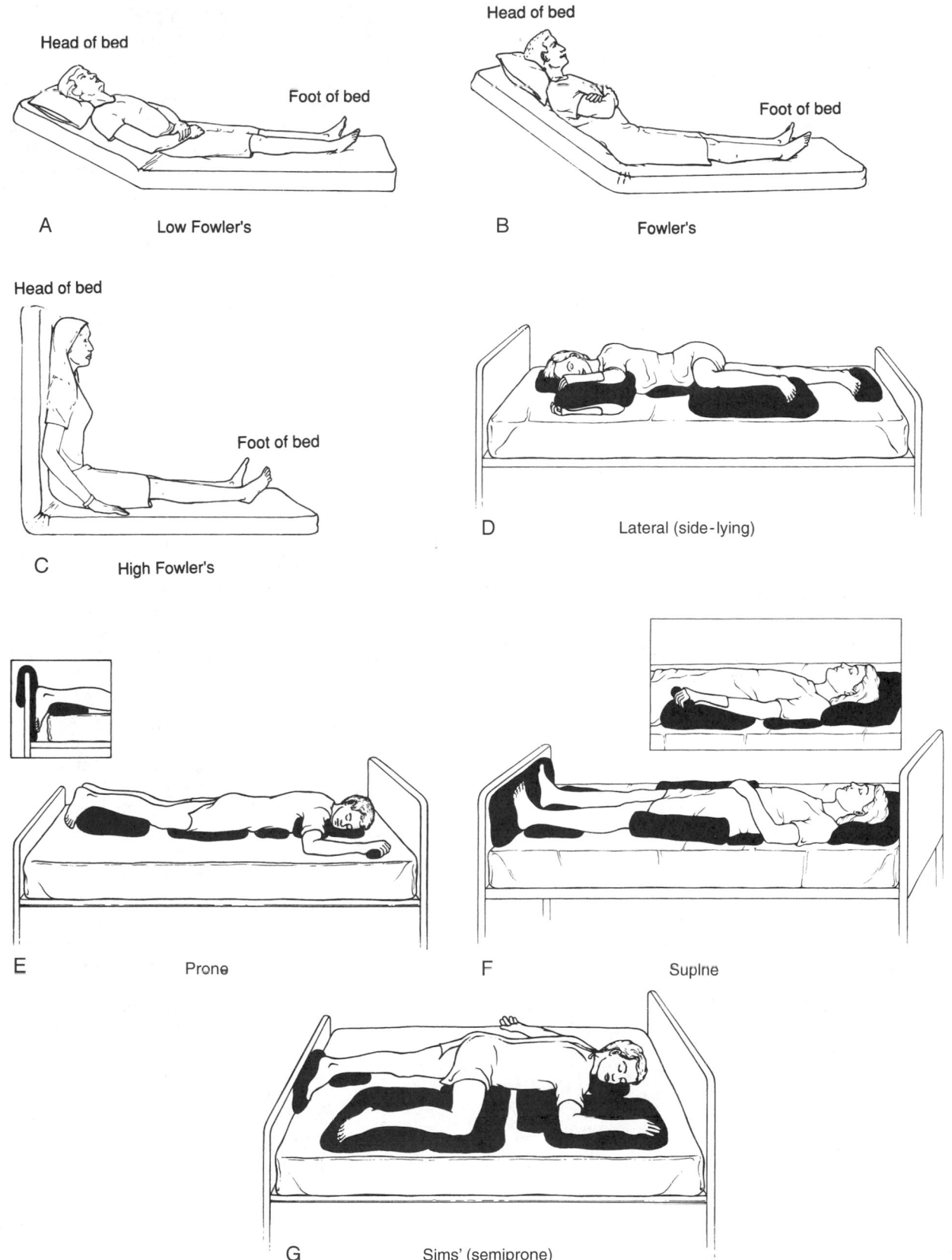

FIGURE 19–1. *A* to *C*, The three Fowler's positions. *D*, Lateral (side-lying) position. *E*, Prone position. *F*, Supine position. *G*, Sims' (semiprone) position. (Reprinted with permission from Lammon, C. B., Foote, A. W., Leli, P. G., et al. (1995). *Clinical nursing skills.* Philadelphia: W. B. Saunders.)

b. This position will prevent pain and bleeding

2. Liver biopsy
   a. During procedure
      (1) Position client **supine**, with the right side of the upper abdomen exposed
      (2) The client's right arm is raised and extended over the left shoulder behind the head
      (3) The liver is located on the right side, and this position provides maximal exposure of the right intercostal space
   b. After procedure
      (1) Assist the client into a right **(lateral) side-lying** position
      (2) Place a small pillow or folded towel under the puncture site for at least 3 hours

3. Intestinal tubes (Miller-Abbott, Cantor, and Harris tubes)
   a. After insertion, place the client on the right side to facilitate passage of the tube into the duodenum
   b. If prescribed, advance the tube 2 to 4 inches at a time, and change the client's position per physician order

4. Nasogastric tube
   a. Inserting
      (1) Position client in **high Fowler's** with the head tilted forward
      (2) This position will close the trachea and open the esophagus
   b. Irrigations and tube feedings
      (1) Elevate the head of the bed 30° **(semi-Fowler's)** to prevent aspiration
      (2) Maintain head elevation for 1 hour after an intermittent feeding
      (3) Head of the bed should remain elevated for continuous feedings

5. Rectal enemas/irrigations
   a. Place client in left **Sims'** position
   b. This position will allow the solution to flow by gravity in the natural direction of the colon

6. Sengstaken-Blakemore, Minnesota, and Linton-Nachlas tubes
   a. Maintain elevation of the head of the bed
   b. This position will enhance lung expansion and reduce portal blood flow, permitting effective compression of the varices

E. Respiratory System
   1. Chronic obstructive pulmonary disease
      a. In advanced disease, position in a sitting position, leaning forward, with the client's arms over several pillows or an overbed table
      b. This position will assist the client to breathe easier
   2. Laryngectomy (radical neck dissection)
      a. Place client in **semi-Fowler's** or **Fowler's** position

b. This position will maintain a patent airway and minimize edema

3. Pneumonectomy
   a. Avoid complete lateral positioning because the mediastinum is no longer held in place on both sides by lung tissue
   b. Extreme turning may cause mediastinal shift and compression of the remaining lung

4. Bronchoscopy postprocedure
   a. Place client in a **semi-Fowler's** position
   b. This position will prevent choking or aspiration because of an impaired ability to swallow

5. Postural drainage: the lung segment to be drained should be in the uppermost position

6. Thoracentesis
   a. During procedure: To facilitate removal of fluid from the chest wall, position client sitting on the edge of bed leaning over the bedside table, with the feet supported on a stool, or lying in bed on the unaffected side with the head of the bed elevated 45° **(Fowler's)**
   b. After procedure: Assist client to a position of comfort

7. Wedge resection of the lung
   a. Elevate the head of the bed 30 to 45° **(semi-Fowler's** to **Fowler's)**
   b. Avoid positioning client on the operative side

F. Cardiovascular System
   1. Abdominal aneurysm resection
      a. Following surgery, limit elevation of the head of the bed to 45° **(Fowler's)** to avoid flexion of the graft
      b. Turn client from side to side regularly
   2. Amputation of the lower extremity
      a. During the first 24 hours after amputation, elevate the foot of the bed (but not the stump itself) to reduce edema, then keep the bed flat to prevent hip flexion contractures
      b. Consult with the physician and then position client **prone** every 3 to 4 hours for a 20- to 30-minute period to stretch muscles and prevent flexion contractures of the hip
      c. In the **prone** position, keep the client's legs close together to prevent abduction
      d. Teach the client to contract the gluteal muscles of the buttocks
   3. Arterial vascular grafting of an extremity
      a. To promote graft patency following the procedure, bed rest is maintained for at least 24 hours, and the affected extremity is kept straight
      b. Limit movement and avoid flexion of the hip and knee
   4. Cardiac catheterization
      a. Keep the extremity of the catheter insertion site extended for 4 to 6 hours, keeping the leg straight to prevent arterial occlusion

b. Maintain strict bed rest for 6 to 12 hours; the client may turn from side to side

c. Do not elevate the head of the bed more than 15°

5. Congestive heart failure

a. Place the client in **high Fowler's** position

b. This position will maximize chest expansion and improve oxygenation

6. Peripheral arterial disease

a. Obtain the physician's order for positioning

b. Because swelling can prevent arterial blood flow, clients may be advised to elevate their feet at rest, but they should not raise their legs above the level of the heart because extreme elevation slows arterial blood flow

7. Pulmonary edema

a. Position client in **high Fowler's**

b. This position will maximize chest expansion and improve oxygenation

8. Thrombophlebitis

a. Place the client on bed rest, with an elevation of the affected extremity

b. No knee gatch or pillow is placed under the knees

9. Vein ligation and stripping

a. Elevate the feet above the level of the heart

b. Instruct the client to avoid leg-dangling and chair-sitting

G. Sensory System

1. Cataract surgery

a. Postoperatively, elevate the head of the bed 30 to 45° **(semi-Fowler's to Fowler's)**

b. Turn client to the back or the nonoperated side to prevent development of edema at the operative site

2. Retinal reattachment

a. If gas or oil has been used to promote retinal reattachment, position the client to allow the gas to float against the retina

b. Most often, the client is positioned on the abdomen, with the head turned to the operated eye so that the client lies with the unaffected eye down

c. This position is maintained for several days until the gas has been absorbed

H. Neurological System

1. Autonomic dysreflexia

a. Elevate the head of the bed to a **high Fowler's** position

b. This position will assist with adequate ventilation and assist in the prevention of hypertensive stroke

2. Cerebral aneurysm

a. Complete bed rest with the head of the bed elevated 30 to 45° **(semi-Fowler's to Fowler's)**

b. This position will prevent pressure on the aneurysm site

3. Cerebral angiography

a. Maintain bed rest for 6 to 24 hours

b. The extremity into which the contrast medium was injected is kept straight and immobilized for approximately the length of the bed rest

4. Cerebrovascular accident (CVA)

a. In clients with hemorrhagic strokes, the head of the bed is elevated to 30° to reduce intracranial pressure (ICP) and facilitate venous drainage

b. For clients with ischemic strokes, the head of the bed is kept flat

c. Maintain the head in a midline, neutral position to facilitate venous drainage from the head

d. Avoid extreme hip and neck flexion

e. Extreme hip flexion may increase intrathoracic pressure, whereas extreme neck flexion prohibits venous drainage from the brain

5. Craniotomy

a. The client should NOT be positioned on the operated site, especially if the bone flap has been removed, because the brain has no bony covering on the affected site

b. Elevate the head of bed 30 to 45° **(semi-Fowler's to Fowler's)** and maintain head in a midline, neutral position to facilitate venous drainage from the head

c. Avoid extreme hip and neck flexion

d. Extreme hip flexion may increase intrathoracic pressure, whereas extreme neck flexion prohibits venous drainage from the brain

6. Laminectomy

a. Logroll the client by turning the client all at once to keep the back as straight as possible

b. When the client is out of bed, the client's back is kept straight and the client is placed in a straight-backed chair, with the feet resting comfortably on the floor

7. Intracranial pressure

a. Elevate head of bed 30 to 45° **(semi-Fowler's to Fowler's)** and maintain head in a midline, neutral position to facilitate venous drainage from the head

b. Avoid extreme hip and neck flexion

c. Extreme hip flexion may increase intrathoracic pressure, whereas extreme neck flexion prohibits venous drainage from the brain

8. Lumbar puncture

a. During procedure: Assist the client to the **lateral (side-lying)** position, with the back bowed at the edge of the examining table, with the knees flexed up to the abdomen, and with the head bent so that the chin is resting on the chest

b. After procedure: Place client in **prone** position for 4 to 12 hours

9. Myelogram postprocedure

a. If a water-based iodine solution is used, a

sitting position with the head of the bed elevated 30 to 45° (**semi-Fowler's** to **Fowler's**) for an 8- to 16-hour period is maintained, to prevent the contrast medium from ascending into the brain; this may be followed by an 8-hour period of a flat-lying **supine** position

b. If an oil-based iodine solution is used, place the client flat in a **supine** position for at least 8 hours, to prevent leakage of cerebrospinal fluid (CSF)

10. Spinal cord injury
   a. Immobilize the client on a spinal backboard, with the head in a neutral position, to prevent incomplete injury from becoming complete
   b. Prevent head flexion, rotation, or extension
   c. Maintain traction and alignment of the head by placing the hand on either side of the head by the ears
   d. Logroll the client; no part of the body should be twisted or turned nor should the client be allowed to assume a sitting position
   e. The head is immobilized with a firm, padded cervical collar

I. Musculoskeletal System
   1. Hip surgery
      a. Avoid extreme positions and acute flexion of the operated hip, and keep the affected leg abducted
      b. Place a pillow between the client's legs to maintain abduction; instruct the client not to cross the legs
      c. Check physician's orders regarding elevation of the head of the bed
      d. Prevent external rotation of the operated leg by placing a trochanter roll beside the external aspect of the thigh and elevate the heels
      e. Turn the client only after checking the physician's orders, as many clients are permitted to turn to the nonoperated side and to the back only

PRACTICE QUESTIONS

1. The client returns to the nursing unit following an above-the-knee amputation of the right leg. The most appropriate client position is which of the following?
   1 Maintain stump flat on the bed
   2 Elevate the foot of the bed
   3 Reverse Trendelenburg
   4 Prone

2. The nurse is caring for a client with a severe burn. The client is scheduled for an autograft to be placed on the lower extremity. Which of the following would be included in the plan of care?
   1 Maintain surgical extremity in a flat position
   2 Keep surgical extremity covered with a blanket

3 Maintain client in a prone position
4 Elevate and immobilize surgical extremity for 3 to 7 days

3. The most appropriate client position/activity following cardiac catheterization is which of the following?
   1 Bed rest with head elevation at 45°
   2 Bed rest with head elevation no greater than 15°
   3 Bed rest with bathroom privileges only
   4 Bed rest in semi-Fowler's position

4. The nurse is providing instructions to a client and family regarding home care following right eye cataract removal. Which of the following statements, if made by the client, would indicate effective teaching?
   1 "I will not sleep on my right side."
   2 "I will not sleep on my left side."
   3 "I will take aspirin if I have any pain."
   4 "I will not wear my glasses until my physician says it is OK."

5. Following a liver biopsy, the nurse plans to place the client in which of the following positions?
   1 Supine
   2 Prone
   3 A left side-lying position with a small pillow or folded towel under the puncture site
   4 A right side-lying position with a small pillow or folded towel under the puncture site

6. The nurse is administering a cleansing enema to a client with a fecal impaction. Prior to administering the enema, the nurse positions the client in which of the following positions?
   1 On the left side of the body, with the head of the bed elevated 45°
   2 On the right side of the body, with the head of the bed elevated 45°
   3 Left Sims' position
   4 Right Sims' position

7. The client is being prepared for a thoracentesis. The nurse assists the client to which of the following positions for the procedure?
   1 Lying in bed on the affected side, with the head of the bed elevated 45°
   2 Lying in bed on the unaffected side, with the head of the bed elevated 45°
   3 Prone, with the head turned to the side and supported by a pillow
   4 Sims' position, with the head of the bed flat

8. The nurse assists the physician with the insertion of a Harris tube in a client with a bowel obstruction. Following insertion of the tube, the nurse assists the client to which of the following positions?
   1 Prone
   2 Supine

3 Right side
4 Left side

9. The client is diagnosed with thrombophlebitis. The appropriate client position/activity is which of the following?
   1 Bed rest, with the affected extremity in a dependent position
   2 Bed rest, with bathroom privileges
   3 Bed rest, keeping the affected extremity flat

4 Bed rest, with elevation of the affected extremity

10. The nurse is caring for a client following a supratentorial craniotomy. The nurse plans to position the client:
   1 Prone
   2 Supine
   3 Semi-Fowler's position
   4 Dorsal recumbent

ANSWERS

1. **2**

Rationale: Edema is controlled by elevating the foot of the bed for the first 24 hours after surgery. Following the first 24 hours, the stump is placed flat on the bed to reduce hip contracture. Edema is also controlled by stump-wrapping techniques.

Test-Taking Strategy: A key issue in this question is that the client has just returned from surgery. Knowledge regarding positioning of the stump during the first 24 hours and thereafter is required to assist you in answering this question. If you had difficulty with this question, take time now to review postoperative positioning following amputation!

Level of Cognitive Ability: Application
Phase of Nursing Process: Planning
Client Needs: Safe, Effective Care Environment
Content Area: Fundamental Skills

Reference
Black, J., & Matassarin-Jacobs, E. (1997). *Medical-surgical nursing: Clinical management for continuity of care* (5th ed.). Philadelphia: W. B. Saunders. p. 1420.

2. **4**

Rationale: Autografts placed over joints or on lower extremities are often elevated and immobilized for 3 to 7 days following surgery. This period of immobilization allows the autograft time to adhere and attach to the wound bed.

Test-Taking Strategy: Read each option carefully and use the process of elimination to select the correct option. Options 2 and 3 can be eliminated first because both a blanket and a prone position can easily disrupt a graft. Note that option 4, the correct answer, is specifically addressing a time frame and immobilization of the extremity.

Level of Cognitive Ability: Application
Phase of Nursing Process: Planning
Client Needs: Physiological Integrity
Content Area: Fundamental Skills

Reference
Black, J., & Matassarin-Jacobs, E. (1997). *Medical-surgical nursing: Clinical management for continuity of care* (5th ed.). Philadelphia: W. B. Saunders. p. 2255.

3. **2**

Rationale: Following cardiac catheterization, the extremity in which the catheter was inserted is kept straight for 4 to 6 hours. If the femoral artery was used, enforce strict bed rest for 6 to 12 hours. The client may turn from side to side. Do not elevate the head of the bed more than 15° to keep the affected leg straight at the groin and prevent arterial occlusion.

Test-Taking Strategy: Use the process of elimination in answering the question. Knowing that the head of the bed should not be elevated greater than 15° will assist you in eliminating options 1 and 4. In semi-Fowler's position, the head of the bed is elevated 30°. Bathroom privileges are not allowed in the immediate postcatheterization period. If you had difficulty with this question, take time now to review postcardiac catheterization care!

Level of Cognitive Ability: Application
Phase of Nursing Process: Implementation
Client Needs: Safe, Effective Care Environment
Content Area: Fundamental Skills

Reference
Black, J., & Matassarin-Jacobs, E. (1997). *Medical-surgical nursing: Clinical management for continuity of care* (5th ed.). Philadelphia: W. B. Saunders. p. 1232.

4. **1**

Rationale: Following cataract surgery, the client should not sleep on the side of the body that was operated on. Clients should be instructed not to take aspirin or medications containing aspirin. Acetaminophen (Tylenol) can be taken as needed for pain. Clients can wear their glasses.

Test-Taking Strategy: Knowledge regarding postoperative instructions to the client following cataract surgery is required to answer this question. If you can remember to instruct clients to stay off the operated side, this will assist you with answering questions related to cataract surgery.

Level of Cognitive Ability: Application
Phase of Nursing Process: Implementation
Client Needs: Health Promotion and Maintenance
Content Area: Fundamental Skills

Reference
Black, J., & Matassarin-Jacobs, E. (1997). *Medical-surgical nursing: Clinical management for continuity of care* (5th ed.). Philadelphia: W. B. Saunders. p. 961.

5. **4**

Rationale: Following a liver biopsy, the client is assisted to assume a right side-lying position with a small pillow or folded towel under the puncture site for at least 3 hours.

Test-Taking Strategy: Knowledge regarding the anatomy of the body will assist you in answering this question. Remember that the liver is on the right side of the body, and that the application of pressure on the right side will minimize the escape of blood or bile through the puncture site.

Level of Cognitive Ability: Application
Phase of Nursing Process: Planning

Client Needs: Safe, Effective Care Environment
Content Area: Fundamental Skills

Reference
Lammon, C., Foote, A., Leli, P., et al. (1995). *Clinical nursing skills.* Philadelphia: W. B. Saunders. p. 169.

6. **3**

Rationale: When administering an enema, the client is placed in a left Sims' position so that the enema solution can flow by gravity in the natural direction of the colon. The Sims' position may also be implemented for immobile clients when repositioning the client. In the Sims' position, the client is lying on the side, with the body turned approximately 45°. The spine is parallel with the mattress, and the shoulders and hips are aligned. The face is supported by a small pillow. The lower arm is behind the body, with the shoulder retracted and hyperextended, and the elbow is slightly flexed. The lower leg is extended, with the upper leg flexed at the hip and knee to a 45 to 90° angle.

Test-Taking Strategy: Knowledge regarding the anatomy of the bowel will assist you in answering the question. From this point, you would be able to eliminate options 2 and 4. Option 1 can be eliminated because the head of the bed should be flat during enema administration.

Level of Cognitive Ability: Application
Phase of Nursing Process: Implementation
Client Needs: Safe, Effective Care Environment
Content Area: Fundamental Skills

Reference
Lammon, C., Foote, A., Leli, P., et al. (1995). *Clinical nursing skills.* Philadelphia: W. B. Saunders. p. 446.

7. **2**

Rationale: To facilitate removal of fluid from the chest wall, position the client sitting on the edge of bed, leaning over the bedside table with the feet supported on a stool, or lying in bed on the unaffected side with the head of the bed elevated 45° **(Fowler's).**

Test-Taking Strategy: Knowledge regarding client positioning during a thoracentesis is required to answer the question. Option 1 can be eliminated because if the client was lying on the affected side it would be very difficult to perform the procedure. Option 4 can be eliminated because the Sims' position is primarily used for rectal enemas or irrigations. In the prone position, the client is lying on the abdomen, which is not an appropriate position for this procedure.

Level of Cognitive Ability: Application
Phase of Nursing Process: Implementation
Client Needs: Safe, Effective Care Environment
Content Area: Fundamental Skills

Reference
Lammon, C., Foote, A., Leli, P., et al. (1995). *Clinical nursing skills.* Philadelphia: W. B. Saunders. p. 175.

8. **3**

Rationale: The Harris tube is a single-lumen, mercury-weighted tube. The weight of the mercury carries the tube by gravity. When a Harris tube is inserted, it is sometimes difficult to get this intestinal tube to pass through the pylorus. To accomplish this, the client is instructed to lie on the right side.

Test-Taking Strategy: Knowledge of the anatomy of the gastrointestinal tract and the Harris tube will assist you in answering this question. Use the process of elimination based on this knowledge. If you had difficulty with this question, take time now to review nursing care related to the client with a Harris tube!

Level of Cognitive Ability: Application
Phase of Nursing Process: Implementation
Client Needs: Physiological Integrity
Content Area: Fundamental Skills

Reference
Black, J., & Matassarin-Jacobs, E. (1997). *Medical-surgical nursing: Clinical management for continuity of care* (5th ed.). Philadelphia: W. B. Saunders. p. 1750.

9. **4**

Rationale: Elevation of the affected leg facilitates blood flow by the force of gravity and also decreases venous pressure, which in turn relieves edema and pain. The foot of the bed is elevated and bed rest is indicated to prevent emboli and to prevent pressure fluctuations in the venous system that occur with walking.

Test-Taking Strategy: Knowledge regarding the pathophysiology related to the venous system will assist you in answering this question. Use the process of elimination along with your nursing knowledge. If you had difficulty with this question, take time now to review nursing care for clients with venous disorders!

Level of Cognitive Ability: Application
Phase of Nursing Process: Implementation
Client Needs: Physiological Integrity
Content Area: Fundamental Skills

Reference
Black, J., & Matassarin-Jacobs, E. (1997). *Medical-surgical nursing: Clinical management for continuity of care* (5th ed.). Philadelphia: W. B. Saunders. p. 1435.

10. **3**

Rationale: In supratentorial surgery (surgery above the brain's tentorium), the client's head is usually elevated 30° to promote venous outflow through the jugular veins. Do not lower the client's head or the head of the bed in the acute phase of care after supratentorial surgery. An exception to this is the client who has undergone evacuation of a chronic subdural hematoma, but a physician's order is required for a position other than head elevation.

Test-Taking Strategy: Knowledge regarding supratentorial surgery and craniotomy is required to answer this question. A helpful hint: supra, above the brain's tentorium, head up. If you had difficulty with this question, take time now to review positioning following craniotomy surgery!

Level of Cognitive Ability: Application
Phase of Nursing Process: Implementation
Client Needs: Safe, Effective Care Environment
Content Area: Fundamental Skills

Reference
Black, J., & Matassarin-Jacobs, E. (1997). *Medical-surgical nursing: Clinical management for continuity of care* (5th ed.). Philadelphia: W. B. Saunders. p. 853.

BIBLIOGRAPHY

Black, J., & Matassarin-Jacobs, E. (1997). *Medical-surgical nursing: Clinical management for continuity of care* (5th ed.). Philadelphia: W. B. Saunders.

Ignatavicius, D., Workman, M. L., & Mishler, M. (1995). *Medical-surgical nursing: A nursing process approach* (2nd ed.). Philadelphia: W. B. Saunders.

Lammon, C., Foote, A., Leli, P., et al. (1995). *Clinical nursing skills.* Philadelphia: W. B. Saunders.

Luckmann, J. (1997). *Saunders manual of nursing care.* Philadelphia: W. B. Saunders.

Potter, P., & Perry, A. (1997). *Fundamentals of nursing: Concepts, process, and practice* (4th ed.). St. Louis: Mosby–Year Book.

Wilson, B., Shannon, M., & Stang, C. (1997). *Nurses drug guide.* Stamford, CT: Appleton & Lange.

CHAPTER 20

Care of a Client with a Tube

PYRAMID TERMS

Chest Tube—Returns negative pressure to the intrapleural space; used to remove abnormal accumulations of air and fluids from the pleural space.

Gastrointestinal (GI) Intubation—Refers to the insertion of a tube into the stomach or intestine.

Endotracheal Tube—Used to maintain a patent airway and is indicated when the client needs mechanical ventilation.

Intestinal Tubes—Passed nasally and designed to enter the small intestine through the pyloric sphincter because of the weight of a small bag of mercury at the end of the tube; used to decompress the bowel or to remove intestinal contents.

Sengstaken-Blakemore Tube—Triple-lumen gastric tube with an inflatable esophageal balloon, an inflatable gastric balloon, and a gastric aspiration lumen; used as a treatment modality for the client with esophageal varices.

Tracheostomy—Artificial opening created into the trachea to establish an airway.

PYRAMID TO SUCCESS

The pyramid to success focuses on the common types of tubes utilized in the clinical setting. NCLEX-RN is likely to address content areas related to the appropriate care of certain tubes and the immediate interventions required if a complication arises. Focus on the specific assessment points related to the specific type of tube. Review procedures for insertion of a particular tube, verifying correct placement, and procedures for administering medications or feedings, if appropriate. Pyramid points also focus on interventions associated with complications or emergencies that may occur.

NURSING PROCESS

ASSESSMENT

Current client condition and prescribed procedures	Elimination patterns
Status of informed consent as appropriate	Mobility restrictions
Vital signs and respiratory status	Level of comfort
Ability to swallow	Ability to communicate verbally
Skin integrity	

ANALYSIS:	Potential for ineffective breathing pattern	Potential for altered elimination patterns
	Risk for aspiration	Potential for injury
	Risk for infection	Impaired physical mobility
	Potential for impaired swallowing	Alteration in comfort
	Potential for impaired skin integrity	Potential for impaired verbal communication

PLANNING

Client will maintain effective breathing patterns. Client will verbalize any difficulty related to swallowing. Client will be free of infection. Protective function of client's skin will be maintained. Elimination patterns will remain normal. Client will remain free from injury. Client will participate in range of motion exercises. Client will be able to communicate. Client will communicate pain control measures.

IMPLEMENTATION

Determine status of informed consent and notify physician if informed consent has not been obtained. Monitor client condition as determined by specific condition and restrictions. Assess vital signs. Monitor respiratory patterns. Monitor ability to swallow. Provide adequate rest, hydration, and intake as determined by condition. Identify the general and specific protective measures for the prescribed procedure or therapy. Notify physician if an elevation in temperature occurs. Observe dressings and insertion sites for bleeding or signs of infection. Monitor skin for redness and signs of breakdown. Monitor elimination patterns. Maintain safety measures as necessary. Place side rails up as required and place client's call bell within reach. Turn and reposition client as indicated based on restrictions related to condition. Initiate active and passive range of motion exercises. Initiate measures to provide comfort. Provide the client with methods to communicate. Document status of client condition.

EVALUATION

Respiratory status remains normal Vital signs remain within normal limits. Insertion sites on the skin remain free of infection. Skin integrity remains intact. Elimination patterns remain normal. Client remains free of injury. Prescribed level of activity is maintained. Interventions employed to provide comfort are effective. Communication methods are effective.

CLIENT NEEDS

SAFE, EFFECTIVE CARE ENVIRONMENT

Advance directives
Advocacy related to client's concerns
Informed consent for invasive procedure
Client rights
Consultations as appropriate
Asepsis in administering care
Standard (universal) precautions
Handling infectious materials

HEALTH PROMOTION AND MAINTENANCE

Disease prevention
Lifestyle changes
Client/family education regarding care at home

PSYCHOSOCIAL INTEGRITY

Unexpected body image changes
Situational role changes
Support systems
Home care services

PHYSIOLOGICAL INTEGRITY

Measures to assure basic care and comfort
Nutrition and hydration
Administering medications through a GI tube
Diagnostic tests to confirm accurate placement of tube
Laboratory values
Potential complications associated with the tube
Emergency interventions for complications

I. Nasogastric (NG) Tubes (Fig. 20–1)

A. Description
  1. Short tubes used to intubate the stomach
  2. Inserted from nose to stomach
B. Types of Tubes
  1. Levin
      a. Single-lumen nasogastric tube
      b. Used to remove gastric contents via intermittent suction, or to provide tube feedings
  2. Salem sump
      a. Double-lumen nasogastric tube with an air vent
      b. Used for decompression with continuous suction
      c. Air vent is not to be clamped and is to be kept above the level of the stomach
      d. If leakage occurs through the air vent, instill 30 mL of air into the air vent and irrigate the main lumen with normal saline (NS)
C. Intubation Procedures
  1. Place client in high Fowler's position
  2. Measure from tip of nose to earlobe to xiphoid process to determine the length of insertion and mark with tape
  3. Lubricate tube about 3 inches with a water-soluble jelly only, to prevent the development of pneumonia if the tube accidentally slips into the bronchus
  4. Instruct client to bend head forward to close the epiglottis and open the esophagus
  5. Insert into nostril, advance backward and through the nasopharynx
  6. Have client take a sip of water and advance tube as client swallows
  7. Do not force tube
  8. If the client experiences any respiratory distress (coughing or choking) during insertion, pull back on the tube and wait until the distress subsides
  9. Advance until the taped mark is reached; tape in place when correct placement is confirmed
  10. If feedings are prescribed, x-ray confirmation should be done prior to initiating feedings

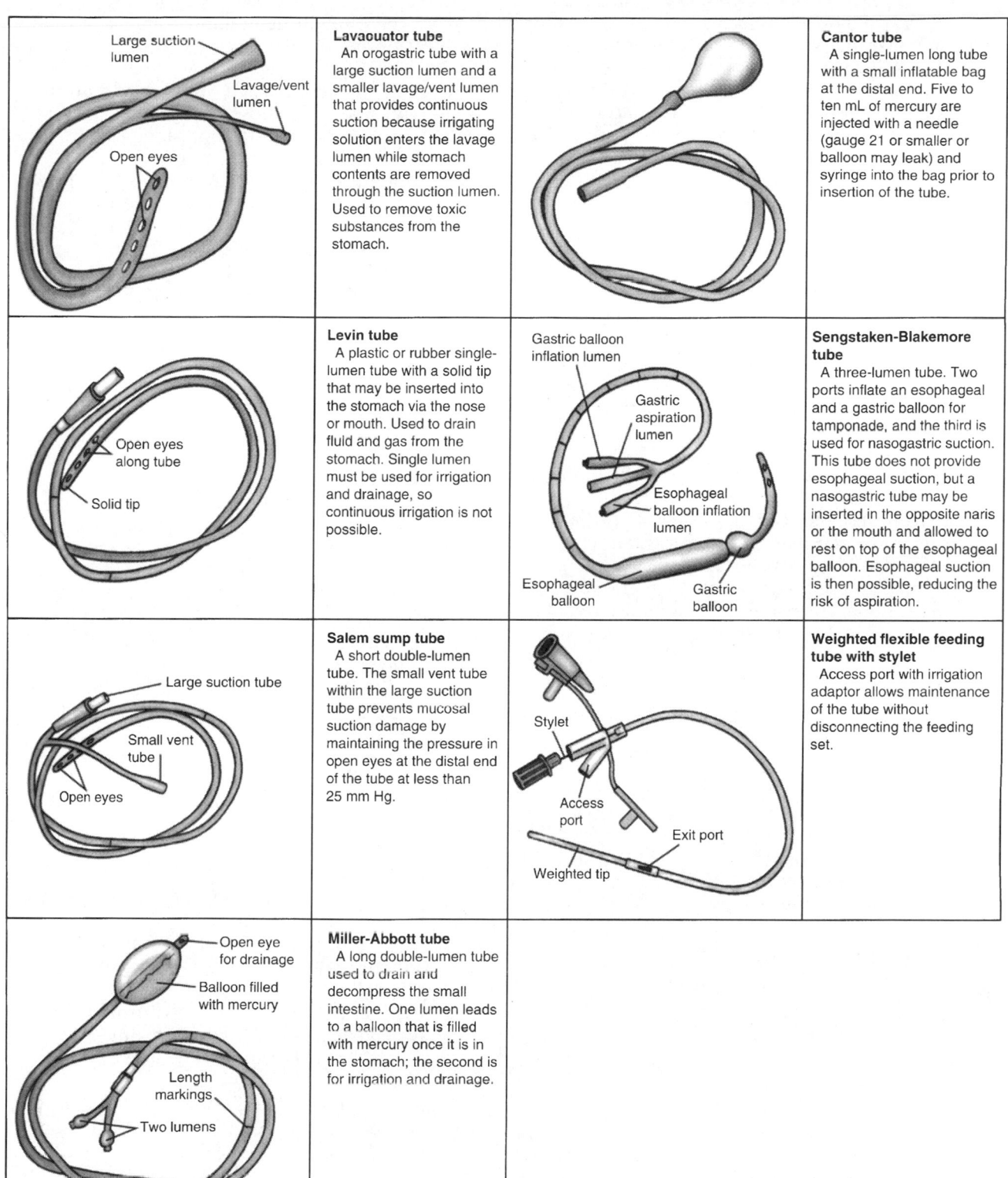

Lavaouator tube
An orogastric tube with a large suction lumen and a smaller lavage/vent lumen that provides continuous suction because irrigating solution enters the lavage lumen while stomach contents are removed through the suction lumen. Used to remove toxic substances from the stomach.

Cantor tube
A single-lumen long tube with a small inflatable bag at the distal end. Five to ten mL of mercury are injected with a needle (gauge 21 or smaller or balloon may leak) and syringe into the bag prior to insertion of the tube.

Levin tube
A plastic or rubber single-lumen tube with a solid tip that may be inserted into the stomach via the nose or mouth. Used to drain fluid and gas from the stomach. Single lumen must be used for irrigation and drainage, so continuous irrigation is not possible.

Sengstaken-Blakemore tube
A three-lumen tube. Two ports inflate an esophageal and a gastric balloon for tamponade, and the third is used for nasogastric suction. This tube does not provide esophageal suction, but a nasogastric tube may be inserted in the opposite naris or the mouth and allowed to rest on top of the esophageal balloon. Esophageal suction is then possible, reducing the risk of aspiration.

Salem sump tube
A short double-lumen tube. The small vent tube within the large suction tube prevents mucosal suction damage by maintaining the pressure in open eyes at the distal end of the tube at less than 25 mm Hg.

Weighted flexible feeding tube with stylet
Access port with irrigation adaptor allows maintenance of the tube without disconnecting the feeding set.

Miller-Abbott tube
A long double-lumen tube used to drain and decompress the small intestine. One lumen leads to a balloon that is filled with mercury once it is in the stomach; the second is for irrigation and drainage.

FIGURE 20–1. Comparison of design and function of selected gastrointestinal tubes. (From Monahan, F. D., & Neighbors, M. (1998). *Medical-surgical nursing: Foundation for clinical practice* (2nd ed.). Philadelphia: W. B. Saunders, p. 977.)

11. When GI tubes are attached to suction, suction may be continuous or intermittent, with a pressure not exceeding 25 mmHg as prescribed by the physician

D. Assessing Placement
  1. Note that the most reliable method to determine placement is by x-ray, which should be performed after initial placement
  2. Assess tube placement every 4 hours and before administering feedings or medications
  3. Assess tube placement by aspirating gastric contents and measuring the pH, which should be 4 or less (pH values greater than 6 indicate intestinal placement)
  4. Inserting 5 to 10 mL of air into the NG tube and listening for the rush of air over the stomach with a stethoscope is an alternative method for assessing placement but is not as reliable as an x-ray or checking gastric pH

E. Assessing Residual
  1. Check residual volumes every 4 hours, before each feeding, or before giving medications
  2. Aspirate all stomach contents (residual) and measure amount
  3. Reinstill residual feeding to prevent excessive fluid and electrolyte losses unless the residual volume appears abnormal
  4. Usually if the residual is less than 100 to 150 mL, feeding, if prescribed, is administered; if greater than 150 mL, hold the feeding

F. Irrigating
  1. Check patency of the tube every 4 hours
  2. Assess placement before irrigating
  3. Gently instill 30 to 50 mL of water or normal saline (NS) (depending on agency policy) with an irrigation syringe
  4. Pull back on the syringe plunger to withdraw the fluid to check patency; repeat if the tube remains sluggish

G. Removal of an NG Tube: Instruct the client to exhale and remove the tube with one very smooth continuous pull

II. GI Tube Feedings

A. Tubes
  1. Nasogastric: Nose to stomach
  2. Nasoduodenal/nasojejunal: Nose to duodenum or jejunum
  3. Gastrostomy: Stomach
  4. Jejunostomy: Jejunum

B. Types of administration
  1. Bolus
    a. Resembles normal meal feeding patterns
    b. Approximately 300 to 400 mL of formula is administered over a 30- to 60-minute period every 3 to 6 hours
  2. Continuous
    a. Administered continuously for 24 hours
    b. An infusion pump regulates the flow
  3. Cyclical

    a. Administered either in the daytime or nighttime for 8 to 16 hours
    b. An infusion pump regulates the flow
    c. Feedings at night allow for more freedom during the day

C. Administering Feedings
  1. Position client in high Fowler's and on the right side if comatose
  2. Warm the feeding to room temperature to prevent diarrhea and cramps
  3. Aspirate all stomach contents (residual), measure the amount, and return the contents to the stomach to prevent electrolyte imbalances
  4. Usually if the residual is less than 100 to 150 mL, feeding is administered; if greater than 150 mL, hold the feeding
  5. Assess tube placement by aspirating gastric contents and measuring the pH (should be 4 or less)
  6. Assess bowel sounds, hold feeding, and notify physician if bowel sounds are absent
  7. Use a feeding pump for continuous or cyclic feedings
  8. Flush tubing with water following feeding to maintain fluid balance and patency of tube
  9. For bolus feeding, leave client in a high Fowler's position for 30 minutes after feeding
  10. For a continuous feeding, keep client in a 30° Fowler's position at all times

D. Precautions
  1. Change feeding container and tubing every 24 hours
  2. Do not hang more solution than will be required for a 4-hour period to prevent bacterial growth
  3. Check the expiration date on the formula prior to administering
  4. Shake the formula well prior to inserting it into the container
  5. Always assess placement of the tube prior to feeding
  6. Always assess bowel sounds, and do not administer any feedings if bowel sounds are absent
  7. If an obstruction occurs, try flushing with water, saline, cranberry juice, gingerale, or cola, if not contraindicated, after checking placement
  8. Add a drop of blue food coloring to the feeding, particularly with clients who have endotracheal or tracheal tubes
  9. Suspect tracheoesophageal fistula when blue gastric contents appear in tracheal excretion; if this occurs, notify physician immediately
  10. Administer feeding at the prescribed rate, or via gravity flow (intermittent, bolus feedings) with a 60-mL syringe with the plunger removed
  11. Gently flush with 30 to 50 mL of water or

NS (depending on agency policy) with the irrigation syringe after the feeding

III. Medications Via NG or Gastrostomy Tube

A. Crush medications or use elixir forms of medications
B. Assure that the medication ordered can be crushed or that the capsule can be opened
C. Dissolve in 5 to 10 mL of water
D. Check placement and residual prior to instilling medications
E. Draw up the medication into a catheter tip syringe, clear excess air, and insert medication into the tube
F. Flush with 30 mL of water (depending on agency policy)
G. Clamp the tube for 30 to 60 minutes (depending on medication and agency policy)

IV. Intestinal Tubes (see Fig. 20–1)

A. Description
   1. Passed nasally into the small intestine
   2. Used to decompress the bowel or to remove intestinal contents
   3. Designed to enter the small intestine through the pyloric sphincter because of the weight of a small bag of mercury at the end
B. Types of tubes
   1. Cantor
      a. Single-lumen tube with a reservoir for 5 to 10 mL of mercury located at its tip, below the level of the drainage holes
      b. Mercury is inserted before the tube is passed through the nose, making the procedure uncomfortable
   2. Miller-Abbott tube
      a. Double-lumen tube
      b. One lumen is for the instillation of mercury once the tube is in the stomach, and the other for irrigation or drainage
C. Implementation
   1. Assess physician's orders and agency policy for advancement and removal of tube
   2. Position client on right side to allow the mercury weights within the tube to facilitate passage through the pylorus of the stomach and into the small intestine
   3. Do not secure the tube to the face with tape until it has reached final placement in the intestines
   4. Allow the tube to advance over several hours
   5. X-ray is performed to verify the desired placement
   6. Monitor drainage from the tube
   7. If the tube becomes blocked, notify the physician; a small amount of air injected into the lumen may be prescribed to clear the tube
   8. Assess the abdomen and measure abdominal girth
   9. To remove, to avoid pulling on the intestines, remove the **intestinal tube** about 6 inches every 10 minutes as prescribed, until it reaches the stomach; then, withdraw as you would an NG tube
   10. Dispose of the mercury in the appropriate manner as per agency policy

V. Esophageal and Gastric Tubes (see Fig. 20–1)

A. Description
   1. Used to apply pressure against esophageal veins to control bleeding
   2. Not used if the client has ulceration or necrosis of the esophagus or had previous esophageal surgery
B. **Sengstaken-Blakemore Tube**
   1. Triple-lumen gastric tube with an inflatable esophageal balloon, an inflatable gastric balloon, and a gastric aspiration lumen
   2. The gastric balloon applies pressure at the cardioesophageal junction to decrease blood flow to esophageal varices and directly compresses gastric varices; traction is applied to maintain the gastric balloon in place
   3. The esophageal balloon directly compresses esophageal varices
   4. If bleeding is not stopped with inflation of the gastric balloon, the esophageal balloon is inflated to 25 to 45 mmHg
   5. An x-ray of the upper abdomen and chest confirms placement
   6. Gastric contents are aspirated by gastric lavage or intermittent suction via the gastric aspiration port
   7. With the **Sengstaken-Blakemore tube**, a nasogastric tube is also inserted in the opposite nares to collect secretions that accumulate above the esophageal balloon
C. Minnesota tube
   1. Four-lumen gastric tube
   2. A modified **Sengstaken-Blakemore tube** with an additional lumen for aspirating esophagopharyngeal secretions
D. Implementation
   1. Check patency and integrity of all balloons prior to insertion
   2. Label each lumen
   3. Place the client upright or in Fowler's position for insertion
   4. Prepare for x-ray immediately after insertion to verify placement
   5. Maintain head elevation once tube is in place
   6. Double-clamp the balloon ports to prevent air leaks
   7. Keep scissors at the bedside at all times
   8. Monitor for respiratory distress and if it occurs, cut tubes to deflate the balloons
   9. Release esophageal pressure as prescribed and per agency policy to prevent ulceration or necrosis of the esophagus

10. Monitor for increased bloody drainage, which may indicate persistent bleeding
11. Monitor for signs of esophageal rupture, which include a drop in blood pressure, increased heart rate, back and upper abdominal pain
12. Esophageal rupture is an emergency and must be reported to the physician immediately

VI. Lavage Tubes

A. Description: Used to remove toxic substances from the stomach
B. Types of Tubes
   1. Lavacuator
      a. An orogastric tube with a large suction lumen and a smaller lavage/vent lumen that provides continuous suction
      b. Irrigation solution enters the lavage lumen while stomach contents are removed through the suction lumen
   2. Ewald's: Reusable single-lumen large tube used for rapid one-time irrigation and evacuation

VII. Urinary and Renal Tubes

A. Routine Urinary Catheter Care
   1. Use gloves and wash the perineal area with warm soapy water
   2. With the nondominant hand, pull back the labia or foreskin to expose the meatus (return foreskin to its normal position)
   3. Cleanse along the catheter with soap and water
   4. Anchor catheter to the thigh
   5. Maintain catheter bag below the level of the bladder
B. Ureteral and Nephrostomy Tubes
   1. Never clamp
   2. Maintain patency
   3. Monitor output closely
   4. Urine output of less than 30 mL per hour or lack of output for more than 15 minutes should be reported to the physician immediately
   5. Irrigate only if prescribed by a physician, using strict aseptic technique
   6. To irrigate, a maximum of 5 mL of sterile NS is instilled with very gentle force
   7. If patency cannot be established with the prescribed irrigation, notify the physician immediately

VIII. Respiratory System Tubes

A. **Endotracheal Tubes**
   1. Description
      a. Used to maintain a patent airway
      b. Indicated when the client needs mechanical ventilation

   2. Orotracheal
      a. Allows use of a larger-diameter tube and reduces the work of breathing
      b. Indicated when the client has a nasal obstruction or a predisposition to epistaxis
      c. Uncomfortable and can be manipulated by the tongue, causing airway obstruction
   3. Nasotracheal
      a. Smaller-sized tube increases resistance and increases client's work of breathing
      b. Discouraged in clients with bleeding disorders
      c. More comfortable for the client, and client is unable to manipulate with tongue
   4. Implementation
      a. Placement confirmed by chest x-ray (correct placement is 1 to 2 cm above the carina)
      b. Placement assessed by auscultating both sides of the chest while manually ventilating with a resuscitation bag
      c. Secure the tube immediately after intubation with adhesive tape
      d. Monitor position of the tube at lip or nose
      e. Monitor skin and mucous membranes
      f. Suction only when needed
      g. Keep a resuscitation (Ambu) bag at the bedside at all times
      h. Maintain cuff inflation, which creates a seal and allows complete mechanical control of respiration
      i. Monitor cuff pressures at least every 8 hours, which should not exceed 20 mmHg
   5. Minimal leak technique
      a. Inflate cuff until a seal is established
      b. No harsh sound should be heard through a stethoscope placed over the trachea when the client breathes in, but a slight leak on peak inspiration is present
      c. Client cannot make sounds, and no air is felt coming out of client's mouth
   6. Minimal occluding volume
      a. Provides an adequate seal in the trachea at the lowest possible cuff pressure
      b. Same procedure as minimal leak technique, without an air leak
B. **Tracheostomy**
   1. Description: Artificial opening created into the trachea to establish an airway
   2. Cuffed tube: Has an outer and inner cannula, obturator, and high-volume, low-pressure cuff
   3. Cuffless tube
      a. Has an outer cannula, an open and a plugged inner cannula, and an obturator
      b. Used for long-term, for evaluating client's ability to breathe through the upper airway during the decannulation process, and for the client no longer at risk for aspiration
   4. Laryngectomy tube
      a. Has an outer and inner cannula and an obturator

b. Used for the client with a permanent stoma

5. Fenestrated tube
   a. Has an opening along the posterior wall of the outer cannula
   b. When the tube is capped, the client can breathe through the upper airway and speak
   c. Cannot be used when the cuff is inflated and the cuff is always deflated before capping the tube with the decannulation cannula

6. Foam-cuffed tube
   a. Cuff is larger than the standard cuffed tube
   b. Is filled with foam, which may apply less pressure to the tracheal mucosa

7. Jackson's metal tube
   a. Has an outer and inner cannula and can be reused after sterilization
   b. Does not have a cuff and is most often used following a permanent **tracheostomy** or laryngectomy

8. Single-cannula tube
   a. Has an outer but no inner cannula
   b. Used for clients with a thick neck or on the client when a standard tube would not enter the trachea

9. Implementation
   a. Assess respirations and for bilateral breath sounds
   b. Monitor arterial blood gases (ABGs) and pulse oximetry
   c. Encourage coughing and deep breathing
   d. Maintain a semi to high Fowler's position
   e. Monitor for bleeding, difficulty in breathing, absence of breath sounds, and crepitus, which are indications of hemorrhage, pneumothorax, and subcutaneous emphysema
   f. Provide respiratory treatments as prescribed
   g. Suction PRN; hyperoxygenate the client before suctioning
   h. If the client is allowed to eat, sit client up for meals and for 30 minutes after meals and assure that the cuff is inflated for meals if the tube is not capped
   i. Monitor cuff pressures as prescribed
   j. Assess the stoma and secretions for blood or purulent drainage
   k. Follow physician orders and agency policy for cleaning the **tracheostomy** site and inner cannula; usually half-strength hydrogen peroxide is used
   l. Administer humidified oxygen as prescribed, because the normal humidification process is bypassed in a client with a **tracheostomy**
   m. Obtain assistance in changing tracheostomy ties; cut and remove the old ties holding the tracheostomy in place
   n. Keep a resuscitation (Ambu) bag, obturator, clamps, and a tracheotomy set at the bedside

IX. Chest Tube Drainage System

A. Description
   1. Returns negative pressure to the intrapleural space
   2. Used to remove abnormal accumulations of air and fluids from the pleural space

B. Collection chamber
   1. Where the **chest tube** from the client connects to the system
   2. Drainage from the tube drains into and collects in a series of calibrated columns in this chamber

C. Water seal chamber
   1. Establishes 2 cm of water pressure
   2. If positive pressure is greater than 2 cm, air or fluid is expelled into the drainage system
   3. Allows for air to move from the pleural space into the drainage system but not back into the chest
   4. Water oscillates (moves up as the client inhales and moves down as the client exhales)
   5. Bubbling indicates an air leak in the chest tube system

D. Suction control chamber
   1. Provides the suction, which can be controlled to provide negative pressure to the chest
   2. This chamber is filled with various levels of water to achieve the desired level of suction; without this control lung tissue could be sucked into the **chest tube**
   3. Gentle bubbling in this chamber indicates that there is suction, and it does not indicate that air is escaping from the pleural space

E. Implementation
   1. An occlusive sterile dressing is maintained at the insertion site
   2. A chest radiograph assesses the position of the tube and determines whether the lung has re-expanded
   3. Assess respiratory status and auscultate lung sounds
   4. Monitor for signs of extended pneumothorax or hemothorax
   5. Keep the drainage system below the level of the chest and free of kinks, dependent loops, or other obstructions
   6. Assure that all connections are secure
   7. Monitor drainage, as it should not exceed 200 mL per hour for 2 consecutive hours
   8. Monitor for fluctuation of the fluid level in the water seal chamber
   9. Fluctuation in the water seal chamber stops if the tube is obstructed, if a dependent loop exists, if suction is not working properly, and if the lung has re-expanded
   10. If the client has a known pneumothorax, intermittent bubbling in the water seal chamber is expected as air is drained from

the chest, but constant bubbling indicates an air leak in the system
11. Encourage coughing and deep breathing
12. Change client position frequently to promote drainage and ventilation
13. Do not milk a **chest tube** unless specifically directed by a physician and if the agency policy allows
14. Keep a clamp and a sterile occlusive dressing at the bedside at all times
15. Mark the **chest tube** drainage in the collection chamber at 1- to 4-hour intervals, using a piece of tape
16. Notify the physician if there is constant bubbling in the water seal chamber or if drainage becomes bright red or increases suddenly
17. If the drainage system is broken or interrupted, clamp the tube or place the end of the tube in a bottle of sterile saline held below the level of the chest and immediately replace the system (determine agency policy for clamping **chest tubes**)
18. If the **chest tube** is accidentally removed, immediately cover the opening in the chest with an occlusive petrolatum gauze dressing
19. When the **chest tube** is removed, the client is asked to perform the Valsalva maneuver; an airtight dressing is taped in place after removal of the **chest tube**

PRACTICE QUESTIONS

1. The nurse is preparing to insert a NG tube. Which of the following supplies would not be used for this procedure?
   1 Half-inch tape
   2 Oil-soluble lubricant
   3 A straw
   4 50-mL catheter tip syringe

2. The registered nurse is observing a new orientee who is inserting an NG tube on an adult client. The new orientee is determining the length of tube insertion. Which of the following observations indicates accurate measurement of the length of the tube to be inserted?
   1 The new orientee places the tube at the tip of the nose and measures by extending the tube to the earlobe and then down to the xiphoid process
   2 The new orientee places the tube at the tip of the nose and measures by extending the tube to the earlobe and then down to the top of the sternum
   3 The new orientee measures the tube and marks it at 20 inches
   4 The new orientee measures the tube and marks it at 32 inches

3. The nurse is inserting an NG tube on an adult client. During the procedure the client begins to cough and have difficulty breathing. Which of the following is the most appropriate nursing action?
   1 Remove the tube and reinsert it when the respiratory distress subsides
   2 Pull back on the tube and wait until the respiratory distress subsides
   3 Quickly insert the tube
   4 Notify the physician immediately

4. The nurse is assessing for correct placement of an NG tube. The nurse aspirates the stomach contents and checks the contents for pH. Which of the following pH values would assure correct placement of the tube?
   1 pH of 7.5
   2 pH of 7.35
   3 pH of 7.0
   4 pH of 4.0

5. The nurse is preparing to remove an NG tube from the client. The nurse would instruct the client to do which of the following?
   1 To perform a Valsalva maneuver
   2 To hold the breath
   3 To exhale
   4 To inhale

6. The nurse is preparing to administer medication through an NG tube that is connected to suction. Which of the following indicates the accurate procedure related to the medication administration?
   1 Aspirate the NG tube following medication administration to maintain patency
   2 Position the client supine to assist in medication absorption
   3 Clamp the NG tube for 30 minutes following administration of the medication
   4 Change the suction setting to low intermittent suction for 30 minutes after medication administration

7. The nurse assists the physician with the insertion of a Miller-Abbott tube. Following insertion of the tube, the nurse would assist the client to which of the following positions?
   1 On the right side
   2 On the left side
   3 Prone
   4 Left lateral Sims'

8. The nurse is caring for a client with esophageal varices. A Sengstaken-Blakemore tube has been inserted. Which of the following items must be kept at the bedside at all times?
   1 An irrigation set
   2 A pair of scissors
   3 A Kelly clamp
   4 An obturator

9. The nurse is inserting an indwelling urinary catheter into the urethra of a male client. As the

nurse inflates the balloon, the client complains of discomfort. The most appropriate nursing action is:

1 Remove the syringe from the balloon; discomfort is normal and temporary

2 Aspirate the fluid, advance the catheter farther, reinflate the balloon

3 Aspirate the fluid, withdraw the catheter slightly, reinflate the balloon

4 Aspirate the fluid, remove the catheter, and reinsert a new catheter

10. The nurse is inserting an indwelling urinary catheter into a male client. As the catheter is inserted into the urethra, urine begins to flow into the tubing. At this point, the nurse:

1 Immediately inflates the balloon

2 Withdraws the catheter approximately 1 inch and inflates the balloon

3 Inserts the catheter until resistance is met and inflates the balloon

4 Inserts the catheter 2.5 to 5 cm and inflates the balloon

11. The nurse is assisting the physician with the insertion of a chest tube. The nurse monitors the client and notes fluctuation of the fluid level in the water seal chamber after the tube is inserted. Based on this assessment, which of the following actions would be most appropriate?

1 Inform the physician

2 Encourage the client to deep breathe

3 Continue to monitor as this is an expected finding

4 Reinforce the occlusive dressing

12. The nurse is caring for a client with a chest tube.

The nurse turns the client to the side and the chest tube accidentally disconnects. The initial nursing action is to:

1 Call the physician

2 Clamp the chest tube

3 Immediately replace the chest tube system

4 Place a sterile dressing over the disconnection site

13. A nurse is assisting the physician with the removal of a chest tube. To remove the chest tube the client is instructed to:

1 Take a deep breath

2 Hold the breath

3 Exhale

4 Perform the Valsalva maneuver

14. A nurse is changing the tapes on a tracheostomy tube. The client coughs and the tube is dislodged. The initial nursing action is to:

1 Cover the tracheostomy site with a sterile dressing to prevent infection

2 Call the physician to reinsert the tracheotomy

3 Place a curved hemostat into the opening to hold the trachea open

4 Call the respiratory therapy department to reinsert the tracheotomy

15. The nurse is caring for the client immediately after removal of the endotracheal tube following radical neck dissection. The nurse plans to report which of the following signs, if experienced by the client?

1 Stridor

2 Occasional pink-tinged sputum

3 Respiratory rate of 24

4 Few basilar crackles on the right

ANSWERS

1. **2**

Rationale: Water-soluble lubricant is used to lubricate 3 inches of the tube at the insertion end. An oil lubricant is not used because if the tube accidentally goes into the bronchus, pneumonia can develop. Half-inch tape is used to secure the tube after correct placement is verified. A 50-mL catheter tip syringe is used to aspirate gastric contents to confirm placement. The client will be asked to take a sip of water through a straw to help with the passage of the tube.

Test-Taking Strategy: Note the key word "not" in the stem of the question. Attempt to visualize the procedure as you answer the question. Remember that water-soluble lubricant must be used to lubricate the tube. If you had difficulty with this question, take time now to review the procedure for inserting an NG tube!

Level of Cognitive Ability: Analysis
Phase of Nursing Process: Planning
Client Needs: Physiological Integrity
Content Area: Adult Health/Gastrointestinal

Reference
Luckmann, J. (1997). *Saunders manual of nursing care*. Philadelphia: W. B. Saunders. p. 1262.

2. **1**

Rationale: Measuring the length of tube needed is done by placing the tube at the tip of the nose and measuring by extending the tube to the earlobe and then down to the xiphoid process. The average length for an adult is about 22 to 26 inches.

Test-Taking Strategy: Attempt to visualize this procedure. Eliminate options 2 and 3 because they are relatively similar. Eliminate option 4 next because 30 inches is rather lengthy. Review the procedure for measuring the length of a nasogastric tube for insertion now, if you had difficulty with this question!

Level of Cognitive Ability: Analysis
Phase of Nursing Process: Evaluation
Client Needs: Physiological Integrity
Content Area: Adult Health / Gastrointestinal

Reference
Luckmann, J. (1997). *Saunders manual of nursing care.* Philadelphia: W. B. Saunders. p. 1262.

3. **2**

Rationale: During insertion of an NG tube, if the client experiences difficulty in breathing or any respiratory distress pull back on the tube and wait until the distress subsides. Options 1 and 4 are unnecessary. Quickly inserting the tube is not an appropriate action because, in this situation, it may be likely that the tube has entered the bronchus.

Test-Taking Strategy: Use the process of elimination to answer the question. Options 3 and 4 can be eliminated first. Visualizing the procedure and anticipating potential complications will assist in eliminating option 1 as an unnecessary action. Review the cautions related to inserting an NG tube now, if you had difficulty with this question!

Level of Cognitive Ability: Application
Phase of Nursing Process: Implementation
Client Needs: Physiological Integrity
Content Area: Adult Health/Gastrointestinal

Reference
Luckmann, J. (1997). *Saunders manual of nursing care.* Philadelphia: W. B. Saunders. p. 1262.

4. **4**

Rationale: If the NG tube is in the stomach, the pH of the contents will be acidic. Option 1 indicates an alkaline pH. Option 2 indicates a neutral pH. Option 3 indicates a slightly acidic pH.

Test-Taking Strategy: Note the key word "assure" in the stem of the question. Recalling that gastric contents are acidic will easily direct you to option 4. If you had difficulty with this question, take time now to review the procedure for assessing NG tube placement!

Level of Cognitive Ability: Analysis
Phase of Nursing Process: Analysis
Client Needs: Physiological Integrity
Content Area: Adult Health / Gastrointestinal

Reference
Lammon, C., Foote, A., Leli, P., et al. (1995). *Clinical nursing skills.* Philadelphia: W. B. Saunders. p. 420.

5. **3**

Rationale: When the nurse discontinues a nasogastric tube, the client is instructed to exhale. This will close the epiglottis and allow for easy withdrawal through the esophagus into the nose. The nurse removes the tube with one very smooth continuous pull.

Test-Taking Strategy: Visualize the procedure as a guide in selecting the correct option. Use the process of elimination, considering what each client action identified in the options would produce. Review the procedure for discontinuing an NG tube now, if you had difficulty with this question!

Level of Cognitive Ability: Application
Phase of Nursing Process: Implementation
Client Needs: Physiological Integrity
Content Area: Adult Health / Gastrointestinal

Reference
Luckmann, J. (1997). *Saunders manual of nursing care.* Philadelphia: W. B. Saunders. p. 1263.

6. **3**

Rationale: If a client has an NG tube connected to suction, the nurse should wait up to 30 minutes before reconnecting the tube to the suction apparatus to allow adequate time for medication absorption. Aspirating the NG tube will remove the medication just administered. Low intermittent suction will also remove the medication just administered. The client should not be placed in the supine position because of the risk for aspiration.

Test-Taking Strategy: Eliminate options 1 and 4 first because these actions are similar and will produce the same effect. Recalling that the client should not be placed in a supine position will assist in eliminating option 2. If you had difficulty with this question, review the procedure for administering medications through an NG tube!

Level of Cognitive Ability: Application
Phase of Nursing Process: Implementation
Client Needs: Physiological Integrity
Content Area: Adult Health / Gastrointestinal

Reference
Leahy, J., & Kizilay, P. (1998). *Foundations of nursing practice: A nursing process approach.* Philadelphia: W. B. Saunders. p. 464.

7. **1**

Rationale: A Miller-Abbott tube is an intestinal tube that has a double lumen, one for a mercury balloon and the other for suction or drainage. Following insertion of the tube, the tube is allowed to advance over several hours. The client is positioned on the right side to facilitate passage through the pylorus of the stomach and into the small intestine.

Test-Taking Strategy: Eliminate options 2 and 4 because they are similar. From the remaining options, recalling the purpose of this tube and the anatomy of the body will assist in directing you to option 1. If you had difficulty with this question, take time now to review care to the client with a Miller-Abbott tube!

Level of Cognitive Ability: Application
Phase of Nursing Process: Implementation
Client Needs: Physiological Integrity
Content Area: Adult Health / Gastrointestinal

Reference
Luckmann, J. (1997). *Saunders manual of nursing care.* Philadelphia: W. B. Saunders. p. 1263.

8. **2**

Rationale: When the client has a Sengstaken-Blakemore tube, a pair of scissors must be kept at the client's bedside at all times. The client needs to be observed for sudden respiratory distress, which occurs if the gastric balloon ruptures and the entire tube moves upward. If this occurs, immediately cut all balloon lumens and remove the tube. An obturator and a Kelly clamp are kept at the bedside of a client with a tracheostomy. An irrigation set may be kept at the bedside, but it is not the priority item.

Test-Taking Strategy: Use knowledge regarding the structure, function, and placement of a Sengstaken-Blakemore tube to answer this question. Note the key word "must" in the stem of the question. This should assist in eliminating options 1, 3, and 4. If you had difficulty with this question, take time now to review nursing care of a client with a Sengstaken-Blakemore tube!

Level of Cognitive Ability: Application
Phase of Nursing Process: Implementation
Client Needs: Safe, Effective Care Environment
Content Area: Adult Health / Gastrointestinal

Reference
Black, J. & Matassarin-Jacobs, E. (1997), *Medical-surgical nursing: Clinical management for continuity of care* (5th ed.). Philadelphia: W. B. Saunders, p. 1185.

9. **2**

Rationale: If the balloon is malpositioned in the urethra, inflating the balloon could produce trauma and pain will occur. If pain occurs, the fluid should be aspirated and the catheter inserted a little farther in order to provide sufficient space to inflate the balloon. The catheter's balloon is behind the opening at the insertion tip. Inserting the catheter the extra distance will ensure that the balloon is inflated inside the bladder and not in the urethra. There is no need to remove the catheter and reinsert a new one. Pain when the balloon is inflated is not normal and will not go away.

Test-Taking Strategy: Knowledge of the proper procedure for inserting an indwelling urinary catheter is helpful in answering this question. Discomfort when inflating the balloon is caused by malposition of the catheter in the urethra. Option 2 will properly position the balloon in the bladder for safe balloon inflation. Option 1 is different from the other three options but can be eliminated since discomfort is neither normal nor temporary when caused by the balloon being inflated. It is not necessary to withdraw the catheter and reinsert a new catheter.

Level of Cognitive Ability: Application
Phase of Nursing Process: Implementation
Client Needs: Safe, Effective Care Environment
Content Area: Adult Health / Renal

Reference
Kozier, B., Erb, G., & Blais, K. (1998). *Fundamentals of nursing: Concepts, process, and practice* (5th ed.). New York: Addison-Wesley. pp. 1256–1257.

10. **4**

Rationale: The catheter's balloon is behind the opening at the insertion tip. The catheter is inserted 2.5 to 5 cm after urine begins to flow in order to provide sufficient space to inflate the balloon. Inserting the catheter the extra distance will ensure that the balloon is inflated inside the bladder and not in the urethra. Inflating the balloon in the urethra could produce trauma.

Test-Taking Strategy: Knowledge of the proper procedure for inserting an indwelling urinary catheter will assist you in answering this question. Note the key phrase "urine begins to flow." Options 2 and 3 can easily be eliminated. Eliminate option 1 next because of the word "immediately." If you had difficulty with this question, take time now to review the procedure for bladder catheterization!

Level of Cognitive Ability: Application
Phase of Nursing Process: Implementation
Client Needs: Safe, Effective Care Environment
Content Area: Adult Health / Renal

Reference
Kozier, B., Erb, G., & Blais, K. (1998). *Fundamentals of nursing: Concepts, process, and practice* (5th ed.). New York: Addison-Wesley. pp. 1256–1257.

11. **3**

Rationale: The presence of fluctuation of the fluid level in the water seal chamber indicates a patent drainage system. With normal breathing, the water level rises with inspiration and falls with expiration. Fluctuation stops if the tube is obstructed, if a dependent loop exists, if the suction is not working properly, and if the lung has re-expanded.

Test-Taking Strategy: Knowledge regarding a chest tube drainage system is required to answer this question. If you had difficulty with this question, take time now to review expected and unexpected assessment findings in the care of a client with a chest tube!

Level of Cognitive Ability: Analysis
Phase of Nursing Process: Implementation
Client Needs: Physiological Integrity
Content Area: Adult Health / Respiratory

Reference
Monahan, F., & Neighbors, M. (1998). *Medical-surgical nursing: Foundations for clinical practice* (2nd ed.). Philadelphia: W. B. Saunders. p. 578.

12. **2**

Rationale: If the drainage system is broken or interrupted, clamp the tube or place the end of the tube in a bottle of sterile saline held below the level of the chest, and then immediately replace the system. Placing a sterile dressing over the disconnection site will not prevent complications resulting from the disconnection. The physician may need to be notified, but this is not the initial action.

Test-Taking Strategy: Note the key word "initial" in the stem of the question. This indicates that a nursing action is required that will prevent a serious complication as a result of the disconnection. Eliminate options 1 and 3 as these actions delay required and immediate intervention. Knowledge of the complications that can occur from a disconnection will easily direct you to option 2. Review interventions related to the complications of a chest tube now, if you had difficulty with this question!

Level of Cognitive Ability: Application
Phase of Nursing Process: Implementation
Client Needs: Physiological Integrity
Content Area: Adult Health / Respiratory

Reference
Monahan, F., & Neighbors, M. (1998). *Medical-surgical nursing: Foundations for clinical practice* (2nd ed.). Philadelphia: W. B. Saunders. p. 578.

13. **4**

Rationale: When the chest tube is removed, the client is asked to perform the Valsalva maneuver (take a deep breath, exhale, and bear down), the tube is quickly withdrawn, and an airtight dressing is taped in place. The pleura seals itself off, and the wound heals in less than a week.

Test-Taking Strategy: Knowledge regarding the procedure for removing a chest tube is required to answer this question. Visualize the procedure as you select an option. If you had difficulty with this question, take time now to review this procedure!

Level of Cognitive Ability: Application
Phase of Nursing Process: Implementation
Client Needs: Physiological Integrity
Content Area: Adult Health / Respiratory

Reference
Monahan, F., & Neighbors, M. (1998). *Medical-surgical nursing: Foundations for clinical practice* (2nd ed.). Philadelphia: W. B. Saunders. p. 579.

14. **3**

Rationale: A replacement tube and obturator should be kept at the bedside along with a curved hemostat that could be used to hold the trachea open if accidental dislodgment occurs. Covering the tracheostomy site will block the airway. Options 2 and 4 will delay treatment in this emergency situation.

Test-Taking Strategy: Eliminate options 2 and 4 first as they are similar. Eliminate option 1 because this action will block the airway. If you had difficulty with this question, take time now to review the intervention required if a tracheostomy tube dislodges!

Level of Cognitive Ability: Application
Phase of Nursing Process: Implementation
Client Needs: Physiological Integrity
Content Area: Adult Health / Respiratory

Reference
Monahan, F., & Neighbors, M. (1998). *Medical-surgical nursing: Foundations for clinical practice* (2nd ed.). Philadelphia: W. B. Saunders. p. 566.

15. **1**

Rationale: The nurse reports stridor to the physician immediately. This is a high-pitched, coarse sound that is heard with the stethoscope over the trachea. It indicates airway edema and places the client at risk for airway obstruction.

Test-Taking Strategy: To answer this question most quickly and accurately, recall that the primary concern after removal of an artificial airway is the client's ability to maintain a patent airway and breathe independently. In comparing each of the options with this risk in mind, all of them must be eliminated with the exception of stridor. Since stridor indicates laryngeal edema and possible airway obstruction, it is the symptom that must be reported immediately!

Level of Cognitive Ability: Analysis
Phase of Nursing Process: Planning
Client Needs: Physiological Integrity
Content Area: Adult Health / Respiratory

Reference
Smeltzer, S., & Bare, B. (1996). *Brunner and Suddarth's textbook of medical-surgical nursing* (8th ed.). Philadelphia: Lippincott-Raven. p. 844.

BIBLIOGRAPHY

Black, J., & Matassarin-Jacobs, E. (1997). *Medical-surgical nursing: Clinical management for continuity of care* (5th ed.). Philadelphia: W. B. Saunders.

Craven, R., & Hirnle, C. (1996). *Fundamentals of nursing: Human health and function* (2nd ed.). Philadelphia: Lippincott-Raven.

Kozier, B., Erb, G., & Blais, K. (1998). *Fundamentals of nursing: Concepts, process, and practice* (5th ed.). New York: Addison-Wesley.

Lammon, C., Foote, A., Leli, P., et al. (1995). *Clinical nursing skills.* Philadelphia: W. B. Saunders.

Leahy, J., & Kizilay, P. (1998). *Foundations of nursing practice: A nursing process approach.* Philadelphia: W. B. Saunders.

Luckmann, J. (1997). *Saunders manual of nursing care.* Philadelphia: W. B. Saunders.

Monahan, F., & Neighbors, M. (1998). *Medical-surgical nursing: Foundations for clinical practice* (2nd ed.). Philadelphia: W. B. Saunders.

Smeltzer, S., & Bare, B. (1996). *Brunner and Suddarth's textbook of medical-surgical nursing* (8th ed.). Philadelphia: Lippincott-Raven.

UNIT V

....

Growth and Development Across the Life Span

PYRAMID TERMS

Accommodation—The ability to change a schema in order to introduce new ideas, objects, or experiences.

Assimilation—The ability to incorporate new ideas, objects, and experiences into the framework of one's thoughts.

Conscious—Includes all experiences that are within an individual's awareness and that the individual is able to control.

Ego—One's "sense of self"; provides such functions as problem-solving, mobilization of defense mechanisms, reality testing, and the capability of functioning independently. The mediator between the Id and the SuperEgo.

Id—Source of all primitive drives and instincts and is thought of as the reservoir of all psychic energy.

Schema—Refers to the child's cognitive structure or framework of thought.

Schemata—Categories that people form in their minds to organize and understand the world.

Subconscious—Often called the preconscious and includes experiences, thoughts, feelings, or desires that might not be in the immediate awareness but can be recalled to consciousness; helps repress unpleasant thoughts or feelings.

SuperEgo—Internal representative of the values, ideals, and moral standards of society.

Unconscious—Memories, feelings, thoughts, or wishes are repressed and are not available to the conscious mind.

PYRAMID TO SUCCESS

Normal growth and development proceeds in an orderly, systematic, and predictable pattern. It provides a basis for identifying and assessing an individual's abilities. Understanding the path of growth and development across the life span assists the nurse in identifying appropriate expected human behavior.

The Pyramid to Success focuses on Sigmund Freud's Theory of Psychosexual Development, Jean Piaget's Theory of Cognitive Development, Erik Erikson's Psychosocial Theory, and Lawrence Kohlberg's Theory of Moral Development.

NURSING PROCESS

ASSESSMENT

Age
Cultural and religious beliefs
Health care beliefs
Family roles
Social networks and supports
Developmental level
Cognitive level
Psychosocial behaviors
Psychosexual behaviors
Moral characteristics

ANALYSIS: Focus on developing a list of actual and potential nursing diagnoses based on data collected from the process of Assessment; Identify age-appropriate or altered development of normal skills; Identify client and family interpretation of the problem and the possible effective measures when developing the nursing diagnoses

PLANNING
Develop the plan of care based on the unique characteristics of the client, considering the identified stage of development; include the client and family in the plan of care as appropriate; consult with client and family as appropriate regarding the plan of care

IMPLEMENTATION
Utilize data gathered during assessment to adjust interventions, in order to meet the unique needs of the client; incorporate interventions that are compatible with the client's cultural, religious, and health care beliefs, educational level, and language; provide care utilizing a nonjudgmental approach; respect client and family needs, based on their preferences

EVALUATION
Determine compatibility of plan with client and family in meeting needs; adjust plan of care as appropriate based on meeting expectations and needs

CLIENT NEEDS

SAFE, EFFECTIVE CARE ENVIRONMENT

Caring
Advocacy
Client rights
Confidentiality
Ethical and legal responsibilities
Consultations and referrals

HEALTH PROMOTION AND MAINTENANCE

Aging process
Developmental stages and transition
Communication
Family planning and family systems
Health and wellness
Health care beliefs
Lifestyle choices

PSYCHOSOCIAL INTEGRITY

Communication
Mental health concepts
Coping mechanisms
Cultural heritage
Religious and spiritual influences on health
Support systems

PHYSIOLOGICAL INTEGRITY

Caring
Communication
Health care preferences
Practices or restrictions related to procedures and treatments

BIBLIOGRAPHY

Ashwill, J., & Droske, S. (1997). *Nursing care of children: Principles and practice.* Philadelphia: W. B. Saunders.

Carson, V., & Arnold, E. (1996). *Mental health nursing: The nurse-patient journey.* Philadelphia: W. B. Saunders.

Leahy, J., & Kizilay, P. (1998). *Foundations of nursing practice: A nursing process approach.* Philadelphia: W. B. Saunders.

Luckmann, J. (1997). *Saunders manual of nursing care.* Philadelphia: W. B. Saunders.

National Council of State Boards of Nursing (eds.) (1997). *Test plan for the national council licensure examination for registered nurses.* Chicago: Author.

Nichols, F., & Zwelling, E. (1997). *Maternal-newborn nursing: Theory and practice.* Philadelphia: W. B. Saunders.

O'Toole, M. (ed.) (1997). *Miller-Keane encyclopedia & dictionary of medicine, nursing, & allied health* (6th ed.). Philadelphia: W. B. Saunders.

Varcarolis, E. (1998). *Foundations of psychiatric mental health nursing* (3rd ed.). Philadelphia: W. B. Saunders.

CHAPTER 21

Theories of Growth and Development

I. Psychosocial Development and Erik Erikson

A. The theory
   1. Describes the human life cycle as a series of eight **Ego** developmental stages spanning birth to death
   2. Each stage presents a psychosocial crisis the goal of which is to integrate physical, maturation, and societal demands
   3. Focuses on psychosocial tasks that are accomplished throughout the life cycle
   4. The **Ego** is separate and liberated from the **Id**, developing across the course of the complete life cycle
   5. **Ego** development is influenced by family, social, and developmental factors
B. Psychosocial development
   1. A lifelong series of conflicts affected by social and cultural factors
   2. Each conflict must be resolved for the child or adult to progress emotionally
   3. Unsuccessful resolution leaves the individual emotionally handicapped
C. Stages of psychosocial development (Table 21–1)

II. Cognitive Development and Jean Piaget

A. The theory
   1. Defines cognitive acts as ways in which the mind organizes and adapts to its environment
   2. **Schema**: Refers to the child's cognitive structure or framework of thought
   3. **Schemata**
      a. Categories that people form in their minds to organize and understand the world
      b. A young child has only a few **schemata** with which to understand the world, and gradually these are increased
      c. Adults use a wide variety of **schemata** to understand the world
   4. **Assimilation**
      a. The ability to incorporate new ideas,

objects, and experiences into the framework of one's thoughts
      b. The growing child will perceive and give meaning to new information according to what is already known and understood
   5. **Accommodation**
      a. The ability to change a **schema** in order to introduce new ideas, objects, or experiences
      b. Changes the mental structure so that new experiences can be added
B. Stages of cognitive development
   1. Sensorimotor stage
      a. 0 to 2 years
      b. Development proceeds from reflex activity to imagining and solving problems through the senses and movement
   2. Preoperational stage
      a. 2 to 7 years
      b. Learning to think in terms of the past, present, and future
      c. The child moves from knowing the world through sensation and movement to prelogical thinking and finding solutions to problems
   3. Concrete operational
      a. 7 to 11 years
      b. Able to classify, order, and sort facts
      c. The child moves from prelogical thought to solving concrete problems through logic
   4. Formal operations
      a. 11 years to adulthood
      b. Able to think abstractly and logically
      c. Logical thinking is expanded to include solving abstract and concrete problems

III. Moral Development and Lawrence Kohlberg

A. Moral development
   1. A complicated process involving the acceptance of the values and rules of society in a way that shapes behavior

Table 21–1. Erik Erikson's Stages of Psychosocial Development

Age	Psychosocial Crisis	Task
Infancy (0–18 months)	Trust vs. Mistrust	Attachment to the mother

Resolution of Crisis
Trust in people; faith and hope about the environment and the future
Unsuccessful Resolution of Crisis
General difficulties relating to people effectively; suspicion; trust-fear conflict, fear of the future

Age	Psychosocial Crisis	Task
Early childhood (18 months to 3 years)	Autonomy vs. Shame and Doubt	Gaining some basic control over self and environment

Resolution of Crisis
Sense of self control and adequacy; will power
Unsuccessful Resolution of Crisis
Independence-fear conflict; severe feelings of self-doubt

Age	Psychosocial Crisis	Task
Late childhood (3–6 years)	Initiative vs. Guilt	Becoming purposeful and directive

Resolution of Crisis
Ability to initiate one's own activities; sense of purpose
Unsuccessful Resolution of Crisis
Aggression-fear conflict; sense of inadequacy or guilt

Age	Psychosocial Crisis	Task
School age (6–12 years)	Industry vs. Inferiority	Developing social, physical, and school skills

Resolution of Crisis
Competence; ability to learn and work
Unsuccessful Resolution of Crisis
Sense of inferiority; difficulty learning and working

Age	Psychosocial Crisis	Task
Adolescence (12–20 years)	Identity vs. Role Confusion	Developing sense of identity

Resolution of Crisis
Sense of personal identity
Unsuccessful Resolution of Crisis
Confusion about who one is; identity submerged in relationships or group memberships

Age	Psychosocial Crisis	Task
Early adulthood (20–35 years)	Intimacy vs. Isolation	Establishing intimate bonds of love and friendship

Resolution of Crisis
Ability to love deeply and commit oneself
Unsuccessful Resolution of Crisis
Emotional isolation, egocentricity

Age	Psychosocial Crisis	Task
Middle adulthood (35–65 years)	Generativity vs. Stagnation	Fulfilling life goals that involve family, career, and society

Resolution of Crisis
Ability to give and care for others
Unsuccessful Resolution of Crisis
Self-absorption; inability to grow as a person

Age	Psychosocial Crisis	Task
Later years (65 years–death)	Integrity vs. Despair	Looking back over one's life and accepting its meaning

Resolution of Crisis
Sense of integrity and fulfillment
Unsuccessful Resolution of Crisis
Dissatisfaction with life

2. Classified in a series of levels and behaviors
B. Levels of moral development (Box 21–1)

IV. Psychosexual Development and Sigmund Freud

A. Components of the theory
1. Levels of awareness
2. Agencies of the mind (**Id, Ego, SuperEgo**)
3. Concept of anxiety and defense mechanisms

4. Psychosexual stages of development
B. Levels of awareness
1. Conscious level of awareness
   a. The **conscious** mind is logical and is regulated by the Reality Principle
   b. Includes all experiences that are within an individual's awareness and that the individual is able to control
   c. Includes all information that is easily remembered and immediately available to an individual

---

BOX 21–1. Moral Development and Lawrence Kohlberg

LEVEL ONE—PRECONVENTIONAL

Stage 0 (0–2 years)
The infant has no awareness of right or wrong.

Stage 1 (2–3 years)
At this stage children cannot reason as mature members of society.

Children view the world in a selfish way, with no real understanding of right or wrong.

The child obeys rules and demonstrates acceptable behavior to avoid punishment, to avoid displeasing those who are in power, and because he or she fears punishment from a superior force such as a parent.

A toddler typically is at the first substage of the preconventional stage, involving punishment and obedience orientation, in which the toddler makes judgments on the basis of avoiding punishment or obtaining a reward.

Physical punishment and withholding privileges tend to give the toddler a negative view of morals.

Withdrawing love and affection as punishment leads to feelings of guilt in the toddler.

Appropriate discipline includes providing simple explanations of why certain behaviors are unacceptable, praising appropriate behavior, and using distractions when the toddler is headed for danger.

Stage 2 (4–7 years)
The child conforms to rules to obtain rewards or have favors returned.

The child's moral standards are those of others, and the child observes them to either avoid punishment or obtain rewards.

A preschooler is in the preconventional stage of moral development.

In this stage, conscience emerges and the emphasis is on external control.

LEVEL TWO—CONVENTIONAL

The child conforms to rules to please others.
The child has increased awareness of others' feelings.
A concern for social order begins to emerge.
A child views good behavior as that which those in authority will approve.
If the behavior is not acceptable, the child feels guilty.

Stage 3 (7–10 years)
Conformity occurs to avoid disapproval or dislike by others.

This stage involves living up to what is expected by individuals close to you or what individuals generally expect of others in their role as son, brother, friend, and so on.

Being good is important and is interpreted as having good motives and showing concerns about others.

It also means maintaining mutual relationships, such as trust, loyalty, respect, and gratitude.

Stage 4 (10–12 years)
The child has more concern with society as a whole.

Emphasis is on obeying laws to maintain social order.

Moral reasoning develops as the child shifts the focus of living to society.

The school-aged child is at the conventional level of the role conformity stage and has an increased desire to please others.

The child observes and to some extent internalizes the standards of others.

The child wants to be considered "good" by those individuals whose opinions matter to the child.

LEVEL THREE—POSTCONVENTIONAL

The individual focuses on individual rights and principles of conscience.

The focus is a concern regarding what is best for all.

Stage 5
Being aware that people hold a variety of values and opinions and that most values and rules are relative to the group.

The adolescent in this stage gives as well as takes, and does not expect to get something without paying for it.

Stage 6
Conformity is based on universal principles of justice and occurs to avoid self condemnation.

This stage involves following self-chosen ethical principles.

The development of the postconventional level of morality occurs in the adolescent at about age 13 years, marked by the development of an individual conscience and a defined set of moral values.

The adolescent can now acknowledge a conflict between two socially accepted standards and try to decide between them.

Control of conduct is now internal, both in standards observed and in reasoning about right and wrong.

2. Preconscious level of awareness
   a. Called the **subconscious**
   b. Includes experiences, thoughts, feelings, or desires that might not be in the immediate awareness but can be recalled to consciousness
   c. The **subconscious** can help repress unpleasant thoughts or feelings and can examine and censor certain wishes and thinking
3. Unconscious level of awareness
   a. The **unconscious** is not logical and is governed by the Pleasure Principle, which refers to seeking immediate tension reduction
   b. Memories, feelings, thoughts, or wishes are repressed and are not available to the **conscious** mind
   c. These repressed memories, thoughts, or feelings, if made prematurely **conscious**, can cause anxiety

C. Agencies of the mind
   1. **Id, Ego**, and **SuperEgo**
      a. The three systems of personality
      b. The psychological processes that follow different operating principles
      c. In a mature and well-adjusted personality, they work together as a team under the leadership of the **Ego**
   2. The **Id**
      a. Source of all drives
      b. Is present at birth
      c. Includes genetic inheritance, reflexes, capacities to respond, instincts, basic drives, needs, and wishes that motivate an individual
      d. It operates according to the Pleasure Principle
      e. The **Id** does not tolerate uncomfortable states and seeks to discharge the tension and return to a more comfortable constant level of energy
      f. The **Id** acts immediately in an impulsive, irrational way and pays no attention to the consequences of its actions, and therefore, often behaves in ways harmful to self and others
      g. The "primary" process is a psychological activity in which the **Id** attempts to reduce tension
      h. The "primary" process can include hallucinating or forming an image of the object that will satisfy its needs and remove the tension
      i. The "primary" process by itself is not capable of reducing tension, therefore a "secondary" psychological process must develop if the individual is to survive; when this occurs, the structure of the second system of the personality, the **Ego**, begins to take form

3. The **Ego**
   a. The functions of the **Ego** include reality testing and problem solving
   b. Begins its development during the 4th or 5th month of life
   c. The **Ego** emerges out of the **Id** and acts as an intermediary between the **Id** and the external world
   d. Emerges because the needs, wishes, and demands of the **Id** require appropriate exchanges with the outside world of reality
   e. Distinguishes between things in the mind and things in the external world
   f. Reality testing is a function of the **Ego**, and the **Ego** uses realistic thinking
   g. The **Ego** follows the Reality Principle and operates by means of the "secondary" process, that is, realistic thinking
   h. The aim of the Reality Principle is to satisfy the **Id's** impulses in the external world with an object that is suitable; determines whether an experience is true or false; and whether it has external existence or not
   i. The **Ego** devises a plan and tests the plan by some kind of action to see if it will work
4. The **SuperEgo**
   a. A necessary part of socialization that develops during the phallic stage during 3 to 5 years of age
   b. It develops from the interactions with one's parents during the extended period of childhood dependency
   c. It includes the internalization of the values, ideals, and moral standards of society
   d. The child internalizes the moral standards of parents and society
   e. The **SuperEgo** consists of the conscience and the **Ego** ideal
   f. The conscience refers to the capacity for self-evaluation and criticism
   g. When moral codes are violated, the conscience punishes the individual by instilling guilt
   h. What parents approve of, and what they reward the child for doing, become incorporated as the **Ego** ideal by the mechanism of introjection
   i. The **SuperEgo** strives for perfection rather than pleasure and represents the ideal rather than the real
   j. Living up to one's **Ego** ideal results in the individual feeling proud and increases self-esteem

D. Anxiety and defense mechanisms
   1. The **Ego** develops defenses or defense mechanisms to fight off anxiety
   2. Defense mechanisms operate on an **unconscious** level, except for suppression, so the individual is not aware of their operation
   3. Defense mechanisms deny, falsify, or distort reality to make it less threatening

BOX 21-2. Freud's Psychosexual Stages of Development

ORAL STAGE (0–1 years)

During this stage, the infant is concerned with his or her own gratification.

The infant is all **Id**, operating on the Pleasure Principle and striving for immediate gratification of needs.

When the infant experiences gratification of basic needs, a sense of trust and security begins.

The **Ego** begins to emerge as the infant begins to see self as separate from the mother; this marks the beginning of the development of a sense of self.

ANAL STAGE (1–3 years)

Toilet training occurs during this period, and the child gains pleasure both from the elimination of the feces and from their retention.

The conflict of this stage is between those demands from society and the parents and the sensations of pleasure associated with the anus.

The child begins to gain a sense of control over instinctive drives and learns to delay immediate gratification to gain a future goal.

PHALLIC STAGE (3–6 years)

The child experiences both pleasurable and conflicting feelings associated wth the genital organs.

The pleasures of masturbation and the fantasy life of children set the stage for the Oedipus complex.

The child's unconscious sexual attraction to and wish to possess the parent of the opposite sex, the hostility and desire to remove the parent of the same sex, and the subsequent guilt for these wishes is the conflict the child faces.

The conflict is resolved when the child identifies with the parent of the same sex.

The emergence of the **SuperEgo** is both the solution to and the result of these intense impulses.

LATENCY STAGE (6–12 years)

A tapering off of **conscious** biological and sexual urges.

The sexual impulses are channeled and elevated into a more culturally accepted level of activity.

Growth of **Ego** functions and the ability to care about and relate to others outside the home is the task of this stage of development.

GENITAL STAGE (12 years and beyond)

Emerges at adolescence with the onset of puberty when the genital organs mature.

The individual gains gratification from his or her own body.

During this stage, the individual develops satisfying sexual and emotional relationships with members of the opposite sex.

The individual plans life goals and gains a strong sense of personal identity.

---

4. An individual cannot survive without defense mechanisms; however, if they become too extreme in distorting reality, then interference in healthy adjustment and personal growth may occur

E. Psychosexual stages of development (Box 21–2)

1. Human development proceeds through a series of stages from infancy to adulthood

2. Each stage is characterized by the inborn tendency of all individuals to reduce tension and seek pleasure

3. Each stage is associated with a particular conflict that must be resolved before the child can move successfully to the next stage

4. Experiences during the early stages determine an individual's adjustment patterns and the personality traits that an individual has as an adult

PRACTICE QUESTIONS

1. The maternity nurse is providing instructions to a new mother regarding the psychosocial development of the infant. Utilizing Erikson's psychosocial development theory, the nurse would instruct the mother to:
   1 Allow the infant to signal a need
   2 Anticipate all the needs of the infant
   3 Avoid the infant during the first 10 minutes of crying
   4 Attend to the infant immediately when crying

2. A mother of a 3-year-old tells the clinic nurse that the child is constantly rebelling and having temper tantrums. The most appropriate instruction to the mother is:
   1 Punish the child every time the child says "no," to change the behavior
   2 Allow the behavior, because this is normal at this age period
   3 Set limits on the child's behavior
   4 Ignore the child when this behavior occurs

3. The home health nurse visits a 70-year-old woman on a weekly basis. At each visit the client reminisces about past life experiences in a positive way. The home health nurse interprets this behavior as:
   1 A normal psychosocial response
   2 Requiring a psychiatric consultation
   3 A mental status alteration
   4 A sensory deficit requiring social activities

4. The mother of an 8-year-old child tells the clinic nurse that she is concerned about the child because the child seems to be more attentive to

friends than anything else. The most appropriate nursing response is which of the following?

1 "You need to be concerned"
2 "You need to monitor the child's behavior closely"
3 "At this age, the child is developing his or her own personality"
4 "You need to provide more praise to the child to stop this behavior"

5. The mother of a 4-year-old child calls the clinic nurse and expresses concern because the child has been masturbating. The most appropriate response by the nurse is which of the following?

1 "The child is very young to begin this behavior and should be brought to the clinic"
2 "This is not normal behavior and the child should be brought to the clinic"
3 "This is a normal behavior at this age"
4 "Children usually begin this behavior at age 8 years"

6. The nursing instructor asks a nursing student to present a clinical conference to peers regarding Freud's psychosexual stages of development, specifically the anal stage. Which of the following most appropriately relates to this stage of development?

1 This stage is associated with toilet training
2 This stage is associated with pleasurable and conflicting feelings about the genital organs
3 This stage is characterized by a tapering-off of conscious biological and sexual urges
4 This stage is characterized by the gratification of self

7. A mother of a 5-year-old child tells the nurse that the child scolds the floor or a table if the child hurts herself on the object. According to

Piaget's theory of cognitive development, this behavior is identified as:

1 Object permanence
2 Egocentric speech
3 Animism
4 Global organization

8. A nursing instructor asks the nursing student to describe the formal operations stage of Piaget's cognitive developmental theory. The most appropriate response by the nursing student is:

1 "The child has the ability to think abstractly"
2 "The child develops logical thought patterns"
3 "The child has difficulty separating fantasy from reality"
4 "The child begins to understand the environment"

9. According to Kohlberg's theory of moral development, in the preconventional level, moral development is thought to be motivated by which of the following?

1 The parents' behavior
2 Peer pressure
3 Social pressures
4 Punishment and reward

10. The nurse educator is conducting a session for the nursing staff regarding the theories of growth and development. Which of the following is not a component of Kohlberg's theory of moral development?

1 Moral development progresses in relationship to cognitive development
2 Individuals move through all six stages in a sequential fashion
3 It provides a framework for understanding how individuals determine a moral code to guide their behavior
4 A person's ability to make moral judgments develops over a period of time

ANSWERS

1. **1**

Rationale: According to Erikson, the caregiver should not try to anticipate the infant's needs at all times but must allow the infant to signal needs. If an infant is not allowed to signal a need, he or she will not learn how to control the environment. Erikson believed that a delayed or prolonged response to an infant's signal would inhibit the development of trust and lead to mistrust of others.

Test-Taking Strategy: Eliminate options 3 and 4 first because of the words "avoid" and "immediately" in these options. Additionally, option 2 can be eliminated because of the absolute term "all."

Level of Cognitive Ability: Application
Phase of Nursing Process: Implementation
Client Needs: Psychosocial Integrity
Content Area: Child Health

Reference
Leahy, J., & Kizilay, P. (1998). *Foundations of nursing practice: A nursing process approach.* Philadelphia: W. B. Saunders. p. 264.

2. **3**

Rationale: According to Erikson, the child focuses on independence between ages 1 and 3 years. Gaining independence often means that the child has to rebel against the parents' wishes. Saying things like "no" or "mine" and having temper tantrums are common during this period of development. Being consistent and setting limits on the child's behavior are necessary elements.

Test-Taking Strategy: Options 2 and 4 can be eliminated first because they are similar. Eliminate option 1 because this action is likely to produce a negative response during this normal developmental pattern. Review psychosocial development of the toddler according to Erikson now, if you had difficulty with this question!

Level of Cognitive Ability: Application
Phase of Nursing Process: Implementation
Client Needs: Psychosocial Integrity
Content Area: Child Health

Reference
Leahy, J., & Kizilay, P. (1998). *Foundations of nursing practice: A nursing process approach.* Philadelphia: W. B. Saunders. p. 264.

3. 1

Rationale: According to Erikson, the later years are 65 years to death. The adult reminisces about past life experiences, viewing them in a positive way. The adult needs to feel good about accomplishments, see successes in life, and feel that he or she has made a contribution to society.

Test-Taking Strategy: Utilize knowledge regarding Erikson's theory of psychosocial development of late adulthood to answer the question. Note the similarity in options 2, 3, and 4. Using Erikson's theory, you will easily be directed to option 1. Review psychosocial development now, if you had difficulty with this question!

Level of Cognitive Ability: Analysis
Phase of Nursing Process: Analysis
Client Needs: Psychosocial Integrity
Content Area: Fundamental Skills

Reference
Varcarolis, E. (1998). *Foundations of psychiatric mental health nursing* (3rd ed.). Philadelphia: W. B. Saunders, p. 44.

4. 3

Rationale: According to Erikson, during middle childhood (ages 7 to 12 years), the child begins to move for support toward peers and friends and away from the parents. The child also begins to develop special interests that reflect his or her own developing personality instead of the parents.

Test-Taking Strategy: Utilize Erikson's psychosocial development theory related to middle childhood to answer the question. Options 1 and 2 can be easily eliminated first. Eliminate option 4 next because, although praising the child for accomplishments is important at this age, the behavior that the child is exhibiting is normal. Review psychosocial development related to middle childhood according to Erikson now, if you had difficulty with this question!

Level of Cognitive Ability: Analysis
Phase of Nursing Process: Implementation
Client Needs: Psychosocial Integrity
Content Area: Child Health

Reference
Varcarolis, E. (1998). *Foundations of psychiatric mental health nursing* (3rd cd.). Philadelphia: W. B. Saunders. p. 44.

5. 3

Rationale: According to Freud's psychosexual stages of development, between the ages of 3 and 6 years the child is in the phallic stage. At this time, children devote much energy to examining their genitalia, masturbating, and expressing interest in sexual concerns.

Test-Taking Strategy: Eliminate options 1 and 2 because they are similar. Use Freud's psychosexual stages of development to answer this question. Knowledge of these stages will easily direct you to option 3. If you had difficulty with this question, take time now to review Freud's psychosocial stages of development!

Level of Cognitive Ability: Analysis
Phase of Nursing Process: Analysis
Client Needs: Psychosocial Integrity
Content Area: Child Health

Reference
Varcarolis, E. (1998). *Foundations of psychiatric mental health nursing* (3rd ed.). Philadelphia: W. B. Saunders. p. 40.

6. 1

Rationale: Generally, toilet training occurs during this period. According to Freud, the child gains pleasure both from the elimination of feces and from their retention. Option 2 relates to the phallic stage. Option 3 relates to the latency period. Option 4 relates to the oral stage.

Test-Taking Strategy: Knowledge regarding Freud's psychosexual stages of development will assist in answering this question. Note the relationship between the words "anal" in the question and "toilet training" in the correct option. If you had difficulty with this question, take time now to review Freud's psychosexual stages of development!

Level of Cognitive Ability: Analysis
Phase of Nursing Process: Analysis
Client Needs: Psychosocial Integrity
Content Area: Child Health

Reference
Varcarolis, E. (1998). *Foundations of psychiatric mental health nursing* (3rd ed.). Philadelphia: W. B. Saunders. pp. 40–42.

7. 3

Rationale: Animism means that all inanimate objects are given living meaning. Object permanence, the realization that something out of sight still exists, occurs in the later stages of the sensorimotor stage of development. Egocentric speech occurs when the child talks just for fun and cannot see another's point of view. Global organization means that if any part of an object or situation changes, the whole thing has changed. Options 2 and 4 occur during the preoperational stage.

Test-Taking Strategy: Attempt to make a relationship with the behavior identified in the question and the correct response. This will easily direct you to option 3. If you had difficulty with this question, take time now to review the concepts of Piaget's theory of cognitive development!

Level of Cognitive Ability: Analysis
Phase of Nursing Process: Analysis
Client Needs: Psychosocial Integrity
Content Area: Child Health

Reference
Leahy, J., & Kizilay, P. (1998). *Foundations of nursing practice: A nursing process approach.* Philadelphia: W. B. Saunders. pp. 266–267.

8. 1

Rationale: In the formal operation stage, the child has the ability to think abstractly and solve hypotheses. Option 2 identifies the concrete operations stage. Option 3 identifies the preoperational stage. Option 4, identifies the sensorimotor stage.

Test-Taking Strategy: Knowledge regarding the characteristics of Piaget's cognitive developmental theory is required to answer this question. If you had difficulty with this question, take time now to review the concepts of Piaget's theory!

Level of Cognitive Ability: Analysis
Phase of Nursing Process: Analysis
Client Needs: Psychosocial Integrity
Content Area: Child Health

Reference
Leahy, J., & Kizilay, P. (1998). *Foundations of nursing practice: A nursing process approach.* Philadelphia: W. B. Saunders. p. 268.

9. 4

Rationale: In the preconventional stage, morals are thought to be motivated by punishment and reward. If the child is obedient and is not punished, then he or she is being moral. The child sees actions as either good or bad. If the child's actions are good, the child is praised. If the child's actions are bad, the child is punished.

Test-Taking Strategy: Eliminate options 2 and 3 because they are similar. Knowledge that the preconventional stage occurs between the ages of 2 and 7 years will assist in directing you to option 4. If you had difficulty with this question, take time now to review Kohlberg's theory of moral development!

Level of Cognitive Ability: Analysis
Phase of Nursing Process: Analysis
Client Needs: Psychosocial Integrity
Content Area: Child Health

Reference
Leahy, J., & Kizilay, P. (1998). *Foundations of nursing practice: A nursing process approach.* Philadelphia: W. B. Saunders. p. 268.

10. 2

Rationale: Kohlberg's theory states that individuals move through the six stages of development in a sequential fashion but that not everyone reaches stages 5 and 6 in their development of personal morality. Options 1, 3, and 4 are correct statements regarding Kohlberg's theory.

Test-Taking Strategy: Note the key word "not" in the stem of the question. Also, note the absolute word "all" in option 2. If you had difficulty with this question, take time now to review Kohlberg's theory!

Level of Cognitive Ability: Analysis
Phase of Nursing Process: Analysis
Client Needs: Psychosocial Integrity
Content Area: Fundamental Skills

Reference
Ashwill, J., & Droske, S. (1997). *Nursing care of children: Principles and practice.* Philadelphia: W. B. Saunders. pp. 36–37.

BIBLIOGRAPHY

Ashwill, J., & Droske, S. (1997). *Nursing care of children: Principles and practice.* Philadelphia: W. B. Saunders.
Carson, V., & Arnold, E. (1996). *Mental health nursing: The nurse-patient journey.* Philadelphia: W. B. Saunders.
Leahy, J., & Kizilay, P. (1998). *Foundations of nursing practice: A nursing process approach.* Philadelphia: W. B. Saunders.

Luckmann, J. (1997). *Saunders manual of nursing care.* Philadelphia: W. B. Saunders.
Nichols, F., & Zwelling, E. (1997). *Maternal-newborn nursing: Theory and practice.* Philadelphia: W. B. Saunders.
O'Toole, M. (1997). *Miller-Keane encyclopedia & dictionary of medicine, nursing, & allied health* (6th ed.). Philadelphia: W. B. Saunders.
Varcarolis, E. (1998). *Foundations of psychiatric mental health nursing* (3rd ed.). Philadelphia: W. B. Saunders.

UNIT VI

....

Maternity Nursing

PYRAMID TERMS

Amniotic Fluid—Fluid that surrounds and protects the fetus; consists of 500 to 1000 mL in amount by the end of pregnancy. The fetus floats in the amniotic fluid, which serves as a cushion against injury from sudden blows or movements and helps maintain a constant body temperature for the fetus.

Ballottement—Rebounding of the fetus against the examiner's finger on palpation. When the cervix is tapped, the fetus floats upward in the amniotic fluid. A rebound is felt by the examiner when the fetus falls back.

Chadwick's Sign—Bluish coloration of the mucous membranes of the cervix, vagina, and vulva.

Delivery—Actual event of birth; the expulsion or extraction of the neonate and fetal membranes at birth.

Fertilization—Takes place when sperm and ovum unite. Occurs within 12 hours of ovulation and within 2 to 3 days of insemination, the average duration of viability for the ovum and sperm.

Goodell's Sign—Softening of the cervix; occurs at the beginning of the second month of gestation and is a probable sign of pregnancy.

Gravida—A pregnant woman; called gravida I (primigravida) during the first pregnancy, gravida II (secundigravida) during the second, and so on.

Hegar's Sign—Compressibility and softening of the lower uterine segment; occurs at about week 6 of gestation; a probable sign of pregnancy.

Implantation—Zygote propels toward the uterus and implants in the uterine wall 6 to 8 days after ovulation.

Infant—A baby born alive; also from 28 days of age until the first birthday.

Labor—Coordinated sequence of involuntary uterine contractions resulting in effacement and dilation of the cervix, followed by expulsion of the products of conception.

Lochia—Discharge from the uterus that consists of blood from the vessels of the placental site and debris from the decidua.

Nagele's Rule—Determines the estimated date of confinement (EDC). Add 7 days to the first day of the last menstrual period (LMP). Subtract 3 months and add 1 year.

Neonate—A human offspring from the time of birth to the 28th day of life; also called newborn.

Newborn—A human offspring from the time of birth to the 28th day of life; also called neonate.

Parity—The number of pregnancies that have been carried to viability.

Placenta—Provides for the exchange of nutrients and waste products between the fetus and mother. Develops by the third month of gestation; also called afterbirth.

Quickening—First perception of fetal movement, appearing usually in the 16th to 18th week of pregnancy.

PYRAMID TO SUCCESS

The Pyramid to Success focuses on the physiological and psychosocial aspects related to the experience of pregnancy. Pyramid points begin with instructing the pregnant client in measures that will promote a healthy environment for both the mother and fetus. Focus on the importance of antenatal follow-up, nutrition, and the interventions for common discomforts that occur during pregnancy. Review the purpose of the commonly prescribed diagnostic tests and procedures in the antenatal period. Focus on disorders that can occur during pregnancy, particularly pregnancy-induced hypertension (PIH) and diabetes. Review the labor and delivery process and the immediate interventions when the mother or fetal status is compromised, such as prolapsed cord or altered fetal heart rate. Review fetal effects from the mother with AIDS or the substance abuse mother. Focus on the normal expectations of the postpartum period and the complications that can occur. Pyramid points also focus on the normal physical assessment findings in the neonate and the early identification of disorders in the neonate.

NURSING PROCESS

ASSESSMENT

Vital signs, weight, and height
Nutritional status
Gestational status
Gravidity and parity
Signs of pregnancy
Physiological changes associated with the pregnancy
Psychological changes associated with the pregnancy
Risk factors or concerns related to the pregnancy
Laboratory and diagnostic studies
Available support systems
Need for support and referral to community agencies

ANALYSIS: Altered Nutrition

PLANNING	IMPLEMENTATION	EVALUATION
Client verbalizes nutritional requirements of pregnancy; client gains weight appropriate for size and pregnancy	Instruct client on nutritional needs and requirements; monitor weight; monitor nutritional status and weight at each prenatal visit; consider religious and cultural considerations when planning care	Client maintains adequate nutritional status during pregnancy

---

ANALYSIS: Altered Physiological and Psychological Processes

PLANNING	IMPLEMENTATION	EVALUATION
Client verbalizes the physiological and psychological changes that may occur; client verbalizes the discomforts that may occur and the appropriate treatments	Instruct client on the physiological and psychological changes that may occur; monitor for physiological and psychological changes; instruct client about the discomforts that may occur and the treatments; inquire regarding existing discomforts	Client obtains relief from treatments implemented for discomforts; vital signs remain within normal limits

---

ANALYSIS: Potential Knowledge Deficit

PLANNING	IMPLEMENTATION	EVALUATION
Client identifies risks associated with pregnancy and the conditions necessitating notifying the physician; client verbalizes the need for and the procedure for any scheduled diagnostic tests or procedures; client verbalizes the need for community resources if necessary	Instruct client on the need for and plan for prenatal visits; instruct client about any scheduled diagnostic tests or procedures; instruct client regarding the need for and when to notify the physician; support and encourage the use of community resources	Client verbalizes the schedule for prenatal visits; client complies with the schedule for prenatal visits; client notifies the physician appropriately; client prepares adequately for scheduled diagnostic tests or procedures; client utilizes community resources as necessary

---

ANALYSIS: Potential for Altered Parenting

PLANNING
Parent(s) verbalize confidence in the care of the neonate and the parenting role; parent(s) demonstrate nurturing behaviors toward the neonate

IMPLEMENTATION
Assist client in identifying parenting skills; encourage expression of feelings regarding parenting role; initiate a plan to assist parents to develop parenting skills; encourage bonding and frequent opportunities for newborn/parent interaction; provide instructions and demonstrate care measures for the neonate; allow ample opportunity for the parents to demonstrate measures to care for the neonate; follow-up with telephone call after discharge or initiate support services for home as appropriate

EVALUATION
Parent(s) demonstrate bonding with the neonate; parent(s) demonstrate appropriate infant care techniques; parent(s) utilize support services as needed

---

ANALYSIS: Potential for Altered Family Processes/Parental Role Conflict

---

PLANNING
Parent(s) verbalize coping patterns; parent(s) verbalize expected changes in family role

IMPLEMENTATION
Encourage parental interaction with the neonate; encourage parent(s) to verbalize feelings related to entry of new family member into the home; assess status of feelings of siblings, if appropriate, regarding potential role changes

EVALUATION
Parent(s) identify role changes; parent(s) and family members acknowledge change in family roles

CLIENT NEEDS

SAFE, EFFECTIVE CARE ENVIRONMENT

Parent rights
Confidentiality
Informed consent for procedures
Continuity of care
Handling infectious materials
Standard (universal) precautions when delivering
  care
Asepsis

HEALTH PROMOTION AND MAINTENANCE

Reproduction and human sexuality
Teaching regarding ante/intra/postpartum care
Expected body image changes
Birthing and parenting issues
Family planning and family systems
Concepts of wellness
Growth and development and health care screening
Lifestyle choices

PSYCHOSOCIAL INTEGRITY

Communication
Cultural and religious influences regarding birth and
  motherhood
Coping mechanisms
Role changes
Support systems

PHYSIOLOGICAL INTEGRITY

Alterations in body systems
Normal expectations during pregnancy
Physiological changes that occur during pregnancy
Nutrition
Labor and delivery process
Commonly prescribed diagnostic tests and procedures
Risk identification during pregnancy
Interventions for unexpected events during the pregnancy

BIBLIOGRAPHY

Ashwill, J., & Droske, S. (1997). *Nursing care of children: Principles and practice*. Philadelphia: W. B. Saunders.

Luckmann, J. (1997). *Saunders manual of nursing care*. Philadelphia: W. B. Saunders.

National Council of State Boards of Nursing (eds.) (1997). *Test Plan for the National Council Licensure Examination for Registered Nurses*. Chicago: Author.

Nichols, F., & Zwelling, E. (1997). *Maternal newborn nursing: Theory and practice*. Philadelphia: W. B. Saunders.

O'Toole, M. (ed.). (1997). *Miller-Keane encyclopedia & dictionary of medicine, nursing and allied health* (6th ed.). Philadelphia: W. B. Saunders.

Reeder, S., Martin, L., & Koniak-Griffin, O. (1997). *Maternity nursing: Family, newborn, and women's health care* (18th ed.). Philadelphia: Lippincott-Raven.

CHAPTER 22

Female Reproductive System

. . . .

I. Organs

A. Ovaries
  1. Formation and expulsion of ova
  2. Secrete estrogen and progesterone
B. Fallopian Tubes
  1. Muscular tubes (oviducts) approximate to the ovaries and connect to the uterus
  2. Propel the ova from the ovaries to the uterus
C. Uterus
  1. Organ in which fetus develops
  2. Organ from which menstruation occurs
D. Cervix
  1. Internal os opens into the body of the uterine cavity
  2. Cervical canal is located between internal os and external os
  3. External os opens into the vagina
E. Vagina
  1. Passageway for menstrual blood
  2. Organ of copulation
  3. Passageway for fetus

II. Menstrual Cycle (Table 22–1)

A. Ovarian Hormones
  1. Include the follicle-stimulating hormone (FSH) and luteinizing hormone (LH)
  2. Released by the anterior pituitary gland
  3. Produce changes in the ovaries
  4. Secretion of ovarian hormones leads to changes in the endometrium
  5. Menstrual cycle, the regularly recurring physiological changes in the endometrium that culminate in its shedding, may vary in length, with the average length approximately 28 days
B. Ovarian Changes
  1. Preovulatory phase
  2. Luteal phase
C. Uterine Changes
  1. Menstrual phase

  2. Proliferative phase
  3. Secretory phase

III. Female Pelvis and Measurements

A. True Pelvis
  1. Lies below pelvic brim
  2. Consists of pelvic inlet, midpelvis, and pelvic outlet
B. False Pelvis
  1. Shallow portion above the pelvic brim
  2. Supports the abdominal viscera
C. Types of Pelvis
  1. Gynecoid
    a. Normal female pelvis
    b. Transversely rounded or blunt
    c. Most favorable for successful labor and birth
  2. Android
    a. Wedge-shaped or angulated
    b. Seen in males
    c. Not favorable for labor
    d. Narrow pelvic planes can cause slow descent and midpelvis arrest
  3. Anthropoid
    a. Oval-shaped
    b. The outlet is adequate, with a normal or moderately narrow pubic arch
  4. Platypelloid
    a. Flat in shape with an oval inlet
    b. Transverse diameter is wide but anteroposterior diameter is short, making the outlet inadequate
D. Pelvic Measurements
  1. Diagonal Conjugate (CD)
    a. Distance between sacral promontory and lower margin of symphysis pubis
    b. Greater than 11.5 cm is adequate
  2. True Conjugate, or Conjugate Vera (CV)
    a. Distance from upper margin of symphysis to sacral promontory

Table 22–1. **Menstrual Cycle**

Ovarian Changes

Preovulatory Phase	Luteal Phase
The hypothalamus releases gonadotropin-releasing hormone (GnRH) through the portal system to the anterior pituitary system Secretion of FSH by the anterior lobe of the pituitary gland stimulates growth of follicles Most follicles die, leaving one to mature into a large graafian follicle Estrogen produced by the follicle stimulates increased secretions of LH by the anterior lobe of the pituitary gland The follicle ruptures and releases an ovum into the peritoneal cavity	Begins with ovulation Body temperature drops and then rises by 0.5 to 1°F around the time of ovulation Corpus luteum is formed from follicle cells that remain in the ovary following ovulation Corpus luteum secretes estrogen and progesterone during the remaining 14 days of the cycle Corpus luteum degenerates if the ovum is not fertilized, and secretion of estrogen and progesterone declines Estrogen and progesterone inhibit secretions of FSH and LH Once corpus luteum degenerates, pituitary secretion of estrogen and progesterone decreases and the ovarian cycle begins again

Uterine Changes

Menstrual Phase	Proliferative Phase	Secretory Phase
Consists of 4 to 6 days of bleeding as endometrium breaks down owing to the decreased amount of estrogen and progesterone FSH rises, enabling the beginning of a new cycle	Estrogen stimulates proliferation and growth of endometrium This phase lasts about 9 days As estrogen increases, it suppresses secretion of FSH and increases secretion of LH LH stimulates ovulation and the development of the corpus luteum Ovulation occurs between day 12 and day 16 Estrogen is high and progesterone is low	This phase lasts about 12 days Follows ovulation Initiated in response to the increase of LH Graafian follicle replaced by corpus luteum Corpus luteum secretes progesterone and estrogen Progesterone prepares the endometrium for pregnancy should a fertilized ovum be implanted

    b. Greater than 11 cm is adequate
  3. Bi-ischial Diameter
    a. Transverse diameter of outlet between the ischial tuberosities
    b. Greater than 8 cm is adequate

IV. Fertilization and Implantation

A. **Fertilization**
  1. Occurs in the upper region of the fallopian tubes
  2. Occurs within 12 hours of ovulation and within 2 to 3 days of insemination, the average durations of viability for the ovum and sperm
  3. Takes place when sperm and ovum unite
  4. Once **fertilized**, the membrane of the ovum undergoes changes that prevent the entry of other sperm
  5. Each reproductive cell carries 23 chromosomes
  6. Sperm carry an X and Y chromosome
  7. When united with the female X chromosome, determines the sex of the child; XY: male, XX: female
B. **Implantation**
  1. Zygote propelled toward uterus
  2. Implants 6 to 8 days after ovulation
  3. Blastocyst secretes chorionic gonadotropin to ensure that the corpus luteum remains viable and secretes estrogen and progesterone for the first 2 to 3 months of gestation

V. Fetal Development (Table 22–2)

A. Embryonic stage from conception to 12 weeks
B. Fetal period from third month to gestation

VI. Fetal Environment

A. Amnion
  1. Encloses the amniotic cavity
  2. Inner membrane that forms about the second week of embryonic development
  3. Forms a fluid-filled sac that surrounds the embryo and later the fetus
B. Chorion
  1. Outer membrane
  2. Becomes vascularized and forms the fetal part of the placenta
C. **Amniotic Fluid**
  1. Consists of 500 to 1000 mL by the end of pregnancy
  2. Surrounds, cushions, and protects the fetus and allows for fetal movement
  3. Maintains the body temperature of the fetus
D. **Placenta**
  1. Provides for exchange of nutrients and waste products between fetus and mother
  2. Develops by the third month
  3. Dependent upon maternal circulation
  4. Large particles such as bacteria cannot pass through **placenta**
  5. In addition to nutrients, drugs, antibodies, and viruses can pass through the placenta

Table 22–2. **Fetal Development**

Embryonic Stage	Fetal Period
Week 1 Free-floating blastocyst	**Week 16** Active movements are present Fetal skin is transparent Lanugo hair begins to develop Skeletal ossification occurs Sex of fetus can be determined at this time
Weeks 2 to 3 2 mm in length Groove formed along middle of back Beginning of blood circulation Heart tubular in shape	**Week 20** 19 cm in length 465 g in weight Lanugo covers the entire body Fetus has nails Muscles developed Enamel and dentin are depositing Heart beat detected by fetoscope
Week 4 4 to 6 mm in length 0.4 g in weight Double heart chambers visible Heart beginning to beat Limb buds	
	Week 24 28 cm in length 780 g in weight Hair on head well formed Skin reddish and wrinkled Reflex hand grasp Vernix caseosa covers entire body Has ability to hear
Week 8 3 cm in length 2 g in weight Eyelids begin to fuse Circulatory system through umbilical cord well established Every organ system present	
Week 12 8 cm in length 45 g in weight Face well formed Limbs long and slender Kidneys begin to form urine Spontaneous movements occur Heart tones detected by electronic devices between 8 and 12 weeks Sex recognizable	**Week 28** 38 cm in length 1200 g in weight Limbs are well flexed Brain develops rapidly Eyelids open and close Lungs sufficiently developed to provide gas exchange (lecithin forming) If born, neonate can breathe at this time
	Week 32 30 cm in length 2000 g in weight Bones are fully developed Subcutaneous fat collected L/S (lecithin/sphingomyelin) ratio switching to 1.2 : 1
	Week 36 42 to 48 cm in length 2500 g in weight Skin pink, body rounded Less wrinkled Lanugo disappearing L/S (lecithin/sphingomyelin) ratio $\geq$ to 2 : 1
	Week 40 48 to 52 cm in length 3000 to 3600 g in weight Skin pinkish and smooth Lanugo present on upper arms and shoulders Vernix caseosa decreases Fingernails extend beyond fingertips Sole (plantar) creases down to heel Testes in scrotum Labia majora well developed

6. In the third trimester, transfer of maternal immunoglobulin provides fetus passive immunity to certain diseases for the first few months after birth
7. By week 8, genetic testing can be done

VII. Fetal Circulation

A. Umbilical Cord
  1. Contains two arteries and one vein
  2. Arteries carry deoxygenated blood and waste products from the fetus
  3. The vein carries oxygenated blood and provides oxygen and nutrients to the fetus
B. Fetal Heart Rate
  1. 120 to 160 beats per minute
  2. Approximately twice the maternal heart rate
C. Fetal Circulation Bypass
  1. Present due to nonfunctioning lungs
  2. Bypasses must close following birth to allow blood to flow through the lungs and liver
  3. Ductus arteriosus connects the pulmonary artery to aorta, bypassing lungs
  4. Ductus venosus connects umbilical vein and inferior vena cava, bypassing fetal liver
  5. Foramen ovale is the opening between right and left atria of heart, bypassing lungs

PRACTICE QUESTIONS

1. The nurse is conducting a prenatal teaching class and is reviewing the functions of the female reproductive system. A client asks the nurse about the purpose of the fallopian tubes. The nurse's response is based on the knowledge that:
   1 Estrogen and progesterone are secreted from the fallopian tubes
   2 The fallopian tubes are the organ of copulation
   3 The fetus develops in the fallopian tubes
   4 Fertilization occurs in the fallopian tubes

2. The nursing student is assigned to care for an adolescent female client in the health care clinic. The instructor reviews the menstrual cycle with the student. The instructor evaluates the student's knowledge regarding the follicle-stimulating hormone (FSH) and the luteinizing hormone (LH). The nursing student accurately responds by stating:
   1 FSH and LH are released from the anterior pituitary gland
   2 FSH and LH are secreted by the corpus luteum of the ovary
   3 FSH and LH are secreted by the adrenal glands
   4 FSH and LH stimulate the formation of milk during pregnancy

3. The nurse, working in a prenatal clinic, reviews a client's chart and notes that the physician documents that the client has a gynecoid pelvis. Based

on this documentation, the nurse determines that this type of pelvis is:
   1 Not favorable for labor
   2 Seen in 25% of women
   3 A wide pelvis with a short diameter
   4 The most favorable for labor and birth

4. The client asks the nurse about the purpose of the placenta. The most appropriate response by the nurse is based on the knowledge that the placenta:
   1 Prevents antibodies and viruses from passing to the fetus
   2 Cushions and protects the fetus
   3 Provides an exchange of nutrients and waste products between the mother and fetus
   4 Maintains the body temperature of the fetus

5. The nurse is describing the process of fetal circulation to a client during a prenatal visit. The nurse describes fetal circulation as:
   1 Consisting of two umbilical veins and one umbilical artery
   2 Consisting of two umbilical arteries and one umbilical vein
   3 Arteries carrying oxygenated blood to the fetus
   4 Veins carrying deoxygenated blood to the fetus

6. The nursing student is assigned to a client in labor. The nursing instructor asks the student to describe fetal circulation, specifically the ductus venosus. The correct student response is:
   1 The ductus venosus connects the pulmonary artery to the aorta
   2 The ductus venosus is an opening between the right and left atria
   3 The ductus venosus connects the umbilical artery to the inferior vena cava
   4 The ductus venosus connects the umbilical vein to the inferior vena cava

7. The nurse is caring for a client during the prenatal period. The client tells the nurse that she wants to know the sex of the fetus as soon as it can be determined. The nurse knows that the sex of the fetus can be determined as early as:
   1 Week 6
   2 Week 8
   3 Week 16
   4 Week 20

8. Surfactant, a substance needed to facilitate neonatal breathing, begins to be produced at approximately which gestational week?
   1 Week 12
   2 Week 18
   3 Week 28
   4 Week 32

9. The nurse is assessing the fetal heart beat using a fetoscope. The fetal heart beat can first be heard with a fetoscope at:
   1 Gestational week 5
   2 Gestational week 10
   3 Gestational week 16
   4 Gestational week 20

10. During the prenatal visit, the nurse assesses the fetal heart rate by fetoscope. Normal fetal heart rate is:
    1 80 to 100 beats per minute
    2 100 to 120 beats per minute
    3 120 to 160 beats per minute
    4 160 to 180 beats per minute

ANSWERS

1. **4**

Rationale: Each fallopian tube is a hollow muscular tube that transports a mature oocyte for final maturation and fertilization. Fertilization typically occurs near the boundary between the ampulla and isthmus of the tube. Estrogen is a hormone produced by the ovarian follicles, corpus luteum, adrenal cortex, and placenta during pregnancy. Progesterone is a hormone secreted by the corpus luteum of the ovary, adrenal glands, and placenta during pregnancy. The vagina is the organ of copulation, and the fetus develops in the uterus.

Test-Taking Strategy: Knowledge of the anatomy and physiology of the female reproductive system is required to answer this question. Use the process of elimination to answer the question. If you had difficulty with this question, take time now to review anatomy and physiology!

Level of Cognitive Ability: Analysis
Phase of Nursing Process: Analysis
Client Needs: Physiological Integrity
Content Area: Maternity

Reference
Martini, F. (1995). *Fundamentals of anatomy and physiology* (3rd ed.). Upper Saddle River, NJ: Prentice-Hall. pp. 1081–1083.

2. **1**

Rationale: FSH and LH, when stimulated by GnRH from the hypothalamus, are released from the anterior pituitary gland to stimulate follicular growth and development, growth of the graafian follicle, and the production of progesterone. Prolactin is the hormone produced by the pituitary gland, which in association with estrogen and progesterone stimulates breast development and the formation of milk during pregnancy.

Test-Taking Strategy: Knowledge of the hormones associated with the menstrual cycle is required to answer the question. Use the process of elimination to answer the question. Option 4 can be eliminated because the question does not address pregnancy. From this point, use your knowledge related to the menstrual cycle to select the correct option. If you had difficulty with this question, review the menstrual cycle now!

Level of Cognitive Ability: Analysis
Phase of Nursing Process: Evaluation
Client Needs: Physiological Integrity
Content Area: Maternity

References
Black, J., & Matassarin-Jacobs, E. (1997). *Medical-surgical nursing: Clinical management for continuity of care* (5th ed.). Philadelphia: W. B. Saunders. p. 2299.

May, K., & Mahlmeister L. (1994). *Maternal & neonatal nursing: Family-centered care* (3rd ed.). Philadelphia: J. B. Lippincott. pp. 74–79.

3. **4**

Rationale: A gynecoid pelvis is a normal female pelvis and is the most favorable for successful labor and birth. An android pelvis, seen in 20% of women, would not be favorable for labor because of the narrow pelvic planes. An anthropoid pelvis has an outlet that is adequate, with a normal or moderately narrow pubic arch, and is seen in 25% of women. The platypelloid pelvis, seen in 5% of women, has a wide transverse diameter, but the anteroposterior diameter is short, making the outlet inadequate.

Test-Taking Strategy: Knowledge regarding pelvic types is required to answer this question. Remember that the gynecoid pelvis is the normal female pelvis. Review pelvic types now, if you had difficulty with this question!

Level of Cognitive Ability: Analysis
Phase of Nursing Process: Assessment
Client Needs: Physiological Integrity
Content Area: Maternity

Reference
Nichols, F., & Zwelling, E. (1997). *Maternal-newborn nursing: Theory and practice.* Philadelphia: W. B. Saunders. p. 177.

4. **3**

Rationale: The placenta provides an exchange of nutrients and waste products between the mother and fetus. The amniotic fluid surrounds, cushions, and protects the fetus and maintains the body temperature of the fetus. Nutrients, drugs, antibodies, and viruses can pass through the placenta.

Test-Taking Strategy: Knowledge regarding the purpose of the placenta and amniotic fluid is required to answer this question. Remember that the placenta provides nutrients. If you had difficulty with this question, take time now to review the structure and function of the placenta and amniotic fluid!

Level of Cognitive Ability: Analysis
Phase of Nursing Process: Analysis
Client Needs: Physiological Integrity
Content Area: Maternity

Reference
Nichols, F., & Zwelling, E. (1997). *Maternal-newborn nursing: Theory and practice.* Philadelphia: W. B. Saunders. pp. 382–385.

5. **2**

Rationale: Blood pumped by the embryo's heart leaves the embryo through two umbilical arteries. Once oxygenated, the blood is then returned by one umbilical vein. The umbilical arteries carry deoxygenated blood and waste products from the fetus, and the vein carries oxygenated blood and provides oxygen and nutrients to the fetus.

Test-Taking Strategy: Knowledge regarding fetal circulation is required to answer this question. Remember that there are three umbilical vessels within an umbilical cord (two arteries and one vein). If you had difficulty with this question, take time now to review fetal circulation!

Level of Cognitive Ability: Analysis
Phase of Nursing Process: Analysis
Client Needs: Physiological Integrity
Content Area: Maternity

Reference
Nichols, F., & Zwelling, E. (1997). *Maternal-newborn nursing: Theory and practice.* Philadelphia: W. B. Saunders. p. 385.

6. **4**

Rationale: The ductus venosus connects the umbilical vein to the inferior vena cava. The foramen ovale is a temporary opening between the right and left atria. The ductus arteriosus joins the aorta and the pulmonary artery.

Test-Taking Strategy: Knowledge regarding fetal circulation is required to answer this question. Review fetal circulation now, if you had difficulty with this question!

Level of Cognitive Ability: Analysis
Phase of Nursing Process: Evaluation
Client Needs: Physiological Integrity
Content Area: Maternity

References
Nichols, F., & Zwelling, E. (1997). *Maternal-newborn nursing: Theory and practice.* Philadelphia: W. B. Saunders. p. 385.
M. O'Toole (ed.) (1997). *Miller-Keane encyclopedia & dictionary of medicine, nursing, & allied health* (6th ed.). Phildadelphia: W.B. Saunders. p. 486.

7. **3**

Rationale: The sex of the fetus is clearly identifiable by gestational weeks 14 to 16.

Test-Taking Strategy: Knowledge regarding fetal development is required to answer this question. It is important to remember that the sex of the fetus can be determined by gestational weeks 14 to 16. If you had difficulty with this question, take time now to review fetal development!

Level of Cognitive Ability: Analysis
Phase of Nursing Process: Assessment
Client Needs: Physiological Integrity
Content Area: Maternity

Reference
Nichols, F., & Zwelling, E. (1997). *Maternal-newborn nursing: Theory and practice.* Philadelphia: W. B. Saunders. p. 378.

8. **3**

Rationale: Surfactant, a substance needed to facilitate neonatal breathing, begins to be produced at approximately week 28.

Test-Taking Strategy: Knowledge regarding neonatal development in relation to the development of surfactant is needed to answer this question. You are likely to encounter questions related to the respiratory status of the fetus and neonate. If you had difficulty with this question, take time now to review information related to surfactant development!

Level of Cognitive Ability: Analysis
Phase of Nursing Process: Analysis
Client Needs: Physiological Integrity
Content Area: Maternity

Reference
Nichols, F., & Zwelling, E. (1997). *Maternal-newborn nursing: Theory and practice.* Philadelphia: W. B. Saunders. p. 379.

9. **4**

Rationale: The fetal heart beat can first be heard with a fetoscope at 18 to 20 weeks' gestation. If a Doppler ultrasound device is used, the fetal heart rate can be detected as early as 10 weeks' gestation.

Test-Taking Strategy: Knowledge regarding assessment of fetal heart sounds is required to answer this question. It is important that you are familiar with detecting fetal heart sounds. If you had difficulty with this question, take time now to review fetal heart assessment!

Level of Cognitive Ability: Analysis
Phase of Nursing Process: Assessment
Client Needs: Physiological Integrity
Content Area: Maternity

Reference
May, K., & Mahlmeister, L. (1994). *Maternal & neonatal nursing: Family-centered care* (3rd ed.). Philadelphia: J. B. Lippincott. p. 285.

10. **3**

Rationale: The normal fetal heart rate is 120 to 160 beats per minute. If the fetal heart rate is less than 100 or more than 160 beats per minute with the uterus at rest, the fetus may be in distress.

Test-Taking Strategy: Knowledge regarding normal fetal heart rate is required to answer this question. The cardiac status of the fetus is an important part of prenatal assessment. Review fetal heart rate now, if you had difficulty with this question!

Level of Cognitive Ability: Analysis
Phase of Nursing Process: Assessment
Client Needs: Physiological Integrity
Content Area: Maternity

Reference
May, K., & Mahlmeister, L. (1994). *Maternal & neonatal nursing: Family-centered care* (3rd ed.). Philadelphia: J. B. Lippincott. p. 286.

BIBLIOGRAPHY

Black, J., & Matassarin-Jacobs, E. (1997). *Medical-surgical nursing: Clinical management for continuity of care* (5th ed.). Philadelphia: W. B. Saunders.

Martini, F. (1995). *Fundamentals of anatomy and physiology* (3rd ed.). Upper Saddle River, NJ: Prentice-Hall.

May, K., & Mahlmeister, L. (1994). *Maternal & neonatal nursing: Family-centered care* (3rd ed.). Philadelphia: J. B. Lippincott.

Nichols, F., & Zwelling, E. (1997). *Maternal-newborn nursing: Theory and practice*. Philadelphia: W. B. Saunders.

O'Toole, M. (ed.) (1997). *Miller-Keane encyclopedia & dictionary of medicine, nursing, & allied health* (6th ed.). Philadelphia: W. B. Saunders.

CHAPTER 23

Obstetrical Assessment

I. Gestation

A. Estimated date of confinement (EDC)
B. Lasts approximately 280 days
C. **Nagele's Rule** for estimating EDC (Box 23–1)
   1. For **Nagele's rule** to be accurate requires that the woman have a regular 28-day menstrual cycle
   2. Add 7 days to the first day of the last menstrual period (LMP), subtract 3 months, and then add 1 year to that date

II. Gravidity and Parity

A. **Gravidity**
   1. **Gravida** refers to a pregnant woman
   2. **Gravidity** refers to the number of pregnancies
   3. **Nulligravida** is a woman who has never been pregnant
   4. **Primigravida** is a woman who is pregnant for the first time
   5. **Multigravida** is a woman in at least her second pregnancy
B. **Parity**
   1. **Parity** is the number of births (not the number of fetuses, e.g., twins) past 20 weeks' gestation, whether the fetus was born alive or not
   2. **Nullipara** is a woman who has not had a birth at more than 20 weeks of gestation
   3. **Primipara** is a woman who has had one birth that occurs after the 20th week of gestation
   4. **Multipara** is a woman who has had two or more pregnancies resulting in viable offspring

---

BOX 23–1. Nagele's Rule for Estimating EDC

First day of LMP: September 11, 1998
Add 7 days: September 18, 1998
Subtract 3 months: June 18, 1998
Add 1 year: June 18, 1999
EDC: June 18, 1999

III. Pregnancy Signs

A. Presumptive Signs
   1. Amenorrhea
   2. Nausea and vomiting
   3. Increased size and increased feeling of fullness in breasts
   4. Pronounced nipples
   5. Urinary frequency
   6. **Quickening:** First perception of fetal movement in 16th to 18th week
   7. Fatigue
   8. Discoloration and thickening of vaginal mucosa
B. Probable Signs
   1. Uterine enlargement
   2. **Hegar's sign:** Softening of the uterus that occurs about Week 6
   3. **Goodell's sign:** Softening of the cervix that occurs at the beginning of the second month
   4. **Chadwick's sign:** Bluish coloration of the mucous membranes of cervix, vagina, and vulva
   5. **Ballottement:** Rebounding of the fetus against the examiner's fingers on palpation
   6. Braxton Hicks contractions
   7. Positive pregnancy test measuring for human chorionic gonadotropin (hCG)
C. Positive Signs
   1. Fetal heart rate by Doppler at 10 to 12 weeks and by fetoscope at 18 to 20 weeks
   2. Active fetal movements palpable
   3. Outline of fetus via radiography or ultrasound

IV. Fundal Height (Box 23–2)

A. Performed to evaluate fetus's gestational age
B. Between 18 and 32 weeks, fundal height in centimeters equals the fetus's age in weeks
C. At 16 weeks, the fundus can be found halfway between the symphysis pubis and the umbilicus
D. At 20 to 22 weeks, the fundus is at the umbilicus
E. At 36 weeks, the fundus is at the xiphoid process

V. Maternal Risk Factors

A. German Measles (Rubella)

BOX 23-2. Measuring Fundal Height

1. Place client in supine position
2. Place end of tape measure at level of symphysis pubis
3. Stretch tape to top of uterine fundus
4. Note and record measurement

---

1. The risk of maternal and fetal or congenital infection is related to the trimester of placental infection
2. Maternal infection during the first 8 weeks of gestation carries the highest rate of maternal and fetal infection

B. Sexually Transmitted Diseases
1. Syphilis
    a. May cross the **placenta**
    b. Usually leads to spontaneous abortions
    c. Increases the incidence of mental subnormality and physical deformities
2. Genital Herpes
    a. May cross **placenta**
    b. Fetus contaminated after membranes rupture or with vaginal **delivery**
3. *Gonorrhea*
    a. Fetus contaminated at the time of **delivery**
    b. May result in postpartum infection
    c. Risks to the neonate include ophthalmia neonatorum, pneumonia, sepsis

◆ C. Human Immunodeficiency Virus (HIV)
1. The virus is transmitted through blood, blood products, and other body fluids such as urine, semen, vaginal fluid
2. Repeated exposure to HIV during pregnancy through unsafe sex practices or intravenous drug use can increase the risk of transmission to the fetus

◆ D. Substance Abuse
1. Many substances cross the **placenta**, therefore no drugs, including over-the-counter medications, should be taken unless prescribed by the physician
2. Substances commonly abused include alcohol, cocaine, crack, marijuana, amphetamines, barbiturates, and heroin
3. Substance abuse threatens normal fetal growth and successful term completion of the pregnancy
4. Substance abuse places the pregnancy at risk for fetal growth retardation, **abruptio placentae**, and fetal bradycardia
5. Physical signs of drug abuse may include dilated or contracted pupils, fatigue, track marks, skin abscesses, inflamed nasal mucosa, and inappropriate behavior by the mother
6. Alcohol during pregnancy may lead to fetal alcohol syndrome and can cause jitteriness, physical abnormalities, congenital anomalies, and growth deficits
7. Smoking leads to low birth weights, a higher incidence of birth defects, and stillbirths

E. Adolescent Pregnancy
1. Factors that result in adolescent pregnancy include the early onset of menarche, changing sexual behaviors in this age group, faulty family development, poverty, and the lack of knowledge of reproduction and birth control
2. The major concerns related to adolescent pregnancy include poor nutritional status, emotional and behavioral difficulties, lack of support systems, increased risk of stillbirth, low-birth-weight newborn infants, fetal mortality, cephalopelvic disproportion, and the increased risk of maternal complications such as hypertension, anemia, prolonged **labor**, and infections

PRACTICE QUESTIONS

1. The client arrives at the prenatal clinic for the first prenatal assessment. The client tells the nurse that the first day of her last menstrual period was September 19, 1998. Utilizing Nagele's rule, the nurse determines the estimated date of confinement as:
   1 July 26, 1999
   2 June 12, 1999
   3 June 26, 1999
   4 July 12, 1999

2. The client is in her second trimester of pregnancy. During her routine prenatal visit, she states that she frequently has calf pain when she walks. Which of the following should the nurse assess to help differentiate the origin of the discomfort?
   1 Chadwick's sign
   2 Leopold's sign
   3 Homan's sign
   4 Kernig's sign

3. The nurse is collecting data during an admission assessment on a client, pregnant with twins. The client also has a 5-year-old child. The nurse would document which gravida and para status on this client?

   1 Gravida III, para II
   2 Gravida II, para II
   3 Gravida I, para I
   4 Gravida II, para I

4. A primipara is being evaluated in the clinic during her second trimester of pregnancy. Which of the following indicates an abnormal physical finding necessitating further testing?
   1 Consistent increase in fundal height
   2 Fetal heart rate of 180
   3 Braxton Hicks contractions
   4 Quickening

5. In planning the care of a pregnant client with

herpes genitalis, the nurse in the clinic would include which of the following measures in the nursing care plan under the teaching component?

1. Daily administration of acyclovir (Zovirax)
2. Total abstinence from sexual intercourse
3. Sitz bath every 4 hours while awake
4. Preparation for a C-section if vaginal lesions are present at the time of labor

6. The client has tested positive for gonorrhea. Which of the following medications would be prescribed based on this finding?
   1. Ceftriaxone sodium (Rocephin) IM
   2. Penicillin G potassium (Pfizerpen) IM
   3. Metronidazole (Flagyl) PO
   4. Clindamycin phosphate (Cleocin) IV

7. A pregnant client tests positive for hepatitis B virus (HBV). The nurse determines that the client understands about this infection when the client says:
   1. "I know my baby will be immune from hepatitis for the first 2 months of life."
   2. "I feel sad that my baby is going to be isolated in the nursery after my delivery."
   3. "Hepatitis B will cause a severe eye infection in my baby."
   4. "I am so glad that I can breast-feed my baby after it has been vaccinated with immune serum globulin."

8. In the prenatal clinic, the nurse is interviewing a new client for the health history information. What is the best way for the nurse to elicit correct responses to questions that refer to sexually transmitted diseases?
   1. Establish a therapeutic relationship between the nurse and pregnant client
   2. Use specific close-ended questions
   3. Omit this area of questions because they are highly personal
   4. Apologize for the embarrassment that these questions will cause the client

9. The pregnant client is positive for the human immunodeficiency (HIV) virus. Based on this information, the nurse determines that:
   1. The client has the herpes simplex virus
   2. HIV antibodies are detected on the ELISA test
   3. The newborn infant will develop this disease after birth
   4. This client has contracted an airborne disease

10. The nurse is interviewing a 16-year-old girl during her initial prenatal clinic visit. She is beginning Week 18 of her first pregnancy. Which of the following statements made by the client indicates an immediate need for further investigation?
    1. "I don't like my face anymore. I always look like I have been crying."
    2. "I don't like my breasts anymore. These silver lines are ugly."
    3. "I don't like my stomach anymore. That brown line is disgusting."
    4. "I don't like my figure anymore. My clothes are all too tight."

ANSWERS

1. **3**

Rationale: Accurate use of Nagele's rule requires that the woman have a regular 28-day menstrual cycle. Add 7 days to the first day of the last menstrual period (LMP), subtract 3 months, and then add 1 year to that date. First day of the LMP: September 19, 1998; add 7 days: September 26, 1998; subtract 3 months: June 26, 1998; add 1 year: June 26, 1999.

Test-Taking Strategy: Knowledge regarding the use of Nagele's rule is required to answer this question. Use caution when following steps to determine the EDC. Avoid taking short-cuts, particularly when math is involved. Read all the options carefully, noting the dates and years in the options before selecting an option. Review Nagele's rule now, if you had difficulty with this question!

Level of Cognitive Ability: Analysis
Phase of Nursing Process: Assessment
Client Needs: Physiological Integrity
Content Area: Maternity

Reference
Nichols, F., & Zwelling, E. (1997). *Maternal-newborn nursing: Theory and practice*. Philadelphia: W. B. Saunders. p. 405.

2. **3**

Rationale: Chadwick's sign is a cervical change and is a presumptive sign of pregnancy. Leopold's sign is a fictitious term. Leopold's maneuvers are a series of abdominal palpation maneuvers that provide information regarding fetal presentation, position, presenting part, attitude, and descent. Kernig's sign tests for meningeal irritability. Homan's sign tests for venous thrombosis of the lower extremity. Pain in the calf during walking could indicate venous thrombosis.

Test-Taking Strategy: Knowledge of the signs related to pregnancy and signs indicating a potential problem are required to answer this question. Review the signs identified in the options now, if you had difficulty with this question!

Level of Cognitive Ability: Application
Phase of Nursing Process: Assessment
Client Needs: Physiological Integrity
Content Area: Maternity

Reference
Gorrie, T., McKinney, E.S., & Murray, S.S. (1998). *Foundations of maternal-newborn nursing* (2nd ed.). Philadelphia: W. B. Saunders. p. 793.

3. **4**

Rationale: Gravida is a term that refers to a woman who is or has been pregnant regardless of the duration of the pregnancy. Para is a term that means the number of pregnancies that have progressed past 20 weeks' gestation. Parity does not reflect the number of fetuses or infants. Therefore, option 4 is the only correct answer for a woman currently pregnant with twins and who has had one other pregnancy past 20 weeks' gestation. Options 1, 2, and 3 are incorrect based on these definitions.

Test-Taking Strategy: Knowledge and understanding of the terms gravida and para is necessary in order to answer this question correctly. If you had difficulty answering this question, review these definitions now!

Level of Cognitive Ability: Application
Phase of Nursing Process: Assessment
Client Needs: Physiological Integrity
Content Area: Maternity

Reference
Gorrie, T., McKinney, E.S., & Murray, S.S. (1998). *Foundations of maternal-newborn nursing* (2nd ed.). Philadelphia: W. B. Saunders. p. 296.

4. **2**

Rationale: The fetal heart rate should be 120 to 160 beats per minute throughout pregnancy. Option 1 is a normal, expected finding. An important factor to assess regarding uterine growth is its constant, steady, predictable increase in size. Option 3 is a normal finding. Uterine contractions begin early in pregnancy and are present throughout the rest of the pregnancy, becoming stronger and harder as the pregnancy advances. These are termed Braxton Hicks contractions. Option 4 is also a normal finding. Fetal movement can be felt by the mother beginning at 18 to 20 weeks of pregnancy and reaches a peak at 29 to 38 weeks.

Test-Taking Strategy: This question asks you to select the response that would indicate that the client needs further testing. Be careful with this type of question. Read each response and eliminate those answers that are inaccurate. Knowledge regarding normal fetal growth and development is essential in answering this question correctly. Also, you need to identify the components of the question. The case situation gives you information about a clinical health problem and the information you need to consider in answering the question. Review normal assessment findings in pregnancy now, if you had difficulty with this question!

Level of Cognitive Ability: Application
Phase of Nursing Process: Assessment
Client Needs: Physiological Integrity
Content Area: Maternity

Reference
Nichols, F., & Zwelling, E. (1997). *Maternal-newborn nursing: Theory and practice.* Philadelphia: W. B. Saunders. pp. 947–948.

5. **4**

Rationale: For women with active lesions, either recurrent or primary, at the time of labor, delivery should be cesarean; therefore, option 4 is correct. The safety of acyclovir has not been established during pregnancy and should be used only when there is a life-threatening infection. Option 2 is incorrect. Clients should be advised to abstain from sexual contact while the lesions are present. If it is an initial infection, they should continue to abstain until they become culture-negative because prolonged viral shedding may occur in such cases. Option 3 is incorrect. Keeping the genital area clean and dry will promote healing.

Test-Taking Strategy: It is necessary to understand the physiology and the treatment plan for the client to answer this question. If you had difficulty with this question, review content related to herpes as a maternal risk factor now!

Level of Cognitive Ability: Application
Phase of Nursing Process: Planning
Client Needs: Safe, Effective Care Environment
Content Area: Maternity

References
Nichols, F., & Zwelling, E. (1997). *Maternal-newborn nursing: Theory and practice.* Philadelphia: W. B. Saunders. p 1496.
Olds, S., London, M., & Ladewig, P. (1996). *Maternal-newborn nursing: A family-centered approach* (5th ed.). Reading, MA: Addison-Wesley. p. 242.

6. **1**

Rationale: Treatment for gonorrhea consists of antibiotic therapy with ceftriaxone IM or oral amoxicillin plus oral doxycycline for 7 days; therefore, option 1 is correct. Option 2 is the treatment for syphilis, option 3 is the treatment for trichomoniasis, and option 4 is the treatment for bacterial vaginosis.

Test-Taking Strategy: The issue of the question is the specific subject content that the question is asking about—in this case, the specific medication required to treat the disease. Review content regarding gonorrhea and the medication used to treat this sexually transmitted disease now, if you had difficulty with this question!

Level of Cognitive Ability: Application
Phase of Nursing Process: Implementation
Client Needs: Physiological Integrity
Content Area: Maternity

Reference
Gorrie, T., McKinney, E.S., & Murray, S.S. (1998). *Foundations of maternal-newborn nursing* (2nd ed.). Philadelphia: W. B. Saunders. p 954.

7. **4**

Rationale: Although HBV is transmitted in breast milk, once serum immune globulin has been administered women may breast feed-without risk to the neonate; therefore, option 4 is correct. Option 1 is incorrect. To reduce the possibility of hepatitis B virus being spread to newborn infants, neonates are now routinely vaccinated at birth. Options 2 and 3 are not true. The neonate should be bathed as soon as possible after birth to remove HBV-infected blood and secretions. Ophthalmia neonatorum is an eye infection present at birth or occurring during the first month, caused most commonly by gonorrhea or chlamydia.

Test-Taking Strategy: This question requires an understanding of hepatitis B virus and its effects on the fetus and neonate. If you had difficulty with this question, review the content related to HBV. It is very likely that you will see questions related to HBV on NCLEX-RN!

Level of Cognitive Ability: Analysis
Phase of Nursing Process: Evaluation
Client Needs: Health Promotion and Maintenance
Content Area: Maternity

Reference
Nichols, F., & Zwelling, E. (1997). *Maternal-newborn nursing: Theory and practice.* Philadelphia: W. B. Saunders. pp 1492–1493.

8. **1**

Rationale: The initial assessment interview establishes the therapeutic relationship between the nurse and the pregnant woman. It is planned, purposeful communication that focuses on specific content. Options 2, 3, and 4 are incorrect and would not lend themselves to eliciting correct responses.

Test-Taking Strategy: Look for the answer to this question that focuses on the client as a worthy human being. Try to visualize the client as you go through the case situation and the question. Read the options carefully and utilize the process of elimination. Remember, establishing a therapeutic relationship is most meaningful!

Level of Cognitive Ability: Application
Phase of Nursing Process: Implementation
Client Needs: Psychosocial Integrity
Content Area: Maternity

Reference
Nichols, F., & Zwelling, E. (1997). *Maternal-newborn nursing: Theory and practice.* Philadelphia: W. B. Saunders. p. 1497.

9. **2**

Rationale: Option 2 is the correct response. Diagnosis depends on serological studies to detect HIV antibodies. The most commonly used test is the enzyme-linked immunosorbent assay (ELISA test). Options 1 and 4 are incorrect because HIV stands for human immunodeficiency virus, and it occurs primarily through the exchange of body fluids. Option 3 is incorrect. A neonate born to an HIV-positive mother has a 20% to 40% risk of developing this disease.

Test-Taking Strategy: Eliminating the incorrect options can be utilized here. Read all of the options very carefully before selecting an answer, and reread the stem of the question before selecting an answer. Knowledge related to HIV is required to answer this question. Review this content now, if you had difficulty with this question. You are very likely to see questions on HIV in the NCLEX-RN exam!

Level of Cognitive Ability: Analysis
Phase of the Nursing Process: Analysis
Client Needs: Physiological Integrity
Content Area: Maternity

Reference
Nichols, F., & Zwelling, E. (1997). *Maternal-newborn nursing: Theory and practice.* Philadelphia: W. B. Saunders. p. 1498.

10. **1**

Rationale: Options 2, 3, and 4 are dealing with body image. Although these comments should not be ignored, the need for follow-up is not urgent. In option 1, there is an implication of periorbital and facial edema that could indicate pregnancy-induced hypertension (PIH). Since this is an adolescent who has not sought early prenatal care, she is at higher risk for the development of PIH.

Test-Taking Strategy: Identify the key words in the question, such as "immediate need." Note the week of the first prenatal visit (Week 18). Set priorities using assessment data without reading more data into the question, and use the process of elimination to select the correct answer. Promote physiological integrity by using assessment factors to suspect a serious condition that could develop pregnancy-induced hypertension. Review assessment signs related to PIH now, if you had difficulty with this question!

Level of Cognitive Ability: Analysis
Phase of Nursing Process: Assessment
Client Needs: Physiological Integrity
Content Area: Maternity

References
Nichols, F., & Zwelling, E. (1997). *Maternal-newborn nursing: Theory and practice.* Philadelphia: W. B. Saunders. p. 645.
Gorrie, T., McKinney, E.S. & Murray, S.S. (1998). *Foundations of maternal-newborn nursing* (2nd ed.). Philadelphia: W. B. Saunders. p. 703.

BIBLIOGRAPHY

Bobak, I., et al. (1995). *Maternity nursing* (4th ed.). St. Louis: Mosby–Year Book.

Gorrie, T., McKinney, E.S., & Murray, S.S. (1994). *Foundations of maternal newborn nursing.* Philadelphia: W. B. Saunders.

Nichols, F., & Zwelling, E. (1997). *Maternal-newborn nursing: Theory and practice.* Philadelphia: W. B. Saunders.

Olds, S., London, M., & Ladewig, P. (1996). *Maternal-newborn nursing: A family-centered approach* (5th ed.). Reading, MA: Addison-Wesley.

Pillitteri, A., (1995). *Maternal and child health nursing: Care of the childbearing and childrearing family* (2nd ed.). Philadelphia: J. B. Lippincott.

CHAPTER 24

Prenatal Period

I. Physiological Maternal Changes

A. Cardiovascular System
   1. Circulating blood volume increases, plasma increases, total volume increases by 40% to 50%
   2. Total red cell volume increases
   3. Physiological anemia occurs as the plasma increase exceeds the increase in red blood cell (RBC) production
   4. Heart size increases with left ventricular hypertrophy
   5. Heart is elevated upward and to the left due to displacement of the diaphragm as the uterus enlarges
   6. Pulse may increase about 10 beats per minute
   7. Blood pressure may decline in the second trimester
   8. Iron requirements are increased
   9. Retention of sodium and water may occur

B. Respiratory System
   1. Oxygen consumption increases by 15% to 20%
   2. Diaphragm is elevated due to the enlarged uterus
   3. Respiratory rate remains unchanged
   4. Shortness of breath may be experienced

C. Gastrointestinal System
   1. Nausea and vomiting may occur due to the secretion of human chorionic gonadotropin (hCG) and which subsides by the third month
   2. Poor appetite may occur due to decreased gastric motility and acidity
   3. Alterations in taste and smell
   4. Constipation due to decreased GI motility or pressure of the uterus
   5. Flatulence and heartburn due to decreased motility and slow emptying of the stomach
   6. Hemorrhoids due to increased venous pressure
   7. Gum tissue may become swollen and bleed easily
   8. Ptyalism (excessive secretion of saliva)

D. Renal System
   1. Frequency of urination occurs in the first and third trimester due to pressure of the enlarging uterus on the bladder
   2. Decreased bladder tone is caused by hormonal changes
   3. Decreased bladder capacity
   4. Renal function increases
   5. Renal threshold for glucose may be reduced

E. Endocrine System
   1. Basal metabolic rate rises
   2. Anterior lobe of the pituitary gland enlarges
   3. Thyroid enlarges slightly, and thyroid activity increases
   4. Aldosterone levels gradually increase
   5. Parathyroid increases in size

F. Reproductive System
   1. Uterus
      a. Uterus enlarges from a weight of 60 g to 1000 g
      b. Size and number of blood vessels and lymphatics increase
      c. Irregular contractions occur
   2. Cervix
      a. Becomes shorter, more elastic, and larger in diameter
      b. Endocervical glands secrete a thick mucus plug, which is expelled from the canal when dilation begins
      c. Increased vascularization causes a softening and blue-purple discoloration **(Chadwick's sign)**
   3. Ovaries
      a. The maturation of new follicles is blocked
      b. The ovaries cease ovum production
   4. Vagina
      a. Hypertrophy and thickening of muscle
      b. Increase in vaginal secretions, and secretions are usually thick, white, and acidic
   5. Breast
      a. Breast size increases
      b. Nipples become more pronounced
      c. Areola becomes darker in color

d. Superficial veins become prominent
e. Hypertrophy of the Montgomery follicles occurs
f. Colostrum may appear from the breast

G. Skin
1. Pigmentation increases
2. A dark streak down the midline of the abdomen may appear (linea nigra)
3. Melasma, or mask of pregnancy, may occur over the forehead, cheeks, and nose
4. Reddish-purple stretch marks (striae) may occur on the abdomen, breasts, thighs, and upper arms
5. Vascular spider nevi may occur on the neck, chest, face, arms, and legs
6. Hair rate growth may decrease

H. Skeletal System
1. Center of gravity changes
2. Postural changes occur as the increased weight of the uterus causes a forward pull of the bony pelvis

I. Metabolism
1. Metabolic functions increase
2. Body weight increases
3. The average expected weight gain during pregnancy is 2 to 4 pounds in the first trimester, and approximately 1 pound per week in the second and third trimesters
4. Water retention is increased, which can contribute to weight gain

II. Psychological Maternal Changes

A. Ambivalence
1. Occurs early in pregnancy even when the pregnancy is planned
2. Mother may experience dependence-independence conflict and ambivalence related to role changes
3. Father may experience ambivalence related to the new role he is assuming, the increased financial responsibilities, and sharing the wife's attention with the child

B. Acceptance
1. Factors that may be related to acceptance of the pregnancy are the woman's readiness for the experience and her identification with the motherhood role
2. When the mother plans and expects the pregnancy, she tends to display pleasure and experience fewer physical discomforts

C. Emotional Lability
1. May be manifested by frequency in the change of emotional states or extremes in emotional states
2. These emotional changes are common, and the mother may feel that these changes are abnormal

D. Body Image Changes
1. The change in a woman's perception of her image during pregnancy occurs gradually and may be either positive or negative
2. The physical changes and symptoms that the woman experiences during pregnancy contribute to her body image

III. Discomforts of Pregnancy

A. Nausea and Vomiting
1. Occurs in the first trimester
2. Due to elevated hCG levels and changes in carbohydrate metabolism
3. Implementation
   a. Eating dry crackers before arising
   b. Eating small, frequent, low-fat meals during the day
   c. Drinking liquids between meals
   d. Avoiding all antiemetics throughout pregnancy
   e. Avoiding fried foods

B. Syncope
1. Usually occurs in the first trimester
2. May be hormonally triggered or caused by increased blood volume, anemia, fatigue, or sudden position changes
3. Implementation
   a. Sitting with the feet up
   b. Changing positions slowly
   c. Changing the position to the left side to relieve the pressure of the uterus on the inferior vena cava

C. Urinary Urgency and Frequency
1. Usually occurs in first and third trimesters
2. Due to pressure of the uterus on the bladder
3. Implementation
   a. Drinking 2 quarts of fluid per day
   b. Limiting fluid intake in the evening
   c. Voiding at regular intervals
   d. Sleeping on the side at night
   e. Wearing perineal pads if necessary

D. Breast Tenderness
1. Can occur from the first through third trimesters
2. Due to increased levels of estrogen and progesterone
3. Implementation
   a. Encouraging the use of a supportive bra with nonelastic straps
   b. Avoiding the use of soap on the nipples and areolar area to prevent drying

E. Increased Vaginal Discharge
1. Can occur from the first through third trimesters
2. Due to hyperplasia of vaginal mucosa and increased mucus production
3. Implementation
   a. Wearing cotton underwear
   b. Avoiding douching
   c. Proper cleansing and hygiene
   d. Advising the client to consult the physician or health care provider if infection is suspected

F. Nasal Stuffiness

1. Occurs during the first through third trimesters
2. Occurs due to increased estrogen that causes swelling of the nasal tissues and dryness
3. Implementation
   a. Encouraging the use of a humidifier
   b. Avoiding the use of nasal sprays or antihistamines

G. Fatigue
1. Occurs usually in the first and third trimesters
2. Usually a result of hormonal changes
3. Implementation
   a. Arranging frequent rest periods throughout the day
   b. Obtaining regular exercise
   c. Avoiding eating and drinking foods containing stimulants throughout pregnancy

H. Heartburn
1. Occurs in the second and third trimesters
2. Results from increased progesterone levels, decreased GI motility and esophageal reflux, and displacement of the stomach by the enlarging uterus
3. Implementation
   a. Eating small, frequent meals
   b. Sitting upright for 30 minutes following a meal
   c. Avoiding fatty and spicy food
   d. Drinking milk between meals
   e. Avoiding antacids and histamine receptor antagonists throughout pregnancy
   f. Administering antacids (Maalox or Mylanta) only when recommended by the physician

I. Ankle Edema
1. Usually occurs in second and third trimesters
2. Occurs due to vasodilation, venous stasis, and increased venous pressure below the uterus
3. Implementation
   a. Elevating legs at least twice a day
   b. Sleeping on the left side
   c. Wearing supportive stockings
   d. Avoiding sitting or standing in one position for long periods of time
   e. Avoiding the use of diuretics during pregnancy

J. Varicose Veins
1. Usually occurs in the second and third trimesters
2. Occurs due to weakening walls of the veins or valves and venous congestion
3. Implementation
   a. Elevating feet when sitting
   b. Using support hose
   c. Sitting or lying with feet and hips elevated
   d. Moving about while standing to improve circulation
   e. Avoiding pressure on the lower thighs

f. Avoiding leg-crossing
g. Avoiding long periods of standing or sitting
h. Avoiding constricting articles of clothing

K. Headache
1. Usually occurs in the second and third trimesters
2. Occurs due to changes in blood volume and vascular tone
3. Implementation
   a. Changing position slowly
   b. Applying a cool cloth to the forehead
   c. Eating a small snack
   d. Using acetaminophen (Tylenol) sparingly, only if prescribed by the physician

L. Hemorrhoids
1. Usually occurs in second and third trimesters
2. Occurs due to increased venous pressure and/or constipation
3. Implementation
   a. Soaking in a warm sitz bath
   b. Sitting on soft pillow
   c. Eating a high-fiber diet and avoiding constipation
   d. Drinking sufficient fluids
   e. Increasing exercise, such as walking
   f. Applying ointments, suppositories, warm compresses as prescribed

M. Constipation
1. Usually occurs in the second and third trimesters
2. Occurs due to decreased intestinal motility, the displacement of the intestines, and taking iron supplements
3. Implementation
   a. Eating high-roughage foods, such as fresh fruits, vegetables, and bran
   b. Drinking plenty of fluids
   c. Exercising regularly
   d. Avoiding mineral oil or castor oil laxatives and using psyllium (Metamucil), senna (Senokot), or 1 teaspoon of milk of magnesia at bedtime sparingly, only as prescribed by the physician

N. Backache
1. Usually occurs in the second and third trimesters
2. Occurs from an exaggerated lumbosacral curve due to the enlarged uterus
3. Implementation
   a. Encouraging rest
   b. Utilizing good body mechanics
   c. Improving posture
   d. Wearing low-heeled shoes
   e. Performing pelvic lift exercises and exercises such as squatting, sitting, and pelvic rocking
   f. Sleeping on a firm mattress

O. Leg Cramps
1. Usually occurs in second and third trimesters
2. Occurs due to an altered calcium-phosphorus

balance and pressure of the uterus on nerves, or from fatigue
   3. Implementation
      a. Getting regular exercise, especially walking
      b. Elevating the feet and dorsiflexing the feet when resting
      c. Increasing calcium intake
P. Shortness of Breath
   1. Can occur in the second and third trimesters
   2. Occurs due to pressure on the diaphragm
   3. Implementation
      a. Allowing frequent rest periods
      b. Sleeping with the head elevated or on the side
      c. Avoiding overexertion

IV. Laboratory Tests (Box 24–1)

A. Blood Type and Rh Factor
   1. ABO typing is performed to determine the woman's blood type
   2. Rh typing is done to determine the presence or absence of Rh antigen (Rh-positive or Rh-negative)
   3. If the client is Rh negative and has a negative antibody screen, the client will need repeat antibody screens and should receive Rh immune globulin at 28 weeks' gestation
B. Rubella Titer
   1. If the client has a negative titer, indicating susceptibility to the rubella virus, the client should receive the appropriate immunization postpartum
   2. The client must be using effective birth control at the time of the immunization and counseled not to become pregnant for 3 months following immunization
C. Hemoglobin and Hematocrit Levels
   1. Hemoglobin and hematocrit levels will drop during gestation as a result of increased plasma volume
   2. An increase in the hematocrit level may indicate the development of pregnancy-induced hypertension (PIH)
   3. A fall in hemoglobin and hematocrit levels indicates anemia
D. Papanicolaou Smear
   1. Done during the initial prenatal examination
   2. Done to screen for cervical neoplasia
E. Gonorrhea Culture
   1. Screening test for gonorrhea
   2. The test may be repeated during the third trimester in high-risk clients

F. Syphilis Screening
   1. Screening test for syphilis
   2. May be repeated during the third trimester in high-risk clients
G. Herpes Cultures
   1. Indicated for clients with a positive history or those with active lesions
   2. Performed to determine the route of **delivery**
   3. Weekly cultures may be done beginning at the 35th or 36th week of pregnancy until delivery
H. Chlamydia Culture
   1. Indicated if the client is in a high-risk group
   2. Indicated if infants from previous pregnancies have developed neonatal conjunctivitis or pneumonia
I. Sickle Cell Screening
   1. Indicated for clients at risk for sickle cell disease
   2. A positive test may indicate a need for further screening
J. Tuberculin Skin Test
   1. Indicated only if all past skin tests have been negative; may not be done until after delivery
   2. A positive skin test indicates the need for chest radiograph (using an abdominal lead shield) to rule out active disease
   3. Converters to positive may be referred for treatment with medication following **delivery**
K. Hepatitis B Surface Antigens
   1. Recommended for all women because of the prevalence of the disease in the general population
   2. Vaccination for nonimmunity for hepatitis B antigen may be indicated specifically for:
      a. Health care workers
      b. Clients born in Asia, Africa, Haiti, or the Pacific islands
      c. Clients with previously undiagnosed jaundice or chronic liver disease
      d. IV drug abusers
      e. Clients with tattoos
      f. Clients with histories of blood transfusions
      g. Clients with histories of multiple episodes of sexually transmitted diseases
      h. Clients who have been previously rejected as blood donors
      i. Clients with histories of dialysis or renal transplantation
      j. Clients from households having hepatitis B–infected members or hemodialysis clients
L. Urinalysis and Urine Culture
   1. A urine specimen for glucose and protein determinations should be obtained at every prenatal visit
   2. Glycosuria is a common result of decreased renal threshold in pregnancy

---

BOX 24–1. Prenatal Visits

Every 4 weeks first 28 to 32 weeks
Every 2 weeks from 32 to 36 weeks
Every week from 36 to 40 weeks

3. If glycosuria persists, this may indicate diabetes
4. White blood cells in the urine may indicate infection
5. Ketonuria may result from insufficient food intake or vomiting
6. Levels of 2+ to 4+ protein in the urine may indicate infection or PIH

V. Diagnostic Tests

A. Ultrasound
1. Outlines and identifies fetal and maternal structures
2. Assists in confirmation of estimated date of **delivery**
3. Implementation
   a. Instruct client to drink 6 to 8 glasses of water before the test and not to void as the test is done with a full bladder
   b. Inform the client that the test presents no known risks to client or fetus

---

BOX 24–2. Nonstress Test (NST)

DESCRIPTION

Performed to assess placental function and oxygenation

Determines fetal well-being

Evaluates fetal heart rate (FHR) in response to fetal movement

IMPLEMENTATION

External ultrasound transducer and the tocodynamometer (toco) are applied to the mother, and a tracing of at least 20 minutes' duration is obtained so that the FHR and the uterine activity can be observed

Obtain baseline blood pressure and monitor BP frequently

Position mother in the left lateral position to avoid vena cava compression

Ask mother to press a button every time she feels fetal movement

The monitor records a mark at each occurrence of fetal movement, which is used as a reference point to assess FHR response

RESULTS

Reactive Nonstress Test (Normal/Negative)
Indicates a healthy fetus
Two or more fetal heart rate accelerations of at least 15 beats per minute, lasting at least 15 seconds from the beginning of the acceleration to the end, in association with fetal movement, during a 20-minute period

Nonreactive Nonstress Test (Abnormal)
No accelerations or accelerations of less than 15 beats per minute or lasting less than 15 seconds in duration during a 40-minute observation

Unsatisfactory
Cannot be interpreted because of the poor quality of the FHR

BOX 24–3. Contraction Stress Test

DESCRIPTION

Assesses placental oxygenation and function

Determines fetal ability to tolerate labor and determines fetal well-being

Fetus is exposed to the stressor of contractions to assess the adequacy of placental perfusion under simulated labor conditions

Performed if nonstress test is abnormal

IMPLEMENTATION

The external fetal monitor is applied to the mother, and a 20- to 30-minute baseline strip is recorded

The uterus is stimulated to contract either by the administration of a dilute dose of oxytocin (Pitocin) or by having the mother use nipple stimulation until 3 palpable contractions with a duration of 40 seconds or more in a 10-minute period have been achieved

Frequent maternal BP readings are done, and the client is monitored closely while increasing doses of oxytocin are given

RESULTS

Negative Contraction Stress Test
Represented by no late or variable decelerations of the fetal heart rate

Positive Contraction Stress Test (Abnormal)
Represented by late or variable decelerations with 50% or more of the contractions in the absence of hyperstimulation of the uterus

Equivocal
Contains decelerations but with less than 50% of the contractions, or the uterine activity shows a hyperstimulated uterus

Unsatisfactory
Adequate uterine contractions cannot be achieved, or the FHR tracing is not of sufficient quality for adequate interpretation

---

B. Alpha-Fetoprotein Screening (AFP)
1. Assesses the quantity of fetal serum proteins; if elevated, is associated with open neural tube and abdominal wall defects
2. Can detect spina bifida and Down's syndrome
3. Implementation
   a. Explain that the level is determined by a single maternal blood sample drawn at 15 to 18 weeks' gestation
   b. If the level is elevated and the gestation is less than 18 weeks, a second sample is drawn
   c. An ultrasound is performed for elevated levels to rule out fetal abnormalities or multiple gestation
C. Chorionic Villus Sampling (CVS)
1. Aspiration of a small sample of chorionic villus tissue at 8 to 12 weeks' gestation

2. Test is performed for the purpose of detecting genetic abnormalities
3. Implementation
   a. Instruct client to drink water to fill the bladder before the procedure to aid in the position of the uterus for catheter insertion
   b. Instruct the client to report bleeding, infection, or leakage of fluid at insertion site after procedure
   c. Rh-negative women may be given RhoGAM for risks related to the procedure

D. Kick Test (Fetal Movement Counting)
   1. Mother lies down on the left side for 1 hour after meals and counts fetal kicks for 30 minutes
   2. Instruct client to notify physician or health care provider if there are fewer than 5 kicks in 1 hour

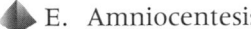 E. Amniocentesis
   1. Aspiration of **amniotic fluid** is done from 14 weeks of pregnancy and on
   2. Performed to determine genetic disorders, the sex of the fetus, and fetal lung maturity
   3. Risks
      a. Maternal hemorrhage
      b. Infection
      c. Rh isoimmunization
      d. Abruptio placentae
      e. Amniotic fluid emboli
   4. Implementation
      a. Instruct client to empty bladder before procedure
      b. Prepare client for ultrasound, which is performed to locate the **placenta**
      c. Obtain baseline vital signs and FHR, and monitor every 15 minutes
      d. Position client supine
      e. Instruct client that if chills, fever, leakage of fluid at the needle insertion site, decreased fetal movement, or uterine contractions occur, to notify the physician or health care provider

F. Fern Test
   1. A microscopic slide test to determine the presence of **amniotic fluid** leakage
   2. Specimen is obtained from the external os of the cervix and vaginal pool
   3. Fluid is examined on a slide under a microscope
   4. A fernlike pattern occurring from the salts of amniotic fluid indicates the presence of **amniotic fluid**
   5. Implementation
      a. Position client in the dorsal lithotomy position
      b. Instruct the client to cough to cause the fluid to leak from the uterus if the membranes are ruptured

G. Nitrazine Test
   1. Use of Nitrazine test strip or cotton swab to detect the presence of **amniotic fluid** in vaginal secretions
   2. Vaginal secretions have a pH of 4.5 to 5.5 and do not affect the yellow Nitrazine strip or swab
   3. Amniotic fluid has a pH of 7.0 to 7.5 and turns the yellow Nitrazine blue
   4. Implementation
      a. Position the client in dorsal lithotomy position
      b. Touch the test tape to the fluid
      c. Assess the test tape for a blue-green, blue-gray, or deep blue color, which indicates that the membranes are probably ruptured

VI. Nutrition

A. General Guidelines (Box 24–4)
   1. The average expected weight gain during pregnancy is 2 to 4 pounds in the first trimester and approximately 1 pound per week in the second and third trimesters
   2. Choose foods from the four basic food groups or food guide pyramid
   3. An increase of about 300 calories per day is needed during pregnancy
   4. A diet consisting of 2500 calories per day, depending on age, should meet the nutritional demands of pregnancy
   5. Calorie needs are greater in the last two trimesters than in the first
   6. An increase of about 500 calories per day is needed during lactation
   7. Encourage a diet high in folic acid with folic acid supplements
   8. A diet rich in folic acid is necessary for all women of childbearing age to prevent neural tube defect
   9. Increase calories, proteins, vitamins, calcium, and other minerals as required
   10. Drink at least 8 glasses of water a day
   11. Sodium is not restricted unless specifically ordered by the physician

---

BOX 24–4. Cultural Considerations in Nutrition

Asian, Chinese, and Japanese
Important diet foods include seafood, rice, vegetables, and fresh fruits
Milk and cheese are used infrequently

Jewish Orthodox
Poultry and some meat of cattle, sheep, goats, and deer are permissible; pork and pork products are not permissible
Milk and cheese may not be eaten with or within 6 hours of a meat meal

Mexican
Food products include corn, chili peppers, and beans
Milk is used infrequently

B. Vegetarianism
   1. During pregnancy, it is necessary to obtain ample and complete proteins from dairy products and eggs
   2. An adequate pure vegetarian diet contains protein from unrefined grains such as brown rice and whole wheat; legumes such as beans, split peas, and lentils; nuts in large quantities; and a variety of cooked and fresh vegetables and fruits
   3. Seeds may provide protein if the quantity is large enough
   4. Vegetarians do not eat any animal products, therefore a daily supplement of 4 μg of vitamin B_{12} is necessary
   5. Complete protein may be obtained by eating any of the following food combinations at the same time:
      a. Legumes and whole grain cereals
      b. Nuts and whole grain cereals
      c. Nuts and legumes
C. Lactose Intolerance
   1. Lactose consumed by an individual with an intolerance can cause abdominal distention, discomfort, nausea, vomiting, loose stool, and cramps
   2. Milk may be tolerated in cooked form, as in custards or fermented dairy products
   3. Cheese and yogurt are sometimes tolerated
   4. Lactase, an enzyme, may be prescribed and is available as a tablet to be chewed before ingesting milk or milk products or as a liquid to add to milk
   5. Lactase-treated milk or lactose-free products are also available commercially
D. Pica
   1. Defined as eating substances that are not ordinarily considered to be edible or to have nutritive value
   2. Practiced in poverty-stricken areas where diets tend to be inadequate, but pica may also be found at other socioeconomic levels
   3. Substances most commonly ingested are dirt, clay, starch, and freezer frost
   4. Iron deficiency anemia occurs as a result of pica

PRACTICE QUESTIONS

1. The client is in her second trimester of pregnancy. She complains of frequent low back pain and ankle edema at the end of the day. Which of the following measures can be recommended by the nurse to help relieve both discomforts?
   1 Lie on the floor with legs elevated onto a couch or padded chair, hips and knees at right angles
   2 Lie on the left side with feet dorsiflexed
   3 Soak feet in hot water after performing 10 pelvic tilt exercises
   4 Lie on the right side with feet elevated on a pillow and heating pad to the back

2. Which of the following nursing orders would be most appropriate to include in the teaching plan for the pregnant woman to strengthen the pelvic floor and decrease the incidence of stress incontinence later in life?
   1 Drink 8 ounces of fluid six times per day
   2 Wipe the perineal area anterior to posterior after toileting
   3 Perform Kegel exercises in 10 repetitions, five times per day
   4 Perform pelvic tilt exercises in 10 repetitions, three times per day

3. The client is 8 weeks pregnant and has waves of nausea accompanied by vomiting throughout the day. Food odors consistently precipitate the nausea. Her husband has an important business dinner planned and she is reluctant to attend due to the nausea and vomiting. This has placed a strain on the husband-wife relationship. Which of the following statements by the nurse indicates an understanding of the problem?
   1 "You feel you are having difficulty fulfilling your role as a wife."
   2 "You are afraid your husband will go to dinner without you."
   3 "You are not physically able to go to dinner and should stay at home."
   4 "You should go to dinner. Others will understand if you don't feel well."

4. The client is beginning Week 30 of gestation. She has come to the clinic for a routine visit. She is wearing hose and flat shoes. Which of the following observations, if made by the nurse, indicates a need for teaching?
   1 Client is wearing panty hose
   2 Client is wearing shoes with arch supports
   3 Client is wearing nonslip shoes
   4 Client is wearing knee-high hose

5. The client is 15 years old. In addition to being pregnant, she is being treated by a dermatologist for acne. Which of the following will most likely be avoided with this client?
   1 Topical erythromycin
   2 Exfoliation
   3 Cleansing with antibacterial soap
   4 Oral tetracycline

6. The plan of care for the pregnant teen should include teaching regarding which of the following concerning dental care?
   1 Use toothpaste with baking soda to decrease plaque build-up
   2 Avoid the use of local anesthetics during dental work
   3 Expect to lose at least one tooth because of calcium and phosphorus leaving the teeth to nourish the fetus
   4 Tell the dentist office staff that she is pregnant

7. A client is admitted to the nursing unit for observation because of suspected preterm labor. During the nurse's initial assessment, hemorrhoids are noted. The client reports that she has been experiencing pain due to the hemorrhoids. Which of the following statements, if made by the client, would identify the need for further teaching regarding hemorrhoids?
   1 "Hemorrhoids are caused by the changes in hormones during pregnancy. They will go away after the baby is born."
   2 "Hemorrhoids are aggravated by standing for long periods of time. I need to lie down periodically during the day to relieve the pressure."
   3 "Hemorrhoids can be gently pushed back inside the body using a lubricant."
   4 "Diet is very important in the treatment of hemorrhoids. Plenty of liquids and a balance of bulk in the diet are needed."

8. A pregnant woman complains of being frequently awakened by leg cramps. Which of the instructions would the nurse implement?
   1 Teach the partner to dorsiflex the client's foot while flexing the knee
   2 Teach the partner to dorsiflex the client's foot while extending the knee
   3 Teach the partner to plantarflex the client's foot while flexing the knee
   4 Teach the partner to plantarflex the client's foot while extending the knee

9. In formulating the plan of care for the alleviation of dyspepsia during pregnancy, the nurse instructs the client to:
   1 Lie down for 30 minutes after eating
   2 Drink decaffeinated coffee and tea
   3 Use spices other than salt when cooking
   4 Eliminate between-meal snacks

10. The client, who is 10 weeks pregnant, states she tires very easily. Her hemoglobin is 11.2 gm/100 ml, and her hematocrit is 28%. Nocturia has become a problem. She has a child 18 months old and works 8 hours per day as a legal secretary. Based on these data, the most accurate nursing diagnosis is:
    1 Fatigue related to altered body chemistry, increased energy requirements
    2 Sleep pattern disturbance related to pregnancy
    3 Ineffective coping related to motherhood
    4 Nutrition, less than body requirements, related to anemia

11. The client is a gravida IV, para III in her final trimester of pregnancy. She does not attend usual social functions due to the fear of stress incontinence. Her oldest child is in a school play that she wants to attend. Which of the following will the nurse discuss with her to promote attendance at the play?
    1 Instruct her to perform Kegel exercises during the play
    2 Instruct her to limit her fluid intake to 500 mL the day of the play
    3 Instruct her to wear a perineal pad to the play
    4 Instruct her to have a friend videotape the play for her

12. Which of the following nursing interventions should be included in the plan of care for the pregnant woman who complains of low back pain?
    1 Instruct her to wear an abdominal support
    2 Instruct her in the technique of pelvic tilt
    3 Instruct her to relax abdominal muscles when standing
    4 Instruct her to wear at least a 2-inch heel on her shoes

13. During a routine prenatal visit, the client complains of gingivitis and gums that bleed easily upon toothbrushing. In the plan of care, the nurse includes a goal that addresses proper nutrition to minimize this problem. The nurse determines that goal achievement has occurred when the client reports which of the following?
    1 "I am eating three servings of cracked-wheat bread each day."
    2 "I am eating fresh fruits and vegetables for snacks and for dessert each day."
    3 "I am drinking 8 ounces of water with each meal."
    4 "I eat two saltine crackers before I get up each morning."

14. The nurse identifies all of the following nursing diagnoses for a client at 37 weeks of gestation. This client has sickle cell anemia. Which diagnosis should receive highest priority?
    1 Activity intolerance
    2 Body image disturbance
    3 Alteration in nutrition, less than body requirements
    4 Fluid volume deficit

15. The nurse is preparing a 36-year-old gravida II, para I for an amniocentesis. She is at 16 weeks' gestation. Which of the following actions will the nurse take prior to the procedure to maintain fetal safety during the procedure?
    1 Require that the client empty her bladder
    2 Test the ultrasound equipment to assure proper functioning
    3 Teach the client the signs and symptoms of labor
    4 Prepare a local anesthetic to be used during the insertion of the spinal needle

16. The client is a gravida III, para O, abortus II. She is placed on bed rest at home due to preterm labor. Which of the following interventions is designed to promote family adaptation?

1 Teach the husband to titrate tocolytic agents
2 Teach the client to perform Kegel exercises
3 Teach the husband to perform passive range of motion exercises and backrubs for his wife
4 Explain to the husband that sexual intercourse probably caused the preterm labor

17. The client of 28 weeks' gestation is Rh-negative and Coombs' antibody–negative. The nurse knows that the client understands what the nurse has taught her about Rh sensitization when the client states:
    1 "I know I can never have another child."
    2 "I will have to have an injection once per month until the baby is born."
    3 "I will tell the nurse at the hospital that I had RhoGAM during pregnancy."
    4 "I am glad I won't have to have these shots if I have another child."

18. During measurement of fundal height, the client (36 weeks' gestation) states she is feeling lightheaded. Based on the nurse's knowledge of pregnancy, the nurse determines that this is most likely due to:
    1 Emotional instability
    2 Compression of the vena cava
    3 A full bladder
    4 Insufficient iron intake

19. The client, age 23, develops melasma during pregnancy. The nurse's focal assessment reveals that the client has started wearing very heavy makeup, is fearful that her mate will reject her, and has decreased her social engagements drastically owing to this change. Which of the following nursing diagnostic stems will best guide the nurse when formulating her plan of care?
    1 Body image disturbance
    2 Anxiety
    3 Social isolation
    4 Altered role performance

20. Which of the following statements by the pregnant client most points to the need for psychological consultation in formulating the plan of care?
    1 "I will never be able to lose my weight and regain a great figure. I feel ugly."
    2 "I don't like the way I look. My husband could never find me attractive again."
    3 "I hate the way I look and feel. The baby has done this to me and I wish I were not pregnant."
    4 "I have terrible mood swings. I will be glad when this is all over."

21. Which of the following midafternoon snacks should be recommended to supply folic acid for the pregnant woman?
    1 1 medium banana
    2 1/2 cup mix of peanuts, sunflower seeds, raisins
    3 1 cup milk with 2 graham crackers
    4 1 cup yogurt

22. The pregnant client tells the nurse that she has been craving "unusual foods." The nurse determines that she has been ingesting daily amounts of white clay dirt from her backyard. Which of the following laboratory results indicates a physiological consequence of this practice?
    1 Hct, 37%
    2 Hgb, 9.1 g/100 ml
    3 Glucose, 86 mg/100 ml
    4 WBC, 12,400/mm³

23. During the first trimester of pregnancy, the client complains of frequent nausea followed by vomiting. During the nursing assessment, which of the following will help differentiate morning sickness from more serious nutritional disorders of pregnancy?
    1 Ketone bodies in urine are negative
    2 Weight compared with last visit is a loss of 2.3 pounds
    3 Patellar reflex is 2+
    4 Chadwick's sign is positive

24. A nonstress test is performed on a client, and the results are documented in the chart. The results are documented as "two or more FHR accelerations of 15 beats per minute, lasting 15 seconds, in association with fetal movement." The nurse interprets these findings as:
    1 A reactive nonstress test
    2 A nonreactive nonstress test
    3 Equivocal
    4 Unsatisfactory

25. A contraction stress test is scheduled for the client. The woman asks the nurse about the test. The most accurate description of the test includes which of the following?
    1 Small amounts of oxytocin (Pitocin) are administered during internal fetal monitoring to stimulate uterine contractions
    2 An external fetal monitor is attached, and the woman ambulates on a treadmill until contractions begin
    3 The uterus is stimulated to contract either by small amounts of oxytocin (Pitocin) or by nipple stimulation
    4 Uterine contractions are stimulated by Leopold's maneuvers

ANSWERS

1. **1**

Rationale: The position described in option 1 will produce the posture of the pelvic tilt while countering gravity as the force that leads to edema of the lower extremities. Although the other options might seem useful, options 3 and 4 identify heat, which should be prescribed by the physician. Option 2 might be helpful for the reduction of hemorrhoids.

Test-Taking Strategy: Identify what the question is asking. Do not select answers that, although helpful for some discomforts of pregnancy, are not pertinent to back pain and ankle edema. Focus on nursing measures, not medical measures such as the application of heat, since the recommendation is being made by the nurse, not the physician.

Level of Cognitive Ability: Analysis
Phase of Nursing Process: Implementation
Client Needs: Physiological Integrity
Content Area: Maternity

Reference
Lowdermilk, D., Perry, S., & Bobak, I. (1997). *Maternity & women's health care* (6th ed.). St. Louis: Mosby–Year Book. pp. 238–239.

2. **3**

Rationale: Option 1 relates to hydration, which is important for normal physiological body functioning. Option 2 will help prevent urinary tract infections from *Escherichia coli.* Pelvic tilt exercises will reduce backache. Kegel exercises strengthen the pelvic floor.

Test-Taking Strategy: Focus on the question that is being asked, which is, how to strengthen the perineal floor muscles. Knowledge of the purpose of Kegel exercises will assist you in selecting the correct option. Review this information now, if you had difficulty with this question!

Level of Cognitive Ability: Application
Phase of Nursing Process: Planning
Client Needs: Health Promotion and Maintenance
Content Area: Maternity

Reference
Gorrie, T., McKinney, E. S., & Murray, S. S. (1998). *Foundations of maternal-newborn nursing* (2nd ed.). Philadelphia: W. B. Saunders. p. 454.

3. **1**

Rationale: There are no data to support the fear that the wife will be left at home. Options 3 and 4 are examples of giving advice and do not lead to open communication with the pregnant woman. Option 1 reflects a feeling that the woman may be having. By naming this feeling, the nurse provides the opportunity for further discussion.

Test-Taking Strategy: Identify what the question is asking, which in this case focuses on the role-relationship of the husband and wife. Apply guidelines for therapeutic communication such as reflection. Note the relationship of the word in the correct option: "role," with the word "relationship" in the question.

Level of Cognitive Ability: Analysis
Phase of Nursing Process: Analysis
Client Needs: Psychosocial Integrity
Content Area: Maternity

Reference
Gorrie, T., McKinney, E. S., & Murray, S. S. (1998). *Foundations of maternal-newborn nursing* (2nd ed.). Philadelphia: W. B. Saunders. p. 168.

4. **4**

Rationale: Varicose veins often develop in the lower extremities during pregnancy. Any constricting clothing such as knee-high hose impedes venous return from the lower legs and thus places the client at higher risk for developing varicosities. Clients should be encouraged to wear support hose. Flat, nonslip shoes with proper support are important to assist the pregnant woman to maintain proper posture and balance and to minimize fall risks.

Test-Taking Strategy: Identify the focus of the stem of the question, which is a knowledge deficit determined through observation of the client. Do not read into the question by guessing why the client is wearing knee-high hose. In this question, a need for teaching indicates that you should look for inappropriate dress by the client that will affect physiological integrity, rather than appropriate dress. Focus on physiological integrity.

Level of Cognitive Ability: Analysis
Phase of Nursing Process: Assessment
Client Needs: Physiological Integrity
Content Area: Maternity

Reference
Nichols, F., & Zwelling, E. (1997). *Maternal-newborn nursing: Theory and practice.* Philadelphia: W. B. Saunders. p. 500.

5. **4**

Rationale: Tetracycline during pregnancy may lead to discoloration of the baby's teeth when they erupt.

Test-Taking Strategy: Focus on the safety factor for the unseen client (fetus). Knowledge regarding medications and safety during pregnancy is required to answer the question. Note the word "avoid" in the question. Look at the options. The only option that addresses oral use of a medication is option 4. This would present the greatest risk to the fetus.

Level of Cognitive Ability: Analysis
Phase of Nursing Process: Analysis
Client Needs: Safe, Effective Care Environment
Content Area: Maternity

Reference
Wilson, B., Shannon, M., & Stang, C. (1998). *Nurses drug guide* (3rd ed.). Stamford, CT: Appleton & Lange. p. 1305.

6. **4**

Rationale: Baking soda may irritate gums, which are more likely to bleed due to hormonal changes of pregnancy. Local anesthetics for minor dental work should not have adverse effects on the fetus. Option 3 supports the erroneous old wives' tale that a tooth is lost for every child. Avoid myths! The dental staff need to know about the pregnancy so that care is taken during examinations and radiographs are avoided.

Test-Taking Strategy: Use the process of elimination to answer the question. Option 4 is the most global option; in this question, the other three options are much more specific. Focus on the safety of the unseen client (fetus).

Level of Cognitive Ability: Application
Phase of Nursing Process: Planning
Client Needs: Safe, Effective Care Environment
Content Area: Maternity

Reference
Nichols, F., & Zwelling, E. (1997). *Maternal-newborn nursing: Theory and practice.* Philadelphia: W. B. Saunders. p. 374.

7. **1**

Rationale: Hemorrhoids are varicosities and are most likely to be precipitated during pregnancy by the pressure of the growing fetus inside the abdominal cavity. Standing aggravates the problem; dietary factors, such as fluids and roughage, and manual reduction are factors that should be included in the plan of care. Hormonal changes are not a factor.

Test-Taking Strategy: Read the stem of the question carefully and note that the question asks for the statement by the client that indicates the need for further teaching. Use knowledge regarding hemorrhoids to assist you in selecting the correct option. If you had difficulty with this question, review content related to hemorrhoids now!

Level of Cognitive Ability: Analysis
Phase of Nursing Process: Evaluation
Client Needs: Health Promotion and Maintenance
Content Area: Maternity

Reference

Reeder, S., Martin, L., & Koniak-Griffin, D. (1997). *Maternity nursing: Family, newborn, and women's health care* (18th ed.). Philadelphia: Lippincott-Raven. p. 421.

8. **2**

Rationale: Leg cramps often occur when the pregnant woman stretches the leg and plantarflexes the foot. Dorsiflexion of the foot while extending the knee stretches the gastrocnemius muscle, prevents the muscle from contracting, and halts the cramping.

Test-Taking Strategy: Knowledge regarding the actions that will alleviate muscle cramps will assist you in answering the question. Including the significant other will foster family closeness, as well as teaching the information. Review these measures now if you had difficulty with this question!

Level of Cognitive Ability: Application
Phase of Nursing Process: Implementation
Client Needs: Physiological Integrity
Content Area: Maternity

Reference

Gorrie, T., McKinney, E. S., & Murray, S. S. (1998). *Foundations of maternal-newborn nursing* (2nd ed.). Philadelphia: W. B. Saunders. p. 156.

9. **2**

Rationale: Lying down is likely to lead to reflux of stomach contents, especially immediately following a meal. Spices tend to trigger heartburn. Eating smaller, more frequent portions is preferred over eating three large meals to control dyspepsia. Caffeine, like spices, may cause heartburn.

Test-Taking Strategy: Providing accurate information to the client is essential. Identify the key issues in the stem of the question which relate to dealing with dyspepsia. Review measures to alleviate dyspepsia now if you had difficulty with this question!

Level of Cognitive Ability: Application
Phase of Nursing Process: Implementation
Client Needs: Physiological Integrity
Content Area: Maternity

Reference

Gorrie, T., McKinney, E. S., & Murray, S. S. (1998). *Foundations of maternal-newborn nursing* (2nd ed.). Philadelphia: W. B. Saunders. p. 155.

10. **1**

Rationale: Anemia and pregnancy are medical diagnoses and are not appropriate in the statement of a nursing diagnosis. The data to support the related factors listed for fatigue are present. There are no data listed to support ineffective coping.

Test-Taking Strategy: Focus on nursing areas, not medical areas such as pregnancy and anemia, which are medical diagnoses. The nurse cannot diagnose or treat these legally. Therefore, eliminate options 2 and 4. Use assessment data to guide analysis. Distinguish between normals in laboratory values for the pregnant woman. Do not read into the question. Although she has nocturia, there is no report of lack of sleep. Focus on the facts. Identify key words in the stem of the question such as "most accurate."

Level of Cognitive Ability: Analysis
Phase of Nursing Process: Analysis
Client Needs: Physiological Integrity
Content Area: Maternity

Reference

Nichols, F., & Zwelling, E. (1997). *Maternal-newborn nursing: Theory and practice.* Philadelphia: W. B. Saunders. p. 502.

11. **3**

Rationale: Kegel exercises are useful to promote long-term bladder tone but will not be effective with one day's use. Limiting fluid intake at bedtime will decrease nocturia but should not be used as a measure during waking hours. A videotape will not satisfy the woman's need to be present at the play. Wearing a perineal pad will give her the security she needs. She should be instructed to remove a damp pad as soon as possible to decrease the incidence of infection.

Test-Taking Strategy: Focus on physiological integrity while meeting a psychosocial need. Even though the stem addresses a psychosocial need to attend a school function, be careful not to select seemingly correct options such as withholding fluids. This could lead to dehydration and preterm labor.

Level of Cognitive Ability: Application
Phase of Nursing Process: Planning
Client Needs: Psychosocial Integrity
Content Area: Maternity

Reference

Lowdermilk, D., Perry, S., & Bobak, I. (1997). *Maternity & women's health care* (6th ed.). St. Louis: Mosby–Year Book. p. 218.

12. **2**

Rationale: Pelvic tilt exercises decrease strain to muscles of the abdomen and lower back caused by the added weight of the abdomen and the shift in the center of gravity. An abdominal support should be worn only if recommended by the physician. Relaxing abdominal muscles will add to the problem. Wearing 2-inch heels on shoes will add to the strain on the muscles and will exaggerate the shift in the center of gravity.

Test-Taking Strategy: Read all options carefully. Focus on nursing strategies rather than medical strategies such as abdominal supports. Keep safety in mind and eliminate responses that are contrary to general safety, such as 2-inch heels on shoes. Review the process of teaching a client the pelvic tilt if you are unfamiliar with this technique!

Level of Cognitive Ability: Application
Phase of Nursing Process: Implementation
Client Needs: Health Promotion and Maintenance
Content Area: Maternity

Reference

Reeder, S., Martin, L., & Koniak-Griffin, D. (1997). *Maternity nursing: Family, newborn, and women's health care* (18th ed.). Philadelphia: J. B. Lippincott. p. 480.

13. **2**

Rationale: Fresh fruits and vegetables will provide vitamins and minerals needed for healthy gums. Cracked-wheat bread may abrade the tender gums; drinking water with meals has no direct effect on gums; eating saltine crackers before arising helps decrease nausea.

Test-Taking Strategy: Identify the issue of the question, which is oral care during pregnancy. Eliminate unlikely options, such as options 1 and 4, which, in general, could produce irritation to fragile gums. This narrows the choices to two options for selection. Review the issue of the question before selecting the option.

Level of Cognitive Ability: Analysis
Phase of Nursing Process: Evaluation
Client Needs: Physiological Integrity
Content Area: Maternity

Reference

Lowdermilk, D., Perry, S., & Bobak, I. (1997). *Maternity & women's health care* (6th ed.). St. Louis: Mosby–Year Book. p. 218.

14. **4**

Rationale: For the client with sickle cell anemia, dehydration will precipitate sickling of the red blood cells. Sickling can lead to life-threatening consequences for the pregnant woman and for the fetus, such as an interruption of blood flow to the respiratory system and placenta.

Test-Taking Strategy: Use Maslow's Hierarchy of Needs to prioritize, remembering that physiological needs come first. Using this principle, eliminate options 1 and 2. Utilize knowledge regarding sickle cell anemia to select the correct option. In this case, the result of sickling presents the physiological priority of fluid volume deficit. Review sickle cell anemia now, if you had difficulty with this question!

Level of Cognitive Ability: Analysis
Phase of Nursing Process: Analysis
Client Needs: Physiological Integrity
Content Area: Maternity

Reference

Gorrie, T., McKinney, E. S., & Murray, S. S. (1998). *Foundations of maternal-newborn nursing* (2nd ed.). Philadelphia: W. B. Saunders. p. 728.

15. **2**

Rationale: Prior to 20 weeks of gestation, it is recommended that an amniocentesis be performed with the bladder full. This pushes the uterus upward for better visualization. After Week 20, the bladder is emptied prior to the test to minimize the risk of puncturing the bladder during the test. The client does need to be taught about the signs and symptoms of labor; this action does not ensure fetal safety. The question asks about safety during the procedure. The local anesthetic makes the insertion of the needle less painful but does not protect the fetus. The use of ultrasound to guide the procedure has greatly decreased the risk of fetal and placental damage during the procedure.

Test-Taking Strategy: Read the question carefully, use the process of elimination to select the correct option. Identify the client in the question, the fetus. Identify key factors and eliminate distracters that do not respond to the question of maintaining fetal safety. Identify key terms such as "during the procedure." Review preparation for amniocentesis now, if you had difficulty with this question. You are likely to see questions related to this procedure on NCLEX-RN!

Level of Cognitive Ability: Application
Phase of Nursing Process: Planning
Client Needs: Safe, Effective Care Environment
Content Area: Maternity

References

Reeder, S., Martin, L., & Koniak-Griffin, D. (1997). *Maternity nursing: Family, newborn, and women's health care* (18th ed.). Philadelphia: J. B. Lippincott. p. 357.
Malarkey, L., & McMorrow, M. (1996). *Nurse's manual of laboratory tests and diagnostic procedures.* Philadelphia: W. B. Saunders. p. 792.

16. **3**

Rationale: Range of motion exercises will help maintain muscle tone during bed rest, and backrubs provide skin-to-skin contact and are comforting. The inclusion of the significant other promotes adaptation and decreases the sense of isolation. Option 4 will lead to guilt and maladaptation. The husband should not be expected to titrate medications. Kegel exercises are beneficial but will not provide the human-to-human contact that promotes family adaptation.

Test-Taking Strategy: Identify the client(s) of the question, the family. Identify the issue of the question, which is adaptation to the woman being placed on bed rest with a history of abortion. Use the process of elimination. Eliminate distracters that are of no value in the situation, such as Kegel exercises. Focus on psychosocial integrity. Placing blame on the husband is of no value. The husband should not be expected to titrate tocolytic agents.

Level of Cognitive Ability: Application
Phase of Nursing Process: Implementation
Client Needs: Psychosocial Integrity
Content Area: Maternity

Reference

Reeder, S., Martin, L., & Koniak-Griffin, D. (1997). *Maternity nursing: Family, newborn, and women's health care* (18th ed.). Philadelphia: J. B. Lippincott. p. 985.

17. **3**

Rationale: It is accepted practice to administer RhoGAM at 28 weeks of gestation to a woman as described here, with a second injection within 72 hours of delivery. This prevents sensitization, which could jeopardize a future pregnancy. For subsequent pregnancies or abortions, the injections must be repeated since immunity is passive.

Test-Taking Strategy: Knowledge regarding the administration of RhoGAM is required to answer the question. From this point, use the process of elimination to select the correct option. Read all options carefully, keeping a focus on the question being asked: evidence from a statement by the client that her knowledge of RhoGAM administration is accurate. Review RhoGAM administration now, if you had difficulty with this question!

Level of Cognitive Ability: Analysis
Phase of Nursing Process: Evaluation
Client Needs: Health Promotion and Maintenance
Content Area: Maternity

References

Lowdermilk, D., Perry, S. & Bobak, I. (1997). *Maternity & women's health care* (6th ed.). St. Louis: Mosby–Year Book. p. 453

Gorrie, T., McKinney, E. S., & Murray, S. S. (1998). *Foundations of maternal-newborn nursing* (2nd ed.). Philadelphia: W. B. Saunders. p. 705.

18. 2

Rationale: Compression of the inferior vena cava and aorta by the uterus may cause supine hypotension syndrome late in pregnancy. Having the woman turn onto her left side or elevating the left buttock during fundal height measurement will correct or prevent the problem.

Test-Taking Strategy: Focus on physiological integrity. Use the ABCs: Airway, Breathing, and Circulation, to answer the question. Be alert to each piece of assessment data presented in light of the question asked. Review vena cava syndrome now, if you had difficulty with this question!

Level of Cognitive Ability: Analysis
Phase of Nursing Process: Assessment
Client Needs: Safe, Effective Care Environment
Content Area: Maternity

Reference

Gorrie, T., McKinney, E. S., & Murray, S. S. (1998). *Foundations of maternal-newborn nursing* (2nd ed.). Philadelphia: W. B. Saunders. p. 126.

19. 1

Rationale: Although the nurse might consider all of these nursing diagnoses initially, the focal assessment points most clearly to body image disturbance. Anxiety would be inaccurate since there is a physical focus for the problem, melasma. The client has decreased social outings, but there is no indication that she has excluded all activities. There are insufficient data to support altered role performance.

Test-Taking Strategy: Use the process of elimination. Identify the focus or issue of the question. Anxiety is not the focus identified in the question. The client might become isolated socially, but there is no evidence of this at the current time. There is no evidence to indicate that her role performance is altered. If the melasma is addressed, along with her psychosocial concerns related to it, body image will be restored and the other diagnoses will not become realities.

Level of Cognitive Ability: Analysis
Phase of Nursing Process: Analysis
Client Needs: Psychosocial Integrity
Content Area: Maternity

Reference

Nichols, F., & Zwelling, E. (1997). *Maternal-newborn nursing: Theory and practice.* Philadelphia: W. B. Saunders. p. 421.

20. 3

Rationale: Options 1, 2, and 4 are feelings about self and body image that many women express during pregnancy. The statement in option 3 is much stronger and places blame on the fetus. The direction of anger to the fetus should be explored. The nurse may find that a psychological referral is appropriate.

Test-Taking Strategy: Identify the key word in the stem: "most." Use the process of elimination to select the correct option. Keep psychosocial assessment as the focus for answering the question.

Level of Cognitive Ability: Analysis
Phase of Nursing Process: Analysis
Client Needs: Psychosocial Integrity
Content Area: Maternity

References

Reeder, S., Martin, L., & Koniak-Griffin, D. (1997). *Maternity nursing: Family, newborn, and women's health care* (18th ed.). Philadelphia: J. B. Lippincott. p. 387.

21. 2

Rationale: All three food items in option 2 contain folic acid. Bananas provide potassium; milk and yogurt supply calcium. Folic acid is needed during pregnancy for healthy cell growth and repair. A pregnant woman should have at least four servings of folic acid–rich foods per day.

Test-Taking Strategy: Note the key words in the stem, which are the "folic acid" source. Knowledge regarding food sources high in folic acid is required to answer the question. Review these food sources now, if you had difficulty with this question!

Level of Cognitive Ability: Application
Phase of Nursing Process: Implementation
Client Needs: Physiological Integrity
Content Area: Maternity

Reference

Reeder, S., Martin, L., & Koniak-Griffin, D. (1997). *Maternity nursing: Family, newborn, and women's health care* (18th ed.). Philadelphia: J. B. Lippincott. p. 460.

22. 2

Rationale: Pica cravings often lead to iron deficiency anemia, resulting in a lowered hemoglobin. The other three laboratory values are within normal limits for the pregnant woman.

Test-Taking Strategy: Knowledge of normal laboratory values and the physiological effects of pica will assist you in selecting the correct option. The process of elimination can then be utilized as the guide to direct you toward the correct option. Review pica and normal laboratory values now, if you had difficulty with this question!

Level of Cognitive Ability: Analysis
Phase of Nursing Process: Evaluation
Client Needs: Physiological Integrity
Content Area: Maternity

Reference

Gorrie, T., McKinney, E. S., & Murray, S. S. (1998). *Foundations of maternal-newborn nursing* (2nd ed.). Philadelphia: W. B. Saunders. p. 211.

23. 2

Rationale: Weight loss along with the symptoms described in the question could indicate hyperemesis gravidarum. Ketone bodies indicate protein wasting; patellar reflexes would be used during magnesium sulfate administration; Chadwick's sign may be an indicator of pregnancy.

Test-Taking Strategy: Identify the focus of the question, which is to select a parameter that will help distinguish morning sickness from excessive loss of body fluid through hyperemesis gravidarum. Identify general responses such as the weight loss, which is a general indicator. Identify normal values of physical examination. Three options are normal and one is not. Even if the correct option to the question is not known, use your knowledge regarding normal signs to assist you in selecting the correct option. Review the findings noted in the options now, if you had difficulty with this question!

Level of Cognitive Ability: Application
Phase of Nursing Process: Assessment
Client Needs: Physiological Integrity
Content Area: Maternity

Reference

Gorrie, T., McKinney, E. S., & Murray, S. S. (1998). *Foundations of maternal-newborn nursing* (2nd ed.). Philadelphia: W. B. Saunders. pp. 138, 689, 696.

24. **1**

Rationale: A reactive nonstress test (normal/negative) indicates a healthy fetus. It is described as two or more fetal heart rate accelerations of at least 15 beats per minute, lasting at least 15 seconds from the beginning of the acceleration to the end in association with fetal movement, during a 20-minute period. A nonreactive nonstress test (abnormal) is described as no accelerations or accelerations of less than 15 beats per minute or lasting less than 15 seconds in duration, for a 40-minute observation. An unsatisfactory test cannot be interpreted because of the poor quality of the FHR.

Test-Taking Strategy: Knowledge regarding the nonstress test is required to answer the question. Remembering that a reactive nonstress test is a normal or negative test may be helpful to answer the question. Read the description of the results in the question carefully to assist you in analyzing the results. If you had difficulty answering this question, take time now to review the nonstress test!

Level of Cognitive Ability: Analysis
Phase of Nursing Process: Analysis
Client Needs: Physiological Integrity
Content Area: Maternity

Reference

Nichols, F., & Zwelling, E. (1997). *Maternal-newborn nursing: Theory and practice.* Philadelphia: W. B. Saunders. pp. 943–945.

25. **3**

Rationale: A contraction stress test assesses placental oxygenation and function, determines fetal ability to tolerate labor, determines fetal well-being, and is performed if the nonstress test is abnormal. The fetus is exposed to the stressor of contractions to assess the adequacy of placental perfusion under simulated labor conditions. An external fetal monitor is applied to the mother and a 20- to 30-minute baseline strip is recorded. The uterus is stimulated to contract either by the administration of a dilute dose of oxytocin (Pitocin) or by having the mother use nipple stimulation until three palpable contractions with a duration of 40 seconds or more in a 10-minute period have been achieved. Frequent maternal BP readings are done, and the client is monitored closely while increasing doses of oxytocin are given.

Test-Taking Strategy: Knowledge regarding the contraction stress test is required to answer the question. Read each option carefully. Remember that in both the nonstress test and the contraction stress test, external monitoring is performed. If you had difficulty answering this question, take time now to review the contraction stress test!

Level of Cognitive Ability: Analysis
Phase of Nursing Process: Analysis
Client Needs: Physiological Integrity
Content Area: Maternity

Reference

Nichols, F., & Zwelling, E. (1997). *Maternal-newborn nursing: Theory and practice.* Philadelphia: W. B. Saunders. pp. 943–945.

BIBLIOGRAPHY

Gorrie, T., McKinney, E. S., & Murray, S. S. (1998). *Foundations of maternal-newborn nursing* (2nd ed.). Philadelphia: W. B. Saunders.

Lowdermilk, D., Perry, S., & Bobak, I. (1997). *Maternity & women's health care* (6th ed.). St. Louis: Mosby–Year Book.

Malarkey, L., & McMorrow, M. (1996). *Nurse's manual of laboratory tests and diagnostic procedures.* Philadelphia: W. B. Saunders.

Nichols, F., & Zwelling, E. (1997). *Maternal-newborn nursing: Theory and practice.* Philadelphia: W. B. Saunders.

Reeder, S., Martin, L., & Koniak-Griffin, D. (1997). *Maternity nursing: Family, newborn, and women's health care* (18th ed.). Philadelphia: J. B. Lippincott.

Wilson, B., Shannon, M., & Stang, C. (1998). *Nurses drug guide* (3rd ed.). Stamford, CT: Appleton & Lange.

CHAPTER 25

Risk Conditions Related to Pregnancy

I. Abortion

A. Description: Termination of pregnancy before the fetus is viable (20 weeks or a weight of 500 g)

B. Types
1. Spontaneous: Pregnancy ends because of natural causes
2. Induced: Therapeutic or elective reasons for terminating the pregnancy
3. Threatened: Developing spontaneous abortion
4. Inevitable: Threatened loss that cannot be prevented
5. Incomplete: Loss of some products of conception and retention of others
6. Complete: Loss of all products of conception
7. Missed: Retention of products of conception in utero after fetal death
8. Habitual: Spontaneous abortions in three or more successive pregnancies

C. Assessment
1. Spontaneous vaginal bleeding
2. Passage of clots
3. Passage of tissue through vagina
4. Low uterine cramping
5. Contractions
6. Hemorrhage and shock

D. Implementation
1. Maintain bed rest
2. Monitor vital signs
3. Monitor cramping and bleeding
4. Count perineal pads to evaluate blood loss
5. Save expelled tissues and clots
6. Provide IV fluids as prescribed to prevent shock
7. Prepare client for Dilatation and Curettage as prescribed for incomplete abortion

◆ II. Acquired Immunodeficiency Syndrome (AIDS)

A. Description
1. The AIDS virus is a causative factor in the development of AIDS

2. Human immunodeficiency virus (HIV) infection is a progressive, severe weakening of the immune system that makes an individual highly susceptible to other infections and certain types of cancer
3. The virus attacks the lymphocytes and produces immune deficiency by destroying the T-helper lymphocytes; this interferes with cell-mediated immunity
4. Develops slowly over years
5. Women infected with the AIDS virus may first demonstrate symptoms at the time of pregnancy or possibly develop life-threatening infections because normal pregnancy involves some suppression of the maternal immune system

B. Transmission
1. All body fluids from an infected host, except perspiration, have been shown to contain the virus
2. Blood, semen, and breast milk have higher concentrations of virus than urine, saliva, vomitus, and stool
3. HIV can cross some membranes such as the **placental** barrier, blood-brain barrier, vaginal mucosa, and (in the neonate) the walls of the gastrointestinal tract
4. Sexual contact
5. Transfusion with blood or blood products
6. Occupational exposure, such as health care workers
7. Shared needles during drug use and using dirty needles
8. Perinatal transmission from infected mother to fetus or newborn infant via transplacental transmission, contamination with maternal blood during birth, or through breast milk

C. Risks to the Mother
1. The mother with HIV is managed as high-risk
2. Frequent complaints of fatigue, shortness of breath, nausea, back pain, urinary frequency, and headaches

3. More vulnerable to postpartum infections
4. May need longer courses of antibiotics for infection
5. AZT (zidovudine), 200 mg PO TID starting in the 14th week of pregnancy to minimize teratogenicity, may be administered to the woman with HIV infection to prevent transmission to the fetus; it may also be necessary to add a second medication to decrease the risk of transmission to the fetus

D. Diagnosis
1. Client may be infected with the virus but not yet have produced antibodies, thereby testing negative but being capable of infecting others
2. Clients who by history may be at risk for possible HIV but test negative for the HIV antibody should be retested; it usually takes 6 to 12 weeks for a host to manufacture detectable HIV antibodies
3. Enzyme-linked immunosorbent assay (ELISA) screening test for AIDS antibody is a very sensitive test but not highly specific; a positive ELISA test indicates the need for further testing using the Western blot

E. Assessment (Table 25–1)
F. Implementation
1. Prenatal
   a. Prevention of opportunistic infections
   b. Instruct client on good handwashing procedure
   c. Avoid persons who are ill
   d. Avoid exposure to cat feces, cat or dog litter, and fish tanks
   e. Avoid undercooked meats, raw eggs, and unpasteurized milk
   f. Prevent further exposure to HIV through sexual contact or use of needles
   g. Initiate recovery from substance abuse
   h. Avoid procedures that increase the risk of perinatal transmission, such as amniocentesis and fetal scalp sampling
2. Intrapartal period
   a. Note that if the fetus has not been exposed to HIV in utero, the highest risk exists during **delivery** through the birth canal
   b. Never use scalp electrodes
   c. Avoid episiotomy to decrease the amount of maternal blood in and around the birth canal
   d. Avoid the administration of oxytocin since oxytocin contractions can be strong, inducing vaginal tears or necessitating the need for episiotomy
   e. Minimize the infant's exposure to maternal blood and body fluids
   f. Place heavy absorbent pads under the mother's hips to absorb **amniotic fluid** and maternal blood
   g. Promptly remove the newborn infant from the mother's blood
   h. Suction the infant promptly
   i. Prepare to administer IV AZT (zidovudine) as prescribed during **delivery**
3. Postpartum
   a. Monitor for signs of infection such as increased temperature and WBC count
   b. Place client in protective isolation to prevent infection if client is experiencing a suppressed immune response
   c. Restrict breast feeding
   d. Identify clients residing in areas with unsafe water supplies and sanitation systems; these clients should avoid breastfeeding to prevent postnatal transmission to a child who may not have been infected in utero
   e. Instruct client how to take temperature and identify symptoms necessitating immediate follow-up
   f. Urge the client to refrain from donating blood or body organs
   g. Advise the client to avoid sharing toothbrushes, razors, or other materials potentially contaminated with blood

G. The Neonate and HIV
1. Description
   a. The fetus of an HIV antibody–positive woman should be monitored closely throughout the pregnancy
   b. Serial ultrasound screenings should be done to identify intrauterine growth restriction
   c. Weekly nonstress testing after 32 weeks

Table 25–1. Assessment of the Stages of AIDS

Stage 1	Stage 2	Stage 3	Stage 4
Fever Myalgia Lymphadenopathy Headache	Active but asymptomatic and may remain so for years May experience an outbreak of herpes zoster (shingles) May experience a transient thrombocytopenia	Symptomatic Evidence of immune dysfunction All body systems can present with signs of immune dysfunction Integumentary and gynecological problems are common	Advanced HIV infection Vulnerable to common bacterial infections Development of opportunistic infections Serious immune compromise

of gestation and biophysical profiles may be necessary

  d. Infants born to HIV-positive clients may test positive because the mother's positive antibodies may persist for as long as 18 months after birth
  e. The use of antiviral medication, reduction of infant exposure to maternal blood and body fluids, and early identification of HIV in pregnancy reduce the risk of transmission to the infant
  f. All infants acquire maternal antibody to HIV infection, but not all acquire infection

 2. Transmission
  a. Across the **placental** barrier
  b. During the process of **labor** and **delivery**
  c. Via breast milk

 3. Implementation
  a. Bathe infant carefully before any invasive procedure, such as the administration of vitamin K, heel sticks, or venipunctures
  b. Infant can room with mother
  c. Prepare to administer AZT (zidovudine) as prescribed for the first 6 weeks of life
  d. All HIV-exposed infants should be treated with medication to prevent infection by *Pneumocystis carinii*
  e. Note that an HIV culture is recommended at age 1 month and after 4 months of age; infants at risk for HIV infection should be seen by the physician at birth, 1 week, 2 weeks, 1 month, and 2 months of life
  f. Infants at risk for HIV infection need to receive all recommended immunizations at the regular schedule
  g. No live immunizations should be administered
  h. Inactivated polio vaccine by injection rather than oral polio vaccine should be administered, because the oral polio vaccine causes a shedding of polio virus in the stool, which may be a risk to the immunocompromised family
  i. Note that the neonate may be asymptomatic for the first several years of life; monitor for early signs of immune deficiency, such as an enlarged spleen or liver, lymphadenopathy, and impairment in growth and development

III. Anemia

A. Description
 1. A condition that can develop as a result of iron deficiency, with a hemoglobin below 10 g/dl or a hematocrit level below 30 g/dL
 2. Anemia predisposes the client to postpartum infection and hemorrhage

B. Assessment
 1. Fatigue
 2. Headache
 3. Pallor
 4. Tachycardia
 5. Hemoglobin below 10 g/dl and hematocrit below 30 g/dl

C. Implementation
 1. Monitor hemoglobin and hematocrit every 2 weeks
 2. Administer and instruct client about iron and folic acid supplements
 3. Instruct client to take iron with a source of vitamin C and to avoid taking iron with tea
 4. Instruct client to eat foods high in iron, folic acid, and protein
 5. Teach client to monitor for signs and symptoms of infections
 6. Prepare to administer injectable iron as prescribed in severe cases
 7. Prepare to administer transfusions if prescribed although they are rarely necessary
 8. Prepare for the administration of oxytoxic drugs as prescribed postpartum to prevent hemorrhage

IV. Cardiac Disease

A. Description
 1. The inability to cope with the added plasma volume and the increased cardiac output
 2. Blood volume is at a maximum during the last weeks of the second trimester

B. Assessment
 1. Signs and symptoms of cardiac decompensation, particularly during the second trimester
 2. Cough
 3. Peripheral edema
 4. Signs of pulmonary edema
 5. Angina type of pain
 6. Dyspnea and fatigue
 7. Palpitations and tachycardia
 8. Signs of respiratory infection

C. Implementation
 1. Monitor vital signs, fetal heart rate, and condition of fetus
 2. Monitor for signs of respiratory infections
 3. Avoid exposure to infections
 4. Plan activity level and stress the need for sufficient rest
 5. Encourage adequate nutrition to prevent anemia
 6. Administer antibiotics as prescribed
 7. Administer cardiac medications as prescribed
 8. Maintain bed rest for client as prescribed during the last weeks of pregnancy
 9. During **labor**
  a. Monitor vital signs frequently
  b. Place client on a cardiac monitor and on an external fetal monitor
  c. Maintain bed rest, with mother lying on side or in semirecumbent position
  d. Administer oxygen

e. Monitor for signs of pulmonary edema and heart failure

f. Provide emotional support

V. Chorioamnionitis

A. Description

1. A bacterial infection of the amniotic cavity, which can occur as a result of premature rupture of the membrane, vaginitis, amniocentesis, or intrauterine procedures

2. Chorioamnionitis causes the development of postpartum endometritis and causes perinatal mortality and maternal morbidity

B. Assessment

1. Uterine tenderness and contractions

2. Elevated temperature

3. Maternal or fetal tachycardia

4. Foul odor to **amniotic fluid**

5. Leukocytosis

C. Implementation

1. Monitor maternal vital signs and fetal heart rate

2. Monitor uterine contractions and activity

3. Monitor results of blood culture

4. Prepare for **amniotic fluid** analysis for Gram stain and leukocyte count by amniocentesis

5. Administer antibiotics as prescribed after cultures are obtained for both mother and fetus

6. Administer oxytoxic agents as prescribed to increase uterine tone

7. Prepare for the **delivery** of the fetus

8. Prepare for neonatal cultures after **delivery**

VI. Chronic Hypertension

A. Description

1. Hypertension that occurs before pregnancy, is diagnosed before the 20th week of gestation, or is diagnosed for the first time during pregnancy and persists beyond the 42nd day postpartum

2. The condition predisposes the client to pregnancy-induced hypertension (PIH)

3. Can cause **abruptio placentae** and intrauterine growth retardation

B. Assessment

1. Headaches

2. Visual changes

3. BP of 140/90 mmHg or greater

4. Delayed fetal growth

5. Oligohydramnios

C. Implementation

1. Monitor blood pressure

2. Monitor fetal activity

3. Monitor fetal growth

4. Encourage frequent rest periods, instructing client to lie in the left lateral position

5. Administer antihypertensive medications as prescribed for diastolic pressures greater than 100

6. Monitor input and output (I&O)

7. Evaluate renal function through prescribed studies such as BUN, serum creatinine, and 24-hour urine levels for creatinine clearance and protein

VII. Diabetes

A. Description

1. A chronic metabolic disease caused by a disturbance in normal production of insulin

2. Pregnancy places demands on carbohydrate metabolism and causes insulin requirements to increase

B. Insulin-Dependent Diabetes

1. Maternal glucose crosses the **placenta** but insulin does not

2. During the first trimester, maternal insulin needs decrease

3. The fetus produces its own insulin and pulls glucose from the mother, which predisposes the mother to hypoglycemic reactions

4. During the second and third trimesters, increases in **placental** hormones cause an insulin-resistant state, requiring an increase in the client's insulin dose

5. After **placental delivery, placental** hormone levels drop abruptly and insulin requirements decrease

C. Diabetes in Pregnancy

1. Diabetes is more difficult to control during pregnancy

2. Premature **delivery** is more frequent

3. The infant of a diabetic mother may be large in size but will have functions related to gestational age rather than size

4. The infant of a diabetic mother is subject to hypoglycemia, hyperbilirubinemia, respiratory distress syndrome, and congenital anomalies

5. Stillborn and neonatal mortality rates are higher in pregnancies of a diabetic woman

6. Conditions that can occur as a result of diabetes include:

a. Acidosis

b. Infection

c. Pregnancy-induced hypertension

d. Hemorrhage

e. Polyhydramnios

f. Fetal death

D. Gestational Diabetes

1. Occurs during the second or third trimester

2. Occurs in pregnancy in clients not previously diagnosed as diabetic and occurs when the pancreas cannot respond to the demand for more insulin

3. Pregnant women should be screened for glucose levels at the 26th week of gestation

4. Glucose levels should remain at 105 mg/dL except for brief periods after meals

5. A 3-hour glucose tolerance test will confirm diabetes when two or more values are above normal

6. Oral hypoglycemic agents are never used during pregnancy
7. Frequently can be treated by diet alone; however, insulin may be needed for some clients
8. Most gestational diabetics convert to normal after **delivery**; however, these individuals have an increased risk of developing diabetes in their lifetime

E. Predisposing Conditions to Gestational Diabetes
   1. Over age 35 years
   2. Obesity
   3. Multiple gestation
   4. Family history of diabetes

F. Assessment
   1. Excessive thirst
   2. Hunger
   3. Weight loss
   4. Blurred vision
   5. Frequent urination
   6. Recurrent urinary tract infections and vaginal yeast infections
   7. Glycosuria and ketonuria
   8. Signs of pregnancy-induced hypertension
   9. Polyhydramnios
   10. Fetus large for gestational age

G. Implementation
   1. Screen clients between the 24th and 28th weeks of pregnancy
   2. Prenatal visits bimonthly for 6 months and weekly thereafter
   3. Monitor for signs of hypoglycemia, and give the client 8 oz of skim milk for hypoglycemic reactions to elevate blood glucose levels gradually
   4. Observe for signs of hyperglycemia
   5. Assess insulin needs
   6. Monitor and maintain blood glucose levels according to gestational week
   7. Monitor for glycosuria and ketonuria
   8. Monitor weight
   9. Insulin administration if diet cannot control blood sugar levels
   10. Assess for signs of pre-eclampsia, which include hypertension, proteinuria, and edema
   11. Check for increased temperature and signs of infection
   12. Instruct client to report burning and pain on urination or vaginal discharge or itching
   13. Assess fetal status
   14. Monitor for signs of premature **labor**
   15. Assess for signs of polyhydramnios
   16. Increase calorie intake to 2000 to 2400 each day as prescribed, with adequate insulin therapy so glucose will move into the cells
   17. Calories in diet should consist of 40% to 50% carbohydrates, 20% to 25% protein, and 30% to 35% fat

H. Implementation During **Labor**
   1. Monitor fetal status continuously for signs of

distress and, if noted, prepare client for immediate cesarean section
   2. Carefully regulate insulin and provide IV glucose as prescribed, since **labor** depletes glycogen

I. Implementation During the Postpartum Period
   1. Observe client closely for an insulin reaction, since a precipitous drop in insulin requirements is usual
   2. The client may not require insulin for the first 24 hours
   3. Reregulate insulin needs as prescribed following the first day according to blood sugar testing
   4. Assess dietary needs based on blood sugar and insulin requirements
   5. Monitor for signs of infection or postpartum hemorrhage

VIII. Disseminated Intravascular Coagulation (DIC)

A. Description
   1. A condition in the mother's body that results in an exaggerated clotting process which increases the formation of clots in microcirculation
   2. Thromboplastin from **placental** tissue and clots enter the blood stream through open vessels at the **placental** site and initiate an exaggeration of the normal clotting process
   3. The rapid and extensive formation of clots causes the platelets and clotting factors to be depleted; this results in bleeding and the potential vascular occlusion of organs from thromboembolus formation

B. Predisposing Conditions
   1. Abruptio placentae
   2. Intrauterine fetal death
   3. **Amniotic fluid** embolism
   4. PIH
   5. Liver disease
   6. Sepsis

C. Assessment
   1. Uncontrolled bleeding
   2. Bruising, purpura, petechiae, and ecchymosis
   3. Presence of occult blood
   4. Hematuria, hematemesis, or vaginal bleeding
   5. Signs of shock
   6. Decreased fibrinogen level and platelet count and hematocrit
   7. Increased prothrombin time (PT) and partial thromboplastin time (PTT), clotting time, and fibrin degradation products

D. Implementation
   1. Monitor vital signs
   2. Administer oxygen
   3. Assess for signs of shock
   4. Administer heparin as prescribed to prevent clot formation and increase available fibrinogen, coagulation factors, and platelets

5. Administer blood or blood products as prescribed as fresh-frozen plasma and/or platelets

IX. Ectopic Pregnancy

A. Description: A pregnancy that occurs in an area other than uterine, with **implantation** usually occurring in fallopian tubes
B. Assessment
    1. Pain unilaterally, with cramping and tenderness
    2. Mass in the adnexa or cul-de-sac
    3. Nausea and vomiting
    4. Slight, dark vaginal bleeding
    5. Fever
    6. Tachycardia
    7. Leukocytosis
    8. Low hemoglobin and hematocrit, elevated erythrocyte sedimentation rate
    9. Profound shock if rupture occurs
C. Implementation
    1. Obtain assessment data rapidly
    2. Obtain vital signs
    3. Initiate measures to prevent shock
    4. Monitor bleeding
    5. Obtain blood for type and cross-match
    6. Prepare for the administration of methotrexate if prescribed, for masses smaller than 4 cm, to induce abortion and preserve the fallopian tube
    7. Prepare client for laparotomy and removal of pregnancy and tube, if necessary, or repair of tube
    8. Administer antibiotics and RhoGam as prescribed
    9. Encourage follow-up care
    10. Encourage counseling for future pregnancies

X. Endometritis

A. Description
    1. An infection of the lining of the uterus following **delivery**, caused by bacteria that invades the uterus at the **placental** site
    2. The infection may spread and involve the entire endometrium and cause peritonitis, pelvic thrombophlebitis, or cellulitis
B. Assessment
    1. Chills
    2. Fever
    3. Increased pulse
    4. Decreased appetite
    5. Headache
    6. Backache
    7. Prolonged, severe afterpains
    8. Tender, large uterus
    9. Foul odor of **lochia** or reddish-brown **lochia**
    10. Ileus
    11. Elevated WBC count with a left shift and immature formed cells
C. Implementation
    1. Position client in Fowler's position to facilitate drainage of **lochia**; monitor vital signs
    2. Provide a private room for the client
    3. Instruct mother that it is not necessary to isolate the newborn infant from the mother
    4. Initiate wound and skin precautions as necessary
    5. Monitor I&O
    6. Encourage fluids
    7. Administer comfort measures such as backrubs and positioning changes
    8. Administer oxytocin medications as prescribed to improve uterine tone
    9. Administer IV antibiotics as prescribed
    10. Administer pain medications as prescribed
    11. Instruct client in proper handwashing techniques

XI. Fetal Death in Utero (FDIU)

A. Description
    1. The death of a fetus after the 20th week of gestation and before birth
    2. DIC can develop if the dead fetus is retained in the uterus for 3 to 4 weeks or more
B. Assessment
    1. Absence of fetal movement
    2. Absence of fetal heart tones
    3. Maternal weight loss
    4. Lack of fetal growth or decrease in fundal height
    5. Lack of cardiac activity and other characteristics suggestive of fetal death noted on the ultrasound
C. Implementation
    1. Prepare for the **delivery** of the fetus
    2. Support the client's decision about **labor**, birth, and the postpartum period
    3. Facilitate grieving process
    4. Allow parents to hold infant after birth
    5. Allow parents to name the infant
    6. Accept such behaviors as anger and hostility from the parents
    7. Refer parents to an appropriate support group

XII. Hepatitis B

A. Description: An inflammation of the liver caused by the hepatitis B virus
B. Transmission to Fetus and Neonate
    1. Transplacental
    2. Intrapartum exposure to infected blood, **amniotic fluid**, or vaginal secretions
    3. Through postpartum exposure
    4. Through breastfeeding
C. Risks to Mother
    1. Maternal fetal risk in uncomplicated hepatitis B is not generally increased unless infection occurs in the third trimester or in the immediate postpartum period
    2. Intrapartum risks include increased risk for prematurity, premature **delivery**, and vertical fetal transmission

3. Postpartum risk for transmission is by horizontal contact, by oral transmission through saliva exchange and kissing, food preparation, and utensils and fomites

D. Risk to Fetus and Neonate
 1. The infant is identified as an HBsAg carrier
 2. Infections in early life are usually asymptomatic
 3. Chronic hepatitis
 4. Associated with glomerulonephritis and nephritis

E. Implementation
 1. Minimize the number of vaginal examinations
 2. Minimize the risk for intrapartum ascending infections
 3. Double-glove for extended periods of blood contact
 4. Administer antibiotics as prescribed during labor to decrease the risk of transmission to the infant, especially if the membranes are ruptured
 5. Remove maternal blood from the neonate immediately after birth
 6. Protect the neonate's scalp integrity
 7. Suction the neonate immediately after birth
 8. Cut the cord with new sterile scissors, not the scissors used on the perineum
 9. Bathe the neonate prior to invasive procedures
 10. Clean and dry the face and eyes before instilling eye prophylaxis
 11. Discourage kissing until the mother and infant have been treated
 12. Support breast-feeding after maternal and neonatal treatment; breast-feeding is not contraindicated if an infected mother and infant are treated
 13. Immune globulin and vaccine are given to all HBsAg-positive neonates within 2 to 12 hours of **delivery**, at least before 24 hours and not more than 7 days after birth
 14. Inform the mother that HBV vaccine will be administered to the neonate, with the first dose given before the infant leaves the hospital; the second dose at 1 month; and the third dose at 6 months
 15. If the mother is identified positive more than 1 month after **delivery**, her HBsAg-negative infant should be treated
 16. Discourage sharing razors and toothbrushes and unprotected intercourse

XIII. Hematoma

A. Description
 1. The formation of a hematoma following the escape of blood into the tissues of the reproductive sac after the **delivery**
 2. Predisposing conditions include operative **delivery** with forceps or injury to a blood vessel

3. A life-threatening condition

B. Assessment
 1. Abnormal, severe pain
 2. Pressure in perineal area
 3. Sensitive tumor in perineal area, with discolored skin
 4. Inability to void
 5. Palpable tumor
 6. Decreased hematocrit and hemoglobin (H&H)
 7. Signs of shock, such as pallor, tachycardia, and hypotension if significant blood loss has occurred

C. Implementation
 1. Monitor vital signs
 2. Monitor client for abnormal pain, especially when forceps **delivery** has occurred
 3. Place ice to the hematoma site
 4. Administer analgesics as prescribed
 5. Monitor I&O
 6. Encourage fluids
 7. Encourage voiding
 8. Prepare for urinary catheterization if the client is unable to void
 9. Administer blood replacements as prescribed
 10. Monitor for signs of infection, such as increased temperature, pulse rate, and WBC count
 11. Administer antibiotics as prescribed since infection is common following hematoma formation
 12. Prepare for incision and evacuation of hematoma if necessary

XIV. Hydatidiform Mole

A. Description
 1. A developmental anomaly of the **placenta** that changes chorionic villi into a mass of clear vesicles
 2. Presents as an edematous grapelike cluster that may be nonmalignant or may develop into choriocarcinoma

B. Assessment
 1. Fetal heart rate not detectable
 2. Vaginal bleeding, which usually occurs by Week 12, of a bright red or dark brown color that may be slight, profuse, or intermittent
 3. Symptoms of PIH, such as elevated blood pressure, edema, and proteinuria, which may be present before Week 20
 4. Fundal height is greater than expected for date
 5. Elevated human chorionic gonadotropin (hCG) levels
 6. Ultrasound shows a characteristic snowstorm pattern

C. Implementation
 1. Monitor vital signs
 2. Monitor fetal heart rate and fetal activity
 3. Prepare mother for uterine evacuation or induced abortion

4. Prepare for hysterectomy if necessary
5. Monitor for postprocedure hemorrhage and infection
6. Monitor hCG levels for 1 year
7. Administer chemotherapeutic agents if necessary and as prescribed
8. Instruct parents regarding birth control measures so pregnancy can be prevented during the 1-year follow-up

XV. Hyperemesis Gravidarum

A. Description: Intractable nausea and vomiting that persists beyond the first trimester and causes disturbances in nutrition, electrolytes, and fluid balance
B. Assessment
   1. Nausea most pronounced on arising; however, it can occur at other times during the day
   2. Persistent vomiting
   3. Thirst
   4. Fever
   5. Hypotension
   6. Tachycardia
   7. Lethargy
   8. Weight loss
   9. Electrolyte imbalances
   10. Ketonuria
   11. Oliguria
   12. Decreased skin turgor and dry skin and mucous membranes
   13. Constipation
   14. Increased hematocrit levels
C. Implementation
   1. Monitor vital signs
   2. Monitor fetal heart rate and fetal activity
   3. Assess fetal growth
   4. Assess skin turgor and texture
   5. Monitor daily weight
   6. Monitor I&O and calorie count
   7. Restriction of PO intake until vomiting subsides
   8. Begin on a dry diet, alternating liquids and solids in small quantities, and advance diet slowly
   9. Monitor urine for ketones
   10. Monitor electrolytes, hemoglobin, and hematocrit levels
   11. Administer IV fluids and electrolytes as prescribed
   12. Administer antiemetics as prescribed

XVI. Incompetent Cervix

A. Description
   1. Premature dilation of cervix, which occurs in the 4th or 5th month of pregnancy
   2. Is associated with cervical trauma as a result of previous surgery or birth
   3. Treatment is surgical
B. Assessment

1. Vaginal bleeding at 18 to 28 weeks of gestation
2. Fetal membranes visible through cervix
C. Implementation
   1. Monitor vital signs
   2. Monitor fetal heart rate
   3. Provide bed rest
   4. Prepare for surgery by pursestring around cervix or stitched through cervix
      a. Pursestring around cervix is called McDonald's procedure
      b. Stitch through cervix is called Shirodkar's procedure
   5. Monitor for postprocedure complications, such as rupture of the membranes or contractions of the uterus
   6. Maintain bed rest for 24 hours postprocedure
   7. Report any postprocedure vaginal bleeding immediately to physician or health care provider
   8. Report increased uterine contractions to physician or health care provider if they occur postprocedure

XVII. Infections

A. Toxoplasmosis (Protozoa)
   1. Produces symptoms of acute, flulike infection in mother
   2. Transmitted through raw meat or handling cat litter of infected cats
   3. Organism passes through **placenta**
   4. Spontaneous abortion likely to occur early in pregnancy
B. Rubella
   1. Organism transmitted across **placenta**
   2. Extremely teratogenic in first trimester
   3. Causes congenital defects of eyes, heart, ears, and brain
   4. Women with low titers should be vaccinated at least 3 months before becoming pregnant or following a delivery
C. Cytomegalovirus (CMV)
   1. Produces flulike or mononucleosis-like symptoms in the mother
   2. Transmitted through the respiratory or sexual route
   3. Organism crosses the **placenta**, or the fetus may be infected through the birth canal
   4. May cause fetal death, retardation, heart defects, deafness
   5. No effective treatment available
D. Genital Herpes
   1. Affects the external genitalia, vagina, and cervix
   2. Causes draining, painful vesicles
   3. Virus is lethal to fetus if it is inoculated during vaginal **delivery**
   4. **Delivery** of the fetus is usually by cesarean section if active lesions are present
   5. Maintain precautions during the vaginal examination

6. Maintain isolation procedures during hospitalization if the disease is active
7. Infant and mother may be separated during the active period, or other special precautionary measures may be used to avoid transmission to neonate

XVIII. Multiple Gestation

A. Description
   1. Caused by double ovulation (fraternal or dizygotic) or a splitting of the fertilized egg (identical or monozygotic)
   2. Complications include spontaneous abortion, anemia, congenital anomalies, hyperemesis gravidarum, intrauterine growth retardation, PIH, polyhydramnios, postpartum hemorrhage, premature rupture of membranes, and preterm **labor** and **delivery**
B. Assessment
   1. Excessive fetal activity
   2. Uterus large for gestational age
   3. Palpation of three or four large parts in uterus
   4. Auscultation of more than one fetal heart rate
   5. Excessive morning sickness
   6. Anemia
   7. Hemorrhoids
   8. Varicosities
   9. Signs of preterm **labor**
   10. Excessive dependent edema
   11. Excessive weight gain
   12. Signs of PIH
C. Implementation
   1. Monitor vital signs
   2. Monitor fetal heart rate and fetal activity
   3. Provide bed rest with client in left lateral position
   4. Monitor for cervical changes
   5. Assess fetal growth
   6. Administer supplemental iron and vitamins as prescribed for anemia
   7. Monitor for preterm **labor** and treat preterm **labor** promptly
   8. Prepare client for ultrasound as prescribed
   9. Prepare for cesarean section for abnormal presentation
   10. Prepare to administer oxytocic drugs after **delivery** to prevent postpartum hemorrhage from uterine overdistention

XIX. Pregnancy-Induced Hypertension (PIH)

A. Description
   1. An acute hypertensive state that develops after the 20th week of gestation
   2. The condition can be mild or severe and can progress to seizures (eclampsia) (Box 25–1)
B. Predisposing Conditions
   1. Primigravida
   2. Teenagers and women over 35 years of age

BOX 25–1. Signs of Worsening PIH or Impending Seizures

BP 160/110 or above	Visual changes
Epigastric pain	Headache
Decreased urinary output	Excessive proteinuria

---

   3. Poor nutrition
   4. Low socioeconomic status
   5. Chronic hypertension
   6. Diabetes
   7. Chronic renal disease
   8. History of PIH
C. Complications of PIH
   1. Abruptio placentae
   2. DIC
   3. Thrombocytopenia
   4. **Placental** insufficiency
   5. Intrauterine fetal death
D. Mild Pre-Eclampsia
   1. Assessment
      a. Hypertension of 15 to 30 mmHg above baseline
      b. Weight gain of 1 lb or more per week in last trimester
      c. Mild, generalized edema
      d. Proteinuria of 1+
   2. Implementation
      a. Provide bed rest and position client in left lateral position
      b. Monitor blood pressure and weight
      c. Monitor neurological status since changes can indicate cerebral hypoxia or impending seizure
      d. Monitor deep tendon reflexes and for the presence of clonus, as hyperreflexia indicates increased central nervous system irritability (Box 25–2)
      e. Provide adequate fluids
      f. Monitor I&O; a urinary output of 30 mL per hour indicates adequate renal perfusion
      g. Increase dietary protein and carbohydrates with no added salt
      h. Administer medications as prescribed to lower blood pressure to prevent a cerebrovascular accident; however, blood pressure should not be lowered drastically because **placental** perfusion can be compromised
E. Severe Pre-Eclampsia
   1. Assessment
      a. Severe hypertension, 30 to 40 mmHg above baseline while on bed rest
      b. Massive, generalized edema and weight gain
      c. Proteinuria 4+
      d. Less than 400 mL output in 24 hours
      e. Severe headache
      f. Dizziness

BOX 25–2. Assessment of Reflexes

Patellar

Position the client with legs dangling over the edge of the examining table or lying on back with legs slightly flexed

Strike the patellar tendon just below the kneecap with the percussion hammer

Normal Response

Extension or kicking out of leg

Biceps

Position your thumb over the client's biceps tendon, supporting the client's elbow with the palm of the hand

Strike a downward blow over the client's thumb with the percussion hammer

Normal Response

Flexion of the arm at the elbow

Clonus

Position the client with legs dangling over the edge of the examining table

Support the leg with one hand and sharply dorsiflex the client's foot with the other hand

Maintain the dorsiflexed position for a few seconds, then release the foot

Normal Response (Negative Clonus Response)

Foot will remain steady in the dorsiflexed position

No rhythmic oscillations or jerking of the foot will be felt

When released, the foot will drop to a plantarflexed position with no oscillations

Abnormal Response (Positive Clonus Response)

Rhythmic oscillations when the foot is dorsiflexed

Similar oscillations will be noted when the foot drops to the plantarflexed position

---

  g. Blurred vision and spots before eyes
  h. Nausea and vomiting
  i. Epigastric pain
  j. Central nervous system irritability
  2. Implementation
    a. Administer magnesium sulfate as prescribed
    b. Administer hydralazine (Apresoline) as prescribed to prevent cerebrovascular accident
    c. Prepare for the induction of **labor**
    d. Plan for the administration of magnesium sulfate for 24 to 48 hours postpartum as prescribed
F. Eclampsia
  1. Assessment
    a. Severe edema
    b. Proteinuria 4+
    c. Sudden large increase in weight
    d. BP greater than 160/110
    e. Cyanosis
    f. Fetal distress
    g. Convulsions
    h. Coma

  2. Implementation
    a. Protect the client from injury
    b. Administer oxygen
    c. Monitor fetal heart rate and contractions
    d. Initiate seizure precautions
    e. Administer seizure medications as prescribed
    f. Prepare for **delivery** after stabilization of client

XX. Pyelonephritis

A. Description
  1. Results from bacterial infections that extend upward from the bladder through the blood vessels and lymphatics
  2. Frequently follows untreated urinary tract infections and is associated with an increased incidence of anemia, low birth weight, PIH, premature **labor** and **delivery**, and premature rupture of membranes
B. Assessment
  1. Flank pain
  2. Burning or painful urination
  3. Increased frequency of urination
  4. Chills, malaise, nausea
  5. Increased temperature, pulse rate, and fetal heart rate
  6. Vomiting
  7. Uterine contractions
  8. Elevated WBC
C. Implementation
  1. Monitor vital signs
  2. Monitor fetal heart rate
  3. Monitor for contractions
  4. Provide fluids
  5. Monitor I&O
  6. Monitor renal function
  7. Administer IV antibiotics as prescribed
  8. Administer antipyretics such as acetaminophen (Tylenol) as prescribed
  9. Obtain urine cultures every 2 to 4 weeks after resolution of infection

XXI. Sexually Transmitted Diseases (STD)

A. *Chlamydia*
  1. Description
    a. Common, sexually transmitted pathogen associated with an increased risk for premature births, stillborns, neonatal conjunctivitis, and newborn chlamydial pneumonia
    b. In the nonpregnant state, it can cause salpingitis, pelvic abscesses, and chronic pelvic pain and infertility
    c. Incubation period is 5 to 10 days or longer, up to 28 days
    d. Diagnostic test is *chlamydia* culture for *Chlamydia trachomatis*
  2. Assessment
    a. Increased vaginal discharge and itching

b. Low-grade temperature

c. Right upper quadrant abdominal pain

d. Bleeding between periods

e. Pain with coitus

f. Dysuria

g. Rectal pain or discharge

h. Mucopurulent cervicitis

i. Cervix that bleeds easily

j. In the neonate, conjunctivitis and pneumonia

3. Implementation

   a. Screen the client to determine whether high risk

   b. Instruct the nonpregnant client about medication; doxycycline is usually prescribed

   c. Instruct the pregnant client about medication; usually erythromycin (E-Mycin), 500 mg PO for 7 days, is prescribed

   d. Instruct mother about medication for the newborn infant; orally administered erythromycin is usually prescribed

   e. Instruct client in the importance of rescreening, because reinfection can occur as the client nears term

   f. Administer appropriate eye prophylaxis to the neonate as prescribed

   g. Monitor neonates for signs and symptoms of pneumonia if at risk

   h. Ensure that the sexual partner is treated

B. Syphilis

1. Description

   a. A chronic infectious disease caused by the organism *Treponema pallidum*

   b. Transmission is by intimate physical contact with syphilitic lesions, which are usually found on the skin or mucous membranes of the mouth and genitals

   c. The incubation period is 2 to 6 weeks following exposure

   d. The infection may cause abortion or premature **labor** and is passed to the fetus after the fourth month of pregnancy as congenital syphilis

2. Assessment (Table 25–2)

3. Implementation

   a. Obtain serum test for syphilis on first prenatal visit

   b. Prepare to repeat serum test for syphilis just before the fourth month as the disease may be acquired after the initial visit

   c. Instruct client that treatment of her partner is necessary if infection occurs

   d. Prepare to administer procaine penicillin G to mother as prescribed

   e. Report all cases to health authorities for treatment of contacts

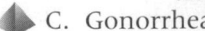 C. Gonorrhea

1. Description

   a. Infection caused by *Neisseria gonorrhoeae*

Table 25–2. Assessment of the Stages of Syphilis

Primary Stage	Secondary Stage	Tertiary Stage
Most infectious stage	Highly infectious stage	Spirochetes enter the internal organs and cause permanent damage
Appearance of ulcerative, painless lesions produced by spirochetes at the point of entry into the body	Lesions appear about 3 weeks after the primary stage and may occur anywhere on the skin and mucous membranes	Symptoms may occur 10 to 30 years following the occurrence of an untreated primary lesion
	Generalized lymphadenopathy occurs	Invades the CNS, causing meningitis, ataxia, general paresis, and progressive mental deterioration
		Affects the aortic valve and aorta

that causes inflammation of the mucous membranes of the genital and urinary tracts

   b. Transmission of organism is by sexual intercourse

   c. Infection may be transmitted to the baby's eyes during **delivery**, causing blindness (ophthalmia neonatorum)

2. Assessment

   a. Female: Usually asymptomatic; vaginal discharge, urinary frequency, and pain possible

   b. Male: Fever, painful urination, pelvic pain, epididymitis with pain, tenderness, and swelling

3. Implementation

   a. Obtain culture for gonorrhea on the first prenatal visit

   b. Prepare to repeat culture for gonorrhea as infection may occur during pregnancy

   c. Administer prophylactic antibiotics: erythromycin or 1% silver nitrate to the newborn infant

   d. Instruct client that treatment of partner is necessary if infection occurs

D. Genital Warts

1. Description

   a. Caused by human papillomavirus (HPV) and affects the cervix, urethra, penis, scrotum, and anus

   b. Appears 1 to 2 months after exposure

   c. Transmitted through sexual contact

   d. There is no cure for HPV

2. Assessment

   a. Small to large wartlike growths on genitals

   b. Cervical cell changes noted because HPV is associated with cervical malignancies

3. Implementation

   a. Encourage yearly Papanicolaou (Pap) smear

b. Limit sexual contacts and use condoms
c. Instruct client regarding potential treatment, including cytotoxic agents, cryotherapy, electrocautery, and surgical excision to remove the lesions

XXII. Tuberculosis

A. Description
  1. A highly communicable disease caused by *Mycobacterium tuberculosis*
  2. It is transmitted by the airborne route
  3. **Tuberculosis** has an insidious onset, and many clients are not aware of symptoms until the disease is well advanced
  4. A **multidrug-resistant strain (MDR-TB)** of **TB** can exist as a result of improper use or noncompliance with treatment programs and the development of mutations in the tubercle bacilli
B. Transmission
  1. Transplacental transmission is rare
  2. Can occur during birth through aspiration of infected **amniotic fluid**
  3. Neonate can become infected from contact with infected individuals
C. Risk to Mother: Active disease during pregnancy has been associated with an increase in hypertensive disorders of pregnancy
D. Diagnosis
  1. If a chest radiograph is required for the mother, a lead shield to the abdomen is required
  2. TB skin testing is safe during pregnancy
E. Assessment
  1. Maternal
    a. May be asymptomatic
    b. Fever and chills
    c. Night sweats
    d. Weight loss
    e. Fatigue
    f. Cough
    g. Green or yellow sputum
    h. Hemoptysis
    i. Dyspnea
    j. Pleural pain
  2. Neonate
    a. Fever
    b. Lethargy
    c. Poor feeding
    d. Failure to thrive
    e. Respiratory distress
    f. Hepatosplenomegaly
    g. Meningitis
    h. Disease may spread to all major organs
F. Implementation
  1. Mother
    a. Administration of isoniazid (INH), ethambutol, and rifampin for 6 to 12 months during and after pregnancy
    b. Pyridoxine should be administered with INH to pregnant women to prevent the development of peripheral neuropathy due to INH
    c. Note that teratogenicity is unknown with rifampin
    d. Promote breastfeeding only if the mother is noninfectious
    e. Breastfeeding is not contraindicated with isoniazid (INH), ethambutol, and rifampin
    f. Note that pregnancy and immunosuppression are contraindications to bacille Calmette-Guérin (BCG) administration
  2. Neonate
    a. If born to a mother with active TB, should be treated with INH for 3 months
    b. Neonates born to infected mothers with active disease can be vaccinated with BCG
    c. Isolate and separate the infant from the mother during active disease until the mother is known to be noninfectious after a minimum of 3 weeks of drug therapy
    d. Administer BCG vaccine to the infant as prescribed
    e. Note that a Mantoux test turns positive after a BCG test is given

XXIII. Urinary Tract Infection (UTI)

A. Description: The most common medical complication of pregnancy, but, if untreated, the client can develop pyelonephritis
B. Predisposing Conditions
  1. History of UTI
  2. Sickle cell trait
  3. Poor hygiene
  4. Anemia
  5. Diabetes
C. Assessment
  1. Burning and pain on urination
  2. Increased frequency of urination
  3. Lower abdominal pain
  4. Costovertebral angle tenderness
  5. Fever
  6. Proteinuria, hematuria, bacteriuria, WBCs in urine
D. Implementation
  1. Monitor vital signs
  2. Monitor fetal heart rate
  3. Increase fluid intake
  4. Monitor I&O
  5. Monitor urine for consistency and odor
  6. Monitor for signs and symptoms of pyelonephritis
  7. Obtain urine for culture and sensitivity
  8. Provide heat to lower abdomen or back
  9. Administer antibiotics as prescribed
  10. Instruct client to complete the course of antibiotics if prescribed
  11. Instruct client regarding the need to repeat the culture after treatment is completed

PRACTICE QUESTIONS

1. Which of the following complications is most likely to be associated with a twin pregnancy?
   1 Maternal anemia
   2 Post-term labor
   3 Oligohydramnios
   4 Gestational diabetes

2. The client with a 38-week twin gestation is admitted to the Birthing Center in early labor. Twin "B" is a breech presentation. Of the following, which will the nurse list as the lowest priority in planning the nursing care of this client?
   1 Attach electronic fetal monitoring
   2 Prepare client for a possible cesarean section
   3 Measure fundal height
   4 Start an IV

3. A stillborn was delivered in the Birthing Suite a few hours ago. After the birth, the family has remained together, holding and touching the baby. Which statement by the nurse would further assist them in their initial period of grief?
   1 "Don't worry, there is nothing you could do to prevent this from happening."
   2 "We need to take the baby from you now so that you can get some sleep."
   3 "What have you named your lovely baby?"
   4 "We will see to it that you have an early discharge so that you don't have to be reminded of this experience."

4. A client has been asked to keep a fetal activity diary. Which of the following responses indicates an adequate understanding of this procedure?
   1 "I will schedule the counting periods approximately 1 hour before meals."
   2 "The best position for counting fetal movement is prone."
   3 "I know my baby is healthy if it moves at least 25 times in 3 hours."
   4 "I should notify my physician if the baby's movements are less than 10 times in 3 hours."

5. A client and her husband are being discharged from the hospital after giving birth to a fetal demise. They ask about the possibility of attending a bereavement support group in the community. The nurse is aware that this is an indication of:
   1 Denial
   2 Prolonged sadness
   3 Normal grieving
   4 Anger

6. Which of the following interventions, if selected by the nurse, is appropriate for the HIV client with the nursing diagnosis of High Risk for Infection?
   1 Offer spiritual support if desired
   2 Provide information on safe sex practices
   3 Enforce total bed rest
   4 Administer magnesium sulfate

7. The nurse is assessing the status of the prenatal client. The nurse determines that which of the following places the prenatal client into the high-risk category for contracting HIV?
   1 Living in an area where HIV infections are minimal
   2 A history of IV drug use in the past year
   3 A history of one sexual partner within the past 10 years
   4 A spouse who is heterosexual and had only one sexual partner in the past 10 years

8. A postpartum client has a nursing diagnosis of High Risk for Infection. A goal has been developed that states "The client will not develop an infection during her hospital stay." Which of the following data supports that the goal has been met?
   1 Presence of chills
   2 Abdominal tenderness
   3 Absence of fever
   4 Loss of appetite

9. A postpartum client suspected of having an infection is informed that she will be unable to have the newborn infant present in the room with her. The client complains and is unhappy about the absence of her infant. Which of the following nursing diagnoses is of the highest priority at this time?
   1 Social Isolation
   2 High Risk for Ineffective Mother-Infant Bonding
   3 Ineffective Individual Coping
   4 Denial

10. The nurse is conducting a clinic visit with a prenatal client with heart disease. The nurse carefully evaluates vital signs, weight gain, and fluid and nutritional status to detect complications caused by:
    1 Hypertrophy and increased contractility
    2 The increase in circulating volume
    3 Fetal cardiomegaly
    4 Rh incompatibility

11. A perinatal client is admitted to the obstetric unit during an exacerbation of a heart condition. When planning for the nutritional requirements of the client, the nurse consults with the dietitian to ensure which of the following?
    1 A low calorie diet to ensure absence of weight gain
    2 A diet low in fluids and fiber to decrease blood volume
    3 A diet high in fluids and fiber to decrease constipation
    4 Unlimited sodium intake to increase circulating blood volume

12. During an office visit, a prenatal client with mitral stenosis states she has been under a lot of stress lately. During the examination, the client questions everything the nurse does and behaves in an anxious manner. The best nursing response/action at this time is to:
    1 Tell her not to worry
    2 Ignore her unfounded concerns and continue
    3 Explain the purpose of the nurse's actions and answer all questions
    4 Refer her to a counselor

13. A perinatal client with a history of heart disease has been instructed on care at home. Which of the following statements, if made by the client, indicates that the client understands her needs?
    1 "There is no restriction on people who visit me."
    2 "I should avoid stressful situations."
    3 "My weight gain is not important."
    4 "I should rest on my right side."

14. A primigravida client comes to the clinic and has been diagnosed with a urinary tract infection. She has repeatedly verbalized concern regarding safety of the fetus. Which of the following nursing diagnoses is most appropriate at this time?
    1 Pain
    2 Impaired Tissue Integrity
    3 Urinary Tract Infection
    4 Fear

15. A prenatal client has acquired the sexually transmitted human papilloma virus that causes condyloma acuminatum. When planning care, which of the following interventions would the nurse consider to be safe for this maternity client?
    1 Laser therapy
    2 Use of cytotoxic agents
    3 Treatment with interferon
    4 All treatment should be avoided

16. The perinatal client is at risk for toxoplasmosis. The nurse would teach the client which of the following to prevent exposure to this disease?
    1 Wash hands only before meals
    2 Eat raw meats
    3 Avoid exposure to litter boxes used by cats
    4 Use topical steroid treatments prophylactically

17. A perinatal client has been instructed on prevention of genital tract infections. Which of the following statements, if made by the client, indicates effective teaching by the nurse?
    1 "I should avoid the use of condoms."
    2 "I can douche anytime I want."
    3 "I can wear my tight-fitting jeans."
    4 "I should choose underwear with a cotton panel liner."

18. During an initial assessment of a maternity client, the nurse notes that the laboratory report shows leukopenia, thrombocytopenia, anemia, and an elevated erythrocyte sedimentation rate. The nurse suspects HIV. Which of the following laboratory tests further supports the presence of HIV?
    1 T-lymphocyte levels
    2 Angiotensin levels
    3 Glomerular filtration rate
    4 Platelet count

19. When caring for the maternal client with HIV, which of the following goals is most appropriate?
    1 The client will not have sexual relations during the remainder of pregnancy
    2 The client will not develop an opportunistic infection during the remainder of pregnancy
    3 The client is advised of an HIV support group
    4 The client is assisted with the grief process

20. A prenatal client diagnosed with anemia has come to the clinic. After assessment, her laboratory values indicate low hemoglobin and hematocrit levels. Which of the following nursing diagnoses do the data best support?
    1 Anxiety
    2 Low Self-Esteem
    3 Cerebral Vascular Accident
    4 High Risk for Infection

21. When planning interventions for counseling the maternal client newly diagnosed with sickle cell anemia, the most important psychosocial intervention at this time is which of the following?
    1 Provide all information regarding the disease initially
    2 Allow the client to be alone if she is crying
    3 Provide emotional support
    4 Avoid the topic of the disease at all costs

22. A client in labor has an underlying diagnosis of sickle cell anemia. During labor, the client is at high risk for sickling crisis. Which of the following is the priority action by the nurse to assist in preventing a crisis from occurring during labor?
    1 Reassure the client
    2 Administer oxygen as prescribed throughout labor
    3 Maintain strict asepsis
    4 Prevent bearing down

23. The nurse has a teaching session with a malnourished client regarding iron supplementation to prevent anemia during pregnancy. Which of the following statements, if made by the client, indicates successful learning?
    1 "The iron is needed to make red blood cells to supply my baby with food."
    2 "Meat does not provide iron and should be avoided."
    3 "Iron supplements will give me diarrhea."
    4 "My body has all the iron it needs and I don't need to take supplements."

24. The nurse is developing goals for the postpartum client who is at risk for infection. Which of the following goals is most appropriate for this diagnosis?
    1 The client will verbalize a reduction of pain
    2 The client will no longer have a positive Homan's sign
    3 The client will report acceptance of the infection
    4 The client will be able to identify measures to prevent infection

25. The nurse is instructing a postpartum client with endometritis about preventing the spread of infection to the newborn infant. Which of the following statements would the nurse make to the client?
    1 Hands should be washed thoroughly before holding the infant
    2 The infant will not be allowed in the room at all
    3 There is no danger of the neonate contracting the disease
    4 Visitors are not allowed to hold the baby

26. The client is a 15-year-old gravida 1 who is 14 weeks pregnant. She comes to the clinic for the first prenatal visit. During the interview, the nurse discovers that the client has been an insulin-dependent diabetic since the age of 9 years. She tells the nurse "I'm trying not to eat much so I won't show, but it is O.K. because I have cut out my insulin." The nurse formulates which of the following most important nursing diagnoses at this time?
    1 Body Image Disturbance, related to fear of gaining weight
    2 Altered Nutrition: Less Than Body Requirements, related to voluntary decrease in food intake
    3 Risk for Impaired Skin Integrity, related to skin stretching from growing uterus
    4 Risk for Injury to Fetus, related to teenage pregnancy

27. The nurse prepares a teaching plan for a newly diagnosed diabetic pregnant client. Which of the following should not be included in the teaching plan?
    1 Effects of diabetes on the pregnancy and fetus
    2 Nutritional requirements for pregnancy and diabetic control
    3 To avoid exercise due to the negative effects on insulin production
    4 To be aware of any infections and report signs of infection immediately to the health care provider

28. The postpartum client with gestational diabetes is scheduled for discharge. During the discharge teaching she asks the nurse "Do I have to worry about this diabetes anymore?" The best response by the nurse is:
    1 "Your blood glucose level is within normal limits now, you will be all right."
    2 "You will only have to worry about the diabetes if you become pregnant again."
    3 "You will be at risk for developing gestational diabetes with your next pregnancy and developing overt diabetes mellitus."
    4 "Once you have gestational diabetes you have overt diabetes and must be treated with medication for the rest of your life."

29. During a prenatal visit, the nurse is explaining dietary management to a client with diabetes. The nurse evaluates that the teaching has been effective when the client states:
    1 "I can eat more sweets now because I need more calories."
    2 "I need more fat in my diet so the baby can gain enough weight."
    3 "I need to eat a high-protein, low-carbohydrate diet now in order to control my blood sugar."
    4 "I need to increase the fiber in my diet to control my blood glucose and prevent constipation."

30. A new prenatal client is 6 months pregnant. On the first prenatal visit, the nurse notes that the client is gravida 4, para 0, aborta 3. The client is 5'6" tall, weighs 130 pounds, and is 25 years old. She states: "I get really tired after working all day and can't keep up with my housework." Which factor in these data lead the nurse to suspect gestational diabetes?
    1 Fatigue
    2 Obesity
    3 Maternal age
    4 Fetal demise

31. A pregnant client is newly diagnosed as having gestational diabetes. She cries during the remainder of the interview and keeps repeating "What have I done to cause this? If I could only live my life over." Which nursing diagnosis should direct nursing care at this time?
    1 Self-Concept Disturbance, related to a complication of pregnancy
    2 Knowledge Deficit, related to diabetic self-care during pregnancy
    3 Body Image Disturbance, related to complications of pregnancy
    4 Risk for Injury to the Fetus, related to maternal distress

32. A primigravida is receiving magnesium sulfate for pregnancy-induced hypertension (PIH). The nurse does assessments every 30 minutes. Which of the following assessments is of most concern to the nurse?

1   Urinary output of 20 mL since the last check
2   Deep tendon reflexes of 2+
3   Respirations of 10 breaths/minute
4   Fetal heart tones of 116 beats/minute

33. During a routine prenatal visit, the client states, "I have not been able to get my wedding ring off for the last 2 days. I guess the heat is making my fingers swell." The nurse needs to further assess the client for:
    1   Blood pressure changes and protein in her urine
    2   Height of the fundus compared with the date of her last visit
    3   Blood glucose level
    4   Any vaginal discharge

34. When a client progresses from pre-eclampsia to eclampsia, the nurse's first action should be to:
    1   Administer IV magnesium sulfate
    2   Assess the blood pressure and fetal heart tones
    3   Clear and maintain an open airway
    4   Administer oxygen by face mask

35. The nurse instructs a client with mild pre-eclampsia on home care. The nurse evaluates that the teaching has been effective concerning assessment of complications when the client states:
    1   "As long as the health nurse is visiting me daily I do not have to keep my next physician's appointment."
    2   "I need to take my blood pressure each morning and alternate arms each time."
    3   "I need to check my weight every day at different times during the day."
    4   "I need to check my urine with a dipstick every day for protein and call the physician if it is 2+ or more."

36. A primigravida is admitted with symptoms of pre-eclampsia. The nurse is aware that the client may be developing HELLP syndrome upon noting which of the following?
    1   A drop in the platelet count to less than 100,000/mm
    2   A drop in the liver enzyme levels
    3   A sudden increase in weight
    4   A deep tendon reflex of 4+ with 1 beat of clonus

37. The nurse is doing a 48-hour postpartum check on a client who was discharged with mild pre-eclampsia. Which of the following data indicate that the PIH is not resolving?
    1   Blood pressure reading has returned to the prenatal baseline
    2   Urinary output has increased
    3   The client complains of a daily headache and developed blurred vision this morning
    4   There is no evidence of dependent edema

38. A client has just had surgery to deliver a nonviable fetus due to abruptio placentae. She has just been told she is developing disseminated intravascular coagulapathy due to these problems. She begins to cry and screams "God, just let me die now!" Which nursing diagnosis should direct care for this client?
    1   Hopelessness, related to loss of baby and personal health
    2   Knowledge Deficit, related to disease process
    3   Self-Esteem Disturbance, related to being ill
    4   Grief, related to loss of the baby

39. A pregnant client has just been admitted with severe pre-eclampsia. The nurse knows it is important to assess for additional complications at this time. Part of the plan of care for this client should be regular assessments for:
    1   Any bleeding, such as in the gums, petechiae and purpura
    2   Enlargement of the breasts
    3   Periods of fetal movement followed by quite periods
    4   Complaints of feeling hot when the room is cool

40. In evaluating the client at risk for DIC, which of the following factors would the nurse consider to be the most significant?
    1   A gravida 6 who delivered 10 hours ago and has lost 450 mL of blood
    2   A gravida 2 who has just been diagnosed with dead fetus syndrome; fetal demise occurred 2 months ago
    3   A primigravida with mild pre-eclampsia
    4   A primigravida who delivered a 10-pound baby 3 hours ago

ANSWERS

1. **1**

Rationale: Maternal anemia occurs because the maternal system is nurturing more than one fetus, thus option 1 is the correct answer. Option 2 is incorrect as the complication that could occur would include preterm labor. The fetus is preterm at a rate 5 to 10 times that of singletons. Option 3 is incorrect. Hydramnios may be associated with a twin pregnancy due to increased renal perfusion from cross-vessel anastomosis with monozygotic twins. Option 4 is not a complication of a twin pregnancy.

Test-Taking Strategy: Analysis questions are the most difficult questions because they require understanding of the principles of physiological responses; in this case, a twin pregnancy and its effect on the mother and the effect of each fetus on the other. The issue of the question is a complication. This is a question, also, that has a true response stem. The key phrase is "most likely," which asks you to select an answer that is true regarding the situation and question. Review complications of multiple gestation now, if you had difficulty with this question!

Level of Cognitive Ability: Analysis
Phase of Nursing Process: Analysis
Client Needs: Physiological Integrity
Content Area: Maternity

Reference

Olds, S., London, M., & Ladewig, P. (1996). *Maternal-newborn nursing: A family-centered approach* (5th ed.). Reading, MA: Addison-Wesley. pp. 723–724.

2. **3**

Rationale: Option 3 is a low priority because fundal height should be measured at each antepartal clinic visit and not as a priority of care in the intrapartum period. Options 1, 2, and 4 are all high priorities. Intrapartal management and assessment require careful attention to maternal and fetal status. The twins should be monitored by dual electronic fetal monitoring, and in so doing, any signs of distress may be reported to the obstetrician. Because most breech presentations are born by cesarean section, many physicians choose C-birth if either of the twins is breech. The mother should have an IV in place in case fluid or blood replacement is required.

Test-Taking Strategy: This question asks you to select a false response item. The key word used here is "lowest," which asks you to select an answer that is not true regarding this particular situation. Also utilize Maslow's Hierarchy of Needs theory to prioritize options in this question. Physiological needs come first!

Level of Cognitive Ability: Application
Phase of Nursing Process: Planning
Client Needs: Safe, Effective Care Environment
Content Area: Maternity

Reference

Olds, S., London, M., & Ladewig, P. (1996). *Maternal-newborn nursing: A family-centered approach* (5th ed.). Reading, MA: Addison-Wesley. pp. 725–726.

3. **3**

Rationale: Nurses should be able to explore measures that assist the family to create memories of an infant so that the existence of the child is confirmed and the parents can complete the grieving process. Option 3 does do this and also demonstrates a caring and empathetic response. Option 1, 2 and 4 are blocks to communication and devalue the parents' feelings.

Test-Taking Strategy: This is a question in which you need to identify the use of a therapeutic communication statement as opposed to a communication block. Always focus on the client's feelings first, which will promote psychosocial adaptation and coping abilities of the client. Choose an option that demonstrates a caring and empathetic response by the nurse, that meets the psychosocial needs of the client/family, and that focuses on the client as a worthy human being—not one that devalues feelings.

Level of Cognitive Ability: Application
Phase of Nursing Process: Implementation
Client Needs: Psychosocial Integrity
Content Area: Maternity

Reference

Gorrie, T., McKinney, E. S., & Murray, S. S. (1998). *Foundations of maternal-newborn nursing* (2nd ed.). Philadelphia: W. B. Saunders. p. 663.

4. **4**

Rationale: Interventions are successful if the woman verbalizes knowledge of why tests are recommended, an idea of how and when they are performed, and her concern about the condition of the fetus. Option 4 is correct. Most healthy fetuses move at least 10 times in 3 hours. Slowing or stopping of fetal movement may be an indication that the fetus needs some attention and evaluation. Option 3 is incorrect based on this rationale. Option 1 is incorrect. In general, women are advised to count fetal movements for 30 to 60 minutes, three times a day (usually after meals when the fetus is more active). Option 2 is incorrect. The client lies down on the left side during the procedure because it provides optimal circulation to the uterus-placenta-fetus unit.

Test-Taking Strategy: Eliminate the incorrect options. Read all the options very carefully before selecting an answer, and reread the stem of the question before selecting the answer. Analysis questions require an understanding of the principles of physiological responses, critical thinking, and therapeutic rationale related to the specific issue of fetal activity. Review normal fetal activity now, if you had difficulty with this question!

Level of Cognitive Ability: Analysis
Phase of Nursing Process: Evaluation
Client Needs: Health Promotion and Maintenance
Content Area: Maternity

References

Olds, S., London, M., & Ladewig, P. (1996). *Maternal-newborn nursing: A family-centered approach* (5th ed.). Reading, MA: Addison-Wesley. p. 376.

5. **3**

Rationale: A perinatal bereavement support group can help the parents work through their pain by nonjudgmental sharing of feelings. It is a necessary part of normal grieving.

Test-Taking Strategy: Read all the options very carefully before selecting an answer, and reread the stem of the question. Use the process of elimination and eliminate the incorrect option. Review the normal grieving process now if you had difficulty with this question!

Level of Cognitive Ability: Analysis
Phase of Nursing Process: Analysis
Client Needs: Psychosocial Integrity
Content Area: Maternity

Reference

Gorrie, T., McKinney, E. S., & Murray, S. S. (1998). *Foundations of maternal-newborn nursing* (2nd ed.). Philadelphia: W. B. Saunders. p. 663.

6. **2**

Rationale: The client can receive infections from partners as well as transmit HIV. Until a vaccine or cure becomes available, the best strategy to prevent the spread of HIV infection is prevention. Prevention can best be accomplished through education. This is an opportunity to discuss ways for the client to protect self, which includes abstinence from sex, making informed choices about partners, and safer sexual practices.

Test-Taking Strategy: Option 1 would be appropriate but not for the diagnosis identified in the stem. Options 3 and 4 are interventions appropriate for pre-eclampsia. Option 2 is the only intervention that addresses the nursing diagnosis identified in the stem. Identify what the question is asking.

Level of Cognitive Ability: Application
Phase of Nursing Process: Implementation
Client Needs: Physiological Integrity
Content Area: Maternity

References

Pillitteri, A. (1995). *Maternal & child health: Nursing care of the childbearing and childrearing family* (2nd ed.). Philadelphia: J. B. Lippincott. pp. 334–336.

7. **2**

Rationale: HIV is not highly contagious but is transmitted by intimate sexual contact, the exchange of body fluids, and exposure to infected blood, as well as transmission from an infected woman to her fetus. Women who fall into the high-risk category for HIV infection include those with persistent and recurrent sexually transmitted diseases or a history of multiple sexual partners and those who use or have used IV drugs.

Test-Taking Strategy: Knowledge regarding risk factors for HIV is necessary to answer the question. The stem asks for a situation that places the client at risk for the disease. Option 2 is the correct answer. Options 1, 3, and 4 are not situations that contribute to the incidence of contracting HIV.

Level of Cognitive Ability: Analysis
Phase of Nursing Process: Analysis
Client Needs: Health Promotion and Maintenance
Content Area: Maternity

References

Lowdermilk, D., Perry, S., & Bobak, I. (1997). *Maternity & women's health care* (6th ed.). St. Louis: Mosby–Year Book. p. 735.

8. **3**

Rationale: Any fever must be considered to have been caused by postpartum infection in the absence of convincing proof of another cause. Chills, abdominal tenderness, and loss of appetite indicate the presence of an infection. Fever is the first indication of an infection.

Test-Taking Strategy: Knowledge of the signs and symptoms of infection is necessary to answer this question. The question is asking for a means of evaluating the effectiveness of a goal. Options 1, 2, and 4 would indicate that the goal had not been met. The only answer that would indicate that the goal had been met is option 3.

Level of Cognitive Ability: Analysis
Phase of Nursing Process: Evaluation
Client Needs: Physiological Integrity
Content Area: Maternity

References

Pillitteri, A. (1995). *Maternal & child health: Nursing care of the childbearing and childrearing family* (2nd ed.). Philadelphia: J. B. Lippincott. p. 714.

9. **2**

Rationale: There is a period shortly after birth that is uniquely important to attachment and mother-infant bonding.

Test-Taking Strategy: The question asks for the priority diagnosis at this time. The stem gives information that supports only option 2. The information provided in the question is insufficient to support the other options.

Level of Cognitive Ability: Analysis
Phase of Nursing Process: Analysis
Client Needs: Psychosocial Integrity
Content Area: Maternity

References

Pillitteri, A. (1995). *Maternal & child health: Nursing care of the childbearing and childrearing family* (2nd ed.). Philadelphia: J. B. Lippincott. pp. 564–565.
Lowdermilk, D., Perry, S., & Bobak, I. (1997). *Maternity & women's health care* (6th ed.). St. Louis: Mosby–Year Book. p. 470.

10. **2**

Rationale: Pregnancy taxes the circulating system of every woman because both the blood volume and cardiac output increase approximately 30%. This is especially important to monitor in the client whose heart may not tolerate this normal increase.

Test-Taking Strategy: Knowledge of the pathophysiology behind the changes that take place in a woman during pregnancy is needed to assist you in answering this question. In option 1, hypertrophy may result in cardiac disease, but the outcome would be a decrease in contractility, not an increase. Options 3 and 4 are directed at the fetus, not the prenatal client identified in the stem. Review pathophysiology in relation to cardiac disease in the maternity client now, if you had difficulty with this question!

Level of Cognitive Ability: Analysis
Phase of Nursing Process: Analysis
Client Needs: Physiological Integrity
Content Area: Maternity

Reference

Gorrie, T., McKinney, E. S., & Murray, S. S. (1998). *Foundations of maternal-newborn nursing* (2nd ed.). Philadelphia: W. B. Saunders. p. 126.

11. **3**

Rationale: Constipation causes the client to utilize the Valsalva maneuver. This causes blood to rush to the heart and overload the cardiac system. Absence of weight gain is not recommended during pregnancy. Diets low in fluid and fiber would cause a decrease in blood volume, which in turn deprives the fetus of nutrients. Too much sodium could cause an overload to the circulating blood volume and contribute to the cardiac condition.

Test-Taking Strategy: If the answer is not evident, try to relate the situation to something you are familiar with. Look for options that would apply to all heart conditions, then use the process of elimination to select the answer. Option 3 is the only correct answer.

Level of Cognitive Ability: Application
Phase of Nursing Process: Planning
Client Needs: Physiological Integrity
Content Area: Maternity

Reference
Lowdermilk, D., Perry, S., & Bobak, I. (1997). *Maternity & women's health care* (6th ed.). St. Louis: Mosby–Year Book. p. 835.

12. 3

Rationale: For the prenatal cardiac client, stress should be reduced as much as possible. Be certain the woman understands the purpose of any test or assessments so she does not worry unnecessarily. Options 1, 2, and 4 are nontherapeutic methods of communication at this time. Explaining the purpose of nursing actions will assist in decreasing the stress level of the client.

Test-Taking Strategy: Remember that therapeutic communication techniques are used to answer questions regarding responses to a client. Therapeutic communication techniques enhance communication. Always select the answer that will enhance communication. Avoid selecting responses that will block communication. Always address the client's concerns and feelings.

Level of Cognitive Ability: Application
Phase of Nursing Process: Implementation
Client Needs: Psychosocial Integrity
Content Area: Maternity

References
Pillitteri, A. (1995). *Maternal & child health: Nursing care of the childbearing and childrearing family* (2nd ed.). Philadelphia: J. B. Lippincott. p. 355.
Gorrie, T., McKinney, E. S., & Murray, S. S. (1998). *Foundations of maternal-newborn nursing* (2nd ed.). Philadelphia: W. B. Saunders. pp. 24–25.

13. 2

Rationale: To avoid infections, visitors with active infections should not be allowed to visit the client. Stress causes increased heart workload. Too much weight gain causes an increase in body requirements and stress on the heart. Resting should be on the left side to promote blood return.

Test-Taking Strategy: Avoid absolute terminology in options such as 1 and 3, where "no" and "not" are used. Knowledge regarding blood return during pregnancy would assist in eliminating option 4.

Level of Cognitive Ability: Analysis
Phase of Nursing Process: Evaluation
Client Needs: Health Promotion and Maintenance
Content Area: Maternity

Reference
Gorrie, T., McKinney, E. S., & Murray, S. S. (1998). *Foundations of maternal-newborn nursing* (2nd ed.). Philadelphia: W. B. Saunders. p. 726.

14. 4

Rationale: The primary concern for this client is safety of her fetus, not herself. The priority nursing diagnosis at this time is option 4. Option 3 is a medical diagnosis and outside the scope of nursing practice. Pain and Impaired Tissue Integrity are commonly seen in clients experiencing urinary tract infections, but the stem includes no data to support either of the options.

Test-Taking Strategy: Avoid medical diagnoses as they are outside the scope of nursing practice. The stem is asking for the priority answer at this time. The data in the stem support only option 4. Always focus on the client's feelings first. The client is determining the priority in this question.

Level of Cognitive Ability: Analysis
Phase of Nursing Process: Analysis
Client Needs: Psychosocial Integrity
Content Area: Maternity

Reference
Lowdermilk, D., Perry, S., & Bobak, I. (1997). *Maternity & women's health care* (6th ed.). St. Louis: Mosby–Year Book. p. 749.

15. 1

Rationale: Laser therapy is the most effective destructive method of treatment that is considered safe for pregnancy. Medications for the disease are considered toxic to the fetus. The primary neonatal effect of the virus is respiratory or laryngeal papillomatosis. The exact route of perinatal transmission is unknown.

Test-Taking Strategy: Eliminate extremes such as "all" in option 4. Medication use during pregnancy is very limited and should not be the first option, therefore eliminate option 2 and 3. This leaves option 1 as the only answer. Review treatment modalities related to condyloma acuminatum (caused by the human papilloma virus) now, if you had difficulty with this question!

Level of Cognitive Ability: Application
Phase of Nursing Process: Planning
Client Needs: Safe, Effective Care Environment
Content Area: Maternity

Reference
Lowdermilk, D., Perry, S., & Bobak, I. (1997). *Maternity & women's health care* (6th ed.). St. Louis: Mosby–Year Book. pp. 741–742.

16. 3

Rationale: Infected house cats transmit the disease through feces. Handling litter boxes can transmit the disease to the maternity client. Meats that are undercooked can harbor microorganisms that can cause infection. Hands should be washed throughout the day when items that could be contaminated are handled. The pharmacological treatment of choice for toxplasmosis is a combination of pyrimethamine and sulfadiazine.

Test-Taking Strategy: Avoid option 1, which uses the key word "only." Option 2 also represents an extreme statement. Knowledge regarding the transmission and treatment of the organism is required to discriminate between options 3 and 4. Review the causes of toxoplasmosis now, if you had difficulty with this question!

Level of Cognitive Ability: Application
Phase of Nursing Process: Implementation
Client Needs: Health Promotion and Maintenance
Content Area: Maternity

References
Lowdermilk, D., Perry, S., & Bobak, I. (1997). *Maternity & women's health care* (6th ed.). St. Louis: Mosby–Year Book. pp. 737–738.

17. 4

Rationale: Condoms should be used to minimize the spread of sexually transmitted infectious diseases. Wearing tight clothes irritates the genital area and does not allow for air circulation. Douching is to be avoided. Wearing items with a cotton panel liner allows for air movement in and around the genital area.

Test-Taking Strategy: This question focuses on how the nurse should monitor or make a judgment concerning a client's response to teaching. Options 1, 2, and 3 are all incorrect statements regarding client self-care. Use the process of elimination and be sure to read the stem of the question and each option carefully before selecting the response!

Level of Cognitive Ability: Analysis
Phase of Nursing Process: Evaluation
Client Need: Health Promotion and Maintenance
Content Area: Maternity

Reference

Lowdermilk, D., Perry, S., & Bobak, I. (1997). *Maternity & women's health care* (6th ed.). St. Louis: Mosby–Year Book. p. 749.

18. 1

Rationale: HIV has a strong affinity for surface marker proteins on lymphocytes. This affinity of HIV for T lymphocytes leads to significant cell destruction. Angiotensin is produced in the kidney. Glomerular filtration rate indicates kidney function. Platelet count is important and an indicator of HIV but has already been identified in the components of the question.

Test-Taking Strategy: Option 4 has already been identified in the components of the question and can be eliminated. Options 2 and 3 are alike in that they are related to kidney function. This leaves option 1. Knowledge regarding clinical manifestations and pathology of the disease is necessary to answer the question. Review this information now, if you had difficulty with this question!

Level of Cognitive Ability: Analysis
Phase of Nursing Process: Analysis
Client Needs: Physiological Integrity
Content Area: Maternity

Reference

Lowdermilk, D., Perry, S., & Bobak, I. (1997). *Maternity & women's health care* (6th ed.). St. Louis: Mosby–Year Book. p. 735.

19. 2

Rationale: The disease is caused by a retrovirus that infects T lymphocytes. This disables the body's ability to fight infection. Nursing goals are directed at the prevention of infections. Sexual relations are not contraindicated with the proper use of protective devices. Options 3 and 4 are the focus of interventions, not goals.

Test-Taking Strategy: The stem asks for a goal. Option 3 and 4 are interventions. Option 1 may be a forced goal that the client may not want to adhere to. Knowledge regarding the infectious nature of HIV is needed to answer the question. Review this information now, if you had difficulty with the question!

Level of Cognitive Ability: Application
Phase of Nursing Process: Planning
Client Needs: Safe, Effective Care Environment
Content Area: Maternity

Reference

Gorrie, T., McKinney, E. S., & Murray, S. S. (1998). *Foundations of maternal-newborn nursing* (2nd ed.). Philadelphia: W. B. Saunders. p. 738.

20. 4

Rationale: Women with anemia have a higher incidence of puerperal complications such as infection than do pregnant women with normal hematological values.

Test-Taking Strategy: Use the process of elimination to select the correct answer. The stem provides the supporting data for only one answer. Options 1 and 2 could occur, but the data needed to support these options are not provided. Option 3 is a medical diagnosis that is not in the scope of nursing practice.

Level of Cognitive Ability: Analysis
Phase of Nursing Process: Analysis
Client Needs: Physiological Integrity
Content Area: Maternity

Reference

Lowdermilk, D., Perry, S., & Bobak, I. (1997). *Maternity & women's health care* (6th ed.). St. Louis: Mosby–Year Book. pp. 845–846.

21. 3

Rationale: Probably the most important of all nursing functions is providing emotional support to the client and family during the counseling process. Option 1 overwhelms the client with information while she is trying to cope with the news of the disease. Option 2 is appropriate only if the client requests to be alone. If not requested, the nurse is abandoning the client in time of need. Option 4 is nontherapeutic. Supportive therapy allows the client to express feelings, explore alternatives, and make decisions in a safe, caring environment.

Test-Taking Strategy: This question addresses the provision that the nurse meets the psychosocial needs of the client in crisis-related situations by promoting psychosocial adaptation and coping in the client. The question is asking for the most important interaction to make. The best answer is option 3. Always address client feelings first!

Level of Cognitive Ability: Application
Phase of Nursing Process: Planning
Client Needs: Psychosocial Integrity
Content Area: Maternity

Reference

Lowdermilk, D., Perry, S., & Bobak, I. (1997). *Maternity & women's health care* (6th ed.). St. Louis: Mosby–Year Book. p. 130.

22. 2

Rationale: An intervention to prevent sickle cell crisis during labor includes administering oxygen as needed. During the labor process the client is at high risk for being unable to meet the oxygen demands of labor and unable to prevent sickling.

Test-Taking Strategy: The question is asking what nursing action would be done first to prevent sickling crisis. Remember that in prioritizing airway is always first. Option 2 addresses airway. Options 1, 3, and 4 are correct answers but not for the situation described in the question. Review sickle cell crisis now, if you had difficulty with this question!

Level of Cognitive Ability: Application
Phase of Nursing Process: Implementation
Client Needs: Physiological Integrity
Content Area: Maternity

Reference

Lowdermilk, D., Perry, S., & Bobak, I. (1997). *Maternity & women's health care* (6th ed.). St. Louis: Mosby–Year Book. pp. 846–847.

23. **1**

Rationale: The nutritional supplement most commonly needed during pregnancy is iron. Anemia of pregnancy is primarily caused by iron deficiency. Iron supplements usually cause constipation. Meats are an excellent source of iron. Iron for the fetus comes from the maternal serum.

Test-Taking Strategy: Options 2 and 4 have absolute terminology, such as "not" and "all." Additionally, identify important words in the stem, such as malnourished. This would eliminate option 4 as a possibility. Knowledge regarding the effects of iron supplements would assist in eliminating option 3 as a possible answer. Review the relationship of nutrition to anemia now, if you had difficulty with this question!

Level of Cognitive Ability: Analysis
Phase of Nursing Process: Evaluation
Client Needs: Physiological Integrity
Content Area: Maternity

Reference
Lowdermilk, D., Perry, S., & Bobak, I. (1997). *Maternity & women's health care* (6th ed.). St. Louis: Mosby–Year Book. pp. 168, 183, 846.

24. **4**

Rationale: The uterus is theoretically sterile during pregnancy until the membranes rupture. It is capable of being invaded by pathogens after that rupture. Puerperal infection is probably the major cause of maternal morbidity and mortality throughout the world.

Test-Taking Strategy: The question asks for a goal appropriate for the diagnosis identified in the stem. Option 3 implies that an infection has been diagnosed and therefore is no longer a high-risk diagnosis. The phase of nursing process this question addresses is planning. Options 1 and 2 are not appropriate for the identified diagnosis but refer to pain and impaired tissue perfusion respectively.

Level of Cognitive Ability: Application
Phase of Nursing Process: Planning
Client Needs: Health Promotion and Maintenance
Content Area: Maternity

References
Pillitteri, A. (1995). *Maternal & child health: Nursing care of the childbearing and childrearing family* (2nd ed.). Philadelphia: J. B. Lippincott. p. 712.
Lowdermilk, D., Perry, S., & Bobak, I. (1997). *Maternity & women's health care* (6th ed.). St. Louis: Mosby–Year Book. p. 750.

25. **1**

Rationale: Transmission of infectious diseases can occur through contaminated items such as hands and bed linens in clients with endometritis. An important method of preventing infection is to break the chain of infection. Infectious processes occur most readily in the very young and the very old. Handwashing is one of the most effective methods of preventing the transmission of infectious diseases.

Test-Taking Strategy: Avoid extreme answers and absolutes such as those used in options 2, 3, and 4. These use the words "not" and "no." Knowledge of the transmission of infection and how to break the chain of infection is necessary to answer the question. Review content related to the transmission of infection now, if you had difficulty with this question!

Level of Cognitive Ability: Application
Phase of Nursing Process: Implementation
Client Needs: Health Promotion and Maintenance
Content Area: Maternity

Reference
Gorrie, T., McKinney, E. S., & Murray, S. S. (1998). *Foundations of maternal-newborn nursing* (2nd ed.). Philadelphia: W. B. Saunders. p. 800.

26. **2**

Rationale: The decrease in nutritional intake during the first trimester of the pregnancy will put the mother and fetus at jeopardy. The mother is prone to developing ketoacidosis, which can be harmful to the infant. Also, specific nutrients, such as folic acid, may produce fetal anomalies if deficient at this time. Body Image Disturbance is a problem for this client; however, nutrition is of a higher priority. The client may have a potential risk for skin integrity; however, this will occur later in the pregnancy. The fetus is at risk, but not because the mother is a teenager.

Test-Taking Strategy: The main strategy with this question is to apply Maslow's Hierarchy of Needs to both the mother and the fetus. Physiological needs are the top priority for both of the clients. The phrase "most important" noted in the stem is a key phrase. The need for proper nutrition is vital for the fetus at this point and also for the diabetic mother. Additionally, the stem asks for the most important nursing diagnosis. Option 2 identifies an actual problem, which is physiological in nature. Options 3 and 4 identify potential problems.

Level of Cognitive Ability: Analysis
Phase of Nursing Process: Analysis
Client Needs: Physiological Integrity
Content Area: Maternity

Reference
Reeder, S., Martin, L., & Koniak-Griffin, D. (1997). *Maternity nursing: Family, newborn, and women's health care* (18th ed.). Philadelphia: Lippincott-Raven. p. 860.

27. **3**

Rationale: Options 1, 2, and 4 are all important points to include in the teaching plan for the new diabetic. Exercise is necessary for the pregnant diabetic. Concepts related to the timing of exercise, control of food intake, and insulin around the time of exercise should be included in the plan.

Test-Taking Strategy: In a planning question, the focus is on nursing action. In this question, the formulation of the nursing care plan is addressed. Understanding points of teaching for a diabetic pregnant client is necessary to answer the question correctly. The stem of the question includes the word "not." It is similar to "avoid" noted in option 3, the correct option for this question as stated. If you had difficulty with this question, review the effects of diet and exercise in diabetes!

Level of Cognitive Ability: Application
Phase of Nursing Process: Planning
Client Needs: Physiological Integrity
Content Area: Maternity

Reference
Reeder, S., Martin, L., & Koniak-Griffin, D. (1997). *Maternity nursing: Family, newborn, and women's health care* (18th ed.). Philadelphia: Lippincott-Raven. p. 86.

28. 3

Rationale: The client is at risk for developing gestational diabetes with each pregnancy. She also has an increased risk of developing overt diabetes and needs to comply with follow-up assessments. She also needs to be taught techniques to lower her risk for developing diabetes, such as weight control. The diagnosis of gestational diabetes indicates that this client has an increased risk for developing overt diabetes; however, with proper care it may not develop.

Test-Taking Strategy: Identify the issue of the question, which is the long-term effects of gestational diabetes. By understanding the long-term effects, the client can better take control of her follow-up care. The client is asking for specific information. When the client receives honest, direct answers, the client can then better cope with future outcomes. Review the long-term effects of gestational diabetes now, if you had difficulty with this question!

Level of Cognitive Ability: Application
Phase of Nursing Process: Implementation
Client Needs: Psychosocial Integrity
Content Area: Maternity

Reference
Lowdermilk, D., Perry, S., & Bobak, I. (1997). *Maternity and women's health care* (6th ed.). St. Louis: Mosby–Year Book. p. 818.

29. 4

Rationale: An increase in calories is needed with pregnancy, but concentrated sugars should be avoided because they may cause hyperglycemia. The fat intake should remain at 30% of the total calories. The fetus of a diabetic mother is prone to macrosomia. The diabetic client needs about 40% to 50% of the diet from carbohydrates and about 20% to 25% of the diet from protein. High-fiber foods will cause blood glucose levels to rise more slowly by delaying gastrointestinal absorption.

Test-Taking Strategy: This is an evaluation question. With evaluation questions, the distracters usually give inaccurate information regarding the issue in the question. In this question, three of the distracters give inaccurate information. Read the options carefully and use the process of elimination to select the answer. Review the key components of the diabetic diet now, if you had difficulty with this question.

Level of Cognitive Ability: Analysis
Phase of Nursing Process: Evaluation
Client Needs: Health Promotion and Maintenance
Content Area: Maternity

Reference
Lowdermilk, D., Perry, S., & Bobak, I. (1997). *Maternity and women's health care* (6th ed.). St. Louis: Mosby–Year Book. p. 816.

30. 4

Rationale: Fatigue is a normal occurrence during pregnancy. At 5'6" tall, 130 pounds does not meet the criteria of 20% over ideal weight. Therefore, the client is not obese. To be at high risk for gestational diabetes, the maternal age should be greater than 30 years. A previous history of unexplained stillbirths or miscarriages puts the client at high risk for gestational diabetes.

Test-Taking Strategy: It is important to reread the stem of the question and compare the stem with the options. In this question, options 2, 3, and 4 are all risk factors for gestational diabetes. However, upon rereading the stem of the question, options 2 and 3 do not apply to this client. Review the risk factors related to gestational diabetes now, if you had difficulty with this question!

Level of Cognitive Ability: Analysis
Phase of Nursing Process: Analysis
Client Needs: Physiological Integrity
Content Area: Maternity

Reference
Lowdermilk, D., Perry, S., & Bobak, I. (1997). *Maternity and women's health care* (6th ed.). St. Louis: Mosby–Year Book. pp. 813–814.

31. 1

Rationale: The client is putting the blame for the diabetes upon herself, lowering her self-concept. She is expressing fear and grief. Knowledge deficit is an important nursing diagnosis for this client, but not immediately. The client will not be able to comprehend information at this time. There are no data to support the nursing diagnoses in options 3 and 4.

Test-Taking Strategy: This question requires analysis of the situation and prioritization of care. The stem of the question asks for the nursing diagnosis that is of the highest priority at this time. Many nursing diagnoses are needed for this client, but further intervention and teaching cannot be done until this initial conflict is resolved. Therefore, the self-concept assumes the highest priority based on the information presented in the question.

Level of Cognitive Ability: Analysis
Phase of Nursing Process: Analysis
Client Needs: Psychosocial Integrity
Content Area: Maternity

Reference
Reeder, S., Martin, L., & Koniak-Griffin, D. (1997). *Maternity nursing: Family, newborn, and women's health care* (18th ed.). Philadelphia: Lippincott-Raven. pp. 855–860.

32. 3

Rationale: Option 1 is adequate because there is 20 mL of urine in 30 minutes. The acceptable criterion is greater than 30 mL/hour. Deep tendon reflexes of 2+ are normal. Magnesium sulfate depresses the respiratory rate. If the rate is less than 12 breaths per minute, the continuation of the medication needs to be reassessed. The fetal heart tone is within normal limits for a resting fetus.

Test-Taking Strategy: It is important to note the key phrase in the stem of the question: "most concern." All the options are actual assessments, so you must analyze the data in order to decide the next proper action. Use the process of elimination to select the correct answer. Review assessment findings in PIH and the effects of magnesium sulfate now, if you had difficulty with this question!

Level of Cognitive Ability: Analysis
Phase of Nursing Process: Analysis
Client Needs: Physiological Integrity
Content Area: Maternity

Reference
Lowdermilk, D., Perry, S., & Bobak, I. (1997). *Maternity and women's health care* (6th ed.). St. Louis: Mosby–Year Book. p. 714.

33. 1

Rationale: Option 1 contains assessments for pregnancy-induced hypertension (PIH). Finger edema is a frequent forerunner of PIH and should be investigated further. Options 2, 3, and 4 are all assessments of other problems, such as diabetes, infections and molar pregnancy.

Test-Taking Strategy: Because it is a planning question, the nurse needs to develop a plan of care according to the data presented. According to the symptoms given by the client, the nurse needs to plan for further assessments in order to develop nursing diagnoses and prioritize care. Use the process of elimination. Select the option that most closely relates to the key in the question: "swelling."

Level of Cognitive Ability: Application
Phase of Nursing Process: Assessment
Client Needs: Physiological Integrity
Content Area: Maternity

Reference
Reeder, S., Martin, L., & Koniak-Griffin, D. (1997). *Maternity nursing: Family, newborn, and women's health care* (18th ed.). Philadelphia: Lippincott-Raven. p. 837.

34. **3**

Rationale: Options 1, 2, and 4 are all procedures that should be done after the convulsion has stopped. It is important as a first action to keep an open airway and prevent injuries to the client.

Test-Taking Strategy: The key to this implementation question is to set priorities for the client. Note the question asks for the "first action." All the options are correct procedures for this client. However, there is a certain order that ought to be followed for the client's safety. Airway is the first priority!

Level of Cognitive Ability: Application
Phase of Nursing Process: Implementation
Client Needs: Physiological Integrity
Content Area: Maternity

Reference
Lowdermilk, D., Perry, S., & Bobak, I. (1997). *Maternity and women's health care* (6th ed.). St. Louis: Mosby–Year Book. p. 715.

35. **4**

Rationale: It is still important to keep physician appointments to assess for any other physical changes in the mother or baby. Blood pressures need to be taken in the same arm, in a sitting position, every day in order to obtain a consistent and accurate reading. The weight needs to be checked at the same time each day, wearing the same clothes, after voiding and before breakfast, in order to obtain reliable weights. Option 4 is a true statement as written.

Test-Taking Strategy: All the options are procedures the client must perform at home. You must then look at the correctness of each procedure. The process of elimination should be used when reading each option. Once all options are read and three have been eliminated, then reread the stem and check to see whether the option selected meets all the criteria asked for in the question stem. Review knowledge regarding the principles of weight and blood pressure measurement now, if you had difficulty with this question.

Level of Cognitive Ability: Analysis
Phase of Nursing Process: Evaluation
Client Needs: Health Promotion and Maintenance
Content Area: Maternity

Reference
Lowdermilk, D., Perry, S., & Bobak, I. (1997). *Maternity and women's health care* (6th ed.). St. Louis: Mosby–Year Book. p. 710.

36. **1**

Rationale: One of the signs of HELLP syndrome is a drop in the platelet count. With HELLP syndrome, there is an elevation of the liver enzyme levels. Options 3 and 4 are both signs of pregnancy-induced hypertension (PIH).

Test-Taking Strategy: It is important to establish the issue of the question prior to answering. This question is asking about the symptoms of HELLP syndrome, not PIH. Once this is realized, two of the distracters can be eliminated, options 3 and 4. The two remaining choices relate to HELLP syndrome, so the issue is to determine which is the correct statement. Review the characteristics of this syndrome now, if you had difficulty with this question!

Level of Cognitive Ability: Analysis
Phase of Nursing Process: Analysis
Client Needs: Physiological Integrity
Content Area: Maternity

Reference
Lowdermilk, D., Perry, S., & Bobak, I. (1997). *Maternity and women's health care* (6th ed.). St. Louis: Mosby–Year Book. pp. 704–705.

37. **3**

Rationale: Options 1, 2, and 4 are all signs that the PIH is being resolved. Option 3 is a symptom of worsening of the pre-eclampsia.

Test-Taking Strategy: It is important to note what the question is specifically asking. The last sentence asks which data do "not" show resolution. Read the question carefully. That will alter how the question is answered. In this question, the distracters are the positive statements. If you had difficulty with this question, review PIH now! You are likely to see questions on NCLEX-RN related to PIH!

Level of Cognitive Ability: Analysis
Phase of Nursing Process: Evaluation
Client Needs: Physiological Integrity
Content Area: Maternity

Reference
Lowdermilk, D., Perry, S., & Bobak, I. (1997). *Maternity and women's health care* (6th ed.). St. Louis: Mosby–Year Book. p. 719.

38. **1**

Rationale: By seeing no way out of the situation except for death, the client meets the criteria for hopelessness. A person who lacks hope feels that life is too much to handle. Option 2 is a possible nursing diagnosis later, but there are not enough data to support it at this point. The data given do not support the nursing diagnosis of Self-Esteem Disturbance. Option 4 is a possible nursing diagnosis at a later time; however, at this time the diagnosis of Hopelessness should take precedence.

Test-Taking Strategy: This question is concerned with formulating and prioritizing nursing diagnoses. One problem you may have with this type of question is reading into the question. The data presented are the only data that need to be analyzed and considered when selecting the correct option!

Level of Cognitive Ability: Analysis
Phase of Nursing Process: Analysis
Client Needs: Psychosocial Integrity
Content Area: Maternity

Reference
McFarland, G., & McFarlane, E. (1997). *Nursing diagnosis & intervention: Planning for patient care* (3rd ed.). St. Louis: Mosby–Year Book. pp. 578–580.

39. **1**

Rationale: Bleeding is an early sign of disseminated intravascular coagulation (DIC) and should be reported. Options 2, 3, and 4 are all normal occurrences in the last trimester of pregnancy.

Test-Taking Strategy: Looking for similarities in the answer may help. In this question, all three distracters are similar as they are all normal occurrences in pregnancy. Therefore, the correct option is the one that is not a normal occurrence. Bleeding does not normally occur with pregnancy.

Level of Cognitive Ability: Application
Phase of Nursing Process: Implementation
Client Needs: Physiological Integrity
Content Area: Maternity

Reference
Reeder, S., Martin, L., & Koniak-Griffin, D. (1997). *Maternity nursing: Family, newborn, and women's health care* (18th ed.). Philadelphia: Lippincott-Raven. p. 830.

40. **2**

Rationale: Hemorrhage is a risk factor with DIC; however, a loss of 450 mL is not considered hemorrhage. Dead fetus syndrome is considered a risk factor for DIC. Severe preeclampsia is considered a risk factor for DIC, a mild case is not. Delivering a large baby is not considered a risk factor for DIC.

Test-Taking Strategy: In some evaluation questions, you may be asked to monitor specific types of clients for responses to previous problems. In this question, understanding risk factors of DIC is required. From here, use the process of elimination. If you had difficulty answering this question, take time now to review the risk factors associated with DIC!

Level of Cognitive Ability: Analysis
Phase of Nursing Process: Evaluation
Client Needs: Physiological Integrity
Content Area: Maternity

Reference
Lowdermilk, D., Perry, S., & Bobak, I. (1997). *Maternity and women's health care* (6th ed.). St. Louis: Mosby–Year Book. p. 792.

BIBLIOGRAPHY

Gorrie, T., McKinney, E. S., & Murray, S. S. (1998). *Foundations of maternal-newborn nursing* (2nd ed.). Philadelphia: W. B. Saunders.

Lowdermilk, D., Perry, S., & Bobak, I. (1997). *Maternity and women's health care* (6th ed.). St. Louis: Mosby–Year Book.

McFarland, G., & McFarlane, E. (1997). *Nursing diagnosis & intervention: Planning for patient care* (3rd ed.). St. Louis: Mosby–Year Book.

Olds, S., London, M., & Ladewig, P. (1996). *Maternal-newborn nursing: A family-centered approach* (5th ed.). Reading, MA: Addison-Wesley.

Pillitteri, A. (1995). *Maternal & child health: Nursing care of the childbearing and childrearing family* (2nd ed.). Philadelphia: J. B. Lippincott.

Reeder, S., Martin, L., & Koniak-Griffin, D. (1997). *Maternity nursing: Family, newborn, and women's health care* (18th ed.). Philadelphia: Lippincott-Raven.

CHAPTER 26

Labor and Delivery

I. The Process of Labor

A. Labor
1. Coordinated sequence of involuntary uterine contractions
2. Results in effacement and dilation of cervix, followed by expulsion of products of conception

B. Delivery: Acutal Event of Birth

C. Passenger: The Fetus

D. Attitude
1. The relationship of the fetal body parts to one another
2. Normal intrauterine attitude is flexion, in which the fetal back is rounded, the head is forward on the chest, and the arms and legs are folded in against the body

E. Lie
1. Relationship of the spine of the fetus to the spine of the mother
2. Longitudinal or vertical
   a. Fetal spine is parallel with the mother's spine
   b. Fetus is either cephalic or breech presentation
3. Transverse or horizontal
   a. Fetal spine is at a right angle, or perpendicular to the mother's spine
   b. Presenting part is the shoulder
   c. **Delivery** by cesarean section
4. Oblique
   a. Fetal spine is at a slight angle from a true horizontal lie
   b. **Delivery** is by cesarean section if uncorrectable

F. Presentation
1. Presenting part: Portion of the fetus that enters the pelvis first
2. Cephalic
   a. The most common presentation
   b. Fetal head presents first
3. Breech
   a. Buttocks present first
   b. **Delivery** by cesarean section may be

required, although it is often possible to deliver vaginally
4. Shoulder
   a. Fetus is in a transverse lie, or the arm, back, abdomen, or side could present
   b. If the fetus does not spontaneously rotate or if it is not possible to turn the fetus manually, a cesarean section may be performed

G. Position: Relationship of Assigned Area of the Presenting Part or Landmark to the Maternal Pelvis (Box 26–1)

H. Station
1. The measurement of the progress of descent in centimeters above or below the midplane from the presenting part to the ischial spines
2. Station 0—at ischial spine
3. Minus station—above ischial spine
4. Plus station—below ischial spine

I. Powers
1. The forces acting to expel the fetus
2. Effacement: Shortening and thinning of the cervix during the first stage of **labor**
3. Dilation: Enlargement of cervical os and cervical canal during first stage

II. Mechanisms of Labor (Table 26–1)

A. Assessment
1. Lightening or dropping: Fetus descends into the pelvis about 2 weeks prior to delivery

---

BOX 26–1. Fetal Positions

ROA—Right occiput anterior
LOA—Left occiput anterior
ROP—Right occiput posterior
LOP—Left occiput posterior
ROT—Right occiput transverse
LOT—Left occiput transverse
RMA—Right mentum anterior
LMA—Left mentum anterior
RMP—Right mentum posterior
LSA—Left sacrum anterior
LSP—Left sacrum posterior

Table 26–1. Mechanisms of Labor

Engagement
Mechanism by which the fetus nestles into the pelvis
Also termed lightening or dropping

Descent
The process that the fetal head undergoes as it begins its journey through the pelvis
A continuous process from the time of engagement until birth, and it is assessed by the measurement called station

Flexion
Process of the fetal head's nodding forward toward the fetal chest

Internal Rotation
Internal rotation of the fetus, most commonly from the occiput transverse position assumed at engagement into the pelvis, to the occiput anterior position while continuously descending

Extension
Enables the head to emerge when the fetus is in a cephalic position
Begins after the head crowns
Is complete when the head passes under the symphysis pubis and occiput, and the anterior fontanel, brow, face, and chin pass over the sacrum and coccyx and are over the perineum

Restitution
Realignment of the fetal head with the body after the head emerges

External Rotation
The shoulders externally rotate after the head emerges and restitution occurs, so that the shoulders are in the anteroposterior diameter of the pelvis

Expulsion
The birth of the entire body

---

2. Braxton Hicks contractions increase
3. Show
4. Vaginal mucosa congested and vaginal mucus increases
5. Brownish or blood-tinged cervical mucus passed
6. Cervix ripens, becomes soft and partly effaced, and may begin to dilate
7. Sudden burst of energy
8. Loss of 1 to 3 lb from water loss resulting from fluid shifts produced by changes in progesterone and estrogen levels
9. Spontaneous rupture of membranes

B. False **Labor**
1. Exaggeration of normal contractions
2. Does not produce dilation, effacement, or descent
3. Contractions irregular without progression
4. Walking has no effect on contractions and often relieves false **labor**

C. True **Labor**
1. Contractions increase in duration and intensity
2. Cervical dilation and effacement are progressive

III. Leopold's Maneuvers

A. Description: To determine position, presentation, and engagement
B. Preparation

1. Ask mother to empty bladder
2. Warm hands and apply them to the abdomen with firm and gentle pressure

C. First Maneuver
1. Determine which part of the fetus is in the fundus
2. Place palms on each side of the upper abdomen and palpate around the fundus
3. If the head is in the fundus, one would feel a hard, round, movable object
4. The buttocks will feel soft and have an irregular shape and are more difficult to move

D. Second Maneuver
1. Move hands downward over each side of the abdomen, applying firm, even pressure
2. The fetus's back, which is a smooth, hard surface, should be felt on one side of the abdomen
3. Irregular knobs and lumps, the hands, feet, elbows, and knees, will be felt on the opposite side of the abdomen

E. Third Maneuver
1. To confirm fetal position
2. Place hand above the symphysis pubis
3. Bring thumb and fingers together and grasp the part of fetus between them, either the head or buttocks

F. Fourth Maneuver
1. Used in the late stage to determine how far the fetus has descended into the pelvic inlet
2. Place hands on the sides of the lower abdomen, close to the midline
3. Slide hands downward and press inward
4. If it has been determined that the buttocks are in the fundus, then feel for the head
5. If the head cannot be felt, it has probably descended

IV. Breathing Techniques

A. Abdominal Breathing
1. Used until **labor** is more advanced
2. The abdomen moves outward during inhalation and downward during exhalation
3. The rate remains slow, with approximately six to nine breaths per minute

B. Pant-Pant-Blow
1. Used in advanced **labor**
2. A more rapid pattern, consisting of two short blows from the mouth followed by a longer blow
3. All exhalations are a blowing motion

V. Fetal Monitoring

A. Description
1. Displays fetal heart rate (FHR)
2. Monitors uterine activity
3. Assess frequency, duration, and intensity of contractions
4. Assess FHR in relation to maternal contractions

5. Baseline FHR is measured between contractions
6. Normal FHR is 120 to 160 beats per minute

B. External Fetal Monitoring
   1. Noninvasive and performed by the use of a tocotransducer or ultrasonic transducer
   2. Perform Leopold's maneuvers to determine on which side the fetal back is located, and place the ultrasound transducer over this area
   3. Place the tocotransducer over the fundus of the uterus
   4. Fasten the transducer to the abdomen
   5. Allow the client to assume a comfortable position, avoiding vena cava compression

C. Internal Fetal Monitoring
   1. Invasive and requires rupturing of the membranes and attaching an electrode to the presenting part of the fetus
   2. Mother must be dilated 2 to 3 cm to perform internal monitoring

D. Patterns
   1. Fetal bradycardia
      a. Less than 120 beats per minute
      b. Change position of the mother and administer oxygen
      c. Notify physician
   2. Fetal tachycardia
      a. Fetal heart rate is greater than 160 beats per minute
      b. Notify physician
      c. Change position of the mother and administer oxygen

E. Variability (Box 26–2)
   1. Description
      a. A change in the baseline FHR in response to fetal sleep and wake states, medications, and hypoxia
      b. A FHR that fluctuates 6 to 25 beats per minute (moderate variability) at the baseline indicates a well-oxygenated, functioning central nervous system (CNS)
   2. Decreased variability
      a. Notify physician
      b. Maintain client in left lateral position
      c. Administer oxygen as prescribed
      d. Discontinue oxytocin if infusing as prescribed

BOX 26–2. Variability

Minimal Variability
Fetal heart rate fluctuates 3–5 beats per minute

Absent Variability
Fetal heart rate fluctuates 0–2 beats per minute

Sinusoidal Pattern
Presence of a uniform, long-term variability with no short-term variability in the fetal heart rate

---

e. Fetal scalp pH to determine a blood pH value
f. Increase IV fluids as prescribed
g. Monitor and maintain blood pressure if hypotension occurs
h. Prepare for cesarean **delivery**

F. Acceleration
   1. A transient rise in FHR of more than 15 beats per minute for more than 15 seconds
   2. May or may not be related to uterine contractions
   3. Marked acceleration (more than 180 beats per minute) may be related to prematurity, maternal fever, hypoxia, fetal infection, or medications

G. Decelerations
   1. Description: A transient decrease in FHR
   2. Early deceleration
      a. Decrease in FHR below baseline
      b. Tracing shows a uniform shape and mirror image of uterine contractions
      c. Starts early in the contraction phase
      d. Can be due to head compression
   3. Variable deceleration
      a. An abrupt decrease in FHR that is variable in duration, intensity, and timing
      b. Can be due to cord compression
      c. Change client's position
      d. Assess for cord prolapse
      e. Notify physician if decelerations are severe and persistent
      f. Administer oxygen as prescribed
      g. Discontinue oxytocin if infusing as prescribed
      h. Increase IV fluids as prescribed
   4. Late deceleration
      a. Decrease in FHR below baseline
      b. Starts late in the contraction phase and recovers well after the end of the contraction
      c. Due to utero**placental** insufficiency
      d. Change client to left lateral position
      e. Notify physician
      f. Administer oxygen as prescribed
      g. Discontinue oxytocin if infusing as prescribed
      h. Increase IV fluids as prescribed
      i. Monitor and maintain BP if hypotension occurs
      j. Fetal scalp pH to determine a blood pH value
      k. Prepare for cesarean **delivery**

H. Hyperstimulation
   1. Increasing resting tone above 15 mmHg or peak contraction pressures above 80 mmHg
   2. Notify physician
   3. Position client in left lateral position
   4. Increase IV fluids as prescribed
   5. Administer oxygen as prescribed
   6. Discontinue oxytocin if infusing as prescribed
   7. Administer tocolytic drugs as prescribed

◆ **VI. Stages of Labor**

A. Stage 1 Latent Phase
1. Assessment
   a. Cervical dilation of 1 to 4 cm
   b. Uterine contractions every 15 to 30 minutes, 15- to 30-seconds' duration of mild intensity
   c. Mother talkative and eager to be in **labor**
2. Implementation
   a. Encourage mother and partner to participate in care
   b. Assist with comfort measures, changes of position, and ambulation
   c. Keep mother and partner informed of progress
   d. Offer fluids and ice chips
   e. Encourage voiding every 1 to 2 hours
B. Stage 1 Active Phase
1. Assessment
   a. Cervical dilation of 4 to 7 cm
   b. Uterine contractions every 3 to 5 minutes, 30- to 60-seconds' duration of moderate intensity
   c. Mother may experience feelings of helplessness
   d. Mother becomes restless and anxious as contractions become stronger
2. Implementation
   a. Encourage maintenance of effective breathing patterns
   b. Provide a quiet environment
   c. Keep mother and partner informed of progress
   d. Promote comfort with backrubs, sacral pressure, pillow support, position changes
   e. Instruct partner in effleurage
   f. Offer ointment for dry lips
   g. Offer fluids and ice chips
   h. Encourage voiding every 1 to 2 hours
C. Stage 1 Transition Phase
1. Assessment
   a. Cervical dilation of 8 to 10 cm
   b. Uterine contractions every 2 to 3 minutes, 45- to 90-seconds' duration of strong intensity
   c. Mother becomes tired, is restless and irritable, and feels out of control
2. Implementation
   a. Encourage rest between contractions
   b. Wake mother at beginning of contraction so she can begin breathing pattern
   c. Keep mother and partner informed of progress
   d. Provide privacy
   e. Offer ointment for dry lips
   f. Offer fluids and ice chips
   g. Encourage voiding every 1 to 2 hours
D. Implementation Throughout Stage 1
1. Monitor maternal vital signs
2. Monitor FHR via ultrasound Doppler, fetoscope, or electronic fetal monitor
3. Assess FHR before, during, and after a contraction, noting that the normal FHR is 120 to 160 beats per minute
4. Monitor uterine contractions by palpation or monitor, determining frequency, duration, and intensity
5. Assess status of cervical dilation and effacement
6. Assess fetal station presentation and position by Leopold's maneuvers
7. Assist with pelvic examination and prepare for a Nitrazine test and a fern test
8. Assess the color of the **amniotic fluid** if the membranes have ruptured, because meconium-stained fluid can indicate fetal distress
E. Stage 2
1. Assessment
   a. Cervical dilation is complete
   b. Progressive **labor** continues, with cervical dilation of 1 cm/hour for primigravidas and 1.5 cm/hour for multigravidas
   c. Fetal descent occurring and demonstrated by change in fetal station
   d. Uterine contractions occur every 2 to 3 minutes, lasting 60 to 75 seconds, and the intensity is strong
   e. Increase in bloody show occurs
   f. Mother may feel out of control, helpless, and panicky
   g. Mother feels urge to bear down; assist mother in pushing efforts
2. Implementation
   a. Perform assessments every 5 minutes
   b. Monitor maternal vital signs
   c. Monitor FHR via ultrasound Doppler, fetoscope, or electronic fetal monitor
   d. Assess FHR before, during, and after a contraction noting that normal FHR is 120 to 160 beats/minute
   e. Monitor uterine contractions by palpation or monitor, determining frequency, duration, and intensity
   f. Provide mother with encouragement and praise
   g. Keep mother and partner informed of progress
   h. Maintain privacy
   i. Provide ice chips
   j. Assist mother into a position that promotes comfort and assists pushing efforts, such as lithotomy, semisitting, kneeling, side-lying, or squatting
   k. Monitor for signs of approaching birth, such as perineal bulging or visualization of the fetal head
   l. Prepare for birth
F. Stage 3
1. Assessment
   a. Contractions occur until **placenta** is born
   b. **Placental** separation and expulsion occur
   c. Birth of **placenta** occurs 5 to 30 minutes after birth of baby

d. Schultze's mechanism: Center portion of **placenta** separates first, and its shiny fetal surface emerges from the vagina

e. Duncan's mechanism: Margin of **placenta** separates, and the dull, red, rough maternal surface emerges from the vagina first

2. Implementation
   a. Assess maternal vital signs
   b. Assess uterine status
   c. Following the birth of the **placenta**, the uterine fundus remains firm and is located 2 fingerbreadths below the umbilicus
   d. Examine the **placenta** for cotyledons and membranes
   e. Assess mother for shivering and provide warmth
   f. Promote parental-neonatal attachment
   g. Initial newborn infant assessment
   h. Assess neonate's Apgar score

G. Stage 4
   1. Description: The period of time from 1 to 4 hours after **delivery**
   2. Assessment
      a. Blood pressure returns to prelabor level
      b. Pulse is slightly lower than during **labor**
      c. Fundus remains contracted, in the midline, 1 to 2 fingerbreadths below the umbilicus
      d. **Lochia** is moderate or scant and is red
   3. Implementation
      a. Maternal assessments every 15 minutes for 1 hour, every 30 minutes for 1 hour, and hourly for 2 hours
      b. Provide warm blankets
      c. Apply ice packs to the perineum
      d. Massage the uterus if needed

VII. Anesthesia

A. Local Anesthesia
   1. Used for blocking pain during episiotomy
   2. Administered just before the birth of the baby
   3. No effect on the fetus
B. Paracervical Block
   1. Used in the first stage of labor
   2. Provides a rapid block of uterine pain
   3. No effect on the perineal area
   4. No effect on the ability to bear down
   5. May cause fetal bradycardia
C. Pudendal Block
   1. Administered just before the birth of the baby
   2. Injection site is at the pudendal nerve through a transvaginal route
   3. Blocks perineal area for episiotomy
   4. Effects last about 30 minutes
   5. No effects on contractions or fetus
D. Epidural Block
   1. Injection site in epidural space at L3–L4

2. Administered during the first stage of **labor**, after 5 to 6 cm dilation or during the second stage
3. Relieves pain from contractions and numbs vagina and perineum
4. May cause hypotension
5. Does not cause headache as the dura mater is not penetrated
6. Assess maternal blood pressure
7. Maintain mother in side-lying position
8. Administer IV fluids as prescribed
9. Increase fluids if hypotension occurs

E. Spinal Block
   1. Injection site in spinal subarachnoid space at L3–L5
   2. Administered just before the birth of the baby
   3. Relieves uterine and perineal pain and numbs the vagina, perineum, and lower extremities
   4. May cause maternal hypotension
   5. May cause postpartum headache
   6. Client must lie flat 8 to 12 hours following spinal injection
   7. Place a rolled blanket under the right hip to displace the uterus from the vena cava
   8. Administer IV fluids as prescribed
F. General Anesthesia
   1. May be used for some surgical interventions
   2. Client not awake
   3. Danger of respiratory depression and vomiting

VIII. Obstetric Procedures

A. Bishop Score (Box 26–3)
   1. Used to determine maternal readiness for **labor**
   2. Evaluates cervical status and fetal position
   3. Indicated before the induction of **labor**
   4. The five factors are assigned a score of 0 to 3, and the total score is calculated
   5. A score of 6 or more indicates a success rate for **labor** induction
B. Induction
   1. A deliberate initiation of uterine contractions that stimulates **labor**
   2. Elective induction may be accomplished by oxytocin infusion
   3. Obtain baseline tracing of uterine contractions and FHR
   4. Increase IV dosage of oxytocin as prescribed only after assessing contractions, FHR, and maternal blood pressure and pulse

BOX 26–3. Factors of the Bishop Score

Dilation of cervix	Position of cervix
Effacement of cervix	Station of presenting
Consistency of cervix	part

5. Do not increase rate of oxytocin once the desired contraction pattern is obtained (contraction frequency of 2 to 3 minutes lasting 60 seconds)

6. Discontinue oxytocin as prescribed if contraction frequency is less than 2 minutes or duration is more than 90 seconds, or if fetal distress is noted

C. Amniotomy
1. Artificial rupture of membranes (AROM) to stimulate **labor**
2. Increases risk of prolapsed cord and infection
3. Monitor FHR before and after AROM
4. Record time of AROM, FHR, and characteristics of fluid
5. Meconium-stained fluid may be associated with fetal distress
6. Bloody fluid may indicate **abruptio placentae** or fetal trauma
7. An unpleasant odor is associated with infection
8. Polyhydramnios is associated with maternal diabetes and certain congenital disorders
9. Oligohydramnios is associated with intrauterine growth retardation (IUGR) and congenital disorders
10. Expect more variable decelerations after rupture of the membranes as a result of cord compression during contractions
11. Limit client activity

D. External Version
1. External manipulation of the fetus from an abnormal position into a normal presentation
2. Indicated for an abnormal presentation that exists after the 34th week
3. Monitor vital signs
4. If mother is Rh-negative, assure that Rh immune globulin was given at 28 weeks' gestation
5. Nonstress test may be performed to evaluate fetal well-being
6. IV fluids and tocolytic therapy may be administered to relax the uterus and permit easier manipulation of fetus
7. Ultrasound is used during the procedure to evaluate fetal position and **placental** placement and guide direction to the fetus
8. Abdominal wall is manipulated to direct fetus into a cephalic presentation if possible
9. Monitor blood pressure to identify vena cava compression
10. Monitor for unusual pain
11. Following procedure:
    a. Perform nonstress test to evaluate fetal well-being
    b. Monitor for uterine activity, bleeding, ruptured membranes, and decreased fetal activity
    c. With Rh-negative clients, perform Kleihauer-Betke test as prescribed to detect the presence and amount of fetal blood in the maternal circulation and to identify clients who need additional Rh immune globulin

E. Episiotomy
1. Incision made into perineum to enlarge vaginal outlet and facilitate **delivery**
2. Check episiotomy site
3. Institute measures to relieve pain
4. Provide ice pack during the first 24 hours
5. Instruct the client in the use of sitz baths
6. Apply analgesic spray or ointment as prescribed
7. Provide perineal care, using clean technique
8. Instruct the client in the proper care of the incision
9. Instruct the client to dry the perineal area from front to back and to blot the area rather than wipe it
10. Instruct the client to shower rather than bathe in the tub
11. Apply a peripad without touching the inside surface of the pad
12. Report any bleeding or discharge to the physician

F. Forceps **Delivery**
1. Two double-crossed, spoonlike articulated blades are used to assist in **delivery** of the fetal head
2. Reassure client and explain the need for forceps
3. Monitor mother and fetus during **delivery**
4. Check neonate and mother after **delivery** for any possible injury
5. Assist with repair of any lacerations

G. Vacuum Extraction
1. A caplike suction device is applied to the fetal head to facilitate extraction
2. Suction is used to assist in **delivery** of the fetal head
3. Traction is applied during uterine contractions until descent of the fetal head is achieved
4. Suction device should not be kept in place any longer than 25 minutes
5. Monitor FHR every 5 minutes if external fetal monitoring is not used
6. Assess newborn infant at birth and throughout the postpartum period for signs of cerebral trauma
7. Caput succedaneum is normal and will resolve in 24 hours

H. Cesarean **Delivery**
1. **Delivery** of the fetus through a transabdominal, low segment incision of the uterus
2. Preoperative
    a. If planned, prepare client and partner
    b. If an emergency, quickly explain the need and procedure to client and partner
    c. Obtain signed informed consent
    d. Make sure that the preoperative diagnostic tests are done, including the Rh factor

e. Prepare to insert an IV line and Foley catheter
f. Prepare abdomen as prescribed
g. Monitor client and fetus continuously for vital signs and signs of **labor**
h. Provide emotional support
i. Administer preoperative medications as prescribed
3. Postoperative
   a. Monitor vital signs
   b. Provide pain relief
   c. Encourage turning, coughing, and deep breathing
   d. Encourage ambulation
   e. Monitor for signs of infection and bleeding
   f. Burning and pain on urination may indicate bladder infection
   g. A tender uterus and foul-smelling **lochia** may indicate endometritis
   h. A productive cough or chills may indicate pneumonia
   i. A positive Homan's sign, pain, or edema of an extremity may indicate thrombophlebitis

PRACTICE QUESTIONS

1. The client has had a cesarean delivery with a low transverse uterine incision. The nurse knows that this type of incision:
   1 Allows a vaginal birth after cesarean (VBAC) to be possible in a subsequent pregnancy
   2 Can be extended if a larger incision is needed
   3 Is the best choice with a placenta previa on the lower anterior uterine wall
   4 Requires that a vertical skin incision be made

2. The nurse is assessing a client scheduled for a repeat cesarean delivery. Which finding needs to be further investigated prior to delivery?
   1 Hemoglobin of 11.5 g/dL
   2 White blood cell count of 35,000/mm³
   3 Maternal pulse rate of 90 beats per minute
   4 Fetal heart rate of 154 beats per minute

3. A client being prepared for a cesarean delivery is brought to the delivery room. In order to maintain optimal perfusion of oxygenated blood to the fetus, the nurse would plan to place the client in a:
   1 Trendelenburg position
   2 Semi-Fowler's position
   3 Supine position with a wedge under the right hip
   4 Prone position

4. The client is having an elective cesarean delivery. The nurse recognizes the need to help allay the client's feelings of anxiety by:
   1 Emphasizing the technical aspects of this type of delivery

2 Deciding how soon the client should see the baby after delivery
3 Decreasing the partner's anxiety by keeping him or her in the waiting area
4 Encouraging the client to discuss her concerns and desires regarding anesthesia options

5. The nurse is preparing the postpartum cesarean delivery client for discharge. Which statement made by the client indicates a need for more information?
   1 "I can start doing abdominal exercises as soon as I get home."
   2 "I will lift nothing heavier than the baby for 2 weeks."
   3 "If I develop a fever, I will call my doctor."
   4 "When getting out of bed, I will turn on my side and push up with my arms."

6. Which priority nursing intervention should be included in the plan of care for a client before performing Leopold's maneuvers?
   1 Locate fetal heart tones before procedure
   2 Have the client drink 8 ounces of water 1 hour before the examination
   3 Warm the sonogram gel before the procedure
   4 Have the client empty her bladder before beginning the examination

7. The nurse places the client in a left side-lying position, provides a bolus of IV fluid, and administers oxygen by face mask for a client with absent long-term and short-term variability. Which criterion should the nurse evaluate to determine the immediate effectiveness of these interventions?
   1 Return of variable decelerations
   2 Decrease in the number of decelerations that are uniform in shape
   3 Improvement in long-term variability
   4 Absence of shoulders before variable decelerations

8. The nurse is placing a client on an external fetal heart rate (FHR) monitor. Which is the best way for the nurse to assess whether the monitor is tracing the maternal heart rate or the FHR?
   1 If the heart rate tracing is above 100 beats per minute, the nurse can be confident that the tracing is the FHR
   2 Palpate the maternal radial pulse while listening to the FHR
   3 Perform Leopold's maneuvers to determine the location of the fetal heart
   4 The maternal heart rate will display a QRS complex

9. A client has been receiving oxytocin (Pitocin) to augment labor. Which sign indicates that the dosage should be decreased?
   1 Contractions every 3 minutes
   2 Fetal tachycardia

3 Soft uterine tone palpated between contractions

4 Increased urinary output

10. The plan of care for a client undergoing an induction of labor with oxytocin (Pitocin) should include strategies to:
    1 Maintain complete bed rest
    2 Notify the neonatal resuscitation team
    3 Administer antibiotics
    4 Maintain continuous electronic fetal monitoring

11. A woman in active labor has contractions lasting 45 seconds every 2 to 3 minutes. The fetal heart rate between contractions is 100 bpm. What is the nurse's priority intervention?
    1 Notify the physician immediately
    2 Encourage relaxation and breathing techniques between contractions
    3 Continue monitoring labor and fetal heart rate
    4 Assess maternal vital signs

12. Which observation should alert the nurse to a serious problem in a client with frequent, severe variable decelerations following rupture of membranes?
    1 Early decelerations
    2 Marked fetal bradycardia
    3 Complaints of increased fetal movement
    4 Fetal scalp blood pH above 7.25

13. Which finding should the nurse expect when assessing the fetal heart rate during labor?
    1 Presence of late decelerations with contractions
    2 Absent long-term variability
    3 A fetal heart rate between 90 and 120 beats per minute
    4 A fetal heart rate between 120 and 160 beats per minute

14. In order to plan effective nursing care for the client being admitted to the Birthing Center in early labor, the nurse would initially plan to:
    1 Assess pelvic adequacy
    2 Administer an analgesic
    3 Estimate fetal size
    4 Determine maternal and fetal vital signs

15. A client arrives at the Birthing Center in active labor. Her membranes are still intact. The nurse-midwife performs an amniotomy. The nurse explains to the client that after this procedure, she will most likely have:
    1 Less pressure on her cervix
    2 Increased efficiency of contractions
    3 A decreased number of contractions
    4 The need for increased BP monitoring

16. A client becomes increasingly more anxious and hyperventilates during the transition phase of labor. The nurse evaluates the situation and recognizes that the client needs:
    1 General anesthesia
    2 To push with her contractions
    3 To be left totally alone
    4 To regain her breathing pattern

17. The nurse performs Leopold's maneuvers. This procedure:
    1 Determines the "lie" and "attitude" of the fetus
    2 Is a systemic method for palpating the fetus through the maternal back
    3 Is a systemic method for palpating the fetus through the maternal abdominal wall
    4 Measures the height of the maternal fundus

18. Based on Leopold's maneuvers, the nurse determines that the fetus is a "cephalic presentation." This is considered:
    1 An abnormal presentation
    2 The least favorable presentation
    3 A presentation associated with prolonged labor
    4 The most common presentation

19. The client has been admitted for a scheduled cesarean section. As she is getting into bed for preliminary preparation for surgery, the client states, "I don't need the cesarean section after all because I think my baby has moved around." The most appropriate response by the nurse is which of the following?
    1 "Tell me what gives you the impression that your baby has moved."
    2 "That would be impossible because babies don't move around this late."
    3 "The physician is all set to go and cannot change the plans now."
    4 "You need to listen to your obstetrician, physicians know what they are doing."

20. What nursing action is indicated when accelerations are noted on the electronic fetal monitor tracing?
    1 Document these data
    2 Take the mother's vital signs
    3 Call the physician as soon as possible
    4 Reposition the mother

21. Umbilical cord compression is suspected during a contraction if which of the following are recorded on the electric monitor tracing?
    1 Early decelerations
    2 Variable decelerations
    3 Late decelerations
    4 Short-term variability

22. The client is in early labor. She is placed on the external electronic fetal monitor. It is important for the nurse to determine first which of the following?
    1 Intensity of contractions

   2 Frequency of contractions
   3 Baseline fetal heart rate
   4 Type of accelerations

23. The client is undergoing electronic fetal monitoring (EFM). Which of the following statements indicates to the nurse that the client correctly understands this procedure?
   1 "I'm getting tired of lying on my back."
   2 "How many volts of electricity are going through my body?"
   3 "What an efficient way to record my baby's heart rate."
   4 "I shut the machine off when I talk on the telephone."

24. The client is in the active stage of labor. The monitor strip shows a late deceleration. The nurse should plan to do which of the following?
   1 Give oxygen via face mask as prescribed
   2 Turn the client on her back
   3 Prepare for immediate birth
   4 Increase the rate of an IV oxytocin infusion

25. Which of the following is the most important data for the nurse to document on a continuous fetal monitor strip?
   1 A temporary interruption in recording
   2 Maternal vital signs
   3 Last menstrual period
   4 Age of client

26. A client tells the nurse her contractions are getting stronger and that she is getting tired. She appears restless, asks the nurse not to leave her alone, and states, "I can't take it anymore." Considering the client's behavior, the nurse suspects she is dilated:
   1 1 to 2 cm
   2 3 to 4 cm
   3 5 to 7 cm
   4 8 to 10 cm

27. The nurse performs Leopold's maneuvers. When the client asks what she is doing, the nurse's best response is that these maneuvers help determine:
   1 Duration of contractions
   2 Fetal heart rate
   3 Fetal position
   4 Frequency of contractions

28. Examination of the client gives the following data: cervix 80% effaced and 3 cm dilated, vertex presentation −2 station, membranes ruptured. The nurse anticipates the activity orders of the client will be:
   1 Ambulation
   2 Bathroom privileges
   3 Complete bed rest
   4 Up in chair

29. The nurse explains the purpose of effleurage to a client in early labor. Which of the following is the nurse's best explanation?
   1 Effleurage is a form of biofeedback to enhance bearing-down efforts during delivery
   2 Effleurage is light stroking of the abdomen to facilitate relaxation during labor
   3 Effleurage is the application of pressure to the sacrum to relieve a backache
   4 Effleurage stimulates uterine activity by contracting a specific muscle group while other parts of the body rest

30. The client asks, "What does it mean that the baby is at minus one?" After providing instruction, the nurse determines the teaching has been effective when the client states that the fetal presenting part is isolated:
   1 1 cm above the ischial spines
   2 1 fingerbreadth below the symphysis pubis
   3 1 inch below the coccyx
   4 1 inch below the iliac crest

31. The nurse observes the fetal monitoring tracing and determines that the heart rate decreases from a baseline of 150 bpm to 110 bpm after the acme of the contraction. The wave is uniform, with the shape resembling the contraction. The nurse recognizes that this finding is a/an:
   1 Early deceleration
   2 Fetal bradycardia
   3 Late deceleration
   4 Variable deceleration

32. The nurse determines the client's cervix is 3 cm dilated, with contractions occurring every 2 to 3 minutes. While assessing the client's psychological status, the nurse anticipates the client to reflect an attitude of:
   1 Excitement
   2 Helplessness
   3 Irritability
   4 Seriousness

33. A client is 6 cm dilated. A fetal scalp blood sample shows a pH of 7.18. Repetitive late decelerations with decreasing variability are observed on the fetal monitor tracing, which do not respond to treatment measures. The most appropriate nursing action at this time is to:
   1 Change the client's position
   2 Increase the oxygen being administered
   3 Prepare for cesarean delivery
   4 Start an intravenous infusion

34. The nurse rechecks a client's blood pressure and determines it has dropped. To decrease the incidence of supine hypotension, the nurse should encourage the client to remain in which position?
   1 Left lateral
   2 Semi-Fowler's
   3 Squatting
   4 Tailor-sitting

35. The nurse instructs the client in active relaxation techniques to help her cope with the discomfort of contractions. The nurse determines that teaching has been effective when the client says active relaxation includes:
    1 Assuming a state of mind that is open to suggestion from a coach
    2 Believing that a supreme power can help relieve the discomfort of contractions
    3 Relaxing uninvolved muscles while the uterus contracts
    4 Understanding the origin of contraction discomfort to be more psychological than physical

36. The nurse observes the client in the second stage of labor crying out in pain with pushing efforts. The nurse recognizes this behavior as:
    1 Exhaustion
    2 Fear of losing control
    3 Involuntary grunting
    4 Valsalva's maneuver

37. A client has been pushing effectively for 1 hour, and the presenting part is at a +2 station. The nurse determines the client's primary physiological need to be:
    1 A change in position
    2 Intravenous analgesia
    3 Oral food and fluids
    4 Rest between contractions

38. A low-risk client is dilated 10 cm and feeling the urge to push with contractions. At this time during labor, the nurse should plan to assess and document the fetal heart rate:
    1 After every contraction
    2 Every 15 minutes
    3 Every 30 minutes
    4 Hourly

39. A primigravida's membranes rupture spontaneously. The nurse's first action is to:
    1 Assess the contraction pattern
    2 Determine the fetal heart rate
    3 Note the amount, color, and odor of the amniotic fluid
    4 Prepare for immediate delivery

40. The nurse tells the client she is now beginning the second stage of labor. The nurse realizes the client understands this stage when she says:
    1 "I'm having bloody show."
    2 "My cervix is completely dilated."
    3 "My membranes are now ruptured."
    4 "The contractions are intense."

41. After a client vaginally delivers a viable newborn infant, the nurse observes the umbilical cord lengthen and a spurt of blood from the vagina. The nurse recognizes these findings as signs of:
    1 Abruptio placentae
    2 Placenta previa
    3 Placental separation
    4 Uterine atony

42. A client delivers a viable male neonate who is given Apgar scores of 8 and 9 at 1 and 5 minutes. The nurse determines the physical condition of the neonate to be:
    1 Critical
    2 Poor
    3 Fair
    4 Good

43. A client has just delivered a viable neonate. The first nursing action to initiate attachment is to:
    1 Complete routine newborn care measures quickly
    2 Determine the parents' desires for contact with the neonate
    3 Encourage immediate breast-feeding
    4 Suggest that the mother hold the newborn infant after the placenta is delivered

44. In providing initial care of the newborn infant following delivery, the most important action of the nurse is to:
    1 Assess gestational age
    2 Identify the infant and mother
    3 Place the newborn infant in a modified Trendelenburg position
    4 Record the number of umbilical vessels

45. A client receives 10 units of oxytocin (Pitocin) intramuscularly at the time of placental expulsion. The nurse determines the medication is effective if the:
    1 Blood pressure decreases
    2 Lochia is heavy and bright red
    3 Pulse rate increases
    4 Uterus is firm at the level of the umbilicus

46. The nurse conducts a physical assessment of a client 1 hour after delivery. The nurse palpates a firm, uterine fundus 2 cm above the umbilicus and displaced to the right. The nurse recognizes that this finding may indicate:
    1 Bladder distention
    2 Endometrial infection
    3 Retained placental fragments
    4 Uterine atony

47. While a client holds, looks at, and talks to her newborn infant immediately following delivery, she begins to cry. The nurse interprets this behavior as indicating the client is:
    1 Disappointed with the baby's gender
    2 Experiencing a normal response to birth
    3 Grieving over the loss of the pregnancy
    4 Likely to demonstrate malattachment

48. A newly delivered client is anxious to establish a relationship with her newborn infant. The most appropriate nursing action at this time is:
    1 Admit the neonate to the nursery
    2 Conduct a gestational age assessment
    3 Delay instillation of ophthalmic antibiotic for 1 hour
    4 Weigh and measure the neonate

49. Care is being provided to a client during the immediate recovery phase, or fourth stage of labor. The nurse's most important action is to:
    1 Assess the uterine fundus and lochia

    2 Assist the client to breast-feed
    3 Encourage food and fluid intake
    4 Provide privacy for the parents and their newborn infant

50. Following the administration of methylergonovine maleate (Methergine) to a client in the immediate postpartum, the nurse evaluates the medication as effective when the client says:
    1 "At least now I can sleep."
    2 "I feel less nauseated."
    3 "My afterpains are really strong."
    4 "The pain is less intense."

ANSWERS

1. **1**

Rationale: A low transverse uterine incision is unlikely to rupture during a subsequent labor and is the only type of uterine incision considered safe for a subsequent VBAC delivery. It cannot be extended laterally owing to the location of the major uterine blood vessels in the lower uterine segment. In the presence of a placenta previa, a classic incision into the body of the uterus would be needed to prevent incising into the placental area. A suprapubic skin incision can be made with a lower uterine transverse incision.

Test-Taking Strategy: The case situation tells you what type of incision the client has had. Knowledge regarding different types of skin and uterine incisions is needed in order to eliminate incorrect options. Read each option carefully and reread the case situation. Review the type of uterine incisions now if you need to!

Level of Cognitive Ability: Analysis
Phase of Nursing Process: Analysis
Client Needs: Physiological Integrity
Content Area: Maternity

Reference
Gorrie, T., McKinney, E., & Murray, S. (1998). *Foundations of maternal-newborn nursing* (2nd ed.). Philadelphia: W. B. Saunders. p. 412.

2. **2**

Rationale: White blood cell counts in a normal pregnancy begin to rise in the second trimester and peak in the third trimester, with a normal range of $11,000/mm^3$ to $15,000/mm^3$ to $18,000/mm^3$. During the immediate postpartum period, the count may be as high as $25,000/mm^3$ to $30,000/mm^3$ due to increased leukocytosis during delivery. A count of $35,000/mm^3$ prior to delivery is abnormal and may indicate infection, which may complicate the delivery. By full term, a normal maternal hemoglobin range is 11 g/dL to 13 g/dL due to the hemodilution caused by an increase in plasma volume during pregnancy. The total volume increases 30% to 50% by the end of the second trimester. Maternal pulse rate during pregnancy increases 10 to 15 beats per minute over prepregnancy readings to facilitate increased cardiac output, oxygen transport, and kidney filtration. A normal fetal heart rate is 120 to 160 beats per minute.

Test-Taking Strategy: The key phrase in the stem is "needs to be further investigated." This is an analysis question that requires you to interpret the assessment findings and determine any abnormalities and their cause. Knowledge of normal laboratory values during pregnancy is needed. Review these laboratory values now if you need to!

Level of Cognitive Ability: Analysis
Phase of Nursing Process: Analysis
Client Needs: Physiological Integrity
Content Area: Maternity

Reference
Nichols, F., & Zwelling, E. (1997). *Maternal-newborn nursing: Theory and practice.* Philadelphia: W. B. Saunders. pp. 415, 926, 947, 984.

3. **3**

Rationale: Vena cava and descending aorta compression by the pregnant uterus impedes blood return from the lower trunk and extremities, therefore decreasing cardiac return, cardiac output, and blood flow to the uterus and subsequently the fetus. The best position to prevent this would be side-lying, with the uterus displaced off the abdominal vessels. There is a belief that left side-lying is optimal due to the slight deviation of the major abdominal vessels to the right side. Positioning for abdominal surgery necessitates a supine position; however a wedge placed under the right hip provides displacement of the uterus. Trendelenburg positioning places pressure from the pregnant uterus on the diaphragm and lungs, decreasing respiratory capacity and oxygenation. A semi-Fowler's or prone position is not practical for this type of abdominal surgery.

Test-Taking Strategy: Look for key words in the stem of the question. "Optimal perfusion" helps you narrow your options and use the process of elimination to choose the best option. If you had difficulty answering this question, review positioning concepts now!

Level of Cognitive Ability: Application
Phases of Nursing Process: Planning
Client Needs: Physiological Integrity
Content Area: Maternity

Reference
Nichols, F., & Zwelling, E. (1997). *Maternal-newborn nursing: Theory and practice.* Philadelphia: W. B. Saunders. pp. 407, 413, 416, 927.

4. **4**

Rationale: Emotional needs of the client and family are best met by assessing their feelings and allowing for verbalization of concerns. Options 1, 2, and 3 involve actions by the nurse that do not involve client input. Those undergoing cesarean delivery often feel disappointment and guilt, even if the procedure is elective. Providing the opportunity for discussion and input into decisions can help alleviate these feelings. Too much technical information may increase the client's anxiety. The presence of a support person is helpful.

Test-Taking Strategy: Remember the nursing process when prioritizing. Always assess before you intervene. Focus on the client's feelings first when dealing with psychosocial issues!

Level of Cognitive Ability: Application
Phase of Nursing Process: Implementation
Client Needs: Psychosocial Integrity
Content Area: Maternity

Reference
Nichols, F., & Zwelling, E. (1997) *Maternal-newborn nursing: Theory and practice.* Philadelphia: W. B. Saunders. p. 927.

5. **1**

Rationale: Abdominal exercises should not start following abdominal surgery until 3 to 4 weeks postoperatively to allow for healing of the incision and decrease of client discomfort. Options 2, 3, and 4 reflect proper understanding of self-care after discharge.

Test-Taking Strategy: Noting the anatomical location of the incision in a cesarean delivery will easily direct you to option 1. Review client teaching points following this procedure now if you had difficulty with this question!

Level of Cognitive Ability: Analysis
Phase of Nursing Process: Evaluation
Client Needs: Health Promotion and Maintenance
Content Area: Maternity

Reference
Nichols, F., & Zwelling, E. (1997). *Maternal-newborn nursing: Theory and practice.* Philadelphia: W. B. Saunders. pp. 1326–1327.

6. **4**

Rationale: An empty bladder contributes to a woman's comfort during the examination. Drinking water to fill the bladder and warming sonogram gel may be performed prior to a sonogram. Often Leopold's maneuvers are performed to aid the examiner in locating the fetal heart tones.

Test-Taking Strategy: Use principles associated with prioritizing when answering this question. Remember Maslow's Hierarchy of Needs and select the answer that addresses the client's need for comfort during the examination. Leopold's maneuvers are often used to help locate fetal heart tones. Sonogram gel is not used during Leopold's maneuvers, though often the client is requested to have a full bladder before ultrasonography.

Level of Cognitive Ability: Application
Phase of Nursing Process: Planning
Client Needs: Physiological Integrity
Content Area: Maternity

Reference
Nichols, F., & Zwelling, E. (1997). *Maternal-newborn nursing: Theory and practice.* Philadelphia: W. B. Saunders. p. 434.

7. **3**

Rationale: When adequate fetal oxygenation is re-established, long-term variability will reappear first, followed by a delayed return of short-term variability.

Test-Taking Strategy: Early and late decelerations do not indicate an improvement in fetal oxygenation. Variable decelerations suggest cord compression. Review content related to variability now, if you had difficulty with this question!

Level of Cognitive Ability: Analysis
Phase of Nursing Process: Evaluation
Client Needs: Physiological Integrity
Content Area: Maternity

Reference
Nichols, F., & Zwelling, E. (1997). *Maternal-newborn nursing: Theory and practice.* Philadelphia: W. B. Saunders. p. 951.

8. **2**

Rationale: The examiner should simultaneously palpate the maternal radial or carotid pulse and auscultate the FHR to differentiate the two. If the FHR and maternal heart rates are similar, the examiner may mistake the maternal heart rate for the FHR.

Test-Taking Strategy: The fetal heart monitor is capable of confusing the maternal heart rate with the FHR. It is possible for the maternal heart rate and the FHR to be in the same range, so it is important to distinguish between the two heart rates. Leopold's maneuvers may help the examiner locate the position of the baby but will not assure a distinction between the two rates. The fetal monitor is assessing heart rate. Each complete cycle of a heart beat is displayed as one dot on the monitor strip. The QRS complex is not visible. Review fetal monitoring now, if you had difficulty with this question!

Level of Cognitive Ability: Application
Phase of Nursing Process: Assessment
Client Needs: Physiological Integrity
Content Area: Maternity

Reference
Nichols, F., & Zwelling, E. (1997). *Maternal-newborn nursing: Theory and practice.* Philadelphia: W. B. Saunders. p. 936.

9. **2**

Rationale: Acute hypoxia is a common cause of fetal tachycardia. The dosage of oxytocin (Pitocin) should be decreased in the presence of fetal tachycardia from excessive uterine activity. The nurse should also assure that the uterus maintains an adequate resting tone between contractions.

Test-Taking Strategy: The goal of labor augmentation is to achieve three good-quality contractions (appropriate intensity and duration) in a 10-minute period. The uterus should return to resting tone between contractions, and there should be no evidence of fetal distress. Use the principles associated with prioritizing when answering this question. Remember your ABCs: Airway, Breathing, and Circulation. Option 2 is the only one that indicates a problem with circulation!

Level of Cognitive Ability: Analysis
Phase of Nursing Process: Analysis
Client Needs: Physiological Integrity
Content Area: Maternity

Reference
Nichols, F., & Zwelling, E. (1997). *Maternal-newborn nursing: Theory and practice.* Philadelphia: W. B. Saunders. p. 915.

10. **4**

Rationale: Assess maternal and fetal well-being before and during oxytocin (Pitocin) administration, including FHR, uterine contractions and tone, and maternal blood pressure.

Test-Taking Strategy: Try not to read into the question. Do not assume complications in the client that are not mentioned in the stem. No evidence of maternal or fetal complications is mentioned in this question that would require antibiotics or complete bed rest, or indicate fetal distress.

Level of Cognitive Ability: Application
Phase of Nursing Process: Planning
Client Needs: Physiological Integrity
Content Area: Maternity

Reference
Nichols, F., & Zwelling, E. (1997). *Maternal-newborn nursing: Theory and practice.* Philadelphia: W. B. Saunders. p. 914.

11. **1**

Rationale: Fetal bradycardia between contractions may indicate the need for immediate medical management. The physician needs to be informed of the nurse's findings.

Test-Taking Strategy: Use principles of prioritizing to answer this question. Note that the woman is in active labor and that the fetal heart rate is below normal. It is imperative that the circulation in the fetus be restored to normal limits!

Level of Client Need: Application
Phase of Nursing Process: Implementation
Client Needs: Physiological Integrity
Content Area: Maternity

Reference
Nichols, F., & Zwelling, E. (1997). *Maternal-newborn nursing: Theory and practice.* Philadelphia: W. B. Saunders. p. 959–960.

12. **2**

Rationale: Frequent variable decelerations may be due to compression of the umbilical cord. Rupture of membranes before engagement may increase the likelihood of cord prolapse. Cord prolapse is a grave situation, which may lead to fetal hypoxia and fetal death.

Test-Taking Strategy: In general, a fetal scalp blood pH above 7.25 is considered normal. Early decelerations are the result of vagal stimulation caused by fetal head compression with the descent of the fetal head and are usually within the normal FHR baseline. Fetal movement is usually a reassuring sign of fetal well-being. Use the process of elimination to answer the question. Note that option 2 is the only option that identifies a serious problem.

Level of Cognitive Ability: Analysis
Phase of Nursing Process: Evaluation
Client Needs: Physiological Integrity
Content Area: Maternity

Reference
Nichols, F., & Zwelling, E. (1997). *Maternal-newborn nursing: Theory and practice.* Philadelphia: W. B. Saunders. p. 884.

13. **4**

Rationale: Normal FHR for a term fetus ranges from 120 to 160 bpm. An FHR between 90 and 110 bpm is considered bradycardia. Late decelerations cause a decrease in fetal PO_2. The absence of long-term variability suggests persistent fetal hypoxia.

Test-Taking Strategy: Use the process of elimination to answer the question. Knowledge regarding the normal FHR is required to answer the question. If you are unfamiliar with the normal FHR, learn it now!

Level of Cognitive Ability: Analysis
Phase of Nursing Process: Assessment
Client Needs: Physiological Integrity
Content Area: Maternity

Reference
Nichols, F., & Zwelling, E. (1997). *Maternal-newborn nursing: Theory and practice.* Philadelphia: W. B. Saunders. pp. 940, 952.

14. **4**

Rationale: To evaluate a woman's physical well-being, assess the temperature, pulse, respirations, and blood pressure, as well as the fetal heart beat, in order to determine the level of risk. Option 2 is incorrect because it would be too premature for an analgesic. Medication given too early tends to slow or stop labor contractions. Options 1 and 3 are incorrect. These assessments should be done by the physician or a nurse midwife during prenatal visits.

Test-Taking Strategy: This question asks you to select the response that prioritizes care. Use the process of elimination to eliminate incorrect options. Also focus on the true response stem, which in this case utilizes the key word "initially." Remember the ABCs! Measuring vital signs is the priority!

Level of Cognitive Ability: Application
Phase of Nursing Process: Planning
Client Needs: Safe, Effective Care Environment
Content Area: Maternity

Reference
Pillitteri, A. (1995). *Maternal and child health nursing: Care of the childbearing and childrearing family* (2nd ed.). Philadelphia: J. B. Lippincott. pp. 493–494.

15. **2**

Rationale: Rupturing of membranes, if they do not rupture spontaneously, allows the fetal head to contact the cervix more directly (more pressure) and may increase the efficiency of contractions. Options 1 and 2 are answered by this rationale. Options 3 and 4 are incorrect. It is not necessary to increase BP readings, but always take the FHR immediately following the rupture of membranes to determine that the fetus does not have a prolapsed umbilical cord as a result of the escape of amniotic fluid.

Test-Taking Strategy: This is a true response stem that utilizes a key phase, "most likely," and asks you to select an answer that is true regarding the situation and question. Knowledge of the effects of amniotomy is required in order to answer this question. If you had difficulty with this question, review this content now!

Level of Cognitive Ability: Application
Phase of Nursing Process: Implementation
Client Needs: Physiological Integrity
Content Area: Maternity

Reference
Pellitteri, A., (1995). *Maternal and child health nursing: Care of the childbearing and childrearing family* (2nd ed.). Philadelphia: J. B. Lippincott. p. 513.

16. 4

Rationale: When the woman enters this phase of labor, her anxiety level tends to increase as she senses the fairly constant intensification of contractions and pain. A general anesthesia may be needed for cesarean birth, and surgical intervention with some obstetrical complications. The nurse encourages the woman to refrain from pushing until the cervix is completely dilated. The client may be terrified of being left alone during the phase of labor. The client may need help regaining focus and her breathing pattern.

Test-Taking Strategy: Note the issue of the question or the specific subject content that the question is asking about. Read the question carefully. Note the relationship of the word "hyperventilates" in the question and "breathing pattern" in the answer!

Level of Cognitive Ability: Analysis
Phase of Nursing Process: Evaluation
Client Needs: Health Promotion and Maintenance
Content Area: Maternity

Reference
Olds, S., London, M., & Ladewig, P. (1996). *Maternal-newborn nursing: A family-centered approach* (5th ed.). Reading, MA: Addison-Wesley. pp. 578–579, 654, 694.

17. 3

Rationale: Option 3 is the correct answer because it is the definition of Leopold's maneuvers. Options 1, 2, and 4 are not determined by this procedure.

Test-Taking Strategy: This question asks you for a true response concerning a specific procedure. That is the issue of the question. Knowledge of Leopold's maneuvers is required to answer this question. If you are unfamiliar with this content, take the time to review it now!

Level of Cognitive Ability: Application
Phase of Nursing Process: Assessment
Client Needs: Physiological Integrity
Content Area: Maternity

Reference
Gorrie, T., McKinney, E., & Murray, S. (1998). *Foundations of maternal-newborn nursing* (2nd ed.). Philadelphia: W. B. Saunders. p. 146.

18. 4

Rationale: The cephalic presentation is more favorable than others and is the most common. Other presentations are associated with prolonged labor or other abnormalities and are more likely to necessitate a cesarean birth.

Test-Taking Strategy: This is an analysis question that requires interpretation of the data based on an assessment. It requires understanding of the procedure that is done and the findings. Additionally, knowledge regarding the types of fetal presentation is required to assist in selecting the correct option. Review this content now, if you had difficulty with this question!

Level of Cognitive Ability: Analysis
Phase of Nursing Process: Analysis
Client Needs: Physiological Integrity
Content Area: Maternity

Reference
Gorrie, T., McKinney, E., & Murray, S. (1998). *Foundations of maternal-newborn nursing* (2nd ed.). Philadelphia: W. B. Saunders. p. 277.

19. 1

Rationale: Anxiety is an expected and normal reaction to surgery and, within limits, is functional. The nurse should remain with the client and let the client express her fears and concerns. Option 1 encourages the client to express concerns because it uses the therapeutic communication tool of paraphrasing, which validates and clarifies. Options 2, 3, and 4 do not and are blocks to communication.

Test-Taking Strategy: This question uses the key words "most appropriate." Option 1 most directly relates to the comment made by the client. Always select a response that encourages the client to express concerns.

Level of Cognitive Ability: Application
Phase of Nursing Process: Implementation
Client Needs: Psychosocial Integrity
Content Area: Maternity

Reference
Gorrie, T., McKinney, E., & Murray, S. (1998). *Foundations of maternal-newborn nursing* (2nd ed.). Philadelphia: W. B. Saunders. p. 413.

20. 1

Rationale: Accelerations are transient increases in the fetal heart rate normally caused by fetal movement or often accompanying contractions. Accelerations are thought to be a sign of fetal well-being and adequate oxygen reserve. Option 1 is correct; therefore, options 2, 3, and 4 are unnecessary actions.

Test-Taking Strategy: Knowledge regarding accelerations is required to assist in answering this question. If you are unfamiliar with this content, take the time to review it now!

Level of Cognitive Ability: Application
Phase of Nursing Process: Implementation
Client Needs: Physiological Integrity
Content Area: Maternity

Reference
Olds, S., London, M., & Ladewig, P. (1996). *Maternal-newborn nursing: A family-centered approach* (5th ed.). Reading, MA: Addison-Wesley. p. 621.

21. 2

Rationale: Early decelerations, in option 1, result from pressure on the fetal head during a contraction. Variable decelerations, in option 2, present on a fetal heart monitor, suggest cord compression (correct option). Option 3, late decelerations, is an ominous pattern in labor because it suggests uteroplacental insufficiency during a contraction. Option 4, short-term variability, refers to the difference between successive heartbeats, identifying that the natural pacemaker activity of the fetal heart is working properly.

Test-Taking Strategy: This question is asking something about a specific subject content—in this case, a potential complication. It is a true response stem. It utilizes a key word, "suspected," and asks you to select an answer that is true regarding the situation and question. Umbilical cord compression is a critical issue. If you are unfamiliar with the signs, review this content now!

Level of Cognitive Ability: Analysis
Phase of Nursing Process: Evaluation
Client Needs: Physiological Integrity
Content Area: Maternity

Reference
Pillitteri, A., (1995). *Maternal and child health nursing: Care of the childbearing and childrearing family* (2nd ed.). Philadelphia: J. B. Lippincott. pp. 506–507.

22. 3

Rationale: Intensity of contractions, in option 1, is assessed by an internal fetal monitor, not an external fetal monitor. Options 2 and 4 are important to assess but not as the first priority. Option 3 is the correct option. Fetal heart rate is evaluated by assessing both baseline and periodic changes. Periodic changes occur in response to the intermittent stress of uterine contractions and the baseline beat-to-beat variability of the FHR. Assessing baseline FHR is important so that abnormal variations of the baseline rate will be identified if they occur.

Test-Taking Strategy: This is a question that requires prioritizing. The word "first" in the stem of the question is a key word. Utilize Maslow's Hierarchy of Needs theory to prioritize. Physiological needs come first, so select an answer that addresses physiological needs. Also utilize the ABCs when selecting an answer. Remember the order of priority of Airway, Breathing, and Circulation. Fetal heart rate reflects the ABCs.

Level of Cognitive Ability: Application
Phase of Nursing Process: Assessment
Client Needs: Physiological Integrity
Content Area: Maternity

Reference
Olds, S., London, M., & Ladewig, P. (1996). *Maternal-newborn nursing: A family-centered approach* (5th ed.). Reading, MA: Addison-Wesley. pp. 617, 621.

23. 3

Rationale: Option 3 is correct. Continuous EFM has a lower false-normal rate than intermittent auscultation of the FHR. Options 1, 2, and 4 are incorrect. The woman is asked to assume a semi-sitting position or a lateral position when undergoing this procedure. This ultrasound transducer acts through the reflection of high-frequency sound waves from a moving interface; in this case, the fetal heart and valves. No electricity or volts are going through the body.

Test-Taking Strategy: Use the process of elimination. Note the relationship of the term "fetal monitoring" in the question and "baby's heart rate" in the correct option, option 3. Review EFM now if you had difficulty with this question!

Level of Cognitive Ability: Analysis
Phase of Nursing Process: Evaluation
Client Needs: Psychosocial Integrity
Content Area: Maternity

Reference
Gorrie, T., McKinney, E. S., & Murray, S. S. (1998). *Foundations of maternal-newborn nursing* (2nd ed.). Philadelphia: W. B. Saunders. p. 342.

24. 1

Rationale: Late decelerations are due to uteroplacental insufficiency as the result of decreased blood flow and oxygen transfer to the fetus through the intervillous space during the uterine contractions. This causes hypoxemia; therefore, oxygen is necessary, making option 1 correct. Option 2 is incorrect because the supine position decreases uterine blood flow to the fetus. The client should be turned onto her side to displace the pressure of the gravid uterus on the inferior vena cava. Option 3 is incorrect. Late decelerations are considered an ominous sign but do not necessarily require immediate birth of the baby. Option 4 is incorrect. Discontinue IV oxytocin infusion when a late deceleration is noted; otherwise, the oxytocin would cause further hypoxemia because of increased uteroplacental insufficiency due to stimulation of contractions caused by the oxytocin.

Test-Taking Strategy: Knowledge related to late decelerations is required to answer this question. As a testing strategy, select option 1 as it addresses oxygen, which is the first priority. Review content related to late decelerations now if you had difficulty with this question!

Level of Cognitive Ability: Application
Phase of Nursing Process: Planning
Client Needs: Physiological Integrity
Content Area: Maternity

Reference
Olds, S., London, M., & Ladewig, P. (1996). *Maternal-newborn nursing: A family-centered approach* (5th ed.). Reading, MA: Addison-Wesley. pp. 624, 630, 765, 768.

25. 2

Rationale: Options 1, 3, and 4 are incorrect. A temporary interruption is noteworthy but not as important as option 2, which is the correct option. Maternal vital signs can influence circulatory exchange with the placenta. Fetal oxygenation depends on a normal flow of oxygenated maternal blood into the placenta and normal uteroplacental exchange.

Test-Taking Strategy: This is a question that requires prioritizing. Note the word "most" in the question. Use Maslow's Hierarchy of Needs theory to prioritize. Physiological needs come first, therefore select the answer that addresses physiological needs. Also, remember the ABCs. Vital signs reflect Airway, Breathing, and Circulation!

Level of Cognitive Ability: Application
Phase of Nursing Process: Implementation
Client Needs: Physiological Integrity
Content Area: Maternity

Reference
Gorrie, T., McKinney, E., & Murray, S. (1998). *Foundations of maternal-newborn nursing* (2nd ed.). Philadelphia: W. B. Saunders. p. 347.

26. 4

Rationale: During the transition phase of the first stage of labor, cervical dilation progresses from 8 to 10 cm. As contractions intensify, women often doubt their ability to cope with labor and fear abandonment.

Test-Taking Strategy: The question asks you to determine the transition phase of labor, based on characteristic behaviors observed. The longer labor has progressed, the more likely these behaviors are to be observed. Therefore, the greatest cervical dilation, 8 to 10 cm, is the correct answer. Review the transition phase of labor now if you had difficulty with this question!

Level of Cognitive Ability: Analysis
Phase of Nursing Process: Assessment
Client Needs: Physiological Integrity
Content Area: Maternity

Reference
Olds, S., London, M., & Ladewig, P. (1996). *Maternal-newborn nursing: A family-centered approach* (5th ed.). Reading, MA: Addison-Wesley. pp. 578–579.

27. 3

Rationale: Leopold's maneuvers are a systematic way to evaluate the maternal abdomen, using inspection and palpation to determine fetal position and presentation.

Test-Taking Strategy: This question requires you to know Leopold's maneuvers, which involve palpation to determine fetal position. Options 1, 2, and 4 could provide data by another means, a fetal monitor. Option 2 is different, and correct. Review Leopold's maneuvers now if you had difficulty with this question!

Level of Cognitive Ability: Application
Phase of Nursing Process: Implementation
Client Needs: Physiological Integrity
Content Area: Maternity

Reference

Olds, S., London, M., & Ladewig, P. (1996). *Maternal-newborn nursing: A family-centered approach* (5th ed.). Reading, MA: Addison-Wesley. pp. 609–610.

28. 3

Rationale: Rupture of the membranes with the presenting part not engaged and firmly down against the cervix can increase the risk of prolapsed cord. Activity and the downward force of gravity with the client upright can increase the risk.

Test-Taking Strategy: This question requires you to know the risk of prolapsed cord in a client with a non-engaged presenting part. Options 1, 2, and 4 are similar and promote activity; therefore, none of these can be correct. Option 3 promotes no activity, reduces risk, and is the correct answer.

Level of Cognitive Ability: Application
Phase of Nursing Process: Planning
Client Needs: Physiological Integrity
Content Area: Maternity

Reference

Olds, S., London, M., & Ladewig, P. (1996). *Maternal-newborn nursing: A family-centered approach* (5th ed.). Reading, MA: Addison-Wesley. p. 579.

29. 2

Rationale: Effleurage is a specific type of cutaneous stimulation involving light stroking of the abdomen and is used prior to transition to promote relaxation and relieve mild to moderate pain.

Test-Taking Strategy: Knowledge of methods of childbirth preparation assists you in answering this question. A point to remember is that all methods promote relaxation and enhance client-coping with the event. Eliminate option 1 because the focus is the client during delivery. Option 4 focuses on promotion of uterine activity rather than relaxation. Eliminate option 3 since not all labor clients experience backache. Review the components of effleurage now if you had difficulty with this question!

Level of Cognitive Ability: Application
Phase of Nursing Process: Implementation
Client Needs: Psychosocial Integrity
Content Area: Maternity

Reference

Olds, S., London, M., & Ladewig, P. (1996). *Maternal-newborn nursing: A family-centered approach* (5th ed.). Reading, MA: Addison-Wesley. pp. 305–306.

30. 1

Rationale: Station is the relationship of the presenting part to an imaginary line drawn between the ischial spines, is measured in centimeters, and noted as a negative number above the line and a positive number below the line.

Test-Taking Strategy: The question requires you to know that station is measured in centimeters and utilizes the ischial spines as a reference point. Only option 1 incorporates this information. Options 2, 3, and 4 are similar in the use of "below," which would be represented by a positive measurement in determining station. Review station now if you had difficulty with this question!

Level of Cognitive Ability: Analysis
Phase of Nursing Process: Evaluation
Client Needs: Physiological Integrity
Content Area: Maternity

Reference

Olds, S., London, M., & Ladewig, P. (1996). *Maternal-newborn nursing: A family-centered approach* (5th ed.). Reading, MA: Addison-Wesley. pp. 567–568.

31. 3

Rationale: A late deceleration due to uteroplacental insufficiency has a smooth, uniform shape that inversely mirrors the contraction but is late in onset and recovery.

Test-Taking Strategy: This question requires you to recognize the characteristics of a late deceleration. The case tells you that the FHR decelerates after the acme, leading you to option 3, a late deceleration. Review decelerations now if you had difficulty with this question!

Level of Cognitive Ability: Analysis
Phase of Nursing Process: Assessment
Client Needs: Physiological Integrity
Content Area: Maternity

Reference

Olds, S., London, M., & Ladewig, P. (1996). *Maternal-newborn nursing: A family-centered approach* (5th ed.). Reading, MA: Addison-Wesley. pp. 623–624.

32. 1

Rationale: In the late phase of the first stage of labor, contractions are usually mild. The woman feels able to cope with the discomfort and may be relieved that labor has begun. Excitement is high as the impending birth moves from fantasy to reality.

Test-Taking Strategy: The question requires you to know the usual psychological state of the client in early labor. Option 1 is different in that it reflects a positive view characteristic of early labor when coping is adequate and discomfort mild. Options 2, 3, and 4 represent similar psychological states often found late in labor when discomfort and fatigue are greater and coping ability may be reduced.

Level of Cognitive Ability: Analysis
Phase of Nursing Process: Assessment
Client Needs: Psychosocial Integrity
Content Area: Maternity

Reference

Olds, S., London, M., & Ladewig, P. (1996). *Maternal-newborn nursing: A family-centered approach* (5th ed.). Reading, MA: Addison-Wesley. p. 577.

33. 3

Rationale: When fetal distress is evident and vaginal birth is not imminent, cesarean birth should be accomplished to promote the safety of the fetus.

Test-Taking Strategy: This question requires the knowledge to recognize severe fetal distress. Options 1, 2, and 4 reflect early treatment measures to correct fetal distress and are similar. Option 3 represents the answer that is different, and correct, when other treatment measures fail to correct the situation.

Level of Cognitive Ability: Application
Phase of Nursing Process: Implementation
Client Needs: Physiological Integrity
Content Area: Maternity

Reference

Olds, S., London, M., & Ladewig, P. (1996). *Maternal-newborn nursing: A family-centered approach* (5th ed.). Reading, MA: Addison-Wesley. pp. 631, 729–730.

34. 1

Rationale: Pressure from the enlarged uterus and the aorta and vena cava when the woman is supine can result in hypotension, which can be relieved by having the woman lie on her left side.

Test-Taking Strategy: This question requires an understanding of the anatomy of the pregnant uterus and the physiological response caused by pressure on the large abdominal vessels. Options 2, 3, and 4 are all similar in that the client is upright. Only option 1 is different, requiring the client to be horizontal and side-lying, and, therefore, the correct answer.

Level of Cognitive Ability: Application
Phase of Nursing Process: Implementation
Client Needs: Physiological Integrity
Content Area: Maternity

Reference

Olds, S., London, M., & Ladewig, P. (1996). *Maternal-newborn nursing: A family-centered approach* (5th ed.). Reading, MA: Addison-Wesley. p. 311.

35. 3

Rationale: The Lamaze method of childbirth preparation includes specific relaxation exercises and conditioned responses as distraction from the discomfort of labor. The woman is an active participant in the use of the technique, which focuses on relaxing uninvolved muscles while the uterus contracts.

Test-Taking Strategy: Knowledge of the Lamaze method of childbirth preparation, which includes active relaxation, assists you in answering this question. The key word in the stem of the question is "active." Option 3 contains an active verb, different from other options, and is the correct answer. Options 1, 2, and 4 are all similar in that the verb is passive.

Level of Cognitive Ability: Analysis
Phase of Nursing Process: Evaluation
Client Needs: Health Promotion and Maintenance
Content Area: Maternity

Reference

Olds, S., London, M., & Ladewig, P. (1996). *Maternal-newborn nursing: A family-centered approach* (5th ed.). Reading, MA: Addison-Wesley. pp. 303–305.

36. 2

Rationale: Pain, helplessness, and fear of losing control are possible responses in the second stage of labor. Whimpering, high-pitched cries, and crying out in pain indicate losing control, whereas low-pitched grunting sounds usually indicate that a woman is working effectively with contractions.

Test-Taking Strategy: This question requires knowledge of psychological responses in the second stage of labor. Options 1, 3, and 4 are similar, represent physiological processes, and cannot be correct. Option 2 is different and correct.

Level of Cognitive Ability: Analysis
Phase of Nursing Process: Assessment
Client Needs: Psychosocial Integrity
Content Area: Maternity

Reference

Olds, S., London, M., & Ladewig, P. (1996). *Maternal-newborn nursing: A family-centered approach* (5th ed.). Reading, MA: Addison-Wesley. pp. 651, 654.

37. 4

Rationale: The birth process expends a great deal of energy. Encouraging rest between contractions conserves maternal energy for facilitating voluntary pushing efforts with contractions. Uteroplacental perfusion is also enhanced, which enhances fetal tolerance of the stress of labor.

Test-Taking Strategy: This question requires knowledge of the need to conserve energy during the second stage of labor. Option 1 is not indicated since the client's current position has been effective. Option 2 is incorrect since delivery is imminent and this would likely cause CNS depression in the infant. Option 3 is incorrect since food and fluids are likely withheld at this time, except for ice chips.

Level of Cognitive Ability: Analysis
Phase of Nursing Process: Analysis
Client Needs: Physiological Integrity
Content Area: Maternity

Reference

Olds, S., London, M., & Ladewig, P. (1996). *Maternal-newborn nursing: A family-centered approach* (5th ed.). Reading, MA: Addison-Wesley. p. 655.

38. 2

Rationale: Practice guidelines recommend auscultation of the fetal heart rate every 15 minutes in low-risk clients during the second stage of labor.

Test-Taking Strategy: The question requires knowledge of nursing standards, which guide nursing practice. Option 2 represents the minimum standard for a low-risk client in stage 2. Options 3 and 4 represent long time intervals at this critical stage of labor. It is not necessary to assess fetal heart rate after every contraction in a low-risk client.

Level of Cognitive Ability: Application
Phase of Nursing Process: Planning
Client Needs: Physiological Integrity
Content Area: Maternity

Reference

Olds, S., London, M., & Ladewig, P. (1996). *Maternal-newborn nursing: A family-centered approach* (5th ed.). Reading, MA: Addison-Wesley. p. 613.

39. 2

Rationale: When the membranes rupture in the birth setting, the nurse immediately assesses the FHR to detect changes associated with prolapse or compression of the umbilical cord.

Test-Taking Strategy: Use principles of prioritizing when answering this question and remember your ABCs. Fetal heart rate is associated with fetal breathing and circulation. Since no information is given to indicate delivery is imminent, option 4 can be eliminated. Option 3 is an appropriate action but not of high priority. Option 1 is appropriate for all labor clients regardless of status and membranes.

Level of Cognitive Ability: Application
Phase of Nursing Process: Implementation
Client Needs: Physiological Integrity
Content Area: Maternity

Reference
Olds, S., London, M., & Ladewig, P. (1996). *Maternal-newborn nursing: A family-centered approach* (5th ed.). Reading, MA: Addison-Wesley. p. 597.

40. 2

Rationale: The second stage of labor begins when the cervix is completely dilated and ends with birth of the infant.

Test-Taking Strategy: The question requires knowledge that the first stage of labor is marked by complete dilation of the cervix. Options 1, 3, and 4 are similar in that they can occur anytime in labor, and are, therefore, incorrect.

Level of Cognitive Ability: Analysis
Phase of Nursing Process: Evaluation
Client Needs: Physiological Integrity
Content Area: Maternity

Reference
Olds, S., London, M., & Ladewig, P. (1996). *Maternal-newborn nursing: A family-centered approach* (5th ed.). Reading, MA: Addison-Wesley. p. 579.

41. 3

Rationale: As the placenta separates, it settles downward into the lower uterine segment, the umbilical cord lengthens, and a sudden trickle or spurt of blood appears.

Test-Taking Strategy: Options 1, 2, and 4 are similar in that they represent complications. Option 3 indicates a normal finding following delivery of the neonate vaginally and is the correct answer. Review this stage of labor now if you had difficulty with this question!

Level of Cognitive Ability: Analysis
Phase of Nursing Process: Assessment
Client Needs: Physiological Integrity
Content Area: Maternity

Reference
Olds, S., London, M., & Ladewig, P. (1996). *Maternal-newborn nursing: A family-centered approach* (5th ed.). Reading, MA: Addison-Wesley. p. 665.

42. 4

Rationale: The Apgar scoring system was designed to evaluate the physical condition of the newborn infant at birth and determine whether immediate need for resuscitation exists. Scores range from 0 to 10. A score of 8 to 10 indicates a newborn infant in good condition who requires only nasopharyngeal suctioning and perhaps oxygen near the face.

Test-Taking Strategy: This question requires knowledge of the Apgar scoring system and the possible scores ranging from 0 to 10. Options 1, 2, and 3 are similar, indicating that additional intervention would be required. Option 4 is different, and correct. Review Apgar scoring now if you had difficulty with this question!

Level of Cognitive Ability: Analysis
Phase of Nursing Process: Analysis
Client Needs: Physiological Integrity
Content Area: Maternity

Reference
Olds, S., London, M., & Ladewig, P. (1996). *Maternal-newborn nursing: A family-centered approach* (5th ed.). Reading, MA: Addison-Wesley. p. 662.

43. 2

Rationale: Although immediate contact may be important for attachment or breast-feeding, the parents' wishes concerning contact with their newborn infant need to be supported and determined first.

Test-Taking Strategy: This question involves the nurse planning for the promotion of psychological adaptation. Option 2 is the correct answer since the client's needs and desires should be determined first in planning nursing care. Remember, assessment is the first step in the nursing process!

Level of Cognitive Ability: Application
Phase of Nursing Process: Planning
Client Needs: Psychosocial Integrity
Content Area: Maternity

Reference
Olds, S., London, M., & Ladewig, P. (1996). *Maternal-newborn nursing: A family-centered approach* (5th ed.). Reading, MA: Addison-Wesley. p. 665.

44. 3

Rationale: The first priority is to maintain respirations. A modified Trendelenburg position will aid the drainage of mucus from the nasopharynx and trachea to facilitate breathing.

Test-Taking Strategy: Use principles of prioritization and remember your ABCs. Option 3 is correct because this position facilitates drainage of mucus and promotes an open airway and effective breathing. Options 1, 2, and 4 are appropriate but can be implemented later.

Level of Cognitive Ability: Application
Phase of Nursing Process: Implementation
Client Needs: Physiological Integrity
Content Area: Maternity

Reference
Olds, S., London, M., & Ladewig, P. (1996). *Maternal-newborn nursing: A family-centered approach* (5th ed.). Reading, MA: Addison-Wesley. p. 662.

45. 4

Rationale: Oxytocin stimulates uterine contractions and is administered to reduce the incidence of third-stage hemorrhage.

Test-Taking Strategy: This question requires knowledge of the action of the medication oxytocin. Options 1, 2, and 3 are similar in that they represent undesirable findings. Option 4 is the correct answer and indicates a desired finding after medication administration. Review the action of oxytocin now, if you had difficulty with this question!

Level of Cognitive Ability: Analysis
Phase of Nursing Process: Evaluation
Client Needs: Physiological Integrity
Content Area: Maternity

Reference
Olds, S., London, M., & Ladewig, P. (1996). *Maternal-newborn nursing: A family-centered approach* (5th ed.). Reading, MA: Addison-Wesley. p. 666.

46. **1**

Rationale: Immediately following expulsion of the placenta, the fundus is firmly contracted, midline, and located one half to two thirds of the way between the symphysis pubis and the umbilicus. Because the uterine ligaments are still stretched, a full bladder can move the uterus.

Test-Taking Strategy: The question requires knowledge of the physiological changes that occur after delivery. Options 2, 3, and 4 are similar and represent complications not usually indicated by a firm but displaced uterus. Option 1 is different and the correct answer.

Level of Cognitive Ability: Analysis
Phase of Nursing Process: Assessment
Client Needs: Physiological Integrity
Content Area: Maternity

Reference
Olds, S., London, M., & Ladewig, P. (1996). *Maternal-newborn nursing: A family-centered approach* (5th ed.). Reading, MA: Addison-Wesley. pp. 1034–1044.

47. **2**

Rationale: The birth of a baby is an emotionally charged moment for new parents. Crying can be a normal expression of emotions surrounding birth. Holding, eye contact, and touch are signs of healthy maternal-newborn attachment.

Test-Taking Strategy: The question requires knowledge of normal attachment behaviors and emotional response at birth. Options 1, 3, and 4 are similar in that they all represent an abnormal response. Option 2 is different and the correct response.

Level of Cognitive Ability: Analysis
Phase of Nursing Process: Analysis
Client Needs: Psychosocial Integrity
Content Area: Maternity

Reference
Olds, S., London, M., & Ladewig, P. (1996). *Maternal-newborn nursing: A family-centered approach* (5th ed.). Reading, MA: Addison-Wesley. pp. 664–665.

48. **3**

Rationale: The initial parental-newborn attachment period can be enhanced if care providers keep routine procedures to a minimum and provide privacy. Delay of eye prophylaxis can enhance eye contact.

Test-Taking Strategy: This question requires knowledge of attachment and actions to facilitate it. Options 1, 2, and 4 are similar in that they separate mother and infant, and are, therefore, incorrect. Option 3 is the correct answer since delaying eye prophylaxis can enhance eye contact, an important aspect of facilitating attachment. Use the process of elimination to answer the question!

Level of Cognitive Ability: Application
Phase of Nursing Process: Implementation
Client Needs: Psychosocial Integrity
Content Area: Maternity

Reference
Olds, S., London, M., & Ladewig, P. (1996). *Maternal-newborn nursing: A family-centered approach* (5th ed.). Reading, MA: Addison-Wesley. p. 665.

49. **1**

Rationale: A potential complication following delivery is hemorrhage. The most significant source of bleeding is the site where the placenta is implanted. It is critical that the uterus remain contracted and vaginal blood flow be monitored every 15 minutes for the first 1 to 2 hours.

Test-Taking Strategy: Use prioritization principles to answer this question. Remembering your ABCs will help you select option 1. Assessing uterine position and consistency, amount and character of lochia provides information about blood loss and circulatory status. Options 2, 3, and 4 are less important at this time.

Level of Cognitive Ability: Application
Phase of Nursing Process: Implementation
Client Needs: Physiological Integrity
Content Area: Maternity

Reference
Olds, S., London, M., & Ladewig, P. (1996). *Maternal-newborn nursing: A family-centered approach* (5th ed.). Reading, MA: Addison-Wesley. p. 667.

50. **3**

Rationale: Methylergonovine maleate is an ergot alkaloid that stimulates smooth muscles. Because the smooth muscle of the uterus is especially sensitive to the medication, it is used postpartally to stimulate the uterus to contract and control excessive blood loss.

Test-Taking Strategy: This question requires knowledge of the action of methylergonovine maleate. Only option 3 reflects the correct medication action: stimulation of smooth muscles, or uterine contractions.

Level of Cognitive Ability: Analysis
Phase of Nursing Process: Evaluation
Client Needs: Physiological Integrity
Content Area: Maternity

Reference
Olds, S., London, M., & Ladewig, P. (1996). *Maternal-newborn nursing: A family-centered approach* (5th ed.). Reading, MA: Addison-Wesley. p. 1069.

BIBLIOGRAPHY

Gorrie, T., McKinney, E., & Murray, S. (1998). *Foundations of maternal-newborn nursing* (2nd ed.). Philadelphia: W. B. Saunders.

Nichols, F., & Zwelling, E. (1997). *Maternal-newborn nursing: Theory and practice.* Philadelphia: W. B. Saunders.

Olds, S., London, M., & Ladewig, P. (1996). *Maternal-newborn nursing: A family-centered approach.* (5th ed.). Reading, MA: Addison-Wesley.

Pillitteri, A., (1995). *Maternal and child health nursing: Care of the childbearing and childrearing family.* (2nd ed.). Philadelphia: J. B. Lippincott.

CHAPTER 27

Problems with Labor and Delivery

I. Dystocia

A. Description
  1. Difficult **labor** that is prolonged or more painful
  2. Occurs because of problems caused by uterine contractions, the fetus, or the bones and tissues of the maternal pelvis
  3. Contractions may be hypotonic or hypertonic
  4. Fetus may be excessively large, malpositioned, or in an abnormal presentation
  5. Can result in:
     a. Fetal injury or death
     b. Maternal dehydration
     c. Infection or injury
B. Assessment
  1. Excessive abdominal pain
  2. Abnormal contraction pattern
  3. Fetal distress
  4. Elevated maternal temperature
  5. Maternal or fetal tachycardia
  6. Lack of progress in **labor**
  7. Ketonuria
  8. Decreased urine output
C. Implementation
  1. Assess fetal heart rate
  2. Monitor uterine contractions
  3. Monitor maternal temperature and heart rate
  4. Monitor for fetal distress
  5. Assist with pelvic examination, measurements, ultrasounds, and other procedures
  6. Administer prophylactic antibiotics as prescribed to prevent infection
  7. Provide rest and administer IV fluids as prescribed
  8. Monitor intake and output (I&O)
  9. Assess for dehydration
  10. Instruct client in breathing techniques and relaxation exercises
  11. Fetal monitoring if oxytocin is prescribed
  12. Monitor color of **amniotic fluid**
  13. Provide comfort as with a normal **delivery**, such as backrubs and position changes
  14. Assess client's fatigue and pain and administer sedatives and pain medications as prescribed
  15. Assess for prolapse of the cord after rupture of the membranes
  16. If prolapse occurs:
     a. Place client in Trendelenburg's or knee-chest position to minimize pressure on the cord
     b. Administer oxygen
     c. Notify physician
     d. Prepare for emergency cesarean section

II. Precipitate Labor and Delivery

A. Description: **labor** lasts less than 3 hours
B. Implementation
  1. Stay with client at all times
  2. Provide emotional support and keep client calm
  3. Encourage mother to pant between contractions
  4. Prepare for rupturing membranes when head crowns if not already ruptured
  5. Do not try to keep fetus from being delivered
  6. Apply gentle pressure to fetal head upward toward the vagina to prevent damage to the fetal head and vaginal lacerations
  7. Deliver fetus between contractions, checking for the cord around the neck
  8. Use restitution to deliver the posterior shoulder
  9. Use gentle downward pressure to move the anterior shoulder under the pubic symphysis
  10. Clear the neonate's mouth
  11. Dry and cover the neonate to keep the body warm
  12. If outside of the hospital, clamp the cord in two places and cut between with a clean knife or scissors after the cord stops pulsating

13. Allow **placenta** to separate naturally
14. Place newborn infant on mother's abdomen or breast to induce uterine contractions

III. Preterm Labor

A. Description
1. **Labor** occurring after the 20th week but before the 37th week
2. Contractions occurring at least once every 10 minutes and lasting 30 seconds or longer
3. Documented cervical change or cervical effacement of 80% or dilatation of 2 cm
B. Assessment
1. Increased or bloody discharge
2. Backache
3. Pressure and cramping
4. Contractions
5. Diarrhea
6. Palpable uterine contractions
C. Implementation
1. Maintain bed rest, a quiet environment, and a lateral recumbent position
2. Administer tocolytic agents as prescribed to suppress **labor**
3. Administration of betamethasone to stimulate fetal lung maturity when preterm **delivery** appears inevitable
4. When administering magnesium sulfate:
   a. Assess effects of drugs on **labor** and fetus
   b. Monitor reflexes
   c. Have antidote (calcium gluconate) available at bedside
   d. Monitor vital signs
   e. Monitor for hypotension
   f. Auscultate lungs and monitor for an increased respiratory rate, which may indicate pulmonary edema
   g. Monitor for fluid overload
   h. Monitor fetal heart rate

IV. Rupture of Uterus

A. Description: Complete or incomplete separation of the uterine tissue due to rupture of the uterus from the stress of **labor**
B. Complete Rupture of the Uterus
1. Pain, which is shearing, excruciating, diffuse, or localized
2. Contractions may stop or fail to progress
3. Relaxation between contractions is incomplete
4. Rigid abdomen
5. Signs of maternal shock
6. Absent fetal heart rate (FHR)
7. Fetus palpated outside the uterus
C. Incomplete Rupture of the Uterus
1. Assessment
   a. Abdominal pain that occurs during contractions
   b. Cervix fails to dilate
   c. Slight vaginal bleeding

   d. FHR absent
D. Implementation
1. Monitor maternal and fetal vital signs
2. Prepare client for cesarean section or hysterotomy with hysterectomy
3. Provide emotional support for client and partner
4. Monitor for and treat signs of shock

V. Placenta Previa

A. Description
1. Improperly implanted **placenta** in the lower uterine segment near or over the internal os of the cervix
2. Complete, total, or central: Internal os covered by **placenta** when cervix is fully dilated
3. Partial: Incomplete coverage of os, marginal or low-lying with only the edge of the **placenta** approaching the internal os
B. Assessment
1. Painless bleeding as early as 7 months
2. Bleeding may be mild to hemorrhage
3. Anemia
4. Soft uterus
5. Abnormal fetal position of breech or transverse lie
6. High presenting part
7. Uterine contractions
C. Implementation
1. Monitor maternal vital signs, FHR, and fetal activity
2. Assess bleeding, including amount and quality
3. Maintain bed rest
4. Position client in left lateral position
5. Administer IV fluids as prescribed
6. Monitor and treat signs of shock
7. Avoid vaginal examination if bleeding is occurring
8. Administer iron supplements or blood transfusions as prescribed to maintain a hematocrit level above 30%
9. Prepare for ultrasound for **placental** localization
10. Prepare to administer Rh immune globulin if the mother is Rh negative and has not been given the injection at 28 weeks' gestation
11. Prepare for premature birth or cesarean section

VI. Abruptio Placentae

A. Description: Premature separation of the **placenta** from the uterine wall after the 20th week of gestation and before the fetus is delivered
B. Assessment
1. Painful vaginal bleeding
2. Hypertonic to tetanic, enlarged uterus
3. Boardlike rigidity of abdomen
4. Abnormal or absent fetal heart tones

5. Hypotension
6. Tachycardia
7. Pallor
8. Cool, moist skin
9. Bloody **amniotic fluid**
10. Rising fundal height from blood trapped behind the **placenta**
11. Signs of shock
12. Manifestations of coagulopathy

C. Implementation
1. Monitor maternal vital signs and FHR
2. Assess for vaginal bleeding, abdominal pain, and increase in fundal height
3. Maintain bed rest
4. Administer oxygen as prescribed
5. Monitor and report any uterine activity
6. Administer IV fluids as prescribed
7. Monitor I&O, because a urine output of less than 30 mL/hour indicates decreased renal perfusion
8. Administer blood and blood products as prescribed
9. Monitor blood studies for impending signs of disseminated intravascular coagulation (DIC), which include low fibrinogen and platelet levels, increased prothrombin time (PT), partial thromboplastin time (PTT), blood-clotting time, and fibrin degradation products
10. Prepare for the **delivery** of the fetus as quickly as possible, with vaginal **delivery** preferable if the fetus is healthy and stable and presenting part is in the pelvis
11. Prepare for emergency cesarean section if the fetus is alive but shows signs of distress
12. Perform Kleihauer-Betke test after **delivery** for Rh-negative clients because fetal maternal hemorrhage is common
13. Monitor for signs of DIC in the postpartum period

VII. Prolapsed Cord

A. Description: The umbilical cord is displaced, either between the presenting part and the amnion or else protruding through the cervix, and causes compression of the cord, compromising fetal circulation

B. Assessment
1. A feeling that something is coming through the vagina
2. Umbilical cord is seen or palpated
3. FHR is irregular and slow
4. Fetal heart monitor will show variable deceleration or bradycardia after rupture of the membranes
5. If fetal hypoxia is severe, violent fetal activity may occur and then cease

C. Implementation
1. Relieve cord pressure immediately
2. Place mother in knee-chest or Trendelenburg's position
3. Elevate the fetal presenting part that is lying on the cord by applying finger pressure with a sterile gloved hand
4. Do not attempt to push the cord into the uterus
5. Monitor FHR
6. Assess fetus for hypoxia
7. Administer oxygen by face mask to the mother as prescribed
8. Prepare for cesarean birth

VIII. Inverted Uterus

A. Description: Uterus turns inside out, usually during **delivery** of the **placenta**

B. Assessment
1. Hemorrhage
2. Severe pain
3. Signs of shock

C. Implementation
1. Monitor vital signs
2. Monitor for signs of shock
3. Prepare the client for a return of the uterus to the correct position via the vagina

IX. Amniotic Fluid Embolism

A. Description
1. The escape of **amniotic fluid** into the maternal circulation
2. The debris containing **amniotic fluid** deposits in the pulmonary arterioles and is usually fatal to the mother

B. Assessment
1. Dyspnea
2. Sudden chest pain
3. Cyanosis
4. Pulmonary edema

C. Implementation
1. Institute emergency measures to maintain life
2. Monitor vital signs
3. Administer oxygen as prescribed
4. Monitor for uncontrolled hemorrhage
5. Prepare to administer digitalis as prescribed for failing cardiac function
6. Prepare to administer fibrinogen as prescribed to replace depleted reserves
7. Prepare to administer heparin as prescribed
8. Prepare to administer blood transfusions as prescribed
9. Prepare for forceps **delivery** if the cervix is dilated

X. Vena Cava Syndrome (Supine Hypotensive Syndrome)

A. Description
1. Occurs when the venous return to the heart is impaired by the weight of the uterus
2. Results in partial occlusion of the vena cava

B. Assessment
1. Signs of shock

2. Hypotension
3. Tachycardia
4. Sweating
5. Nausea and vomiting
6. Air hunger
7. Fetal distress

C. Implementation
1. Monitor vital signs
2. Monitor FHR
3. Administer oxygen as prescribed
4. Position client by turning to the left side to shift the weight of the fetus off the inferior vena cava
5. Assess for shock caused by reduced cardiac output

◆ XI. Fetal Distress

A. Assessment
1. Fetal heart rate above 160 or below 120 beats per minute
2. Meconium-stained fluid
3. Fetal hyperactivity
4. Variable deceleration pattern
5. Late deceleration
6. Fetal pH below 7.2

B. Implementation
1. Monitor vital signs
2. Discontinue oxytocin as prescribed
3. Position mother by turning to the left side
4. Administer oxygen via face mask as prescribed
5. Elevate legs
6. Increase IV to correct hypotension
7. Prepare for emergency cesarean section

PRACTICE QUESTIONS

1. For the previous 4 hours, a client in labor has been experiencing contractions every 2 minutes, lasting 60 to 70 seconds, and strong to palpation. She is 2 cm dilated and complaining of severe pain. Which type of labor dystocia is this describing?
   1 Hyptonic
   2 Precipitate
   3 Hypertonic
   4 Protracted active phase

2. A client is admitted 9 cm dilated and experiencing precipitate labor. A priority nursing action is to:
   1 Obtain an order for an oxytocin infusion
   2 Keep the client in a side-lying position
   3 Prepare the client for an epidural anesthesia
   4 Encourage the client to start pushing with the contractions

3. Which of the following assessment findings place a pregnant client at risk for preterm labor?
   1 A 26-year-old primigravida
   2 A single-fetus pregnancy

   3 A hemoglobin of 13.5 g/dL
   4 A diagnosed urinary tract infection

4. The nurse recognizes that the risks for uterine rupture during labor and delivery include:
   1 Hypotonic contractions
   2 Shoulder dystocia
   3 Being pregnant for the first time (primigravida)
   4 Weak bearing-down efforts

5. A client is admitted to the labor suite complaining of painless vaginal bleeding. A routine labor procedure that is contraindicated with this client's situation is:
   1 Leopold's maneuvers
   2 External electronic FHR monitoring
   3 Manual pelvic examination
   4 Hemoglobin and hematocrit evaluation

6. The nurse assessing the antepartal client with vaginal bleeding is aware that an abruptio placentae is accompanied by which of the following assessment findings?
   1 Abdomen soft upon palpation
   2 No complaint of abdominal pain
   3 Lack of uterine irritability or tetanic contractions
   4 Uterine tenderness upon palpation

7. The nurse establishes that which of the following, if found in the client in labor, least indicates dystocia?
   1 High level of maternal fear or anxiety
   2 Failure of fetus to descend
   3 Progressive changes in the cervix
   4 Signs of fetal distress

8. The mother experiencing dystocia looks alarmed and asks: "What's going on? Why are you all poking and prodding? Is my baby OK?" Based on this information and your knowledge of a difficult delivery, which nursing diagnosis would you assign to this client?
   1 Anxiety, related to knowledge deficit
   2 Powerlessness, related to dysfunctional labor process
   3 Risk for altered parenting, related to painful delivery
   4 Sensory overload, related to need for rapid and multiple interventions

9. The nurse planning care for the client experiencing dystocia considers the highest nursing priority to be frequent:
   1 Explanations to family members about what is happening in this situation
   2 Comfort measures, change of position, and touch
   3 Reinforcement of breathing techniques learned in childbirth preparatory classes

4 Monitoring for changes in physical and emotional condition of mother and fetus

10. Precipitous labor and delivery may have a number of consequences. The nurse caring for the nulliparous woman in labor would be aware and alert the physician if which one of the following became apparent?
    1 Decreased periods of uterine relaxation between contractions
    2 Dilation of the cervix of >1.2 and <5 cm/hour during the active phase
    3 Descent of <1 to 2 cm/hour
    4 Latent phase of <6 hours

11. After a precipitate delivery, the nurse assesses that the woman is passive and touches her newborn baby only briefly with her fingertips. The nurse would do which of the following first to help the woman process what has happened?
    1 Encourage the mother to breast-feed soon after birth
    2 Consider the cultural characteristics of the woman
    3 Write a complete account of the parent's reaction on the birth record
    4 Support the mother no matter what her reaction to the newborn infant is

12. In a precipitous delivery, the nurse waits for the placenta to separate before attempting to deliver it. The nurse assesses for which of the following signs that indicate the placenta has separated?
    1 Shortening of the umbilical cord
    2 Decrease in blood loss from the introitus
    3 Change in the uterine contour
    4 Sudden sharp abdominal pain

13. The woman at risk of preterm labor has been told that she is to restrict activity. The nurse asks the client to say what this means to her. The nurse evaluates that the client has the least correct understanding of what is intended if the client stated that activity restriction:
    1 May include any activity as long as it is carried out in bed
    2 Means a variety of things depending on the mother's condition and physician preference
    3 Instructions may change at various times throughout the pregnancy
    4 May encompass instructions on mobility, bathroom activities, and sexual relations

14. The nurse is planning to develop a standardized teaching plan about preterm labor to use with pregnant clients. The nurse considers which of the following variables as the least important when developing this plan?
    1 Women may use coping mechanisms such as denial and waiting to deal with preterm labor
    2 Symptoms of preterm labor are ambiguous

and may be attributed to the normal discomforts of pregnancy
    3 It is most cost effective to give information only to women who obtain high scores on the risk assessment tools
    4 Early detection may make the interventions more effective

15. The nurse is teaching the client about preterm labor. The nurse does which of the following as the most effective method for teaching the client to assess preterm uterine contractions?
    1 Palpate for uterine contractions at the same time as the client
    2 Provide a simple pamphlet with multiple illustrations
    3 Ask about contractions at each visit
    4 Attach the monitor to the client's abdomen and have her palpate at the same time

16. A woman at 20 weeks of gestation calls the physician's office and speaks to a clinic nurse. The client states that she is having subtle but persistent changes in her vaginal discharge, menstruation-like cramps, and diarrhea. What of the following is the least helpful response of this nurse?
    1 "This is an emergency; you should come to the clinic within the hour."
    2 "Drink 3 glasses of water and lie on your left side for 1 hour."
    3 "Palpate for contractions for 1 hour or for four contractions, whichever comes first."
    4 "Tell me about your activity, food, fluid, and medication intake for the last 24 hours."

17. The client has experienced uterine rupture. The nurse formulates which of the following as the first priority nursing diagnosis for the client?
    1 Fear, related to outcome
    2 Acute pain
    3 Impaired gas exchange
    4 Anticipatory grieving

18. When a complete uterine rupture has occurred, the outcome may be fetal death. If fetal death occurs, after the physiological needs of the woman have been met the nurse should plan to do which of the following next?
    1 Avoid talking about the dead fetus
    2 Encourage the husband and wife to think about future childbearing
    3 Allow family members to see and hold the dead baby if they wish
    4 Determine what the family perceived of the event

19. The client has a placenta previa. The nurse avoids doing a cervical examination on this woman primarily because it could:
    1 Increase the chance of infection
    2 Initiate premature labor
    3 Cause profound hemorrhage

4 Rupture the fetal membranes

20. A woman has delivered a baby after a pregnancy with a placenta previa. The nurse assesses the client carefully, knowing that the client is at risk for:
    1 Postpartum hemorrhage
    2 Chronic hypertension
    3 Postpartum infection
    4 Coagulopathy

21. Which of the following is the first priority goal for the client experiencing placenta previa?
    1 There are no signs of fetal distress
    2 Mother expresses understanding of her condition
    3 Mother identifies and uses available support systems
    4 Client demonstrates compliance with activity limitations

22. Abruptio placentae can trigger disseminated intravascular coagulopathy (DIC). The nurse would suspect this in a client if the nurse observes:
    1 Pain and swelling of the calf of one leg
    2 Rapid clotting times
    3 Laboratory values indicating increased platelets
    4 Petechiae, oozing from injection sites, and hematuria

23. Severe separation of the placenta is always an emergency. The first priority of the nurse to assist the client psychosocially is to:
    1 Work with family members to modify escalating anxiety
    2 Encourage the woman to express beliefs why this happened
    3 Elicit support for the woman from significant others
    4 Explain the plan of treatment to the woman and her partner

24. The nurse is planning to teach preventive measures for abruptio placentae in the antenatal clinic. The nurse, using current research, especially targets as the focus of this teaching session women who:
    1 Smoke or use cocaine
    2 Engage in moderate exercise
    3 Are in their mid-twenties
    4 Are primiparas

25. The client with abruptio placentae begins to develop shock. A first-priority nursing action is:
    1 Turn client onto her side
    2 Monitor maternal vital signs
    3 Monitor urinary output
    4 Begin fetal monitoring

ANSWERS

1. **3**

Rationale: The client is 2 cm dilated and in the latent phase of labor. The most common type of dysfunctional labor at this point is hypertonic. A normal pattern during the latent phase of labor is contractions every 5 to 10 minutes, lasting 30 to 45 seconds, and mild in intensity. Precipitate labor is that which lasts in its entirety for 3 hours or less. The client has already been in labor for at least 4 hours. Hypotonic labor contractions are short, irregular, weak, and usually occur during the active phase of labor.

Test-Taking Strategy: Pay attention to the defining information in the case situation. Read every word. One of the key factors here is that the client is 2 cm dilated. This, along with her contraction pattern, tells you what phase of labor she is in. Be sure to read the options carefully. "Hypo" and "hyper" are easily mistaken for one another when reading quickly. If you are not clear about the characteristics of the types of contractions, review them now!

Level of Cognitive Ability: Analysis
Phase of Nursing Process: Assessment
Client Needs: Physiological Integrity
Content Area: Maternity

Reference
Nichols, F., & Zwelling, E. (1997). *Maternal-newborn nursing: Theory and practice.* Philadelphia: W. B. Saunders. p. 742.

2. **2**

Rationale: Priority care of this client includes promotion of fetal oxygenation. Precipitate labor progresses quickly, with frequent contractions and short periods of relaxation between contractions. This does not allow for maximal reperfusion of the placenta with oxygenated blood. A side-lying position can assist in blood flow to the uterus by preventing vena cava and abdominal aorta compression. Further stimulation with oxytocin is contraindicated. There may not be enough time to administer an epidural anesthesia prior to delivery with such quick progression. The chance of an unattended birth is possible. Pushing with contractions is not indicated at 8 cm of dilation, especially with this type of labor. Controlled delivery of the baby is essential to prevent maternal and fetal injury.

Test-Taking Strategy: The key word in the case situation is "precipitate." The key word in the stem is "priority." Using Maslow's Hierarchy of Needs theory, physiological integrity needs to be dealt with first. Also, think of the ABCs when prioritizing, including the baby's needs as well as the client's. Options 1, 3, and 4 contain information contradictory to caring for this client.

Level of Cognitive Ability: Application
Phase of Nursing Process: Implementation
Client Needs: Physiological Integrity
Content Area: Maternity

Reference
Gorrie, T., McKinney, E. S., & Murray, S. S. (1998). *Foundations of maternal-newborn nursing* (2nd ed.). Philadelphia: W. B. Saunders. p. 755.

3. **4**

Rationale: One risk factor for preterm labor is the presence of a genitourinary infection. The connection is not clearly understood. One hypothesis involves the release of prostaglandins by the pathogens, which may contribute to the initiation of contractions. Other risk factors include a multifetal pregnancy that contributes to overdistention of the uterus, anemia that decreases oxygen supply to the uterus, and age less than 15 years or first pregnancy over the age of 35 years.

Test-Taking Strategy: Knowledge of preterm labor and theories regarding its cause are needed. Look for the option that is outside of the norm. Options 1, 2, and 3 are all average findings. By the process of elimination, option 4 is the only deviation from normal.

Level of Cognitive Ability: Analysis
Phase of the Nursing Process: Analysis
Client Needs: Physiological Integrity
Content Area: Maternity

Reference
Gorrie, T., McKinney, E. S., & Murray, S. S. (1998). *Foundations of maternal-newborn nursing* (2nd ed.). Philadelphia: W. B. Saunders. p. 759.

4. **2**

Rationale: Shoulder dystocia at delivery causes increased pressure in the thin, lower uterine segment and subsequently the risk for spontaneous rupture. Statistically, rupture is more common in multigravidas, especially when combined with the use of oxytocin. Hypotonic contractions and weak bearing-down efforts alone do not add to the risk of rupture since they do not add to the stress on the uterine wall.

Test-Taking Strategy: By the process of elimination, look at which option provides an additional source of pressure to the uterus and would be most likely to add to the risk of rupturing, or "tearing," the uterus. Option 2 is the only option that would provide an additional source of pressure to the uterus.

Level of Cognitive Ability: Application
Phase of Nursing Process: Assessment
Client Needs: Physiological Integrity
Content Area: Maternity

Reference
Nichols, F., & Zwelling, E. (1997). *Maternal-newborn nursing: Theory and practice.* Philadelphia: W. B. Saunders. p. 893.

5. **3**

Rationale: Painless vaginal bleeding is a sign of a possible placenta previa. Digital examination of the cervix can lead to maternal and fetal hemorrhage. Leopold's maneuvers can reveal a nonengaged presenting part or malpresentation, both of which often accompany placenta previa owing to the placenta filling the lower uterine segment. The nurse could also assess at the same time for uterine tenderness or hardness, which is consistent with a placental abruption, and assist in making a differential diagnosis. Hemoglobin and hematocrit values help estimate the amount of blood loss. Electronic fetal monitoring (external) is crucial in evaluating the status of the fetus who is at risk for severe hypoxia.

Test-Taking Strategy: Knowledge of the signs and symptoms of placenta previa is necessary. Review this content now if you had difficulty with this question! Option 3 is

the only procedure that is invasive to the pregnancy and endangers the physiological safety of the client and fetus.

Level of Cognitive Ability: Analysis
Phase of Nursing Process: Implementation
Client Needs: Physiological Integrity
Content Area: Maternity

Reference
Nichols, F., & Zwelling, E. (1997). *Maternal-newborn nursing: Theory and practice.* Philadelphia: W. B. Saunders. p. 872.

6. **4**

Rationale: Vaginal bleeding in a pregnant client most often is caused by placenta previa or a placental abruption. Uterine tenderness accompanies placental abruption, especially with a central abruption and trapped blood behind the placenta. The abdomen will feel hard and boardlike upon palpation as the blood penetrates the myometrium and causes uterine irritability. A sustained tetanic contraction can occur if the client is in labor and the uterine muscle cannot relax.

Test-Taking Strategy: Read carefully so you are aware of which disorder you are investigating. It can be easy to confuse a placenta previa and abruption. Remember, the difference involves the presence of uterine pain and tenderness with an abruption, as opposed to painless bleeding with a previa. Options 1, 2, and 3 describe the absence of a sign or symptom of abruptio placentae, whereas option 4 is the only one that describes the presence of one. Review this content now, if you had difficulty with this question!

Level of Cognitive Ability: Application
Phase of Nursing Process: Assessment
Client Needs: Physiological Integrity
Content Area: Maternity

Reference
Nichols, F., & Zwelling, E. (1997). *Maternal-newborn nursing: Theory and practice.* Philadelphia: W. B. Saunders. pp. 874–875.

7. **3**

Rationale: Progressive changes in the cervix are a reassuring pattern in labor. Abnormal labor patterns are assessed according to the nature of the cervical dilation and fetal descent.

Test-Taking Strategy: Read all four options. Be careful not to read into the question. Use your nursing knowledge to choose correctly among the possible choices. The wording of the question guides you to look for a response that is a normal finding in labor.

Level of Cognitive Ability: Analysis
Phase of Nursing Process: Assessment
Client Needs: Physiological Integrity
Content Area: Maternity

Reference
Lowdermilk, D., Perry, S., & Bobak, I. (1997). *Maternity & women's health care* (6th ed.). St. Louis: Mosby–Year Book. p. 952.

8. **1**

Rationale: The etiologies for all the nursing diagnoses except option 1 are out of the control of nursing intervention. The nurse cannot change or independently intervene for dysfunctional labor process, painful delivery, or the need for rapid and multiple interventions. The nurse can independently intervene with knowledge deficit. The other problem statements have a potential for being true, but they are either not clearly written or do not suggest specific nursing actions. Also, they are not amenable to change by the nurse.

Test-Taking Strategy: Nursing diagnoses must be clearly stated. The problem portion of the statement must fit the defining characteristics of the problem statement, and the etiology must be changeable by someone, must clearly suggest nursing actions, and must be part of the independent function of nursing. By applying these criteria, each of the incorrect options can be eliminated.

Level of Cognitive Ability: Analysis
Phase of Nursing Process: Analysis
Client Needs: Psychosocial Integrity
Content Area: Maternity

References

Lowdermilk, D., Perry, S., & Bobak, I. (1997). *Maternity & women's health care* (6th ed.). St. Louis: Mosby–Year Book. pp. 954–955.
Carpenito, L. (1997). *Handbook of nursing diagnosis* (7th ed.). Philadelphia: Lippincott-Raven. pp. 9–15, 216–221, 260–263, 279–282, 357–360.

9. **4**

Rationale: All the answers are correct and would be used during the care of the client. However, the first priority is to monitor for changes in physiological integrity. Each of the others would be considered of somewhat lesser priority than option 4.

Test-Taking Strategy: In questions requiring priority setting, physiological and safety needs come first. Using this concept, each of the incorrect options may be systematically eliminated.

Level of Cognitive Ability: Application
Phase of Nursing Process: Planning
Client Needs: Physiological Integrity
Content Area: Maternity

Reference

Lowdermilk, D., Perry, S., & Bobak, I. (1997). *Maternity & women's health care* (6th ed.). St. Louis: Mosby–Year Book. p. 954.

10. **1**

Rationale: Signs of possible need for emergency intervention are indicated by inadequate uterine relaxation between contractions. Inadequate relaxation interferes with the transfer of oxygen and nutrients to the fetus through the mother's placenta. All other options are within normal limits for a nulliparous woman. By definition, a precipitate labor lasts less than 3 hours.

Test-Taking Strategy: Use nursing knowledge about the normal parameters of labor to answer this question. Apply knowledge of physiology to the case situation. If you had difficulty with this question, review content related to precipitous labor and delivery now!

Level of Cognitive Ability: Analysis
Phase of Nursing Process: Analysis
Client Needs: Physiological Integrity
Content Area: Maternity

Reference

Lowdermilk, D., Perry, S., & Bobak, I. (1997). *Maternity & women's health care* (6th ed.). St. Louis: Mosby–Year Book, p. 384.

11. **4**

Rationale: There may be many reactions to the birth of a baby. The mother may be exhausted, in pain, stunned by the rapid nature of the delivery, or following her cultural norms. The mother may want to process what has happened and will need time to assimilate all that happened. A therapeutic nurse-client relationship will be formed or enhanced with a nurturing and accepting attitude.

Test-Taking Strategy: The correct answer incorporates the other three answers and also stresses the fact that the nurse's role is to provide a caring, psychologically safe environment for the client. The nurse values clients in their growth process and thus facilitates further growth.

Level of Cognitive Ability: Application
Phase of Nursing Process: Implementation
Client Needs: Psychosocial Integrity
Content Area: Maternity

Reference

Lowdermilk, D., Perry, S., & Bobak, I. (1997). *Maternity & women's health care* (6th ed.). St. Louis: Mosby–Year Book. p. 414.

12. **3**

Rationale: Signs of placental separation include lengthening of the umbilical cord, a sudden gush of dark blood from the introitus, a firmly contracted uterus, and the uterus changing from a discoid to globular shape. The client may experience vaginal fullness, but not sudden and sharp abdominal pain.

Test-Taking Strategy: The stem asks for the correct response. Use your nursing knowledge to eliminate the incorrect responses. Knowledge of the signs of placental separation will guide you to the only correct choice. Review this content now, if you had difficulty with this question!

Level of Cognitive Ability: Analysis
Phase of Nursing Process: Assessment
Client Needs: Physiological Integrity
Content Area: Maternity

Reference

Lowdermilk, D., Perry, S., & Bobak, I. (1997). *Maternity & women's health care* (6th ed.). St. Louis: Mosby–Year Book. p. 413.

13. **1**

Rationale: What the client may interpret as activity restrictions may differ from what the health care provider may have planned. Careful information must be given to ensure that a clear understanding exists between the nurse and the client.

Test-Taking Strategy: Use teaching and learning strategies. Options 2, 3, and 4 have a common theme. Options that are similar are unlikely to be correct. Option 1 stands alone and addresses the issue of bed rest. Additionally, use the process of elimination to answer the question!

Level of Cognitive Ability: Analysis
Phase of Nursing Process: Evaluation
Client Needs: Health Promotion and Maintenance
Content Area: Maternity

Reference

Lowdermilk, D., Perry, S., & Bobak, I. (1997). *Maternity & women's health care* (6th ed.). St. Louis: Mosby–Year Book. p. 942.

14. **3**

Rationale: The predictive value of most risk assessment systems is low. In 70% to 80% of cases of preterm labor, no risk factors can be identified. Symptomatology of preterm labor should be taught to all pregnant women.

Test-Taking Strategy: The question is worded to make you seek an incorrect statement. The answer to the question is stated in absolute terms. Absolute terminology tends to make the statement false.

Level of Cognitive Ability: Analysis
Phase of Nursing Process: Planning
Client Needs: Health Promotion and Maintenance
Content Area: Maternity

References

Lowdermilk, D., Perry, S., & Bobak, I. (1997). *Maternity & women's health care* (6th ed.). St. Louis: Mosby–Year Book. p. 943.

15. **1**

Rationale: Option 1 uses teaching and learning principles. It includes the most direct way to assess the level of client understanding. The client may not be able to read well. The client may not understand what to feel for and may answer only to please you. A monitor would be cost prohibitive and does not give human feedback.

Test-Taking Strategy: Use teaching and learning theory. The correct answer provides for demonstration and return demonstration as teaching methods, and promotes interaction between the nurse and client.

Level of Cognitive Ability: Application
Phase of Nursing Process: Implementation
Client Needs: Health Promotion and Maintenance
Content Area: Maternity

References

Nichols, F., & Zwelling, E. (1997). *Maternal-newborn nursing: Theory and practice.* Philadelphia: W. B. Saunders. p. 777.

16. **1**

Rationale: If the woman is active, it may be helpful for her to lie on her side, drink fluids, and keep her bladder empty to eliminate uterine hypoxia and thereby decrease uterine activity. If the woman continues to have persistent uterine activity after 1 hour or counts four or more contractions in less than an hour, she should be seen for further evaluation.

Test-Taking Strategy: Option number 1 stands out from the other three in that it may alarm the client, and it does not seek further clarification through the assessment phase of the nursing process. The presenting symptoms are vague and may or may not signal an emerging problem. Since the wording of the question guides you to look for an incorrect response on the part of the nurse, option 1 is chosen as the least helpful.

Level of Cognitive Ability: Application
Phase of Nursing Process: Implementation
Client Needs: Health Promotion and Maintenance
Content Area: Maternity

Reference

Lowdermilk, D., Perry, S., & Bobak, I. (1997). *Maternity & women's health care* (6th ed.). St. Louis: Mosby–Year Book. p. 943.

17. **3**

Rationale: The correct option deals with a physiological need and impacts on the ABCs (Airway, Breathing, Circula-

tion). The other nursing diagnoses, although appropriate, must assume a lesser priority than Impaired Gas Exchange.

Test-Taking Strategy: When answering this type of question, use priority-setting strategies, and remember that physiological needs come first!

Level of Cognitive Ability: Analysis
Phase of Nursing Process: Analysis
Client Needs: Physiological Integrity
Content Area: Maternity

Reference

Lowdermilk, D., Perry, S., & Bobak, I. (1997). *Maternity & women's health care* (6th ed.). St. Louis: Mosby–Year Book. pp. 975–976.

18. **4**

Rationale: The nurse should first plan to assess the level of anxiety, recovery from anesthesia, and the ability of the person to take in and process information. Information given before anxiety reduction or recovery would be ineffective and wasted effort. This event was sudden and catastrophic and much of the information may not have been perceived. The nurse should first assess before deciding how to intervene.

Test-Taking Strategy: Knowledge of how the nurse might respond in a crisis for this family is essential to answer this question. Use the steps of the nursing process to select the correct option, remembering that assessment comes first!

Level of Cognitive Ability: Application
Phase of Nursing Process: Planning
Client Needs: Psychosocial Integrity
Content Area: Maternity

References

Nichols, F., & Zwelling, E. (1997). *Maternal-newborn nursing: Theory and practice.* Philadelphia: W. B. Saunders. p. 636.

19. **3**

Rationale: Since the placenta is implanted low in the uterus, cervical examination could cause the disruption of the placenta and initiate profound hemorrhage. The other options are also correct, but the profound hemorrhage is of the greatest concern in this instance.

Test-Taking Strategy: Look for key words. The stem asks for the primary reason. Understanding the principles involved in this condition is helpful in answering this question. All the options are a possible outcome of cervical examination in the pregnant woman; however, understanding the mechanism of the placenta previa would lead to the correct option.

Level of Cognitive Ability: Application
Phase of Nursing Process: Implementation
Client Needs: Physiological Integrity
Content Area: Maternity

Reference

Lowdermilk, D., Perry, S., & Bobak, I. (1997). *Maternity & women's health care* (6th ed.). St. Louis: Mosby–Year Book. pp. 773–778.

20. **1**

Rationale: Because the placenta is implanted in the lower uterine segment that does not contain the same intertwining musculature as the fundus of the uterus, this site is more prone to bleeding. The nurse then has to assess the client carefully for signs of postpartum hemorrhage.

Test-Taking Strategy: The answer to this question depends upon understanding the normal physiology of the uterus and the site of implantation. This knowledge allows you to eliminate each of the incorrect options systematically. Review the complications associated with placenta previa now, if you had difficulty with this question!

Level of Cognitive Ability: Application
Phase of Nursing Process: Assessment
Client Needs: Physiological Integrity
Content Area: Maternity

Reference

Lowdermilk, D., Perry, S., & Bobak, I. (1997). *Maternity & women's health care* (6th ed.). St. Louis: Mosby–Year Book. p. 776.

21. **1**

Rationale: Options 2, 3, and 4 may be carried out, but the physiological integrity and safety of the mother-neonate dyad is the priority. These other options may contribute to this ultimate outcome.

Test-Taking Strategy: Options 2, 3, and 4 have a common theme. They deal with the psychosocial aspects of care while option 1 deals with physiological and safety issues. In options 2, 3, and 4 also, the focus of the goal is the mother, whereas the focus of the goal in option 1 is the fetus. For both these reasons, option 1 is different from the others, making it the most likely choice as the correct answer.

Level of Cognitive Ability: Application
Phase of Nursing Process: Planning
Client Needs: Physiological Integrity
Content Area: Maternity

Reference

Lowdermilk, D., Perry, S., & Bobak, I. (1997). *Maternity & women's health care* (6th ed.). St. Louis: Mosby–Year Book. p. 776.

22. **4**

Rationale: DIC is a state of diffuse clotting in which clotting factors are consumed. This leads to widespread bleeding. Platelets are decreased because they are consumed by the process; coagulation studies show no clot formation (and are thus prolonged); and fibrin plugs may clog the microvasculature diffusely, rather than in an isolated area.

Test-Taking Strategy: Option 1 is eliminated first, based on the knowledge that DIC is a widespread problem, not a localized one. Options 2 and 3 contain a similar theme, and therefore by elimination the fourth option (because it is different) is the likely option. Review the signs related to DIC now, if you had difficulty with this question!

Level of Cognitive Ability: Analysis
Phase of Nursing Process: Assessment
Client Needs: Physiological Integrity
Content Area: Maternity

Reference

Lowdermilk, D., Perry, S., & Bobak, I. (1997). *Maternity & women's health care* (6th ed.). St. Louis: Mosby–Year Book. pp. 792–793.

23. **1**

Rationale: Anxiety is the key concept being tested in this question. Anxiety interferes with processing, learning about, and coping with the situation. Anxiety must be reduced before the woman can process, before significant others can support, and before learning can take place.

Test-Taking Strategy: Identify the key word. In this instance, the question asks for the first priority. The avoidance of anxiety is the key issue!

Level of Cognitive Ability: Analysis
Phase of Nursing Process: Planning
Client Needs: Psychosocial Integrity
Content Area: Maternity

Reference

Gorrie, T., McKinney, E. S., & Murray, S. S. (1998). *Foundations of maternal-newborn nursing* (2nd ed.). Philadelphia: W. B. Saunders. p. 685.

24. **1**

Rationale: The literature suggests that the highest incidence of abruptio placentae occurs in women who smoke, or who use alcohol, cocaine, and caffeine during pregnancy. Women who have had more than five pregnancies, who are of advanced age, and who do heavy physical labor are also at risk.

Test-Taking Strategy: Knowledge regarding the risk factors associated with abruptio placentae is required to answer this question. Use the process of elimination, however, and eliminate the options that are nonmodifiable risks as in options 3 and 4. Review the risk factors associated with abruptio placentae now, if you had difficulty with this question!

Level of Cognitive Ability: Application
Phase of Nursing Process: Planning
Client Needs: Health Promotion and Maintenance
Content Area: Maternity

Reference

Lowdermilk, D., Perry, S., & Bobak, I. (1997). *Maternity & women's health care* (6th ed.). St. Louis: Mosby–Year Book. pp. 778–780.

25. **1**

Rationale: With a client in shock, the nurse would want to increase perfusion to the placenta. A simple way, requiring no equipment, would be to turn the mother on her side. This would increase blood flow to the placenta by relieving pressure from the gravid uterus on the great vessels. The other options would follow quickly.

Test-Taking Strategy: This question requires the nurse to set a priority. In this question, note the phrase "A first-priority." Read each option carefully. The first action would be option 1, followed by both maternal and FHR monitoring.

Level of Cognitive Ability: Application
Phase of Nursing Process: Implementation
Client Needs: Physiological Integrity
Content Area: Maternity

Reference

Lowdermilk, D., Perry, S., & Bobak, I. (1997). *Maternity & women's health care* (6th ed.). St. Louis: Mosby–Year Book. pp. 788–792.

BIBLIOGRAPHY

Carpenito, L. (1997). *Handbook of nursing diagnosis* (7th ed.). Philadelphia: Lippincott-Raven.

Gorrie, T., McKinney, E. S., & Murray, S. S. (1998). *Foundations of maternal-newborn nursing* (2nd ed.). Philadelphia: W. B. Saunders.

Lowdermilk, D., Perry, S., & Bobak, I. (1997). *Maternity & women's health care* (6th ed.). St. Louis: Mosby–Year Book.

Nichols, F., & Zwelling, E. (1997). *Maternal-newborn nursing: Theory and practice*. Philadelphia: W. B. Saunders.

CHAPTER 28

The Postpartum Period

I. Postpartum

A. Description: Period when the reproductive tract returns to the normal, nonpregnant state

B. Postpartum Period: Starts immediately after **delivery** and is completed usually by Week 6 following delivery

II. Physiological Maternal Changes

A. Involution
   1. Description
      a. The rapid decrease in the size of the uterus as it returns to the nonpregnant state
      b. Clients who breast-feed may experience a more rapid involution
   2. Assessment
      a. Weight of the uterus decreases from 2 lb to 2 oz in 6 weeks
      b. Endometrium regenerates
      c. Fundus steadily descends into the pelvis
      d. Fundal height decreases about 1 fingerbreadth (1 cm) per day
      e. A flaccid fundus indicates uterine atony and should be massaged until firm
      f. A tender fundus indicates an infection
      g. By 10 days postpartum, uterus cannot be palpated abdominally

B. **Lochia**
   1. Description: discharge from the uterus that consists of blood from the vessels of the **placental** site and debris from the decidua
   2. Assessment
      a. Rubra: bright red discharge that occurs from **delivery** day to Day 3
      b. Serosa: Brownish-pink discharge that occurs from Days 4 to 10
      c. Alba: White discharge that occurs from Days 10 to 14
      d. Normally, the discharge has a fleshy odor
      e. Discharge decreases daily in amount
      f. Discharge increases with ambulation

C. Cervix: Cervical involution, and after 1 week the muscle begins to regenerate

D. Vagina: Vaginal distention decreases, although muscle tone is never restored completely to the pregravid state

E. Ovarian Function and Menstruation
   1. Ovarian function depends on the rapidity with which the pituitary function is restored
   2. Menstrual flow resumes within 8 weeks in nonbreast-feeding mothers
   3. Menstrual flow usually resumes within 3 to 4 months in breast-feeding mothers
   4. Breast-feeding mothers may experience amenorrhea during the entire period of lactation
   5. Woman may ovulate without menstruating, so breast-feeding should not be considered a form of birth control

F. Breasts
   1. Breasts continue to secrete colostrum
   2. A decrease of estrogen and progesterone levels after **delivery** stimulate increased prolactin levels, which promotes breast milk production
   3. Breasts become distended with milk on the third day
   4. Breast-feeding will relieve engorgement
   5. Engorgement occurs in 48 to 72 hours in nonbreast-feeding mothers

G. Urinary Tract
   1. May have urinary retention due to loss of elasticity and tone and loss of sensation in the bladder from trauma, medications, anesthesia, and lack of privacy
   2. Diuresis usually begins within first 12 hours after **delivery**

H. Gastrointestinal Tract
   1. Women are usually very hungry after **delivery**
   2. Constipation can occur
   3. Hemorrhoids are common

I. Vital Signs
   1. Temperature may be elevated during the first 24 hours due to dehydration
   2. Bradycardia is common during the first week, with a range of 50 to 70 beats per minute
   3. Blood pressure remains unchanged

III. Postpartum Implementation

A. Assessment
   1. Monitor vital signs
   2. Assess height, consistency, and location of the fundus
   3. Monitor color, amount, and odor of **lochia**
   4. Assess breasts for engorgement
   5. Monitor perineum for swelling or discoloration
   6. Monitor episiotomy for healing
   7. Assess incisions or dressings of cesarean birth client
   8. Monitor bowel status
   9. Monitor input and output (I&O)
   10. Encourage frequent voiding
   11. Encourage ambulation
   12. Administer RhoGam as prescribed within 72 hours postpartum to the Rh-negative client who is not sensitized
   13. Assess bonding with the newborn infant
   14. Assess emotional status
B. Client Teaching
   1. Initiate counseling client in discharge instructions
   2. Demonstrate newborn care skills as necessary
   3. Provide the opportunity for the mother to bathe the newborn infant
   4. Instruct on feeding technique
   5. Instruct mother to avoid heavy lifting for at least 3 weeks
   6. Instruct mother to plan at least one rest period per day
   7. Instruct mother that contraception should begin after **delivery** or with the initiation of coitus
   8. Instruct mother on the importance of follow-up, which should be scheduled at 4 to 6 weeks
   9. Instruct mother to report any signs of chills, fever, increased **lochia**, or depressed feelings to the physician immediately

IV. Postpartum Discomforts

A. Afterbirth Pains
   1. Occur due to contractions of the uterus
   2. Are more common in multiparas, breast-feeding mothers, clients treated with oxytocin (Pitocin), and clients who had an overdistended uterus during pregnancy
B. Perineal Discomfort
   1. Apply ice packs to the perineum during the first 24 hours to reduce swelling
   2. After the first 24 hours, apply warmth by sitz baths
C. Episiotomy
   1. Instruct client to administer perineal care after each voiding
   2. Encourage the use of an analgesic spray as prescribed

   3. Administer analgesic as prescribed if comfort measures are unsuccessful
D. Breast Discomfort from Engorgement
   1. Encourage wearing a support bra at all times, even while sleeping
   2. Encourage the use of ice packs if not breast-feeding
   3. Encourage the use of warm soaks before feeding for breast-feeding mother
   4. Administer analgesics as prescribed if comfort measures are unsuccessful
E. Postpartum Blues (Table 28–1)
   1. Condition is caused by physiological and emotional stress
   2. The mother may feel upset and depressed at times
   3. Verbalization should be encouraged
   4. Postpartum blues may progress to postpartum depression if unresolved

V. Nutritional Counseling

A. Discuss caloric intake for breast-feeding and nonbreast-feeding mothers
B. Nutritional needs depend on prepregnancy weight, ideal weight for height, and whether the mother is breast-feeding
C. If the mother is breast-feeding, calorie needs increase by approximately 500 calories per day, and the mother may require increased fluids and the continuance of prenatal vitamins and minerals

VI. Breast-Feeding

A. General Principles/Considerations
   1. Put baby to breast as soon as mother and baby's conditions are stable; on **delivery** table if possible
   2. Stay with the client each time she nurses until she feels secure or confident with the baby and her feelings

Table 28–1. Rubin's Postpartum Phases of Regeneration

Taking-In Phase: First 3 Days
Mother focuses on her own primary needs, such as sleep and food
Important for nurse to listen and help mother interpret the events of delivery to make them more meaningful
Not an optimum time to teach the mother about baby care

Taking Hold Phase: Days 3–10
More in control of independence
Begins to assume the tasks of mothering
An optimum time to teach the mother about baby care

Letting Go Phase
Mother may feel deep loss over separation of the baby from part of the body and may grieve over the loss
Mother may be caught in a dependent/independent role, wanting to feel safe and secure yet wanting to make decisions
Teenage mothers need special consideration because of the conflict taking place within them as part of adolescence

3. Uterine cramping may occur the first day after **delivery** while nursing, when oxytocin simulation causes the uterus to contract
4. Use general hygiene and wash the breasts once daily
5. Do not use soap as it tends to remove natural oils, which increases the chances of cracking
6. Bra should be well fitted and supporting
7. Breasts may leak between feedings or during coitus; place breast pad in bra
8. Calories should be increased by 500 per day, and the diet should include additional fluids; prenatal vitamins should be taken as prescribed
9. Baby's stools will be light yellow, watery, and frequent
10. Medications should be avoided unless prescribed
11. Gas-producing foods and caffeine should be avoided
12. Birth control pills should not be taken
13. Baby will develop her or his own feeding schedule

B. Breast-feeding Procedure for Mother
   1. Wash hands and assume comfortable position
   2. Start with the breast that the last feeding ended with
   3. Brush newborn infant's lower lip with nipple
   4. Tickle lips to have baby open mouth wide
   5. Guide nipple and surrounding areola into baby's mouth
   6. After baby has nursed, release suction by depressing the newborn infant's chin or inserting a clean finger into the baby's mouth
   7. Burp baby after first breast
   8. Repeat procedure on the second breast until the baby stops nursing
   9. Burp baby again
   10. Instruct mother to listen for audible sucking and swallowing

C. Engorgement
   1. Breast-feed frequently
   2. Apply warm packs before feeding
   3. Apply ice packs between feedings

D. Cracked Nipples
   1. Expose nipples to air for 10 to 20 minutes after feeding
   2. Rotate position of the baby for each feeding

PRACTICE QUESTIONS

1. A postpartum client who delivered at 32 weeks' gestation wishes to breast-feed her preterm infant. At this point the infant is on gavage feedings only. What is the nurse's best response to the mother?
   1 "There is no need to prepare for breast-feeding at this point since the infant is on gavage feedings."
   2 "You can prepare your breast by pinching and rolling the nipples and hand-expressing colostrum."
   3 "You can begin pumping as soon as possible after delivery with an electric breast pump."
   4 "You need to pump every 6 hours to establish a good milk supply."

2. The hospital experience strongly influences the process of breast-feeding. Which one of the following factors is the most significant in teaching a client to breast-feed?
   1 Brief separation of infant and mother after birth to allow the mother to rest
   2 A client with previous breast-feeding experience
   3 A physician who encourages clients to breast-feed
   4 A positive nurse-client relationship

3. The nurse palpates the fundus and notes the character of the lochia in the fourth stage of labor. The expected finding during this stage is:
   1 White
   2 Pink
   3 Serosanguineous
   4 Dark red

4. Following episiotomy and delivery of a newborn infant, the nurse performs a perineal assessment on the mother. The nurse notes a trickle of bright red blood coming from the perineum. The nurse assesses the fundus and notes that it is firm. The nurse determines that:
   1 This is a normal expectation following episiotomy
   2 The perineal assessment should be performed more frequently
   3 The bright red bleeding is abnormal and should be reported
   4 The mother should be allowed bathroom privileges only

5. During the postpartum period, a client asks the nurse what the term involution means. The nurse's response is based on which of the following?
   1 Involution is a progressive descent of the uterus into the pelvic cavity, occurring approximately 1 cm per day
   2 Involution refers to the gradual reversal of the uterine muscle into the abdominal cavity
   3 Involution refers to the descent of the uterus into the pelvic cavity, occurring at a rate of 2 cm daily
   4 Involution refers to the inverted uterus that is beginning to return to normal

6. The client is breast-feeding her newborn infant. She complains to the nurse that she is experiencing nipple soreness. Which of the following suggestions would the nurse provide to the client?

1 Avoid rotating breast-feeding positions so that the nipple will toughen

2 Stop nursing during the period of nipple soreness to allow the nipples to heal

3 Nurse the baby less frequently and substitute a bottle feeding until the nipples become less sore

4 Position the infant with the ear, shoulder, and hip in straight alignment and with the baby's stomach against the mother's

7. The mother is breast-feeding her newborn baby and experiences breast engorgement. Which of the following measures will provide comfort for the engorgement?

1 Encouraging the mother to breast-feed only during the daytime hours

2 Encouraging the mother to apply cold compresses to the breasts

3 Encouraging the mother to massage the breasts before feeding to stimulate let-down

4 Encouraging the mother to avoid the use of a bra while the breasts are engorged

8. The nurse develops a plan of care for the client in the fourth stage of labor. Which of the following nursing diagnoses would be most appropriate for this stage?

1 Pain related to the process of labor or birth

2 Anxiety related to childbirth

3 Fatigue related to physical exertion during labor

4 Urinary retention related to loss of sensation to void and rapid bladder filling

9. Following delivery, the nurse assesses the uterine fundus. The position of the fundus would most likely be noted:

1 At the level of the umbilicus

2 Above the level of the umbilicus

3 One fingerbreadth above the symphysis pubis

4 To the right of the abdomen

10. Four hours postpartum, the client's temperature is 101°F. The most appropriate nursing action is:

1 Continue to monitor the temperature

2 Notify the physician

3 Apply cool packs to the abdomen

4 Remove the blanket from the client's bed

ANSWERS

1. **3**

Rationale: Prematurity usually causes a delay before the baby can be fed at the breast. Mothers must initiate and maintain their milk supply with an electric breast pump.

Test-Taking Strategy: Option 1 is incorrect. Milk expression by electric pump needs to begin as soon as possible after delivery and continue eight or more times each 24 hours. This explains why option 4 is incorrect, because four times a day is less than the eight or more times recommended. Hand-expression is not as effective as using an electric pump, so option 2 is incorrect. Review the concepts related to breast-feeding now, if you had difficulty with this question!

Level of Cognitive Ability: Application
Phase of Nursing Process: Implementation
Client Needs: Psychosocial Integrity
Content Area: Maternity

Reference
Nichols, F., & Zwelling, E. (1997). *Maternal-newborn nursing: Theory and practice.* Philadelphia: W. B. Saunders. pp. 1238–1239.

2. **4**

Rationale: Because hospital stays are short, all contacts with the mother become teachable moments. The nurse-client relationship becomes a growth-fostering experience so that the mother feels confident in her ability to breast-feed. Brief separation decreases the chance of correct latch and suck in the immediate postpartum period. Infants should be placed at the breast immediately after delivery. Uninterrupted contact after birth decreases crying and startling in neonates, reduces BP, and stabilizes temperature and respirations faster than when the infant is left alone in a bassinet.

Test-Taking Strategy: Use the process of elimination when answering the question. Noting the key words "most significant" will assist in directing you to option 4. The most significant factor is a positive nurse-client relationship.

Level of Cognitive Ability: Analysis
Phase of Nursing Process: Planning
Client Needs: Health Promotion and Maintenance
Content Area: Maternity

Reference
Nichols, F., & Zwelling, E. (1997). *Maternal-newborn nursing: Theory and practice.* Philadelphia: W. B. Saunders. pp. 1238–1239.

3. **4**

Rationale: In assessment of the perineum, the lochia is assessed for amount, color, and the presence of clots. The color of the lochia during the fourth stage of labor is dark red.

Test-Taking Strategy: Knowledge regarding the color, amount, and consistency of lochia following delivery is required to answer the question. Note that the question refers to the fourth stage of labor. This is a key phrase to indicate that option 4 is the correct option. Review perineal assessments now, if you had difficulty with this question!

Level of Cognitive Ability: Analysis
Phase of Nursing Process: Assessment
Client Needs: Physiological Integrity
Content Area: Maternity

Reference
Nichols, F., & Zwelling, E. (1997). *Maternal-newborn nursing: Theory and practice.* Philadelphia: W. B. Saunders. p. 768.

4. **3**

Rationale: Lochial flow should be distinguished from bleeding originating from a laceration or episiotomy, which is usually brighter red than lochia and presents as a continuous trickle of bleeding even though the fundus of the uterus is firm. This bright red bleeding is abnormal and needs to be reported.

Test-Taking Strategy: Knowledge regarding lochial flow and complications associated with episiotomy are required to answer the question. The key phrase in the question is "bright red." This should be an indication that the flow is not normal. Review lochial flow and complications associated with episiotomy now, if you had difficulty with this question!

Level of Cognitive Ability: Analysis
Phase of Nursing Process: Assessment
Client Needs: Physiological Integrity
Content Area: Maternity

Reference
Nichols, F., & Zwelling, E. (1997). *Maternal-newborn nursing: Theory and practice.* Philadelphia: W. B. Saunders. p. 768.

5. **1**

Rationale: Involution is a progressive descent of the uterus into the pelvic cavity. After birth, descent occurs approximately 1 fingerbreadth, or approximately 1 cm, per day.

Test-Taking Strategy: Knowledge regarding the definition and process of involution is required to answer this question. Use medical terminology to assist you in defining the term and selecting the correct option. If you had difficulty with this question, take time now to review the term involution!

Level of Cognitive Ability: Analysis
Phase of Nursing Process: Analysis
Client Needs: Physiological Integrity
Content Area: Maternity

Reference
Luckmann, J. (1997). *Saunders manual of nursing care.* Philadelphia: W. B. Saunders. p. 462.

6. **4**

Rationale: Comfort measures for nipple soreness include positioning the newborn infant with the ear, shoulder, and hip in straight alignment and with the baby's stomach against the mother's; rotating breast-feeding positions; breaking suction with the little finger; nursing frequently; beginning feeding on the less sore nipple; not allowing the infant to chew on the nipple or to sleep holding the nipple in the mouth; and applying teabags soaked in warm water to the nipple.

Test-Taking Strategy: Use the process of elimination to answer the question. Knowledge regarding the self-care measures to promote comfort to the mother with nipple soreness is required to answer the question. If you had difficulty answering the question, take time now to review these measures!

Level of Cognitive Ability: Application
Phase of Nursing Process: Implementation
Client Needs: Health Promotion and Maintenance
Content Area: Maternity

Reference
Luckmann, J. (1997). *Saunders manual of nursing care.* Philadelphia: W. B. Saunders. p. 463.

7. **3**

Rationale: Comfort measures for breast engorgement include massaging the breasts before feeding to stimulate letdown; wearing a supportive, well-fitting bra at all times; taking a warm shower just before feeding or applying warm compresses; alternating breasts during feeding.

Test-Taking Strategy: Use the process of elimination to answer the question. Knowledge regarding the self-care measures to promote comfort to the mother with breast engorgement is required to answer the question. If you had difficulty answering the question, take time now to review these measures!

Level of Cognitive Ability: Application
Phase of Nursing Process: Implementation
Client Needs: Health Promotion and Maintenance
Content Area: Maternity

Reference
Luckmann, J. (1997). *Saunders manual of nursing care.* Philadelphia: W. B. Saunders. p. 463.

8. **4**

Rationale: The fourth stage of labor is composed of the first hour postpartum when the woman's body begins to readjust and relax. Options 1 and 2 relate to the first stage of labor. Option 3 relates to the second stage of labor. Option 4, the correct answer, is related to the third and fourth stages of labor.

Test-Taking Strategy: Recalling the stages of labor and the processes that occur will assist you in answering the question. Remembering that the fourth stage of labor is the last stage will direct you toward the correct option. Review the stages of labor now, if you had difficulty with this question!

Level of Cognitive Ability: Analysis
Phase of Nursing Process: Planning
Client Needs: Physiological Integrity
Content Area: Maternity

Reference
Nichols, F., & Zwelling, E. (1997). *Maternal-newborn nursing: Theory and practice.* Philadelphia: W. B. Saunders. p. 769.

9. **1**

Rationale: Immediately after delivery, the uterine fundus should be at the level of the umbilicus or 1 to 3 fingerbreadths below it and in the midline of the abdomen. If the fundus is above the umbilicus, this may indicate that there are blood clots in the uterus that need to be expelled by fundal massage.

Test-Taking Strategy: Knowledge regarding normal postdelivery assessment findings in the mother is required to answer this question. Knowledge regarding normal anatomy will assist in directing you to the correct option. If you had difficulty with this question, take time now to review postdelivery assessment findings!

Level of Cognitive Ability: Analysis
Phase of Nursing Process: Assessment
Client Needs: Physiological Integrity
Content Area: Maternity

Reference
Nichols, F., & Zwelling, E. (1997). *Maternal-newborn nursing: Theory and practice.* Philadelphia: W. B. Saunders. p. 768.

10. **2**

Rationale: Vital signs return to normal within the first hour postpartum if no complications arise. If the temperature is greater than 2°F above normal, this may indicate infection and the physician should be notified.

Test-Taking Strategy: Knowledge regarding the expected vital signs following delivery is required to answer this question. Use the process of elimination to select the correct answer. It is most appropriate in this situation to notify the physician, as a temperature of 101°F can indicate infection.

Level of Cognitive Ability: Analysis
Phase of Nursing Process: Implementation
Client Needs: Physiological Integrity
Content Area: Maternity

Reference
Nichols, F., & Zwelling, E. (1997). *Maternal-newborn nursing: Theory and practice.* Philadelphia: W. B. Saunders. p. 767.

BIBLIOGRAPHY

Ashwill, J., & Droske, S. (1997). *Nursing care of children: Principles and practice.* Philadelphia: W. B. Saunders.

Carpenito, L. (1997). *Handbook of nursing diagnosis* (7th ed.). Philadelphia: Lippincott-Raven.

Lowdermilk, D., Perry, S., & Bobak, I. (1997). *Maternity & women's health care* (6th ed.). St. Louis: Mosby–Year Book.

Luckmann, J. (1997). *Saunders manual of nursing care.* Philadelphia: W. B. Saunders.

Nichols, F., & Zwelling, E. (1997). *Maternal-newborn nursing: Theory and practice.* Philadelphia: W. B. Saunders.

CHAPTER 29

Postpartum Complications

I. Cystitis

A. Description: An infection of the bladder
B. Assessment
   1. Burning and pain on urination
   2. Lower abdominal pain
   3. Increased frequency of urination
   4. Costovertebral angle tenderness
   5. Fever
   6. Proteinuria, hematuria, bacteriuria, WBCs in urine
C. Implementation
   1. Palpate bladder for distention
   2. Palpate fundus
   3. Obtain urine specimen for culture and sensitivity if prescribed
   4. Institute measures to assist the client to void
   5. Encourage frequent and complete emptying of the bladder
   6. Force fluids to 3000 mL per day
   7. Administer antibiotics as prescribed after the urine culture is obtained
   8. Instruct client in the methods of prevention and treatment of cystitis

II. Hematoma

A. Description
   1. The formation of a hematoma occurs following the escape of blood into the tissues of the reproductive sac after the **delivery**
   2. Predisposing conditions include operative **delivery** with forceps or injury to a blood vessel
   3. Can be a life-threatening condition
B. Assessment
   1. Abnormal severe pain
   2. Pressure in perineal area
   3. Sensitive tumor in perineal area with discolored skin
   4. Inability to void
   5. Palpable tumor
   6. Decreased hematocrit and hemoglobin (H&H)
   7. Signs of shock, such as pallor; tachycardia; and hypotension if significant blood loss has occurred
C. Implementation
   1. Monitor vital signs
   2. Monitor client for abnormal pain, especially when forceps **delivery** has occurred
   3. Place ice to the hematoma site
   4. Administer analgesics as prescribed
   5. Monitor intake and output (I&O)
   6. Encourage fluids
   7. Encourage voiding
   8. Prepare for urinary catheterization if client is unable to void
   9. Administer blood replacements as prescribed
   10. Monitor for signs of infection, such as increased temperature, pulse rate, and WBC count
   11. Administer antibiotics as prescribed, as infection is common following hematoma formation
   12. Prepare for incision and evacuation of hematoma if necessary

III. Hemorrhage

A. Description: Bleeding of 500 mL or more following **delivery**
B. Assessment
   1. Early
      a. Hemorrhage occurs during first 24 hours after **delivery**
      b. Caused by uterine atony, lacerations, or inversion of uterus
   2. Late
      a. Hemorrhage occurs after the first 24 hours following **delivery**
      b. Caused by retained **placental** fragments
C. Implementation
   1. Monitor vital signs and fundus every 5 to 15 minutes
   2. Remain with client
   3. Assess and estimate blood loss by pad count

4. Massage fundus, with care not to overmassage
5. Notify physician or health care provider if hemorrhage occurs
6. Assess level of consciousness
7. Monitor I&O
8. Monitor fluid replacement
9. Monitor hemoglobin and hematocrit
10. Maintain asepsis since hemorrhage predisposes to infection
11. Prepare for the administration of oxytocin if prescribed
12. Prepare for the administration of blood transfusions if prescribed

IV. Infection

A. Description: Any infection of the reproductive organs that occurs within 28 days of **delivery** or abortion
B. Assessment
  1. Fever
  2. Chills
  3. Anorexia
  4. Pelvic discomfort or pain
  5. Vaginal discharge
  6. Elevated WBC count
C. Implementation
  1. Monitor vital signs and temperature every 2 to 4 hours
  2. Make client as comfortable as possible, and position for comfort and to promote drainage
  3. Keep mother warmed if chilled
  4. Isolate baby from mother only if mother is infected
  5. Provide nutritious, high-caloric, protein diet
  6. Monitor I&O
  7. Force fluids of 3000 to 4000 mL, if not contraindicated
  8. Encourage frequent voiding
  9. Monitor culture results if cultures were prescribed
  10. Administer antibiotics according to organism, as prescribed

V. Mastitis

A. Description
  1. Inflammation of the breast as a result of infection
  2. Primarily seen in breast-feeding mothers 2 to 3 weeks after **delivery**
B. Assessment
  1. Localized heat and swelling
  2. Pain
  3. Elevated temperature
  4. Complaints of flulike symptoms
C. Implementation
  1. Promote comfort of the client
  2. Instruct mother in good handwashing and breast hygiene techniques
  3. Apply heat or cold to site as prescribed

4. Maintain lactation in breast-feeding mothers
5. Encourage manual expression of breast milk or use of breast pump every 4 hours
6. Encourage mother to support breasts with supportive bra
7. Administer analgesics as prescribed
8. Administer antibiotics as prescribed

VI. Pulmonary Embolism

A. Description: The passage of thrombus, often originating in one of the uterine or other pelvic veins, into the lungs, where it disrupts the circulation of blood
B. Assessment
  1. Dyspnea
  2. Tachypnea
  3. Cough
  4. Tachycardia
  5. Rales
  6. Hemoptysis
  7. Pleuritic chest pain
  8. Feeling of impending doom
C. Implementation
  1. Administer oxygen as prescribed
  2. Position client with the head of the bed elevated to promote comfort
  3. Monitor vital signs frequently
  4. Frequently assess respiratory rate and breath sounds, and for signs of increasing hypoxemia
  5. Monitor for signs of respiratory distress, such as tachypnea, tachycardia, restlessness, cool and clammy skin, cyanosis, and the use of accessory muscles
  6. Increase IV fluids as prescribed
  7. Administer anticoagulants as prescribed
  8. Prepare to assist physician to administer streptokinase to dissolve the clot if prescribed

VII. Subinvolution

A. Description: Incomplete involution or failure of the uterus to return to its normal size and condition
B. Assessment
  1. Uterine pain on palpation
  2. Uterus is larger than expected
  3. Greater than normal vaginal bleeding
C. Implementation
  1. Assess vital signs
  2. Assess uterus and fundus
  3. Monitor for vaginal bleeding
  4. Elevate the legs to promote venous return
  5. Encourage frequent voiding
  6. Monitor H&H
  7. Prepare to administer methylergonovine maleate (Methergine) or ergonovine maleate (Ergotrate) as prescribed

VIII. Thrombophlebitis

A. Description

Table 29–1. **Assessment of the Types of Thrombophlebitis**

Superficial	*Femoral*	*Pelvic*
Tenderness and pain in the affected lower extremity	Chills and fever	Severe chills
Warm and pinkish-red color over thrombus area	Malaise	Dramatic body temperature changes
Palpable thrombus that feels bumpy and hard	Pain, stiffness, and swelling of the affected leg	Occurrence of pulmonary embolism may be first sign
Slightly elevated pulse rate	Shiny, white skin over the affected area	
	Positive Homan's sign	
	Diminished peripheral pulses	

    1. A condition in which a clot forms in a vessel wall secondary to the inflammation of a vessel wall
    2. A partial obstruction of the vessel can occur
    3. Increased blood-clotting factors in the postpartum period place the client at risk
B. Types
    1. Superficial thrombophlebitis
    2. Femoral thrombophlebitis
    3. Pelvic thrombophlebitis
C. Assessment (Table 29–1)
    1. Superficial
      a. Tenderness and pain in the affected lower extremity
      b. Warm and pinkish-red color over thrombus area
      c. Palpable thrombus that feels bumpy and hard
      d. Slightly elevated pulse rate
    2. Femoral
      a. Chills and fever
      b. Malaise
      c. Pain, stiffness, and swelling of the affected leg
      d. Shiny, white skin over the affected area
      e. Positive Homan's sign (indicates deep vein thrombosis)
      f. Diminished peripheral pulses
    3. Pelvic
      a. Severe chills
      b. Dramatic body temperature changes
      c. The occurrence of pulmonary embolism may be the first sign
D. Implementation
    1. Assess lower extremities for edema, tenderness, varices, and increased skin temperature
    2. Evaluate legs for Homan's sign by extending the legs with the knees slightly flexed and dorsiflexing the foot
    3. Maintain bed rest
    4. Elevate the affected leg
    5. Apply a bed cradle and keep bedclothes off affected leg
    6. Never massage the leg
    7. Monitor for manifestations of pulmonary embolism
    8. Superficial thrombosis
      a. Provide rest
      b. Apply hot packs to the affected site as prescribed

      c. Apply elastic stockings
      d. Administer analgesics as prescribed
    9. Femoral thrombophlebitis
      a. Provide bed rest
      b. Elevate affected leg
      c. Apply moist heat continuously to affected area if prescribed to alleviate discomfort
      d. Administer analgesics as prescribed
      e. Administer antibiotics if prescribed
      f. Prepare to administer intravenous heparin to prevent further thrombus formation if prescribed
    10. Pelvic thrombophlebitis
      a. Provide bed rest
      b. Administer analgesics as prescribed
      c. Administer antibiotics if prescribed
      d. Prepare to administer intravenous heparin
E. Client Education (Box 29–1)

PRACTICE QUESTIONS

1. An indicator of a hematoma in a postpartum woman who has received epidural anesthesia is best identified by which of the following?
  1 Complaints of a tearing sensation
  2 Complaints of intense pressure
  3 Changes in vital signs
  4 Signs of heavy bruising

2. In planning care for the postpartum woman with small vulvar hematomas, the nurse plans to:
  1 Assess vital signs every 4 hours
  2 Inform the care provider of assessment findings
  3 Measure fundal height every 4 hours
  4 Prepare an ice pack for application to the area

BOX 29–1. Client Education for Thrombophlebitis

- Avoid pressure behind the knees
- Avoid prolonged sitting
- Avoid constrictive clothing
- Avoid crossing the legs
- Never massage the leg
- Know how to apply support hose if prescribed
- Understand the importance of anticoagulant therapy as prescribed
- Understand the importance of follow-up with the health care provider

3. The new mother received epidural anesthesia during labor and had a forceps delivery after pushing for 2 hours. At 6 hours postpartum, her systolic blood pressure has dropped 20 points, her diastolic blood pressure has dropped 10 points, and her pulse is 120. The client is very anxious and restless. Upon further assessment, a vulvar hematoma is verified. After notifying the care provider, the delivery nurse should plan to:
   1 Monitor fundal height
   2 Apply perineal pressure
   3 Prepare the client for surgery
   4 Reassure the client

4. After surgical evacuation and repair of a paravaginal hematoma, the 3-day postpartum mother is discharged. The nurse knows that the new mother needs further discharge instructions when the new mother states:
   1 "Because I am so sore, I will nurse the baby while lying on my side."
   2 "I will probably need my mother to help me with housekeeping."
   3 "My husband and I will not have intercourse until the stitches are healed."
   4 "The only medications I will take are prenatal vitamins and stool softeners."

5. A 45-year-old woman delivered her first baby by cesarean section 5 days ago. The postpartum recovery has been complicated by thrombophlebitis in her left leg. She cries frequently and requests to have her newborn infant stay in the nursery. The nurse analyzes that the mother may have intensified postpartum "blues" because:
   1 She is an older first-time mother
   2 She is considering giving the baby up for adoption
   3 She is required to stay on bed rest
   4 She is unable to nurse the baby

6. To prevent thrombophlebitis, the nurse should encourage the woman recovering from cesarean delivery to:
   1 Ambulate frequently
   2 Apply warm, moist packs to the legs
   3 Remain on bed rest with legs elevated
   4 Wear support stockings

7. A postpartum client has developed thrombophlebitis. The nurse knows that the affected extremity should be elevated 8 inches above the level of the heart by:
   1 Elevating the affected extremity on a pillow
   2 Elevating the foot of the bed
   3 Placing the bed in reverse Trendelenburg position
   4 Placing the bed in Trendelenburg position

8. The postpartum client is being treated for thrombophlebitis. The nurse knows that the client's response to treatment will be evaluated by regularly assessing the client for:
   1 Dysuria
   2 Epistaxis, hematuria, and dysuria
   3 Hematuria, ecchymosis, and epistaxis
   4 Hematuria, ecchymosis, and vertigo

9. A postpartum client who has had complications of thrombophlebitis suddenly complains of chest pain and dyspnea. Prior to informing the care provider, the nurse should assess the client's:
   1 Level of consciousness
   2 Fundal height
   3 Homan's sign
   4 Vital signs

10. A nursing goal for the postpartum client with thromboembolic disease is to prevent the complication of pulmonary embolism. In planning care to assist in meeting this goal, the nurse should:
    1 Administer and monitor anticoagulant therapy
    2 Assess breath sounds frequently
    3 Enforce strict bed rest
    4 Monitor vital signs frequently

11. The nurse suspects the client has a pulmonary embolism. The most important anticipated action is to:
    1 Administer oxygen by face mask as prescribed at 8 to 10 liters/minute
    2 Elevate the head of the bed to 30 to 45 degrees
    3 Initiate an IV line if one is not already in place
    4 Monitor vital signs frequently

12. The postpartum client with a pulmonary embolism is returning to the maternity unit after being in ICU for 3 days. Which evaluation by the nurse shows the need for further nursing intervention?
    1 The client nurses her newborn infant in the side-lying position
    2 The client needs the head of the bed elevated for comfort
    3 The newborn baby prefers the bottle over breast milk
    4 The client turns herself from side to side

13. The nurse assesses that the 4-hour postpartum client has cool, clammy skin and is restless and excessively thirsty. The nurse should:
    1 Assess for hypovolemia and notify the health care provider
    2 Assess vital signs and begin hourly pad counts
    3 Begin fundal massage and start oxygen by mask
    4 Elevate the head of the bed and assess vital signs

14. The client is experiencing uterine hemorrhage. In planning care for the client, the nurse should:
    1 Keep the woman and her family members informed of her condition
    2 Monitor vital signs every 2 hours

3 Notify the health care provider if cramping occurs

4 Perform firm fundal massage every 2 hours

15. The nurse is caring for a woman who is gravida 6. In anticipation of this delivery, the nurse should:
    1 Begin fundal massage
    2 Ensure that medications that facilitate uterine contractions are available
    3 Initiate a large-bore IV access
    4 Verify that a blood sample has been sent for cross-match

16. The postpartum client has lost 700 mL of blood, and the vital signs indicate hypovolemia. Because the uterus remains atonic in spite of interventions, the nurse should:
    1 Administer blood products
    2 Administer oxytocin (Pitocin)
    3 Prepare for emergency surgery
    4 Perform fundal massage

17. The new mother attempting breast-feeding for the first time has developed mastitis. She is discouraged and states that she fears she will transmit the infection to the baby. She considers discontinuing breast-feeding. A priority nursing diagnosis for this client is:
    1 Alteration in Body Image, related to inflammation and engorgement
    2 Alteration in Newborn Nutrition, related to decreased milk quality
    3 Alteration in Self-Concept, related to inability to breast-feed

4 Potential for Injury to the newborn, related to maternal transmission of infection

18. Breast-feeding instructions for the postpartum mother should include avoidance of soaps on the nipples, frequent changing of breast pads, intermittent exposure of nipples to air, and handwashing before handling breasts and before breast-feeding. These measures are specific to the prevention of:
    1 Engorgement
    2 Newborn colic
    3 "Let-down" reflex
    4 Mastitis

19. The nurse is caring for the woman who is being treated with antibiotics for mastitis. Teaching should include the importance of:
    1 Continuation of breast-feeding
    2 Completion of entire antibiotic regimen
    3 Wearing a supportive bra
    4 Applying heat packs to promote circulation

20. The new breast-feeding mother is being discharged from the hospital after being treated for mastitis. The nurse knows that she needs further teaching when the mother states:
    1 "I need to change my breast pads when they are wet."
    2 "I will wash my breasts gently with plain water."
    3 "My left breast is sore, so I will offer the right breast frequently for breast feeding."
    4 "When my breasts feel engorged, I will use an ice pack for the pain."

ANSWERS

1. **3**

Rationale: Changes in vital signs indicate hypovolemia in the anesthetized postpartum woman with vulvar hematoma.

Test-Taking Strategy: Because the woman is anesthetized, she cannot feel pain or pressure. Therefore, option 3 is correct. Option 4 (heavy bruising) may be visualized, but vital sign changes indicate hematoma caused by blood collection in the perineal tissues. Utilize the ABCs in selecting an option!

Level of Cognitive Ability: Analysis
Phase of Nursing Process: Analysis
Client Needs: Physiological Integrity
Content Area: Maternity

Reference
Nichols, F., & Zwelling, E. (1997). *Maternal-newborn nursing: Theory and practice.* Philadelphia: W. B. Saunders. p. 1287.

2. **4**

Rationale: Application of ice will reduce swelling caused by hematoma formation in the vulvar area.

Test-Taking Strategy: This question specifically asks about the planning phase of the nursing process. Option 4 is correct because it speaks to the plan of care. The other interventions are not specific to the woman with the complication of hematoma. Review nursing care to the client with a hematoma now, if you had difficulty with this question!

Level of Cognitive Ability: Application
Phase of Nursing Process: Planning
Client Needs: Physiological Integrity
Content Area: Maternity

Reference
Nichols, F., & Zwelling, E. (1997). *Maternal-newborn nursing: Theory and practice.* Philadelphia: W. B. Saunders. p. 1288.

3. **3**

Rationale: Epidural anesthesia, a prolonged second stage, and forceps delivery are predisposing factors for hematoma formation, with collection of up to 500 mL of blood in the vaginal area. Surgery to stop the bleeding is indicated for this severe complication.

Test-Taking Strategy: Knowledge of predisposing factors for hematoma is necessary to analyze that this emergency situation requires immediate surgery to stop the bleeding. In this case, option 3 is correct because it is the answer that provides the most global response. Review nursing content related to vulvar hematomas now, if you had difficulty with this question!

Level of Cognitive Ability: Application
Phase of Nursing Process: Planning
Client Needs: Physiological Integrity
Content Area: Maternity

Reference
Nichols, F., & Zwelling, E. (1997). *Maternal-newborn nursing: Theory and practice.* Philadelphia: W. B. Saunders. p. 1288.

4. **4**

Rationale: The postoperative client will need an antibiotic because she is at increased risk for infection due to the break in skin integrity and collection of blood at the hematoma site.

Test-Taking Strategy: Knowledge of the need for an antibiotic in this high-risk situation is necessary in eliminating the client responses that need no further instruction. Option 4 shows that the client needs further instruction about her medication. Read the stem of the question carefully. Use the process of elimination in answering the question. Review treatment plans associated with hematoma now, if you had difficulty with this question!

Level of Cognitive Ability: Analysis
Phase of Nursing Process: Evaluation
Client Needs: Health Promotion and Maintenance
Content Area: Maternity

Reference
Nichols, F., & Zwelling, E. (1997). *Maternal-newborn nursing: Theory and practice.* Philadelphia: W. B. Saunders. p. 1288.

5. **3**

Rationale: Clients with thrombophlebitis are placed on bed rest with elevation of the affected extremity. Bed rest restricts normal neonatal care, feeding, and parenting and will require interventions that promote attachment.

Test-Taking Strategy: Read the question carefully. Option 3, bed rest, is the only correct answer because the other options are unfounded assumptions about the client's situation. Avoid reading into the question. Review interventions related to thrombophlebitis now, if you had difficulty answering this question!

Level of Cognitive Ability: Analysis
Phase of Nursing Process: Analysis
Client Needs: Psychosocial Integrity
Content Area: Maternity

Reference
Nichols, F., & Zwelling, E. (1997). *Maternal-newborn nursing: Theory and practice.* Philadelphia: W. B. Saunders. p. 1293.

6. **1**

Rationale: Stasis is believed to be the strongest single predisposing factor in the development of thrombophlebitis. Because cesarean delivery is a risk factor, new mothers should ambulate early and frequently to promote circulation and prevent stasis.

Test-Taking Strategy: The question asks about the prevention of thrombophlebitis. Ambulating frequently (option 1) is correct whereas options 2, 3, and 4 should be planned for the client who has been diagnosed with thrombophlebitis. Read the question carefully. Review content related to the prevention of thrombophlebitis in the postoperative period now, if you had difficulty with this question!

Level of Cognitive Ability: Application
Phase of Nursing Process: Implementation
Client Needs: Health Promotion and Maintenance
Content Area: Maternity

Reference
Nichols, F., & Zwelling, E. (1997). *Maternal-newborn nursing: Theory and practice.* Philadelphia: W. B. Saunders. p. 1291.

7. **4**

Rationale: Placing the bed in Trendelenburg position (option 4) rather than flexing the leg at the hip promotes venous drainage.

Test-Taking Strategy: The test-taker should have knowledge of the different bed positions to answer this question correctly. Trendelenburg position (option 4) promotes venous drainage. Elevating the extremity by using a pillow (option 1) or elevating the foot of the bed (option 2) will cause flexion at the hip, thus impeding venous drainage. Option 3 does not promote venous drainage. Review these concepts now, if you had difficulty answering this question!

Level of Cognitive Ability: Application
Phase of Nursing Process: Implementation
Client Needs: Physiological Integrity
Content Area: Maternity

Reference
Nichols, F., & Zwelling, E. (1997). *Maternal-newborn nursing: Theory and practice.* Philadelphia: W. B. Saunders. p. 1292.

8. **3**

Rationale: The treatment for thrombophlebitis is anticoagulant therapy. The nurse is responsible for assessing for the adverse effects of anticoagulants, which include hematuria, ecchymosis, and epistaxis. All symptoms are a result of excess bleeding caused by heparin or anticoagulation overdosage.

Test-Taking Strategy: Be careful in answering questions in which several options are similar in content. It is important to know the signs of excess bleeding in answering this question about the client being treated for thrombophlebitis. It is important to know that thrombophlebitis is treated with anticoagulation therapy. Also, note that option 3 is the only option that addresses bleeding in all its components. Also note that option 1 is also a component of option 2; therefore, eliminate both these options.

Level of Cognitive Ability: Analysis
Phase of Nursing Process: Evaluation
Client Needs: Physiological Integrity
Content Area: Maternity

Reference
Nichols, F., & Zwelling, E. (1997). *Maternal newborn nursing: Theory and practice.* Philadelphia: W. B. Saunders. p. 1293.

9. **4**

Rationale: In many cases thrombophlebitis precedes pulmonary embolism, which is heralded by the symptom of dyspnea. Option 4, vital signs, will be one of the first changes to occur with pulmonary embolism as pulmonary blood flow is compromised.

Test-Taking Strategy: Fundal height (option 2) and Homan's sign (option 3) are not priority assessments at this time. Level of consciousness (option 1) may be affected in pulmonary embolism, but vital sign changes will be detected before the other choices. Remember ABCs!

Level of Cognitive Ability: Analysis
Phase of Nursing Process: Analysis
Client Needs: Physiological Integrity
Content Area: Maternity

Reference
Nichols, F., & Zwelling, E. (1997). *Maternal-newborn nursing: Theory and practice.* Philadelphia: W. B. Saunders. p. 1294.

10. **1**

Rationale: The purpose of anticoagulant therapy is to prevent the clot from moving to another area. Option 1 is the correct choice for preventing pulmonary embolism.

Test-Taking Strategy: Anticoagulant therapy is the only intervention listed that will prevent the clot from traveling to the pulmonary circulation. The question speaks to prevention. Anticoagulant therapy is the only choice that will prevent the complication of pulmonary embolism.

Level of Cognitive Ability: Application
Phase of Nursing Process: Planning
Client Needs: Physiological Integrity
Content Area: Maternity

Reference
Nichols, F., & Zwelling, E. (1997). *Maternal-newborn nursing: Theory and practice.* Philadelphia: W. B. Saunders. p. 1295.

11. **1**

Rationale: Because pulmonary circulation is compromised in the presence of an embolus, cardiorespiratory support is initiated by oxygen administration.

Test-Taking Strategy: Remember the ABCs of care in a question regarding anticipated action. In this case, the airway and breathing are adequate, but circulation of oxygenated blood can best be supported with oxygen administration (option 1). Note that the stem of the question states "most important anticipated action." This should direct you to the correct option, option 1.

Level of Cognitive Ability: Application
Phase of Nursing Process: Implementation
Client Needs: Physiological Integrity
Content Area: Maternity

Reference
Gorrie, T., McKinney, E. S., & Murray, S. S. (1998). *Foundations of maternal-newborn nursing* (2nd ed.). Philadelphia: W. B. Saunders. p. 796.

12. **3**

Rationale: Breast-feeding will be compromised and the newborn infant may begin to prefer the bottle over the breast if the mother and baby are separated for an extended period. When the mother's condition is stable after being separated, re-establishing breast-feeding should be a nursing priority.

Test-Taking Strategy: Options 1, 2, and 4 refer to the "client." Option 3 is different in that it refers to the newborn infant. In this case, the correct answer is the one that has a different sentence structure. Also, use the process of elimination in answering the question.

Level of Cognitive Ability: Analysis
Phase of Nursing Process: Evaluation
Client Needs: Psychosocial Integrity
Content Area: Maternity .

Reference
Nichols, F., & Zwelling, E. (1997). *Maternal-newborn nursing: Theory and practice.* Philadelphia: W. B. Saunders. p. 1295.

13. **1**

Rationale: Hypovolemia symptoms include cool, clammy, pale skin; sensations of anxiety or impending doom; restlessness; and thirst. When these symptoms are present, the nurse should analyze that the client may be hypovolemic and should further assess vital signs, which would show tachycardia and tachypnea. The health care provider should then be notified.

Test-Taking Strategy: Knowledge of the symptoms of shock due to blood loss is necessary in answering this question, which identifies the symptoms of hypovolemia. Option 1 is correct because it is the most global response and is most appropriate for this high-risk condition. Options 2, 3, and 4 list specific interventions that should be implemented only after the health care provider has been notified.

Level of Cognitive Ability: Analysis
Phase of Nursing Process: Implementation
Client Needs: Physiological Integrity
Content Area: Maternity

Reference
Gorrie, T., McKinney, E. S., & Murray, S. S. (1998). *Foundations of maternal-newborn nursing* (2nd ed.). Philadelphia: W. B. Saunders. p. 790.

14. **1**

Rationale: Firm fundal massage for uterine atony is painful and may cause fear and distress as large clots may be expelled. Keeping the woman and her family informed of her condition while controlling bleeding will help minimize fear and apprehension and will maximize cooperation.

Test-Taking Strategy: Read this question and options carefully. It asks about planning care for the client with hemorrhage. Option 1 is the only correct answer, as options 2, 3, and 4 are routine interventions for the postpartum client. Additionally, with a client experiencing a uterine hemorrhage, vital signs would be taken more frequently than every 2 hours (option 2).

Level of Cognitive Ability: Application
Phase of Nursing Process: Planning
Client Needs: Psychosocial Integrity
Content Area: Maternity

Reference
Gorrie, T., McKinney, E. S., & Murray, S. S. (1998). *Foundations of maternal-newborn nursing* (2nd ed.). Philadelphia: W. B. Saunders. p. 791.

15. **3**

Rationale: The client is a gravida 6 and is at risk for possible uterine atony. IV access is a priority action in this case so that blood and medication can be administered if necessary.

Test-Taking Strategy: Remember the ABCs of care. In this case, IV access is key to maintaining circulation in the event of hemorrhage. Fundal massage (option 1) will not be necessary until after delivery. Options 2 and 4 are incorrect answers because their implementation will not be possible until the IV access is made. Review the risk factors related to uterine atony now, if you had difficulty with this question!

Level of Cognitive Ability: Application
Phase of Nursing Process: Implementation
Client Needs: Safe, Effective Care Environment
Content Area: Maternity

Reference
Nichols, F., & Zwelling, E. (1997). *Maternal-newborn nursing: Theory and practice.* Philadelphia: W. B. Saunders. p. 1287.

16. **3**

Rationale: When uterine atony cannot be reversed, the nurse should notify the health care provider and nurse anesthetist in preparation for surgery.

Test-Taking Strategy: Options 1, 2, and 4 are all interventions to reverse uterine atony, but read the question carefully. The question states that the uterus remains atonic in spite of interventions. Therefore, the best answer is to prepare for surgery.

Level of Cognitive Ability: Application
Phase of Nursing Process: Implementation
Client Needs: Physiological Integrity
Content Area: Maternity

Reference
Nichols, F., & Zwelling, E. (1997). *Maternal-newborn nursing: Theory and practice.* Philadelphia: W. B. Saunders. p. 1287.

17. **1**

Rationale: Inflammation and engorgement are major symptoms of mastitis that may alter the new breast-feeding mother's body image. Mastitis does not decrease milk quality or transmit infection, nor does it cause the mother to be unable to breast-feed.

Test-Taking Strategy: Incorrect options can be eliminated because they wrongly assume decreased milk quality (option 2), inability to breast-feed (option 3), and that infection can be transmitted to the newborn baby (option 4). Read the nursing diagnosis in its entirety. Inflammation and engorgement (option 1) is directly related to mastitis.

Level of Cognitive Ability: Analysis
Phase of Nursing Process: Analysis
Client Needs: Psychosocial Integrity
Content Area: Maternity

Reference
Nichols, F., & Zwelling, E. (1997). *Maternal-newborn nursing: Theory and practice.* Philadelphia: W. B. Saunders. p. 1302.

18. **4**

Rationale: Mastitis is an infection frequently associated with a break in the skin surface of the nipple. The measures described are personal hygiene measures to help prevent mastitis.

Test-Taking Strategy: Knowledge of the cause and preven-tion of mastitis is required to answer this question correctly. Read the question carefully. If you had difficulty with this question, review content related to mastitis now!

Level of Cognitive Ability: Analysis
Phase of Nursing Process: Analysis
Client Needs: Health Promotion and Maintenance
Content Area: Maternity

Reference
Gorrie, T., McKinney, E. S., & Murray, S. S. (1998). *Foundations of maternal-newborn nursing* (2nd ed.). Philadelphia: W. B. Saunders. p. 801.

19. **2**

Rationale: Because treatment of mastitis begins with antibiotic therapy, it is essential that the client complete the regimen of 10 days, even though symptoms will be reduced in 24 to 48 hours.

Test-Taking Strategy: Read the question carefully. Each option is a correct intervention for mastitis, but the question addresses the client who is being treated with antibiotics. Therefore, option 2 is correct because it is similar to the thought in the question. Also it is the most global response, in that the other interventions will be ineffective unless antibiotics are completed. Remember, with antibiotic therapy, it is critical that the client be informed about the importance of completing the antibiotics.

Level of Cognitive Ability: Application
Phase of Nursing Process: Implementation
Client Needs: Physiological Integrity
Content Area: Maternity

Reference
Nichols, F., & Zwelling, E. (1997). *Maternal-newborn nursing: Theory and practice.* Philadelphia: W. B. Saunders. p. 1301.

20. **3**

Rationale: Failure to nurse equally on both sides will decrease the flow of milk through the breast, causing engorgement of the breast offered less frequently.

Test-Taking Strategy: Look for the response that is an inaccurate statement and reflects the need for further teaching. Options 1, 2, and 4 are adequate responses by the client, whereas option 3 requires prior knowledge of breast-feeding physiology to know that there is need for further teaching. If you had difficulty with this question, review the concepts related to breast feeding now!

Level of Cognitive Ability: Analysis
Phase of Nursing Process: Evaluation
Client Needs: Health Promotion and Maintenance
Content Area: Maternity

Reference
Gorrie, T., McKinney, E. S., & Murray, S. S. (1998). *Foundations of maternal-newborn nursing* (2nd ed.). Philadelphia: W. B. Saunders. p. 801.

BIBLIOGRAPHY

Carpenito, L. (1997). *Handbook of nursing diagnosis* (7th ed.). Philadelphia: Lippincott-Raven.
Gorrie, T., McKinney, E. S., & Murray, S. S. (1998). *Foundations of maternal-newborn nursing* (2nd ed.). Philadelphia: W. B. Saunders.
Lowdermilk, D., Perry, S., & Bobak, I. (1997). *Maternity & women's health care* (6th ed.). St. Louis: Mosby–Year Book.
Nichols, F., & Zwelling, E. (1997). *Maternal-newborn nursing: Theory and practice.* Philadelphia: W. B. Saunders.

CHAPTER 30

Care of the Newborn

I. Initial Care of the Newborn

A. Assessment
1. Observe or assist with initiation of respirations
2. Assess Apgar score
3. Note characteristics of cry
4. Obtain vital signs
5. Monitor for nasal flaring, grunting, retractions, abnormal respirations
6. Observe **newborn** for signs of hypothermia or hyperthermia
7. Assess for gross anomalies

B. Implementation
1. Suction mouth, then nares, with bulb syringe
2. Dry **newborn** and stimulate crying by rubbing
3. Maintain temperature stability
4. Wrap **newborn** in warm blankets
5. Place stockinette cap on **newborn's** head
6. Keep **newborn** with mother to facilitate bonding
7. Place **newborn** at mother's breast if breast-feeding is planned, or place on mother's abdomen
8. Place **newborn** in warmer
9. Position **newborn** on side or abdomen or modified Trendelenburg position to facilitate drainage of mucus
10. Ensure **newborn's** proper identification
11. Footprint **newborn** and fingerprint mother on identification sheet
12. Place matching identification bracelets on mother and **newborn**

C. Apgar Scoring System
1. Perform and record Apgar score at 1 minute and at 5 minutes
2. If the score is less than 7 at 5 minutes, the Apgar score should be performed at 10 minutes
3. Assess each of the five items to be scored and assign values of 0 (very poor) to 2 (excellent) for each item

4. Add the points to determine the **newborn's** total score
   a. A score of 7 to 10 indicates a healthy **newborn** infant
   b. A score of 3 to 6 is considered moderately depressed
   c. A score of 0 to 2 is severely depressed
5. Five vital indicators (Table 30–1):
   a. Heart rate
   b. Respiratory rate
   c. Muscle tone
   d. Reflex irritability
   e. Skin color
6. Implementation (Table 30–2)

II. Initial Physical Examination

A. General Guidelines
1. Keep **newborn** warm during the examination
2. Begin with general observations and proceed to detailed findings
3. Perform assessments that are least disturbing to the **newborn** first
4. Initiate nursing interventions for abnormal findings
5. Document all abnormal findings

B. Vital Signs
1. Heart rate: 120 to 160 (apical); assess for a full minute due to irregularities after birth
2. Respirations: 30 to 60 breaths per minute; assess for a full minute
3. Axillary temperature: 36.4°C to 37°C (97.6°F to 98.6°F)
4. Blood pressure: 60/40 to 80/50 mmHg

C. Body Measurements
1. Length: 45 to 55 cm (18 to 22 inches)
2. Weight: 2500 to 4300 g (5.5 to 9.5 lb)
3. Head circumference: 33 to 35.5 cm (13 to 14 inches)
4. Chest circumference: 30 to 33 cm (12 to 13 inches) and should be equal to or 2 to 3 cm less than the head circumference

TABLE 30–1. **Apgar Scoring**

Indicator	0 Points	1 Point	2 Points
Heart rate	Absent	Less than 100	More than 100
Respiratory rate	Absent	Slow, irregular, weak cry	Good vigorous cry
Muscle tone	Flaccid, limp	Some flexion of extremities	Good flexion, active motion
Reflex irritability	No response	Weak cry and grimace	Vigorous cry, cough, sneeze
Skin color	Blue	Body skin normal, extremities blue	Body and extremity skin color normal

D. Head
  1. 25% of the body length (cephalocaudal development)
  2. Bones of the skull are not fused
  3. Palpable sutures (connective tissue between the skull bones)
  4. Fontanels: Unossified membranous tissue at the junction of the sutures (Table 30–3)
  5. Molding
     a. Asymmetry of head due to pressure in birth canal
     b. Disappears in about 72 hours
  6. Masses from birth trauma
     a. Caput succedaneum: Edema of the soft tissue over bone (crosses over suture line); subsides within a few days
     b. Cephalohematoma: Swelling caused by bleeding into an area between the bone and its periosteum (does not cross over suture line); usually absorbed within 6 weeks with no treatment
  7. Head lag
     a. Common when pulling **newborn** to a sitting position
     b. When prone, **newborn** should be able to lift head slightly and turn head from side to side

E. Eyes
  1. Slate gray (light skin) or brown-gray (dark skin) in color
  2. Symmetrical and clear
  3. Pupils equal, round, and react to light by accommodation
  4. Blink reflex present
  5. Eyes cross due to weak extraocular muscles
  6. Able to track and fixate momentarily
  7. Red reflex present
  8. Eyelids often edematous due to pressure during the birth process and the effects of eye medication

F. Ears
  1. Symmetrical
  2. Firm cartilage with recoil
  3. Pinna should be on or above line drawn from canthus of eye
  4. Low-set ears associated with Down's syndrome

G. Nose
  1. Flat, broad, in center of face
  2. Obligatory nose breathing
  3. Occasional sneezing to remove obstructions

H. Mouth
  1. Pink, moist gums
  2. Soft and hard palates intact
  3. Epstein's pearls (small, white cysts) may be present on hard palate
  4. Uvula in midline
  5. Tongue moves freely, is symmetrical, has short frenulum
  6. Sucking and crying movements symmetrical
  7. Able to swallow
  8. Gag reflex present

I. Neck
  1. Short and thick
  2. Head held in midline
  3. Trachea on midline

Table 30–2. **Apgar Score Implementation**

Score	Implementation
7 to 10	Rarely needs resuscitation
3 to 6	Requires resuscitation Suction Dry quickly Maintain warmth Ventilate 30 to 50 times a minute until heart rate is above 100, color is pink, and spontaneous respirations begin Provide oxygen Careful observation needed during the first few days of life
0 to 2	Requires intensive resuscitation Clear airway Insert endotracheal tube Use Ambu bag if necessary Ventilate with 100% oxygen at 40 to 60 breaths per minute Initiate full CPR as needed at 1:5 (breaths to chest compressions) ratio Maintain body temperature Support parents

Table 30–3. **Fontanels**

Fontanel	Characteristics	Closure
Anterior	Soft, flat, diamond-shaped 3–4 cm wide by 2–3 cm long	Closes between 12 and 18 months
Posterior	Triangular 0.5–1 cm wide Located between occipital and parietal bones	Closes between birth and 8–12 weeks of age

4. Raises head momentarily when prone
5. Good range of motion (ROM) and is able to flex and extend

J. Chest
  1. Appears circular since anteroposterior and lateral diameters are about equal
  2. Respirations appear diaphragmatic
  3. Bronchial sounds heard on auscultation
  4. Nipples prominent and often edematous
  5. Milky secretion (witch's milk) common
  6. Breast tissue present
  7. Clavicles need to be palpated to assess for fractures

K. Skin
  1. Pinkish-red (light-skinned **newborn**) to pinkish-brown or pinkish-yellow (dark-skinned **newborn**)
  2. Vernix caseosa
  3. Lanugo
  4. Milia
  5. Dry, peeling skin
  6. Dark red color common in premature **newborns**
  7. Cyanosis common with hypothermia, infection, and hypoglycemia and with cardiac, respiratory, or neurological abnormalities
  8. Acrocyanosis may be due to compromised peripheral circulation
  9. Assess for ecchymosis and petechiae due to trauma of birth
  10. Assess skin turgor over the abdomen to determine hydration status
  11. Observe for forceps marks
  12. Harlequin sign
    a. Deep red color develops over one side of the **newborn's** body while the other side remains pale due to vasomotor disturbance
    b. Skin resembles a clown's suit
  13. Birthmarks (Table 30–4)

L. Abdomen
  1. Umbilical cord
    a. Three vessels, two arteries, and one vein in cord; if less than three vessels are noted, notify the physician
    b. Small, thin cord may be associated with poor fetal growth
    c. Assess for intact cord and ensure that clamp is secured
    d. Cord should be clamped for at least the first 24 hours after birth; clamp can be removed when the cord is dried and occluded
    e. Note any bleeding or drainage from the cord
    f. Triple dye may be applied for initial cord care because it minimizes microorganisms and promotes drying; use a cotton-tipped applicator to paint the dye, one time, on the cord and on 1 inch of surrounding skin
    g. Application of 70% isopropyl alcohol to

the cord minimizes microorganisms and promotes drying
    h. If symptoms of infection such as moistness, oozing, discharge, and a reddened base occur, antibiotic treatment is prescribed
  2. Gastrointestinal
    a. Monitor cord for meconium staining
    b. Assess for umbilical hernia
    c. Note abdominal depression associated with diaphragmatic hernia
    d. Assess for abdominal distention associated with obstruction, mass, or sepsis
    e. Monitor bowel sounds, which should occur within 1 to 2 hours after birth
  3. Anus
    a. Anal opening patent
    b. First-stool meconium should pass within first 24 hours

M. Genitals
  1. Female
    a. Labia edematous, clitoris enlarged
    b. Smegma present (thick, white mucus discharge)
    c. Pseudomenstruation possible (blood-tinged mucus)
    d. Hymen tag may be visible
    e. First voiding should occur within 24 hours
  2. Male
    a. Prepuce (foreskin) covers glans penis
    b. Scrotum edematous
    c. Meatus at tip of penis
    d. Testes descended but may retract on cold
    e. Assess for hernia or hydrocele
    f. First voiding should occur within 24 hours

N. Spine
  1. Straight

Table 30–4. Birthmarks

Birthmark	Characteristics
Telangiectatic nevi (stork bites)	Pale pink or red, flat, dilated capillaries
	On eyelids, nose, lower occipital bone, and nape
	Blanch easily
	More noticeable during crying periods
	Disappears by age 2 years
Nevus flammeus (port-wine stain)	Capillary angioma directly below epidermis
	Nonelevated, sharply demarcated, red to purple, dense areas of capillaries
	Commonly appears on face
	Does not fade with time
	May require surgery in the future
Nevus vasculosus (strawberry mark)	Capillary hemangioma
	Raised, clearly delineated, dark red, with a rough surface
	Common in head region
	Disappears by age 7 to 9 years
Mongolian spots	Bluish-black pigmentation
	On lumbar dorsal area and buttocks
	Gradually fade during first and second years of life
	Common in Asian and dark-skinned races

2. Posture flexed
3. Supports head momentarily when prone
4. Arms and legs flexed
5. Chin flexed on upper chest
6. Sporadic movements that are well coordinated
7. Degree of hypotonicity or hypertonicity is indicative of central nervous system (CNS) damage

O. Extremities
1. Flexed
2. Full ROM
3. Movements symmetrical
4. Fists clenched
5. Fingers and toes should be 10 each in number and separate
6. Legs bowed
7. Major gluteal folds even
8. Creases on soles of feet
9. Assess for hip dysplasia
10. When thighs are rotated outward, no clicks should be heard
11. Pulses palpable (radial, brachial, femoral)
12. Assess for fractures (especially clavicle) or dislocations (hip)
13. Slight tremors are common but could be a sign of hypoglycemia or drug withdrawal

III. Body Systems Assessment

A. Cardiovascular System
1. Keep **newborn** warm
2. Take apical heart rate for 1 full minute
3. Listen for murmurs
4. Palpate pulses
5. Assess for cyanosis
6. Blanch skin on trunk and extremities to assess circulation
7. Observe cord stump for bleeding
8. Document inability to feed without cardiac distress

B. Respiratory System
1. Position **newborn** on side
2. Suction as necessary
   a. Use a bulb syringe for upper airway suctioning (compress bulb before insertion)
   b. Use a French catheter for deeper suctioning
3. Observe for respiratory distress and hypoxemia
   a. Nasal flaring
   b. Increasingly severe retractions
   c. Grunting
   d. Cyanosis
   e. Bradycardia
   f. Low body temperature
   g. Periods of apnea lasting longer than 15 seconds
4. Administer oxygen via hood if necessary as prescribed

C. Hepatic System
1. Normal or physiological jaundice appears after the first 24 hours in full-term **neonates** and after the first 48 hours in premature **neonates**; jaundice occurring prior to this time (pathological jaundice) may indicate early hemolysis of RBCs and must be reported to the physician
2. Physiological jaundice peaks about the fifth day of life (indirect bilirubin levels: 6 to 7 mg/dL)
3. Monitor serum bilirubin levels
4. Feed early to stimulate intestinal activity and to keep bilirubin level low
5. For **neonates** with jaundice on breast milk, feed early and every 2 hours to stimulate intestinal activity and keep bilirubin level low
6. Temporarily discontinue breast-feeding for 48 hours if bilirubin levels exceed 15 to 20 mg/dL
7. Prevent chilling, as hypothermia can cause acidosis that interferes with bilirubin conjugation and excretion
8. Liver stores iron passed from the mother for 5 to 6 months
9. Glycogen storage occurs in liver
10. **Newborn** is at risk for hemorrhagic disorders; coagulation factors synthesized in the liver are dependent on vitamin K, which is not synthesized until intestinal bacteria are present
11. Handle **newborn** carefully and monitor for any bruising or bleeding episodes
12. Watch for meconium passage and subsequent stools
13. Administer one dose of vitamin K (AquaMEPHYTON), 0.5 to 1.0 mg IM to the **neonate** in the vastus lateralis muscle as prescribed to aid in blood coagulation
14. Assess **newborn's** hemoglobin and blood glucose level

D. Renal System
1. The immature kidneys are unable to concentrate urine
2. A weight loss of 5% to 15% during the first week of life occurs due to voiding and limited intake
3. Weigh **newborn** daily
4. Monitor intake and output (I&O)
5. Weigh diapers if necessary
6. Measure specific gravity if necessary
7. Assess for signs of dehydration
   a. Dry mucous membranes
   b. Sunken eyeballs
   c. Poor skin turgor
   d. Sunken fontanels

E. Immune System
1. Passive immunity via the **placenta** (IgG)
2. Passive immunity from colostrum (IgA)
3. Elevations in IgM indicate infection in utero
4. Use aseptic technique when caring for the **newborn**
5. Observe universal precautions when handling **newborn**

6. Ensure meticulous handwashing
7. Wear gowns when caring for the **newborn**
8. Ensure that an infection-free staff cares for the **newborn**
9. Monitor **newborn's** temperature
10. Observe for any cracks or openings in the skin
11. Administer eye medication within 1 hour after birth to prevent ophthalmia neonatorum
    a. Erythromycin (0.5%) ophthalmic ointment or drops; also prevents *Chlamydia trachomatis*
    b. Tetracycline (1%) ophthalmic ointment or drops
    c. Silver nitrate solution; not often used because it is not effective against *C. trachomatis*; causes chemical conjunctivitis
12. Provide cord care
    a. Umbilical clamp can be removed after 24 hours
    b. Keep cord clean and dry by wiping with alcohol
    c. Keep diaper from covering cord; fold diaper below cord
    d. Assess cord for odor, swelling, or discharge
    e. Teach mother how to perform cord care
13. Provide circumcision care
    a. Apply petroleum jelly gauze to the penis except when a Plastibell is used
    b. Remove petroleum jelly gauze, if applied, after first voiding following circumcision
    c. Observe for swelling, infection, or bleeding from the circumcision site
    d. Monitor for urinary retention
    e. Teach mother care of circumcision site

F. Metabolic System and Gastrointestinal System
1. **Newborns** are able to digest simple carbohydrates but are unable to digest fats due to the lack of lipase
2. Proteins may be only partially broken down, so may serve as antigens and provoke an allergic reaction
3. The **newborn** has a small stomach capacity (about 90 mL), with rapid intestinal peristalsis (bowel emptying time is 2.5 to 3 hours)
4. Most breast-fed **newborns** are put to breast soon after birth
5. Feedings are initiated when readiness for feedings is determined and vital signs are stable
6. Start with a feeding of 10 to 15 mL of sterile water to assess patency of swallowing and integrity of the GI tract; once a small amount is fed to the **newborn**, the remainder of the feeding is finished with either formula or breast milk
7. Observe feeding reflexes, such as rooting, sucking, and swallowing
8. Assist mother with breast-feeding or formula feeding

9. Burp **newborn** during and after feeding
10. Assess for regurgitations or vomiting
11. Position **newborn** on right side after feeding
12. Observe for the passage of meconium
13. Observe for normal stool
    a. Soft, yellow stools for breast-fed **newborns**
    b. Seedy, yellow stools for formula-fed **newborns**
14. Perform **newborn** phenylketonuria (PKU) screening test before discharge and as an outpatient after sufficient protein intake occurs; the **newborn** should be on formula or breast milk for 24 hours before screening, and screening must be repeated in 7 to 14 days

G. Neurological System
1. **Newborn** head size is proportionally larger than that of adults due to cephalocaudal development
2. Myelinization of nerve fibers is incomplete, so primitive reflexes are present
3. Fontanels open to allow for brain growth
4. Assess for an abnormal size and bulging or depressed fontanels
5. Measure and graph head circumference in relation to chest circumference and length
6. Assess **newborn's** movements, noting symmetry, posture, and abnormal movements
7. Observe for jitteriness, marked tremors, and seizures
8. Test **newborn's** reflexes
9. Assess for lethargy
10. Assess pitch of cry

H. Thermal Regulatory System
1. **Newborns** do not shiver to produce heat
2. **Newborns** have brown fat deposits that produce heat
3. Heat is dissipated through vasodilation
4. Prevent heat loss due to evaporation by keeping **newborn** dry and well-wrapped
5. Prevent heat loss due to radiation by keeping **newborn** away from cold objects and outside walls
6. Prevent heat loss due to convection by shielding the **newborn** from drafts
7. Prevent heat loss due to conduction by performing all treatments on a warm, padded surface
8. Keep temperature in room warm
9. Take **newborn's** axillary temperature every hour for the first 4 hours of life, every 4 hours for the remainder of the first 24 hours, and then every shift

I. Reflexes
1. Sucking and rooting
    a. Touch the **newborn's** lip, cheek, or corner of mouth with a nipple
    b. **Newborn** turns head toward the nipple, opens the mouth, takes hold of the nipple, and sucks

c. Usually disappears after 3 to 4 months but may persist for up to 1 year
2. Swallowing
    a. Occurs spontaneously after sucking and obtaining fluids
    b. **Newborn** swallows in coordination with sucking without gagging, coughing, or vomiting
3. Tonic neck or fencing
    a. While the **newborn** is falling asleep or sleeping, gently and quickly turn the head to one side
    b. As the **newborn** faces the left side, the left arm and leg extend outward while the right arm and leg flex
    c. When turned to the right side, the right arm and leg extend while the left arm and leg flex
    d. Usually disappears within 3 to 4 months
4. Palmar-plantar grasp
    a. Place a finger in the palm of the **newborn's** hand, then place a finger at the base of the toes
    b. The **newborn's** fingers curl around the examiner's finger and the **newborn's** toes curl downward
    c. Palmar response lessens within 3 to 4 months
    d. Plantar response lessens within 8 months
5. Moro's reflex
    a. Hold the **newborn** in a semisitting position, then allow the head and trunk to fall backward to at least a 30° angle, or place the **newborn** on a flat surface and strike the flat surface to startle the **newborn**
    b. The **newborn** symmetrically abducts and extends the arms
    c. The **newborn** fans the fingers out and forms a C with the thumb and the forefinger
    d. The **newborn** adducts the arms to an embracing position and returns to a relaxed flexion state
    e. Present at birth; a complete response may occur up to 8 weeks
    f. A body jerk motion occurs from 8 to 18 weeks
    g. No response may be noted by 6 months as long as neurological maturation has not been delayed
    h. A persistent response lasting more than 6 months may indicate the occurrence of brain damage during pregnancy
6. Startle reflex
    a. The response is best elicited if the **newborn** is at least 24 hours old
    b. Make a loud noise or clap hands to elicit the response
    c. The **newborn's** arms adduct while the elbows flex
    d. The hands stay clenched

e. The reflex should disappear within 4 months
7. Pull-to-sit
    a. Pull the **newborn** up from the wrist while the **newborn** is in the prone position
    b. The head will lag until the **newborn** is in an upright position, then the head will be level with the chest and shoulders momentarily before falling forward
    c. The head will then lift for a few minutes
    d. The response depends on the **newborn's** general muscle tone and condition as well as maturity levels
8. Babinski's sign—plantar
    a. Beginning at the heel of the foot, gently stroke upward along the lateral aspect of the sole, then the examiner moves the finger along the ball of the foot
    b. The **newborn's** toes hyperextend while the big toe dorsiflexes
    c. Reflex disappears after the **newborn** is 1 year old
    d. Absence of this reflex indicates the need for a neurological examination
9. Stepping or walking
    a. Hold the **newborn** in a vertical position, allowing one foot to touch a table surface
    b. The **newborn** simulates walking, alternately flexing and extending the feet
    c. The reflex is usually present for 3 to 4 months
10. Crawling
    a. Place the **newborn** on the abdomen
    b. The **newborn** begins making crawling movements with the arms and legs
    c. The reflex usually disappears after about 6 weeks

IV. Parent Teaching

A. Formula Feeding
    1. Teach sterilization techniques if the water supply is located in areas where the purification process of the water is questionable
    2. Remind mother not to heat the bottle of formula in the microwave oven
    3. Teach the mother that formula is a sufficient diet for the first 4 to 6 months
    4. Assess the mother's ability to burp the **newborn**
B. Breast-Feeding
    1. Assess the **newborn's** ability to attach to the mother's breast and suck
    2. Teach the mother about engorgement
    3. Teach the mother how to pump her breasts and how to store breast milk properly
    4. Teach the mother that breast milk is a sufficient diet for the first 4 to 6 months
    5. Give the mother the phone number of the

local organizations that offer support to breast-feeding mothers

C. Bathing
  1. Bathe **newborn** in a warm room before feeding
  2. Have all equipment for bathing available
  3. Use a mild soap (not on the face)
  4. Proceed from the cleanest area to the dirtiest
  5. Clean eyes from the inner canthus outward
  6. Special care should be taken to clean under the folds of the neck, underarms, groin, and genitals
  7. Make bath time enjoyable for both the **newborn** and mother

D. Clothing
  1. Assess diaper and clothing needs for the **newborn** with the mother
  2. Instruct the mother that the **newborn's** head should be covered in cold weather to prevent heat loss
  3. Instruct mother to layer **newborn's** clothing in cooler weather

E. Cord Care
  1. Clean cord with alcohol after each diaper change and at least two to three times daily
  2. Keep the diaper folded below the cord
  3. Sponge-bathe the **newborn** until the cord falls off
  4. Cord should fall off within 2 weeks

F. Circumcision
  1. Remove petroleum jelly gauze if applied after first voiding following circumcision
  2. Cleanse penis after each voiding by squeezing warm water over the penis
  3. Observe for swelling, infection, drainage, or bleeding from the circumcision site
  4. A milky covering over the glans penis is normal and should not be disrupted

V. Preterm Newborn

A. Description
  1. A **neonate** born before 37 weeks' gestation
  2. The primary concern relates to immaturity of all body systems

B. Assessment
  1. Respirations irregular with periods of apnea
  2. Body temperature is below normal
  3. **Newborn** has poor suck and swallow reflexes
  4. Bowel sounds are diminished
  5. Increased or decreased urinary output
  6. Extremities are thin, with minimal creasing on soles and palms
  7. **Newborn** extends extremities and does not maintain flexion
  8. Lanugo, on skin and in the hair on the **newborn's** head, is present in woolly patches
  9. Skin is thin, with visible blood vessels and minimal subcutaneous fat pads
  10. Skin may appear jaundiced

  11. Testes are undescended in boys
  12. Labia are narrow in girls

C. Implementation
  1. Monitor vital signs every 2 to 4 hours
  2. Maintain cardiopulmonary functions
  3. Administer oxygen and humidification as prescribed
  4. Monitor I&O and electrolyte balance
  5. Assess intake closely
  6. Monitor daily weight
  7. Maintain **newborn** in a warming device
  8. Position every 1 to 2 hours, and handle **newborn** carefully
  9. Avoid exposure to infections
  10. Provide **newborn** with appropriate stimulation, such as touch

VI. Post-Term Newborn

A. Description: A **neonate** born after 42 weeks of gestation

B. Assessment
  1. Hypoglycemia
  2. Parchment-like skin without lanugo
  3. Dry and cracked skin
  4. Fingernails long and extended over ends of fingers
  5. Profuse scalp hair
  6. Body is long and thin
  7. Extremities show wasting of fat and muscle
  8. Meconium staining may be present on nails and umbilical cord

C. Implementation
  1. Provide normal **newborn** care
  2. Monitor for hypoglycemia
  3. Maintain **newborn's** temperature
  4. Monitor for meconium aspiration
  5. Initiate seizure precautions

VII. Small for Gestational Age

A. Description: A **neonate** who is plotted at or below the 10th percentile on the intrauterine growth curve

B. Assessment
  1. Fetal distress
  2. Gestational age and physical maturity
  3. Lowered or elevated body temperature
  4. Physical abnormalities
  5. Hypoglycemia
  6. Signs of polycythemia
    a. Ruddy appearance
    b. Cyanosis
    c. Jaundice
  7. Signs of infection
  8. Signs of aspiration of meconium

C. Implementation
  1. Maintain airway
  2. Maintain temperature
  3. Observe for signs of respiratory distress
  4. Monitor for signs of infection
  5. Monitor glucose levels

6. Monitor for signs of hypoglycemia
7. Initiate feedings and monitor for signs of aspiration
8. Provide stimulation, such as touch and cuddling

VIII. Large for Gestational Age

A. Description: A **neonate** who is plotted at or above the 90th percentile on the intrauterine growth curve
B. Assessment
　1. Gestational age
　2. Birth trauma or injury
　3. Respiratory distress
　4. Ilypoglycemia
C. Implementation
　1. Monitor vital signs
　2. Monitor glucose levels
　3. Observe for signs of hypoglycemia
　4. Initiate early feedings
　5. Monitor for infection and initiate measures to prevent sepsis
　6. Provide touch and cuddling for the **newborn**

◆ IX. Respiratory Distress Syndrome (RDS)

A. Description: A serious lung disorder caused by immaturity and inability to produce surfactant, resulting in hypoxia and acidosis
B. Assessment
　1. Tachypnea
　2. Flaring nares
　3. Expiratory grunting
　4. Retractions
　5. Decreased breath sounds
　6. Apnea
　7. Pallor and cyanosis
　8. Hypothermia
　9. Poor muscle tone
C. Implementation
　1. Monitor color, respiratory rate, and degree of effort in breathing
　2. Support respirations as prescribed
　3. Monitor blood gases and oxygen saturation levels (blood gases from umbilical artery)
　4. Monitor blood gases so oxygen administered to the **newborn** is at the lowest possible concentration necessary to maintain adequate arterial oxygenation
　5. Schedule any premature **newborn** who required oxygen support for an eye examination before discharge to assess for retinal damage
　6. Suction every 2 hours or more often as necessary
　7. Position **newborn** on side or back, with neck slightly extended
　8. Administer respiratory therapy (percussion and vibration) as prescribed; use padded small plastic cup or small oxygen mask for percussion; use electric toothbrush for vibration
　9. Provide nutrition
　10. Support bonding
　11. Prepare parents for short- to long-term period of oxygen dependency if necessary
　12. Encourage mother to pump breasts for future breast-feeding if she so desires
　13. Encourage as much participation in **newborn's** care as condition allows

X. Hyperbilirubinemia ◆

A. Description
　1. At any serum bilirubin level, the appearance of jaundice during the first day of life indicates a pathological process
　2. Evaluation is indicated when serum levels are over 12 mg/dL in the term **newborn**
　3. Therapy is aimed at preventing kernicterus, which results in permanent neurological damage from the deposition of bilirubin in the brain cells
B. Assessment
　1. Jaundice
　2. Elevated serum bilirubin levels
　3. Enlarged liver
　4. Poor muscle tone
　5. Lethargy
　6. Poor sucking reflex
C. Implementation
　1. Monitor for presence of jaundice
　　a. Examine the baby's skin color in natural light
　　b. Press finger over a bony prominence or tip of the **newborn's** nose to press out capillary blood from the tissues
　　c. Note that jaundice starts at the head first, spreads to the chest, then abdomen; then the arms and legs, followed by the hands and feet, which are the last to be jaundiced
　2. Keep **newborn** well-hydrated to maintain blood volume and encourage excretion of bilirubin
　3. Facilitate early, frequent feeding to hasten passage of meconium
　4. Report any signs of jaundice in the first 24 hours and any abnormal signs and symptoms to the physician
　5. Prepare for phototherapy and monitor the **newborn** closely during the treatment
D. Phototherapy
　1. Description
　　a. Use of intense fluorescent lights to reduce serum bilirubin levels in the **newborn**
　　b. Injury from treatment, such as eye damage, dehydration, or sensory deprivation, can occur
　2. Implementation
　　a. Expose as much of the **newborn's** skin as possible
　　b. Cover the genital area, and monitor the

genital area for skin irritation or breakdown

   c. Cover the **newborn's** eyes with eye shields

   d. Make sure eyelids are closed when patches are applied

   e. Remove the shields at least once per shift to inspect the eyes for infection or irritation and to allow eye contact

   f. Measure the quantity of light every 8 hours

   g. Monitor skin temperature closely

   h. Increase fluids to compensate for water loss

   i. Expect loose green stools and green urine

   j. Monitor **newborn's** skin color with the fluorescent light turned off every 4 to 8 hours

   k. Monitor the skin for bronze baby syndrome, a grayish-brown discoloration of the skin

   l. Reposition **newborn** every 2 hours

  m. Provide stimulation

  n. After treatment, continue monitoring for signs of hyperbilirubinemia, as rebound elevations are normal after therapy is discontinued

XI. Erythroblastosis Fetalis

A. Description

  1. Destruction of RBCs that results from an antigen-antibody reaction

  2. Characterized by hemolytic anemia or hyperbilirubinemia

  3. Exchange of fetal and maternal blood takes place primarily when the **placenta** separates at birth

  4. Rh antigens from the baby's blood enter the maternal blood stream

  5. The mother's blood does not contain Rh factor, so the mother produces anti-Rh antibodies

  6. Antibodies are harmless to the mother but attach to the erythrocytes in the fetus and cause hemolysis

  7. Sensitization is rare with first pregnancy

  8. ABO incompatibility is usually less severe

B. Assessment

  1. Anemia

  2. Jaundice that develops rapidly after birth and before 24 hours

  3. Edema

C. Implementation

  1. Administer RhoGAM to the mother during the first 72 hours after **delivery** if the Rh-negative mother delivers an Rh-positive fetus but remains unsensitized

  2. Assist with exchange transfusion after birth or intrauterine transfusion as prescribed

  3. The baby's blood is replaced with Rh-negative blood to stop the destruction of the baby's red cells; the Rh-negative blood is replaced with the baby's own blood gradually

  4. Reassure the mother that the **newborn** will suffer no untoward effects from the condition

XII. Sepsis

A. Description: Generalized infection resulting from the presence of bacteria in the blood

B. Assessment

  1. Pallor

  2. Tachypnea

  3. Tachycardia

  4. Poor feeding

  5. Abdominal distention

C. Implementation

  1. Assess for periods of apnea or irregular respirations

  2. Stimulate if apnea is present by gently rubbing chest or foot

  3. Administer oxygen as prescribed

  4. Monitor vital signs

  5. Maintain warmth in an Isolette

  6. Provide isolation as necessary

  7. Assess for low-grade fever

  8. Monitor I&O

  9. Monitor daily weight

  10. Monitor for diarrhea

  11. Assess feeding, which may be poor

  12. Assess sucking reflex, which may be poor

  13. Assess for jaundice

  14. Assess for irritability and lethargy

  15. Administer antibiotics as prescribed and observe carefully for toxicity, because a **newborn's** liver and kidney are immature

XIII. TORCH Syndrome

A. Description

  1. Refers to infections of the fetus or **newborn**

  2. Caused by one of the following

   a. **T**-oxoplasmosis

   b. **O**-ther viruses

   c. **R**-ubella

   d. **C**-ytomegalovirus

   e. **H**-erpes

B. Infections (Table 30–5)

XIV. Syphilis

A. Description

  1. Sexually transmitted disease

  2. Congenital syphilis can result in premature **delivery**, skin lesions, abnormal skeletal development

  3. The organism *Treponema pallidum*, a spirochete, is able to cross the **placenta** throughout pregnancy and infect the fetus, usually after 18 weeks' gestation

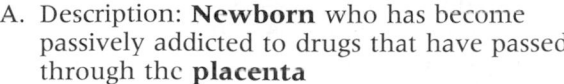

Table 30–5. Infections Comprising TORCH Syndrome

Infection	Characteristics
Toxoplasmosis	Protozoan infection Produces no serious effects in the mother Can be transmitted to the fetus Can result in severe physical and developmental abnormalities Common carriers include cat feces and raw beef
Other Infections	Such as syphilis
Rubella	Systemic viral infection Causes congenital rubella syndrome, which includes congenital heart disease, cataracts, growth retardation, and pneumonia if the mother becomes infected within the first trimester Deafness and some learning disabilities can occur if the mother becomes infected during the first trimester
Cytomegalovirus	A viral infection that persists in the body indefinitely, with periods of reactivation without symptoms Can infect the fetus or infant during delivery or after birth through breast milk, blood transfusions, or contact with infected secretions May cause microcephaly, blindness, deafness and mental and motor retardation
Herpes simplex	Sexually transmitted disease caused by a virus Periods of reactivation Neonate is commonly infected during delivery by direct contact with lesions in the genital tract Can cause neurological impairment or death

4. Risks include preterm birth, stillbirth, and low birth weight
5. Congenital effects are irreversible and may include CNS damage and hearing loss

B. Assessment
  1. Hepatosplenomegaly
  2. Joint swelling
  3. Rash
  4. Anemia
  5. Jaundice
  6. Snuffles
  7. Ascites
  8. Pneumonitis
  9. Cerebrospinal fluid changes

C. Implementation
  1. Monitor **newborn** for signs of syphilis
  2. Monitor for palmar rash and snuffles
  3. Prepare **newborn** for serological testing if prescribed
  4. Administer antibiotic therapy as prescribed
  5. Use drainage/secretion precautions with suspected congenital syphilis
  6. Wear gloves when handling **neonate** until 24 hours of antibiotic therapy has been administered
  7. Provide psychological support to the mother and provide instructions regarding follow-up care to the **newborn**

XV. The Addicted Newborn

A. Description: **Newborn** who has become passively addicted to drugs that have passed through the **placenta**

B. Addicting Drugs
  1. Heroin
    a. **Newborn** may appear normal at birth, with a low birth weight
    b. Withdrawal occurs within 12 to 24 hours and may last 5 to 7 days
  2. Methadone
    a. Withdrawal occurs within 1 to 2 days to 1 week or more, is most evident at 48 to 72 hours, and may last 6 days to 8 weeks
    b. **Newborn** appears very ill
    c. May develop jaundice due to prematurity
  3. Cocaine
    a. Causes decreased interactive behavior
    b. Feeding problems are present
    c. Irregular sleep patterns and diarrhea
    d. Major deformities will occur, especially in the renal system

C. Assessment
  1. Irritability
  2. Tremors
  3. Hyperactivity
  4. Hypertonicity
  5. Respiratory distress
  6. Vomiting
  7. High-pitched cry
  8. Sneezing
  9. Fever
  10. Diarrhea
  11. Excessive sweating
  12. Poor feeding
  13. Extreme sucking of fists
  14. Convulsions

D. Implementation
  1. Monitor respiratory and cardiac status frequently
  2. Monitor temperature and vital signs
  3. Hold **newborn** firm and close to the body during feeding and when giving care
  4. Initiate seizure precautions
  5. Pad sides of crib
  6. Provide small frequent feedings and allow a longer period for feeding
  7. Monitor I&O
  8. Administer IV hydration if prescribed
  9. Protect **neonate's** skin from injury that can be caused by the constant rubbing from hyperactive jitters
  10. Swaddle **newborn**
  11. Place **newborn** in a quiet room and reduce stimulation
  12. Allow mother to ventilate feelings of anxiety and guilt
  13. Refer mother for treatment of substance abuse problem

XVI. Fetal Alcohol Syndrome

A. Description

1. Caused by maternal alcohol use during pregnancy
2. Most serious cause of teratogenesis
3. Causes mental and physical retardation

B. Assessment
1. Facial changes
   a. Short palpebral fissures
   b. Hypoplastic philtrum
   c. Short, upturned nose
   d. Flat midface
   e. Thin upper lip
   f. Low nasal bridge
2. Abnormal palmar creases
3. Congenital heart disorders
4. Respiratory distress
5. Apnea
6. Cyanosis
7. Irritability
8. Tremors
9. Poor feeding
10. Hypersensitivity to stimuli
11. Seizures

C. Implementation
1. Monitor for respiratory distress
2. Position **newborn** on side to facilitate drainage of secretions
3. Keep resuscitation equipment at the bedside
4. Assess for hypoglycemia
5. Assess suck and swallow reflex
6. Administer small feedings and burp well
7. Suction as necessary, especially following feedings
8. Monitor I&O
9. Monitor weight and head circumference
10. Decrease environmental stimuli

◆ **XVII. Newborn with Acquired Immunodeficiency Syndrome (AIDS)**

A. Description
1. The fetus of a human immunodeficiency virus (HIV) antibody–positive woman should be monitored closely throughout the pregnancy
2. Serial ultrasound screenings should be done to identify intrauterine growth restriction
3. Weekly nonstress testing after 32 weeks of gestation and biophysical profiles may be necessary
4. **Neonates** born to HIV-positive clients may test positive because the mother's positive antibodies may persist for as long as 18 months after birth
5. The use of antiviral medication, the reduction of **neonatal** exposure to maternal blood and body fluids, and the early identification of HIV in pregnancy reduce the risk of transmission to the **newborn**
6. All **neonates** acquire maternal antibody to HIV infection, but not all acquire the infection

7. The **neonate** may be asymptomatic for the first several years of life

B. Transmission
1. Across **placental** barrier
2. During **labor** and **delivery**
3. Breast milk

C. Assessment
1. May have no outward signs for the first several months of life
2. Signs of immune deficiency
3. Hepatomegaly
4. Splenomegaly
5. Lymphadenopathy
6. Impairment in growth and development

D. Implementation
1. Cleanse **newborn's** skin carefully before any invasive procedure, such as the administration of vitamin K, heel sticks, or venipunctures
2. Circumcisions are not done on **newborns** with HIV-positive mothers until the **newborn's** status is determined
3. **Newborn** can room with mother
4. All HIV-exposed **newborns** should be treated with medication to prevent infection by *Pneumocystis carinii*
5. Administer zidovudine (AZT) as prescribed for the first 6 weeks of life
6. Monitor for early signs of immune deficiency, such as enlarged spleen or liver, lymphadenopathy, and impairment in growth and development
7. **Newborns** at risk for HIV infection should be seen by the physician at birth, 1 week, 2 weeks, 1 month, and 2 months of life
8. Inform mother that an HIV culture is recommended at age 1 month and after 4 months of age

E. Immunizations
1. **Newborns** at risk for HIV infection need to receive all recommended immunizations at the regular schedule
2. Inactivated polio vaccine by injection rather than oral polio vaccine should be administered because the oral polio vaccine causes a shedding of polio virus in the stool, which may be a risk to the immunocompromised family
3. Immunizations with live vaccines, such as oral polio, and measles-mumps-rubella (MMR), should not be done until the **neonate's, infant's**, or child's status is confirmed
4. If a child is infected, live vaccine will not be given

XVIII. Newborn of Diabetic Mother

A. Description
1. **Neonate** born to an insulin-dependent mother or gestational diabetic mother
2. High incidence of congenital anomalies

3. High incidence of hypoglycemia, respiratory distress, hypocalcemia, and hyperbilirubinemia
B. Assessment
   1. Excessive size and weight due to excess fat and glycogen in tissues
   2. Edema or puffiness in the face and cheeks
   3. Signs of hypoglycemia, such as twitching, difficulty in feeding, lethargy, apnea, seizures, and cyanosis
   4. Hyperbilirubinemia
   5. Signs of respiratory distress, tachypnea, cyanosis, retractions, grunting, nasal flaring
C. Implementation
   1. Monitor for signs of respiratory distress
   2. Monitor bilirubin and blood glucose levels
   3. Monitor weight
   4. Feed early, with 10% glucose water, breast milk, or formula
   5. Administer IV glucose if necessary
   6. Monitor for edema
   7. Monitor for tremors, seizures, apnea, and acidosis

◆ **XIX. Hypoglycemia**

A. Description
   1. Abnormally low level of glucose in the blood (less than 30 mg/dL in the first 72 hours or below 45 mg/dL after the first 3 days of life)
   2. Normal blood glucose level is 40 to 60 mg/dL in 1-day-old neonate and 50 to 90 mg/dL in neonate older than 1 day
B. Assessment
   1. Increased respiratory rate
   2. Twitching, nervousness, or tremors
   3. Unstable temperature
   4. Cyanosis
C. Implementation
   1. Prevent low blood glucose through early feedings
   2. Administer glucose orally or IV
   3. Monitor blood glucose values as prescribed
   4. Monitor for feeding problems
   5. Evaluate apneic periods
   6. Assess for shrill or intermittent cries
   7. Evaluate lethargy and poor muscle tone

PRACTICE QUESTIONS

1. To bathe a newborn, a mother should be taught to:
   1 Start with the dirtiest area first
   2 Begin with the eyes and face
   3 Begin with the feet and work upward
   4 Only wash the diaper area, since this is the only part of the baby that gets soiled

2. Following birth, the nurse should prevent hypothermia caused by evaporation in the neonate by:
   1 Warming the crib pad
   2 Turning on the overhead radiant warmer

   3 Closing the doors to the room
   4 Drying the baby with a warm blanket

3. The nurse is teaching cord care to a new mother. Which of the following principles is of greatest importance?
   1 Cord care is done only at birth to control bleeding
   2 Alcohol is the best agent used to clean the cord
   3 The process of keeping the cord clean and dry will decrease bacterial growth
   4 It takes 21 days for the cord to dry up and fall off

4. The nurse provides a class to new mothers on newborn care. In teaching cord care, which of the following suggestions is best?
   1 If triple dye has been applied to the cord, it is not necessary to do anything else to it
   2 Apply alcohol to the cord, ensuring that all areas around the cord are cleaned two to three times a day
   3 Gently apply alcohol to the cord, being careful not to move the cord because it will cause the newborn pain
   4 All that is necessary is to wash the cord with antibacterial soap once a day, allowing it to air dry

5. Clients should be taught how to perform appropriate cord care and to monitor for infection at home when the newborn is discharged. Which of the following suggests signs of an infection?
   1 A darkened, drying stump
   2 A moist cord with discharge
   3 A purple stump that shows pinkness around the base
   4 A purple stump that shows some moistness at the base

6. A male neonate has just been circumcised. The nurse would expect the surgical site to appear:
   1 Pink, without drainage
   2 Reddened, with a small amount of bloody drainage
   3 Reddened, with a large amount of bloody drainage that requires a dressing change every 30 minutes
   4 Reddened, with a small amount of yellow exudate on the glans

7. The parents of a male neonate who is not circumcised request information on how to clean the newborn's penis. The best response is:
   1 "Retract the foreskin and cleanse the glans when bathing the neonate."
   2 "Do not retract the foreskin to cleanse as this may cause adhesions."
   3 "Retract the foreskin no farther than it will easily go and replace over the glans after cleaning."
   4 "Retract the foreskin and cleanse with every diaper change."

8. A newly delivered client is attempting to breast-feed for the first time. The nurse notices that the client has inverted nipples. What nursing action can the nurse take to assist the client in breast-feeding the newborn?
   1 Provide breast shells and assist the mother with using a breast pump before each feeding to make the nipples easier for the newborn to grasp
   2 Have the mother grasp the nipples between the thumb and forefinger and tug firmly to get the nipple to protrude
   3 Massage the breast, applying gentle pressure on the areola
   4 Take a cool shower, allowing the water to run over the breasts, as this will encourage the nipples to protrude

9. The home care nurse's assignment is to visit a new mother at home 24 to 48 hours after discharge. What finding would the nurse expect in a healthy breast-feeding mother and newborn?
   1 A mother breast-feeding every 3 to 4 hours without signs of cracked nipples, with the newborn in a tummy-to-tummy position; the baby demonstrates bursts of sucking followed by a pause and swallow
   2 A mother breast-feeding the newborn with the newborn's head turned toward her breast and the body flat in her arms; mother has sore nipples; baby has a suck blister and is wetting three to four diapers a day
   3 A mother complaining of breast engorgement, breast-feeding every 6 to 8 hours, with the newborn demonstrating difficulty in latching on to the breast
   4 A mother with cracked nipples feeding the newborn with a supplemental bottle

10. In caring for a preterm newborn's skin, the nurse must understand the special characteristics that exist. These include:
    1 A thin and gelatinous skin, with decreased amounts of subcutaneous fat and open posture
    2 A thin and gelatinous skin, with flexed posture and decreased subcutaneous fat
    3 A thin and gelatinous skin, with flexed posture and increased amounts of brown fat
    4 Fine, downy hair on a thin epidermal and dermal layer, with flexed posture and increased amounts of brown fat

11. Preterm newborns are at risk for developing respiratory distress syndrome (RDS). The clinical signs of RDS are:
    1 Cyanosis, tachypnea, retractions, and expiratory grunt
    2 Acrocyanosis, apnea, pnuemothorax, and grunting
    3 Barrel-shaped chest, hypotension, bradycardia
    4 Acrocyanosis, emphysema, and interstitial edema

12. Which of the following actions is recommended for a neonate who is being breast-fed when diagnosed with hyperbilirubinemia?
    1 Alternate feeding with supplemental formula
    2 Stop breast-feeding for 48 hours, and have mother pump breasts
    3 Add additional feeding with bottled glucose
    4 Increase the frequency of breast-feeding

13. The nurse observes slight facial jaundice in a 2-day-old full-term neonate during a postpartum home visit. The nurse interprets this finding using which one of the following assessment guidelines?
    1 Facial jaundice is common from birth to 5 days of age
    2 Bilirubin is produced at minimal rates in the neonate immediately following delivery
    3 Jaundice is visible on the skin of a neonate at levels from 4 to 6 mg/dL, which are not abnormal in a 2-day-old neonate
    4 The neonate possesses an adequate supply of liver enzymes to conjugate excess bilirubin following delivery

14. A 4-day-old newborn is receiving phototherapy at home for a bilirubin level of 14 mg/dL. The nurse should plan to include which of the following in the plan of care during the home visit to the client?
    1 Having minimal contact with the neonate to prevent stimulation
    2 Advising parents to limit newborn PO intake during phototherapy
    3 Applying lotions to exposed newborn skin
    4 Assessing skin integrity, and fluid and electrolyte status of the neonate

15. The nurse is completing a newborn assessment on a neonate whose mother had an elevated temperature during a prolonged labor. Which intervention(s) would be important to include and document in the newborn's plan of care?
    1 Maintain routine vital signs assessment
    2 Promote early maternal-newborn interaction
    3 Delay feeding the newborn for 4 hours
    4 Observe vital signs and central nervous system status frequently during the first 2 days

16. The nurse assesses hypotonia, irritability, and a poor sucking reflex in a full-term neonate upon admission to the nursery. The nurse interprets that which of the following additional sign(s) would be consistent with fetal alcohol syndrome (FAS)?
    1 Head circumference appropriate for gestational age
    2 Birth weight of 6 pounds 14 ounces
    3 Length of 19 inches
    4 Microcephaly and increased respiratory effort

17. The nurse is caring for the neonate with fetal alcohol syndrome (FAS). The nurse would plan to include which of the following priority interventions in the care of this baby?
    1 Monitor neonatal response to feedings and weight gain pattern
    2 Encourage frequent handling of neonate by staff and parents
    3 Maintain neonate in a brightly lighted area of the nursery
    4 Allow neonate to establish own sleep/rest pattern

18. A pregnant HIV-positive woman successfully delivers a baby. The nurse provides guidance to help the client in decision-making regarding newborn care. Which statement would not be included in the teaching plan for this client?
    1 Be sure to wash hands prior to and following bathroom use
    2 The infant needs to receive the recommended immunizations
    3 Breast-feeding is encouraged, especially for the first 6 weeks postpartum
    4 The newborn should be on antiviral medications for the first 6 weeks after delivery

19. A pregnant woman in her second trimester calls the prenatal clinic nurse to report a recent exposure to a child with rubella. Which of the following responses by the nurse is most appropriate?
    1 "There is no need to be concerned if you don't have a fever or rash within the next 2 days."
    2 "Be sure to tell the doctor on your next prenatal visit, but there is little risk in the second trimester."
    3 "You should avoid all school-aged children during pregnancy."
    4 "You were wise to call. I will check your rubella titer screening results and we can identify immediately whether future interventions are needed."

20. A pregnant woman has a positive history of genital herpes but has not had lesions during this pregnancy. The nurse should plan to provide which of the following information to the client?
    1 "You will be isolated from your newborn following delivery."
    2 "You will be evaluated at the time of delivery for herpetic genital tract lesions. If present, a cesarean delivery will be needed."
    3 "There is little risk to your baby during this pregnancy, the birth, and following delivery."
    4 "Vaginal deliveries can reduce neonatal infection risks even if you have an active lesion at birth."

21. The nurse administers erythromycin ointment (0.5%) to the eyes of the newborn. The mother asks the nurse why this is performed. The nurse tells the client that this is routinely done to:

1 Minimize spread of microorganisms to the neonate from invasive procedures during labor
2 Protect the neonate's eyes from possible infections acquired while hospitalized
3 Prevent ophthalmia neonatorum from occurring postdelivery to a neonate born to a woman with an untreated gonococcal infection
4 Prevent cataracts in the newborn born to a woman who is rubella susceptible

22. The client asks the nurse why her newborn baby needs an injection of vitamin K. The best response by the nurse is:
    1 "Your baby needs vitamin K to develop immunity."
    2 "The vitamin K will protect your baby from being jaundiced."
    3 "Newborns are deficient in vitamin K. This injection prevents your baby from abnormal bleeding."
    4 "Newborns have sterile bowels. Vitamin K will help the bowel become colonized with the necessary bacteria."

23. A childbirth educator teaches a class of expectant parents that it is standard routine to instill a medication into the eyes of a newborn as a preventive measure against ophthalmia neonatorum. The educator tells the class that the most common medication currently used in the United States for the prophylaxis of ophthalmia neonatorum is:
    1 Erythromycin
    2 Neomycin
    3 Penicillin
    4 Silver nitrate

24. The nursing management of an HIV-infected newborn should include which nursing goal?
    1 Instruct breast-feeding mothers regarding the treatment of their nipples with nystatin
    2 Monitor the newborn's vital signs routinely
    3 Maintain universal standards at all times while caring for the newborn
    4 Initiate referral to evaluate for blindness, deafness, and learning or behavioral problems

25. Which specific instruction should be included in the teaching plan for a mother whose newborn is HIV positive?
    1 Instruct the mother and family to provide meticulous skin care to the newborn and to change the newborn's diaper after each voiding or stool
    2 Instruct the mother to feed the neonate in an upright position, with head and chest tilted slightly back to avoid aspiration
    3 Instruct the mother to feed the newborn with a special nipple and burp the newborn frequently to decrease the tendency to swallow air

4 Instruct the mother to check the anterior fontanel for bulging and the sutures for widening each day

26. Which statement by a pregnant client with AIDS indicates her understanding of the risk to her newborn during delivery?
    1 There is a risk of transmission from HIV-positive mothers to the baby, although the newborn may be asymptomatic at birth
    2 There is no risk to the neonate of an AIDS-infected mother during delivery
    3 Newborns who contract AIDS during delivery will show immediate symptoms
    4 Newborns who are HIV positive after delivery will remain HIV positive for life

27. The nurse in the newborn nursery receives word to prepare for the admission of a 43-week-gestation neonate with Apgar scores of 1 and 4. In planning for admission of this newborn, the nurse's highest priority should be to:
    1 Connect the resuscitation bag to the oxygen outlet
    2 Turn on the apnea and cardiorespiratory monitor
    3 Set up the intravenous line with 10% dextrose in water
    4 Set up the radiant warmer control temperature at 36.5°C (97.6°F)

28. The nursery nurse teaches discharge instructions to the mother of a 5-day-old post-term newborn who required ventilatory support for 3 days for meconium aspiration. Which of the following statements, if made by the mother, indicates that the mother needs further teaching?
    1 "If my baby's hands and feet are blue in color, it usually means that they are cold."
    2 "My baby should be drinking 2.5 to 3 ounces every 4 hours."
    3 "I understand that my baby will be susceptible to respiratory infections throughout childhood."
    4 "A bluish discoloration around my baby's mouth is a sign of hypoxia."

29. The nurse is caring for a post-term, small for gestational age (SGA) neonate immediately after admission to the nursery. The priority nursing action is to monitor:
    1 Urinary output
    2 Total bilirubin levels
    3 Blood glucose levels
    4 Hemoglobin and hematocrit

30. The nurse receives a report that a large for gestational age (LGA) newborn will be admitted to the nursery. Which of the following neonatal descriptions would the nurse anticipate seeing in an LGA newborn?
    1 Weight, 3600 g; 42 weeks' gestation; absent vernix; cracked, thin skin, with yellow staining of the nailbeds and umbilical cord
    2 Weight, 3800 g; 40 weeks' gestation; flexed posture
    3 Weight, 3200 g; 34 weeks' gestation; smooth, pink skin; visible veins; abundant lanugo; and an anterior plantar crease
    4 Weight, 3400 g; 38 weeks' gestation; pink skin; rare, visible veins; and raised areola with a 4-mm breast bud

31. The nurse is performing an initial assessment on a large for gestational age (LGA) newborn. Which physical assessment technique would the nurse perform to assess for evidence of birth trauma?
    1 Palpate the clavicles for a fracture
    2 Auscultate the heart for a cardiac defect
    3 Blanch the skin for evidence of jaundice
    4 Perform Ortolani's maneuver for hip dislocation

32. The nurse is caring for a newborn with respiratory distress syndrome (RDS). Which of the following assessment data obtained by the nurse indicates a potential complication associated with this disorder?
    1 No visible bowel loops; abdomen soft with active bowel sounds
    2 No seizure activity; anterior fontanel soft and flat
    3 No audible murmur; pulse rate between 135 and 145 BPM
    4 No audible breath sounds in left lung; heart sounds louder in right side of chest

33. The nurse receives the following arterial blood gas report on a newborn with respiratory distress syndrome (RDS) who was recently weaned from the ventilator and placed in an Oxyhood at 50% oxygen: "pH 7.25, PaO$_2$ 70 mmHg, PaCO$_2$ 50 mmHg, and HCO$_3^-$ 24 mEq/L." The nurse evaluates the blood gas report as indicating:
    1 Respiratory acidosis
    2 Respiratory alkalosis
    3 Metabolic acidosis
    4 Metabolic alkalosis

34. The nurse collects a bilirubin level on a 2-day-old jaundiced term newborn. The results are total bilirubin, 7.2 mg/dL; direct bilirubin, 1.2 mg/dL; and indirect bilirubin, 6.0 mg/dL. The newborn's mother verbalizes concern over the bilirubin results. After analyzing the bilirubin results, the nurse's response includes an explanation that the bilirubin level is:
    1 Within acceptable ranges
    2 Indicative of Rh incompatibility
    3 Lower than normal for the newborn's age
    4 Indicative of a need for phototherapy

35. The nurse is caring for a newborn whose mother

is Rh negative. In planning the newborn's care, it would be most important for the nurse to:
1 Prepare for an exchange transfusion
2 Set up a phototherapy unit

3 Request the newborn's blood type and direct Coombs' test result
4 Administer an injection of vitamin K to prevent isoimmunization

ANSWERS

1. **2**

Rationale: Bathing should start at the eyes and face, usually the cleanest area. Next, the external ear and behind the ears are cleansed. The newborn's neck should be washed because formula, lint, or breast milk will often accumulate in the folds of the neck. Hands and arms are then washed. The baby's legs are washed, and the diaper area is washed last.

Test-Taking Strategy: Remember the basic techniques of bathing a client. Remember, when bathing an adult or baby, start with the cleanest part of the body and proceed to the dirtiest part. Options 1, 3, and 4 are incorrect.

Level of Cognitive Ability: Application
Phase of Nursing Process: Implementation
Client Needs: Health Promotion and Maintenance
Content Area: Maternity

Reference
Nichols, F., & Zwelling, E. (1997). *Maternal-newborn nursing: Theory and practice.* Philadelphia: W. B. Saunders. pp. 1159–1161.

2. **4**

Rationale: Evaporation of moisture from wet body surfaces dissipates heat along with the moisture. By keeping the baby dry (by drying the wet baby at birth), evaporation is prevented.

Test-Taking Strategy: There are four methods of heat loss. Conduction occurs when the baby is on a cold surface, such as a pad. Convection occurs as air moves across the baby's skin from an open door and heat is transferred to the air. Radiation occurs when heat from the body radiates to a colder surface. Evaporation occurs when moisture from the newborn's wet body surface dissipates heat along with moisture. Preventing heat loss in a newborn is an important nursing intervention. Review these concepts now, if you had difficulty with this question!

Level of Cognitive Ability: Application
Phase of Nursing Process: Planning
Client Needs: Physiological Integrity
Content Area: Maternity

Reference
Nichols, F., & Zwelling. E. (1997). *Maternal-newborn nursing: Theory and practice.* Philadelphia: W. B. Saunders. pp. 1072–1073.

3. **3**

Rationale: The cord should be kept clean and dry to decrease bacterial growth. This includes keeping the diaper folded below the cord to keep urine away from the cord. The cord should be cleansed two to three times a day. It usually falls off within 7 to 14 days. Agents other than alcohol may be used to clean the cord.

Test-Taking Strategy: Use the process of elimination in answering the question. Option 1 is incorrect. Cord care is required until the cord dries up and falls off between 7 and 14 days. Agents other than alcohol may be used on the cord. Option 4 is incorrect: the cord should fall off between 7 and 14 days. Option 3 is the most global and correct answer. Use the process of elimination to answer the questions. Review the concepts of cord care now, if you had difficulty answering the question!

Level of Cognitive Ability: Analysis
Phase of Nursing Process: Analysis
Client Needs: Physiological Integrity
Content Area: Maternity

Reference
Nichols, F., & Zwelling, E. (1997). *Maternal-newborn nursing: Theory and practice.* Philadelphia: W. B. Saunders. p. 1147.

4. **2**

Rationale: The cord and base should be cleaned two to three times per day. The steps are to lift the cord, wipe around it starting at the top, clean the base of the cord, and fold the diaper below the umbilical cord to allow the cord to air dry.

Test-Taking Strategy: Use the process of elimination in answering the question. Option 1 is incorrect. Continuation of cord care is necessary until the cord falls off within 7 to 14 days. Option 3 is incorrect. The cord needs to be cleansed with alcohol thoroughly. The baby does not feel pain in this area. Option 4 is incorrect. Water and soap are not necessary; in fact, the cord should be kept from getting wet. Review the principles related to cord care now, if you had difficulty with this question!

Level of Cognitive Ability: Application
Phase of Nursing Process: Implementation
Client Needs: Health Promotion and Maintenance
Content Area: Maternity

Reference
Nichols, F., & Zwelling. E. (1997). *Maternal-newborn nursing: Theory and practice.* Philadelphia: W. B. Saunders. p. 1147.

5. **2**

Rationale: Symptoms of infection are moistness, oozing, discharge, and a reddened base. If symptoms of infection occur, notify health care providers. Antibiotic treatment is necessary.

Test-Taking Strategy: Use the process of elimination in answering the question. The word "discharge" in option 2 is the key to indicating infection. Options 1 and 3 are normal signs. Option 4 may suggest signs of infection, but option 2 signifies definite signs of infection. Review the signs and symptoms of infection now, if you had difficulty with this question!

Level of Cognitive Ability: Analysis
Phase of Nursing Process: Evaluation
Client Needs: Physiological Integrity
Content Area: Maternity

Reference
Nichols, F., & Zwelling. E. (1997). *Maternal-newborn nursing: Theory and practice*. Philadelphia: W. B. Saunders. p. 1147.

6. **2**

Rationale: The glans penis is normally dark red. A small amount of bloody drainage is expected. During the healing process, the glans becomes covered with a yellow exudate in 24 hours. This is a part of normal healing. If excessive bleeding is noted from the circumcision, the nurse applies gentle pressure to the site of bleeding with a sterile, folded 4×4. If bleeding is not controlled, a blood vessel may need to be ligated. The nurse notifies the physician.

Test-Taking Strategy: Read the question carefully. The question asks for an expected appearance. Use the process of elimination. A small amount of bloody drainage is expected. Option 1 indicates the appearance of a healed circumcision. Option 3 is incorrect, as there should be only a slight amount of bleeding. Option 4 indicates how the site should appear 24 hours after the circumcision. Review the procedure related to circumcision now, if you had difficulty with this question!

Level of Cognitive Ability: Analysis
Phase of Nursing Process: Assessment
Client Needs: Physiological Integrity
Content Area: Maternity

Reference
Lowdermilk, D., Perry, S., & Bobak, I. (1997). *Maternity & women's health care* (6th ed.). St. Louis: Mosby–Year Book. p. 585.

7. **2**

Rationale: In newborn boys, the prepuce is continuous with the epidermis of the glans and is nonretractable. Forced retraction may cause adhesions to develop. Current recommendations are to allow separation to occur naturally, which will occur between 3 years of age and puberty. Most foreskins are retractable by 3 years of age and should be pushed back gently for cleaning once a week.

Test-Taking Strategy: Look for the option that is different. Options 1, 3, and 4 are incorrect because retracting the foreskin is not recommended in an uncircumcised male. Option 2 is the only different option, stating that the foreskin should not be retracted.

Level of Cognitive Ability: Application
Phase of Nursing Process: Implementation
Client Needs: Health Promotion and Maintenance
Content Area: Maternity

Reference
Reeder, S., Martin, L., & Koniak-Griffin, D. (1997). *Maternity nursing: Family, newborn, and women's health care* (18th ed.). Philadelphia: Lippincott-Raven. p. 747.

8. **1**

Rationale: Wearing breast shells and using a breast pump before each feeding will make it easier for the newborn to grasp the nipple.

Test-Taking Strategy: True inverted nipples will retract if the areola is pressed between the thumb and forefinger, making option 2 incorrect. Option 3 is good advice for mothers suffering from engorgement. Option 4 will only make the mother cold and has no effect on inverted nipples. Use the process of elimination to assist with answering this question. Review the concepts related to breast-feeding if you had difficulty with this question!

Level of Cognitive Ability: Application
Phase of Nursing Process: Implementation
Client Needs: Physiological Integrity
Content Area: Maternity

Reference
Reeder, S., Martin, L., & Koniak-Griffin, D., (1997). *Maternity nursing: Family, newborn and women's health care* (18th ed.). Philadelphia: Lippincott-Raven. p. 779.

9. **1**

Rationale: The baby should be positioned completely facing the mother, with head, neck, and spine aligned. Poor positioning increases the number of attempts for latching on.

Test-Taking Strategy: Option 2 is incorrect because it demonstrates improper positioning. Options 3 and 4 are the result of improper positioning. Additionally, options 2, 3, and 4 all identify complications (sore nipples, breast engorgement, cracked nipples). Option 1 is the only option that identifies a normal expectation.

Level of Cognitive Ability: Analysis
Phase of Nursing Process: Evaluation
Client Needs: Health Promotion and Maintenance
Content Area: Maternity

Reference
Nichols, F., & Zwelling, E. (1997). *Maternal-newborn nursing: Theory and practice*. Philadelphia: W. B. Saunders. pp. 1217–1220.

10. **1**

Rationale: The skin of a newborn plays a significant role in thermoregulation and as a barrier against infection. The skin is immature in contrast to that of a term newborn. The skin of a preterm newborn is thin and gelatinous. There are decreased amounts of subcutaneous fat, brown fat, and glycogen stores. In addition, preterm newborns lose heat because of the high body surface area in relation to their weight and because their posture is more relaxed with less flexion. For these reasons, preterm newborns are less able to generate heat. This places the preterm newborn at risk for increased heat loss and increased fluid requirements.

Test-Taking Strategy: Options 2, 3, and 4 are incorrect. Preterm newborns have open posture (option 1), which contributes to heat loss. Also, they have decreased amounts of subcutaneous and brown fat. Option 4 is partially correct in that they may have fine, downy hair, considering their gestational age, but the remainder of this option is incorrect. Review the characteristics of a preterm newborn now, if you had difficulty with this question!

Level of Cognitive Ability: Analysis
Phase of Nursing Process: Analysis
Client Needs: Physiological Integrity
Content Area: Maternity

Reference
Nichols, F., & Zwelling. E. (1997). *Maternal-newborn nursing: Theory and practice*. Philadelphia: W. B. Saunders. p. 1348.

11. **1**

Rationale: The neonate with RDS may present with clinical signs of cyanosis, tachypnea, or apnea, nasal flaring, chest wall retractions, or an audible expiratory grunt. Acrocyanosis is a normal finding in a neonate. It is the bluish discoloration of the hands or feet. Option 3 is incorrect.

Test-Taking Strategy: Read all the components of each option carefully. Remembering that acrocyanosis is a normal sign in a newborn will assist in eliminating options 2 and 4. Option 1 is the best choice because all the signs present in this option are related to the respiratory system.

Level of Cognitive Ability: Analysis
Phase of Nursing Process: Assessment
Client Needs: Physiological Integrity
Content Area: Maternity

Reference
Nichols, F., & Zwelling, E. (1997). *Maternal-newborn nursing: Theory and practice.* Philadelphia: W. B. Saunders. p. 1342.

12. **4**

Rationale: Supplementation with water does not reduce hyperbilirubinemia. The greater the number of breast-feedings, the lower the bilirubin. Breast-feeding should be initiated early and be frequent. Discourage water, dextrose H_2O, or formula supplements.

Test-Taking Strategy: Use the process of elimination in answering the question. Options 1 and 2 are incorrect as these options do not encourage continuation of breast-feeding and can cause nipple confusion in the newborn. Option 3 is incorrect; bilirubin is excreted in the stool and the addition of glucose water will only cause an increase in urination. Review hyperbilirubinemia now, if you had difficulty with this question!

Level of Cognitive Ability: Application
Phase of Nursing Process: Implementation
Client Needs: Physiological Integrity
Content Area: Maternity

Reference
Ashwill, J., & Droske, S. (1997). *Nursing care of children: Principles and practice.* Philadelphia: W. B. Saunders. p. 65.

13. **3**

Rationale: Neonatal bilirubin levels below 12 mg/dL on the second to seventh day following birth are considered normal in the full-term neonate. Jaundice is visible in the skin at levels from 4 to 6 mg/dL. Options 1, 2, and 4 are incorrect.

Test-Taking Strategy: A thorough understanding of the principles of normal physiological jaundice in the full-term neonate is necessary to answer this question correctly. In addition, you can assume that all other physiological parameters of the neonate, such as cardiopulmonary functioning, were normal at birth since the newborn was discharged early following delivery. If you had difficulty with this question, take the time now to review the content related to normal physiological jaundice!

Level of Cognitive Ability: Analysis
Phase of Nursing Process: Analysis
Client Needs: Physiological Integrity
Content Area: Maternity

Reference
Nichols, F., & Zwelling, E. (1997). *Maternal-newborn nursing: Theory and practice.* Philadelphia: W. B. Saunders. pp. 1070–1071.

14. **4**

Rationale: Safe care for the newborn during phototherapy requires shielding the eyes, using a soft eye shield to prevent retinal damage; keeping the newborn skin exposed except for a diaper; and changing position frequently. No lotions should be used to minimize skin breakdown and enhance the therapeutic effect of light in subcutaneous tissue. Adequate oral fluids are essential to prevent dehydration, since diarrhea is a common side effect of therapy. Contact with the neonate is important.

Test-Taking Strategy: Use the process of elimination in answering this question. The nursing care plan for safe home therapy of the newborn is guided by the principles of maintaining adequate skin integrity, parental bonding, and neonatal fluid and electrolyte balance. Recalling these principles allows you to eliminate each of the incorrect options successfully. If you had difficulty with this question, take the time now to review the content related to phototherapy!

Level of Cognitive Ability: Application
Phase of Nursing Process: Planning
Client Needs: Health Promotion and Maintenance
Content Area: Maternity

Reference
Reeder, S., Martin, L., & Koniak-Griffin, D. (1997). *Maternity nursing: Family, newborn and women's health* (18th ed.). Philadelphia: Lippincott-Raven. pp. 1214–1216.

15. **4**

Rationale: During the postnatal period, the time of onset of suspicious signs is crucial. Onset of symptoms within the first 48 hours of life is more often associated with prenatal or perinatal risk factors. Clinical signs of sepsis in the newborn include temperature instability, tachycardia, respiratory changes, and central nervous symptoms, such as lethargy, irritability, or hypotonia.

Test-Taking Strategy: To answer this question correctly, you need to know the early neonatal signs of sepsis. Note that the question concerns a mother who had an elevated temperature during a prolonged labor. This provides a clue that neonatal assessments need to be more frequent than the routine. This would eliminate option 1. Promoting early maternal-newborn interaction is always important but is not directly related to answering this question. Delaying a feeding is not appropriate. Frequent assessment of vital signs and central nervous system adaptation ensures that caregivers will recognize signs early and, it is hoped, avert further compromise to the airway, breathing, and circulatory status of a newborn. Option 4 is the most specific and thorough option.

Level of Cognitive Ability: Application
Phase of Nursing Process: Planning
Client Needs: Physiological Integrity
Content Area: Maternity

Reference
Lowdermilk, D., Perry, S., & Bobak, I. (1997). *Maternity and women's health care* (6th ed.). St. Louis: Mosby–Year Book. p. 1084.

16. **4**

Rationale: Features of neonates at birth who are eventually diagnosed with FAS include craniofacial abnormalities, cleft lip or palate, intrauterine growth retardation (IUGR), cardiac abnormalities, abnormal palmar creases, and irregular hair distribution. Microcephaly, limb anomalies, and increased respiratory effort during the transition to extrauterine life are also frequently noted by caregivers.

Test-Taking Strategy: Knowledge regarding normal assessment findings in the full-term newborn and FAS is required to answer this question. This question asks the nurse to analyze the characteristics observed in the neonate and to continue to collect data based upon the knowledge of the physiological changes that can occur in the neonate exposed to alcohol during pregnancy. Use the process of elimination in answering this question. The other distracters represent normal assessment findings in the full-term newborn and can be eliminated as options. If you had difficulty with this question, take the time now to review the content related to normal newborn assessment findings and FAS!

Level of Cognitive Ability: Analysis
Phase of Nursing Process: Assessment
Client Needs: Physiological Integrity
Content Area: Maternity

Reference

Lowdermilk, D., Perry, S., & Bobak, I. (1997). *Maternity and women's health care* (6th ed.). St. Louis: Mosby–Year Book. pp. 1094–1096.

17. 1

Rationale: A primary nursing goal for the neonate diagnosed with FAS is to establish nutritional balance following delivery. These neonates may exhibit hyperirritability, vomiting, diarrhea, or an uncoordinated sucking and swallowing ability. A quiet environment with minimal stimuli and handling will help establish appropriate sleep/rest cycles in the neonate as well.

Test-Taking Strategy: Utilize Maslow's hierarchy of needs theory to assist in answering this question. Option 1 addresses physiological needs most directly, ensures the safest environment for the neonate, and minimizes potential side effects from aspiration or vomiting.

Level of Cognitive Ability: Application
Phase of Nursing Process: Planning
Client Needs: Physiological Integrity
Content Area: Maternity

Reference

Nichols, F., & Zwelling, E. (1997). *Maternal-newborn nursing: Theory and practice.* Philadelphia: W. B. Saunders. pp. 1359–1361.

18. 3

Rationale: Handwashing is an important preventative measure. The infant will need to receive all recommended immunizations. HIV acquisition can occur during breast-feeding, thus HIV-positive clients should be encouraged to bottle-feed their neonates. Neonates of HIV-positive clients are recommended to receive a dose of zidovudine (AZT) suspension, 2 mg/kg PO every 6 hours for the first 6 weeks of life.

Test-Taking Strategy: The correct response to this question requires that the nurse apply appropriate knowledge of the transmission of HIV and universal precautions to the postpartum guidance of an HIV-infected mother. Options 1 and 2 can be easily eliminated using principles of aseptic techniques and health promotion measures. Knowledge that HIV can be transmitted via breast milk will easily direct you to option 3. The guidance provides safe, effective care to minimize viral transmission following birth.

Level of Cognitive Ability: Application
Phase of Nursing Process: Implementation
Client Needs: Safe, Effective Care Environment
Content Area: Maternity

Reference

Nichols, F., & Zwelling, E. (1997). *Maternal-newborn nursing: Theory and practice.* Philadelphia: W. B. Saunders. pp. 1500–1501.

19. 4

Rationale: Rubella virus is spread by aerosol droplet transmission through the upper respiratory tract and has an incubation period of 14 to 21 days. Rubella can be asymptomatic in up to 50% of cases. The risks of maternal and subsequent fetal infection during the second trimester include hearing loss and congenital anomalies. Rubella titer determination is a standard antenatal test for childbearing women during their initial screening and entry into the health care delivery system.

Test-Taking Strategy: Knowledge regarding the transmission of rubella virus to the fetus is required to answer this question. Option 4 reconfirms maternal behavior and helps clarify maternal concerns with accurate information based upon the acquisition of rubella infection and potential fetal side effects. Use the process of elimination. The remaining interventions are incorrect and are systematically eliminated as possible choices.

Level of Cognitive Ability: Application
Phase of Nursing Process: Implementation
Client Needs: Physiological Integrity
Content Area: Maternity

Reference

Nichols, F., & Zwelling, E. (1997). *Maternal-newborn nursing: Theory and practice.* Philadelphia: W. B. Saunders. pp. 1509–1510.

20. 2

Rationale: The following recommendations have been endorsed by the Infectious Disease Society for Obstetrics-Gynecology for women with a positive history of genital herpes during childbearing: In the absence of genital lesions, vaginal delivery is indicated unless there are other indications for cesarean delivery. For herpetic genital lesions in labor or with ruptured membranes, cesarean delivery can reduce neonatal infection risks. Maternal isolation is not necessary, but potentially exposed neonates should be cultured on the day of delivery.

Test-Taking Strategy: The appropriate response of the nurse is based upon applying the knowledge of the course of transmission of the herpesvirus from an infected mother to the neonate during the childbearing period. This response also assists the client to plan for the future realistically. If you had difficulty with this question, utilize the reference source listed and take the time to review this content now!

Level of Cognitive Ability: Application
Phase of Nursing Process: Planning
Client Needs: Health Promotion and Maintenance
Content Area: Maternity

Reference

Nichols, F., & Zwelling, E. (1997). *Maternal-newborn nursing: Theory and practice.* Philadelphia: W. B. Saunders. pp. 1495–1496.

21. 3

Rationale: During the labor of a woman with gonococcal infection, ascending infection can occur following the rupture of membranes. Contamination can also occur as the neonate passes through the birth canal. The organism may invade fetal mucosal surfaces such as conjunctiva, rectal mucosa, and pharynx. Erythromycin ophthalmic ointment (0.5%) is an acceptable prophylactic treatment following delivery (1% silver nitrate may also be administered).

Test-Taking Strategy: This question tests your knowledge of standard nursing protocols of care for all newborns following delivery. The application of knowledge related to the spread of gonococcal infection during the childbearing period is also needed. Knowledge of these areas guides you to eliminate each of the other incorrect options. If you had difficulty with this question, take the time now to review initial care of the newborn!

Level of Cognitive Ability: Application
Phase of Nursing Process: Implementation
Client Needs: Physiological integrity
Content Area: Maternity

Reference
Lowdermilk, D., Perry S., & Bobak, I. (1997). *Maternity and women's health care* (6th ed.). St. Louis: Mosby–Year Book. p. 1086.

22. **3**

Rationale: Vitamin K is administered to the neonate to prevent abnormal bleeding. Newborns are vitamin K–deficient because their bowels are sterile. The normal flora in the intestinal tract produces vitamin K. The neonate's bowel does not support the normal production of vitamin K until bacteria adequately colonize it. The bowel becomes colonized by bacteria as food is ingested. Vitamin K is necessary for the body to synthesize coagulation factors. Parenteral administration of vitamin K is a well-substantiated measure to correct the neonate's lag in vitamin K production and prevent hemorrhagic disease of the newborn caused by vitamin K deficiency.

Test-Taking Strategy: A knowledge of the action of vitamin K and the physiology of the gastrointestinal tract is necessary to answer this question. Use the process of elimination to eliminate incorrect options. Because jaundice and immunity are not related to the action of vitamin K, options 1 and 2 should be eliminated. The issue of the question is about the action of a medication. Note the similar words: "injection" in the question and "injection" in the correct option. If you had difficulty with this question, review the purpose of vitamin K injection in the neonate now!

Level of Cognitive Ability: Application
Phase of Nursing Process: Implementation
Client Needs: Physiological Integrity
Content Area: Maternity

Reference
Nichols, F. H., Zwelling, E. (1997). *Maternal-newborn nursing; Theory and practice*. Philadelphia: W. B. Saunders. pp. 1141–1142, 1152.

23. **1**

Rationale: Ophthalmic erythromycin 0.5% ointment is a broad-spectrum antibiotic and is used prophylatically to prevent ophthalmia neonatorum, an eye infection acquired from the baby's passage through the birth canal. Ophthalmia neonatorum is caused mostly by the presence of gonococci and/or chlamydia. Infection from these organisms can cause blindness or serious eye damage. Erythromycin is effective against both chlamydia and gonococci. None of the other choices are effective against both bacteria.

Test-Taking Strategy: Knowledge of medications and ophthalmia neonatorum is necessary to answer this question. A knowledge of medications given routinely to the neonate is a priority. If you had difficulty with this question, take the time now to review initial care of the newborn!

Level of Cognitive Ability: Application
Phase of Nursing Process: Implementation
Client Needs: Physiological Integrity
Content Area: Maternity

Reference
Lowdermilk, D., Perry S., & Bobak, I. (1997). *Maternity and women's health care* (6th ed.). St. Louis: Mosby–Year Book. p. 1086.

24. **3**

Rationale: The HIV-infected newborn must be cared for with strict attention to universal standards (precautions). This prevents the transmission of AIDS from the newborn to others and prevents transmission of other infectious agents to the immunocompromised newborn.

Test-Taking Strategy: Use the process of elimination to answer this question. Identify the client of the question. The client of the question is the newborn; therefore, option 1 can be eliminated because it addresses care to the mother. Remember priorities of nursing care. In reviewing the options to this question, the priority is to ensure universal standards are maintained. The nurse would maintain universal standards first!

Level of Cognitive Ability: Application
Phase of Nursing Process: Implementation
Client Needs: Safe, Effective Care Environment
Content Area: Maternity

Reference
Olds, S., London, M., & Ladewig, P. (1996). *Clinical handbook for maternal-newborn nursing: A family-centered approach* (5th ed.). Reading, MA: Addison-Wesley. p. 195.

25. **1**

Rationale: Meticulous skin care helps protect the HIV-positive newborn from secondary infections. Feeding the newborn in an upright position, using a special nipple, and bulging fontanels are unrelated to the pathology associated with HIV.

Test-Taking Strategy: Read the question carefully. The question specifically asks for instructions to be given to the mother regarding HIV. Although options 2, 3, and 4 may be correct or partially correct in substance, the content does not specifically relate to care to the newborn that is HIV positive.

Level of Cognitive Ability: Application
Phase of Nursing Process: Planning
Client Needs: Safe, Effective Care Environment
Content Area: Maternity

Reference
Olds, S., London, M., & Ladewig, P. (1996). *Clinical handbook for maternal-newborn nursing: A family-centered approach* (5th ed.). Reading, MA: Addison-Wesley. p. 195.

26. **1**

Rationale: There is a risk of transmission of HIV/AIDS to newborns at delivery when the pregnant woman is HIV positive. Newborns may not exhibit symptoms for 18 months or more.

Test-Taking Strategy: Knowledge regarding the risk of transmission of HIV/AIDS to newborns at delivery is necessary to answer this question. Understanding the risk of transmission of HIV is an extremely important issue. If you had difficulty answering this question or are unsure of this content area, take the time now to review this material!

Level of Cognitive Ability: Analysis
Phase of Nursing Process: Evaluation
Client Needs: Health Promotion and Maintenance
Content Area: Maternity

Reference
Olds, S., London, M., & Ladewig, P. (1996). *Clinical handbook for maternal-newborn nursing: A family-centered approach* (5th ed.). Reading, MA: Addison-Wesley. pp. 54–55, 194–195.

27. **1**

Rationale: First priority on admission to the nursery for a newborn with low Apgar scores is airway, which would involve preparing respiratory resuscitation equipment. The remaining options are also important, although they are of somewhat lower priority. Setting up an IV with 5% dextrose in water will provide circulatory support. The radiant warmer will provide an external heat source, which is necessary to prevent further respiratory distress. Monitoring devices may be important for assessment but do not provide support measures.

Test-Taking Strategy: This question asks you to prioritize care planning based on information about a newborn's condition. Remember the ABCs (Airway, Breathing, Circulation). A method of planning for airway support is to have the resuscitation bag connected to an oxygen source.

Level of Cognitive Ability: Application
Phase of Nursing Process: Planning
Client Needs: Physiological Integrity
Content Area: Maternity

Reference
Pillitteri, A. (1995). *Maternal & child health nursing: Care of the childbearing and childrearing family* (2nd ed.). Philadelphia: Lippincott-Raven. pp. 760–761.

28. **3**

Rationale: Option 3 is not true for the post-term newborn. Once the meconium aspiration syndrome is resolved, the newborn should be cared for like any other newborn. Options 1, 2, and 4 are true statements and reflect understanding of discharge instructions.

Test-Taking Strategy: This question asks you to identify the option that is incorrect, therefore requiring additional instructions to the mother. Options 1, 2, and 4 are correct statements. Option 3 is incorrect. You must utilize theory knowledge of postdischarge care of the post-term newborn to answer this question.

Level of Cognitive Ability: Analysis
Phase of Nursing Process: Evaluation
Client Needs: Health Promotion and Maintenance
Content Area: Maternity

Reference
Pillitteri, A. (1995). *Maternal & child health nursing: Care of the childbearing and childrearing family* (2nd ed.). Philadelphia: Lippincott-Raven. pp. 760–761.

29. **3**

Rationale: The most common metabolic complication in the SGA newborn is hypoglycemia, which can produce central nervous system abnormalities and mental retardation if not corrected immediately. Urinary output, although important, is not the highest priority action because the post-term SGA neonate is typically dehydrated due to placental dysfunction. Hemoglobin and hematocrit levels are monitored because the post-term SGA neonate exhibits polycythemia, although this also does not require immediate attention. The polycythemia contributes to increased bilirubin levels, usually beginning on the second day after delivery.

Test-Taking Strategy: This question asks you to identify the priority nursing action. Knowledge of initial problems in the post-term SGA newborn is also needed to answer this question. Review the SGA newborn content now, if you had difficulty with this question!

Level of Cognitive Ability: Application
Phase of Nursing Process: Implementation
Client Needs: Physiological Integrity
Content Area: Maternity

Reference
Olds, S., London, M., and Ladewig, P. (1996). *Maternal-newborn nursing: A family-centered approach* (5th ed.). Reading, MA: Addison-Wesley. pp. 924, 926–928.

30. **3**

Rationale: Option 3 describes the characteristics of a preterm (34 weeks) LGA newborn. The weight of 3200 grams is above the 90th percentile on an intrauterine growth chart, which is a definitive criterion for the LGA newborn. Option 1 describes a post-term newborn whose weight is within the 10th and 90th percentiles. Options 2 and 4 describe term newborns whose weights are within the 10th and 90th percentiles.

Test-Taking Strategy: This question asks you to recognize the LGA newborn by weight, gestational age, and description. Options 1, 2, and 4 can be grouped together as not meeting LGA criteria because of the closeness in gestational age and weights. Option 3 can also be compared with option 4, noting that the 200-gram weight difference does not equate to a 4-week-gestation time span. Use the process of elimination and look at each component in each option to answer the question!

Level of Cognitive Ability: Analysis
Phase of Nursing Process: Assessment
Client Needs: Physiological Integrity
Content Area: Maternity

Reference
Reeder, S., Martin, L., & Koniak-Griffin, D. (1997). *Maternity nursing: Family, newborn, and women's health care* (18th ed.). Philadelphia: Lippincott-Raven. pp. 716, 1121–1122.

31. **1**

Rationale: Because of the neonate's large size, there is an increased risk for shoulder dystocia. This may result in fractured clavicles and/or brachial plexus palsy. Other complications related to birth trauma include facial paralysis, phrenic nerve palsy, depressed skull fractures, hematomas, and bleeding. Option 2 is not related to birth trauma even though there is an increase in cardiac defects in the LGA newborn. Option 3 would not be present initially. Hip dislocation is congenital and is not caused by birth trauma.

Test-Taking Strategy: The question asks you to identify an assessment technique that would be used in assessing for birth trauma. Think of trauma as an injury. Option 1 is the only option that identifies an injury. Knowledge of evidence of birth trauma is required to answer this question correctly.

Level of Cognitive Ability: Application
Phase of Nursing Process: Assessment
Client Needs: Physiological Integrity
Content Area: Maternity

Reference
Pillitteri, A. (1995). *Maternal & child health nursing: Care of the childbearing and childrearing family* (2nd ed.). Philadelphia: Lippincott-Raven. p. 773.

32. **4**

Rationale: Pneumothorax, intraventricular hemorrhage (IVH), patent ductus arteriosus (PDA), and necrotizing enterocolitis (NEC) are complications associated with RDS. Clinical signs of pneumothorax include a sudden rapid deterioration in condition, tachypnea, grunting, pallor, cyanosis, decreased breath sounds in affected lung, shifting of the cardiac apex away from an affected lung, bradycardia, and hypertension. In IVH, the newborn may exhibit a dramatic change in condition, showing apnea, bradycardia, hypotension, seizures, decerebrate posturing, bulging anterior fontanel, and temperature instability. PDA usually presents with a murmur, wide pulse pressures, tachycardia, bounding pulses, signs and symptoms of pulmonary edema, retractions, and rales. Signs found in NEC include lethargy, abdominal distention, temperature instability, retention of feedings, and visible bowel loops.

Test-Taking Strategy: This question asks you to identify signs and symptoms of potential complications of RDS. Knowledge of these complications is required. Three of the options (1, 2, and 3) can also be grouped together because they each contain normal assessment findings, which leaves option 4 as the correct answer. Additionally, option 4 is the option that identifies respiratory signs.

Level of Cognitive Ability: Analysis
Phase of Nursing Process: Assessment
Client Needs: Physiological Integrity
Content Area: Maternity

Reference
Reeder, S., Martin, L., & Koniak-Griffin, D. (1997). *Maternity nursing: Family, newborn, and women's health care* (18th ed.). Philadelphia: Lippincott-Raven. p. 1169.

33. **1**

Rationale: In normal acid-base balance, the pH is 7.35 to 7.45. Normal PaO_2 is 50 to 80 mmHg, and normal $PaCO_2$ is 35 to 45 mmHg. A decreased pH with an increased $PaCO_2$ indicates a respiratory acidosis. Respiratory alkalosis is defined as a pH above 7.45 and a $PaCO_2$ below 35 mmHg. Metabolic acidosis exists with a pH below 7.35 and an HCO_3^- below 20 mEq/L. Metabolic alkalosis is defined as a pH above 7.45, along with an HCO_3^- above 24 mEq/L. Normal HCO_3^- is 20 to 24 mEq/L.

Test-Taking Strategy: This question requires that you possess knowledge about arterial blood gas interpretation. Begin by identifying the difference between acidosis and alkalosis, then progress to differentiate between respiratory and metabolic causes. Knowledge of the normal ranges for blood gas results is also necessary. Take the time now to review the steps in reading and interpreting blood gases if you had difficulty with this question!

Level of Cognitive Ability: Analysis
Phase of Nursing Process: Evaluation
Client Needs: Physiological Integrity
Content Area: Maternity

Reference
Olds, S., London, M., & Ladewig, P. (1996). *Maternal-newborn nursing: A family-centered approach* (5th ed.). Reading, MA: Addison-Wesley. pp. 998–1000.

34. **1**

Rationale: Total bilirubin levels tend to peak on the second and third days after birth. These levels are between 5 and 10 mg/dL in the healthy newborn. The range given is normal for a 2-day-old newborn, and there are no data to support an Rh incompatibility. Term newborns are not treated with phototherapy until their bilirubin is above 12 mg/dL.

Test-Taking Strategy: This question asks you to analyze bilirubin results in a 2-day-old jaundiced term newborn. Knowledge about normal levels will assist in eliminating options 3 and 4. You could eliminate option 2 because specific blood-type information is not provided. Review these concepts now, if you had difficulty with this question!

Level of Cognitive Ability: Analysis
Phase of Nursing Process: Analysis
Client Needs: Physiological Integrity
Content Area: Maternity

Reference
Reeder, S., Martin, L., & Koniak-Griffin, D. (1997). *Maternity nursing: Family, newborn, and women's health care* (18th ed.). Philadelphia: Lippincott-Raven. pp. 1213–1215.

35. **3**

Rationale: To further assess and plan for the newborn's care, the newborn's blood type and direct Coombs' test result must be known. If the newborn's blood type is Rh negative, or if the newborn's blood type is Rh positive with a negative direct Coombs' test, then there is no concern about Rh incompatibility. If the newborn's blood type is Rh positive and the direct Coombs' is positive, then Rh incompatibility exists. Options 1 and 2 are inappropriate at this time because additional data are needed. Option 4 is incorrect because vitamin K is given to prevent hemorrhagic disease of the newborn.

Test-Taking Strategy: This question asks you to select the most important plan based on the mother's Rh blood type. Use the nursing process to prioritize, and remember, assessment is the first step! Additional data are required before any additional nursing plans can be formalized.

Level of Cognitive Ability: Application
Phase of Nursing Process: Planning
Client Needs: Physiological Integrity
Content Area: Maternity

Reference
Pillitteri, A. (1995). *Maternal & child health nursing: Care of the childbearing and childrearing family* (2nd ed.). Philadelphia: Lippincott-Raven. pp. 415–417, 768–769.

BIBLIOGRAPHY

Ashwill, J., & Droske, S. (1997). *Nursing care of children: Principles and practice*. Philadelphia: W. B. Saunders.

Lowdermilk, D., Perry, S., & Bobak, I. (1997). *Maternity & women's health care* (6th ed.). St. Louis: Mosby–Year Book.

Luckmann, J. (1997). *Manual of nursing care*. Philadelphia: W. B. Saunders.

Nichols, F., & Zwelling, E. (1997). *Maternal-newborn nursing: Theory and practice*. Philadelphia: W. B. Saunders.

Olds, S., London, M., & Ladewig, P. (1996). *Clinical handbook for maternal-newborn nursing: A family-centered approach* (5th ed.). Reading, MA: Addison-Wesley.

O'Toole, M. (ed.). (1997). *Miller-Keane encyclopedia & dictionary of medicine, nursing, & allied health* (6th ed.). Philadelphia: W. B. Saunders.

Pillitteri, A. (1995). *Maternal & child health nursing: Care of the childbearing and childrearing family* (2nd ed.). Philadelphia: Lippincott-Raven.

Reeder, S., Martin, L., & Koniak-Griffin, D. (1997). *Maternity nursing: Family, newborn, and women's health care* (18th ed.). Philadelphia: Lippincott-Raven.

CHAPTER 31

Maternity and Newborn Medications

....

I. Beractant (Survanta)

A. Description
1. Lung surfactant
2. Used to prevent or treat respiratory distress syndrome
3. Replenishes surfactant and restores surface activity to the lungs
B. Implementation
1. Monitor for bradycardia and decreased oxygen saturation during administration
2. Assess lung sounds for rales and moist breath sounds

II. Betamethasone (Celestone)

A. Description
1. Corticosteroid
2. Increases production of surfactant
3. Used for client in preterm **labor** between 28 and 32 weeks whose **labor** can be inhibited for 48 hours without jeopardizing mother or fetus
4. Medication crosses **placenta**
5. Distributed in breast milk
B. Implementation
1. Decreases mother's resistance to infection
2. Monitor mother for infection
3. Monitor WBC count
4. Breast-feeding is contraindicated during medication administration
5. Chronic use of the medication during the first trimester may cause cleft palate

III. Butorphanol Tartrate (Stadol)

A. Description
1. Exerts an analgesic effect
2. Is a narcotic agonist-antagonist
3. Used to relieve moderate to severe pain associated with **labor**
4. Readily crosses **placenta**
5. Distributed in breast milk
B. Implementation
1. Use cautiously in clients delivering preterm infants
2. Do not administer during advanced **labor** if the neonate is expected to be delivered before the medication is adequately removed from fetal circulation, because respiratory depression can occur
3. If the woman has a pre-existing narcotic dependency, the antagonist effect of these compounds will cause her to exhibit symptoms of narcotic withdrawal immediately
4. Assess fetal heart tones and uterine contractions
5. Not recommended if the client is breast-feeding

IV. Ergonovine Maleate (Ergotrate)

A. Description
1. Directly stimulates uterine muscle and increases the force and frequency of contractions
2. Produces a firm, tetanic contraction of the uterus
3. Produces arterial vasoconstriction and can cause vasospasm of the coronary arteries
4. Used to prevent or treat postpartum and postabortal hemorrhage due to atony or involution
5. Contraindicated during pregnancy
B. Implementation
1. Not to be used before the **delivery** of the newborn
2. Monitor blood pressure closely, because the medication produces vasoconstriction; if a rise is noted, withhold the medication and notify the physician
3. Monitor uterine contractions (frequency, strength, and duration) frequently
4. Assess extremities for color, warmth, movement, and pain
5. Monitor for chest pain, and if it occurs, notify the physician

6. Analgesics may be required, because the medication produces painful uterine contractions

V. Erythromycin Ophthalmic Ointment (0.5% Ilotycin)

A. Description: Used prophylactically against gonococcal and chlamydial conjunctivitis in **neonates**

B. Implementation
1. Instill into each of the **neonate's** conjunctival sacs within 1 hour after **delivery**
2. Cleanse the **neonate's** eyes before instilling ointment
3. Do not flush eyes after instillation

VI. Hepatitis B Vaccine

A. Description
1. Administered at birth, between 1 and 4 months of age, and between 6 and 18 months of age
2. Contraindicated if sensitivity to vaccine exists, and for those with an allergy to yeast, a severely compromised cardiopulmonary status, a moderate to severe illness, or an immune deficiency condition

B. Implementation
1. Monitor for fever, headache, fatigue, and vertigo
2. Monitor for soreness, induration, redness, swelling, pain, and itching at the injection site

VII. Methylergonovine (Methergine)

A. Description
1. Oxytocic
2. Directly stimulates uterine muscle
3. Increases strength and frequency of contractions and decreases uterine bleeding
4. Used to prevent and treat postpartum and postabortion hemorrhage due to atony or involution
5. Contraindicated during pregnancy
6. Small amounts may occur in breast milk

B. Implementation
1. Monitor maternal vital signs
2. Assess for bleeding prior to administration
3. Monitor uterine tone
4. Assess extremities for color, warmth, movement, or pain
5. Monitor for chest pain
6. Monitor for increased cramping or foul-smelling lochia

VIII. Oxytocin (Pitocin)

A. Description
1. Stimulates the smooth muscle of the uterus
2. Increases the force and frequency of contractions

3. Enhances milk ejection from the breasts

B. Implementation
1. Given by IV infusion via an infusion pump to control the rate of flow carefully
2. Should be piggybacked into the main IV line as close to the IV site as possible
3. Monitor dose being administered carefully
4. Monitor vital signs every 15 to 30 minutes
5. Internal fetal scalp electrode should be utilized to monitor for fetal heart rate (FHR) changes
6. Monitor FHR and uterine activity (frequency, duration, and intensity) every 15 minutes
7. Administer oxygen if prescribed
8. Monitor intake and output (I&O) hourly
9. Monitor for water intoxication as evidenced by nausea, vomiting, tachycardia, or cardiac dysrhythmias
10. Palpate uterine contractions, monitoring for hypertonic contractions that could cause fetal hypoxia, uterine rupture, or abruptio placentae
11. Use may increase the risk of postpartum hemorrhage owing to hypersensitivity, and the uterus may become atonic when the medication wears off
12. Minimal cervical change is usually noted until the active phase is achieved
13. Notify physician if contractions last less than 1 minute, occur more frequently than every 2 minutes, or stop
14. Stop medication if uterine hyperstimulation or nonreassuring FHR occurs; turn client on side, increase IV, and administer oxygen via face mask
15. Document the dose of the medication, and the time the medication was started, increased, maintained, and discontinued
16. Keep the family informed of the client's progress
17. Terbutaline or magnesium sulfate should be readily available in case hyperstimulation occurs
18. Breast-feeding is not recommended while the mother is on the medication

IX. Magnesium Sulfate

A. Description
1. Anticonvulsant
2. CNS depressant
3. Smooth muscle relaxant
4. Used to prevent and control seizures in pre-eclamptic and eclamptic client
5. Used to treat preterm **labor**
6. Readily crosses **placenta**
7. Distributed in breast milk for 24 hours after magnesium therapy is discontinued

B. Implementation
1. Medication is piggybacked into the IV at the connector nearest the client
2. Continuous infusion pump must be used

3. Monitor deep tendon reflexes hourly for signs of developing toxicity, because suppressed reflexes may be a sign of impending respiratory arrest
4. Patellar reflex must be present, and respiratory rate must be greater than 16 breaths per minute before each parenteral dose
5. Monitor fluid intake
6. Monitor I&O hourly
7. Output should be maintained at 30 mL per hour as the medication is eliminated through the kidneys
8. Client may complain of flushing, sensation of warmth, or sweating
9. Monitor vital signs every 30 to 60 minutes, especially respirations
10. Call physician if respirations are less than 12, indicating respiratory depression
11. Monitor renal function, magnesium levels, and cardiac function
12. Monitor magnesium levels, as the target range is 4 to 7 mEq/L
13. If a rise in the magnesium level occurs (confusion, irregular heart beat, cramping, unusual tiredness or weakness, lightheadedness or dizziness), notify physician
14. Keep calcium gluconate on hand in case of a magnesium sulfate overdose, because calcium gluconate antagonizes the effect of magnesium sulfate
15. Magnesium sulfate is continued for the first 12 to 24 hours postpartum if it is used for pre-eclampsia
16. Continuous IV infusion increases the risk of magnesium toxicity in the neonate
17. IV administration should not be used for 2 hours preceding delivery

X. Meperidine Hydrochloride (Demerol)

A. Description
1. Narcotic analgesic
2. Used to relieve moderate to severe pain associated with **labor**
3. Administered by IM or IV route
4. Crosses **placenta**
5. Distributed in breast milk
B. Implementation
1. Used cautiously in clients delivering preterm infants
2. Do not give in early **labor** as it may slow the **labor** process
3. Do not give in advanced **labor** if the neonate is to be delivered before the medication is adequately removed from the fetal circulation—may cause respiratory depression
4. Should not be given within 1 hour of delivery because it is circulated to the fetus

5. May cause maternal hypotension
6. May produce nausea when administered alone; therefore, may be given with promethazine (Phenergan)
7. Monitor respiratory status
8. Do not administer if maternal respirations are depressed
9. Regular use of opiates during pregnancy may produce withdrawal symptoms in the neonate

XI. Naloxone Hydrochloride (Narcan)

A. Description
1. Narcotic antagonist
2. Prevents or reverses the effects of opioids, including respiratory depression
3. Used to reverse narcotic depression
4. Unknown whether medication crosses **placenta** or is distributed in breast milk
B. Implementation
1. Maintain patent airway
2. Monitor the heart rate and the depth and rhythm of respirations until the effects of the narcotics wear off
3. Administer cautiously in newborns of clients who are known or are suspected to be physically dependent on opioid drugs

XII. RhoGAM

A. Description
1. Prevents isoimmunization in Rh-negative clients who are exposed or potentially exposed to Rh-positive red blood cells by transfusion, termination of pregnancy, amniocentesis, chorionic villus sampling (CVS), abdominal trauma, or bleeding during pregnancy or the birth process
2. Prevention of anti-Rh (D) antibody formation is most successful if the medication is administered twice: at 28 weeks of gestation and again within 72 hours after **delivery**
3. Should be administered within 72 hours after potential or actual exposure to Rh-positive blood
4. Must be given with each subsequent exposure or potential exposure to Rh-positive blood
5. Of no benefit once the client has developed a positive antibody titer to the Rh antigen
B. Implementation
1. Side effects are uncommon and mild
2. Temperature may rise slightly
3. Tenderness at the injection site
4. Contraindicated for Rh-positive women
5. Administer by IM injection to the mother within 72 hours after delivery
6. Never administer by IV
7. Not to be administered to a **newborn**

XIII. Ritodrine (Yutopar)

A. Description
1. Uterine relaxant
2. Relaxes uterine muscle and suppresses uterine contractions
3. Used to prolong gestation by inhibiting uterine contractions in preterm **labor**
4. Medication crosses the **placenta**
5. Unknown whether the medication is distributed in breast milk
6. Contraindicated before Week 20 of gestation

B. Implementation
1. Assess vital signs and FHR every 15 minutes
2. Monitor uterine contractions every 15 minutes during infusion
3. Assess lungs for rales
4. Monitor for pulmonary edema
5. Monitor potassium and glucose levels

◆ XIV. Rubella Virus Vaccine

A. Description
1. Induces the production of rubella antibodies to achieve active immunity
2. Used for postpartum clients not immune to rubella
3. Contraindicated in pregnant women
4. Contraindicated in immunosuppressed clients

B. Implementation
1. Monitor the client's prenatal record for rubella status
2. For clients not demonstrating immunity, obtain an order to administer the vaccine
3. Educate client about avoiding becoming pregnant for 3 months after receiving vaccine
4. Administration of blood or blood products, or RhoGAM, may alter the body's response to vaccine
5. Postpone vaccination until 3 months after the administration of blood products, or obtain documentation of immunity 6 to 8 weeks after vaccination
6. Breast-feeding mothers can be vaccinated

◆ XV. Silver Nitrate Ophthalmic Solution 1%

A. Description
1. Used to prevent gonorrheal ophthalmia neonatorum
2. Does not destroy chlamydia

B. Implementation
1. Instill 2 drops of 1% solution into each of the **newborn's** eyes within 1 hour after **delivery** if prescribed
2. Separate the **newborn's** upper and lower lids and place a pool of solution between them
3. Allow solution to pool at least 30 seconds, making sure it comes in contact with all areas of the conjunctiva
4. Remove excess medication to prevent skin discoloration

5. Use a separate ampule for each eye
6. Do not irrigate eyes after instilling silver nitrate
7. Can cause chemical conjunctivitis

XVI. Terbutaline Sulfate (Brethine)

A. Description
1. Sympathomimetic
2. Delays premature labor in pregnancies between 20 and 34 weeks
3. Hypokalemia, pulmonary edema, hypoglycemia may occur if given during labor
4. Hypoglycemia may be noted in **neonate**
5. Distributed in breast milk

B. Implementation
1. Assess maternal heart rate, blood pressure, glucose, and fluid and electrolyte status
2. Monitor FHR
3. Assess uterine contractions for intensity, frequency, and duration
4. Note that contractions may resume when client is on oral therapy
5. Instruct client to contact physician if 4 to 6 contractions per hour occur

XVII. Vitamin K (AquaMEPHYTON)

A. Description
1. Used for prophylaxis and to treat hemorrhagic disease of the **newborn**
2. Necessary for aiding in the production of active prothrombin
3. **Newborns** are deficient in vitamin K for the first 5 to 8 days of life because of the lack of intestinal flora that is necessary to absorb vitamin K

B. Implementation
1. Administer during the early neonatal period
2. Protect the medication from light
3. Monitor for jaundice, and monitor the bilirubin level because the medication can cause hyperbilirubinemia in the **newborn**
4. Monitor for bruising at the injection site and for bleeding from the cord
5. Administer in the vastus lateralis muscle of the thigh, in the lateral aspect of the anterior portion

PRACTICE QUESTIONS

1. The nurse may safely administer butorphanol tartrate (Stadol) to the laboring woman:
   1 Any time during labor
   2 Up to 30 minutes before anticipated delivery
   3 Up to 90 minutes before anticipated delivery
   4 Up to 2 to 3 hours before anticipated delivery

2. When epidural analgesia is given to a woman for pain relief after a cesarean birth, the nurse should have which one of the following medications readily available for the immediate reversal of respiratory depression?

1 Betamethasone (Celestone)
2 Morphine sulfate
3 Meperidine hydrochloride (Demerol)
4 Naloxone (Narcan)

3. After delivery, a woman is determined to be a candidate for a RhoGAM [anti-Rh₀(D) gamma globulin] injection. The nurse determines that the teaching the client received about the purpose of RhoGAM was effective when the client states that RhoGAM will protect her next baby from which of the following?
   1 Being affected by Rh incompatibility
   2 Having Rh-positive blood
   3 Developing a rubella infection
   4 Developing physiological jaundice

4. A woman is to receive ergonovine maleate (Methergine) by mouth during the first and second postpartum days. Prior to administering Methergine, it is most important to check the woman's:
   1 Lochia
   2 Blood pressure
   3 Deep tendon reflexes
   4 Uterine tone

5. Two days ago, a woman was admitted to the hospital in preterm labor at 32 weeks' gestation. The expectant parents are very anxious and fearful about giving birth to a premature infant. The nurse realizes that the couple's coping may be assisted by explaining to them that upon admission the expectant mother received an injection of betamethasone (Celestone) that will:
   1 Stop the premature uterine contractions
   2 Delay delivery for at least 48 hours
   3 Enhance fetal lung maturity
   4 Prevent premature closure of the ductus arteriosus

6. A client is to receive a rubella vaccine on the second postpartum day. Included in the teaching plan are the potential risks of the vaccine. Based on these risks, the nurse cautions the client to avoid:
   1 Sunlight for 3 days
   2 Scratching the injection site
   3 Pregnancy for 2 to 3 months after the vaccination
   4 Sexual intercourse for 2 to 3 months after the vaccination

7. When oxytocin (Pitocin) is used for the induction of labor, the nurse will immediately discontinue the oxytocin infusion if which one of the following events occurs?
   1 Severe drowsiness
   2 Uterine atony
   3 Early decelerations of the fetal heart rate
   4 Uterine hyperstimulation

8. A pregnant teenager is receiving magnesium sulfate therapy for the management of pre-eclampsia. The nurse determines that the client has developed an unwanted outcome of magnesium toxicity when which of the following signs occurs?
   1 Deep tendon reflexes of +3/4
   2 Serum magnesium level of 6 mEq/L
   3 Proteinuria of +3
   4 Respirations of 10 per minute

9. In developing a nursing care plan for a pregnant woman with HIV (human immunodeficiency virus), the nurse knows the current recommendation regarding zidovudine (AZT) therapy is:
   1 Intravenous AZT every 4 hours
   2 One dose of AZT intramuscularly immediately postpartum
   3 Oral AZT daily starting at 14 weeks' gestation
   4 Oral AZT for 6 weeks postpartum

10. A pre-eclamptic woman is receiving magnesium sulfate intravenously. The nurse determines that the magnesium sulfate therapy is effective if:
    1 Ankle clonus is noted
    2 Blood pressure is decreased
    3 Eclampsia is prevented
    4 Scotomas are present

ANSWERS

1. **4**

Rationale: Parenteral analgesia can be administered during the first stage of labor, up to 2 to 3 hours before the anticipated delivery. If given after this point in labor, the neonate may be born with respiratory depression because of placental exchange of the medication.

Test-Taking Strategy: Knowledge of the stage of labor, placental exchange of medication, and the effect on the neonate is necessary to answer the question. Assessment of the stage of labor is necessary for the appropriate administration of analgesics, since these medications are administered according to stages of labor and estimated delivery time. Avoid the selection of option 1 because of the words "any time." From the remaining options, select option 4 because of the time frame.

Level of Cognitive Ability: Application
Phase of Nursing Process: Implementation
Client Needs: Physiological Integrity
Content Area: Pharmacology

Reference
Nichols, F. H., & Zwelling, E. (1997). *Maternal-newborn nursing: Theory and practice.* Philadelphia: W. B. Saunders. pp. 840, 841.

2. **4**

Rationale: Narcotics are used for epidural analgesia. An adverse reaction of epidural analgesia is a delayed respiratory depression. Respirations are monitored for 24 hours after administration of epidural analgesia. Naloxone (Narcan) is a narcotic antagonist that reverses the effects of narcotics and is given if respirations fall below 6 to 8 per minute. Morphine and Demerol are narcotics and are contraindicated. Celestone is a steroid administered to enhance fetal lung maturity.

Test-Taking Strategy: A general knowledge of medication actions and epidural analgesia is necessary to find this answer. Identify key words in the question that indicate the need for you to prioritize; in this question the key word is "immediate." Review the purposes and actions of these medications now, if you had difficulty with this question!

Level of Cognitive Ability: Application
Phase of Nursing Process: Planning
Client Needs: Physiological Integrity
Content Area: Pharmacology

Reference
Hodgson, B., & Kizior, R. (1998). *Saunders nursing drug handbook 1998.* Philadelphia: W. B. Saunders. pp. 719–721.

3. **1**

Rationale: Rh incompatibility can occur when an Rh-negative mother becomes sensitized to the Rh antigen. Sensitization may develop when an Rh-negative woman becomes pregnant with a fetus who is Rh positive. During pregnancy and at delivery, some of the baby's Rh-positive blood can enter the maternal circulation, causing the woman's immune system to form antibodies against Rh-positive blood. Administration of RhoGAM prevents the woman from developing antibodies against Rh-positive blood by providing passive antibody protection against the Rh antigen.

Test-Taking Strategy: This question asks you to evaluate the client's knowledge about the purpose of a medication. Read each response and eliminate those answers that are inaccurate statements by the client. A knowledge of Rh incompatibility will assist you in answering this question correctly. If the words "anti-Rh₀(D) gamma globulin" in the stem are unfamiliar, try to figure out the meaning by breaking down the words using your medical terminology knowledge. If you need to select an answer and are not quite sure, select a response that has similarity to a thought in the question. In this case "anti-Rh₀(D) gamma globulin" indicates an immune response that is similar to "Rh incompatibility" found in option 1.

Level of Cognitive Ability: Analysis
Phase of Nursing Process: Evaluation
Client Needs: Physiological Integrity
Content Area: Pharmacology

Reference
Nichols, F. H., & Zwelling, E., (1997). *Maternal-newborn nursing: Theory and practice.* Philadelphia: W. B. Saunders. pp. 652–653.

4. **2**

Rationale: Methylergonovine maleate (Methergine), a synthetic ergot preparation, is an agent that is used to prevent or control postpartum hemorrhage by contracting the uterus. The immediate dose is usually given intramuscularly, and then, if needed, it is given by mouth. It causes constant uterine contractions and may elevate blood pressure. A priority assessment prior to administration of Methergine is blood pressure. Methergine is to be administered very cautiously in the presence of hypertension, and the physician should be notified if hypertension is present.

Test-Taking Strategy: A knowledge of the action and adverse effects of medications is needed here. The key words indicating the need to prioritize are "most important." Utilize the ABCs (Airway, Breathing, Circulation) when selecting an answer. Blood pressure is a method of assessing circulation. Lochia and uterine tone are similar distracters as they are directly related to one another; therefore, neither of these options can be the answer. Deep tendon reflexes are assessed with the use of magnesium sulfate.

Level of Cognitive Ability: Application
Phase of Nursing Process: Assessment
Client Needs: Physiological Integrity
Content Area: Pharmacology

Reference
Nichols, F. H., & Zwelling, E. (1997). *Maternal-newborn nursing: Theory and practice.* Philadelphia: W. B. Saunders. p. 781.

5. **3**

Rationale: Betamethasone (Celestone), an anti-inflammatory steroid, is given to increase the fetus' surfactant level and increase lung maturity, reducing the incidence of respiratory distress syndrome. Surfactant production does not become stable until after 32 weeks' gestation, and if adequate amounts of surfactant are not present in the lungs, respiratory distress and death are a possible consequence. Delivery of the baby needs to be delayed for at least 48 hours after administration of Celestone in order to allow time for the lungs to mature. By discussing Celestone with the parents, the nurse may alleviate some of their anxieties and fears.

Test-Taking Strategy: Knowledge of the medication's action is necessary to answer this question. A knowledge of premature infants will also assist in answering this question. Knowing that respiratory distress syndrome caused by immature lungs is a major problem of prematurity and therefore a major concern for the expectant parents will help make the correct option apparent. Giving information and providing anticipatory guidance to clients reduces stress and promotes psychosocial adaptation. A similarity exists between options 1 and 2 as they both relate to stopping labor. When a similarity exists in the answers, neither option is likely to be correct.

Level of Cognitive Ability: Analysis
Phase of Nursing Process: Analysis
Client Needs: Psychosocial Integrity
Content Area: Pharmacology

Reference
Nichols, F. H., & Zwelling, E. (1997). *Maternal-newborn nursing: Theory and practice.* Philadelphia: W. B. Saunders. p. 1342.

6. **3**

Rationale: Rubella vaccine is a live, attenuated virus that evokes an antibody response that provides immunity for 15 years. Because rubella is a live vaccine, it will act as the virus and is potentially teratogenic in the organogenesis phase of fetal development. The client needs to be informed about the potential effects that this vaccine may have and the need to avoid becoming pregnant for a period of 2 to 3 months afterward. Abstinence from sexual intercourse is not necessary, unless another form of effective contraception is not being utilized. The vaccine may cause local or systemic reactions, but all are mild and short lived. Sunlight has no effect on the person who is vaccinated.

Test-Taking Strategy: A knowledge of the effect of live vaccines on pregnancy and fetal development is necessary to answer this question. Knowing that most vaccinations are either contraindicated or given with caution will help you answer the question. Also realizing that the viruses can cross the placental barrier will also assist you in choosing the correct answer. Use all your nursing knowledge to assist you in answering this question.

Level of Cognitive Ability: Application
Phase of Nursing Process: Implementation
Client Needs: Physiological Integrity
Content Area: Pharmacology

Reference
Nichols, F. H., & Zwelling, E. (1997). *Maternal-newborn nursing: Theory and practice.* Philadelphia: W. B. Saunders. pp. 1510–1511.

7. 4

Rationale: Induction of labor is the initiation of labor through mechanical or pharmacological intervention. Oxytocin is a synthetic hormone that stimulates uterine contractions and is one of the common pharmacological methods of inducing labor. A major danger associated with oxytocin induction of labor is hyperstimulation of uterine contractions. Fetal distress may occur when the uterus is hyperstimulated owing to decreased placental perfusion. Therefore, oxytocin infusion must be stopped when there are any signs of uterine hyperstimulation. Early decelerations of the fetal heart rate are a reassuring sign and do not indicate fetal distress.

Test-Taking Strategy: A knowledge of commonly used medications during labor and delivery is necessary to answer this question. Knowing that induction of labor involves the stimulation of uterine contractions will help you answer this question. Using your knowledge about the effect of uterine contractions on uteroplacental circulation should guide you in recognizing that hyperstimulation of contractions would compromise fetal oxygenation, a primary physiological need. If there are words that you are unfamiliar with (e.g., atony), break down the word using your medical terminology skills.

Level of Cognitive Ability: Application
Phase of Nursing Process: Implementation
Client Need: Physiological Integrity
Content Area: Pharmacology

Reference
Nichols, F. H., & Zwelling, E. (1997). *Maternal-newborn nursing: Theory and practice.* Philadelphia: W. B. Saunders. pp. 912–913.

8. 4

Rationale: Magnesium toxicity is a danger of magnesium sulfate therapy. Signs of magnesium sulfate toxicity are related to the central nervous system (CNS) depressant effects of the medication and include respiratory depression, loss of deep tendon reflexes, sudden drop in fetal heart rate, and/or maternal heart rate and blood pressure. Magnesium is excreted through the kidneys. If renal impairment is present, magnesium toxicity can develop very quickly. The target range for the serum level of magnesium is 4 to 7 mEq/L. Proteinuria is a sign of pre-eclampsia.

Test-Taking Strategy: A knowledge of medications will assist in answering this question. Knowing that magnesium sulfate is a CNS depressant will make the correct option apparent. A similarity exists between options 1 and 3 in that they are both signs of pre-eclampsia. When a similarity exists in the options, then neither one is likely to be the correct answer.

Level of Cognitive Ability: Analysis
Phase of Nursing Process: Evaluation
Client Needs: Physiological Integrity
Content Area: Pharmacology

Reference
Hodgson, B., & Kizior, R. (1998). *Saunders nursing drug handbook 1998.* Philadelphia: W. B. Saunders. p. 619.

9. 3

Rationale: It is recommended that pregnant women with HIV take oral AZT starting in the 14th week of gestation. Starting AZT therapy prior to 14 weeks' gestation is not recommended because of potentially teratogenic effects. During labor, a bolus of AZT is given intravenously, and the neonate is treated for 6 weeks after birth.

Test-Taking Strategy: A knowledge of current research and pharmacological therapy for AIDS is helpful in answering this question. Realizing that AIDS is a chronic disease requiring long-term therapy should assist you in eliminating the incorrect options that are related to short-term treatment. Knowing that the fetus is most vulnerable to the effects of medications and chemicals during the period of organogenesis will assist you in selecting the correct answer.

Level of Cognitive Ability: Analysis
Phase of Nursing Process: Planning
Client Needs: Physiological Integrity
Content Area: Pharmacology

Reference
Nichols, F. H., & Zwelling, E. (1997). *Maternal-newborn nursing: Theory and practice.* Philadelphia: W. B. Saunders. p. 1499.

10. 3

Rationale: When caring for a client with pre-eclampsia, the goal of care is directed at preventing eclampsia (seizures). Magnesium sulfate is an anticonvulsant; it is not an antihypertensive agent. Although a decrease in blood pressure may be noted initially, this effect is usually transient. Ankle clonus indicates hyperreflexia and may precede the onset of eclampsia. Scotomas are areas of complete or partial blindness. Visual disturbances, such as scotomas, often precede an eclamptic convulsion.

Test-Taking Strategy: Knowing that magnesium sulfate is an anticonvulsant or that avoiding eclamptic seizures is a desired outcome of therapy will allow you to answer this question. Knowing the warning signs that precede an eclamptic seizure will also assist you in eliminating incorrect options. Unusual or highly technical language, such as clonus and scotoma, typically indicates that the option is not correct.

Level of Cognitive Ability: Analysis
Phase of Nursing Process: Evaluation
Client Needs: Physiological Integrity
Content Area: Pharmacology

Reference
Nichols, F. H., & Zwelling, E. (1997). *Maternal-newborn nursing: Theory and practice.* Philadelphia: W. B. Saunders. p. 651.

BIBLIOGRAPHY

Clark, J., Queener, S., & Karb, V. (1997). *Pharmacologic basis of nursing practice* (5th ed.). St. Louis: Mosby–Year Book.

Hodgson, B., & Kizior, R. (1998). *Saunders nursing drug handbook 1998*. Philadelphia: W. B. Saunders.

Lehne, R. (1998). *Pharmacology for nursing care* (3rd ed.). Philadelphia: W. B. Saunders.

Nichols, F. H., & Zwelling, E. (1997). *Maternal-newborn nursing: Theory and practice*. Philadelphia: W. B. Saunders.

UNIT VII

··

Pediatric Nursing

PYRAMID TERMS

Abuse—Includes nonaccidental physical injury or the nonaccidental act of omission by a parent or person responsible for the care of the child.

Active Immunity—The protection that can last months, years, or even a lifetime and forms in response to exposure to antigens in nature or vaccines.

Atresia—Congenital absence or closure of a body orifice.

Attenuated Vaccines—Vaccines derived from microorganisms or viruses whose virulence has been weakened due to passage through another host.

Cephalocaudal—Growth and development that proceeds from head to toe.

Chronological Age—Age in years.

Developmental Age—Age based on functional behavior and ability to adapt to the environment. It does not necessarily correspond to chronological age.

Encopresis—Fecal incontinence after age 4.

Functional Age—The age equivalent at which the child is actually able to perform specific self-care or related tasks.

Growth—Measurable physical and physiologic changes that occur over time.

Growth Spurts—Brief periods of rapid increase in growth rate.

Hereditary—The transmission of genetic characteristics from parent to offspring.

Inactivated Vaccines—Vaccines that contain killed microorganisms.

Intelligence—What an individual can do relative to learning, thinking, and problem solving.

Learning—Behavior changes that occur as a result of both maturation and experience with the environment.

Nasal Flaring—A serious sign of air hunger. A widening of the nares to enable the child to take in more oxygen.

Passive Immunity—Antibody transfer from a person with active immunity to a person who does not have that antibody.

Puberty—The period of time during which the adolescent experiences a growth spurt, develops secondary sex characteristics, and achieves reproductive maturity.

Regression—Behavior that is more appropriate to an earlier stage of development and is often used to cope with stress or anxiety.

Regurgitation—An abnormal backward flow of body fluid.

Retractions—An abnormal movement of the chest walls during inspiration.

Separation Anxiety—Distress and apprehension caused by being removed from parents, home, or familiar surroundings.

Shunt—Abnormal blood flow from one side of the heart to the other.

Stenosis—The narrowing or constriction of an opening.

Stridor—A shrill harsh sound heard during inspiration or expiration, or both, that is produced by the flow of air through a narrowed segment of the respiratory tract.

Wheezing—High-pitched musical whistles heard with or without a stethoscope.

PYRAMID TO SUCCESS

Pyramid points focus on psychosocial, cognitive, psychosexual, and moral stages of growth and development. Growth and development includes physical characteristics, nutritional behaviors, skills, play, and specific safety measures relevant to a particular age group. Pyramid points focus on safety and the age-appropriate measures to ensure a safe and hazard-free environment for the child. Additional pyramid points focus on acute disorders that can occur in children. Focus on specific feeding techniques, positioning techniques, and interventions that will provide and maintain adequate airway, breathing, and circulation patterns in the child. On NCLEX-RN, be alert to the age of the client, if the age is presented in a question!

NURSING PROCESS

ASSESSMENT

Vital signs
Age and developmental status
Routines and rituals
Family process and unit
Cultural and religious patterns
Nutritional intake
Feeding patterns
Patterns of urinary and bowel elimination
Sleep patterns
Diversional activities

ANALYSIS: Altered Nutrition

PLANNING	IMPLEMENTATION	EVALUATION
The child's nutritional intake will meet the metabolic needs for the age group.	Assess the current nutritional status and compare with age-appropriate requirements. Obtain height and weight. Identify cultural and religious dietary needs. Identify favorite foods and eating rituals. Allow the child to select food if appropriate. Offer frequent snacks and small meal portions using small utensils. Allow the child to eat with other children if the parents are not present. Encourage the parents to bring food in from home if appropriate.	The child maintains appropriate nutritional intake. The child maintains body weight during hospitalization.

ANALYSIS: Self-Care Deficit

PLANNING	IMPLEMENTATION	EVALUATION
The child will participate in age-appropriate feeding, dressing, toileting, and bathing.	Offer choices and involve the child in care when appropriate.	The child performs activities that maintain independence as much as possible.

ANALYSIS: Sleep Pattern Disturbance

PLANNING	IMPLEMENTATION	EVALUATION
The child will maintain a balance of sleep and activity.	Determine the child's usual sleep routines. Plan care to allow time for periods of sleep.	The child takes naps and sleeps an appropriate amount of time based on age requirements.

ANALYSIS: Altered Family Process

PLANNING

Parents participate in the care of the child.

IMPLEMENTATION

Prepare for all procedures and encourage the parents to stay with the child as much as possible. Provide the parents with information about support systems. Teach the child, if appropriate, or the parents about prescribed medications or other treatments required after discharge.

EVALUATION

Family support is available and the parents seek resources when necessary.

ANALYSIS: Ineffective Individual Coping

PLANNING

The child will maintain current level of development.

IMPLEMENTATION

Follow home routines as much as possible. Assess normal urinary and bowel elimination patterns. Follow home routines of elimination if possible. Do not scold the child if incontinent.

EVALUATION

The child maintains the appropriate level of growth and development. The child maintains age-appropriate and condition-appropriate self-care.

ANALYSIS: Diversional Activity Deficit

PLANNING

The child becomes involved in play activities.

IMPLEMENTATION

Provide a safe environment for the child. Provide play activities based on the child's developmental level. Encourage the parents to bring in a favorite toy. Introduce the child to other children on the unit. Encourage peer contact if appropriate.

EVALUATION

The child plays and communicates with others.

ANALYSIS: Anxiety

PLANNING

The child will display decreased signs of distress if any are present.

IMPLEMENTATION

Orient the child and parents to the hospital and routines. Provide opportunities for the child to express his or her feelings. Provide a consistent caregiver as much as possible.

EVALUATION

The child separates from the parents in an appropriate manner during hospitalization.

CLIENT NEEDS

SAFE, EFFECTIVE CARE ENVIRONMENT

Parent and child rights
Confidentiality
Informed consent in regard to minors
Continuity of care
Protective measures
Accident prevention
Environmental and personal safety related to the developmental age of the child
Spread and control of infectious agents particularly with regard to communicable diseases

HEALTH PROMOTION AND MAINTENANCE

Developmental stages
Family systems
Disease prevention
Health promotion programs
Immunizations
Communicable diseases
Instructions to the child and parents regarding care at home
Protection of the child and other contacts to prevent illness

PSYCHOSOCIAL INTEGRITY

Play
Communication
Cultural, religious, and spiritual influences
Family and support systems
Child abuse and neglect

PHYSIOLOGICAL INTEGRITY

Age-appropriate normal body structure and function
Elimination
Nutrition
Rest and sleep
Medication administration
Comfort measures
Intrusive procedures
Responses to therapies

BIBLIOGRAPHY

Ashwill, J., & Droske, S. (1997). *Nursing care of children: Principles and practice*. Philadelphia: W. B. Saunders.

Hodgson, B., & Kizior, R. (1999). *Saunders nursing drug handbook 1999*. Philadelphia: W. B. Saunders.

Luckmann, J. (1997). *Saunders manual of nursing care*. Philadelphia: W. B. Saunders.

National Council of State Boards of Nursing (eds.) (1997). Test Plan for the National Council Licensure Examination for Registered Nurses. Chicago: Author.

Nichols, F., & Zwelling, E. (1997). *Maternal newborn nursing: Theory and practice*. Philadelphia: W. B. Saunders.

O'Toole, M. (ed.). (1997). *Miller-Keane encyclopedia & dictionary of medicine, nursing, & allied health* (6th ed.). Philadelphia: W. B. Saunders.

CHAPTER 32

Growth and Development

I. The Hospitalized Infant and Toddler

A. **Separation Anxiety**
   1. Protest
      a. Cries, screams, searches for a parent; avoids and rejects contact with strangers
      b. Verbal attack on others
      c. Physical fighting; kicks, fights, hits, pinches
   2. Despair
      a. Withdrawn, depressed, disinterested in the environment
      b. Loss of newly learned skills
   3. Detachment
      a. If the separation from the parent continues, the child enters the detachment phase
      b. During the phase, the child again becomes interested in the environment and begins to play
      c. If the parents return during this stage, the child may ignore them and the parents may think that the child does not want to see them
      d. This reaction is a coping mechanism that the child uses to protect self from further emotional pain related to separation

B. Fear of Injury and Pain: Affected by Previous Experiences, Separation from Parents, and Preparation for the Experience

C. Loss of Control
   1. Hospitalization with its own set of rituals and routines can severely disrupt the life of a toddler
   2. The lack of control is often exhibited in behaviors related to feeding, toileting, playing, and bedtime
   3. The child may demonstrate **regression**

D. Implementation
   1. Provide swaddling and soft talking to the infant
   2. Provide opportunities for sucking and oral stimulation for the infant using a pacifier if the infant is NPO
   3. Provide stimulation if appropriate for the infant, using contrasting colors and textures
   4. Provide routines and rituals as close as possible to what the child is used to at home
   5. Provide choices as much as possible to the child to provide some control
   6. Approach with a positive attitude
   7. Allow the toddler to express feelings of protest
   8. Encourage toddlers to talk about parents or others in their lives
   9. Accept regressive behavior without ridiculing the child
   10. Provide the child with favorite and comforting objects
   11. Allow the toddler as much mobility as possible
   12. Anticipate temper tantrums and maintain a safe environment for physical acting out
   13. Employ pain-reduction techniques as appropriate

II. The Hospitalized Preschooler

A. **Separation Anxiety**
   1. Generally less obvious and less serious than in the toddler
   2. As stress increases, the preschooler's ability to separate from the parents decreases
   3. Protest
      a. Less direct and aggressive than the toddler
      b. May displace feelings on others
   4. Despair
      a. Similar to the toddler
      b. Quietly withdrawn, depressed, disinterested in the environment
      c. Loss of newly learned skills
      d. Child becomes generally uncooperative, refusing to eat or take medication

e. The child repeatedly asks when the parents will be visiting

5. Detachment
   a. If the separation from the parent continues, the child enters the detachment phase
   b. During this phase, the child again becomes interested in the environment and begins to play
   c. If the parents return during this stage, the child may ignore them, and the parents may think that the child does not want to see them
   d. This reaction is a coping mechanism that the child uses to protect self from further emotional pain related to separation

B. Fear of Injury and Pain
  1. The preschooler has a general lack of understanding of body integrity
  2. Fears invasive procedures and mutilation
  3. Imagines things to be much worse than they are
  4. Preschoolers believe that they are ill because of something they did or thought

C. Loss of Control
  1. Likes familiar routines and rituals and may show **regression** if not allowed to maintain some control
  2. Has attained a good deal of independence and self-care at home and may expect that to continue in the hospital

D. Implementation
  1. Provide a safe and secure environment
  2. Take time for communication
  3. Allow the child to express anger
  4. Acknowledge fears and anxieties
  5. Accept regressive behavior
  6. Assist the child in moving from regressive to appropriate behaviors according to age
  7. Encourage rooming-in or leave favorite toy
  8. Allow mobility
  9. Provide play and diversional activities
  10. Place the child with other children of the same age if possible
  11. Encourage the child to be independent
  12. Explain procedures simply on the child's level
  13. Avoid intrusive procedures when possible
  14. Allow to wear underpants

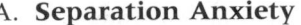

III. The Hospitalized School-Aged Child

A. **Separation Anxiety**
  1. Accustomed to periods of separation from the parents but as stressors are added the separation becomes more difficult
  2. More concerned with missing school and the fear that their friends will forget them
  3. Usually do not see the stage of behavior of protest, despair, and detachment with school-aged child

B. Fear of Injury and Pain
  1. Fear of bodily injury and pain
  2. Fear of illness itself, disability, death, and intrusive procedures in genital areas
  3. Uncomfortable with any type of sexual exam
  4. Groans or whines, holds rigidly still, communicates about pain

C. Loss of Control
  1. Are usually highly social, independent, and involved with activities
  2. Seek information
  3. Ask relevant questions about tests and procedures and their illness
  4. Associate their actions as the cause of the illness
  5. May feel helpless and dependent if physical limitations occur

D. Implementation
  1. Encourage rooming-in
  2. Focus on the child's abilities and needs
  3. Encourage the child to become involved with his or her own care
  4. Accept **regression** but encourage independence
  5. Provide choices to the child
  6. Allow expression of feelings both verbally and nonverbally
  7. Acknowledge fears and concerns and allow for discussion
  8. Explain all procedures using body diagrams or outlines
  9. Provide privacy
  10. Avoid intrusive procedures if possible
  11. Allow the child to wear underpants
  12. Involve the child in activities appropriate to developmental level and conditions
  13. Provide individualized recreation
  14. Encourage the child to contact friends
  15. Provide for educational needs
  16. Employ appropriate interventions to relieve pain

IV. The Hospitalized Adolescent

A. **Separation Anxiety**
  1. Not sure whether they want their parents with them when they are hospitalized
  2. Separation from friends is a source of anxiety
  3. Become upset if friends go on with their lives, excluding them

B. Fear of Injury and Pain
  1. Fear of being different from others and their peers
  2. May give the impression that they are not afraid even though they are terrified
  3. Become guarded when any areas related to sexual development are examined

C. Loss of Control
  1. Behaviors exhibited include anger, withdrawal, and uncooperativeness
  2. Seek help and then reject it

D. Implementation
1. Encourage questions about appearance and effects of the illness on the future
2. Explore feelings about the hospital and significance the illness might have on relationships
3. Encourage to wear own clothes and perform normal grooming
4. Allow favorite foods to be brought in if possible
5. Provide privacy
6. Use medical terminology and body diagrams to prepare for procedures
7. Introduce the child to other adolescents on the unit
8. Encourage maintaining contact with peer groups
9. Provide for educational needs

10. Identify formation of future plans
11. Help develop positive coping mechanisms

V. Communication Approaches

A. General Guidelines
1. Allow the child to feel comfortable with you
2. Communicate through the use of objects
3. Allow the child to express fears and concerns
4. Speak clearly in a quiet, unhurried voice
5. Offer choices when possible
6. Be honest with the child
7. Set limits with the child as appropriate
B. Infants
1. Infants respond to nonverbal communication behaviors of adults such as holding, rocking, patting, and touching
2. Use a slow approach and allow the infant to get to know you
3. Use a calm, soft, soothing voice
4. Be responsive to cries
5. Talk and read to infants
6. Allow security objects such as blankets and pacifiers if the infant has them
C. Toddlers
1. Approach the toddler cautiously
2. Remember that toddlers accept verbal communications of others literally
3. Learn the toddler's words for common items and use them in conversations
4. Use short, concrete terms
5. Prepare toddlers for procedures immediately before the event
6. Repeat explanations and descriptions
7. Use play for demonstrations
8. Use visual aids such as picture books, puppets, and dolls
9. Allow the child to handle instruments
10. Explain what the instrument does and how it feels
11. Encourage the use of comfort objects
D. Preschooler
1. Seek opportunities to offer choices
2. Speak in simple sentences

3. Be concise and limit the length of explanations
4. Allow to ask questions
5. Describe procedures as they are about to be performed
6. Use play to explain procedures and activities
7. Allow to handle the equipment, which will ease fear and help to answer questions
E. School-Aged Child
1. Establish limits
2. Provide reassurance to help in alleviating fears and anxieties
3. Engage in conversations that encourage thinking
4. Use medical play techniques
5. Use photographs, books, teaching dolls, and videos to explain procedures
6. Explain in clear terms
7. Allow time for composure and privacy
F. The Adolescent
1. Remember that the adolescent may be preoccupied with body image
2. Encourage and support independence
3. Provide privacy and confidentiality
4. Use photographs, books, and videos to explain procedures
5. Engage in conversations about adolescent interests
6. Avoid becoming too abstract, too detailed, and too technical
7. Avoid responding to less than desirable social behaviors by prying, confrontation, or judgmental attitudes

VI. Developmental Characteristics

A. The Infant
1. Physical
   a. Height increases by 3/4 inch per month
   b. Weight is doubled at 5 to 6 months and tripled at 12 months
   c. At birth, head circumference is 2 cm greater than chest circumference
   d. By 1 to 2 years of age, size of head circumference and chest circumference are equal
   e. Anterior fontanel closes at 12 to 18 months
   f. Posterior fontanel closes by 2 to 3 months
   g. Ten upper and 10 lower deciduous teeth by 1 to 2 years of age
   h. Lower central incisors present by 6 to 8 months
   i. Reflexes such as rooting, tonic neck, palmar grasp, moro, and stepping disappear by 4 months of age, with sucking lasting through infancy
   j. Sleeps most of the time
2. Vital signs (Table 32–1)
3. Nutrition
   a. The infant may breast- or bottle-feed depending on the mother's choice

Table 32–1. Vital Signs

Infant	1-Year-Old
Temperature: axillary 96.8°–99°F	Temperature: axillary 96.8°–99°F
Apical rate: 120–160 beats per minute	Apical rate: 80–160 beats per minute
Respirations: 30–60 breaths per minute	Respirations: 20–40 breaths per minute
Blood pressure: 46–92/38–71 mmHg	Blood pressure: 96/65 mmHg

    b. Calorie requirements are 110 to 120 kcal/kg/day

    c. Give no more than 30 oz of formula per day

    d. Iron stores from birth are depleted by 4 months

    e. Do not give skim milk, as fatty acids are required

    f. Introduce solids at 4 to 6 months

    g. Introduce foods one at a time, with sequence as follows: rice cereal; fruits and vegetables starting with yellow and then green; meats; and then egg yolks, avoiding egg whites

    h. Avoid nuts, foods with seeds, raisins, and popcorn

    i. Never mix food and/or medications with formula

    j. Avoid honey or syrup in milk or water to prevent botulism

    k. By 12 to 14 months child should drink from a cup

  4. Skills (Table 32–2)

  5. Play

    a. Solitary

Table 32–2. Infant Skills

2–3 Months	8–9 Months
Smiles	Sits steadily unsupported
Turns head side to side	Crawls
Cries	May stand while holding on
Follows objects	Begins to stand without help
Holds head in midline	**10–11 Months**
4–5 Months	Can change from prone to sitting position
Grasps objects	Walks holding onto furniture
Switches objects from hands	Stands securely
Rolls over for the first time	Entertains self for periods of time
Enjoys social interaction	**12–13 Months**
Begins to show memory	
Aware of unfamiliar surroundings	Walks with one hand held
	Can take a few steps without falling
6–7 Months	**14–15 Months**
Creeps	Walks alone
Sits with support	Can crawl upstairs
Imitates	Show emotions as anger and affection
Exhibits fear of strangers	
Holds arms out	Will explore away from mother in familiar surroundings
Frequent mood swings	
Waves bye-bye	

    b. Birth to 3 months: verbal, visual, and tactile stimuli

    c. 4 to 6 months: initiates actions and recognizes new experiences

    d. 6 to 12 months: aware of self; imitates, repeats pleasurable actions

    e. Enjoy soft stuffed animals, crib mobiles with contrasting colors, squeeze toys, rattles, musical toys, water toys during the bath, large picture books, and push toys after they begin to walk

  6. Safety

    a. Baby-proof home

    b. Infants who weigh up to 20 lb should be restrained in a car seat in the middle backseat in a semireclined, rear-facing position

    c. Use safety straps for infant seats

    d. Guard the infant when on the bed or changing table

    e. Use gates to protect the infant from stairs

    f. Never shake or vigorously jiggle a baby's head

    g. Be sure that bathwater is not hot

    h. Do not leave unattended in the bath

    i. Do not hold the infant while drinking or working near hot liquids

    j. Cool vaporizers should be used instead of steam to prevent burn injuries

    k. Avoid food that is round and similar to the size of the airway to prevent choking

    l. Be sure toys have no small pieces

    m. Hanging toys or mobiles over the crib should be well out of reach to prevent strangulation

    n. Avoid placing large toys in the crib as an older infant may use them as steps to climb

    o. Cribs should be positioned away from curtain and blind cords

    p. Cover electrical outlets

    q. Remove hazardous objects from low, reachable places

    r. Remove chemicals, poisons, and plants from the infant's reach

    s. Keep syrup of ipecac and the poison control number available

B. The Toddler

  1. Physical

    a. Height and weight increase in a step-like fashion reflecting **growth spurts** and lags

    b. Head circumference increases about 1 inch between ages 1 and 2

    c. Thereafter, head circumference increases about 1/2 inch per year until age 5

    d. Anterior fontanel closes between ages 12 to 18 months

    e. Weight changes are slower than in infancy by about 4 to 6 lb per year

    f. By age 2, the average weight is 27 lb

    g. Normal height changes include a **growth** of about 3 inches per year

BOX 32–1. The Toddler's Vital Signs

Temperature: axillary 97.5°–98.6°F
Apical rate: 80–125 beats per minute
Respirations: 25–35 breaths per minute
Blood pressure: average 72–110/40–73 mmHg

   h. The average height of the toddler is 34 inches at age 2 years
   i. Lordosis is evident with a "potbelly"
   j. Should begin brushing the teeth with a small soft-bristle toothbrush around age 2, with dentist visits beginning around age 2½
   k. Typically sleeps through the night and has one daytime nap and discontinues the daytime nap at about age 3
   l. A consistent bedtime ritual helps prepare the toddler for sleep
   m. Security objects at bedtime may assist in sleep
2. Vital signs (Box 32–1)
3. Nutrition
   a. Calorie requirements are 100 kcal/kg/day
   b. Most toddlers prefer to feed themselves
   c. The toddler generally does best by eating several small nutritious meals each day rather than three large meals
   d. Offer a limited number of foods at any one time
   e. Limit concentrated sweets and empty calories
   f. At risk for aspiration of small foods that are not easily chewed, such as peanuts and popcorn
   g. Physiological anorexia is normal owing to the alternating periods of fast and slow **growth**
   h. Sit the toddler in a high chair at the family table
   i. Allow sufficient time to eat but remove food when toddler begins playing with it
   j. The toddler drinks well from a cup held with both hands
   k. The toddler is skillful at handling finger foods
   l. Avoid using food as a reward or punishment
4. Skills
   a. The toddler begins to walk by age 12 to 15 months
   b. Runs by age 2 years and walks backward and hops on one foot by age 3 years
   c. The toddler usually cannot alternate feet when climbing stairs
   d. The toddler begins to master fine-motor skills for building, undressing, and drawing lines
   e. Often uses "no" even when the toddler means "yes" to assert independence

   f. Begins to use short sentences and has a vocabulary of about 300 words by age 2
   g. Tends to ask many "why" questions
5. Bowel and bladder control
   a. Signs that a toddler is ready for toilet-training include muscle coordination with walking, communicating with parents, awareness of a wet or soiled diaper, holding urine for 2 hours, and interest in pleasing parents
   b. Bowel control develops before bladder control
   c. By age 3, the toddler achieves fairly good bowel and bladder control
   d. The toddler may stay dry during the day but may need a diaper at night until age 4
6. Play
   a. The major socializing mechanism is parallel play, and therapeutic play can begin at this age
   b. Short attention span causes toddler to change toys often
   c. Explores body parts of self and others
   d. Typical toys include push/pull toys, blocks, sand, finger paints and bubbles, large balls, crayons, trucks and dolls, containers, Play-Doh, toy telephones, cloth books, wooden puzzles
7. Safety
   a. Toddlers are eager to explore the world around them
   b. The toddler should be supervised at play
   c. Once toddlers are able to sit up alone they should be restrained in an upright, forward-facing position in a car seat until they weigh 40 lb
   d. Lock car doors
   e. Use back burners on the stove to prepare a meal, and turn pot handles inward and toward the middle of the stove
   f. Keep dangling cords from small appliances away from toddlers
   g. Place inaccessible locks on windows and doors, and keep furniture away from windows
   h. Secure screens on all windows
   i. Place gates at stairways
   j. Do not permit the toddler to sleep or play in an upper bunk bed
   k. Never leave the child alone near a bathtub, pail of water, swimming pool, or any other body of water
   l. Keep toilet lids closed
   m. Keep all medicines, poisons, household plants, and toxic products high and locked out of reach
   n. Keep syrup of ipecac and the poison control number available
C. The Preschooler
  1. Physical
   a. Grows 2½ to 3 inches per year

BOX 32–2. The Preschooler's Vital Signs
Temperature: axillary 97.5°–98.6°F Apical rate: 90–100 beats per minute Respirations: 25 breaths per minute Blood pressure: average 85/60–90/70 mmHg

    b. Average height is 37 inches at age 3

    c. Is 40½ inches at age 4 and 43 inches at age 5

    d. Gains 5 lb per year

    e. Average weight of 32 lb at age 5

    f. Requires about 12 hours of sleep each day

    g. A security object and nightlight assist with sleeping

    h. Can use a toothbrush properly and should brush twice a day

2. Vital signs (Box 32–2)

3. Nutrition

    a. Daily calorie requirement is 85 kcal/kg or about 1700 kcal/day

    b. Exhibits food fads and strong taste preferences

    c. By 5 years old, tends to focus on social aspects of eating, table conversations, manners, and willingness to try new foods

4. Skills

    a. Has good posture

    b. Develops fine-motor coordination

    c. Can hop, skip, and run more smoothly

    d. Athletic abilities develop

    e. Demonstrates increased skills in balancing

    f. Alternates feet when climbing stairs

    g. Can tie shoelaces

    h. May talk continuously and ask many "why" questions

    i. Vocabulary increases to about 900 words by age 3 and 2100 words by age 5

    j. By age 3 usually talks in three- or four-word sentences and speaks in short phrases

    k. By age 4 speaks five- or six-word sentences and by age 5 speaks in longer sentences that contain all parts of speech

    l. Can be readily understood by others and can clearly understand what others are saying

5. Bowel and bladder control

    a. By age 4, the child has daytime control of bowel and bladder but may experience bed-wetting accidents at night

    b. By age 5, the preschooler achieves both bowel and bladder control, although accidents may occur in stressful situations

6. Play

    a. Cooperative

    b. Imaginary playmates

    c. Likes to build and create things, and play is simple and imaginative

    d. Understands sharing and is able to interact with peers

    e. Requires regular socialization with age mates

    f. Play activities include a large space for running and jumping

    g. Dress-up clothes, paints, paper, and crayons for creative expressions

    h. Swimming and sports for **growth** development

    i. Puzzles and toys aid with fine development

7. Safety

    a. Preschoolers are active and inquisitive

    b. Because of their magical thinking, they may believe that daring feats seen in cartoons are possible and they may attempt them

    c. Can learn simple safety practices because they can follow simple and verbal directions and their attention span is lengthened

    d. Once the child has outgrown the car safety seat (weight more than 40 lb), the child should be placed and restrained in a booster seat that raises the child high enough to allow car seat belts to be correctly positioned over the child's chest and pelvis

    e. Teach the child basic safety rules to ensure safety when playing in a playground near swings and ladders

    f. Never allow the child to play with matches or lighters

    g. The child should be taught what to do in the event of a fire or if clothes catch fire

    h. Fire drills should be practiced with the child

    i. Guns should be stored unloaded and secured under lock and key

    j. The child should be taught to leave an area immediately if a gun is seen, and to tell an adult

    k. A child should be taught never to point a toy gun at another person

    l. Teach the child that if another person touches his or her body in an inappropriate way to tell an adult

    m. Teach the child to avoid speaking to strangers and never to accept a ride, toys, or gifts from a stranger

    n. Teach children their full name, address, parents' names, and telephone number

    o. Keep syrup of ipecac and the poison control number available

    p. Teach the child how to dial 911 in an emergency situation

D. The School-Aged Child

1. Physical

    a. Girls usually grow faster than boys

BOX 32–3. The School-Aged Child's Vital Signs

Temperature: oral 97.5°–98.6°F
Apical rate: 70–110 beats per minute
Respirations: 16–22 breaths per minute
Blood pressure: average 83–121/45–79 mmHg

   b. **Growth** of about 2 inches per year between ages 6 and 12
   c. Height ranges from 45 inches at age 6 to 59 inches at age 12
   d. Weight gain of 4½ to 6½ lb per year
   e. Average weight of 46 lb at age 6 and 88 lb at age 12
   f. Permanent teeth erupt around age 6, and deciduous teeth are gradually lost
   g. Brush teeth at least twice a day
   h. Regular dentist visits should be stressed
   i. Sleep requirements range from 10 to 12 hours a night
  2. Vital signs (Box 32–3)
  3. Nutrition
   a. Increased **growth** needs
   b. Balanced diet from basic four food groups
   c. May still be a picky eater but willing to try new foods
  4. Skills
   a. Refinement of fine-motor skills
   b. Continued development of gross motor skills
   c. Increase in strength and endurance
  5. Play
   a. Play is more competitive
   b. Rules and rituals are important aspects of play and games
   c. Enjoys drawing, collecting items, dolls, pets, guessing games, board games, listening to the radio, TV, reading, and video and computer games
   d. Participates in team sports
   e. Participates in secret clubs, gang activities, scout organizations
  6. Safety
   a. Experiences less fear in play activities and frequently imitates real life by using tools and household items
   b. Adjust car seat belts so that the lap belt fits snugly over the bony pelvis and the shoulder harness is positioned across the chest
   c. Place the shoulder harness of the seat belt behind the shoulder if it crosses the face or soft tissue of the neck
   d. Major causes of injuries include bicycles, skateboards, and team sports as the child increases motor abilities and independence
   e. Children should always wear a helmet when riding a bike, inline skates, or skateboards
   f. Teach the child water safety rules
   g. Instruct the child to avoid teasing or playing roughly with animals
   h. Never allow the child to play with matches or lighters
   i. Children should be taught what to do in the event of a fire or if their clothes catch fire
   j. Fire drills should be practiced with the child
   k. Guns should be stored unloaded and secured under lock and key
   l. The child should be taught to leave an area immediately if a gun is seen, and to tell an adult
   m. Teach children that if another person touches their body in an inappropriate way, they should tell an adult
   n. Teach the child to avoid speaking to strangers and never to accept a ride, toys, or gifts from a stranger
   o. Teach traffic safety rules
   p. Teach the child how to dial 911 in an emergency situation
   q. Keep syrup of ipecac and the poison control number available
E. The Adolescent
  1. Physical
   a. In girls, **puberty** begins between ages 8 and 14
   b. In boys, **puberty** begins between the ages of 9 and 16
   c. Body mass increases to adult size
   d. Sebaceous and sweat glands become active and fully functional
   e. Body hair distribution occurs
   f. Increase in height, weight, breast development, and pelvic girth in girls
   g. Menstrual periods occur about 2½ years after the onset of **puberty**
   h. In boys, increase in height, weight, muscle mass, and penis and testicle size
   i. Voice deepens in boys
   j. Normal weight gain during **puberty**
   k. Girls gain 15 to 55 lb
   l. Boys gain 15 to 65 lb
   m. Careful brushing and care of the teeth are important, and many adolescents must wear braces
   n. Sleep patterns include a tendency to stay up late; therefore, in an attempt to catch up on missed sleep, adolescents sleep late at every opportunity
  2. Vital signs (Box 32–4)
  3. Nutrition
   a. Average daily requirements in girls is 38 to 48 kcal/kg/day
   b. Average daily requirements in boys is 42 to 60 kcal/kg/day
   c. Basic four food groups are important

BOX 32–4. The Adolescent's Vital Signs

Temperature: oral 97.5°–98.6°F
Apical rate: 55–90 beats per minute
Respirations: 15–20 breaths per minute
Blood pressure: average 93–131/49–85 mmHg

---

   d. Typically eat whenever they have a break in activities
   e. Calcium and protein needed to aid in bone and muscle **growth**

4. Skills
   a. Gross and fine-motor skills are well developed
   b. Strength and endurance increase
5. Play
   a. Games and athletics are the most common forms of play
   b. Competition is important
   c. Strict rules are important
   d. Enjoy activities such as sports, videos, movies, reading, parties, hobbies, computer games, music, and experimenting with makeup and hairstyles
6. Safety
   a. Risk takers
   b. Have a natural urge to experiment and be independent
   c. Instruct in the dangers related to drugs and alcohol
   d. Help to recognize that there are choices when difficult or potentially dangerous situations arise
   e. Advocate the use of seat belts
   f. Instruct in the consequences of injuries that motor vehicle accidents can cause
   g. Instruct in water safety and emphasize that they should enter the water feet first as opposed to diving, especially when the depth of the water is unknown
   h. Instruct about the dangers associated with violence and gangs

PRACTICE QUESTIONS

1. The parents of a 2-year-old arrive at the hospital to visit the child. The child is in the playroom and ignores the parents during the visit. This 2-year-old behavior indicates:
   1 The child is withdrawn
   2 The child is more interested in playing with other children
   3 The child has adjusted to the hospital setting
   4 A normal pattern

2. A mother arrives at the clinic with her toddler and tells the nurse that she has a difficult time getting the child to go to bed at night. Which of the following is most appropriate for the nurse to suggest to the mother?
   1 Inform the child of bedtime a few minutes before it is time for bed
   2 Allow the child to have temper tantrums
   3 Allow the child to set bedtime limits
   4 Avoid a nap during the day

3. The most appropriate toy for a 3-year-old is which of the following?
   1 A farm set
   2 A golf set
   3 A puzzle
   4 A wagon

4. The clinic nurse provides information to the mother of a toddler regarding toilet-training. Which of the following is not a component of the information session?
   1 Waiting until the child is 24 to 30 months old makes the task considerably easier
   2 Bladder control is usually achieved before bowel control
   3 The child should never be forced to sit on the potty for long periods
   4 The ability of the child to remove his or her clothing is a sign of physical readiness

5. The mother of a 3-year-old is concerned because the child is still insisting on a bottle at naptime and at bedtime. Which of the following is the most appropriate suggestion to the mother?
   1 Do not allow the child to have the bottle
   2 Allow the bottle during naps but not at bedtime
   3 Allow the bottle if it contains juice
   4 Allow the bottle if it contains water

6. The nurse assesses the vital signs of an infant with a respiratory infection. The respiratory rate is 50 breaths per minute. Which of the following actions are most appropriate?
   1 Notify the physician
   2 Administer oxygen
   3 Reassess the respiratory rate in 15 minutes
   4 Document the findings

7. The nurse prepares to take a blood pressure on a school-aged child. To obtain an accurate measurement, the blood pressure cuff should cover:
   1 One half of the distance between the antecubital fossa and the shoulder
   2 One third of the distance between the antecubital fossa and the shoulder
   3 Two thirds of the distance between the antecubital fossa and the shoulder
   4 One quarter of the distance between the antecubital fossa and the shoulder

8. The nurse provides instructions to the parents of a newborn regarding car travel and safety seats.

Which of the following are the most appropriate information related to the safety of the infant?
1 Restrain in a car seat in the front seat in a semireclined, rear-facing position
2 Restrain in a car scat in the front seat in a semireclined, forward-facing position
3 Restrain in a car seat in the middle backseat in a semireclined, rear-facing position
4 Restrain in a car seat in the middle backseat in a semireclined, forward-facing position

9. The nurse is monitoring a 3-month-old infant for increased intracranial pressure. On palpation of the fontanels, the nurse notes that the anterior fontanel has not closed and is soft and flat. Which of the following actions should the nurse take?
1 Elevate the head of the bed to 90 degrees
2 Notify the physician
3 Increase oral fluids
4 Document the findings

10. The nurse is evaluating the developmental level of a 2-year-old. Which of the following does the nurse expect to observe in this child?
1 Uses a fork to eat
2 Holds a cup in one hand
3 Uses a knife for cutting food
4 Pours own milk into a cup

11. The nurse is caring for a 5-year-old who has been placed in traction following a fracture to the femur. Which of the following is the most appropriate activity for this child?
1 Large picture books
2 A radio
3 A sports video
4 Finger paints

12. The mother of a 16-year-old tells the nurse that she is concerned because the child sleeps until noon every weekend, and whenever the child has a day off from school. The most appropriate nursing response is which of the following?
1 "The child should have a blood test to check for anemia."
2 "Adolescents love to sleep late in the morning."
3 "The child shouldn't be staying up so late at night."
4 "If the child eats properly, that shouldn't be happening."

13. A 4-year-old diagnosed with leukemia is hospitalized for chemotherapy. The child is fearful of the hospitalization. Which of the following nursing interventions are the most appropriate to alleviate the child's fears?
1 Advise the family to visit only during the scheduled visiting hours
2 Encourage play with other children of the same age

3 Provide a private room, allowing the child to bring the favorite toys from home
4 Encourage the child's parents to stay with the child

14. A 16-year-old is admitted to the hospital for acute appendicitis, and an appendectomy is performed. Which of the following interventions is most appropriate to facilitate normal growth and development?
1 Allow the family to bring in favorite computer games
2 Encourage the parents to room-in with the child
3 Encourage the child to rest and read
4 Allow the child to participate in activities with other individuals in the same age group when the condition permits

15. The nurse prepares to administer digoxin (Lanoxin) to a 3-year-old with a diagnosis of congestive heart failure. The nurse notes that the apical rate is 125 beats per minute (bpm). Which of the following nursing actions is most appropriate?
1 Administer the digoxin
2 Recheck the apical rate in 15 minutes
3 Notify the physician
4 Hold the medication

16. A 2-year-old is treated in the emergency room for a burn to the chest and abdomen. The child sustained the burn from grabbing a cup of hot coffee that was left on the kitchen counter. The nurse reviews safety principles with the parents before discharge. Which of the following statements, if made by the parents, indicates an understanding of the measures to provide safety in the home?
1 "I guess my children need to understand what the word 'hot' means."
2 "We will install a safety gate as soon as we get home so the children can't get into the kitchen."
3 "We will be sure that the children stay in their rooms when we work in the kitchen."
4 "We will be sure not to leave hot liquids unattended."

17. The clinic nurse provides instructions to a parent of a toddler experiencing physiological anorexia. Which of the following is not a component of the teaching plan?
1 Do not force-feed the child
2 Limit juice to 6 oz per day
3 Feed the child if he or she will not eat
4 Limit to two nutritious snacks per day and give only at the toddler's request

18. A mother of a 4-year-old expresses concern because her hospitalized child began thumb sucking. The mother states that this behavior began 2

days after hospital admission. The most appropriate nursing response is which of the following?
1 "A 4-year-old is too old for this type of behavior."
2 "Your child is acting like a baby."
3 "The doctor will need to be notified."
4 "It is best to ignore the behavior."

19. The clinic nurse assesses a 6-month-old infant. Which of the following does the nurse expect to note in this infant?
1 The use of simple words such as "Mama"
2 Single-consonant babbling
3 Waves bye-bye
4 Uses gestures to communicate

20. The mother of a toddler asks the nurse when it is safe to place the car safety seat in a forward-facing position. The best nursing response is which of the following?
1 Once the toddler is able to sit up alone
2 The seat should not be faced forward unless there are safety locks in the car
3 The seat should never be placed in a forward-facing position because of the risk of the child unbuckling the harness
4 When the height of the toddler is 27 inches

ANSWERS

1. **4**

Rationale: The toddler is particularly vunerable to separation. A toddler often shows anger at being left by ignoring the parent or by pretending to be more interested in play than in going home. Parents of hospitalized toddlers are frequently distressed by such behavior. The toddler engages in parallel play and plays alongside, but not with other children.

Test-Taking Strategy: Option 3 can be easily eliminated first. There are no data in the question to support option 1. From the remaining options, knowledge regarding separation anxiety in the toddler will direct you to option 4.

Level of Cognitive Ability: Analysis
Phase of Nursing Process: Analysis
Client Needs: Psychosocial Integrity
Content Area: Child Health

Reference
Ashwill, J., & Droske, S. (1997). *Nursing care of children: Principles and practice.* Philadelphia: W. B. Saunders. pp. 101–102.

2. **1**

Rationale: Most toddlers take an afternoon nap, and until their second birthday, some also require a morning nap. Toddlers often resist going to bed. Firm consistent limits are needed for temper tantrums or when toddlers try stalling tactics. Bedtime protests may be reduced by warning the child of bedtime a few minutes before the time.

Test-Taking Strategy: Options 3 and 4 can be easily eliminated. From the remaining two options, select option 1 over option 2 because preparing the toddler for an event will minimize resistive behavior.

Level of Cognitive Ability: Application
Phase of Nursing Process: Implementation
Client Needs: Health Promotion and Maintenance
Content Area: Child Health

Reference
Ashwill, J., & Droske, S. (1997). *Nursing care of children: Principles and practice.* Philadelphia: W. B. Saunders. p. 103.

3. **4**

Rationale: Toys for the toddler must be strong, safe, and too large to swallow or place in the ear or nose. Toddlers need supervision at all times. Push/pull toys, large balls, large crayons, trucks, and dolls are some of the appropriate toys. A farm set and a golf set may contain items that the child could swallow. Only a large puzzle is appropriate.

Test-Taking Strategy: Options 1 and 2 can be easily eliminated because they contain items that could be swallowed by the child. From the remaining options, the most appropriate toy is a wagon. Remember that large and strong toys are safest for the toddler.

Level of Cognitive Ability: Analysis
Phase of Nursing Process: Implementation
Client Needs: Psychosocial Integrity
Content Area: Child Health

Reference
Ashwill, J., & Droske, S. (1997). *Nursing care of children: Principles and practice.* Philadelphia: W. B. Saunders. pp. 102, 179.

4. **2**

Rationale: Waiting until the child is 24 to 30 months old makes the task considerably easier, because toddlers of this age are less negative and usually more willing to control their sphincters to please their parents. Bowel control is usually achieved before bladder control. The child should not be forced to sit for long periods. The ability to remove clothing is one of the physical signs of readiness.

Test-Taking Strategy: Note the key word "not" in the stem of the question. Option 3 can be easily eliminated. Knowledge of physiology will assist in eliminating options 1 and 4 and direct you to the correct option. Review the task of toilet-training now, if you had difficulty with this question!

Level of Cognitive Ability: Application
Phase of Nursing Process: Implementation
Client Needs: Health Promotion and Maintenance
Content Area: Child Health

Reference
Ashwill, J., & Droske, S. (1997). *Nursing care of children: Principles and practice.* Philadelphia: W. B. Saunders. p. 104.

5. **4**

Rationale: A toddler should never be allowed to fall asleep with a bottle because of the risk of bottle mouth caries. If the bottle is allowed in bed, it should contain only water.

Test-Taking Strategy: Eliminate options 1 and 2 because they are similar. Recalling that bottle mouth caries is a risk in children will assist in directing you to option 4.

Level of Cognitive Ability: Application
Phase of Nursing Process: Implementation
Client Needs: Health Promotion and Maintenance
Content Area: Child Health

Reference

Ashwill, J., & Droske, S. (1997). *Nursing care of children: Principles and practice.* Philadelphia: W. B. Saunders. p. 108.

6. **4**

Rationale: The normal respiratory rate in an infant is 30 to 60 breaths per minute. The normal apical rate is 120 to 160 bpm and the average blood pressure is 46 to 92/38 to 71 mmHg. The nurse documents the findings.

Test-Taking Strategy: Knowledge regarding the normal vital signs of an infant is required to answer this question. If you had difficulty with this question, take time now to review these normal parameters!

Level of Cognitive Ability: Analysis
Phase of Nursing Process: Analysis
Client Needs: Physiological Integrity
Content Area: Child Health

Reference

Ashwill, J., & Droske, S. (1997). *Nursing care of children: Principles and practice.* Philadelphia: W. B. Saunders. p. 212.

7. **3**

Rationale: The size of the BP cuff is important. Cuffs that are too small will cause falsely elevated values and those that are too large will cause inaccurate low values. The cuff should cover two thirds of the distance between the antecubital fossa and the shoulder.

Test-Taking Strategy: Attempt to visualize the placement measurements described in each of the options. This may assist in directing you to option 3. If you had difficulty with this question, take time now to review BP assessments in children!

Level of Cognitive Ability: Application
Phase of Nursing Process: Planning
Client Needs: Physiological Integrity
Content Area: Child Health

Reference

Ashwill, J., & Droske, S. (1997). *Nursing care of children: Principles and practice.* Philadelphia: W. B. Saunders. p. 213.

8. **3**

Rationale: Infants should be placed in a bucket-type car seat that faces backward in the backseat until they weigh 18 to 20 lb. The infant should never face forward or ride in the front seat.

Test-Taking Strategy: Visualize each of the descriptions in the options with a focus on safety. This should easily direct you to option 3. If you had difficulty with this question, take time now to review safety measures for the infant!

Level of Cognitive Ability: Application
Phase of Nursing Process: Implementation
Client Needs: Health Promotion and Maintenance
Content Area: Child Health

Reference

Ashwill, J., & Droske, S. (1997). *Nursing care of children: Principles and practice.* Philadelphia: W. B. Saunders. p. 290.

9. **4**

Rationale: The anterior fontanel is diamond shaped and located on the top of the head. It should be soft and flat in a normal infant, and it normally closes by 18 to 24 months of age. The posterior fontanel closes by 2 to 3 months of age.

Test-Taking Strategy: Note the key phrase "soft and flat." This should provide you with the clue that this is a normal finding. A bulging or tense fontanel may result from crying or increased ICP. If you had difficulty with this question, review normal assessment findings in an infant!

Level of Cognitive Ability: Application
Phase of Nursing Process: Implementation
Client Needs: Physiological Integrity
Content Area: Child Health

Reference

Ashwill, J., & Droske, S. (1997). *Nursing care of children: Principles and practice.* Philadelphia: W. B. Saunders. p. 57.

10. **2**

Rationale: By age 2 years, the child can hold a cup in one hand and use a spoon well. By ages 3 to 4, the child begins to use a fork. By the end of the preschool period, the child should begin to use a knife for cutting.

Test-Taking Strategy: Note the age of the child. Option 3 can be easily eliminated. Think about the fine-motor skills that need to be developed in selecting the correct option. With this in mind eliminate options 1 and 4. If you had difficulty with this question, review the developmental skills of a 2-year-old!

Level of Cognitive Ability: Analysis
Phase of Nursing Process: Evaluation
Client Needs: Health Promotion and Maintenance
Content Area: Child Health

Reference

Ashwill, J., & Droske, S. (1997). *Nursing care of children: Principles and practice.* Philadelphia: W. B. Saunders. p. 280.

11. **4**

Rationale: In the preschooler, play is simple and imaginative, and includes activities such as dressing up, finger paints, clay, pasting, and simple board and card games. Large picture books are most appropriate for the infant. A radio and sports video is most appropriate for the adolescent.

Test-Taking Strategy: Note the age of the child and think about the age-related activity that would be most appropriate. Eliminate options 2 and 3 knowing that they are most appropriate for the adolescent. From the remaining options, the word "large" in option 1 should provide you with the clue that this activity is more appropriate for a child younger than age 5. If you had difficulty with this question, review the appropriate activities for a preschooler!

Level of Cognitive Ability: Analysis
Phase of Nursing Process: Implementation
Client Needs: Psychosocial Integrity
Content Area: Child Health

Reference

Ashwill, J., & Droske, S. (1997). *Nursing care of children: Principles and practice.* Philadelphia: W. B. Saunders. p. 179.

12. **2**

Rationale: Sleep patterns in the adolescent vary according to individual need. Adolescents love to sleep late in the morning but they should be encouraged to be responsible for waking themselves, particularly in time to get ready for school.

Test-Taking Strategy: The question asks for the most appropriate nursing response. Options 3 and 4 can be eliminated first. From the remaining options, there is no indication that a physiological alteration is present; therefore, option 2 is most appropriate. Review adolescent sleep patterns now if you had difficulty with this question!

Level of Cognitive Ability: Application
Phase of Nursing Process: Implementation
Client Needs: Physiological Integrity
Content Area: Child Health

Reference
Luckmann, J. (1997). *Saunders manual of nursing care.* Philadelphia: W. B. Saunders. p. 509.

13. **4**

Rationale: Although the preschooler may already be spending some time away from parents at a day care center or preschool, illness adds a stressor that makes separation more difficult. The child may repeatedly ask when parents will be coming for a visit or may be constantly wanting to call the parents. Options 1 and 3 will increase stress related to separation anxiety. Option 2 is unrelated to the issue of the question and additionally may not be appropriate for a child at risk for immunocompromise.

Test-Taking Strategy: Note that the issue relates to the child's fear. Options 1 and 3 will further increase anxiety and fear, and should be eliminated. Bearing the issue of the question in mind, and considering the child's diagnosis, you should easily be directed toward option 4.

Level of Cognitive Ability: Application
Phase of Nursing Process: Implementation
Client Needs: Psychosocial Integrity
Content Area: Child Health

Reference
Ashwill, J., & Droske, S. (1997). *Nursing care of children: Principles and practice.* Philadelphia: W. B. Saunders. pp. 353–354.

14. **4**

Rationale: Adolescents often are not sure whether they want their parents with them when they are hospitalized. Because of the importance of the peer group, separation from friends is a source of anxiety. Ideally, the peer group will support their ill friend. Options 1, 2, and 3 isolate the child from the peer group.

Test-Taking Strategy: Consider the psychosocial needs of the adolescent when answering the question. Options 1, 2, and 3 are similar in that they isolate the child from his or her own peer group. If you had difficulty with this question, take time now to review the psychosocial needs of the adolescent!

Level of Cognitive Ability: Analysis
Phase of Nursing Process: Implementation
Client Needs: Psychosocial Integrity
Content Area: Child Health

Reference
Ashwill, J., & Droske, S. (1997). *Nursing care of children: Principles and practice.* Philadelphia: W. B. Saunders. p. 355.

15. **1**

Rationale: The normal apical rate for a 3-year-old is 80 to 125 bpm. Since the apical rate is within normal range, options 2, 3, and 4 are inappropriate.

Test-Taking Strategy: Knowledge of the normal vital signs is required to answer this question. Additionally, knowledge of the parameters related to the administration of digoxin will assist in directing you to option 1. If you had difficulty with this question, take time now to review these normal vital signs!

Level of Cognitive Ability: Analysis
Phase of Nursing Process: Implementation
Client Needs: Physiological Integrity
Content Area: Child Health

Reference
Ashwill, J., & Droske, S. (1997). *Nursing care of children: Principles and practice.* Philadelphia: W. B. Saunders. p. 212.

16. **4**

Rationale: Toddlers, with their increased mobility and developing motor skills, can reach hot water, open fires, or hot objects placed on counters and stoves above their eye level. Parents should be encouraged to remain in the kitchen when preparing a meal and reminded to use the back burners on the stove, and to turn pot handles inward and toward the middle of the stove. Hot liquids should never be left unattended, and the toddler should always be supervised. Options 1, 2, and 3 do not reflect an adequate understanding of the principles of safety.

Test-Taking Strategy: Option 1 can be easily eliminated. Options 2 and 3 are similar in that they isolate the child from the environment. Option 4 is the only option that reflects an understanding of safety principles by the parents.

Level of Cognitive Ability: Analysis
Phase of Nursing Process: Evaluation
Client Needs: Health Promotion and Maintenance
Content Area: Child Health

Reference
Ashwill, J., & Droske, S. (1997). *Nursing care of children: Principles and practice.* Philadelphia: W. B. Saunders. p. 295.

17. **3**

Rationale: A toddler has the skills required to feed self. Do not feed children who can feed themselves. Do not force-feed a child. To increase nutritious intake, limit juice intake to 6 oz per day, and milk intake to 16 to 24 oz per day. Additionally, limit to two nutritious snacks per day and give only at the toddler's request.

Test-Taking Strategy: Note the key word "not" in the stem of the question. Bearing in mind that the goal is to provide a nutritious intake should direct you to option 3. Additionally, feeding children if they will not eat will impair independence.

Level of Cognitive Ability: Application
Phase of Nursing Process: Implementation
Client Needs: Physiological Integrity
Content Area: Child Health

Reference
Ashwill, J., & Droske, S. (1997). *Nursing care of children: Principles and practice.* Philadelphia: W. B. Saunders. p. 281.

18. **4**

Rationale: In the hospitalized preschooler, it is best to accept regression if it occurs. Regression is most often due to the stress of the hospitalization. Parents may be overly concerned about regression and should be told that their child may continue the behavior at home. There is no need to call the physician. Options 1 and 2 are inappropriate.

Test-Taking Strategy: Note the key phrase "most appropriate." Options 1, 2, and 3 will cause additional stress and concern in the parent. If you had difficulty with this question, review the psychosocial issues related to the hospitalized preschool child!

Level of Cognitive Ability: Analysis
Phase of Nursing Process: Implementation
Client Needs: Psychosocial Integrity
Content Area: Child Health

Reference
Ashwill, J., & Droske, S. (1997). *Nursing care of children: Principles and practice*. Philadelphia: W. B. Saunders. pp. 355, 357.

19. **2**

Rationale: Single-consonant babbling occurs between 6 and 8 months. Between 8 and 9 months, the infant begins to understand and obey simple commands such as "wave bye-bye." Simple words such as "Mama" and the use of gestures to communicate begin between 9 and 12 months.

Test-Taking Strategy: Knowledge of language and communication developmental milestones is required to answer the question. Pay attention to the age of the infant identified in the question. This should assist in directing you to

option 2. Take time now to review these milestones if you had difficulty with this question!

Level of Cognitive Ability: Analysis
Phase of Nursing Process: Assessment
Client Needs: Physiological Integrity
Content Area: Child Health

Reference
Ashwill, J., & Droske, S. (1997). *Nursing care of children: Principles and practice*. Philadelphia: W. B. Saunders. p. 85.

20. **1**

Rationale: Once a toddler is able to sit up alone, car safety seats can be adjusted to face forward in an upright position. The car safety seat is suitable for the growing toddler until the toddler reaches the weight of 40 lb. Options 2, 3, and 4 are incorrect.

Test-Taking Strategy: Knowledge regarding car safety and the toddler is required to answer this question. Review these safety principles now if you had difficulty with this question!

Level of Cognitive Ability: Application
Phase of Nursing Process: Implementation
Client Needs: Health Promotion and Maintenance
Content Area: Child Health

Reference
Ashwill, J., & Droske, S. (1997). *Nursing care of children: Principles and practice*. Philadelphia: W. B. Saunders. p. 294.

BIBLIOGRAPHY

Ashwill, J., & Droske, S. (1997). *Nursing care of children: Principles and practice*. Philadelphia: W. B. Saunders.
Carson, V., & Arnold, E. (1996). *Mental health nursing: The nurse-patient journey*. Philadelphia: W. B. Saunders.
Hodgson, B., & Kizior, R. (1999). *Saunders nursing drug handbook 1999*. Philadelphia: W. B. Saunders.
Luckmann, J. (1997). *Saunders manual of nursing care*. Philadelphia: W. B. Saunders.
Nichols, F., & Zwelling, E. (1997). *Maternal newborn nursing: Theory and practice*. Philadelphia: W. B. Saunders.
O'Toole, M. (ed.). (1997). *Miller-Keane encyclopedia & dictionary of medicine, nursing, & allied health* (6th ed.). Philadelphia: W. B. Saunders.

CHAPTER 33

Neurological, Cognitive, and Psychosocial Disorders

. . . .

I. Head Injury

A. Description
1. The pathological result of any mechanical force to the skull, scalp, meninges, or brain
2. Multiple trauma is the leading cause of death in children beyond infancy
3. Manifestations depend on the type of injury and the subsequent amount of increased intracranial pressure (ICP)

◆ B. Assessment
1. Increased ICP in infants
   a. Poor feeding or vomiting
   b. Irritability or restlessness
   c. Lethargy
   d. Bulging fontanel
   e. Increased head circumference
   f. Separation of cranial sutures
   g. Distended scalp veins
   h. Eyes deviated downward (sunset sign)
   i. Increased or decreased response to pain
2. Increased ICP in children
   a. Headache
   b. Diplopia
   c. Mood swings
   d. Slurred speech
   e. Papilledema
   f. Altered level of consciousness (LOC)
   g. Nausea and vomiting
3. Late signs of increased ICP
   a. Tachycardia leading to bradycardia
   b. Apnea
   c. Systolic hypertension
   d. Widening pulse pressure
   e. Decorticate/decerebrate posturing

◆ C. Implementation
1. Monitor the airway
2. Assess neurological function
3. Assess vital signs
4. Monitor for decreased responsiveness to pain as a significant sign of altered LOC
5. Provide seizure precautions
6. Assess injuries
7. Immobilize the neck if a cervical injury is suspected
8. Administer oxygen and IV fluids as prescribed
9. Monitor for nose or ear drainage, which could indicate leakage of cerebrospinal fluid (CSF)
10. Monitor intake and output (I&O) and electrolyte status
11. Avoid nasotracheal suction in a child with a basal or skull fracture
12. Assess wound dressings for the presence of drainage

II. Hydrocephalus

A. Description
1. An imbalance of CSF absorption or production, caused by malformations, tumors, hemorrhage, infections, or trauma
2. Results in head enlargement and increased ICP
B. Types
1. Communicating
   a. Occurs as a result of impaired absorption within the subarachnoid space
   b. No interference of CSF within the ventricular system occurs
2. Noncommunicating: obstruction of CSF flow within the ventricular system occurs
C. Assessment
1. Infant
   a. Increased head circumference
   b. Bones of the head are thin and widely separated

    c. Anterior fontanel tense, bulging, and nonpulsating

    d. Scalp veins dilated

    e. Frontal bossing

    f. Sunsetting eyes

  2. Child

    a. Behavior changes such as irritability and lethargy

    b. Headache upon awakening

    c. Nausea and vomiting

    d. Ataxia

    e. Nystagmus

    f. High, shrill cry and seizure activity are late signs

D. Surgical Implementation

  1. The goal of surgical treatment is to prevent further CSF accumulation by bypassing the blockage and draining the fluid from the ventricles where it may be reabsorbed

  2. Ventriculoperitoneal **shunt** (VP **shunt**): CSF drains into the peritoneal cavity from the lateral ventricle

  3. Atrioventricular **shunt** (AV **shunt**): CSF drains into the right atrium of the heart from the lateral ventricle bypassing the obstruction

E. Implementation Postoperatively

  1. Monitor vital signs

  2. Monitor for signs of infection and assess dressings for drainage

  3. For the first 2 days, position on nonoperated side as prescribed so that no weight is placed on the valve

  4. The child is kept flat as prescribed to avoid rapid reduction of intracranial fluid

  5. Observe for increased ICP

  6. If increased ICP occurs, elevate the head of the bed to 15 to 30 degrees to enhance gravity flow through the **shunt**

  7. Measure head circumference

  8. Monitor I&O

  9. Provide comfort measures

  10. Administer medications as prescribed, which may include diuretics, antibiotics, or anticonvulsants

  11. Instruct parents how to recognize **shunt** infection or malfunction

III. Spina Bifida

A. Description

  1. Central nervous system (CNS) defect that occurs as a result of neural tube failure to close during embryonic development

  2. Associated deficits include sensory or motor disturbance, dislocated hips, and club feet and hydrocephalus

  3. Defect closure usually done during infancy

B. Types

  1. Spina bifida occulta

    a. Posterior vertebral arches fail to close in the lumbosacral area

    b. Spinal cord remains intact and usually is not visible

    c. Meninges are not exposed on skin surface

    d. Neurological deficits are not usually present

  2. Spina bifida cystica

    a. Protrusion of the spinal cord and/or its meninges

    b. Results in incomplete closure of the vertebral and neural tubes resulting in a sac-like protrusion in the lumbar or sacral area, with varying degrees of nervous tissue involvement

    c. Can include meningocele, myelomeningocele, lipomeningocele and lipomeningomyelocele

  3. Meningocele

    a. Protrusion involves meninges and a sac-like cyst that contains CSF in the midline of the back, usually in the lumbosacral area

    b. No involvement of spinal cord

    c. Neurological deficits are usually not present

  4. Myelomeningocele

    a. Protrusion of meninges, CSF, nerve roots, and a portion of the spinal cord

    b. The sac is covered by a thin membrane that is prone to leakage or rupture

    c. Neurological deficits are evident

  5. Assessment

    a. Depends on spinal cord involvement

    b. Visible spinal defect

    c. Flaccid paralysis of the legs

    d. Altered bladder and bowel function

    e. Hip and joint deformities

  6. Implementation

    a. Evaluate the sac and measure the lesion

    b. Perform neurological assessment

    c. Monitor for ICP

    d. Measure the head circumference

    e. Assess the anterior fontanel for fullness

    f. Protect the sac

    g. Place in a prone position to avoid stress or pressure on the sac

    h. Use an aseptic technique to prevent infection

    i. Cover sac with sterile saline dressing to maintain the moisture of the sac and contents

    j. Change the dressing whenever soiled because of the risk of infection

    k. Assess the sac for redness or clear or purulent drainage

    l. Assess for physical impairments

    m. Prepare the child and family for surgery

    n. Administer antibiotics as prescribed to prevent infection

    o. Administer anticholinergics to improve urinary continence, antispasmodics to control bladder spasms, and laxatives to achieve bowel continence as prescribed

IV. Reye's Syndrome

A. Description
1. Acute encephalopathy characterized by a viral infection leading to hepatic, metabolic, and neurologic failure
2. The exact cause is not clear
3. It is recommended that aspirin not be administered to children with varicella or influenza because of its association with Reye's syndrome
4. Acetaminophen (Tylenol) is considered the medication of choice for pediatric clients
5. The goal of treatment is to maintain effective cerebral perfusion and control increasing ICP

B. Assessment
1. History of systemic viral illness 4 to 7 days before the onset of symptoms
2. Malaise
3. Nausea
4. Vomiting
5. Progressive neurological deterioration

C. Implementation
1. Assess neurological status
2. Monitor for signs of ICP
3. Monitor cardiac and respiratory status
4. Monitor hydration status
5. Maintain fluid and electrolyte balance
6. Monitor for signs of bleeding, which can occur with hepatic involvement

V. Meningitis

A. Description
1. An infectious process of the CNS caused by bacteria and viruses that may be acquired as a primary disease or as a result of complications of neurosurgery, trauma, infection of the sinus or ears, or systemic infections
2. Diagnosis is made by testing CSF obtained by lumbar puncture, which shows increased pressure, cloudy CSF, high protein, and low glucose
3. Meningococcal meningitis is transmitted primarily by droplet infection
4. Viral meningitis is associated with viruses such as mumps, paramyxovirus, herpes virus and enterovirus

B. Assessment
1. Signs and symptoms vary depending on the age of the child and the duration of the preceding illness, and there is no one classic sign or symptom
2. Fever
3. Vomiting
4. Diarrhea
5. Poor feeding or anorexia
6. Headache
7. Poor or high-pitched cry
8. Altered level of consciousness such as lethargy or irritability
9. Nuchal rigidity
10. Bulging anterior fontanel in the infant
11. Kernig's sign and Brudzinski's sign in children and adolescents
12. Muscle or joint pain

C. Implementation
1. Provide isolation and maintain for at least 24 hours after antibiotics are initiated
2. Administer antibiotics as prescribed
3. Perform neurological assessment
4. Assess for personality changes and irritability
5. Monitor I&O
6. Assess nutritional status
7. Determine close contacts of the child with meningitis because they will need prophylactic treatment

VI. Seizures

A. Description
1. Sudden, transient alterations in brain function resulting from excessive levels of electrical activity in the brain
2. Classified as either partial or generalized, depending on the area of the brain involved

B. Assessment
1. Obtain information from parents about the time of onset, precipitating events, and behavior before and after the seizure
2. Determine child's history related to seizures

C. Implementation
1. Ensure patency of the airway
2. Stay with the child during a seizure
3. Assess skin color, respiratory rate, and signs of respiratory distress
4. Monitor breathing during and after the seizure
5. Do not restrain the child or place anything in the child's mouth
6. Place in side-lying position with side rail up, protecting the child
7. Loosen clothing around the child's neck
8. Pad crib or bed
9. Remove sharp objects from the bed
10. Administer anticonvulsants as prescribed
11. Instruct parents in the administration and side effects of the prescribed anticonvulsants

VII. Cerebral Palsy

A. Description: A chronic disability characterized by a difficulty in controlling the muscles due to an abnormality in the extrapyramidal or pyramidal motor system

B. Assessment
1. Irritability
2. Feeding difficulties
3. Delayed development
4. Poor motor development
5. Abnormal posturing
6. Ataxic gait
7. Poor muscle tone
8. Persistence of infant reflexes

C. Implementation
1. The goal to management is early recognition and intervention to maximize the child's abilities
2. A multidisciplinary team approach is implemented to meet the many needs of the child
3. Assess the child's developmental level and **intelligence**
4. Encourage early intervention and participation in school programs
5. Encourage communication and interaction with the child on a functional level not **chronological age** level
6. Provide a safe environment by removing sharp objects, using a protective helmet if the child falls frequently, and implementing seizure precautions if necessary
7. Provide safe, appropriate toys for age and developmental level
8. Position upright after meals
9. Reinforce speech therapy techniques, nonverbal methods to communicate, proper feeding techniques, and jaw control

VIII. Mental Retardation

A. Description
1. Subaverage general intellectual functioning along with a deficit in adaptation in behavior
2. Down syndrome is a congenital condition that results in moderate to severe retardation and has been linked to an extra group G chromosome, chromosome 21 (trisomy 21)
B. Assessment
1. Cognitive skills and level of adaptive functioning
2. Delays in fine and gross motor skills
3. Speech delays
4. Decreased spontaneous activity
5. Nonresponsiveness
6. Irritability
7. Poor eye contact during feeding
C. Implementation
1. Medical strategies are focused on preventing and treating infections, correcting structural deformities, and treating associated behaviors
2. Implement community and educational services using a multidisciplinary approach
3. Promote care skills as much as possible
4. Assist with communication and socialization skills
5. Facilitate appropriate play time
6. Initiate safety precautions as necessary
7. Assist the family with decisions regarding care
8. Provide information regarding support services and community agencies

IX. Autism

A. Description
1. A severe mental disorder beginning in infancy or toddlerhood
2. Apparent to the parents before the age of 3
3. Characterized by impairment in reciprocal social interaction and in verbal and nonverbal communication
4. The cause is unknown and the prognosis may be poor
5. Diagnosis is established on the basis of symptoms and through the use of specialized autism assessment tools
6. Also called infantile autism
B. Assessment
1. Disturbance in the rate and appearance of physical, social, and language skills
2. Abnormal responses of body sensations
3. Thinking capacity, but with absent or delayed speech and language
4. Abnormal ways of relating to people, objects, and events
5. There are no delusions, hallucinations, or incoherence, and the facies is intelligent and responsive
6. The child is self-absorbed and unable to relate to others
7. The child may play happily alone for hours, but have temper tantrums if interrupted
8. Language disturbance often includes repetition of previously heard speech and reversal of the pronouns "I" and "you"
9. If the child can talk, the child uses speech not for communication but to repeat words or phrases meaninglessly
10. The child may develop an unusual attachment to a significant object and display frequent rocking, spinning, twirling, or other bizarre behaviors
C. Implementation
1. Determine the child's routines, habits, and preferences and maintain consistency as much as possible
2. Determine the specific ways in which the child communicates
3. Facilitate communication through the use of picture boards
4. Evaluate the child for safety
5. Implement safety precautions as necessary for self-injurious behaviors such as head banging
6. Monitor for stress and anxiety
7. Avoid placing demands on the child
8. Initiate referrals to special programs as required
9. Provide support to parents

X. Attention Deficit Hyperactivity Disorder (ADHD)

A. Description
1. A developmental disorder characterized by developmentally inappropriate degrees of inattention, overactivity, and impulsivity
2. One of the most common reasons for referral of children to mental health services

3. Childhood problems include lowered intellectual development, some minor physical abnormalities, sleeping disturbances, behavioral or emotional disorders, and difficulty in social relationships

4. Diagnosis is established on the basis of self-reports, parent and teacher reports, and psychological assessments

B. Assessment
1. Fidgets with the hands or feet or squirms in the seat
2. Easily distracted with external or internal stimuli
3. Difficulty with following through on instructions
4. Poor attention span
5. Shifts from one uncompleted activity to another
6. Talks excessively
7. Interrupts or intrudes others
8. Engages in physically dangerous activities without considering the possible consequences

C. Implementation
1. Provide environmental and physical safety measures
2. Enhance capabilities and self-esteem
3. Encourage support groups for parents
4. Administer methylphenidate (Ritalin) as prescribed
5. Instruct the child and parents regarding medication administration
6. Inform the child and parents that positive effects of medication will be seen within 1 to 2 weeks if taken as prescribed

XI. Tourette's Disorder

A. Description: Appears between ages 2 and 15 and is characterized by recurrent involuntary and rapid movements affecting various parts of the body accompanied by vocal noises such as barks, grunts, or profanities

B. Implementation
1. Establish a trusting one-on-one relationship
2. Protect the client from harm by providing a helmet or protective padding
3. Allow the child to have a favorite toy or other object
4. Provide positive reinforcement for appropriate behaviors
5. Maintain eye contact
6. Assess suicide potential
7. Remove dangerous objects from the environment
8. Set limits on socially inappropriate or manipulative behaviors
9. Encourage the client to confront tension and frustration before they emerge as inappropriate behaviors
10. Provide noncompetitive group situations

XII. Child Abuse

A. Description: Involves emotional or physical **abuse** or neglect, as well as sexual exploitation or molestation by caretakers or other individuals

B. Assessment
1. Physical **abuse**
   a. Unexplained bruises, burns, or fractures
   b. Bald spots on the scalp
   c. Apprehensive child
   d. Extreme aggressiveness or withdrawal
   e. Fear of the parents
   f. Lack of crying when approached by a stranger
2. Physical neglect
   a. Inadequate weight gain
   b. Poor hygiene
   c. Consistent hunger
   d. Inconsistent school attendance
   e. Constant fatigue
   f. Reports of lack of child supervision
   g. Delinquency
3. Emotional **abuse**
   a. Speech disorders
   b. Habit disorders such as sucking, biting, rocking
   c. Psychoneurotic reactions
   d. **Learning** disorders
   e. Suicide attempts
4. Sexual **abuse**
   a. Difficulty walking or sitting
   b. Torn, stained, or bloody underclothing
   c. Pain, swelling, or itching of the genitals
   d. Bruises, bleeding, or lacerations in the genital or anal area
   e. Unwillingness to change clothes or unwillingness to participate in gym activities
   f. Poor peer relations
   g. Delinquency
   h. Changes in sleep performance
   i. Self-disruptive behavior

C. Implementation
1. Assess the parents' strengths and weaknesses, normal coping mechanisms, and presence or absence of support systems
2. Support the child during a thorough physical assessment
3. Assess injuries
4. Report cases of suspected **abuse**
5. Place the child in an environment that is safe, thereby preventing further injury
6. Document in an objective manner information related to the suspected **abuse**
7. Assist the family in identifying stressors, support systems, and resources
8. Refer the family to appropriate support groups

PRACTICE QUESTIONS

1. The nurse is performing an admission assessment on a 6-month-old infant with a diagnosis of hydrocephalus. The nurse assesses for the major

symptom associated with hydrocephalus when the nurse:

1 Tests the urine for protein
2 Takes the apical pulse
3 Palpates the anterior fontanel
4 Takes the blood pressure

2. The nurse recognizes that the infant with the diagnosis of hydrocephalus has a head that is heavier than the average infant. The nurse also recognizes that special safety precautions are needed when moving the infant with hydrocephalus. Which of the following statements should the nurse include in the discharge teaching with the parents to reflect this safety need?

1 "When picking 'up your infant, support the infant's neck and head with the open palm of your hand."
2 "Feed your infant in a side-lying position."
3 "Place a helmet on your infant when in bed."
4 "Hyperextend your infant's head and place a rolled towel under the neck area."

3. The nurse is evaluating the parent's understanding of discharge care including the functioning of the infant's ventricular peritoneal shunt. Which of the following statements, if made by the parent, indicates accurate assessment of shunt complications?

1 "If the baby has a high-pitched cry, I should call the doctor."
2 "I should position my baby on the side with the shunt when sleeping."
3 "My baby will pass urine more often now that the shunt is in place."
4 "I should call my doctor if my baby refuses purees."

4. The nurse is performing an admission assessment on a newborn with the diagnosis of spina bifida (meningomyelocele type). The nurse assesses for a major symptom associated with this type of spina bifida when the nurse:

1 Checks the capillary refill on the nailbeds of the upper extremities
2 Tests the urine for blood
3 Palpates the abdomen for masses
4 Checks for responses to painful stimuli from the torso downward

5. A mother arrives at the emergency room with her 5-year-old child. The mother states that the child fell off a bunk bed. A head injury is suspected. The nurse assesses the child for signs of increased intracranial pressure (ICP). Which of the following is a late sign of increased ICP?

1 Bulging fontanel
2 Altered level of consciousness
3 Nausea
4 Widening pulse pressure

6. The nurse is caring for a newborn with spina bifida (meningomyelocele type). The newborn is scheduled for the removal of the gibbus (sac on the back filled with cerebrospinal fluid, meninges, and some of the spinal cord). In the preoperative period, the priority nursing action is to monitor:

1 Blood pressure
2 Moisture of the normal saline dressing on the gibbus area
3 Specific gravity
4 Anterior fontanel for depression

7. The community health nurse visits an infant with spina bifida (meningomyelocele type) at home. The nurse is part of the early intervention program team. The nurse has done primary teaching with the parents for home care. Which of the following statements, if made by the parents, indicates further teaching is necessary?

1 "Our baby needs to be supported in a baby seat when being fed."
2 "Our baby is putting toys in her mouth."
3 "Our baby's legs are floppy, so we haven't been doing the exercises."
4 "Our baby cannot crawl, but pulls herself around the carpet."

8. The nurse is caring for a child with spina bifida who has a neurogenic bladder. As part of the nursing care plan, the nurse monitors for urinary tract infections. The nurse anticipates that the most likely medication to be prescribed prophylactically is:

1 Prednisone
2 Furosemide (Lasix)
3 Sulfisoxazole (Gantrisin)
4 Immune globulin IV

9. The nurse is caring for a child with Reye's syndrome. The nurse assesses for the major symptom associated with Reye's syndrome when the nurse notes:

1 Persistent vomiting
2 Protein in the urine
3 A history of a staphylococcus infection
4 Symptoms of hyperglycemia

10. The child is diagnosed with Reye's syndrome. The nurse prepares a nursing care plan for this child and, in the planning, the nurse includes:

1 Providing a quiet atmosphere with dimmed lights
2 Assessing hearing loss
3 Monitoring output
4 Changing body position every 2 hours

11. The physician prescribes home health nurse visits for the child discharged home with Reye's syndrome. During a home visit, the nurse instructs the parents concerning the residual effects of Reye's syndrome. Which of the following statements, if made by the parents, indicates a need for further instruction?

1 "We need to decrease the stimuli at home to prevent intracranial pressure."

2 "We need to give frequent, small, nutritious meals to decrease the amount of vomiting."

3 "We need to have the child nap during the day to provide rest."

4 "We need to check for jaundiced skin and eyes every day."

12. The nurse is performing an admission assessment on a child with seizures. The nurse is interviewing the child's parents to establish their adjustment to caring for a child with a chronic illness. Which of the following statements, if made by parents, indicates a need for further teaching?

1 "Our child is involved in a swim program with neighbors and friends."

2 "Our child sleeps in our bedroom at night."

3 "Our baby-sitter just completed CPR training."

4 "We worry about injuries when our child has a seizure."

13. Which of the following assessment data indicates a potential complication associated with a seizure?

1 Blood on the pillow

2 Blanched toenails

3 Migraine headaches

4 High-pitched cry

14. The nurse plans for a safe environment when caring for an infant at risk for a grand mal seizure. In the plan of care, the seizure precautions most appropriately include placing which of the following items at the bedside?

1 A suction apparatus and an airway

2 Oxygen with a tracheotomy set

3 Emergency cart

4 Airway and a tracheotomy set

15. The nurse is caring for a child with grand mal seizures. Phenytoin sodium (Dilantin) is prescribed for the child. Which of the following should most appropriately be included in the plan of care for this child?

1 Monitoring intake and output every shift

2 Checking the blood pressure before the administration of medications

3 Providing oral hygiene, especially care of the gums, every shift

4 Administer medications a half hour before food intake

16. Adolescents with seizure disorders need special teaching regarding their care. The nurse is performing discharge teaching to an adolescent with a history of grand mal seizures, who is on an anticonvulsant medication. Which of the following statements, if made by the adolescent, indicates an understanding of the teaching?

1 "I will never be able to drive a car."

2 "My anticonvulsant medication will clear up my skin."

3 "I can't drink alcohol while I am taking my medication."

4 "If I forget my morning medication, I can take two pills at bedtime."

17. The nurse is performing an admission assessment on a child admitted with a diagnosis of grand mal seizures. The nurse assesses for causes of the seizure activity when the nurse:

1 Tests the child's urine for specific gravity

2 Obtains a family history of psychiatric illness

3 Obtains a history of any factors that might precipitate seizure activity

4 Asks the child what happens during a seizure

18. Anticonvulsant medications have therapeutic values that are monitored to evaluate their prevention of seizure activity. The nurse is caring for a child on carbamazepine (Tegretol). Which of the following serum drug levels are therapeutic for this medication?

1 0 to 6 mcg/mL

2 2 to 8 mcg/mL

3 4 to 12 mcg/mL

4 10 to 12 mcg/mL

19. The nurse is caring for a child recently diagnosed with cerebral palsy. The parents of the child ask the nurse about the disorder. The nurse bases the response to the parents on the understanding that cerebral palsy is:

1 A chronic disability characterized by a difficulty in controlling the muscles

2 An infectious disease of the central nervous system

3 An inflammation of the brain as a result of a viral illness

4 A congenital condition that results in moderate to severe retardation

20. The nurse is caring for a child with cerebral palsy. The primary goal to be included in the plan of care is to:

1 Eliminate the cause of the disease

2 Prevent the occurrence of emotional disturbances

3 Maximize the child's assets and minimize the limitations caused by the disease

4 Improve muscle control and coordination

21. The nurse is caring for a child diagnosed with Down syndrome. In describing the disorder to the parents, the nurse bases the explanation on the fact that Down syndrome is a:

1 Condition characterized by above average intellectual functioning with deficits in adaptive behavior

2 Condition characterized by average intellectual functioning and the absence of deficits in adaptive behavior

3 Congenital condition that results in moderate

to severe retardation and has been linked to an extra group G chromosome

4 Condition characterized by subaverage intellectual functioning with the absence of deficits in adaptive behavior

22. The nurse is caring for an 8-year-old child with a basilar skull fracture. Which of the following physician orders does the nurse question?
1 Restrict fluid intake
2 Keep an IV line patent
3 Insert an indwelling urinary catheter
4 Suction PRN

23. A lumbar puncture is performed on a child suspected of having bacterial meningitis. Cerebrospinal fluid (CSF) is obtained for analysis. Which of the following results verify the diagnosis?
1 Cloudy CSF with low protein and low glucose
2 Cloudy CSF with high protein and low glucose
3 Clear CSF with high protein and low glucose
4 Decreased pressure, cloudy CSF with high protein

24. The nurse is caring for a child with meningococcal meningitis. Based on the mode of transmission of this infection, which of the following is included in the plan of care?
1 No precautions are required as long as antibiotics have been started
2 Maintain enteric precautions
3 Maintain isolation precautions for at least 24 hours after the initiation of antibiotics
4 Maintain neutropenic precautions

25. The nurse develops a plan of care for the child with meningitis. Which of the following is the priority nursing diagnosis for this child?
1 Altered cerebral tissue perfusion
2 Parental knowledge deficit
3 Altered family process
4 Alteration in comfort

26. The nurse assessing for an early sign of meningitis in a child attempts to elicit Kernig's sign. The appropriate procedure to elicit Kernig's sign is to:

1 Bend the head toward the knees and hips and assess for pain
2 Tap the facial nerve and assess for spasm
3 Compress the upper arm and assess for tetany
4 Extend the leg and knee and assess for pain

27. The clinical nurse is observing a child diagnosed with autism. The primary characteristics of autism include which of the following?
1 Consistent imitation of the actions of others
2 Normal social play
3 Lack of social interaction and awareness
4 Normal verbal but abnormal nonverbal communication

28. Following assessment of the child with autism, the nurse develops a plan of care. The priority nursing diagnosis included in the plan of care is which of the following?
1 Impaired social interaction
2 Risk for injury
3 Altered thought processes
4 Impaired verbal communication

29. The emergency room nurse is performing an assessment on a child suspected of being sexually abused. Which of the following assessment data most likely indicate this suspicion?
1 Poor hygiene
2 Bald spots on the scalp
3 Fear of the parents
4 Swelling of the genitals

30. The nurse performs an admission assessment on a child and suspects physical abuse. Which of the following is a primary and legal nursing responsibility?
1 Document the child's physical assessment findings accurately and thoroughly
2 Report the case in which the abuse is suspected
3 Refer the family to the appropriate support groups
4 Assist the family in identifying resources and support systems

ANSWERS

1. **3**

Rationale: An elevated or bulging anterior fontanel indicates an increase in cerebrospinal fluid (CSF) collection in the cerebral ventricle. Proteinuria, apical pulse, and blood pressure changes are not specific to increasing CSF in the brain tissue.

Test-Taking Strategy: Use the principles associated with excessive fluid build-up in the cranial cavity when answering the question. Fluid accumulation in the cranial cavity will exert pressure on the soft brain tissue. This will cause the anterior fontanel to expand. A method of assessing fluid collection in the cranial cavity is to palpate this anterior fontanel. A full or bulging fontanel will indicate increasing amounts of fluid accumulation. Additionally, correlate "hydrocephalus" in the question, with "anterior fontanel" in option 3, the correct option. If you had difficulty with this question, take time to review the symptoms associated with hydrocephalus!

Level of Cognitive Ability: Application
Phase of Nursing Process: Assessment
Client Needs: Physiological Integrity
Content Area: Child Health

Reference

Wong, D., & Whaley, L. (1996). *Clinical manual of pediatric nursing* (4th ed.). St. Louis: Mosby–Year Book. pp. 472–473.

2. **1**

Rationale: Hydrocephalus is a condition characterized by an enlargement of the cranium as a result of an abnormal accumulation of cerebrospinal fluid within the cerebral ventricular system. This characteristic causes the increase in the weight of the infant's head. The infant's head becomes top-heavy. Supporting the infant's head and neck, when picking it up, will prevent the hyperextension of the neck area and the infant from falling backward. Options 2, 3, and 4 are incorrect. The infant should be fed with the head elevated for proper motility of food processing. A helmet could suffocate an unattended infant during rest and sleep times, and hyperextension of the infant's head can put pressure on the neck vertebrae, causing injury.

Test-Taking Strategy: This question asks you to select the parent teaching that would provide prevention of injury when moving the infant with an enlarged head. There is only one correct answer. Options 2, 3, and 4 are unsafe practices and additionally do not specifically address the issue of the question, moving the infant. If you had difficulty with this question, take time now to review care of the infant with hydrocephalus!

Level of Cognitive Ability: Application
Phase of Nursing Process: Planning
Client Needs: Safe, Effective Care Environment
Content Area: Child Health

Reference

O'Toole, M. (ed.). (1997). *Miller-Keane encyclopedia & dictionary of medicine, nursing, & allied health* (6th ed.). Philadelphia: W. B. Saunders. p. 762.

3. **1**

Rationale: If the shunt is broken or malfunctioning, the fluid from the ventricle part of the brain will not be diverted to the peritoneal cavity. The cerebrospinal fluid will build up in the cranial area. The result is intracranial pressure that then causes a high-pitched cry in the infant. Option 2 is incorrect. The baby should not have pressure when on the shunt side. Skin breakdown and possible compressions to the apparatus could result. Option 3 is incorrect. This type of shunt affects the gastrointestinal system, not the genitourinary system. Option 4 is only a concern if the baby becomes malnourished or dehydrated, which could then raise the body temperature. Otherwise, refusal to eat purees has no direct relationship to the shunt's functioning.

Test-Taking Strategy: Knowledge regarding a ventricular peritoneal shunt is required to answer the question. Use the process of elimination based on this knowledge to answer the question. Remember that a high-pitched cry in an infant indicates a concern or problem. If you had difficulty with this question, take time now to review assessment findings that indicate a complication with a shunt!

Level of Cognitive Ability: Analysis
Phase of Nursing Process: Evaluation
Client Needs: Health Promotion and Maintenance
Content Area: Child Health

Reference

Ashwill, J., & Droske, S. (1997). *Nursing care of children: Principles and practice*. Philadelphia: W. B. Saunders. pp. 1237–1240.

4. **4**

Rationale: Newborns with spina bifida (meningomyelocele type) demonstrate lack of nerve innervation from below the site of the gibbus (sac containing the meninges and spinal cord with excess cerebrospinal fluid). They therefore show diminished or no responses to painful stimuli in these areas below the gibbus. Options 1, 2, and 3 are incorrect because the area above the gibbus is not affected. The capillary refill is normal. The urine will not have blood present. If the kidneys are affected, proteinuria could be present but not generally in the newborn period. No masses are present besides the gibbus on the back area, externally protruding from the vertebral deformity.

Test-Taking Strategy: Use the knowledge of the complications of diminished or absent nerve innervation, to the area below the gibbus, to answer this assessment question regarding spina bifida (meningomyelocele type). This problem, with nerve innervation, is caused by the compression of the spinal cord where the space between two vertebrae occurs. If the spinal cord is traumatized, it is irreversible. If it is compressed, surgical intervention will relieve the pressure and increase the transmission of nerve impulses to the areas that were affected. If you had difficulty with this question, take time now to review the symptoms associated with meningomyelocele!

Level of Cognitive Ability: Application
Phase of Nursing Process: Assessment
Client Needs: Physiological Integrity
Content Area: Child Health

Reference

Ashwill, J., & Droske, S. (1997). *Nursing care of children: Principles and practice*. Philadelphia: W. B. Saunders. p. 1234.

5. **4**

Rationale: Late signs of increased ICP include tachycardia leading to bradycardia, apnea, systolic hypertension, widening pulse pressure, and posturing. A bulging fontanel is a sign of increased ICP in an infant. Nausea and altered level of consciousness are signs of increased ICP in a child. Options 1, 2, and 3 are not late signs.

Test-Taking Strategy: Note the age of the child and that the question asks for the "late" sign. Option 1 can be eliminated because the fontanels are closed in a child. Knowledge of the early and late signs will direct you to the correct option.

Level of Cognitive Ability: Analysis
Phase of Nursing Process: Assessment
Client Needs: Physiological Integrity
Content Area: Child Health

Reference

Ashwill, J., & Droske, S. (1997). *Nursing care of children: Principles and practice*. Philadelphia: W. B. Saunders. p. 1259.

6. **2**

Rationale: The newborn is at risk for infection before closure of the gibbus. A sterile normal saline dressing is placed over the gibbus to maintain moisture of the gibbus and its contents. This prevents tearing or breakdown of the skin integrity at the site. Blood pressure is difficult to assess during the newborn period and is not the best indicator of infection. Urine concentration is not well developed in the newborn stage of development. Depression of the anterior fontanel is a sign of dehydration. With spina bifida, an increase in intracranial pressure is more of a priority. A complication of spina bifida demonstrates a bulging or taut anterior fontanel.

Test-Taking Strategy: Knowledge of the characteristics of spina bifida and the potential complications is needed to correctly answer this question. Read the question carefully. The question asks for a preoperative priority nursing action. Blood pressure and specific gravity are common preoperative assessments but are not as reliable an indicator of changes in newborn status, as they would be for an older child. Knowledge of the newborn development of organ maturity and body functioning is also needed to make the correct selection from the options present. Option 2 is the only correct choice. Review preoperative care now if you had difficulty with this question!

Level of Cognitive Ability: Application
Phase of Nursing Process: Implementation
Client Needs: Physiological Integrity
Content Area: Child Health

Reference
Ashwill, J., & Droske, S. (1997). *Nursing care of children: Principles and practice.* Philadelphia: W. B. Saunders. p. 1234.

7. **3**

Rationale: The parents need additional information concerning the importance of doing passive range of motion to the flaccid extremities to prevent contractures. Range of motion and proper positioning will maintain functional positions of the extremities for further bracing and maintenance of skin integrity. With spina bifida (meningomyelocele type), the child will not regain full neurological functioning because of the spinal cord damage already done. Option 1 demonstrates knowledge of an unsteady body posture and inadequate muscle control, characteristics common to this type of spina bifida. Options 2 and 4 reflect normal infant development milestones with some adaptations by the infant when trying to crawl.

Test-Taking Strategy: Knowledge of normal infant growth and development, as well as adaptive skills the infant with special needs (flaccid muscles) can employ to gain a milestone, is required to answer the question. With this knowledge you can determine appropriate behaviors and responses of the parents to their baby's care and achievements. Options 1, 2, and 4 all reflect appropriate activities that will promote normal growth and development of their infant. Option 3 demonstrates a lack of rationale for doing range of motion exercises with their baby. Further teaching is needed to increase compliance with this part of the home care plan. Review parent education teaching points now if you had difficulty with this question!

Level of Cognitive Ability: Analysis
Phase of Nursing Process: Evaluation
Client Needs: Health Promotion and Maintenance
Content Area: Child Health

Reference
Ashwill, J., & Droske, S. (1997). *Nursing care of children: Principles and practice.* Philadelphia: W. B. Saunders. p. 1236.

8. **3**

Rationale: The most likely medication to be prescribed to prevent urinary tract infection is an antibiotic. A common prescribed medication is sulfisoxazole. The neurogenic bladder prevents the bladder from completely emptying owing to the decrease in muscle tone. Prednisone relieves allergic reactions and inflammation rather than preventing infec-

tion. Furosemide promotes diuresis and decreases edema caused by congestive heart failure. Immune globulin IV assists with antibody production with immune compromised clients. Option 3 is the correct answer.

Test-Taking Strategy: Knowledge of the actions and uses of these medications is required to assist you in answering this question. The question asks about prophylactic medications used to prevent the occurrence of urinary tract infections. If you are unfamiliar with these medications, take time now to review their actions and purposes!

Level of Cognitive Ability: Application
Phase of Nursing Process: Implementation
Client Needs: Physiological Integrity
Content Area: Pharmacology

Reference
Lehne, R. (1998). *Pharmacology for Nursing Care.* (3rd ed.). Philadelphia: W. B. Saunders. p. 892.

9. **1**

Rationale: Persistent vomiting is a major symptom associated with intracranial pressure. Intracranial pressure and encephalopathy are major symptoms of Reye's syndrome. Options 2, 3, and 4 are incorrect. Protein is not present in the urine. Reye's syndrome is related to a history of viral infections, and hypoglycemia is a symptom of this disease.

Test-Taking Strategy: This question asks you to select the response that identifies the characteristic symptom of intracranial pressure common to Reye's syndrome. Use the process of elimination to answer the question. The nurse should monitor feeding tolerance and vomiting episodes. A history of viral infection and hypoglycemia is also diagnostic to Reye's syndrome. If you had difficulty with this question, take time now to review the symptoms of Reye's syndrome and the signs of intracranial pressure!

Level of Cognitive Ability: Application
Phase of Nursing Process: Assessment
Client Needs: Physiological Integrity
Content Area: Child Health

Reference
O'Toole, M. (ed.). (1997). *Miller-Keane encyclopedia & dictionary of medicine, nursing, & allied health* (6th ed.). Philadelphia: W. B. Saunders. p. 1411.

10. **1**

Rationale: The major elements of care are to maintain effective cerebral perfusion and control intracranial pressure. Decreasing stimuli in the environment decreases the stress on the cerebral tissue and neuron responses. Cerebral edema is a progressive part of this disease process. Hearing loss and output are not affected. Changing the body position every 2 hours does not affect the cerebral edema and intracranial pressure directly. The child should be in a head-elevated position to decrease the progression of the cerebral edema and promote drainage of cerebrospinal fluid.

Test-Taking Strategy: The question asks for the nursing plan needed to decrease the progression of intracranial pressure for the child with Reye's syndrome. Knowledge of the effect of environmental stimuli and the responses of the brain cells to stimuli is required to recognize how cerebral edema can result. If you had difficulty with this question, take time now to review the appropriate plan of nursing care for the child with Reye's syndrome!

Level of Cognitive Ability: Application
Phase of Nursing Process: Planning
Client Needs: Physiological Integrity
Content Area: Child Health

Reference
Ashwill, J., & Droske, S. (1997). *Nursing care of children: Principles and practice.* Philadelphia: W. B. Saunders. p. 1251.

11. **2**

Rationale: The vomiting that occurs in Reye's syndrome is caused by cerebral edema and is a symptom of intracranial pressure. Small, frequent meals will not affect the amount of vomiting. Options 1, 3, and 4 are all correct. Decreasing stimuli and providing rest decrease stress on the brain tissue. Checking for jaundice will assist in identifying the presence of liver complications, which are characteristic of Reye's syndrome. If you had difficulty with this question, take time now to review the parent teaching points associated with the care of the child with Reye's syndrome!

Test-Taking Strategy: The question asks you to select the response that indicates that the parents need further instruction. These types of questions can be confusing. Read each response and eliminate those answers that are accurate statements made by the parents. Look for the response that is an inaccurate statement as this would reflect the need for further education. Knowledge regarding the causes of vomiting with Reye's syndrome will assist you in answering this question correctly. Options 1 and 3 are correct statements for home care. Option 4 is a correct statement because it describes further assessment of complications. Your only incorrect statement is option 2.

Level of Cognitive Ability: Analysis
Phase of Nursing Process: Evaluation
Client Needs: Health Promotion and Maintenance
Content Area: Child Health

Reference
Ashwill, J. W., and Droske, S. C. (1997). *Nursing care of children: Principles and practice.* Philadelphia: W. B. Saunders. p. 251.

12. **2**

Rationale: Parents are especially concerned about seizures that might go undetected at night. The nurse should suggest a baby monitor. Reassurance by the nurse should ensure parental confidence. The nurse needs to decrease parental overprotection. Options 1 and 3 demonstrate the parents' ability to choose respite care and activities appropriately. Option 4 is a common concern. The parents need to be reminded that as the child grows they can not always observe their child, but that their knowledge of seizure activity and care are appropriate to minimize complications.

Test-Taking Strategy: Remember that the therapeutic communication techniques are the answers to your questions regarding parent and child responses. Therapeutic techniques enhance communication. Always listen to the parents' and child's statements. Always address feelings, but identify incorrect practices without making the parents feel guilty about their choices or behaviors. Option 2 identifies a need to provide the parents with an alternate manner to monitor for night seizures.

Level of Cognitive Ability: Analysis
Phase of Nursing Process: Evaluation
Client Needs: Health Promotion and Maintenance
Content Area: Child Health

Reference
Ashwill, J., & Droske, S. (1997). *Nursing care of children: Principles and practice.* Philadelphia: W. B. Saunders. p. 1258.

13. **1**

Rationale: The complications associated with seizures include airway compromise, extremity and teeth injuries, tongue lacerations, and lowered self-esteem. Night seizures can cause the child to bite down on the tongue. Option 2 is incorrect. Cyanosis can occur during the tonic-clonic part of the seizure activity, but blanching does not occur. Option 3, migraine headaches, is not common in children with seizures. Option 4 is incorrect. Seizures do not cause a high-pitched cry, unless a tumor or intracranial pressure is the cause of the seizure diagnosis.

Test-Taking Strategy: Use your knowledge of tonic-clonic activity and the involuntary tightening of all the body muscles that occurs during seizure activity when answering this question. The tongue can get easily caught by the child's teeth when the seizure activity occurs. This causes injury, swelling, and bleeding of the tongue tissue. Knowledge of the potential complications of seizures will assist in eliminating options 2, 3, and 4. If you had difficulty with this question, take time now to review the complications associated with seizures!

Level of Cognitive Ability: Analysis
Phase of Nursing Process: Assessment
Client Needs: Physiological Integrity
Content Area: Child Health

Reference
Sommers, M., & Johnson, S. (1997). *Davis's manual of nursing therapeutics for diseases and disorders.* Philadelphia: F. A. Davis. p. 396.

14. **1**

Rationale: Grand mal seizures cause tightening of all body muscles followed by tremors. Obstructive airway and increased oral secretions are the major complications during and following the seizure. Options 2 and 4 are incorrect because performing a tracheotomy is not done. Suctioning is helpful to prevent choking and cyanosis. Option 3 (emergency cart) is incorrect, because this cart would not be left at the bedside, but would be available in the treatment room or on the nursing unit.

Test-Taking Strategy: Knowing that grand mal seizures produce excessive oral secretions and airway obstruction assists in selecting the correct option. Note the key phrase in the question "most appropriately." Use the process of elimination to answer the question. Oxygen is not effective if the airway is not patent. Tracheotomies are not performed during the seizure activity because of tremors and muscle contractions. An emergency cart would be helpful during an active seizure but would not be placed at the bedside. Grand mal seizures are not continuous, but are intermittent and unpredictable in occurrence. If you had difficulty with this question, take time now to review the plan of care associated with seizure precautions!

Level of Cognitive Ability: Application
Phase of Nursing Process: Planning
Client Needs: Safe, Effective Care Environment
Content Area: Child Health

Reference
Sommers, M., & Johnson, S. (1997). *Davis's manual of nursing therapeutics for diseases and disorders.* Philadelphia: F. A. Davis. pp. 394–395.

15. 3

Rationale: Phenytoin sodium causes gum bleeding and hypertrophy, and, therefore, soft toothbrushes and gum massage should be instituted to diminish this complication and prevent further trauma. Options 1 and 2 are incorrect because the intake and output, as well as blood pressure are not affected by this drug. Option 4 is not correct because directions for administration of this medication include to administer with food to minimize gastrointestinal upset.

Test-Taking Strategy: Knowledge of the side effects and method of administering oral phenytoin sodium is required to answer this question. If you had difficulty with this question, take time now to review the side effects of this important medication!

Level of Cognitive Ability: Application
Phase of Nursing Process: Planning
Client Needs: Physiological Integrity
Content Area: Pharmacology

Reference

Hodgson, B., & Kizior, R. (1999). *Saunders nursing drug handbook 1999.* Philadelphia: W. B. Saunders. pp. 823–825.

16. 3

Rationale: Alcohol, marijuana, and street drugs will lower the seizure threshold. These substances should be avoided. The adolescent can attain a driver's license in most states when they are seizure-free for 1 year. Anticonvulsants cause acne and oily skin; therefore, a dermatologist may need to be consulted. If an anticonvulsant medication is missed, the physician should be notified.

Test-Taking Strategy: Use the process of elimination to answer the question. Knowledge of drug administration, side effects, and the interactions of anticonvulsants with other medications and substances is needed. Laws of each state vary, but most consider 1-year seizure-free activity as adequate to obtain a driver's license. Prescribed medications, if missed, require a physician or pharmacist's guidance. If you had difficulty with this question, take time now to review the client education points related to anticonvulsants!

Level of Cognitive Ability: Analysis
Phase of Nursing Process: Evaluation
Client Needs: Health Promotion and Maintenance
Content Area: Pharmacology

Reference

Ashwill, J., & Droske, S. (1997). *Nursing care of children: Principles and practice.* Philadelphia: W. B. Saunders. p. 1257.

17. 3

Rationale: Specific gravity is not a reliable test as it changes depending on the existing condition. Psychiatric illness has no impact on seizure occurrence or cause. Children do not remember what happened during the seizure. Of the options given, option 3 is the only option that provides you with the causes of seizure activity.

Test-Taking Strategy: Focusing on the key words "assesses for causes" should easily direct you to option 3, the only option that relates specifically to causes of seizures.

Level of Cognitive Ability: Application
Phase of Nursing Process: Assessment
Client Needs: Physiological Integrity
Content Area: Child Health

Reference

Wong, D., & Whaley, L. (1996). *Clinical manual of pediatric nursing* (4th ed.). St. Louis: Mosby–Year Book. p. 476.

18. 3

Rationale: When carbamazepine is administered, blood levels need to be drawn periodically to check for the child's absorption of the medication. The amount of the medication prescribed is based on the blood level achieved. Carbamazepine's therapeutic serum range is 4 to 12 mcg/mL.

Test-Taking Strategy: Using knowledge of the correct range of a therapeutic serum level for anticonvulsant medications will assist you in choosing the correct option. Each child's size, age, and muscle mass will alter the absorption of certain anticonvulsant medications. Growth, as well as other medications, has an impact on therapeutic levels attained. Children should have a baseline serum level taken and then periodic levels drawn, based on growth changes and seizure activity occurrence. If you had difficulty with this question, take time now to review the therapeutic serum drug level of carbamazepine!

Level of Cognitive Ability: Analysis
Phase of Nursing Process: Assessment
Client Needs: Health Promotion and Maintenance
Content Area: Pharmacology

Reference

Hodgson, B., & Kizior, R. (1999). *Saunders nursing drug handbook 1999.* Philadelphia: W. B. Saunders. pp. 144–146.

19. 1

Rationale: Cerebral palsy is a chronic disability characterized by difficulty in controlling the muscles owing to an abnormality in the extrapyramidal or pyramidal motor system. Meningitis is an infectious process of the central nervous system. Encephalitis is an inflammation of the brain that occurs as a result of viral illness or CNS infection. Down's syndrome is an example of a congenital condition that results in moderate to severe retardation.

Test-Taking Strategy: Use the process of elimination to answer the question. Eliminate options 2 and 3 first, noting that they are similar and basically stating a similar statement. Note the relationship between "palsy" in the question and "muscles" in option 1, the correct option. If you had difficulty with this question, take time now to review the characteristics associated with cerebral palsy!

Level of Cognitive Ability: Analysis
Phase of Nursing Process: Analysis
Client Needs: Physiological Integrity
Content Area: Child Health

Reference

Ashwill, J., & Droske, S. (1997). *Nursing care of children: Principles and practice.* Philadelphia: W. B. Saunders. p. 1241.

20. 3

Rationale: The goal of managing the child with cerebral palsy is early recognition and intervention to maximize the child's abilities. The cause of the disease cannot be eliminated. The disease is caused by damage to the motor system that can occur during the prenatal, perinatal, and postnatal periods. It is best to minimize emotional disturbances if possible, but not prevent them, as it is healthy for the child to express emotions. Improvement of muscle control and coordination is a component of the plan, but the primary goal is to maximize the child's assets and minimize the limitations caused by the disease.

Test-Taking Strategy: Use knowledge regarding cerebral palsy and the process of elimination to answer the question.

Eliminate options 1 and 2 first, as the cause of the disease cannot be eliminated and emotional disturbances cannot be prevented. From the remaining two options, identify the option that is more global, option 3.

Level of Cognitive Ability: Application
Phase of Nursing Process: Implementation
Client Needs: Psychosocial Integrity
Content Area: Child Health

Reference
Ashwill, J., & Droske, S. (1997). *Nursing care of children: Principles and practice.* Philadelphia: W. B. Saunders. p. 1242.

21. **3**

Rationale: Down syndrome is a form of mental retardation. It is a congenital condition that results in moderate to severe mental retardation. A high percentage of cases is linked to an extra group G chromosome, chromosome 21 (trisomy 21).

Test-Taking Strategy: Use the process of elimination to answer the question. Eliminate options 1 and 2 first because average and above average intelligence is not associated with this disorder. Eliminate option 4 because deficits in adaptive behavior do occur with Down syndrome. Knowing that Down syndrome is associated with an extra chromosome will assist in directing you to the correct option. If you had difficulty with this question, take time now to review the characteristics associated with Down syndrome!

Level of Cognitive Ability: Analysis
Phase of Nursing Process: Analysis
Client Needs: Physiological Integrity
Content Area: Child Health

Reference
Ashwill, J., & Droske, S. (1997). *Nursing care of children: Principles and practice.* Philadelphia: W. B. Saunders. p. 1316.

22. **4**

Rationale: Nasotracheal suctioning is contraindicated in a child with a basilar skull fracture. Because of the nature of the injury, the suction catheter may be introduced into the brain. The child may need a urinary catheter for accurate monitoring of I&O. Fluids are restricted to prevent fluid overload. An IV line is maintained to administer fluids or medications if necessary.

Test-Taking Strategy: Knowledge regarding care of a child with a basilar skull fracture is required to answer this question. Note that options 1, 2, and 3 are similar in that they all address the issue of fluid intake or output. If you had difficulty with this question, take time now to review the care of a child with this type of skull fracture!

Level of Cognitive Ability: Analysis
Phase of Nursing Process: Analysis
Client Needs: Physiological Integrity
Content Area: Child Health

Reference
Ashwill, J., & Droske, S. (1997). *Nursing care of children: Principles and practice.* Philadelphia: W. B. Saunders. p. 1261.

23. **2**

Rationale: A diagnosis of meningitis is made by testing CSF obtained by lumbar puncture. In the case of bacterial meningitis, findings usually include increased pressure, cloudy CSF, high protein, and low glucose.

Test-Taking Strategy: Use the process of elimination and knowledge regarding the diagnostic findings in meningitis to assist in answering the question. Eliminate options 3 and 4 first, as clear CSF and decreased pressure are not likely to be found if an infectious process such as meningitis is suspected. From this point, knowledge that high protein indicates a possible diagnosis of meningitis is helpful. If you had difficulty with this question, take time now to review this diagnostic test!

Level of Cognitive Ability: Analysis
Phase of Nursing Process: Analysis
Client Needs: Physiological Integrity
Content Area: Child Health

Reference
Ashwill, J., & Droske, S. (1997). *Nursing care of children: Principles and practice.* Philadelphia: W. B. Saunders. p. 1246.

24. **3**

Rationale: Meningococcal meningitis, caused by *Neisseria*, usually occurs in older children and adolescents. Because it is transmitted primarily by droplet infection, the risk increases as the number of contacts increase. Isolation is begun and maintained for at least 24 hours after antibiotics are given.

Test-Taking Strategy: Knowledge regarding the mode of transmission of meningococcal meningitis is required to answer this question. Use the process of elimination. Both enteric and neutropenic precautions, options 2 and 4, are unrelated to the mode of transmission. Knowledge that it takes approximately 24 hours for antibiotics to reach a therapeutic blood level will assist in the selection of option 3 over option 2. If you had difficulty with this question, take time now to review the mode of transmission of meningococcal meningitis!

Level of Cognitive Ability: Application
Phase of Nursing Process: Implementation
Client Needs: Safe, Effective Care Environment
Content Area: Child Health

Reference
Ashwill, J., & Droske, S. (1997). *Nursing care of children: Principles and practice.* Philadelphia: W. B. Saunders. pp. 1245–1246.

25. **1**

Rationale: Altered cerebral tissue perfusion is the priority nursing diagnosis for the child with meningitis. Pain related to meningeal irritation and altered family process related to a child with an acute illness may also be appropriate nursing diagnoses, but are not the priority. Parental knowledge deficit related to the seriousness of meningitis and the possible residual neurologic deficits would be a secondary nursing diagnosis.

Test-Taking Strategy: Knowledge regarding the risk of intracranial pressure in the child with meningitis would assist in answering the question. Utilize the ABCs, Airway, Breathing, and Circulation, to assist in answering the question. Tissue perfusion relates to circulation!

Level of Cognitive Ability: Application
Phase of Nursing Process: Planning
Client Needs: Physiological Integrity
Content Area: Child Health

Reference
Ashwill, J., & Droske, S. (1997). *Nursing care of children: Principles and practice.* Philadelphia: W. B. Saunders. p. 1247.

26. 4

Rationale: A child can easily extend the leg when in the supine position; however, when the thigh is flexed toward the abdomen, pain prevents complete extension of the leg. Kernig's sign is pain that occurs with extension of the leg and knee. Brudzinski's sign occurs when flexion of the head causes flexion of the hips and knees. Chvostek's sign, seen in tetany, is a spasm of the facial muscles elicited by tapping the facial nerve in the region of the parotid gland. Trousseau's sign is a sign for tetany in which carpal spasm can be elicited by compressing the upper arm and causing ischemia to the nerves distally.

Test-Taking Strategy: Knowledge regarding the appropriate procedure to elicit Kernig's sign is required to answer the question. If you had difficulty with this question, take time now to review these signs, their significance, and the procedure to elicit these signs!

Level of Cognitive Ability: Application
Phase of Nursing Process: Implementation
Client Needs: Physiological Integrity
Content Area: Child Health

References
Ashwill, J., & Droske, S. (1997). *Nursing care of children: Principles and practice.* Philadelphia: W. B. Saunders. p. 1247.
O'Toole, M. (ed.). (1997). *Miller-Keane encyclopedia & dictionary of medicine, nursing, & allied health* (6th ed.). Philadelphia: W. B. Saunders. pp. 328, 1658.

27. 3

Rationale: Autism is a severe developmental disorder that begins in infancy or toddlerhood. The primary characteristic is lack of social interaction and awareness. Social behaviors in autism include lack of or abnormal imitation of others' actions, and the lack of or abnormal social play. Additional characteristics include lack of or impaired verbal communication and markedly abnormal nonverbal communication.

Test-Taking Strategy: Use knowledge of the characteristics of autism and the process of elimination to answer the question. Eliminate options 2 and 4 first, as they address normal behaviors. Knowledge that the autistic child lacks social interaction and awareness will direct you to selecting option 3. If you had difficulty with this question, take time now to review the characteristics associated with autism!

Level of Cognitive Ability: Analysis
Phase of Nursing Process: Assessment
Client Needs: Psychosocial Integrity
Content Area: Child Health

Reference
Ashwill, J., & Droske, S. (1997). *Nursing care of children: Principles and practice.* Philadelphia: W. B. Saunders. pp. 1322–1324.

28. 2

Rationale: Risk for injury related to an inability to anticipate danger, a tendency for self-mutilation, and sensory perceptual deficits is the priority nursing diagnosis. Impaired social interaction, altered thought processes, and impaired verbal communication are also appropriate nursing diagnoses for the child with autism, but the priority is the risk for injury.

Test-Taking Strategy: Use Maslow's hierarchy of needs theory to answer this question. Physiological needs take priority. When a physiological need does not exist, safety needs are the priority. None of the options address a physiological need. Option 2 addresses the safety need!

Level of Cognitive Ability: Application
Phase of Nursing Process: Planning
Client Needs: Safe, Effective Care Environment
Content Area: Child Health

Reference
Ashwill, J., & Droske, S. (1997). *Nursing care of children: Principles and practice.* Philadelphia: W. B. Saunders. p. 1324.

29. 4

Rationale: The most likely assessment findings in sexual abuse include difficulty walking or sitting; torn, stained, or bloody underclothing; pain, swelling, or itching of the genitals; and bruises, bleeding, or lacerations in the genital or anal area. Poor hygiene may be indicative of physical neglect. Bald spots on the scalp and fear of the parents are most likely associated with physical abuse.

Test-Taking Strategy: Read the question carefully noting the key phrase "sexually abused." The only option that specifically addresses an assessment finding related to sexual abuse is option 4. If you had difficulty with this question, take time now to review the assessment findings in a child suspected of abuse!

Level of Cognitive Ability: Analysis
Phase of Nursing Process: Assessment
Client Needs: Physiological Integrity
Content Area: Child Health

Reference
Ashwill, J., & Droske, S. (1997). *Nursing care of children: Principles and practice.* Philadelphia: W. B. Saunders. pp. 1287–1290.

30. 2

Rationale: The primary legal nursing responsibility when child abuse is suspected, is to report the case. All 50 states require health care professionals to report all cases of suspected abuse. Although documenting assessment findings, assisting the family and referring the family to appropriate resources, and support groups are important, the primary legal responsibility is to report the case.

Test-Taking Strategy: Use the process of elimination noting the key phrase "primary and legal" to answer the question. In addition to the many implications associated with child abuse, abuse is a crime. With this in mind, option 2, reporting the case of abuse, is the primary responsibility. If you had difficulty with this question, take time now to review the responsibilities of the nurse when child abuse is suspected!

Level of Cognitive Ability: Application
Phase of Nursing Process: Implementation
Client Needs: Safe, Effective Care Environment
Content Area: Child Health

Reference
Ashwill, J., & Droske, S. (1997). *Nursing care of children: Principles and practice.* Philadelphia: W. B. Saunders. pp. 1294–1295.

BIBLIOGRAPHY

Ashwill, J., & Droske, S. (1997). *Nursing care of children. Principles and practice.* Philadelphia: W. B. Saunders.

Carson, V., & Arnold, E. (1996). *Mental health nursing: The nurse patient journey.* Philadelphia: W. B. Saunders.

Hodgson, B., & Kizior, R. (1999). *Saunders nursing drug handbook 1999.* Philadelphia: W. B. Saunders.

Luckmann, J. (1997). *Saunders manual of nursing care.* Philadelphia: W. B. Saunders.

Nichols, F., & Zwelling, E. (1997). *Maternal newborn nursing: Theory and practice.* Philadelphia: W. B. Saunders.

O'Toole, M. (ed.). (1997). *Miller-Keane encyclopedia & dictionary of medicine, nursing, & allied health* (6th ed.). Philadelphia: W. B. Saunders.

Sommers, M., & Johnson, S. (1997). *Davis's manual of nursing therapeutics for diseases and disorders.* Philadelphia: F. A. Davis.

Wong, D., & Whaley, L. (1996). *Clinical manual of pediatric nursing* (4th ed.). St. Louis: Mosby–Year Book.

CHAPTER 34

Eye, Ear, and Throat Disorders

I. Strabismus

A. Description
1. Called "squint" or "lazy eye"
2. A condition in which the eyes are not aligned because of lack of coordination of the extraocular muscles
3. Most often as a result of muscle imbalance or paralysis of extraocular muscles, but may also result from conditions such as a brain tumor, myasthenia gravis, or infection
4. Normal in the young infant but should not be present after about age 4 months

B. Assessment
1. Amblyopia if not treated early
2. Permanent loss of vision if not treated early
3. Loss of binocular vision
4. Impairment of depth perception
5. Frequent headaches
6. Squints or tilts head to see

C. Implementation
1. Corrective lenses as indicated
2. Instruct the parents regarding eye-patching of the "good" eye to strengthen the weak eye
3. Prepare for surgery to realign the weak muscles if prescribed
4. Prepare for botulinum toxin (Botox) injection into the eye muscle, which produces temporary paralysis and allows muscles opposite the paralyzed muscle to straighten the eye
5. Inform the parents the injection of Botox wears off in about 2 months, and if successful, correction will occur
6. Instruct the parents in the need for follow-up visits

II. Conjunctivitis

A. Description
1. Also known as "pink eye"
2. Inflammation of the conjunctiva
3. Usually caused by allergy, infection, or trauma

4. Bacterial and viral conjunctivitis is extremely contagious
5. Chlamydial conjunctivitis is rare in older children and if diagnosed in a nonsexually active child, the child should be assessed for possible sexual **abuse**

B. Assessment
1. Itching, burning, or scratchy eyelids
2. Redness
3. Edema
4. Discharge

C. Implementation
1. Instruct in infection control measures such as good handwashing and not sharing towels and washcloths
2. Administer antibiotic or antiviral eye drops or ointment as prescribed if infection is present
3. Administer antihistamines as prescribed if an allergy is present
4. Instruct the child and parents in the administration of the prescribed medications
5. Instruct the parents that child should be kept home from school or day care until antibiotic eye drops have been administered for 24 hours
6. Instruct the child to avoid rubbing the eye to prevent injury
7. Instruct the child wearing contact lenses to discontinue wearing them and to obtain new lenses to eliminate the chance of reinfection
8. Instruct the adolescent that eye makeup should be discarded and replaced
9. Instruct in the use of cool compresses to lessen irritation, and in wearing dark glasses for photophobia

III. Otitis Media

A. Description
1. Infection of the middle ear occurring from a

blocked eustachian tube, which prevents normal drainage

2. Otitis media is a common complication of an acute respiratory infection
3. Infants and children are more prone to otitis media because their eustachian tubes are shorter, wider, and straighter

B. Assessment
1. Fever
2. Irritability
3. Restlessness
4. Rolling of head from side to side
5. Pulling or rubbing ear
6. Earache or pain
7. Loss of appetite
8. Hearing loss
9. Purulent drainage
10. Red, opaque, bulging, or retracting tympanic membrane

C. Implementation
1. Encourage fluids
2. Teach the parents to feed infants in an upright position
3. Instruct the child to avoid chewing during the acute period as chewing increases pain
4. Provide local heat and have the child lie with the affected ear down
5. Instruct the parents in the appropriate procedure to clean drainage from the ear with sterile cotton swabs
6. Instruct in the administration of analgesics or antipyretics such as acetaminophen (Tylenol) to decrease fever and pain
7. Instruct the parents in the administration of the prescribed antibiotics emphasizing that the 10- to 14-day period is necessary to eradicate positive organisms
8. Instruct the parents that screening for hearing loss may be necessary
9. If ear drops are prescribed, instruct the parents to pull the earlobe down and back in children younger than age 3, and to pull the pinna up and back for a child older than 3 years

D. Myringotomy
1. Description: insertion of tympanostomy tubes into the middle ear to equalize pressure and keep ear aerated
2. Implementation postoperatively
   a. Instruct the parents and child to keep ears dry
   b. Ear plugs should be worn during bathing, shampooing, and swimming
   c. Diving and submerging under water is not allowed

IV. Tonsillectomy and Adenoidectomy

A. Description
1. "Tonsillitis" is a term commonly used to describe an inflammation and infection of the tonsils

2. Adenoiditis refers to infection and inflammation of the adenoids

B. Assessment
1. Persistent or recurrent sore throat
2. Enlarged bright red tonsils that may be covered with white exudate
3. Difficulty swallowing
4. Mouth breathing and an unpleasant mouth odor
5. Fever
6. Cough
7. Enlarged adenoids may cause nasal quality of speech, mouth breathing, hearing difficulty, snoring, or obstructive sleep apnea

C. Implementation Preoperatively
1. Assess for signs of active infection
2. Assess bleeding and clotting studies as throat is very vascular
3. Prepare the child for sore throat postoperatively and inform that he or she will need to drink liquids
4. Assess for any loose teeth to decrease the risk of aspiration during surgery

D. Implementation Postoperatively
1. Position prone or side-lying to facilitate drainage
2. Have suction equipment available but do not suction unless there is an airway obstruction
3. Monitor for signs of hemorrhage; if hemorrhage occurs, turn the child to the side and notify the physician
4. Discourage coughing or clearing the throat
5. Provide clear, cool, noncitrus and noncarbonated fluids
6. Avoid milk products initially as they will coat the throat
7. Avoid red liquids, which will indicate the appearance of blood if the child vomits
8. Do not give the child any straws, forks, or sharp objects that can be put in the mouth
9. Administer acetaminophen for sore throat as prescribed
10. Instruct the parents to notify the physician if bleeding, persistent earache, or fever occurs
11. Instruct the parents to keep the child away from crowds until healing has occurred

PRACTICE QUESTIONS

1. The mother arrives at a well baby clinic with her 1-month-old infant. She expresses concern because one of the infant's eyes appears to be crossed. The most appropriate response by the nurse is which of the following?
   1 "The infant will probably need surgery."
   2 "This condition is probably permanent."
   3 "It bears watching because the other eye may do the same thing."
   4 "This is normal in the young infant but should not be present after about age 4 months."

2. The day care nurse is observing a 2-year-old child. The nurse suspects that the child may have

strabismus. Which of the following observations might be indicative of this condition?

1 The child consistently tilts the head to see
2 The child consistently turns the head to see
3 The child does not respond when spoken to
4 The child has difficulty hearing

3. The physician has told the mother of a newborn diagnosed with strabismus that surgery will be necessary to realign the weakened eye muscles. The mother asks the nurse when the surgery might be performed. The most appropriate response is which of the following?

1 "Surgery will be performed immediately."
2 "Surgery will be performed shortly before the child starts school."
3 "Surgery will be performed before the child is 2 years old."
4 "Surgery will be performed before the child begins to read."

4. The physician prescribes "patching" for a child with strabismus of the right eye. The nurse instructs the mother regarding this procedure. Which of the following is included in the teaching plan?

1 Place the patch on the right eye
2 Place the patch on both eyes
3 Place the patch on the left eye
4 Alternate the patch from the right to left eye hourly

5. The mother of a 6-year-old arrives at the clinic because the child has been experiencing scratchy, red, and swollen eyes. The nurse notes a discharge from the eyes and a culture is sent to the laboratory for analysis. Chlamydial conjunctivitis is diagnosed. Based on this diagnosis, which of the following requires further investigation?

1 The presence of an allergy
2 Possible trauma
3 Possible sexual abuse
4 The presence of a respiratory infection

6. The nurse prepares a teaching plan for a mother of a child diagnosed with bacterial conjunctivitis. Which of the following, if stated by the mother, indicates a need for further education?

1 "I need to wash my hands frequently."
2 "I need to clean the eye as prescribed."
3 "I need to give the eye drops as prescribed."
4 "It is OK to share towels and washcloths."

7. A 7-year-old child is diagnosed with viral conjunctivitis. Antibiotic eye drops are prescribed for the child. The mother asks the nurse when the child can return to school. The most appropriate response is:

1 "The child can return to school immediately."
2 "The child should be kept home until the antibiotic eye drops have been administered for 24 hours."
3 "The child should be kept home until the antibiotic eye drops have been administered for 48 hours."
4 "The child cannot return to school until seen by the physician in 1 week."

8. An adolescent is diagnosed with conjunctivitis. The child asks the nurse if it is OK to wear contact lenses. Which of the following is not an appropriate instruction?

1 Contacts can be worn if they are cleaned as directed
2 Contact lenses should not be worn
3 New contact lenses should be obtained
4 Old contact lenses should be discarded

9. A 4-year-old child is diagnosed with otitis media. The mother asks the nurse about the causes of this illness. Which of the following is not an associated risk factor related to otitis media?

1 Household smoking
2 Bottle-feeding
3 Exposure to illness in other children
4 A history of urinary tract infections (UTIs)

10. The nurse provides instructions to parents regarding the methods that will decrease the risk of recurrent otitis media in infants. Which of the following is included in the instructions?

1 Feed the infant in an upright position
2 Allow the infant to have a bottle during naptime
3 Maintain bottle-feeding as long as possible
4 Discontinue breast-feeding as soon as possible

11. The nurse is caring for a child following myringotomy with insertion of tympanostomy tubes. The nurse notes a small amount of reddish drainage from the child's ear following the surgery. Which of the following is the most appropriate nursing action?

1 Notify the physician
2 Change the ear tubes so that they do not become blocked
3 Document the findings
4 Check the ear drainage for the presence of cerebrospinal fluid (CSF)

12. The mother of a child who had a myringotomy with insertion of tympanostomy tubes calls the nurse and tells the nurse that the tubes fell out. Which of the following is the most appropriate response to the mother?

1 "Replace the tubes immediately so that the created opening does not close."
2 "This is an emergency and requires immediate intervention. Bring the child to the emergency room."
3 "This is not an emergency. I will speak to the physician and call you right back."
4 "Place the tubes into hydrogen peroxide for 1 hour before replacing them in the child's ears."

13. Antibiotics are prescribed for the child following a myringotomy with insertion of tympanostomy tubes. The nurse provides discharge instructions to the parents regarding the administration of the antibiotics. Which of the following statements, if made by the parents, indicates that they understood the instructions?
    1 "Administer the antibiotics if the child has a fever."
    2 "Administer the antibiotics until the child feels better."
    3 "Administer the antibiotics until they are gone."
    4 "Begin to taper the antibiotics after 3 days of a full course."

14. The mother of a child who underwent a myringotomy with insertion of tympanostomy tubes calls the nurse and reports that the child is complaining of discomfort. Which of the following is the most appropriate response?
    1 "Give the child children's aspirin for the discomfort."
    2 "Give the child Tylenol for the discomfort."
    3 "You need to speak to the physician because the child should not be having any discomfort."
    4 "I will speak to the physician so that a narcotic can be prescribed."

15. The nurse prepares a teaching plan regarding the administration of ear drops for the parents of a 6-year-old child. Which of the following is included in the plan?
    1 Pull the ear up and back
    2 Wear gloves when administering the medication
    3 Hold the child in a sitting position when administering the ear drops
    4 Pull the ear down, back, and out

16. The nurse provides discharge instructions to the mother of a child following a myringotomy with insertion of tympanostomy tubes. Which of the following is not included in the plan?
    1 Be sure the child uses soft tissues to blow the nose
    2 Place ear plugs with petroleum jelly in the ears during baths and showers
    3 Swimming in deep water is prohibited
    4 Swimming in lake water needs to be avoided

17. The nurse is reviewing the laboratory results of a child scheduled for a tonsillectomy. Which of the following laboratory values is most significant to review?
    1 Prothrombin time
    2 Sedimentation rate
    3 Blood urea nitrogen (BUN)
    4 Creatinine

18. The child is scheduled for a tonsillectomy. Which of the following presents the highest risk of aspiration during surgery?
    1 Difficulty swallowing
    2 The presence of loose teeth
    3 Bleeding during surgery
    4 Exudate in the throat area

19. The most appropriate position for a child following a tonsillectomy is which of the following?
    1 Supine
    2 Trendelenburg
    3 Side-lying
    4 High Fowler's

20. Following tonsillectomy, which of the following physician orders does the nurse question?
    1 Clear, cool liquids when awake
    2 No milk or milk products
    3 Monitor for bleeding
    4 Suction PRN

21. The nurse is caring for a child following a tonsillectomy. Which of the following may indicate that the child is bleeding?
    1 A decreased pulse rate
    2 An elevation in blood pressure (BP)
    3 Complaints of discomfort
    4 Frequent swallowing

22. Following tonsillectomy, the child begins to vomit bright red blood. The most appropriate initial nursing action is to:
    1 Administer the prescribed antiemetic
    2 Turn the child to the side
    3 Notify the physician
    4 Maintain a nothing by mouth (NPO) status

23. Following tonsillectomy, which of the following fluid or food items is most appropriate to offer to the child?
    1 Cool cherry Kool-Aid
    2 Vanilla pudding
    3 Cold ginger ale
    4 Jell-O

24. The child is scheduled for a tonsillectomy in the day stay surgical unit. On the day following surgery, the mother calls the surgical unit and expresses concern because the child has a very bad mouth odor. Which of the following responses is most appropriate?
    1 "The child probably has an infection."
    2 "You need to contact the physician immediately."
    3 "Bad mouth odor is normal and may be relieved by drinking more liquids."
    4 "Have the child gargle with mouthwash every 4 hours."

25. The nurse is providing discharge instructions to the mother of an 8-year-old child who had a tonsillectomy. The mother tells the nurse that the child loves tacos and asks when the child can safely eat one. The most appropriate response is:

1 "In 1 week."
2 "In 3 weeks."
3 "Two days following surgery."
4 "When the physician says it's OK."

ANSWERS

1. 4

Rationale: Strabismus, also called "lazy eye," is a condition in which the eyes are not aligned because of lack of coordination of the extraocular muscles. It is normal in the young infant but should not be present after about age 4 months.

Test-Taking Strategy: Knowledge regarding this condition is required to answer this question. Note that the question asks for the "most appropriate" response. This may assist you in eliminating options 1, 2, and 3. If you had difficulty with this question, take time now to review this disorder!

Level of Cognitive Ability: Analysis
Phase of Nursing Process: Implementation
Client Needs: Physiological Integrity
Content Area: Child Health

Reference
Ashwill, J., & Droske, S. (1997). *Nursing care of children: Principles and practice.* Philadelphia: W. B. Saunders. p. 1333.

2. 1

Rationale: The nurse may suspect strabismus in a child when the child complains of frequent headaches, squints, or tilts the head to see. Options 2, 3, and 4 are not indicative of this condition.

Test-Taking Strategy: Begin by eliminating options 3 and 4 because they are similar. Knowledge regarding the signs of this condition will assist in directing you to option 1. Review these signs now if you had difficulty with this question!

Level of Cognitive Ability: Analysis
Phase of Nursing Process: Assessment
Client Needs: Physiological Integrity
Content Area: Child Health

Reference
Ashwill, J., & Droske, S. (1997). *Nursing care of children: Principles and practice.* Philadelphia: W. B. Saunders. p. 1333.

3. 3

Rationale: In a child diagnosed with strabismus, surgery may be indicated to realign the weakened muscles. It is most often indicated when amblyopia (decreased vision in the deviated eye) is present. The surgery should be performed before the child is 2 years old.

Test-Taking Strategy: Option 1 can be easily eliminated. Options 2 and 4 can be eliminated next because they address a similar time frame. If you had difficulty with this question, take time now to review the treatment for strabismus!

Level of Cognitive Ability: Analysis
Phase of Nursing Process: Implementation
Client Needs: Physiological Integrity
Content Area: Child Health

Reference
Ashwill, J., & Droske, S. (1997). *Nursing care of children: Principles and practice.* Philadelphia: W. B. Saunders. p. 1333.

4. 3

Rationale: Patching may be used in the treatment of strabismus to strengthen the weak eye. In this treatment, the "good" eye is patched. This encourages the child to use the weaker eye. It is most successful when done during the preschool years. The schedule for patching is individualized and is prescribed by the ophthalmologist.

Test-Taking Strategy: Knowledge regarding the physiology associated with strabismus is helpful in answering this question. Remembering that this condition is a "lazy eye" will direct you to the correct option. It makes sense to patch the unaffected eye in order to strengthen the muscles in the affected eye. Review the procedure for patching now if you had difficulty with this question!

Level of Cognitive Ability: Application
Phase of Nursing Process: Implementation
Client Needs: Physiological Integrity
Content Area: Child Health

Reference
Ashwill, J., & Droske, S. (1997). *Nursing care of children: Principles and practice.* Philadelphia: W. B. Saunders. p. 1333.

5. 3

Rationale: A diagnosis of chlamydial conjunctivitis in a nonsexually active child should signal the health care provider to assess the child for possible sexual abuse. Allergy, infection, and trauma can cause conjunctivitis but the causative organism is not likely to be chlamydia. Chlamydial conjunctivitis may also be suspected in a sexually active adolescent with chronic infection that is unresponsive to other treatment.

Test-Taking Strategy: Note the age of the child and the organism that is identified in the question. This may assist in directing you to option 3. Options 1, 2, and 4 should be recognized as the common causes of conjunctivitis. These options are similar in that they all relate to a physiological problem. Review the content related to chlamydial conjunctivitis now if you had difficulty with this question!

Level of Cognitive Ability: Analysis
Phase of Nursing Process: Assessment
Client Needs: Psychosocial Integrity
Content Area: Child Health

Reference
Ashwill, J., & Droske, S. (1997). *Nursing care of children: Principles and practice.* Philadelphia: W. B. Saunders. p. 1337.

6. 4

Rationale: Bacterial conjunctivitis is highly contagious and infection control measures should be taught. These include good handwashing and not sharing towels and washcloths. Options 2 and 3 are correct treatment measures.

Test-Taking Strategy: Knowledge that bacterial conjunctivitis is highly contagious will assist in answering this question. Options 1, 2, and 3 can be easily eliminated. If you had difficulty with this question, take time now to review infection control measures for bacterial conjunctivitis!

Level of Cognitive Ability: Analysis
Phase of Nursing Process: Evaluation
Client Needs: Health Promotion and Maintenance
Content Area: Child Health

Reference
Ashwill, J., & Droske, S. (1997). *Nursing care of children: Principles and practice*. Philadelphia: W. B. Saunders. p. 1337.

7. **2**

Rationale: Viral conjunctivitis is extremely contagious. The child should be kept home from school or day care until the child has received antibiotic eye drops for 24 hours.

Test-Taking Strategy: Knowledge that viral conjunctivitis is highly contagious will assist in eliminating option 1. Eliminate option 4 next as this time frame is rather lengthy. Knowledge regarding the action of antibiotics will assist in directing you to option 2. Review infection control measures related to viral conjunctivitis if you had difficulty with this question!

Level of Cognitive Ability: Application
Phase of Nursing Process: Implementation
Client Needs: Health Promotion and Maintenance
Content Area: Child Health

Reference
Ashwill, J., & Droske, S. (1997). *Nursing care of children: Principles and practice*. Philadelphia: W. B. Saunders. p. 1337.

8. **1**

Rationale: If the child wears contact lenses the child should be instructed to discontinue wearing them until the infection has completely cleared. Securing new contact lenses will eliminate the chance of reinfection from contaminated contact lenses and will also lessen the risk of a corneal ulceration.

Test-Taking Strategy: Note the key word "not" in the stem of the question. Options 2, 3, and 4 are similar in that they relate to avoiding the use of contact lenses during infection. If you had difficulty with this question, take time now to review treatment measures for conjunctivitis!

Level of Cognitive Ability: Application
Phase of Nursing Process: Implementation
Client Needs: Health Promotion and Maintenance
Content Area: Child Health

Reference
Ashwill, J., & Droske, S. (1997). *Nursing care of children: Principles and practice*. Philadelphia: W. B. Saunders. p. 1337.

9. **4**

Rationale: Factors that increase the risk of otitis media include exposure to illness in other children in day care centers, household smoking, bottle-feeding, and congenital conditions such as Down's syndrome and cleft palate. The use of a pacifier beyond age 6 months has also been identified as a risk factor. Allergies are also thought to precipitate otitis media.

Test-Taking Strategy: Note the key word "not" in the stem of the question. Careful reading of each of the options will

quickly direct you to option 4. If you had difficulty with this question, take time now to review the risk factors associated with otitis media!

Level of Cognitive Ability: Analysis
Phase of Nursing Process: Analysis
Client Needs: Health Promotion and Maintenance
Content Area: Child Health

Reference
Ashwill, J., & Droske, S. (1997). *Nursing care of children: Principles and practice*. Philadelphia: W. B. Saunders. p. 824.

10. **1**

Rationale: To decrease the risk of recurrent otitis media, parents should be encouraged to breast-feed during infancy, discontinue bottle-feeding as soon as possible, feed the infant in an upright position, and never give the infant a bottle in bed. Parents should be told not to smoke in the child's presence because passive smoking increases the incidence of otitis media.

Test-Taking Strategy: Knowledge of the physiology related to otitis media will assist in answering the question. Option 2 can be easily eliminated. Recalling that breast-feeding offers some protection by providing maternal antibodies will assist in eliminating options 3 and 4. Review measures that will assist in preventing otitis media if you had difficulty with this question!

Level of Cognitive Ability: Application
Phase of Nursing Process: Implementation
Client Needs: Health Promotion and Maintenance
Content Area: Child Health

Reference
Ashwill, J., & Droske, S. (1997). *Nursing care of children: Principles and practice*. Philadelphia: W. B. Saunders. p. 825.

11. **3**

Rationale: Postoperatively, following myringotomy with insertion of tympanostomy tubes, the child is monitored for ear drainage. A small amount of reddish drainage is normal for the first few days after surgery. Any heavy bleeding or bleeding that occurs after 3 days should be reported. The nurse should document the findings. Options 1, 2, and 4 are not necessary.

Test-Taking Strategy: Note the key phrase "small amount" in the question. Considering both the anatomical location of the surgery and the key phrase, you should easily be directed to the correct option. Review postoperative assessment following this type of surgery now if you had difficulty with this question!

Level of Cognitive Ability: Analysis
Phase of Nursing Process: Implementation
Client Needs: Physiological Integrity
Content Area: Child Health

Reference
Ashwill, J., & Droske, S. (1997). *Nursing care of children: Principles and practice*. Philadelphia: W. B. Saunders. p. 824.

12. **3**

Rationale: The size and appearance of the tympanostomy tubes should be described to the parents following surgery. They should be reassured that if the tubes fall out, it is not an emergency but that the physician should be notified.

Test-Taking Strategy: Option 2 should be eliminated first because this will cause concern in the parent. Next, eliminate options 1 and 4 as they are similar and relate to replacing the tubes. Take time now to review parent instructions following this procedure if you had difficulty with this question!

Level of Cognitive Ability: Application
Phase of Nursing Process: Implementation
Client Needs: Physiological Integrity
Content Area: Child Health

Reference
Ashwill, J., & Droske, S. (1997). *Nursing care of children: Principles and practice.* Philadelphia: W. B. Saunders. p. 825.

13. **3**

Rationale: Antibiotics need to be taken as prescribed and the full course needs to be completed. It is important that parents are instructed regarding the administration of antibiotics. Options 1, 2, and 4 are incorrect. Antibiotics are not tapered but administered until they are completed.

Test-Taking Strategy: Knowledge regarding the administration of antibiotics is required to answer this question. Recall that antibiotics must be taken for the full course regardless if the child is feeling better. Review concepts related to the administration of antibiotics now if you had difficulty with this question!

Level of Cognitive Ability: Analysis
Phase of Nursing Process: Evaluation
Client Needs: Physiological Integrity
Content Area: Child Health

Reference
Ashwill, J., & Droske, S. (1997). *Nursing care of children: Principles and practice.* Philadelphia: W. B. Saunders. p. 824.

14. **2**

Rationale: Following myringotomy with insertion of tympanostomy tubes, the child may experience some discomfort. Tylenol can be given to relieve the discomfort. A narcotic is not necessary and aspirin should not be administered to a child.

Test-Taking Strategy: Options 1 and 4 can be easily eliminated. It seems reasonable that the child may have some discomfort following this surgical procedure; therefore, eliminate option 3. If you had difficulty with this question, review postoperative care following this procedure!

Level of Cognitive Ability: Analysis
Phase of Nursing Process: Implementation
Client Needs: Physiological Integrity
Content Area: Child Health

Reference
Ashwill, J., & Droske, S. (1997). *Nursing care of children: Principles and practice.* Philadelphia: W. B. Saunders. p. 824.

15. **4**

Rationale: To administer ear drops in a child, the ear should be pulled down, back, and out. In adults, the ear is pulled up and back. Gloves do not need to be worn by the parents, but handwashing before and after the procedure needs to be performed. The child needs to be in a side-lying position with the affected ear facing upward to facilitate the flow of medication down the ear canal by gravity.

Test-Taking Strategy: Options 2 and 3 can be eliminated first. From the remaining options, recalling the anatomy of the child's ear canal will direct you to option 4. Review this procedure now if you had difficulty with this question!

Level of Cognitive Ability: Application
Phase of Nursing Process: Implementation
Client Needs: Health Promotion and Maintenance
Content Area: Child Health

Reference
Lammon, C., Foote, A., Leli, P., et al. (1995). *Clinical nursing skills.* Philadelphia: W. B. Saunders. p. 580.

16. **1**

Rationale: Parents need to be instructed that the child should not blow the nose for 7 to 10 days. Bath- and lake water are potential sources of bacterial contamination. Diving and swimming deeply under water are prohibited. The child's ears need to be kept dry. Options 2, 3, and 4 are appropriate instructions.

Test-Taking Strategy: Note the key word "not" in the stem of the question. Options 2, 3, and 4 are similar and all relate to the concept of keeping the ears dry. Option 1 may cause disruption of the surgical site. Review parent discharge instructions following this procedure if you had difficulty with this question!

Level of Cognitive Ability: Application
Phase of Nursing Process: Planning
Client Needs: Physiological Integrity
Content Area: Child Health

Reference
Ashwill, J., & Droske, S. (1997). *Nursing care of children: Principles and practice.* Philadelphia: W. B. Saunders. p. 825.

17. **1**

Rationale: Before the surgical procedure the child is assessed for signs of active infection and for redness and exudate of the throat. Because the tonsillar area is so vascular, postoperative bleeding is a concern. The prothrombin time (PT), partial thromboplastin time (PTT), platelet count, hematocrit and hemoglobin (H&H), white blood count (WBC), and urinalysis are performed preoperatively. The PT results identify a potential for bleeding. The BUN, creatinine, and sedimentation rate do not determine the potential for bleeding.

Test-Taking Strategy: The issue of the question relates to the potential for bleeding. Options 3 and 4 can be eliminated because they relate to kidney function. Similarly, option 2 can be eliminated because it is unrelated to the issue of the question.

Level of Cognitive Ability: Analysis
Phase of Nursing Process: Assessment
Client Needs: Physiological Integrity
Content Area: Child Health

Reference
Ashwill, J., & Droske, S. (1997). *Nursing care of children: Principles and practice.* Philadelphia: W. B. Saunders. p. 830.

18. **2**

Rationale: In the preoperative period, the child should be observed for the presence of loose teeth to decrease the risk of aspiration during surgery. Options 1 and 4 are incorrect. Bleeding during surgery will be controlled via packing and suction as needed.

Test-Taking Strategy: The issue of the question relates to aspiration. Note the key word "highest" in the stem of the question. Options 1 and 4 can be easily eliminated. Recalling that the tonsillar area is vascular, anticipation of bleeding during surgery is expected and will be controlled. Review preoperative assessment procedures related to tonsillectomy now if you had difficulty with this question!

Level of Cognitive Ability: Analysis
Phase of Nursing Process: Assessment
Client Needs: Physiological Integrity
Content Area: Child Health

Reference
Ashwill, J., & Droske, S. (1997). *Nursing care of children: Principles and practice.* Philadelphia: W. B. Saunders. p. 830.

19. **3**

Rationale: The child should be placed in a prone or side-lying position following tonsillectomy to facilitate drainage. Options 1, 2, and 4 will not achieve this goal.

Test-Taking Strategy: Visualize each of the positions described in the options. Keeping in mind that the goal is to facilitate drainage will easily direct you to option 3. Review positioning procedures following tonsillectomy now if you had difficulty with this question!

Level of Cognitive Ability: Application
Phase of Nursing Process: Implementation
Client Needs: Physiological Integrity
Content Area: Child Health

Reference
Ashwill, J., & Droske, S. (1997). *Nursing care of children: Principles and practice.* Philadelphia: W. B. Saunders. p. 831.

20. **4**

Rationale: Following tonsillectomy, suction equipment should be available, but do not suction unless there is an airway obstruction. Clear cool liquids are encouraged. Milk and milk products are avoided initially because they coat the throat, cause the child to clear the throat, and increase the risk of bleeding. Option 3 is an important nursing intervention following any type of surgery.

Test-Taking Strategy: Option 3 can be eliminated first because this is a nursing rather than medical prescription. Consider the anatomical location of the surgery to assist in answering the question. This should easily direct you to option 4. Review postoperative care following tonsillectomy now if you had difficulty with this question!

Level of Cognitive Ability: Analysis
Phase of Nursing Process: Analysis
Client Needs: Safe, Effective Care Environment
Content Area: Child Health

Reference
Ashwill, J., & Droske, S. (1997). *Nursing care of children: Principles and practice.* Philadelphia: W. B. Saunders. p. 831.

21. **4**

Rationale: Frequent swallowing, restlessness, a fast and thready pulse, and vomiting bright red blood are signs of bleeding. An elevated BP is not an indication of bleeding.

Test-Taking Strategy: Use the concepts related to the signs of shock to assist in answering the question. These concepts should assist in eliminating options 1 and 2. From the remaining options, knowing that discomfort does not indicate bleeding will direct you to option 4. Review the signs of bleeding now if you had difficulty with this question!

Level of Cognitive Ability: Analysis
Phase of Nursing Process: Assessment
Client Needs: Physiological Integrity
Content Area: Child Health

Reference
Ashwill, J., & Droske, S. (1997). *Nursing care of children: Principles and practice.* Philadelphia: W. B. Saunders. p. 831.

22. **2**

Rationale: Following tonsillectomy, if bleeding occurs, the child is turned to the side and the physician is notified. An NPO status is maintained and an antiemetic may be prescribed; however, the initial nursing action is to turn the child to the side.

Test-Taking Strategy: Note the key word "initial" in the stem of the question. Although all of the options may be appropriate, to maintain physiological integrity the initial action is to turn the child to the side.

Level of Cognitive Ability: Application
Phase of Nursing Process: Implementation
Client Needs: Physiological Integrity
Content Area: Child Health

Reference
Ashwill, J., & Droske, S. (1997). *Nursing care of children: Principles and practice.* Philadelphia: W. B. Saunders. p. 831.

23. **4**

Rationale: Following tonsillectomy, clear cool liquids should be administered. Citrus, carbonated, and extremely hot or cold liquids need to be avoided because they may irritate the throat. Red liquids need to be avoided because they give the appearance of blood if the child vomits. Milk and milk products (pudding) are avoided because they coat the throat, cause the child to clear the throat, and thus increase the risk of bleeding.

Test-Taking Strategy: Knowledge regarding the foods and fluids that should be avoided following tonsillectomy is required to answer this question. Avoiding foods and fluids that may irritate or cause bleeding is the concern. This will assist in eliminating options 2 and 3. The word "cherry" in option 1 should be the clue that this is not an appropriate food item. Review dietary measures following tonsillectomy if you had difficulty with this question!

Level of Cognitive Ability: Application
Phase of Nursing Process: Implementation
Client Needs: Physiological Integrity
Content Area: Child Health

Reference
Ashwill, J., & Droske, S. (1997). *Nursing care of children: Principles and practice.* Philadelphia: W. B. Saunders. p. 831.

24. **3**

Rationale: Bad mouth odor is normal following tonsillectomy and may be relieved by drinking more liquids. Options 1, 2, and 4 are incorrect. Additionally, mouthwash gargles will irritate the throat.

Test-Taking Strategy: Eliminate option 4 first, knowing that mouthwash gargles will irritate the surgical site. Options 1 and 2 are similar, incorrect, and will cause additional concern in the mother. Review postoperative expectations following tonsillectomy now if you had difficulty with this question!

Level of Cognitive Ability: Application
Phase of Nursing Process: Implementation
Client Needs: Physiological Integrity
Content Area: Child Health

Reference
Ashwill, J., & Droske, S. (1997). *Nursing care of children: Principles and practice.* Philadelphia: W. B. Saunders. p. 831.

25. **2**

Rationale: Citrus juices, which irritate the throat, need to be avoided for 10 days. Red liquids are avoided because they will give the appearance of blood if the child vomits.

The mother is instructed to add full liquids on the second day and soft foods as the child tolerates them. Rough or scratchy foods or spicy foods are to be avoided for 3 weeks.

Test-Taking Strategy: Knowledge regarding the specific instructions related to food and fluids following tonsillectomy is required to answer this question. Review the dietary instructions now if you had difficulty with this question!

Level of Cognitive Ability: Application
Phase of Nursing Process: Implementation
Client Needs: Health Promotion and Maintenance
Content Area: Child Health

Reference
Ashwill, J., & Droske, S. (1997). *Nursing care of children: Principles and practice.* Philadelphia: W. B. Saunders. p. 831.

BIBLIOGRAPHY

Ashwill, J., & Droske, S. (1997). *Nursing care of children: Principles and practice.* Philadelphia: W. B. Saunders.

Hodgson, B., & Kizior, R. (1999). *Saunders nursing drug handbook 1999.* Philadelphia: W. B. Saunders.

Lammon, C., Foote, A., Leli, P., et al. (1995). *Clinical nursing skills.* Philadelphia: W. B. Saunders.

Luckmann, J. (1997). *Saunders manual of nursing care.* Philadelphia: W. B. Saunders.

Nichols, F., & Zwelling, E. (1997). *Maternal newborn nursing: Theory and practice.* Philadelphia: W. B. Saunders.

O'Toole, M. (ed.). (1997). *Miller-Keane encyclopedia & dictionary of medicine, nursing, & allied health* (6th ed.). Philadelphia: W. B. Saunders.

CHAPTER 35

Respiratory Disorders

....

I. Epiglottitis

A. Description
1. A bacterial form of croup
2. An inflammation of the epiglottis most commonly caused by *Haemophilus influenzae* type B or *Streptococcus pneumoniae*
3. Occurs most frequently in age groups 3 to 7
4. The onset is abrupt and occurs most often in the winter
5. Considered an emergency situation

B. Assessment
1. High fever
2. Sore throat
3. Red and inflamed throat
4. Difficulty swallowing
5. Drooling
6. Muffled voice
7. Inspiratory **stridor**
8. Absence of spontaneous cough
9. Tripod positioning; while supporting the body with the hands, the child thrusts the chin forward and opens the mouth in an attempt to widen the airway

C. Implementation
1. Monitor airway status
2. Assess respiratory status and breath sounds noting **nasal flaring**, the use of accessory muscles, and the presence of **stridor**
3. Assess vital signs by taking the temperature by axillary not oral route
4. Do not leave the child unattended
5. Do not force the child to lie down
6. Do not restrain the child
7. NO attempts should be made to visualize the posterior pharynx or to obtain throat culture to prevent spasm of the epiglottis and airway occlusion
8. Maintain NPO status
9. Monitor hydration status and input and output (I&O) status
10. Prepare the child for lateral neck films to confirm the diagnosis
11. Administer IV fluids and antibiotics as prescribed

12. Administer analgesics and antipyretics (acetaminophen [Tylenol]) to reduce fever and throat pain as prescribed
13. Provide cool-mist oxygen therapy as prescribed
14. Provide high humidification to cool the airway and decrease swelling
15. Have resuscitation equipment available
16. Prepare for enotracheal intubation or tracheotomy for severe respiratory distress
17. Question the physician regarding the need for immunization (*Haemophilus* type B) to prevent reccurrence

II. Laryngotracheobronchitis—croup

A. Description
1. Inflammation of larynx, trachea, and bronchi
2. May be viral or bacterial
3. Has a gradual onset and may be preceded by an upper respiratory infection

B. Assessment
1. Fever
2. Irritability
3. Restlessness
4. Hoarse voice
5. Seal bark and brassy cough
6. Inspiratory **stridor** and labored respirations
7. Use of accessory muscles for breathing
8. Crackles and **wheezing**
9. Anorexia, nausea, and vomiting
10. Signs of anoxia and carbon dioxide retention
11. Cyanosis

C. Implementation
1. Maintain a patent airway
2. Assess respiratory status, monitoring for **nasal flaring**, sternal retraction, and inspiratory **stridor**
3. Monitor for cyanosis or pallor
4. Monitor vital signs
5. Elevate the head of the bed and provide bed rest
6. Provide humidified oxygen via cool-mist tent
7. Provide fluids

8. Administer IVs as prescribed to maintain hydration status
9. Administer acetaminophen to reduce fever
10. Avoid cough syrups and cold medicines, which may dry and thicken secretions
11. Administer antibiotics as prescribed, noting that they are not indicated unless a bacterial infection is present
12. Administer bronchodilators if prescribed to relax smooth muscles and relieve **stridor**
13. Administer corticosteroids if prescribed for anti-inflammatory effect
14. Have resuscitation equipment available

III. Bronchitis

A. Description: Infection of the major bronchi
B. Assessment
    1. Fever
    2. Hacking and productive cough
    3. Rhonchi and rales
C. Implementation
    1. Monitor for respiratory distress
    2. Monitor vital signs
    3. Provide humidified air
    4. Monitor for signs of dehydration such as sunken fontanel, poor skin turgor, and decreased and concentrated urinary output
    5. Increase fluid intake
    6. Monitor weight
    7. Administer acetaminophen for fever
    8. Administer respiratory treatments as prescribed

IV. Bronchiolitis

A. Description
    1. An inflammation of the bronchioles that causes a thick production of mucus that occludes bronchiole tubes and small bronchi
    2. Respiratory syncytial virus (RSV) is a common cause
    3. RSV, although not airborne, is highly communicable and is usually transferred by the hands
B. Assessment
    1. Upper respiratory infection (URI) symptoms
    2. Fever
    3. Nasal drainage
    4. Tachypnea
    5. **Nasal flaring**
    6. Increased difficulty in breathing
    7. **Retractions**
    8. Expiratory wheeze and grunt
    9. Harsh cough
    10. Irritability
C. Implementation
    1. Maintain a patent airway
    2. Monitor vital signs
    3. Position at a 30- to 40-degree angle with the neck slightly extended to maintain an open

airway and decrease pressure on the diaphragm
    4. Provide cool, humidified oxygen
    5. Assess for signs of dehydration such as sunken fontanel, poor skin turgor, and decreased and concentrated urinary output
D. The Child with RSV
    1. Isolate in a single room or place in a room with another RSV child
    2. Maintain good handwashing procedures
    3. Ensure that nurses caring for these children do not care for other high-risk children
    4. Wear gowns when soiling of clothing may occur
    5. Administer ribavirin (Virazole), an antiviral respiratory medication, if prescribed
    6. The nurse wearing contact lenses should wear goggles when coming in contact with ribavirin because the mist may dissolve soft lenses

V. Asthma

A. Description
    1. Includes bronchospasm, edema, and inflammation of the bronchial airways
    2. Is commonly caused by physical and chemical irritants such as foods, pollens, dust, smoke, animal dander, temperature changes, URI, activity, and stress
B. Assessment
    1. Dyspnea
    2. Expiratory **wheezing**
    3. Hacking, nonproductive cough
    4. Hoarse, loud breath sounds
    5. Tachycardia
    6. Orthopnea
    7. Apprehension and restlessness
C. Implementation
    1. Acute episode
        a. Assess cardiac, respiratory, and pulse oximetry by monitor
        b. Initiate an IV line
        c. Prepare the child for chest x-ray
        d. Administer humidified oxygen by nasal prongs or face mask as prescribed
        e. Administer bronchodilator via nebulizer as prescribed
        f. Prepare to administer bronchodilatory and corticosteroids by IV if prescribed
        g. Prepare to obtain blood gases and serum electrolytes
        h. Prepare to administer subcutaneous epinephrine if the child does not respond to treatment
        i. Administer IV sodium bicarbonate as prescribed to correct acidosis
        j. Be alert to decreased **wheezing** or a silent chest, which may signal the inability to move air
    2. Long-term management
        a. Eliminate or avoid allergens or

environmental factors that can precipitate an attack

b. Avoid exposure to individuals with a viral respiratory infection

c. Instruct the child how to recognize early symptoms of an asthma attack, which may include itchy chest or chin, cough, irritability or tired feeling, increased breathing rate, dry mouth, or unusual dark circles under the eyes

d. Instruct in the administration of bronchodilators and anti-inflammatory medications as prescribed

e. Encourage adequate rest, sleep, and a well-balanced diet

f. Instruct in the importance of adequate fluid intake to liquefy secretions

g. Assist in developing an exercise program

h. Instruct in the procedure for respiratory treatments and exercises as prescribed

i. Encourage the parents to keep immunizations up to date

j. Inform other health care providers of the asthma condition

k. Allow the child to take control of self-care measures based on age appropriateness

VI. Pneumonia

A. Description: Inflammation of the alveoli caused by bacteria, virus, organisms, and aspiration

B. Assessment
   1. Pneumococcal pneumonia
      a. Fever
      b. Increased pulse and respiratory rate
      c. **Retractions**
      d. Productive cough
   2. Viral pneumonia
      a. Follows URI
      b. Low-grade fever
      c. Nonproductive cough
      d. Increased respiratory rate
   3. Staphylococcal pneumonia
      a. Fever
      b. Cough
      c. Respiratory distress
      d. Cyanosis

C. Implementation
   1. Assess breath sounds and respiratory rate
   2. Monitor vital signs
   3. Elevate the head of the bed
   4. Monitor cardiac, respiratory, and pulse oximetry via monitor
   5. Provide humidified oxygen as prescribed
   6. Assess for restlessness
   7. Monitor I&O and weight
   8. Monitor for signs of dehydration
   9. Encourage fluid intake of warm liquids to loosen secretions
   10. Administer antipyretics (acetaminophen) for fever
   11. Administer antibiotics as prescribed

12. Assist with coughing and deep breathing
13. Schedule chest physiotherapy before meals and bedtime
14. Monitor for tension pneumothorax or empyema with staphylococcal pneumonia
15. Maintain isolation with pneumococcal and staphylococcal pneumonia
16. Avoid the use of infant seats because pressure may be placed on the diaphragm, decreasing lung expansion

VII. Cystic Fibrosis (CF)

A. Description
   1. A chronic multisystem disorder affecting exocrine gland function
   2. The mucus produced by the exocrine glands is abnormally thick, causing obstruction of the small passageways of these organs
   3. An autosomal recessive trait disorder

B. Assessment
   1. Respiratory system
      a. **Wheezing** and dry nonproductive cough
      b. Repeated episodes of bronchitis and pneumonia
      c. Purulent and copious sputum with infections
      d. Crackles and diminished breath sounds
      e. Accessory muscle use
      f. **Retractions**
      g. Hypoxia
      h. Cyanosis
      i. Barrel chest
      j. Clubbing of fingers
      k. Emphysema and atelectasis as the airways become increasingly obstructed
      l. Cor pulmonale and congestive heart failure (CHF), spontaneous pneumothorax, or hemoptysis as the disease progresses
   2. Gastrointestinal system
      a. Steatorrhea
      b. Malnutrition and **growth** failure
      c. Protuberant abdomen
      d. Meconium ileus in the neonate
      e. Rectal prolapse and intussusception
      f. Biliary cirrhosis, portal hypertension, and esophageal varices as a result of obstruction of bile ducts
   3. Integumentary system
      a. Abnormally high concentrations of sodium and chloride in sweat
      b. Electrolyte imbalances especially during hot weather
      c. Dry mouth
      d. Increased susceptibility to infection
   4. Reproductive system
      a. An average of 2 years' delay in development
      b. Difficulty becoming pregnant because of thick cervical mucus

    c. Increases incidence of fetal loss and preterm birth

C. Sweat Test

1. Sweating is stimulated on the child's forearm with pilocarpine, and the amount of sodium and chloride is measured
2. A chloride level greater than 60 mEq/L is a positive test result
3. A chloride level of 40 mEq/L is suggestive of CF and requires a repeat test

D. Implementation

1. Assess respiratory status
2. Elevate the head of the bed or support the child in an upright position if he or she is having difficulty breathing
3. Administer humidified low-flow oxygen
4. Encourage coughing and deep breathing
5. Teach the child forced expiratory technique to mobilize secretions
6. Perform respiratory treatments as prescribed
7. Administer chest physiotherapy (CPT) before meals
8. Assess weight
9. Promote optimal nutrition and hydration
10. Administer expectorants and bronchodilators as prescribed to facilitate thinning and mobilization of secretions
11. Instruct the parents not to give cough suppressants as they will inhibit expectoration of secretions and promote infection
12. Protect the child from exposure to infections
13. Instruct the parents to be sure immunizations are up to date
14. Administer pancreatic enzymes as prescribed within 30 minutes of eating meals and snacks
15. Do not mix pancreatic enzymes with hot or starchy foods but with a small amount of nonfat, nonprotein food
16. Enteric coated pancreatic enzymes should not be crushed or chewed
17. Pancreatic enzymes should not be given if the child is nothing by mouth (NPO)
18. Administer multivitamins and iron supplements as prescribed
19. Supplement the child's diet with salt during extremely hot weather or if the child has a fever
20. Instruct in the administration of antibiotics if prescribed
21. Instruct in the use of mucolytics, bronchodilators, hydrating agents, and steroids as prescribed

VIII. Sudden Infant Death Syndrome (SIDS)

A. Description

1. Unexpected death of an apparently healthy infant under age 1 year for which a rough autopsy fails to demonstrate an adequate cause of death
2. The cause is not known

B. Characteristics

1. Maternal risk factors
   a. Maternal smoking
   b. Younger mothers
   c. Any condition that places the mother at risk during pregnancy increases the risk of SIDS
2. Birth factors
   a. Prematurity
   b. Low-birth-weight infants
   c. Multiple births
   d. Infants with central nervous system (CNS) problems
3. Time of year: most frequently during winter months
4. Time of death: usually occurs during sleep
5. Age: most frequently occurs during ages 2 to 4 months
6. Sex/race
   a. Higher in males
   b. Higher in Native Americans

C. Appearance when found

1. Apneic
2. Blue
3. Lifeless
4. Frothy blood-tinged fluid in nose and mouth
5. May be found in any position
6. May be clutching bedding

D. Prevention

1. Healthy infants should be placed for sleep on their sides or backs rather than prone
2. Soft bedding should be avoided because the infant may suffocate by rebreathing CO_2 expired air

IX. Tuberculosis (TB) in Children

A. Description

1. A reportable contagious disease caused by *Mycobacterium tuberculosis*
2. The route of transmission is through inhalation of droplets from an individual with active TB
3. Most children are infected by a family member or by another individual with whom they have frequent contact, such as a baby-sitter

B. Assessment

1. Children ages 3 to 15 are usually asymptomatic, have normal chest x-ray results, and can be diagnosed only through a positive skin test
2. Some children develop malaise, fever, cough, weight loss, anorexia, and lymphadenopathy

C. Mantoux Test

1. In most children, skin testing will produce a positive reaction 3 to 6 weeks after the initial infection and occasionally as long as 3 months after infection

2. An area of induration of 15 mm or greater is considered to be a positive sign in all children

3. Induration measuring 10 mm or greater is considered to be a positive result in children younger than 4 years of age and in those with chronic illness or high risk for exposure to TB

4. A reaction of 5 mm or greater is considered to be positive for the highest risk groups

D. Sputum Test: Because children often swallow sputum rather than expectorate, gastric washings may be done to obtain swallowed sputum

E. Implementation

1. Bacillus Calmette-Guérin vaccine (BCG), the vaccine used to prevent TB, is used mainly for children with negative chest x-ray and skin test results who have had repeated exposures to TB, and for asymptomatic human immunodeficiency virus (HIV)-infected children who are at increased risk for developing TB

2. Antituberculin medication for 9 months and for 12 months if the child has an HIV infection

3. Stress the importance of adequate rest and adequate diet

4. Instruct in measures to prevent transmission of TB to others

PRACTICE QUESTIONS

1. The nurse is caring for a 2-year-old child diagnosed with croup. The nursing student asks the nurse about the clinical manifestations associated with croup. Which of the following is not associated with this illness?
   1 Symptoms usually worsen at night and are better during the day
   2 Symptoms usually worsen during the day and are relieved during sleep
   3 The cough is harsh and metallic
   4 Inspiratory stridor and a low-grade fever may be present

2. The home care nurse provides instructions to the mother of a child with croup. The mother expresses concern regarding the occurrence of an acute spasmodic episode. Which of the following suggestions are not provided to the mother regarding management if an acute episode occurs?
   1 Place a steam vaporizer in the child's room
   2 Place the child in a closed bathroom and allow the child to inhale steam from hot running water
   3 Place a cool-mist humidifier in the child's room
   4 Take the child out into the cool, humid night air

3. The child with croup is being discharged from the hospital. The nurse provides instructions to the mother and advises the mother to bring the child to the emergency room if the child:
   1 Appears tired
   2 Takes fluids poorly
   3 Is irritable
   4 Develops stridor

4. A hospitalized 2-year-old child with croup is receiving corticosteroid therapy. The mother asks the nurse why the physician did not prescribe antibiotics. The most appropriate response is:
   1 "The child is too young to receive antibiotics."
   2 "The child still has the maternal antibodies from birth and does not need antibiotics."
   3 "Antibiotics are not indicated unless a bacterial infection is present."
   4 "The child may be allergic to antibiotics."

5. The child with croup is placed in a cool-mist tent. The mother becomes concerned because the child is frightened, consistently cries, and tries to climb out of the tent. The most appropriate nursing action is to:
   1 Call the physician and obtain an order for a mild sedative
   2 Tell the mother that the child must stay in the tent
   3 Place a toy in the tent to make the child feel more comfortable
   4 Let the mother hold the child and direct a cool mist over the child's face

6. A child with croup is placed in a cool-mist tent. The mother asks if the child can have a security blanket inside the tent. The most appropriate response is:
   1 "Objects from home are not allowed to be brought to the hospital."
   2 "The child may have the security blanket inside the tent."
   3 "The blanket is not allowed because it will harbor bacteria."
   4 "The blanket is not allowed, but the child may have a toy from the hospital play room."

7. The nurse provides discharge instructions to the mother of a child hospitalized with croup. Which of the following statements, if made by the mother, indicate a need for further instruction?
   1 "I will give my child cough syrup if a cough develops."
   2 "I will be sure that my child drinks at least 2 to 4 glasses of fluids every day."
   3 "I will give Tylenol if my child develops a fever."
   4 "Sips of warm fluid will help if my child develops a croup attack."

8. The mother arrives at the emergency room with her child, and a diagnosis of epiglottitis is documented. Which of the following physician orders are most important for the nurse to question?

1 Obtain a throat culture
2 Take the axillary temperature
3 Administer humidified oxygen
4 Administer antipyretics for fever

9. The emergency room nurse is caring for a child diagnosed with epiglottitis. Indications that the child may be experiencing airway obstruction include which of the following?
   1 The child is leaning backward supporting self with the hands and arms
   2 A low-grade fever and complaints of a sore throat
   3 The child is leaning forward with the chin thrust out
   4 Nasal flaring and bradycardia

10. The emergency room nurse is caring for a child suspected of epiglottitis. The nurse has ensured that the child has a patent airway. The next priority in the care of this child is to:
    1 Prepare the child for an x-ray
    2 Assist the physician with intubation
    3 Prepare the child for tracheotomy
    4 Prepare to administer epinephrine

11. The nurse is caring for an infant with bronchiolitis. Diagnostic tests have confirmed respiratory syncytial virus (RSV). Based on this finding, which of the following is the most appropriate nursing action?
    1 Move the infant to another room with another RSV child
    2 Leave the infant in the present room because RSV is not contagious
    3 Inform the staff that they must wear a mask when caring for the child
    4 Initiate strict enteric precautions

12. The nurse caring for an infant with bronchiolitis is monitoring for signs of dehydration. Which of the following is the most reliable method of determining fluid loss?
    1 Monitoring I&O
    2 Monitoring for sunken fontanel
    3 Monitoring for dry mucous membranes
    4 Monitoring body weight

13. Ribavirin (Virazole) is prescribed for the hospitalized child with RSV. The nurse prepares to administer this medication via which of the following routes?
    1 Subcutaneous
    2 Intramuscular
    3 Via oxygen tent
    4 Orally

14. Which of the following precautions will the nurse specifically take during the preparation and administration of ribavirin to a child with RSV?
    1 Handwashing
    2 Wear goggles

3 Wear a gown
4 Wear a gown and mask

15. A 10-year-old child with asthma is treated for acute exacerbation in the emergency room. Which of the following is not an indication that the condition is improving?
    1 Increased wheezing
    2 Decreased wheezing
    3 Warm dry skin
    4 A pulse rate of 90 beats per minute (bpm)

16. A child arrives in the emergency room for treatment of an acute asthma attack. The nurse prepares to administer which of the following medications first?
    1 Subcutaneous epinephrine
    2 Subcutaneous terbutaline
    3 IV corticosteroid
    4 A bronchodilator via nebulizer

17. The mother arrives at the clinic with her 3-year-old child. The mother tells the nurse that the child has had a fever and a cough for the past 2 days, and this morning the child began to wheeze. Viral pneumonia is diagnosed. Which of the following does the nurse anticipate as a component of the treatment plan?
    1 Oral antibiotics
    2 Hospitalization and IV antibiotics
    3 Supportive treatment
    4 IV fluid administration

18. The mother of an 8-year-old child being treated for right lower lobe pneumonia at home calls the clinic nurse. The mother tells the nurse that the child has discomfort on the right side and that the acetaminophen (Tylenol) is not very effective. The most appropriate suggestion by the nurse is to:
    1 Increase the dose of the acetaminophen
    2 Increase the frequency of the acetaminophen
    3 Encourage the child to lie on the right side
    4 Encourage the child to lie on the left side

19. The charge nurse of the newborn nursery is providing a teaching session to new employees regarding sudden infant death syndrome (SIDS). Which of the following would be included in the teaching session?
    1 SIDS usually occurs during sleep and is more common in infants from lower socioeconomic groups
    2 SIDS usually occurs during sleep and is more common in girls
    3 SIDS usually occurs during sleep and most frequently occurs between 8 and 10 months of age
    4 SIDS usually occurs during sleep and is more common in high-birth-weight infants

20. A new mother expresses concern to the nurse regarding SIDS. She asks the nurse how to position her new infant for sleep. The most appropriate response is:
    1 The infant should be placed on its side or back rather than on the stomach
    2 The infant should be placed on its side or prone
    3 The infant should be placed on its side or stomach with the face turned
    4 The infant should be placed on its back or prone

21. A mother of a child with cystic fibrosis (CF) asks the clinic nurse about the disease. The nurse bases the response on which of the following?
    1 It is a disease that causes the formation of multiple cysts in the lungs
    2 It is a chronic multisystem disorder affecting the exocrine glands
    3 It is transmitted as an autosomal dominant trait
    4 It is a disease that causes dilation of the passageways of many organs

22. A sweat test is performed on a child with a suspected diagnosis of CF. Which of the following test results is positive for CF?
    1 Chloride level of 20 mEq/L
    2 Chloride level of 30 mEq/L
    3 Chloride level of 40 mEq/L
    4 Chloride level of 70 mEq/L

23. The clinic nurse is providing instructions to a mother of a child with CF regarding the immunization schedule for the child. Which of the following statements does the nurse make to the mother?
    1 "The immunization schedule will need to be altered."
    2 "The child will receive all of the immunizations except for the polio series."
    3 "The child will receive the recommended basic series of immunizations along with a yearly influenza vaccination."
    4 "The child should not receive any hepatitis vaccines."

24. The home health nurse is instructing the mother of a child with CF about the appropriate dietary measures. Which of the following diets are included in the instructions?
    1 Low-calorie, low-fat diet
    2 High-calorie, high-protein diet
    3 High-calorie, low-protein diet
    4 High-calorie, restricted fat diet

25. The nurse prepares to administer a pancreatic enzyme powder to the child with CF. Which of the following food items does the nurse mix with the medication?
    1 Apple sauce
    2 Tapioca
    3 Mashed potatoes
    4 Hot oatmeal

26. The home health nurse teaches a child with CF how to perform the "huff" maneuver. Which of the following instructions does the nurse provide to the child?
    1 Take a deep breath, hold it for 15 seconds, then exhale slowly whispering the word "huff"
    2 Take a shallow breath then exhale rapidly, whispering the word "huff"
    3 Take a deep breath, then exhale rapidly, whispering the word "huff"
    4 Take a shallow breath, hold it for 10 seconds, then exhale rapidly, whispering the word "huff"

27. The mother of a child with CF asks the home health nurse when the postural drainage should be performed. On further assessment, the mother states that the child eats meals at 8:00 A.M., 12 noon and at 6:00 P.M. Which of the following times should the postural drainage be performed?
    1 10:00 A.M., 2:00 P.M., and 8:00 P.M.
    2 9:00 A.M., 1:00 P.M., and 6:00 P.M.
    3 8:00 A.M., 12:00 noon, and 6:00 P.M.
    4 8:00 A.M., 2:00 P.M., and 6:00 P.M.

28. The clinic nurse reads the results of a Mantoux test on a 3-year-old child. The results indicate an area of induration measuring 10 mm. The nurse interprets these results as:
    1 Negative
    2 Positive
    3 Inconclusive
    4 Definitive, requiring a repeat test

29. The nurse educator provides a teaching session to staff nurses regarding the BCG vaccine. Which of the following is included in the teaching?
    1 It is used for children with a positive Mantoux test
    2 It is used for children with both a positive Mantoux test and positive chest x-ray
    3 It is used for all children to prevent tuberculosis
    4 It is used for asymptomatic HIV infected children who are at increased risk for developing TB

30. Isoniazid (INH) is prescribed for a 2-year-old child with a positive Mantoux test. The mother of the child asks the nurse how long the child will need to take the medication. The most appropriate response is:
    1 Six months
    2 Nine months
    3 Twelve months
    4 Eighteen months

ANSWERS

1. 2

Rationale: Croup often begins at night and may be preceded by several days of URI symptoms. It is characterized by a sudden onset of a harsh, metallic cough, sore throat, and inspiratory stridor. Symptoms usually worsen at night and are better in the day. It is usually accompanied by a low-grade fever, but occasionally the fever may be as high as 104°F.

Test-Taking Strategy: Note the key word "not" in the stem of the question. Eliminate option 4 first because of the word "may." Knowledge of the manifestations associated with this illness will assist in eliminating options 1 and 3. If you had difficulty with this question, take time now to review this disorder!

Level of Cognitive Ability: Analysis
Phase of Nursing Process: Analysis
Client Needs: Physiological Integrity
Content Area: Child Health

Reference
Ashwill, J., & Droske, S. (1997). *Nursing care of children: Principles and practice.* Philadelphia: W. B. Saunders. p. 833.

2. 1

Rationale: Steam from hot running water in a closed bathroom and cool mist from a bedside humidifier are effective in reducing mucosal edema. Cool-mist humidifiers are recommended over steam vaporizers, which present a danger of scald burns. Taking the child out into the cool, humid night air may also relieve mucosal swelling. Remember, however, that a cold mist may precipitate bronchospasm.

Test-Taking Strategy: The issue of the question is twofold: to reduce mucosal edema and to provide a safe environment. Note the key word "not" in the question. Option 1 is the option that would provide an unsafe environment for the child. Review management of acute spasmodic croup now if you had difficulty with this question!

Level of Cognitive Ability: Application
Phase of Nursing Process: Implementation
Client Needs: Safe, Effective Care Environment
Content Area: Child Health

Reference
Ashwill, J., & Droske, S. (1997). *Nursing care of children: Principles and practice.* Philadelphia: W. B. Saunders. p. 833.

3. 4

Rationale: The mother should be instructed that if the child develops stridor at rest, cyanosis, severe agitation or fatigue, moderate to severe retractions, or is unable to take oral fluids, to bring the child to the emergency room.

Test-Taking Strategy: Utilize the ABCs, Airway, Breathing, and Circulation, to answer the question. This should easily direct you to option 4.

Level of Cognitive Ability: Application
Phase of Nursing Process: Implementation
Client Needs: Physiological Integrity
Content Area: Child Health

Reference
Ashwill, J., & Droske, S. (1997). *Nursing care of children: Principles and practice.* Philadelphia: W. B. Saunders. p. 833.

4. 3

Rationale: Antibiotics are not indicated in the treatment of croup unless a bacterial infection is present. Options 1, 2, and 4 are incorrect. Additionally, there are no supporting data in the question to indicate that the child may be allergic to antibiotics.

Test-Taking Strategy: Avoid reading into the question. Eliminate option 4 as there are no supporting data in the question regarding the potential for allergies. Noting the age of the child will assist in eliminating both options 1 and 2. Review the indications for the use of antibiotics now if you had difficulty with this question!

Level of Cognitive Ability: Analysis
Phase of Nursing Process: Analysis
Client Needs: Physiological Integrity
Content Area: Child Health

Reference
Ashwill, J., & Droske, S. (1997). *Nursing care of children: Principles and practice.* Philadelphia: W. B. Saunders. p. 833.

5. 4

Rationale: If the use of a tent or hood is causing distress, treatment may be more effective if the child is held by the parent and a cool mist is directed toward the child's face. A mild sedative should not be administered to the child. Crying will aggravate laryngospasm and increase hypoxia, which may cause airway obstruction. Options 2 and 3 will not alleviate the child's fear.

Test-Taking Strategy: Options 1, 2, and 3 will not alleviate the child's fear. Additionally, they are all similar in that they do not address the fear. Option 4 is the option that addresses the issue of the question.

Level of Cognitive Ability: Analysis
Phase of Nursing Process: Implementation
Client Needs: Psychosocial Integrity
Content Area: Child Health

Reference
Ashwill, J., & Droske, S. (1997). *Nursing care of children: Principles and practice.* Philadelphia: W. B. Saunders. p. 835.

6. 2

Rationale: Familiar objects provide a sense of security for children in the strange hospital environment. The child should be allowed to have a favorite toy or blanket while in the mist tent.

Test-Taking Strategy: Knowledge regarding care to the child while in a mist tent is required to answer this question. Option 1 can be easily eliminated. Next eliminate options 3 and 4 because they are similar. Review care to the child in a mist tent now if you had difficulty with this question!

Level of Cognitive Ability: Application
Phase of Nursing Process: Implementation
Client Needs: Psychosocial Integrity
Content Area: Child Health

Reference
Ashwill, J., & Droske, S. (1997). *Nursing care of children: Principles and practice.* Philadelphia: W. B. Saunders. p. 836.

7. 1

Rationale: Cough syrups and cold medicines are not to be given because they may dry and thicken secretions. Adequate hydration of 500 to 1000 mL of fluids daily is important in thinning secretions. Acetaminophen is used if a fever develops. Sips of warm fluids during a croup attack help relax the vocal cords and thin mucus.

Test-Taking Strategy: Note the key phrase "a need for further instruction." Options 2 and 3 can be easily eliminated. Recalling that warm fluids can relax membranes and thin secretions will assist in directing you to option 1. Review the effects of cough medicines now if you had difficulty with this question!

Level of Cognitive Ability: Analysis
Phase of Nursing Process: Evaluation
Client Needs: Physiological Integrity
Content Area: Child Health

Reference
Ashwill, J., & Droske, S. (1997). *Nursing care of children: Principles and practice.* Philadelphia: W. B. Saunders. p. 838.

8. 1
Rationale: The throat of a child with suspected epiglottitis should not be examined or cultured, because any stimulation with a tongue depressor or culture swab could cause laryngospasm and complete airway obstruction. Humidified oxygen and antipyretics are components of management. Axillary rather than oral temperatures should be taken.

Test-Taking Strategy: Knowledge regarding the high potential for complete airway obstruction in a child with epiglottitis is required to answer this question. This knowledge will quickly direct you to option 1.

Level of Cognitive Ability: Analysis
Phase of Nursing Process: Analysis
Client Needs: Physiological Integrity
Content Area: Child Health

Reference
Ashwill, J., & Droske, S. (1997). *Nursing care of children: Principles and practice.* Philadelphia: W. B. Saunders. p. 840.

9. 3
Rationale: Clinical manifestations suggestive of airway obstruction include tripod positioning (leaning forward supported by arms, chin thrust out, mouth open), nasal flaring, tachycardia, a high fever, and sore throat.

Test-Taking Strategy: Eliminate option 4 first because tachycardia rather than bradycardia will occur in a child experiencing respiratory distress. Eliminate option 2 next, knowing that a high fever occurs with epiglottitis. From the remaining options, visualize the descriptions in each, and determine which position would best assist a child experiencing respiratory distress. You should easily be directed to option 3.

Level of Cognitive Ability: Analysis
Phase of Nursing Process: Assessment
Client Needs: Physiological Integrity
Content Area: Child Health

Reference
Ashwill, J., & Droske, S. (1997). *Nursing care of children: Principles and practice.* Philadelphia: W. B. Saunders. p. 838.

10. 1
Rationale: When epiglottitis is suspected, the priorities are to maintain a patent airway and to obtain an x-ray to confirm the diagnosis. If epiglottitis is present, the child is taken promptly to the operating room for tracheal intuba-

tion or immediate surgical airway. Epinephrine is not used in the treatment of epiglottitis.

Test-Taking Strategy: Note the key word "suspected" in the question. This should assist in directing you to option 1. Confirmation of the diagnosis is necessary to determine the appropriate management. If you had difficulty with this question, take time now to review the treatment of this life-threatening condition!

Level of Cognitive Ability: Analysis
Phase of Nursing Process: Planning
Client Needs: Physiological Integrity
Content Area: Child Health

Reference
Luckmann, J. (1997). *Saunders manual of nursing care.* Philadelphia: W. B. Saunders. p. 1716.

11. 1
Rationale: RSV is a highly communicable disorder. It is not transmitted via the airborne route. It is usually transferred by the hands, and meticulous handwashing is necessary to decrease the spread of organisms. The infant with RSV is isolated in a single room or placed in a room with another RSV child. Enteric precautions are not necessary; however, the nurse should wear a gown when soiling of clothing may occur.

Test-Taking Strategy: Knowledge regarding the transmission of RSV is required to answer this question. Take time now to review the care of the child with RSV if you had difficulty with this question!

Level of Cognitive Ability: Application
Phase of Nursing Process: Implementation
Client Needs: Safe, Effective Care Environment
Content Area: Child Health

Reference
Ashwill, J., & Droske, S. (1997). *Nursing care of children: Principles and practice.* Philadelphia: W. B. Saunders. p. 842.

12. 4
Rationale: Body weight is the most reliable method of measurement of body fluid loss or gain. One kilogram of weight change represents 1 L of fluid loss or gain.

Test-Taking Strategy: Note the key phrase "most reliable." Options 2 and 3 can be easily eliminated first. From the remaining options, recall that it would be very difficult to obtain an accurate output on an infant. This concept should easily direct you toward option 4.

Level of Cognitive Ability: Analysis
Phase of Nursing Process: Analysis
Client Needs: Physiological Integrity
Content Area: Child Health

Reference
Ashwill, J., & Droske, S. (1997). *Nursing care of children: Principles and practice.* Philadelphia: W. B. Saunders. p. 844.

13. 3
Rationale: Ribavirin is an antiviral respiratory medication that is used mainly in hospitalized children with severe RSV and in high-risk children. Administration is via hood, face mask, or oxygen tent over 12 to 18 hours for a minimum of 3 and a maximum of 7 days. The medication is most effective if administered within the first 3 days of the disease.

Test-Taking Strategy: Knowledge regarding the administration of this medication is required to answer this question. If you are unfamiliar with this medication, take time now to review its method of administration!

Level of Cognitive Ability: Application
Phase of Nursing Process: Planning
Client Needs: Physiological Integrity
Content Area: Child Health

Reference

Ashwill, J., & Droske, S. (1997). *Nursing care of children: Principles and practice.* Philadelphia: W. B. Saunders. p. 842.

14. **2**

Rationale: Some caregivers experience headaches, burning nasal passages and eyes, and crystallization of soft contact lenses as a result of administration of ribavirin. Specific to this medication is the use of goggles. A mask may be worn. Handwashing is to be performed before and after any child contact. A gown is not necessary.

Test-Taking Strategy: Knowledge regarding the effects of this medication is required to answer this question. Note the key word "specifically" in the question. This should assist in directing you to the correct option. If you had difficulty with this question, take time now to review the concepts related to the administration of this medication!

Level of Cognitive Ability: Application
Phase of Nursing Process: Implementation
Client Needs: Safe, Effective Care Environment
Content Area: Child Health

Reference

Ashwill, J., & Droske, S. (1997). *Nursing care of children: Principles and practice.* Philadelphia: W. B. Saunders. p. 842.

15. **2**

Rationale: Decreased wheezing in a child who otherwise is not improving clinically may be incorrectly interpreted as a positive sign when, in fact, it may signal an inability to move air. A "silent chest" is an ominous sign during an asthma episode. With treatment, increased wheezing may actually signal that the child's condition is improving. The normal pulse rate in a 10-year-old is 70 to 110 BPM. Warm, dry skin indicates an improvement in condition as the child is normally diaphoretic during exacerbation.

Test-Taking Strategy: Note the key word "not" in the stem of the question. Options 3 and 4 can be easily eliminated. From the remaining options, it is necessary to know the signs of improvement in a child treated for asthma. Review these clinical manifestations now if you had difficulty with this question!

Level of Cognitive Ability: Analysis
Phase of Nursing Process: Assessment
Client Needs: Physiological Integrity
Content Area: Child Health

Reference

Ashwill, J., & Droske, S. (1997). *Nursing care of children: Principles and practice.* Philadelphia: W. B. Saunders. p. 867.

16. **4**

Rationale: In treating an acute asthma attack, a bronchodilator (usually albuterol) is administered via a powdered nebulizer first. IV corticosteroids may also be administered following the bronchodilator. Subcutaneous epinephrine or terbutaline may then be given if the child is not responding to treatment.

Test-Taking Strategy: Knowledge that asthma is a reversible obstructive airway disease should assist in directing you to option 4. It would seem logical that the first action would be to dilate the bronchi. If you had difficulty with this question, take time now to review the treatment for an acute asthma episode!

Level of Cognitive Ability: Application
Phase of Nursing Process: Planning
Client Needs: Physiological Integrity
Content Area: Child Health

Reference

Ashwill, J., & Droske, S. (1997). *Nursing care of children: Principles and practice.* Philadelphia: W. B. Saunders. pp. 868–870.

17. **3**

Rationale: With viral pneumonia, treatment is supportive. More severely ill children may be hospitalized and given oxygen, chest physiotherapy, and IV fluids. Antibiotics are not given. Bacterial pneumonia, however, is treated with antibiotic therapy.

Test-Taking Strategy: Note the key word "viral" in the question. Recalling that antibiotics are not effective in treating viruses will assist in eliminating options 1 and 2. There are no data in the question to support the need for IV fluid administration. This leaves option 3 as the correct answer. It is also the most global response.

Level of Cognitive Ability: Analysis
Phase of Nursing Process: Planning
Client Needs: Physiological Integrity
Content Area: Child Health

Reference

Ashwill, J., & Droske, S. (1997). *Nursing care of children: Principles and practice.* Philadelphia: W. B. Saunders. p. 849.

18. **3**

Rationale: Splinting of the affected side by lying on that side may decrease discomfort. It is inappropriate to advise the mother to increase the dose or frequency of acetaminophen. Lying on the left side will not be helpful in alleviating discomfort.

Test-Taking Strategy: Options 1 and 2 can be easily eliminated. Recalling the principles related to splinting an incision in the postoperative client will assist in directing you to option 3. These principles can be applied in this situation.

Level of Cognitive Ability: Application
Phase of Nursing Process: Implementation
Client Needs: Physiological Integrity
Content Area: Child Health

Reference

Ashwill, J., & Droske, S. (1997). *Nursing care of children: Principles and practice.* Philadelphia: W. B. Saunders. p. 850.

19. **1**

Rationale: SIDS usually occurs during sleep. It most frequently occurs between the second and fourth months of life. It is more common in boys, low-birth-weight infants, and infants from lower socioeconomic groups. It occurs more often during the winter months. The highest incidence is in Native Americans followed by African-Americans.

Test-Taking Strategy: Knowledge regarding the characteristics related to etiology and incidence of SIDS is required to answer this question. If you are unfamiliar with this information, take time now to review!

Level of Cognitive Ability: Application
Phase of Nursing Process: Implementation
Client Needs: Health Promotion and Maintenance
Content Area: Child Health

Reference
Ashwill, J., & Droske, S. (1997). *Nursing care of children: Principles and practice.* Philadelphia: W. B. Saunders. p. 856.

20. 1

Rationale: Nurses should encourage parents to place healthy infants on their sides or backs for sleep, and they should provide the rationale for the parents to increase compliance.

Test-Taking Strategy: Eliminate options 2 and 3 first because they are similar. From the remaining options, utilize principles related to safe positioning techniques in selecting the correct option. Review positioning for the healthy infant now if you had difficulty with this question.

Level of Cognitive Ability: Application
Phase of Nursing Process: Implementation
Client Needs: Safe, Effective Care Environment
Content Area: Child Health

Reference
Ashwill, J., & Droske, S. (1997). *Nursing care of children: Principles and practice.* Philadelphia: W. B. Saunders. p. 856.

21. 2

Rationale: CF is a chronic multisystem disorder affecting the exocrine glands. The mucus produced by these glands (particularly those of the bronchioles, small intestine, and the pancreatic and bile ducts) is abnormally thick, causing obstruction of the small passageways of these organs. It is transmitted as an autosomal recessive trait.

Test-Taking Strategy: Knowledge regarding the physiology associated with CF is required to answer this question. If you knew that it was a multisystem disorder, you would easily be directed toward option 2. Additionally, option 2 is the most global response. If you are unfamiliar with this disease, take time now to review!

Level of Cognitive Ability: Analysis
Phase of Nursing Process: Analysis
Client Needs: Physiological Integrity
Content Area: Child Health

Reference
Ashwill, J., & Droske, S. (1997). *Nursing care of children: Principles and practice.* Philadelphia: W. B. Saunders. p. 887.

22. 4

Rationale: In a sweat test, sweating is stimulated on the child's forearm with pilocarpine, the sample is collected on absorbent material, and the amount of sodium and chloride is measured. A sample of at least 50 mg of sweat is required for accurate results. A chloride level greater than 60 mEq/L is considered to be a positive test result. A chloride level of 40 mEq/L is suggestive of CF and requires a repeat test.

Test-Taking Strategy: Knowledge regarding diagnostic results related to the sweat test is required to answer this question. If you had difficulty with this question or are unfamiliar with this test, take time now to review!

Level of Cognitive Ability: Analysis
Phase of Nursing Process: Analysis
Client Needs: Physiological Integrity
Content Area: Child Health

Reference
Ashwill, J., & Droske, S. (1997). *Nursing care of children: Principles and practice.* Philadelphia: W. B. Saunders. p. 890.

23. 3

Rationale: It is essential that children with CF be adequately protected from communicable diseases by immunization. It is recommended that in addition to the basic series of immunizations, children with CF should also receive yearly influenza vaccines.

Test-Taking Strategy: Eliminate options 1, 2, and 4 because they are similar. Recalling the importance of protection from communicable diseases, particularly in children with such a disorder as CF, will assist in directing you to option 3.

Level of Cognitive Ability: Application
Phase of Nursing Process: Implementation
Client Needs: Health Promotion and Maintenance
Content Area: Child Health

Reference
Ashwill, J., & Droske, S. (1997). *Nursing care of children: Principles and practice.* Philadelphia: W. B. Saunders. p. 891.

24. 2

Rationale: Children with CF are managed with a high-calorie, high-protein diet. Pancreatic enzyme replacement therapy, and fat-soluble vitamin supplements are administered. If nutritional problems are severe, nighttime gastrostomy feedings or total parenteral nutrition (TPN) is administered. Fats are not restricted unless steatorrhea cannot be controlled by increased pancreatic enzymes.

Test-Taking Strategy: Knowledge regarding the appropriate diet in the child with CF is required to answer this question. If you are unfamiliar with this diet plan, take time now to review!

Level of Cognitive Ability: Application
Phase of Nursing Process: Implementation
Client Needs: Physiological Integrity
Content Area: Child Health

Reference
Ashwill, J., & Droske, S. (1997). *Nursing care of children: Principles and practice.* Philadelphia: W. B. Saunders. p. 891.

25. 1

Rationale: Pancreatic enzyme powders are not to be mixed with hot foods or foods containing tapioca or other starches. Enzyme powder should be mixed with nonfat, nonprotein foods such as apple sauce. Pancreatic enzymes are inactivated by heat and are partially degraded by gastric acids.

Test-Taking Strategy: Eliminate option 4 first because of the word "hot." Knowledge regarding the administration of pancreatic enzymes is helpful in making the correct selection. If you had difficulty with this question, be sure to review the procedures for administering pancreatic enzyme powder!

Level of Cognitive Ability: Application
Phase of Nursing Process: Planning
Client Needs: Physiological Integrity
Content Area: Child Health

Reference
Ashwill, J., & Droske, S. (1997). *Nursing care of children: Principles and practice.* Philadelphia: W. B. Saunders. p. 891.

26. **3**

Rationale: The "huff" maneuver (forced expiratory technique) is used to mobilize secretions. This technique reduces the likelihood of bronchial collapse. The child is taught to cough with an open glottis by taking a deep breath, then exhaling rapidly, whispering the word "huff."

Test-Taking Strategy: Eliminate options 2 and 4 first, recalling that shallow breathing is ineffective in promoting the mobilization of secretions. Select option 3 over option 1 based on the knowledge that exhaling rapidly will assist in reducing bronchial collapse and mobilize secretions. Holding the breath will not achieve this physiological function. Review this technique now if you had difficulty with this question!

Level of Cognitive Ability: Application
Phase of Nursing Process: Implementation
Client Needs: Health Promotion and Maintenance
Content Area: Child Health

Reference
Ashwill, J., & Droske, S. (1997). *Nursing care of children: Principles and practice.* Philadelphia: W. B. Saunders. p. 892.

27. **1**

Rationale: Respiratory treatments should be performed at least 1 hour before meals or 2 hours after meals to prevent vomiting. In some children with CF, treatments are prescribed every 2 hours, particularly if infection is present. It is also important to perform the treatment before bedtime to clear airways and facilitate rest.

Test-Taking Strategy: Visualize the procedure of postural drainage in answering the question. Knowledge that this position may induce vomiting will assist in eliminating options 2, 3, and 4. If you had difficulty with this question, take time now to review this procedure!

Level of Cognitive Ability: Analysis
Phase of Nursing Process: Implementation
Client Needs: Health Promotion and Maintenance
Content Area: Child Health

Reference
Ashwill, J., & Droske, S. (1997). *Nursing care of children: Principles and practice.* Philadelphia: W. B. Saunders. p. 892.

28. **2**

Rationale: Induration measuring 10 mm or greater is considered to be a positive result in children younger than 4 years of age and in those with chronic illness or high risk for environmental exposure to tuberculosis. A reaction of 5 mm or greater is considered to be a positive result for the highest risk groups.

Test-Taking Strategy: Knowledge regarding a positive Mantoux test in children is required to answer this question. Option 4 can be easily eliminated first. Note the child's age in the question to determine the correct option from the remaining three. If you had difficulty with this question, take time now to review the analysis of a Mantoux test in children!

Level of Cognitive Ability: Analysis
Phase of Nursing Process: Analysis
Client Needs: Physiological Integrity
Content Area: Child Health

Reference
Ashwill, J., & Droske, S. (1997). *Nursing care of children: Principles and practice.* Philadelphia: W. B. Saunders. p. 899.

29. **4**

Rationale: In the United States, the BCG vaccine is used mainly for children with a negative chest x-ray and skin test results, who have had repeated exposures to TB and for asymptomatic HIV-infected children who are at increased risk for developing TB. BCG is the only vaccine available for use in the prevention of TB.

Test-Taking Strategy: Knowledge that BCG is a preventative vaccine will assist in eliminating options 1 and 2. From the remaining options, eliminate option 3 because of the word "all" in this option. Review the indications for the use of this vaccine now if you had difficulty with this question!

Level of Cognitive Ability: Application
Phase of Nursing Process: Implementation
Client Needs: Health Promotion and Maintenance
Content Area: Child Health

Reference
Ashwill, J., & Droske, S. (1997). *Nursing care of children: Principles and practice.* Philadelphia: W. B. Saunders. p. 900.

30. **2**

Rationale: INH is given to prevent TB infection from progressing to active disease. A chest x-ray film is obtained before initiation of preventative therapy. In infants and children the recommended duration of INH therapy is 9 months. For children with HIV infection, a minimum of 12 months is recommended.

Test-Taking Strategy: Knowledge regarding treatment with INH in a 2-year-old child is required to answer this question. If you are unfamiliar with treatment plans for TB in children, take time now to review!

Level of Cognitive Ability: Application
Phase of Nursing Process: Implementation
Client Needs: Health Promotion and Maintenance
Content Area: Child Health

Reference
Ashwill, J., & Droske, S. (1997). *Nursing care of children: Principles and practice.* Philadelphia: W. B. Saunders. p. 899.

BIBLIOGRAPHY

Ashwill, J., & Droske, S. (1997). *Nursing care of children: Principles and practice.* Philadelphia: W. B. Saunders.

Hodgson, B., & Kizior, R. (1999). *Saunders nursing drug handbook 1999.* Philadelphia: W. B. Saunders.

Lammon, C., Foote, A., Leli, P., et al. (1995). *Clinical nursing skills.* Philadelphia: W. B. Saunders.

Luckmann, J. (1997). *Saunders manual of nursing care.* Philadelphia: W. B. Saunders.

Nichols, F., & Zwelling, E. (1997). *Maternal newborn nursing: Theory and practice.* Philadelphia: W. B. Saunders.

O'Toole, M. (ed.). (1997). *Miller-Keane encyclopedia & dictionary of medicine, nursing, & allied health* (6th ed.). Philadelphia: W. B. Saunders.

CHAPTER 36

Cardiovascular Disorders

I. Congestive Heart Failure

A. Description
1. Inability of the heart to pump sufficiently to meet the metabolic needs of the body
2. In infants and children, inadequate cardiac output is most commonly caused by congenital heart defects that produce an excessive volume or pressure load on the myocardium
3. In children a combination of both left-sided and right-sided heart failure is usually present

B. Assessment of Early Symptoms
1. Tachypnea during feeding
2. Poor feeding
3. Diaphoresis during feeding

C. Implementation
1. Elevate the head of the bed
2. Administer oxygen as prescribed during stressful periods such as bouts of crying or invasive procedures
3. Feed in a relaxed environment
4. Provide small frequent feedings, which will be less tiring
5. Monitor input and output (I&O) and daily weight to assess for fluid retention
6. Weigh diapers
7. A weight gain of more than 50 g/day may indicate fluid overload
8. Monitor for facial or peripheral edema, auscultate lung sounds, and report weight gain to the physician
9. Monitor electrolyte levels
10. Administer digoxin (Lanoxin) and furosemide (Lasix) as prescribed
11. Administer vasodilators or angiotensin-converting enzyme (ACE) inhibitors as prescribed
12. Prostaglandin E_1 (PGE_1) may be administered in the neonatal period for ductal-dependent congenital heart defects with cardiovascular collapse to maintain patency of the ductus arteriosus before surgery
13. Instruct the parents regarding description of diagnosis and administration of medications
14. Instruct the parents in cardiopulmonary resuscitation (CPR)

II. Intracardiac Shunt

A. Description: Occurs when the blood flow is forced by a higher pressure to go through an opening that is not normally present

B. Left-to-Right **Shunts**
1. Description
   a. Blood is shunted to the right side of the heart because the left side is normally functioning under a higher pressure than the right
   b. Oxygenated and unoxygenated blood mix, which results in increased pulmonary blood flow because the opening sends more blood to the right side of the heart than normal
2. Assessment
   a. May be asymptomatic
   b. May show signs and symptoms of congestive heart failure (CHF)
   c. May exhibit failure to thrive
   d. **Growth** retardation
   e. Diaphoresis
   f. Fatigue
   g. Tachypnea
   h. Poor eating
   i. Dyspnea
   j. Hypoxemia
3. Types (Table 36–1)
4. Implementation
   a. Assess respiratory status for the presence of **nasal flaring** and use of accessory muscles
   b. Auscultate the lungs for the presence of crackles and rhonchi

Table 36–1. Types of Left-to-Right Shunts

Type	Management Approach
Atrial-septal defect (ASD)	Surgical closure done at age 4 to 5 years
Ventricular septal defect (VSD)	May close spontaneously; if closure does not occur, surgical closure will be performed before school age; if pulmonary hypertension is present, closure is necessary by age 1
Patent ductus arteriosus (PDA)	May close spontaneously; congestive heart failure must be treated; can be closed by surgical or nonsurgical measures
Atrioventricular canal defect (AVCD)	Surgical closure of septal defects; possible mitral valve replacement for severe defects and reconstruction of atrioventricular (AV) valve tissue

    c. Assess for signs of CHF such as fluid retention in the eyes, hands, feet, and chest
    d. Assess for diuresis
    e. Assess urine output; weighing diapers is necessary
    f. Assess calorie intake
    g. Plan interventions to allow maximal rest for the child
    h. Allow the parent or child, if appropriate, to verbalize feelings and concerns regarding disorder
C. Right-to-Left **Shunts**
  1. Description
    a. Occur when blood is shunted to the left side of the heart because one of the right heart chambers has a higher pressure
    b. Oxygenated blood mixes with unoxygenated blood; cyanosis occurs
    c. May be treated with prostaglandin E_1, which temporarily maintains patency of ductus arteriosus until surgery is performed.
  2. Assessment
    a. Symptoms occur in the first week of life
    b. Dyspnea after feeding, crying, or other activities
    c. Hypercyanotic or "tet spells" characterized by increased respiratory rate and depth and increased hypoxemia with tetralogy of Fallot
    d. Squatting episodes with tetralogy of Fallot
    e. Signs of CHF
    f. Respiratory distress
    g. Clubbing of the digits
    h. Poor **growth**
    i. Tachycardia
  3. Types (Table 36–2)
  4. Implementation
    a. Monitor vital signs
    b. Monitor respiratory status, notifying the physician if any changes occur

    c. Auscultate breath sounds for crackles or rales
    d. Keep the child as stress-free as possible
    e. If respiratory effort is increased, place the child in a reverse Trendelenburg (elevate the head and upper body) to decrease the work of breathing
    f. Monitor for hypercyanosis and place the child in knee-chest position and notify the physician if it occurs
    g. Administer humidified oxygen as prescribed
    h. Provide an endotracheal tube and ventilator care as prescribed and restrain the hands of an intubated child
    i. Monitor for signs of CHF
    j. Monitor body weight
    k. Monitor I&O and notify the physician if a decrease in urine output occurs
    l. Palpate the liver, noting enlargement, which is an indication of right-sided heart failure
    m. Administer diuretics as prescribed
    n. Administer propranolol (Inderal) for hypercyanotic episodes as prescribed and monitor glucose levels, notifying the physician if glucose level is less than 60 mg/dL

III. Stenotic Lesions

A. Description: Narrowing or constriction of an opening in a valve or vessel that results in obstruction of blood flow through the area
B. Assessment
  1. Murmurs
  2. Signs of CHF
  3. Tachycardia
  4. Tachypnea
  5. Dyspnea
  6. Pallor
  7. Decreased peripheral pulses
  8. Cardiomegaly
C. Types (Table 36–3)
D. Implementation
  1. Monitor vital signs
  2. Measure blood pressure in all four extremities

Table 36–2. Types of Right-to-Left Shunts

Type	Management Approach
Tetralogy of Fallot	Medical management and corrective surgery by age 1
Transposition of the great arteries	Surgical correction performed in the first few weeks of life
Truncus arteriosus	Medical and surgical management
Pulmonary atresia	Medical and surgical management
Tricuspid atresia	Palliative and corrective surgery
Hypoplastic left heart syndrome	Surgical correction or cardiac transplantation

Table 36–3. **Types of Stenotic Lesions**

Type	Management Approach
Aortic stenosis	Balloon angioplasty and/or commissurotomy to open the valve; valve replacement may be required at a later time
Coarctation of the aorta	Aggressive congestive heart failure management; surgical repair by 2 years of age if possible
Pulmonary stenosis	Balloon angioplasty and/or surgical valvotomy

3. Assess peripheral pulses
4. Administer oxygen as prescribed
5. Monitor for signs of CHF
6. Monitor I&O
7. Maintain fluid restriction
8. Obtain daily weight
9. Administer cardiac medications and diuretics as prescribed

IV. Cardiac Surgery

A. Implementation Postoperatively
1. Monitor vital signs frequently
2. Monitor temperature and notify the physician if a fever occurs
3. Maintain aseptic technique
4. Monitor for signs of sepsis such as fever, chills, diaphoresis, lethargy, and altered levels of consciousness
5. Monitor lines, tubes, or catheters that are in place and remove promptly as prescribed when no longer needed, to prevent infection
6. Assess for signs of discomfort such as irritability, changes in heart rate, respiratory rate and blood pressure, and inability to sleep
7. Administer pain medications as prescribed, noting effectiveness
8. Administer antibiotics and antipyretics as prescribed
9. Encourage rest periods
10. Facilitate parent-child contact as soon as possible

B. Postoperative Home Care (Box 36–1)

V. Rheumatic Fever

A. Description
1. An inflammatory autoimmune disease that affects the connective tissues of the heart, joints, subcutaneous tissues, and/or blood vessels of the central nervous system (CNS)
2. The most serious complication is rheumatic heart disease, which affects the cardiac valves
3. Presents 2 to 6 weeks following an untreated or partially treated group A beta hemolytic streptococcal infection of the upper respiratory tract
4. Jones criteria are utilized in determining diagnosis

B. Assessment
1. Edema, inflammation of large joints
2. Joint pain
3. Fever
4. Erythematous macular rash on trunk and extremities
5. Chorea
6. Subcutaneous nodules in the joints, scalp, and spine
7. Arthritis
8. Aschoff bodies causing endocarditis
9. Fibrosis of mitral and aortic valves
10. Elevated antistreptolysin O titer
11. Elevated sedimentation rate
12. Elevated C-reactive protein

C. Implementation
1. Assess vital signs
2. Assess skin lesions
3. Control joint pain and inflammation with massage and alternating hot and cold applications as prescribed
4. Provide bed rest during an acute febrile phase
5. Eradicate infection
6. Administer penicillin as prescribed
7. Administer anti-inflammatory agents as prescribed, and if aspirin is prescribed it should not be given to a child who has chickenpox or other viral infections

---

BOX 36–1. Home Care Postoperative Cardiac Surgery

- Omit play outside for several weeks
- Avoid activities where the child could fall, such as bike riding, for 2 to 4 weeks
- Avoid crowds for 1 week after discharge
- Follow a no-added-salt diet if prescribed
- Do not add any new foods to the infant's eating schedule
- Do not place creams, lotions, or powders on the incision until completely healed
- The child may return to school the third week after discharge starting with half days
- No physical education for 2 months
- Instruct the parents to discipline the child normally
- Instruct the parents about the importance of the 2-week follow-up
- Avoid immunizations, invasive procedures, and dental visits for 2 months
- Advise the parents regarding the importance of a dental visit every 6 months after age 3 and to inform the dentist of the cardiac problem so that antibiotics can be prescribed if necessary
- Inform the parents to call the physician when coughing, tachypnea, cyanosis, vomiting, diarrhea, anorexia, pain, fever, or any swelling, redness, or drainage occurs at the site of the incision

8. Monitor for signs of carditis including shortness of breath, edema of the face, abdomen or ankles, and precordial pain

9. Limit physical exercise in a child with carditis

10. Initiate seizure precautions if the child is experiencing chorea

11. Advise the child to inform parents if anyone in school develops a strep throat

PRACTICE QUESTIONS

1. The nurse caring for an infant with congestive heart failure (CHF) is monitoring the infant closely for early signs of exacerbation. Which of the following alerts the nurse of the development of CHF?
   1 Bradycardia during feeding
   2 Diaphoresis during feeding
   3 Slow and shallow breathing
   4 Pallor

2. The physician has prescribed oxygen PRN for the child with CHF. In which of the following situations does the nurse administer the oxygen to the child?
   1 During feeding
   2 When the mother is holding the child
   3 When changing the child's diapers
   4 When drawing blood for electrolyte values

3. The infant with CHF is receiving diuretic therapy. Which of the following is the most appropriate method to assess urine output?
   1 Insert a Foley catheter
   2 Weigh the diapers
   3 Compare intake with output
   4 Measure the amount of water added to the formula

4. The nurse is monitoring the daily weight on an infant with CHF. Which of the following alerts the nurse to suspect fluid overload and the need to call the physician?
   1 A daily weight gain of more than 20 g in a 24-hour period
   2 A daily weight gain of more than 30 g in a 24-hour period
   3 A daily weight gain of more than 40 g in a 24-hour period
   4 A daily weight gain of more than 50 g in a 24-hour period

5. The nurse provides home care instructions to the parents of a child with CHF regarding the procedure for administration of digoxin (Lanoxin). Which of the following is not a component of the plan?
   1 If the child vomits after medication administration, repeat the dose
   2 Take the child's pulse before administering the medication

3 Do not mix the medication with food
4 If more than one dose is missed, call the physician

6. The nurse reviews the chart of an infant admitted to the intensive care unit. The diagnosis is documented as a left-to-right cardiac shunt. Which of the following physiological alterations occurs in this condition?
   1 Blood is shunted to the left side of the heart
   2 The right side of the heart functions under greater pressure than the left side
   3 Oxygenated and unoxygenated blood mix
   4 Oxygenated and unoxygenated blood do not mix

7. The nurse is caring for a child with a diagnosis of a right-to-left shunt. The most common assessment finding in this disorder is which of the following?
   1 Cyanosis
   2 Diaphoresis
   3 Growth retardation
   4 These children are asymptomatic

8. A child with transposition of the great arteries and patent ductus arteriosus (PDA) receives prostaglandin E_1 (PGE_1). The mother of the child is a registered nurse and asks the nurse why the child needs the medication. The most appropriate response is:
   1 "To maintain an adequate hormonal level."
   2 "To maintain the position of the great arteries."
   3 "To maintain patency of the ductus arteriosus."
   4. "To prevent cyanosis."

9. The child with a right-to-left shunt is maintained on an NPO status. Propranolol (Inderal) is being administered to the child. Which of the following laboratory values is most important to monitor in this child?
   1 BUN
   2 Creatinine
   3 Glucose
   4 Electrolytes

10. The nurse is caring for an infant with tetralogy of Fallot. The nurse recognizes that the infant is experiencing a hypercyanotic episode. The initial nursing action is to:
    1 Call the physician
    2 Place the infant in a knee-chest position
    3 Elevate the head of the bed
    4 Administer carbon dioxide whiffs

11. The clinic nurse reviews the record of a child just seen by the physician. The physician has documented a diagnosis of a suspected stenotic lesion. Which of the following symptoms docu-

mented in the record is most commonly found in this disorder?

1 Subclavian bruit
2 Cardiac murmur
3 Pallor
4 Gastric regurgitation

12. The nurse provides home care instructions to the mother of a child who is being discharged following heart surgery. The nurse describes the activity guidelines to the mother. Which of the following is not included in the instructions?

1 Avoid large crowds of people for at least 1 month following surgery
2 Resume regular nap and sleep schedules
3 Omit play outside, allowing inside play as tolerated
4 Avoid activities where the child could fall for 2 to 4 weeks

13. The nurse receives a telephone call from the admitting office and is told that a child with rheumatic fever (RF) will be arriving at the nursing unit for admission. The initial nursing assessment during admission includes which of the following?

1 History of sore throat or unexplained fever within the past 2 months
2 History of unexplained nausea or vomiting
3 History of unexplained headaches
4 History of back pain

14. Acetylsalicylic acid (aspirin) is prescribed for the child with RF. The nurse questions this order if the child has which of the following?

1 A viral infection
2 Joint pain
3 Facial edema
4 Arthralgia

15. Which of the following laboratory studies assists in confirming the diagnosis of RF?

1 White blood cell (WBC) count
2 Red blood cell (RBC) count
3 Immunoglobulin
4 Antistreptolysin O titer

ANSWERS

1. **2**

Rationale: The early symptoms of CHF include tachypnea, poor feeding, and diaphoresis during feeding. Tachycardia rather than bradycardia occurs during feeding. Pallor may be noted in the infant with CHF, but it is not an early symptom.

Test-Taking Strategy: Think about the physiology and the effects on the heart when fluid overload occurs. These concepts will assist in directing you to option 2. If you had difficulty with this question, take time now to review the early signs of CHF in an infant!

Level of Cognitive Ability: Analysis
Phase of Nursing Process: Assessment
Client Needs: Physiological Integrity
Content Area: Child Health

Reference
Ashwill, J., & Droske, S. (1997). *Nursing care of children: Principles and practice.* Philadelphia: W. B. Saunders. p. 949.

2. **4**

Rationale: Oxygen administration may be ordered for stressful periods especially during bouts of crying or invasive procedures.

Test-Taking Strategy: Recall the situations that would place stress and an increased workload on the heart. This concept should easily direct you to option 4. Drawing blood is an invasive procedure that would likely cause the child to cry.

Level of Cognitive Ability: Analysis
Phase of Nursing Process: Implementation
Client Needs: Physiological Integrity
Content Area: Child Health

Reference
Ashwill, J., & Droske, S. (1997). *Nursing care of children: Principles and practice.* Philadelphia: W. B. Saunders. p. 950.

3. **2**

Rationale: The most appropriate method to assess urine output in an infant on diuretic therapy is to weigh the diapers. Comparing intake with output does not provide an accurate measure of urine output. Measuring the amount of water added to formula is unrelated to the amount of output. Although Foley catheter drainage is most accurate in determining output, it is not the most appropriate method in an infant.

Test-Taking Strategy: Eliminate options 3 and 4 first because they will not provide an indication of urine output. From the remaining two options, note the phrase "most appropriate" in the stem of the question. This phrase should direct you to option 2.

Level of Cognitive Ability: Analysis
Phase of Nursing Process: Assessment
Client Needs: Physiological Integrity
Content Area: Child Health

Reference
Ashwill, J., & Droske, S. (1997). *Nursing care of children: Principles and practice.* Philadelphia: W. B. Saunders. p. 950.

4. **4**

Rationale: A weight gain of more than 50 g/day may indicate fluid overload. The nurse should assess urine output, evaluate for evidence of facial or peripheral edema, auscultate lung sounds, and report the weight gain to the physician.

Test-Taking Strategy: Knowledge regarding fluid overload and the abnormal parameters requiring physician notification in an infant with CHF is required to answer this question. Take time now to review these parameters if you had difficulty with this question!

Level of Cognitive Ability: Analysis
Phase of Nursing Process: Analysis
Client Needs: Physiological Integrity
Content Area: Child Health

Reference
Ashwill, J., & Droske, S. (1997). *Nursing care of children: Principles and practice*. Philadelphia: W. B. Saunders. p. 950.

5. 1

Rationale: The parents need to be instructed that if the child vomits after the digoxin is administered, they are not to repeat the dose. Options 2, 3, and 4 are accurate instructions regarding the administration of this medication. Additionally, the parents should be instructed that if a dose is missed and it is not identified until 4 or more hours later, the dose should not be administered.

Test-Taking Strategy: Note the key word "not" in the stem of the question. General knowledge regarding digoxin administration will assist in eliminating option 2. Principles related to administering medications to children will assist in eliminating option 3. From the remaining options, select option 1 over option 4 because if the child vomits it would be difficult to determine if the medication was also vomited or absorbed by the body.

Level of Cognitive Ability: Application
Phase of Nursing Process: Implementation
Client Needs: Health Promotion and Maintenance
Content Area: Child Health

Reference
Ashwill, J., & Droske, S. (1997). *Nursing care of children: Principles and practice*. Philadelphia: W. B. Saunders. p. 955.

6. 3

Rationale: In a left-to-right cardiac shunt, blood is shunted to the right side of the heart because the left side is normally functioning under higher pressure than the right side. This shunting allows oxygenated and unoxygenated blood to mix. This results in increased pulmonary blood flow because the abnormal communication or opening sends more blood to the right side of the heart (through the opening) than normal.

Test-Taking Strategy: The key phrase is "left-to-right." Bear this phrase in mind in eliminating options 1 and 2. Recalling that unoxygenated blood returns to the right side of the heart from the body, it would make sense that oxygenated and unoxygenated blood would mix in this disorder. This concept will assist in directing you to option 3.

Level of Cognitive Ability: Analysis
Phase of Nursing Process: Analysis
Client Needs: Physiological Integrity
Content Area: Child Health

Reference
Ashwill, J., & Droske, S. (1997). *Nursing care of children: Principles and practice*. Philadelphia: W. B. Saunders. p. 842.

7. 1

Rationale: The child with a right-to-left shunt will be considerably sicker than a child with a left-to-right shunt. Many of these children will present with symptoms in the first week of life. The most common assessment finding in these children is cyanosis. The child may also become dyspneic after feeding, crying, and other exertional activities. Many children with a left-to-right shunt may remain asymptomatic.

Test-Taking Strategy: Knowledge regarding the physiology associated with a right-to-left shunt will easily direct you to option 1. If you had difficulty with this question, take time now to review the manifestations associated with this disorder!

Level of Cognitive Ability: Analysis
Phase of Nursing Process: Assessment
Client Needs: Physiological Integrity
Content Area: Child Health

Reference
Ashwill, J., & Droske, S. (1997). *Nursing care of children: Principles and practice*. Philadelphia: W. B. Saunders. p. 923.

8. 3

Rationale: A child with transposition of the great arteries and PDA may receive prostaglandin E_1 before surgery to maintain patency of the ductus arteriosus.

Test-Taking Strategy: Use knowledge regarding the purpose of this medication to answer the question. Understanding the physiology associated with the disorder will direct you to option 3. Review the purpose of this medication in this condition now if you had difficulty with this question!

Level of Cognitive Ability: Analysis
Phase of Nursing Process: Implementation
Client Needs: Physiological Integrity
Content Area: Child Health

Reference
Ashwill, J., & Droske, S. (1997). *Nursing care of children: Principles and practice*. Philadelphia: W. B. Saunders. p. 926.

9. 3

Rationale: Propranolol, a beta blocker, is used in the palliative treatment of hypercyanotic episodes. It can cause hypoglycemia if administered in a child that is NPO or hypovolemic. The nurse should monitor glucose levels every 4 to 6 hours if the child is NPO or hypovolemic and receiving propranolol. The physician should be notified if the glucose level is less than 60 mg/dL.

Test-Taking Strategy: Eliminate options 1 and 2 because they are similar and both relate to renal function studies. From the remaining two options, you may be tempted to select option 4, but familiarity with the medication will direct you to the correct option. Review this important medication now if you had difficulty answering!

Level of Cognitive Ability: Analysis
Phase of Nursing Process: Assessment
Client Needs: Physiological Integrity
Content Area: Child Health

Reference
Ashwill, J., & Droske, S. (1997). *Nursing care of children: Principles and practice*. Philadelphia: W. B. Saunders. p. 928.

10. 2

Rationale: If a hypercyanotic episode occurs, place the child in a knee-chest position and then notify the physician. This position is thought to increase pulmonary blood flow by increasing systemic vascular resistance. This position also improves systemic arterial oxygen saturation by decreasing venous return, so that smaller amounts of highly saturated blood reach the heart. Toddlers and children squat to obtain this position and relieve chronic hypoxia.

Test-Taking Strategy: Note the key word "initial" in the stem of the question. Eliminate option 4 first. Next, eliminate option 1 because a nursing intervention is required before notifying the physician. Remembering that a toddler or child squats to achieve this position will assist in directing you to option 2.

Level of Cognitive Ability: Application
Phase of Nursing Process: Implementation
Client Needs: Physiological Integrity
Content Area: Child Health

Reference
Ashwill, J., & Droske, S. (1997). *Nursing care of children: Principles and practice*. Philadelphia: W. B. Saunders. p. 928.

11. **2**

Rationale: The child with a stenotic lesion will have varying symptoms, depending on the type and degree of the stenotic lesion. Most of them will have murmurs when first seen in the health care setting. Pallor may be noted, but is not specific to this type of disorder alone. Options 1 and 4 are not related to this disorder.

Test-Taking Strategy: Note the similarity of "stenotic lesion" in the question and "cardiac murmur" in the option. This may assist in directing you to the correct option. Review the manifestations associated with stenotic lesions now if you had difficulty with this question!

Level of Cognitive Ability: Analysis
Phase of Nursing Process: Assessment
Client Needs: Physiological Integrity
Content Area: Child Health

Reference
Ashwill, J., & Droske, S. (1997). *Nursing care of children: Principles and practice*. Philadelphia: W. B. Saunders. p. 930.

12. **1**

Rationale: The mother should be instructed that the child needs to avoid large crowds of people for 1 week following discharge. This includes day care centers and church. Options 2, 3, and 4 are accurate instructions regarding activity following heart surgery.

Test-Taking Strategy: Note the key word "not" in the stem of the question. Options 2 and 3 can easily be eliminated first. From the remaining two options, note the time frame in option 1. This seems rather lengthy. Therefore, select option 1 as the answer to the question as it is stated. Review child activity guidelines following heart surgery now if you had difficulty with this question!

Level of Cognitive Ability: Application
Phase of Nursing Process: Implementation
Client Needs: Health Promotion and Maintenance
Content Area: Child Health

Reference
Ashwill, J., & Droske, S. (1997). *Nursing care of children: Principles and practice*. Philadelphia: W. B. Saunders. p. 922.

13. **1**

Rationale: RF characteristically presents 2 to 6 weeks following an untreated or partially treated group A beta-hemolytic streptococcal infection of the upper respiratory tract. Initially the nurse determines whether any family members have had a sore throat or unexplained fever within the past 2 months.

Test-Taking Strategy: Options 2, 3, and 4 are unrelated to RF. Note the similarity between rheumatic "fever" in the question and the word "fever" in the correct option. If you had difficulty with this question, take time now to review the etiology related to RF!

Level of Cognitive Ability: Analysis
Phase of Nursing Process: Assessment
Client Needs: Physiological Integrity
Content Area: Child Health

Reference
Ashwill, J., & Droske, S. (1997). *Nursing care of children: Principles and practice*. Philadelphia: W. B. Saunders. pp. 657, 659.

14. **1**

Rationale: Prescribed anti-inflammatory agents including aspirin may be given to the child with RF. Aspirin should not be given to a child who has chickenpox or other viral infections. Options 2 and 4 are clinical manifestations of RF. Facial edema may be associated with the development of a cardiac complication.

Test-Taking Strategy: Options 2 and 4 can be eliminated because they are similar. Knowledge that facial edema may indicate a cardiac complication will assist in eliminating this option. Review the contraindications related to the use of aspirin if you had difficulty with this question!

Level of Cognitive Ability: Analysis
Phase of Nursing Process: Assessment
Client Needs: Physiological Integrity
Content Area: Child Health

Reference
Ashwill, J., & Droske, S. (1997). *Nursing care of children: Principles and practice*. Philadelphia: W. B. Saunders. p. 658.

15. **4**

Rationale: A diagnosis of RF is confirmed by the presence of two major manifestations or one major and two minor manifestations from the Jones criteria. Additionally, evidence of a recent streptococcal infection is confirmed by a positive antistreptolysin O titer, streptozyme, or an anti-DNAase B assay.

Test-Taking Strategy: Knowledge that RF is characteristically associated with streptococcal infection will easily direct you to option 4. If you had difficulty with this question, take time now to review the Jones criteria!

Level of Cognitive Ability: Analysis
Phase of Nursing Process: Assessment
Client Needs: Physiological Integrity
Content Area: Child Health

Reference
Ashwill, J., & Droske, S. (1997). *Nursing care of children: Principles and practice*. Philadelphia: W. B. Saunders. p. 658.

BIBLIOGRAPHY

Ashwill, J., & Droske, S. (1997). *Nursing care of children: Principles and practice*. Philadelphia: W. B. Saunders.
Hodgson, B., & Kizior, R. (1999). *Saunders nursing drug handbook 1999*. Philadelphia: W. B. Saunders.
Lammon, C., Foote, A., Leli, P., et al. (1995). *Clinical nursing skills*. Philadelphia: W. B. Saunders.
Luckmann, J. (1997). *Saunders manual of nursing care*. Philadelphia: W. B. Saunders.
Nichols, F., & Zwelling, E. (1997). *Maternal newborn nursing: Theory and practice*. Philadelphia: W. B. Saunders.
O'Toole, M. (ed.). (1997). *Miller-Keane encyclopedia & dictionary of medicine, nursing, & allied health* (6th ed.). Philadelphia: W. B. Saunders.

CHAPTER 37

Gastrointestinal Disorders

. . . .

I. Vomiting

A. Description
   1. The major concerns when a child is vomiting are the risk of dehydration, the loss of fluid, and electrolytes, and the development of metabolic alkalosis
   2. Additional concerns include aspiration, atelectasis, and the development of pneumonia
B. Assessment
   1. Signs of aspiration
   2. Character of vomitus
   3. Abdominal cramping
   4. Pain
   5. Dehydration
   6. Fluid and electrolyte imbalances
   7. Metabolic alkalosis
   8. Diarrhea
   9. Headache
C. Implementation
   1. Monitor vital signs
   2. Monitor the character, amount, and frequency of vomiting
   3. Assess the force of the vomiting, as projectile vomiting is indicative of pyloric **stenosis** or increased intracranial pressure
   4. Maintain a patent airway
   5. Position the child on the side to prevent aspiration
   6. Monitor input and output (I&O)
   7. Assess for signs of dehydration
   8. Monitor electrolyte levels
   9. Maintain NPO status and then provide adequate fluid intake as tolerated and as prescribed
   10. Start feeding slowly with small amounts of fluid at frequent intervals
   11. Assess for diarrhea or abdominal pain
   12. Advise the parents to inform the physician when signs of dehydration, blood in vomitus, forceful vomiting, or abdominal pain is present

II. Diarrhea

A. Description: The major concerns when a child is having diarrhea are the risk of dehydration, the loss of fluid and electrolytes, and the development of metabolic acidosis
B. Assessment
   1. Diarrhea
   2. Abdominal cramping
   3. Pain
   4. Dehydration
   5. Fluid and electrolyte imbalances
   6. Metabolic acidosis
C. Implementation
   1. Monitor vital signs
   2. Monitor the character, amount, and frequency of diarrhea
   3. Monitor skin integrity
   4. Monitor I&O
   5. Assess for dehydration
   6. Monitor electrolyte levels
   7. Maintain NPO status to place the bowel at rest and then provide adequate fluid intake as tolerated and as prescribed
   8. Slowly refeed the child with fluids, and as diarrhea resolves begin easily digestible foods
   9. Provide fluid and electrolyte replacement as prescribed
   10. If potassium is prescribed by IV, ensure that the child has voided before administering
   11. Provide isolation as required
   12. Instruct the parents in good handwashing technique

III. Cleft Lip and Cleft Palate

A. Description
   1. A congenital anomaly that occurs as a result

of failure of soft tissue or bony structure to fuse during embryonic development

2. Involves abnormal openings in the lip or palate that may occur unilaterally or bilaterally and are readily apparent at birth

3. Causes include genetic, **hereditary**, and environmental factors; exposure to radiation or rubella virus; chromosome abnormalities; and teratogenic factors

4. Surgical correction requires several stages

5. Cleft lip repair is usually performed by age 4 weeks

6. In some cases, cleft lip repair is performed in the first 2 to 3 days of life, with cosmetic modifications performed at ages 4 to 5 years

7. Cleft palate repair is performed between the ages of 6 months to 2 years as early closure facilitates speech development

B. Assessment

1. Cleft lip can range from a slight notch to a complete separation from the floor of the nose

2. Cleft palate can include nasal distortion, midline or bilateral cleft, with variable

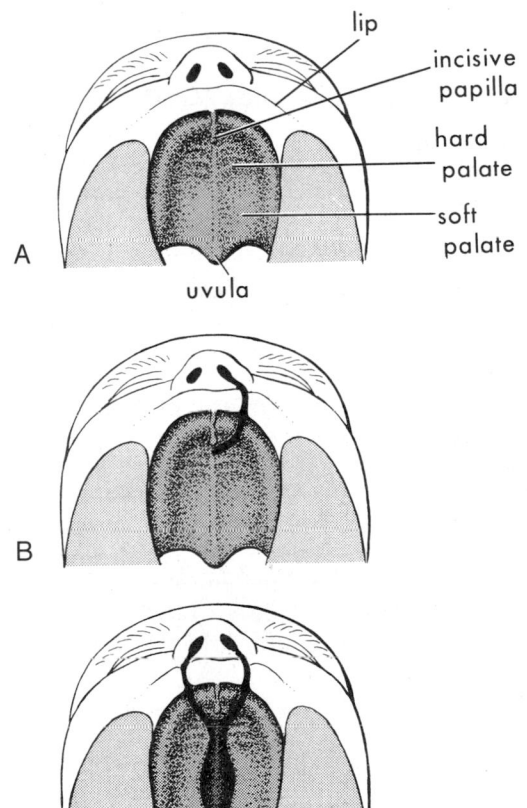

FIGURE 37–1. Drawings of various types of cleft lip and cleft palate. *A,* Normal lip and palate. *B,* Complete unilateral cleft of the lip and alveolar process of the maxilla with a unilateral cleft of the anterior or primary palate. *C,* Complete bilateral cleft of the lip and alveolar processes of the maxillae with complete bilateral cleft of the anterior and posterior plate. (From Betz, C. L., Hunsberger, M. M., & Wright, S. [1994]. *Family-centered nursing care of children.* Philadelphia: W. B. Saunders.)

BOX 37–1. ESSR Method of Feeding

ENLARGE the nipple so that the food is delivered to the back of the throat without sucking
STIMULATE sucking by rubbing the nipple on the lower lip
SWALLOW
REST to allow the child to finish swallowing what has been placed in the mouth

---

extension from the uvula and soft and hard palate (Fig. 37–1)

C. Implementation

1. Assess the ability to suck, swallow, and breathe without distress

2. Assess the ability to handle normal secretions

3. Encourage the parents to describe their feelings related to deformity

4. Modify feeding techniques to allow adequate **growth**

5. Teach the parents special feeding or suctioning techniques

6. Plan to use specialized feeding techniques, obturators, and special nipples and feeders for the child unable to adequately suck on a standard nipple

7. Hold the child in an upright position and direct the formula to the side and back of the mouth to prevent aspiration

8. Feed small amounts gradually

9. Burp frequently

10. Encourage breast-feeding if appropriate

11. Reassure the parents that surgery usually is successful

12. Teach the parents the ESSR (enlarge, stimulate, swallow, rest) method of feeding (Box 37–1)

D. Implementation Postoperatively

1. Position infant on the side lateral to repair or on the back

2. Avoid the prone position to prevent rubbing of the surgical site on mattress

3. Restrain with soft elbow or jacket restraints to keep the child from touching the repair site

4. Remove the restraints every 2 hours for skin care and range of motion exercises

5. Monitor the surgical site for redness, swelling, excessive bleeding, drainage, and monitor for fever

6. Provide analgesics for pain

7. Avoid contact with sharp objects near the surgical site

8. Keep pacifiers, straws, spoons, forks, or fingers away from the mouth for 7 to 10 days

9. Avoid oral suction or placing objects in the mouth such as a tongue depressor or thermometer

10. Advance the diet as prescribed from clear liquids to normal soft diet within 48 hours
11. For cleft palate repair provide short nipples that don't rest on palatal sutures and give baby food or baby food mixed with water
12. Prevent sucking
13. If a palate repair was required, avoid inserting the spoon into the mouth, which may disrupt sutures
14. After feeding place the infant on his or her side lateral to repair with the head elevated
15. Cleanse the lip suture line with sterile water after feeding and rinse the mouth with water after feedings to clean palate repair
16. Apply antibacterial ointment to the surgical site as prescribed using a cotton-tipped applicator
17. Do not brush the child's teeth for 1 to 2 weeks
18. Encourage the parents to hold the child
19. Initiate appropriate referrals for speech impairment or language-based **learning** difficulties

IV. Esophageal Atresia and Tracheoesophageal Fistula

A. Description
   1. The esophagus terminates before it reaches the stomach and/or a fistula is present that forms an unnatural connection with the trachea
   2. The condition causes oral intake to enter the lungs or a large amount of air to enter the stomach, and choking, coughing, and severe abdominal distention can occur
   3. Aspiration pneumonia and severe respiratory distress will develop, and death will occur without surgical intervention
   4. Surgical repair includes ligation of the fistula with anastomosis of the **atresia** to decrease the severity of stricture formation
B. Assessment
   1. Cough and choking with feedings
   2. Difficulty swallowing
   3. Excessive oral secretions
   4. **Regurgitation** and vomiting
   5. **Nasal flaring** and **retractions**
   6. Cyanosis
   7. Abdominal distention
   8. Failure to pass a suction catheter or nasogastric (NG) tube
C. Implementation Preoperatively
   1. Place in a supine or prone position with the head of the bed elevated
   2. Keep the child warm and administer humidified oxygen to relieve respiratory distress
   3. Maintain nothing by mouth (NPO) status
   4. Assist with placement of NG tube and aspirate every 5 to 10 minutes to keep the proximal pouch clear of secretions
   5. Maintain IV fluids as prescribed

D. Implementation Postoperatively
   1. Monitor respiratory status
   2. Maintain IV fluids, antibiotics, and parenteral nutrition as prescribed
   3. Monitor I&O
   4. Monitor weight daily
   5. Assess for dehydration and possible fluid overload
   6. Provide care to the chest tube if in place
   7. Assess for signs of pain
   8. Assess esophagostomy site for redness, breakdown, or exudate
   9. If cervical esophagostomy was performed, keep the area covered with gauze to absorb saliva and provide skin care with half-strength hydrogen peroxide as prescribed
   10. Provide gastrostomy tube feedings when prescribed
   11. Maintain elevation of the gastrostomy tube, which allows gastric contents to pass to the small intestine and air to escape, thus decreasing the risk of leakage at the anastomosis
   12. Do not offer a pacifier to the child until he or she can tolerate oral secretions
   13. Instruct the parents in the techniques of gastrostomy tube feedings and skin site care

V. Gastroesophageal Reflux (GER)

A. Description
   1. Backflow of gastric contents into the esophagus, as a result of relaxation or incompetence of the lower esophageal or cardiac sphincter
   2. Complications include esophagitis, esophageal strictures, aspiration of gastric contents, and aspiration pneumonia
   3. Treatment includes diet, positioning, medications, and surgery; however, surgery is considered as the last resort in treatment
B. Assessment
   1. Forceful chronic vomiting
   2. Apnea with cyanosis
   3. Aspiration
   4. Hematemesis and melena
   5. Weight loss and failure to thrive
   6. Recurrent respiratory infections
   7. Abdominal pain
   8. Bitter taste as described in older children
C. Implementation
   1. Assess amount and characteristics of emesis
   2. Assess the relation of vomiting to the time of feedings and infant activity
   3. Burp the infant frequently when feeding
   4. Handle the child minimally after feedings
   5. Monitor breath sounds before and after feedings
   6. Suction equipment at bedside
   7. Monitor I&O
   8. Monitor for signs and symptoms of dehydration

9. Maintain IV fluids as prescribed
10. Cardiac and apnea monitor as prescribed

D. Positioning
   1. Place the infant in an upright angle 24 hours a day
   2. Position at a 60-degree upright angle when supine and a 30-degree upright angle when prone until asymptomatic

E. Diet
   1. Provide small, frequent feedings
   2. For infants, thicken formula by adding 1 to 3 teaspoons of rice cereal per ounce of formula and cross-cut the nipple
   3. For toddlers, feed solids first, followed by liquids

F. Medications
   1. Schedule medications around meal times
   2. Administer antacids as prescribed for symptom relief
   3. Administer H_2receptor antagonists to decrease acid secretions
   4. Administer prokinetic agents to accelerate gastric emptying

G. Surgery
   1. If surgery is prescribed, it will require a procedure known as fundoplication, in which a wrap to the stomach fundus is made around the distal esophagus
   2. Instruct the parents that the child's ability to burp or vomit will eventually return
   3. Instruct the parents about the possibility of dumping syndrome, which begins 30 minutes after a feeding and may include diaphoresis, palpitations, weakness, syncope, abdominal fullness, nausea, or diarrhea

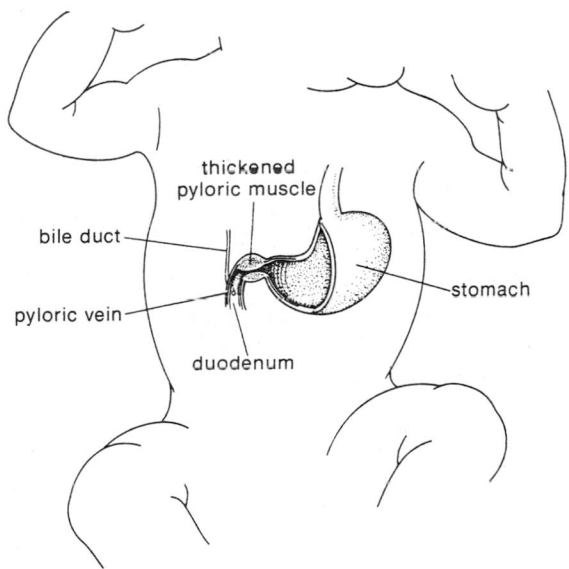

FIGURE 37–2. Pyloric stenosis. (From Betz, C. L., Hunsberger, M. M., & Wright, S. [1994]. *Family-centered nursing care of children.* Philadelphia: W. B. Saunders.)

VI. Pyloric Stenosis (Fig. 37–2)

A. Description: Hypertrophy of the circular muscles of the pylorus causes narrowing of the pyloric canal between the stomach and the duodenum

B. Assessment
   1. Vomiting that progresses from mild **regurgitation** to projectile and usually occurs after a feeding
   2. Vomitus contains gastric contents; may contain mucus, may be blood-tinged, and does not usually contain bile
   3. Constant hunger
   4. Fussiness and frequent crying
   5. Decrease in size and number of stools
   6. Failure to gain weight
   7. Upper abdominal distention
   8. Peristaltic waves visible from left to right across epigastrium during or immediately following a feeding
   9. Dehydration and malnutrition
   10. Electrolyte imbalances
   11. Metabolic alkalosis

C. Implementation
   1. Monitor vital signs
   2. Monitor I&O
   3. Monitor weight
   4. Monitor for signs of dehydration
   5. Monitor for signs of electrolyte imbalances
   6. Monitor stools
   7. Administer antacids as prescribed to neutralize the acidity of refluxed contents and to prevent esophageal tissue damage
   8. Administer medications as prescribed to promote gastric emptying or pyloric sphincter relaxation
   9. Prepare the child and parents for pyloromyotomy if prescribed

D. Pyloromyotomy
   1. Description: an incision through the muscle fibers of the pylorus
   2. Implementation preoperatively
      a. Assess frequency and amount of vomiting after feeding
      b. Prevent aspiration
      c. Monitor hydration status by daily weights, I&O, and urine for specific gravity
      d. Correct fluid and electrolyte imbalances
      e. Administer IV fluids as prescribed
      f. Assist and maintain the gastric tubes if inserted
   3. Implementation postoperatively
      a. Maintain a patent airway
      b. Monitor vital signs
      c. Monitor for signs of shock
      d. Begin clear liquids 4 to 6 hours postoperatively as prescribed
      e. Advance the diet to dilute then full-strength formula as prescribed

f. Feed infant slowly, burping frequently
g. Position in high-Fowler's on the right side after feedings
h. Handle the infant minimally after feedings
i. Monitor for abdominal distention
j. Monitor the surgical wound and for signs of infection
k. Instruct the parents about wound care, feeding, and positioning

VII. Lactose Intolerance

A. Description: Inability to tolerate lactose as a result of an absence or deficiency of lactase, an enzyme found in the secretions of the small intestine that is required for the digestion of lactose
B. Assessment
1. Diarrhea
2. Abdominal distention
3. Crampy abdominal pain
4. Excessive flatus
C. Implementation
1. Provide a lactose-free diet
2. Encourage the breast-feeding mother to limit dairy products
3. Gradually add food containing small amounts of lactose such as yogurt, hard cheeses, and small amounts of milk to assess the child's reaction
4. Instruct the parents regarding alternative sources of calcium

VIII. Celiac Disease

A. Description
1. Intolerance to gluten, the protein component of wheat, barley, rye, and oats
2. Symptoms of the disorder occur 3 to 6 months following the introduction of gluten-containing grains into the diet
3. It results in the accumulation of the amino acid glutamine, which is toxic to intestinal mucosal cells
4. Intestinal villi atrophy, which affects absorption of ingested nutrients
B. Assessment
1. Steatorrhea: frequent, bulky, greasy malodorous stools with a frothy appearance because of fat in stool
2. Abdominal distention
3. Weight loss
4. Signs of malnutrition
5. **Growth** failure
6. Irritability and apathy
7. Anemia
C. Celiac Crisis
1. Precipitated by infection, fasting, and ingestion of gluten
2. Can lead to electrolyte imbalance, rapid dehydration, and severe acidosis

---

BOX 37–2. Basics of a Gluten-Free Diet

FOODS ALLOWED

Meat such as beef, pork, and poultry, fish, eggs, milk and dairy products, vegetables, fruits, grains, rice, corn, gluten-free wheat flour, puffed rice, corn flakes, corn meal, precooked gluten-free cereals

FOODS PROHIBITED

Commercially prepared ice cream; malted milk; prepared puddings; grains, including anything made from wheat, rye, oats, or barley such as breads, rolls, cookies, cakes, crackers, cereal, spaghetti, macaroni, beer, and ale

---

3. Causes profuse watery diarrhea and vomiting
D. Implementation
1. Gluten-free diet and substituting corn and rice as a grain source
2. Lifelong elimination of gluten sources as wheat, rye, oats, and barley
3. Mineral and vitamin supplements including fat-soluble supplements A, D, E, and K
4. Teach the parents about a gluten-free diet (Box 37–2)
5. Instruct in measures to prevent celiac crisis
6. Instruct in the importance of preventing infection

IX. Appendicitis

A. Description
1. Inflammation of the appendix
2. When the appendix becomes inflamed or infected, rupture may occur within a matter of hours, leading to peritonitis and sepsis
B. Assessment
1. Pain in periumbilical area that descends to right lower quadrant
2. Abdominal pain that is most intense at McBurney's point
3. Rebound tenderness and abdominal rigidity
4. Elevated white blood cell (WBC) count
5. Side-lying position with abdominal guarding with legs flexed
6. Low-grade fever
7. Anorexia, nausea, and vomiting
8. Constipation or diarrhea
C. Ruptured Appendix/Peritonitis
1. Description: inflammation of the peritoneum
2. Assessment
a. Increased fever
b. Progressive abdominal distention and abdominal pain
c. Right guarding of abdomen
d. Tachycardia
e. Tachypnea
f. Pallor
g. Chills
h. Restlessness

D. Appendectomy
   1. Description: surgical removal of the appendix
   2. Implementation preoperatively
      a. Maintain NPO status
      b. Administer IV fluids to prevent dehydration
      c. Monitor for signs of ruptured appendix and peritonitis
      d. Administer antibiotics as prescribed
      e. Monitor for changes in level of pain
      f. Monitor bowel sounds
      g. Position right side-lying or low to semi-Fowler's position to promote comfort
      h. Apply ice packs to abdomen for 20 minutes every hour as prescribed
      i. Avoid application of heat to abdomen
      j. Avoid laxatives or enemas
   3. Implementation postoperatively
      a. Monitor temperature for signs of infection
      b. Maintain NPO status until bowel function has returned
      c. Advance diet gradually as tolerated when bowel sounds return
      d. Assess incision for signs of infection such as redness, swelling, and pain
      e. If rupture of the appendix has occurred, expect a Penrose drain to be inserted or incision may be left open to heal from the inside out
      f. Expect that drainage from Penrose may be profuse for the first 12 hours
      g. Position the client in right side-lying or low to semi-Fowler's position with legs flexed to facilitate drainage
      h. Change the dressing as prescribed and record type and amount of drainage
      i. Perform wound irrigations if prescribed
      j. Maintain NG suction and patency of NG tube as prescribed
      k. Administer antibiotics and analgesics as prescribed

X. Hirschsprung's Disease (Fig. 37–3)

A. Description
   1. A congenital anomaly also known as congenital aganglionosis or megacolon
   2. Occurs as the result of an absence of ganglion cells in the rectum and upward in the colon
   3. Results in mechanical obstruction from inadequate motility in an intestinal segment
   4. May be a familial congenital defect or may be associated with other anomalies such as Down's syndrome and genital urinary abnormalities
   5. Treatment for mild or moderate disease is based on relieving the chronic constipation with stool softeners and rectal irrigations
   6. Treatment for moderate to severe disease involves a two-step surgical procedure
   7. Initially, in the neonatal period, the obstruction is relieved by a temporary colostomy
   8. A complete surgical repair is performed when the child weighs 8 to 10 kg (17.6–22 pounds) via a pull-through procedure to excise portions of the bowel; at this time, the colostomy is closed

B. Assessment
   1. In newborns, failure to pass meconium stool within 48 hours after birth
   2. Constipation
   3. Ribbon-like and foul-smelling stools
   4. Abdominal distention
   5. Bowel obstruction
   6. In infants, failure to thrive
   7. Reluctance to ingest fluids
   8. Bile-stained vomitus
   9. In toddlers and older children, chronic constipation
   10. Visible peristalsis
   11. Palpable fecal mass
   12. Signs of enterocolitis such as fever, severe prostration, or explosive watery diarrhea

C. Implementation
   1. Administer stool softeners as prescribed
   2. Dietary management and cleansing enemas until the child is able to tolerate surgery

D. Implementation Preoperatively
   1. Assess bowel function
   2. Administer bowel preparation as prescribed
   3. Maintain NPO status
   4. Provide IV fluids as prescribed for hydration
   5. Administer antibiotics as prescribed to sterilize the bowel
   6. Monitor I&O and weight
   7. Monitor hydration and fluid and electrolyte status
   8. Measure abdominal girth
   9. Avoid rectal temperatures
   10. Monitor for respiratory distress associated with abdominal distention

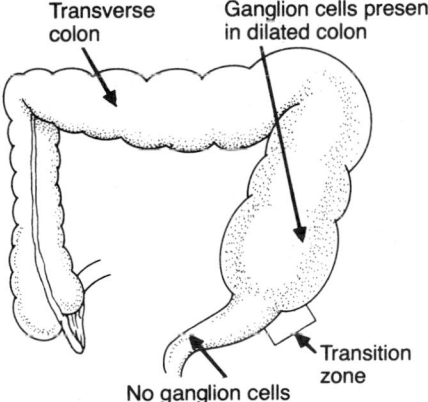

FIGURE 37–3. Hirschsprung's disease. Lack of ganglion cells in a segment of colon prevents transmission of normal peristaltic waves and results in intestinal obstruction. (From Betz, C. L., Hunsberger, M. M., & Wright, S. [1994]. *Family-centered nursing care of children.* Philadelphia: W. B. Saunders.)

E. Implementation Postoperatively
1. Monitor vital signs, avoiding rectal temperatures
2. Measure abdominal circumference
3. Assess the surgical site for redness, swelling, and drainage
4. Assess the stoma for bleeding or skin breakdown
5. Assess the anal area for the presence of stool, redness, or discharge
6. Maintain NPO status until bowel signs return or flatus is passed
7. Monitor for bowel sounds, which usually return within 48 to 72 hours
8. Maintain NG to intermittent suction until peristalsis returns
9. Maintain IV until the child tolerates appropriate PO intake
10. Begin the diet with clear liquids, advancing to regular as tolerated and as prescribed
11. Assess for dehydration and fluid overload
12. Monitor I&O and weight
13. Assess pain and provide comfort measures as required
14. Provide the parents with instructions regarding colostomy care, skin care, and colostomy irrigations as required
15. Teach the parents about appropriate diet and adequate fluid intake

XI. Intussusception

A. Description
1. Telescoping of one portion of the bowel into another portion
2. Results in an obstruction to the passage of intestinal contents
B. Assessment
1. Colicky abdominal pain
2. Pain causes the child to scream and draw knees to abdomen
3. Vomiting of gastric contents
4. Bile-stained fecal emesis
5. Currant jelly–like stools containing blood and mucus
6. Hypoactive or hyperactive bowel sounds
7. Tender distended abdomen, possibly with a palpable mass
8. Lethargy
C. Implementation
1. Monitor hydration status and for signs of dehydration
2. Assess skin turgor and mucous membranes
3. Monitor I&O and weight
4. Maintain NPO status and NG tube if distention is present
5. Maintain IV fluids as prescribed
6. Monitor for signs of sepsis or peritonitis as evidenced by fever, increased heart rate, changes in level of consciousness (LOC) or blood pressure, and respiratory distress, and report immediately

7. Prepare for hydrostatic reduction if prescribed
8. Following hydrostatic reduction, administer clear fluids and advance the diet gradually as prescribed
9. Monitor for the passage of barium and the characteristics of stool
10. Monitor for the return of normal bowel signs
11. If surgery is performed, maintain NPO status until bowel function returns, then begin clear liquids, advancing as tolerated as prescribed

XII. Abdominal Wall Defects

A. Description
1. Can include umbilical hernia, inguinal hernia, or hydrocele
2. A hernia is a protrusion of the bowel through an abnormal opening in the abdominal wall
3. In children, a hernia most commonly occurs at the umbilicus and through the inguinal canal
4. A hydrocele is the presence of abdominal fluid in the scrotal sac
B. Assessment
1. Umbilical hernia: soft swelling or protrusion around the umbilicus that is usually reducible with the finger
2. Inguinal hernia
   a. Painless inguinal swelling that is reducible
   b. Swelling may disappear during periods of rest and is most noticeable when the infant cries or coughs
3. Incarcerated hernia
   a. When the descended portion becomes tightly caught in the hernial sac compromising blood supply
   b. A medical emergency requiring surgical repair
   c. Irritability
   d. Tenderness at the site
   e. Anorexia
   f. Abdominal distention
   g. Difficulty defecating
   h. May lead to complete intestinal obstruction and gangrene
4. Noncommunicating hydrocele
   a. Occurs when residual peritoneal fluid is trapped with no communication to the abdominal cavity
   b. Usually disappears by age 1 year
5. Communicating hydrocele
   a. Associated with a hernia that remains open from the scrotum to the abdominal cavity
   b. Assessment includes a bulge in the inguinal area or the scrotum that increases with crying or straining and decreases when the child is at rest
C. Implementation Postoperatively (Hernia)
1. Monitor vital signs

2. Assess for wound infection
3. Monitor for redness or drainage
4. Monitor hydration status
5. Monitor I&O
6. Advance the diet as tolerated
7. Administer analgesics as prescribed

D. Implementation Postoperatively (Hydrocele)
  1. Provide ice bags and a scrotal support to relieve pain and swelling
  2. Instruct to avoid tub bathing until incision heals
  3. Instruct to avoid strenuous physical activities

XIII. Constipation/Encopresis

A. Description
  1. Constipation is the infrequent and difficult passage of dry, hard stools
  2. **Encopresis** is fecal incontinence and children often complain that soiling is involuntary and occurs without warning
  3. If the child does not have a neurological or anatomic disorder, **encopresis** is usually the result of fecal impaction and an enlarged rectum caused by chronic constipation

B. Assessment
  1. Constipation
     a. Abdominal pain and cramping without distention
     b. Palpable movable fecal masses
     c. Normal or decreased bowel sounds
     d. Malaise
     e. Anorexia
     f. Headache
     g. Nausea and vomiting
  2. **Encopresis**
     a. Evidence of soiled clothing
     b. Scratching or rubbing of anal area
     c. Fecal odor
     d. Social withdrawal

C. Implementation
  1. Simple constipation may resolve using only dietary changes or methods to change the habit of retention
  2. Severe **encopresis** may require intervention to be continued over a period of 3 to 6 months
  3. Overcoming withholding
     a. Administer enemas as prescribed until impaction is cleared
     b. Monitor for hypernatremia or hyperphosphatemia when administering repeated enemas
     c. Administer stool softener or laxative as prescribed
     d. Administer mineral oil 30 to 75 mL BID as prescribed
     e. Administer mineral oil chilled or mixed with cold drinks to disguise the taste
  4. Dietary changes
     a. Increase water and fiber intake
     b. Decrease sugar and milk intake
     c. Administer fat-soluble vitamins during the use of mineral oil because the oil can interfere with vitamin absorption in the small intestine
  5. Changing the retention habit: have the child sit on the toilet for 5 to 10 minutes approximately 20 to 30 minutes after breakfast and dinner to assist with defecation

XIV. Irritable Bowel Syndrome

A. Description
  1. Occurs as a result of increased motility that can lead to spasm and pain
  2. The diagnosis is based on the elimination of pathology
  3. It is a self-limiting, intermittent problem with no definitive treatment
  4. Stress and emotional factors may contribute to its occurrence

B. Assessment
  1. Diffuse abdominal pain unrelated to meals or activity
  2. Alternating constipation and diarrhea with the presence of undigested food and mucus in the stool
  3. Normal **growth**

C. Implementation
  1. Reassure that the problem is self-limiting and intermittent and will resolve
  2. Encourage the maintenance of a healthy well-balanced, moderate-fiber diet
  3. Encourage health promotion activities such as exercise and school activities
  4. Inform the parents of psychosocial resources if required

XV. Imperforate Anus

A. Description: Incomplete development or absence of the anus in its normal position in the perineum

B. Assessment
  1. Failure to pass meconium stool
  2. Absence or **stenosis** of the anal rectal canal
  3. Anal membrane
  4. External fistula to the peritoneum

C. Implementation
  1. Determine patency of the anus
  2. Monitor for the presence of stool in the urine and vagina and report immediately

D. Implementation Postoperatively
  1. Monitor the skin for signs of infection
  2. Position side-lying with legs flexed or a prone position to keep hips elevated to reduce edema and pressure on the surgical site
  3. Keep the anal surgical incision clean and dry and monitor for redness, swelling, or drainage
  4. Maintain NPO status and NG tube if in place
  5. Maintain IV fluids until gastrointestinal (GI) motility returns

6. Provide colostomy care if prescribed
7. Colostomy site should be pink without drainage, swelling, or skin breakdown
8. A fresh colostomy stoma will be red and edematous, but this should decrease with time
9. Instruct the parents to perform anal dilatation if prescribed to achieve and maintain bowel patency
10. Instruct parents to use only dilators supplied by the physician, a water-soluble lubricant, and to insert the dilator no more than 1 to 2 cm into the anus to prevent damage to the mucosa

XVI. Viral Hepatitis

A. Description
  1. An acute or chronic inflammation of the liver
  2. The most effective means of preventing hepatitis is immunization
  3. The most common mode of transmission of hepatitis A (HAV) is person-to-person by fecal-oral route
  4. Hepatitis B (HBV) is primarily transmitted parenterally or by sexual contact
  5. Children who have had direct contact with a person infected with HAV should receive immune globulin as soon as possible after exposure
  6. Cases of hepatitis should be reported promptly to local public health officials
B. Assessment
  1. A history of exposure to jaundiced children, confirmed outbreaks in day care centers or schools, or exposure to blood or body fluids should raise the suspicion of hepatitis
  2. Right upper quadrant tenderness
  3. Hepatomegaly
  4. Pale clay-colored stools
  5. Dark and frothy urine
  6. Jaundice, which is best assessed in the sclera, nailbeds, and mucous membranes
  7. Hepatitis A: in infants and preschool children, is usually either asymptomatic or causes mild nonspecific symptoms such as anorexia, malaise, and easy fatigability
  8. Hepatitis B: may cause a wide range of symptoms ranging from asymptomatic infection to fatal acute fulminant hepatitis
C. Implementation
  1. Prevention of the spread of infection
  2. Instruct on good handwashing
  3. Instruct to thoroughly disinfect diaper-changing surfaces with a solution of 1/4 cup bleach to a gallon of water
  4. Provide enteric precautions for at least 1 week after the onset of jaundice with HAV
  5. Maintain comfort and provide adequate rest and sleep

6. Provide a low-fat balanced diet
7. Instruct the parents that because hepatitis A is not infectious within 1 week after the onset of jaundice, the child may return to school at that time if feeling well enough
8. Instruct the parents that jaundice may get worse before it resolves
9. Instruct the parents in the signs indicating a worsening of the child's condition such as changes in the neurological status, bleeding, and fluid retention

XVII. Ingestion of Poisons

A. Lead Poisoning
  1. Description: excessive accumulation of lead in the blood
  2. Causes
    a. Ingestion of lead through paint chips, soil contaminated with lead, canned food products, lead used in plumbing, vinyl miniblinds, and improperly glazed pottery
    b. A diet high in fat and low in iron and calcium increases lead absorption
  3. Diagnostic test
    a. Erythrocyte protoporphyrin (EP) levels are used to screen children for lead levels and anemia
    b. An EP level greater than 9 μg/dL indicates the need for more frequent screening
    c. An EP level greater than 15 μg/dL indicates the need for nutritional and educational interventions and environmental investigation
    d. An EP level greater than 20 μg/dL requires pharmacological intervention
  4. Assessment
    a. Anorexia
    b. Malaise and headache
    c. Constipation or diarrhea
    d. Failure to thrive
    e. Abdominal pain
    f. Lead lines in gums around teeth
    g. Tachycardia
    h. Hypertension or hypotension
    i. Lacrimation and nasal congestion
    j. Muscle pains
    k. Renal toxicity
  5. Complications
    a. Cerebral edema
    b. Renal toxicity
    c. CNS toxicity
  6. Implementation
    a. Remove child from lead source
    b. Administer chelating agents (calcium EDTA [calcium disodium versenate] with dimercaprol [BAL in oil])
    c. Monitor kidney function for nephrotoxicity when medication is given
    d. Monitor calcium levels because medication enhances excretion of calcium

e. Administer anticonvulsants as prescribed
f. Administer oral or IM iron as prescribed
g. Follow-up lead levels to monitor progress

B. Acetaminophen (Tylenol)
   1. Description: seriousness of ingestion is determined by amount ingested and length of time before intervention
   2. Assessment
      a. First 24 hours: malaise, nausea, vomiting, sweating, pallor, weakness
      b. One to three days: elevated liver enzymes and bilirubin, right upper quadrant pain, prolonged prothrombin time (PT)
      c. One week: jaundice, liver necrosis, possible death from hepatic failure
   3. Implementation
      a. Induce vomiting or gastric lavage depending on the amount ingested
      b. Administer activated charcoal or antidote acetylcysteine (Mucomyst)
      c. Administer acetylcysteine with juice or cola or via NG tube
      d. Do not administer charcoal if a prescribed antidote is anticipated, as charcoal will make an antidote ineffective
      e. Administer IV fluids as prescribed
      f. Provide sodium restricted, high-calorie, high-protein diet

C. Salicylates
   1. Description
      a. Most common cause of drug poisoning in children
      b. Toxic dose: single dose exceeding 200 to 280 mg/kg
      c. Peak gastric absorption occurs within 2 hours of ingestion
   2. Assessment
      a. GI effects: nausea, vomiting, thirst
      b. Central nervous system (CNS) effects: hyperventilation, confusion, seizures, coma, respiratory failure, circulatory collapse
      c. Renal effects: oliguria
      d. Hematopoietic effects: bleeding tendencies
      e. Metabolic effects: sweating, dehydration, fever, hyponatremia, hypokalemia, dehydration, hypoglycemia
   3. Implementation
      a. Induce vomiting with syrup of ipecac or perform gastric lavage
      b. Administer activated charcoal to decrease absorption of salicylate
      c. Administer IVs, sodium bicarbonate, electrolytes, or volume expanders as prescribed
      d. Administer vitamin K for bleeding tendencies as prescribed
      e. Administer glucose for hypoglycemia as prescribed
      f. Prepare the child for dialysis as prescribed if the child is unresponsive to therapy

PRACTICE QUESTIONS

1. The nurse is caring for an 18-month-old child who has been vomiting. The most appropriate position for the child during naps and sleep time is:
   1 Side-lying position
   2 Prone with the face turned to the side
   3 Supine
   4 Prone with the head elevated

2. A 3-year-old child is hospitalized because of persistent vomiting. Which of the following conditions does the nurse expect to occur in this child?
   1 Diarrhea
   2 Metabolic acidosis
   3 Metabolic alkalosis
   4 Hyperactive bowel sounds

3. The nurse is monitoring for fluid volume deficit in an infant who is vomiting and having diarrhea. The nurse weighs the infant's diaper after each voiding and stool and carefully calculates fluid volume knowing that:
   1 Each gram of diaper weight is equivalent to 0.5 mL of urine
   2 Each gram of diaper weight is equivalent to 1 mL of urine
   3 Each gram of diaper weight is equivalent to 2 mL of urine
   4 Each gram of diaper weight is equivalent to 2.5 mL of urine

4. The nurse is monitoring for signs of dehydration in a 1-year-old child who has been hospitalized for diarrhea. The nurse prepares to take the child's temperature. Which of the following methods should be avoided?
   1 Tympanic measurement
   2 Axillary measurement
   3 Rectal measurement
   4 Electronic measurement

5. The parents of a child with a cleft lip are concerned and ask the nurse when the lip will be repaired. The nurse bases the response on the knowledge that:
   1 Cleft lip repair is usually performed between 6 months and 2 years
   2 Cleft lip repair is usually performed by 6 months of age
   3 Cleft lip repair is usually performed by 4 weeks of age
   4 Cleft lip cannot be repaired

6. The home care nurse provides instructions to the mother of an infant with cleft palate regarding feeding. Which of the following is not a component of the instruction?

1 Use a nipple with a small hole to prevent choking
2 Stimulate sucking by rubbing the nipple on the lower lip
3 Allow the infant time to swallow
4 Allow the infant to rest frequently to provide time to swallow what has been placed in the mouth

7. Following a cleft lip repair, the nurse instructs the parents regarding cleaning of the lip repair site. Which of the following solutions does the nurse use in demonstrating this procedure to the parents?
1 Tap water
2 Sterile water
3 Full-strength hydrogen peroxide
4 Half-strength hydrogen peroxide

8. An infant returns to the nursing unit following a surgical repair of a cleft lip located on the right side of the lip. The best position to place this infant at this time is:
1 On the right side
2 On the left side
3 Prone
4 Supine

9. The clinic nurse reviews the record of an infant seen in the clinic. The nurse notes that a diagnosis of esophageal atresia with tracheoesophageal fistula (TEF) is suspected. Which of the following assessment findings would not be noted in this disorder?
1 Severe projectile vomiting
2 Coughing
3 Choking
4 Cyanosis

10. An infant returns to the nursing unit following surgery for a diagnosis of esophageal atresia with TEF. The infant is receiving IV fluids and a gastrostomy tube is in place. Following assessment, the nurse positions the infant and:
1 Places the gastrostomy tube to gravity flow
2 Attaches the gastrostomy tube to low suction
3 Tapes the gastrostomy tube to the bed linens
4 Elevates the gastrostomy tube

11. The nurse provides feeding instructions to a mother of an infant diagnosed with gastroesophageal reflux (GER). To assist in reducing the episodes of emesis, the best instruction is which of the following?
1 Thin the feedings by adding water to the formula
2 Thicken the feedings by adding rice cereal to the formula
3 Provide less frequent, larger feedings
4 Burp less frequently during feedings

12. The nurse prepares a teaching plan for the parents of an infant with GER regarding proper positioning to manage reflux. The nurse prepares the plan with which of the following goals in mind?
1 The infant should be maintained in a 30-degree angle when supine
2 The infant should be maintained in a 60-degree angle when prone
3 The infant should be maintained in an upright angle 24 hours a day
4 The infant should be maintained in a 20-degree angle when side-lying

13. The nurse admits a child to the hospital with a diagnosis of pyloric stenosis. On admission assessment, which of the following data does the nurse expect to obtain when asking the mother about the child's symptoms?
1 Vomiting large amounts of bile
2 Watery diarrhea
3 Increased urine output
4 Projectile vomiting

14. The nurse is caring for a child with hypertrophic pyloric stenosis. The child is scheduled for pyloromyotomy. In which of the following positions does the nurse place the child during the preoperative period?
1 Prone with the head of the bed elevated
2 Prone with the head of the bed lowered to promote drainage
3 Supine with the head of the bed at a 30-degree angle
4 Supine with the head of the bed at a 45-degree angle

15. The home care nurse instructs the mother about dietary measures for a 5-year-old child with lactose intolerance. Which of the following supplements is required because of the necessity of avoidance in the diet?
1 Zinc
2 Protein
3 Calcium
4 Fat

16. The breast-feeding mother of an infant with lactose intolerance asks the nurse about dietary measures. Which of the following foods does the nurse instruct the mother to avoid?
1 Hard cheeses
2 Green leafy vegetables
3 Dried beans
4 Egg yolks

17. The nurse reviews the record of a 1-year-old child seen in the clinic and notes that the physician has documented a diagnosis of celiac crisis. Which of the following symptoms does the nurse expect to note in this condition?
1 Anorexia
2 Joint pain
3 Profuse watery diarrhea
4 Constipation

18. The nurse provides home care instructions to the parents of a child with celiac disease. Which of the following food items does the nurse advise the parents to include in the child's diet?
    1 Rice
    2 Rye toast
    3 Oatmeal
    4 Wheat bread

19. The nurse is caring for a child who is scheduled for an appendectomy. When the nurse reviews the physician's preoperative orders, which of the following is questioned?
    1 Initiate IV line
    2 Maintain NPO status
    3 Administer Fleet enema
    4 Administer preoperative medication on call

20. The nurse is assessing the child with a diagnosis of suspected appendicitis. In assessing the intensity and progression of the pain, the nurse palpates the child at McBurney's point. In performing this assessment the nurse knows that McBurney's point is located:
    1 Midway between the right anterior inferior iliac crest and the umbilicus
    2 Midway between the left anterior superior iliac crest and the umbilicus
    3 Midway between the right anterior superior iliac crest and the umbilicus
    4 Midway between the left anterior superior iliac crest and the umbilicus

21. The mother of an infant diagnosed with Hirschsprung's disease asks the nurse about the disorder. The nurse bases the response on which of the following?
    1 It is a congenital aganglionosis or megacolon
    2 It is a complete small intestinal obstruction
    3 It is a condition that causes the pyloric valve to remain open
    4 It is a severe inflammation of the gastrointestinal tract

22. The clinic nurse reviews the record of a 3-week-old infant and notes that the physician has documented a diagnosis of suspected Hirschsprung's disease. Which of the following symptoms most likely led the mother to seek health care for the infant?
    1 Diarrhea
    2 Projectile vomiting
    3 Regurgitation of feedings
    4 Foul smelling pellet-like stools

23. The nurse is monitoring a newborn with a suspected diagnosis of imperforate anus. Which of the following is not a clinical manifestation associated with this disorder?
    1 The presence of stool in the urine
    2 Failure to pass a rectal thermometer

    3 Failure to pass meconium in the first 24 hours after birth
    4 The passage of currant jelly–like stools

24. The nurse is caring for a newborn with a colostomy that was created during surgical intervention for imperforate anus. When the newborn returns from surgery, the nurse assesses the stoma and notes that it is red and edematous. Which of the following is the most appropriate nursing intervention?
    1 Call the physician
    2 Document the findings
    3 Apply ice immediately
    4 Elevate the buttocks

25. The nurse provides home care instructions to the parents of an infant following surgical intervention for imperforate anus. The nurse instructs about the procedure for anal dilatation. Which of the following is not a component of the instructions?
    1 Use only dilators supplied by the physician
    2 Use a water-soluble lubricant
    3 Insert the dilator no more than 1 to 2 cm into the anus
    4 Insert a glycerin suppository prior to the dilatation

26. A 1-year-old child is diagnosed with intussusception. The mother of the child asks the nurse to describe the disorder. The nurse responds that this disorder is:
    1 An acute bowel obstruction
    2 A condition in which a proximal segment of the bowel prolapses into a distal segment of the bowel
    3 A condition in which a distal segment of the bowel prolapses into a proximal segment of the bowel
    4 A condition that causes an acute inflammatory process in the bowel

27. The nurse is caring for a child with a diagnosis of intussusception. Which of the following symptoms does the nurse expect to note in this child?
    1 Bright red blood and mucus in the stools
    2 Profuse projectile vomiting
    3 Watery diarrhea
    4 Ribbon-like stools

28. A child with a diagnosis of umbilical hernia has been scheduled for surgical repair in 2 weeks. The clinic nurse instructs the parents about the signs of possible hernial strangulation. Which of the following signs requires physician notification by the parents?
    1 Fever
    2 Diarrhea
    3 Constipation
    4 Vomiting

29. A 3-year-old child is seen in the health care clinic and a diagnosis of encopresis is made. Which of the following is a sign of this disorder?
    1 Nausea and vomiting
    2 Diarrhea
    3 Evidence of soiled clothing
    4 Malaise and anorexia

30. The pediatric nurse educator provides a teaching session to the nursing staff regarding hepatitis in children. Which of the following is not a component of the teaching session?
    1 Vaccines are available to prevent hepatitis A (HAV) and hepatitis B (HBV)
    2 Cases of hepatitis should be promptly reported to health care officials
    3 Enteric precautions are necessary for HBV but not for HAV
    4 The child's stools will be pale and clay-colored

31. The clinic nurse is assessing the status of jaundice in a child with hepatitis. Which assessment will provide the best data regarding the presence of jaundice?
    1 The nailbeds
    2 The skin in the abdominal area
    3 The skin in the sacral area
    4 The membranes in the ear canal

32. The nurse provides home care instructions to the family of a child with hepatitis regarding care of the child and the prevention of transmission of the virus. Which of the following is not a component of the teaching?
    1 Handwashing techniques
    2 Cleaning household surfaces with bleach
    3 Providing a well-balanced, high-fat diet to the child
    4 The use of gloves

33. An erythrocyte protoporphyrin (EP) level is drawn on a child to screen for lead poisoning. The results indicate a level of 9 μg/dL. The nurse interprets this value as:
    1 Inconclusive
    2 Normal
    3 Positive
    4 Requiring a repeat test

34. A child is hospitalized with a diagnosis of lead poisoning. The nurse caring for the child administers which of the following medications?
    1 Activated charcoal
    2 Sodium bicarbonate
    3 Ipecac syrup
    4 Calcium EDTA (calcium disodium versenate) with dimercaprol (BAL in oil)

35. The child is receiving EDTA with BAL in oil for the treatment of lead poisoning. Which of the following laboratory studies is most important to monitor?
    1 Potassium level
    2 White blood cell (WBC) count
    3 Red blood cell (RBC) count
    4 Calcium level

36. The emergency room nurse prepares to treat a child with acetaminophen (Tylenol) overdose. Which of the following does the nurse anticipate to be prescribed?
    1 Vitamin K (AquaMEPHYTON)
    2 Protamine sulfate
    3 EDTA with BAL in oil
    4 Acetylcysteine (Mucomyst)

37. A child is brought to the emergency room by the mother who reports that she found the child sitting on the floor with an open bottle of aspirin beside the child. The mother reports that the bottle contained 5 aspirin and that the bottle was empty when she found the child. The nurse determines that the child may have received a toxic dose of the medication if the child consumed more than:
    1 50 mg/kg of the child's body weight
    2 100 mg/kg of the child's body weight
    3 150 mg/kg of the child's body weight
    4 200 mg/kg of the child's body weight

38. The emergency nurse is caring for a child brought to the emergency room following the ingestion of approximately one-half bottle of aspirin. The nurse anticipates that the most likely initial treatment will be:
    1 The administration of syrup of ipecac
    2 The administration of sodium bicarbonate
    3 The administration of vitamin K
    4 Dialysis

ANSWERS

1. **1**

Rationale: The vomiting child should be placed in an upright or side-lying position to prevent aspiration. Options 2, 3, and 4 will place the child at risk for aspiration if vomiting occurs.

Test-Taking Strategy: Eliminate options 2 and 4 first because they are similar. Additionally, these positions would place the child at risk for aspiration if vomiting occurred. Visualize the remaining two positions in selecting the correct option. Option 3 is also inappropriate and would cause aspiration. Review appropriate positioning techniques now if you had difficulty with this question!

Level of Cognitive Ability: Application
Phase of Nursing Process: Implementation
Client Needs: Physiological Integrity
Content Area: Child Health

Reference

Ashwill, J., & Droske, S. (1997). *Nursing care of children: Principles and practice*. Philadelphia: W. B. Saunders. p. 692.

2. **3**

Rationale: Vomiting will cause the loss of hydrochloric acid and subsequent metabolic alkalosis. Metabolic acidosis would occur in a child experiencing diarrhea because of the loss of bicarbonate. Diarrhea may not accompany vomiting. Hyperactive bowel sounds are not necessarily associated with vomiting.

Test-Taking Strategy: Recalling that gastric fluids are acidic and that the loss of these fluids will lead to alkalosis will assist in answering the question. There are no supporting data in the question to support options 1 and 4. Review the manifestations that occur with vomiting now if you had difficulty with this question!

Level of Cognitive Ability: Analysis
Phase of Nursing Process: Assessment
Client Needs: Physiological Integrity
Content Area: Child Health

Reference

Ashwill, J., & Droske, S. (1997). *Nursing care of children: Principles and practice*. Philadelphia: W. B. Saunders. p. 694.

3. **2**

Rationale: When monitoring for fluid-volume deficit, the nurse should weigh the infant's diaper after each voiding and stool. Each gram of diaper weight is equivalent to 1 mL of urine.

Test-Taking Strategy: Specific knowledge regarding the measurements related to monitoring for fluid-volume deficit is required to answer this question. If you are unfamiliar with these measures and values, take time now to review!

Level of Cognitive Ability: Analysis
Phase of Nursing Process: Assessment
Client Needs: Physiological Integrity
Content Area: Child Health

Reference

Ashwill, J., & Droske, S. (1997). *Nursing care of children: Principles and practice*. Philadelphia: W. B. Saunders. p. 687.

4. **3**

Rationale: Rectal temperature measurements should be avoided if diarrhea is present. Use of a rectal thermometer can stimulate peristalsis and cause more diarrhea. Axillary and tympanic measurements of temperature would be acceptable. Most measurements are done via electronic devices.

Test-Taking Strategy: Eliminate option 4 first because most methods of temperature measurement are done through an electronic device. Note the diagnosis stated in the question. This should easily direct you toward option 3 as the measure to avoid.

Level of Cognitive Ability: Analysis
Phase of Nursing Process: Planning
Client Needs: Physiological Integrity
Content Area: Child Health

Reference

Ashwill, J., & Droske, S. (1997). *Nursing care of children: Principles and practice*. Philadelphia: W. B. Saunders. p. 687.

5. **3**

Rationale: Cleft lip repair is usually performed by age 4 weeks and in some situations in the first 2 to 3 days of life. Early repair may improve bonding and makes feeding much easier. Some cosmetic modifications may be needed at ages 4 to 5 years.

Test-Taking Strategy: Knowledge regarding the repair of cleft lip is required to answer the question. Option 4 can be easily eliminated first. Eliminate options 1 and 2 next, because they are similar. Review the management of cleft lip repair now if you had difficulty with this question!

Level of Cognitive Ability: Analysis
Phase of Nursing Process: Analysis
Client Needs: Psychosocial Integrity
Content Area: Child Health

Reference

Ashwill, J., & Droske, S. (1997). *Nursing care of children: Principles and practice*. Philadelphia: W. B. Saunders. p. 703.

6. **1**

Rationale: Teach the mother the ESSR method of feeding the child with a cleft palate. ENLARGE the nipple by crosscutting a hole so that food is delivered to the back of the throat without sucking. STIMULATE sucking by rubbing the nipple on the lower lip. SWALLOW. REST to allow the infant to finish swallowing what has been placed in the mouth.

Test-Taking Strategy: Note the key word "not" in the stem of the question. Eliminate options 3 and 4 first, because they are similar. Use basic principles regarding the methods to stimulate sucking to eliminate option 2. Review teaching guidelines for the child with cleft lip or palate now if you had difficulty with this question!

Level of Cognitive Ability: Application
Phase of Nursing Process: Implementation
Client Needs: Physiological Integrity
Content Area: Child Health

Reference

Ashwill, J., & Droske, S. (1997). *Nursing care of children: Principles and practice*. Philadelphia: W. B. Saunders. p. 704.

7. 2

Rationale: The lip repair site is cleansed with sterile water using a cotton swab or saline, after feeding and as prescribed. The parents should be instructed to use a rolling motion from the suture line out. The parents should also demonstrate performance of the correct procedure to the nurse.

Test-Taking Strategy: Eliminate options 3 and 4 first because they are similar. From the remaining options, recall the importance of asepsis to a surgical site. This concept will direct you to option 2. Review this procedure now if you had difficulty with this question!

Level of Cognitive Ability: Application
Phase of Nursing Process: Implementation
Client Needs: Physiological Integrity
Content Area: Child Health

Reference
Ashwill, J., & Droske, S. (1997). *Nursing care of children: Principles and practice.* Philadelphia: W. B. Saunders. p. 706.

8. 2

Rationale: Following cleft lip repair, the infant should be positioned supine or on the side lateral to the repair to prevent the contact of the suture lines with the bed linens. It is best to place the infant on the left side rather than supine immediately after surgery, to prevent the risk of aspiration if the infant vomits.

Test-Taking Strategy: Consider the anatomical location of the surgical site and the key phrase "right side" in answering this question. You should easily be directed to the correct option using these concepts. Review postoperative positioning techniques now if you had difficulty with this question!

Level of Cognitive Ability: Application
Phase of Nursing Process: Implementation
Client Needs: Physiological Integrity
Content Area: Child Health

Reference
Ashwill, J., & Droske, S. (1997). *Nursing care of children: Principles and practice.* Philadelphia: W. B. Saunders. p. 706.

9. 1

Rationale: Any child who exhibits the "3 Cs" of coughing, choking with feedings, and cyanosis should be suspected of TEF. Failure to pass a suction catheter or nasogastric tube at birth, excessive oral secretions, vomiting, abdominal distention, and an airless, scaphoid abdomen (atresia without fistula) are also clinical manifestations.

Test-Taking Strategy: Recalling the "3 Cs" associated with this disorder will assist in directing you to the correct option. Review the clinical manifestations associated with this disorder now if you had difficulty with this question!

Level of Cognitive Ability: Analysis
Phase of Nursing Process: Assessment
Client Needs: Physiological Integrity
Content Area: Child Health

Reference
Ashwill, J., & Droske, S. (1997). *Nursing care of children: Principles and practice.* Philadelphia: W. B. Saunders. p. 708.

10. 4

Rationale: In the immediate postoperative period, the gastrostomy tube is elevated, allowing gastric contents to pass to the small intestine and air to escape. This promotes comfort and decreases the risk of leakage at the anastomosis. Options 1, 2, and 3 are incorrect.

Test-Taking Strategy: Option 3 can be easily eliminated because this action could cause accidental removal of the tube. Option 2 can be eliminated next, with the concept that suction on a surgical site could disrupt the repair. Knowledge that gastrostomy tubes are not normally attached to gravity flow will assist in directing you to the correct option. Review postoperative nursing care now if you had difficulty with this question!

Level of Cognitive Ability: Application
Phase of Nursing Process: Implementation
Client Needs: Physiological Integrity
Content Area: Child Health

Reference
Ashwill, J., & Droske, S. (1997). *Nursing care of children: Principles and practice.* Philadelphia: W. B. Saunders. p. 711.

11. 2

Rationale: Small, more frequent feedings with frequent burping are often tried as the first line of treatment in GER. Feedings thickened with rice cereal may reduce episodes of emesis. If thickened formula is used, 1 to 3 teaspoons of rice cereal per ounce of formula is most commonly used and may require cross-cutting of the nipple. Thinning the feeding is incorrect.

Test-Taking Strategy: Use basic principles related to feeding an infant to assist in eliminating options 3 and 4. Noting the key phrase "reducing the episodes of emesis" will assist in directing you to select option 2 over option 1. Review therapeutic interventions associated with this disorder now if you had difficulty with this question!

Level of Cognitive Ability: Application
Phase of Nursing Process: Implementation
Client Needs: Physiological Integrity
Content Area: Child Health

Reference
Ashwill, J., & Droske, S. (1997). *Nursing care of children: Principles and practice.* Philadelphia: W. B. Saunders. pp. 714–715.

12. 3

Rationale: Proper positioning is one of the mainstays of reflux management. Ideally, the goal is to maintain the infant in an upright angle 24 hours a day, at a 60-degree angle when supine, and at a 30-degree angle when prone. This position is maintained until the infant remains asymptomatic for 6 weeks.

Test-Taking Strategy: Knowledge that an upright position will prevent reflux will assist in answering the question. Bearing this concept in mind, you should easily be directed to option 3. Review positioning for GER now if you had difficulty with this question!

Level of Cognitive Ability: Analysis
Phase of Nursing Process: Planning
Client Needs: Physiological Integrity
Content Area: Child Health

Reference
Ashwill, J., & Droske, S. (1997). *Nursing care of children: Principles and practice.* Philadelphia: W. B. Saunders. p. 715.

13. 4

Rationale: Clinical manifestations of pyloric stenosis include projectile nonbilious vomiting, irritability, hunger and crying, constipation, and signs of dehydration including a decrease in urine output.

Test-Taking Strategy: Considering the anatomical location of this disorder and its potential effects, will assist in eliminating options 2 and 3. Recalling that a major clinical manifestation is projectile nonbilious vomiting will assist in directing you to option 4. Review these clinical manifestations now if you had difficulty with this question!

Level of Cognitive Ability: Analysis
Phase of Nursing Process: Assessment
Client Needs: Physiological Integrity
Content Area: Child Health

Reference
Ashwill, J., & Droske, S. (1997). *Nursing care of children: Principles and practice.* Philadelphia: W. B. Saunders. p. 718.

14. **1**

Rationale: In the preoperative period, the infant is positioned prone with the head of the bed elevated to reduce the risk of aspiration. Options 2, 3, and 4 are inappropriate positions to prevent this risk.

Test-Taking Strategy: Visualize each of the positions to select the correct option. Keeping in mind that aspiration is the concern will easily direct you to option 1. Review preoperative care for pyloromyotomy now, if you had difficulty with this question!

Level of Cognitive Ability: Application
Phase of Nursing Process: Implementation
Client Needs: Physiological Integrity
Content Area: Child Health

Reference
Ashwill, J., & Droske, S. (1997). *Nursing care of children: Principles and practice.* Philadelphia: W. B. Saunders. p. 719.

15. **3**

Rationale: Lactose intolerance is the inability to tolerate lactose, the sugar found in dairy products. Removing milk from the diet can provide enough relief from symptoms. Additional dietary changes may be required to provide adequate sources of calcium and in the infant, protein and calories.

Test-Taking Strategy: Knowledge that lactose is the sugar found in dairy products will easily direct you to option 3 since dairy products contain high sources of calcium. Review the dietary management for lactose intolerance now if you had difficulty with this question!

Level of Cognitive Ability: Application
Phase of Nursing Process: Implementation
Client Needs: Health Promotion and Maintenance
Content Area: Child Health

Reference
Ashwill, J., & Droske, S. (1997). *Nursing care of children: Principles and practice.* Philadelphia: W. B. Saunders. p. 731.

16. **1**

Rationale: Breast-feeding mothers need to be encouraged to limit dairy products. Cheese is a dairy product. Alternative calcium sources include egg yolks, green leafy vegetables, dried beans, cauliflower, and molasses.

Test-Taking Strategy: Note the key word "avoid" in the stem of the question. Knowledge that lactose is the sugar found in dairy products will easily direct you to option 1. Review the dietary management for lactose intolerance now if you had difficulty with this question!

Level of Cognitive Ability: Application
Phase of Nursing Process: Implementation
Client Needs: Health Promotion and Maintenance
Content Area: Child Health

Reference
Ashwill, J., & Droske, S. (1997). *Nursing care of children: Principles and practice.* Philadelphia: W. B. Saunders. p. 731.

17. **3**

Rationale: Clinical manifestations associated with celiac crisis include profuse watery diarrhea and vomiting that quickly lead to severe dehydration and metabolic acidosis. The cause of the crisis is usually infection or hidden sources of gluten. The child may require IV sources to correct fluid and acid-base imbalances, albumin to treat shock, and corticosteroids to decrease severe mucosal inflammation.

Test-Taking Strategy: Knowledge regarding the clinical manifestations associated with celiac crisis is required to answer the question. If you know that celiac disease causes diarrhea, then it is likely that crisis will lead to exaggeration of this symptom. Review this disorder now if you had difficulty with this question!

Level of Cognitive Ability: Analysis
Phase of Nursing Process: Assessment
Client Needs: Physiological Integrity
Content Area: Child Health

Reference
Ashwill, J., & Droske, S. (1997). *Nursing care of children: Principles and practice.* Philadelphia: W. B. Saunders. p. 733.

18. **1**

Rationale: Dietary management is the mainstay of treatment in celiac disease. All wheat, rye, barley, and oats should be eliminated from the diet and replaced with corn and rice. Vitamin supplements, especially fat-soluble vitamins and folate, may be needed in the early period of treatment to correct deficiencies. These restrictions are likely to be lifelong, although small amounts of grains may be tolerated after the ulcerations have healed.

Test-Taking Strategy: Knowledge regarding the dietary management in celiac disease is required to answer this question. Recalling that corn and rice are substitute food replacements in this disease will easily direct you to option 1. Review the dietary management in this disorder now if you had difficulty with this question!

Level of Cognitive Ability: Application
Phase of Nursing Process: Implementation
Client Needs: Health Promotion and Maintenance
Content Area: Child Health

Reference
Ashwill, J., & Droske, S. (1997). *Nursing care of children: Principles and practice.* Philadelphia: W. B. Saunders. p. 733.

19. **3**

Rationale: In the preoperative period, enemas or laxatives should not be administered. No heat should be applied to the abdomen because this may increase the chance of perforation secondary to vasodilation. IV fluids are started and the child is NPO. Prescribed preoperative medications most likely are administered on call to the operating room.

Test-Taking Strategy: Consider the anatomical location and the concern of rupture in this disorder. Options 1, 2, and 4 are standard preoperative measures. Option 3 places the child at risk for a perforated appendix. Review preoperative care in the child with appendicitis now if you had difficulty with this question!

Level of Cognitive Ability: Analysis
Phase of Nursing Process: Implementation
Client Needs: Physiological Integrity
Content Area: Child Health

Reference
Ashwill, J., & Droske, S. (1997). *Nursing care of children: Principles and practice.* Philadelphia: W. B. Saunders. p. 755.

20. **3**

Rationale: McBurney's point is midway between the right anterior superior iliac crest and the umbilicus. It is usually the location of greatest pain in the child with appendicitis.

Test-Taking Strategy: Knowledge that the appendix is located in the right side of the abdomen will assist in eliminating options 2 and 4. From this point, attempt to visualize this assessment procedure. This will assist in directing you to option 3. Take time now to review the location of McBurney's point if you had difficulty with this question!

Level of Cognitive Ability: Analysis
Phase of Nursing Process: Assessment
Client Needs: Physiological Integrity
Content Area: Child Health

Reference
Ashwill, J., & Droske, S. (1997). *Nursing care of children: Principles and practice.* Philadelphia: W. B. Saunders. p. 755.

21. **1**

Rationale: Hirschsprung's disease, also known as congenital aganglionosis or megacolon, is the result of an absence of ganglion cells in the rectum and to varying degrees upward in the colon.

Test-Taking Strategy: Knowledge regarding the pathophysiology associated with Hirschsprung's disease is required to answer this question. If you are unfamiliar with this disorder take time now to review!

Level of Cognitive Ability: Analysis
Phase of Nursing Process: Analysis
Client Needs: Physiological Integrity
Content Area: Child Health

Reference
Ashwill, J., & Droske, S. (1997). *Nursing care of children: Principles and practice.* Philadelphia: W. B. Saunders. p. 735.

22. **4**

Rationale: Chronic constipation beginning in the first month of life resulting in pellet-like or ribbon stools that are foul smelling is a clinical manifestation of this disorder. Delayed passage or absence of meconium stool in the neonatal period is the cardinal sign. Bowel obstruction, especially in the neonatal period, abdominal pain and distention, and failure to thrive are also clinical manifestations.

Test-Taking Strategy: Knowledge regarding the clinical manifestations associated with Hirschsprung's disease is required to answer this question. If you are unfamiliar with these symptoms take time now to review!

Level of Cognitive Ability: Analysis
Phase of Nursing Process: Assessment
Client Needs: Physiological Integrity
Content Area: Child Health

Reference
Ashwill, J., & Droske, S. (1997). *Nursing care of children: Principles and practice.* Philadelphia: W. B. Saunders. pp. 735–736.

23. **4**

Rationale: During the newborn assessment, this defect should be easily identified on-site. However, a rectal thermometer or tube may be necessary to determine patency if meconium is not passed in the first 24 hours after birth. The presence of stool in the urine, vagina, or in a skin dimple should be reported immediately as an indication of abnormal anorectal development. Currant jelly–like stools is not a clinical manifestation of this disorder.

Test-Taking Strategy: Use the definition of the word "imperforate" to assist in answering this question. Note the key word "not" in the stem of the question. This should easily direct you to option 4 as the answer to this question as it is stated. Review the important assessment data associated with this disorder now if you had difficulty with this question!

Level of Cognitive Ability: Analysis
Phase of Nursing Process: Assessment
Client Needs: Physiological Integrity
Content Area: Child Health

Reference
Ashwill, J., & Droske, S. (1997). *Nursing care of children: Principles and practice.* Philadelphia: W. B. Saunders. p. 748.

24. **2**

Rationale: A fresh colostomy stoma will be red and edematous but this will decrease with time. The colostomy site should be pink without evidence of abnormal drainage, swelling, or skin breakdown. The nurse should document these findings since this is a normal expectation. Options 1, 3, and 4 are inappropriate interventions.

Test-Taking Strategy: Knowledge regarding the normal expected findings in a fresh colostomy is required to answer this question. Note the key phrase "returns from surgery." You should expect redness and edema at this time. Review postoperative colostomy assessment now if you had difficulty with this question!

Level of Cognitive Ability: Analysis
Phase of Nursing Process: Implementation
Client Needs: Physiological Integrity
Content Area: Child Health

Reference
Ashwill, J., & Droske, S. (1997). *Nursing care of children: Principles and practice.* Philadelphia: W. B. Saunders. p. 748.

25. **4**

Rationale: Following this surgery, anal dilatation at home by the parents is necessary to achieve and maintain bowel patency. Inserting a glycerin suppository before the dilatation is not a component of this procedure. Options 1, 2, and 3 are accurate instructions and will prevent damage to the rectal mucosa.

Test-Taking Strategy: Note the key word "not" in the stem of the question. Use knowledge regarding this procedure to assist in answering the question. Review this important procedure now if you had difficulty with this question!

Level of Cognitive Ability: Application
Phase of Nursing Process: Implementation
Client Needs: Health Promotion and Maintenance
Content Area: Child Health

Reference
Ashwill, J., & Droske, S. (1997). *Nursing care of children: Principles and practice*. Philadelphia: W. B. Saunders. p. 748.

26. **2**

Rationale: Intussusception occurs when a proximal segment of the bowel prolapses into a distal segment of the bowel. It is a common cause of acute bowel obstruction in infants and young children. It is not an inflammatory process.

Test-Taking Strategy: Knowledge regarding the pathophysiology associated with intussusception is required to answer this question. Recalling that this condition is a telescoping of the bowel will assist in eliminating options 1 and 4. Remember the principles of gravity to assist in directing you to the correct option. Review this disorder now if you had difficulty with this question!

Level of Cognitive Ability: Analysis
Phase of Nursing Process: Analysis
Client Needs: Physiological Integrity
Content Area: Child Health

Reference
Bowden, V., Dickey, S., & Greenberg, C. (1998). *Children and their families: The continuum of care*. Philadelphia: W. B. Saunders. p. 1072.

27. **1**

Rationale: The child with intussusception classically presents with severe abdominal pain that is crampy and intermittent, causing the child to draw in the knees to the chest. Vomiting may be present but it is not projectile. Bright red blood and mucus are passed through the rectum and are commonly described as currant jelly–like stools. Ribbon-like stools are not a manifestation of this disorder.

Test-Taking Strategy: Knowledge related to the clinical manifestations associated with intussusception is required to answer this question. Recalling that a classic manifestation is currant jelly–like stools will assist in directing you to option 1. Review this disorder now if you had difficulty with this question!

Level of Cognitive Ability: Analysis
Phase of Nursing Process: Assessment
Client Needs: Physiological Integrity
Content Area: Child Health

Reference
Bowden, V., Dickey, S., & Greenberg, C. (1998). *Children and their families: The continuum of care*. Philadelphia: W. B. Saunders. p. 1073.

28. **4**

Rationale: The parents of a child with an umbilical hernia need to be instructed in the signs of strangulation. These signs include vomiting, pain, and irreducible mass at the umbilicus. The parents should be instructed to contact the physician immediately if strangulation is suspected.

Test-Taking Strategy: Use the definition of the word "strangulation" to assist in answering this question. This will eliminate options 1 and 2. From the remaining options, use knowledge regarding these signs to assist in answering the question. Review the signs of strangulation now if you had difficulty with this question!

Level of Cognitive Ability: Application
Phase of Nursing Process: Implementation
Client Needs: Physiological Integrity
Content Area: Child Health

Reference
Ashwill, J., & Droske, S. (1997). *Nursing care of children: Principles and practice*. Philadelphia: W. B. Saunders. p. 743.

29. **3**

Rationale: Encopresis is defined as fecal incontinence and is a major concern if the child is constipated. Signs include evidence of soiling clothing, scratching or rubbing the anal area because of irritation, fecal odor without apparent awareness by the child, and social withdrawal.

Test-Taking Strategy: Knowledge regarding the definition of encopresis will easily direct you to option 3. If you are unfamiliar with this disorder, take time now to review!

Level of Cognitive Ability: Analysis
Phase of Nursing Process: Assessment
Client Needs: Physiological Integrity
Content Area: Child Health

Reference
Ashwill, J., & Droske, S. (1997). *Nursing care of children: Principles and practice*. Philadelphia: W. B. Saunders. p. 741.

30. **3**

Rationale: Prevention of the spread of infection is an essential intervention for HAV. This should include enteric precautions for at least 1 week after the onset of jaundice and excellent handwashing. Options 1, 2, and 4 are accurate regarding hepatitis.

Test-Taking Strategy: Note the key word "not" in the stem of the question. Knowledge regarding the routes of transmission for HAV and HBV is required to answer this question. If you are unfamiliar with the routes of transmission, take time now to review. You are likely to find a question related to these concepts on NCLEX-RN!

Level of Cognitive Ability: Application
Phase of Nursing Process: Implementation
Client Needs: Health Promotion and Maintenance
Content Area: Child Health

Reference
Ashwill, J., & Droske, S. (1997). *Nursing care of children: Principles and practice*. Philadelphia: W. B. Saunders. pp. 765–766.

31. **1**

Rationale: Jaundice, if present, is best assessed in the sclera, nailbeds, and mucous membranes. Generalized jaundice will appear in the skin throughout the body. Option 4 is not an appropriate assessment area for the presence of jaundice.

Test-Taking Strategy: Note the key word "best" in the stem of the question. Options 2 and 3 can be eliminated first because jaundice present in the skin is generalized. From the remaining options, recalling that skin discoloration can best be assessed in the nailbeds will direct you to option 1. Review assessment findings related to jaundice now if you had difficulty with this question!

Level of Cognitive Ability: Analysis
Phase of Nursing Process: Assessment
Client Needs: Physiological Integrity
Content Area: Child Health

Reference
Ashwill, J., & Droske, S. (1997). *Nursing care of children: Principles and practice*. Philadelphia: W. B. Saunders. p. 765.

32. 3

Rationale: The child with hepatitis should consume a well-balanced, low-fat diet in order to provide rest to the liver. Options 1, 2, and 4 are components of the home care instructions to the family of a child with hepatitis. Additionally, diapers should not be changed on or near surfaces used for preparing or serving food.

Test-Taking Strategy: Note the key word "not" in the stem of the question. Options 1, 2, and 4 can be easily eliminated by using the basic principles related to standard precautions. If you had difficulty with this question, take time now to review home care instructions to the family of a child with hepatitis!

Level of Cognitive Ability: Application
Phase of Nursing Process: Implementation
Client Needs: Safe, Effective Care Environment
Content Area: Child Health

Reference

Ashwill, J., & Droske, S. (1997). *Nursing care of children: Principles and practice.* Philadelphia: W. B. Saunders. p. 766.

33. 2

Rationale: An EP level equal to or less than 9 µg/dL is considered normal. A level greater than 9 µg/dL is indicative of more frequent screening. A level greater than 15 µg/dL requires nutritional and educational interventions and environmental investigation. A level greater than 20 µg/dL requires pharmacological treatment.

Test-Taking Strategy: Eliminate options 1 and 4 first because they are similar. Knowledge regarding the normal EP level will assist in directing you to option 2. Review these levels now if you are unfamiliar with them!

Level of Cognitive Ability: Analysis
Phase of Nursing Process: Analysis
Client Needs: Physiological Integrity
Content Area: Child Health

Reference

Ashwill, J., & Droske, S. (1997). *Nursing care of children: Principles and practice.* Philadelphia: W. B. Saunders. pp. 337–340.

34. 4

Rationale: EDTA in combination with BAL is a chelating agent that is administered IM for 5 days. It causes lead to be deposited in the bone and excreted via the kidneys. Sodium bicarbonate may be used in salicylate poisoning. Ipecac syrup is used in poisonings to induce vomiting. Activated charcoal is used to decrease absorption in certain poisoning situations.

Test-Taking Strategy: Knowledge regarding the treatment related to lead poisoning is required to answer this question. Review this treatment now if you are unfamiliar with it!

Level of Cognitive Ability: Application
Phase of Nursing Process: Implementation
Client Needs: Physiological Integrity
Content Area: Child Health

Reference

Ashwill, J., & Droske, S. (1997). *Nursing care of children: Principles and practice.* Philadelphia: W. B. Saunders. pp. 337–340.

35. 4

Rationale: The calcium level should be monitored because EDTA enhances the excretion of calcium. Additionally, kidney function tests should be monitored because EDTA is nephrotoxic.

Test-Taking Strategy: Knowledge regarding the adverse effects of this medication is required to answer this question. If you are unfamiliar with this medication, take time now to review!

Level of Cognitive Ability: Analysis
Phase of Nursing Process: Analysis
Client Needs: Physiological Integrity
Content Area: Child Health

Reference

Ashwill, J., & Droske, S. (1997). *Nursing care of children: Principles and practice.* Philadelphia: W. B. Saunders. pp. 337–340.

36. 4

Rationale: Acetylcysteine is the antidote for acetaminophen overdose. It is administered PO with juice of cola or via NG tube. Vitamin K is the antidote for warfarin (Coumadin). Protamine sulfate is the antidote for heparin. EDTA is used in the treatment of lead poisoning.

Test-Taking Strategy: Knowledge regarding the antidote for acetaminophen overdose is required to answer this question. Learn the major antidotes for medication overdose now if you are unfamiliar with them. You are likely to find questions related to antidotes on NCLEX-RN!

Level of Cognitive Ability: Analysis
Phase of Nursing Process: Planning
Client Needs: Physiological Integrity
Content Area: Child Health

Reference

Ashwill, J., & Droske, S. (1997). *Nursing care of children: Principles and practice.* Philadelphia: W. B. Saunders. pp. 337–340.

37. 4

Rationale: The ingestion of salicylates is the most common cause of poisoning in children. A toxic dose is a single dose exceeding 200 to 280 mg/kg. Peak gastric absorption occurs within 2 hours of ingestion.

Test-Taking Strategy: Knowledge regarding the toxic dose of salicylates is required to answer this question. If you had to make a selection and were not sure, it is best in this type of question to select the highest value. Review salicylate toxicity now if you had difficulty with this question. You are likely to find a question related to this type of poisoning on NCLEX-RN!

Level of Cognitive Ability: Analysis
Phase of Nursing Process: Analysis
Client Needs: Physiological Integrity
Content Area: Child Health

Reference

Ashwill, J., & Droske, S. (1997). *Nursing care of children: Principles and practice.* Philadelphia: W. B. Saunders. pp. 337–340.

38. **1**

Rationale: Initial treatment of salicylate overdose includes inducing vomiting with syrup of ipecac or gastric lavage. Activated charcoal may be administered to decrease absorption. IV fluids and sodium bicarbonate may be administered to enhance excretion but would not be the initial treatment. Dialysis is used in extreme cases if the child is unresponsive to therapy. Vitamin K is the antidote for warfarin (Coumadin) overdose.

Test-Taking Strategy: Knowledge regarding the treatment for aspirin overdose is required to answer this question.

Note the key word "initial" in the stem of the question. This key word will assist in directing you to option 1. Review the treatment for this common overdose now if you had difficulty with this question!

Level of Cognitive Ability: Analysis
Phase of Nursing Process: Planning
Client Needs: Physiological Integrity
Content Area: Child Health

Reference
Ashwill, J., & Droske, S. (1997). *Nursing care of children: Principles and practice.* Philadelphia: W. B. Saunders. pp. 337–340.

BIBLIOGRAPHY

Ashwill, J., & Droske, S. (1997). *Nursing care of children: Principles and practice.* Philadelphia: W. B. Saunders.
Bowden, V., Dickey, S., & Greenberg, C. (1998). *Children and their families: The continuum of care.* Philadelphia: W. B. Saunders.
Hodgson, B., & Kizior, R. (1999). *Saunders nursing drug handbook 1999.* Philadelphia: W. B. Saunders.

Lammon, C., Foote, A., Leli, P., et al. (1995). *Clinical nursing skills.* Philadelphia: W. B. Saunders.
Luckmann, J. (1997). *Saunders manual of nursing care.* Philadelphia: W. B. Saunders.
Nichols, F., & Zwelling, E. (1997). *Maternal newborn nursing: Theory and practice.* Philadelphia: W. B. Saunders.
O'Toole, M. (ed.). (1997). *Miller-Keane encyclopedia & dictionary of medicine, nursing, & allied health* (6th ed.). Philadelphia: W. B. Saunders.

CHAPTER 38

Metabolic and Endocrine Disorders

I. Fever

A. Description
1. An abnormal body temperature elevation
2. A child's temperature can vary depending on activity, emotional stress, the type of clothing the child is wearing, and the temperature of the environment
3. Assessment findings associated with fever provide important indications of the seriousness of the fever

B. Assessment
1. Temperature elevation
2. Flushed skin
3. Diaphoresis
4. Chills
5. Restlessness or lethargy

C. Implementation
1. Monitor vital signs
2. Administer a sponge bath with lukewarm water for 20 to 30 minutes
3. Administer antipyretics such as acetaminophen (Tylenol) as prescribed
4. Do not administer aspirin (acetylsalicylic acid, ASA) because of the risk of Reye's syndrome
5. Retake the temperature 30 to 60 minutes after the antipyretic is administered
6. Provide adequate fluid intake as tolerated and as prescribed
7. Monitor for dehydration and fluid and electrolyte imbalance
8. Instruct the parents how to take the temperature, how to safely medicate their child, and when it is necessary to call the physician

II. Dehydration (Box 38–1)

A. Description
1. Dehydration is the most common fluid and electrolyte imbalance in children

2. Infants and children are more vulnerable to fluid-volume deficit because a greater amount of their body water is in the extracellular fluid compartment
3. In infants and children, the organs that conserve water are immature, placing them at risk for fluid-volume deficit
4. The causes can include decreased fluid intake, diaphoresis, vomiting, diarrhea, burns, or malnutrition

B. Assessment
1. Weight loss
2. Dry mucous membranes and decrease in skin turgor
3. Sunken eyeballs and depressed fontanels
4. Decreased urine output and increased urine-specific gravity
5. Absence of tears
6. Decreased blood pressure
7. Tachycardia and tachypnea
8. Excessive thirst
9. Prolonged capillary refill time and increased hemoglobin and hematocrit

C. Implementation
1. Monitor vital signs
2. Monitor skin turgor and for signs of dehydration
3. Monitor weight and monitor for changes including fluid gains and losses

---

BOX 38–1. Types of Dehydration

ISOTONIC DEHYDRATION

Electrolyte and water deficits occur in approximately balanced proportions

HYPERTONIC DEHYDRATION

Water loss exceeds electrolyte loss

HYPOTONIC DEHYDRATION

Electrolyte deficit exceeds water deficit

4. Monitor I&O and urine for specific gravity
5. Administer intravenous (IV) fluids and electrolyte replacements as prescribed if the child is unable to ingest sufficient fluids orally
6. Withhold a full diet until the child is well hydrated and the cause of the dehydration is under control
7. Provide clear liquids orally in small quantities such as 1 to 2 oz every hour

III. Phenylketonuria (PKU)

A. Description
   1. Genetic disorder that results in central nervous system (CNS) damage from toxic levels of phenylalanine in the blood
   2. An autosomal recessive disorder
   3. PKU is characterized by serum phenylalanine levels greater than 25 mg/dL (normal level is less than 2 mg/dL)
   4. All 50 states require routine screening of all newborns for PKU

B. Assessment
   1. In all children
      a. Digestive problems and vomiting
      b. Seizures
      c. Musty or mousy odor of the urine
      d. Mental retardation
   2. In older children
      a. Eczema
      b. Hypertonia
      c. Hypopigmentation of the hair, skin, and irises
      d. Hyperactive behavior

C. Implementation
   1. Screening of newborns for PKU
   2. If initial screening is positive, further diagnostic evaluation is required to verify the diagnosis
   3. Rescreen infants by 14 days of age if initial screen was done before 24 to 48 hours of age
   4. Restrict phenylalanine intake
   5. Monitor physical, neurological, and intellectual development
   6. Stress the importance of follow-up treatment
   7. Encourage parents to express feelings about the diagnosis and the risk of PKU in future children

IV. Insulin-Dependent Diabetes Mellitus (Type 1 DM)

A. Description
   1. Type 1 DM or juvenile-onset diabetes is caused by the partial or complete lack of secretory capacity of the beta cells of the pancreas, resulting in insulin deficiency
   2. Complete insulin deficiency requires the use of exogenous insulin to promote appropriate glucose use and to prevent complications

related to elevated blood glucose levels such as hyperglycemia, diabetic ketoacidosis, and death

B. Assessment
   1. Polyuria, polydipsia, polyphagia
   2. Hyperglycemia
   3. Weight loss
   4. Fruity odor to breath
   5. Dehydration
   6. Blurred vision
   7. Slow wound healing
   8. Weakness
   9. Changes in level of consciousness (LOC)

C. Long-Term Effects
   1. Failure to grow at a normal rate
   2. Delayed maturation
   3. Recurrent infections
   4. Neuropathy
   5. Cardiovascular disease
   6. Retinal microvascular disease
   7. Renal microvascular disease

D. Complications
   1. Hyperglycemia
   2. Hypoglycemia
   3. Diabetic ketoacidosis
   4. Coma
   5. Hypokalemia
   6. Hyperkalemia
   7. Microvascular changes
   8. Cardiovascular changes

E. Diet
   1. Total amount of calories are individualized based on the child's age and **growth** expectations
   2. As prescribed by the physician, the child may be instructed to follow the food exchange from the American Diabetic Association diet or the dietary guidelines for Americans (Food Guide Pyramid) issued by the U.S. Departments of Agriculture and Health Services
   3. Incorporate the diet into the individual child's needs, likes and dislikes, lifestyle, cultural, and socioeconomic patterns
   4. Allow the child to participate in making food choices to provide a sense of control

F. Exercise
   1. Instruct the child in dietary adjustments when exercising
   2. Extra food needs to be consumed for increased activity, usually 10 to 15 g of carbohydrate for every 30 to 45 minutes of activity
   3. Instruct the child to monitor blood glucose before exercising
   4. Plan with the child an appropriate exercise regimen incorporating the developmental stage

G. Insulin
   1. Diluted insulin may be required for some infants to provide small enough dosages to avoid hypoglycemia

2. Diluted insulin should be clearly labeled to avoid dosage errors

3. To prevent dosage errors, be certain that there is a match of the insulin concentration with the calibration of units on the insulin syringe

4. Illness, infection, and stress increase the need for insulin, and insulin should not be withheld during illness, infection, or stress because hyperglycemia and ketoacidosis can result

5. Instruct the parents and child to recognize symptoms of hypoglycemia and hyperglycemia

6. Orange juice; sugar-sweetened beverages, or hard candy should be kept available and administered if a hypoglycemic reaction occurs

7. Instruct the child and parents in the administration of the insulin

8. Instruct the parents in administering glucagon by injection if the child has a hypoglycemic reaction and is unable to drink sugar-containing fluid

9. Instruct the parents to always have a spare bottle of insulin available

10. Advise the parents to obtain a Medic-Alert bracelet indicating the type and daily insulin dosage

H. Blood Glucose Monitoring
   1. Results provide the parents with information to maintain good glycemic control
   2. More accurate than urine testing
   3. Requires children to prick themselves several times a day as prescribed
   4. Instruct the parents and child in the proper procedure for obtaining the blood glucose level
   5. Inform the parents and child that the procedure must be done precisely to obtain accurate results
   6. Stress the importance of handwashing before and after performing the procedure to prevent infection
   7. Stress the importance of following the manufacturer's instructions
   8. Instruct the parents and child to calibrate the monitor as instructed by the manufacturer
   9. Instruct the parents and child to check the expiration date on the test strips
   10. Instruct the parents and child that if blood glucose results do not seem reasonable, reread the instructions, reassess technique, check the expiration date of the test strips, and perform the procedure again to verify results

I. Urine Testing
   1. Instruct the parents and child in the procedure for testing urine for ketones and glucose
   2. Teach the child that the second voided urine specimen is most accurate

3. The presence of ketones may indicate impending ketoacidosis

4. Urine glucose testing is not recommended as the only means of monitoring the child who is taking insulin, because it is a less reliable indicator compared with blood glucose monitoring

J. Hypoglycemia
   1. Description
      a. Described as a blood glucose level below 60 mg/dL
      b. Occurs as a result of too much insulin, not enough food, or excessive activity
   2. Mild hypoglycemia
      a. Provide 15 g of carbohydrate and repeat the treatment in 10 to 15 minutes if symptoms do not subside
      b. Instruct the child to eat additional food or the next scheduled meal in 15 to 30 minutes
   3. Moderate hypoglycemia
      a. Provide 15 to 30 g of carbohydrate and repeat the treatment in 10 to 15 minutes if symptoms do not subside
      b. Instruct the child to eat additional food such as low-fat milk or cheese after 15 to 30 minutes
   4. Severe hypoglycemia (loss of consciousness)
      a. Administer intramuscular (IM) or subcutaneous (SC) glucagon or dextrose IV as prescribed
      b. Administer a second dose if the child remains unconscious
      c. Provide a small meal when the child wakes up and is no longer nauseated
      d. Instruct the parents on the administration of glucagon

K. Hyperglycemia
   1. Description: elevated blood glucose level over 200 mg/dL
   2. Implementation: instruct the parents to notify the physician when blood sugar results are greater than 200 mg/dL, when moderate or high ketonuria is present, when unable to take food or fluids, and when illness persists

L. Diabetic Ketoacidosis (DKA)
   1. Description
      a. A complication of diabetes mellitus that develops when a severe insulin deficiency occurs
      b. DKA is a life-threatening condition
      c. Hyperglycemia that progresses to metabolic acidosis occurs
      d. It develops over a period of several hours to days
      e. Serum glucose level over 300 mg/dL and urine and serum ketones positive
   2. Implementation
      a. Restore circulating volume and protect against cerebral, coronary, or renal hypoperfusion

- Always give insulin even if the child does not have an appetite, or contact the physician for specific instructions
- Test blood glucose levels at least every 4 hours
- Test for urinary ketones with each voiding
- Notify the physician if moderate or large amounts of urinary ketones are present
- Follow the child's usual meal plan
- Encourage calorie-free liquids to aid in clearing ketones
- Encourage rest, especially if urinary ketones are present
- Notify the physician if vomiting, fruity odor to the breath, deep rapid respirations, decreasing level of consciousness, or persistent hyperglycemia occurs

b. Correct hyperglycemia with IV regular insulin administration as prescribed
c. Monitor vital signs, urine output, and mental status closely
d. Correct dehydration with IV infusions of 0.9%, or 0.45% normal saline as prescribed
e. Correct acidosis
f. Correct electrolyte imbalance
g. Administer oxygen as prescribed
h. Monitor blood glucose closely
i. Monitor the child closely for signs of fluid overload
j. Monitor potassium closely because when the child receives insulin to lower the blood sugar level, the serum potassium will decrease as the acidosis improves, and potassium replacement may then be required
k. IV dextrose is added as prescribed when the blood sugar reaches an appropriate level
l. Treat the cause of hyperglycemia (Box 38–2)

PRACTICE QUESTIONS

1. The nurse is gathering supplies in preparation to administer a tepid bath to a child with a fever. Which of the following items is not necessary?
   1 Washcloths and towels
   2 A bottle of alcohol
   3 Toys
   4 Lightweight pajamas

2. A cooling blanket is prescribed for a child with a fever. The nurse caring for the child has never used this type of equipment. The charge nurse provides instructions to the nurse and assists the nurse assigned to the child. Which of the following is not a part of the instructions in the use of the cooling blanket?
   1 Place the cooling blanket on the bed and cover it with a sheet
   2 Check the skin condition of the child before, during, and after the use of the cooling blanket
   3 Keep the child uncovered to assist in reducing the fever
   4 Keep the child dry while on the cooling blanket to prevent the risk of frostbite

3. A nursing student is assigned to admit a child that has been experiencing vomiting and diarrhea. The physician documents a diagnosis of gastroenteritis and isotonic dehydration. The nursing instructor asks the student to describe isotonic dehydration. The appropriate response is:
   1 "It occurs when water and electrolytes are lost in approximately the same proportion as they exist in the body."
   2 "It occurs when the loss of electrolytes is greater than the loss of water."
   3 "It occurs when the loss of water is greater than the loss of electrolytes."
   4 "It causes the serum sodium level to rise above 150 mEq/L."

4. The clinic nurse is assessing a child for dehydration. The nurse documents that the child is moderately dehydrated. Which of the following symptoms is included in determining this assessment finding?
   1 Flat fontanels
   2 Dry mucous membranes
   3 Pale skin color
   4 Oliguria

5. The physician orders IV potassium for a child with hypertonic dehydration. Which of the following assessments is of the highest priority before administering the potassium?
   1 Temperature
   2 Blood pressure
   3 Weight
   4 Urine output

6. The pediatric nurse educator provides a teaching session to the nursing staff regarding phenylketonuria (PKU). Which of the following is included in the teaching session?
   1 PKU is an autosomal dominant disorder
   2 Treatment includes dietary restriction of tyramine
   3 All 50 states require routine screening of all newborns for PKU
   4 PKU primarily affects the gastrointestinal system

7. The mother brings her 3-week-old infant to the clinic for a PKU rescreening blood test. The results of the test indicate a serum phenylalanine level of 1 mg/dL. The nurse interprets these results as:
   1 Inconclusive
   2 Requiring rescreening at age 6 weeks
   3 Positive
   4 Negative

8. A school-aged child with insulin-dependent diabetes mellitus, (type 1 DM) has soccer practice three afternoons a week. The school nurse provides instructions regarding how to prevent hypoglycemia during practice. Which of the following is the most appropriate instruction?
   1 To take one half of the amount of prescribed insulin on practice days
   2 To eat twice the amount normally eaten at lunchtime
   3 To take the prescribed insulin at noontime rather than in the morning
   4 To eat six graham crackers or a cup of orange juice before soccer practice

9. An adolescent with diabetes is attending a dance in the school gym. The child becomes flushed and complains of hunger and dizziness. The school nurse is at the dance. The nurse takes the child to the nurse's office and performs a blood glucose level that measures 60 mg/dL. The most appropriate intervention is:
   1 Send the child home
   2 Call the physician
   3 Give the child a glass of juice
   4 Let the child rest until the dizziness subsides

10. The home care nurse is teaching an adolescent with type 1 DM regarding insulin administration and rotation sites. Which of the following statements, if made by the adolescent, indicates effective teaching?
   1 "I need to use one major site for the morning injection and another site for the evening injection for 2 to 3 weeks before changing major sites."
   2 "I need to use a different site for each insulin injection."
   3 "I need to use the same site for 1 month before rotating to another site."
   4 "I should use my stomach and my thighs only for injections."

11. The mother of a 6-year-old type 1 DM calls the clinic nurse and tells the nurse that the child has been sick. The mother reports that she checked the child's urine and it showed positive ketones. Which of the following does the nurse instruct the mother to do?
    1 Come to the clinic immediately
    2 Hold the next dose of insulin
    3 Administer an additional dose of regular insulin
    4 Encourage the child to drink calorie-free liquids

12. A diabetic child is brought to the emergency room by the mother, who states that the child has been complaining of abdominal pain and has a fruity odor on the breath. Diabetic ketoacidosis (DKA) is diagnosed. The nurse prepares to administer:
    1 5% dextrose IV infusion
    2 0.9% normal saline IV infusion
    3 NPH insulin IV
    4 Potassium IV

ANSWERS

1. 2

Rationale: Alcohol should never be used for bathing the child with a fever because it can cause rapid cooling, peripheral vasoconstriction, and chilling, thus elevating the temperature further. Washcloths can be used to squeeze water over the child's body. Towels are used to dry the child. Toys, especially water toys can be used to provide distraction during the bath. Lightweight clothing should be placed on the child after the child is dried.

Test-Taking Strategy: Options 1 and 4 can be easily eliminated. From the remaining options, select option 2 over option 3 because of the harmful effects of alcohol and the effect of potentially elevating the temperature. Review the procedure for administering a tepid bath now if you had difficulty with this question!

Level of Cognitive Ability: Application
Phase of Nursing Process: Implementation
Client Needs: Physiological Integrity
Content Area: Child Health

Reference
Ashwill, J., & Droske, S. (1997). *Nursing care of children: Principles and practice.* Philadelphia: W. B. Saunders. p. 458.

2. 3

Rationale: While on a cooling blanket, the child should be covered lightly to maintain privacy and reduce shivering. Options 1, 2, and 4 are important interventions to prevent shivering, frostbite, and skin breakdown.

Test-Taking Strategy: Knowledge regarding the physiological response associated with fever is helpful in answering this question. Use the process of elimination to assist in directing you to option 3. Review the procedure associated with the use of a cooling blanket now if you had difficulty with this question!

Level of Cognitive Ability: Application
Phase of Nursing Process: Implementation
Client Needs: Physiological Integrity
Content Area: Child Health

Reference
Ashwill, J. & Droske, S. (1997). *Nursing care of children: Principles and practice.* Philadelphia: W. B. Saunders. p. 459.

3. 1

Rationale: Isotonic dehydration occurs when water and electrolytes are lost in approximately the same proportion as they exist in the body. In this type of dehydration, the serum sodium levels remain normal (135–145 mEq/L). Option 2 describes hypotonic dehydration, and in this type the serum sodium level is less than 130 mEq/L. Options 3 and 4 describe hypertonic dehydration.

Test-Taking Strategy: Knowledge regarding the various types of dehydration is required to answer this question. However, thinking about the terms "hypotonic" and "hypertonic" and relating these terms to losses or excesses, may assist you to eliminate options 2, 3, and 4. Review these types of dehydration now if you had difficulty with this question!

Level of Cognitive Ability: Analysis
Phase of Nursing Process: Evaluation
Client Needs: Physiological Integrity
Content Area: Child Health

Reference

Bowden, V., Dickey, S., & Greenberg, C. (1998). *Children and their families: The continuum of care.* Philadelphia: W. B. Saunders. p. 1000.

4. 4

Rationale: In moderate dehydration, the fontanels are slightly sunken, the mucous membranes are very dry, and the skin color is dusky. Options 1, 2, and 3 describe mild dehydration. In mild dehydration, urine output is decreased but oliguria is not present.

Test-Taking Strategy: Note the key word "moderately." This key phrase will assist in eliminating options 1, 2, and 3. Knowing that dehydration is classified as mild, moderate, or severe will direct you to selecting option 4, which is the clinical manifestation of greatest concern from those presented in all options. Review the manifestations related to mild, moderate, and severe dehydration now if you had difficulty with this question!

Level of Cognitive Ability: Analysis
Phase of Nursing Process: Assessment
Client Needs: Physiological Integrity
Content Area: Child Health

Reference

Ashwill, J., & Droske, S. (1997). *Nursing care of children: Principles and practice.* Philadelphia: W. B. Saunders. p. 681.

5. 4

Rationale: The priority assessment is to assess the status of urine output. Potassium should never be administered in the presence of oliguria or anuria. If urine output is less than 1 to 2 mL/kg/hour, it should not be administered.

Test-Taking Strategy: Knowledge regarding the effects of potassium on various organ systems is required to answer the question. Knowledge that the kidneys play a key role in the excretion and reabsorption of potassium will easily direct you to option 4. Review this important medication now if you had difficulty with this question!

Level of Cognitive Ability: Analysis
Phase of Nursing Process: Assessment
Client Needs: Physiological Integrity
Content Area: Child Health

Reference

Ashwill, J., & Droske, S. (1997). *Nursing care of children: Principles and practice.* Philadelphia: W. B. Saunders. p. 681.

6. 3

Rationale: PKU is an autosomal recessive disorder. Treatment includes dietary restriction of phenylalanine intake.

PKU is a genetic disorder that results in central nervous system (CNS) damage from toxic levels of phenylalanine in the blood. Option 3 is accurate.

Test-Taking Strategy: Knowledge regarding PKU is required to answer the question. Recalling that PKU is a recessive disorder will assist in eliminating option 1. Reading option 2 carefully will direct you to eliminate this option because tyramine is restricted in clients on monoamine oxidase inhibitors (MAOIs), not in PKU. Recalling that PKU affects the CNS will direct you in selecting option 3. Review the characteristics associated with this disorder now if you had difficulty with this question!

Level of Cognitive Ability: Application
Phase of Nursing Process: Implementation
Client Needs: Physiological Integrity
Content Area: Child Health

Reference

Ashwill, J., & Droske, S. (1997). *Nursing care of children: Principles and practice.* Philadelphia: W. B. Saunders. p. 565.

7. 4

Rationale: PKU is characterized by serum phenylalanine levels greater than 25 mg/dL. A normal level is less than 2 mg/dL. A result of 1 mg/dL is a negative test result.

Test-Taking Strategy: Knowledge regarding the normal serum phenylalanine level is required to answer this question. Note that the level identified in the question is a low level. This should assist in directing you to option 4. Review this important screening test now if you had difficulty with this question!

Level of Cognitive Ability: Analysis
Phase of Nursing Process: Analysis
Client Needs: Physiological Integrity
Content Area: Child Health

Reference

Ashwill, J., & Droske, S. (1997). *Nursing care of children: Principles and practice.* Philadelphia: W. B. Saunders. p. 566.

8. 4

Rationale: An extra snack of 15 to 30 g of carbohydrate eaten before activities such as soccer practice will prevent hypoglycemia. Six graham crackers or a cup of orange juice will provide 15 to 30 g of carbohydrate. The child or parents should not be instructed to adjust the amount or time of insulin administration. Meal amounts should not be doubled.

Test-Taking Strategy: Options 1 and 3 can be eliminated first because insulin dosages and times should not be adjusted. From the remaining options, recalling the manifestations and treatment associated with hypoglycemia will direct you to option 4. Review treatment to prevent hypoglycemia now if you had difficulty with this question!

Level of Cognitive Ability: Application
Phase of Nursing Process: Implementation
Client Needs: Physiological Integrity
Content Area: Child Health

Reference

Ashwill, J., & Droske, S. (1997). *Nursing care of children: Principles and practice.* Philadelphia: W. B. Saunders. p. 1199.

9. 3

Rationale: A blood glucose below 70 mg/dL indicates hypoglycemia. The child is attending an activity that is different from the normal routine at school. Insulin requirements change with unfamiliar situations. When signs of hypoglycemia occur, the child needs an immediate source of sugar. Options 1, 2, and 4 do not address the hypoglycemic state immediately.

Test-Taking Strategy: Identify the issue of the question, which is a hypoglycemic state and the key phrase "most appropriate." The stem of the question is requiring you to interpret the situation as a hypoglycemic state and determining the appropriate action. Options 1, 2, and 4 do not address treatment of the hypoglycemic state. If you had difficulty with this question, take time now to review the assessment data associated with hypoglycemia!

Level of Cognitive Ability: Application
Phase of Nursing Process: Implementation
Client Needs: Physiological Integrity
Content Area: Child Health

Reference
Ashwill, J., & Droske, S. (1997). *Nursing care of children: Principles and practice.* Philadelphia: W. B. Saunders. p. 1197.

10. 1

Rationale: To help decrease variations in absorption from day to day, the child should use one location within a major site for the morning injection, rotating to another site for the evening injection, and a third site for the bedtime injection for a period of 2 to 3 weeks before changing major sites.

Test-Taking Strategy: Eliminate option 4 first because of the word "only." From the remaining options, it is necessary to know the physiology associated with absorption of insulin. If you had difficulty with this question, take time now to review insulin administration!

Level of Cognitive Ability: Analysis
Phase of Nursing Process: Evaluation
Client Needs: Physiological Integrity
Content Area: Child Health

Reference:
Ashwill, J., & Droske, S. (1997). *Nursing care of children: Principles and practice.* Philadelphia: W. B. Saunders. p. 1200.

11. 4

Rationale: When the child is sick, the mother should test the child for urinary ketones with each voiding. If ketones are present, liquids are essential to aid in clearing. The child should be encouraged to drink calorie-free liquids. It is not necessary to bring the child to the clinic immediately. Insulin doses should not be adjusted or changed.

Test-Taking Strategy: Eliminate options 2 and 3 first because insulin doses should not be adjusted or changed. From the remaining options, note the phrase "positive ketones." This finding does not require immediate physician referral. Review home care instructions for the sick diabetic child now if you had difficulty with this question!

Level of Cognitive Ability: Application
Phase of Nursing Process: Implementation
Client Needs: Physiological Integrity
Content Area: Child Health

Reference
Ashwill, J., & Droske, S. (1997). *Nursing care of children: Principles and practice.* Philadelphia: W. B. Saunders. p. 1208.

12. 2

Rationale: Rehydration is the initial step in resolving DKA. Normal saline is the initial IV rehydration fluid. NPH insulin is never administered by IV. Dextrose solutions are added to the treatment when the blood glucose levels reach an acceptable level. IV potassium may be required depending on the potassium levels, but is not part of the initial treatment.

Test-Taking Strategy: Eliminate option 1, knowing that dextrose would not be administered in a hyperglycemic state. Eliminate option 3 next, knowing that NPH insulin is never administered by IV. Knowledge that hydration is the initial treatment in DKA will easily direct you to option 2. Review the treatment for this important condition now if you had difficulty with this question!

Level of Cognitive Ability: Analysis
Phase of Nursing Process: Planning
Client Needs: Physiological Integrity
Content Area: Child Health

Reference
Ashwill, J., & Droske, S. (1997). *Nursing care of children: Principles and practice.* Philadelphia: W. B. Saunders. p. 1209.

BIBLIOGRAPHY

Ashwill, J., & Droske, S. (1997). *Nursing care of children: Principles and practice.* Philadelphia: W. B. Saunders.
Bowden, V., Dickey, S., & Greenberg, C. (1998). *Children and their families: The continuum of care.* Philadelphia: W. B. Saunders.
Hodgson, B., & Kizior, R. (1999). *Saunders nursing drug handbook 1999.* Philadelphia: W. B. Saunders.

Lammon, C., Foote, A., Leli, P., et al. (1995). *Clinical nursing skills.* Philadelphia: W. B. Saunders.
Luckmann, J. (1997). *Saunders manual of nursing care.* Philadelphia: W. B. Saunders.
Nichols, F., & Zwelling, E. (1997). *Maternal newborn nursing: Theory and practice.* Philadelphia: W. B. Saunders.
O'Toole, M. (ed.). (1997). *Miller-Keane encyclopedia & dictionary of medicine, nursing, & allied health* (6th ed.). Philadelphia: W. B. Saunders.

CHAPTER 39

Renal and Urinary Disorders

I. Glomerulonephritis

A. Description
1. A term that includes a variety of disorders, most of which are caused by an immunological reaction
2. It results in proliferative and inflammatory changes within the glomerular structure
3. Destruction, inflammation, and sclerosis of the glomeruli of both kidneys occur
4. Inflammation of the glomeruli results from an antigen-antibody reaction produced from an infection elsewhere in the body
5. Loss of kidney function develops

B. Causes
1. Immunological diseases
2. Autoimmune diseases
3. Streptococcal infection, group A beta-hemolytic
4. History of pharyngitis or tonsillitis 2 to 3 weeks prior to symptoms

C. Types
1. Acute: Occurs 2 to 3 weeks after a streptococcal infection
2. Chronic: Can occur after the acute phase or slowly over time

D. Complications
1. Heart failure
2. Hypertensive encephalopathy
3. Pulmonary edema
4. Renal failure

E. Assessment
1. Client is pale and irritable
2. Gross hematuria or dark, smoky, cola-colored or red-brown urine
3. Proteinuria that produces a persistent and excessive foam in the urine
4. Oliguria or anuria
5. Urinary debris, mid to high specific gravity, low urinary pH
6. Increased BUN and creatinine
7. Increased antistreptolysin O titer (used to diagnose disorders caused by streptococcal infections)
8. Shortness of breath
9. Headache
10. Chills and fever
11. Fatigue and weakness
12. Anorexia, nausea, and vomiting
13. Reduced visual acuity
14. Abdominal or flank pain
15. Edema in the face and periorbital area, feet, or generalized
16. Hypertension
17. Ascites, pleural effusion, and congestive heart failure (CHF)

F. Implementation
1. Monitor vital signs
2. Monitor intake and output (I&O) and urine closely
3. Restrict fluid intake as prescribed
4. Monitor daily weight
5. Restrict sodium intake as prescribed if edema is present
6. Provide a high-calorie and low-protein diet
7. Monitor for edema and fluid overload, ascites, pulmonary edema, and CHF
8. Provide bed rest and limited activity
9. Administer diuretics, antihypertensives, and antibiotics as prescribed
10. Monitor for signs of renal failure, cardiac failure, and hypertensive encephalopathy
11. Initiate seizure precautions as indicated
12. Provide safety measures
13. Instruct parents to report signs of bloody urine, headache, or edema
14. Instruct parents that child needs to obtain treatment for infections, specifically sore throats and upper respiratory infections

II. Nephrotic Syndrome

A. Description: A set of clinical manifestations

469

arising from protein wasting secondary to diffuse glomerular damage

B. Assessment
   1. Pale, irritable, and fatigued child
   2. Child gains weight
   3. Decreased urine output
   4. Dark, frothy urine; hematuria may be present
   5. Abdominal ascites
   6. Proteinuria
   7. Hypoalbuminemia
   8. Edema
   9. Hyperlipidemia
   10. Waxy pallor of the skin
   11. Hypertension
   12. Anorexia
   13. Anemia
   14. Amenorrhea or abnormal menses

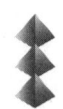

C. Implementation
   1. Monitor vital signs
   2. Monitor I&O and daily weights
   3. Maintain bed rest if severe edema is present
   4. Provide normal to low-protein diet as prescribed, with adequate carbohydrate and calorie intake
   5. Provide a mild sodium restriction as prescribed
   6. Monitor the potassium level; potassium may be restricted from the diet if the potassium level rises, or it may be added to the diet if the level falls because of the administration of diuretics
   7. Administer diuretics as prescribed
   8. Administer steroids and cytotoxic medications as prescribed
   9. Administer plasma volume expanders such as albumin, plasma, and dextran as prescribed to raise the osmotic pressure

III. Enuresis

A. Description
   1. Refers to a condition in which the child is unable to control bladder function although the child has reached an age at which control of voiding is expected
   2. By age 5 years, most children are aware of bladder fullness and are able to control voiding
B. Primary Nocturnal Enuresis
   1. A child who has not been dry at night for a prolonged period of time
   2. Common in children, and most children will eventually outgrow bed-wetting without therapeutic intervention
   3. The child is not able to sense a full bladder and does not awaken to void
   4. The child may have delayed maturation of the central nervous system (CNS)
C. Secondary or Acquired Enuresis
   1. The child who starts having problems with wetting when previously the child has been dry

   2. The child may have problems with daytime control and complaints of dysuria, urgency, or frequency
   3. The child should be assessed for urinary tract infections
D. Assessment
   1. Normal daytime voiding pattern
   2. History of bed-wetting with no prolonged period of dryness in a child older than age 5 years
E. Implementation
   1. Obtain urinalysis and urine culture as prescribed to rule out infection or existing disorder
   2. Involve child in caring for the wet sheets and changing the bed, to assist the child to take ownership of the problem
   3. Limit fluid intake at night, and encourage the child to void just before going to bed
   4. Assist the family with identifying a treatment plan that will best fit their needs
   5. Provide reward systems as appropriate for the child
   6. Incorporate behavioral conditioning techniques
   7. Encourage follow-up to determine the effectiveness of the treatment

IV. Cryptorchidism

A. Description: Occurs when one or both testes fail to descend through the inguinal canal into the scrotal sac
B. Assessment: Testes not palpable nor easily guided into the scrotum
C. Implementation
   1. Monitor during the first 12 months of life to determine whether spontaneous descent occurs
   2. After age 1 year, medical or surgical treatment may be instituted
   3. Human chorionic gonadotropin (hCG), a pituitary hormone that stimulates the production of testosterone, may be prescribed
   4. Surgical correction is done by orchiopexy
   5. Monitor for bleeding and infection if surgery is performed

V. Hypospadias/Epispadias

A. Description: Congenital defects involving abnormal placement of the urethral orifice of the penis
B. Assessment
   1. Hypospadias: Urethral orifice located below the glans penis along the ventral surface
   2. Epispadias: Urethral orifice located on the dorsal surface of the penis
   3. Surgical implementation
      a. Done before the age of toilet training
      b. Children with hypospadias should not be circumcised because the foreskin may be used in surgical reconstruction

4. Implementation postoperatively
   a. The child will have some type of urinary diversion to allow time for healing of the meatus
   b. Monitor vital signs
   c. Encourage high fluid intake
   d. Monitor urine for cloudiness or a foul smell
   e. Restrict activity for several days
   f. Instruct parents in the care of the urinary diversion if present

VI. Bladder Exstrophy

A. Description
   1. A congenital anomaly characterized by extrusion of the urinary bladder to the outside of the body through a defect in the lower abdominal wall
   2. The cause is not known
   3. Treatment requires surgical management and occurs in a series of staged reconstructions
   4. Initial surgery for closure of the abdominal defect should occur within the first few days of life
   5. The goal of subsequent operations is to reconstruct the bladder and genitalia and enable the child to achieve urinary continence
B. Assessment
   1. Exposed bladder mucosa
   2. Displaced anal opening
   3. Widened symphysis pubis
   4. Defects of the external genitalia
C. Implementation
   1. Assess patency of the anus
   2. Monitor adequacy of urine output
   3. Maintain integrity of the exposed bladder mucosa until surgical closure is performed
   4. Assess for urinary continence and history of urinary tract infections (UTIs) in the older child
   5. At birth, care should be taken to protect the exposed bladder tissue from drying while allowing the drainage of urine
   6. Cover the bladder with a nonadhering plastic wrap
   7. Avoid the use of petroleum jelly gauze because this type of dressing can dry out, adhere to the mucosa, and damage the delicate tissues when the dressing is removed
   8. Monitor laboratory values and urinalysis to assess for renal function
   9. Administer antibiotics as prescribed
   10. Provide emotional support to the parents
   11. Encourage parents to verbalize their fears and concerns

PRACTICE QUESTIONS

1. The nurse interviews the parents of a child recently diagnosed with glomerulonephritis. Which finding collected by the nurse is most often associated with the diagnosis of glomerulonephritis?
   1 Strep throat 2 weeks prior to diagnosis
   2 Child fell off a bike onto the handlebars
   3 Nausea and vomiting for the last 24 hours
   4 Urticaria and itching for 1 week prior to diagnosis

2. The nurse completes a history and physical assessment and reviews the laboratory findings on a child admitted for suspected glomerulonephritis. Which of the following findings is associated with the diagnosis of glomerulonephritis?
   1 Elevated BUN
   2 Postural hypotension
   3 Low urinary specific gravity
   4 Dark brown or rust-colored urine

3. The nurse is caring for a 7-year-old child diagnosed with acute glomerulonephritis. A priority nursing intervention that should be included in the nursing care plan is:
   1 Promote adequate bed rest while providing for quiet play
   2 Catheterize the child to monitor intake and output strictly
   3 Force oral fluids to prevent hypovolemic shock
   4 Encourage classmates to visit and to keep the child informed of school events

4. A nurse is caring for a seven-year old child with glomerulonephritis and discusses the plan of care with the parents. A common reaction of parents to the diagnosis of glomerulonephritis is:
   1 Fear of the complicated treatment regimen
   2 Anger at the child for requiring hospitalization
   3 Guilt that they did not seek treatment more quickly
   4 Depression that the child may not be able to play sports

5. The nurse is performing an admission assessment on a 2-year-old child who has been diagnosed with nephrotic syndrome. The nurse assesses for the most common characteristic associated with nephrotic syndrome, which is:
   1 Generalized edema
   2 Frank blood in urine
   3 Increased urinary output
   4 Hypotension

6. The nurse is preparing a 2-year-old child with suspected nephrotic syndrome for a renal biopsy to confirm the diagnosis. The mother asks the nurse, "Will my child ever look thin again?" How should the nurse respond?
   1 "Wearing loose-fitting clothing should help conceal the extra weight."
   2 "In most cases, medication and diet will control fluid retention."
   3 "Do you feel guilty because you didn't notice the weight gain?"
   4 "When children are little, it's expected they'll look a little chubby."

7. The nurse is preparing a care plan for a 4-year-old child hospitalized with nephrotic syndrome. Which intervention regarding diet therapy is most appropriate?
   1 Provide a high-protein, high-salt diet
   2 Discourage visitors at mealtimes
   3 Encourage the child to eat in the playroom with others
   4 Maintain a full liquid diet during the acute phase

8. The nurse is caring for a 6-year-old child with nephrotic syndrome. As part of the care plan to reduce proteinuria, the nurse would most likely administer which prescribed medication?
   1 Prazosin hydrochloride (Minipress)
   2 Furosemide (Lasix)
   3 Prednisone (Deltasone)
   4 Cyclophosphamide (Cytoxan)

9. A 7-year-old child is seen in the clinic, and the primary health care provider documents a diagnosis of primary nocturnal enuresis. The mother asks the nurse about the diagnosis. The nurse bases the response on the fact that primary nocturnal enuresis:
   1 Requires surgical intervention to improve the problem
   2 Is caused by a psychiatric problem
   3 Is common and most children will outgrow bed-wetting without therapeutic intervention
   4 Does not respond to treatment

10. The nurse is caring for an 8-month-old infant. A urinalysis has been ordered, and the nurse plans to collect the specimen. Which of the following methods is most appropriate?
    1 Catheterize the infant, using a No. 5 French Foley
    2 Obtain the specimen from the diaper, using a syringe, after the infant voids
    3 Attach a urinary collection device to the infant's perineum
    4 Monitor the urinary patterns and prepare to collect the specimen into a cup when the infant voids

11. The nurse is caring for an infant with cryptorchidism. The nurse anticipates that the most likely diagnostic studies to be prescribed are those that assess:
    1 Kidney function
    2 Babinski's reflex
    3 DNA synthesis
    4 Chromosomal analysis

12. The child with cryptorchidism is being discharged following orchiopexy, which was performed on an outpatient basis. What care measure should take priority in the plan of care at home?

   1 Administration of analgesics
   2 Measurement of intake and output
   3 Application of cold to surgical site
   4 Prevention of infection at surgical site

13. The nurse is caring for a 2-year-old child who has been admitted to correct cryptorchidism. The highest priority in the postoperative nursing care for this child is to:
    1 Force oral fluids
    2 Prevent tension on the suture
    3 Test urine for glucose
    4 Encourage coughing

14. The nurse has completed discharge instructions for a 2-year-old child who has had an orchiopexy to correct cyptorchidism. Which of the following statements, if made by the mother of the child, indicates that further teaching is necessary?
    1 "I'll check his temperature and report a fever of 102°F."
    2 "I'll let him decide when to return to his usual activities."
    3 "I'll give him medication so he'll be comfortable."
    4 "I'll check his voiding to be sure there's no problem."

15. The nurse collects a urine specimen preoperatively from a child with epispadias who is scheduled for surgical repair. When analyzing the results of the urinalysis, which of the following will the nurse most likely expect to note?
    1 Hematuria
    2 Proteinuria
    3 Bacteriuria
    4 Glucosuria

16. A 1-year-old child with hypospadias is scheduled for surgery to correct this condition. The nurse prepares a nursing care plan for this child and understands that this surgery is taking place at a time when:
    1 Fears of separation and mutilation are great
    2 Sibling rivalry will cause regression to occur
    3 Embarrassment about voiding irregularities is common
    4 Concern over the size and function of the penis is present

17. An 18-month-old child is being discharged following surgical repair of hypospadias. Which postoperative nursing care measure should the nurse stress to the parents as they prepare to take this child home?
    1 Encourage toilet-training to ensure that the flow of urine is normal
    2 Restrict fluid intake to reduce urinary output for the first few days
    3 Caution parents not to hold the child by straddling him on their hips
    4 Leave diapers off for the first 48 hours to allow the site to heal

18. The nurse is reviewing the treatment plan for a newborn infant with hypospadias. The infant is being discharged with the parents. Which statement by the parents indicates their understanding of the eventual outcome?
    1 "Circumcision has been delayed to save tissue for surgical repair."
    2 "Catheterization will be necessary when the baby does not void."
    3 "Caution should be used when straddling the infant on a hip."
    4 "Vital signs should be taken daily to check for bladder infection."

19. The parents of a newborn have been told that their child was born with bladder exstrophy. The parents ask the nurse about this condition. The nurse bases the response on knowledge that this condition is:
    1 Caused by the use of medications taken by the mother during pregnancy
    2 A hereditary disorder that occurs in every other generation
    3 A condition in which the urinary bladder is abnormally located in the pelvic cavity

4 An extrusion of the urinary bladder to the outside of the body through a defect in the lower abdominal wall

20. Following an assessment of an infant with bladder exstrophy, the nurse prepares the plan of care. Which of the following nursing diagnoses is the priority for an infant with this disorder?
    1 Alteration in Elimination
    2 Impaired Tissue Integrity
    3 Parental Knowledge Deficit
    4 Potential for Infection

21. The nurse is caring for an infant with a diagnosis of bladder exstrophy. The most appropriate intervention to protect the exposed bladder tissue from drying is to:
    1 Cover the bladder with petroleum jelly gauze
    2 Keep the bladder tissue dry by covering it with dry sterile gauze
    3 Cover the bladder with a nonadhering plastic wrap
    4 Apply sterile distilled water dressings over the bladder mucosa

ANSWERS

1. **1**

Rationale: Group A beta-hemolytic streptococcal infection is a cause of glomerulonephritis. Often the child becomes ill with streptococcal infection of the upper respiratory tract and then develops symptoms of acute poststreptococcal glomerulonephritis after an interval of 1 to 2 weeks. The assessment data in options 2, 3, and 4 are unrelated to a diagnosis of glomerulonephritis.

Test-Taking Strategy: Knowledge regarding the causes of glomerulonephritis is required to answer the question. Use the process of elimination and this knowledge to answer the question. Option 2 relates to a kidney injury. Options 3 and 4 are not related to the diagnosis of glomerulonephritis. A strep infection 1 to 2 weeks prior to the development of glomerulonephritis is the classic assessment finding. If you had difficulty with this question, take time now to review the causes of glomerulonephritis!

Level of Cognitive Ability: Analysis
Phase of Nursing Process: Assessment
Client Needs: Physiological Integrity
Content Area: Child Health

Reference
Luckmann, J. (1997). *Saunders manual of nursing care.* Philadelphia: W. B. Saunders. p. 1200.

2. **4**

Rationale: Gross hematuria resulting in dark brown or rust-colored urine is a classic symptom of glomerulonephritis. Hypertension is also common. BUN levels are elevated only when there is an 80% decrease in glomerular filtration rate. A mid to high urinary specific gravity is associated with glomerulonephritis.

Test-Taking Strategy: Knowledge regarding the assessment findings associated with glomerulonephritis is required to answer this question. Eliminate options 2 and 3 first because hypertension and a high specific gravity are most likely to occur in this kidney disorder. Knowledge that BUN levels elevate only when there is an 80% decrease in the glomerular filtration rate will assist in directing you to the correct option, option 4. If you had difficulty with this question, take time now to review the clinical manifestations associated with glomerulonephritis.

Level of Cognitive Ability: Analysis
Phase of Nursing Process: Analysis
Client Needs: Physiological Integrity
Content Area: Child Health

Reference
Luckmann, J. (1997). *Saunders manual of nursing care.* Philadelphia: W. B. Saunders. p. 1201.

3. **1**

Rationale: Bed rest is required during the acute phase, and activity is gradually increased as the condition improves. Providing for quiet play according to the developmental stage of the child is important. Catheterization may cause a risk of infection. Fluids should not be forced. Visitors should be limited to allow for adequate rest.

Test-Taking Strategy: Use the process of elimination to answer the question. Option 4 may be accurate for many illnesses and the developmental needs of the sick child should always be considered, but in this case, rest is the priority over socialization. Monitoring of intake and output is essential, but the risk of infection could occur with catheterization. Although fluids should be offered throughout the day, intake must reflect output and should not be restricted or forced. Review the appropriate nursing interventions for the child with glomerulonephritis, if you had difficulty with this question!

Level of Cognitive Ability: Application
Phase of Nursing Process: Implementation
Client Needs: Physiological Integrity
Content Area: Child Health

Reference
Ashwill, J., & Droske, S. (1997). *Nursing care of children: Principles and practice.* Philadelphia: W. B. Saunders. p. 785.

4. **3**

Rationale: Guilt is a common reaction of the parents of a child diagnosed with glomerulonephritis. They blame themselves for not responding more quickly to the child's initial symptoms, or they may believe they could have prevented the development of glomerular damage.

Test-Taking Strategy: Use the process of elimination to answer the question. The question asks about the common reaction of the parents. Options 1 and 2 may be plausible, but are not the likely concerns. In option 4, the parents may feel somewhat depressed at the prospect of restricted activities, but again, this is not the common concern.

Level of Cognitive Ability: Application
Phase of Nursing Process: Implementation
Client Needs: Psychosocial Integrity
Content Area: Child Health

Reference
Ashwill, J., & Droske, S. (1997). *Nursing care of children: Principles and practice.* Philadelphia: W. B. Saunders. p. 785.

5. **1**

Rationale: Massive edema resulting in dramatic weight gain is a characteristic finding in nephrotic syndrome. Urine is dark, foamy, and frothy, but only microscopic hematuria is present; frank bleeding does not occur. Urine output is decreased, and hypertension is likely to be present.

Test-Taking Strategy: Use knowledge regarding the characteristics of nephrotic syndrome and the process of elimination to answer the question. Eliminate options 3 and 4 first, as urine output is most likely to be decreased in a renal disorder, and hypertension is more likely to be present. Associate generalized edema with nephrotic syndrome, as this will be helpful to you if you encounter a similar question on NCLEX-RN. If you had difficulty with this question, take time now to review the characteristics of nephrotic syndrome!

Level of Cognitive Ability: Application
Phase of Nursing Process: Assessment
Client Needs: Physiological Integrity
Content Area: Child Health

Reference
Ashwill, J., & Droske, S. (1997). *Nursing care of children: Principles and practice.* Philadelphia: W. B. Saunders. p. 789.

6. **2**

Rationale: Most children experience remission with treatment and corticosteroids. Diuretics may also be a component of the treatment plan, and a restricted sodium diet is recommended. It is important to give the parent information in a matter-of-fact manner and address the issue that is the parent's concern. Options 1, 3, and 4 do not address the parent's concern.

Test-Taking Strategy: The client of the question is the parent. Options 1 and 3 are nontherapeutic, adding to the mother's guilt and putting down her concern. Option 4 doesn't acknowledge the concern and is a stereotypical answer. Utilize therapeutic communication techniques and always address the client's feelings and concerns.

Level of Cognitive Ability: Application
Phase of Nursing Process: Implementation
Client Needs: Psychosocial Integrity
Content Area: Child Health

Reference
Ashwill, J., & Droske, S. (1997). *Nursing care of children: Principles and practice.* Philadelphia: W. B. Saunders. p. 790.

7. **3**

Rationale: Mealtimes should center on pleasurable socialization. Encourage the child to eat meals with other children on the unit. A diet that is normal in protein with a mild sodium restriction is normally prescribed.

Test-Taking Strategy: Use the process of elimination to answer the question. Eliminate options 1 and 4 first. A diet that is normal in protein with a mild sodium restriction is normally prescribed. Option 2 diminishes the importance of socialization at mealtime. This leaves option 3 as the correct option. If you had difficulty with this question, take time now to review the diet normally prescribed for the child with nephrotic syndrome!

Level of Cognitive Ability: Application
Phase of Nursing Process: Planning
Client Needs: Psychosocial Integrity
Content Area: Child Health

Reference
Luckmann, J. (1997). *Saunders manual of nursing care.* Philadelphia: W. B. Saunders. p. 1205.

8. **2**

Rationale: The child is usually placed on diuretic therapy until protein loss is controlled. Corticosteroids, such as prednisone, may be prescribed to decrease inflammation. Corticosteroids also suppress the autoimmune response and stimulate vascular reabsorption of edema. Cyclophosphamide is an alkylating agent and may be used in maintaining remission. Prazosin hydrochloride (Minipress) is most commonly used to control hypertension.

Test-Taking Strategy: Use the process of elimination and knowledge regarding the actions of the medications to answer the question. Take time now to review the pharmacological treatments associated with nephrotic syndrome, if you had difficulty with this question. Additionally, review the actions and purposes of the medications listed in the options if you are unfamiliar with them!

Level of Cognitive Ability: Application
Phase of Nursing Process: Implementation
Client Needs: Physiological Integrity
Content Area: Child Health

References
Luckmann, J. (1997). *Saunders manual of nursing care.* Philadelphia: W. B. Saunders. p. 1204.
Ashwill, J., & Droske, S. (1997). *Nursing care of children: Principles and practice.* Philadelphia: W. B. Saunders. p. 790.

9. **3**

Rationale: Primary nocturnal enuresis occurs in a child who has not been dry at night for a prolonged period. It is common in children, and most children will eventually outgrow bed-wetting without therapeutic intervention. The child is not able to sense a full bladder and does not awaken to void. The child may have delayed maturation of the central nervous system. It is not caused by a psychiatric problem.

Test-Taking Strategy: Knowledge regarding the characteristics of enuresis is required to answer the question. Enuresis is common in children and, based on this knowledge, you would be directed to the correct option. If you had difficulty with this question, take time now to review the characteristics associated with enuresis!

Level of Cognitive Ability: Application
Phase of Nursing Process: Implementation
Client Needs: Physiological Integrity
Content Area: Child Health

Reference
Ashwill, J., & Droske, S. (1997). *Nursing care of children: Principles and practice.* Philadelphia: W. B. Saunders. pp. 794–795.

10. **3**

Rationale: Although many methods have been used to collect urine from an infant, the most reliable method is the urine collection device. This device is a plastic bag with an opening lined with adhesive so that it may be attached to the perineum. Urine for certain tests, such as specific gravity, may be obtained from a diaper. Urinary catheterization is not to be done unless specifically prescribed because of the risk of infection. It is not reasonable to monitor urinary patterns and attempt to collect the specimen in a cup when the infant voids.

Test-Taking Strategy: Use the process of elimination to answer the question. Note the key phrase "most appropriate." Eliminate option 4, as this is unrealistic. Eliminate option 1, as catheterization is not prescribed and the risk of infection exists with this procedure. Eliminate option 2, because only certain tests can be obtained from the urine in a diaper. If you had difficulty with this question, take time now to review the procedure for collecting urine specimens from an infant and an incontinent child!

Level of Cognitive Ability: Application
Phase of Nursing Process: Implementation
Client Needs: Safe, Effective Care Environment
Content Area: Child Health

Reference
Ashwill, J., & Droske, S. (1997). *Nursing care of children: Principles and practice.* Philadelphia: W. B. Saunders. pp. 443–445.

11. **1**

Rationale: Cryptorchidism may be the result of hormone deficiency, intrinsic abnormality of a testis, or a structural problem. Diagnostic tests would assess kidney function, since the kidneys and testes arise from the same germ tissue. Babinski's reflex tests neurological function. DNA synthesis and a chromosomal analysis are unrelated to this diagnosis.

Test-Taking Strategy: Use the process of elimination and your knowledge regarding the anatomical occurrence of cryptorchidism to answer the question. Cryptorchidism, undescended or hidden testicles, relates to the genitourinary system. Option 2 relates to neurological function. Options 3 and 4 relate to the structure of cells. Option 1 is the only option that relates to the genitourinary system!

Level of Cognitive Ability: Analysis
Phase of Nursing Process: Analysis
Client Needs: Physiological Integrity
Content Area: Child Health

Reference
Ball, J., & Bindler, R. (1995). *Pediatric nursing: Caring for children.* Norwalk, CT: Appleton & Lange. p. 624.

12. **4**

Rationale: The most common complications associated with orchiopexy are bleeding and infection. Discharge instruction should include demonstration of proper wound cleansing and dressing, and teaching parents to identify signs of infection such as redness, warmth, swelling, or discharge. Testicles will be held in a position to prevent movement, and great care should be taken to prevent contamination of the suture line.

Test-Taking Strategy: Note the word "priority" in the stem of the question. Utilize Maslow's Hierarchy of Needs theory to answer the question. Of the options presented, the potential for infection is the physiological priority. Option 1 is important, but not the priority, given the options listed. Use of cold, as suggested in option 3 is not necessary. Measurement of intake and output in option 2 is not required.

Level of Cognitive Ability: Application
Phase of Nursing Process: Planning
Client Needs: Safe, Effective Care Environment
Content Area: Child Health

Reference
Ashwill, J., & Droske, S. (1997). *Nursing care of children: Principles and practice.* Philadelphia: W. B. Saunders. p. 798.

13. **2**

Rationale: When a child returns from surgery, the testicle is held in position by an internal suture that passes through the testes and scrotum and is attached to the thigh. It is important not to dislodge this suture, and it should be immobilized for 1 week.

Test-Taking Strategy: Read the question carefully, noting that the priority nursing action is specific to this type of surgery. Knowledge regarding this type of surgery would be helpful in answering the question. Depending on the type of anesthesia used, option 4 may be appropriate, but it is not the priority. Although it is important to maintain adequate hydration, it is not necessary to force fluids. Testing urine for glucose is also not related to surgery. If you had difficulty with this question, take time now to review nursing care following the surgical correction of cryptorchidism!

Level of Cognitive Ability: Application
Phase of Nursing Process: Implementation
Client Needs: Physiological Integrity
Content Area: Child Health

Reference
Ashwill, J., & Droske, S. (1997). *Nursing care of children: Principles and practice.* Philadelphia: W. B. Saunders. p. 798.

14. **2**

Rationale: The child's activity should be restricted for 3 to 7 days after surgery to promote healing and prevent injury. This will prevent dislodging of the suture, which is internal. Normally, 2 year olds will want to be very active, and it may be difficult to restrict activities. The parent should be taught to monitor the temperature, provide analgesics as needed, and monitor the urine output.

Test-Taking Strategy: Read the stem of the question carefully, and use the process of elimination to identify the correct option to this question, as stated. Option 1 is an important action in order to recognize signs of infection. Option 3 is appropriate to keep pain to a minimum. Option 4 monitors the voiding pattern, which is also important following surgery. If you had difficulty with this question, take time now to review the discharge instructions following surgical correction of cryptorchidism!

Level of Cognitive Ability: Analysis
Phase of Nursing Process: Evaluation
Client Needs: Health Promotion and Maintenance
Content Area: Child Health

Reference
Ashwill, J., & Droske, S. (1997). *Nursing care of children: Principles and practice.* Philadelphia: W. B. Saunders. p. 798.

15. **3**

Rationale: Epispadias is a congenital malformation with absence of the upper wall of the urethra. The urethral opening is located anywhere on the dorsum of the penis. This anatomical characteristic leads to the easy entry of bacteria into the urine.

Test-Taking Strategy: Use knowledge regarding the anatomical characteristic of epispadias and the process of elimination to answer the question. Options 1, 2, and 4 do not relate to the potential for infection that is present in the condition of epispadias. If you had difficulty with this question, take time now to review the diagnostic findings associated with epispadias!

Level of Cognitive Ability: Analysis
Phase of Nursing Process: Analysis
Client Needs: Physiological Integrity
Content Area: Child Health

Reference
O'Toole, M. (ed.) (1997). *Miller-Keane encyclopedia & dictionary of medicine, nursing and allied health* (6th ed.). Philadelphia: W. B. Saunders. p. 547.

16. **1**

Rationale: At the age of 1 year, a child's fears of separation and mutilation are great, since the child is facing the developmental task of trusting others. As the child gets older, fears about virility and reproductive ability may surface.

Test-Taking Strategy: Use knowledge regarding the stages of growth and development to answer the question. Do not read into the question. The question does not provide enough data to determine that siblings exist. Options 3 and 4 may be issues when the child is older. If you had difficulty with this question, take time now to review the stages of growth and development. Questions related to growth and development are likely to appear on NCLEX-RN!

Level of Cognitive Ability: Application
Phase of Nursing Process: Planning
Client Needs: Psychosocial Integrity
Content Area: Child Health

Reference
Ashwill, J., & Droske, S. (1997). *Nursing care of children: Principles and practice.* Philadelphia: W. B. Saunders. p. 353.

17. **3**

Rationale: Parent teaching following hypospadias repair includes restricting the child from activities that put pressure on the surgical site. The parents should be instructed to use double diapers to hold the stent in place and should be instructed how to hold the child during the postoperative period. Fluids should be encouraged to maintain hydration. Toilet-training should not be an issue during this stressful period.

Test-Taking Strategy: Use the process of elimination to answer the question. Option 1 is incorrect since toilet-training should not be initiated during times of stress, such as following surgery. Option 2 is inappropriate since fluids should be encouraged rather than restricted. Option 4 is not the best answer since contamination of the surgical site could occur. Double diapers is better to hold the stent in place. If you had difficulty with this question, take time now to review the postoperative care following surgical repair of hypospadias!

Level of Cognitive Ability: Application
Phase of Nursing Process: Implementation
Client Needs: Health Promotion and Maintenance
Content Area: Child Health

Reference
Ashwill, J., & Droske, S. (1997). *Nursing care of children: Principles and practice.* Philadelphia: W. B. Saunders. p. 799.

18. **1**

Rationale: The infant should not be circumcised because the dorsal foreskin tissue will be used for surgical repair of the hypospadias. This defect will most likely be corrected during the first year of life to limit the psychological effects on the child.

Test-Taking Strategy: Read the question carefully, recalling that surgery will be planned for this infant during the first year of life. Option 3 is important in the postoperative period, not before surgery. Vital signs do not need to be taken daily. Catheterization, option 2, will only increase the risk of infection. Take time now to review the surgical procedure related to the repair of the hypospadias, if you had difficulty with this question!

Level of Cognitive Ability: Analysis
Phase of Nursing Process: Evaluation
Client Needs: Physiological Integrity
Content Area: Child Health

Reference
Ashwill, J., & Droske, S. (1997). *Nursing care of children: Principles and practice.* Philadelphia: W. B. Saunders. p. 799.

19. **4**

Rationale: Bladder exstrophy is a congenital anomaly characterized by the extrusion of the urinary bladder to the outside of the body through a defect in the lower abdominal wall. The cause is not known, and a higher incidence occurs in the male.

Test-Taking Strategy: Use knowledge regarding the characteristics of bladder exstrophy to answer the question. If you are unfamiliar with this condition, note the relationship of "ex"strophy to the word "ex"trusion in the correct option. This should provide you with the hint that this condition is located external to the body. If you had difficulty with this question, take time now to review the characteristics of bladder exstrophy!

Level of Cognitive Ability: Application
Phase of Nursing Process: Implementation
Client Needs: Physiological Integrity
Content Area: Child Health

Reference
Ashwill, J., & Droske, S. (1997). *Nursing care of children: Principles and practice.* Philadelphia: W. B. Saunders. pp. 800–801.

20. **2**

Rationale: In bladder exstrophy, the bladder is exposed and external to the body. The highest priority is impaired tissue integrity related to the exposed bladder mucosa. Although the infant needs to be monitored for elimination patterns and kidney function, this is not the priority concern for this condition. Parental knowledge deficit related to the diagnosis and treatment of the condition will need to be addressed, but again is not the priority. Although infection related to the anatomically located defect is an appropriate nursing diagnosis, it is a potential problem and not an actual one.

Test-Taking Strategy: Use the process of elimination to answer the question. Eliminate option 4 first as this addresses a potential problem rather than an actual one. Eliminate option 3 next because physiological needs take precedence over psychosocial needs. Knowledge that the bladder mucosa is exposed in this condition should direct you to the correct answer from the remaining two options.

Level of Cognitive Ability: Analysis
Phase of Nursing Process: Planning
Client Needs: Physiological Integrity
Content Area: Child Health

Reference
Ashwill, J., & Droske, S. (1997). *Nursing care of children: Principles and practice.* Philadelphia: W. B. Saunders. p. 801.

21. **3**

Rationale: Care should be taken to protect the exposed bladder tissue from drying while allowing drainage of urine. This is best accomplished by covering the bladder with a nonadhering plastic wrap. The use of petroleum jelly gauze should be avoided because this type of dressing can dry out, adhere to the mucosa, and damage the delicate tissue when removed. Dry sterile dressings and dressings soaked in solutions can also dry out and damage the mucosa when removed.

Test-Taking Strategy: Use the process of elimination in answering the question. Note the similarities in options 1, 2, and 4. These types of dressings can dry out and cause damage to the bladder mucosa. Note the key word in the correct option, "nonadhering." If you had difficulty with this question, take time now to review care to the infant with bladder exstrophy!

Level of Cognitive Ability: Application
Phase of Nursing Process: Implementation
Client Needs: Physiological Integrity
Content Area: Child Health

Reference
Ashwill, J., & Droske, S. (1997). *Nursing care of children: Principles and practice.* Philadelphia: W. B. Saunders. pp. 794–795.

BIBLIOGRAPHY

Ashwill, J., & Droske, S. (1997). *Nursing care of children: Principles and practice.* Philadelphia: W. B. Saunders.

Ball, J., & Bindler, R. (1995). *Pediatric nursing: Caring for children.* Norwalk, CT: Appleton & Lange.

Luckmann, J. (1997). *Saunders manual of nursing care.* Philadelphia: W. B. Saunders.

O'Toole, M. (ed.) (1997). *Miller-Keane encyclopedia & dictionary of medicine, nursing and allied health* (6th ed.). Philadelphia: W. B. Saunders.

CHAPTER 40

Integumentary Disorders

I. Eczema

A. Description
   1. A superficial inflammatory process involving primarily the epidermis
   2. A common allergic reaction in children
   3. Childhood eczema often begins in infancy, and the rash appears on the face, neck, and folds of elbows and knees
   4. May persist for several years or return after the child is older
   5. Sometimes caused by an allergic sensitivity to foods such as milk, fish, or eggs
B. Assessment
   1. Redness
   2. Itching
   3. Minute papules and vesicles
   4. Weeping, oozing, and crusting of lesions
C. Implementation
   1. Identify cause
   2. Alleviate itching by soothing baths or moisturizing creams
   3. Administer topical steroids and oral antihistamines as prescribed

II. Impetigo

A. Description
   1. Incubation period: 7 to 10 days
   2. Infectious period: during the course of the infection
   3. Transmission: contact
   4. Season: summer
B. Assessment
   1. Small, red macules that progress to vesicles and rupture and release serous fluid
   2. Located around the mouth and nose and may be present on the extremities
C. Implementation
   1. Contact isolation
   2. Apply topical antibiotics and administer oral antibiotics as prescribed

III. Pediculosis Capitis (Lice)

A. Description
   1. Incubation period: eggs incubate for about 1 week and lice reach sexual maturity in about 2 weeks
   2. Infectious period: during infestation before treatment
   3. Transmission: direct contact with infected person and indirect contact with infected person's belongings
   4. Season: nonspecific, a common problem in schools
B. Assessment
   1. Adult lice are difficult to see, and are small gray specks that may crawl very fast
   2. Nits are visible and firmly attached to the hair shaft near the scalp, and are tiny silver or gray specks resembling dandruff
   3. Implementation: antilice shampoo and medications

IV. Scabies

A. Description
   1. Incubation period
      a. Female mite burrows into epidermis, lays eggs, and dies in the burrow after 4 to 5 weeks
      b. The eggs hatch in 3 to 5 days and larvae migrate to the skin to mature and complete their life cycle
   2. Infectious period: during the course of the infestation
   3. Transmission: by personal contact with infected person
   4. Season: any time of year
B. Assessment
   1. Intense pruritus, especially at night
   2. Burrows (fine grayish red lines that may be difficult to see) on the skin

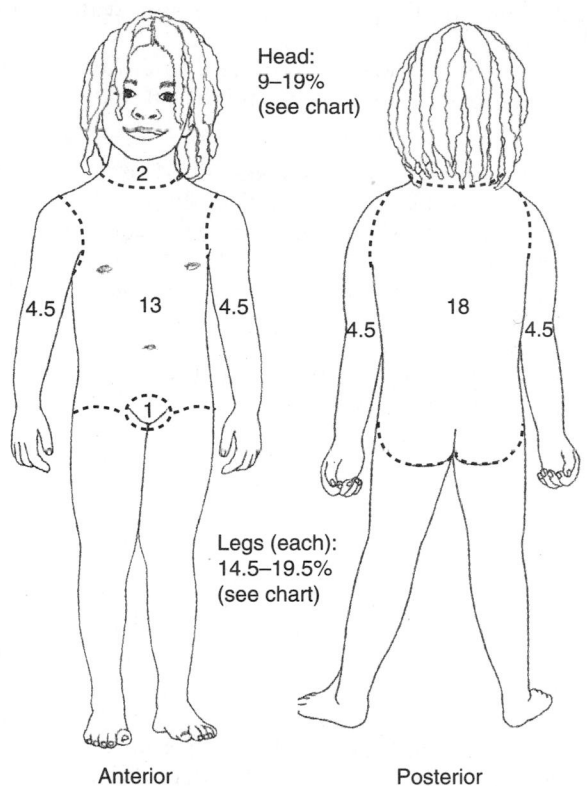

Head:
9–19%
(see chart)

4.5   13   4.5

2

1

18

4.5   4.5

Legs (each):
14.5–19.5%
(see chart)

Anterior   Posterior

Child Burn Size Estimation Table
(percent total body surface area)

Burn area	Age (years)				
	1	1–4	5–9	10–14	15
Head	19	17	13	11	9
Neck	2	2	2	2	2
Anterior trunk	13	13	13	13	13
Posterior trunk	18	18	18	18	18
Genitalia	1	1	1	1	1
Upper extremity (each)	9	9	9	9	9
Lower extremity (each)	14.5	15.5	17.5	18.5	19.5

FIGURE 40–1. Calculating total body surface area (TBSA) burned in children. The standard Rule of Nines and standard body surface charts must be adapted because of the difference in body proportions between adults and children. (Child Burn Size Estimation Table reprinted from Lund, C. C., & Browder, N. C. [1944]. Estimation of burn size. Surg Gynecol Obstet 79: 352–358. By permission of Surgery, Gynecology, and Obstetrics, now known as the *Journal of the American College of Surgeons*.)

C. Implementation
　　1. Topical application of either lindane cream (Kwell, Scabene) crotamiton (Eurax), or permethrin 5% (Elimite)
　　2. Lindane cream (Kwell, Scabene), should not be used in children younger than age 2 because of the risk of neurotoxicity
　　3. Contacts of the infected individual need to be treated

V. The Burned Child

A. Pediatric Differences
　　1. Very young children who have been severely burned have a higher mortality rate than older children and adults with comparable burns
　　2. Lower burn temperatures and shorter exposure to heat can cause a more severe burn in a child than in an adult because a child's skin is thinner
　　3. Severely burned children are at increased risk for fluid and heat loss, dehydration, and metabolic acidosis than in an adult
　　4. The higher proportion of body fluid to mass in children increases the risk of cardiovascular problems
　　5. Burns involving greater than 10% total body surface area (TBSA) require some form of fluid resuscitation
　　6. Infants and children are at increased risk for protein and calorie deficiency because they have smaller muscle mass and lower body fat than adults
　　7. Scarring is more severe in a child
　　8. An immature immune system presents an increased risk of infection for infants and young children
　　9. A delay in **growth** may occur following a burn
B. Extent of Burn Injury
　　1. The Rule of Nines gives an inaccurate estimate because of the differences in body proportion between children and adults (Fig. 40–1)
　　2. The Lund and Browder method to estimate the extent of burn injury provides a body surface chart corrected for age
C. Parkland Formula of Fluid Resuscitation (Box 40–1)

BOX 40–1. Parkland Formula of Fluid Resuscitation

4 mL Ringer's lactate solution × kg of body weight × % TBSA burned

One half of the total is administered in the first 8 hours postburn

One quarter of the total is administered in the second 8 hours postburn

One quarter of the total is administered in the third 8 hours postburn

Time is calculated from the time of injury, not the time of admission

The criterion for successful burn, shock, and fluid resuscitation is based on an hourly urine output of 1 mL/1 kg/hour in children

PRACTICE QUESTIONS

1. Corticream is prescribed by the physician for a child with atopic dermatitis (eczema). The nurse instructs the mother how to appropriately apply the cream. Which of the following instructions does the nurse provide to the mother?
   1 Avoid cleansing the area before applying the cream
   2 Apply the cream over the entire body
   3 Apply a thin layer of cream and rub into the area thoroughly
   4 Apply a thick layer of cream in affected areas only

2. The school nurse provides an instructional session to parents of the children attending the school regarding impetigo. Which of the following is not a component of the instructional session?
   1 It is most common in humid weather
   2 It begins in an area of broken skin, such as an insect bite
   3 It is extremely contagious
   4 Lesions are most often located on the arms and chest

3. The clinic nurse provides instructions to the mother of a child with impetigo regarding the application of antibiotic ointment. The mother asks the nurse when the child can return to school. The most appropriate response is:
   1 Twenty-four hours after using antibiotic ointment
   2 Forty-eight hours after using antibiotic ointment
   3 One week after using antibiotic ointment
   4 Ten days after using antibiotic ointment

4. The school nurse prepares instructions regarding the use of permethrin 1% (Nix) for the parents of the children diagnosed with pediculosis (head lice). Which of the following is not included in the instructions?
   1 The Nix can be obtained over-the-counter in a local pharmacy
   2 It is applied to the hair after shampooing and left on for 24 hours
   3 It is applied to the hair after shampooing, left on for 10 minutes, and then rinsed out
   4 The hair should not be shampooed for 24 hours following treatment

5. The school nurse prepares a list of home care instructions for the parents of the school children diagnosed with pediculosis. Which of the following is included in this list?
   1 Use antilice sprays on all bedding and furniture
   2 Take all bedding and linens to the cleaners to be dry cleaned

3 Boil combs and brushes in hot water for 1 hour
4 Vacuum floors, play areas, and furniture to remove any hairs that might carry live nits

6. The mother of a 3-year-old child arrives at the clinic and tells the nurse that the child has been continuously scratching the skin and has developed a rash. The nurse assesses the child and suspects the presence of scabies. Which of the following most accurately describes the presence of this infestation?
   1 Clusters of fluid-filled vesicles
   2 Fine thread-like lines
   3 Purple-colored lesions
   4 Thick, honey-colored crusts

7. Permethrin 5% (Elimite) is prescribed for a 4-year-old child with a diagnosis of scabies. The clinic nurse instructs the mother regarding the use of this treatment. Which of the following instructions does the nurse provide to the mother?
   1 The lotion should be applied from head to toe
   2 Apply the lotion and leave on for 4 hours
   3 Apply the lotion to cool dry skin at least ½ hour after bathing
   4 Avoid clothing the child while the lotion is in place

8. A 2-year-old child is admitted to the burn unit with partial and full-thickness burns over 35% of the body. Following admission assessment, the priority nursing intervention focuses on:
   1 Sedating with morphine sulfate
   2 Restricting IV fluids
   3 Inserting a nasogastric tube
   4 Inserting a Foley catheter

9. A 10-kg child sustains a burn from a house fire and the total body surface area (TBSA) is determined to be 50%. The Parkland formula of fluid resuscitation is used to determine the amount of fluid that this child requires. How many milliliters of fluid will the child receive in the first 8 hours from the time of the injury?
   1 250 mL
   2 500 mL
   3 750 mL
   4 1000 mL

10. The nurse is monitoring a burned child during treatment for burn shock. Which of the following assessments provides the most accurate guide to the adequacy of fluid resuscitation?
    1 Skin turgor
    2 Level of edema at burn site
    3 Adequacy of peripheral pulses
    4 Neurological assessment

ANSWERS

1. **3**

Rationale: Corticream is a topical corticosteroid. It should be applied sparingly and rubbed into the area thoroughly. The affected area should be cleansed gently before application. It should not be applied over extensive areas. Systemic absorption is more likely to occur with extensive application.

Test-Taking Strategy: Knowledge regarding the application of steroid cream is required to answer this question. Eliminate option 1 because it does not make sense not to cleanse an affected area. Eliminate option 2 because cream should be applied only to areas that are affected. Eliminate option 4 because of the word "thick." Review the procedure for application of this cream now if you had difficulty with this question!

Level of Cognitive Ability: Application
Phase of Nursing Process: Implementation
Client Needs: Physiological Integrity
Content Area: Pharmacology

Reference
Hodgson, B., & Kizior, R. (1999). *Saunders nursing drug handbook 1999.* Philadelphia: W. B. Saunders. pp. 498–500.

2. **4**

Rationale: Impetigo is most common during hot, humid summer months. It begins in an area of broken skin, such as an insect bite, scabies, or atopic dermatitis. It may be caused by *Staphylococcus aureus,* group A betahemolytic streptococci, or a combination of these bacteria. It is extremely contagious. Lesions are usually located around the mouth and nose, but may be present on the extremities.

Test-Taking Strategy: Knowledge regarding the etiology and manifestations are required to answer this question. Impetigo is the most common skin infection of childhood, and if you are unfamiliar with this disorder take time now to review!

Level of Cognitive Ability: Application
Phase of Nursing Process: Implementation
Client Needs: Health, Promotion and Maintenance
Content Area: Child Health

Reference
Ashwill, J., & Droske, S. (1997). *Nursing care of children: Principles and practice.* Philadelphia: W. B. Saunders. p. 1032.

3. **2**

Rationale: The child should not attend school for 24 to 48 hours after the initiation of systemic antibiotics or 48 hours after using antibiotic ointment. The school should be notified of the diagnosis.

Test-Taking Strategy: Use knowledge related to the administration of antibiotics to answer the question. Eliminate options 3 and 4 first as the time frames are closely related and rather lengthy. Note the key word "ointment" in the stem of the question; this should assist in directing you to option 2.

Level of Cognitive Ability: Application
Phase of Nursing Process: Implementation
Client Needs: Safe, Effective Care Environment
Content Area: Child Health

Reference
Ashwill, J., & Droske, S. (1997). *Nursing care of children: Principles and practice.* Philadelphia: W. B. Saunders. p. 1032.

4. **2**

Rationale: Nix is an over-the-counter antilice product that kills both lice and eggs with one application and has residual activity for 10 days. It is applied to the hair after shampooing and left for 10 minutes before rinsing out. The hair should not be shampooed for 24 hours after the treatment.

Test-Taking Strategy: Note the key word "not" in the stem of the question. This should assist in directing you, by the process of elimination, to option 2. If you are unfamiliar with this treatment, take time now to review. Pediculosis is one of the largest and most exasperating problems in schools!

Level of Cognitive Ability: Application
Phase of Nursing Process: Implementation
Client Needs: Physiological Integrity
Content Area: Child Health

Reference
Ashwill, J., & Droske, S. (1997). *Nursing care of children: Principles and practice.* Philadelphia: W. B. Saunders. p. 1042.

5. **4**

Rationale: Antilice sprays are unnecessary. Additionally, they should never be used on a child. Bedding and linens should be washed with hot water and dried on a hot setting. Items that cannot be washed should be dry cleaned or sealed in plastic bags in a warm place for 3 weeks. Combs and brushes should be boiled or soaked in antilice shampoo or hot water for 15 minutes. Thorough home cleaning is necessary to remove any remaining lice or nits.

Test-Taking Strategy: Eliminate option 1, knowing that antilice sprays should not be used. Knowing that bedding and linens can be washed will eliminate option 2. The time for boiling in option 3 is rather lengthy; therefore, eliminate this option. If you had difficulty with this question, take time now to review these important home care instructions!

Level of Cognitive Ability: Application
Phase of Nursing Process: Implementation
Client Needs: Safe, Effective Care Environment
Content Area: Child Health

Reference
Ashwill, J., & Droske, S. (1997). *Nursing care of children: Principles and practice.* Philadelphia: W. B. Saunders. p. 1042.

6. **2**

Rationale: Scabies appears as burrows or fine, grayish thread-like lines. They may be difficult to see if they are obscured by excoriation and inflammation. Clusters of fluid-filled vesicles are seen in herpesvirus. Thick, honey-colored crusts are characteristic of impetigo. Purple-colored lesions may be indicative of various disorders, including systemic conditions.

Test-Taking Strategy: Knowledge that scabies infestation produces burrows will assist in directing you to option 2. If you are unfamiliar with the clinical manifestations associated with scabies, take time now to review!

Level of Cognitive Ability: Analysis
Phase of Nursing Process: Assessment
Client Needs: Physiological Integrity
Content Area: Child Health

Reference
Ashwill, J., & Droske, S. (1997). *Nursing care of children: Principles and practice*. Philadelphia: W. B. Saunders. p. 1043.

7. 3

Rationale: Permethrin is applied from the neck downward, making sure the soles of the feet, behind the ears, and under the toenails and fingernails are covered. The lotion should be kept on for 8 to 14 hours, and then the child should be given a bath. The lotion should not be applied for at least one-half hour after bathing and should be applied only to cool, dry skin. The child should be clothed during treatment.

Test-Taking Strategy: Options 1 and 4 can be easily eliminated. Knowledge regarding the treatment time will assist in directing you to option 3. Take time now to review this treatment if you had difficulty with this question!
Level of Cognitive Ability: Application
Phase of Nursing Process: Implementation
Client Needs: Physiological Integrity
Content Area: Child Health

Reference
Ashwill, J., & Droske, S. (1997). *Nursing care of children: Principles and practice*. Philadelphia: W. B. Saunders. p. 1044.

8. 4

Rationale: A Foley catheter is inserted into the child's bladder so that urine output can be accurately measured on an hourly basis. Although pain medication may be required, the child should not be sedated. IV fluids are not restricted and are administered at a rate sufficient to keep the child's urine output at 1 mL/kg of body weight per hour, thus reflecting adequate tissue perfusion. A nasogastric tube may or may not be required but is not the priority intervention.

Test-Taking Strategy: Option 1 can be eliminated first because the child should not be sedated. Eliminate option 2 next, knowing that fluid resuscitation is an important component of therapy to prevent burn shock. From the remaining options, knowledge that urine output reflects adequate tissue perfusion will direct you to option 4. Review the treatment of burns now if you had difficulty with this question!

Level of Cognitive Ability: Analysis
Phase of Nursing Process: Implementation
Client Needs: Physiological Integrity
Content Area: Child Health

Reference
Bowden, V., Dickey, S., & Greenberg, C. (1998). *Children and their families: The continuum of care*. Philadelphia: W. B. Saunders. p. 1787.

9. 4

Rationale: The Parkland formula is calculated as 4 mL Ringer's lactate (RL) solution × kg of body weight ×% TBSA burn. One half of the total is administered in the first 8 hours postburn. One fourth of the total is administered in the second 8 hours postburn. One fourth of the total is administered in the third 8 hours postburn; 4 mL × 10 kg × 50% TBSA burn = 2000 mL RL in 24 hours. The child receives 1000 mL in the first 8 hours at 125 mL/hour, 500 mL in the second 8 hours at 62 mL/hour and 500 mL in the third 8 hours at 62 mL/hour.

Test-Taking Strategy: Knowledge regarding the calculation of amount of fluid required by the Parkland formula is required to answer this question. If you are unfamiliar with this method of calculation, take time now to review!

Level of Cognitive Ability: Analysis
Phase of Nursing Process: Analysis
Client Needs: Physiological Integrity
Content Area: Child Health

Reference
Bowden, V., Dickey, S., & Greenberg, C. (1998). *Children and their families: The continuum of care*. Philadelphia: W. B. Saunders. p. 1787.

10. 4

Rationale: Sensorium is an important guide to the adequacy of fluid resuscitation. The burn injury itself does not affect the sensorium, so the child should be alert and oriented. Any alteration in sensorium should be evaluated further. A neurological assessment determines the level of sensorium in the child. Options 1, 2, and 3 do not provide an accurate assessment of the adequacy of fluid resuscitation.

Test-Taking Strategy: Note the key phrase "most accurate" in the stem of the question. Although options 1, 2, and 3 may provide some information related to fluid volume, in a burn injury, from the options provided, neurological assessment is most accurate. Review assessments during fluid resuscitation and treatment for burn shock now if you had difficulty with this question!

Level of Cognitive Ability: Analysis
Phase of Nursing Process: Assessment
Client Needs: Physiological Integrity
Content Area: Child Health

Reference
Bowden, V., Dickey, S., & Greenberg, C. (1998). *Children and their families: The continuum of care*. Philadelphia: W. B. Saunders. p. 1787.

BIBLIOGRAPHY

Ashwill, J., & Droske, S. (1997). *Nursing care of children: Principles and practice*. Philadelphia: W. B. Saunders.

Bowden, V., Dickey, S., & Greenberg, C. (1998). *Children and their families: The continuum of care*. Philadelphia: W. B. Saunders.

Hodgson, B., & Kizior, R. (1999). *Saunders nursing drug handbook 1999*. Philadelphia: W. B. Saunders.

Lammon, C., Foote, A., Leli, P., et al. (1995). *Clinical nursing skills*. Philadelphia: W. B. Saunders.

Luckmann, J. (1997). *Saunders manual of nursing care*. Philadelphia: W. B. Saunders.

Nichols, F., & Zwelling, E. (1997). *Maternal newborn nursing: Theory and practice*. Philadelphia: W. B. Saunders.

O'Toole, M. (ed.). (1997). *Miller-Keane encyclopedia & dictionary of medicine, nursing, & allied health* (6th ed.). Philadelphia: W. B. Saunders.

CHAPTER 41

Musculoskeletal Disorders

I. Dysplasia of the Hip

A. Description
1. A condition in which the head of the femur is improperly seated in the acetabulum or hip socket of the pelvis
2. Can range from very mild to severely dislocated
3. Can be congenital or develop after birth

B. Assessment (Fig. 41–1)
1. Neonates: laxity of the ligaments around the hip, which allows the femoral head to be displaced from the acetabulum upon manipulation
2. Infants beyond the newborn period
   a. Asymmetry of the gluteal skinfolds when placed prone and the legs are extended against the examining table
   b. Limited range of motion (ROM) in the affected hip
   c. Asymmetric abduction of the affected hip when placed supine with the knees and hips flexed
   d. Apparent short femur on the affected side (Galeazzi sign)
3. The walking child: minimal to pronounced variations in gait with lurching toward the affected side
4. Positive Barlow or Ortolani's maneuver

C. Implementation
1. In the neonatal period, splinting of the hips with Pavlik harness to maintain flexion and abduction and external rotation
2. Following the neonatal period, traction, and/or surgery to release muscles and tendons
3. Positioning and immobilization in a spica cast following surgery until healing is achieved
4. Osteotomy following traction in profoundly affected children
5. Instruct parents regarding proper care of a Pavlik harness or spica cast (Fig. 41–2)

II. Congenital Clubfoot

A. Description
1. A congenital malformation of the lower extremities
2. The defect may be unilateral or bilateral
3. Defects are rigid and cannot be manipulated into a neutral position
4. Long-term interval follow-up is required until the child reaches skeletal maturity

B. Assessment: the foot is plantar flexed with an inverted heel and adducted forefoot

C. Implementation
1. Treatment begins as soon after birth as possible
2. Serial manipulation and casting are performed weekly, and if correction is not achieved in 3 to 6 months, surgery is indicated
3. Monitor for pain
4. Monitor neurovascular status of the toes
5. Instruct parents in cast care and signs of neurovascular impairment requiring physician notification

III. Scoliosis

A. Description
1. A lateral curvature of the spine
2. Surgical and nonsurgical interventions are employed and the type of treatment depends on the degree of curvature, the age of the child, and the amount of **growth** that is anticipated
3. Long-term monitoring is essential to detect any progression of the curve

B. Assessment
1. Visible curve fails to straighten when child bends forward and hangs arms down toward feet
2. Hips, ribs, and shoulders are asymmetrical
3. Apparent leg length discrepancy

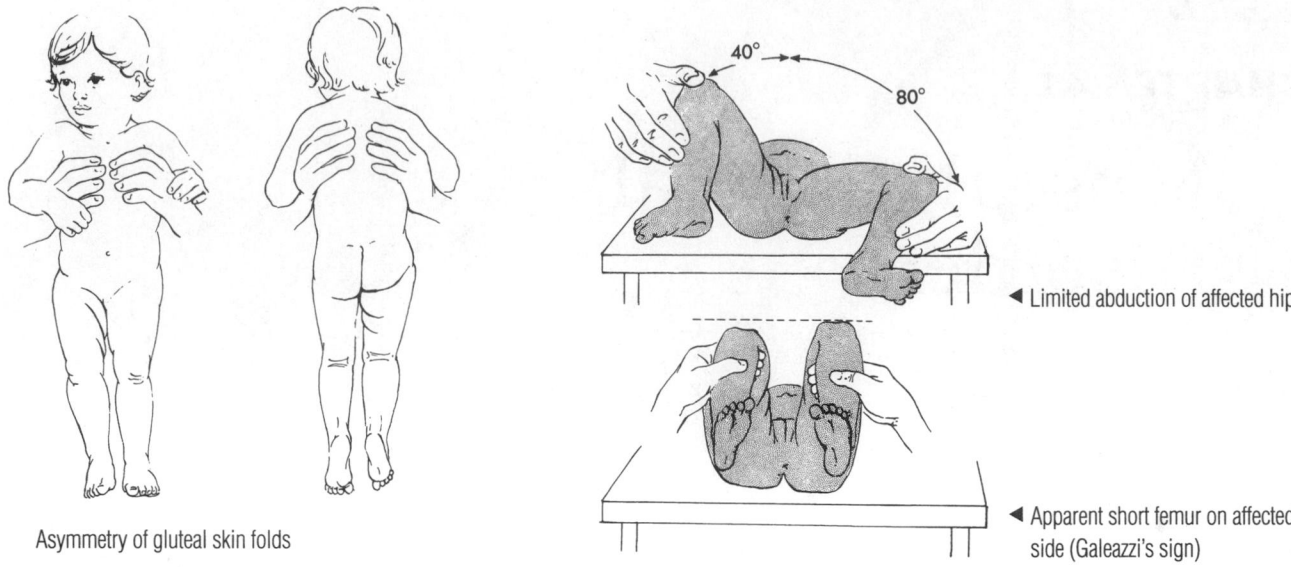

Asymmetry of gluteal skin folds

◀ Limited abduction of affected hip

◀ Apparent short femur on affected side (Galeazzi's sign)

FIGURE 41–1. Physical findings in unilateral congenital dislocation of the hip. (From Tachdjian, M. O. [1990]. *Pediatric orthopedics* [2nd ed.]. Philadelphia: W. B. Saunders. p. 326.)

C. Implementation
   1. Monitor progression of the curvature
   2. Prepare the child for the use of a brace if prescribed
   3. Prepare the child and parents for surgery (spinal fusion) if prescribed
   4. Prepare the child and parents for surgery (placement of internal instrumentation rods) if prescribed
D. Implementation Postoperatively
   1. Maintain flat position
   2. Log-roll the child when turning to maintain alignment

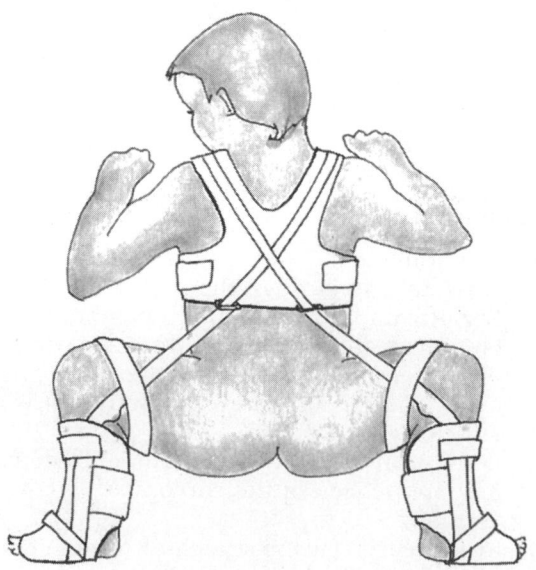

FIGURE 41–2. The child in a Pavlik harness. (From Tachdjian, M. O. [1990]. *Pediatric orthopedics* [2nd ed.]. Philadelphia: W. B. Saunders. p. 336.)

3. Assess extremities for neurovascular status
4. Encourage coughing and deep breathing and use of incentive spirometry
5. Assess pain and administer prescribed analgesics
6. Monitor for incontinence
7. Instruct in activity restrictions
8. Instruct the child to roll from a side-lying position to a sitting position and assist with ambulation

E. Braces
   1. Instruct the child to wear a brace as prescribed
   2. Inspect the skin for signs of redness or breakdown
   3. Keep the skin clean and dry, avoiding lotions and powders
   4. Advise the child to wear soft nonirritating clothing under the brace
   5. Instruct in prescribed exercises
   6. Encourage verbalization about body image

IV. Juvenile Rheumatoid Arthritis (JRA)

A. Description
   1. An autoimmune inflammatory disease affecting the joints
   2. The cause is unknown
   3. Juvenile onset is diagnosed before 16 years of age
   4. A leading cause of blindness and disability in children
   5. Treatment is supportive and directed toward preserving joint function, controlling inflammation, minimizing deformity, and reducing the impact that the disease may have on the development of the child
   6. Therapy includes medications, physical and occupational therapies, and family education

Table 41–1. **Assessment of JRA**

Systemic JRA	*Pauciarticular JRA*	*Polyarticular JRA*
Fever	Mild joint pain and swelling	Morning joint stiffness
Salmon-pink rash	Affects large joints	Low-grade fever
Affects five or more joints	Affects no more than four joints	Affects weight-bearing joints
May also have anorexia, anemia, fatigue	Iridocyclitis	Affects five or more joints

7. Surgical intervention may be implemented when the child has problems with joint contractures and unequal **growth** of extremities

B. Assessment (Table 41–1)

C. Implementation
   1. Facilitate social, emotional, and developmental **growth**
   2. Instruct the parents and child in the administration of medications as prescribed, such as nonsteroidal anti-inflammatory drugs (NSAIDs) and antirheumatic medications
   3. Assist the child with ROM exercises and instruct in prescribed exercises
   4. Instruct the parents and child in the use of hot or cold packs, splinting, and positioning the affected joint in a neutral position during painful episodes
   5. Encourage and support prescribed physical and occupational therapy
   6. Instruct in the importance of preventive eye care
   7. Instruct in the importance of reporting visual disturbances
   8. Assess the child's perception regarding the chronic illness
   9. Encourage normal performance of activities of daily living (ADL)

V. Fractures (Fig. 41–3)

A. Description
   1. A break in the continuity of the bone caused by trauma, twisting, or bone decalcification
   2. Fractures in children usually result from increased mobility and inadequate or immature motor and cognitive skills
   3. Fractures in children may be caused by trauma or bone diseases
   4. Fractures in infancy are generally rare and warrant further investigation to rule out the possibility of child **abuse**
   5. The most frequently seen fracture in children is in the forearm

B. Assessment
   1. Pain or tenderness over the involved area
   2. Loss of function
   3. Obvious deformity
   4. Crepitation
   5. Ecchymosis
   6. Erythema
   7. Edema
   8. Muscle spasm

C. Initial Care of a Fracture
   1. Immobilize affected extremity
   2. If compound fracture exists, splint the extremity and cover the wound with a sterile dressing

D. Implementation
   1. Reduction
      a. Restoring the bone to proper alignment
      b. Closed reduction: accomplished by manual alignment of the fragments followed by immobilization
      c. Open reduction: requires the surgical insertion of internal fixation devices such as rods, wires, or pins that help maintain alignment while healing occurs
   2. Retention: the application of traction or a cast to maintain alignment until healing occurs

E. Traction
   1. Cervical skin traction
      a. Relieves muscle spasms and compression in upper extremities and neck
      b. Uses a head halter and a pad chin to attach the traction

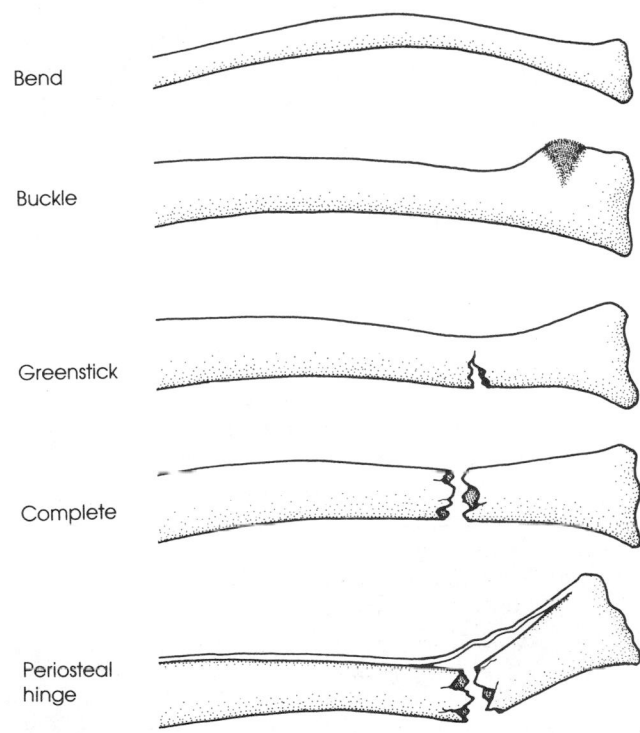

FIGURE 41–3. Types of childhood fractures. Children's bones are more easily injured than adult bones, but since they are more porous, they tend to bend, buckle, or break in a greenstick manner, rather than to fracture completely. A greenstick fracture occurs when the compressed side of the bone bends and the side under tension gives way, resulting in an incomplete fracture. In a complete fracture, the bone fragments are divided, although they may be superficially linked by the periosteal hinge. (From Marlow, S. R., & Redding, B. A. [1988]. *Textbook of pediatric nursing* [6th ed.]. Philadelphia: W. B. Saunders.)

c. Uses powder to protect the ears from friction rub

d. Position the child with the head of the bed elevated 20 to 30 degrees and attach the weights to a pulley system over the head of the bed

2. Bryant's skin traction

a. Used to stabilize a fractured femur

b. Used to correct a congenital hip in children

c. Position the child flat with a 90-degree hip flexion

3. Russell's skin traction

a. Used to stabilize a fractured femur before surgery

b. Similar to Buck's traction but provides a double pull with the use of a knee sling

c. Traction pulls at the knee and foot

d. Position the child with the foot of the bed slightly elevated

4. Balanced suspension

a. Used with skin or skeletal traction

b. Used to approximate fractures of femur, tibia, or fibula

c. Produced by a counterforce other than the child

d. Types include Thomas splint with Pearson attachment, Steinmann pin, Kirschner wires

e. Position child in low Fowler's position, either on the side or back

f. Maintain a 20-degree angle from the thigh to the bed

g. Protect the skin from breakdown

h. Provide pin care if pins are used with the skeletal traction

i. Clean pin site with normal saline and hydrogen peroxide or Betadine as prescribed

F. Casts

1. Description

a. Made of plaster or fiberglass to provide immobilization of bone and joints after a fracture or injury

b. Fractures of the hip and knee may require a body or spica cast

2. Implementation

a. Examine the cast for pressure areas

b. Monitor the extremity for circulatory impairment such as pain, swelling, discoloration, tingling, numbness, or coolness or diminished pulse

c. Notify the physician if circulatory compromise occurs

d. Prepare for bivaling or cutting the cast if circulatory impairment occurs

e. Instruct the child not to stick objects down the cast

f. Teach the child to keep the cast clean and dry

g. Instruct the child on isometric exercises to prevent muscle atrophy

PRACTICE QUESTIONS

1. A 6-month-old infant is seen in the clinic and is diagnosed with unilateral hip dysplasia. Which of the following assessment findings is not noted in this condition?

   1 An apparent short femur on the affected side

   2 Limited range of motion (ROM) in the affected hip

   3 Asymmetric adduction of the affected hip when placed supine with the knees and hips flexed

   4 Asymmetry of the gluteal skinfolds when the infant is placed prone and the legs are extended against the examining table

2. The nurse is assisting a physician during the examination of an infant with hip dysplasia. The physician performs the Ortolani's maneuver. The nurse determines that this maneuver is performed to:

   1 Push the unstable femoral head out of the acetabulum

   2 Reduce the dislocated femoral head back into the acetabulum

   3 Determine the extent of ROM

   4 Assess for asymmetry on the affected side

3. The clinic nurse provides instructions to the parents of an infant with hip dysplasia regarding care of the Pavlik harness. Which of the following does the nurse include in the instructions?

   1 The harness should be worn 12 hours a day

   2 The harness needs be removed for diaper changes and for feeding

   3 The harness should be removed only to check the skin, and for bathing

   4 The infant should not be moved when out of the harness

4. The mother brings her 2-week-old infant to the clinic for treatment following a diagnosis of clubfoot made at the time of birth. Which of the following statements, if made by the mother, indicates a need for further education regarding this disorder?

   1 "I need to bring my child back to the clinic in 1 month for a new cast."

   2 "Treatment needs to be started as soon as possible."

   3 "I need to come to the clinic every week with my child for the casting."

   4 "I realize my child will require follow-up care until full-grown."

5. The nurse is caring for a child following spinal fusion for the treatment of scoliosis. The child complains of abdominal discomfort and begins to have episodes of vomiting. On further assessment, the nurse notes abdominal distention. Which of the following nursing actions is most appropriate?

    1 Administer an antiemetic
    2 Place the child in a side-lying Sims' position
    3 Notify the physician
    4 Increase the IV fluids

6. The nurse is providing instructions to the parents of a child with scoliosis regarding the use of a brace. Which of the following is not a component of the instructions?
    1 Apply lotion under the brace to prevent skin breakdown
    2 Avoid the use of powder because it will cake under the brace
    3 Have the child wear a soft fabric under the brace
    4 Encourage the child to perform prescribed exercises

7. The pediatric nurse educator provides a teaching session to the nursing staff regarding juvenile rheumatoid arthritis (JRA). Which of the following is not included in the teaching session?
    1 It most often occurs before the age of 16
    2 It is twice as likely to occur in boys than in girls
    3 It is the leading cause of blindness and disability in children
    4 Clinical manifestations include morning stiffness and painful, stiff, swollen joints

8. The mother of a child with JRA calls the clinic nurse because the child is experiencing a painful exacerbation of the disease. The mother asks the nurse if the child should perform ROM exercises at this time. The most appropriate nursing response is:

    1 "The ROM exercises must be performed every day."
    2 "Avoid all exercise during painful periods."
    3 "Administer additional pain medication before performing ROM exercises."
    4 "Have the child perform simple isometric exercises during this time."

9. A 2-year-old child is placed in Bryant's traction for treatment of a fractured femur. The nurse develops a plan of care for the child. Which of the following is not a component of the plan?
    1 Restrain the child to maintain a supine position
    2 Place the child supine with the legs flexed slightly less than 90 degrees
    3 Ensure that the sacrum is resting on the mattress
    4 Ensure the use of a footplate to keep the traction straps away from the child's ankles

10. A 4-year-old child sustains a fall at home and is brought to the emergency room by the mother. Following x-ray, it has been determined that the child has a fractured arm and a plaster cast is applied. The nurse provides instructions to the mother regarding cast care for the child. Which of the following statements, if made by the mother, indicates a need for further education?
    1 "The cast may feel warm as the cast dries."
    2 "If the cast becomes wet, a blow drier set on the cool setting may be used to dry the cast."
    3 "A small amount of white shoe polish can touch up a soiled white cast."
    4 "I can use lotion or powder around the cast edges to relieve itching."

ANSWERS

1. **3**

Rationale: Asymmetric abduction of the affected hip, when placed supine with the knees and hips flexed, is an assessment finding in hip dysplasia in infants beyond the newborn period. Options 1, 2, and 4 are accurate assessment findings in this disorder.

Test-Taking Strategy: Attempt to visualize each of the assessment findings described in the options. This will assist in directing you to option 3. If you had difficulty with this question, take time now to review the assessment finding in hip dysplasia!

Level of Cognitive Ability: Analysis
Phase of Nursing Process: Assessment
Client Needs: Physiological Integrity
Content Area: Child Health

Reference
Ashwill, J., & Droske, S. (1997). *Nursing care of children: Principles and practice.* Philadelphia: W. B. Saunders. p. 1151.

2. **2**

Rationale: In the Barlow maneuver, the examiner pushes the unstable femoral head out of the acetabulum. In the Ortolani's maneuver, the examiner reduces the dislocated femoral head back into the acetabulum. A positive finding is a palpable clink upon entry or exit of the femoral head over the acetabular ring. Options 3 and 4 are done to assess for hip dysplasia.

Test-Taking Strategy: Knowledge regarding assessment findings and these maneuvers is required to answer this question. Review these maneuvers now if you had difficulty with this question. Remember that these maneuvers should be performed only by a physician or trained health care provider!

Level of Cognitive Ability: Analysis
Phase of Nursing Process: Assessment
Client Needs: Physiological Integrity
Content Area: Child Health

Reference
Ashwill, J., & Droske, S. (1997). *Nursing care of children: Principles and practice.* Philadelphia: W. B. Saunders. p. 1151.

3. **3**

Rationale: The harness should be worn 23 hours a day and should be removed only to check the skin, and for bathing. The hips and buttocks should be supported carefully when the infant is out of the harness. The harness does not need to be removed for diaper changes or feedings.

Test-Taking Strategy: Attempt to visualize this harness in answering the question. This will assist in eliminating options 2 and 4. Select option 3 over option 1 because the time frame in option 1 is rather low. Review home care instruction regarding this harness now if you had difficulty with this question!

Level of Cognitive Ability: Application
Phase of Nursing Process: Implementation
Client Needs: Health Promotion and Maintenance
Content Area: Child Health

Reference
Ashwill, J., & Droske, S. (1997). *Nursing care of children: Principles and practice.* Philadelphia: W. B. Saunders. p. 1152.

4. **1**

Rationale: Treatment for clubfoot is started as soon as possible after birth. Serial manipulation and casting are performed at least weekly. If sufficient correction is not achieved in 3 to 6 months, surgery is usually indicated. Because clubfoot can recur, all children with clubfoot require long-term interval follow-up until they reach skeletal maturity to ensure an optimal outcome.

Test-Taking Strategy: Knowledge regarding the treatment plan for clubfoot is required to answer the question. Note the key phrase "indicates a need for further education." This may assist in eliminating options 2 and 4. Recalling that serial manipulations and casting are required weekly will assist in directing you to option 1. Review these treatment procedures now if you had difficulty with this question!

Level of Cognitive Ability: Analysis
Phase of Nursing Process: Analysis
Client Needs: Physiological Integrity
Content Area: Child Health

Reference
Ashwill, J., & Droske, S. (1997). *Nursing care of children: Principles and practice.* Philadelphia: W. B. Saunders. pp. 1162–1164.

5. **3**

Rationale: A complication following surgical treatment of scoliosis is superior mesenteric artery syndrome. This disorder is caused by mechanical changes in the position of the child's abdominal contents, resulting from lengthening of the child's body. It results in a syndrome of emesis and abdominal distention similar to that which occurs with intestinal obstruction or paralytic ileus. Postoperative vomiting in children with body casts or those who have undergone spinal fusion warrants attention because of the possibility of superior mesenteric artery syndrome.

Test-Taking Strategy: Eliminate option 4 first because it should not be implemented without a prescribed order. Eliminate option 2 next because this child requires log rolling, and the Sims' position may cause injury following surgery. From the remaining options, note the assessment signs and symptoms in the question. These should alert you that physician notification is necessary. Review superior mesenteric artery syndrome now if you had difficulty with this question!

Level of Cognitive Ability: Analysis
Phase of Nursing Process: Implementation
Client Needs: Physiological Integrity
Content Area: Child Health

Reference
Ashwill, J., & Droske, S. (1997). *Nursing care of children: Principles and practice.* Philadelphia: W. B. Saunders. p. 1142.

6. **1**

Rationale: The use of lotions or powders should be avoided as they can become sticky or cake under the brace, causing irritation. Options 2, 3, and 4 are appropriate instructions to the parents of a child with a brace.

Test-Taking Strategy: Note the key word "not" in the stem of the question. Careful reading of the options will assist in directing you to option 1. Review home care instructions regarding the care of a child in a brace now if you had difficulty with this question!

Level of Cognitive Ability: Application
Phase of Nursing Process: Implementation
Client Needs: Health Promotion and Maintenance
Content Area: Child Health

Reference
Ashwill, J., & Droske, S. (1997). *Nursing care of children: Principles and practice.* Philadelphia: W. B. Saunders. p. 1143.

7. **2**

Rationale: JRA is twice as likely to occur in girls than in boys. Options 1, 3, and 4 are accurate regarding this disorder.

Test-Taking Strategy: Note the key word "not" in the stem of the question. Knowledge regarding the etiology and clinical manifestations associated with JRA is required to answer this question. This knowledge will easily direct you to option 2. Review this disorder now if you are unfamiliar with JRA!

Level of Cognitive Ability: Analysis
Phase of Nursing Process: Analysis
Client Needs: Physiological Integrity
Content Area: Child Health

Reference
Ashwill, J., & Droske, S. (1997). *Nursing care of children: Principles and practice.* Philadelphia: W. B. Saunders. p. 1124.

8. **4**

Rationale: During painful episodes, hot or cold packs, and splinting and positioning the affected joint in a neutral position help reduce the pain. Although resting the extremity is appropriate, it is important to begin simple isometric or tensing exercises as soon as the child is able. These exercises do not involve joint movement.

Test-Taking Strategy: Eliminate options 1, 2, and 3 because of the words "must," "all," and "additional" in each of these options. Review pain management and care during exacerbations now if you had difficulty with this question!

Level of Cognitive Ability: Application
Phase of Nursing Process: Implementation
Client Needs: Physiological Integrity
Content Area: Child Health

Reference
Ashwill, J., & Droske, S. (1997). *Nursing care of children: Principles and practice.* Philadelphia: W. B. Saunders. p. 1127.

9. **3**

Rationale: In Bryant's traction, the sacrum should be off the mattress. Options 1, 2, and 4 are accurate interventions in the use of this traction.

Test-Taking Strategy: Note the key word "not" in the stem of the question. Attempt to visualize this type of traction in selecting the correct response. Review this type of traction and the associated nursing interventions now if you had difficulty with this question!

Level of Cognitive Ability: Application
Phase of Nursing Process: Planning
Client Needs: Physiological Integrity
Content Area: Child Health

Reference
Ashwill, J., & Droske, S. (1997). *Nursing care of children: Principles and practice.* Philadelphia: W. B. Saunders. p. 1100.

10. **4**

Rationale: The mother needs to be instructed not to use lotion or powders on the skin around the cast edges or inside the cast. Lotions or powders can become sticky or caked and cause skin irritation. Options 1, 2, and 3 are appropriate instructions.

Test-Taking Strategy: Note the key phrase "indicates a need for further education." Knowledge regarding routine cast care should easily direct you to option 4. Review home care instructions regarding cast care now if you had difficulty with this question!

Level of Cognitive Ability: Analysis
Phase of Nursing Process: Evaluation
Client Needs: Health Promotion and Maintenance
Content Area: Child Health

Reference
Bowden, V., Dickey, S., & Greenberg, C. (1998). *Children and their families: The continuum of care.* Philadelphia. W. B. Saunders. pp. 1234–1235.

BIBLIOGRAPHY

Ashwill, J., & Droske, S. (1997). *Nursing care of children: Principles and practice.* Philadelphia: W. B. Saunders.

Bowden, V., Dickey, S., & Greenberg, C. (1998). *Children and their families: The continuum of care.* Philadelphia: W. B. Saunders.

Hodgson, B., & Kizior, R. (1999). *Saunders nursing drug handbook 1999.* Philadelphia: W. B. Saunders.

Lammon, C., Foote, A., Leli, P., et al. (1995). *Clinical nursing skills.* Philadelphia: W. B. Saunders.

Luckmann, J. (1997). *Saunders manual of nursing care.* Philadelphia: W. B. Saunders.

Nichols, F., & Zwelling, E. (1997). *Maternal newborn nursing: Theory and practice.* Philadelphia: W. B. Saunders.

O'Toole, M. (ed.). (1997). *Miller-Keane encyclopedia & dictionary of medicine, nursing, & allied health* (6th ed.). Philadelphia: W. B. Saunders.

CHAPTER 42

Acquired Immunodeficiency Syndrome

I. Acquired Immunodeficiency Syndrome

A. Description
1. A disorder caused by the human immunodeficiency virus (HIV) and is characterized by a generalized dysfunction of the immune system
2. Both the cellular and the humoral immunity are compromised
3. Treatment includes a modified immunization schedule to prevent disease and to provide prophylaxis against opportunistic infections especially *Pneumocystis carinii* pneumonia (PCP)
4. Medical therapy includes the administration of antiretroviral medications to inhibit viral reproduction and the aggressive use of medications to treat infections

B. Assessment
1. During neonatal period
   a. Lymphadenopathy
   b. Hepatosplenomegaly
   c. Opportunistic infections
   d. Progressive encephalopathy
   e. Microcephaly
2. Infants
   a. Failure to thrive
   b. Developmental delays
   c. Oral candidiasis
   d. Diarrhea
   e. Hepatosplenomegaly
   f. Chronic interstitial pneumonia and cough
   g. Chronic otitis media
3. Children/adolescent
   a. Malaise and fatigue
   b. Night sweats
   c. Weight loss
   d. Diarrhea
   e. Fever
   f. **Regression** of developmental milestones
   g. Generalized lymphadenopathy
   h. Nephropathy
   i. Interstitial pneumonitis and *Pneumocystis carinii* pneumonia
   j. Encephalopathy

C. Diagnostic Tests
1. ELISA
   a. Enzyme linked immunosorbent assay (ELISA) determines response of antibodies to HIV virus
   b. Used in children older than 18 months
2. Western blot
   a. Confirms the presence of HIV antibodies
   b. Useful in children older than 18 months of age
   c. A positive HIV antibody test in children younger than 18 months of age indicates only that the mother is infected
3. p24 antigen
   a. Used to detect HIV antigen in children younger than 18 months
   b. Test can be useful at any age
   c. Only a positive result is significant
   d. Two or more positive results are diagnostic for HIV infection
4. CD4+: used to assess a child's immune status, risk for disease progression, and the need for PCP prophylaxis after 1 year of age

II. Care to the Child with AIDS

A. Prophylaxis
1. Provide prophylaxis as prescribed against PCP at 4 to 6 weeks of age if exposed perinatally to HIV
2. Provide continued prophylaxis through 12 months of age for children diagnosed with HIV

3. For HIV-infected children older than 12 months continued prophylaxis is based on CD4+ counts and whether PCP has previously occurred

B. Parent Instructions
   1. Frequent handwashing
   2. Assess for fever, malaise, fatigue, weight loss, vomiting and diarrhea, altered activity level, and oral lesions and notify the physician if these occur
   3. The signs and symptoms of opportunistic infections
   4. The administration of antiretroviral medications as prescribed
   5. The child should avoid exposure to other illnesses
   6. Keep immunizations up to date
   7. Keep the child home when sick
   8. Do not kiss babies on the mouth
   9. Monitor weight
   10. Provide high-calorie and high-protein diet
   11. Do not share eating utensils
   12. Wash eating utensils in the dishwasher
   13. Cover unused food and formula and refrigerate
   14. Discard unused refrigerated formula after 24 hours
   15. Wear gloves for care, especially when in contact with body fluids and when changing diapers
   16. Change diapers frequently away from food areas
   17. Fold soiled disposable diapers inward and tab and dispose in a tightly covered plastic-lined container
   18. Dispose of trash daily
   19. Cover sandboxes when not in use to create a barrier to germs
   20. Clean up spills with bleach solution (10:1 ratio of water to bleach)

C. Immunizations: inactivated poliovirus (IPV) is substituted for oral poliovirus (OPV) in the regular immunization schedule

PRACTICE QUESTIONS

1. The pediatric nurse educator provides a teaching session to the nursing staff regarding acquired immunodeficiency syndrome (AIDS). Which of the following is included in the teaching session?
   1 Most newborns of HIV-positive women test positive for HIV virus
   2 HIV primarily attacks the hematological system
   3 The B cells are depleted and cannot signal T4 cells to form protective antibodies
   4 The virus attacks the immune system by destroying T lymphocytes

2. A newborn of an HIV-positive mother is tested for the presence of HIV antibodies. An enzyme linked immunosorbent assay (ELISA) test is performed and the results are positive. The nurse interprets these results as:
   1 Positive for HIV virus
   2 Indicating the presence of maternal infection
   3 Indicating the absence of maternal infection
   4 Negative for HIV virus

3. The physician prescribes laboratory studies on an infant of an HIV-positive women to determine the presence of HIV infection. Which of the following laboratory studies does the nurse expect to be prescribed?
   1 Western blot
   2 Chest x-ray for PCP
   3 CD4 count
   4 p24 antigen assay

4. A mother with HIV infection brings her 10-month-old infant to the clinic for a routine check-up. The physician has documented that the infant is asymptomatic for HIV infection. Following the check-up, the mother tells the nurse that she is so pleased that the infant will not get HIV. The most appropriate nursing response to the mother is:
   1 "I am so pleased also that everything has turned out fine"
   2 "Everything looks great, but be sure that you return with your infant next month for the scheduled visit"
   3 "Most children infected with HIV develop symptoms within the first 9 months of life and some become symptomatic sometime before age 3"
   4 "Since symptoms have not developed, it is unlikely that the infant will develop HIV infection"

5. A child with an HIV-infected mother is seen in the clinic on a monthly basis and is being monitored for symptoms indicative of acquired immunodeficiency syndrome (AIDS). The nurse understands that the most common disease indicative of AIDS in children is:
   1 Gastroenteritis
   2 Meningitis
   3 *Pneumocystis carinii* pneumonia (PCP)
   4 Lymphoid interstitial pneumonia (LIP)

6. The clinic nurse is instructing the mother of a child with HIV regarding immunizations. Which of the following does the nurse include in the instructions?
   1 Household members need to avoid receiving the influenza vaccine
   2 Siblings need to receive inactivated polio vaccine
   3 The hepatitis B vaccine is not to be given to the child
   4 A Western blot needs to be evaluated before immunizations

7. A child with AIDS is hospitalized for the treatment of PCP. The child will be receiving nebulizer treatments at home when discharged. The nurse instructs the parents regarding the maintenance of the nebulizer equipment. Which of the following is included in the instructions?
   1 Clean the nebulizer pieces after each treatment with 1/4 strength bleach and water
   2 Soak the nebulizer pieces in white vinegar and water for 30 minutes at the end of each day
   3 Boil the nebulizer pieces for 15 minutes after each treatment
   4 Clean the mouthpiece with alcohol after each use and soak in alcohol for 30 minutes at the end of each day

8. The child with HIV infection is receiving zidovudine (AZT, Retrovir). Which of the following laboratory studies indicates that the child is experiencing an adverse reaction for the medication?
   1 Sedimentation rate
   2 Complete blood count (CBC)
   3 Calcium level
   4 Potassium level

9. The nurse is caring for a 4-year-old child with a diagnosis of HIV infection. In planning care to address the psychosocial issues, the nurse expects that this child:
   1 Is unable to grasp the concept of illness and death
   2 Begins to understand something is wrong
   3 Begins to conceptualize the death process involving physical harm
   4 Expresses fear, withdrawal, and denial

10. The home care nurse provides instructions regarding basic infection control to the parents of a child with HIV infection. Which of the following is not a component of these instructions?
    1 Carefully wash all fresh fruits and vegetables
    2 Wash baby bottles, nipples, and pacifiers in the dishwasher
    3 Discard any unused food and formula immediately
    4 Rub the inside of the nipple with salt and rinse well if it becomes slimy

ANSWERS

1. **4**

Rationale: Children born to HIV-positive women test positive for HIV antibody. This is actually a measure of maternal antibody and not indicative of true infection. HIV attacks the immune system. T4 cells are depleted in number and cannot signal B cells to form protective antibodies to fight off the invading virus. The virus attacks the immune system by destroying T lymphocytes.

Test-Taking Strategy: Eliminate option 2 first, knowing that HIV attacks the immune system. Eliminate option 1 next with the knowledge that newborns test positive for HIV antibody but not the virus. Recalling that T4 cells are depleted will assist in eliminating option 3. Review the physiological occurrences in AIDS now if you had difficulty with this question!

Level of Cognitive Ability: Application
Phase of Nursing Process: Implementation
Client Needs: Physiological Integrity
Content Area: Child Health

Reference:
Bowden, V., Dickey, S., & Greenberg, C. (1998). *Children and their families: The continuum of care.* Philadelphia: W. B. Saunders. pp. 1645–1646.

2. **2**

Rationale: A positive antibody test in a child younger than 18 months of age indicates only that the mother is infected, as maternal IgG antibodies persist in infants for 6 to 9 months and, in some cases, as long as 18 months. A positive ELISA is not indicative of true infection.

Test-Taking Strategy: Knowledge regarding the purpose of the ELISA test is required to answer the question. Noting the key word "newborn" in the question may also assist in directing you to the correct option. Review tests associated with HIV infection now if you had difficulty with this question!

Level of Cognitive Ability: Analysis
Phase of Nursing Process: Analysis
Client Needs: Physiological Integrity
Content Area: Child Health

Reference:
Ashwill, J., & Droske, S. (1997). *Nursing care of children: Principles and practice.* Philadelphia: W. B. Saunders. p. 645.

3. **4**

Rationale: True infections in infants are confirmed by the detection of HIV, by a p24 antigen assay, culture of HIV or polymerase chain reaction (PCR). A Western blot confirms the presence of HIV antibodies. The CD4 count indicates how well the immune system is working. A chest x-ray for PCP evaluates the presence of other manifestations of HIV infection.

Test-Taking Strategy: Knowledge regarding the laboratory studies used to determine the presence of HIV infection is required to answer this question. If you are unfamiliar with these laboratory studies, take time now to review them. Specific laboratory tests to review include the ELISA, Western blot, CD4 counts, and p24 antigen assay!

Level of Cognitive Ability: Analysis
Phase of Nursing Process: Analysis
Client Needs: Physiological Integrity
Content Area: Child Health

Reference
Bowden, V., Dickey, S., & Greenberg, C. (1998). *Children and their families: The continuum of care.* Philadelphia: W. B. Saunders. p. 1645.

4. 3

Rationale: Most children infected with HIV develop symptoms within the first 9 months of life. The remainder become symptomatic sometime before age 3. Children, with their immature immune systems, have a much shorter incubation period than adults.

Test-Taking Strategy: Options 1, 2, and 4 can be eliminated because they are similar in content. Option 3 is the only option that provides specific and accurate data regarding HIV infection in the infant. Review assessment findings associated with HIV infection now if you had difficulty with this question!

Level of Cognitive Ability: Application
Phase of Nursing Process: Implementation
Client Needs: Psychosocial Integrity
Content Area: Child Health

Reference
Bowden, V., Dickey, S., & Greenberg, C. (1998). *Children and their families: The continuum of care.* Philadelphia: W. B. Saunders. p. 1646.

5. 3

Rationale: PCP is one of the most common diseases indicative of AIDS in children. Along with PCP, children may experience at least two serious bacterial infections in 2 years. These infections are sepsis, otitis media, chronic sinusitis, meningitis, gastroenteritis, and pneumonia. LIP is a form of chronic pneumonitis. Children with LIP usually have acquired HIV infection perinatally. LIP can progress to severe respiratory compromise.

Test-Taking Strategy: Knowledge regarding the most common indications related to AIDS is required to answer this question. Take time now to review the common manifestations associated with AIDS if you had difficulty with this question!

Level of Cognitive Ability: Analysis
Phase of Nursing Process: Assessment
Client Needs: Physiological Integrity
Content Area: Child Health

Reference
Bowden, V., Dickey, S., & Greenberg, C. (1998). *Children and their families: The continuum of care.* Philadelphia: W. B. Saunders. pp. 1646–1647.

6. 2

Rationale: A child with HIV will receive the same immunizations as other children except for the polio vaccine. The child with HIV and the siblings receive inactivated polio vaccine. All household members receive the influenza vaccine. Option 4 is not necessary and is inaccurate.

Test-Taking Strategy: Option 4 can be easily eliminated. From the remaining options, recalling that inactivated polio vaccine needs to be administered to the child with HIV and siblings will assist in directing you to option 2. Review immunizations in the immunodeficient child now if you had difficulty with this question!

Level of Cognitive Ability: Application
Phase of Nursing Process: Implementation
Client Needs: Health Promotion and Maintenance
Content Area: Child Health

Reference
Ashwill, J., & Droske, S. (1997). *Nursing care of children: Principles and practice.* Philadelphia: W. B. Saunders. p. 649.

7. 2

Rationale: Nebulizer pieces are cleaned with warm water after each treatment and left to air dry. They are soaked in white vinegar and water for 30 minutes at the end of each day. Options 1, 3, and 4 are inaccurate and would damage the nebulizer equipment.

Test-Taking Strategy: Options 1 and 4 should be eliminated first because these cleaning agents are very strong and will damage the equipment. Next eliminate option 3 because the boiling process may also cause damage. Review home care instructions regarding respiratory treatments now if you had difficulty with this question!

Level of Cognitive Ability: Application
Phase of Nursing Process: Implementation
Client Needs: Health Promotion and Maintenance
Content Area: Child Health

Reference
Reference: Ashwill, J., & Droske, S. (1997). *Nursing care of children: Principles and practice.* Philadelphia: W. B. Saunders. p. 651.

8. 2

Rationale: AZT effectively interferes with HIV replication but can cause bone marrow suppression. Anemia occurs most commonly after 4 to 6 weeks of therapy. Hematology studies need to be monitored for anemia and granulocytopenia. Renal and liver function tests should also be monitored.

Test-Taking Strategy: Knowledge regarding the adverse effects related to this medication is required to answer this question. If you can recall, however, that anemia is a concern, you will easily be directed to option 2. Review the adverse effects related to this medication now if you had difficulty with this question!

Level of Cognitive Ability: Analysis
Phase of Nursing Process: Analysis
Client Needs: Physiological Integrity
Content Area: Pharmacology

Reference
Hodgson, B., & Kizior, R. (1999). *Saunders nursing drug handbook 1999.* Philadelphia: W. B. Saunders. pp. 1067–1069.

9. 3

Rationale: The preschool child will begin to conceptualize the death process involving physical harm. A child from birth to 2 years of age will be unable to grasp the concept of illness and death. A school-aged child will begin to understand something is wrong. An adolescent will express fear, withdrawal, and denial.

Test-Taking Strategy: Noting the age of the child will assist in directing you to the correct option. Use concepts of growth and development and the related psychosocial issues to answer the question. Review these concepts now if you had difficulty with this question!

Level of Cognitive Ability: Analysis
Phase of Nursing Process: Analysis
Client Needs: Psychosocial Integrity
Content Area: Child Health

Reference
Bowden, V., Dickey, S., & Greenberg, C. (1998). *Children and their families: The continuum of care.* Philadelphia: W. B. Saunders. p. 1652.

10. **3**

Rationale: The parents should be instructed to cover unused food and formula and refrigerate. They should also be informed to discard unused refrigerated food or formula after 24 hours. Options 1, 2, and 4 are accurate instructions related to basic infection control.

Test-Taking Strategy: Knowledge regarding basic infection control measures is required to answer this question. Note the key word "not" in the stem of the question. This may assist in directing you to option 3. Review these important infection control measures now if you had difficulty with this question!

Level of Cognitive Ability: Application
Phase of Nursing Process: Implementation
Client Needs: Health Promotion and Maintenance
Content Area: Child Health

Reference
Ashwill, J., & Droske, S. (1997). *Nursing care of children: Principles and practice*. Philadelphia: W. B. Saunders. p. 649.

BIBLIOGRAPHY

Ashwill, J., & Droske, S. (1997). *Nursing care of children: Principles and practice*. Philadelphia: W. B. Saunders.

Bowden, V., Dickey, S., & Greenberg, C. (1998). *Children and their families: The continuum of care*. Philadelphia: W. B. Saunders.

Hodgson, B., & Kizior, R. (1999). *Saunders nursing drug handbook 1999*. Philadelphia: W. B. Saunders.

Lammon, C., Foote, A., Leli, P., et al. (1995). *Clinical nursing skills*. Philadelphia: W. B. Saunders.

Luckmann, J. (1997). *Saunders manual of nursing care*. Philadelphia: W. B. Saunders.

Nichols, F., & Zwelling, E. (1997). *Maternal newborn nursing: Theory and practice*. Philadelphia: W. B. Saunders.

O'Toole, M. (ed.). (1997). *Miller-Keane encyclopedia & dictionary of medicine, nursing, & allied health* (6th ed.). Philadelphia: W. B. Saunders.

CHAPTER 43

Hematological Disorders

I. Sickle Cell Anemia

A. Description
1. Caused by the inheritance of a gene for a structurally abnormal portion of the hemoglobin (Hgb) chain
2. The sickle hemoglobin is hemoglobin S (HbS)
3. HbS is sensitive to changes in the oxygen content of the red blood cell
4. Insufficient oxygen causes the cells to assume a sickle shape and the cells become rigid and clumped together, obstructing capillary blood flow
5. Situations that precipitate sickling include hypoxia, low environmental or body temperature, acidosis, strenuous exercise, dehydration, infections, or anesthesia
6. Risk factors include having parents heterozygous for HbS or being African-American
7. The process is reversible but after repeated sickling, the cell becomes permanently sickled
8. Treatment focuses on the prevention and treatment of crisis

B. Assessment
1. Susceptibility to infections
2. Delayed **growth** and development
3. The clinical hallmark of sickle cell disease is the acute pain crisis, which is secondary to vaso-occlusion
4. Other significant crisis events are infections, acute splenic sequestration, and bone marrow aplasia
5. Pain crisis with pain in the back, ribs, and extremities
6. Sequestration crisis in which blood is sequestered in the spleen and causes splenomegaly, hypotension, and shock
7. Acute chest syndrome caused by occlusion of the pulmonary vessels causing chest pain,

pulmonary infiltrates, and pneumonia, leukocytosis, and hypoxia
8. Cardiac ischemia causing chest pain, congestive heart failure (CHF), and myocardial infarction (MI)
9. Abdominal pain
10. Joint pain
11. Peripheral blood smear showing classic distorted sickled erythrocytes
12. Positive HbS screening test
13. Anemia
14. Renal ischemia causing decreased urine concentration

C. Implementation
1. Instruct the child and parents about the importance of avoiding activities that lead to hypoxia
2. Instruct the parents and child to recognize the early signs and symptoms of crisis
3. Inform the parents of the **hereditary** aspects of the disorder

D. Sickle Cell Crisis
1. Administer oxygen as prescribed
2. Administer pain medication as prescribed
3. Maintain adequate hydration and maintenance of blood flow with intravenous (IV) normal saline as prescribed and with oral fluids
4. Remove any constrictive clothing
5. Maintain a position so that the child keeps the extremities extended to promote venous return
6. Do not raise the knee gatch of the bed
7. Elevate the head of the bed no more than 30 degrees
8. Maintain room temperature at or above 72°F
9. Assess circulation in the extremities frequently
10. Assess peripheral pulses, color, sensation, motion, and capillary refill of the extremities
11. Assess pulse oximetry

II. Iron Deficiency Anemia

A. Description
1. Iron stores are depleted followed by a reduction in hemoglobin resulting in small red blood cells (RBCs)
2. Results in a decreased supply of iron for the manufacture of hemoglobin in RBCs
3. Commonly results from blood loss, increased metabolic demands, syndromes of gastrointestinal (GI) malabsorption, and dietary inadequacy

B. Assessment
1. Mild to marked manifestations of anemia
2. Weakness
3. Pallor

C. Implementation
1. Increase the oral intake of iron
2. Instruct the parents and child in food choices that are high in iron (Box 43–1)
3. Administer iron supplements as prescribed

III. Aplastic Anemia

A. Description
1. A deficiency of circulating erythrocytes resulting from arrested development of RBCs within the bone marrow
2. The cause is associated with chronic exposure to myelotoxic agents

B. Assessment: pancytopenia (a deficiency of erythrocytes, leukocytes, and thrombocytes)

C. Implementation
1. Administer blood transfusions as prescribed
2. Note that transfusions are discontinued as soon as the bone marrow begins to produce RBCs
3. Administer immunosuppressive therapy as prescribed
4. Prepare the child for splenectomy, if prescribed for the child with an enlarged spleen that is destroying normal RBCs or suppressing their development

IV. Hemophilia

A. Description
1. An X-linked recessive trait
2. Hemophilia A (classic hemophilia) results from a deficiency of factor VIII

BOX 43–1. Iron-Rich Foods

Liver, especially pork and lamb
Red and organ meats
Kidney beans
Whole wheat breads and cereals
Green leafy vegetables
Carrots
Egg yolks
Raisins

---

3. Hemophilia B (Christmas disease) is a deficiency of factor IX
4. Males inherit hemophilia from their mothers and females inherit the carrier status from their fathers
5. Some females who are carriers have an increased tendency to bleed, and, although it is rare, females can have hemophilia if their fathers have the disorder and their mothers are carriers of the genetic disorder

B. Assessment
1. Abnormal bleeding in response to trauma or surgery
2. Joint and muscle hemorrhage
3. Tendency to bruise easily
4. Prolonged prothrombin time and a normal bleeding time

C. Implementation
1. Prepare to administer by intravenous (IV) factor VIII cryoprecipitate
2. Monitor for bleeding
3. Maintain bleeding precautions
4. Monitor for joint pain
5. Immobilize affected extremity if joint pain occurs
6. Instruct the parents and child regarding iron-rich foods
7. Instruct the parents to obtain a Medic-Alert bracelet for the child
8. Instruct the parents regarding activities for the child, emphasizing the avoidance of contact sports

V. β-Thalassemia Major

A. Description
1. An autosomal recessive disorder
2. Also called Cooley's anemia and includes a group of disorders characterized by reduced production of one of the globin chains in the synthesis of hemoglobin
3. The incidence is highest in individuals of Mediterranean descent

B. Assessment
1. Severe anemia
2. Pallor
3. Small size for age
4. Fever
5. Bone pain
6. Microcytic, hypochromic RBCs
7. Hypoxia

C. Implementation
1. Instruct in the administration of folic acid (vitamin B_9) as prescribed, which stimulates the production of blood cells
2. Administer transfusion therapy as prescribed
3. Administer chelation therapy with deferoxamine (Desferal) as prescribed, to prevent organ damage from the elevated levels of iron cause by multiple transfusion therapy
4. Provide genetic counseling

PRACTICE QUESTIONS

1. The community health nurse has been providing educational sessions at schools and community centers in a large city. In one particular area of the city, the topic of the session is focused on sickle cell disease (SCD). In describing the etiology of the disease, which of the following is included in the educational session?
   1 SCD is an autosomal dominant disease
   2 If each parent carries the trait, the children will inherit the trait
   3 Children with the HbS (sickle hemoglobin) will be symptomatic
   4 If one parent has the HbS trait and the other parent is normal, there is a 50% chance that each offspring will inherit the trait

2. A child suspected of SCD is seen in the clinic and laboratory studies are performed. Which of the following is noted in this disease?
   1 Decrease white blood cell (WBC) count
   2 Elevated erythrocyte count
   3 Elevated reticulocyte count
   4 Increased hemoglobin count

3. The pediatric nursing instructor asks the nursing student to describe the cause of the clinical manifestations that occur in SCD. Which of the following is the appropriate response?
   1 Sickled cells increase the blood flow through the body and cause a great deal of pain
   2 The sickled cells mix with the unsickled cells and cause the immune system to become depressed
   3 Bone marrow depression occurs because of the development of sickled cells
   4 Sickled cells are unable to flow easily through the microvasculature, and their clumping obstructs blood flow

4. A child with SCD is admitted to the hospital for treatment of vaso-occlusive pain crisis. The oxygen saturation level is 92%. The nurse prepares to administer care for the child. Which of the following is not a component of the plan of care?
   1 The administration of IV fluids for rehydration
   2 The administration of meperidine (Demerol) for pain management
   3 The administration of oxygen
   4 The administration of increased fluid intake

5. The clinic nurse instructs the mother of a child with SCD regarding the precipitating factors related to pain crisis. Which of the following is not a precipitating factor?
   1 Infection
   2 Trauma
   3 Fluid overload
   4 Stress

6. Laboratory studies are performed on a child suspected of iron deficiency anemia (IDA). Which of the following laboratory results indicates this type of anemia?
   1 An elevated hemoglobin level with a low hematocrit level
   2 A decreased reticulocyte count
   3 An elevated red blood cell (RBC) count
   4 RBCs that are microcytic and hypochromic

7. Oral iron supplements are prescribed for the 6-year-old child with IDA. The nurse instructs the mother to administer the iron with which of the following food items?
   1 Water
   2 Milk
   3 Apple juice
   4 Orange juice

8. The home care nurse is instructing the parents of a child with IDA regarding the administration of a liquid oral iron supplement. Which of the following is included in the teaching plan?
   1 Administer the iron through a straw
   2 Administer the iron at mealtimes
   3 Add the iron to the formula for easy administration
   4 Mix the iron with cereal to administer

9. The nurse caring for a child with aplastic anemia reviews the laboratory results and notes a WBC count of 6000/μL and a platelet count of 27,000/mm^3. Which of the following nursing interventions does the nurse incorporate into the plan of care?
   1 Maintain strict isolation precautions
   2 Encourage naps
   3 Encourage a diet high in iron
   4 Encourage quiet play activities

10. The pediatric nurse educator provides a teaching session to the nursing staff regarding hemophilia. Which of the following regarding this disorder does the nurse plan to include in the discussion?
   1 Hemophilia is a Y-linked hereditary disorder
   2 Males inherit hemophilia from their fathers
   3 Females inherit hemophilia from their mothers
   4 Hemophilia A results from deficiency of factor VIII

11. The nurse provides instructions regarding home care to the parents of a 3-year-old child hospitalized with hemophilia. Which of the following is not a component of the teaching plan?
   1 Supervise the child closely
   2 Pad corners of the furniture
   3 Remove household items that can easily fall over
   4 Avoid immunizations and dental hygiene

12. The nurse analyzes the laboratory results of a child with hemophilia. Which of the following is most likely to be abnormal in this child?
    1 Bleeding time
    2 Platelet count
    3 Prothrombin time (PT)
    4 Partial thromboplastin time (PTT)

13. The nurse is providing home care instructions to the mother of a 10-year-old child with hemophilia. Which of the following activities does the nurse suggest that the child could safely participate with peers?
    1 Basketball
    2 Swimming
    3 Soccer
    4 Field hockey

14. A nursing student is presenting a clinical conference and discusses the etiology related to β-thalassemia. The nursing student informs the group that the child at greatest risk of developing this disorder is:
    1 A child whose intake of iron is extremely poor
    2 A breast-fed child by a mother with chronic anemia
    3 A child of Mediterranean descent
    4 A child of Mexican descent

15. The child with β-thalassemia is receiving chronic transfusion therapy for the treatment of this disorder. Chelation therapy is prescribed in order to prevent organ damage from too much iron in the body, as a result of the transfusions. Which of the following medications does the nurse anticipate to be prescribed in chelation therapy?
    1 Dalteparin sodium (Fragmin)
    2 Meropenem (Merrem)
    3 Molindone HCl (Moban)
    4 Deferoxamine (Desferal)

ANSWERS

1. 4

Rationale: SCD is an autosomal recessive disease. Children with the HbS trait are not symptomatic. Option 4 is correct. Additionally, if each parent carries the trait, there is a 25% chance that their offspring will be normal, a 50% chance that the child will carry the trait, and a 25% chance that each child will have the disease.

Test-Taking Strategy: Knowledge regarding the etiology related to SCD is necessary to answer this question. It is important that you review this information if you are unfamiliar with it. You are likely to find questions related to this disease on NCLEX-RN!

Level of Cognitive Ability: Application
Phase of Nursing Process: Implementation
Client Needs: Physiological Integrity
Content Area: Child Health

Reference
Ashwill, J., & Droske, S. (1997). *Nursing care of children: Principles and practice.* Philadelphia: W. B. Saunders. p. 968.

2. 3

Rationale: A laboratory diagnosis is established on the basis of a complete blood count (CBC), examination for sickled RBCs in the peripheral smear, and hemoglobin electrophoresis. Laboratory studies will show a decreased hemoglobin, hematocrit, and platelet count, increased reticulocyte count, and the presence of nucleated red blood cells. Elevated reticulocyte counts occur in children with SCD because the life span of their sickled RBCs is shortened.

Test-Taking Strategy: Recalling the pathophysiology associated with SCD will assist in answering this question. Review the laboratory tests that are diagnostic of this disorder now if you had difficulty with this question!

Level of Cognitive Ability: Analysis
Phase of Nursing Process: Assessment
Client Needs: Physiological Integrity
Content Area: Child Health

References
Ashwill, J., & Droske, S. (1997). *Nursing care of children: Principles and practice.* Philadelphia: W. B. Saunders. p. 968.
Bowden, V., Dickey, S., & Greenberg, C. (1998). *Children and their families: The continuum of care.* Philadelphia: W. B. Saunders. p. 1567.

3. 4

Rationale: All of the clinical manifestations of SCD are a result of the sickled cells being unable to flow easily through the microvasculature, and their clumping obstructs blood flow. With reoxygenation most of the sickled RBCs resume their normal shape.

Test-Taking Strategy: Recalling that sickled cells clump will assist in directing you to the correction option. Review the pathophysiology associated with SCD now if you had difficulty with this question!

Level of Cognitive Ability: Analysis
Phase of Nursing Process: Evaluation
Client Needs: Physiological Integrity
Content Area: Child Health

Reference
Ashwill, J., & Droske, S. (1997). *Nursing care of children: Principles and practice.* Philadelphia: W. B. Saunders. p. 969.

4. 2

Rationale: Management of severe pain that occurs with vaso-occlusive crisis includes the use of strong narcotic analgesics such as morphine sulfate and hydromorphone. Demerol is contraindicated because of its side effects and increased risk of seizures. Oxygen is administered when hypoxia is present and the oxygen saturation level is less than 95%.

Test-Taking Strategy: Note the key word "not" in the stem of the question. Noting that the oxygen saturation level is 92% will assist in eliminating option 3. Eliminate options 1 and 4, knowing that hydration is necessary and because these options are similar. Review care to the client with SCD now if you had difficulty with this question!

Level of Cognitive Ability: Application
Phase of Nursing Process: Planning
Client Needs: Physiological Integrity
Content Area: Child Health

References
Ashwill, J., & Droske, S. (1997). *Nursing care of children: Principles and practice* Philadelphia: W. B. Saunders. p. 972.
Bowden, V., Dickey, S., & Greenberg, C. (1998). *Children and their families: The continuum of care.* Philadelphia: W. B. Saunders. p. 1578.

5. 3

Rationale: Pain crisis may be precipitated by infection, dehydration, hypoxia, trauma, or general stress. The mother of a child with sickle cell disease should encourage fluid intake of 1 1/2 to 2 times the daily requirement to prevent dehydration.

Test-Taking Strategy: Note the key word "not" in the stem of the question. Recalling that fluids are a main component of treatment in SCD to prevent pain crisis, will direct you to option 3. Fluids are required to prevent dehydration. Review precipitating factors of pain crisis now if you had difficulty with this question!

Level of Cognitive Ability: Analysis
Phase of Nursing Process: Analysis
Client Needs: Health Promotion and Maintenance
Content Area: Child Health

Reference
Ashwill, J., & Droske, S. (1997). *Nursing care of children: Principles and practice.* Philadelphia: W. B. Saunders. pp. 971, 974.

6. 4

Rationale: The results of a CBC in children with IDA will show low hemoglobin levels and microcytic and hypochromic RBCs. The reticulocyte count is usually normal or slightly elevated.

Test-Taking Strategy: Eliminate options 1 and 3 first, knowing that the CBC and hemoglobin counts will be decreased. From the remaining two options, select option 4 over option 2 because of the relationship between anemia and RBCs.

Level of Cognitive Ability: Analysis
Phase of Nursing Process: Analysis
Client Needs: Physiological Integrity
Content Area: Child Health

Reference
Ashwill, J., & Droske, S. (1997). *Nursing care of children: Principles and practice.* Philadelphia: W. B. Saunders. p. 965.

7. 4

Rationale: Vitamin C increases the absorption of iron by the body. The mother should be instructed to administer the medication with a citrus fruit or juice high in vitamin C.

Test-Taking Strategy: Recalling that vitamin C increases the absorption of iron will assist in eliminating options 1 and 2. From the remaining options, select option 4 because this food item contains the highest amount of vitamin C.

Level of Cognitive Ability: Application
Phase of Nursing Process: Implementation
Client Needs: Health Promotion and Maintenance
Content Area: Pharmacology

Reference
Ashwill, J., & Droske, S. (1997). *Nursing care of children: Principles and practice.* Philadelphia: W. B. Saunders. p. 967.

8. 1

Rationale: Oral iron supplement should be administered through a straw or medicine dropper placed at the back of the mouth because it will stain the teeth. The parents should be instructed to brush or wipe the teeth after administration. Iron is administered between meals because absorption is decreased if there is food in the stomach. Iron requires an acidic environment to facilitate its absorption in the duodenum.

Test-Taking Strategy: Eliminate options 3 and 4 first because they are similar and because medication should not be added to formula and food. Note the key word "liquid" in the question. This should assist in recalling that liquid iron stains teeth. Review the teaching points related to this medication now if you had difficulty with this question!

Level of Cognitive Ability: Application
Phase of Nursing Process: Implementation
Client Needs: Health Promotion and Maintenance
Content Area: Pharmacology

Reference
Ashwill, J., & Droske, S. (1997). *Nursing care of children: Principles and practice.* Philadelphia: W. B. Saunders. p. 967.

9. 4

Rationale: Precautionary measures to prevent bleeding should be taken when a child has a low platelet count. These include no injections, no rectal temperatures, use of a soft toothbrush, and abstinence from contact sports or activities that could cause an injury. Strict isolation is required if the WBC count is low. Options 2 and 3 are unrelated to the risk of bleeding.

Test-Taking Strategy: Note that the WBC count is normal and that the platelet count is low. Recall that a low platelet count places the client at risk for bleeding. This will assist in eliminating options 1, 2, and 3. Review normal WBC and platelet counts now if you had difficulty with this question!

Level of Cognitive Ability: Analysis
Phase of Nursing Process: Planning
Client Needs: Physiological Integrity
Content Area: Child Health

Reference
Chernecky, C., & Berger, B. (1997). *Laboratory tests and diagnostic procedures* (2nd ed.). Philadelphia: W. B. Saunders. p. 815.

10. 4

Rationale: Males inherit hemophilia from their mothers and females inherit the carrier status from their fathers. Some females who are carriers have an increased tendency to bleed, and, although it is rare, females can have hemophilia if their fathers have the disorder and their mothers are carriers of the genetic disorder. Hemophilia is inherited in a recessive manner via a genetic defect on the X chromosome. Hemophilia A results from a deficiency of factor VIII. Hemophilia B (Christmas disease) is a deficiency of factor IX.

Test-Taking Strategy: Knowledge regarding hemophilia and its related etiology is required to answer the question. Take time to review this important disorder now if you had difficulty with this question!

Level of Cognitive Ability: Analysis
Phase of Nursing Process: Planning
Client Needs: Physiological Integrity
Content Area: Child Health

Reference
Bowden, V., Dickey, S., & Greenberg, C. (1998). *Children and their families: The continuum of care.* Philadelphia: W. B. Saunders. p. 1535.

11. 4

Rationale: The nurse needs to stress the importance of immunizations, dental hygiene, and routine well-child care. Options 1, 2, and 3 are appropriate. The parents are also instructed regarding care in the event of blunt trauma, especially trauma involving the joints, and to apply prolonged pressure to superficial wounds until the bleeding has stopped.

Test Taking Strategy: Note the key word "not" in the stem of the question. Knowledge that bleeding is a concern in this disorder will assist in eliminating options 1, 2, and 3, which include measures of protection and safety for the child. If you had difficulty with this question, take time now to review care to the child with hemophilia!

Level of Cognitive Ability: Application
Phase of Nursing Process: Implementation
Client Needs: Health Promotion and Maintenance
Content Area: Child Health

Reference
Ashwill, J., & Droske, S. (1997). *Nursing care of children: Principles and practice.* Philadelphia: W. B. Saunders. p. 981.

12. 4

Rationale: PTT measures the activity of thromboplastin, which is dependent on intrinsic factors. In hemophilia, the intrinsic clotting factor VIII (antihemophilic factor) is deficient, resulting in a prolonged PTT. Options 1, 2, and 3 are not necessarily abnormal.

Test-Taking Strategy: Knowledge regarding the laboratory tests used to monitor hemophilia is required to answer this question. Review these laboratory tests now if you had difficulty with this question!

Level of Cognitive Ability: Analysis
Phase of Nursing Process: Analysis
Client Needs: Physiological Integrity
Content Area: Child Health

Reference
Bowden, V., Dickey, S., & Greenberg, C. (1998). *Children and their families: The continuum of care.* Philadelphia: W. B. Saunders. p. 1540.

13. 2

Rationale: Children with hemophilia need to avoid contact sports and to take precautions such as wearing elbow and knee pads and helmets with other sports. The safest activity that will prevent injury is swimming.

Test-Taking Strategy: Note the key word "safely" in the stem of the question. Recalling that bleeding is a major concern in this condition will assist in directing you to option 2. Eliminate options 1, 3, and 4 because these activities present the potential for injury.

Level of Cognitive Ability: Analysis
Phase of Nursing Process: Implementation
Client Needs: Health Promotion and Maintenance
Content Area: Child Health

Reference
Ashwill, J., & Droske, S. (1997). *Nursing care of children: Principles and practice.* Philadelphia: W. B. Saunders. 981.

14. 3

Rationale: β-thalassemia is inherited by an autosomal recessive pattern. This disorder is found primarily in individuals of Mediterranean descent. The disease has been reported in the Asian and African population as well.

Test-Taking Strategy: Knowledge regarding the etiology associated with this disorder is required to answer this question. If you are unfamiliar with this disorder, take time now to review the information associated with its incidence and etiology!

Level of Cognitive Ability: Analysis
Phase of Nursing Process: Analysis
Client Needs: Physiological Integrity
Content Area: Child Health

Reference
Ashwill, J., & Droske, S. (1997). *Nursing care of children: Principles and practice.* Philadelphia: W. B. Saunders. p. 975.

15. 4

Rationale: The major complication of chronic transfusion therapy is hemosiderosis. In order to prevent organ damage from too much iron in the blood, chelation therapy with a medication called deferoxamine (Desferal) is used. Deferoxamine is classified as an antidote for acute iron toxicity. Dalteparin sodium (Fragmin) is an anticoagulant used as prophylaxis of postoperative deep vein thrombosis. Meropenem (Merrem) is an antibiotic. Molindone HCl (Moban) is an antipsychotic.

Test-Taking Strategy: Knowledge regarding the antidote for iron toxicity is required to answer this question. Familiarity with the medications identified in the options will also assist in directing you to option 4. If you had difficulty with this question, take time now to review these medications!

Level of Cognitive Ability: Analysis
Phase of Nursing Process: Analysis
Client Needs: Physiological Integrity
Content Area: Pharmacology

References
Ashwill, J., & Droske, S. (1997). *Nursing care of children: Principles and practice.* Philadelphia: W. B. Saunders. p. 975.
Hodgson, B., & Kizior, R. (1999). *Saunders nursing drug handbook 1999.* Philadelphia: W. B. Saunders. pp. 281, 289, 642, 700.

BIBLIOGRAPHY

Ashwill, J., & Droske, S. (1997). *Nursing care of children: Principles and practice.* Philadelphia: W. B. Saunders.
Chernecky, C., & Berger, B. (1997). *Laboratory tests and diagnostic procedures* (2nd ed.). Philadelphia: W. B. Saunders.
Hodgson, B., & Kizior, R. (1999). *Saunders nursing drug handbook 1999.* Philadelphia: W. B. Saunders.

Lammon, C., Foote, A., Leli, P., et al. (1995). *Clinical nursing skills.* Philadelphia: W. B. Saunders.
Luckmann, J. (1997). *Saunders manual of nursing care.* Philadelphia: W. B. Saunders.
Nichols, F., & Zwelling, E. (1997). *Maternal newborn nursing: Theory and practice.* Philadelphia: W. B. Saunders.
O'Toole, M. (ed.). (1997). *Miller-Keane encyclopedia & dictionary of medicine, nursing, & allied health* (6th ed.). Philadelphia: W. B. Saunders.

CHAPTER 44

Oncological Disorders

I. Leukemia

A. Description (Table 44–1)
1. Malignant exacerbation in the number of leukocytes, usually at an immature stage, in the bone marrow
2. Affects the bone marrow causing anemia, leukopenia, the production of immature cells, thrombocytopenia, and a decline in immunity
3. The cause is unknown and appears to involve gene damage of cells, leading to the transformation of cells from a normal state to a malignant state
4. Risk factors include genetic, viral, immunological, and environmental factors and exposure to radiation, chemicals, and medications
5. Risk factors in children include those with Down syndrome or a twin of a child who has had leukemia
6. Peak incidence is age 3 to 5 for acute lymphocytic leukemia (ALL)
7. Is more common in boys than girls after age 1 year

B. Assessment
1. Anorexia, fatigue, weakness, weight loss
2. Pallor and anemia
3. Bruising and bleeding from the nose or gums, rectal bleeding, hematuria
4. Prolonged bleeding after minor abrasions or lacerations
5. Petechiae
6. Elevated temperature

Table 44–1. Classification of Leukemia

Acute Lymphocytic Leukemia (ALL)	Acute Myelogenous Leukemia (AML)
Mostly lymphoblasts present in bone marrow	Mostly myeloblasts present in bone marrow
Age of onset is less than 15 years	Age of onset is between 15 and 39 years

7. Lymphadenopathy, splenomegaly
8. Palpitations and tachycardia
9. Orthostatic hypotension
10. Dyspnea on exertion
11. Headache
12. Bone pain and joint swelling
13. Normal, elevated or a decline in a white blood cell (WBC) count
14. Decreased hemoglobin and hematocrit levels
15. Decreased platelet count
16. Positive bone marrow biopsy identifying leukemic blast phase cells

C. Infection (Box 44–1)
1. A major cause of death in the immunosuppressed child
2. Can occur through autocontamination or cross-contamination
3. Most common sites of infection are the skin, respiratory tract, and gastrointestinal (GI) tract

D. Bleeding (Box 44–2)
1. During the period of greatest bone marrow suppression (the nadir), the platelet count may be extremely low
2. Children with platelet counts below 20,000/mm^3 may need a platelet transfusion
3. For children with severe blood loss, packed red blood cells may be prescribed

E. Fatigue and Nutrition
1. Assist the child in selecting a well-balanced diet
2. Provide small meals that require little chewing
3. Assist the child in self-care and mobility activities
4. Allow adequate rest periods during care
5. Do not perform activities unless they are essential

F. Chemotherapy
1. Monitor for severe bone marrow suppression
2. Monitor for infection and bleeding
3. Protect the child from life-threatening infections for at least 2 to 3 weeks following chemotherapy

---

BOX 44–1. Protecting the Child from Infection

- Initiate protective isolation procedures
- Maintain the child in a private room and a room with high efficiency particulate air (HEPA) filtration or laminar airflow system if possible
- Maintain frequent and thorough handwashing
- Use strict aseptic technique for all nursing procedures
- Limit the number of caregivers entering the child's room and ensure that anyone entering the child's room is wearing a mask
- Keep supplies for the child separate from supplies for other children
- Reduce exposure to environmental organisms by eliminating raw fruits and vegetables and fresh flowers and by not leaving standing water in the child's room
- Be sure that the child's room is cleaned daily
- Assist the child with daily bathing using an antimicrobial soap
- Assist the child to perform oral hygiene frequently
- Use strict aseptic technique with IV administration, changing IV tubing every 48 hours
- Initiate a bowel program to prevent constipation and rectal trauma
- Avoid invasive procedures such as injections, rectal temperatures, and urinary catheterization
- Assess for signs and symptoms of infection
- Monitor temperature, pulse, and blood pressure

- Change wound dressings daily and inspect wounds for redness, swelling, or drainage
- Assess urine for color and cloudiness
- Assess the skin and oral mucous membranes for signs of infection
- Auscultate lung sounds
- Encourage the child to cough and deep breathe
- Monitor the WBC and neutrophil count
- Notify the physician if signs of infection are present and prepare to obtain specimens for culture of open lesions, urine, and sputum
- Administer prescribed antibiotic, antifungal, and antiviral medications as prescribed
- Instruct the parents to keep the child away from crowds and those with infections
- Instruct the parents that the child should not receive immunization with a live virus
- Instruct the parents that siblings should receive inactivated polio vaccine but may receive live measles-mumps-rubella (MMR) vaccine
- Keep any child with chickenpox or any child who has been exposed to the virus away from the child with leukemia
- Instruct the parents to inform the teacher that they should be notified immediately if a case of chickenpox occurs in another child at school

---

4. Monitor for nausea, vomiting, and diarrhea
5. Assess oral mucous membranes for stomatitis
6. Monitor for renal, hepatic, and cardiac toxicity
7. Instruct the parents in signs and symptoms to monitor following chemotherapy and when to notify the physician
8. Inform the parents that hair loss may occur from chemotherapy
9. Instruct the parents about the care of central venous access devices as necessary
10. Listen and encourage the child and family to verbalize their feelings and express their concerns
11. Introduce the family to other families of children with cancer
12. Consult social services and chaplains as necessary

II. Hodgkin's Disease (Box 44–3)

A. Description
  1. A malignancy of the lymph nodes that originates in a single lymph node or a single chain of nodes
  2. Metastasis occurs to other adjacent lymph structures and eventually invades nonlymphoid tissue
  3. Usually involves lymph nodes, tonsils, spleen, and bone marrow
  4. Characterized by the presence of Reed-Sternberg cells in the lymph nodes
  5. Possible causes include viral infections and previous exposure to alkalating chemical agents
  6. Prognosis is dependent on the stage of disease
  7. Occurs more often in boys in children under age 15
  8. Diagnosis is usually made in the teenage to adult years

B. Assessment
  1. Persistent fever
  2. Night sweats
  3. Loss of appetite and significant weight loss

4. Fatigue and weakness
5. Pruritus
6. Anemia
7. Thrombocytopenia
8. Enlarged lymph nodes, spleen, and liver
9. Positive biopsy of lymph nodes, with cervical nodes most often affected first
10. Presence of Reed-Sternberg cells
11. Positive computed tomography (CT) scan of liver and spleen

C. Implementation (Box 44–4)
1. For stages 1 and 2 without mediastinal node involvement, the treatment of choice is extensive external radiation of involved lymph node regions
2. With more extensive disease, radiation along with multiagent chemotherapy is used
3. Monitor for drug-induced pancytopenia, which increases the risk for infection, bleeding, and anemia
4. Monitor for signs of infection and bleeding
5. Protect the child from infection
6. Provide a safe, hazard-free environment
7. Monitor for side effects related to chemotherapy or radiation

---

BOX 44–2. Protecting the Child from Bleeding

- Examine the child for signs and symptoms of bleeding
- Handle the child gently
- Measure abdominal girth, which can indicate internal hemorrhage
- Instruct the child to use a soft toothbrush and to avoid dental floss
- Provide soft foods that are cool to warm in temperature
- Avoid injections if possible to prevent trauma to the skin and bleeding
- Apply firm and gentle pressure to a needle-stick site for at least 10 minutes
- Pad side rails and sharp corners of the bed and furniture
- Discourage the child from engaging in activities involving the use of sharp objects
- Instruct the child to avoid constrictive or tight clothing
- Use caution when taking blood pressure to prevent skin injury
- Instruct the child to avoid blowing the nose
- Avoid rectal suppositories, enemas, and thermometers
- Examine all body fluids and excrement for the presence of blood
- Count the number of pads or tampons used if the female adolescent is menstruating
- Instruct the child in the signs and symptoms of bleeding
- Instruct the parents to avoid administering nonsteroidal anti-inflammatory drugs (NSAIDs) and products that contain aspirin to the child

---

BOX 44–3. Staging of Hodgkin's Disease

STAGE I

Involvement of a single lymph node region or a extralymphatic organ or site

STAGE II

Involvement of two or more lymph node regions on the same side of the diaphragm or localized involvement of an extralymphatic organ or site

STAGE III

Involvement of lymph node regions on both sides of the diaphragm or localized involvement of an extralymphatic organ or site or spleen or both

STAGE IV

Diffuse or disseminated involvement of one or more extralymphatic organs with or without associated lymph node involvement

---

8. Monitor for nausea and vomiting and administer antiemetics as prescribed
9. Monitor for skin irritation and breakdown as a result of radiation therapy

III. Nephroblastoma (Wilms' Tumor)

A. Description
1. A tumor of the kidney that may present unilaterally and localized or bilaterally, sometimes with metastasis to other organs
2. Average age of occurrence is between 2 and 6 years
3. This tumor grows very rapidly and prognosis depends on the stage of the disease at the time of diagnosis
4. Treatment may include chemotherapy alone or in combination with radiation and nephrectomy

B. Assessment
1. Mobile abdominal mass
2. Abdominal pain
3. Urinary retention and/or hematuria
4. Hypertension
5. Fever
6. Malaise
7. Anemia

C. Implementation Preoperatively
1. Monitor vital signs
2. Measure abdominal girth
3. Avoid palpation of the abdomen

BOX 44–4. MOPP Therapy for Hodgkin's Disease

Mechlorethamine (Mustargen)
Vincristine sulfate (Oncovin)
Procarbazine (Matulane)
Prednisone

4. Place a sign at bedside "Do Not Palpate Abdomen"

D. Implementation Postoperatively
1. Monitor vital signs
2. Monitor for changes in blood pressure
3. Monitor for signs of hemorrhage and infection
4. Maintain strict I&O measurements
5. Monitor urine output closely
6. Monitor for abdominal distention
7. Monitor bowel sounds

IV. Neuroblastoma

A. Description
1. An embryonal tumor found in children that arises from the neural crest
2. Typically, the tumor infringes on adjacent normal tissue and organs
3. Most commonly seen in the chest and neck, abdomen, and adrenal glands
4. A 24-hour urine will be collected to assess for elevated catecholamines (vanillylmandelic acid [VMA])

B. Assessment
1. Profuse diarrhea
2. Weight loss
3. Irritability
4. Fatigue and malaise
5. Anorexia
6. Palpable mass
7. Symptoms related to a neck and chest mass such as cough, respiratory dysfunction, and neck and facial edema
8. Symptoms related to bone marrow involvement such as anemia, bleeding, and infection
9. Symptoms related to cervical and thoracic masses
10. Neurological symptoms and paralysis related to pressure of the mass on the spinal column

C. Implementation
1. Treatment depends on the presence and extent of metastasis
2. Early stage disease without metastasis may only require surgical excision of the tumor and follow-up evaluations
3. Children with later-stage disease may receive radiation to tumor sites and systemic chemotherapy for several months

D. Implementation Preoperatively
1. Monitor for signs and symptoms related to the location of the tumor
2. Monitor vital signs
3. Monitor neurological status
4. Monitor for signs of increased intracranial pressure (ICP)
5. Obtain abdominal and cranial measurements
6. Monitor for signs of infection
7. Provide emotional support to the child and parents

E. Implementation Postoperatively
1. Monitor vital signs
2. Monitor abdominal girth and cranial measurements
3. Monitor neurological status
4. Maintain fluid and electrolyte balance
5. Monitor I&O
6. Monitor for signs of fluid overload
7. Elevate the head of the bed to semi-Fowler's position
8. Monitor for signs of infection
9. Provide pain relief measures
10. Instruct the parents about long-term management
11. Refer the parents to appropriate community services

V. Osteogenic Sarcoma

A. Description
1. An aggressive tumor and the most common bone malignancy in children
2. Usually found in the metaphysis of long bones, especially in the lower extremities
3. Symptoms in its earliest stage are almost always attributed to extremity injury or normal growing pains
4. Peak age of incidence is in the teenage years

B. Assessment
1. Progressive intermittent pain
2. Palpable mass
3. Limping if weight-bearing limb is affected
4. Progressive limited range of motion
5. Pathological fractures at the tumor site

C. Implementation
1. Prepare the child and family for prescribed treatment modalities, which may include surgical resection by limb salvage to remove affected tissue, amputation, and chemotherapy
2. Provide honesty and support for the child and family
3. Prepare for prosthetic fitting as necessary
4. Assist the child in dealing with problems of self image

VI. Ewing's Sarcoma

A. Description
1. A tumor that invades the soft tissue around the bone, especially the femur, vertebrae, ribs, and pelvic bones
2. Peak incidence is age 7 to 12 years

B. Assessment
1. Pain
2. Soft tissue swelling around the affected bone
3. Neurological symptoms if a vertebral tumor is present
4. Respiratory symptoms if a rib tumor is present
5. Anorexia, fever, malaise, fatigue, and weight loss if metastatic disease is present

C. Implementation: Prepare the child and family for treatments that may include chemotherapy, radiation, or excision of the tumor

VII. Brain Tumors

A. Description
   1. The most common solid tumor and the second most common type of cancer in children after leukemia
   2. The cause is unknown, but heredity and environmental factors are both associated
   3. Treatment can be devastating to the child's cognition and overall developmental progress
B. Assessment
   1. Vomiting on arising, which becomes progressively more projectile
   2. Headaches that worsen on arising and improve during the day
   3. Ataxia
   4. Visual changes
   5. Lethargy
   6. Papilledema
   7. Seizures
   8. Positive Babinski's sign
   9. Cranial enlargement in infants
   10. Bulging fontanel in infants
   11. Nuccal rigidity
   12. Behavioral changes
C. Implementation
   1. Initial intervention is "debulking" or removal of as much of the tumor as possible while minimally disturbing the surrounding brain tissue
   2. A ventriculoperitoneal **shunt** may be inserted to relieve symptoms of hydrocephalus
   3. Dexamethasone (Decadron) may be administered to reduce brain tissue swelling that occurs during surgery
   4. Radiation and chemotherapy may be instituted
D. Implementation Preoperatively
   1. Perform neurological assessment
   2. Institute safety measures
   3. Assess weight loss and nutritional status
   4. Initiate seizure precautions
   5. Prepare the child as much as possible
   6. The child's head will be shaved
   7. Provide a favorite cap or hat for the child
   8. Prepare the child to wake up with a large head dressing
E. Implementation Postoperatively
   1. Monitor vital signs and neurological status frequently
   2. Monitor for signs of increased ICP or hemorrhage
   3. Monitor temperature, which may be elevated because of hypothalamus or brain stem involvement during surgery
   4. Maintain a cooling blanket by the bedside
   5. Monitor the back of the head dressing for posterior pooling of blood
   6. Monitor for colorless drainage, which may indicate cerebrospinal fluid (CSF) and should be reported immediately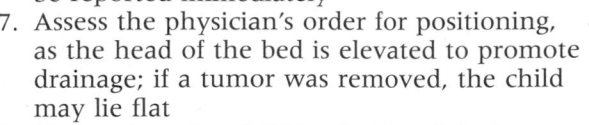
   7. Assess the physician's order for positioning, as the head of the bed is elevated to promote drainage; if a tumor was removed, the child may lie flat
   8. Never place the child in the Trendelenburg position
   9. Provide a quiet environment
   10. Administer analgesics as prescribed
   11. Assess for functional deficits

PRACTICE QUESTIONS

1. The pediatric nurse clinician is discussing the pathophysiology related to childhood leukemia to a class of nursing students. Which of the following is not associated with this type of cancer?
   1 Normal bone marrow is replaced by blast cells
   2 Red blood cell (RBC) and platelet production become affected
   3 The reticuloendothelial system is affected
   4 The presence of Reed-Sternberg cells is found on biopsy

2. A 4-year-old child is admitted to the hospital for abdominal pain. The mother reports that the child has been pale, excessively tired, and is bruising very easily. On physical examination, lymphadenopathy and hepatosplenomegaly are noted. Diagnostic studies are being performed on the child because acute lymphocytic leukemia (ALL) is suspected. Which of the following laboratory studies confirms this diagnosis?
   1 White blood cell count
   2 A lumbar puncture
   3 Bone marrow biopsy
   4 A platelet count

3. The pediatric nurse assists the physician in performing a lumbar puncture on a 3-year-old child with leukemia suspected of central nervous system (CNS) disease. In which of the following positions does the nurse place the child during this procedure?
   1 Prone with the knees flexed to the abdomen and the head bent with the chin resting on the chest
   2 Modified Sims' position
   3 Lateral recumbent with the knees flexed to the abdomen and the head bent with the chin resting on the chest
   4 Lithotomy position

4. The pediatric nurse is caring for a 9-year-old child with leukemia who is hospitalized for the administration of combination chemotherapy. In monitoring for CNS involvement, which of the following does the nurse include in the assessment?

1 Color, motion, and sensation of the extremities
2 Pupillary reaction
3 Level of consciousness
4 The presence of petechiae in the sclera

5. The nurse instructs the parents of a child with leukemia regarding measures related to monitoring for infection. Which of the following is not a component in the instructions?
   1 Proper handwashing techniques
   2 Taking a rectal temperature daily
   3 Inspecting the skin daily for redness
   4 Inspecting the mouth daily for lesions

6. A hospitalized child with leukemia has received intravenous (IV) chemotherapy, and discharge to home is being planned. Laboratory values indicate that the child is neutropenic. During the course of the chemotherapy, the IV infiltrated. The child has a small open area at the site of infiltration that is being treated daily by cleansing and the application of a topical antibiotic. The nurse instructs the mother regarding the signs of infection at this affected site. Which of the following statements, if made by the mother, indicates that teaching was effective?
   1 "If I see pus at the site I will know that an infection is present."
   2 "If I see redness at the site, I don't need to worry as long as there is no pus."
   3 "I will clean the site and apply the topical ointment every day."
   4 "If the temperature is elevated, I don't need to be concerned because this is normal with affected white blood cells."

7. A 6-year-old child with leukemia is hospitalized and is receiving combination chemotherapy. Laboratory results indicate that the child is neutropenic, and protective isolation procedures are initiated. The grandmother of the child visits and brings a fresh bouquet of flowers picked from her garden and asks the nurse for a vase for the flowers. Which of the following is the most appropriate response to the grandmother?
   1 "I have a vase in the utility room and I will get it for you."
   2 "The flowers from your garden are beautiful but should not be placed in the child's room at this time."
   3 "I will get the vase and wash it well before you put the flowers in it."
   4 "When you bring the flowers into the room, place them on the bedside stand as far away from the child as possible."

8. A 9-year-old child with leukemia is in remission and has returned to school. The school nurse calls the mother of the child and tells the mother that a classmate has just been diagnosed with chickenpox. The mother immediately calls the clinic nurse because the leukemic child has never had chickenpox. The most appropriate response to the mother is:
   1 "Monitor the child for an elevated temperature and call the clinic if a temperature occurs."
   2 "Keep the child out of school for a 2-week period."
   3 "There is no need to be concerned."
   4 "Bring the child into the clinic for a vaccine."

9. The nurse analyzes the laboratory values on a child with leukemia receiving chemotherapy. The nurse notes that the platelet count is 20,000/mm³. Based on this laboratory result, which of the following does the nurse incorporate in the plan of care?
   1 Initiate protective isolation precautions
   2 Monitor the temperature every 4 hours
   3 Monitor closely for signs of infection
   4 Use toothettes for mouth care

10. A child with leukemia is complaining of nausea. The nurse suspects that the nausea is related to the medication therapy. The nurse, concerned about the child's nutritional status, most appropriately offers which of the following during this episode of nausea?
    1 The child's favorite foods
    2 Cool, clear liquids
    3 Low-protein foods
    4 Low-calorie foods

11. A 12-year-old child is seen in the clinic and a diagnosis of Hodgkin's disease is suspected. Several diagnostic studies are performed to determine the presence of this disease. When evaluating the diagnostic results, the nurse expects to note which of the following if this child has Hodgkin's disease?
    1 The presence of blast cells in the bone marrow
    2 The presence of Reed-Sternberg cells
    3 The presence of Epstein-Barr virus
    4 Elevated catecholamines (vanillylmandelic acid [VMA]) urinary levels

12. The nurse is performing an assessment on a 10-year-old child suspected of having Hodgkin's disease. Which of the following data, if collected by the nurse, are most characteristic of this disease?
    1 Painful, enlarged inguinal lymph nodes
    2 Fever and malaise
    3 Painless, firm, and movable adenopathy in the cervical area
    4 Anorexia and weight loss

13. A 6-year-old child has just been diagnosed with localized Hodgkin's disease and chemotherapy is planned to begin immediately. The mother of the child asks the nurse about radiation therapy because it was not prescribed as a part of treat-

ment. The most appropriate response to the mother is:

1 "I'm not sure. I'll discuss it with the physician."
2 "The child is too young to have radiation therapy."
3 "It's very costly, and chemotherapy works just as well."
4 "The physician would prefer that you discuss treatment options with the oncologist."

14. The pediatric nurse is assigned to care for a child with a diagnosis of Wilms' tumor. In planning care for the child, the nurse understands that this tumor is:

1 An abdominal tumor
2 A renal tumor
3 A brain tumor
4 A bone tumor

15. The mother of a 4-year-old child brings the child to the clinic and tells the pediatric nurse specialist that the child's abdomen seems to be very swollen. On further assessment of subjective data, the mother tells the nurse that the child is eating well and that the activity level of the child is unchanged. The nurse, suspecting the possibility of Wilms' tumor, avoids which of the following during the physical assessment?

1 Palpating the abdomen for a mass
2 Assessing the urine for the presence of hematuria
3 Monitoring the temperature for the presence of fever
4 Monitoring the blood pressure for the presence of hypertension

16. The pediatric nurse is caring for a child who has just returned from the recovery room following a nephrectomy for Wilms' tumor. The physician prescribed replacement of IV fluids based on nasogastric (NG) tube drainage. The nurse calculates the amount of IV fluid replacement by:

1 Dividing the total 4-hour NG output by 4 and adding this amount to the current IV fluid
2 Dividing the total 8-hour NG output by 4 and adding this amount to the current IV fluid
3 Multiplying the total 4-hour NG output by 2 and adding this amount to the current IV fluid
4 Multiplying the total 8-hour NG output by 2 and adding this amount to the current IV fluid

17. A diagnostic workup is being performed on a 1-year-old child suspected of a diagnosis of neuroblastoma. Which of the following diagnostic findings is most specifically related to this type of tumor?

1 Elevated VMA levels in the urine
2 The presence of blast cells in the bone marrow
3 Projectile vomiting occurring most often in the morning
4 Positive Babinski's sign

18. The pediatric nurse specialist is providing a teaching session to the nursing staff regarding osteogenic sarcoma. Which of the following is not a component of the information provided during this session?

1 The symptoms of the disease in the early stage are almost always attributed to normal growing pains
2 The femur is the most common site of this sarcoma
3 Limping, if a weight-bearing limb is affected, is a clinical manifestation
4 The child does not experience pain at the primary tumor site

19. A 13-year-old child is diagnosed with a Ewing's sarcoma of the femur. Following a course of chemotherapy, it has been decided that leg amputation is necessary. Following the amputation, the child becomes very frightened because of aching and cramping felt in the missing limb. Which of the following is the most appropriate nursing statement to assist in alleviating the child's fear?

1 "This aching and cramping are normal and temporary and will subside."
2 "This normally occurs after the surgery and we will teach you ways to deal with it."
3 "The pain medication that I give you will take these feelings away."
4 "This pain is not real pain, and relaxation exercises will help it go away."

20. The nursing instructor assigns a student nurse to present a clinical conference to the student group about brain tumors in children. The nursing student prepares for the conference and includes which of the following in the presentation?

1 Surgery is not normally performed because of the risk of functional deficits occurring
2 Head shaving is no longer required before removal of the brain tumor
3 The most common site of metastasis is the kidneys
4 The most significant symptoms are headaches and morning vomiting

21. A brain tumor is suspected in a 9-year-old child and magnetic resonance imaging (MRI) and a positron emission tomography (PET) scan are ordered. Sedation before these procedures is prescribed for the child. Which of the following medications does the nurse anticipate will be prescribed for this child prior to these procedures?

1 Ondansetron HCl (Zofran)
2 Dexamethasone (Decadron)
3 Chloral hydrate (Noctec)
4 Ofloxacin (Floxin)

22. A child with a brain tumor is admitted to the hospital for "debulking" of the tumor. To ensure

a safe environment for this child, which of the following is included in the plan of care?

1 Assisting the child with ambulation at all times
2 Avoiding contact with other children on the nursing unit
3 Initiating seizure precautions
4 Using a wheelchair for out-of-bed activities

23. The child with a brain tumor returns from the recovery room following "debulking" of the tumor. Which of the following signs indicates that brain stem involvement occurred during the surgical procedure?
    1 Elevated temperature
    2 Orthostatic hypotension
    3 Inability to swallow
    4 Altered hearing ability

24. The nurse is assessing for bleeding in a child following surgery for removal of a brain tumor. The nurse checks the head dressing for the presence of blood and notes a colorless drainage on the back of the dressing. Which of the following is the most appropriate nursing intervention?
    1 Circle the area of drainage and continue to monitor
    2 Reinforce the dressing
    3 Notify the physician
    4 Document the findings and continue to monitor

25. Following surgical removal of a brain tumor, the physician writes an order to maintain the child in a flat position. In the postoperative period, the nurse is monitoring the child and notes that the child is restless, the pulse rate is elevated, and the blood pressure has dropped significantly from the baseline value. The nurse suspects that the child is in shock. Which of the following is the most appropriate nursing action?
    1 Place the child in the Trendelenburg position
    2 Elevate the head of the bed
    3 Increase the IV fluids
    4 Notify the physician

ANSWERS

1. **4**

Rationale: In leukemia, normal bone marrow is replaced by malignant blast cells. As the blast cells take over the bone marrow, eventually RBC and platelet production are affected and the child becomes anemic and thrombocytopenic. The reticuloendothelial system is affected, thus disturbing the body's defense system and rendering these children unable to fight infections normally. The Reed-Sternberg cell is found in Hodgkin's disease.

Test-Taking Strategy: Note the key word "not" in the stem of the question. Recalling that the Reed-Sternberg cell is found in Hodgkin's disease will easily direct you to option 4. Review the pathophysiology related to leukemia now if you had difficulty with this question!

Level of Cognitive Ability: Analysis
Phase of Nursing Process: Analysis
Client Needs: Physiological Integrity
Content Area: Child Health

Reference
Ashwill, J., & Droske, S. (1997). *Nursing care of children: Principles and practice.* Philadelphia: W. B. Saunders. p. 1001.

2. **3**

Rationale: The confirmatory test for leukemia is microscopic examination of bone marrow obtained by bone marrow aspirate and biopsy. A lumbar puncture may be done to look for blast cells in the spinal fluid that are indicative of CNS disease. The white blood cell (WBC) count may be high or low in leukemia. An altered platelet count occurs as a result of chemotherapy or the disease process.

Test-Taking Strategy: Note the key word "confirm" in the stem of the question. Use this key word and knowledge that the bone marrow is affected in leukemia to answer this question. If you had difficulty with this question, review the significance of the bone marrow biopsy now!

Level of Cognitive Ability: Analysis
Phase of Nursing Process: Assessment
Client Needs: Physiological Integrity
Content Area: Child Health

Reference
Ashwill, J., & Droske, S. (1997). *Nursing care of children: Principles and practice.* Philadelphia: W. B. Saunders. p. 1000.

3. **3**

Rationale: A lateral recumbent with knees flexed to the abdomen and head bent with chin resting on the chest is assumed for a lumbar puncture. This position separates the spinal processes and facilitates needle insertion into the subarachnoid space.

Test-Taking Strategy: Note the key word "lumbar" in the question. Visualize each of the descriptions of positions described in the options. This will assist in directing you to option 3. If you are unfamiliar with this procedure, review this child position now!

Level of Cognitive Ability: Application
Phase of Nursing Process: Implementation
Client Needs: Physiological Integrity
Content Area: Child Health

Reference
Lammon, C., Foote, A., Leli, P., et al. (1995). *Clinical nursing skills.* Philadelphia: W. B. Saunders. p. 170.

4. **3**

Rationale: The CNS is assessed because of the risk of infiltration of blast cells into the CNS. The child's level of consciousness as well as signs of irritability, vomiting, and lethargy are assessed. Color, motion, and sensation of the extremities are neurovascular assessments. Changes in pupillary reaction are most often noted in conditions related to increased intracranial pressure. The presence of petechiae in the sclera is an objective sign of leukemia.

Test-Taking Strategy: Note the key phrase "central nervous system" in the question. Eliminate options 1 and 4 first because they do not relate to the CNS. Select option 3 over option 2 because level of consciousness (LOC) will determine CNS function. Option 3 is also the most global option.

Level of Cognitive Ability: Application
Phase of Nursing Process: Assessment
Client Needs: Physiological Integrity
Content Area: Child Health

Reference

Ashwill, J., & Droske, S. (1997). *Nursing care of children: Principles and practice.* Philadelphia: W. B. Saunders. p. 1003.

5. **2**

Rationale: The risk of injury to fragile mucous membranes is so great in the child with leukemia that only oral or axillary temperatures should be taken. Rectal abscesses can easily occur to damaged rectal tissue. No rectal temperatures should be taken. Additionally oral temperatures should be avoided if the child has oral ulcers. Options 1, 3, and 4 are appropriate teaching measures.

Test-Taking Strategy: Note the key word "not" in the stem of the question. Options 1 and 3 can be easily eliminated first. From the remaining options, note the word "rectal" in option 2. Recalling that rectal temperatures should be avoided will direct you to this option. Review home care instructions related to infection in the leukemic child now if you had difficulty with this question!

Level of Cognitive Ability: Application
Phase of Nursing Process: Implementation
Client Needs: Health Promotion and Maintenance
Content Area: Child Health

Reference

Ashwill, J., & Droske, S. (1997). *Nursing care of children: Principles and practice.* Philadelphia: W. B. Saunders. p. 1003.

6. **3**

Rationale: Some neutropenic children will not produce purulent drainage. Because pus is made of WBCs, drainage cannot be used as a sign of infection. Redness may be the only sign. An elevated temperature is a sign of infection. Option 3 is the only correct statement.

Test-Taking Strategy: Note the key phrase "teaching was effective" in the stem of the question. Recalling the physiology associated with leukemia will assist in eliminating options 1, 2, and 4. Additionally, note that option 3 clearly rephrases the treatment to the affected site, as stated in the question.

Level of Cognitive Ability: Analysis
Phase of Nursing Process: Evaluation
Client Needs: Health Promotion and Maintenance
Content Area: Child Health

Reference

Ashwill, J., & Droske, S. (1997). *Nursing care of children: Principles and practice.* Philadelphia: W. B. Saunders. p. 1003.

7. **2**

Rationale: For the hospitalized neutropenic child, flowers or plants should not be kept in the room because standing water and damp soil harbor *Aspergillus* and *Pseudomonas*, to which these children are very susceptible. Additionally, fruits and vegetables not peeled before being eaten harbor molds and should be avoided until the WBC count rises.

Test-Taking Strategy: Knowledge regarding protective isolation procedures required in a neutropenic child will assist in answering this question. Note that options 1 and 3 are similar and should be eliminated first. From the remaining two options, select option 2 over option 4 because this nursing response maintains the procedure required. Review protective isolation procedures for the neutropenic child now if you had difficulty with this question!

Level of Cognitive Ability: Application
Phase of Nursing Process: Implementation
Client Needs: Safe, Effective Care Environment
Content Area: Child Health

Reference

Ashwill, J., & Droske, S. (1997). *Nursing care of children: Principles and practice.* Philadelphia: W. B. Saunders. p. 1005.

8. **4**

Rationale: Immunocompromised children are unable to adequately fight varicella. Chickenpox can be deadly to the immunocompromised child. If an immunocompromised child who has not had chickenpox is exposed to someone with varicella, the child should receive VZIG (varicella-zoster immune globulin) within 96 hours of exposure.

Test-Taking Strategy: Note the key phrase "never had chickenpox" in the question. Recall that a child with leukemia is immunocompromised and is unable to fight infection. This should assist you in eliminating options 1, 2, and 3. Review protective procedures for the immunocompromised child now if you had difficulty with this question!

Level of Cognitive Ability: Application
Phase of Nursing Process: Implementation
Client Needs: Physiological Integrity
Content Area: Child Health

Reference

Ashwill, J., & Droske, S. (1997). *Nursing care of children: Principles and practice.* Philadelphia: W. B. Saunders. p. 1004.

9. **4**

Rationale: If a child is severely thrombocytopenic, with a platelet count less than 20,000/mm³, precautions need to be taken because of the increased risk of bleeding. The precautions include limiting activity that could result in head injury, using soft toothbrushes or toothettes, checking urine and stools for blood, and administering stool softeners to prevent straining with constipation. Additionally, suppositories and rectal temperatures are avoided. Options 1, 2, and 3 are related to the prevention of infection rather than bleeding.

Test-Taking Strategy: Knowledge of the normal platelet count will assist in answering this question. Noting that the platelet count is low, and that a low platelet count places the child at risk for bleeding will assist in directing you to option 4. Additionally, note that options 1, 2, and 3 are similar because they all relate to the prevention of and monitoring for infection.

Level of Cognitive Ability: Analysis
Phase of Nursing Process: Planning
Client Needs: Physiological Integrity
Content Area: Child Health

Reference

Ashwill, J., & Droske, S. (1997). *Nursing care of children: principles and practice.* Philadelphia: W. B. Saunders. p. 1005.

10. **2**

Rationale: When the child is nauseated, it is best to offer cool, clear liquids because they are soothing and better tolerated. It is best not to offer favorite foods when the child is nauseated because foods eaten during times of nausea will be associated with being sick. Offer small, frequent meals of high-protein and high-calorie content.

Test-Taking Strategy: The issue of the question relates to nutritional status in a child with nausea. You should easily be able to eliminate options 3 and 4. From the remaining two options, you may be tempted to select option 1. Recalling the issue related to nausea will assist in directing you to option 2. Review interventions related to these issues now if you had difficulty with this question!

Level of Cognitive Ability: Analysis
Phase of Nursing Process: Implementation
Client Needs: Physiological Integrity
Content Area: Child Health

Reference
Ashwill, J., & Droske, S. (1997). *Nursing care of children: Principles and practice.* Philadelphia: W. B. Saunders. p. 1005.

11. **2**

Rationale: Hodgkin's disease is a neoplasm of lymphatic tissue. The presence of giant, multinucleated cells (Reed-Sternberg cells) is the hallmark of this disease. The presence of blast cells in the bone marrow is indicative of leukemia. Infectious mononucleosis and the Epstein-Barr virus have been associated with Hodgkin's disease, but would not determine the presence of Hodgkin's. Elevated VMA urinary levels are found in children with neuroblastoma.

Test-Taking Strategy: Recalling that the Reed-Sternberg cell is characteristic of Hodgkin's disease will easily direct you to option 2. Review the clinical manifestations associated with Hodgkin's disease now if you had difficulty with this question!

Level of Cognitive Ability: Analysis
Phase of Nursing Process: Assessment
Client Needs: Physiological Integrity
Content Area: Child Health

Reference
Ashwill, J., & Droske, S. (1997). *Nursing care of children: Principles and practice.* Philadelphia: W. B. Saunders. p. 1011.

12. **3**

Rationale: Clinical manifestations specifically associated with Hodgkin's disease include a painless firm and movable adenopathy in the cervical and supraclavicular area. Hepatosplenomegaly is also noted. Although anorexia, weight loss, fever, and malaise are associated with Hodgkin's disease, these manifestations are seen in many disorders.

Test-Taking Strategy: Note the key word "most" in the stem of the question. Eliminate options 2 and 4 first because these symptoms are general and vague. Recalling that painless adenopathy is associated with Hodgkin's disease will direct you to option 3. Review the clinical manifestations related to Hodgkin's disease now, if you had difficulty with this question!

Level of Cognitive Ability: Analysis
Phase of Nursing Process: Assessment
Client Needs: Physiological Integrity
Content Area: Child Health

Reference
Ashwill, J., & Droske, S. (1907). *Nursing care of children: Principles and practice.* Philadelphia: W. B. Saunders. pp. 1011–1012.

13. **2**

Rationale: Radiotherapy is usually delayed until a child is 8 years of age whenever possible to prevent retardation of bone growth and soft tissue development.

Test-Taking Strategy: Note the age of the child in the question. Additionally, use therapeutic communication techniques and knowledge regarding the effects of radiation to answer this question. Options 1 and 4 are nontherapeutic and place the mother's inquiry on hold. Use the child's age as a guide in directing you to option 2.

Level of Cognitive Ability: Application
Phase of Nursing Process: Implementation
Client Needs: Psychosocial Integrity
Content Area: Child Health

Reference
Bowden, V., Dickey, S., & Greenberg, C. (1998). *Children and their families: The continuum of care.* Philadelphia: W. B. Saunders. p. 1494.

14. **2**

Rationale: Wilms' tumor, or nephroblastoma, is the most common renal tumor in children. Arising from the renal parenchyma of the kidney, this tumor grows very rapidly. It may be present unilaterally and localized or bilaterally, sometimes with metastasis to other organs.

Test-Taking Strategy: Knowledge regarding the location of Wilms' tumor is required to answer this question. If you are unfamiliar with this type of tumor, take time now to review!

Level of Cognitive Ability: Analysis
Phase of Nursing Process: Planning
Client Needs: Physiological Integrity
Content Area: Child Health

Reference
Ashwill, J., & Droske, S. (1997). *Nursing care of children: Principles and practice.* Philadelphia: W. B. Saunders. p. 1010.

15. **1**

Rationale: If Wilms' tumor is suspected, the tumor mass should not be palpated during the initial assessment by the practitioner. Excessive manipulation can cause seeding of the tumor and cause spread of the cancerous cells. Fever, hematuria, and hypertension are clinical manifestations associated with Wilms' tumor.

Test-Taking Strategy: Note the key word "avoids" in the stem of the question. Knowledge that this tumor is located in the kidney will assist in eliminating options 2, 3, and 4 because of the relationship of these options to renal function. If you are unfamiliar with significant assessment procedures in the child with Wilms' tumor, take time now to review!

Level of Cognitive Ability: Application
Phase of Nursing Process: Implementation
Client Needs: Physiological Integrity
Content Area: Child Health

Reference
Ashwill, J., & Droske, S. (1997). *Nursing care of children: Principles and practice.* Philadelphia: W. B. Saunders. pp. 1010–1011.

16. 1

Rationale: Following nephrectomy, the child will have an NG tube in place with an order for replacement IV fluid for NG drainage. Typically NG tube output is totaled every 4 hours. This total is divided by 4 and either the resulting number is added to the current IV fluid or another IV solution is hung so that the amount lost by NG drainage is replaced over the next 4 hours. The process is repeated until the NG drainage has slowed enough so that it does not affect overall fluid and electrolyte balance.

Test-Taking Strategy: Noting that the child has just returned from the recovery room will assist in eliminating options 2 and 4 because NG tube drainage is assessed more frequently than every 8 hours. From the remaining two options, select option 1 over option 3 because the amount of fluid replacement calculated by the procedure described in option 3 is quite excessive. Review fluid replacement requirements following nephrectomy in the child with Wilms' tumor now if you had difficulty with this question!

Level of Cognitive Ability: Application
Phase of Nursing Process: Implementation
Client Needs: Physiological Integrity
Content Area: Child Health

Reference
Ashwill, J., & Droske, S. (1997). *Nursing care of children: Principles and practice.* Philadelphia: W. B. Saunders. p. 1011.

17. 1

Rationale: Neuroblastoma is a solid tumor found only in children. It arises from neural crest cells, which develop into the sympathetic nervous system and the adrenal medulla. Typically the tumor infringes on adjacent normal tissue and organs. Neuroblastoma cells may excrete catecholamines and their metabolites. Urine samples will indicate elevated VMA levels. The presence of blast cells in the bone marrow occurs in leukemia. Projectile vomiting occurring most often in the morning and a positive Babinski's sign are clinical manifestations of a brain tumor.

Test-Taking Strategy: Use the process of elimination in answering this question. If you are unfamiliar with this type of tumor, recall that blast cells are noted in leukemia, and eliminate option 2. Next eliminate options 3 and 4, noting that these manifestations are found in the child with a brain tumor. Review the manifestations associated with neuroblastoma now if you had difficulty with this question!

Level of Cognitive Ability: Analysis
Phase of Nursing Process: Assessment
Client Needs: Physiological Integrity
Content Area: Child Health

Reference
Ashwill, J., & Droske, S. (1997). *Nursing care of children: Principles and practice.* Philadelphia: W. B. Saunders. p. 1018.

18. 4

Rationale: A clinical manifestation of osteogenic sarcoma is progressive insidious intermittent pain at the tumor site. By the time these children receive medical attention, they may be in considerable pain from the tumor. Options 1, 2, and 3 are accurate regarding osteogenic sarcoma.

Test-Taking Strategy: Note the key word "not" in the stem of the question. Knowledge that osteogenic sarcoma is a malignant tumor of the bone will easily direct you to option 4. Review the clinical manifestations associated with osteogenic sarcoma now if you had difficulty with this question!

Level of Cognitive Ability: Application
Phase of Nursing Process: Implementation
Client Needs: Physiological Integrity
Content Area: Child Health

Reference
Ashwill, J., & Droske, S. (1997). *Nursing care of children: Principles and practice.* Philadelphia: W. B. Saunders. p. 1019.

19. 1

Rationale: Following amputation, phantom limb pain is a temporary condition that some children may experience. This sensation of burning, aching, or cramping in the missing limb is most distressing to the child. The child needs to be reassured that the condition is normal and only temporary.

Test-Taking Strategy: Use therapeutic communication techniques to answer this question. Note that the issue of the question relates to alleviating the child's fear. Option 1 is the only option that will alleviate fear. Options 2, 3, and 4 infer that this pain may be permanent.

Level of Cognitive Ability: Application
Phase of Nursing Process: Implementation
Client Needs: Psychosocial Integrity
Content Area: Child Health

Reference
Ashwill, J., & Droske, S. (1997). *Nursing care of children: Principles and practice.* Philadelphia: W. B. Saunders. p. 1020.

20. 4

Rationale: The hallmark symptoms of children with brain tumors are headache and morning vomiting related to the child getting out of bed. Initial intervention is "debulking" or operating to remove as much of the tumor as possible while minimally disturbing the surrounding brain tissue so that the child's neurological functioning is preserved as much as possible. Before surgery, the child's head will be shaved, although every effort is made to shave only as much hair as is necessary. Depending on the type of tumor, a myelogram may be done to determine metastatic disease in the spinal cord.

Test-Taking Strategy: Knowledge regarding the clinical manifestations and therapeutic interventions associated with a brain tumor is required to answer this question. This knowledge will assist in eliminating options 1, 2, and 3. If you are unfamiliar with the clinical manifestations and therapeutic interventions, take time now to review!

Level of Cognitive Ability: Analysis
Phase of Nursing Process: Planning
Client Needs: Physiological Integrity
Content Area: Child Health

Reference
Ashwill, J., & Droske, S. (1997). *Nursing care of children: Principles and practice.* Philadelphia: W. B. Saunders. pp. 1016–1017.

21. 3

Rationale: Ondansetron hydrochloride is an antiemetic used during chemotherapy. Chloral hydrate is a sedative and the medication used most often to sedate young children. Dexamethasone is administered to reduce some of the brain tissue swelling that occurs from the manipulation of tissue during surgery. Ofloxacin is an anti-infective medication.

Test-Taking Strategy: Knowledge related to the actions and effects of the medications identified in the options will assist in directing you to option 3. If you are unfamiliar with these medications, it is important to take the time now to review!

Level of Cognitive Ability: Analysis
Phase of Nursing Process: Analysis
Client Needs: Physiological Integrity
Content Area: Child Health

References
Ashwill, J., & Droske, S. (1997). *Nursing care of children: Principles and practice.* Philadelphia: W. B. Saunders. p. 1016.
Hodgson, B., & Kizior, R. (1999). *Saunders nursing drug handbook 1999.* Philadelphia: W. B. Saunders. pp. 198, 766, 772

22. **3**

Rationale: Seizure precautions should be considered for any child with a brain tumor both preoperatively and postoperatively. A thorough neurological assessment should be performed on the child, and the child's safety should be assessed prior to allowing the child to get out of bed without help. Options 1 and 4 are not required unless functional deficits exist. Option 2 is not necessary.

Test-Taking Strategy: Note the key phrase "safe environment" in the stem of the question. Eliminate options 1 and 4 first because they are similar. Additionally, note the phrase "all times" in option 1. Eliminate option 2 because it is unnecessary. If you had difficulty with this question, review nursing interventions related to the child with a brain tumor!

Level of Cognitive Ability: Application
Phase of Nursing Process: Planning
Client Needs: Safe, Effective Care Environment
Content Area: Child Health

Reference
Ashwill, J., & Droske, S. (1997). *Nursing care of children: Principles and practice.* Philadelphia: W. B. Saunders. p. 1016.

23. **1**

Rationale: Vital signs and neurological status are assessed frequently. Special attention is paid to the child's temperature, which may be elevated because of hypothalamus or brain stem involvement during surgery. A cooling blanket should either be in place on the bed or readily available if the child becomes hyperthermic. Options 3 and 4 are related to functional deficits following surgery. An elevated blood pressure and a widened pulse pressure may be associated with increasing intracranial pressure (ICP).

Test-Taking Strategy: Recalling the function of the hypothalamus and brain stem will easily direct you to option 1.

If you had difficulty with this question, review the complications that can occur following debulking of a brain tumor!

Level of Cognitive Ability: Analysis
Phase of Nursing Process: Assessment
Client Needs: Physiological Integrity
Content Area: Child Health

Reference
Ashwill, J., & Droske, S. (1997). *Nursing care of children: Principles and practice.* Philadelphia: W. B. Saunders. p. 1017.

24. **3**

Rationale: Colorless drainage on the dressing indicates the presence of cerebrospinal fluid and should be reported to the physician immediately.

Test-Taking Strategy: Note the key phrase "colorless drainage." This should quickly alert you to the possibility of the presence of cerebrospinal fluid. You should easily be able to eliminate options 1, 2, and 4. If you had difficulty with this question, review the significance of the presence of colorless drainage following cranial surgery!

Level of Cognitive Ability: Analysis
Phase of Nursing Process: Implementation
Client Needs: Physiological Integrity
Content Area: Child Health

Reference
Ashwill, J., & Droske, S. (1997). *Nursing care of children: Principles and practice.* Philadelphia: W. B. Saunders. p. 1017.

25. **4**

Rationale: The child is never placed in the Trendelenburg position because it increases ICP and the risk of bleeding. In the event of shock the physician is notified immediately before changing the child's position or increasing IV fluids. Increasing IV fluids can cause an increase in ICP.

Test-Taking Strategy: Recall the complications associated with cranial surgery to answer this question. Eliminate option 1 because this position increases ICP. Eliminate option 2 because this intervention will not assist in alleviating shock. In fact, this action could cause harm to the child. Eliminate option 3 because this action could increase ICP. Additionally, the nurse should not increase IV fluids in this child without a physician's order.

Level of Cognitive Ability: Application
Phase of Nursing Process: Implementation
Client Needs: Physiological Integrity
Content Area: Child Health

Reference
Ashwill, J., & Droske, S. (1997). *Nursing care of children: Principles and practice.* Philadelphia: W. B. Saunders. p. 1017.

BIBLIOGRAPHY

Ashwill, J., & Droske, S. (1997). *Nursing care of children: Principles and practice.* Philadelphia: W. B. Saunders.
Bowden, V., Dickey, S., & Greenberg, C. (1998). *Children and their families: The continuum of care.* Philadelphia: W. B. Saunders.
Hodgson, B., & Kizior, R. (1999). *Saunders nursing drug handbook 1999.* Philadelphia: W. B. Saunders.

Lammon, C., Foote, A., Leli, P., et al. (1995). *Clinical nursing skills.* Philadelphia: W. B. Saunders.
Luckmann, J. (1997). *Saunders manual of nursing care.* Philadelphia: W. B. Saunders.
Nichols, F., & Zwelling, E. (1997). *Maternal newborn nursing: Theory and practice.* Philadelphia: W. B. Saunders.
O' Toole, M. (ed.). (1997). *Miller-Keane encyclopedia & dictionary of medicine, nursing, & allied health* (6th ed.). Philadelphia: W. B. Saunders.

CHAPTER 45

Infectious and Communicable Diseases

I. Rubeola

A. Description
   1. Incubation period: 7 to 14 days
   2. Infectious period: 1 to 2 days before onset of symptoms to 4 days after rash appears
   3. Transmission: Airborne, or direct contact with infectious droplets
   4. Season: Winter, spring
B. Assessment
   1. Koplik's spots—small, bright red spots with a bluish-white speck in the center of each; they are located on the mucosa and last 3 days
   2. Rash is red and maculopapular, blanches easily with pressure, gradually turns a brownish color, and lasts 6 to 7 days
   3. Rash begins behind the ears and spreads downward to the feet
C. Implementation
   1. Respiratory isolation if hospitalized
   2. Restrict to quiet activities and bed rest

II. Roseola

A. Description
   1. Incubation period: 5 to 15 days
   2. Infectious period: Unknown, but thought to extend from the febrile stage to the time the rash first appears
   3. Transmission: Saliva
   4. Season: Spring and fall
B. Assessment
   1. Fever for 3 to 5 days, followed by a rash, composed of rose-pink maculas, that blanches with pressure
   2. Rash is found on the neck and trunk and is surrounded by a whitish ring
   3. Rash lasts 24 to 48 hours before fading
C. Implementation: Supportive

III. Rubella (German Measles)

A. Description
   1. Incubation period: 14 to 21 days
   2. Infectious period: 10 days before onset of symptoms to 15 days after rash appears
   3. Transmission
      a. Airborne, or direct contact with infectious droplets
      b. Transplacental
   4. Season: Winter, spring
B. Assessment
   1. Pinkish-rose maculopapular rash that begins on the face and spreads to the entire body
   2. Petechial spots may occur on the soft palate
C. Implementation
   1. Contact isolation
   2. Supportive treatment

IV. Mumps

A. Description
   1. Incubation period: 16 to 18 days but may extend to 25 days
   2. Infectious period: Usually 1 to 2 days (7 days prior to swelling to 9 days after onset)
   3. Transmission
      a. Airborne droplets
      b. Saliva and possibly urine
   4. Season: Late winter, spring
B. Assessment: Fever, muscular pain, headache, and malaise, followed by parotid glandular swelling
C. Implementation: Respiratory isolation is indicated until 9 days after the onset of parotid swelling

V. Chickenpox

A. Description
   1. Incubation period: 10 to 21 days
   2. Infectious period: 1 to 2 days before the onset

of rash to 5 days after the onset of lesions and crusting of lesions
   3. Transmission: Direct contact, droplet, airborne particles
   4. Season: Late winter through early spring
B. Assessment
   1. Elevated temperature, malaise, and anorexia, followed by a macular rash that first appears on the trunk and scalp and moves to the extremities
   2. The lesions become pustules, begin to dry, and develop a crust
   3. They appear on the mucous membranes of the mouth, genital area, and rectum
C. Implementation
   1. In the hospital setting, strict isolation
   2. In the home setting, the child is isolated from all individuals susceptible to infection

VI. Pertussis (Whooping Cough)

A. Description
   1. Incubation period: 6 to 20 days
   2. Infectious period: Catarrhal stage (1 to 2 weeks) until the 4th week
   3. Transmission: Direct contact or respiratory droplets from coughing
   4. Season: Can occur during any season
B. Assessment: Symptoms of respiratory infection followed by increased severity of cough
C. Implementation
   1. Hospitalized child is placed in respiratory isolation
   2. Supportive therapy
   3. Antibiotics

VII. Diphtheria

A. Description
   1. Incubation period: 2 to 5 days
   2. Infectious period: Ranges from 2 weeks or less up to several months in an untreated individual
   3. Transmission: Contact with carrier or disease droplets
   4. Season: Fall and winter
B. Assessment
   1. Foul-smelling mucopurulent nasal discharge
   2. Gray membrane on tonsils and pharynx
   3. Neck edema
C. Implementation
   1. Respiratory isolation
   2. Supportive therapy
   3. Antibiotics

VIII. Poliomyelitis

A. Description
   1. Incubation period
      a. 3 to 6 days for abortive
      b. 7 to 21 days for paralytic
   2. Infectious period

   a. Shortly before the onset of illness
   b. The virus is shed in the pharynx for 1 week after onset, and in the feces for several weeks to months
   3. Transmission: Fecal-oral, oral-oral
   4. Season: Summer and fall
B. Assessment
   1. Fever, malaise, anorexia, nausea, headache, sore throat
   2. Abdominal pain, followed by soreness and stiffness of the trunk, neck, and limbs, which progresses to flaccid paralysis
C. Implementation
   1. Enteric precautions
   2. Supportive treatment
   3. Monitor for respiratory paralysis

IX. Scarlet Fever

A. Description
   1. Incubation period: 1 to 7 days
   2. Infectious period: Acute stage until 36 hours after antibiotic therapy is started
   3. Transmission: Airborne, direct contact
   4. Season: Late fall, winter, spring
B. Assessment
   1. A fine, red, papular rash in the axilla, groin, and neck, which spreads to cover the entire body
   2. The rash blanches with pressure except in areas of deep creases (Pastia's sign)
   3. The tongue is coated with a white furry covering, which progresses to a red, swollen tongue (white strawberry tongue, strawberry tongue)
   4. Tonsils are edematous and covered with a gray-white exudate
   5. Petechial hemorrhage covers the soft palate
C. Implementation
   1. Antibiotics
   2. Supportive therapy

X. Infectious Mononucleosis (Epstein-Barr Virus)

A. Description
   1. Incubation period: 4 to 7 weeks
   2. Infectious period: Unknown; virus is shed before onset of disease until 6 months or longer after recovery
   3. Transmission: Saliva; close, intimate contact; blood
   4. Season: Can occur during any season
B. Assessment
   1. Fever, pharyngitis, malaise, headache, fatigue, nausea, abdominal pain
   2. Lymphadenopathy and hepatosplenomegaly
C. Implementation
   1. Supportive
   2. Monitor for signs of splenic rupture, which include abdominal pain, left upper quadrant pain, or left shoulder pain

◆ XI. Rocky Mountain Spotted Fever

A. Description
1. Incubation period: 2–14 days
2. Transmission: Bite of infected tick
3. Season: April through September

B. Assessment
1. Headache, fever, anorexia, restlessness, maculopapular or petechial rash that begins on the palms and soles and spreads to the rest of the body
2. Hemorrhagic and necrotic lesions can occur
3. Periorbital edema progressing to generalized edema

C. Implementation
1. Antibiotic therapy
2. Preventive teaching regarding the risk of exposure to ticks
3. Antibiotics and supportive care for presenting symptoms

XII. *Enterobius* (Pinworm)

A. Transmission
1. Ingestion or inhalation of eggs
2. Hands to mouth
3. Fecal-oral

B. Assessment: Nocturnal anal itching, sleeplessness

C. Implementation
1. Scotch tape test to identify
2. Enteric precautions
3. Anthelmintic medications

XIII. Immunizations

A. Immunization schedule (Box 45–1)
◆ B. Contraindications to immunizations
1. Severe febrile illness
2. Suppressed immune system (NO LIVE VACCINES)
3. Siblings and household contacts of

immunosuppressed children should not receive the oral polio vaccine (OPV) but may be given the inactivated poliovirus vaccine (IPV)
4. Received gamma globulin within past 6 weeks
5. Allergic to contents of immunization (prior to the administration of measles-mumps-rubella [MMR] vaccine, assess for known history of allergy to eggs, neomycin, or related antibiotics)
6. Recent chemotherapy

PRACTICE QUESTIONS

1. A child with measles (rubeola) is being admitted to the hospital. In preparing for the admission of the child, which of the following will the nurse include in the plan of care?
   1 Contact precautions
   2 Enteric precautions
   3 Respiratory isolation
   4 Protective isolation

2. Several children have contracted measles (rubeola) in a local school. The school nurse conducts a teaching session for the mothers of the school children. Which of the following would not be a part of the teaching regarding this communicable disease?
   1 Respiratory symptoms, such as a profuse, runny nose, cough, and fever, occur prior to the development of a rash
   2 Small blue-white spots with a red base may appear in the mouth
   3 The rash usually begins behind the ears, at the hairline, on the forehead, and on the upper part of the neck
   4 The infectious period ranges from 10 days before the onset of symptoms to 15 days after the rash appears

3. The mother of a 15-month-old child brings the child to the clinic and reports that the child has a fever and has developed a rash on the neck and trunk of the body. Roseola is diagnosed. The mother is concerned that her other children will contract the disease. Which of the following instructions will the nurse provide to the mother regarding the prevention of transmission of the disease?
   1 The disease is transmitted through the urine and feces, so the other children should use a separate bathroom
   2 The disease is transmitted through saliva, so the other children should not share eating utensils
   3 The disease is transmitted through the respiratory tract, so the child should be isolated from the other children as much as possible
   4 The disease is transmitted by contact with body fluids, so any items contaminated with body fluids need to discarded in a separate receptacle

---

BOX 45–1. Recommended Immunization Schedule for Healthy Infants and Children

Birth	Hepatitis B
1 month	Hepatitis B
2 months	OPV, DTP, HIB
4 months	DTP, HIB, OPV
6 months	DTP, HIB, hepatitis B
12 months	HIB, OPV
15 months	MMR
18 months	DTP
12–18 months	Varicella vaccine
4–6 years	DTP, OPV, MMR
11–12 years	MMR (if not administered at 4–6 years)
11–16 years	TD booster

DTP, diphtheria, tetanus toxoids, and pertussis; HIB, *Haemophilus influenzae* type B; MMR, measles-mumps-rubella; OPV, oral poliovirus vaccine; TD, tetanus-diphtheria.

4. The pediatric nurse is caring for a hospitalized child with a diagnosis of rubella (German measles). The nurse reviews the physician's progress notes and reads that the child has developed Forschheimer's sign. Based on this documentation, which of the following would the nurse expect to note in the child?
   1 Petechial spots located on the palate
   2 Small blue-white spots noted on the buccal mucosa
   3 A fiery red edematous rash on the cheeks
   4 Swelling of the parotid gland

5. The nurse is assigned to care for a child with rubella (German measles). Which of the following protective measures will not be necessary when providing direct care to the child?
   1 Mask
   2 Gloves
   3 Gown
   4 Goggles

6. The nurse provides instructions to the mother of a child with mumps regarding respiratory isolation procedures. The mother asks the nurse about the length of time required for the respiratory isolation. The most appropriate nursing response is:
   1 "Respiratory isolation is not necessary."
   2 "Mumps is not transmitted by the respiratory system."
   3 "Respiratory isolation is indicated for 9 days following the onset of parotid swelling."
   4 "Respiratory isolation is indicated for 18 days following the onset of parotid swelling."

7. The pediatric nurse specialist provides an educational session to the nursing students about childhood communicable diseases. A nursing student asks the pediatric nurse specialist to describe the signs and symptoms associated with the most common complication of mumps. Which of the following signs or symptoms is indicative of the most common complication of this communicable disease?
   1 A red, swollen testicle
   2 Nuchal rigidity
   3 Pain
   4 Deafness

8. The parents of a child with mumps express concern that their child will develop orchitis as a result of having mumps. The parents ask the nurse about the complication and about the signs that may indicate this complication. Which of the following would not be a part of the nurse's response to the parents?
   1 Abrupt onset of pain
   2 Headache and vomiting
   3 Fever and chills
   4 Difficulty in urinating

9. The mother brings her 6-year-old child to the clinic because the child has developed a rash on the trunk and on the scalp. The mother reports that the child has had a low-grade temperature, has not felt like eating, and has been generally tired. The child is diagnosed with chickenpox. The mother inquires about the infectious period associated with chickenpox. The nurse bases the response on which of the following?
   1 The infectious period is unknown
   2 The infectious period is 1 to 2 days before the onset of rash to 5 days after the onset of lesions and the crusting of lesions
   3 The infectious period is 10 days before the onset of symptoms to 15 days after the appearance of the rash
   4 The infectious period ranges from 2 weeks or less up to several months

10. The nurse provides home care instructions to the parents of a child hospitalized with pertussis. The child is in the convalescent stage and is being prepared for discharge. Which of the following will not be a component of the teaching plan?
    1 Maintain respiratory isolation and a quiet environment for at least 2 weeks
    2 Coughing spells may be triggered by noises or episodes of fright
    3 Encourage fluid intake
    4 Good handwashing techniques must be instituted to prevent spreading the disease to others

11. A 6-month-old infant receives a DTP (diphtheria, tetanus, pertussis) immunization at the well baby clinic. The mother returns home and calls the clinic to report that the infant has developed swelling and redness at the site of injection. The most appropriate suggestion to the mother is:
    1 Apply a warm pack to the injection site
    2 Bring the infant back to the clinic
    3 Apply an ice pack to the injection site
    4 Monitor the infant for a fever

12. A nursing instructor asks a nursing student about the contraindications associated with the administration of oral poliovirus vaccine (OPV). The student is asked to identify the rationale regarding the administration of OPV to siblings of an immunocompromised child. The most appropriate response by the nursing student is:
    1 "The viruses in OPV multiply in the vaccinee's respiratory tract and can then be transmitted with breathing and coughing."
    2 "OPV is not contraindicated in siblings of an immunocompromised child."
    3 "The viruses in OPV multiply in the vaccinee's gastrointestinal (GI) tract and can then be transmitted in saliva and feces."
    4 "OPV is not contraindicated as long as the siblings and immunocompromised child do not share food or utensils."

13. A child diagnosed with scarlet fever is being cared for at home. The home health nurse visits the child and performs an assessment. Which of the following is not a clinical manifestation associated with this disease?
    1 Pastia's sign
    2 White strawberry tongue
    3 Petechial hemorrhages on the soft palate
    4 Koplik's spots

14. The home health nurse visits a child with Epstein-Barr virus (mononucleosis) and provides home care instructions to the parents. Which of the following would be included in the instructions?
    1 Maintain bed rest for 2 weeks
    2 Maintain respiratory isolation precautions for 1 week
    3 Notify the physician if the child develops a fever
    4 Notify the physician if abdominal pain or left shoulder pain occurs

15. A 5-year-old child is hospitalized with Rocky Mountain spotted fever (RMSF). The nursing assessment reveals that the child was bitten by a tick 2 weeks ago. The child presents with complaints of headache, fever, and anorexia. The nurse notes a rash on the child's palms and soles of the feet. The nurse reviews the physician's orders and anticipates which of the following will be prescribed?
    1 Tetracycline (Achromycin)
    2 Amphotericin B (Abelcet)
    3 Ganciclovir (Vitrasert)
    4 Amantadine (Symmetrel)

16. The mother of a preschooler who attends day care calls the clinic nurse and tells the nurse that the child is constantly scratching the perianal area and that the area is irritated. The nurse suspects the possibility of pinworm infection (enterobiasis). The nurse instructs the mother to obtain a cellophane tape rectal specimen. Which

of the following is the appropriate instruction regarding obtaining this specimen?
    1 Obtain the specimen when the child is put to bed
    2 Obtain the specimen after toileting
    3 Obtain the specimen after bathing
    4 Obtain the specimen in the morning when the child awakens

17. The clinic nurse prepares to administer an MMR (measles-mumps-rubella) vaccine to a 5-year-old child. The nurse would administer this vaccine:
    1 Intramuscularly in the anterolateral aspect of the thigh
    2 Intramuscularly in the deltoid muscle
    3 Subcutaneously into the outer aspect of the upper arm
    4 Subcutaneously in the gluteal muscle

18. The clinic nurse of a well baby clinic prepares to administer immunizations. Which of the following conditions, if present in a child, would be a contraindication for receiving an immunization?
    1 Cold
    2 Otitis media
    3 Diarrhea
    4 Fever

19. A mother brings her 4-month-old infant to the well baby clinic for immunizations. The nurse would prepare to administer which of the following immunizations to this infant?
    1 DTP, MMR, OPV
    2 MMR, HIB, DTP
    3 DTP, HIB, OPV
    4 Varicella and hepatitis B vaccines

20. The clinic nurse obtains a health history from a mother of a 15-month-old child prior to administering an MMR vaccine. Which of the following assessment findings would be of highest priority prior to the administration of this vaccine?
    1 Allergy to eggs
    2 A recent cold
    3 The presence of diarrhea
    4 Any recent ear infections

ANSWERS

1. **3**

Rationale: Rubeola is transmitted via airborne particles or direct contact with infectious droplets. Respiratory isolation is required, and a mask should be worn by those in contact with the child. Gowns and gloves are not indicated. Articles that are contaminated should be bagged and labeled. Options 1, 2, and 4 are not indicated in rubeola.

Test-Taking Strategy: Knowledge of the route of transmission is required to answer this question. This knowledge will easily direct you to option 3. Review the route of

transmission and therapeutic management now, if you had difficulty with this question!
Level of Cognitive Ability: Application
Phase of Nursing Process: Planning
Client Needs: Safe, Effective Care Environment
Content Area: Child Health
Reference
Ashwill, J., & Droske, S. (1997). *Nursing care of children: Principles and practice.* Philadelphia: W. B. Saunders. pp. 597, 599.

2. **4**

Rationale: The infectious period for rubeola ranges from 1 to 2 days before the onset of symptoms to 4 days after the rash appears. Options 1, 2, and 3 are accurate descriptions of rubeola. The small, blue-white spots found in this communicable disease are called Koplik's spots. Option 4 describes the infectious period for rubella.

Test-Taking Strategy: Note the key word "not" in the stem of the question. Recalling that the infectious period ranges from 1 to 2 days before the onset of symptoms to 4 days after rash appearance will direct you to option 4. If you are unfamiliar with the clinical manifestations associated with rubeola, take time now to review!

Level of Cognitive Ability: Application
Phase of Nursing Process: Implementation
Client Needs: Health Promotion and Maintenance
Content Area: Child Health

Reference
Ashwill, J., & Droske, S. (1997). *Nursing care of children: Principles and practice*. Philadelphia: W. B. Saunders. p. 597.

3. **2**

Rationale: Roseola is transmitted via saliva. Therefore, others should not share eating utensils. Options 1, 3, and 4 are not accurate transmission routes of roseola.

Test-Taking Strategy: Eliminate options 1 and 4 first because they are similar. For the remaining two options, recalling that roseola is transmitted via saliva will assist in directing you to option 2. Review the route of transmission of roseola now, if you had difficulty with this question!

Level of Cognitive Ability: Application
Phase of Nursing Process: Implementation
Client Needs: Health Promotion and Maintenance
Content Area: Child Health

Reference
Ashwill, J., & Droske, S. (1997). *Nursing care of children: Principles and practice*. Philadelphia: W. B. Saunders. p. 600.

4. **1**

Rationale: Forschheimer's sign refers to petechial spots, which are reddish, pinpoint, and located on the soft palate. Small, blue-white spots noted on the buccal mucosa are known as Koplik's spots and are seen in rubeola. A fiery red edematous rash on the cheeks, also called "slapped cheek," is seen in erythema infectiosum. Swelling of the parotid gland is seen in mumps.

Test-Taking Strategy: Knowledge regarding the clinical manifestations of rubella is required to answer this question. If you were familiar with the clinical manifestations of other communicable diseases, you would be able to eliminate options 2, 3, and 4. If you are unfamiliar with Forschheimer's sign, take time now to review!

Level of Cognitive Ability: Analysis
Phase of Nursing Process: Assessment
Client Needs: Physiological Integrity
Content Area: Child Health

Reference
Ashwill, J., & Droske, S. (1997). *Nursing care of children: Principles and practice*. Philadelphia: W. B. Saunders. p. 599.

5. **4**

Rationale: Care of the child with rubella involves contact isolation. Contact isolation requires masks, gowns, and gloves for contact with any infectious material. Contaminated articles must be bagged and labeled per agency protocol.

Test-Taking Strategy: Note the key words "not" and "direct" in the stem of the question. Recalling that rubella is transmitted via airborne particles or direct contact with infectious droplets will assist in directing you to option 4 as the item not required when providing direct care to this child. If you had difficulty with this question, take time now to review the modes of transmission for rubella!

Level of Cognitive Ability: Application
Phase of Nursing Process: Implementation
Client Needs: Safe, Effective Care Environment
Content Area: Child Health

Reference
Ashwill, J., & Droske, S. (1997). *Nursing care of children: Principles and practice*. Philadelphia: W. B. Saunders. p. 600.

6. **3**

Rationale: Mumps is transmitted via airborne droplets, by salivary secretions, and possibly by contact with the urine. Uncomplicated mumps may require only symptomatic care. Respiratory isolation is indicated for 9 days following the onset of parotid swelling.

Test-Taking Strategy: Knowledge regarding the infectious period for mumps is required to answer this question. Options 1 and 2 can be eliminated first because they are similar. From the remaining two options, select option 3, because the time frame indicated in option 4 seems rather lengthy. Review the infectious period related to mumps now, if you had difficulty with this question!

Level of Cognitive Ability: Application
Phase of Nursing Process: Implementation
Client Needs: Safe, Effective Care Environment
Content Area: Child Health

Reference
Ashwill, J., & Droske, S. (1997). *Nursing care of children: Principles and practice*. Philadelphia: W. B. Saunders. p. 603.

7. **2**

Rationale: The most common complication of mumps is aseptic meningitis, with the virus being identified in the cerebrospinal fluid. Common signs include nuchal rigidity, lethargy, and vomiting. A red, swollen testicle may be indicative of orchitis. Although this complication appears to cause most concern among parents, it is not the most common complication. Mumps is one of the leading causes of unilateral nerve deafness, but it does not occur frequently. Muscular pain, parotid pain, or testicular pain may occur, but pain does not indicate a sign of a common complication.

Test-Taking Strategy: Knowledge that aseptic meningitis is the most common complication of mumps will easily direct you to option 2. If you had difficulty with this question, review the complications associated with mumps now!

Level of Cognitive Ability: Analysis
Phase of Nursing Process: Assessment
Client Needs: Physiological Integrity
Content Area: Child Health

Reference
Ashwill, J., & Droske, S. (1997). *Nursing care of children: Principles and practice*. Philadelphia: W. B. Saunders. p. 603.

8. **4**

Rationale: Unilateral orchitis occurs more frequently that bilateral orchitis. About 1 week after the appearance of parotitis, there is an abrupt onset of testicular pain, tenderness, fever, chills, headache, and vomiting. The affected testicle becomes red, swollen, and tender. Atrophy resulting in sterility occurs only in a small number of cases. Difficulty in urinating is not a sign of this complication.

Test-Taking Strategy: Note the key word "not" in the stem of the question. Knowledge regarding the signs associated with orchitis is required to answer this question. If you had difficulty identifying these signs, take time now to review orchitis!

Level of Cognitive Ability: Application
Phase of Nursing Process: Implementation
Client Needs: Physiological Integrity
Content Area: Child Health

Reference
Ashwill, J., & Droske, S. (1997). *Nursing care of children: Principles and practice.* Philadelphia: W. B. Saunders. p. 603.

9. **2**

Rationale: The infectious period for chickenpox is 1 to 2 days before the onset of rash to 5 days after the onset of lesions and the crusting of lesions. In roseola, the infectious period is unknown. Option 3 describes rubella. Option 4 describes diphtheria.

Test-Taking Strategy: Knowledge regarding the infectious period associated with chickenpox is required to answer this question. Option 1 can be easily eliminated. Eliminate options 3 and 4 next because the time frames in these two options seem rather lengthy. If you had difficulty with this question, take time now to review the infectious period associated with chickenpox!

Level of Cognitive Ability: Analysis
Phase of Nursing Process: Analysis
Client Needs: Physiological Integrity
Content Area: Child Health

Reference
Ashwill, J., & Droske, S. (1997). *Nursing care of children: Principles and practice.* Philadelphia: W. B. Saunders. pp. 599, 600, 604, 612.

10. **1**

Rationale: Pertussis is transmitted by direct contact or respiratory droplets from coughing. The infectious period occurs during the catarrhal stage (1 to 2 weeks) until the fourth week. Respiratory isolation is not required during the convalescent phase. Options 2, 3, and 4 are components of home care instruction. Additionally, a quiet environment is encouraged.

Test-Taking Strategy: Note the key word "not" in the stem of the question. Options 3 and 4 can be easily eliminated because they are general interventions associated with convalescence. Knowing that coughing spells are associated with pertussis will assist in directing you to option 1. Additionally, 2 weeks of respiratory isolation is not required. If you had difficulty with this question, review home care instructions for the child with pertussis!

Level of Cognitive Ability: Application
Phase of Nursing Process: Implementation
Client Needs: Health Promotion and Maintenance
Content Area: Child Health

Reference
Ashwill, J., & Droske, S. (1997). *Nursing care of children: Principles and practice.* Philadelphia: W. B. Saunders. p. 613.

11. **3**

Rationale: Occasionally, tenderness, redness, or swelling may occur at the site of the injection. This can be relieved with ice packs for the first 24 hours, followed by warm compresses if the inflammation persists. It is not necessary to bring the infant back to the clinic. Option 4 may be an appropriate intervention but is not specific to the issue of the question.

Test-Taking Strategy: Note the key phrase "most appropriate" in the stem of the question. Option 4 can be eliminated first because it does not relate specifically to the issue of the question. Eliminate option 2 next as an unnecessary intervention. From the remaining two options, general principles related to the effects of heat and cold will easily direct you to option 3.

Level of Cognitive Ability: Application
Phase of Nursing Process: Implementation
Client Needs: Physiological Integrity
Content Area: Child Health

Reference
Bowden, V., Dickey, S., & Greenberg, C. (1998). *Children and their families: The continuum of care.* Philadelphia: W. B. Saunders. p. 341.

12. **3**

Rationale: Immunocompetent persons receiving OPV represent a risk for persons who are immunocompromised. The viruses in OPV multiply in the vaccinee's GI tract and can then be transmitted in saliva and feces. The risk of transmission can be reduced by avoiding contact with saliva and by practicing rigorous hygiene, especially handwashing.

Test-Taking Strategy: Options 2 and 4 can be eliminated first, knowing that OPV is contraindicated in siblings of an immunocompromised child. From the remaining two options, knowledge that the virus in OPV can be transmitted in saliva and feces will easily direct you to option 3. Review the contraindications associated with the administration of OPV vaccine now, if you had difficulty with this question!

Level of Cognitive Ability: Analysis
Phase of Nursing Process: Analysis
Client Needs: Physiological Integrity
Content Area: Child Health

Reference
Lehne, R. (1998). *Pharmacology for nursing care* (3rd ed.). Philadelphia: W. B. Saunders. p. 743.

13. **4**

Rationale: Pastia's sign describes a rash that will blanch with pressure except in areas of deep creases. The tongue is initially coated with a white furry covering with red projecting papillae (white strawberry tongue). By the fourth day, the white strawberry tongue sloughs off, leaving a red swollen tongue (strawberry tongue). The tonsils are edematous, and petechial hemorrhages cover the soft palate. Koplik's spots are associated with rubeola.

Test-Taking Strategy: Note the key word "not" in the stem of the question. Knowledge that Koplik's spots are associated with rubeola will assist in answering this question. If you are unfamiliar with the clinical manifestations associated with scarlet fever, take time now to review!

Level of Cognitive Ability: Analysis
Phase of Nursing Process: Assessment
Client Needs: Physiological Integrity
Content Area: Child Health

Reference
Ashwill, J., & Droske, S. (1997). *Nursing care of children: Principles and practice*. Philadelphia: W. B. Saunders. pp. 597, 614, 615.

14. **4**

Rationale: The parents need to be instructed to notify the physician if abdominal pain, especially in the left upper quadrant, or left shoulder pain occurs because this may indicate splenic rupture. Children with enlarged spleens are also instructed to avoid contact sports until splenomegaly resolves. Bed rest is not necessary, and children usually self-limit their activity. No isolation precautions are required, although transmission can occur via saliva, close intimate contact, or contact with infected blood. Fever is treated with acetaminophen (Tylenol).

Test-Taking Strategy: Knowledge regarding the organs affected in mononucleosis will assist in answering this question. Options 1 and 2 can be eliminated first because they are unnecessary interventions in this disease. From the remaining two options, knowledge that splenic rupture is a concern will direct you to option 4.

Level of Cognitive Ability: Application
Phase of Nursing Process: Implementation
Client Needs: Physiological Integrity
Content Area: Child Health

Reference
Bowden, V., Dickey, S., & Greenberg, C. (1998). *Children and their families: The continuum of care*. Philadelphia: W. B. Saunders. p. 1662.

15. **1**

Rationale: The nursing care of a child with RMSF includes the administration of tetracycline. An alternative medication is chloramphenicol, a fluoroquinolone. Amphotericin B is used for fungus infections. Ganciclovir is used to treat cytomegalovirus. Amantadine is used to treat influenza A virus.

Test-Taking Strategy: Knowledge regarding the treatment plan associated with RMSF is required to answer this question. If you are unfamiliar with this treatment plan or with the medications identified in the options, take time now to review!

Level of Cognitive Ability: Analysis
Phase of Nursing Process: Analysis
Client Needs: Physiological Integrity
Content Area: Child Health

Reference
Lehne, R. (1998). *Pharmacology for nursing care* (3rd ed.). Philadelphia: W. B. Saunders. p. 844.

16. **4**

Rationale: Diagnosis is confirmed by direct visualization of the worms. Parents can view the sleeping child's anus with a flashlight. The worm is white, thin, about 0.5 inch long, and it moves. A simple technique, the cellophane tape slide method, is used to capture worms and eggs. Transparent adhesive tape is lightly touched to the anus and then applied to a slide for examination. The best specimens are obtained as the child awakens, before toileting or bathing.

Test-Taking Strategy: Knowledge regarding the procedure related to the cellophane tape slide for the diagnosis of pinworm is required to answer this question. If you are unfamiliar with this procedure, take time now to review!

Level of Cognitive Ability: Application
Phase of Nursing Process: Implementation
Client Needs: Physiological Integrity
Content Area: Child Health

Reference
Bowden, V., Dickey, S., & Greenberg, C. (1998). *Children and their families: The continuum of care*. Philadelphia: W. B. Saunders. p. 1673.

17. **3**

Rationale: MMR is administered subcutaneously into the outer aspect of the upper arm. Each child should receive two vaccinations, the first between 12 and 15 months of age and the second between 4 and 6 years or 11 and 12 years.

Test-Taking Strategy: Knowledge that MMR is administered subcutaneously will assist in eliminating options 1 and 2. From the remaining two options, recalling that the gluteal muscle is most often used for intramuscular injections will assist in directing you to option 3. Review the procedures related to the administration of MMR now, if you had difficulty with this question!

Level of Cognitive Ability: Application
Phase of Nursing Process: Planning
Client Needs: Physiological Integrity
Content Area: Child Health

Reference
Lehne, R. (1998). *Pharmacology for nursing care* (3rd ed.). Philadelphia: W. B. Saunders. p. 742

18. **4**

Rationale: High fevers and severe illness are reasons to delay immunization, but only until the child has recovered from the acute stage of the illness. Minor illnesses such as a cold, otitis media, or mild diarrhea without fever are not contraindications to immunization.

Test-Taking Strategy: Utilize the process of elimination to answer this question. Recalling that high fevers and severe illnesses are contraindications to receiving immunizations will easily direct you to option 4. If you had difficulty with this question, take time now to review the contraindications associated with immunizations!

Level of Cognitive Ability: Analysis
Phase of Nursing Process: Analysis
Client Needs: Physiological Integrity
Content Area: Child Health

Reference
Bowden, V., Dickey, S., & Greenberg, C. (1998). *Children and their families: The continuum of care*. Philadelphia: W. B. Saunders. p. 341.

19. **3**

Rationale: DTP, HIB, and OPV are administered at 4 months of age. MMR is administered between 12 and 15 months of age and repeated at age 4 to 6 or at age 11 to 12 years. Varicella vaccine is administered between 12 and 18 months of age. Hepatitis B is administered at birth, 1 month, and 6 months of age.

Test-Taking Strategy: Knowledge regarding the immunization schedule for infants and children is required to answer this question. Noting the age of the infant in the question will assist in directing you to option 3. If you are unfamiliar with the immunization schedule, learn it now. You are likely to find a question related to immunizations on NCLEX-RN!

Level of Cognitive Ability: Application
Phase of Nursing Process: Planning
Client Needs: Physiological Integrity
Content Area: Child Health

Reference
Lehne, R. (1998). *Pharmacology for nursing care* (3rd ed.). Philadelphia: W. B. Saunders. p. 741.

20. **1**

Rationale: Prior to the administration of MMR vaccine, a thorough health history needs to be obtained. MMR is used with caution in a child with a history of an allergy to gelatin, eggs, or neomycin, because the live measles vaccine is produced by chick embryo cell culture. MMR also contains a small amount of the antibiotic neomycin. Options 2, 3, and 4 are not contraindications to administering immunizations.

Test-Taking Strategy: Note the key word "highest" in the stem of the question. Knowledge that options 2, 3, and 4 are not contraindications to administering immunizations will assist in answering this question. Additionally, the key word "highest" should assist in directing you to option 1. If you had difficulty with this question, review the nursing implications related to the administration of MMR!

Level of Cognitive Ability: Analysis
Phase of Nursing Process: Assessment
Client Needs: Physiological Integrity
Content Area: Child Health

Reference
Lehne, R. (1998). *Pharmacology for nursing care* (3rd ed.) Philadelphia: W. B. Saunders. pp. 740–741.

BIBLIOGRAPHY

Ashwill, J., & Droske, S. (1997). *Nursing care of children: Principles and practice.* Philadelphia: W. B. Saunders.

Bowden, V., Dickey, S., & Greenberg, C. (1998). *Children and their families: The continuum of care.* Philadelphia: W. B. Saunders.

Hodgson, B., & Kizior, R. (1999). *Saunders nursing drug handbook 1999.* Philadelphia: W. B. Saunders.

Lehne, R. (1998). *Pharmacology for nursing care* (3rd ed.). Philadelphia: W. B. Saunders.

Luckmann, J. (1997). *Saunders manual of nursing care.* Philadelphia: W. B. Saunders.

Nichols, F., & Zwelling, E. (1997). *Maternal-newborn nursing: Theory and practice.* Philadelphia: W. B. Saunders.

O'Toole, M. (ed.). (1997). *Miller-Keane encyclopedia & dictionary of medicine, nursing & allied health* (6th ed.). Philadelphia: W. B. Saunders.

UNIT VIII

....

Pediatric Medications and Calculations

PYRAMID TO SUCCESS

Medication dosages for children differ significantly from those for adults because of the existing physiological differences. Neonates and infants have immature liver and kidney function, which delays the metabolism and elimination of many medications. Toxicity can occur in neonates and infants receiving medications that are highly bound to protein, because they have a lower concentration of plasma proteins. The slowed gastric emptying time in neonates also affects medication absorption. Altered medication absorption also occurs in children under the age of 3 years because of decreased gastric secretion. The amount of total body fat and total body water in children also affects medication dosage.

Awareness of the factors affecting medication administration in children is critical in ensuring that a child receives an accurate dose of a medication. When calculating a medication dosage, the nurse evaluates whether the answer is within reason and makes sense. In the clinical setting, the nurse should always seek verification regarding the dosage to be administered. Short cuts should not be used when calculating medication dosages. The medication problem and answer should be labeled with the correct measurement. Be careful with decimal points when calculating a medication dosage.

On CAT NCLEX-RN, it is important to check the calculation before selecting the answer to the question. REMEMBER, on CAT NCLEX-RN, the correct answer will be on the screen. Following the formula for medication calculations, placing the decimal points in the correct places, and checking the accuracy of the calculation will assure selection of the correct answer!

PRACTICE MAKES PERFECT!

NURSING PROCESS

ASSESSMENT

Physician's order
The five rights: right drug, right dose, right child, right route, and right time
History of allergies
Child's current condition and the purpose for the medication or intravenous solution
Child's developmental level and understanding of the need for medication
Parent's understanding of the need for medication
Need for conversion when calculating the correct dose of medication
Verification of accurate dosage

ANALYSIS: Potential for Injury

PLANNING	IMPLEMENTATION	EVALUATION
Child will remain free of injury.	Assess physician's order. Ask parents about a history of allergies in the child. Assess child's current condition. Assess the need for conversion when calculating the correct dose of medication. Once dosage is determined, verify dosage calculation with another nurse. Prepare and administer the medication or IV solution once the correct dosage is determined.	Correct dosage is determined and administered to the child.

ANALYSIS: Risk for Infection

PLANNING	IMPLEMENTATION	EVALUATION
Child will remain free of infection.	Monitor vital signs. Monitor child for signs of infection.	Child's vital signs remain within normal limits. Child does not develop an infection.

ANALYSIS: Risk for Fluid Volume Excess

PLANNING	IMPLEMENTATION	EVALUATION
Child will maintain fluid balance	Monitor child for signs of fluid overload. Monitor intake and output (I&O). Carefully calculate IV infusion amounts, including amount of IV flush.	Child does not develop an infection or fluid overload. Fluid balance is maintained.

ANALYSIS: Knowledge Deficit

PLANNING	IMPLEMENTATION	EVALUATION
Parents will verbalize purpose of medication or IV solution	Determine parents' understanding regarding the prescribed medication. Teach parents about the medication. Document the administration of the prescribed therapy and child's tolerance to the therapy.	Child tolerates medication or intravenous solution. Parent verbalizes purpose of prescribed therapy.

CLIENT NEEDS

SAFE, EFFECTIVE CARE ENVIRONMENT

Parent and child rights
Informed consent from parent for treatments and procedures
Confidentiality regarding child's condition
Continuity of child care
Protective measures
Error prevention related to medication administration
Safe and accurate preparation and administration of medications to the child
Asepsis with medication administration
Environmental and personal safety related to the developmental age of the child
Handling hazardous and infectious materials

HEALTH PROMOTION AND MAINTENANCE

Developmental stage of the child
Family systems
Disease prevention
Protection of the child to prevent illness
Instructions to child and parent regarding purpose for the prescribed medication, administering the prescribed medication, and the importance of follow-up care

PSYCHOSOCIAL INTEGRITY

Play
Communication
Cultural and religious considerations
Family and support systems

PHYSIOLOGICAL INTEGRITY

Age-appropriate normal body structure and function
Child allergies
Intrusive procedures
Safe administration of medications and parenteral fluids
Use of special equipment
Purpose of the prescribed medication
Vital signs and significant laboratory values prior to the administration of the medication
Monitoring for untoward side effects of medications
Documenting the expected and unexpected responses to the prescribed medication

BIBLIOGRAPHY

Ashwill, J., & Droske, S. (1997). *Nursing care of children: Principles and practice*. Philadelphia: W. B. Saunders.

Leahy, J., & Kizilay, P. (1998). *Foundations of nursing practice: A nursing process approach*. Philadelphia: W. B. Saunders.

Lehne, R. (1998). *Pharmacology for nursing care* (3rd ed.). Philadelphia: W. B. Saunders.

National Council of State Boards of Nursing (eds) (1997). *Test plan for the National Council Licensure Examination for Registered Nurses*. Chicago: Author.

O'Toole, M. (ed.). (1997). *Miller-Keane encyclopedia & dictionary of medicine, nursing & allied health* (6th ed.). Philadelphia: W. B. Saunders.

CHAPTER 46

Pediatric Medications and Calculations

. . . .

I. Administering Oral Medication

A. Most oral pediatric medications are in liquid or suspension form since children usually are not able to swallow a tablet

B. Solutions may be measured using an oral syringe; if an oral syringe is not available, hypodermic syringes without the needle can be used for dosage measurement

C. When volumes are extremely small, oral liquids are measured using a calibrated medication dropper

D. Be alert to liquid medications prepared as suspensions because a medication in suspension settles to the bottom of the bottle between uses, and thorough mixing is required prior to pouring the medication

E. Suspensions must be administered immediately after measurement to prevent settling and administering an incomplete dosage

F. Administer oral medications with the child sitting in an upright position, with the head elevated, to prevent aspiration if the child cries or resists

G. Never pinch the child's nostrils when administering medication

H. Do not place medication in a nursing bottle

I. Draw the required dose of an unpleasant medication into a small syringe and place the syringe into the side and toward the back of an infant's mouth; administer the medication slowly, allowing the infant to swallow

J. Place the small child sideways on the lap; the child's closest arm should be placed under the adult's arm and behind the adult's back; cradle the child's head and hold the child's hand and administer the medication slowly with a plastic spoon or small plastic cup

K. Mix liquid medications with less than an ounce of fluid to disguise the taste if necessary. Crush tablets if necessary and mix with 1 teaspoon of puréed fruit or flavored syrup

L. Check the child's mouth if a tablet or capsule has been administered to assure that it has been swallowed; if swallowing is a problem, some tablets can be crushed and given in small amounts of foods

M. Enteric-coated and timed-release tablets or capsules cannot be crushed

II. Administering Parenteral Medications

A. Subcutaneous (SC) and intramuscular (IM) medications

1. Medications most often given via the subcutaneous route are insulin and most immunizations

2. Any site with sufficient subcutaneous tissue may be used; the upper arm is the site of choice for most immunizations

3. The intramuscular site of choice for infants and small children is the vastus lateralis or the rectus femoris of the thigh

4. Usually not more than 1 mL is injected per IM or SC sites, and sites are rotated regularly

5. Pediatric dosages for SC and IM administration are calculated to the nearest hundredth and measured using a tuberculin syringe

6. Usually a 5/8-inch needle is used to administer SC and IM injections to small infants

7. One-inch needles are appropriate for most IM injections in children

8. Place an adhesive bandage or decorated bandage over the puncture site, particularly for toddlers and preschoolers

B. IV medications

1. IV medications are diluted for administration

2. When a child is receiving an IV medication, the IV site needs to be assessed for signs of infiltration and inflammation immediately before, during, and after completion of each medication administration

3. Signs of inflammation include redness, heat, swelling, and tenderness
4. Signs of infiltration include swelling, coldness, pain, and lack of blood return
5. If infiltration or inflammation occurs, the IV is discontinued and restarted at a new site
6. IV medication may be administered on a continuous basis by adding the medication to an IV solution bag and infusing it through a primary infusion line
7. IV medications may be administered on an intermittent basis, involving several dosages within a 24-hour period

C. Intermittent IV medication administration
1. Children receiving IV medications on an intermittent basis may or may not have a primary IV
2. If a primary IV exists, the medication may be administered by IV piggyback (IVPB) via a secondary line
3. If a primary line does not exist, an indwelling infusion catheter is used for medication administration
4. All intermittent medication administrations are preceded and followed by a flush to assure that the medication has cleared the IV tubing and that the total dosage has been administered
5. The flush volume is added to the medication volume for flow rate calculations
6. Determine agency guidelines related to the volume of flush for peripheral lines and for central lines
7. Electronic controllers and pumps are used to regulate and administer intermittent IV medications

D. Special IV administration sets
1. Special IV administration sets, referred to by their trade names (Burretrol, Soluset, Volutrol), may be used for medication preparation and administration
2. These special sets are all microdrip sets calibrated to deliver 60 drops (gtt) per mL
3. The total capacity of these special IV administration sets is between 100 and 150 mL, calibrated in 1-mL increments so that exact measurement of small volumes is possible
4. The medication is mixed with the appropriate amount of diluent and added to the special IV administration set, and the medication is allowed to infuse at the prescribed rate
5. Label the special IV administration set to identify the medication and fluid dosage added
6. Attach a label that states "medication infusing" during the medication infusion time
7. Attach a label stating "flush infusing" during the flush infusion time

E. Retrograde IV injection
1. The medication is mixed with the appropriate amount of diluent in a syringe
2. The IV tubing is clamped close to the child, the medication is injected through the port in the direction of the burette, the tubing is unclamped, and the medication is allowed to infuse over the prescribed time

F. Syringe pump for IV medication administration
1. A syringe containing the medication is fitted into a pump that is connected to the IV tubing through a Y-connector
2. The medication is administered over the prescribed time

III. Calculation of Medication Dosage by Body Weight

A. **Conversion** of body weight
1. Pounds (lb) to kilograms (kg)
   a. 1 kg = 2.2 lb
   b. To convert from pounds to kilograms, divide by 2.2
   c. The answer, in kilograms, will be smaller than the pounds you are converting, since you are dividing
   d. Answers are expressed to the nearest tenth
2. Kilograms (kg) to pounds (lb)
   a. 1 kg = 2.2 lb
   b. To convert from kilograms to pounds, multiply by 2.2
   c. The answer, in pounds, will be larger than the kilograms you are converting, since you are multiplying
   d. Express weight to the nearest tenth

B. Calculating daily dosages
1. Dosages are expressed in terms of mg/kg/day, or mg/lb/day
2. The total daily dosage is usually administered in divided (more than one) doses per day
3. Express the child's body weight in kilograms or pounds to correlate with the dosage specifications
4. Calculate the total daily dosage
5. Divide the total daily dosage by the number of doses to be administered in 1 day

IV. Calculation of Body Surface Area (BSA)

A. The **body surface area** is determined by comparing body weight and height with averages or norms on a graph called a nomogram
B. Not all children are the same size at the same age; therefore, the nomogram chart is used to determine the **BSA** of a child
C. Look at the nomogram chart (Fig. 46–1), and note that heights are on the lefthand side of the chart and weights are on the righthand side
D. Place a ruler on the chart
E. Line up the left side of the ruler on the height and the right side of the ruler on the weight. Read the **BSA** where the point of the straight edge of the ruler intersects with the surface area (SA) column
F. This gives the estimated SA in square meters (m²)

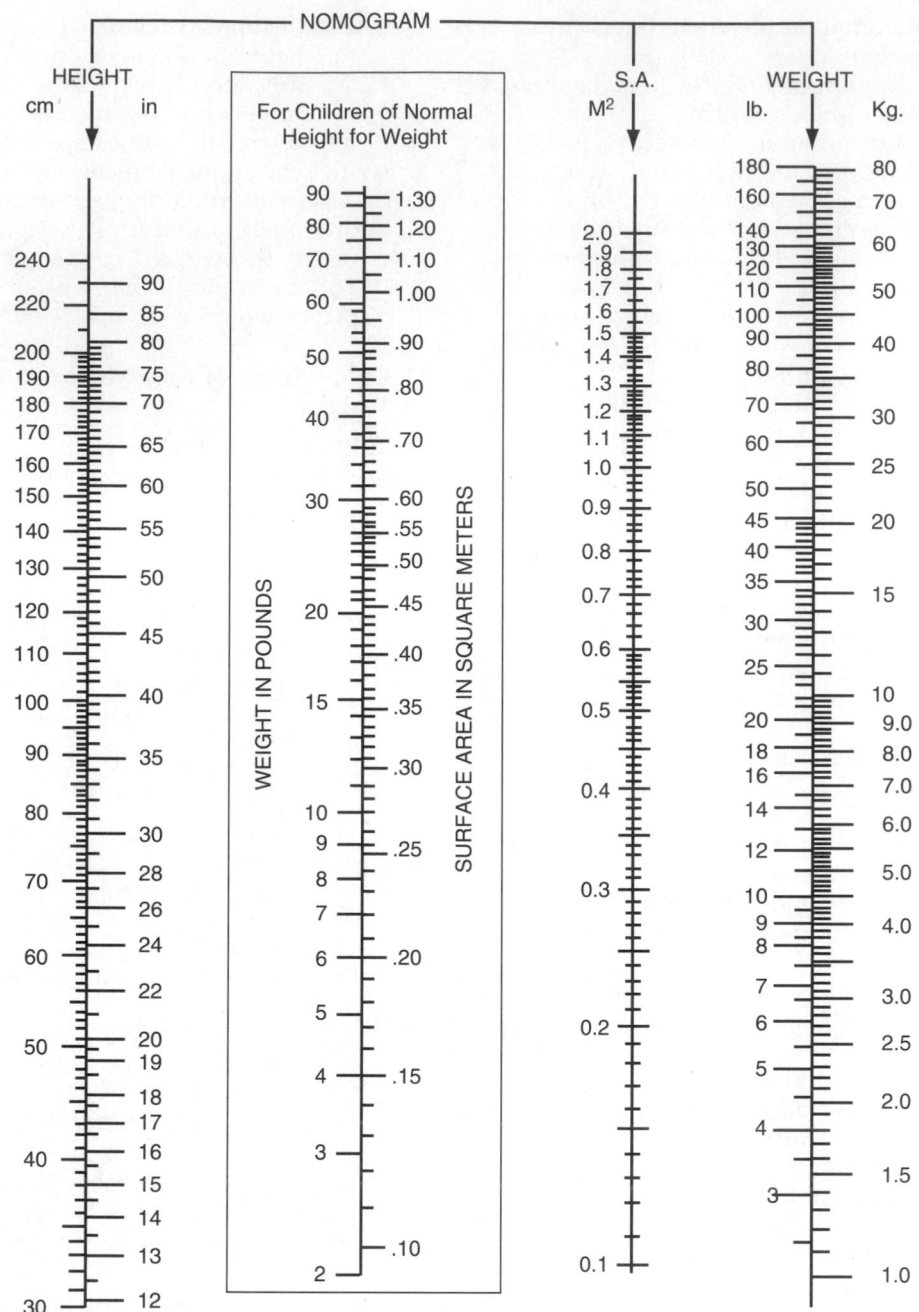

FIGURE 46–1. West nomogram for infants and children. *Directions*: (1) Find height. (2) Find weight. (3) Draw a straight line connecting the height and the weight; where the line intersects on the SA column is the body surface area (m²). (Modified from data of Boyd, E., West, C. D. *in* Behrman, R.E. & Vaughan, V. C. [1996]. Nelson textbook of pediatrics [15th ed.]. Philadelphia: W. B. Saunders.)

EXAMPLE:

Use the nomogram and calculate the **BSA** for a child whose height is 58 inches and weight is 12 kg.

ANSWER:

0.66 m²

V. Calculation Based on BSA

A. When dosage recommendations for children specify milligrams or units per square meter, calculating the dosage is simple multiplication

EXAMPLE:

The dosage recommendation is 4 mg per m². The child has a **BSA** of 1.1 m². What is the dosage to be administered?

ANSWER:

$1.1 \times 4 \text{ mg} = 4.4 \text{ mg}$

B. When dosages are specified only for adults, a formula is used to calculate a child's dosage from the adult dosage

EXAMPLE:

The physician has prescribed an antibiotic for a child. The average adult dose is 250 mg. The child has a **BSA** of 0.41 m². What is the dose for the child?

ANSWER:

Formula:

$$\frac{\text{BSA of child}}{1.7\,\text{m}^2} \times \text{adult dose} = \text{child's dose}$$

$$\frac{0.41}{1.7} \times 250\,\text{mg} = 60.29\,\text{mg}$$

PRACTICE QUESTIONS

1. Penicillin V (Veetids), 250 mg PO every 8 hours, is prescribed for a child with a respiratory infection. The child's weight is 45 pounds. The safe pediatric dose is 25 to 50 mg/kg/day. The nurse determines that:
   1 The dose is too low
   2 The dose is too high
   3 The dose is within the safe range
   4 There is not enough information to determine the safe dose

2. Penicillin V (Pen-Vee K), 250 mg PO every 8 hours, is prescribed for a child with a respiratory infection. The medication label reads: Penicillin, 125 mg per 5 mL. The nurse has determined that the dosage prescribed is a safe dose for the child. How many milliliters will the nurse administer to the child per dose?
   1 2 mL
   2 4 mL
   3 8 mL
   4 10 mL

3. The physician has prescribed phenobarbital sodium (Luminal Sodium), 25 mg PO BID, for a child with febrile seizures. The child's weight is 7.2 kg. The safe pediatric dose is 1 to 6 mg/kg/day. The nurse determines that:
   1 The dose is too low
   2 The dose is too high
   3 The dose is within the safe range
   4 There is not enough information to determine the safe dose

4. The physician has prescribed phenobarbital sodium (Luminal Sodium), 25 mg PO BID, for a child with febrile seizures. The medication label reads: Phenobarbital, 20 mg per 5 mL. The nurse has determined that the dosage prescribed is a safe dose for the child. How many milliliters will the nurse administer to the child per dose?
   1 2 mL
   2 4.5 mL
   3 6.25 mL
   4 7.0 mL

5. Cloxacillin (Tegopen), 100 mg PO q6h, is prescribed for a child with an elevated temperature who is suspected of having a respiratory tract infection. The child weighs 17 lb. The safe pediatric dose is 50 mg/kg/day. The nurse determines that:
   1 The dose is too low
   2 The dose is too high
   3 The dose is within the safe range
   4 There is not enough information to determine the safe dose

6. Cloxacillin (Tegopen), 100 mg PO QID, is prescribed for a child with an infection. The medication label reads: 125 mg per 5 mL. The nurse has determined that the dosage prescribed is a safe dose for the child. How many milliliters will the nurse administer to the child per dose?
   1 2 mL
   2 4 mL
   3 6 mL
   4 7 mL

7. Sulfisoxazole (Gantrisin), 1.5 lg PO QID, is prescribed for an adolescent with a urinary tract infection. The medication label reads: 500-mg tablets. The nurse has determined that the dosage prescribed is safe. How many tablets will the nurse administer to the child?
   1 0.5 tablet
   2 1 tablet
   3 2 tablets
   4 3 tablets

8. Diphenhydramine hydrochloride (Benadryl), 25 mg PO every 6 hours, is prescribed for a child with an allergic reaction. The child weighs 25 kg. The safe pediatric dose is 5 mg/kg/day. The nurse determines that:
   1 The dose is too low
   2 The dose is too high
   3 The dose is within the safe range
   4 There is not enough information to determine the safe dose

9. Promethazine hydrochloride (Phenergan), 20 mg IM every 6 hours, is prescribed for the child with nausea. The medication label reads: 25 mg per mL. The nurse has determined that the dosage prescribed is safe. How many milliliters will the nurse administer to the child per dose?
   1 0.4 mL
   2 0.8 mL
   3 1 mL
   4 1.2 mL

10. Penicillin G procaine (Wycillin, 1,000,000 U IM, has been prescribed for the child with a strep throat. The child's weight is 62 lb. The safe pediatric dose is greater than 60 lb: 600,000 to 1,200,000 U daily. The nurse determines that:
    1 The dose is too low
    2 The dose is too high
    3 The dose is within the safe range
    4 There is not enough information to determine the safe dose

11. Atropine sulfate, 0.2 mg IM, is prescribed for the child preoperatively. The medication label reads: 0.4 mg per mL. The nurse has determined that the dosage prescribed is safe. How many milliliters will the nurse administer to the child per dose?
    1 0.5 mL
    2 0.8 mL
    3 1 mL
    4 1.2 mL

12. Penicillin G procaine (Wycillin), 1,000,000 U IM, is prescribed for the child with an infection. The medication label reads: 1,200,000 U per 2 mL. The nurse has determined that the dosage prescribed is safe. How many milliliters will the nurse administer to the child per dose?
    1 0.8 mL
    2 1.2 mL
    3 1.44 mL
    4 1.66 mL

13. Morphine sulfate, 2.5 mg, IV piggyback, is prescribed for a child with cancer. The safe pediatric dose is 0.05–0.1 mg/kg. The child weighs 50 kg. The nurse determines that:
    1 The dose is too low
    2 The dose is too high
    3 The dose is within the safe range
    4 There is not enough information to determine the safe dose

14. Morphine sulfate, 2.5 mg, IV piggyback, in 10 mL of normal saline (NS) is prescribed for a child postoperatively. The medication label reads: 1/15 gr per mL. The nurse has determined that the dosage is safe. How many milliliters will the nurse prepare to administer to the child?
    1 0.62 mL
    2 0.8 mL
    3 1.0 mL
    4 1.62 mL

15. The nurse is checking postoperative orders and planning care for a 110-pound child after spinal fusion. Morphine sulfate, 8 mg SC every 4 hours PRN for pain, is ordered. The pediatric drug reference states that the safe dose is 0.1 to 0.2 mg/kg/dose every 2 to 4 hours. From this information, the nurse determines that:
    1 The dose is too low
    2 The dose is too high
    3 The dose is within the safe range
    4 There is not enough information to determine the safe dose

16. The physician's order reads: ampicillin (Omnipen), 125 mg IV every 6 hours. The medication label reads: 1 g and reconstitute with 7.4 mL of bacteriostatic water. How many milliliters will the nurse draw up for one dose?
    1 0.54 mL
    2 0.92 mL
    3 1.1 mL
    4 7.4 mL

17. The physician's order reads: tobramycin sulfate (Nebcin), 7.5 mg IM BID. The medication label reads: 10 mg/mL. How many milliliters will the nurse give to administer one dose?
    1 0.25 mL
    2 0.50 mL
    3 0.75 mL
    4 1.33 mL

18. The physician's order reads: piperacillin sodium (Pipracil), 650 mg IV every 6 hours. The medication label reads: 2 g and reconstitute with 5 mL of bacteriostatic water. How many milliliters will the nurse draw up for one dose?
    1 0.62 mL
    2 1.0 mL
    3 1.62 mL
    4 5.0 mL

19. The physician's order reads: theophylline timed-release capsules (Slo-bid), 100 mg PO every 6 hours. The medication label reads: 50-mg capsules. How many capsules will the nurse give to administer one dose?
    1 1 capsule
    2 2 capsules
    3 3 capsules
    4 4 capsules

20. The physician's order reads: acetaminophen (Tylenol) liquid, 450 mg PO every 4 hours PRN for pain. The medication label reads: 160 mg/5 mL. How many milliliters will the nurse give to administer one dose?
    1 0.1 mL
    2 5 mL
    3 10 mL
    4 14 mL

21. The pediatric client with ventricular septal defect repair is placed on a maintenance dosage of digoxin (Lanoxin) elixir. The dosage is 0.07 mg/kg/day, and the client's weight is 7.2 kg. The physician orders the Lanoxin to be given BID. How much Lanoxin should the client receive at each dose?
    1 0.25 mg
    2 0.37 mg
    3 0.50 mg
    4 2.50 mg

ANSWERS

1. **3**

Rationale:

Pounds to kilograms: 45 lb divided by 2.2 lb/kg
= 20.45 kg

Dosage parameters: 25 mg/kg × 20.45 kg
= 511.25 mg/day

50 mg/kg × 20.45 kg
= 1022.50 mg/day

Dosage frequency: 250 mg × 3 doses = 750 mg/day

Dosage is safe.

Test-Taking Strategy: Identify the key components of the question and what the question is asking. In this case, the question asks for the safe dosage range of the medication. Follow the formula steps. Change pounds to kilograms. Calculate the dosage parameters using the safe dose range identified in the question and the child's weight in kg. Remember to determine the total daily dosage prior to selecting an option.

Level of Cognitive Ability: Analysis
Phase of Nursing Process: Analysis
Client Needs: Safe, Effective Care Environment
Content Area: Child Health

References
Ashwill, J., & Droske, S. (1997). *Nursing care of children: Principles and practice.* Philadelphia: W. B. Saunders. p. 491.
Kee, J., & Marshall, S. (1996). *Clinical calculations* (3rd ed.). Philadelphia: W. B. Saunders. pp. 199–212.

2. **4**

Rationale: Formula:

$$\frac{\text{Desired}}{\text{Available}} \times \text{Volume} = \frac{250 \text{ mg}}{125 \text{ mg}} \times 5 \text{ mL}$$

$$= 10 \text{ mL per dose}$$

Test-Taking Strategy: Identify the key components of the question and what the question is asking. In this case, the question asks for the milliliters per dose. Use the formula and follow the formula to determine the correct dosage. Label the answer before selecting an option!

Level of Cognitive Ability: Application
Phase of Nursing Process: Implementation
Client Needs: Safe, Effective Care Environment
Content Area: Child Health

References
Leahy, J., & Kizilay, P. (1998). *Foundations of nursing practice: A nursing process approach.* Philadelphia: W. B. Saunders. p. 453.
Kee, J., & Marshall, S. (1996). *Clinical calculations* (3rd ed.). Philadelphia: W. B. Saunders. pp. 199–212.

3. **2**

Rationale:

Dosage parameters: 1 mg/kg/day × 7.2 kg = 7.2 mg/day

6 mg/kg/day × 7.2 kg
= 43.2 mg/day

Dosage frequency: 25 mg × 2 doses = 50 mg/day

Dosage is high.

Test-Taking Strategy: Identify the key components of the question and what the question is asking. In this case, the question asks for the safe dosage range of the medication. Follow the formula steps. Calculate the dosage parameters, using the safe dose range identified in the question and the child's weight in kilograms. Remember to determine the total daily dosage prior to selecting an option.

Level of Cognitive Ability: Analysis
Phase of Nursing Process: Analysis
Client Needs: Safe, Effective Care Environment
Content Area: Child Health

References
Ashwill, J., & Droske, S. (1997). *Nursing care of children: Principles and practice.* Philadelphia: W. B. Saunders. p. 491.
Kee, J., & Marshall, S. (1996). *Clinical calculations* (3rd ed.). Philadelphia: W. B. Saunders. pp. 199–212.

4. **3**

Rationale: Formula:

$$\frac{\text{Desired}}{\text{Available}} \times \text{Volume} = \frac{25 \text{ mg}}{20 \text{ mg}} \times 5 \text{ mL}$$

$$= 6.25 \text{ mL per dose}$$

Test-Taking Strategy: Identify the key components of the question and what the question is asking. In this case, the question asks for the milliliters per dose. Use the formula and follow the formula to determine the correct dosage. Label the answer before selecting an option!

Level of Cognitive Ability: Application
Phase of Nursing Process: Implementation
Client Needs: Safe, Effective Care Environment
Content Area: Child Health

References
Leahy, J., & Kizilay, P. (1998). *Foundations of nursing practice: A nursing process approach.* Philadelphia: W. B. Saunders. p. 453.
Kee, J., & Marshall, S. (1996). *Clinical calculations* (3rd ed.). Philadelphia: W. B. Saunders. pp. 199–212.

5. **3**

Rationale:

Pounds to kilograms: 17 lb divided by 2.2 lb/kg
= 7.72 kg

Dosage parameters: 50 mg/kg × 7.72 kg = 386 mg/day

Dosage frequency: 100 mg × 4 doses = 400 mg/day

Dosage is safe.

Test-Taking Strategy: Identify the key components of the question and what the question is asking. In this case, the question asks for the safe dosage range of the medication. Follow the formula steps. Change pounds to kilograms. Calculate the dosage parameters, using the safe dose range identified in the question and the child's weight in kilograms. Remember to determine the total daily dosage prior to selecting an option.

Level of Cognitive Ability: Analysis
Phase of Nursing Process: Analysis
Client Needs: Safe, Effective Care Environment
Content Area: Child Health

References
Ashwill, J., & Droske, S. (1997). *Nursing care of children: Principles and practice.* Philadelphia: W. B. Saunders. p. 491.
Kee, J., & Marshall, S. (1996). *Clinical calculations* (3rd ed.). Philadelphia: W. B. Saunders. pp. 199–212.

6. **2**

Rationale: Formula:

$$\frac{\text{Desired}}{\text{Available}} \times \text{Volume} = \frac{100 \text{ mg}}{125 \text{ mg}} \times 5 \text{ mL}$$

$$= 4 \text{ mL per dose}$$

Test-Taking Strategy: Identify the key components of the question and what the question is asking. In this case, the question asks for the milliliters per dose. Use the formula and follow the formula to determine the correct dosage. Label the answer before selecting an option!

Level of Cognitive Ability: Application
Phase of Nursing Process: Implementation
Client Needs: Safe, Effective Care Environment
Content Area: Child Health

References

Leahy, J., & Kizilay, P. (1998). *Foundations of nursing practice: A nursing process approach.* Philadelphia: W. B. Saunders. p. 453.
Kee, J., & Marshall, S. (1996). *Clinical calculations* (3rd ed.). Philadelphia: W. B. Saunders. pp. 199–212.

7. **3**

Rationale:

Change 1 g to mg

1000 mg = 1 g

When converting from gm to mg, larger to smaller, move the decimal point 3 places to the right.

1 g = 1000 mg

Formula:

$$\frac{\text{Desired}}{\text{Available}} \times \text{Tablet} = \frac{1000 \text{ mg}}{500 \text{ mg}} \times 1 \text{ Tablet} = 2 \text{ Tablets}$$

Test-Taking Strategy: Identify the key components of the question and what the question is asking. In this case, the question asks for tablets per dose. Change grams to milligrams first. Then, use the formula and follow the formula to determine the correct dosage. Label the answer before selecting an option!

Level of Cognitive Ability: Application
Phase of Nursing Process: Implementation
Client Needs: Safe, Effective Care Environment
Content Area: Child Health

References

Ashwill, J., & Droske, S. (1997). *Nursing care of children: Principles and practice.* Philadelphia: W. B. Saunders. p. 491.
Kee, J., & Marshall, S. (1996). *Clinical calculations* (3rd ed.). Philadelphia: W. B. Saunders. pp. 199–212.

8. **3**

Rationale:

Dosage parameters: 5 mg/kg × 25 kg = 125 mg/day

Dosage frequency: 25 mg × 4 doses = 100 mg/day

Dosage is safe.

Test-Taking Strategy: Identify the key components of the question and what the question is asking. In this case, the question asks for the safe dosage range of the medication. Follow the formula steps. Calculate the dosage parameters using the safe dose range identified in the question and the child's weight in kilograms. Remember to determine the total daily dosage prior to selecting an option.

Level of Cognitive Ability: Analysis
Phase of Nursing Process: Analysis
Client Needs: Safe, Effective Care Environment
Content Area: Child Health

References

Ashwill, J., & Droske, S. (1997). *Nursing care of children: Principles and practice.* Philadelphia: W. B. Saunders. p. 491.
Kee, J., & Marshall, S. (1996). *Clinical calculations* (3rd ed.). Philadelphia: W. B. Saunders. pp. 199–212.

9. **2**

Rationale: Formula:

$$\frac{\text{Desired}}{\text{Available}} \times \text{Volume} = \frac{20 \text{ mg}}{25 \text{ mg}} \times 1 \text{ mL}$$

$$= 0.8 \text{ mL per dose}$$

Test-Taking Strategy: Identify the key components of the question and what the question is asking. In this case, the question asks for the milliliters per dose. Use the formula and follow the formula to determine the correct dosage. Label the answer before selecting an option!

Level of Cognitive Ability: Application
Phase of Nursing Process: Implementation
Client Needs: Safe, Effective Care Environment
Content Area: Child Health

References

Leahy, J., & Kizilay, P. (1998). *Foundations of nursing practice: A nursing process approach.* Philadelphia: W. B. Saunders. p. 453.
Kee, J., & Marshall, S. (1996). *Clinical calculations* (3rd ed.). Philadelphia: W. B. Saunders. pp. 199–212.

10. **3**

Rationale: Dosage parameters: The child's weight is 62 lb, which falls within the safe pediatric dose range. Dosage is safe.

Test-Taking Strategy: Identify the key components of the question and what the question is asking. In this case, the question asks for the safe dosage range of the medication. Calculation is not required because the information required is identified in the question. Read the question carefully!

Level of Cognitive Ability: Analysis
Phase of Nursing Process: Analysis
Client Needs: Safe, Effective Care Environment
Content Area: Child Health

References

Ashwill, J., & Droske, S. (1997). *Nursing care of children: Principles and practice.* Philadelphia: W. B. Saunders. p. 491.
Kee, J., & Marshall, S. (1996). *Clinical calculations* (3rd ed.). Philadelphia: W. B. Saunders. pp. 199–212.

11. **1**

Rationale: Formula:

$$\frac{\text{Desired}}{\text{Available}} \times \text{Volume} = \frac{0.2 \text{ mg}}{0.4 \text{ mg}} \times 1 \text{ mL}$$

$$= 0.5 \text{ mL per dose}$$

Test-Taking Strategy: Identify the key components of the question and what the question is asking. In this case, the question asks for the milliliters per dose. Use the formula and follow the formula to determine the correct dosage. Label the answer before selecting an option!

Level of Cognitive Ability: Application
Phase of Nursing Process: Implementation
Client Needs: Safe, Effective Care Environment
Content Area: Child Health

References
Leahy, J., & Kizilay, P. (1998). *Foundations of nursing practice: A nursing process approach.* Philadelphia: W. B. Saunders. p. 453.
Kee, J., & Marshall, S. (1996). *Clinical calculations* (3rd ed.). Philadelphia: W. B. Saunders. pp. 199–212.

12. **4**
Rationale: Formula:

$$\frac{\text{Desired}}{\text{Available}} \times \text{Volume} = \frac{1,000,000}{1,200,000} \times 2\ \text{mL}$$
$$= 1.66\ \text{mL per dose}$$

Test-Taking Strategy: Identify the key components of the question and what the question is asking. In this case, the question asks for the milliliters per dose. Use the formula and follow the formula to determine the correct dosage. Label the answer before selecting an option!

Level of Cognitive Ability: Application
Phase of Nursing Process: Implementation
Client Needs: Safe, Effective Care Environment
Content Area: Child Health

References
Leahy, J., & Kizilay, P. (1998). *Foundations of nursing process approach.* Philadelphia: W. B. Saunders. p. 453.
Kee, J., & Marshall, S. (1996). *Clinical calculations* (3rd ed.). Philadelphia: W. B. Saunders. pp. 199–212.

13. **3**
Rationale:

Dosage parameters: 0.05 mg/kg/dose × 50 kg = 2.5 mg/dose

0.1 mg/kg/dose × 50 kg = 5 mg/dose

Dosage is safe.

Test-Taking Strategy: Identify the key components of the question and what the question is asking. In this case, the question asks for the safe dosage range of the medication. Follow the formula steps. Calculate the dosage parameters, using the safe dose range identified in the question and the child's weight in kilograms. Remember to label the answer!

Level of Cognitive Ability: Analysis
Phase of Nursing Process: Analysis
Client Needs: Safe, Effective Care Environment
Content Area: Child Health

References
Ashwill, J., & Droske, S. (1997). *Nursing care of children: Principles and practice.* Philadelphia: W. B. Saunders. p. 491.
Kee, J., & Marshall, S. (1996). *Clinical calculations* (3rd ed.). Philadelphia: W. B. Saunders. pp. 199–212.

14. **1**
Rationale: Convert grains to milligrams:

60 mg = 1 gr

1/15 gr × 60 mg = 4 mg

Formula:

$$\frac{\text{Desired}}{\text{Available}} \times \text{Volume} = \frac{2.5\ \text{mg}}{4\ \text{mg}} \times 1\ \text{mL}$$
$$= 0.62\ \text{mL}$$

Test-Taking Strategy: Identify the key components of the question and what the question is asking. In this case, the question asks for the milliliters per dose. Begin by converting grains to milligrams. Use the formula and follow the formula to determine the correct dosage. Label the answer before selecting an option!

Level of Cognitive Ability: Application
Phase of Nursing Process: Implementation
Client Needs: Safe, Effective Care Environment
Content Area: Child Health

References
Leahy, J., & Kizilay, P. (1998). *Foundations of nursing practice: A nursing process approach.* Philadelphia: W. B. Saunders. p. 453.
Kee, J., & Marshall, S. (1996). *Clinical calculations* (3rd ed.). Philadelphia: W. B. Saunders. pp. 199–212.

15. **3**
Rationale: Convert pounds to kilograms by dividing by 2.2, because 1 kg = 2.2 lb.

110 lb divided by 2.2 = 50 kg

Dosage parameters: 0.1 mg/kg × 50 kg = 5 mg

0.2 mg/kg × 50 kg = 10 mg

The dose is safe.

Test-Taking Strategy: It is very important to identify the components of the question. The case study provides you with a medication order, a child's weight, and safe dose information. The stem asks you to solve a math problem. Remember to convert to the same unit of measure. Your safe dose is given in milligrams per kilograms and the child's weight is given in pounds. You should know that your conversion factor is 2.2. Since pounds are smaller than kilograms, you divide the number of pounds by the conversion factor. Conversely, when going from a larger to a smaller unit of measure, you multiply by the conversion factor. Calculate the dosage parameters using the safe dose range identified in the question and the child's weight in kilograms.

Level of Cognitive Ability: Analysis
Phase of Nursing Process: Analysis
Client Needs: Safe, Effective Care Environment
Content Area: Child Health

Reference
Pickar, G. (1996). *Dosage calculations* (5th ed.). Albany, NY: Delmar. p. 174.

16. **2**
Rationale: Convert 1 g to milligrams. In the metric system, to convert larger to smaller multiply by 1000 or move the decimal 3 places to the right.

1 g = 1000 mg

Formula:

$$\frac{\text{Desired}}{\text{Available}} \times \text{Volume} = \frac{125\ \text{mg}}{1000\ \text{mg}} \times 7.4\ \text{mL}$$
$$= 0.925\ \text{mL} = 0.92\ \text{mL per dose}$$

Dosage to give is 0.92 mL

Test-Taking Strategy: Convert grams to milligrams first. Next, set up a formula, knowing that 1000 mg = 7.4 mL. Desired is 125 mg, available is 1000 mg in 7.4 mL. Be careful with decimal points!

Level of Cognitive Ability: Application
Phase of Nursing Process: Planning
Client Needs: Safe, Effective Care Environment
Content Area: Fundamental Skills

Reference
Leahy, J., & Kizilay, P. (1998). *Foundations of nursing practice: A nursing process approach.* Philadelphia: W. B. Saunders. p. 453.

17. **3**

Rationale: Formula:

$$\frac{\text{Desired}}{\text{Available}} \times \text{Volume} = \frac{7.5 \text{ mg}}{10 \text{ mg}} \times 1.0 \text{ mL} = 0.75 \text{ mL}$$

Dosage to give is 0.75 mL.

Test-Taking Strategy: Set up the formula knowing that desired is 7.5 mg, available is 10 mg in 1 mL. Be careful with decimal points!

Level of Cognitive Ability: Application
Phase of Nursing Process: Implementation
Client Needs: Safe, Effective Care Environment
Content Area: Fundamental Skills

Reference
Ashwill, J., & Droske, S. (1997). *Nursing care of children: Principles and practice.* Philadelphia: W. B. Saunders. p. 491.

18. **3**

Rationale: Convert 2 gm to mg. In the metric system, to convert larger to smaller, multiply by 1000 or move the decimal 3 places to the right.

2 gm = 2000 mg

Formula:

$$\frac{\text{Desired}}{\text{Available}} \times \text{Volume} = \frac{650 \text{ mg}}{2000 \text{ mg}}$$

$$\times 5.0 \text{ mL} = 1.625 \text{ mL} = 1.62 \text{ mL}$$

Dosage to give is 1.62 mL.

Test-Taking Strategy: Convert grams to milligrams first. Next, set up the formula, knowing that 2000 mg = 5.0 mL. Desired is 650 mg, available is 2000 mg in 5 mL. Be careful with decimal points!

Level of Cognitive Ability: Application
Phase of Nursing Process: Implementation
Client Needs: Safe, Effective Care Environment
Content Area: Fundamental Skills

Reference
Leahy, J., & Kizilay, P. (1998). *Foundations of nursing practice: A nursing process approach.* Philadelphia: W. B. Saunders. p. 453.

19. **2**

Rationale: Formula:

$$\frac{\text{Desired}}{\text{Available}} \times \text{Capsule} = \frac{100 \text{ mg}}{50 \text{ mg}} \times 1 \text{ Capsule} = 2 \text{ Capsules}$$

Dosage to give is 2 capsules.

Test-Taking Strategy: Set up the formula knowing that desired is 100 mg, available is 50 mg in 1 capsule.

Level of Cognitive Ability: Application
Phase of Nursing Process: Implementation
Client Needs: Safe, Effective Care Environment
Content Area: Fundamental Skills

Reference
Leahy, J., & Kizilay, P. (1998). *Foundations of nursing practice: A nursing process approach.* Philadelphia: W. B. Saunders. p. 453.

20. **4**

Rationale: Formula:

$$\frac{\text{Desired}}{\text{Available}} \times \text{Volume} = \frac{450 \text{ mg}}{160 \text{ mg}} \times 5 \text{ mL} = 14 \text{ mL}$$

Dosage to give is 14 mL.

Test-Taking Strategy: Set up the formula knowing that desired is 450 mg, available is 160 mg per 5 mL.

Level of Cognitive Ability: Application
Phase of Nursing Process: Implementation
Client Needs: Safe, Effective Care Environment
Content Area: Child Health

Reference
Leahy, J., & Kizilay, P. (1998). *Foundations of nursing practice: A nursing process approach.* Philadelphia: W. B. Saunders. p. 453.

21. **1**

Rationale: Calculate dosage by weight first:

0.07 mg/day × 7.2 kg = 0.50 mg/day.

The physician orders Lanoxin BID; therefore, 2 doses in 24 hours will be administered.

0.50 mg/day divided by 2 doses
= 0.25 mg for each dose

Test-Taking Strategy: Read the question carefully, noting that the question states "BID" and "each dose." Options 2 and 4 would result from miscalculation. Option 3 is the dosage for 24 hours/day, but the question requests BID, which would require 2 doses in 24 hours.

Level of Cognitive Ability: Application
Phase of Nursing Process: Implementation
Client Needs: Safe, Effective Care Environment
Content Area: Child Health

Reference
Leahy, J., & Kizilay, P. (1998). *Foundations of nursing practice: A nursing process approach.* Philadelphia: W. B. Saunders. p. 453.

BIBLIOGRAPHY

Ashwill, J., & Droske, S. (1997). *Nursing care of children: Principles and practice*. Philadelphia: W. B. Saunders.

Hodgson, B., & Kizior, R. (1998). *Saunders nursing drug handbook 1998*. Philadelphia: W. B. Saunders.

Kee, J., & Marshall, S. (1996). *Clinical calculations* (3rd ed.). Philadelphia: W. B. Saunders. pp. 199–212.

Kuhn, M. (1998). *Pharmaco-therapeutics: A nursing process approach* (4th ed.). Philadelphia: F. A. Davis.

Leahy, J., & Kizilay, P. (1998). *Foundations of nursing practice: A nursing process approach*. Philadelphia: W. B. Saunders.

Lehne, R. (1998). *Pharmacology for nursing care* (3rd ed.). Philadelphia: W. B. Saunders.

Luckmann, J. (1997). *Saunders manual of nursing care*. Philadelphia: W. B. Saunders.

Monahan, F., & Neighbors, M. (1998). *Medical-surgical nursing: Foundations for clinical practice* (2nd ed.). Philadelphia: W. B. Saunders.

O'Toole, M. (1997). *Miller-Keane encyclopedia & dictionary of medicine, nursing, & allied health* (6th ed.). Philadelphia: W. B. Saunders.

Pickar, G. (1996). *Dosage calculations* (5th ed.). Albany, NY: Delmar.

UNIT IX

....

The Adult Client with an Integumentary Disorder

PYRAMID TERMS

Burns—Cell destruction of the layers of the skin and the resultant depletion of fluid and electrolytes.

Carbon Monoxide Poisoning—Carbon monoxide is a colorless, odorless, and tasteless gas that has an affinity for hemoglobin 200 times greater than that of oxygen. Oxygen molecules are displaced and carbon monoxide reversibly binds to hemoglobin to form carboxyhemoglobin. Tissue hypoxia occurs.

Chemical Burns—Caused by tissue contact with strong acids, alkalis, or organic compounds. Systemic toxicity from cutaneous absorption can occur.

Electrical Burns—Caused by heat generated by an electrical energy as it passes through the body. Results in internal tissue damage.

Fourth-Degree Burn—Involves injury to the muscle and bone. Injured area appears black. Edema is absent.

Full-Thickness (Third-Degree) Burn—Deep red, black, white, or brown area. Injured surface appears dry. Tissue disruption is noted, with fat exposed. Skin is edematous.

Partial-Thickness (Second-Degree) Burn—Mottled red base and broken epidermis with a wet, shiny and weeping surface. Large blisters cover an extensive area. Skin is edematous and painful.

Smoke Inhalation Injury—Results when the victim is trapped in an enclosed, smoke-filled space.

Superficial (First-Degree) Burn—Mild to severe erythema, and the skin blanches with pressure.

Thermal Burns—Caused by exposure to flames, hot liquids, steam, or hot objects.

Decubitus—Localized area of skin breakdown that occurs as a result of poor circulation to the area; also called pressure ulcer.

Herpes Zoster (Shingles)—An acute viral infection of the nerve structure caused by varicella-zoster. Herpes zoster is contagious to individuals who have not had chickenpox.

Kaposi's Sarcoma—Skin lesions that occur in individuals with a compromised immune system.

Lyme Disease—An infection acquired from a tick bite. Ticks live in wooded areas and survive by attaching to a host.

Skin Cancer—A malignant lesion of the skin that may or may not metastasize. Causes include chronic friction and irritation to a skin area and exposure to ultraviolet rays. Diagnosis is confirmed by a skin biopsy that is positive for cancer cells.

PYRAMID TO SUCCESS

The Pyramid to Success focuses on the concept that the integumentary system provides the first line of defense against infections. Focus on the protective measures necessary to prevent infection. Pyramid points address the risk factors related to the development of integumentary disorders, the preventive measures related to skin cancer, and the content related to Kaposi's sarcoma and Lyme disease. Focus on the emergency measures related to a client with a burn, fluid resuscitation, monitoring for complications, and skin grafting. Psychosocial issues relate to the body image disturbances that can occur as a result of the integumentary disorder.

NURSING PROCESS

ASSESSMENT

Change in skin color, texture, temperature, sensation, and turgor
Itching
Fever
Hair loss
Cleanliness
Trophic changes of the skin, hair, and nails
Skin integrity and lesions
Nevi and scars

ANALYSIS: Impaired Skin Integrity

PLANNING	IMPLEMENTATION	EVALUATION
Skin integrity will remain intact.	Assess client for risk for the development of alteration in skin integrity. Monitor skin condition. Monitor skin for breakdown or lesions. Initiate skin protective measures to prevent breakdown.	Client's skin remains intact and shows no signs of infection or drainage.

ANALYSIS: Potential for Infection

PLANNING	IMPLEMENTATION	EVALUATION
The client will not develop an infection.	Monitor temperature and for signs of infection. Monitor any lesions for drainage. Initiate body and fluid precautions as required.	Temperature remains within normal limits.

ANALYSIS: Alteration in Nutrition

PLANNING	IMPLEMENTATION	EVALUATION
The client will maintain an adequate nutritional intake.	Encourage a well balanced diet. Encourage adequate fluid intake. Monitor intake and output (I&O). Obtain weights. Monitor laboratory values.	Hydration and nutritional status of client is adequate.

ANALYSIS: Alteration in Comfort

PLANNING	IMPLEMENTATION	EVALUATION
Client will verbalize a need for pain medication.	Administer pain medication as prescribed. Monitor and document effectiveness of pain medication.	Client verbalizes reasonable comfort from pain medication.

ANALYSIS: Altered Tissue Perfusion

PLANNING	IMPLEMENTATION	EVALUATION
Client reports sensation in extremities.	Monitor neurovascular status; assess color, motion, and sensation of affected area. Assess peripheral pulses.	Neurovascular status remains intact.

ANALYSIS: Body Image Disturbance

PLANNING	IMPLEMENTATION	EVALUATION
The client acknowledges the actual change in body appearance. Client verbalizes the impact of the situation on existing personal relationships and life style.	Encourage client to verbalize concerns regarding the skin disorder. Provide care in a nonjudgmental manner, maintaining the client's privacy and dignity.	Client verbalizes concerns related to skin disorder. Client verbalizes personal strengths. Client verbalizes available community resources.

ANALYSIS: Knowledge Deficit

PLANNING	IMPLEMENTATION	EVALUATION
The client will verbalize appropriate care to the skin.	Instruct client regarding the prescribed treatment plan. Allow client to demonstrate procedures related to the treatment plan.	Client demonstrates appropriate procedures for caring for skin disorder.

CLIENT NEEDS

SAFE, EFFECTIVE CARE ENVIRONMENT

Informed consent for treatments and procedures
Confidentiality related to disorder
Asepsis
Handling infectious materials
Standard (universal) precautions

HEALTH PROMOTION AND MAINTENANCE

Physical assessment of the integumentary system
Disease prevention measures
Health promotion programs
Instructions to the client regarding care to integumentary disorder

PSYCHOSOCIAL INTEGRITY

Body image changes
Utilizing coping mechanisms
Adapting to role changes
Use of support systems

PHYSIOLOGICAL INTEGRITY

Basic care and comfort
Adequate nutrition for healing
Comfort interventions
Expected effects of treatments
Monitoring laboratory values
Fluid and electrolyte imbalances
Monitoring for complications
Providing emergency care

BIBLIOGRAPHY

Black, J., & Matassarin-Jacobs, E. (1977). *Medical surgical nursing: Clinical management for continuity of care* (5th ed.). Philadelphia: W. B. Saunders.
Luckmann, J. (1997). *Saunders manual of nursing care*. Philadelphia: W. B. Saunders.

National Council of State Boards of Nursing. (1997). *Plan for the National Licensure Examination for Registered Nurses*. Chicago: Author.
O'Toole, M. (ed.) (1997). *Miller-Keane encyclopedia & dictionary of medicine, nursing, allied health* (6th ed.). Philadelphia: W. B. Saunders.

CHAPTER 47

Integumentary System

I. Anatomy and Physiology

A. The skin is the largest sensory organ of the body
B. Functions
  1. First line of defense against infections
  2. Protects underlying tissues and organs
  3. Receives stimuli from the external environment
  4. Maintains normal body temperature
  5. Excretes salts, water, and organic wastes
  6. Protects the body from dehydration
  7. Synthesizes vitamin D_3, that converts to calcitriol, for normal calcium metabolism
  8. Stores nutrients
  9. Protects the internal organs from injury
  10. Detects touch, pressure, pain, and temperature stimuli and relays that information to the nervous system
C. Layers
  1. Epidermis
  2. Dermis
  3. Subcutaneous fat
D. Accessory Structures
  1. Nails
  2. Hair
  3. Glands
    a. Sebaceous
    b. Sweat
E. Normal Bacterial Flora
  1. A pH of 4.2 to 5.6 halts the growth of bacteria
  2. Organisms are shed with normal exfoliation
  3. Normal bacterial flora
    a. Gram-positive and gram-negative staphylococcus
    b. Pseudomonas
    c. Streptococcus

II. Risk Factors

A. Exposure to chemical and environmental pollutants
B. Exposure to radiation
C. Exposure to the sun
D. Lack of personal hygiene habits
E. Use of cosmetics and harsh soaps
F. Medications, such as long-term steroid and/or anticoagulant therapy
G. Nutritional deficiencies
H. Moderate to severe emotional stress
I. Infection, with injured areas as potential entry points
J. Changes associated with developmental stages and aging

III. Psychosocial Impact

A. Change in body image
B. Fear of rejection
C. Social isolation (from embarrassment about changes in skin appearance)
D. Decreased self-esteem
E. Restrictions in physical activity
F. Pain
G. Disruption or loss of employment
H. Cost of medications, if prescribed
I. Cost of hospitalizations and follow-up care, including dressing supplies

IV. Diagnostic Tests

A. Skin Biopsy
  1. Description: Obtaining a small piece of skin tissue for histopathologic study
  2. Implementation preprocedure
    a. Obtain informed consent
    b. Cleanse site as prescribed
  3. Implementation postprocedure
    a. Place specimen when obtained by physician in the appropriate container and send to pathology laboratory for analysis
    b. Use surgically aseptic technique for biopsy site dressings
    c. Assess the biopsy site for bleeding and infection
B. Skin Cultures
  1. Description
    a. Noninvasive procedure

b. A small skin culture sample is obtained, using a sterile applicator

c. Sample is sent to laboratory to identify an existing organism

2. Implementation: Obtain skin culture samples prior to instituting antibiotic therapy

3. Implementation postprocedure: Send skin culture sample to the laboratory

C. Wood's Light Examination

1. Description: Skin is viewed under ultraviolet light through a special glass (Wood's glass) to identify superficial infections of the skin

2. Implementation preprocedure: Darken room prior to the examination

3. Implementation postprocedure: Assist client while adjustment from darkened room occurs

D. Skin Testing

1. Description

a. The administration of an allergen to the skin's surface or into the dermis

b. Administered by patch, scratch, or intradermal techniques

2. Implementation preprocedure

a. Discontinue systemic corticosteroids or antihistamine therapy for 48 hours prior to test as prescribed

b. Obtain informed consent

c. Have resuscitation equipment available if a scratch test is performed, as it may induce an anaphylactic reaction

3. Implementation postprocedure

a. Instruct client to keep skin-testing patch area dry

b. Instruct client to avoid activities that may produce sweating if a patch test was performed

c. Record the site, date, and time of the test

d. Record the date and the time for follow-up site reading

e. Inspect the site for erythema, papules, vesicles, edema, and induration

f. Provide client with a list of potential allergens, if identified

V. Skin Disorders

A. Contact Dermatitis

1. Description: An inflammatory response of the skin that produces skin changes after contact with a specific antigen

2. Assessment

a. Pruritus and burning

b. Edema

c. Erythema at point of contact

d. Signs of infection

e. Vesicles with drainage

3. Implementation

a. Elevation of extremity to reduce edema

b. Application of cool, wet dressings and tepid baths as prescribed

c. Maintain a cool environment

d. Protect affected area from trauma

e. Prevent scratching and rubbing of affected area

f. Assist with skin testing, as prescribed, to determine allergen(s)

g. Instruct client to avoid contact with the allergen when determined

h. Instruct client to avoid harsh soaps

i. Instruct client to avoid using heating pads or blankets

j. Administer antibiotic for infection as prescribed

k. Administer antipruritic or antihistamine, as prescribed, for itching

l. Administer corticosteroids for inflammation as prescribed

B. Poison Ivy, Poison Oak, and Poison Sumac

1. Description: A dermatitis that develops from contact with urushiol from poison ivy, oak, or sumac plants

2. Assessment

a. Papulovesicular lesions

b. Severe itching

3. Implementation

a. Cleanse the skin of plant oils

b. Apply cool, wet dressings with Burow's solution, as prescribed, to relieve the itching

c. Apply lotion or topical steroids as prescribed

d. Administer oral corticosteroids as prescribed

C. **Lyme Disease** (Table 47–1)

1. Description

a. An infection caused by *Borrelia burgdorferi*, acquired from a tick bite

b. Ticks live in wooded areas and survive by attaching to a host

2. Assessment

3. Implementation

a. Gently remove the tick with tweezers or fingers, wash skin with antiseptic, and dispose of tick by flushing it down the toilet

Table 47–1. **Stages of Lyme Disease**

First Stage	Second Stage	Third Stage
Symptoms can occur several days to months following the bite	Occurs several weeks following the tick bite	Large joints become involved
A small red pimple develops that spreads into a ring-shaped rash	Joint pain Neurological complications	Arthritis progresses
Rash may be large or small or may not occur at all	Heart disease symptoms	
Flulike symptoms occur, such as headaches, stiff neck, muscle aches, and fatigue		

b. Obtain a blood test 4 to 6 weeks after a bite to detect the presence of the disease (testing before this time is not reliable)
c. Instruct client in the administration of antibiotics, as prescribed, if the disease is confirmed
d. Instruct client to avoid areas that contain ticks, such as wooded grassy areas, especially in the summer months
e. Instruct client to wear tight-fitting clothing while outside and to spray body with tick repellent before going outside
f. Instruct client to examine body when returning inside

D. Erysipelas and Cellulitis
1. Description
   a. Erysipelas is an acute, superficial, rapidly spreading inflammation of the dermis and lymphatics caused by beta-hemolytic streptococcus group A, that enters the tissue via an abrasion, bite, trauma, or wound
   b. Cellulitis is skin infection into the deeper dermis and subcutaneous fat, and the causative organism is usually *Streptococcus pyogenes*
2. Assessment
   a. Pain
   b. Itching
   c. Swelling
   d. Redness
   e. Warmth
   f. Nodules
3. Implementation
   a. Promote rest
   b. Apply warm compresses as prescribed to promote circulation and to decrease discomfort, erythema, and edema
   c. Administer antibiotics as prescribed for infection following a culture of the area

E. Psoriasis
1. Description
   a. A chronic, noninfectious skin inflammation involving keratin synthesis that results in psoriatic patches
   b. Possible causes of the disorder include stress, trauma, infection, and changes in climate
   c. The disorder may also be exacerbated by the use of certain medications
   d. Koebner's phenomenon is the development of psoriatic lesions at a site of injury, such as a scratched or sunburned area
2. Assessment
   a. Pruritus
   b. Shedding, silvery white, scaling plaques; usually affect the scalp, knees, shins, elbows, and sacral regions
   c. A yellow discoloration, pitting, and thickening of the nails
   d. Joint inflammation

3. Implementation
   a. Administer and instruct the client regarding daily soaks and tepid, wet compresses as prescribed to the affected areas
   b. Assist client to remove the scales during the soak
   c. Apply corticosteroids and cover areas with warm moist dressings or occlusive dressing as prescribed to decrease infection
   d. Use Saran wrap or plastic bags as the occlusive dressing, and apply rubber gloves on the client's hands
   e. Utilize a bed cradle to keep covers off the client's skin
   f. Instruct the client not to scratch the affected areas
   g. Monitor for and instruct the client to recognize the signs and symptoms of infection
   h. Administer antipsoriatics as prescribed, anticipating the use of anthralin (Anthra-Derm)(coal tar), followed by exposure to ultraviolet light
   i. Prepare the client for photochemotherapy (PUVA [psoralen and ultraviolet A] therapy) as prescribed, anticipating the administration of methoxsalen (Oxsoralen) 2 hours prior to the ultraviolet light
   j. Prepare to administer keratolytics and antimicrobials as prescribed
   k. Administer tar preparations as prescribed to suppress mitotic activity and produce an anti-inflammatory effect
   l. Instruct client to wear light cotton clothing over affected areas
   m. Instruct client to avoid over-the-counter medications
   n. Instruct client regarding prescribed treatments and medications
   o. Assist the client to identify ways to reduce stress

F. **Skin Cancer** (Box 47–1)
1. Description
   a. A malignant lesion of the skin, which may or may not metastasize
   b. Causes include chronic friction and irritation to a skin area and exposure to ultraviolet rays
   c. Diagnosis is confirmed by a skin biopsy that is positive for cancer cells

---

BOX 47–1. Appearance of Skin Cancer Lesions

A waxy nodule
An irregular, circular, bordered lesion with hues of tan, black, or blue
A small, red, nodular lesion
An oozing, bleeding, crusting lesion

2. Types
    a. Basal cell: The most common form, arising from the basal cells contained in the epidermis
    b. Squamous cell: The second most common **skin cancer** in whites; it is a tumor of the epidermal keratinocytes and can infiltrate surrounding structures, metastasize to lymph nodes, and be subsequently fatal
    c. Malignant melanoma: Cancer of the melanocytes that can metastasize to the brain, lungs, bone, liver, and skin and is ultimately fatal

3. Assessment
    a. Change in color, size, or shape of pre-existing lesion
    b. Pruritus
    c. Local soreness

4. Implementation
    a. Instruct client regarding preventive measures
    b. Instruct client to monitor for lesions that do not heal or that change characteristics
    c. Instruct client to have moles or lesions removed that are subject to chronic irritation
    d. Instruct client to avoid contact with chemical irritants
    e. Instruct client to use sun-screening lotions and layered clothing when outdoors
    f. Assist with surgical excision of lesion as prescribed

◆ G. **Kaposi's Sarcoma**
1. Description: Skin lesions that occur primarily in individuals with a compromised immune system
2. Assessment
    a. Purplish, reddish-brown lesions on skin
    b. Raised, oblong, tender, or nontender and slow-growing skin tumors
    c. Organ involvement includes the lymph nodes, airways or lungs, or any part of the gastrointestinal tract from the mouth to the anus
3. Implementation
    a. Maintain body fluid precautions
    b. Provide protective isolation if the immune system is depressed
    c. Prepare client for radiation as prescribed
    d. Prepare client for chemotherapy as prescribed
    e. Administer immunotherapy, as prescribed, to stabilize the immune system

◆ H. **Herpes Zoster (Shingles)**
1. Description
    a. An acute viral infection of the dorsal nerve root ganglion, caused by the varicella-zoster virus
    b. Can be caused by the reactivation of the varicella-zoster virus or exposure to varicella-zoster or can occur during any immunocompromised state
    c. Diagnosis is determined by visual examination, skin cultures, and skin stains that identify the organism, and by an antinuclear antibody (ANA) blood test that will produce a positive result
    d. A culture provides the definitive diagnosis
    e. **Herpes zoster** is contagious to individuals who have not had chickenpox
2. Assessment
    a. Unilaterally clustered skin vesicles along peripheral sensory nerves on the trunk, thorax, or face
    b. Fever
    c. Burning and neuralgia
    d. Pruritus
    e. Paresthesia
3. Implementation
    a. Isolate client, because exudate from lesions contains the virus
    b. Maintain strict wound and skin precautions
    c. Monitor vital signs
    d. Assess neurovascular status and seventh cranial nerve function
    e. Assess for signs and symptoms of infection
    f. Keep blisters intact if formed
    g. Assist client with acetic acid compresses and tepid baths as prescribed
    h. Prepare to assist physician with a nerve block using lidocaine (Xylocaine) if prescribed
    i. Administer antiviral agents, analgesics, antianxiety agents, antipruritics and corticosteroids as prescribed
    j. Use an air mattress and a bed cradle on the client's bed
    k. Prevent client from scratching and rubbing the affected area
    l. Instruct client to wear light-weight, loose cotton clothing and to avoid wool and synthetic clothing

I. Paronychia
1. Description
    a. An infection of the tissue around the nailplate
    b. The disorder most commonly occurs in middle-aged women and in diabetics
2. Assessment
    a. Redness and swelling around the nailbed
    b. Soreness at the nailbed
3. Implementation
    a. Monitor temperature
    b. Monitor for infection around nails
    c. Monitor for cellulitis in the affected area
    d. Assist client with warm soaks as prescribed
    e. Prepare to assist with incision and drainage of infected area if prescribed

f. Administer antibiotic or fungicidal ointments as prescribed

J. Impetigo
  1. Description: A bacterial infection of the skin caused by streptococcus or staphylococcus or both
  2. Assessment
     a. Skin lesions that appear as vesicles
     b. Lesions progress to crusted pustules
  3. Implementation
     a. Allow lesions to dry by air exposure
     b. Assist client with cleansing with hexachlorophene soap as prescribed
     c. Assist with compresses as prescribed to remove crusts and to allow for healing
     d. Apply and instruct client in the use of antibiotic ointments as prescribed
     e. Apply and instruct client in the use of emollients as prescribed to prevent the skin from cracking
     f. Instruct client in methods to prevent the spread of the disease
     g. Instruct client in the use of separate towels, linens, and dishes

K. Boils
  1. Description
     a. A deep bacterial inflammation of a hair follicle caused by staphylococcus
     b. Commonly occur on the face, neck, arms, legs, and groin
  2. Assessment
     a. Redness on skin
     b. Tender and painful furuncle
     c. Skin swelling at the site
     d. A yellow or white center at the furuncle
  3. Implementation
     a. Instruct client good handwashing technique to prevent the spread of infection
     b. Apply hot moist compresses until drainage occurs
     c. Assist the physician in incision and drainage, which relieves the pain and allows the escape of purulent drainage
     d. Instruct client in the use of separate bath linens
     e. Instruct the client in daily cleanliness
     f. Instruct client in the administration of antibiotics if prescribed

L. Frostbite
  1. Description
     a. Damage to tissues and blood vessels as a result of prolonged exposure to cold
     b. Fingers, toes, nose, and ears are often affected
  2. Assessment
     a. Numbness
     b. Paresthesia
     c. Pallor
     d. Severe pain, swelling, erythema, and blistering occur once the client is in a warm environment

e. Necrosis and gangrene may develop in severe cases
  3. Implementation
     a. Handle the tissues gently
     b. Rewarm the affected part with tepid water, about 105° F
     c. Do not massage the area, as this may result in further tissue damage
     d. Do not debride blisters
     e. Apply bulky dressings to permit drainage from blisters and provide protection

M. Scabies
  1. Description
     a. A parasitic skin disorder caused by an infestation of the *Sarcoptes scabiei* (itch mite)
     b. Is endemic among school children and institutionalized populations because of the close personal contact
     c. Risk factors include close personal contact with an infected person or contaminated article
     d. There is a 1-month delay between the initial infestation and the onset of pruritus in the host
     e. Common sites are the hands, feet, finger webs, nipples, umbilicus, penis, soles, and palms
  2. Assessment
     a. Erythematous papules and pustules
     b. Threadlike, brownish, linear burrows up to 1 cm long
     c. Secondary lesions consist of vesicles, crusts, reddish-brown nodules, and excoriations
     d. Intense pruritus that worsens at night
  3. Implementation
     a. Administer antihistamines or topical steroids to relieve itching as prescribed
     b. Apply topical antiscabies creams or lotions such as Kwell cream or Eurax, as prescribed, to kill the mites
     c. Instruct the client to apply antiscabies preparations to the entire body from the neck down and to leave on for 6 to 24 hours, as prescribed
     d. Instruct client to apply antiscabies creams to dry skin, because moist skin increases absorption and the potential for side effects
     e. Following treatment with antiscabies preparations instruct the client to remove the medication by washing with soap and water

N. Acne Vulgaris
  1. Description
     a. A common, self-limiting, multifactorial disorder
     b. Requires active treatment for control until it spontaneously resolves
     c. The types of lesions are comedones (open

and closed), pustules, papules, and nodules

   d. The exact cause is unknown

   e. There is no evidence that consumption of foods such as chocolate, nuts, or fatty foods affect acne

   f. Exacerbations coincide with the menstrual cycle from hormonal activity

   g. Heat, humidity, and excessive perspiration have a role in increased acne

2. Assessment

   a. Closed comedones: Whiteheads and noninflamed lesions that develop as a follicle, enlarge with retention of horny cells

   b. Open comedones: Blackheads that result from continuing accumulation of horny cells and sebum, which dilate the follicles

   c. Pustules and papules result as the inflammatory process progresses

   d. Nodules result from total disintegration of a comedo and subsequent collapse of the follicle

   e. Deep scarring can result from nodules

3. Implementation

   a. Instruct client in the administration of topical antibiotics, such as clindamycin (Cleocin) and erythromycin (E.E.S.) or tretinoin (Retin-A), as prescribed

   b. Provide client with written instructions regarding the use of the medications

   c. Instruct client that improvement may not be apparent for 4 to 6 weeks

   d. Instruct client in the use of isotretinoin (Accutane), if prescribed, to inhibit inflammation

   e. Instruct client about the adverse effects of isotretinoin (Accutane), which include elevated triglycerides, skin dryness, cheilitis (lip inflammation), and eye discomfort

   f. Instruct client to stop taking vitamin A supplements during treatment with isotretinoin (Accutane)

   g. Instruct client in appropriate skin-cleansing methods, with emphasis on not scrubbing the face and using only the agreed-upon topicals

   h. Instruct client not to squeeze, prick, or pick at lesions

   i. Instruct client to use products labeled noncomedogenic and cosmetics that are water based, and to avoid contact with products that are excessively oil-based

   j. Instruct client on the importance of follow-up treatment

O. **Decubiti** (Table 47–2)

1. Description

   a. An impairment of skin integrity

   b. Localized areas of necrosis of the skin and subcutaneous tissue due to pressure

   c. Prevention of skin breakdown is a major role of the nurse, particularly in caring for the bedridden or immobile client

2. Risk factors

   a. Malnutrition

   b. Incontinence

   c. Immobility

   d. Decreased sensory perception

   e. Skin-shearing

3. Assessment

4. Implementation

   a. Institute measures to prevent **decubiti**

   b. Assess the nutritional status of the client

   c. Provide adequate nutritional intake to promote tissue integrity

   d. Monitor for an alteration in skin integrity

   e. Relieve or remove pressure on the skin

   f. Turn and reposition the immobile client every 2 hours, or more frequently if necessary

   g. Ambulate the client

   h. Provide active and passive exercises every 8 hours

   i. Keep the skin clean and dry and the sheets wrinkle-free

   j. Apply a moisture barrier as prescribed to protect the skin

   k. Use assistive devices to prevent pressure, such as an alternating air pressure mattress or sheepskin padding

   l. Apply medications or dressings to the wound as prescribed

---

Table 47–2. **Stages of Decubiti**

Stage 1	Stage 2	Stage 3	Stage 4
A reddened area that returns to normal skin color after 15 to 20 minutes of pressure relief, such as turning the client to another position The skin is intact Area is red and does not blanch with external pressure	Area in which the top layer of skin is missing The ulcer usually is shallow with a pink to red base; a white or yellow eschar may be present	Deep ulcers that extend into the dermis and subcutaneous tissues White, gray, or yellow eschar usually is present at the bottom of the ulcer, and the ulcer crater may have a lip or edge Purulent drainage is common	Deep ulcers that extend into muscle and bone Foul-smelling Brown or black eschar Purulent drainage is common

◆ **VI. Burn Injuries**
A. Description: Cell destruction of the layers of the skin and the resultant depletion of fluid and electrolytes
B. **Burn Size**
1. **Small burns**: The body's response to injury is localized to the injured area
2. **Large or extensive burns**
   a. Consist of 25% or more of the total body surface area (TBSA)
   b. The body's response to the injury is systemic
   c. Affects all the major systems of the body
C. Description of Extent of **Burn** Injury
1. **Minor burns**
   a. The **burn** extent is no greater than 15% of the TBSA in the adult
   b. Full thickness injuries that are less than 2% of the TBSA
   c. **Burn** areas do not involve the eyes, hands, face, feet, or perineum
   d. The client is an adult younger than 50 years of age
   e. The client has no pre-existing medical condition at the time of the **burn** injury
   f. No other injury occurred with the **burn**
2. **Moderate burns**
   a. The **burn** extent is no greater than 25% of the TBSA in the adult
   b. Full-thickness injuries that are less than 10% of the TBSA
   c. **Burn** areas do not involve the eyes, hands, face, feet, or perineum
   d. The client is an adult younger than 50 years of age
   e. The client has no pre-existing medical condition at the time of the **burn** injury
   f. No other injury occurred with the **burn**
3. **Major burns**
   a. The **burn** extent is more than 25% of the TBSA in the adult
   b. Full-thickness injuries are more than 10% of the TBSA
   c. **Burn** areas involve the eyes, hands, face, feet, or perineum
   d. The **burn** injury was caused by electricity
   e. The client is older than 50 years of age
   f. The client has a pre-existing medical condition at the time of the **burn** injury
   g. **Burns** are accompanied by other injuries or inhalation **burns**
◆ D. Estimating the Extent of Injury (Table 47–3)
E. **Burn Depth**
1. Superficial—first degree
   a. Mild to severe erythema
   b. Skin blanches with pressure
   c. Painful
   d. Tingling
   e. Pain is eased by cooling
   f. Discomfort lasts about 48 hours
   g. Healing occurs in about 3 to 7 days
   h. Skin grafts are not required
2. Partial thickness—second degree

Table 47–3. Methods to Estimate Extent of Burn Injury

Rule of Nines/Adult		Lund and Browder Method
Head and neck	9%	Modifies percentages for body segments according to age
Anterior trunk	18%	
Posterior trunk	18%	Provides a more accurate estimate of the burn size
Arms (9%)	18%	
Legs (18%)	36%	Uses a diagram of the body divided into sections, with the representative % of the TBSA for ages greater than 1 year
Perineum	1%	
		Should be re-evaluated after initial wound debridement

TBSA, total body surface area.

   a. Large blisters covering an extensive area
   b. Edema
   c. Mottled red base and broken epidermis, with a wet, shiny, and weeping surface
   d. Painful
   e. Injured area is sensitive to cold air
   f. Superficial partial thickness heals in 14 to 21 days
   g. Deep partial thickness heals in 21 to 28 days
   h. Grafts may be used if the healing process is prolonged
3. Full thickness—third degree
   a. Deep red, black, white, or brown area
   b. Injured surface appears dry
   c. Edema
   d. Tissue disruption with fat exposed
   e. Little pain
   f. Spontaneous healing will not occur
   g. Requires removal of eschar and split- or full-thickness skin-grafting
   h. Scarring and wound contractures are likely to develop without preventive measures
   i. Healing takes weeks to months
4. Fourth degree
   a. Involves injury to the muscle and bone
   b. Injured area appears black
   c. Edema is absent
   d. Pain is absent
   e. No blisters
   f. Eschar is hard and inelastic
   g. Healing time takes weeks to months
   h. Grafts are required
F. Age and General Health
1. Mortality rates are higher for children less than 4 years of age, particularly in the 0- to 1-year age group, and for clients over the age of 65 years
2. Debilitating disorders, such as cardiac, respiratory, endocrine, and renal disorders, influence the client's response to injury and treatment
3. Mortality rate is higher when the client has a pre-existing disorder at the time of the **burn** injury

G. **Burn Location**
1. **Burns** of head, neck, and chest are associated with pulmonary complications
2. **Burns** of face are associated with corneal abrasion
3. **Burns** of ear are associated with auricular chondritis
4. Hands and joints require intensive therapy to prevent disability
5. The perineal area is prone to autocontamination by urine and feces
6. Circumferential **burns** of the extremities can produce a tourniquet-like effect and lead to vascular compromise
7. Circumferential thoracic **burns** lead to inadequate chest wall expansion and pulmonary insufficiency

VII. Types of Burns

A. **Thermal Burns**: Caused by exposure to flames, hot liquids, steam, or hot objects
B. **Chemical Burns**
1. Caused by tissue contact with strong acids, alkalis, or organic compounds
2. Systemic toxicity from cutaneous absorption can occur
C. **Electrical Burns**
1. Caused by heat generated by an electrical energy as it passes through the body
2. Result in internal tissue damage
3. Cutaneous **burns** cause muscle and soft tissue damage that may be extensive, particularly in high-voltage electrical injuries
4. The voltage, type of current, contact site, and duration of contact are important to identify
5. Alternating current is more dangerous than direct current as it is associated with cardiopulmonary arrest, ventricular fibrillation, tetanic muscle contractions, and long bone or vertebral fractures
D. **Radiation Burns**: Caused by exposure to a radioactive source

VIII. Inhalation Injuries

A. **Smoke Inhalation Injury**
1. Description: Results when the victim is trapped in an enclosed, smoke-filled space
2. Assessment
   a. **Facial burns**
   b. Erythema
   c. Swelling of oropharynx and nasopharynx
   d. Singed nasal hairs
   e. Agitation and anxiety
   f. Tachycardia
   g. Flaring nostrils
   h. Stridor, wheezing, and dyspnea
   i. Hoarse voice
   j. Sooty sputum and cough

B. **Carbon Monoxide Poisoning** (Table 47–4)
1. Description
   a. **Carbon monoxide** is a colorless, odorless, and tasteless gas that has an affinity for hemoglobin 200 times greater than that of oxygen
   b. Oxygen molecules are displaced and carbon monoxide reversibly binds to hemoglobin to form carboxyhemoglobin
   c. Tissue hypoxia occurs
2. Assessment
C. Smoke Poisoning
1. Description
   a. Caused by the inhalation of the by-products of combustion
   b. A localized inflammatory reaction occurs and causes a decrease in bronchial ciliary action and a decrease in surfactant
2. Assessment
   a. Mucosal edema in the airways
   b. Wheezing on auscultation
   c. After several hours, sloughing of the tracheobronchial epithelium may occur, and hemorrhagic bronchitis may develop
   d. Adult respiratory distress syndrome (ARDS) can result
D. Direct Thermal Heat Injury
1. Description
   a. Can occur to the lower airways by the inhalation of steam or explosive gases or the aspiration of scalding liquids
   b. Can occur to the upper airways, which appear erythematous and edematous, with mucosal blisters and ulcerations
   c. Mucosal edema can lead to upper airway obstruction, especially during first 24 to 48 hours
   d. All clients with head or neck **burns** should be monitored closely for the development of airway obstruction and are immediately considered for endotracheal intubation if obstruction occurs
2. Assessment
   a. Erythema and edema of upper airways
   b. Mucosal blisters and ulcerations
   c. Mucosal edema

Table 47–4. Carbon Monoxide Poisoning

Blood Level (%)	Clinical Manifestation
5–10	Impaired visual acuity
11–20	Flushing
21–30	Nausea
	Impaired dexterity
31–40	Vomiting
	Dizziness
	Syncope
41–50	Tachypnea
	Tachycardia
Greater than 50	Coma and death

IX. Pathophysiology of Burns

A. Following the **burn**, vasoactive substances are released from the injured tissue, and these substances cause an increase in the capillary permeability, allowing the plasma to seep to the surrounding tissues

B. The direct injury to the vessels increases capillary permeability

C. The direct injury to the cell membranes permits sodium entry and potassium exit

D. Extensive **burns** result in generalized body edema and a decrease in circulating intravascular blood volume

E. The heart rate increases

F. The hematocrit levels increase

G. Evaporative fluid losses through the **burn** wound are greater than normal, and the losses continue until complete wound closure occurs

H. The fluid losses result in a decrease in organ perfusion

I. If the intravascular space is not replenished with IV fluids, hypovolemic shock and ultimately death will occur

J. Capillary permeability decreases 18 to 26 hours post**burn** but does not normalize until 2 to 3 weeks following the injury

K. Cardiac output returns to normal and increases to meet the hypermetabolic needs of the body at 24 hours post**burn**

L. The initial rise in the hematocrit level falls to below normal at the third to fourth day post**burn** because of the red blood cell (RBC) loss and damage at the time of injury

M. Initially, the body shunts blood from the kidneys, causing oliguria

N. The body then begins to reabsorb fluid, and diuresis of the excess fluids occurs over the next days to weeks

O. Blood flow to the gastrointestinal tract is diminished, leading to intestinal ileus and gastrointestinal dysfunction

P. Immune system function is depressed, resulting in immunosuppression and thus increasing the risk of infection and sepsis

Q. Pulmonary hypertension can develop, resulting in a decrease in the arterial oxygen tension level and a decrease in lung compliance

X. Management of the Burn Injury (Box 47–2)

A. Emergent Phase

1. Description

a. Begins at the time of injury and ends with the restoration of capillary permeability, usually at 48 to 72 hours following the injury; includes resuscitative phase

b. The primary goal is to prevent hypovolemic shock and preserve vital organ functioning

2. Prehospital care

a. Begins at the scene of the accident and ends when emergency care is obtained

b. Remove the victim from the source of the **burn**

c. Remove the source of heat

d. Assess airway, breathing, and circulation

e. Assess for associated trauma

f. Conserve body heat

g. Cover **burns** with sterile or clean cloths

h. Remove constricting jewelry and clothing

i. Assess the need for intravenous fluids

j. Transport

3. Emergency Room care: Continuation of care administered at the scene of the injury

4. **Major burns**

a. Evaluate the degree and extent of the **burn** and treat life-threatening conditions

b. A patent airway is established and 100% oxygen is administered as prescribed if the **burn** occurred in an enclosed area

c. Monitor for respiratory distress and assess need for intubation

---

BOX 47–2. Phases of Management of Burn Injury

EMERGENT PHASE

Begins at the time of injury and ends with the restoration of capillary permeability, usually at 48–72 hours following the injury

The primary goal is to prevent hypovolemic shock and preserve vital organ functioning

Includes prehospital care and emergency room care

RESUSCITATIVE PHASE

Begins with the initiation of fluids and ends when capillary integrity returns to near-normal levels and the large fluid shifts have decreased

The amount of fluid administered is based on client's weight and extent of injury

Most fluid replacement formulas are calculated from the time of injury and not from the time of arrival at the hospital

The goal is to prevent shock by maintaining adequate circulating blood volume and maintaining vital organ perfusion

ACUTE PHASE

Begins when the client is hemodynamically stable, capillary permeability is restored, and diuresis has begun

Usually begins 48–72 hours after the time of injury

Emphasis during this phase is placed on restorative therapy, and the phase continues until wound closure is achieved

The focus is on infection control, wound care, wound closure, nutritional support, pain management, and physical therapy

REHABILITATIVE PHASE

Final phase of burn care

Overlaps the acute care phase and goes well beyond hospitalization

Goals of this phase are designed so that the client can gain independence and achieve maximal function

d. Assess oropharynx for blisters and erythema

e. Monitor arterial blood gases (ABGs) and carboxyhemoglobin levels

f. For an inhalation injury, administer 100% oxygen via a tight-fitting non-rebreather face mask as prescribed until carboxyhemoglobin levels fall below 15%

g. Assess for hypovolemia and prepare for the administration of IV fluids to maintain fluid balance

h. Initiate peripheral IV access to nonburned skin proximal to any extremity **burn**, or prepare for the insertion of a central venous pressure line as prescribed

i. Monitor vital signs closely

j. Insert a Foley catheter as prescribed, and maintain urine output at 50 mL per hour

k. Maintain NPO status

l. Insert a nasogastric tube as prescribed to prevent paralytic ileus, to prevent vomiting, and to reduce risk of aspiration

m. Administer tetanus toxoid as prescribed

n. Administer pain medication, as prescribed, by IV route

o. Prepare client for an escharotomy or fasciotomy as prescribed

5. **Minor burns**

a. Administer pain medication with small doses of morphine sulfate or meperidine (Demerol) as prescribed

b. Instruct client in the use of oral analgesics as prescribed

c. Prepare to administer tetanus toxoid booster as prescribed if client has not received tetanus within the past 5 years; clients not immunized should receive tetanus human immune globulin and the first series of active immunizations with tetanus toxoid

d. Administer wound care as prescribed, which may include cleansing, debriding loose tissue, and removing any damaging agents, followed by application of topical antimicrobial cream and a sterile dressing

e. Instruct client in follow-up care, including active range of motion exercises and wound care treatments

B. Resuscitative Phase

1. Description

a. Begins with the initiation of fluids and ends when capillary integrity returns to near-normal levels, and the large fluid shifts have decreased

b. The amount of fluid administered is based on client's weight and extent of injury

c. Most fluid replacement formulas are calculated from the time of injury and not from the time of arrival at the hospital

d. The goal is to prevent shock by maintaining adequate circulating blood volume and maintaining vital organ perfusion

2. Fluid Resuscitation (Table 47–5)

a. The amount of fluid administered depends on how much intravenous fluid per hour is required to maintain a urinary output of 30–50 mL per hour

b. Successful fluid resuscitation is evaluated by stable vital signs, an adequate urine output, palpable peripheral pulses, and a clear sensorium

c. Urinary output is the most common and most sensitive noninvasive assessment parameter for cardiac output and tissue perfusion

d. Adjustment of the rate of administration of IV fluid on the basis of urinary output plus serum electrolyte levels is known as titration of fluid to meet the needs of the **burn** client

3. Implementation

a. Monitor for tracheal or laryngeal edema and administer respiratory treatments as prescribed

b. Monitor pulse oximetry and prepare for ABGs and carboxyhemoglobin (COHB) levels if inhalation injury is suspected

c. Elevate the head of the bed for **burns** of face and head

d. Initiate ECG monitoring

e. Monitor temperature and assess for infection

f. Shave or cut body hair around wound margins

g. Monitor daily weights, expecting a weight gain of 15 to 20 lb in the first 72 hours

h. Monitor gastric output and pH levels and for gastric discomfort and bleeding, indicating a stress ulcer

i. Administer antacids, H_2-receptor antagonists, and the antiulcer medication sucralfate (Carafate), as prescribed

j. Auscultate bowel sounds for ileus and monitor for abdominal distention and gastrointestinal dysfunction

Table 47–5. Brooke and Parkland (Baxter) Fluid Resuscitation Formulas for First 24 Hours After a Burn Injury

Formula	Solution	Infusion Rate
Brooke		
2 mL/kg/% BSA burn + 2000 mL/24 hr (maintenance)	¾ crystalloid, ¼ colloid D5W maintenance	½ in first 8 hours ½ in next 16 hours
Parkland (Baxter)		
4 mL/kg/% BSA burn for 24-hr period	Crystalloid only (lactated Ringer's)	½ in first 8 hours ½ in next 16 hours

BSA, body surface area.

k. Monitor stools for occult blood
l. Obtain urine specimen for myoglobin and hemoglobin levels
m. Monitor IV fluids closely and hourly input and output (I&O) to determine adequacy of the amounts of IV fluids
n. Monitor for renal failure and notify physician if urine output is less than 30 or greater than 50 mL per hour
o. Elevate circumferential **burns** of the extremities on pillows above the level of the heart to reduce dependent edema
p. Monitor pulses and capillary refill of the affected extremities and assess perfusion of the distal extremity with a circumferential **burn**
q. Prepare for a chest radiograph and other radiographs to rule out fractures or associated trauma
r. Keep room temperature warm
s. Place client on an air-fluidized bed and use a bed cradle to keep sheets off the client's skin

4. Pain management
a. Administer morphine sulfate or meperidine (Demerol), as prescribed, by the IV route
b. Medicate client prior to painful procedures
c. Avoid IM or SC routes because absorption through the soft tissue is unreliable when hypovolemia and large fluid shifts are occurring
d. Avoid administering medication by the oral route because of the possibility of GI dysfunction

5. Nutrition
a. Essential to promote wound-healing and prevent infection
b. The basal metabolic rate (BMR) is 40 to 100 times higher than normal
c. Maintain nothing by mouth (NPO) status until bowel sounds are heard, then advance to clear liquids as prescribed
d. Nutrition may be provided via enteral tube feeding, peripheral parenteral nutrition, or total parenteral nutrition
e. Provide a diet high in protein, carbohydrates, fats, and vitamins
f. Monitor calorie intake

6. Escharotomy
a. A lengthwise incision is made through the **burn** eschar to relieve constriction and pressure and to improve circulation
b. Performed for circulatory compromise due to circumferential **burns**
c. Performed at the bedside without anesthesia because nerve endings have been destroyed by the **burn** injury
d. Escharotomy can be performed on the thorax to improve ventilation
e. Following the escharotomy, assess pulses,

color, movement, and sensation of affected extremity, and control any bleeding with pressure
f. Apply topical antimicrobial agents and dressings to the area as prescribed following the procedure

7. Fasciotomy
a. An incision is made extending through the subcutaneous tissue and fascia
b. The procedure is performed if adequate tissue perfusion does not return following an escharotomy
c. Performed in the operating room with the client under general anesthesia
d. Following the procedure, assess pulses, color, movement, and sensation of affected extremity, and control any bleeding with pressure
e. Apply topical antimicrobial agents and dressings to the area, as prescribed, following the procedure

C. Acute Phase
1. Description
a. Begins when the client is hemodynamically stable, capillary permeability is restored, and diuresis has begun
b. The acute phase usually begins 48 to 72 hours after the time of injury
c. Emphasis during this phase is placed on restorative therapy, and the phase continues until wound closure is achieved
d. The focus is on infection control, wound care, wound closure, nutritional support, pain management, and physical therapy

2. Implementation
a. Provide protective isolation techniques
b. Maintain strict handwashing
c. Use sterile sheets and linens when caring for the client
d. Use gloves, cap, masks, shoe covers, scrub clothes, and plastic aprons when caring for the client
e. Provide wound care as prescribed and prepare for wound closure
f. Provide pain management
g. Provide adequate nutrition as prescribed
h. Prepare client for rehabilitation

D. Wound Care
1. Description: The cleansing, debridement, and dressing of the **burn** wounds
2. Hydrotherapy
a. Wounds are cleansed by immersion, showering, or spraying
b. Hydrotherapy occurs for 30 minutes or less to prevent increased sodium loss through the **burn** wound, heat loss, pain, and stress
c. Hydrotherapy is generally not used for clients who are hemodynamically unstable or those with new skin grafts
d. Care is taken to minimize bleeding and

Table 47–6. Debridement

Mechanical	Enzymatic	Surgical
Use of scissors and forceps to lift and trim away loose eschar Wet to dry or wet to wet dressing changes A painful procedure	Application of prepared proteolytic and fibrinolytic topical enzymes that digest necrotic tissue, which facilitates eschar removal Requires a moist environment to be effective; they are applied directly to the burn wound Pain and bleeding are major problems	Excision of eschar and coverage of wound *Tangential*: Very thin layers of eschar are shaved until viable tissue is reached *Fascial*: Used for very deep burns and removal of burn tissue and underlying fat down to the fascia

BOX 47–3. Temporary Wound Coverings

BIOLOGICAL

Amnion
Amniotic membranes from human placenta
Dressing is changed every 48 hours with amnion

Allograft Homograft
Donated human cadaver skin is harvested within 24 hr after death
Rejection can occur within 24 hr
Monitor for wound exudate and signs of infection

Xenograft Heterograft
Porcine skin is harvested after slaughter and preserved for storage
Rejection can occur within 24–72 hr
Xenograft over granulation tissue is replaced every 2–5 days until the wound heals naturally or until closure with autograft is complete

BIOSYNTHETIC AND SYNTHETIC

Visual inspection of wound is possible as dressings are transparent or translucent
Monitor for wound exudate and signs of infection

maintain body temperature during the procedure
 e. If hydrotherapy is not used, wounds are washed and rinsed in bed prior to application of antimicrobial agents
 3. Debridement (Table 47–6)
  a. Removal of eschar to prevent bacterial proliferation under the eschar and to promote wound healing
  b. Debridement may be mechanical, enzymatic, or surgical
 4. Deep Partial or Full-Thickness Burns
  a. Wound is cleansed and debrided
  b. Topical antimicrobial agents applied once or twice daily
E. Wound Closure (Table 47–7)
 1. Description
  a. Prevents infection and loss of fluid
  b. Promotes healing
  c. Prevents contractures
  d. Performed on the 5th to 21st day, depending on the extent of the **burn**
 2. Temporary wound coverings (Box 47–3)
  a. Biologic
  b. Biosynthetic and synthetic
 3. Autografting (Box 47–4)
  a. Permanent wound coverage
  b. Surgical removal of a thin layer of the client's own unburned skin and application of the client's skin to the excised **burn** wound
  c. Performed in the operating room under anesthesia
  d. Can be applied in a sheet graft or mesh graft, which are referred to as split-thickness skin grafts
  e. Monitor for bleeding following the graft, because bleeding beneath an autograft can prevent adherence
  f. Small amounts of blood or serum can be removed by gently rolling the fluid from

Table 47–7. Open Method Versus Closed Method of Wound Care

Method	Advantages	Disadvantages
Open		
Antimicrobial cream is applied, and wound is left open to the air without a dressing Antimicrobial cream is applied every 12 hr	Visualization of the wound Easier mobility and joint range of motion Simplicity in wound care	Increased chance of hypothermia from exposure
Closed		
Gauze dressings are carefully wrapped from the distal to the proximal area of the extremity to ensure that circulation is not compromised No two burn surfaces should be allowed to touch; touching can promote webbing of digits, contractures, and poor cosmetic outcome Dressings are changed every 8–12 hr	Decreases evaporative fluid and heat loss Aids in debridement	Mobility limitations Prevents effective range of motion exercises Wound assessment is limited

BOX 47–4. Types of Skin Grafts

SPLIT THICKNESS

Graft of half of the epidermis

FULL THICKNESS

Graft consisting of epidermis and dermis

PINCH GRAFT

Graft of a small piece of skin

SHEET GRAFT

Used to graft burns in visible areas
Applied to the wound without alteration in its integrity

MESH GRAFT

Contains many little slits that allow for expansion of donor skin
Can cover large areas or irregularly shaped wounds
Allows for drainage from bleeding wounds
When healed, the mesh pattern of the skin graft remains visible
Used on hidden body areas

the center of the graft to the periphery, where it can be absorbed with a sterile gauze pad
   g. For large accumulations of blood, the physician will aspirate the blood using a small-gauge needle and syringe
   h. Autografts are immobilized following surgery for 3 to 7 days to allow time to adhere and attach to the wound bed
   i. Position for immobilization and elevation of graft site to prevent movement and shearing of the graft

4. Care to the graft site
   a. Elevate and immobilize the graft site
   b. Keep site free from pressure
   c. Avoid weight-bearing
   d. When graft takes, roll a cotton-tipped applicator over the graft to remove exudate, because exudate can lead to infection and prevent graft adherence
   e. Monitor for foul-smelling drainage, increased temperature, increased WBCs, hematoma, fluid accumulation
   f. Instruct client to avoid using fabric softeners and harsh detergents in laundry
   g. Instruct client to lubricate healing skin with cocoa butter
   h. Instruct client to protect the affected area from sunlight
   i. Instruct client to use splints and support garments as prescribed

5. Care to the donor site
   a. The fine-mesh gauze dressing is allowed to dry
   b. Cover with nonadherent dressing and absorbent gauze as prescribed

   c. Nonadherent dressing will separate as healing occurs
   d. The gauze can be gently lifted and trimmed away as new epithelium forms below it
   e. Keep site dry, open to air, and free from pressure
   f. Prevent client from scratching donor site
   g. Apply lubricating lotions to soften area and reduce itching after the donor site is healed
   h. Donor site can be reused once healing has occurred

F. Physical Therapy
1. An individualized program of splinting, positioning, exercises, ambulation, activities of daily living, and physical therapy is implemented early in the acute phase of recovery to maximize functional and cosmetic outcomes
2. Perform range of motion exercises as prescribed to reduce edema and maintain strength and joint function
3. Ambulate client as prescribed to maintain strength of the lower extremities
4. Apply splints as prescribed to maintain proper joint position and prevent contractures
   a. Static splints immobilize the joint and are applied for periods of immobilization, during sleeping, and for clients who cannot maintain proper positioning
   b. Dynamic splints exercise the affected joint
   c. Do not apply pressure to skin areas with splints, which could lead to further tissue and nerve damage
5. Scarring is controlled by elastic wraps and bandages that apply continuous pressure to the healing skin during the period of time when the skin is vulnerable to shearing
6. Antiburn scar support garments are worn 23 hours a day until the **burn** scar tissue has matured, which takes 18 months to 2 years

G. Rehabilitative Phase (Box 47–5)
1. Description
   a. Final phase of **burn** care
   b. Overlaps the acute-care phase and goes well beyond hospitalization
   c. Goals of this phase are designed so that the client can gain independence and achieve maximal function

BOX 47–5. Surgical Options for Contractures and Scarring

Split-thickness and full-thickness skin grafts
Skin flaps
Z-plasties
Tissue expansion

2. Goals
   a. Promoting wound-healing
   b. Minimizing deformities
   c. Increasing strength and function
   d. Providing emotional support

PRACTICE QUESTIONS

1. Which of the following individuals is at the greatest risk for development of an integumentary disorder?
   1 An elderly female
   2 An adolescent
   3 An outdoor construction worker
   4 A physical education teacher

2. The client scheduled for a skin biopsy asks the nurse how painful the procedure is. The most appropriate response by the nurse is:
   1 "There is no pain associated with this procedure."
   2 "There is some pain, but the physician will prescribe an analgesic following the procedure."
   3 "The local anesthetic may cause a burning or stinging sensation."
   4 "A preoperative medication will be given so you will be sleeping and not feel any pain."

3. The nurse is reviewing the discharge instructions for the client who had a skin biopsy. Which of the following statements, if made by the client, indicates a need for further instruction?
   1 "I will call the physician if I see any drainage from the wound."
   2 "I will return in 7 days to have the sutures removed."
   3 "I will use the antibiotic ointment as prescribed."
   4 "I will remove the dressing when I get home and wash my skin with tap water."

4. The nurse prepares to assist the physician in examining the client's skin with a Wood light. Which of the following would be included in the plan for this procedure?
   1 Obtain an informed consent
   2 Darken the room for the examination
   3 Shave the skin and scrub with Betadine solution
   4 Prepare a local anesthetic

5. The nurse is assessing for the presence of cyanosis in a dark-skinned client. Which body area provides the best assessment?
   1 Back of the hands
   2 Earlobes
   3 Palms
   4 Sacrum

6. The clinic nurse provides instructions to a client who is to return to the clinic in 1 week for a patch test. The patch test will be done to identify the allergen causing the dermatitis. Which of the following instructions is most appropriate to provide to this client?
   1 Remain NPO prior to the test
   2 Shower on the morning of the test, using an antibacterial soap
   3 Discontinue the prescribed antihistamine 2 days before the test
   4 Consume fluids only on the day of the test

7. The nurse provides discharge instructions to a client following patch testing. Which of the following statements, if made by the client, indicates the need for further instruction?
   1 "I will return to the clinic in 2 days for the initial reading."
   2 "If the patch comes off, I need to reapply it."
   3 "I need to avoid activities that will cause me to sweat."
   4 "I need to keep the test sites dry at all times."

8. The clinic nurse implements a teaching plan for the client who has complained of chronic dry skin and episodes of pruritus. Which of the following, if stated by the client, would indicate a need for further teaching?
   1 "I should drink 8 to 10 glasses of water a day."
   2 "I need to avoid using astringents on my skin."
   3 "I should limit myself to one shower a day and apply emollient to my skin after the shower."
   4 "I should use a dehumidifier, especially during the winter months."

9. The camp nurse instructs a group of children about Lyme disease. Which of the following information would the nurse include in the instructions?
   1 Can be contagious by skin contact with an infected individual
   2 Can be caused by the inhalation of spores from bird droppings
   3 Is caused by contamination from cat feces
   4 Is caused by a tick carried by deer

10. The client is diagnosed with stage I of Lyme disease. Which of the following is a characteristic of this stage?
    1 Signs of neurological disorders
    2 Enlarged and inflamed joints
    3 Arthralgias
    4 Flulike symptoms

11. Following assessment and diagnostic evaluation, it has been determined that the client has Lyme disease, stage II. Which of the following is most indicative of this stage?
    1 Erythematous rash
    2 Neurological deficits
    3 Arthralgias
    4 Joint enlargements

12. The clinic nurse reads the chart of a client who was seen by the physician and notes that the physician has documented that the client has Lyme disease, stage III. Which of the following clinical manifestations would the nurse expect to note in the client?
    1 A generalized skin rash
    2 A cardiac dysrhythmia
    3 Enlarged and inflamed joints
    4 Paralysis in the extremity where the tick bite occurred

13. A female client arrives at the health care clinic and tells the nurse that she was just bitten by a tick and would like to be tested for Lyme disease. The client tells the nurse that she removed the tick and flushed it down the toilet. Which of the following nursing actions is most appropriate?
    1 Refer the client for a blood test immediately
    2 Inform the client that there is no test available for Lyme disease
    3 Instruct the client to return in 4 to 6 weeks to be tested because testing before this time is not reliable
    4 Tell the client that testing is not necessary unless arthralgia develops

14. Following diagnosis of Lyme disease, stage I, the nurse would anticipate that which of the following will be part of the treatment plan for the client?
    1 No treatment unless symptoms develop
    2 A 3-week course of oral antibiotic therapy
    3 Treatment with IV penicillin G
    4 Daily oatmeal baths for a period of 2 weeks

15. A cub scout leader is preparing a group of cub scouts for an overnight camping trip. The leader provides the scouts with a list of methods to prevent Lyme disease. Which of the following would not be part of this list?
    1 Avoid the use of insect repellents as they will attract the ticks
    2 Wear long-sleeved tops and long pants
    3 Bring a hat to wear during the trip
    4 Wear closed shoes and socks that can be pulled up over the pants

16. A male client calls the emergency room and tells the nurse that he has been cleaning a wooded area in the back yard and has discovered that he came directly in contact with poison ivy shrubs. The client tells the nurse that he cannot see anything on the skin and asks the nurse what to do. Which of the following is the most appropriate nursing response?
    1 "Come to the emergency room."
    2 "It is not necessary to do anything if you cannot see anything on your skin."
    3 "Take a shower immediately, lathering and rinsing several times."

    4 "Apply calamine lotion immediately to the exposed skin areas."

17. The client with AIDS is diagnosed with cutaneous Kaposi's sarcoma. Based on this diagnosis, the nurse understands that this has been determined by which of the following?
    1 Appearance of reddish blue lesions noted on the skin
    2 Swelling in the lower extremities
    3 Punch biopsy of the cutaneous lesions
    4 Swelling in the genital area

18. Which of the following individuals is least likely at risk for the development of Kaposi's sarcoma?
    1 A man with a history of same-sex partners
    2 A renal transplant client
    3 A client receiving antineoplastic medications
    4 An individual working in an environment where exposure to asbestos exists

19. The nurse prepares to bathe and change the bed linens of a client with cutaneous Kaposi's sarcoma lesions. The lesions are open and draining a scant amount of serous fluid. Which of the following would the nurse most appropriately incorporate in the plan during the bathing of this client?
    1 Wearing a gown, gloves, and a mask
    2 Wearing a gown and gloves
    3 Wearing gloves
    4 Wearing a gown and gloves to change the bed linens and gloves only for the bath

20. The client is being admitted to the hospital for treatment of acute cellulitis of the lower left leg. The client asks the admitting nurse to explain what cellulitis means. The nurse bases the response on the understanding that the characteristics of cellulitis include:
    1 A skin infection into the deep dermis and subcutaneous fat
    2 An acute superficial infection
    3 An inflammation of the epidermis
    4 An epidermal infection caused by staphylococcus

21. The nurse prepares to care for a client with acute cellulitis of the lower leg. Which of the following would the nurse anticipate to be prescribed for the client?
    1 Warm compresses to the affected area
    2 Cold compresses to the affected area
    3 Intermittent heat lamp treatments four times daily
    4 Alternating hot and cold compresses continuously

22. Which of the following individuals is least likely to be at risk for the development of psoriasis?
    1 A 32-year-old African-American
    2 A client with a family history of the disorder

3 An individual who has experienced a significant amount of emotional distress

4 A woman experiencing menopause

23. The clinic nurse assesses the skin of a client with a diagnosis of psoriasis. Which of the following characteristics is not associated with this skin disorder?

   1 A discoloration and pitting of the nails

   2 Silvery white, scaly patches on the scalp, elbows, knees, and sacral regions

   3 Complaints of pruritus

   4 Red-purplish, scaly lesions

24. Ultraviolet light (UVL) therapy is prescribed as a component of the treatment plan for a client with psoriasis. Which of the following is not a component of the plan of care related to this light treatment?

   1 Eye goggles need to be worn to prevent exposure to UVL

   2 The face needs to be shielded with a loosely applied covering

   3 The client will stand in a light treatment chamber for 30 minutes

   4 Only the area requiring treatment should be exposed to the UVL

25. The clinic nurse notes that the physician has documented a diagnosis of herpes zoster in the client's chart. Based on an understanding of the cause of this disorder, the nurse would determine that this definitive diagnosis was made following which diagnostic test?

   1 Skin biopsy

   2 Wood's light examination

   3 Culture of the lesion

   4 Patch test

26. The nurse is assigned to care for a client with herpes zoster. Which of the following characteristics does the nurse expect to note when assessing the lesions of this infection?

   1 A generalized body rash

   2 Small, blue-white spots with a red base

   3 A fiery red, edematous rash on the cheeks

   4 Clustered skin vesicles

27. The nurse manager is planning the clinical assignments for the day. Which of the following staff members would not be assigned to the client with herpes zoster?

   1 The nurse who never had mumps

   2 An experienced RN who never had chickenpox

   3 The nurse who never had roseola

   4 The nurse who never had German measles

28. A client returns to the clinic for follow-up treatment following a skin biopsy of a suspicious lesion performed 1 week ago. The biopsy report indicates that the lesion is a melanoma. Which of the following describes the characteristic of this type of lesion?

   1 Is highly metastatic

   2 Metastasis is rare

   3 Is characterized by local invasion

   4 Is encapsulated

29. When assessing a lesion diagnosed as malignant melanoma, the nurse would most likely expect to note which of the following?

   1 A small papule with a dry, rough scale

   2 A firm, nodular lesion topped with a crust

   3 A pearly papule with a central crater and a waxy border

   4 An irregularly shaped lesion

30. The nurse prepares discharge instructions following cryosurgery for treatment of a malignant skin lesion. Which of the following would the nurse include in the plan of care?

   1 To clean the site with hydrogen peroxide to prevent infection

   2 To apply ice to the site to prevent discomfort

   3 To apply alcohol-soaked dressings twice a day

   4 To avoid showering for 7 to 10 days

31. The health education nurse provides instructions to a group of clients regarding measures that will assist in preventing skin cancer. Which of the following would not be a part of this teaching plan?

   1 Use sunscreen when participating in outdoor activities

   2 Examine the body monthly for any lesions that may be suspicious

   3 Wear a hat, opaque clothing, and sunglasses when in the sun

   4 Avoid sun exposure after 3:00 P.M.

32. The clinic nurse reviews the client's chart and notes that the physician has documented a diagnosis of paronychia. Based on this diagnosis, which of the following does the nurse expect to note during the assessment?

   1 Swelling of the skin near the parotid gland

   2 Red, shiny skin around the nailbed

   3 White, silvery patches on the elbows

   4 White, taut skin in the popliteal area

33. The nurse provides home care instructions to a client diagnosed with impetigo. Which of the following would not be included in the teaching plan?

   1 Continue with antibiotics as prescribed

   2 Wash client's dishes separately from those of other household members

   3 It is not necessary to separate client's laundry from that of other household members

   4 Wash hands thoroughly and frequently throughout the day

34. The client arrives at the emergency room and has experienced frostbite to the right hand. Which of the following does the nurse note on assessment of the client's hand?
    1 A fiery red skin with edema in the nailbeds
    2 A pink, edematous hand
    3 Black fingertips surrounded by an erythematous rash
    4 A white color to the skin, which is insensitive to touch

35. The nurse prepares to treat a client with frostbite of the toes. Which of the following does the nurse anticipate to be prescribed for this condition?
    1 Rapid and continuous rewarming of the toes in a warm water bath until flushing of the skin occurs
    2 Rapid and continuous rewarming of the toes in hot water for 15 to 20 minutes
    3 Rapid and continuous rewarming of the toes when flushing occurs
    4 Rapid and continuous rewarming of the toes in cold water for 45 minutes

36. The evening nurse reviews the nursing documentation in the client's chart and notes that the day nurse has documented that the client has a stage II pressure ulcer (decubitus) in the sacral area. Which of the following would the nurse expect to note on assessment of the client's sacral area?
    1 Skin is intact
    2 Partial thickness skin loss of the epidermis
    3 A deep, crater-like appearance
    4 The presence of sinus tracts

37. Which of the following conditions is least likely to be a risk factor for the development of skin breakdown?
    1 A client who is unable to move about and is confined to bed
    2 A client incontinent of urine and feces
    3 A client with chronic nutritional deficiencies
    4 A client with a lowered mental awareness status

38. The nurse inspects the oral cavity of a client with candidiasis (thrush). Which of the following does the nurse expect to note?
    1 The presence of numerous small, red pinpoint lesions
    2 The presence of blisters
    3 The presence of white patches
    4 The presence of purple-colored patches

39. The nurse plans to instruct a client with candidiasis (thrush) of the oral cavity about how to care for the disorder. Which of the following is not a component of the instructions?
    1 To rinse the mouth four times daily with a commercial mouthwash
    2 To avoid spicy foods
    3 To avoid citrus juices and hot liquids
    4 To eat foods that are liquid or pureed

40. The nurse is caring for a client with a diagnosis of pemphigus. A hallmark sign characteristic of this condition is:
    1 Homan's sign
    2 Chvostek's sign
    3 Trousseau's sign
    4 Nikolsky's sign

41. The nurse is implementing a teaching plan to a group of adolescents regarding the causes of acne. Which of the following is the most appropriate statement regarding the cause of this disorder?
    1 It is caused by eating chocolate, nuts, and fatty foods
    2 It is caused by oily skin
    3 The exact cause is not known
    4 It is caused by exposure to heat and humidity

42. Isotretinoin (Accutane) is prescribed for a client with severe cystic acne. Which of the following, if stated by the client, would indicate a need for further teaching regarding this medication?
    1 "I need to continue to take my vitamin A supplements."
    2 "I need to use emollients and lip balms for my dry skin."
    3 "The medication may cause dryness and burning in my eyes."
    4 "I will need to return for a blood test to check my triglyceride level."

43. The clinic nurse inspects the skin of a client suspected of having scabies. Which of the following assessment findings would the nurse note if this disorder were present?
    1 The appearance of vesicles or pustules with a thick, honey-colored crust
    2 The presence of white patches scattered about the trunk
    3 Multiple straight or wavy, threadlike lines beneath the skin
    4 Patchy hair loss and round red macules with scales

44. The home health nurse visits a client suspected of having scabies. Which of the following precautions will the nurse institute during the assessment of the client?
    1 Wear a mask and gloves
    2 Wear gloves only
    3 Wear a gown and gloves
    4 Avoid touching the client's home furnishings

45. The adult client was burned as a result of an explosion. The burn initially affected the client's entire face (anterior half of the head), and the upper half of the anterior torso, and there were circumferential burns to the lower half of both arms. The client's clothes caught on fire, and the client ran, causing subsequent burn injuries to the posterior surface of the head and the upper half of the posterior torso. Using the Rule of

Nines, the extent of the burn injury is which of the following?
1 31.5%
2 36%
3 40.5%
4 45%

46. The client was burned at 7:00 A.M. The client states that before the burn, the body weight was 198 pounds (90 kg). Using the Lund and Browder method, the physician has estimated that the total body surface area (TBSA) burned is 83%. Using the Parkland (Baxter) formula, the total amount of intravenous lactated Ringer's solution that the client will receive by 3:00 P.M. of the same day that the burn occurred is which of the following?
1 3735 mL
2 7470 mL
3 14,940 mL
4 29,880 mL

47. A 38-year-old client was injured when gasoline ignited the client's clothing, causing partial thickness burns to the anterior torso and forearms. Using the Lund and Browder chart, the estimated TBSA burned is 12%. According to the American Burn Association guidelines, this burn would be classified as a:
1 Superficial burn
2 Minor burn
3 Moderate burn
4 Major burn

48. The client was admitted 7 days ago with a diagnosis of 45% TBSA partial thickness burns. Treatment for the wounds has included cleaning the wounds and applying Silvadene dressings twice daily. Which of the following descriptions of the wound indicate that the wound is healing as optimally as possible?
1 Blisters are intact
2 Beefy red granulation tissue is totally covering the wounds
3 Epithelial cell growth is present and is spontaneously closing the wounds
4 Grafts are pink and adherent without exudate

49. The nurse is caring for a 2-year-old who just arrived in the emergency department following flame burns to the face and chest. The nurse notes a hoarse cough that produces sputum with black flecks. Eyelashes and eyebrows have been singed. The child's eyelids are swollen. The child becomes restless and the color becomes dusky. The nurse interprets these assessment data to indicate which of the following?
1 The child is afraid and is having a panic attack due to the unfamiliar surroundings
2 Pain from the burn injury is causing the child to act out
3 Hypotension is causing vertigo

4 The burn has probably caused laryngeal edema that has occluded the airway

50. Which of the following is the anticipated therapeutic outcome of an escharotomy procedure performed for a third-degree circumferential arm burn?
1 Brisk bleeding from the site
2 Formation of granulation tissue
3 Decreasing edema formation
4 Return of distal pulses

51. The client sustained a burn from cutaneous exposure to lye. At the site of injury, copious irrigation to the site was performed for 1 full hour. On admission to the emergency department, the nurse assesses the burn site. Which of the following indicates that the chemical burn process is continuing?
1 Thick, leathery eschar
2 Liquefied, soapy necrosis
3 Cherry-red, firm tissue
4 Intact blisters surrounded by erythema

52. The client is undergoing radiation therapy to treat lung cancer. Following the treatment, the nurse notes that the chest and neck are red, and the client is complaining of pain at the radiation site. The nurse interprets these assessment data as:
1 A superficial injury to tissue from the radiation
2 An allergic reaction to the radiation
3 A cutaneous reaction to products formed by the lysis of the neoplastic cells
4 An ischemic injury, much like decubitus formation, due to pressure from the linear accelerator

53. The nurse is caring for a client who sustained second- and third-degree burns on the anterior lower legs and anterior thorax. Which of the following does the nurse expect to note during the emergent phase of the burn injury?
1 Decreased heart rate
2 Decreased blood pressure
3 Elevated hematocrit levels
4 Increased urinary output

54. The nurse is caring for a client who suffered an inhalation injury from a wood stove. The carbon monoxide level reveals a level of 12%. Based on this level, the nurse anticipates which of the following signs in the client?
1 Flushing
2 Dizziness
3 Tachycardia
4 Coma

55. The client arrives at the emergency department following a burn injury that occurred in the basement at home. An inhalation injury is suspected. Which of the following does the nurse anticipate to be prescribed for the client?

1 100% oxygen via a tight-fitting rebreather face mask
2 Oxygen via nasal cannula at 15 liters
3 100% oxygen via a tight-fitting, non-rebreather face mask
4 Oxygen via nasal cannula at 10 liters

56. The nurse is administering IV fluids as prescribed to a client who sustained second- and third-degree injuries of the back and legs. In evaluating the adequacy of fluid resuscitation, which of the following provides the most reliable indicator for determining the adequacy?
1 Vital signs
2 Urine output
3 Peripheral pulses
4 Mental status

57. The nurse is caring for a client with circumferential burns of both legs. Which of the following leg positions is most appropriate for this type of a burn?
1 In a dependent position
2 Flat without elevation
3 Elevation above the level of the heart
4 Elevation of the knee gatch on the bed

58. The nurse is caring for a burn client in protective isolation. Which of the following is not a component of protective isolation techniques?

1 Using sterile sheets and linens
2 Strict handwashing
3 Wearing gloves and a gown only when caring for the client
4 Wearing protective garb, including a mask, cap, shoe covers, and plastic aprons

59. The nurse is caring for a client following an autograft and grafting to a burn wound on the right knee. Which of the following does the nurse anticipate to be prescribed for the client?
1 Immobilization for 3 to 7 days
2 Placing the affected leg flat
3 Placing the affected leg in a dependent position
4 Immobilization for 24 hours

60. The nurse provides discharge instructions regarding skin care to a client following hospitalization for grafting to burn injuries sustained to the left chest and left arm. Which of the following is not a component of the discharge teaching plan?
1 Bathe using a mild soap and rinse thoroughly
2 Avoid the use of lanolin products to the newly healed skin area
3 Avoid direct sunlight to the newly healed skin area
4 Never wear warm clothing over the newly healed skin area

ANSWERS

1. **3**

Rationale: Prolonged exposure to the sun, unusual cold, or other conditions can damage the skin. The outdoor construction worker fits into a high-risk category for the development of an integumentary disorder. Although an elderly client may be at higher risk than a younger individual, immobility and lack of nutrition increase the elder person's risk. An adolescent may be prone to the development of acne, but this does not occur in all adolescents. The physical education teacher is at low or no risk of developing an integumentary problem.

Test-Taking Strategy: Avoid reading into both the question and each of the options, and read the information in each of the options carefully. Note the key phrase "greatest risk." Eliminate option 4 first. Eliminate options 1 and 2 next because not all elderly or adolescents are at risk for the development of integumentary disorders. Note the qualifier, "outdoor," in the correct option. This should provide you with the key that this is the correct option. If you had difficulty with this question, take time now to review the risk factors associated with integumentary disorders!

Level of Cognitive Ability: Analysis
Phase of Nursing Process: Assessment
Client Needs: Health Promotion and Maintenance
Content Area: Adult Health/Integumentary

Reference
Black, J., & Matassarin-Jacobs, E. (1997). *Medical-surgical nursing: Clinical management for continuity of care* (5th ed.). Philadelphia: W. B. Saunders, p. 2182.

2. **3**

Rationale: Depending on the size and location of the lesion, a biopsy is usually a quick and almost painless procedure. The most common source of pain is the initial local anesthetic, which can produce a burning or stinging sensation.

Test-Taking Strategy: Use the process of elimination to answer the question. Eliminate option 1 first. Eliminate option 2 because this option addresses postprocedure, which is not the issue of the client's question to the nurse. Eliminate option 4 because a preoperative medication that puts the client to sleep is not a part of the procedure for a skin biopsy. If you had difficulty with this question, take time now to review the procedure related to a skin biopsy!

Level of Cognitive Ability: Application
Phase of Nursing Process: Implementation
Client Needs: Psychosocial Integrity
Content Area: Adult Health/Integumentary

Reference
Black, J., & Matassarin-Jacobs, E. (1997). *Medical-surgical nursing: Clinical management for continuity of care* (5th ed.). Philadelphia: W. B. Saunders, p. 2195.

3. **4**

Rationale: Following a skin biopsy, the nurse instructs the client to keep the dressing dry and in place for a minimum of 8 hours. After the dressing is removed, the site is cleaned once a day with tap water or saline to remove any dry blood or crusts. The physician may prescribe an antibiotic ointment to minimize local bacterial colonization. The nurse instructs the client to report any redness or excessive drainage at the site. Sutures are usually removed 7 to 10 days after biopsy.

Test-Taking Strategy: Use the process of elimination to answer the question. Eliminate option 3 first as the client verbalizes a physician's prescription. Eliminate options 1 and 2 next. A client needs to report signs of drainage and needs to return to the physician for follow-up and suture removal. Consider the alteration in skin integrity that occurs with a skin biopsy. This should assist in directing you to the correct option!

Level of Cognitive Ability: Analysis
Phase of Nursing Process: Evaluation
Client Needs: Health Promotion and Maintenance
Content Area: Adult Health/Integumentary

Reference

Ignatavicius, D., Workman, M., & Mishler, M. (1995). *Medical-surgical nursing: A nursing process approach* (2nd ed.). Philadelphia: W. B. Saunders, p. 1926.

4. **2**

Rationale: Examination of the skin under a Wood light is always carried out in a darkened room. This is a noninvasive examination, therefore an informed consent is not required. A hand-held long-wavelength ultraviolet light or a Wood light is used. The skin does not need to be shaved nor is a local anesthetic necessary. Areas of blue-green or red fluorescence are associated with certain skin infections. The procedure is painless.

Test-Taking Strategy: Knowledge about the procedure for examining the skin with a Wood light is required to answer the question. Knowing that this is a noninvasive procedure will assist in eliminating options 1, 3, and 4. Take time to review this procedure if you had difficulty answering this question!

Level of Cognitive Ability: Application
Phase of Nursing Process: Planning
Client Needs: Safe, Effective Care Environment
Content Area: Adult Health/Integumentary

Reference

Black, J., & Matassarin-Jacobs, E. (1997). *Medical-surgical nursing: Clinical management for continuity of care* (5th ed.). Philadelphia: W. B. Saunders, p. 2194.

5. **3**

Rationale: In a dark-skinned client, the nurse examines the lips, tongue, nailbeds, conjunctiva, and palms and soles at regular intervals for subtle color changes. In a client with cyanosis, the lips and tongue are gray, and the palms, soles, conjunctiva, and nailbeds have a bluish tinge.

Test-Taking Strategy: Knowledge regarding assessment of skin color in a dark-skinned client is required to answer the question. Assessing for cyanosis in a client reflects the ABCs: Airway, Breathing, and Circulation. Take time now to review this important assessment technique if you had difficulty with this question!

Level of Cognitive Ability: Application
Phase of Nursing Process: Assessment
Client Needs: Physiological Integrity
Content Area: Adult Health/Integumentary

Reference

Ignatavicius, D., Workman, M., & Mishler, M. (1995). *Medical-surgical nursing: A nursing process approach* (2nd ed.). Philadelphia: W. B. Saunders, p. 1294.

6. **3**

Rationale: Client preparation for a patch test includes informing the client to discontinue the administration of systemic corticosteroids or antihistamines for at least 48 hours before the test. These medications must be discontinued to prevent suppression of the inflammatory response to an allergen. Topical steroid therapy may be continued as long as the agent is not applied on the area to be tested.

Test-Taking Strategy: Use the process of elimination to answer the question. Eliminate options 1 and 4 first. These options are similar, and there is no need to restrict fluids or remain NPO prior to the procedure. A "patch" test does not require a body shower with an antibacterial soap. Note the relationship between "allergen" in the question and "antihistamine" in the response. This should assist in directing you to the correct option.

Level of Cognitive Ability: Application
Phase of Nursing Process: Implementation
Client Needs: Physiological Integrity
Content Area: Adult Health/Integumentary

Reference

Ignatavicius, D., Workman, M., & Mishler, M. (1995). *Medical-surgical nursing: A nursing process approach* (2nd ed.). Philadelphia: W. B. Saunders, p. 1926.

7. **2**

Rationale: The nurse instructs the client to keep the test sites dry at all times. The nurse also discourages excessive physical activity that will result in sweating. If the client reapplies patches that come loose, this can interfere with an accurate interpretation of the allergic reactions. The nurse reinforces the necessity of removing loose or nonadherent test patches for reapplication at a later date. The initial reading is performed 2 days after application, and the final reading is performed 2 to 5 days later.

Test-Taking Strategy: Use the process of elimination. Eliminate options 3 and 4 first, since keeping the test site dry and avoiding sweating are similar. Knowledge that follow-up is important after any procedure should assist in directing you to option 2, the correct option for this question as it is stated. If you had difficulty with this question, take time now to review the client-teaching points following a patch test!

Level of Cognitive Ability: Analysis
Phase of Nursing Process: Evaluation
Client Needs: Health Promotion and Maintenance
Content Area: Adult Health/Integumentary

Reference

Ignatavicius, D., Workman, M., & Mishler, M. (1995). *Medical-surgical nursing: A nursing process approach* (2nd ed.). Philadelphia: W. B. Saunders, p. 1926–1927.

8. **4**

Rationale: The client should avoid using a dehumidifier because this will further dry room air. Instead, the client should use a room humidifier during the winter months or whenever the furnace is in use. The client should be taught to maintain a daily fluid intake of 3000 mL, unless contraindicated, and should avoid alcohol and caffeine ingestion. The client should avoid applying rubbing alcohol, astringents, or other drying agents to the skin. One bath or one shower per day for 15 to 20 minutes with warm water and a mild soap should be immediately followed by the application of an emollient to prevent evaporation of water from the hydrated epidermis.

Test-Taking Strategy: Use the process of elimination, but read each option carefully. Knowledge that a dehumidifier is going to dry the air in the environment will assist in directing you to option 4, the correct option for this question as stated. If you had difficulty with this question, take time now to review client-teaching points related to dry skin and pruritus!

Level of Cognitive Ability: Analysis
Phase of Nursing Process: Evaluation
Client Needs: Health Promotion and Maintenance
Content Area: Adult Health/Integumentary

Reference

Black, J., & Matassarin-Jacobs, E. (1997). *Medical-surgical nursing: Clinical management for continuity of care* (5th ed.). Philadelphia: W. B. Saunders, p. 2204.

9. **4**

Rationale: Lyme disease is a multisystem infection that results from a bite by a tick carried by several species of deer. Persons bitten by the *Ixodes* ticks are infected with the spirochete *Borrelia burgdorferi*. Histoplasmosis is caused by the inhalation of spores from bat or bird droppings. Toxoplasmosis is caused from the ingestion of cysts from contaminated cat feces. Lyme disease cannot be transmitted from one person to another.

Test-Taking Strategy: Knowledge regarding the cause of Lyme disease is required to answer this question. Knowing that this disease is caused by a bite will assist in eliminating the incorrect options. If you had difficulty with this question, take time now to review the cause of Lyme disease!

Level of Cognitive Ability: Application
Phase of Nursing Process: Implementation
Client Needs: Health Promotion and Maintenance
Content Area: Adult Health/Integumentary

References

Black, J., & Matassarin-Jacobs, E. (1997). *Medical-surgical nursing: Clinical management for continuity of care* (5th ed.). Philadelphia: W. B. Saunders, pp. 416–417.
Luckmann, J. (1997). *Saunders manual of nursing care.* Philadelphia: W. B. Saunders, p. 1654.

10. **4**

Rationale: The hallmark of stage I is the development of a skin rash within 2 to 30 days of infection, generally at the site of the tick bite. The rash develops into a concentric ring, giving it a bull's eye appearance. The lesion enlarges up to 50 to 60 cm, and smaller lesions develop farther away from the original tick bite. In stage I, most infected persons develop flulike symptoms that last 7 to 10 days, and these symptoms may recur later.

Test-Taking Strategy: Use the process of elimination and eliminate options 2 and 3 first, as they are similar. Next, note that the question asks for the characteristic of stage I. From the remaining two options, select the least serious

since the issue of the question relates to stage I. Expect neurological disorders to occur with progression of the disease. If you had difficulty with this question, take time now to review the stages of Lyme disease!

Level of Cognitive Ability: Analysis
Phase of Nursing Process: Assessment
Client Needs: Physiological Integrity
Content Area: Adult Health/Integumentary

Reference

Luckmann, J. (1997). *Saunders manual of nursing care.* Philadelphia: W. B. Saunders, pp. 1654–1656.

11. **2**

Rationale: Stage II of Lyme disease develops within 1 to 6 months in the majority of untreated individuals. The most serious problems include cardiac conduction defects and neurological disorders such as Bell's palsy and paralysis. These problems are not usually permanent. Arthralgias and joint enlargements are noted in stage III. A rash appears in stage I.

Test-Taking Strategy: Knowledge regarding the clinical manifestations that occur in the stages of Lyme disease is helpful in answering the question. Eliminate options 3 and 4 first as they are similar. Knowledge that a rash appears initially following the tick bite will assist in eliminating option 1. If you had difficulty with this question, take time now to review the clinical manifestations associated with each stage of Lyme disease!

Level of Cognitive Ability: Analysis
Phase of Nursing Process: Assessment
Client Needs: Physiological Integrity
Content Area: Adult Health/Integumentary

Reference

Luckmann, J. (1997). *Saunders manual of nursing care.* Philadelphia: W.B. Saunders, p. 1656.

12. **3**

Rationale: Stage III develops within a month to several months after initial infection. It is characterized by arthritic symptoms, such as arthralgias and enlarged or inflamed joints, which can persist for several years after the initial infection. Cardiac and neurological dysfunction occur in stage II. A rash occurs in stage I. Paralysis of the extremity where the tick bite occurred is not a directly related characteristic of Lyme disease.

Test-Taking Strategy: Knowledge regarding the stages of Lyme disease is helpful in answering the question. Remember that a rash occurs in stage I, cardiac and neurological disorders in stage II, and joint involvement in stage III. If you had difficulty with this question, take time now to review the clinical manifestations associated with Lyme disease!

Level of Cognitive Ability: Analysis
Phase of Nursing Process: Assessment
Client Needs: Physiological Integrity
Content Area: Adult Health/Integumentary

Reference

Luckmann, J. (1997). *Saunders manual of nursing care.* Philadelphia: W. B. Saunders, p. 1654.

13. **3**

Rationale: A blood test is available to detect Lyme disease; however, it is not a reliable test if performed prior to 4 to 6 weeks following the tick bite. Antibody formation takes place in the following manner: IgM is detected 3 to 4 weeks after Lyme disease onset, peaks at 6 to 8 weeks, then gradually disappears; IgG is detected 2 to 3 months after infection and may remain elevated for years.

Test-Taking Strategy: Use the process of elimination. Eliminate option 1 first. "Immediately" should indicate that this is potentially an incorrect option. A blood test is available, therefore eliminate option 2. Eliminate option 4, because treatment should begin before the arthralgia develops. If you had difficulty with this question, take time now to review the method of diagnosing Lyme disease!

Level of Cognitive Ability: Application
Phase of Nursing Process: Implementation
Client Needs: Physiological Integrity
Content Area: Adult Health/Integumentary

References
Fischbach, F. (1996). *A manual of laboratory & diagnostic tests* (5th ed.). Philadelphia: Lippincott-Raven, p. 522.
Ignatavicius, D., Workman, M., & Mishler, M. (1995). *Medical-surgical nursing: A nursing process approach* (2nd ed.). Philadelphia: W. B. Saunders, p 496.

14. **2**

Rationale: Prevention, public education, and early diagnosis are vital to the control and treatment of Lyme disease. A 3-week course of oral antibiotic therapy is recommended during stage I. Later stages of Lyme disease may require therapy with intravenous antibiotics, such as penicillin G.

Test-Taking Strategy: Knowledge regarding the treatment associated with Lyme disease is helpful to answer the question. Note that the question states stage I. Eliminate option 3, because IV antibiotics will not be administered in this stage. Eliminate option 4, because although oatmeal baths may be helpful for pruritus, they would not be helpful in a systemic disorder. Waiting for symptoms to develop is an incorrect option. Take time to review the treatment associated with Lyme disease now, if you had difficulty with this question!

Level of Cognitive Ability: Analysis
Phase of Nursing Process: Analysis
Client Needs: Physiological Integrity
Content Area: Adult Health/Integumentary

Reference
Luckmann, J. (1997). *Saunders manual of nursing care.* Philadelphia: W. B. Saunders, p. 1656.

15. **1**

Rationale: In the prevention of Lyme disease, individuals need to be instructed to use an insect repellent on the skin and clothes when in an area where ticks are likely to be found. Long-sleeved tops and long pants, closed shoes, and a hat or cap should be worn. If possible, heavily wooded areas or areas with thick underbrush should be avoided. Socks can be pulled up and over pant legs to prevent ticks from entering under clothing.

Test-Taking Strategy: Note the key phrase "would not be part of this list." Use the process of elimination in answering the question. Note that option 1 uses the word "avoid." Reading carefully will assist in directing you to the correct option. If you had difficulty with this question, take time now to review measures to prevent contact with ticks!

Level of Cognitive Ability: Application
Phase of Nursing Process: Implementation
Client Needs: Health Promotion and Maintenance
Content Area: Adult Health/Integumentary

Reference
Ignatavicius, D., Workman, M., & Mishler, M. (1995). *Medical-surgical nursing: A nursing process approach* (2nd ed.). Philadelphia: W. B. Saunders, p. 496.

16. **3**

Rationale: When an individual comes in contact with a poison ivy plant, the sap from the plant forms an invisible film upon the human skin. The client should be instructed to immediately shower and that the skin should be lathered several times and rinsed each time in running water. Calamine lotion is a treatment that is used if dermatitis develops. It is not necessary for the client to be seen in the emergency room at this time.

Test-Taking Strategy: Use the process of elimination to answer the question. Knowledge that dermatitis can develop from contact with an allergen will assist in selecting the correct answer. Also, knowledge that contact with poison ivy results in an invisible film will assist in directing you to option 3. Take time now to review the immediate treatment for contact with poison ivy, if you had difficulty with this question!

Level of Cognitive Ability: Application
Phase of Nursing Process: Implementation
Client Needs: Health Promotion and Maintenance
Content Area: Adult Health/Integumentary

Reference
O'Toole, M. (ed.). (1997). *Miller-Keane encyclopedia & dictionary of medicine, nursing, & allied health* (6th ed.). Philadelphia: W. B. Saunders, pp. 1274–1275.

17. **3**

Rationale: Kaposi's sarcoma lesions begin as red, dark blue, or purple macules on the lower legs that change into plaques. These large plaques ulcerate, or open and drain. The lesions spread by metastasis through the upper body, then to the face and oral mucosa. They can move to the lymphatic system, lungs, and GI tract. Late disease results in swelling and pain in the lower extremities, penis, scrotum, or face. Diagnosis is made by punch biopsy of cutaneous lesions and biopsy of pulmonary and GI lesions.

Test-Taking Strategy: Use the process of elimination, eliminating options 2 and 4 first. These symptoms occur late in the development of Kaposi's sarcoma. Note the key phrase "diagnosis has been determined." From the remaining two options, this phrase should assist in directing you to the option that will confirm the diagnosis, which will be the biopsy of the lesions!

Level of Cognitive Ability: Analysis
Phase of Nursing Process: Assessment
Client Needs: Physiological Integrity
Content Area: Adult Health/Integumentary

References
Black, J., & Matassarin-Jacobs, E. (1997). *Medical-surgical nursing: Clinical management for continuity of care* (5th ed.). Philadelphia: W. B. Saunders, p. 2230.
Luckmann, J. (1997). *Saunders manual of nursing care.* Philadelphia: W. B. Saunders, p. 1936.

18. **4**

Rationale: Kaposi's sarcoma is a vascular malignancy that presents as a skin disorder. It is a common AIDS indicator. It is seen most frequently in men with a history of same-sex partners. Although the cause of Kaposi's sarcoma is not known, it is considered to be due to an alteration or failure in the immune system. The renal transplant client and the client receiving antineoplastic medications are at risk for immunosuppression. Exposure to asbestos is not related to the development of Kaposi's sarcoma.

Test-Taking Strategy: Read the question carefully, noting the phrase "least likely at risk." You can easily eliminate option 1. Note the similarity between options 2 and 3. These clients are at risk for immunosuppression. With this in mind, these options can be eliminated, leaving option 4 as the correct option. If you had difficulty with this question, take time now to review the risk factors associated with Kaposi's sarcoma!

Level of Cognitive Ability: Analysis
Phase of Nursing Process: Assessment
Client Needs: Physiological Integrity
Content Area: Adult Health/Integumentary

References
Black, J., & Matassarin-Jacobs, E. (1997). *Medical-surgical nursing: Clinical management for continuity of care* (5th ed.). Philadelphia: W. B. Saunders, p. 2230.
Luckmann, J. (1997). *Saunders manual of nursing care.* Philadelphia: W. B. Saunders, p. 1936.

19. **2**

Rationale: Gowns and gloves are required if the nurse anticipates contact with soiled items, such as from wound drainage, and in caring for a client who is incontinent with diarrhea or has an ileostomy or colostomy. Masks are not required unless droplet or airborne precautions are necessary. Regardless of the amount of wound drainage, a gown and gloves must be worn.

Test-Taking Strategy: Think about the method of transmission when answering a question of this type. Read the question, noting the task that is presented; in this case, it is bathing and changing linens. Eliminate option 1 because the method of transmission is not respiratory in nature. Eliminate options 3 and 4 since neither provide adequate protection based on the method of transmission. If you had difficulty with this question, take time now to review standard precautions!

Level of Cognitive Ability: Application
Phase of Nursing Process: Planning
Client Needs: Safe, Effective Care Environment
Content Area: Adult Health/Integumentary

Reference
Leahy, J., & Kizilay, P. (1998). *Foundations of nursing practice: A nursing process approach.* Philadelphia: W. B. Saunders, p. 1237.

20. **1**

Rationale: Cellulitis is a skin infection into deeper dermis and subcutaneous fat that results in deep red erythema without sharp borders; which spreads widely through tissue spaces. The skin is erythematous, edematous, tender, and sometimes nodular. Erysipelas is an acute, superficial, rapidly spreading inflammation of the dermis and lymphatics.

Test-Taking Strategy: Knowledge regarding the characteristics of cellulitis is required to answer the question. If you

had difficulty with this question, take time now to review the characteristics of cellulitis and erysipelas!

Level of Cognitive Ability: Analysis
Phase of Nursing Process: Analysis
Client Needs: Physiological Integrity
Content Area: Adult Health/Integumentary

Reference
Black, J., & Matassarin-Jacobs, E. (1997). *Medical-surgical nursing: Clinical management for continuity of care* (5th ed.). Philadelphia: W. B. Saunders, p. 2222.

21. **1**

Rationale: Warm compresses may be used to decrease the discomfort, erythema, and edema. After tissue and blood culture results are obtained, antibiotics will be initiated. The nurse should provide supportive care as prescribed to manage symptoms such as fatigue, fever, chills, headache, and myalgia.

Test-Taking Strategy: Use the process of elimination, noting that option 1, the correct option, is different from the other options. Heat lamps can cause more disruption to already inflamed tissue. Cold and hot are not the best measures. Option 1, the correct option, addresses "warm" compresses. If you had difficulty with this question, take time now to review the treatment associated with cellulitis!

Level of Cognitive Ability: Analysis
Phase of Nursing Process: Analysis
Client Needs: Physiological Integrity
Content Area: Adult Health/Integumentary

Reference
Luckmann, J. (1997). *Saunders manual of nursing care.* Philadelphia: W. B. Saunders, p. 1613.

22. **1**

Rationale: Psoriasis occurs equally among women and men, although the incidence is lower in darker-skinned races. The disorder may begin at any time throughout the life span but most commonly affects persons aged 10 to 40 years. Emotional distress, trauma, systemic illness, seasonal changes, and hormonal changes are linked to exacerbations.

Test-Taking Strategy: Use knowledge regarding what psoriasis is and the etiology associated with the disorder to answer the question. If you had difficulty with the question, take time now to review the causes of the disorder and the factors that affect exacerbations!

Level of Cognitive Ability: Analysis
Phase of Nursing Process: Assessment
Client Needs: Health Promotion and Maintenance
Content Area: Adult Health/Integumentary

References
Ignatavicius, D., Workman, M., & Mishler, M. (1995). *Medical-surgical nursing: A nursing process approach* (2nd ed.). Philadelphia: W. B. Saunders, p. 1957.
Luckmann, J. (1997). *Saunders manual of nursing care.* Philadelphia: W. B. Saunders, p. 1639.

23. **4**

Rationale: Psoriatic patches are covered with silvery white scales. Affected areas include the scalp, elbows, knees, shins, sacral area, and trunk. Thickening, pitting, and discoloration of the nails occur. Pruritus may occur. The lesions in psoriasis are not red-purplish, scaly lesions.

Test-Taking Strategy: Knowledge regarding the clinical manifestations associated with psoriasis is required to answer the question. From this knowledge, you should be able to identify that option 4 is not associated with this condition. If you had difficulty with this question, take time now to review the manifestations associated with psoriasis!

Level of Cognitive Ability: Analysis
Phase of Nursing Process: Assessment
Client Needs: Physiological Integrity
Content Area: Adult Health/Integumentary

Reference
Luckmann, J. (1997). *Saunders manual of nursing care.* Philadelphia: W. B. Saunders, p. 1639.

24. **3**

Rationale: Safety precautions are required during UVL therapy. Most UVL treatments require the person to stand in a light treatment chamber for up to 15 minutes. It is best to expose to the UVL only those areas requiring treatment. Protective wrap-around goggles prevent exposure of the eyes to UVL. The face should be shielded with a loosely applied pillow case if it is unaffected. Direct contact with the light bulbs of the treatment unit should be avoided to prevent burning of the skin.

Test-Taking Strategy: Note the key phrase "would not be a component of the plan." Note that option 3, the correct option in the question as stated, addresses a time frame of 30 minutes, which is an extensive time period for exposure to UVL. If you had difficulty with this question, take time now to review client education for UVL treatments!

Level of Cognitive Ability: Application
Phase of Nursing Process: Planning
Client Needs: Physiological Integrity
Content Area: Adult Health/Integumentary

Reference
Luckmann, J. (1997). *Saunders manual of nursing care.* Philadelphia: W. B. Saunders, p. 1640.

25. **3**

Rationale: With classic presentation of herpes zoster, the clinical examination is diagnostic. A viral culture of the lesion provides the definitive diagnosis. Herpes zoster is caused by a reactivation of the varicella-zoster virus, the cause of the virus for chickenpox. In a Wood light examination, the skin is viewed under ultraviolet light to identify superficial infections of the skin. A patch test is a skin test that involves the administration of an allergen to the skin's surface to identify specific allergies.

Test-Taking Strategy: Knowledge that herpes zoster is caused by a virus will assist in the process of elimination and in directing you toward the correct option. Eliminate options 2 and 4 first. From the remaining two options, remember that a biopsy will determine tissue type whereas a culture will identify an organism!

Level of Cognitive Ability: Analysis
Phase of Nursing Process: Assessment
Client Needs: Physiological Integrity
Content Area: Adult Health/Integumentary

Reference
Luckmann, J. (1997). *Saunders manual of nursing care.* Philadelphia: W. B. Saunders, p. 1635.

26. **4**

Rationale: The primary lesion of herpes zoster is a vesicle. The classic presentation is grouped vesicles on an erythematous base along a dermatome. Because they follow nerve pathways, the lesions do not cross the body's midline.

Test-Taking Strategy: Knowledge regarding the characteristics of herpes zoster lesions is required to answer the question. Remembering that these lesions occur as grouped vesicles along a nerve pathway will assist in answering the question. If you had difficulty with this question, take time now to review the characteristics of herpes zoster lesions!

Level of Cognitive Ability: Analysis
Phase of Nursing Process: Assessment
Client Needs: Physiological Integrity
Content Area: Adult Health/Integumentary

Reference
Black, J., & Matassarin-Jacobs, E. (1997). *Medical-surgical nursing: Clinical management for continuity of care* (5th ed.). Philadelphia: W. B. Saunders, p. 2223.

27. **2**

Rationale: Herpes zoster is caused by a reactivation of the varicella-zoster virus, the causative virus for chickenpox. Individuals who have not been exposed to the varicella-zoster virus are susceptible to chickenpox. Health care workers who are unsure of their immune status should have varicella titers done before exposure to a person with herpes zoster.

Test-Taking Strategy: Knowledge that herpes zoster is caused by a reactivation of the varicella-zoster virus, the causative virus for chickenpox, will assist in answering the question. Determining a relationship between herpes zoster and chickenpox will direct you toward the correct option!

Level of Cognitive Ability: Analysis
Phase of Nursing Process: Planning
Client Needs: Safe, Effective Care Environment
Content Area: Adult Health/Integumentary

Reference
Luckmann, J. (1997). *Saunders manual of nursing care.* Philadelphia: W. B. Saunders, p. 1636.

28. **1**

Rationale: Melanomas are pigmented, malignant lesions originating in the melanin-producing cells of the epidermis. This skin cancer is highly metastatic, and a person's survival depends on early diagnosis and treatment. Basal cell carcinomas arise in the basal cell layer of the epidermis. Early malignant basal cell lesions often go unnoticed, and although metastasis is rare, underlying tissue destruction can progress to include vital structures. Squamous cell carcinomas are malignant neoplasms of the epidermis. They are characterized by local invasion and the potential for metastasis.

Test-Taking Strategy: Knowledge regarding the various types of skin cancers is required to answer this question. Knowledge that melanomas are highly metastatic will assist in directing you to the correct option. If you had difficulty with this question, take time now to review the characteristics of skin cancers!

Level of Cognitive Ability: Analysis
Phase of Nursing Process: Analysis
Client Needs: Physiological Integrity
Content Area: Adult Health/Integumentary

Reference

Ignatavicius, D., Workman, M., & Mishler, M. (1995). *Medical-surgical nursing: A nursing process approach* (2nd ed.). Philadelphia: W. B. Saunders, p. 1961.

29. **4**

Rationale: A melanoma is an irregularly shaped, pigmented papule or plaque with a red-, white-, or blue-toned color. Basal cell carcinoma appears as a pearly papule with a central crater and rolled waxy border. Squamous cell carcinoma is a firm, nodular lesion topped with a crust or a central area of ulceration. Actinic keratosis, a premalignant lesion, appears as a small macule or papule with dry, rough, adherent yellow or brown scale.

Test-Taking Strategy: Knowledge regarding the characteristics of melanoma is required to answer this question. Remembering that irregularly shaped lesions are a cause for concern will assist you in answering the question. If you had difficulty with this question, take time now to review the characteristics of malignant skin lesions!

Level of Cognitive Ability: Analysis
Phase of Nursing Process: Assessment
Client Needs: Physiological Integrity
Content Area: Adult Health/Integumentary

Reference

Ignatavicius, D., Workman, M., & Mishler, M. (1995). *Medical-surgical nursing: A nursing process approach* (2nd ed.). Philadelphia: W. B. Saunders, p. 1962.

30. **1**

Rationale: Cryosurgery involves the local application of liquid nitrogen to isolated lesions and causes cell death and tissue destruction. The nurse prepares the client for swelling and increased tenderness of the treated area when the skin thaws. Tissue freezing is followed in 1 to 2 days by hemorrhagic blister formation. The nurse instructs the client to clean the treatment site with hydrogen peroxide to prevent secondary infection. A topical antibiotic may also be prescribed. Application of a warm, damp washcloth intermittently to the site will provide relief from any discomfort. Alcohol-soaked dressings will cause irritation. It is not necessary to avoid showering.

Test-Taking Strategy: Use the process of elimination to answer the question. Eliminate option 4 first because there is no reason for the client to avoid showers. Eliminate option 3 (alcohol-soaked dressing) next. From the remaining two options, note that option 1 addresses the prevention of infection. This is the best option to select. If you had difficulty with this question, take time now to review client education following cryosurgery!

Level of Cognitive Ability: Application
Phase of Nursing Process: Implementation
Client Needs: Health Promotion and Maintenance
Content Area: Adult Health/Integumentary

Reference

Black, J., & Matassarin-Jacobs, E. (1997). *Medical-surgical nursing: clinical management for continuity of care* (5th ed.). Philadelphia: W. B. Saunders, p. 2225.

31. **4**

Rationale: The client should be instructed to avoid sun exposure between the hours of 11:00 A.M. and 3:00 P.M. Sunscreen, a hat, opaque clothing, and sunglasses should be worn for outdoor activities. The client should be instructed to examine the body monthly for the appearance of any possible cancerous or precancerous lesions.

Test-Taking Strategy: Read the question carefully. Note the key phrase "would not be a part of this teaching plan." This phrase will assist in directing you to the correct option. Take time to review client education in the prevention of skin cancer now, if you had difficulty with this question!

Level of Cognitive Ability: Application
Phase of Nursing Process: Implementation
Client Needs: Health Promotion and Maintenance
Content Area: Adult Health/Integumentary

Reference

Ignatavicius, D., Workman, M., & Mishler, M. (1995). *Medical-surgical nursing: A nursing process approach* (2nd ed.). Philadelphia: W. B. Saunders, p. 1963.

32. **2**

Rationale: Paronychia, or infection around the nail, is characterized by red, shiny skin, often associated with painful swelling. These infections frequently result from trauma, picking at the nail, or disorders such as dermatitis. Often these become secondarily infected with bacteria or fungus, which later involves the nail. Warm soaks three to four times a day may reduce pain and pressure; however, incision and drainage of the inflamed site is frequently required.

Test-Taking Strategy: Knowledge regarding the characteristics of paronychia is required to answer the question. If you knew that this disorder related to an infection of the nail, you would easily be directed toward the correct option. If you had difficulty with this question, take time now to review the definition of this disorder!

Level of Cognitive Ability: Analysis
Phase of Nursing Process: Assessment
Client Needs: Physiological Integrity
Content Area: Adult Health/Integumentary

Reference

Black, J., & Matassarin-Jacobs, E. (1997). *Medical-surgical nursing: Clinical management for continuity of care* (5th ed.). Philadelphia: W. B. Saunders, p. 2223.

33. **3**

Rationale: The nurse would not tell a client that it is not necessary to separate laundry from that of other household members. Thorough handwashing, separating laundry, and separate washing of the client's dishes are required because the infection is contagious as long as skin lesions are present. Antibiotics are administered and should be continued as prescribed.

Test-Taking Strategy: Knowledge regarding the transmission of impetigo is required to answer the question. Note the key phrase "would not be included" in the stem of the question. This should assist in directing you to the correct option. If you had difficulty with this question, take time now to review client teaching related to home care and the prevention of transmission!

Level of Cognitive Ability: Application
Phase of Nursing Process: Implementation
Client Needs: Health Promotion and Maintenance
Content Area: Adult Health/Integumentary

Reference

Black, J., & Matassarin-Jacobs, E. (1997). *Medical-surgical nursing: Clinical management for continuity of care* (5th ed.). Philadelphia: W. B. Saunders, p. 2221.

34. 4

Rationale: Assessment findings in frostbite include a white or blue color, and the skin will be hard, cold, and insensitive to touch. As thawing occurs, flushing of the skin, the development of blisters or blebs, or tissue edema appears. Gangrene may develop within 9 to 15 days.

Test-Taking Strategy: Knowledge regarding the characteristics of frostbite is required to answer the question. The key to the correct answer is in option 4, the correct option. The phrase "insensitive to touch" should assist in directing you toward this option. If you had difficulty with this question, take time now to review the characteristics associated with frostbite!

Level of Cognitive Ability: Analysis
Phase of Nursing Process: Assessment
Client Needs: Physiological Integrity
Content Area: Adult Health/Integumentary

References

Ignatavicius, D., Workman, M., & Mishler, M. (1995). *Medical-surgical nursing: A nursing process approach* (2nd ed.). Philadelphia: W. B. Saunders, p. 1967.
Luckmann, J. (1997). *Saunders manual of nursing care.* Philadelphia: W. B. Saunders, p. 1736.

35. 1

Rationale: Acute frostbite is ideally treated with rapid and continuous rewarming of the tissue in a warm water bath for 15 to 20 minutes or until flushing of the skin occurs. Slow thawing or interrupted periods of warmth are avoided, because this can contribute to increased cellular damage. Thawing can cause considerable pain, and the nurse administers analgesics as prescribed.

Test-Taking Strategy: Use the process of elimination to answer the question. Eliminate options 2 and 4 first. Avoid options that address "hot" or "cold." Eliminate option 3 because intervention would begin immediately. If you had difficulty with this question, take time now to review the interventions associated with frostbite!

Level of Cognitive Ability: Application
Phase of Nursing Process: Implementation
Client Needs: Physiological Integrity
Content Area: Adult Health/Integumentary

Reference

Luckmann, J. (1997). *Saunders manual of nursing care.* Philadelphia: W. B. Saunders, p. 1736.

36. 2

Rationale: In a stage II pressure ulcer, the skin is not intact. There is partial thickness skin loss of the epidermis or dermis. The ulcer is superficial and may be characterized as an abrasion, blister, or shallow crater. The skin is intact in stage I. A deep, crater-like appearance occurs in stage III, and sinus tracts develop in stage IV.

Test-Taking Strategy: Use the process of elimination, utilizing knowledge of the characteristics associated with each stage of pressure ulcers. If you had difficulty with this question, take time now to review the characteristics associated with each stage of pressure ulcers!

Level of Cognitive Ability: Analysis
Phase of Nursing Process: Assessment
Client Needs: Physiological Integrity
Content Area: Adult Health/Integumentary

Reference

Ignatavicius, D., Workman, M., & Mishler, M. (1995). *Medical-surgical nursing: A nursing process approach* (2nd ed.). Philadelphia: W. B. Saunders, p. 1936

37. 4

Rationale: Bed or chair confinement, inability to move, loss of bowel or bladder control, poor nutrition, absent or inconsistent care giving, and a lowered mental awareness can all contribute to the development of skin breakdown. The least likely risk, as presented in the options, is the lowered mental awareness status. Options 1, 2, and 3 identify physiological conditions that are the risk priorities.

Test-Taking Strategy: Utilize Maslow's Hierarchy of Needs theory to answer the question. Remember that physiological needs are the priority. This will assist you in eliminating options 1, 2, and 3 and in selecting option 4 as the correct option to this question, as it is stated!

Level of Cognitive Ability: Analysis
Phase of Nursing Process: Assessment
Client Needs: Physiological Integrity
Content Area: Adult Health/Integumentary

Reference

Luckmann, J. (1997). *Saunders manual of nursing care.* Philadelphia: W. B. Saunders, p. 194.

38. 3

Rationale: Assessment of candidiasis (thrush) reveals white patches on the tongue, palate, and buccal mucosa. The lesions adhere firmly to the tissues and are difficult to remove. The lesions are often referred to as milk curds because of their appearance. Clients often describe the lesions as dry and hot.

Test-Taking Strategy: Remembering that candidiasis (thrush) presents as white patches will assist in answering the question. If you had difficulty with this question, take time now to review the characteristics associated with candidiasis (thrush)!

Level of Cognitive Ability: Analysis
Phase of Nursing Process: Assessment
Client Needs: Physiological Integrity
Content Area: Adult Health/Integumentary

Reference

Black, J., & Matassarin-Jacobs, E. (1997). *Medical surgical nursing: Clinical management for continuity of care* (5th ed.). Philadelphia: W. B. Saunders, p. 1725.

39. 1

Rationale: Clients cannot tolerate commercial mouthwashes because the high alcohol concentration in these products can cause pain and discomfort to the lesions. A solution of warm water, half strength peroxide, or mouthwash formulas without alcohol is better tolerated and may promote healing. A change in diet to liquid or pureed food often eases the discomfort of eating. The client should avoid spicy foods, citrus juices, and hot liquids.

Test-Taking Strategy: Note the key phrase "is not a component of the instructions." From this point, use knowledge regarding the characteristics of candidiasis (thrush) and the process of elimination to answer the question. Take time now to review the teaching points of client education related to candidiasis (thrush) if you had difficulty with this question!

Level of Cognitive Ability: Application
Phase of Nursing Process: Planning
Client Needs: Health Promotion and Maintenance
Content Area: Adult Health/Integumentary

Reference

Black, J., & Matassarin-Jacobs, E. (1997). *Medical-surgical nursing: Clinical management for continuity of care* (5th ed.). Philadelphia: W. B. Saunders, p. 1726.

40. **4**

Rationale: A hallmark sign of pemphigus is Nikolsky's sign. Nikolsky's sign is when the epidermis can be rubbed off by slight friction or injury. Other characteristics include flaccid bullae that rupture easily and emit a foul-smelling drainage, leaving crusted, denuded skin. The lesions are common on the face, back, chest, groin, and umbilicus. Even slight pressure on an intact blister may cause spread to adjacent skin. Trousseau's sign is a sign for tetany, in which carpal spasm can be elicited by compressing the upper arm and causing ischemia to the nerves distally. Chvostek's sign, seen in tetany, is a spasm of the facial muscles elicited by tapping the facial nerve in the region of the parotid gland. Homan's sign, a sign of thrombosis in the leg, is discomfort behind the knee on forced dorsiflexion of the foot.

Test-Taking Strategy: Knowledge regarding the various definitions of the signs identified in the options will assist you in answering the question. If you knew that Homan's sign was related to thrombophlebitis and that Chvostek's sign and Trousseau's sign were related to tetany, then by the process of elimination, you would select option 4. If you had difficulty with this question, take time now to review these various signs!

Level of Cognitive Ability: Analysis
Phase of Nursing Process: Assessment
Client Needs: Physiological Integrity
Content Area: Adult Health/Integumentary

References

Black, J., & Matassarin-Jacobs, E. (1997). *Medical-surgical nursing: Clinical management for continuity of care* (5th ed.). Philadelphia: W. B. Saunders, p. 2220.
O'Toole, M. (ed.) (1997). *Miller-Keane Encyclopedia & dictionary of medicine, nursing, & allied health* (6th ed.). Philadelphia: W. B. Saunders, pp. 328, 751, 1658.

41. **3**

Rationale: The exact cause of acne is unknown. There is no scientific evidence that consumption of foods such as chocolate, nuts, or fatty foods affects acne. Exacerbation of acne that coincides with the menstrual cycle results from hormonal activity. Heat, humidity, and excessive perspiration also play a role in increased acne.

Test-Taking Strategy: Read the stem carefully and note that it asks for the "cause." Use the process of elimination and knowledge regarding the cause and factors that exacerbate acne. Options 1, 2, and 4 relate specifically to factors that exacerbate acne. Take time now to review the cause of and factors that exacerbate acne, if you had difficulty with this question!

Level of Cognitive Ability: Analysis
Phase of Nursing Process: Implementation
Client Needs: Physiological Integrity
Content Area: Adult Health/Integumentary

Reference

Black, J., & Matassarin-Jacobs, E. (1997). *Medical-surgical nursing: Clinical management for continuity of care* (5th ed.). Philadelphia: W. B. Saunders, p. 2212.

42. **1**

Rationale: In severe cystic acne, isotretinoin (Accutane) is used to inhibit inflammation. Adverse effects include elevated triglycerides, skin dryness, eye discomfort such as dryness and burning, and cheilitis (lip inflammation). Close medical follow-up is required, and dry skin and cheilitis can be decreased by the use of emollients and lip balms. Vitamin A supplements are stopped during this treatment.

Test-Taking Strategy: Knowledge regarding the adverse effects related to this medication is required to answer this question. If you had difficulty with this question take time now to review the action, side effects, and adverse effects related to this medication!

Level of Cognitive Ability: Analysis
Phase of Nursing Process: Evaluation
Client Needs: Physiological Integrity
Content Area: Pharmacology

Reference

Black, J., & Matassarin-Jacobs, E. (1997). *Medical-surgical nursing: Clinical management for continuity of care* (5th ed.). Philadelphia: W. B. Saunders, p. 2212.

43. **3**

Rationale: Scabies can be identified by the multiple straight or wavy, threadlike lines noted beneath the skin. The skin lesions are caused by the female, which burrows beneath the skin and lays its eggs. The eggs hatch in a few days, and the baby mites find their way to the skin surface where they mate and complete the life cycle.

Test-Taking Strategy: Knowledge that the scabies mite burrows beneath the skin surface will assist in the process of elimination and provide direction toward selection of the correct option. If you had difficulty with this question, take time now to review the characteristics associated with scabies!

Level of Cognitive Ability: Analysis
Phase of Nursing Process: Assessment
Client Needs: Physiological Integrity
Content Area: Adult Health/Integumentary

Reference

Black, J., & Matassarin-Jacobs, E. (1997). *Medical-surgical nursing: Clinical management for continuity of care* (5th ed.). Philadelphia: W. B. Saunders, p. 2221.

44. **3**

Rationale: The Centers for Disease Control and Prevention recommends the wearing of gowns and gloves for close contact with a person infested with scabies. Masks are not necessary. Transmission via clothing and other inanimate objects is uncommon. Scabies is usually transmitted from person to person by direct skin contact. All contacts that the client has had should be treated at the same time.

Test-Taking Strategy: Consider the mode of transmission of scabies and use the process of elimination in answering the question. Since scabies is transmitted by direct skin contact, eliminate options 1, 2, and 4. If you had difficulty with the question, take time now to review standard precautions and the transmission mode of scabies!

Level of Cognitive Ability: Application
Phase of Nursing Process: Implementation
Client Needs: Safe, Effective Care Environment
Content Area: Adult Health/Integumentary

Reference
O'Toole, M. (ed.) (1997). *Miller-Keane encyclopedia & dictionary of medicine, nursing & allied health* (6th ed.). Philadelphia: W. B. Saunders, p. 1444.

45. **2**

Rationale: According to the Rule of Nines, with the initial burn, the anterior half of the head equals 4.5%, the upper half of the anterior torso equals 9%, and the lower half of both arms equals 9%. The subsequent burn included the posterior half of the head, equaling 4.5%, and the upper half of the posterior torso, equaling 9%. This totals 36%.

Test-Taking Strategy: Knowledge regarding the Rule of Nines is required to answer this question. The entire head equals 9%, each entire arm equals 9% (both arms 18%), the anterior or posterior torso each equals 18% (36% for entire torso), each entire leg equals 18% (both legs equal 36%), and the perineum equals 1%. Remember: 9 (head), 18 (arms), 36 (thorax), 36 (legs), equaling 99. If you had difficulty with this question, take time now to review the Rule of Nines!

Level of Cognitive Ability: Analysis
Phase of Nursing Process: Assessment
Client Needs: Physiological Integrity
Content Area: Adult Health/Integumentary

Reference
Black, J., & Matassarin-Jacobs, E. (1997). *Medical-surgical nursing: Clinical management for continuity of care* (5th ed.). Philadelphia: W. B. Saunders, p. 2239.

46. **3**

Rationale: The Parkland (Baxter) formula for estimating fluid requirements is 4 mL × kg × %TBSA. Half of this total is administered in the first 8 hours following the burn. Therefore, 4 × 90 × 83/2 = 14,940 mL.

Test-Taking Strategy: Knowledge regarding the Parkland (Baxter) formula is required to answer the question. Take the time now to become familiar with this formula, if you had difficulty with this question!

Level of Cognitive Ability: Analysis
Phase of Nursing Process: Analysis
Client Needs: Physiological Integrity
Content Area: Adult Health/Integumentary

Reference
Ignatavicius, D., Workman, M., & Mishler, M. (1995). *Medical-surgical nursing: A nursing process approach* (2nd ed.). Philadelphia: W. B. Saunders, p. 1989.

47. **2**

Rationale: Partial thickness burn injuries are classified as first-degree burns and second-degree burns. Minor burns are considered to be burns of less than 15% TBSA in adults under 40 years of age, burns of less than 10% in children under 10 years of age, or burns less than 10% in adults older than 40 years. In minor burns, no risk of cosmetic injury, functional impairment, or disability exists.

Test-Taking Strategy: Knowledge regarding the criteria for classifying a burn is required to answer the question. Remembering that a client is considered to have a major burn if it involves special care areas, or significant concurrent injuries, may assist you in answering these kinds of questions. If you had difficulty with this question, take time now to review the classification system!

Level of Cognitive Ability: Analysis
Phase of Nursing Process: Assessment
Client Needs: Physiological Integrity
Content Area: Adult Health/Integumentary

Reference
Luckmann, J. (1997). *Saunders manual of nursing care*. Philadelphia: W. B. Saunders, p. 1669.

48. **3**

Rationale: In partial thickness burns, the wound should re-epithelialize spontaneously from intact basal cells interspersed throughout the wound. Basal cell lining structures, such as hair follicles and sweat glands, which extend deep into the dermal-epidermal junction, are the primary sources for epithelialization, leading to the punctate appearance of the wound. Option 1 is incorrect because blisters are usually removed during early wound debridement. Option 2 is incorrect because granulation tissue forms in wounds that are not able to re-epithelialize spontaneously. The tissue forms owing to budding of capillaries in the wound. The presence of granulation tissue, however, is a positive sign in wounds that are not expected to re-epithelialize spontaneously. Option 4 is incorrect because partial thickness wounds are not generally grafted unless the wound depth increases because of factors such as poor perfusion, infection, and inadequate nutrition.

Test-Taking Strategy: Knowledge regarding the process of wound healing following a burn injury is required to answer the question. Remembering that partial thickness wounds should heal spontaneously in the absence of complicating factors may assist in answering questions similar to this one. If you had difficulty with the question, take time now to review the process of wound healing!

Level of Cognitive Ability: Analysis
Phase of Nursing Process: Evaluation
Client Needs: Physiological Integrity
Content Area: Adult Health/Integumentary

Reference
Black, J., & Matassarin-Jacobs, E. (1997). *Medical-surgical nursing: Clinical management for continuity of care* (5th ed.). Philadelphia: W. B. Saunders, p. 2257.

49. **4**

Rationale: Pediatric populations are at very high risk of airway occlusion due to laryngeal edema. The child exhibited several warning signs of an inhalation injury, namely, a history of flame burn to the face, hoarseness, cough, carbonaceous sputum, singed facial hair, facial edema, and then color change. Additionally, one of the cardinal signs of hypoxia is restlessness and anxiety.

Test-Taking Strategy: Utilize the A, B, Cs to answer the question. The only option that addresses airway is option 4. If you had difficulty with this question, take time now to review the clinical manifestations associated with burns to the face!

Level of Cognitive Ability: Analysis
Phase of Nursing Process: Assessment
Client Needs: Physiological Integrity
Content Area: Child Health

Reference
Ashwill, J., & Droske, S. (1997). *Nursing care of children: Principles and practice*. Philadelphia: W. B. Saunders, pp. 1070–1071.

50. 4

Rationale: Escharotomies are performed to alleviate the compartment syndrome that can occur when edema forms under nondistensible eschar in a circumferential third-degree burn. Escharotomies are performed through avascular eschar to subcutaneous fat. Although bleeding may occur from the site, it is considered a complication rather than an anticipated therapeutic outcome. Usually, direct pressure with a bulky dressing and elevation will control the bleeding, but occasionally an artery is damaged that may require ligation. Formation of granulation tissue is not the intent of an escharotomy. Escharotomy will not affect the formation of edema.

Test-Taking Strategy: Utilize the A, B, Cs to answer the question. The only option that addresses circulation is option 4. If you had difficulty with this question, take time now to review the purpose of an escharotomy!

Level of Cognitive Ability: Analysis
Phase of Nursing Process: Evaluation
Client Needs: Physiological Integrity
Content Area: Adult Health/Integumentary

Reference

Black, J., & Matassarin-Jacobs, E. (1997). *Medical-surgical nursing: Clinical management for continuity of care* (5th ed.). Philadelphia: W. B. Saunders, p. 2250.

51. 2

Rationale: Alkalis, such as lye, cause a liquefaction necrosis, and exposure to fat forms a soapy coagulum. Thick, leathery eschar forms with exposure to acids or heat. Cherry-red, firm tissue can occur as a result of thermal injury. Intact blisters indicate a partial thickness thermal injury, and erythema could result from cellulitis.

Test-Taking Strategy: Remembering that acid burns form a leathery eschar as a result of coagulation necrosis and that alkali burns form a soapy coagulum will assist in answering the question. If you had difficulty with this question, take time now to review assessment findings in chemical burns!

Level of Cognitive Ability: Analysis
Phase of Nursing Process: Assessment
Client Needs: Physiological Integrity
Content Area: Adult Health/Integumentary

Reference

Black, J., & Matassarin-Jacobs, E. (1997). *Medical-surgical nursing: Clinical management for continuity of care* (5th ed.). Philadelphia: W. B. Saunders, p. 2241.

52. 1

Rationale: Cutaneous injury from radiation can manifest with erythema (probably due to capillary damage), hyperpigmentation (from stimulation of melanocytes), dry desquamation (due to basal cell destruction), and/or moist desquamation (also due to basal cell destruction). Moist desquamation is comparable to a second-degree burn in histology, appearance, and sensation.

Test-Taking Strategy: Knowledge regarding the physiological manifestations that occur with radiation burns is helpful to answer this question. Option 1 addresses a superficial injury. The word "superficial" is the key to the correct option. If you had difficulty with this question, take time now to review the effects of radiation burns!

Level of Cognitive Ability: Analysis
Phase of Nursing Process: Assessment
Client Needs: Physiological Integrity
Content Area: Adult Health/Integumentary

Reference

Black, J., & Matassarin-Jacobs, E. (1997). *Medical-surgical nursing: Clinical management for continuity of care* (5th ed.). Philadelphia: W. B. Saunders, p. 2234.

53. 3

Rationale: During the emergent phase, the hematocrit increases to above normal because of hemoconcentration from the large fluid shifts. Hematocrit levels of 50% to 55% are expected during the first 24 hours after injury, with return to normal by 36 hours after injury. Initially, blood is shunted away from the kidneys, and renal perfusion and glomerular filtration are decreased, resulting in low urine output. Pulse rates are typically higher than normal; the blood pressure is normal or slightly elevated unless hypovolemia is severe. The emergent phase begins at the time of injury and ends with the restoration of capillary permeability, usually at 48 to 72 hours following the injury.

Test-Taking Strategy: Knowledge regarding the pathophysiology related to burn injuries during the emergent phase is required to answer the question. Use the process of elimination by thinking about how the body would react in such a traumatizing event. Eliminate options 1 and 4 first. Knowledge that the blood pressure would drop only in severe hypovolemia will assist in directing you to the correct option. Take time now to review pathophysiology related to burn injuries if you had difficulty with this question!

Level of Cognitive Ability: Analysis
Phase of Nursing Process: Assessment
Client Needs: Physiological Integrity
Content Area: Adult Health/Integumentary

Reference

Luckmann, J. (1997). *Saunders manual of nursing care.* Philadelphia: W. B. Saunders, pp. 1669–1672.

54. 1

Rationale: Carbon monoxide levels between 5% and 10% result in impaired visual acuity; levels of 11% to 20% result in flushing and headache; levels of 21% to 30% result in nausea and impaired dexterity. Levels of 31% to 40% result in vomiting, dizziness, and syncope, levels of 41% to 50% result in tachypnea and tachycardia, and levels greater than 50% result in coma and death.

Test-Taking Strategy: Knowledge regarding the clinical manifestations of carbon monoxide poisoning is required to answer this question. If you had difficulty with this question, take time now to review these clinical manifestations!

Level of Cognitive Ability: Analysis
Phase of Nursing Process: Assessment
Client Needs: Physiological Integrity
Content Area: Adult Health/Integumentary

Reference

Black, J., & Matassarin-Jacobs, E. (1997). *Medical-surgical nursing: Clinical management for continuity of care* (5th ed.). Philadelphia: W. B. Saunders, p. 2237.

55. 3

Rationale: If inhalation injury is suspected, administration of 100% oxygen via a tight-fitting non-rebreather mask is prescribed until carboxyhemoglobin levels fall below 15%. In inhalation injuries, the oropharynx is inspected for evidence of erythema, blisters, or ulcerations. The need for endotracheal intubation is also assessed.

Test-Taking Strategy: Knowledge that 100% oxygen is required following an inhalation injury will assist in eliminating options 2 and 4. With a tight-fitting mask, a nonrebreather is preferred so that the client will not rebreathe exhaled air. If you had difficulty with this question, take time now to review care to the client following an inhalation injury!

Level of Cognitive Ability: Analysis
Phase of Nursing Process: Analysis
Client Needs: Physiological Integrity
Content Area: Adult Health/Integumentary

Reference

Black, J., & Matassarin-Jacobs, E. (1997). *Medical-surgical nursing: Clinical management for continuity of care* (5th ed.). Philadelphia: W. B. Saunders, p. 2242.

56. 2

Rationale: Successful or adequate fluid resuscitation in the adult is signaled by stable vital signs, adequate urine output, palpable peripheral pulses, and clear sensorium. The most reliable indicator for determining adequacy of fluid resuscitation is the urine output. For an adult, the hourly urine volume should be 30 to 50 mL.

Test-Taking Strategy: Note the key phrase in the stem of the question, "most reliable." The question is addressing fluid resuscitation. Select the option that is similar to the issue of the question. Urinary output is most similar to the issue of administering fluids.

Level of Cognitive Ability: Analysis
Phase of Nursing Process: Evaluation
Client Needs: Physiological Integrity
Content Area: Adult Health/Integumentary

Reference

Black, J., & Matassarin-Jacobs, E. (1997). *Medical-surgical nursing: Clinical management for continuity of care* (5th ed.). Philadelphia: W. B. Saunders, p. 2249.

57. 3

Rationale: Circumferential burns of the extremities may compromise circulation. Elevating injured extremities above the level of the heart and active exercise help reduce dependent edema formation.

Test-Taking Strategy: Use the process of elimination, remembering that when an injury occurs, such as a burn, edema occurs. The correct option, option 3, is the only option that addresses a position that will reduce edema. If you had difficulty with this question, take time now to review care to the client experiencing this type of burn injury!

Level of Cognitive Ability: Application
Phase of Nursing Process: Implementation
Client Needs: Physiological Integrity
Content Area: Adult Health/Integumentary

Reference

Black, J., & Matassarin-Jacobs, E. (1997). *Medical-surgical nursing: Clinical management for continuity of care* (5th ed.). Philadelphia: W. B. Saunders, p. 2250.

58. 3

Rationale: Thorough handwashing should be done before and after each contact with the burn-injured client. Sterile sheets and linens are used. Protective garb, including gloves, cap, mask, shoe covers, scrub clothes, and plastic aprons, needs to be worn when caring for the client.

Test-Taking Strategy: Use the process of elimination, noting the key word "not" in the stem of the question. Option 2 can easily be eliminated. Select option 3 because this is the least thorough technique to prevent infection. If you had difficulty with this question, take time now to review protective isolation techniques when caring for a burn client!

Level of Cognitive Ability: Application
Phase of Nursing Process: Implementation
Client Needs: Safe, Effective Care Environment
Content Area: Adult Health/Integumentary

Reference

Black, J., & Matassarin-Jacobs, E. (1997). *Medical-surgical nursing: Clinical management for continuity of care* (5th ed.). Philadelphia: W. B. Saunders, p. 2252.

59. 1

Rationale: Autografts placed over joints or on the lower extremities are often elevated and immobilized following surgery for 3 to 7 days. This period of immobilization allows the autograft time to adhere and attach to the wound bed.

Test-Taking Strategy: Eliminate options 2 and 3 first because they are similar. Read the question carefully, noting that the autograft was placed over a joint. This should direct you toward the correct option of selecting the longer period of immobilization for this type of graft. If you had difficulty with this question, take time now to review care to an autograft placed over a joint!

Level of Cognitive Ability: Analysis
Phase of Nursing Process: Analysis
Client Needs: Physiological Integrity
Content Area: Adult Health/Integumentary

Reference

Black, J., & Matassarin-Jacobs, E. (1997). *Medical-surgical nursing: Clinical management for continuity of care* (5th ed.). Philadelphia: W. B. Saunders, p. 2255.

60. 4

Rationale: Newly healed skin is more sensitive to the cold, and the client should be instructed to wear warm clothing. The client should wash using a mild soap, rinsing thoroughly, and patting the skin dry using a clean towel. Newly healed skin sunburns easily, and direct sunlight needs to be avoided. Products that contain perfume, alcohol, or lanolin should be avoided because they tend to irritate newly healed skin.

Test-Taking Strategy: Read each option carefully, noting that the correct option utilizes the absolute term "never." Absolute terms need to be avoided. If you had difficulty with this question, take time now to review home care instructions regarding skin care!

Level of Cognitive Ability: Application
Phase of Nursing Process: Planning
Client Needs: Physiological Integrity
Content Area: Adult Health/Integumentary

Reference

Black, J., & Matassarin-Jacobs, E. (1997). *Medical-surgical nursing: Clinical management for continuity of care* (5th ed.). Philadelphia: W. B. Saunders, p. 2263.

BIBLIOGRAPHY

Ashwill, J., & Droske, S. (1997). *Nursing care of children: Principles and practice.* Philadelphia: W. B. Saunders.

Black, J., & Matassarin-Jacobs, E. (1997). *Medical-surgical nursing: Clinical management for continuity of care* (5th ed.). Philadelphia: W. B. Saunders.

Fischbach, F. (1996). *A manual of laboratory & diagnostic tests* (5th ed.). Philadelphia: Lippincott-Raven.

Hodgson, B., & Kizin, R. (1999). *Saunders nursing drug handbook 1999.* Philadelphia: W. B. Saunders.

Ignatavicius, D., Workman, M., & Mishler, M. (1995). *Medical-surgical nursing: A nursing process approach* (2nd ed.). Philadelphia: W. B. Saunders.

Lehne, R. (1998). Pharmacology for nursing care (3rd ed.). Philadelphia: W. B. Saunders.

Luckmann, J. (1997). *Saunders manual of nursing care.* Philadelphia: W. B. Saunders.

O'Toole, M. (ed.) (1997). *Miller-Keane encyclopedia & dictionary of medicine, nursing & allied health* (6th ed.). Philadelphia: W. B. Saunders.

Richard, R., & Staley, M. (1994). *Burn care and rehabilitation: Principles and practice.* Philadelphia: F. A. Davis.

CHAPTER 48

Integumentary Medications

I. Emollients and Lotions

A. Emollients (Box 48–1)
   1. Oily or fatty substances that soften and soothe irritated skin by allowing the skin to retain water
   2. Available as creams or ointments
   3. Used for dry, scaly, itchy inflammatory conditions
B. Lotions (Box 48–2)
   1. Liquid suspensions or dispersions
   2. Require shaking before application
   3. Although lotions are predominantly water, they have a drying effect on the skin when the water evaporates
   4. Used as a wash for the skin, as soaks, or as wet dressings on ulcers or **burns**
   5. Used for subacute inflammatory lesions after the severe exudative phase has ceased
   6. Medicated lotions are often used as anti-inflammatory agents because they provide a drying, protective, and cooling effect

II. Rubs and Liniments (Box 48–3)

A. Used for the temporary relief of muscular aches, rheumatism, arthritis, sprains, and neuralgia
B. Over-the-counter (OTC) products contain combinations of antiseptics, local anesthetics, analgesics, and counterirritants
C. Some products contain salicylates and, if used over a large area of the skin, may cause salicylate side effects such as tinnitus, nausea, or vomiting

D. A heating pad is not used with these products as irritation or burning of the skin may occur

III. Anti-Infective Agents

A. Description
   1. Includes antiseptics and antibacterial, antifungal, antiviral, and antiparasitic medications
   2. Topical antibiotics are safe and effective in certain conditions; extensive use may encourage the emergence of resistant bacteria
B. Antiseptics
   1. Sodium hypochlorite (Dakin solution)
      a. A chloride solution that loosens, dissolves, and deodorizes necrotic tissue and blood clots
      b. It kills most common bacteria, including spores, amebas, fungi, protozoal viruses, and yeast
      c. It is used for irrigating and cleaning necrotic or purulent wounds
      d. Loses its potency during storage, so fresh solution is prepared frequently
      e. It should not be in contact with healing or normal tissue
   2. Chlorhexidine gluconate (Hibiclens)
      a. Effective for cleaning wounds caused by staphylococci and other gram-positive bacteria
      b. Used for irrigating and cleansing wounds, but not for packing wounds because it may cause contact dermatitis

---

BOX 48–1. Emollients

Glycerin	Cold cream
Petrolatum	Zinc ointment
Lanolin	

BOX 48–2. Lotions

Calamine lotion (Caladryl lotion)
Aluminum acetate solution (Burrow's solution)
Potassium permanganate solution
Zinc stearate

BOX 48–3. Rubs and Liniments

Aspercreme   Ben-Gay
Myoflex   Deep-Down Rub
Hot cream/balm/stick

3. Acetic acid
   a. Effective for irrigating, cleansing, and packing wounds infected by *Pseudomonas aeruginosa*
   b. Healthy skin surrounding the wound must be protected with a petroleum barrier because it excoriates the skin
4. Hydrogen peroxide
   a. As a 3% solution, has effervescent action that releases gas and breaks up necrotic tissue
   b. It is used to irrigate and clean necrotic tissue and pus from open wounds
   c. It is not used to pack wounds because it decomposes too rapidly
   d. When epithelial tissue begins to form, hydrogen peroxide is discontinued because it inhibits tissue formation
5. Hexachlorophene (pHisoHex, Septisol)
   a. A combination of hexachlorophene and alcohol
   b. Hexachlorophene is a bacterial static agent with activity against staphylococci and other gram-positive bacteria
   c. Hexachlorophene is heavily absorbed through broken skin and can cause neurotoxicity; it should not be used on wounds
   d. Alcohol dries and irritates tissue, is not a very effective germicide, and forms a film that can actually promote infection
   e. All hexachlorophene products are well rinsed from the skin after their use to prevent systemic absorption
C. Antibacterials (Box 48–4)
   1. Description
      a. Not effective for acute, superficial, or relatively localized infections
      b. Applied one to five times daily to the infected area and covered if needed
   2. Mupirocin (Bactroban)
      a. Topical antibacterial active against impetigo cause by staphylococcus or streptococcus species
      b. Applied three times daily

BOX 48–4. Antibacterials

Bacitracin   Mycitracin Triple Antibiotic
Neomycin   Triple Antibiotic
Polymyxin B   Neo-Polycin ointment
Mity-Mycin

BOX 48–5. Antipruritics

Corn starch or oatmeal baths
Calamine or phenol
Solutions of potassium permanganate, aluminum subacetate, boric acid, or normal saline

   c. If improvement is not observed within 3 to 5 days, it is discontinued
D. Antifungals
   1. May cause erythema, stinging, blistering, peeling, pruritus, urticaria, and general skin irritation
   2. Client is re-evaluated if no results are obtained after 4 weeks of treatment
E. Antivirals
   1. Acyclovir (Zovirax) inhibits DNA replication in the virus
   2. Used for herpes simplex types 1 and 2, varicella-zoster, Epstein-Barr virus, and cytomegalovirus
   3. Can cause mild pain and transient burning and stinging
   4. Applied completely over the lesion every 3 hours six times daily for 1 week
   5. Rubber gloves are used to apply the ointment to prevent the spread of infection
F. Antiparasitics
   1. Used to treat scabies (mites) and pediculosis (lice)
   2. May be harmful during pregnancy and in young children
   3. May irritate the skin, eyes, and mucous membranes
   4. May cause allergic reactions

IV. Antipruritics (Box 48–5)

A. Used to allay itching
B. Applied as wet dressings, pastes, lotions, creams, or ointments
C. Persons with dry skin should be instructed to bathe less frequently

V. Keratolytics (Box 48–6)

A. Description
   1. Preparations that dissolve keratin
   2. Soften scales and loosen the horny layer of

BOX 48–6. Keratolytics

Salicylic acid (Wart-Off, Freezone, Compound W)
Resorcinol (Fostex Medicated Cleansing Bar, Meted-2, Sebulex)
Podophyllum resin (Pod-Ben-25)
Podofilox (Condylox)
Cantharidin (Cantharone)
Masoprocol (Actinex)

skin, resulting in minimal peeling or extensive desquamation

3. Used to treat superficial fungal infections, dermatitis, psoriasis, and localized dermatitis

B. Salicylic acid
1. Used to treat seborrheic dermatitis, acne, and psoriasis, and to thin and remove calluses
2. Can be absorbed systematically and can cause salicylism, characterized by dizziness and tinnitus; is not applied to large surface areas or open wounds

C. Podophyllum resin
1. Used for various types of **skin cancer**
2. Causes lesions to slough off, leaving a superficial ulcer and moderate dermatitis
3. After the therapy is discontinued, the lesions are dressed with a mild antiseptic ointment; healing usually occurs within a few days

D. Cantharidin (Cantharone)
1. Is used in treating warts
2. Has an exfoliation effect only on the epidermal cells
3. May cause tingling, itching, and burning
4. Site may be very tender for a period of 2 to 6 days

E. Masoprocol (Actinex)
1. Has antiproliferative activity against keratinocytes and is used to treat keratosis
2. Occlusive dressings are not to be used
3. Transient burning may be experienced after administration

VI. Stimulants and Irritants (Box 48–7)

A. Description: Produce a mild irritation to the surface of the skin, causing hyperemia and inflammation that promote the healing process

B. Coal tar
1. Used in treating psoriasis, seborrheic dermatitis, and atopic dermatitis
2. Has an unpleasant odor and frequently stains the skin and hair
3. Can cause phototoxicity

C. Compound benzoin tincture
1. Protects the skin when the client has bed sores, ulcers, cracked nipples, and fissures of any orifice
2. Causes a mild irritation that produces increased blood flow and healing

VII. Protectives (Box 48–8)

A. Description
1. Preparations that form a film on the skin to

BOX 48–7. **Stimulants and Irritants**
Coal tar
Compound benzoin tincture

BOX 48–8. **Protectives**	
Tegaderm	Uniflex
DuoDerm	Mediskin and Silver
PolySkin	Zinc oxide paste
Ensure-It (Deseret)	(Unna's boot)
Op-Site	Vigilon
Tegasorb	

protect it from irritations such as light, moisture, air, and dust

2. Promote natural healing without the usual formation of dry crust over the wound; hydrate the wound surface
3. Allow exudate to collect beneath the dressing, forming an artificial blister
4. Uniflex, PolySkin, and Ensure-It may be used to cover central and peripheral IV sites
5. Op-Site, Tegasorb, Mediskin and Silver and Vigilon may be used for skin **burns**

B. Sunscreens
1. Act by absorbing ultraviolet rays
2. The best sunscreens contain PABA (para-aminobenzoic acid)
3. Most effective when applied about 30 minutes to 1 hour before exposure to the sun; should be reapplied after swimming or sweating
4. Can cause contact dermatitis and photosensitivity reactions

VIII. Growth Factors

A. Description
1. Used to promote wound healing
2. Stimulate cells to divide and migrate, which results in wound healing, formation of granulation tissue, and new epidermis

B. Procuren solution
1. Promotes healing by actively stimulating growth and granulation tissue, capillaries, and epithelium
2. Applied to the wound and covered with petrolatum-impregnated gauze
3. The material is left in place for 12 hours and then washed off with tap water irrigation; during the remaining 12 hours of the day, the wound is covered with sulfadiazine (Silvadene)

IX. Enzymes

A. Description
1. Used to promote healing of wounds and to debride skin ulcers
2. Reduce inflammation resulting from trauma and infection
3. Dissolve fibrin clots, which helps reduce the size of surface hematomas
4. To be effective, must be in contact with affected tissue in adequate concentrations for a sufficient length of time

BOX 48–9. Enzymes that Promote Wound Healing

Papain (Panafil) (Panafil White)
Hyaluronidase (Wydase)

    5. Wound may need to be surgically debrided prior to application; if not administered to a clean, debrided wound, healing may be delayed
B. Enzymes that promote wound healing (Box 48–9)
    1. Papain (Panafil) (Panafil White)
      a. Does not injure or affect healthy tissue or cells
      b. Enzyme must be in immediate contact with the purulent wound material
      c. Wounds are cleansed with prescribed irrigating solution between doses
      d. Hydrogen peroxide cannot be used to irrigate the wound, because it inactivates the papain
      e. Light dressings and cellophane wrap may be used over the wound to prevent soiling of clothing
      f. Dressings are changed frequently to prevent contamination and to remove necrotic debris
    2. Hyaluronidase (Wydase)
      a. Facilitates the absorption of fluids given by subcutaneous hypodermoclysis
      b. Can be injected SC into an infiltrated IV site when a potent vasoconstrictor such as norepinephrine (Levophed) or metaraminol (Aramine) has infiltrated
      c. It reduces the sloughing of tissue likely to occur secondarily to infiltration
C. Enzymes to remove exudates (Box 48–10)
    1. Description
      a. They alter the thick, purulent drainage to a thin, liquid material that can be easily wiped or irrigated off the wound
      b. Enzyme contact with the wound is necessary to promote wound healing
      c. Wound needs to be cleansed, and cross-hatching of eschar on **burns** is performed prior to application
    2. Sutilains (Travase)
      a. Used to remove nonviable or necrotic tissue and purulent enzymes from second- or **third-degree burns,** ulcers, traumatic injury, and peripheral vascular disease wounds

BOX 48–10. Enzymes to Remove Exudates

Sutilains (Travase)
Collagenase (Santyl)
Fibrinolysin and desoxyribonuclease (Elase)

      b. Inactive on viable tissue
    3. Collagenase (Santyl)
      a. Used as a topical debriding agent
      b. Provides effective debridement of the collagen tissue at the wound edges where necrotic tissue is anchored
      c. Encourages the formation of granulation tissue at the wound edges and quicker epithelization of wounds
      d. Apply with tongue depressor directly into deep wounds
      e. Prior to application, cleanse wound of debris by gently rubbing with a gauze pad with sterile water or Dakin solution, followed by sterile saline
      f. Remove all excess ointment each time dressing is changed
      g. Apply only to injured area; causes erythema in healthy tissues
      h. Protect healthy tissue with zinc oxide paste
      i. Terminate use when necrotic tissue is gone
    4. Fibrinolysin and desoxyribonuclease (Elase)
      a. Used to debride wounds, including **burns, decubitus** ulcers, and inflamed or infected lesions
      b. Clean wound with sterile water, pat dry
      c. Flush away necrotic debris with saline
      d. Apply thin layer and cover with petrolatum gauze
D. Dextranomer (Debrisan)
    1. Not a debriding agent but is a cleansing agent that actually absorbs peptides and proteins
    2. Effective in wet wounds only
    3. Do pack Debrisan into wounds tightly, because maceration of surrounding tissue may occur

X. Corticosteroids

A. Have anti-inflammatory, antipruritic, and vasoconstrictive actions
B. Contraindications
    1. Clients demonstrating previous sensitivity to steroids
    2. Those with current systemic fungal, viral, or bacterial infections
    3. Those with current complications related to steroid therapy
C. Local adverse effects
    1. Hypopigmentation
    2. Acneform eruptions
    3. Contact dermatitis
    4. Burning, dryness, irritation, itching
    5. Overgrowth of bacteria, fungi, and viruses
    6. Skin atrophy
D. Systemic adverse effects
    1. Occur rarely
    2. Adrenal suppression
    3. Cushing's syndrome
    4. Striae, skin atrophy
    5. Ocular effects (glaucoma and cataracts)

E. Topical steroids
1. Monitor plasma cortisol levels if prolonged therapy is necessary
2. Apply products sparingly in a light film, rubbing gently
3. Wash area just prior to application to increase medication penetration
4. May apply to skin alone or with dry occlusive dressing
5. Monitor for toxic reactions, liver dysfunction, or worsening of condition
6. Instruct client to report burning, irritation, and infection to physician

XI. Acne Products (Box 48–11)

A. Description
1. Mild acne can be treated with bar soaps, soap-free cakes, liquid cleansers, lotions, gels, and creams
2. For moderate acne, topical anti-inflammatory medication such as benzoyl peroxide, tretinoin (Retin-A), isotretinoin (Accutane), azelaic acid (Azelex), and adapalene (Differin) may be prescribed; antibiotics may also be prescribed
3. Side effects can include excessive redness, extreme dryness of the skin leading to blistering and crusting, temporary pigmentation changes, and peeling of the skin
4. All products are kept away from the eyes, inside the nose, mucous membranes, and hair
B. Benzoyl peroxide: A keratolytic agent that is bacteriostatic and may decrease the production of irritant free fatty acids in the follicle
C. Tretinoin (Retin-A) and adapalene (Differin): Acids of vitamin A that are used to treat acne vulgaris, **skin cancer,** and aging of the skin
D. Tretinoin (Retin-A)
1. Decreases cohesiveness of the epithelial cells, increasing cell mitosis and turnover; potentially irritating, particularly when used correctly
2. Within 48 hours of use, the skin generally becomes red and begins to peel
3. Temporary hyperpigmentation and hypopigmentation can occur
4. Client should avoid sun exposure, as photosensitivity may occur

5. Apply liberally to the skin; the hands are washed thoroughly immediately after applying
6. Therapeutic results should be seen after 2 to 3 weeks but may not be optimal until after 6 weeks
7. Client may use cosmetics, but the skin needs to be cleaned thoroughly before applying
E. Isotretinoin (Accutane)
1. A metabolite of vitamin A
2. Used to treat severe cystic acne, and its use is reserved for persons who have not responded to other therapies, including systemic antibiotics
3. Can cause xerosis and facial desquamation, palmoplantar desquamation, pruritus, brittle nails, and hair loss
4. Is administered with meals two times daily for a 15- to 20-week course
5. If another course of therapy is needed, an 8-week lapse of time should occur
6. Photosensitivity may occur, so the client needs to be instructed to decrease sun exposure
7. Alcohol consumption should be eliminated during therapy, as alcohol may potentiate the serum triglyceride elevation
F. Local antibiotics
1. Used to treat acne; include clindamycin (Cleocin T), erythromycin, tetracycline (Topicycline), and meclocycline (Meclan)
2. Therapeutic response generally requires 6 to 12 weeks of therapy
3. Side effects include acute contact dermatitis, transient stinging or burning, staining of the skin, erythema, and skin tenderness

XII. Poison Ivy Treatment. See Box 48–12

XIII. Burn Products

A. Nitrofurazone (Furacin)
1. Applied topically to the **burn** as a solution, ointment, or cream
2. Has a broad spectrum of antibacterial activity
3. Used in **second- or third-degree burns** when bacterial resistance to other agents is a problem
4. Topical: Apply 1/16″ film directly to burn
5. Side effects: Contact dermatitis, rash
6. Less common side effects: Pruritius, local edema
B. Mafenide (Sulfamylon)
1. A water-soluble cream that is bacteriostatic for

BOX 48–11. Acne Products

CLEANSERS	DRYING AGENTS
Acnomel	Acnomel
Brasivol	Dry and Clear
Clearasil Medicated	Ionax
Astringent	Listerex
Fostex	
pHisoDerm	
Stri-Dex	

BOX 48–12. Poison Ivy Treatment Products

Calamine	Ivy-Rid
Calomox	Ivy-Chex
Rhuli cream/spray/gel	

both gram-negative and gram-positive organisms
2. Is used to treat **second- and third-degree** burns to reduce the bacteria present in avascular tissues
3. Diffuses through the devascularized areas of the skin; may precipitate metabolic acidosis, usually compensated by hyperventilation
4. Apply 1/16″ film
5. Side effects can include local pain, rash
6. Systemic effects include bone marrow depression, hemolytic anemia, hyperventilation
7. Keep burn covered with mafenide at all times
8. Notify physician if hyperventilation occurs; if acidosis develops, mafenide is washed off skin

C. Silver sulfadiazine (Flint SSD, Silvadene)
1. Has a broad spectrum of activity against gram-negative bacteria, gram-positive bacteria, and yeast
2. Released slowly from the cream, which is selectively toxic to bacteria
3. Used primarily to prevent sepsis in clients with **second- and third-degree burns**
4. Is not a carbonic anhydrase inhibitor and therefore does not cause acidosis
5. Rash and itching do occur from topical application
6. Apply 1/16″ film (keep burn covered at all times with silver sulfadiazine)
7. Side effects include rash, itching
8. Systemic effects include leukopenia, interstitial nephritis
9. Monitor complete blood count (CBC), particularly the white blood cells (WBC), frequently; if leukopenia develops, the medication is discontinued

D. Silver nitrate
1. An antiseptic solution active against gram-negative bacteria
2. Dressings are applied to the burn, which are then kept moist with silver nitrate, which stains anything brown or black that it comes in contact with; this discoloration is not usually permanent
3. Used on extensive **burns** that may precipitate fluid and electrolyte imbalances
4. Apply to dressing; do not apply to wounds, cuts, or broken skin

PRACTICE QUESTIONS

1. The female client tells the clinic nurse that her skin is very dry and irritated. Which of the following products would the nurse suggest that the client apply to the dry skin?
   1 A glycerin emollient
   2 Aspercreme
   3 Myoflex
   4 Acetic acid solution

2. The physician has prescribed Myoflex topical cream for a client with a diagnosis of rheumatism who is complaining of muscular aches. Which of the following instructions will the nurse provide to the client regarding this medication?
   1 Apply a heating pad to the area after applying the medication
   2 The medication acts by decreasing muscle spasms
   3 The medication is prescribed to cause the skin to peel
   4 The medication will act as a local anesthetic

3. An outbreak of pediculosis capitis has occurred at the local school. The school nurse is providing instructions to the mothers of the children attending the school regarding the application of permethrin (Nix, Elimite). Which of the following instructions will the nurse provide?
   1 Apply at bedtime and rinse off in the morning
   2 Apply prior to washing the hair
   3 Avoid saturating the hair and scalp when applying
   4 Allow to remain on hair 10 minutes and then rinse with water

4. A client is seen in the clinic for complaints of skin itchiness that has been persistent over the past several weeks. Following an assessment, it has been determined that the client has scabies. Lindane (Kwell) is prescribed, and the nurse provides instructions to the client regarding the use of the medication. Which of the following instructions will the nurse provide to the client?
   1 Leave cream on for 8 to 12 hours and then remove by washing
   2 Apply a thick layer of cream to the entire body
   3 Apply the cream as prescribed for 2 days in a row
   4 Apply to the entire body and scalp, excluding the face

5. Lindane (Kwell) is prescribed for the treatment of scabies. This medication therapy is contraindicated in which of the following clients?
   1 A 42-year-old woman
   2 An elderly client
   3 A 6-year-old child
   4 A 52-year-old man with hypertension

6. A topical glucocorticoid is prescribed for the client with dermatitis. The nurse provides instructions to the client regarding the use of the medication. Which of the following, if stated by the client, would indicate a need for further instruction?
   1 "I need to apply the medication in a thin film."
   2 "I should gently rub the medication into the skin."
   3 "I should place a bandage over the site after applying the medication."
   4 "The medication will help to relieve the inflammation and itching."

7. The nurse is applying a topical glucocorticoid to a client with eczema. The nurse would be concerned about the potential for systemic absorption of the medication if the medication was being applied to which of the following body areas?
   1 Back
   2 Axilla
   3 Palms
   4 Soles

8. The hospitalized client with severe seborrheic dermatitis is receiving treatments of topical glucocorticoid applications followed by the application of an occlusive dressing. Which systemic effect can occur as a result of this treatment?
   1 Adrenal suppression
   2 Adrenal hyperactivity
   3 Local infection
   4 Thinning of the skin

9. Salicylic acid is prescribed for a client with a diagnosis of psoriasis. Which of the following indicates the presence of a systemic toxicity from this medication?
   1 Decreased respirations
   2 Diarrhea
   3 Constipation
   4 Tinnitus

10. The client is diagnosed with herpes simplex type 1. The physician prescribes a topical medication for treatment. The nurse anticipates that which of the following medications will be prescribed?
    1 Triple antibiotic
    2 Acyclovir (Zovirax)
    3 Mupirocin (Bactroban)
    4 Masoprocol (Actinex)

11. The client with psoriasis is using coal tar as prescribed by the physician. Which of the following characteristics is not associated with this treatment?
    1 The medication has an unpleasant odor
    2 The medication can stain the skin and hair
    3 The medication can cause systemic effects
    4 The medication can cause phototoxicity

12. The camp nurse asks the children preparing to swim in the lake if they have applied sunscreen. Chemical sunscreens are most effective when applied:
    1 One hour before exposure to the sun
    2 Immediately before exposure to the sun
    3 15 minutes before exposure to the sun
    4 Immediately after swimming

13. DuoDerm is prescribed for a client with a leg ulcer. The home health nurse is preparing a plan of care for the client. Which of the following is most appropriate to include in the plan?
    1 Change DuoDerm daily
    2 Apply DuoDerm over a dry, sterile dressing

3 Change DuoDerm weekly
4 Apply DuoDerm over a normal saline–soaked dressing

14. The nurse is caring for a client with a burn injury to the lower legs. Nitrofurazone (Furacin) is prescribed to be applied to the sites of injury. Which of the following indicates the appropriate method to apply this medication?
    1 Apply saline-soaked dressings over the medication
    2 Apply 1″ film directly to the burn sites
    3 Apply 1/16″ film directly to the burn sites
    4 Apply 1/2″ film directly to the burn sites after cleansing the wounds

15. Mafenide (Sulfamylon) is prescribed for the client with a burn injury. When applying the medication, the client complains of local discomfort and burning. Which of the following is the most appropriate nursing action?
    1 Discontinue the medication
    2 Notify the physician
    3 Apply a thinner film than prescribed to the burn site
    4 Inform the client that this is normal

16. The burn client is receiving treatments of topical mafenide (Sulfamylon) to the site of injury. Which of the following indicates that a systemic effect has occurred?
    1 Local pain at the burn site
    2 Local rash at the burn site
    3 Hyperventilation
    4 Elevated blood pressure

17. A Vigilon burn dressing is prescribed for the client with a partial thickness burn to the arm. The home health nurse assigned to this client will plan home visits to change the dressing:
    1 Daily
    2 Every 2 days
    3 Weekly
    4 Twice weekly

18. Sodium hypochlorite (Dakin) solution is prescribed for a client with a leg wound containing purulent drainage. Which of the following is not be a component of the treatment plan with the use of this solution?
    1 Avoid contact with normal skin tissue
    2 Rinse off immediately following irrigation
    3 Soak sterile dressing with solution and pack into the wound
    4 Prepare solution prior to use

19. Tretinoin (Retin-A) is prescribed for a client with acne. The client calls the clinic nurse and tells the nurse that the skin has become very red and is beginning to peel. Which of the following nursing statements to the client is most appropriate?
    1 "Come to the clinic immediately."
    2 "Discontinue the medication."

3 "Notify the physician."
4 "This is a normal occurrence with the use of this medication."

20. The nurse provides instructions to a client regarding the use of tretinoin (Retin-A). Which of the following is not a component of the instructions regarding the use of this medication?
    1 Wash hands thoroughly after applying medication
    2 Optimal results will be seen after 6 weeks
    3 Apply a thin layer to the skin
    4 Cleanse the skin thoroughly before applying the medication

21. Isotretinoin (Accutane) is prescribed for a client to treat severe cystic acne. The length of the usual prescribed course of treatment is:
    1 1 month
    2 8 weeks
    3 15 to 20 weeks
    4 1 year

22. Isotretinoin (Accutane) is prescribed for a client with severe acne. Prior to the administration of this medication, the nurse would anticipate that which laboratory test will be prescribed?
    1 Complete blood count
    2 White blood cell count
    3 Triglyceride level
    4 Platelet count

23. A client with severe acne is seen in the clinic. The physician prescribes isotretinoin (Accutane). The nurse reviews the client's record. Which of the following medications if noted on the client's record would require physician notification?
    1 Digoxin (Lanoxin)
    2 Phenytoin (Dilantin)
    3 Vitamin A
    4 Furosemide (Lasix)

24. Fibrinolysin and desoxyribonuclease (Elase) dry powder are prescribed to treat a skin ulcer. Which of the following nursing interventions is not a component of the plan of care regarding this treatment?
    1 Clean wound with a sterile solution prior to applying Elase
    2 Prepare solution just prior to use
    3 Apply a thick layer of medication and cover with a dry, sterile dressing
    4 Apply a thin layer of medication and cover with a petrolatum gauze

25. The registered nurse is observing a newly hired nurse perform a dressing change on a client with a leg ulcer. Sutilains (Travase) is prescribed. Which of the following observations indicate an inaccurate procedure regarding this treatment?

1 The nurse cleans the wound with a sterile solution
2 The nurse covers the Travase application with a dry, sterile dressing
3 The nurse moistens the wound with sterile normal saline and then applies the Travase
4 The nurse places the Travase in the refrigerator following use

26. Dextranomer (Debrisan) is prescribed for a client with a decubitus ulcer. Which of the following is not accurate regarding this medication?
    1 It is effective in wet wounds only
    2 It should be packed lightly into the wound
    3 Maceration of tissue surrounding the wound can occur from the medication
    4 The wound bed must be thoroughly dried prior to applying the medication

27. Minoxidil solution (Rogaine) is prescribed for the client to treat hair loss. The usual dosage for this medication is:
    1 0.5 mL applied two times daily
    2 1 mL applied at bedtime
    3 1 mL applied two times a day
    4 1 mL applied four times a day

28. The clinic nurse is performing an admission assessment on a client. The nurse notes that the client is taking azelaic acid (Azelex). Because of the medication prescription, the nurse suspects that the client is being treated for:
    1 Herpes simplex
    2 Acne
    3 Eczema
    4 Hair loss

29. Collagenase (Santyl) is prescribed for a client with a severe burn of the hand. The home care nurse provides instructions to the client regarding the use of the medication. Which of the following indicates an accurate understanding of the use of this medication?
    1 "I will apply the ointment once a day and leave it open to the air."
    2 "I will apply the ointment once a day and cover it with a sterile dressing."
    3 "I will apply the ointment twice a day and leave it open to the air."
    4 "I will apply the ointment at bedtime and in the morning and cover it with a sterile dressing."

30. Minoxidil (Rogaine) is prescribed for the client to treat hair loss. The client asks the nurse if the hair will continue to grow when the medication is stopped. The most appropriate nursing response is:
    1 "The hair will continue to grow."
    2 "Newly gained hair is lost in 3 to 4 months."
    3 "It depends on how long you have been taking the Rogaine."
    4 "I'm not sure, you need to ask your physician."

ANSWERS

1. **1**

Rationale: Glycerin is an emollient that is used for dry, cracked, and irritated skin. Aspercreme and Myoflex are used to treat muscular aches. Acetic acid solution is used for irrigating, cleansing, and packing wounds infected by *Pseudomonas aeruginosa.*

Test-Taking Strategy: Note the key words "skin is very dry and irritated." These key words and knowledge of the products indicated in the options will assist in directing you to option 1. Review these products now, if you had difficulty with this question!

Level of Cognitive Ability: Application
Phase of Nursing Process: Implementation
Client Needs: Health Promotion and Maintenance
Content Area: Pharmacology

Reference
Kuhn, M. (1998). *Pharmacotherapeutics: A nursing process approach* (4th ed.). Philadelphia: F. A. Davis. p. 988.

2. **4**

Rationale: Myoflex is one of the many product used for the temporary relief of muscular aches, rheumatism, arthritis, sprains, and neuralgia. These types of products contain combinations of antiseptics, local anesthetics, analgesics, and counterirritants. They are not prescribed to cause the skin to peel, and if this sort of reaction occurs the physician should be notified. The medication does not act in a systemic manner. A heating pad should not be applied because irritation or burning of the skin may occur.

Test-Taking Strategy: Noting the key words "topical cream" may assist in eliminating option 2. Eliminate option 3 knowing that this is not an expected therapeutic effect. Recalling the principles related to heat application will assist in eliminating option 1.

Level of Cognitive Ability: Application
Phase of Nursing Process: Implementation
Client Needs: Health Promotion and Maintenance
Content Area: Pharmacology

Reference
Kuhn, M. (1998). *Pharmacotherapeutics: A nursing process approach* (4th ed.). Philadelphia: F. A. Davis. p. 988.

3. **4**

Rationale: The instructions for the use of Nix include wash, rinse, and towel dry hair; apply sufficient volume to saturate hair and scalp; allow to remain on hair 10 minutes and then rinse with water.

Test-Taking Strategy: Knowledge regarding the use of this medication is required to answer this question. Note that both options 1 and 4 address a time frame for allowing the medication to remain on the hair. Recognizing this may provide you with the clue that one of these options is correct. If you are unfamiliar with the use of this treatment, review now!

Level of Cognitive Ability: Application
Phase of Nursing Process: Implementation
Client Needs: Health Promotion and Maintenance
Content Area: Pharmacology

Reference
Kuhn, M. (1998). *Pharmacotherapeutics: A nursing process approach* (4th ed.). Philadelphia: F. A. Davis. p. 991.

4. **1**

Rationale: Kwell is applied in a thin layer to the entire body below the head. No more than 30 g (1 oz) should be used. The medication is removed by washing 8 to 12 hours later. As a rule, only one application is required.

Test-Taking Strategy: Knowledge regarding the use of Kwell is required to answer this question. If you are unfamiliar with the use of this medication, take time now to review!

Level of Cognitive Ability: Application
Phase of Nursing Process: Implementation
Client Needs: Health Promotion and Maintenance
Content Area: Pharmacology

Reference
Lehne, R. (1998). *Pharmacology for nursing care* (3rd ed.). Philadelphia: W. B. Saunders. p. 1003.

5. **3**

Rationale: Lindane can penetrate the intact skin and can cause convulsions if absorbed in sufficient quantities. Clients at highest risk for convulsions are premature infants, children, and clients with pre-existing seizure disorders. Lindane should not be used on pediatric clients unless safer medications have failed to control infection.

Test-Taking Strategy: Knowledge regarding the contraindications associated with the use of Lindane is required to answer this question. If you are unfamiliar with these contraindications, learn them now!

Level of Cognitive Ability: Analysis
Phase of Nursing Process: Analysis
Client Needs: Physiological Integrity
Content Area: Pharmacology

Reference
Lehne, R. (1998). *Pharmacology for nursing care* (3rd ed.). Philadelphia: W. B. Saunders. p. 1003.

6. **3**

Rationale: Clients should be advised not to use occlusive dressings (bandages or plastic wraps) to cover the affected site following the application of the topical glucocorticoid, unless the physician specifically prescribes wound coverage. Options 1, 2, and 4 are accurate statements related to the use of this medication.

Test-Taking Strategy: Note the key words "need for further instruction." Eliminate option 4 knowing that this is the action for glucocorticoids. The words "thin" in option 1 and "gently" in option 2 should assist you in eliminating these options. If you had difficulty with this questions, take time now, to review this medication!

Level of Cognitive Ability: Analysis
Phase of Nursing Process: Evaluation
Client Needs: Health Promotion and Maintenance
Content Area: Pharmacology

Reference
Lehne, R. (1998). *Pharmacology for nursing care* (3rd ed.). Philadelphia: W. B. Saunders. p. 1055.

7. **2**

Rationale: Topical glucocorticoids can be absorbed into the systemic circulation. Absorption is higher from regions where the skin is especially permeable (scalp, axilla, face, eyelids, neck, perineum, genitalia), and lower from regions where penetrability is poor (back, palms, soles).

Test-Taking Strategy: Focus on the issue of the question "permeability and the potential for systemic absorption." Eliminate options 3 and 4 because these body areas are similar in terms of skin substance. From the remaining options, think about permeability of the skin area. This should direct you to option 2.

Level of Cognitive Ability: Analysis
Phase of Nursing Process: Analysis
Client Needs: Physiological Integrity
Content Area: Pharmacology

Reference
Lehne, R. (1998). *Pharmacology for nursing care* (3rd ed.). Philadelphia: W. B. Saunders. p. 1055.

8. **1**

Rationale: Topical glucocorticoids can be absorbed in sufficient amounts to produce systemic toxicity. Principal concerns are growth retardation (in children) and adrenal suppression in all age groups. Systemic toxicity is more likely under extreme conditions of use, such as with prolonged therapy in which extensive surfaces are treated with high doses of high-potency agents in conjunction with occlusive dressings.

Test-Taking Strategy: Options 3 and 4 can be eliminated first because they are local reactions. From the remaining two options, knowledge regarding the concerns related to systemic toxicity is required to answer the question. Review these systemic effects now, if you had difficulty with this question!

Level of Cognitive Ability: Analysis
Phase of Nursing Process: Analysis
Client Needs: Physiological Integrity
Content Area: Pharmacology

Reference
Lehne, R. (1998). *Pharmacology for nursing care* (3rd ed.). Philadelphia: W. B. Saunders. p. 1055.

9. **4**

Rationale: Salicylic acid is readily absorbed through the skin, and systemic toxicity (salicylism) can result. Symptoms include tinnitus, hyperpnea, dizziness, and psychologic disturbances. Constipation and diarrhea are not associated with salicylism.

Test-Taking Strategy: Noting the name of the medication will assist in directing you to the correct option if you can recall the toxic effects that occur with acetyl "salicylic" acid (aspirin). If you are unfamiliar with the toxic effects of salicylic acid, take time now to review!

Level of Cognitive Ability: Analysis
Phase of Nursing Process: Assessment
Client Needs: Physiological Integrity
Content Area: Pharmacology

Reference
Lehne, R. (1998). *Pharmacology for nursing care* (3rd ed.). Philadelphia: W. B. Saunders. p. 1056.

10. **2**

Rationale: Acyclovir is a topical antiviral agent that inhibits DNA replication in the virus. It has activity against herpes simplex types 1 and 2, varicella-zoster, Epstein-Barr virus and cytomegalovirus. Triple antibiotic would not be effective in treating herpesvirus. Bactroban is a topical antibacterial active against impetigo caused by staphylococcus or streptococcus. Actinex is a keratolytic.

Test-Taking Strategy: Knowledge that herpes simplex is a virus will direct you to the option that identifies an antiviral medication. If you are not familiar with these medications, take time now to review!

Level of Cognitive Ability: Analysis
Phase of Nursing Process: Analysis
Client Needs: Physiological Integrity
Content Area: Pharmacology

Reference
Kuhn, M. (1998). *Pharmacotherapeutics: A nursing process approach* (4th ed.). Philadelphia: F. A. Davis. p. 989.

11. **3**

Rationale: Coal tar is used to treat psoriasis and other chronic disorders of the skin. It suppresses DNA synthesis, mitotic activity, and cell proliferation. It has an unpleasant odor, can frequently stain the skin and hair, and can cause phototoxicity. Systemic toxicity does not occur.

Test-Taking Strategy: Note the key word "not" in the stem of the question. The name of the medication will assist in eliminating options 1 and 2. It is necessary to know that the medication does not cause systemic effects to answer this question correctly. If you had difficulty with this question, review this treatment now!

Level of Cognitive Ability: Analysis
Phase of Nursing Process: Assessment
Client Needs: Physiological Integrity
Content Area: Pharmacology

References
Lehne, R. (1998). *Pharmacology for nursing care* (3rd ed.). Philadelphia: W. B. Saunders. p. 1059.
Kuhn, M. (1998). *Pharmacotherapeutics: A nursing process approach* (4th ed.). Philadelphia: F. A. Davis. p. 989.

12. **1**

Rationale: Sunscreens are most effective when applied about 30 minutes to 1 hour before exposure to the sun so that they can penetrate the skin. All sunscreens should be reapplied after swimming or sweating.

Test-Taking Strategy: Knowledge that sunscreens need to penetrate the skin will assist in eliminating options 2 and 3. Noting the key words "most effective" will assist in directing you to option 1. Review protective skin measures now, if you had difficulty with this question!

Level of Cognitive Ability: Analysis
Phase of Nursing Process: Implementation
Client Needs: Health Promotion and Maintenance
Content Area: Pharmacology

Reference
Kuhn, M. (1998). *Pharmacotherapeutics: A nursing process approach* (4th ed.). Philadelphia: F. A. Davis. p. 993.

13. **3**

Rationale: DuoDerm contains hydroactive particles embedded in a polymer base, which are softened by wound moisture and act as a protective gel over healing tissue. It is applied directly to the wound and can be left in place up to 7 days.

Test-Taking Strategy: Knowledge regarding the use of DuoDerm is required to answer this question. If you are unfamiliar with this type of protective dressing, take time now to review!

Level of Cognitive Ability: Application
Phase of Nursing Process: Planning
Client Needs: Physiological Integrity
Content Area: Pharmacology

Reference
Kuhn, M. (1998). *Pharmacotherapeutics: A nursing process approach* (4th ed.). Philadelphia: F. A. Davis. p. 993.

14. **3**

Rationale: Furacin is applied topically to the burn and has a broad spectrum of antibiotic activity. It is used in second- or third-degree burns in which bacterial resistance to other agents is a real or potential problem. A film of 1/16″ is applied directly to the burn. Saline-soaked dressings are not used.

Test-Taking Strategy: Knowledge regarding the use of this medication is required to answer this question. Option 1 can be eliminated because infection is a major concern with the burn client and a wet dressing can more easily harbor bacteria. Recalling that a very thin film is required will easily direct you to option 3. Review the use of this medication for burn therapy now, if you had difficulty with this question!

Level of Cognitive Ability: Application
Phase of Nursing Process: Implementation
Client Needs: Physiological Integrity
Content Area: Pharmacology

Reference
Kuhn, M. (1998). *Pharmacotherapeutics: A nursing process approach* (4th ed.). Philadelphia: F. A. Davis. p. 998.

15. **4**

Rationale: Mafenide is bacteriostatic for both gram-negative and gram-positive organisms and is used to treat second- and third-degree burns to reduce bacteria present in avascular tissues. The client should be informed that the medication will cause local discomfort and burning.

Test-Taking Strategy: Eliminate options 1 and 3 because it is not within the scope of nursing practice to alter or discontinue a medication therapy. Knowledge that this is a normal expected occurrence will easily direct you to option 4. If you had difficulty with this question, take time now to review!

Level of Cognitive Ability: Application
Phase of Nursing Process: Implementation
Client Needs: Physiological Integrity
Content Area: Pharmacology

Reference
Kuhn, M. (1998). *Pharmacotherapeutics: A nursing process approach* (4th ed.). Philadelphia: F. A. Davis. p. 998.

16. **3**

Rationale: Sulfamylon is a strong carbonic anhydrase inhibitor and can suppress renal excretion of acid, thereby causing acidosis. Clients receiving this treatment should be monitored for acid-base status, and if the acidosis becomes severe the medication should be discontinued for 1 to 2 days. Options 1 and 2 describe local rather than systemic effects. An elevated blood pressure may be expected in the client with pain.

Test-Taking Strategy: Note the key words "systemic effect." Options 1 and 2 can be eliminated because these are local rather than systemic effects. From the remaining options, recall that the client in pain would already likely have an elevated blood pressure. This should direct you to option 3 as the correct answer to this question. Review the systemic effects of this medication now, if you had difficulty with this question!

Level of Cognitive Ability: Analysis
Phase of Nursing Process: Assessment
Client Needs: Physiological Integrity
Content Area: Pharmacology

Reference
Kuhn, M. (1998). *Pharmacotherapeutics: A nursing process approach* (4th ed.). Philadelphia: F. A. Davis. p. 998.

17. **1**

Rationale: A Vigilon dressing is used to clean small partial-thickness burns. It is a colloidal suspension on a polyethylene mesh support, is permeable to gases and water vapor, and provides a moist environment. It is changed daily.

Test-Taking Strategy: Eliminate options 2 and 4 first because they are similar time frames. Knowledge regarding the use of this type of burn covering will assist in directing you to option 1. If you are unfamiliar with this type of burn covering, take time now to review!

Level of Cognitive Ability: Application
Phase of Nursing Process: Planning
Client Needs: Health Promotion and Maintenance
Content Area: Pharmacology

Reference
Kuhn, M. (1998). *Pharmacotherapeutics: A nursing process approach* (4th ed.). Philadelphia: F. A. Davis. p. 999.

18. **3**

Rationale: Dakin solution is a chloride solution that is used for irrigating and cleaning necrotic or purulent wounds. It can be used for packing necrotic wounds. It cannot be used to pack purulent wounds since the solution is inactivated by copious pus. It should not come in contact with healing or normal tissue, and it should be rinsed off immediately if used for irrigation. Solutions are unstable and must be prepared fresh for each use.

Test-Taking Strategy: Note the key word "not" in the stem of the question. Eliminate options 1 and 2 first because they are similar and indicate avoiding healthy tissue. It makes sense to prepare the solution prior to use; therefore, eliminate option 4. If you are unfamiliar with the use of this solution, take time now to review!

Level of Cognitive Ability: Application
Phase of Nursing Process: Planning
Client Needs: Physiological Integrity
Content Area: Pharmacology

Reference
Kuhn, M. (1998). *Pharmacotherapeutics: A nursing process approach* (4th ed.). Philadelphia: F. A. Davis. p. 988.

19. 4

Rationale: Tretinoin decreases cohesiveness of the epithelial cells, increasing cell mitosis and turnover. It is potentially irritating, particularly when used correctly. Within 48 hours of use, the skin generally becomes red and begins to peel.

Test-Taking Strategy: Options 1 and 3 can be eliminated first because they are similar. Eliminate option 2 next because it is not within the scope of nursing practice to advise a client to discontinue a medication. If you are unfamiliar with the use of this medication, take time now to review!

Level of Cognitive Ability: Application
Phase of Nursing Process: Implementation
Client Needs: Physiological Integrity
Content Area: Pharmacology

Reference
Kuhn, M. (1998). *Pharmacotherapeutics: A nursing process approach* (4th ed.). Philadelphia: F. A. Davis. p. 997.

20. 3

Rationale: Tretinoin is applied liberally to the skin. The hands are washed thoroughly immediately after applying. Therapeutic results should be seen after 2 to 3 weeks but may not be optimal until after 6 weeks. The skin needs to be cleansed thoroughly before applying the medication.

Test-Taking Strategy: Note the key word "not" in the stem of the question. Eliminate options 1 and 4 first, using the principles of asepsis. Knowledge regarding the use of the medication will assist in directing you to option 3. Review this medication now if you had difficulty with this question!

Level of Cognitive Ability: Application
Phase of Nursing Process: Implementation
Client Needs: Health Promotion and Maintenance
Content Area: Pharmacology

Reference
Kuhn, M. (1998). *Pharmacotherapeutics: A nursing process approach* (4th ed.). Philadelphia: F. A. Davis. p. 997.

21. 3

Rationale: Isotretinoin is administered two times daily for 15 to 20 weeks. The usual adult dosage is 0.5 to 1 mg/kg/day. If needed, a second course may be given, but not until 2 months have elapsed after completing the first course.

Test-Taking Strategy: Knowledge regarding the use of this medication is required to answer this question. If you are unfamiliar with this treatment, take time now to review!

Level of Cognitive Ability: Analysis
Phase of Nursing Process: Analysis
Client Needs: Physiological Integrity
Content Area: Pharmacology

Reference
Lehne, R. (1998). *Pharmacology for nursing care* (3rd ed.). Philadelphia: W. B. Saunders. p. 1059.

22. 3

Rationale: Accutane can elevate triglyceride levels. Blood triglyceride content should be measured prior to treatment and periodically thereafter until effects of triglycerides have been evaluated.

Test-Taking Strategy: Eliminate options 1 and 2 first because a complete blood count will also measure the white blood cell count. From the remaining options, it is necessary to know that the medication can affect the triglyceride level in the client. Review this medication now, if you had difficulty with this question!

Level of Cognitive Ability: Analysis
Phase of Nursing Process: Analysis
Client Needs: Physiological Integrity
Content Area: Pharmacology

Reference
Lehne, R. (1998). *Pharmacology for nursing care* (3rd ed.). Philadelphia: W. B. Saunders. p. 1059.

23. 3

Rationale: Vitamin A, being a relative of isotretinoin, can produce generalized intensification of isotretinoin toxicity. Because of the potential for increased toxicity, vitamin A supplements should be discontinued prior to isotretinoin therapy.

Test-Taking Strategy: Knowledge that isotretinoin is a derivative of vitamin A will easily direct you to the correct option. If you are unfamiliar with this medication, take time now to review the contraindications associated with its use!

Level of Cognitive Ability: Analysis
Phase of Nursing Process: Implementation
Client Needs: Physiological Integrity
Content Area: Pharmacology

Reference
Lehne, R. (1998). *Pharmacology for nursing care* (3rd ed.). Philadelphia: W. B. Saunders. p. 1059.

24. 3

Rationale: The wound should be cleansed with a sterile solution and gently patted dry. A thin layer of Elase is applied and covered with a petrolatum gauze. If a dry powder is used for best effects, the solution should be prepared just prior to use.

Test-Taking Strategy: Note the word "not" in the stem of the question. Noting this key word should assist in directing you to option 3. Review the method of application of Elase now if you had difficulty with this question!

Level of Cognitive Ability: Application
Phase of Nursing Process: Planning
Client Needs: Physiological Integrity
Content Area: Pharmacology

Reference
Kuhn, M. (1998). *Pharmacotherapeutics: A nursing process approach* (4th ed.). Philadelphia: F. A. Davis. p. 1010.

25. 2

Rationale: The wound should be cleansed with a sterile solution prior to treatment. The nurse then should thoroughly moisten the wound with normal saline or sterile water and apply a loose thin dressing after applying a thin film of Travase extending 1/4 to 1/2 inch beyond the area to be debrided. The ointment should be refrigerated.

Test-Taking Strategy: Note the word "inaccurate" in the stem of the question. Knowledge regarding the use of this medication is required to answer the question. Review the method of application of Travase now, if you had difficulty with this question!

Level of Cognitive Ability: Analysis
Phase of Nursing Process: Evaluation
Client Needs: Physiological Integrity
Content Area: Pharmacology

Reference
Kuhn, M. (1998). *Pharmacotherapeutics: A nursing process approach* (4th ed.). Philadelphia: F. A. Davis. p. 1010.

26. 4

Rationale: Debrisan is a cleansing rather than a debriding agent. It is effective in wet wounds only. It should not be packed into wounds tightly because maceration of surrounding tissue may result.

Test-Taking Strategy: Knowledge regarding the use of this medication is required to answer this question. If you are unfamiliar with the use of Debrisan, take time now to review!

Level of Cognitive Ability: Analysis
Phase of Nursing Process: Analysis
Client Needs: Physiological Integrity
Content Area: Pharmacology

Reference
Kuhn, M. (1998). *Pharmacotherapeutics: A nursing process approach* (4th ed.). Philadelphia: F. A. Davis. p. 1012.

27. 3

Rationale: A 2% minoxidil solution is used for topical treatment of baldness. The usual dosage is 1 mL applied two times a day.

Test-Taking Strategy: Knowledge regarding the usual dosage for minoxidil solution is required to answer this question. If you are unfamiliar with this medication, take time now to review!

Level of Cognitive Ability: Analysis
Phase of Nursing Process: Analysis
Client Needs: Physiological Integrity
Content Area: Pharmacology

Reference
Lehne, R. (1998). *Pharmacology for nursing care* (3rd ed.). Philadelphia: W. B. Saunders. p. 1061.

28. 2

Rationale: Azelex is a topical medication used to treat mild to moderate acne. It appears to work by suppressing growth of *Propionibacterium acnes* and by decreasing proliferation of keratinocytes.

Test-Taking Strategy: Knowledge regarding the use of Azelex is required to answer this question. It is a relatively new medication used to treat mild to moderate acne. If you are unfamiliar with this medication, take time now to review!

Level of Cognitive Ability: Analysis
Phase of Nursing Process: Analysis
Client Needs: Physiological Integrity
Content Area: Pharmacology

Reference
Lehne, R. (1998). *Pharmacology for nursing care* (3rd ed.). Philadelphia: W. B. Saunders. p. 1058.

29. 2

Rationale: Santyl is used to promote debridement of dermal lesions and severe burns. It is applied once daily and covered with a sterile dressing.

Test-Taking Strategy: Note the key word "accurate" in the stem of the question. Knowledge regarding the use of this medication is required to answer this question. If you are unfamiliar with this medication, take time now to review!

Level of Cognitive Ability: Analysis
Phase of Nursing Process: Evaluation
Client Needs: Health Promotion and Maintenance
Content Area: Pharmacology

Reference
Lehne, R. (1998). *Pharmacology for nursing care* (3rd ed.). Philadelphia: W. B. Saunders. p. 1061.

30. 2

Rationale: Hair regrowth is most likely when baldness has developed recently and has been limited to a small area. Upon discontinuation of the medication, newly gained hair is lost in 3 to 4 months, and the natural progression of hair loss resumes.

Test-Taking Strategy: Option 4 can be easily eliminated because it places the client's question on hold. Knowledge regarding the clinical response and effects of this medication is required to select the correct answer from the remaining options. If you are unfamiliar with this medication, take time now to review!

Level of Cognitive Ability: Application
Phase of Nursing Process: Implementation
Client Needs: Psychosocial Integrity
Content Area: Pharmacology

Reference
Lehne, R. (1998). *Pharmacology for nursing care* (3rd ed.). Philadelphia: W. B. Saunders. p. 1061.

BIBLIOGRAPHY

Black J., & Matassarin-Jacobs, E. (1997). *Medical-surgical nursing: Clinical management for continuity of care* (5th ed.). Philadelphia: W. B. Saunders.

Hodgson, B., & Kizior, R. (1998). *Saunders nursing drug handbook 1998.* Philadelphia: W. B. Saunders.

Kuhn, M. (1998). *Pharmacotherapeutics: A nursing process approach* (4th ed.). Philadelphia: F. A. Davis.

Lehne, R. (1998). *Pharmacology for nursing care* (3rd ed.). Philadelphia: W. B. Saunders.

Luckmann, J. (1997). *Saunders manual of nursing care.* Philadelphia: W. B. Saunders.

Monahan, F., & Neighbors, M. (1998). *Medical-surgical nursing: Foundations for clinical practice* (2nd ed.). Philadelphia: W. B. Saunders.

O'Toole, M. (ed.) (1997). *Miller-Keane encyclopedia & dictionary of medicine, nursing, & allied health* (6th ed.). Philadelphia: W. B. Saunders.

UNIT X

....

The Adult Client with an Oncological Disorder

PYRAMID TERMS

Benign—Usually refers to growths that are encapsulated, remain localized, and are slow growing.

Cancer—A neoplastic disorder that can involve all body organs. Cells lose their normal growth-controlling mechanism, and the growth of cells is uncontrolled.

Carcinogen—A physical, chemical, or biological stressor that causes neoplastic changes in normal cells.

Carcinoma in Situ—A lesion with all the histological characteristics of malignancies, except invasion.

Carcinomas—Originate from epithelial cells, solid tumors, the skin, GI tract, lungs, uterus, breast and other organs.

Hospice—A concept of care for terminally ill clients that includes the concepts of intensive caring rather than intensive care. The family and client are the focus of nursing care, and the goal is to relieve pain and facilitate the optimal quality of life.

Lymphomas—Originate from lymphoid tissue.

Leukemias or Myelomas—Originate from blood-forming organs.

Malignant—Refers to growths that are not encapsulated but metastasize and grow. A cancerous lesion having the characteristics of disorderly, uncontrolled, and chaotic proliferation of cells.

Metastasis—The transfer of disease from one organ or part to another not directly connected with it. Secondary malignant lesions, originating from the primary tumor, are located in anatomically distant places.

Nadir—The period of time when an antineoplastic medication has its most profound effects on the bone marrow.

Neoplasia—A new growth, which may be benign or malignant.

Sarcomas—Originate from muscle, bone, fat, or the lymph system or from connective tissues.

Staging—A method of classifying malignancies based on the presence and extent of the tumor within the body.

Tumor Markers—Specific bodily substances that seem to indicate tumor progression or regression.

Undifferentiated Cells—Cells that have lost the capacity for specialized functions.

PYRAMID TO SUCCESS

Pyramid points focus on treatment modalities related to an oncological disorder, such as pain management, internal and external radiation, and chemotherapy, and on oncological disorders such as skin cancer, leukemia, breast cancer, and lung cancer. Specific focus relates to the nursing care related to these treatment modalities and disorders, and to client adaptation and the impact of the treatment or disorder. Specifically, focus on the complications related to chemotherapy and the nursing measures required in monitoring for these complications, and in preventing life-threatening conditions such as infection and bleeding. Specific laboratory values include the white blood cell count and the platelet count.

NURSING PROCESS

ASSESSMENT

Risk factors
Dietary factors
Pain or discomfort
Change in bowel or bladder habits
Any sore that does not heal
Recurrent infections
Unusual bleeding or discharge
Thickening or lump in breast or elsewhere in the body
Anorexia, nausea, indigestion, or vomiting
Unexplained weight loss
Obvious change of wart or mole
Nagging cough or hoarseness
Expectorating or vomiting blood
Blood in the urine or stools

ANALYSIS: Alteration in Nutrition

PLANNING	IMPLEMENTATION	EVALUATION
The client consumes an adequate intake of food and fluids. The client remains free of nausea.	Monitor and document food intake. Monitor laboratory values. Develop a meal plan to include schedule of meals and high-quality foods incorporating client's likes and dislikes.	The client maintains weight. The client consumes a balanced diet. The client is free of nausea and vomiting. The client tolerates the prescribed diet.

ANALYSIS: Alteration in Comfort

PLANNING	IMPLEMENTATION	EVALUATION
The client requests medication for discomfort. The client verbalizes relief of pain from comfort measures and medication.	Rate the client's pain on a scale of 0 to 10. Provide comfort measures and pain medications as required. Assess and document the effects of pain control measures and pain medications. Describe pain management regimen to client and family.	The client verbalizes ability to cope with pain and measures for pain relief. The client obtains effective relief of pain.

ANALYSIS: Self-Care Deficit

PLANNING	IMPLEMENTATION	EVALUATION
The client acknowledges the need for care. The client is able to perform independent self-care activities.	Include the client in determining the care routine. Encourage independence in the performance of self-care as much as possible. Instruct client and family in alternative methods for self-care.	The client participates in self-care to the optimum level.

ANALYSIS: Altered Body Image

PLANNING	IMPLEMENTATION	EVALUATION
The client verbalizes body image changes.	Encourage the client to verbalize the effects of physical and emotional changes. Actively listen to client and family and acknowledge the reality of concerns about treatments, progress, and prognosis.	The client describes actual change in body function.

ANALYSIS: Social Isolation

PLANNING	IMPLEMENTATION	EVALUATION
The client identifies behaviors that will reduce social isolation.	Identify with the client factors that might contribute to feelings of social isolation. Reinforce efforts by the client, family, and friends to maintain interactions and relationships.	The client identifies resources and support systems that will assist in decreasing social isolation.

ANALYSIS: Ineffective Individual Coping

PLANNING	IMPLEMENTATION	EVALUATION
The client identifies personal strengths that may promote effective coping.	Assist client to identify personal strengths. Encourage client to express concerns related to problem solving.	The client utilizes support systems. The client verbalizes a plan for accepting the personal health care situation.

ANALYSIS: Fear of Death and Dying

PLANNING	IMPLEMENTATION	EVALUATION
The client verbalizes fears related to prognosis.	Encourage and assist client and family to express fears. Initiate and mobilize support services such as hospice for client and family.	The client demonstrates behaviors that reduce fear.

CLIENT NEEDS

SAFE, EFFECTIVE CARE ENVIRONMENT

Advance directives
Advocacy related to client's decisions
Client rights
Confidentiality regarding diagnosis
Informed consent for treatments and procedures
Oncology-related consultations and referrals
Handling hazardous and infectious materials related to radiation and chemotherapy
Asepsis
Standard and protective precautions

HEALTH PROMOTION AND MAINTENANCE

Expected body image changes related to chemotherapy and treatments
Prevention of disease related to infection
Health-screening measures for cancer
Health promotion programs regarding risks for cancer
Lifestyle choices
Instructions regarding monthly self-breast or self-testicular examinations
Client lifestyle choices
Client and family instructions regarding home care

PSYCHOSOCIAL INTEGRITY

Ability to cope, adapt, and/or problem solve during illness or stressful events
Grief and loss related to death and the dying process
Religious and cultural preferences
Assisting the client and family to cope with alteration in body image
Mobilizing appropriate support and resource systems
Promoting a positive environment to maintain optimal quality of life

PHYSIOLOGICAL INTEGRITY

Providing basic care and comfort
Promoting nutrition
Managing pain
Administration of blood and blood products
Central venous access devices
Diagnostic tests and laboratory values such as white blood cell and platelet counts
Chemotherapy
Radiation therapy
Monitoring for the expected and unexpected responses to radiation and chemotherapy
Protecting the client from the life-threatening side effects of treatments

BIBLIOGRAPHY

Black, J., & Matassarin-Jacobs, E. (1997). *Medical-surgical nursing. Clinical management for continuity of care* (5th ed.). Philadelphia: W. B. Saunders.

Luckmann, J. (1997). *Saunders manual of nursing care*. Philadelphia: W. B. Saunders.

National Council of State Boards of Nursing (eds) (1997). *Test plan for the National Council Licensure Examination for Registered Nurses*. Chicago: Author.

CHAPTER 49

Oncological Disorders

. . . .

I. Cancer

A. Description
1. A neoplastic disorder that can involve all body organs
2. Cells lose their normal growth-controlling mechanism, and the growth of cells is uncontrolled
B. **Metastasis**: Can occur through the lymphatics, the blood stream, seeding, or transfer and spread from one site to another
C. **Staging** (Box 49–1)
1. A method used to describe the tumor
2. Includes the extent of the tumor, the extent to which malignancy has increased in size, the involvement of regional nodes, and metastatic development
D. Risk factors
1. Chemical **carcinogens**
2. Radiation **carcinogens**, such as sunlight or x-rays
3. Viral factors
4. Genetic factors
5. Demographic/geographical factors
6. Dietary factors such as obesity, use of alcohol, high-fat and low-fiber diets
7. Psychological factors, such as stress
E. Prevention
1. Avoid obesity
2. Decrease fat intake
3. Increase total fiber in diet
4. Increase vitamins A, C, and E
5. Decrease alcohol consumption
6. Avoid salt-cured/nitrate-cured foods
7. Avoid exposure to **carcinogens**
8. Obtain adequate rest and exercise to decrease stress
F. Early detection (Box 49–2)
1. Mammography
2. Papanicolaou ("Pap") test
3. Stools for occult blood
4. Sigmoidoscopy
5. Breast self-examination
6. Testicular self-examination
7. Skin inspection

II. Breast Self-Examination (BSE)

A. Performing BSE
1. Perform 7 to 10 days after menses
2. Postmenopausal clients or clients who have had a hysterectomy should select a specific

---

BOX 49–1. Tumor Staging

EXTENT OF TUMOR

T = Primary tumor
N = Regional nodes
M = Metastasis

EXTENT TO WHICH MALIGNANCY HAS INCREASED IN SIZE

T0 = No evidence of primary tumor
TIS = Carcinoma in situ
T1, T2, T3, T4 = Progression of increase in tumor, size, and involvement
TX = Tumor cannot be assessed

INVOLVEMENT OF REGIONAL NODES

N0 = Regional nodes not abnormal
N1, N2, N3, N4 = Increasing degree of abnormal regional lymph nodes

METASTATIC DEVELOPMENT

M0 = No evidence of distant metastasis
M1, M2, M3 = Increasing degree of distant metastasis

BOX 49–2. Warning Signs of Cancer

Change in bowel or bladder habits
Any sore that does not heal
Unusual bleeding or discharge
Thickening or lump in breast or elsewhere
Indigestion
Obvious change of wart or mole
Nagging cough or hoarseness

day of the month and perform BSE monthly on that day

B. Procedure
 1. Before a mirror
    a. Inspect with arms at the side
    b. Raise arms overhead to inspect for changes in size or contour, dimpling, or changes in the nipple
    c. Inspect by resting the palms on the hips and pressing down firmly to flex chest muscles
 2. Lying down
    a. Place a pillow under the right breast
    b. Use the pads of the middle three fingers of the left hand, press firmly, and feel for lumps or changes using a rubbing, circular pattern to cover all breast tissue
    c. Gently squeeze the nipple, looking for discharge
    d. Perform BSE on the left breast using the same method
 3. In the shower
    a. With fingers flat, move gently over every part of each breast
    b. Check for lumps or thickening

III. Testicular Self-Examination (TSE)

A. Select a day of the month and perform the examination on the same day each month
B. Perform after a warm bath or shower
C. Hold the scrotum in one hand
D. Examine each testicle separately by gently rolling it between the thumb and fingers of the other hand
E. Check for hard lumps or knots

IV. Diagnostic Tests

A. Tomography
 1. Description
    a. X-ray films showing details of structures otherwise hidden by overlying radiopaque bone
    b. Allows views of tissues at various planes as if slices have been made through the tissue
 2. Implementation: No special preparation is required
B. Computed tomography (CT scan)
 1. Description
    a. X-ray technique that produces sequential cross-sectional body images at progressive depths
    b. Can differentiate **normal tissue from abnormal** masses and accurately identify their size and location
    c. An oral or IV contrast agent may be administered to increase the sensitivity of the CT scan
 2. Implementation
    a. Obtain informed consent if a dye is injected

b. Assess client for allergies to the dye
c. Clients should be told that they will lie on a table and the x-ray machine will move around them
d. Clients should be told that the test is painless unless an IV contrast dye is used, which may cause a burning sensation on injection
e. Inform client that the dye may cause nausea, vomiting, flushing, itching, and a bitter taste in the mouth
f. Client should be told that the x-ray machine can be very noisy

C. Ultrasound
 1. Description
    a. Uses high-frequency sound waves to visualize organs and masses
    b. A noninvasive method of identifying and following the growth of neoplasms without radiation exposure
 2. Implementation
    a. Test preparation may include cleansing the bowel with enemas if the abdominal area is to be tested, and having the client drink 6 to 8 glasses of water without voiding before the test
    b. Inform clients that they may not be allowed to void until after the test
    c. Inform clients that the test is painless and that only a slight pressure may be felt
    d. Inform clients that lubricant gel is applied to the area but is easily wiped off after the test

D. Magnetic resonance imaging (MRI)
 1. Description
    a. Identifies abnormalities by creating sectional images of the body without the use of contrast dye or radiation; however, a dye may be used in some situations
    b. Provides clear images of internal structures in response to the magnetic field created by harmless, low-energy radio waves
    c. Used to detect localized and staged malignancies of the central nervous system (CNS), spine, head, neck, and musculoskeletal system
 2. Implementation
    a. Remove all items before the test that might be affected by a magnet
    b. Note that the test cannot be performed if any items affected by a magnet cannot be removed, such as a pacemaker or surgical clip
    c. Note that the test is painless, although some clients may feel somewhat claustrophobic because of the narrow tunnel in the machine where they must lie
    d. Assess the client for claustrophobia
    e. Administer medications as prescribed if the client is claustrophobic
    f. Instruct the client that the machine makes a loud hammering sound during the test

g. If an IV contrast dye is used to enhance the image, ask whether client tends to become nauseated easily; adjust food and fluids accordingly

E. Radioisotope scans
   1. Description
      a. Radioisotopes are used to locate tumors and lesions within the brain, kidneys, liver, lungs, pericardium, and bones
      b. When the radioisotope enters the client's body, the fate of the radioisotope can be followed or traced by the scanning machine
      c. Abnormal tissue appears different on the scan because the isotope is metabolized differently by this tissue
      d. A scan of the organ will reveal a high uptake of the radioisotope at the site of a tumor, and the area in which the concentration of the radioisotope is unusually high is called a hot spot
      e. The areas of less concentration of a radioactive isotope are called cold spots
   2. Implementation
      a. The client receives a tracer dose of the appropriate radioisotope, either orally or by injection
      b. Before the scanning procedure can be performed, the radioisotope must be assimilated by the organ under study; the length of time for organ assimilation of the radioisotope will vary
      c. During the procedure the client is asked to lie still and breathe normally while the scanner measures the radioactivity concentrated in the organ under study and records its findings
      d. Sedation before this procedure may be prescribed for the restless, agitated, or anxious client

F. Lymphangiogram
   1. Description
      a. Examines the lymphatic system, the primary site of **metastasis** for tumors with good lymphatic drainage
      b. The test is performed by injecting blue dye into the interdigital webs of the feet
      c. The skin on each foot over the lymphatics is anesthetized and a cutdown is performed so that cannulas can be inserted to infuse the dye
      d. The dye is picked up by the lymphatic system; the dye may take several hours to infuse into the lymphatics of the abdomen
      e. X-ray studies are then obtained
   2. Implementation
      a. Note that the test cannot be performed for 48 hours after another contrast study
      b. Inform the client that the test is fairly long and uncomfortable
      c. Instruct the client to drink plenty of fluids after the test

d. Inform the client that the dye may continue to discolor the urine for several days
e. Inform the client that the feet will remain tinted blue for a long time after the test
f. Inform clients that they must return the following day for follow-up x-ray studies

G. Biopsy
   1. Description
      a. Surgical incision of a small piece of tissue for microscopic examination
      b. Used to rule out or confirm a diagnosis of malignancy
      c. A total type of biopsy excises the entire tumor for examination
      d. An excisional type of biopsy excises only a part of the tumor
      e. Following excision, a frozen section or a permanent paraffin section is done in order to examine the specimen
      f. The advantage of the frozen section is the speed with which the section can be prepared and the diagnosis made, as only minutes are required for this test
      g. Permanent paraffin section takes about 24 hours; however, it provides clearer details than does the frozen section
   2. Implementation
      a. The procedure is usually performed in an outpatient surgical setting
      b. Prepare the client for the surgery following the physician's instructions
      c. Obtain a signed informed consent form

H. Blood studies
   1. Routine tests do not test for a specific type of **cancer** but indicate the presence of any number of problems
   2. Other blood tests, such as **tumor markers** and biochemical tests, identify the extent of a particular type of **cancer**
   3. These specific tests are not used to make the diagnosis of **cancer** but only to check its progression

V. Pain Control

A. Causes of pain
   1. Bone destruction
   2. Obstruction of an organ
   3. Compression of peripheral nerves
   4. Infiltration/distention of tissue
   5. Inflammation/necrosis
   6. Psychological, such as fear or anxiety
B. Implementation
   1. Collaborate with other members of the health care team to develop a pain management program
   2. Administer oral preparations if possible and if they provide adequate relief of pain
   3. Mild and moderate pain may be treated with salicylates, acetaminophen (Tylenol), and

nonsteroidal anti-inflammatory drugs (NSAIDs)
4. Severe pain is treated with narcotics, such as codeine sulfate, meperidine (Demerol), morphine sulfate, and hydromorphone hydrochloride (Dilaudid)
5. Continuous IV and subcutaneous infusions of narcotics provide superior pain control
6. Monitor for side effects of medications
7. Monitor for effectiveness of medication
8. Provide nonpharmacological techniques of pain control, such as relaxation, guided imagery, biofeedback, and diversion
9. Do not undermedicate the **cancer** client who is in pain

VI. Surgery

A. Description: Used to diagnose, stage, and treat **cancer**
B. Curative surgery
1. For **cancer** that is localized to the organ of origin and regional lymph nodes
2. **Cancers** that recur locally can be excised, resulting in occasional cure or remission or both
3. Metastatic lesions that appear in the lungs, liver, or brain can be removed to attempt a surgical cure
4. Excision of a metastatic lesion is considered if no other evidence of disease exists and the metastatic lesion appeared after a relatively long disease-free period
C. Palliative surgery
1. Performed if the risk/benefit ratio is favorable and if it can benefit the client and improve quality of life
2. Reduces pain, relieves airway obstruction, relieves obstructions in the GI and urinary tract
3. Performed to relieve pressure on the brain and spinal cord
4. Performed to prevent hemorrhage
5. Performed to remove infected and ulcerated tumors and drain abscesses
D. Reconstructive surgery: Performed to improve the quality of life by restoring maximal function and appearance
E. Preventive surgery
1. Performed in clients with multiple high-risk factors
2. Performed in certain conditions that may increase the risk of **cancer**, such as polyps or ulcerative colitis

◆ VII. Chemotherapy

A. Description
1. Kills or inhibits the reproduction of neoplastic cells
2. The effect of antineoplastic medications may

not be limited to neoplastic cells, and normal cells are also affected by the medication
3. Cell cycle phase-specific medications affect cells only during a certain phase of the reproductive cycle
4. Cell cycle phase-nonspecific medications affect cells in any phase of the reproductive cycle
5. Usually several medications are used in combination to increase the therapeutic response and minimize toxicity
6. Antineoplastic therapy may be combined with other treatments, such as surgery and radiation
7. The routes of antineoplastic medication administration can vary
B. Anaphylactic reactions
1. Precautions
a. Obtain an allergy history
b. Administer a test dose when prescribed by the physician
c. Stay with the client during administration of the medication
d. Have emergency equipment and medications readily available
e. Obtain vital signs
f. Provide an IV line for administration of emergency medications if needed
2. Signs of anaphylactic reaction
a. Dyspnea
b. Chest tightness or pain
c. Pruritus/urticaria
d. Tachycardia
e. Dizziness
f. Anxiety/agitation
g. Inability to speak
h. Nausea and abdominal pain
i. Hypotension
j. Decreased sensorium
k. Flushed appearance
l. Cyanosis
3. Implementation for anaphylactic reaction
a. Stop medication
b. Maintain airway
c. Maintain IV access with 0.9% normal saline (NS)
d. Notify physician
e. Place client in the supine position with the legs elevated, if not contraindicated
f. Monitor vital signs
g. Administer prescribed medications

VIII. Radiation Therapy

A. Description
1. Used as a primary, adjunctive, or palliative modality
2. Involves therapeutic application of high-energy rays to tumors
3. Damage to normal cells is the primary cause of side effects and toxicity
B. External radiation

1. Description: Radiation delivered from an external source
2. Side effects
   a. Headache
   b. Nausea, vomiting, and diarrhea
   c. Skin irritation or injury
   d. Erythema and dryness of the skin
   e. Change or loss of taste
   f. Dry mouth
   g. Esophagitis
   h. Cystitis
   i. Decreased white blood cell (WBC) count and platelets
3. Implementation
   a. Monitor for signs of skin breakdown
   b. Monitor for signs of complications, including cystitis, diarrhea, and nutritional alterations
   c. Increase fluids
   d. Provide a high-protein, high-carbohydrate, high-caloric diet and provide dietary supplements as prescribed
   e. Instruct client not to eat before a treatment if nausea occurs
   f. Administer antiemetics as prescribed and needed
   g. Do not wash off therapy markings
   h. Note that radiodermatitis occurs 3 to 6 weeks after treatments
   i. Avoid creams, lotions, or perfume on irradiated areas
   j. Wash irradiated areas with lukewarm water and mild soap and pat dry
   k. Avoid exposure to sunlight or artificial heat
   l. Monitor for moist desquamation
4. Moist desquamation
   a. Weeping of the skin due to the loss of the upper layer of the skin
   b. Cleanse the area with warm water and pat dry
   c. Apply antibiotic ointment or steroid cream as prescribed
   d. Expose the site to air
C. Internal radiation (Box 49–3)
   1. Description
      a. May be known as brachytherapy
      b. Intracavitary implants involve the temporary insertion of a sealed source into a body cavity
      c. Radioactive isotopes that are "sealed" are placed inside wires, needles, catheters, or seeds in interstitial implants to position the radioactive source directly into the tumor and surrounding tissue
   2. Implementation
      a. Organize nursing tasks to minimize exposure to the client
      b. Maintain strict isolation and radiation precautions
      c. Place the client in a private room
      d. Maintain on bed rest, lying on the back,

with head either flat or at less than 45° to prevent dislodging of the radiation source
   e. Restrict visitors
   f. Nurses who are pregnant or attempting pregnancy should not be assigned to the client
   g. Avoid direct contact around the implant site; provide direct care from the head, foot, or side of the bed, depending on the source of the radiation
   h. Encourage increased fluids and maintain a patent Foley catheter
   i. Monitor for skin eruption, discharge, or abnormal vaginal bleeding
   j. Monitor for dehydration or paralytic ileus
   k. Place a sealed lead container with a long-handled forceps in the client's room
   l. Monitor for dislodging of the radiation source (Box 49–4)
   m. Note that body secretions are considered

BOX 49–3. Time, Distance, and Shielding Principles for Internal Radiation

- Nursing assignments to a client with a radiation implant should be rotated
- Limit time to one half hour per care provider per shift
- Wear lead shields to reduce the transmission of radiation
- A nurse should never care for more than one client with a radiation implant at one time
- The nurse can spend more time with the client if he or she maintains a distance of 20 feet from the client, where exposure will be minimal
- Communicate to the client from a distance
- Stand as far away from the radiation source as possible
- Provide nursing care by standing at the client's shoulder for cervical implants and at the foot of the bed for head and neck implants
- Identify the room with appropriate radiation signs
- Wear a dosimeter badge to monitor the amount of radiation exposure
- A cumulative radiation dose should not exceed 1250 rad every 3 months
- Visitors should stand 6 feet away from the client
- Pregnant women or individuals under 18 years of age should not go into the client's room

---

BOX 49–4. A Dislodged Radiation Source

- Do not touch a dislodged radiation source with the bare hands
- If the radiation source dislodges, use long-handled forceps, place the source in the lead container, and call the physician
- If unable to locate the radiation source, bar visitors and notify the physician

contaminated, and special techniques per agency policy are required for disposal of body secretions with unsealed sources

n. With sealed sources, the radioisotopes cannot circulate through the body or contaminate body secretions

o. Save dressings and linens until the radiation is removed, then dispose of in the usual manner

3. Internal radiation removal
   a. The client is no longer radioactive
   b. Allow the client to be out of bed
   c. A normal diet may be resumed
   d. Sexual partners cannot "catch" **cancer**
   e. Provide Betadine douche if prescribed if the implant was placed in the cervix
   f. Administer Fleet enema as prescribed
   g. Inform clients that they may resume sexual intercourse after 7 to 10 days if the implant was cervical or vaginal
   h. Advise the client to notify the physician if nausea, vomiting, diarrhea, frequent urination, excessive vaginal bleeding, rectal bleeding, hematuria, abdominal pain or distention, or raised temperature occurs

IX. Bone Marrow Transplantation

A. Description
   1. Used in the treatment of **leukemia** for clients who have closely matched donors and who are experiencing temporary remission with chemotherapy
   2. The goal of treatment is to rid the client of all leukemic or other **malignant** cells through treatment with high doses of chemotherapy and whole body irradiation
   3. Since these treatments are lethal to bone marrow, without the replacement of bone marrow function through transplantation the client would die of infection or hemorrhage

B. Types of donor marrow
   1. Allogeneic: Marrow donor is usually a sibling or parent with a similar tissue type
   2. Syngeneic: Uses bone marrow from an identical twin
   3. Autologous
      a. Most common type
      b. The marrow donor is also the recipient
      c. Marrow is harvested during disease remission and is stored frozen to be reinfused later

C. Procedure
   1. Harvest
      a. Marrow is harvested through multiple aspirations from the iliac crest to retrieve sufficient bone marrow for the transplant
      b. Approximately 500 to 1000 mL of marrow is aspirated
      c. Marrow is filtered for any residual **cancer**

cells or to deplete T cells that may cause graft versus host disease

d. Allogeneic marrow is transfused immediately: autologous marrow is frozen for later use

e. Harvest is obtained before the initiation of the conditioning regimen

2. Conditioning: Conditioning refers to an immunosuppression therapy regimen used to eradicate all **malignant** cells, provide a state of immunosuppression, and create space in the bone marrow for the engraftment of the new marrow

3. Transplantation
   a. Bone marrow is administered through the client's central line in a manner similar to a blood transfusion
   b. Marrow is infused over a 30-minute period or may be administered by IV push directly into the central line

4. Engraftment
   a. The transfused bone marrow cells move to the marrow-forming sites of the recipient's bones
   b. When successful, the engraftment process takes 2 to 5 weeks
   c. Engraftment occurs when the white blood cells, erythrocyte, and platelet counts begin to rise

D. Post-transplantation period
   1. The client remains without any natural immunity until the donor marrow begins to proliferate and engraftment occurs
   2. Infection and severe thrombocytopenia are major concerns until engraftment occurs

E. Complications
   1. Failure to engraft: If the transplanted bone marrow fails to engraft, the client will die unless another transplantation is attempted and is successful
   2. Graft versus host disease (GVHD)
      a. Although the recipient cannot recognize the donated bone marrow cells as foreign or non-self because of the total immunosuppression, the immune competent cells of the donated marrow recognize the client's cells as foreign and mount an immune offense against them
      b. The graft is actually trying to attack the host
      c. GVHD is managed with immunosuppressive agents, with caution to avoid suppressing the new immune system to the extent that the client becomes more susceptible to infection, or the transplanted cells stop engrafting
   3. Veno-occlusive disease
      a. Involves occlusion of the hepatic venules by thrombosis or phlebitis
      b. Signs include right upper quadrant abdominal pain, jaundice, ascites, weight gain, and hepatomegaly

c. Early detection is critical because there is no known way to open the hepatic vessels

d. The client will be treated with fluids and supportive therapy

◆ X. Skin Cancer

A. Description
1. A **malignant** lesion of the skin, which may or may not metastasize
2. Causes include chronic friction and irritation to a skin area and exposure to ultraviolet rays
3. Diagnosis is confirmed by a skin biopsy that is positive for **cancer** cells

B. Assessment
1. Change in color, size, or shape of pre-existing lesion
2. Pruritus
3. Local soreness
4. Lesions
   a. A waxy nodule
   b. An irregular, circular bordered lesion with hues of tan, black, or blue
   c. A small, red, nodular lesion
   d. An oozing, bleeding, crusting lesion

C. Implementation
1. Instruct client to monitor for lesions that do not heal or that change characteristics
2. Instruct client to have moles or lesions removed that are subject to chronic irritation
3. Instruct client to avoid contact with chemical irritants
4. Use sun-screening lotions and layered clothing when outdoors
5. Assist with surgical excision of the lesion as prescribed

◆ XI. Leukemia (Box 49–5)

A. Description
1. **Malignant** exacerbation in the number of leukocytes, usually at an immature stage, in the bone marrow
2. May be acute, with a sudden onset and short duration, or chronic, with a slow onset and persistent symptoms over a period of years
3. Affects the bone marrow, causing anemia, leukopenia, the production of immature cells, thrombocytopenia, and a decline in immunity
4. The cause is unknown and appears to involve gene damage of cells, leading to the transformation of cells from a normal state to a **malignant** state
5. Risk factors include genetic, viral, immunological, and environmental factors and exposure to radiation, chemicals, and medications

◆ B. Assessment
1. Anorexia, fatigue, weakness, weight loss
2. Anemia
3. Nosebleeds
4. Increased menstrual flow

> **BOX 49–5. Classification of Leukemia**
>
> **ACUTE LYMPHOCYTIC LEUKEMIA (ALL)**
> Mostly lymphoblasts present in bone marrow
> Age of onset is less than 15 years
>
> **ACUTE MYELOGENOUS LEUKEMIA (AML)**
> Mostly myeloblasts present in bone marrow
> Age of onset is between 15 and 39 years
>
> **CHRONIC MYELOGENOUS LEUKEMIA (CML)**
> Mostly granulocytes present in bone marrow
> Age of onset after 50 years of age
>
> **CHRONIC LYMPHOCYTIC LEUKEMIA (CLL)**
> Mostly lymphocytes present in bone marrow
> Age of onset is after 50 years of age

5. Bleeding from the gums
6. Rectal bleeding
7. Hematuria
8. Petechiae
9. Prolonged bleeding after minor abrasions or lacerations
10. Elevated temperature
11. Lymphadenopathy and splenomegaly
12. Palpitations and tachycardia
13. Orthostatic hypotension
14. Pallor and dyspnea on exertion
15. Headache
16. Bone pain and joint swelling
17. Normal, elevated, or reduced WBC count
18. Decreased hemoglobin and hematocrit levels
19. Decreased platelet count
20. Positive bone marrow biopsy identifying leukemic blast phase cells

C. Infection
1. A major cause of death in the immunosuppressed client
2. Can occur through autocontamination or cross-contamination
3. Common sites of infection are the skin, respiratory tract, and GI tract
4. Initiate protective isolation procedures
5. Frequent and thorough handwashing
6. Ensure that anyone entering the client's room is wearing a mask
7. Strict aseptic technique for all procedures
8. Keep supplies for the client separate from supplies for other clients
9. Limit the number of caregivers entering the client's room
10. Maintain the client in a private room
11. Place the client in a room with high-efficiency particulate air (HEPA) filtration or a laminar air flow system if possible
12. Reduce exposure to environmental organisms by eliminating raw fruits and

vegetables and fresh flowers and by not leaving standing water in the client's room

13. Be sure that the client's room is cleaned daily
14. Assist the client with daily bathing, using an antimicrobial soap
15. Assist the client to perform oral hygiene frequently
16. Use strict aseptic technique with IV administration, changing IV tubing every 48 hours
17. Initiate a bowel program to prevent constipation and prevent rectal trauma
18. Avoid invasive procedures such as injections, rectal temperatures, and urinary catheterization
19. Assess for signs and symptoms of infection
20. Change wound dressings daily, and inspect wounds for redness, swelling, or drainage
21. Assess urine for color and cloudiness
22. Assess skin and oral mucous membranes for signs of infection
23. Auscultate lung sounds, and encourage the client to cough and deep breathe
24. Monitor temperature, pulse, and blood pressure
25. Monitor WBC and neutrophil count
26. Notify physician if signs of infection are present, and prepare to obtain specimens for culture of open lesions, urine, and sputum
27. Administer prescribed antibiotic, antifungal, and antiviral medication as prescribed
28. Instruct client to avoid crowds and those with infections
29. Instruct clients that neither they nor their household contacts should receive immunization with a live virus

D. Bleeding
1. During the period of greatest bone marrow suppression (the **nadir**), the platelet count may be extremely low, less than 10,000/mm³
2. The client is at risk for bleeding when the platelet count falls below 50,000/mm³, and spontaneous bleeding frequently occurs when the platelet count is lower than 20,000/mm³
3. Clients with platelet counts below 20,000/mm³ may need a platelet transfusion
4. For clients with severe blood loss, packed red blood cells (RBC) may be prescribed
5. Monitor laboratory values
6. Examine the client for signs and symptoms of bleeding
7. Handle the client gently
8. Measure abdominal girth, which can indicate internal hemorrhage
9. Instruct the client to use a soft toothbrush and avoid dental floss
10. Instruct the client to use an electric razor only for shaving
11. Provide soft foods that are cool to warm in temperature

12. Avoid injections if possible to prevent trauma to the skin and bleeding
13. Apply firm and gentle pressure to a needlestick site for at least 10 minutes
14. Pad side rails and sharp corners of the bed and furniture
15. Discourage the client from engaging in activities involving the use of sharp objects
16. Instruct the client to avoid constrictive or tight clothing
17. Use caution when taking blood pressures to prevent skin injury
18. Instruct the client to avoid blowing the nose
19. Avoid rectal suppositories, enemas, and thermometers
20. Examine all body fluids and excrement for the presence of blood
21. If the female client is menstruating, count the number of pads or tampons used
22. Instruct client to avoid NSAIDs and products that contain aspirin
23. Administer blood products as prescribed

E. Fatigue and nutrition
1. Assist the client in selecting a well-balanced diet
2. Provide small meals that require little chewing
3. Assist the client in self-care and mobility activities
4. Allow adequate rest periods during care
5. Do not perform activities unless they are essential
6. Administer blood products as prescribed

F. Chemotherapy
1. Monitor for severe bone marrow suppression
2. Monitor for infection and bleeding
3. Protect the client from life-threatening infections
4. Monitor for nausea, vomiting, and diarrhea
5. Assess oral mucous membranes for stomatitis
6. Monitor for renal, hepatic, and cardiac toxicity
7. Instruct the client in signs and symptoms to monitor for following chemotherapy and when to notify the physician
8. Inform client that hair loss may occur from chemotherapy

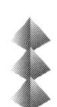

XII. Hodgkin's Disease

A. Description
1. A malignancy of the lymph nodes that originates in a single lymph node or a single chain of nodes
2. **Metastasis** occurs to other adjacent lymph structures and eventually invades nonlymphoid tissue
3. Usually involves lymph nodes, tonsils, spleen, and bone marrow and is characterized by the presence of Reed-Sternberg cells in the lymph nodes
4. Possible causes include viral infections and

BOX 49–6. Staging in Hodgkin's Disease

STAGE I

Involvement of a single lymph node region or an extralymphatic organ or site

STAGE II

Involvement of two or more lymph node regions on the same side of the diaphragm or localized involvement of an extralymphatic organ or site

STAGE III

Involvement of lymph node regions on both sides of the diaphragm or localized involvement of an extralymphatic organ or site, or spleen or both

STAGE IV

Diffuse or disseminated involvement of one or more extralymphatic organs with or without associated lymph node involvement

---

previous exposure to alkylating chemical agents
5. Prognosis is dependent on the stage of the disease (Box 49–6)

B. Assessment
   1. Persistent fever
   2. Night sweats
   3. Loss of appetite and significant weight loss
   4. Fatigue and weakness
   5. Pruritus
   6. Anemia and thrombocytopenia
   7. Enlarged lymph nodes, spleen, and liver
   8. Positive biopsy of lymph nodes, with cervical nodes most often affected first
   9. Presence of Reed-Sternberg cells
   10. Positive CT scan of liver and spleen

C. Implementation
   1. For stages I and II without mediastinal node involvement, the treatment of choice is extensive external radiation of involved lymph node regions
   2. With more extensive disease, radiation along with multiagent chemotherapy is utilized (Box 49–7)
   3. Monitor for side effects related to chemotherapy or radiation
   4. Monitor for drug-induced pancytopenia, which increases the risk for infection, bleeding, and anemia
   5. Monitor for signs of infection and bleeding
   6. Protect client from infection

BOX 49–7. MOPP Therapy for Hodgkin's Disease

Mechlorethamine (Mustargen)
Vincristine sulfate (Oncovin)
Procarbazine (Matulane)
Prednisone

---

7. Provide safe, hazard-free environment
8. Monitor for nausea and vomiting and administer antiemetics as prescribed
9. Monitor for skin irritation and breakdown due to radiation therapy
10. Discuss the possibility of sterility with the male client receiving radiation and inform the client of options related to sperm banks

XIII. Multiple Myeloma

A. Description
   1. A **malignant** proliferation of plasma cells and tumors within the bone
   2. Causes destruction to bone tissue, decreased production of immunoglobulin and antibodies, and increased levels of uric acid and calcium, which can lead to renal failure
   3. The cause is unknown

B. Assessment
   1. Bone (skeletal) pain, especially in the pelvis, spine, and ribs
   2. Weakness and fatigue
   3. Signs of respiratory infection
   4. Anemia
   5. Elevated temperature
   6. Elevated calcium and uric acid levels
   7. Decreased platelet count
   8. Bone fractures
   9. Spinal cord compression and paraplegia
   10. Renal failure

C. Implementation
   1. Monitor for signs of infection
   2. Protect the client from infection
   3. Force fluids, up to 3 to 4 liters a day, to maintain an adequate output
   4. Administer IVs and diuretics as prescribed to increase renal excretion of calcium
   5. Encourage ambulation to prevent renal problems and to slow down bone resorption
   6. Provide skeletal support during moving, turning, and ambulating to prevent pathological fractures
   7. Provide a hazard-free environment
   8. Monitor for signs of bleeding, infection, and skeletal fractures
   9. Administer chemotherapy as prescribed
   10. Administer analgesics as prescribed to control pain
   11. Administer antibiotics as prescribed for infection
   12. Instruct the client to recognize signs and symptoms of infection

XIV. Testicular Cancer

A. Description
   1. Arises from germinal epithelium from the sperm-producing germ cells or from nongerminal epithelium from other structures in the testicles
   2. Most often occurs between ages of 20 and 40 years

3. **Metastasis** occurs to the lung, liver, bone, and adrenal glands (Box 49–8)
B. Prevention: Routine testicular self-examination
C. Assessment
   1. Painless testicular swelling
   2. Dragging sensation in scrotum
   3. Abdominal masses
   4. Palpable lymphadenopathy
   5. Gynecomastia
   6. Infertility
   7. Late signs include back or bone pain and respiratory symptoms
D. Implementation
   1. Administer chemotherapy as prescribed
   2. Prepare the client for radiation therapy as prescribed
   3. Prepare the client for unilateral orchiectomy if prescribed for diagnosis and primary surgical management
   4. Prepare the client for radical retroperitoneal lymph node dissection if prescribed to stage the disease and reduce tumor volume so that chemotherapy and radiation therapy are more effective
   5. Discuss reproduction, sexuality, and fertility information and options with the client
   6. Identify with the client such reproductive options as sperm storage, donor insemination, and adoption
E. Postoperative implementation
   1. Monitor vital signs
   2. Monitor for signs of bleeding
   3. Monitor for signs of wound infection
   4. Monitor intake and output (I&O)
   5. Notify the physician if chills, fever, increasing pain or tenderness at the incision site, or drainage of the incision occurs
   6. Instruct clients that they may resume normal activities except for lifting objects heavier than 20 pounds or stair climbing
   7. Instruct the client to perform monthly testicular self-examination on the remaining testis

XV. Cervical Cancer

A. Description
   1. Preinvasive **cancer** is limited to the cervix (Box 49–9)
   2. Invasive **cancer** is in the cervix and other pelvic structures

---

BOX 49–9. Preinvasive Cancers

CERVICAL INTRAEPITHELIAL NEOPLASIA (CIN)

CIN I—Mild dysplasia
CIN II—Moderate dysplasia
CIN III—Severe dysplasia to cancer in situ (CIS)

---

3. **Metastasis** is usually confined to the pelvis, but distant **metastasis** occurs through lymphatic spread
4. **Premalignant** changes are described on a continuum from dysplasia, which is the earliest premalignancy change, to **carcinoma in situ** (CIS), the most advanced **premalignant** change
B. Precipitating factors
   1. Low socioeconomic groups
   2. Early first marriage
   3. Early and frequent intercourse
   4. Multiple sex partners
   5. High parity
   6. Poor hygiene
C. Assessment
   1. Painless vaginal bleeding postmenstrually and postcoitally
   2. Foul-smelling or serosanguineous vaginal discharge
   3. Pelvic, lower back, leg, or groin pain
   4. Anorexia and weight loss
   5. Leakage of urine and feces from the vagina
   6. Dysuria
   7. Hematuria
   8. Cytological changes on Papanicolaou test
D. Implementation (Box 49–10)
E. Laser therapy
   1. Used when all boundaries of the lesion are visible during colposcopic examination
   2. Energy from the beam is absorbed by fluid in the tissues, causing them to vaporize
   3. Minimal bleeding is associated with the procedure
   4. Slight vaginal discharge is expected following the procedure, and healing occurs in 6 to 12 weeks
F. Cryosurgery
   1. Freezing of the tissues by a probe with subsequent necrosis

---

BOX 49–8. Types of Testicular Cancer

GERMINAL TUMORS

Seminomas
Nonseminomas

NONGERMINAL TUMORS

Interstitial cell tumors
Androblastoma

BOX 49–10. Treatment for Cervical Cancer

NONSURGICAL	SURGICAL
External radiation	Conization
Internal radiation implants (intracavitary)	Hysterectomy
	Pelvic exenteration
Chemotherapy	
Laser therapy	
Cryosurgery	

2. No anesthesia is required, although cramping may occur during the procedure
3. A heavy, watery discharge will occur for several weeks following the procedure
4. Instruct the client to avoid intercourse and the use of tampons while the discharge is present

G. Conization
1. A cone-shaped area of cervix is removed
2. Performed in women who desire further childbearing
3. Long-term follow-up care is needed as new lesions can develop
4. The risks of the procedure include hemorrhage, uterine perforation, incompetent cervix, cervical stenosis, and preterm labor in future pregnancies

H. Hysterectomy
1. Description
   a. For microinvasive **cancer** if childbearing is not desired
   b. A vaginal approach is most commonly performed
   c. A radical hysterectomy and bilateral lymph node dissection may be performed for **cancer** that has spread beyond the cervix but not to the pelvic wall
2. Postoperative implementation
   a. Monitor vital signs
   b. Assist with coughing and deep-breathing exercises
   c. Assist with range of motion (ROM) exercises and provide early ambulation
   d. Apply antiembolism stockings as prescribed
   e. Monitor I&O and hydration status
   f. Monitor bowel sounds
   g. Monitor vaginal bleeding
   h. Note that more than one saturated pad per hour may indicate excessive bleeding
   i. Assess incision site for signs of infection
   j. Monitor Foley catheter drainage
   k. Administer pain medication as prescribed
   l. Instruct client to avoid and limit stair climbing for 1 month and to avoid tub baths and sitting for long periods
   m. Avoid strenuous activity or lifting anything weighing more than 10 to 20 pounds
   n. Instruct client to consume foods that aid in the healing
   o. Instruct client to avoid sexual intercourse for 3 to 6 weeks
   p. Instruct client in the signs associated with complications

I. Pelvic exenteration (Box 49–11)
1. Description
   a. A radical surgical procedure performed for recurrent **cancer** if there is no evidence of tumor outside the pelvis and no lymph node involvement
   b. When the bladder is removed, an ileal conduit will be created and located on the right side of the abdomen to divert urine

---

BOX 49–11. Types of Pelvic Exenteration

ANTERIOR
Removal of uterus, ovaries, fallopian tubes, vagina, bladder, urethra, pelvic lymph nodes

POSTERIOR
Removal of uterus, ovaries, fallopian tubes, descending colon, rectum, and anal canal

TOTAL
Combination of anterior and posterior

---

   c. A colostomy may need to be created and will be located of the left side of the abdomen for the passage of feces
2. Postoperative implementation
   a. Monitor vital signs
   b. Monitor for atelectasis and pneumonia
   c. Assist with coughing and deep-breathing exercises
   d. Monitor for hemorrhage, shock, and deep vein thrombosis
   e. Apply antiembolism stockings
   f. Administer prophylactic heparin as prescribed
   g. Monitor bowel sounds
   h. Monitor I&O and IVs and for signs of dehydration
   i. Monitor incision site for infection
   j. Administer perineal irrigations with half-strength NS and hydrogen peroxide as prescribed
   k. Provide sitz baths as prescribed
   l. Administer analgesics as prescribed for pain
   m. Instruct client to avoid strenuous activity for 6 months
   n. Instruct client that the perineal opening, if present, may drain for several months
   o. Instruct client in the care of the ileal conduit and colostomy
   p. Provide sexual counseling, as vaginal intercourse is not possible after anterior and total pelvic exenteration

XVI. Ovarian Cancer

A. Description
1. Grows rapidly, spreads fast, and is often bilateral
2. **Metastasis** occurs by direct spread to the organs in the pelvis, by distal spread through lymphatic drainage, or by peritoneal seeding
3. Prognosis is usually poor because the tumor is usually detected late
4. An exploratory laparotomy is performed to diagnose and stage the tumor

B. Assessment
1. Abdominal discomfort or swelling
2. GI disturbances
3. Dysfunctional vaginal bleeding

4. Abdominal mass
C. Implementation
   1. External radiation is used if the tumor has invaded other organs
   2. Chemotherapy is used postoperatively for all stages of ovarian **cancer**
   3. Intraperitoneal chemotherapy, which involves the instillation of chemotherapy into the abdominal cavity
   4. Immunotherapy, which alters the immunological response of the ovary and promotes tumor resistance
   5. Total abdominal hysterectomy and bilateral salpingo-oophorectomy

XVII. Endometrial Cancer

A. Description
   1. A slow-growing tumor associated with the menopausal years
   2. **Metastasis** occurs through the lymphatic system to the ovaries and pelvis; via the blood to the lungs, liver, and bone, or intra-abdominal to the peritoneal cavity
B. Precipitating factors
   1. History of uterine polyps
   2. Nulliparity
   3. Polycystic ovary disease
   4. Estrogen stimulation
   5. Late menopause
   6. Family history
C. Assessment
   1. Postmenopausal bleeding
   2. Watery, serosanguineous discharge
   3. Low back, pelvic, or abdominal pain
   4. Enlarged uterus in advanced stages
D. Nonsurgical implementation
   1. External radiation or internal radiation used alone or in combination with surgery, depending on the stage of **cancer**
   2. Chemotherapy to treat advanced and recurrent disease
   3. Progestational therapy with medroxyprogesterone (Depo-Provera) or megestrol acetate (Megace) for estrogen-dependent tumors
   4. Tamoxifen (Nolvadex), an antiestrogen, may also be prescribed
E. Surgical implementation: Total abdominal hysterectomy and bilateral salpingo-oophorectomy

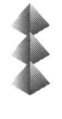 XVIII. Breast Cancer

A. Description
   1. Classified as invasive when it penetrates the tissue surrounding the mammary duct and grows in an irregular pattern
   2. **Metastasis** occurs via lymph nodes
   3. Common sites of metastatic disease are bone, lungs, brain, and liver
   4. Diagnosis is made by breast biopsy through a needle aspiration or by surgical removal of the tumor with microscopic examination made for **malignant** cells
B. Precipitating factors
   1. Family history
   2. Early menarche and late menopause
   3. Previous **cancer** of breast, uterus, or ovaries
   4. Nulliparity
   5. Obesity
   6. High-dose radiation exposure to the chest
C. Assessment
   1. Mass felt during BSE
   2. Mass usually felt in the upper outer quadrant or beneath the nipple
   3. A fixed, irregular, nonencapsulated mass
   4. A painless mass except in the very late stages
   5. Nipple retraction or elevation
   6. Asymmetry, with affected breast being higher
   7. Bloody or clear nipple discharge
   8. Skin dimpling, retraction, or ulceration
   9. Skin edema or peau d'orange skin
   10. Axillary lymphadenopathy
   11. Lymphedema of affected arm
   12. Symptoms of bone or lung **metastasis**
   13. Presence of lesion on mammography
D. Prevention: Monthly BSE
E. Nonsurgical implementation
   1. Chemotherapy
   2. Radiation therapy
   3. Hormonal manipulation via the use of estrogen in postmenopausal women or tamoxifen (Nolvadex) for estrogen receptor–positive tumors
F. Surgical implementation
   1. Surgical breast procedures (Box 49–12)
   2. Oophorectomy for estrogen receptive–positive tumors
   3. Ablative therapy with adrenalectomy or chemical ablation, which blocks production of cortisol, androstenedione, and aldosterone
G. Postoperative implementation
   1. Monitor vital signs
   2. Position in semi-Fowler's on the back or unaffected side, with the affected arm elevated above the level of the heart to promote drainage and prevent lymphedema
   3. Turn client only to back and unaffected side
   4. Encourage coughing and deep breathing
   5. If a Hemovac is in place, maintain suction and record the amount of drainage and drainage characteristics
   6. Assess operative sites for swelling or the presence of fluid collection under the skin flaps
   7. Monitor for signs of infection
   8. Place a sign above the bed stating, "NO IVs, NO IMs, NO BPs, NO VENIPUNCTURES"
   9. Provide the use of a pressure sleeve as prescribed if edema is severe
   10. Administer diuretics as prescribed for severe lymphedema

---

BOX 49–12. Surgical Breast Procedures

LUMPECTOMY

Excision and removal of the tumor
Lymph node dissection may also be performed

SIMPLE MASTECTOMY

Removal of the breast with no lymph node removal
The breast tissue is removed, but the anterior skin, axillary lymph nodes, and underlying muscles are left intact

PARTIAL MASTECTOMY

The tumor is removed along with a small amount of surrounding tissue

MODIFIED RADICAL MASTECTOMY

The breast tissue and nipple are totally removed, with partial excision of the skin, lymph nodes, and surrounding tissue

RADICAL MASTECTOMY

All breast tissue and nipple are removed, along with partial removal of the overlying skin, chest muscles, axillary lymph tissue, and nearby adipose tissue

---

11. Provide a low-salt diet as prescribed for severe lymphedema
12. Monitor the site for restriction of dressing, impaired sensation, color changes of skin
13. Consult with the physician and physical therapists regarding the appropriate exercise program
14. Assist with exercise as prescribed to decrease lymphedema and muscle weakness
15. See Box 49–13

XIX. Gastric Cancer

A. Description
   1. An abnormal **malignant** growth in the stomach
   2. Risk factors include a diet high in complex carbohydrates, grains, and salt and low in fresh, green leafy vegetables and fresh fruit; smoking; alcohol; the use of nitrates; and a history of gastric ulcers
   3. Complications include hemorrhage, obstruction, **metastasis**, and dumping syndrome
   4. The goal of treatment is to remove the tumor and provide a nutritional program
B. Assessment
   1. Fatigue
   2. Anorexia and weight loss
   3. Nausea and vomiting
   4. Indigestion and epigastric discomfort
   5. A sensation of pressure in the stomach
   6. Dysphagia
   7. Anemia
   8. Ascites

9. Palpable mass
C. Implementation
   1. Monitor vital signs
   2. Monitor hemoglobin and hematocrit and administer blood transfusion as prescribed
   3. Monitor weight
   4. Assess nutritional status
   5. Encourage small, bland, easily digestible meals with vitamin and mineral supplements
   6. Administer pain medication as prescribed
   7. Prepare the client for chemotherapy or radiation therapy as prescribed
   8. Prepare the client for surgical resection of the tumor as prescribed (Box 49–14)
D. Postoperative implementation
   1. Monitor vital signs
   2. Fowler's position for comfort and to promote drainage
   3. Administer fluids and electrolyte replacement IVs as prescribed
   4. Maintain NPO status as prescribed for 1 to 3 days until peristalsis returns
   5. Monitor nasogastric (NG) suction
   6. Do not irrigate or remove the NG tube
   7. Assist physician with NG irrigation or removal of NG tube
   8. Monitor I&O
   9. Assess bowel sounds
   10. Advance the diet from NPO to sips of clear water to six small bland meals a day as prescribed

---

BOX 49–13. Client Instructions Following Mastectomy

- Avoid overuse of the arm during the first few months
- To prevent lymphedema, keep the affected arm elevated
- Incision care with lanolin to soften and prevent wound contracture
- Encourage use of Reach for Recovery volunteers
- Encourage the client to perform breast self-examination on the remaining breast
- Protect affected hand and arm
- Avoid strong sunlight to the arm
- Do not let the arm hang dependent
- Do not carry a pocketbook or anything heavy over the affected arm
- Avoid trauma, cuts, bruises, or burns to the affected side
- No constricted clothing or jewelry on affected side
- Wear gloves when gardening
- Use oven mitts when cooking
- Use a thimble when sewing
- Apply lanolin hand cream several times daily
- Use cream cuticle remover
- Call the physician if signs of inflammation occur in the affected arm
- Wear Medic-Alert bracelet stating lymphedema arm

> **BOX 49–14. Surgical Implementation for Gastric Cancer**
>
> **TOTAL GASTRECTOMY**
> Also called esophagojejunostomy
> Removal of the stomach with attachment of the esophagus to the jejunum or duodenum
>
> **VAGOTOMY**
> Surgical division of the vagus nerve to eliminate the vagal impulses that stimulate hydrochloric acid secretion in the stomach
>
> **GASTRIC RESECTION**
> Also called antrectomy
> Involves removal of the lower half of the stomach and usually includes a vagotomy
>
> **BILLROTH I**
> Also called gastroduodenostomy
> Partial gastrectomy, and the remaining segment is anastomosed to the duodenum
>
> **BILLROTH II**
> Also called gastrojejunostomy
> Partial gastrectomy, with remaining segment anastomosed to the jejunum
>
> **PYLOROPLASTY**
> Enlarges the pylorus to prevent or decrease pyloric obstruction, thereby enhancing gastric emptying

11. Monitor for complications of hemorrhage, dumping syndrome, diarrhea, hypoglycemia, and vitamin B_{12} deficiency

XX. Intestinal Tumors

A. Description
   1. **Malignant** lesions that develop in the cells lining the bowel wall or develop as polyps in the colon or rectum
   2. Complications include bowel perforation with peritonitis, abscess and/or fistula formation, frank hemorrhage, and complete intestinal obstruction
   3. Metastasis occurs via the circulatory or lymphatic system, or by direct extension to other areas in the colon or other organs
B. Assessment
   1. Blood in stools
   2. Anorexia
   3. Vomiting and weight loss
   4. Malaise
   5. Anemia
   6. Abnormal stools
      a. Ascending colon tumor: Diarrhea
      b. Descending colon tumor: Constipation or some diarrhea, or flat, ribbon-like stool due to a partial obstruction
      c. Rectal tumor: Alternating constipation and diarrhea

7. Guarding or abdominal distention
8. Abdominal mass (a late sign)
9. Cachexia (a late sign)
C. Implementation
   1. Monitor for signs of complications, which include bowel perforation with peritonitis, abscess and/or fistula formation, frank hemorrhage, and complete intestinal obstruction
   2. Monitor for signs of intestinal perforation, including low blood pressure (BP), rapid and weak pulse, distended abdomen, and elevated temperature
   3. Monitor for signs of intestinal obstruction, which may include vomiting (may be fecal contents), pain, constipation, and abdominal distention
   4. Note that an early sign of intestinal obstruction includes increased peristaltic activity, which produces an increase in bowel sounds; as the obstruction progresses, hypoactive sounds are heard
   5. Prepare for radiation preoperatively to facilitate surgical resection, and postoperatively to decrease the risk of recurrence or to reduce pain, hemorrhage, bowel obstruction, or **metastasis**
   6. Chemotherapy is used postoperatively to assist in the control of symptoms and spread of the disease
D. Surgical implementation: Bowel resection and creation of a colostomy or ileostomy
E. Colostomy/ileostomy
   1. Preoperative implementation
      a. Consult with the enterostomal therapist to assist in identifying optimal placement of the ostomy
      b. Instruct client to eat a low-residue diet for a day or two prior to surgery as prescribed
      c. Administer intestinal antiseptics and antibiotics as prescribed to decrease the bacterial content of the colon and to reduce the risk of infection from the surgical procedure
      d. Administer laxatives and enemas as prescribed
   2. Postoperative colostomy
      a. Place a petroleum jelly gauze over the stoma to keep it moist, followed by a dry sterile dressing if a pouch system is not in place
      b. Place a pouched system on the stoma as soon as possible
      c. Monitor the stoma for size, unusual bleeding, or necrotic tissue
      d. Monitor for color changes in the stoma
      e. Note that the normal stoma color is red or pink, indicating high vascularity
      f. Note that a pale pink stoma indicates low hemoglobin and hematocrit levels, and a purple-black stoma indicates compromised circulation, requiring physician notification

g. Monitor the pouch system for proper fit and signs of leakage

h. Assess the functioning of the colostomy

i. Expect that stool is liquid immediately postoperative but becomes more solid depending on the area of the colostomy

j. Ascending colon colostomy: Expect liquid stool

k. Transverse colon colostomy: Expect loose to semiformed stool

l. Descending colon colostomy: Expect close to normal stool

m. Fecal matter should not be allowed to remain on the skin

n. Empty pouch when one third full

o. Administer analgesics and antibiotics as prescribed

p. Irrigate the perineal wound if prescribed and monitor for signs of infection

q. Instruct client to avoid foods that cause excess gas formation and odor

r. Instruct client on stoma care and irrigations as prescribed

s. Instruct client that normal activities may be resumed when approved by the physician

3. Postoperative ileostomy

a. Healthy stoma is red

b. Color change to dark blue or black should be reported to the physician

c. Postoperative drainage will be dark green and progress to yellow as the client begins to eat

d. Stool is liquid

e. Risk for dehydration and electrolyte imbalance

f. Do not give suppositories through the ileostomy

XXI. Lung Cancer

A. Description

1. **Malignant** tumor of the lung that may be primary or metastatic

2. The lungs are a common target for **metastasis** from other organs

3. Bronchiogenic carcinoma spreads through direct extension and lymphatic dissemination

4. The four major types of lung **cancer** include small cell (oat cell), epidermal (squamous cell), adenocarcinoma, and large cell anaplastic carcinoma

5. Diagnosis is made by a chest radiograph, which will show a lesion or mass, and bronchoscopy and sputum studies, which will demonstrate a positive cytology for **cancer** cells

B. Causes

1. Cigarette smoking

2. Exposure to environmental pollutants

3. Exposure to occupational pollutants

C. Assessment

1. Cough

2. Dyspnea

3. Hoarseness

4. Hemoptysis

5. Chest pain

6. Anorexia

7. Weakness

8. Weight loss

D. Implementation

1. Monitor vital signs

2. Assess breathing patterns and breath sounds and for signs of respiratory impairment

3. Assess for tracheal deviation

4. Administer analgesics as prescribed for pain management

5. Position client upright for ease in breathing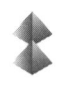

6. Administer oxygen as prescribed and humidification to moisten and loosen secretions

7. Monitor pulse oximetry

8. Provide respiratory treatments as prescribed

9. Administer bronchodilators and steroids as prescribed to decrease bronchospasm, inflammation, and edema

10. Provide a high-protein, high-calorie diet

11. Provide activity as tolerated, rest periods, and active and passive ROM exercises

12. Monitor for bleeding, infection, and electrolyte imbalance

E. Nonsurgical implementation

1. Radiation therapy for localized intrathoracic lung **cancers**

2. Chemotherapy to promote tumor regression

3. Immunotherapy directed at enhancing an effective response, which favorably affects the course of disease

4. Nonspecific immune therapy with bacille Calmette-Guérin vaccine (BCG) as prescribed

F. Surgical implementation

1. Laser therapy: To relieve endobronchial obstruction

2. Thoracotomy with pneumonectomy: Surgical removal of a lung for bronchiogenic carcinoma

3. Thoracotomy with lobectomy: Surgical removal of one lobe of the lung for tumors confined to a single lobe

4. Thoracotomy with segmental resection: Surgical removal of a lobe segment for clients unable to tolerate lobectomy or pneumonectomy

G. Preoperative implementation

1. Explain the potential postoperative need for chest tubes

2. Note that a chest tube is not inserted for a pneumonectomy, and the serum fluid that accumulates in the empty thoracic cavity eventually consolidates, preventing shifts of the mediastinum, heart, and remaining lung

H. Postoperative implementation

1. Monitor vital signs

2. Assess cardiac and respiratory status

3. Maintain chest tube drainage system, which will drain air and/or blood that accumulates in the pleural space

4. Monitor for the absence and presence of lung sounds

5. Assess chest tube insertion site for crepitus (subcutaneous air) and drainage

6. Administer oxygen as prescribed

7. Monitor pulse oximetry

8. Provide activity as tolerated

9. Encourage performance of ROM exercises of operative shoulder as prescribed

10. Maintain client position based on procedure performed (Box 49–15)

XXII. Laryngeal Cancer

A. Description
  1. A **malignant** tumor of the larynx
  2. Laryngeal **cancer** presents as **malignant** ulcerations with underlying filtration
  3. **Metastasis** to the lung is common
  4. Diagnosis is made by laryngoscopy and biopsy showing a positive cytology for **cancer** cells

B. Causes
  1. Cigarette smoking
  2. Alcohol abuse
  3. Exposure to environmental pollutants
  4. Exposure to radiation
  5. Voice strain

C. Assessment
  1. Persistent hoarseness
  2. Persistent sore throat
  3. Painless neck mass
  4. A feeling of a lump in the throat
  5. Burning sensation in the throat
  6. Dysphagia
  7. Change in voice quality
  8. Dyspnea
  9. Hemoptysis
  10. Weakness and weight loss
  11. Foul breath

D. Implementation
  1. Fowler's position to promote optimal air exchange
  2. Monitor respiratory status

---

3. Monitor for signs of aspiration of food and fluid

4. Provide activity as tolerated

5. Provide a high-calorie, high-vitamin, high-protein diet

6. Provide nutritional support via total parenteral nutrition (TPN), NG tube feedings, and gastrostomy as prescribed

7. Administer oxygen as prescribed

8. Provide respiratory treatments as prescribed

9. Administer analgesic as prescribed

E. Nonsurgical implementation
  1. Radiation therapy if the **cancer** is limited to a small area in one vocal cord
  2. Chemotherapy, which may be done in combination with radiation and surgery

F. Surgical implementation
  1. Small tumor excision or total laryngectomy: Performed for infiltrate tumors that involve vocal cord paralysis and for tumors that do not respond to radiation therapy
  2. Radical neck dissection: Performed when lymph node involvement is present and involves a laryngectomy and tracheostomy

G. Preoperative implementation
  1. Establish methods of communication for the client
  2. Encourage the client to express feelings about changes in body image and loss of voice
  3. Describe the rehabilitation program and information about the tracheotomy and suctioning

H. Postoperative implementation
  1. Monitor vital signs
  2. Assess respiratory status
  3. Position client in high Fowler's position
  4. Monitor airway patency and provide frequent suctioning to remove bloody secretions
  5. Maintain mechanical ventilator support or a tracheostomy collar with humidification as prescribed
  6. Monitor pulse oximetry
  7. Maintain surgical drains in the neck area if present
  8. Observe for hemorrhage and edema in the neck
  9. Monitor IV fluids or TPN until nutrition is administered via an NG, gastrostomy, or jejunostomy tube
  10. Provide oral hygiene
  11. Assess gag and cough reflex and ability to swallow
  12. Increase intake in fluids as prescribed
  13. Increase activity, as tolerated
  14. Assess the color, amount, and consistency of sputum
  15. Provide stoma and laryngectomy care (Box 49–16)
  16. Provide consultation with speech and language pathologist as prescribed

---

BOX 49–15. Positioning Following Lung Surgery

PNEUMONECTOMY

Avoid complete lateral positioning because the mediastinum is no longer held in place on both sides by lung tissue

Extreme turning may cause mediastinum shift and compression of the remaining lung

SEGMENTAL (WEDGE) RESECTION

Elevate the head of the bed 30 to 45 degrees and avoid positioning client on the operative side

---

BOX 49–16. Stoma Care Following Laryngectomy

- Teach the client clean suctioning technique
- Instruct client how to clean incision and provide stoma care
- Protect neck from injury
- Avoid swimming, showering, and using aerosol sprays
- Demonstrate ways to prevent debris from entering the stoma
- Instruct client to wear a stoma guard to shield the stoma
- Advise client to wear loose-fitting, high-collar clothing to hide the stoma
- Advise client to increase humidity in the home
- Instruct in ROM exercises for arms, shoulders, and neck daily as prescribed
- Avoid exposure to people with infections
- Alternate rest periods with activity
- Increase fluid intake to 3000 mL/day
- Advise client to obtain a Medic-Alert bracelet

---

17. Prepare the client for rehabilitation and speech therapy through the use of an artificial larynx followed by esophageal speech
18. Reinforce method of communication established preoperatively

XXIII. Cancer of the Prostate

A. Description
   1. A slow-growing **cancer** of the prostate gland, which is usually an androgen-dependent type of adenocarcinoma
   2. The risk increases in men with each decade after age 50 years
   3. **Metastasis** occurs via direct invasion of surrounding tissues, spread through the blood stream and lymphatics, and via **metastasis** to the bony pelvis and spine
   4. Bone **metastasis** is a concern
B. Assessment
   1. Asymptomatic in early stages
   2. Hard, pea-sized nodule palpated on rectal examination
   3. Hematuria
   4. Late symptoms include weight loss, urinary obstruction, and pain radiating from the lumbosacral area down the leg
   5. Prostate-specific antigen (PSA) test does not necessarily indicate malignancy and is used routinely to monitor the client's response to therapy
   6. Elevated serum acid phosphatase level indicates spread
C. Nonsurgical implementation
   1. Prepare the client for hormone manipulation therapy as prescribed
   2. Administer leuprolide acetate (Lupron), flutamide (Eulexin), or diethylstilbestrol (DES)

as prescribed to slow the rate of growth of the tumor
   3. Prepare the client for radiation (internal or external), which may be prescribed alone or in conjunction with surgery and may be prescribed pre- or postoperatively to reduce the lesion and limit **metastasis**
   4. Prepare the client for the administration of chemotherapy in hormone-resistant tumors
D. Surgical implementation
   1. Prepare the client for orchiectomy if prescribed, which will limit the production of testosterone
   2. Prepare the client for TUR or prostatectomy if prescribed
E. Transurethral resection (TUR)
   1. Insertion of a scope into the urethra to excise prostatic tissue
   2. Bleeding is common following TUR, and monitoring for hemorrhage is an important nursing intervention
   3. A continuous bladder irrigation (CBI) will be prescribed postoperatively to maintain the urine at a pink color
   4. Bladder spasms are common following surgery, and antispasmodics for the bladder spasms may be prescribed
   5. Dribbling or incontinence may occur postoperatively, and it is important for the nurse to instruct the client to monitor for recurrence
   6. Sterility may or may not occur following the surgical procedure
F. Suprapubic prostatectomy
   1. Removal of the prostate by an abdominal incision with a bladder incision
   2. The client will have an abdominal dressing that may drain copious amounts of urine, and the abdominal dressing will need to be changed frequently
   3. Severe hemorrhage is possible, and monitoring for blood loss is an important nursing intervention
   4. Bladder spasms are common, and antispasmodics may be prescribed for the bladder spasms
   5. CBI will be prescribed and administered to keep the urine pink in color
   6. A longer healing process is involved compared with the TUR
   7. Sterility occurs with this procedure
G. Retropubic prostatectomy
   1. Removal of the prostate gland by a low abdominal incision without opening the bladder
   2. Less bleeding occurs with this procedure, as compared with suprapubic, and the client experiences fewer bladder spasms
   3. There is minimal abdominal drainage
   4. CBI may be used
   5. Sterility occurs with this procedure

H. Perineal prostatectomy
  1. The prostate gland is removed through an incision made between the scrotum and anus
  2. Minimal bleeding occurs with this procedure
  3. The client needs to be monitored closely for infection, as the risk of infection is increased with this type of prostatectomy
  4. Urinary incontinence is common
  5. The procedure causes sterility
  6. It is important to teach the client how to perform perineal exercises
  7. It is important to avoid inserting rectal tubes and taking the temperature rectally
  8. The administration of enemas also needs to be avoided
I. Postoperative implementation (Box 49–17)
  1. Monitor vital signs
  2. Monitor urinary output
  3. Increase fluids to 2400 to 3000 mL a day unless contraindicated
  4. Ambulate client as early as possible and as soon as the urine begins to clear
  5. Monitor urine for hemorrhage and clots
  6. Monitor for arterial bleeding as evidenced by bright red urine with numerous clots, and if it occurs, increase CBI and notify the physician immediately
  7. Monitor for venous bleeding as evidenced by a burgundy-colored urine output; if it occurs, inform the physician, who may apply traction on the catheter
  8. Monitor hemoglobin and hematocrit levels
  9. Expect red to light-pink urine for 24 hours, turning to amber in 3 days
  10. Inform client that a continuous feeling of an urge to void is normal
  11. Instruct client to avoid attempts to void around the catheter as it will cause bladder spasms
  12. Administer antibiotics, analgesics, stool softeners, and antispasmodics as prescribed
  13. Monitor the three-way Foley catheter, which will have a 30- to 45-mL retention balloon
  14. Maintain CBI with NS or prescribed solution to keep the catheter free of obstruction
J. Postoperative suprapubic prostatectomy
  1. Monitor suprapubic and Foley catheter drainage

BOX 49–17. Postoperative Care Following TUR

CONTINUOUS BLADDER IRRIGATION (CBI)

A three-way (lumen) irrigation to decrease bleeding and to keep the bladder free from clots:
  One lumen for inflating balloon (30 mL)
  One lumen for outflow
  One lumen for instillation (inflow)

IMPLEMENTATION

- Maintain traction of the catheter if applied to prevent bleeding by pulling the catheter taut and taping it to the abdomen or thigh
- Instruct client to keep leg straight if traction is applied to catheter and taped to the thigh
- Catheter traction is not released without a physician's order
- Catheter traction is usually released after any bright red drainage has diminished
- Use NS or prescribed solution only, to prevent water intoxication
- Run the solution at a rate as prescribed to keep the urine pink
- Run the solution rapidly if bright red drainage or clots are present
- Run solution at about 40 gtt/min when bright red drainage clears
- If urinary catheter becomes obstructed, turn off CBI and irrigate catheter with 30 to 50 mL of normal saline if prescribed; notify physician if obstruction does not resolve
- Monitor for TUR syndrome or severe hyponatremia (water intoxication) caused by the excessive absorption of bladder irrigation
- Monitor for altered mental status, bradycardia, increased blood pressure, and confusion as indicative of signs of TUR syndrome
- Discontinue CBI and Foley catheter as prescribed, which is usually 24 to 48 hours postoperatively

- Monitor for continence and retention when the catheter is removed
- Inform client that some burning, frequency, and dribbling may occur following catheter removal
- Inform client that he may pass small clots and tissue debris for several days
- Inform client that he should be voiding 150 to 200 mL of clear yellow urine every 3 to 4 hours by 3 days postoperatively
- Teach client to avoid heavy lifting, stressful exercise, driving, Valsalva's maneuver, and sexual intercourse for 2 to 6 weeks to prevent strain, and to call the physician if bleeding occurs or there is a decrease in urinary stream
- Instruct client to drink 12 to 14 glasses of water each day, preferably before 8 P.M.
- Instruct client to avoid alcohol, caffeinated beverages, and spicy foods to avoid overstimulation of the bladder
- Instruct client that if urine becomes bloody, to rest and increase fluid intake, and that if the bleeding does not subside, to notify the physician

2. Monitor CBI if prescribed
3. Note that the Foley catheter will be removed 2 to 4 days postoperatively if the client has a suprapubic catheter
4. Clamp the suprapubic catheter after the Foley catheter is removed, and instruct the client to attempt to void
5. After the client has voided, assess the residual urine in the bladder by unclamping the suprapubic catheter
6. Prepare for removal of the suprapubic catheter when the client consistently empties the bladder and the residual urine is 75 mL or less
7. Monitor the suprapubic incision dressing, which may become saturated with urine, until the incision heals

K. Postoperative retropubic prostatectomy
1. Note that since the bladder is not entered, there is no urinary drainage on the abdominal dressing
2. Monitor for infection
3. Assess for urinary or purulent drainage on the dressing, and if this occurs notify the physician
4. Monitor for fever and increased pain, which may indicate an infection

L. Postoperative perineal prostatectomy
1. Note that the client will have an incision, which may or may not have a drain
2. Avoid rectal thermometers, rectal tubes, and enemas, as they may cause trauma and bleeding

XXIV. Bladder Cancer

A. Description
1. Papillomatous growths in the bladder urothelium that undergo **malignant** changes and that may infiltrate the bladder wall
2. Predisposing factors include cigarette smoking, exposure to industrial chemicals, and exposure to radiation
3. Common sites of **metastasis** include the liver, bones, and lungs
4. As the tumor progresses, it can extend into the rectum, vagina, other pelvic soft tissues, and retroperitoneal structures

B. Assessment
1. Gross, painless hematuria
2. Frequency
3. Urgency
4. Dysuria
5. Clot-induced obstruction
6. Bladder biopsy confirms diagnosis

C. Radiation
1. Most bladder **cancers** are poorly radiosensitive and require high doses of radiation
2. Radiation therapy is more acceptable for advanced disease that cannot be eradicated by surgery
3. Palliative radiation may be used to relieve

pain and bowel obstruction and control potential hemorrhage and leg edema secondary to venous or lymphatic obstruction
4. Intracavitary radiation may be prescribed, which protects adjacent tissue
5. External radiation combined with chemotherapy or surgery may be prescribed because the external radiation alone may be ineffective
6. Complications of radiation
   a. Abacterial cystitis
   b. Proctitis
   c. Fistula formation
   d. Ileitis or colitis
   e. Bladder ulceration and hemorrhage

D. Chemotherapy
1. Intravesical instillation
   a. An alkylating chemotherapeutic agent is instilled in the bladder
   b. This method provides a concentrated topical treatment with little systemic absorption
   c. Chemotherapeutic agents used are thiotepa, mitomycin, doxorubicin (Adriamycin), and cyclophosphamide or BCG
   d. The medication is injected into a urethral catheter and retained for 2 hours
   e. Following instillation, the client's position is rotated every 15 to 30 minutes, starting in the supine position to avoid lying on a full bladder
   f. After 2 hours, the client voids in a sitting position and is instructed to increase fluids to flush the bladder
   g. Treat the urine as a biohazard and send it to the radioisotope laboratory for monitoring
   h. For 6 hours following intravesical chemotherapy, disinfect the toilet with household bleach after voiding
2. Systemic chemotherapy
   a. Used to treat inoperable or late tumors
   b. Agents used include cisplatin (Platinol), doxorubicin, methotrexate, cyclophosphamide, and pyridoxine
3. Complications of chemotherapy
   a. Bladder irritation
   b. Hemorrhagic cystitis

E. Surgical implementation
1. TUR
   a. Local resection and fulguration (destruction of tissue by electrical current through electrodes placed in direct contact with the tissue)
   b. Performed for very early tumors for cure or for inoperable tumors for palliation
2. Partial cystectomy
   a. The removal of up to half the bladder
   b. Done in early tumors and for clients who cannot tolerate a radical cystectomy
   c. During the initial postoperative period,

bladder capacity is markedly reduced to about 60 mL; however, as the bladder tissue expands, the capacity increases to 200 to 400 mL

d. Maintenance of a continuous output of urine following surgery is critical to prevent bladder distention and stress on the suture line

e. A urethral and suprapubic catheter may be in place, and the suprapubic catheter may be left in place for 2 weeks until healing occurs

3. Cystectomy and urinary diversion

a. Removal of the bladder and urethra in women and the bladder, urethra, and usually prostate and seminal vesicles in men

b. When the bladder and urethra are removed, permanent urinary diversion is required

c. The surgery may be performed in two stages if the tumor is extensive, with the creation of the urinary diversion first and the cystectomy several weeks later

d. If a radical cystectomy is performed, lower extremity lymphedema may occur due to lymph node dissection, and impotence may occur in the male client

4. Ileal conduit

a. Also called ureteroileostomy or Bricker's procedure

b. Ureters are implanted into a segment of the ileum, with the formation of an abdominal stoma

c. The urine flows into the conduit and is continually propelled out through the stoma by peristalsis

d. The client is required to wear an appliance over the stoma to collect the urine

e. Complications include obstruction, pyelonephritis, leakage at the anastomosis site, stenosis, hydronephrosis, calculi, skin irritation and ulceration, and stomal defects

5. Kock pouch

a. A continent internal ileal reservoir created from a segment of the ileum and ascending colon

b. The ureters are implanted into the side of the reservoir, and a special nipple valve is constructed to attach the reservoir to the skin

c. Postoperatively, the client will have a 24 to 26 Foley catheter in place to drain urine continuously until the pouch has healed

d. The catheter is irrigated gently with normal saline to prevent obstruction from mucus or clots

e. Following removal of the catheter, the client is instructed how to self-catheterize

and drain the reservoir at 4- to 6-hour intervals

6. Indiana pouch

a. A continent reservoir is created from the ascending colon and terminal ileum, making a pouch larger than the Kock pouch

b. Postoperatively, the client will have a 24 to 26 Foley catheter in place to drain urine continuously until the pouch has healed

c. The catheter is irrigated gently with NS to prevent obstruction from mucus or clots

d. Following removal of the catheter, the client is instructed how to self-catheterize and drain the reservoir at 4- to 6-hour intervals

7. Creation of a neobladder

a. Similar to the creation of an internal reservoir, with the difference being that instead of emptying through an abdominal stoma, it empties through a pelvic outlet into the urethra

b. The client empties the neobladder by relaxing the external sphincter and creating abdominal pressure or by intermittent self-catheterization

8. Percutaneous nephrostomy or pyelostomy

a. Used when the **cancer** is inoperable, to prevent obstruction

b. Involves a percutaneous or surgical insertion of a nephrostomy tube into the kidney for drainage

c. Nursing implementation involves stabilizing the tube to prevent dislodgment and monitoring output

9. Ureterostomy

a. May be performed as a palliative procedure if the ureters are obstructed by the tumor

b. The ureters are attached to the surface of the abdomen, where the urine flows directly into a drainage appliance without a conduit

c. Potential problems include infection, skin irritation, and obstruction to urinary flow due to strictures at the opening

10. Vesicostomy

a. The bladder is sutured to the abdomen, and a stoma is created in the bladder wall

b. The bladder empties through the stoma

F. Preoperative implementation

1. Administer bowel preparation as prescribed, which may include clear liquid diet, laxatives and enemas, and antibiotics to lower the bacterial count in the bowel

2. Assist the surgeon and enterostomal nurse in selecting an appropriate skin site for creation of the abdominal stoma

3. Encourage the client to talk about feelings related to the stoma creation

G. Postoperative implementation
   1. Monitor vital signs
   2. Assess incision site
   3. Assess stoma (should be red and moist) every hour for the first 24 hours (Box 49–18)
   4. Note edema in the stoma, which may be present in the immediate postoperative period
   5. If the stoma appears dark and dusky, notify the physician immediately as this indicates necrosis
   6. Monitor for prolapse or retraction of the stoma
   7. Assess for return of bowel function

BOX 49–18. Urinary Stoma Care

- Instruct client to change appliance in the morning when urinary production is slowest
- Collect equipment, remove collection bag, use water or commercial solvent to loosen adhesive
- Hold a rolled gauze pad against stoma to collect and absorb urine during procedure
- Cleanse skin around stoma and under drainage bag with mild nonresidue soap and water
- Inspect skin for excoriation and instruct the client to prevent urine from coming in contact with the skin
- After skin is dry, apply skin adhesive around the appliance
- Instruct client to cut the stoma opening of the skin barrier just large enough to fit over the stoma (no more that 3 mm larger than the stoma)
- Instruct client that the stoma will shrink, requiring a smaller stoma opening on the skin barrier
- Apply skin barrier before attaching the pouch or faceplate
- Place appliance over stoma and secure in place
- Encourage self-care; teach client to use mirror
- Instruct client that the pouch may be drained by a bedside bag or leg bag, especially at night
- Instruct client to empty the urinary collection bag when it is one third to one half full to prevent pulling of the appliance and leakage
- Instruct client to check the appliance seal if perspiring occurs
- Instruct client to leave the urinary pouch in place as long as it is not leaking, and change every 5 to 7 days
- During appliance changes, leave the skin open to air as long as possible
- Use a nonkaraya gum product as urine erodes karaya gum
- To control odor, instruct the client to drink adequate fluids, to wash appliance thoroughly with soap and lukewarm water, to soak collection pouch in dilute white vinegar for 20 to 30 minutes, or to place a special deodorant tablet into the pouch while it is being worn
- Instruct clients who take baths to keep the level of the water below the stoma and avoid oily soaps
- If the client plans to shower, instruct client to direct the flow of water away from the stoma

---

BOX 49–19. Self-Irrigation and Catheterization of Stoma

IRRIGATION

Instruct client to wash hands and use clean technique

Instruct client to use a catheter and syringe to instill 60 mL of NS or water into the reservoir and to gently aspirate or allow to drain

Instruct client to irrigate until the drainage remains free of mucus but to be cautious not to overirrigate

CATHETERIZATION

Instruct client to wash hands and use a clean technique

Initially, the client is taught to insert a catheter every 2 to 3 hours to drain the reservoir; during each week thereafter, the interval is increased by 1 hour until the catheterization is done every 4 to 6 hours

Lubricate catheter well with water-soluble lubricant and instruct the client never to force the catheter into the reservoir

If resistance is met, instruct the client to pause, rotate the catheter, and apply gentle pressure to insert

Instruct the client to notify the physician if unable to insert catheter

When urine has stopped, instruct client to take several deep breaths and move the catheter in and out 2 to 3 inches to ensure that the pouch is empty

Instruct the client to withdraw the catheter slowly, and to pinch the catheter when withdrawn so that it does not leak urine

Instruct clients to carry catheterization supplies with them

---

8. Monitor for peristalsis, which will return in 3 to 4 days
9. Maintain NPO status as prescribed until bowel sounds return
10. Monitor urine flow, which is continuous (30 to 60 mL per hour) following surgery
11. Notify physician if the urine output is less than 30 mL an hour or if there is no urine output for more than 15 minutes
12. Ureteral stents or catheters may be in place for 2 to 3 weeks or until healing occurs
13. Maintain stability with catheters to prevent dislodgment
14. Following a continent diversion or creation of a neobladder, monitor urinary output closely and irrigate the catheter gently to prevent obstruction, as prescribed, with 60 mL of normal saline (Box 49–19)
15. Monitor for hematuria
16. Monitor for signs of peritonitis
17. Monitor for bladder distention following a partial cystectomy
18. Monitor for shock, hemorrhage, thrombophlebitis, and lower extremity lymphedema following a radical cystectomy

19. Monitor the urinary drainage pouch for leaks, and check skin integrity
20. Monitor the pH of the urine (do not place the dipstick in the stoma), as strong alkali urine can cause skin irritation and facilitate crystal formation
21. Instruct the client regarding the potential for urinary tract infection (UTI) or the development of calculi
22. Instruct the client to assess the skin for irritation and to monitor the urinary drainage pouch for any leakage
23. Encourage the client to express feelings about changes in body image, embarrassment, and sexual dysfunction

PRACTICE QUESTIONS

1. The nurse is instructing the client how to perform a testicular self-examination. Which instruction is correct?
   1 Examine the testicles while lying down
   2 The best time for the examination is after a shower
   3 Gently feel the testicle with one finger to feel for a growth
   4 Testicular examinations should be done at least every 6 months

2. The community nurse is conducting a health promotion program at a local school. Which of the following will not be identified as a risk factor associated with cancer?
   1 Viral factors
   2 Stress
   3 Low-fat and high-fiber diets
   4 Exposure to radiation

3. The client with cancer is receiving chemotherapy and develops thrombocytopenia. Which goal should be given the highest priority in the nursing plan of care?
   1 Ambulation three times daily
   2 Monitoring temperature
   3 Monitoring hemoglobin and hematocrit
   4 Monitoring for pathological fractures

4. The nurse assesses the oral cavity of a client with cancer and notes white patches on the mucous membranes. The nurse determines that this occurrence:
   1 Is common
   2 Is characteristic of a thrush infection
   3 Indicates that oral hygiene needs to be improved
   4 Suggests that the client is anemic

5. The nurse is monitoring the laboratory results of a client preparing to receive chemotherapy. The nurse determines that the WBC count is normal if which of the following results is present?
   1 3000 to 8000 mm³
   2 4000 to 9000 mm³
   3 7000 to 15,000 mm³
   4 2000 to 5000 mm³

6. The community health nurse is instructing a group of female clients about breast self-examination. The nurse instructs the clients to perform the examination:
   1 At the onset of menstruation
   2 One week after menstruation begins
   3 Every month during ovulation
   4 Weekly at the same time of day

7. During breast self-examination instruction, the nurse instructs the client to lie down and to examine the left breast. The nurse instructs the client that while examining the left breast she should place a pillow:
   1 Under the right shoulder
   2 Under the left shoulder
   3 Under the small of the back
   4 Under the right scapula

8. The nurse is teaching BSE to a client who had a hysterectomy. The most appropriate instruction regarding when the BSE should be performed is:
   1 7 to 10 days after menses
   2 Just before menses begins
   3 At ovulation time
   4 At a specific day of the month and on that same day every month thereafter

9. A client suspected of having an abdominal tumor is scheduled for a CT scan with dye injection. Which of the following is an accurate description of the scan?
   1 The test may be painful
   2 The dye injected may cause a warm, flushing sensation
   3 Fluids will be restricted following the test
   4 The test takes approximately 2 hours

10. The 32-year-old female client has a history of fibrocystic disorder of the breasts. The nurse interviewing the client asks whether the breast lumps are more noticeable:
    1 In the spring months
    2 In the autumn
    3 After menses
    4 Before menses

11. The client has undergone mastectomy. The nurse interprets that the client is making the best adjustment to the loss of the breast if which of the following behaviors is observed?
    1 Participating in the care of the surgical drain
    2 Reading a postoperative care booklet
    3 Refusing to look at the wound
    4 Asking for pain medication when needed

12. The client is preparing for discharge 10 days after radical vulvectomy. The nurse plans to teach this client that which of the following activities is

acceptable after discharge because it will not precipitate complications?

1 Sexual activity
2 Walking
3 Sitting for lengthy periods
4 Driving a car

13. The client has undergone vaginal hysterectomy. The nurse avoids which of the following in the care of this client?

1 Removal of antiembolism stockings twice daily
2 Assisting with range of motion leg exercises
3 Elevating the knee gatch on the bed
4 Checking placement of pneumatic compression boots

14. The client suspected of an ovarian tumor is scheduled for a pelvic ultrasound. Client preparation for the ultrasound includes which of the following?

1 NPO prior to the procedure
2 A light breakfast only
3 Drinking 6 to 8 glasses of water without voiding prior to the test
4 Wearing comfortable clothing and shoes for the procedure

15. The client is diagnosed as having a bowel tumor. Several diagnostic tests are prescribed. Which of the following tests will confirm the diagnosis of malignancy?

1 Magnetic resonance imaging (MRI)
2 CT scan
3 Abdominal ultrasound
4 Biopsy of the tumor

16. A client is diagnosed with multiple myeloma. The client asks the nurse about the diagnosis. The nurse bases the response on which of the following?

1 Malignant exacerbation in the number of leukocytes
2 Altered red blood cell production
3 Altered production of lymph cells
4 Malignant proliferation of plasma cells and tumors within the bone

17. The nurse is reviewing the laboratory results of a client diagnosed with multiple myeloma. Which of the following would the nurse expect to note specifically with this diagnosis?

1 Decreased number of plasma cells in the bone marrow
2 Increased white blood cells
3 Increased calcium level
4 Decreased BUN

18. The nurse is developing a plan of care for the client with multiple myeloma. A priority nursing intervention includes which of the following?

1 Coughing and deep breathing
2 Forcing fluids

3 Monitoring the red blood cell count
4 Providing frequent oral care

19. The oncology nurse specialist is preparing an educational session regarding the characteristics of Hodgkin's disease. Which of the following is not a characteristic of this disease?

1 Presence of Reed-Sternberg cells
2 Involvement of lymph nodes, spleen, and liver
3 Occurs most often in older adults
4 Prognosis depends on the stage of the disease

20. The oncology nurse is preparing to administer chemotherapy to the client with Hodgkin's disease. A multiagent medication regimen known as MOPP is prescribed. The medications included in this therapy are:

1 Bleomycin, Oncovin, vincristine, prednisone
2 Adriamycin, vincristine, Oncovin, prednisone
3 Adriamycin, Cytoxan, prednisone, Oncovin
4 Procarbazine, mechlorethamine, Oncovin, prednisone

21. The community health nurse is conducting a health promotion program for community members regarding testicular cancer. Which of the following is not a sign of testicular cancer?

1 Painless testicular swelling
2 Heavy sensation in the scrotum
3 Alopecia
4 Back pain

22. The nurse is analyzing the laboratory results of a client with leukemia who received a regimen of chemotherapy. Which of the following laboratory values does the nurse note specifically as a result of the massive cell destruction that occurred from the chemotherapy?

1 Anemia
2 Decreased platelets
3 Decreased leukocyte count
4 Increased uric acid level

23. The nurse is preparing a client with a bowel tumor for surgery. The physician has informed the client that the surgery is palliative in the treatment of the tumor. The nurse understands that this type of surgery is performed to:

1 Restore maximal function and appearance
2 Eliminate high-risk factors
3 Reduce pain
4 Cure the client

24. The client is receiving external radiation to the neck for cancer of the larynx. The most likely side effect to be expected is:

1 Constipation
2 Dyspnea
3 Sore throat
4 Diarrhea

25. The nurse assesses the skin of a client receiving external radiation therapy and documents a

finding noted as moist desquamation. The most appropriate description of moist desquamation is which of the following?
1 Reddened skin
2 A rash
3 Weeping of the skin
4 Dermatitis

26. The nurse is providing instructions to the client receiving external radiation therapy. Which of the following is not a component of the instructions?
1 Avoid exposure to sunlight
2 Wash the skin with a mild soap and pat dry
3 Apply pressure on the irritated area to prevent bleeding
4 Eat a high-protein diet

27. The nurse is caring for a client with an internal radiation implant. When caring for the client, the nurse observes which of the following principles?
1 Limit the time with the client to 1 hour per shift
2 Do not allow pregnant women into the client's room
3 Individuals under 16 years of age may be allowed to go into the room as long as they are 6 feet away from the client
4 Remove the dosimeter badge when entering the client's room

28. The client was hospitalized for a cervical radiation implant. The implant is removed and the client is to be discharged. Which of the following is not a component of the discharge instructions?
1 Cream may be used to relieve dryness or itching
2 Foul-smelling vaginal discharge is a sign of an infection
3 Sexual intercourse may be resumed after 7 to 10 days
4 Some vaginal bleeding is expected for 1 to 3 months

29. A cervical radiation implant is placed in the client for treatment of cervical cancer. What activity order is most appropriate for this client?
1 Out of bed in a chair only
2 Ambulate to the bathroom only
3 Bed rest
4 Out of bed ad lib

30. The nurse teaches skin care to the client receiving external radiation therapy. Which of the following statements, if made by the client, indicates the need for further instruction?
1 "I will handle the area gently."
2 "I will avoid the use of deodorants."
3 "I will limit sun exposure to 1 hour daily."
4 "I will wear loose-fitting clothing."

31. The client is hospitalized for insertion of an internal cervical radiation implant. While giving care, the nurse finds the radiation implant in the bed. The initial action by the nurse is to:
1 Call the physician
2 Pick up the implant with gloved hands and flush down the toilet
3 Reinsert the implant into the vagina immediately
4 Pick up the implant with long-handled forceps and place it in a lead container

32. The nurse is caring for a client experiencing hematological toxicity as a result of chemotherapy. The nurse develops a plan of care for the client. Which of the following would be included in the plan of care?
1 Restriction of all visitors
2 Restriction of fluid intake
3 Insertion of an indwelling urinary catheter to prevent skin breakdown
4 Restriction of fresh fruits and vegetables in the diet

33. The nurse is reviewing the laboratory results of a client receiving chemotherapy. The platelet count is 10,000/mm^3. Based on this laboratory value, the priority nursing assessment is which of the following?
1 Assess level of consciousness
2 Assess temperature
3 Assess bowel sounds
4 Assess skin turgor

34. The home health care nurse is caring for a client with cancer. The client is complaining of acute pain. The most appropriate nursing assessment of the client's pain includes which of the following?
1 The client's pain rating
2 The nurse's impression of the client's pain
3 Nonverbal cues from the client
4 Pain relief after appropriate nursing intervention

35. The community nurse is conducting a teaching session to a group of community members regarding the risks of cervical cancer. Which of the following is not a risk factor associated with this type of cancer?
1 Intercourse with circumcised males
2 Early, frequent intercourse
3 Multiple sexual partners
4 History of genital herpes

36. The nurse is caring for a client who is 4 days postoperative after a pelvic exenteration. The physician has changed the client's diet from NPO to clear liquids. The nurse makes which priority assessment before administering the diet?
1 Ability to ambulate
2 Urine specific gravity
3 Incision appearance
4 Bowel sounds

37. The client is admitted to the hospital with a diagnosis of suspected Hodgkin's disease. Which of the following assessment signs would the nurse most likely expect to note in the client?
   1 Weakness
   2 Fatigue
   3 Weight gain
   4 Enlarged lymph nodes

38. During the admission assessment of a client with ovarian cancer, the nurse recognizes which symptom as typical of the disease?
   1 Hypermenorrhea
   2 Abdominal distention
   3 Diarrhea
   4 Abnormal bleeding

39. The nurse is reviewing the complications of conization with a client who has microinvasive cervical cancer. Which of the following complications is not associated with this procedure?
   1 Infection
   2 Infertility
   3 Ovarian perforation
   4 Hemorrhage

40. When assessing the laboratory results of the client with bladder cancer and bone metastasis, the nurse notes a calcium level of 12 mg/dL. The nurse recognizes that this is consistent with which oncologic emergency?
   1 Hyperkalemia
   2 Spinal cord compression
   3 Superior vena caval syndrome
   4 Hypercalcemia

41. The nurse is conducting a diet history with an elderly client living alone. The nurse finds that the client's typical 24-hour food intake consists of eggs and sausage for breakfast, a fast-food lunch of hamburger and French fries, take-out fried chicken for dinner, and ice cream in the evening. To decrease the risk of cancer, what information will the nurse provide to the client?
   1 "You should not eat eggs."
   2 "You should not eat sausage."
   3 "Drinking a lot of alcohol increases the risk of liver cancer."
   4 "A high-fat diet increases your risk for colon cancer."

42. The client reports to the nurse that when performing testicular self-examination, he found a lump the size and shape of a pea. The most appropriate response to the client is which of the following?
   1 "That's important to report even though it might not be serious."
   2 "That could be cancer. I'll ask the doctor to examine you."
   3 "Let me know if it gets bigger next month."
   4 "Lumps like that are normal, don't worry."

43. The hospice nurse visits a client dying of ovarian cancer. During the visit, the client expresses that "If I can just live long enough to attend my daughter's graduation, I'll be ready to die." Which phase of coping is this client experiencing?
   1 Denial
   2 Bargaining
   3 Depression
   4 Anger

44. The nurse is caring for a client following a modified radical mastectomy. Which of the following assessment findings indicates that the client is experiencing a complication related to the surgery?
   1 Sanguineous drainage in the drainage tube
   2 Pain at the incisional site
   3 Complaints of decreased sensation near the operative site
   4 Arm edema on the operative side

45. The nurse is admitting a client with laryngeal cancer to the nursing unit. The nurse assesses for which of the following as the most common risk factor for this type of cancer?
   1 Use of chewing tobacco
   2 Cigarette smoking
   3 Urban living
   4 Alcohol abuse

46. The nurse is teaching the client who had laryngectomy for laryngeal cancer how to use an artificial larynx. The nurse tells the client to:
   1 Insert the device into the tracheostomy
   2 Hold the device alongside the neck
   3 Hold the device over the upper portion of the sternum
   4 Swallow air into the esophagus to use in making speech

47. The female client who has been receiving radiation therapy for bladder cancer tells the nurse that it feels as though she is voiding through the vagina. The nurse interprets that the client may be experiencing:
   1 Extreme stress due to the diagnosis of cancer
   2 Altered perineal sensation as a side effect of radiation therapy
   3 The development of a vesicovaginal fistula
   4 Rupture of the bladder

48. The client with leukemia is receiving busulfan (Myleran). Allopurinol (Zyloprim) is prescribed for the client. The purpose of the allopurinol (Zyloprim) is to:
   1 Prevent gouty arthritis
   2 Prevent hyperuricemia
   3 Prevent stomatitis
   4 Prevent diarrhea

49. The client receiving chemotherapy is experiencing stomatitis. The nurse advises the client to use

which of the following as the best substance with which to rinse the mouth?
1 Hydrogen peroxide mixture
2 Weak salt and sodium bicarbonate mouth rinse
3 Lemon-flavored mouthwash
4 Alcohol-based mouthwash

50. The community nurse is conducting a health promotion program, and the topic of the discussion relates to the risk factors of gastric cancer. Which of the following is not associated with the incidence of this type of cancer?
1 History of gastric polyps
2 History of pernicious anemia
3 A diet of smoked or highly salted and spiced food
4 High meat and carbohydrate consumption

51. A gastrectomy is performed on a client with gastric cancer. In the immediate postoperative period, the nurse notes bloody drainage from the NG tube. Which of the following is the most appropriate nursing intervention?
1 Notify the physician
2 Continue to monitor the drainage
3 Measure abdominal girth
4 Irrigate the NG tube

52. The nurse is reviewing the medical history of a client admitted to the hospital with a diagnosis of colorectal cancer. Which of the following is not an associated risk factor of this type of cancer?
1 A history of inflammatory bowel disease
2 Family history of colon cancer
3 A high-fiber diet
4 A diet high in fats and carbohydrates

53. The nurse is performing an admission assessment on a client diagnosed with a right colon tumor. Which of the following is a characteristic symptom of this type of tumor?
1 Diarrhea
2 Flat, ribbon-like stools
3 Dull abdominal pain exacerbated by walking
4 Crampy gas pains

54. The nurse is reviewing the preoperative orders of a client with a colon tumor who is scheduled for abdominal perineal resection. The nurse notes that the physician has prescribed neomycin (Mycifradin) for the client. The nurse determines that this medication has been prescribed:
1 Because the client has an infection
2 To prevent an infection
3 To decrease the bacteria in the bowel
4 Because the client is allergic to penicillin

55. The nurse is assessing the perineal wound in a client who has returned from the operating room following an abdominal perineal resection. The nurse notes serosanguineous drainage from the wound. Which of the following nursing interventions is most appropriate?
1 Notify the physician
2 Change the dressing as prescribed
3 Clamp the Penrose drain
4 Remove and replace the perineal packing

56. The nurse is assessing the colostomy of a client who had an abdominal perineal resection for a bowel tumor. Which of the following assessment findings indicates that the colostomy is beginning to function?
1 Blood drainage from the colostomy
2 The client's ability to tolerate food
3 Absent bowel sounds
4 The passage of flatus

57. The nurse is caring for a client following a radical neck dissection and creation of a tracheostomy performed for laryngeal cancer. The nurse is providing discharge instructions to the client. Which of the following is not a component of the teaching plan regarding care of the stoma?
1 Apply a thin layer of petrolatum to the skin around the stoma to prevent cracking
2 Protect the stoma from water
3 Use an air conditioner to provide cool air to assist in breathing
4 Keep powders and sprays away from the stoma site

58. The nurse is caring for a client with a suspected diagnosis of cancer of the prostate. The nurse analyzes the laboratory values and notes that the serum acid phosphatase titer is elevated. The nurse determines that this laboratory test is most often useful in determining:
1 The diagnosis of prostate cancer
2 Complications associated with cancer
3 The progression or regression of the cancer
4 The likelihood of associated bone cancer

59. Hormone therapy is prescribed as the mode of treatment for a client with prostatic cancer. The nurse understands that the goal of this form of treatment is to:
1 Limit the amount of circulating androgens
2 Increase the amount of circulating androgens
3 Increase testosterone levels
4 Increase prostaglandin levels

60. The nurse is caring for a client with cancer of the prostate following a prostatectomy. Discharge instructions are provided to the client. Which of the following instructions does the nurse provide to the client?
1 Notify the physician if blood clots are noticed during urination
2 Driving in a car may be resumed in 1 week
3 Restrict fluid intake to prevent incontinence
4 Avoid lifting objects heavier than 20 pounds for at least 6 weeks

61. The oncology nurse is providing a teaching session to a group of nursing students regarding the risks and causes of bladder cancer. Which of the following is not associated with this type of cancer?
    1 It most often occurs in women
    2 It is generally seen in clients older than age 40 years
    3 Environmental health hazards have been attributed as a cause
    4 Using cigarettes, artificial sweeteners, and drinking coffee can increase the risk

62. The nurse is reviewing the history of a client with bladder cancer. The most common symptom of this type of cancer is which of the following?
    1 Frequency of urination
    2 Urgency on urination
    3 Hematuria
    4 Dysuria

63. The nurse is caring for a client following intravesical instillation of an alkylating chemotherapeutic agent into the bladder for the treatment of bladder cancer. Following the instillation, the nurse most appropriately instructs the client to:
    1 Urinate immediately
    2 Maintain strict bed rest
    3 Retain the instillation fluid for 30 minutes
    4 Change position every 15 minutes from side to side

64. The nurse is assessing the stoma of a client following a ureterostomy. Which of the following does the nurse expect to note?
    1 A pale stoma
    2 A red and moist stoma
    3 A dry stoma
    4 A dark-colored stoma

65. The nurse is caring for a client following a radical mastectomy. Which of the following nursing interventions would assist in preventing lymphedema of the affected arm?
    1 Placing cool compresses on the affected arm
    2 Elevating the affected arm on a pillow above heart level
    3 Maintaining an IV site below the antecubital area on the affected side

4 Avoiding arm exercises in the immediate post-operative period

66. The nurse is caring for a client with a lung tumor. A pneumonectomy is scheduled. Which of the following is not a component of the postoperative plan of care?
    1 Monitoring the closed-chest drainage system
    2 Encouraging coughing and deep breathing
    3 Assessing the surgical dressing for drainage
    4 Avoiding complete lateral positioning

67. The nurse is preparing a client for a mammography. Which of the following is an accurate instruction regarding the procedure?
    1 Mammography takes about 1 hour
    2 Avoid the use of deodorants, powders, or creams on the day of the test
    3 There is no discomfort associated with the procedure
    4 Maintain an NPO status on the day of the test

68. A client is scheduled for a Papanicolaou smear at the next scheduled clinic visit. The nurse provides instructions to the client regarding preparation for this test. Which of the following is an accurate instruction?
    1 The test can be performed during menstruation
    2 Fluids are restricted on the day of the test
    3 The test is painless
    4 Vaginal douching is required 2 hours before the test

69. A nurse is monitoring a client for signs and symptoms related to vena caval syndrome. Which of the following is an early sign of this oncologic emergency?
    1 Periorbital edema
    2 Arm edema
    3 Mental status changes
    4 Cyanosis

70. The nurse is caring for a client with metastatic breast cancer. The client develops a new and sudden sharp pain in the back. The most appropriate nursing intervention is to:
    1 Reposition the client
    2 Medicate the client for pain
    3 Encourage ambulation
    4 Notify the physician

ANSWERS

1. **2**

Rationale: The TSE is recommended monthly after a warm bath or shower when the scrotal skin is relaxed. The client should stand to examine the testicles. Using both hands, with fingers under the scrotum and thumbs on top, the client should gently roll the testicles, feeling for any lumps.

Test-Taking Strategy: Read each option carefully. Eliminate option 4 first because of the phrase "6 months." Next eliminate option 3 because of the word "one." From the remaining options, eliminate option 1 by trying to visualize the process of the self-examination. If you had difficulty with this question, take time now to review this important examination!

Level of Cognitive Ability: Application
Phase of Nursing Process: Implementation
Client Needs: Health Promotion and Maintenance
Content Area: Adult Health/Oncology

Reference

Leahy, J., & Kizilay, P. (1998). *Foundations of nursing practice: A nursing process approach.* Philadelphia: W. B. Saunders. p. 334.

2. **3**

Rationale: Viruses may be one of multiple agents acting to initiate carcinogenesis and have been associated with several types of cancer. Increased stress has been associated with causing the growth and proliferation of cancer cells. Two forms of radiation, ultraviolet and ionizing, can lead to cancer. High-fiber diets may reduce the risk of colon cancer. A diet high in fat may be a factor in the development of breast, colon, and prostate cancers.

Test-Taking Strategy: Note the key word "not" in the stem of the question. Read each option carefully, utilizing the process of elimination. Familiarity with the risk factors related to cancer will easily direct you to option 3. Review these risk factors now, if you had difficulty with this question!

Level of Cognitive Ability: Application
Phase of Nursing Process: Implementation
Client Needs: Health Promotion and Maintenance
Content Area: Adult Health/Oncology

Reference

Black, J., & Matassarin-Jacobs, E. (1997). *Medical-surgical nursing: Clinical management for continuity of care* (5th ed.). Philadelphia: W. B. Saunders. pp. 539–541.

3. **3**

Rationale: Thrombocytopenia indicates a decrease in the number of platelets in the circulating blood. A major concern is monitoring for and preventing bleeding. Option 2 relates to monitoring for infection, particularly if leukopenia is present. Options 1 and 4, although important in the plan of care, are not directly related to thrombocytopenia.

Test-Taking Strategy: Note the key word "thrombocytopenia" in the question. Recalling that this condition places the client at risk of bleeding will assist in eliminating options 1, 2, and 4. If you are unfamiliar with the nursing interventions related to this disorder, review now!

Level of Cognitive Ability: Application
Phase of Nursing Process: Planning
Client Needs: Physiological Integrity
Content Area: Adult Health/Oncology

Reference

O'Toole, M. (1997). *Miller-Keane encyclopedia & dictionary of medicine, nursing, & allied health* (6th ed.). Philadelphia: W. B. Saunders. p. 1610.

4. **2**

Rationale: Candidiasis is a fungal infection caused by *Candida albicans.* In the mouth, it is called thrush and appears as white plaques with an underlying red base with fissures on the corners of the mouth. Although it can occur in an immunocompromised client, it is not considered to be common. Options 3 and 4 are not accurate regarding this infection.

Test-Taking Strategy: Options 1 and 3 can be eliminated first. Recalling that the anemic client is more likely to ex-hibit pallor will direct you to option 2. If you are unfamiliar with the manifestations associated with thrush, take time now to review!

Level of Cognitive Ability: Analysis
Phase of Nursing Process: Assessment
Client Needs: Physiological Integrity
Content Area: Adult Health/Oncology

Reference

Black, J., & Matassarin-Jacobs, E. (1997). *Medical-surgical nursing: Clinical management for continuity of care* (5th ed.). Philadelphia: W. B. Saunders. p. 2221.

5. **2**

Rationale: The normal WBC count ranges from 4000 to 9000 mm³. Option 1 indicates a low value of 3000 mm³. Options 3 and 4 indicate elevated values.

Test-Taking Strategy: Knowledge regarding the normal WBC count is required to answer this question. If you are not familiar with this value, learn it now!

Level of Cognitive Ability: Analysis
Phase of Nursing Process: Analysis
Client Needs: Physiological Integrity
Content Area: Adult Health/Oncology

Reference

Black, J., & Matassarin-Jacobs, E. (1997). *Medical-surgical nursing: Clinical management for continuity of care* (5th ed.). Philadelphia: W. B. Saunders. p. 2221.

6. **2**

Rationale: The BSE should be performed monthly several days after the menstrual period. It is not recommended to perform the examination weekly. At the onset of menstruation and during ovulation, hormonal changes occur that may alter breast tissue.

Test-Taking Strategy: Option 4 can be easily eliminated because of the word "weekly." Eliminate options 1 and 3 next because of the similarity that exists in regards to the hormonal changes that occur during these times. If you are unfamiliar with the procedure for performing BSE, review this important self-examination now!

Level of Cognitive Ability: Application
Phase of Nursing Process: Implementation
Client Needs: Health Promotion and Maintenance
Content Area: Adult Health/Oncology

Reference

Leahy, J., & Kizilay, P. (1998). *Foundations of nursing practice: A nursing process approach.* Philadelphia: W. B. Saunders. pp. 332–333.

7. **2**

Rationale: The nurse would instruct the client to lie down and place a towel or pillow under the shoulder on the side of the breast to be examined. If the left breast is to be examined, the pillow would be placed under the left shoulder.

Test-Taking Strategy: Attempt to visualize this procedure to select the correct option. Remember, to examine the left, the pillow is placed under the left; to examine the right, the pillow is placed under the right. If you are unfamiliar with the procedure for performing BSE, review this important self-examination now!

Level of Cognitive Ability: Application
Phase of Nursing Process: Implementation
Client Needs: Health Promotion and Maintenance
Content Area: Adult Health/Oncology

Reference
Leahy, J., & Kizilay, P. (1998). *Foundations of nursing practice: A nursing process approach.* Philadelphia: W. B. Saunders. pp. 332–333.

8. **4**

Rationale: If the client has had a hysterectomy or is no longer menstruating, the BSE should be performed on the same day every month. Options 1 and 2 are inappropriate because the client who had a hysterectomy would not be menstruating. It is best not to perform the BSE at ovulation time because of the hormonal changes that occur.

Test-Taking Strategy: Note the key word "hysterectomy" in the question. Options 1 and 2 can be easily eliminated. Eliminate option 3 because of the hormonal changes that occur at this time. If you are unfamiliar with the procedure for performing BSE, review this important self-examination now!

Level of Cognitive Ability: Application
Phase of Nursing Process: Implementation
Client Needs: Health Promotion and Maintenance
Content Area: Adult Health/Oncology

Reference
Leahy, J., & Kizilay, P. (1998). *Foundations of nursing practice: A nursing process approach.* Philadelphia: W. B. Saunders. pp. 332–333.

9. **2**

Rationale: The CT scan causes no pain and can last for 15 to 60 minutes. The dye may cause a warm, flushing sensation when injected. Fluids are encouraged following the procedure. If an iodine dye is used, the client should be asked about allergies to seafood or iodine.

Test-Taking Strategy: Note the key words "dye injection" in the question. This should provide you with the clue that the issue relates to the dye. If you are unfamiliar with this diagnostic test, review the important teaching points related to it now!

Level of Cognitive Ability: Analysis
Phase of Nursing Process: Analysis
Client Needs: Physiological Integrity
Content Area: Adult Health/Oncology

Reference
Leahy, J., & Kizilay, P. (1998). *Foundations of nursing practice: A nursing process approach.* Philadelphia: W. B. Saunders. pp. 755–756.

10. **4**

Rationale: The nurse assesses the client with fibrocystic breast disorder for worsening of symptoms (breast lumps, painful breasts, and possible nipple discharge) before the onset of menses. This is associated with cyclical hormone changes.

Test-Taking Strategy: The key words in the question are "more noticeable." This implies that there is a predictable variation in symptoms. Use knowledge of the effects of various hormones in the body to analyze the options and choose correctly.

Level of Cognitive Ability: Application
Phase of Nursing Process: Assessment
Client Needs: Physiological Integrity
Content Area: Adult Health/Oncology

Reference
Beare, P., & Myers, J. (1998). *Adult health nursing* (3rd ed.). St. Louis: Mosby–Year Book. p. 1685.

11. **1**

Rationale: Clients demonstrates the best adaptation by participating in their own care. This would include care of surgical drains that would be in place for a short time after discharge. Asking for pain medication is also an action-oriented option, but it does not relate to acceptance of the loss of the breast. Reading the postoperative care booklet is useful but is not the best of the options presented here. Refusing to look at the wound indicates no adaptation to the loss.

Test-Taking Strategy: Note that the key word in the question is "best." This tells you that more than one or all of the options may be partially or totally correct. Use prioritizing ability to determine the best option of those presented, keeping in mind the issue "best adjustment."

Level of Cognitive Ability: Analysis
Phase of Nursing Process: Analysis
Client Needs: Psychosocial Integrity
Content Area: Adult Health/Oncology

Reference
Beare, P., & Myers, J. (1998). *Adult health nursing* (3rd ed.). St. Louis: Mosby–Year Book. p. 1692.

12. **2**

Rationale: The client should resume activity slowly, but walking is a beneficial activity. The client should know to rest when fatigue occurs. Activities to be avoided include driving, heavy housework, wearing tight clothing, crossing the legs, and prolonged standing or sitting. Sexual activity is prohibited for 4 to 6 weeks after surgery.

Test-Taking Strategy: Read the question carefully. Note the key phrase in the stem, which is "not precipitate complications." With this in mind, evaluate each of the options in terms of the stress or harm it could cause to the perineal area. This should help you systematically eliminate each of the incorrect options. Review home care measures following vulvectomy now, if you had difficulty with this question!

Level of Cognitive Ability: Application
Phase of Nursing Process: Planning
Client Needs: Health Promotion and Maintenance
Content Area: Adult Health/Oncology

Reference
Beare, P., & Myers, J. (1998). *Adult health nursing* (3rd ed.). St. Louis: Mosby–Year Book. p. 1684.

13. **3**

Rationale: The client is at risk of deep vein thrombosis or thrombophlebitis after this surgery, as for any other major surgery. For this reason, the nurse implements measures that will prevent this complication. Range of motion exercises, antiembolism stockings, and pneumatic compression boots are all helpful. The nurse should avoid using the knee gatch in the bed, which inhibits venous return, thus placing the client at greater risk for deep vein thrombosis or thrombophlebitis.

Test-Taking Strategy: Note that the key word in this question is "avoids." This tells you that the correct answer to the question is an incorrect nursing action. Use the process of elimination and basic nursing knowledge to choose correctly. Review postoperative nursing interventions now, if you had difficulty with this question!

Level of Cognitive Ability: Application
Phase of Nursing Process: Implementation
Client Needs: Physiological Integrity
Content Area: Adult Health/Oncology

Reference
Beare, P., & Myers, J. (1998). *Adult health nursing* (3rd ed.). St. Louis: Mosby–Year Book. p. 1669.

14. **3**

Rationale: A pelvic ultrasound requires the ingestion of large volumes of water just prior to the procedure. A full bladder is necessary so that this organ will be visualized as such and not mistaken as a possible pelvic growth. An abdominal ultrasound may require that the client abstain from food or fluid for several hours before the procedure. Option 4 is unrelated to this specific procedure.

Test-Taking Strategy: Note the key word "pelvic" in the question. You should easily be able to eliminate option 4. From the remaining options, focusing on the key word will assist in directing you to option 3. Review preparation for a pelvic ultrasound now, if you had difficulty with this question!

Level of Cognitive Ability: Application
Phase of Nursing Process: Planning
Client Needs: Physiological Integrity
Content Area: Adult Health/Oncology

Reference
Leahy, J., & Kizilay, P. (1998). *Foundations of nursing practice: A nursing process approach*. Philadelphia: W. B. Saunders. p. 151.

15. **4**

Rationale: A biopsy is done to determine whether a tumor is malignant or benign. An MRI, CT scan, and ultrasound will visualize the presence of a mass but will not confirm a diagnosis of malignancy.

Test-Taking Strategy: Note the key word "confirm" in the stem of the question. This key word should easily direct you to option 4. If you are unfamiliar with the purpose of the tests identified in the options, review them now!

Level of Cognitive Ability: Analysis
Phase of Nursing Process: Analysis
Client Needs: Physiological Integrity
Content Area: Adult Health/Oncology

Reference
O'Toole, M. (1997). *Miller-Keane encyclopedia & dictionary of medicine, nursing, & allied health* (6th ed.). Philadelphia: W. B. Saunders. p. 194.

16. **4**

Rationale: Multiple myeloma is a B-cell neoplastic condition characterized by abnormal, malignant proliferation of plasma cells and the accumulation of mature plasma cells in the bone marrow. Option 1 describes the leukemic process. Options 2 and 3 are not characteristics of multiple myeloma.

Test-Taking Strategy: Knowledge regarding the pathophysiology associated with this disorder is required to answer the question. Review this information now, if you are unfamiliar with this oncological disorder!

Level of Cognitive Ability: Analysis
Phase of Nursing Process: Analysis
Client Needs: Physiological Integrity
Content Area: Adult Health/Oncology

Reference
Black, J., & Matassarin-Jacobs, E. (1997). *Medical-surgical nursing: Clinical management for continuity of care* (5th ed.). Philadelphia: W. B. Saunders. p. 1498.

17. **3**

Rationale: Findings indicative of multiple myeloma are an increased number of plasma cells in the bone marrow, anemia, hypercalcemia due to the release of calcium from the deteriorating bone tissue, and an elevated BUN. An increased WBC count may or may not be present and is not specifically related to multiple myeloma.

Test-Taking Strategy: Knowledge regarding the pathophysiology associated with this disorder and the effects it produces on the body is required to answer the question. Review this information now, if you are unfamiliar with this oncological disorder!

Level of Cognitive Ability: Analysis
Phase of Nursing Process: Analysis
Client Needs: Physiological Integrity
Content Area: Adult Health/Oncology

Reference
O'Toole, M. (1997). *Miller-Keane encyclopedia & dictionary of medicine, nursing, & allied health* (6th ed.). Philadelphia: W. B. Saunders. p. 1024.

18. **2**

Rationale: Hypercalcemia secondary to bone destruction is a priority concern in the client with multiple myeloma. The nurse should administer fluids in amounts adequate to maintain an output of 1.5 to 2.0 L/day. Clients require about 3 to 4 L of fluid per day. The fluid is needed not only to dilute the calcium overload but also to prevent protein from precipitating in the renal tubules. Options 1, 3, and 4 may be a component of the plan of care but are not the priority in this client.

Test-Taking Strategy: Knowledge regarding the clinical manifestations that occur in multiple myeloma is required to answer the question. Recalling that forcing fluids is specific to the care of a client with this disorder will direct you to option 2. Review the specific manifestations of this disorder now, if you had difficulty with this question!

Level of Cognitive Ability: Analysis
Phase of Nursing Process: Planning
Client Needs: Physiological Integrity
Content Area: Adult Health/Oncology

Reference
Black, J., & Matassarin-Jacobs, E. (1997). *Medical-surgical nursing: Clinical management for continuity of care* (5th ed.). Philadelphia: W. B. Saunders. p. 1500.

19. **3**

Rationale: Hodgkin's disease is a disorder of young adults and primarily occurs between the ages of 20 and 40 years. Options 1, 2, and 4 are characteristics of this disease.

Test-Taking Strategy: Note the key word "not" in the stem of the question. Recalling that Hodgkin's occurs in the young adult will easily direct you to option 3. Review the characteristics of this disorder now, if you had difficulty with this question!

Level of Cognitive Ability: Analysis
Phase of Nursing Process: Planning
Client Needs: Physiological Integrity
Content Area: Adult Health/Oncology

Reference

Black, J., & Matassarin-Jacobs, E. (1997). *Medical-surgical nursing: Clinical management for continuity of care* (5th ed.). Philadelphia: W. B. Saunders. pp. 1500–1501.

20. **4**

Rationale: MOPP therapy includes mechlorethamine, Oncovin (vincristine), procarbazine, and prednisone. It is the treatment of choice and is the most widely used regimen in stages IIB, III, and IV of Hodgkin's Disease.

Test-Taking Strategy: MOPP is an abbreviation for the medications used in this therapy. Use the letters M, O, P, and P to assist in selecting the medications used in this therapy. If you are unfamiliar with this therapy, review now!

Level of Cognitive Ability: Analysis
Phase of Nursing Process: Analysis
Client Needs: Physiological Integrity
Content Area: Adult Health/Oncology

Reference

Black, J., & Matassarin-Jacobs, E. (1997). *Medical-surgical nursing: Clinical management for continuity of care* (5th ed.). Philadelphia: W. B. Saunders. p. 1502.

21. **3**

Rationale: Alopecia is not an assessment finding in testicular cancer. It may, however, occur as a result of radiation or chemotherapy. Options 1, 2, and 4 are assessment findings in testicular cancer. Back pain may indicate metastasis to the retroperitoneal lymph nodes.

Test-Taking Strategy: Note the key word "not" in the stem of the question. Use the process of elimination, remembering that alopecia occurs as a result of chemotherapy rather than from the disease. Review the manifestations associated with testicular cancer now, if you had difficulty with this question!

Level of Cognitive Ability: Application
Phase of Nursing Process: Implementation
Client Needs: Health Promotion and Maintenance
Content Area: Adult Health/Oncology

Reference

Black, J., & Matassarin-Jacobs, E. (1997). *Medical-surgical nursing: Clinical management for continuity of care* (5th ed.). Philadelphia: W. B. Saunders. p. 2374.

22. **4**

Rationale: Hyperuricemia is especially common following treatment for leukemias and lymphomas, since the therapy results in massive cell kill. Although options 1, 2, and 3 may also be noted, an increased uric acid level is specifically related to cell destruction.

Test-Taking Strategy: Note the key phrase "massive cell destruction" in the question. Recalling the cell response to destruction will assist in directing you to option 4. Review this concept now, if you had difficulty with this question!

Level of Cognitive Ability: Analysis
Phase of Nursing Process: Analysis
Client Needs: Physiological Integrity
Content Area: Adult Health/Oncology

Reference

Lehne, R. (1998). *Pharmacology for nursing care* (3rd ed.). Philadelphia: W. B. Saunders. p. 1017.

23. **3**

Rationale: Use of surgery in palliative care is carefully considered and used only if the risk-benefit ratio is favorable. Palliative surgery that can benefit the client with cancer and improve quality of life includes procedures that reduce pain, relieve airway obstructions, relieve obstructions in the GI and urinary tracts, relieve pressure on the brain and spinal cord, and prevent hemorrhage. Options 1, 2, and 4 do not describe palliative surgery.

Test-Taking Strategy: Note the key word "palliative" in the question. Knowledge of the definition of this word will assist in directing you to option 3. Review the various types of surgery now, if you had difficulty with this question!

Level of Cognitive Ability: Analysis
Phase of Nursing Process: Analysis
Client Needs: Physiological Integrity
Content Area: Adult Health/Oncology

Reference

Black, J., & Matassarin-Jacobs, E. (1997). *Medical-surgical nursing: Clinical management for continuity of care* (5th ed.). Philadelphia: W. B. Saunders. p. 569.

24. **3**

Rationale: In general, only the area in the treatment field is affected by the radiation. Skin reactions, fatigue, nausea, and anorexia may occur with radiation to any site, whereas other side effects occur only when specific areas are involved in treatment. A client receiving radiation to the larynx is most likely to experience a sore throat. Options 1 and 4 may occur with radiation to the GI tract. Dyspnea may occur with lung involvement.

Test-Taking Strategy: Eliminate options 1 and 4 first as they are similar and GI related. Consider the anatomical location of the radiation therapy to assist you in selecting option 3. Review the effects of radiation therapy now, if you had difficulty with this question!

Level of Cognitive Ability: Analysis
Phase of Nursing Process: Assessment
Client Needs: Physiological Integrity
Content Area: Adult Health/Oncology

Reference

Black, J., & Matassarin-Jacobs, E. (1997). *Medical-surgical nursing: Clinical management for continuity of care* (5th ed.). Philadelphia: W. B. Saunders. p. 571.

25. **3**

Rationale: Moist desquamation occurs when the basal cells of the skin are destroyed. The dermal level is exposed, which results in the leakage of serum. Reddened skin, a rash, and dermatitis may occur with external radiation but are not described as a moist desquamation.

Test-Taking Strategy: Noting the key word "moist" will easily direct you to option 3. Options 1, 2, and 4 are eliminated because they are similar and describe a dry rather than a moist skin alteration. Review the signs associated with a moist desquamation now, if you had difficulty with this question!

Level of Cognitive Ability: Analysis
Phase of Nursing Process: Assessment
Client Needs: Physiological Integrity
Content Area: Adult Health/Oncology

Reference

Monahan, F., & Neighbors, M. (1998). *Medical-surgical nursing: Foundations for clinical practice* (2nd ed.). Philadelphia: W. B. Saunders. p. 1520.

26. **3**

Rationale: The client should avoid pressure on the irritated area and should wear loose-fitting clothing. Specific physician instructions would be necessary to obtain if an alteration in skin integrity occurred as a result of the radiation therapy. Options 1, 2, and 4 are accurate instructions regarding radiation therapy.

Test-Taking Strategy: Note the key word "not" in the stem of the question. Use the process of elimination in selecting the correct option. The word "pressure" should be an indication that this is an inappropriate measure. Review client teaching points related to skin care and radiation therapy now, if you had difficulty with this question!

Level of Cognitive Ability: Application
Phase of Nursing Process: Implementation
Client Needs: Health Promotion and Maintenance
Content Area: Adult Health/Oncology

Reference

Monahan, F., & Neighbors, M. (1998). *Medical-surgical nursing: Foundations for clinical practice* (2nd ed.). Philadelphia: W. B. Saunders. p. 1523.

27. **2**

Rationale: The time that the nurse spends in the room of a client with an internal radiation implant is 30 minutes per 8-hour shift. The dosimeter badge must be worn when in the client's room. Children younger than 16 years of age and pregnant women are not allowed in the client's room.

Test-Taking Strategy: Utilize the process of elimination. Option 4 can be eliminated first. Knowledge of the time frame related to exposure to the client will assist in eliminating option 1. From the remaining options, select option 2 because of the possible risks associated with exposure to the mother and fetus. Review these important principles now, if you had difficulty with this question!

Level of Cognitive Ability: Application
Phase of Nursing Process: Implementation
Client Needs: Safe, Effective Care Environment
Content Area: Adult Health/Oncology

Reference

Monahan, F., & Neighbors, M. (1998). *Medical-surgical nursing: Foundations for clinical practice* (2nd ed.). Philadelphia: W. B. Saunders. p. 1519.

28. **2**

Rationale: Foul-smelling vaginal discharge is expected and will occur for some time following removal of a cervical radiation implant. Options 1, 3, and 4 are accurate discharge instructions.

Test-Taking Strategy: Note the key word "not" in the stem of the question. Knowledge regarding the client teaching points related to radiation implants is required to answer the question. Review these points now, if you had difficulty with this question!

Level of Cognitive Ability: Application
Phase of Nursing Process: Implementation
Client Needs: Health Promotion and Maintenance
Content Area: Adult Health/Oncology

Reference

Monahan, F., & Neighbors, M. (1998). *Medical-surgical nursing: Foundations for clinical practice* (2nd ed.). Philadelphia: W. B. Saunders. p. 1835.

29. **3**

Rationale: The client with a cervical radiation implant should be maintained on bed rest in the dorsal position to prevent movement of the radiation source. The head of the bed is elevated to a maximum of 10 to 45 degrees for comfort. Avoid turning the client on the side. If turning is absolutely necessary, place a pillow between the knees and, with the body in straight alignment, log roll the client.

Test-Taking Strategy: Consider the anatomical location of the implant and the risk of dislodgment to answer the question. Additionally, note that options 1, 2, and 4 are similar. If you had difficulty with this question, take time now to review care to the client with a radiation implant!

Level of Cognitive Ability: Application
Phase of Nursing Process: Implementation
Client Needs: Safe, Effective Care Environment
Content Area: Adult Health/Oncology

Reference

Monahan, F., & Neighbors, M. (1998). *Medical-surgical nursing: Foundations for clinical practice* (2nd ed.). Philadelphia: W. B. Saunders. p. 1835.

30. **3**

Rationale: The client needs to be instructed to avoid exposure to the sun. Options 1, 2, and 4 are accurate measures in the care of a client receiving external radiation therapy.

Test-Taking Strategy: Note the key phrase "need for further instruction." Eliminate option 1 because of the word "gently" and option 4 because of the word "loose." From the remaining options, recalling that sun exposure is to be avoided will assist in answering the question. Review skin care measures for the client receiving external radiation now, if you had difficulty with this question!

Level of Cognitive Ability: Analysis
Phase of Nursing Process: Evaluation
Client Needs: Health Promotion and Maintenance
Content Area: Adult Health/Oncology

Reference

Monahan, F., & Neighbors, M. (1998). *Medical-surgical nursing: Foundations for clinical practice* (2nd ed.). Philadelphia: W. B. Saunders. p. 1523.

31. **4**

Rationale: A lead container and long-handled forceps should be kept in the client's room at all times during internal radiation therapy. If the implant becomes dislodged, the nurse should pick up the implant with the long-handled forceps and place it in the lead container. Options 1, 2, and 3 are inaccurate interventions.

Test-Taking Strategy: Note the key word "initial" in the stem of the question. Option 3 is not an appropriate action. Eliminate option 2 next because the implant would not be discarded. Although the physician would be notified, the initial action is option 4. Review the measures related to a dislodged implant now, if you had difficulty with this question!

Level of Cognitive Ability: Application
Phase of Nursing Process: Implementation
Client Needs: Safe, Effective Care Environment
Content Area: Adult Health/Oncology

Reference
Monahan, F., & Neighbors, M. (1998). *Medical-surgical nursing: Foundations for clinical practice* (2nd ed.). Philadelphia: W. B. Saunders. p. 1519.

32. **4**

Rationale: In the immunocompromised client, a low-bacteria diet is implemented. This includes avoiding fresh fruits and vegetables and thorough cooking of all foods. Not all visitors are restricted, but the client is protected from people with known infections. Fluids should be encouraged. Invasive measures such as an indwelling urinary catheter should be avoided to prevent infections.

Test-Taking Strategy: Eliminate option 1 because of the word "all." Next, eliminate option 2 because it is not reasonable to eliminate fluids in a client receiving chemotherapy at risk for fluid and electrolyte imbalances. Eliminate option 3 because of the risk of infection that exists with this measure. Review interventions for the client with hematological toxicity now, if you had difficulty with this question!

Level of Cognitive Ability: Application
Phase of Nursing Process: Planning
Client Needs: Safe, Effective Care Environment
Content Area: Adult Health/Oncology

Reference
Monahan, F., & Neighbors, M. (1998). *Medical-surgical nursing: Foundations for clinical practice* (2nd ed.). Philadelphia: W. B. Saunders. pp. 1536–1537.

33. **1**

Rationale: A high risk of hemorrhage exists when the platelet count is less than 20,000/mm³. Fatal central nervous system (CNS) hemorrhage or massive GI hemorrhage can occur when the platelet count is less than 10,000/mm³. The client should be assessed for changes in level of consciousness, which may be an early indication of an intracranial hemorrhage. Option 2 is a priority nursing assessment when the WBC count is low and the client is at risk for an infection. Although options 3 and 4 are important to assess, they are not the priority in this situation.

Test-Taking Strategy: Note the key word "priority" in the stem of the question. Recalling the normal platelet count and determining that a low count places the client at risk for bleeding will assist in eliminating options 2, 3, and 4 as assessment measures for bleeding. Review the normal platelet count and the nursing interventions for a client with a low count now, if you had difficulty with this question!

Level of Cognitive Ability: Analysis
Phase of Nursing Process: Assessment
Client Needs: Physiological Integrity
Content Area: Adult Health/Oncology

Reference
Black, J., & Matassarin-Jacobs, E. (1997). *Medical-surgical nursing: Clinical management for continuity of care* (5th ed.). Philadelphia: W. B. Saunders. p. 582.

34. **1**

Rationale: The client's self-report is a critical component of pain assessment. The nurse should ask the client about the description of the pain and listen carefully to the client's words used to describe the pain. Nonverbal cues from the client are important but are not the most appropriate pain assessment measure. The nurse's impression of the client's pain is not appropriate in determining the client's level of pain. Assessing pain relief is an important measure, but this option is not related to the issue of the question.

Test-Taking Strategy: Noting the issue of the question will assist in eliminating option 4. Eliminate option 2 because the nurse is not the client of the question. From the remaining two options, the subjective data from the client will provide the most accurate description of the pain!

Level of Cognitive Ability: Analysis
Phase of Nursing Process: Assessment
Client Needs: Physiological Integrity
Content Area: Adult Health/Oncology

Reference
Monahan, F., & Neighbors, M. (1998). *Medical-surgical nursing: Foundations for clinical practice* (2nd ed.). Philadelphia: W. B. Saunders. p. 1556.

35. **1**

Rationale: Risk factors associated with cervical cancer include intercourse with uncircumcised males, early and frequent intercourse with multiple sexual partners, multiparity, chronic cervicitis, and a history of genital herpes or human papilloma virus infection. The rate of cervical cancer is also higher in the black race.

Test-Taking Strategy: Note the key word "not" in the stem of the question. Read the options carefully in selecting the correct option. If you had difficulty with this question, review the risks of cervical cancer now!

Level of Cognitive Ability: Application
Phase of Nursing Process: Implementation
Client Needs: Health Promotion and Maintenance
Content Area: Adult Health/Oncology

Reference
Black, J., & Matassarin-Jacobs, E. (1997). *Medical-surgical nursing: Clinical management for continuity of care* (5th ed.). Philadelphia: W. B. Saunders. p. 542.

36. **4**

Rationale: The client is kept NPO until peristalsis returns, usually in 4 to 6 days. When signs of bowel function return, clear fluids are given to the client. If no distention occurs, the diet is advanced as tolerated. The most important assessment is to assess bowel sounds prior to feeding the client. Options 1, 2, and 3 are unrelated to the issue of the question.

Test-Taking Strategy: Note the key word "priority" and the key phrase "NPO to clear liquid" in the stem of the question. Knowledge regarding general postoperative care measures will assist in selecting the correct option. Option 4 is the only option that relates to GI function, which is the issue of the question!.

Level of Cognitive Ability: Application
Phase of Nursing Process: Assessment
Client Needs: Physiological Integrity
Content Area: Adult Health/Oncology

Reference

Monahan, F., & Neighbors, M. (1998). *Medical-surgical nursing: Foundations for clinical practice* (2nd ed.). Philadelphia: W. B. Saunders. p. 1832

37. **4**

Rationale: Hodgkin's disease is a chronic, progressive neoplastic disorder of lymphoid tissue characterized by the painless enlargement of lymph nodes with progression to extralymphatic sites such as the spleen and liver. Weight loss is most likely to be noted. Fatigue and weakness may occur but are not significantly related to the disease.

Test-Taking Strategy: Knowledge that Hodgkin's disease affects the lymph nodes will easily direct you to option 4. Option 3 can be easily eliminated first because in such a disorder, weight loss is most likely to occur. Options 1 and 2 are similar and rather vague symptoms that can occur in many disorders. Review the manifestations associated with Hodgkin's disease now, if you had difficulty with this question!

Level of Cognitive Ability: Analysis
Phase of Nursing Process: Assessment
Client Needs: Physiological Integrity
Content Area: Adult Health/Oncology

Reference

Black, J., & Matassarin-Jacobs, E. (1997). *Medical-surgical nursing: Clinical management for continuity of care* (5th ed.). Philadelphia: W. B. Saunders. p. 1500.

38. **2**

Rationale: Clinical manifestations of ovarian cancer include abdominal distention, urinary frequency and urgency. Pleural effusion, malnutrition, pain from pressure caused by the growing tumor and the effects of urinary or bowel obstruction such as constipation, ascites with dyspnea, and ultimately general severe pain can occur. Abnormal bleeding, often resulting in hypermenorrhea, is associated with uterine cancer.

Test-Taking Strategy: Eliminate options 1 and 4 first because they are similar. From the remaining options, consider the anatomical location of the diagnosis. This will assist in directing you to option 2. Review the manifestations associated with ovarian cancer now, if you had difficulty with this question!

Level of Cognitive Ability: Analysis
Phase of Nursing Process: Assessment
Client Needs: Physiological Integrity
Content Area: Adult Health/Oncology

Reference

Black, J., & Matassarin-Jacobs, E. (1997). *Medical-surgical nursing: Clinical management for continuity of care* (5th ed.). Philadelphia: W. B. Saunders. pp. 2401, 2413.

39. **3**

Rationale: Conization is generally not performed on women who desire to bear children because it can lead to incompetence of the cervix or infertility. Complications of the procedure include hemorrhage, infection, and, less frequently, cervical stenosis.

Test-Taking Strategy: Note the key words "not" and "cervical cancer" in the question. Select option 3 because this option addresses an "ovarian" condition, not a cervical one. Review the complications associated with this procedure now, if you had difficulty with this question!

Level of Cognitive Ability: Analysis
Phase of Nursing Process: Assessment
Client Needs: Physiological Integrity
Content Area: Adult Health/Oncology

Reference

Monahan, F., & Neighbors, M. (1998). *Medical-surgical nursing: Foundations for clinical practice* (2nd ed.). Philadelphia: W. B. Saunders. p. 1784.

40. **4**

Rationale: Hypercalcemia is a serum calcium ion level greater than 11 mg/dL or 5.5 mEq/L. It most often occurs in clients who have bone metastasis and is a late manifestation of extensive malignancy. The presence of cancer in the bone causes the bone to release calcium into the blood stream.

Test-Taking Strategy: Knowledge regarding the normal calcium level will easily direct you to option 4. Note the relationship of "calcium level" in the question and "hypercalcemia" in the correct option. Review oncological emergencies now, if you had difficulty with this question!

Level of Cognitive Ability: Analysis
Phase of Nursing Process: Assessment
Client Needs: Physiological Integrity
Content Area: Adult Health/Oncology

Reference

Ignatavicius, D., Workman, M., & Mishler, M. (1995). *Medical surgical nursing: A nursing process approach* (2nd ed.). Philadelphia: W. B. Saunders. p. 583.

41. **4**

Rationale: A diet high in fat may be a factor in the development of breast, colon, and prostate cancer. High-fiber diets may reduce the risk of colon cancer. Excessive alcohol may increase the risk of cancer of the mouth, larynx, throat, esophagus, and liver.

Test-Taking Strategy: Eliminate option 3 first because the question does not address alcohol. Although the food items identified in options 1 and 2 are addressed in the question, option 4 is the global response and addresses both options 1 and 2!

Level of Cognitive Ability: Application
Phase of Nursing Process: Implementation
Client Needs: Health Promotion and Maintenance
Content Area: Adult Health/Oncology

Reference

Black, J., & Matassarin-Jacobs, E. (1997). *Medical-surgical nursing: Clinical management for continuity of care* (5th ed.). Philadelphia: W. B. Saunders. p. 541.

42. **1**

Rationale: Testicular cancer almost always occurs in only one testicle and is usually a pea-sized, painless lump. It is highly curable when found early. The client should report the finding to the physician when found.

Test-Taking Strategy: Eliminate option 4 because it does not address the client's concern and is a block to communication. Option 3 places the client's concern on hold and is an inappropriate and inaccurate response. Option 2 is nontherapeutic and may cause concern in the client. Review the TSE and therapeutic communication techniques now, if you had difficulty with this question!

Level of Cognitive Ability: Application
Phase of Nursing Process: Implementation
Client Needs: Psychosocial Integrity
Content Area: Adult Health/Oncology

Reference
Monahan, F., & Neighbors, M. (1998). *Medical-surgical nursing: Foundations for clinical practice* (2nd ed.). Philadelphia: W. B. Saunders. p. 334.

43. **2**

Rationale: Denial, bargaining, anger, depression, and acceptance are recognized stages that a person facing a life-threatening illness experiences. Denial is expressed as shock and disbelief and may be the first response to hearing bad news. Depression may be manifested by hopelessness, weeping openly, or remaining quiet or withdrawn. Anger may also be a first response to upsetting news, and the predominant theme is, "Why me?" or the blaming of others.

Test-Taking Strategy: Focus on the client's statement as identified in the question to assist in selecting the correct option. From this point, you should easily be able to eliminate options 1, 3, and 4. Review these stages now, if you had difficulty with this question!

Level of Cognitive Ability: Analysis
Phase of Nursing Process: Analysis
Client Needs: Psychosocial Integrity
Content Area: Adult Health/Oncology

Reference
Leahy, J., & Kizilay, P. (1998). *Foundations of nursing practice: A nursing process approach.* Philadelphia: W. B. Saunders. pp. 1148–1149.

44. **4**

Rationale: Arm edema on the operative side (lymphedema) is a complication following mastectomy and can occur immediately postoperatively, or secondary edema may occur months or even years after surgery. Options 1, 2, and 3 are expected occurrences following mastectomy and do not indicate a complication.

Test-Taking Strategy: Use the process of elimination, considering the normal, expected occurrences following a mastectomy. You should easily be able to eliminate options 1, 2, and 3. If you had difficulty with this question, take time now to review the complications following mastectomy!

Level of Cognitive Ability: Analysis
Phase of Nursing Process: Assessment
Client Needs: Physiological Integrity
Content Area: Adult Health/Oncology

Reference
Black, J., & Matassarin-Jacobs, E. (1997). *Medical-surgical nursing: Clinical management for continuity of care* (5th ed.). Philadelphia: W. B. Saunders. pp. 2440–2441.

45. **2**

Rationale: The most common risk factor associated with laryngeal cancer is cigarette smoking. Approximately three quarters of those diagnosed with this form of cancer smoke currently or have smoked in the past. Alcohol abuse seems to have a synergistic effect with cigarette smoking. Air pollution is also a contributing cause, as well as chronic laryngitis and voice abuse.

Test-Taking Strategy: Note the key words "most common" in the question. Begin to answer this question by eliminating options 3 and 4. Since cancer of the upper and lower airway is most often related to tobacco, these are the options that are most likely correct. To discriminate between the last two options, knowing that cigarettes are the most harmful guides you to choose this option over the chewing tobacco!

Level of Cognitive Ability: Application
Phase of Nursing Process: Assessment
Client Needs: Physiological Integrity
Content Area: Adult Health/Oncology

Reference
Black, J., & Matassarin-Jacobs, E. (1997). *Medical-surgical nursing: Clinical management for continuity of care* (5th ed.). Philadelphia: W. B. Saunders. p. 1082.

46. **2**

Rationale: The artificial larynx is an electronic device that assists clients to produce speech after laryngectomy. There are two types: one is held at the side of the neck and the other is inserted into the mouth. The vibration produces a mechanical-sounding speech that is monotone in quality but is intelligible.

Test-Taking Strategy: To answer this question accurately, it is necessary to be generally familiar with these devices. If you did not answer this question correctly, take a few moments to review this concept and the available devices that assist with speech!

Level of Cognitive Ability: Application
Phase of Nursing Process: Implementation
Client Needs: Physiological Integrity
Content Area: Adult Health/Respiratory

Reference
Black, J., & Matassarin-Jacobs, E. (1997). *Medical-surgical nursing: Clinical management for continuity of care* (5th ed.). Philadelphia: W. B. Saunders. p. 1093.

47. **3**

Rationale: A vesicovaginal fistula is a genital fistula that occurs between the bladder and the vagina. The fistula is an abnormal opening between these two body parts, and if this occurs, the client may experience drainage of urine through the vagina. The client's complaint is not associated with options 1, 2, and 4.

Test-Taking Strategy: Noting the key phrase "voiding through the vagina" should easily direct you to option 3. Review the symptoms associated with vesicovaginal fistula now, if you had difficulty with this question!

Level of Cognitive Ability: Analysis
Phase of Nursing Process: Analysis
Client Needs: Physiological Integrity
Content Area: Adult Health/Oncology

Reference
Monahan, F., & Neighbors, M. (1998). *Medical-surgical nursing: Foundations for clinical practice* (2nd ed.). Philadelphia: W. B. Saunders. p. 1821.

48. 2

Rationale: Allopurinol decreases uric acid production and reduces uric acid concentrations in both serum and urine. In the client receiving chemotherapy, uric acid levels elevate as a result of the massive cell destruction that occurs from the chemotherapy. This medication prevents or treats hyperuricemia secondary to chemotherapy. Although the medication is used to treat gout, it is not the purpose in this client situation. This medication is not used to prevent stomatitis or diarrhea.

Test-Taking Strategy: Knowledge regarding the action of this medication is required to answer this question. Recalling that hyperuricemia occurs as a result of chemotherapy will assist in directing you to option 2. If you had difficulty with this question or are unfamiliar with the action of this medication, take time now to review!

Level of Cognitive Ability: Analysis
Phase of Nursing Process: Analysis
Client Needs: Physiological Integrity
Content Area: Adult Health/Oncology

Reference
Hodgson, B., & Kizior, R. (1998). *Saunders nursing drug handbook 1998.* Philadelphia: W. B. Saunders. pp. 24–25.

49. 2

Rationale: An acidic environment in the mouth is favorable for bacterial growth, in an area already compromised from chemotherapy. Therefore, the client is advised to rinse the mouth at least before every meal and at bedtime with a weak salt and sodium bicarbonate mouth rinse. This lessens the growth of bacteria and limits plaque formation. The other substances are irritating to oral tissue, which is already at risk. If hydrogen peroxide must be used due to severe plaque, it should be a very weak solution, because it dries the mucous membranes.

Test-Taking Strategy: Specific knowledge of this complication of radiation and chemotherapy is needed to answer this question correctly. Options 3 and 4 can be eliminated first because of the irritating effects of these solutions. From the remaining options, note the word "weak" in the correct option. If needed, take a few moments now to review the treatment measures for stomatitis!.

Level of Cognitive Ability: Application
Phase of Nursing Process: Implementation
Client Needs: Physiological Integrity
Content Area: Adult Health/Oncology

Reference
Monahan, F., & Neighbors, M. (1998). *Medical-surgical nursing: Foundations for clinical practice* (2nd ed.). Philadelphia: W. B. Saunders. pp. 1529–1530.

50. 4

Rationale: High meat and carbohydrate consumption plays a role in the development of cancer of the pancreas. Options 1, 2, and 3 are risk factors related to gastric cancer. Additionally, an increased risk exists in the male population in clients 50 years of age and older and in clients with a history of precancerous lesions and chronic gastritis.

Test-Taking Strategy: Note that the question asks about the risk factors associated with gastric cancer. Note the key word "not" in the stem of the question. Eliminate options 1 and 2 because they are directly related to gastric disorders. Eliminate option 3 knowing that spicy foods cause gastric irritation. Review the risk factors associated with gastric cancer now, if you had difficulty with this question!

Level of Cognitive Ability: Application
Phase of Nursing Process: Implementation
Client Needs: Health Promotion and Maintenance
Content Area: Adult Health/Oncology

Reference
Monahan, F., & Neighbors, M. (1998). *Medical-surgical nursing: Foundations for clinical practice* (2nd ed.). Philadelphia: W. B. Saunders. pp. 1058, 1126.

51. 2

Rationale: Following gastrectomy, drainage from the NG tube is normally bloody for 24 hours postoperatively and then changes to brown-tinged and then to yellow or clear. Since bloody drainage is expected in the immediate postoperative period, the nurse should continue to monitor the drainage. There is no need to notify the physician at this time. Measuring abdominal girth is performed to detect the development of distention. Following gastrectomy, an NG tube should not be irrigated unless there are specific physician's orders to do so.

Test-Taking Strategy: Note the key words "immediate" and "most appropriate" in the question. These key items should easily direct you to option 2. If you had difficulty with this question, take time now to review the expected postoperative findings following gastrectomy!

Level of Cognitive Ability: Application
Phase of Nursing Process: Implementation
Client Needs: Physiological Integrity
Content Area: Adult Health/Oncology

Reference
Monahan, F., & Neighbors, M. (1998). *Medical-surgical nursing: Foundations for clinical practice* (2nd ed.). Philadelphia: W. B. Saunders. p. 999.

52. 3

Rationale: Colorectal cancer most often occurs in populations with diets low in fiber and high in refined carbohydrates, fats, and meats. Other risk factors include a family history of the disease, rectal polyps, and active inflammatory disease of at least 10 years' duration.

Test-Taking Strategy: Note the key word "not" in the stem of the question. Eliminate options 1 and 2 because they are similar and directly related to the issue of colorectal cancer. Knowledge that a high-fiber diet is recommended as a preventive measure will assist in selecting the correct option. Review the risk factors associated with colorectal cancer now, if you had difficulty with this question!

Level of Cognitive Ability: Analysis
Phase of Nursing Process: Analysis
Client Needs: Physiological Integrity
Content Area: Adult Health/Oncology

Reference

Monahan, F., & Neighbors, M. (1998). *Medical-surgical nursing: Foundations for clinical practice* (2nd ed.). Philadelphia: W. B. Saunders. p. 1100.

53. **3**

Rationale: Characteristic symptoms of right colon tumors include vague, dull abdominal pain exacerbated by walking, and dark red or mahogany-colored blood mixed in the stool. Options 1, 2, and 4 are symptoms associated with left colon tumors.

Test-Taking Strategy: Knowledge regarding the signs of right and left colon tumors is required to answer this question. If you are not familiar with the differences, take time now to review!

Level of Cognitive Ability: Analysis
Phase of Nursing Process: Assessment
Client Needs: Physiological Integrity
Content Area: Adult Health/Oncology

Reference

Monahan, F., & Neighbors, M. (1998). *Medical-surgical nursing: Foundations for clinical practice* (2nd ed.). Philadelphia: W. B. Saunders. p. 1100.

54. **3**

Rationale: To reduce the risk of contamination at the time of surgery, the bowel is emptied and cleansed. Laxatives and enemas are given to empty the bowel. Intestinal anti-infectives such as neomycin or kanamycin are administered to decrease the bacteria in the bowel.

Test-Taking Strategy: Knowledge regarding the purpose of administering anti-infectives prior to bowel surgery is required to answer the question. Eliminate options 1 and 4 first because no reference is made to this information in the question. Recalling the concepts related to the flora of the intestinal tract will assist in directing you to option 3 as the primary purpose of this medication. Review this important preoperative intervention now, if you had difficulty with this question!

Level of Cognitive Ability: Analysis
Phase of Nursing Process: Analysis
Client Needs: Physiological Integrity
Content Area: Adult Health/Oncology

Reference

Monahan, F., & Neighbors, M. (1998). *Medical-surgical nursing: Foundations for clinical practice* (2nd ed.). Philadelphia: W. B. Saunders. p. 1101.

55. **2**

Rationale: Immediately after surgery, profuse serosanguineous drainage from the perineal wound is expected. There is no need to notify the physician at this time. A Penrose drain should not be clamped because this action will cause the accumulation of drainage within the tissue. Both Penrose drains and packing are removed gradually over a period of 5 to 7 days. The nurse should not remove the perineal packing.

Test-Taking Strategy: Note the key words "most appropriate." Eliminate options 3 and 4 knowing that these are inappropriate interventions. Knowledge of the normal expectations following this type of surgery will assist in directing you to select option 2 as the most appropriate action. Review postoperative expectations following abdominal perineal resection now, if you had difficulty with this question!

Level of Cognitive Ability: Application
Phase of Nursing Process: Implementation
Client Needs: Physiological Integrity
Content Area: Adult Health/Oncology

Reference

Monahan, F., & Neighbors, M. (1998). *Medical-surgical nursing: Foundations for clinical practice* (2nd ed.). Philadelphia: W. B. Saunders. pp. 1101–1102.

56. **4**

Rationale: Following abdominal perineal resection, the nurse would expect the colostomy to begin to function within 72 hours after surgery, although it may take up to 5 days. The nurse should assess for a return of peristalsis, listen for bowel sounds, and check for the passage of flatus. Absent bowel sounds do not indicate the return of peristalsis. The client would remain NPO until bowel sounds return and the colostomy is functioning. Bloody drainage is not expected from a colostomy.

Test-Taking Strategy: Note the key phrase "beginning to function." This key phrase should assist in eliminating option 3. Knowledge of general postoperative measures will assist in eliminating option 2. Focus on the issue of the question to assist in eliminating option 1 as a correct option. Review postoperative care of a client following abdominal perineal resection now, if you had difficulty with this question!

Level of Cognitive Ability: Analysis
Phase of Nursing Process: Assessment
Client Needs: Physiological Integrity
Content Area: Adult Health/Oncology

Reference

Monahan, F. & Neighbors, M. (1998). *Medical-surgical nursing: Foundations for clinical practice* (2nd ed.). Philadelphia: W. B. Saunders. p. 1103.

57. **3**

Rationale: Air conditioners need to be avoided to protect from excessive coldness. A humidifier in the home should be used if excessive dryness is a problem. Options 1, 2, and 4 are appropriate interventions regarding stoma care following radical neck dissection and creation of a tracheostomy.

Test-Taking Strategy: Note the key word "not' in the stem of the question. You should easily be able to eliminate options 2 and 4. From the remaining options, recalling that a humidifier rather than an air conditioner is recommended will assist you in selecting the correct option. If you had difficulty with this question, take time now to review discharge instructions following radical neck dissection!

Level of Cognitive Ability: Application
Phase of Nursing Process: Implementation
Client Needs: Health Promotion and Maintenance
Content Area: Adult Health/Oncology

Reference
Monahan, F., & Neighbors, M. (1998). *Medical-surgical nursing: Foundations for clinical practice* (2nd ed.). Philadelphia: W. B. Saunders. p. 631.

58. **3**

Rationale: Serum acid phosphatase titers are elevated in clients with prostatic cancer because acid phosphatase, which is produced by the acinar cells, is absorbed into the circulation rather than secreted into the seminal fluid and kept in the prostate. This makes measurement of serum acid phosphatase a useful biochemical test for monitoring the progression or regression of prostatic cancer.

Test-Taking Strategy: Option 1 can be eliminated first knowing that biopsy is necessary to confirm the diagnosis of cancer. From the remaining options, select option 3 because it is the most global response. Review this serum test now, if you had difficulty with this question!

Level of Cognitive Ability: Analysis
Phase of Nursing Process: Analysis
Client Needs: Physiological Integrity
Content Area: Adult Health/Oncology

Reference
Monahan, F., & Neighbors, M. (1998). *Medical-surgical nursing: Foundations for clinical practice* (2nd ed.). Philadelphia: W. B. Saunders. p. 1757.

59. **1**

Rationale: Hormone therapy (androgen deprivation) is a mode of treatment for prostatic cancer. The goal is to limit the amount of circulating androgens because prostate cells depend on androgen for cellular maintenance. Deprivation of androgen can often lead to regression of disease and improvement of symptoms.

Test-Taking Strategy: Knowledge regarding the physiology associated with the prostate gland will assist in answering the question. Note that options 2, 3, and 4 all indicate an "increase." Your best selection, if you need to make an educated guess, is to select option 1. Review the goal of this form of therapy now, if you had difficulty with this question!

Level of Cognitive Ability: Analysis
Phase of Nursing Process: Analysis
Client Needs: Physiological Integrity
Content Area: Adult Health/Oncology

Reference
Monahan, F., & Neighbors, M. (1998). *Medical-surgical nursing: Foundations for clinical practice* (2nd ed.). Philadelphia: W. B. Saunders. p. 1759.

60. **4**

Rationale: Small pieces of tissue or blood clots can be passed during urination for up to 2 weeks after surgery. Driving a car and sitting for long periods of time are restricted for at least 3 weeks. A high daily fluid intake of 2 to 2.5 L/day should be maintained to limit clot formation and prevent infection. Option 4 is an accurate discharge instruction following prostatectomy.

Test-Taking Strategy: Option 3 can be easily eliminated first. Eliminate option 2 next, because 1 week is a rather short time period. Recalling that blood clots are expected following this type of surgery will assist in directing you to option 4. Review client teaching points following prostatectomy now, if you had difficulty with this question!

Level of Cognitive Ability: Application
Phase of Nursing Process: Implementation
Client Needs: Health Promotion and Maintenance
Content Area: Adult Health/Oncology

Reference
Monahan, F., & Neighbors, M. (1998). *Medical-surgical nursing: Foundations for clinical practice* (2nd ed.). Philadelphia: W. B. Saunders. p. 1720.

61. **1**

Rationale: The incidence of bladder cancer is three times greater in men than in women and affects the Caucasian population twice as often as African-Americans. Options 2, 3, and 4 are associated with the incidence of bladder cancer.

Test-Taking Strategy: Knowledge regarding the risk factors associated with bladder cancer is required to answer the question. Basic information regarding the risks associated with cancer will assist in eliminating options 3 and 4. If you had difficulty with this question, take time now to review these risks!

Level of Cognitive Ability: Application
Phase of Nursing Process: Implementation
Client Needs: Health Promotion and Maintenance
Content Area: Adult Health/Oncology

Reference
Monahan, F., & Neighbors, M. (1998). *Medical-surgical nursing: Foundations for clinical practice* (2nd ed.). Philadelphia: W. B. Saunders. p. 1419.

62. **3**

Rationale: The most common symptom in clients with cancer of the bladder is hematuria. The client may also experience irritative voiding symptoms such as frequency, urgency, and dysuria, and these symptoms are often associated with cancer in situ.

Test-Taking Strategy: Note the key words "most common" in the stem of the question. Options 1, 2, and 4 are symptoms that are also associated with bladder infection. If you need to make an educated guess, prioritize the options in a physiological manner and select option 3. Review the clinical manifestations associated with bladder cancer now, if you had difficulty with this question!

Level of Cognitive Ability: Analysis
Phase of Nursing Process: Assessment
Client Needs: Physiological Integrity
Content Area: Adult Health/Oncology

Reference
Monahan, F., & Neighbors, M. (1998). *Medical-surgical nursing: Foundations for clinical practice* (2nd ed.). Philadelphia: W. B. Saunders. p. 1419.

63. **4**

Rationale: Normally the medication is injected into the bladder through a urethral catheter, the catheter is clamped or removed, and the client is asked to retain the fluid for 2 hours. The client is to change position every 15 to 30 minutes from side to side and from supine to prone, or to resume all activity immediately. The client then voids and is instructed to drink water to flush the bladder.

Test-Taking Strategy: Knowledge regarding post-treatment care is required to answer this question. If you are unfamiliar with this treatment measure, take time now to review!

Level of Cognitive Ability: Application
Phase of Nursing Process: Implementation
Client Needs: Physiological Integrity
Content Area: Adult Health/Oncology

Reference

Black, J., & Matassarin-Jacobs, E. (1997). *Medical-surgical nursing: Clinical management for continuity of care* (5th ed.). Philadelphia: W. B. Saunders. p. 1584.

64. **2**

Rationale: Following ureterostomy, the stoma should be red and moist. A pale stoma may indicate an inadequate amount of vascular supply. A dry stoma may indicate body fluid deficit. Any sign of darkness or duskiness in the stoma may mean loss of vascular supply and must be corrected immediately or necrosis can occur.

Test-Taking Strategy: You should easily be able to eliminate options 1 and 4. From the remaining options, note the key word "moist" in option 2. This should indicate that this is an expected and positive assessment. If you had difficulty with this question, take time now to review expected and unexpected findings following ureterostomy!

Level of Cognitive Ability: Analysis
Phase of Nursing Process: Assessment
Client Needs: Physiological Integrity
Content Area: Adult Health/Oncology

Reference

Black, J., & Matassarin-Jacobs, E. (1997). *Medical-surgical nursing: Clinical management for continuity of care* (5th ed.). Philadelphia: W. B. Saunders. p. 1587.

65. **2**

Rationale: Following mastectomy, the arm should be elevated above the level of the heart. Arm exercises should be encouraged. No BP readings, injections, IV lines, or blood draws should be performed on the affected arm. Cool compresses are not a suggested measure to prevent lymphedema from occurring.

Test-Taking Strategy: Note the key phrase "assist in preventing." Use the process of elimination and note the relationship between the words "lymphedema" in the question and "elevating" in the correct option. Review these important measures now, if you had difficulty with this question!

Level of Cognitive Ability: Application
Phase of Nursing Process: Implementation
Client Needs: Physiological Integrity
Content Area: Adult Health/Oncology

Reference

Black, J., & Matassarin-Jacobs, E. (1997). *Medical-surgical nursing: Clinical management for continuity of care* (5th ed.). Philadelphia: W. B. Saunders. p. 2443.

66. **1**

Rationale: Closed-chest drainage is not usually used following pneumonectomy. The serous fluid that accumulates in the empty thoracic cavity eventually consolidates. The consolidation prevents shifts of the mediastinum, heart, and remaining lung. Complete lateral positioning is avoided because the mediastinum is no longer held in place on both sides by lung tissue, and extreme turning may cause mediastinal shift and compression of the remaining lung. Options 2 and 3 are general postoperative measures.

Test-Taking Strategy: Eliminate options 2 and 3 first. Attempt to visualize the effects of the surgical procedure in selecting the correct option. If you had difficulty with this question, take time now to review postoperative care of this important surgical procedure!

Level of Cognitive Ability: Application
Phase of Nursing Process: Implementation
Client Needs: Physiological Integrity
Content Area: Adult Health/Oncology

Reference

Black, J., & Matassarin-Jacobs, E. (1997). *Medical-surgical nursing: Clinical management for continuity of care* (5th ed.). Philadelphia: W. B. Saunders. pp. 1156, 1161.

67. **2**

Rationale: Mammography takes about 15 to 30 minutes to complete. Some discomfort may be experienced because of the breast compression required to obtain a clear image. There is no reason to maintain an NPO status prior to the procedure. Option 2 is an accurate instruction.

Test-Taking Strategy: Note the key word "accurate" in the question. Eliminate options 3 and 4 first. Attempt to visualize the procedure to assist in selecting the correct option. If you are unfamiliar with this important screening test, take time now to review!

Level of Cognitive Ability: Application
Phase of Nursing Process: Implementation
Client Needs: Physiological Integrity
Content Area: Adult Health/Oncology

Reference

Black, J., & Matassarin-Jacobs, E. (1997). *Medical-surgical nursing: Clinical management for continuity of care* (5th ed.). Philadelphia: W. B. Saunders. p. 2328.

68. **3**

Rationale: A Pap smear is usually painless. The test cannot be performed during menstruation. The client needs to be instructed to avoid douching for at least 24 hours prior to the test. There is no reason to restrict fluids on the day of the test.

Test-Taking Strategy: Knowledge regarding the Pap test is required to answer the question. Eliminate option 2 first as an unlikely preparation measure. Eliminate options 1 and 4 next because both menstruation and douching will affect the results of the test. Review client preparation for a Pap test now, if you had difficulty with this question!

Level of Cognitive Ability: Application
Phase of Nursing Process: Implementation
Client Needs: Physiological Integrity
Content Area: Adult Health/Oncology

Reference

Black, J., & Matassarin-Jacobs, E. (1997). *Medical-surgical nursing: Clinical management for continuity of care* (5th ed.). Philadelphia: W. B. Saunders. pp. 2320–2321.

69. **1**

Rationale: Vena caval syndrome occurs when the superior vena cava is compressed or obstructed by tumor growth. Early signs and symptoms generally occur in the morning and include edema of the face, especially around the eyes, and client complaints of tightness of a shirt or blouse collar. As the compression worsens, the client experiences edema of the hands and arms. Mental status changes and cyanosis are late signs.

Test-Taking Strategy: Note the key word "early" in the stem of the question. This key word should assist in eliminating options 2, 3, and 4. If you are unfamiliar with vena caval syndrome, take time now to review this important oncologic emergency!

Level of Cognitive Ability: Analysis
Phase of Nursing Process: Assessment
Client Needs: Physiological Integrity
Content Area: Adult Health/Oncology

Reference

Ignatavicius, D., Workman, M., & Mishler, M. (1995). *Medical-surgical nursing: A nursing process approach* (2nd ed.). Philadelphia: W. B. Saunders. p. 583.

70. **4**

Rationale: Spinal cord compression should be suspected in a client with metastatic disease, particularly when a new and sudden onset of back pain occurs. Spinal cord compression causes back pain before neurological changes occur. Spinal cord compression is an oncologic emergency, and the physician should be notified.

Test-Taking Strategy: The key phrase "new and sudden" should easily direct you to option 4. If you had difficulty with this question or are unfamiliar with spinal cord compression, take time now to review this oncologic emergency!

Level of Cognitive Ability: Application
Phase of Nursing Process: Implementation
Client Needs: Physiological Integrity
Content Area: Adult Health/Oncology

Reference

Ignatavicius, D., Workman, M., & Mishler, M. (1995). *Medical-surgical nursing: A nursing process approach* (2nd ed.). Philadelphia: W. B. Saunders. p. 582.

BIBLIOGRAPHY

Beare, P., & Myers, J. (1998). *Adult health nursing* (3rd ed.). St. Louis: Mosby–Year Book.

Black, J., & Matassarin-Jacobs, E. (1997). *Medical-surgical nursing. Clinical management for continuity of care* (5th ed.). Philadelphia: W. B. Saunders.

Chernecky, C., & Berger, B. (1997). *Laboratory tests and diagnostic procedures* (2nd ed.). Philadelphia: W. B. Saunders.

Hodgson, B., & Kizior, R. (1998). *Saunders nursing drug handbook 1998*. Philadelphia: W. B. Saunders.

Ignatavicius, D., Workman, M., & Mishler, M. (1995). *Medical-surgical nursing: A nursing process approach* (2nd ed.). Philadelphia: W. B. Saunders.

Kuhn, M. (1998). *Pharmaco-therapeutics: A nursing process approach* (4th ed.). Philadelphia: F. A. Davis.

Leahy, J., & Kizilay, P. (1998). *Foundations of nursing practice: A nursing process approach*. Philadelphia: W. B. Saunders.

Lehne, R. (1998). *Pharmacology for nursing care* (3rd ed.). Philadelphia: W. B. Saunders.

Luckmann, J. (1997). *Saunders manual of nursing care*. Philadelphia: W. B. Saunders.

Monahan, F., & Neighbors, M. (1998). *Medical-surgical nursing: Foundations for clinical practice* (2nd ed.). Philadelphia: W. B. Saunders.

O'Toole, M. (ed) (1997). *Miller-Keane encyclopedia & dictionary of medicine, nursing, & allied health* (6th ed.). Philadelphia: W. B. Saunders.

CHAPTER 50

Antineoplastic Medications

I. **Antineoplastic Medications**

A. Description
1. Kill or inhibit the reproduction of neoplastic cells
2. The effect of antineoplastic medications may not be limited to neoplastic cells; normal cells are also affected by the medication
3. Cell cycle phase-specific medications affect cells only during a certain phase of the reproductive cycle
4. Cell cycle phase-nonspecific medications affect cells in any phase of the reproductive cycle
5. Usually several medications are used in combination to increase the therapeutic response and minimize toxicity
6. Antineoplastic therapy may be combined with other treatments, such as surgery and radiation
7. The routes of antineoplastic medication administration can vary
8. Side effects result from the effects of the antineoplastic medication on normal cells

B. Side Effects
1. Mucositis/stomatitis
2. Alopecia
3. Anorexia
4. Nausea and vomiting
5. Diarrhea
6. Anemia
7. Low white blood cell (WBC) count (neutropenia)
8. Thrombocytopenia
9. Infertility

C. Implementation
1. Physiological Integrity
    a. Monitor complete blood count (CBC), WBC count, platelet count, and electrolytes
    b. Initiate bleeding precautions if thrombocytopenia occurs
    c. Monitor for petechiae, ecchymosis, bleeding of the gums, and nosebleeds as the decreased platelet count can precipitate bleeding tendencies
    d. Initiate neutropenic precautions if WBC count decreases
    e. Monitor for fever, sore throat, unusual bleeding, or signs and symptoms of infection
    f. Inform client that loss of appetite may also be due to a bitter taste in the mouth from the medications
    g. Monitor for nausea and vomiting and provide a high-calorie diet with protein supplements
    h. Administer antiemetics several hours before chemotherapy and for 12 to 48 hours after as prescribed, as antineoplastic medications stimulate the vomiting center
    i. Encourage hydration by IV fluids before and during therapy
    j. Promote a fluid intake of at least 2000 mL a day to maintain adequate renal function
    k. Administer allopurinol (Zyloprim) as prescribed to lower the serum uric acid that occurs from the rapid destruction of cells by the antineoplastic medications
2. Safe, Effective Care Environment
    a. Prepare IV chemotherapy solution in a vented space to ensure safety
    b. Wear gloves, a gown, and a mask when handling IV medications
    c. Monitor for phlebitis with IV administration, as these medications irritate veins
    d. Monitor for extravasation, which causes tissue necrosis; if this occurs, apply an ice pack and call physician
    e. Prepare to administer in short, high-dose, intermittent courses as prescribed to

maximize antineoplastic effects while allowing normal cells to recover
  f. Discard IV equipment in designated containers
  g. Avoid IM injections and venipunctures as much as possible to prevent bleeding
 3. Psychosocial Integrity
  a. Instruct client in the potential hair loss and that varying degrees of hair loss may occur after the first or second treatment
  b. Discuss the purchase of a wig before treatment starts
  c. Inform client that new hair growth will occur several months after the final treatment
  d. Instruct client about the need for contraception as these medications have teratogenic effects
  e. Discuss the potential effect of infertility, which may be irreversible
  f. Encourage pretreatment counseling
 4. Health Promotion and Maintenance
  a. Instruct client that if diarrhea is a problem, avoid hot foods and high-fiber foods, which increase peristalsis
  b. Instruct client to inspect oral mucosa for erythema and ulcers and to rinse mouth after meals and provide good oral hygiene
  c. Instruct client to use saline or sodium bicarbonate mouth rinses for mouth sores
  d. Instruct client in the use of antifungal medications for mouth sores, if prescribed for the development of a superinfection
  e. Instruct client to avoid crowds and persons with infections and to report signs of infection
  f. Instruct client to report any fever, chills, or sore throat
  g. Instruct individuals with colds or infections to wear a mask or avoid visiting the client
  h. Instruct client to use a soft toothbrush and an electric razor to minimize the risk of bleeding
  i. Instruct client to avoid alcohol to minimize the risk of toxicity
  j. Instruct client to avoid aspirin-containing products to minimize the risk of bleeding
  k. Instruct client to consult the physician before receiving vaccinations

II. Alkylating Medications (Box 50–1)

A. Description
 1. Affect the synthesis of DNA by causing cross-linking of DNA to inhibit cell reproduction
 2. Cell cycle phase-nonspecific medications
B. Side Effects
 1. Anorexia
 2. Nausea
 3. Vomiting
 4. Stomatitis

BOX 50–1. Alkylating Medications

NITROGEN MUSTARDS

Chlorambucil (Leukeran)
Cyclophosphamide (Cytoxan)
Estramustine phosphate sodium (Emcyt)
Ifosfamide (Ifex)
Mechlorethamine HCl (Mustargen)
Melphalan (Alkeran)
Uracil mustard

NITROSOUREAS

Busulfan (Myleran)
Carmustine (BiCNU)
Lomustine (CeeNu)
Streptozocin (Zanosar)

ALKYLATING-LIKE MEDICATIONS

Altretamine (Hexalen)
Carboplatin (Paraplatin)
Cisplatin (Platinol)
Dacarbazine (DTIC)
Triethylenethiophosphoramide (thiotepa)

---

 5. Skin rash
 6. Pain during IV administration
 7. Busulfan (Myleran) may cause hyperuricemia
 8. Chlorambucil (Leukeran) may cause gonadal suppression and hyperuricemia
 9. Cisplatin (Platinol) may cause ototoxicity, tinnitus, hypokalemia, hypocalcemia, hypomagnesemia, and nephrotoxicity
 10. Cyclophosphamide (Cytoxan) may cause alopecia, gonadal suppression, hemorrhagic cystitis, and hematuria
 11. Mechlorethamine HCl (Mustargen) may cause gonadal suppression and hyperuricemia
C. Implementation
 1. Assess vital signs and temperature for signs of infection
 2. Monitor CBC, WBC, platelets, uric acid, and electrolyte counts
 3. Withhold medication if platelet count is less than 75,000 cells/μL or WBC count is less than 4000 cells/μL, and notify physician
 4. Assess results of pulmonary function tests
 5. Assess results of chest radiographs and renal and liver function studies
 6. Hydrate client with IV and/or oral fluids before administering medication as prescribed
 7. Administer antiemetic 30 to 60 minutes before medication as prescribed
 8. Reduce pain with IV administration as prescribed by altering IV rates, diluting the medication, or warming the injection site to distend the vein and increase blood flow
 9. Monitor IV site for irritation and phlebitis
 10. When administering cisplatin (Platinol),

assess client for dizziness, tinnitus, hearing loss, incoordination, and numbness or tingling of extremities

11. Monitor for signs of hemorrhagic cystitis, such as hematuria or dysuria, during cyclophosphamide (Cytoxan) or ifosfamide (Ifex) therapy, and encourage client to drink increased fluids
12. Instruct client that cyclophosphamide (Cytoxan), when prescribed orally, is administered without food
13. Instruct client to increase fluids to 2 to 3 liters per day
14. Instruct client to follow a diet low in purines to alkalize the urine
15. Advise client to avoid citric acid
16. Instruct client to report signs of infection or bleeding
17. Instruct client how to avoid infection
18. Instruct client about good oral hygiene with a soft toothbrush

III. Antitumor Antibiotic Medications
(Box 50–2)

A. Description
 1. Interfere with DNA and ribonucleic acid synthesis
 2. Cell cycle phase-nonspecific medication
B. Side Effects
 1. Nausea and vomiting
 2. Fever
 3. Bone marrow depression
 4. Skin rash
 5. Alopecia
 6. Stomatitis
 7. Gonadal suppression
 8. Hyperuricemia
 9. Vesication (blistering of tissue at IV site)
 10. Plicamycin (Mithracin) affects bleeding time
 11. Daunorubicin (Cerubidine) may cause congestive heart failure (CHF) and dysrhythmias
 12. Doxorubicin (Adriamycin) and idarubicin (Idamycin) may cause cardiotoxicity, cardiomyopathy, and ECG changes
 13. Pulmonary toxicity can occur with bleomycin sulfate (Blenoxane)

BOX 50–2. Antitumor Antibiotic Medications

Bleomycin sulfate (Blenoxane)
Dactinomycin (actinomycin D, Cosmegen)
Daunorubicin (Cerubidine)
Doxorubicin (Adriamycin)
Idarubicin (Idamycin)
Mitomycin (Mutamycin)
Mitoxantrone (Novantrone)
Plicamycin (Mithracin)

C. Implementation
 1. Assess vital signs and temperature for signs of infection
 2. Monitor CBC, WBC, platelets, uric acid, bleeding time, and electrolyte counts
 3. Withhold medication if platelets are less than 75,000 cells/μL or WBC count is less than 4000 cells/μL, and notify physician
 4. Assess results of pulmonary function tests
 5. Monitor for ECG changes
 6. Assess lung sounds for rales
 7. Assess for signs of CHF, including dyspnea, crackles, peripheral edema, and weight gain
 8. Assess results of chest radiographs and renal and liver function studies
 9. Hydrate client with IV and/or oral fluids before administering medication as prescribed
 10. Administer antiemetic 30 to 60 minutes before medication as prescribed
 11. Reduce pain with IV administration as prescribed by altering IV rates, diluting the medication, or warming the injection site to distend the vein and increase blood flow
 12. Monitor IV site for irritation, phlebitis, and vesication
 13. Assess for myocardial toxicity, dyspnea, dysrhythmias, hypotension, and weight gain when administering doxorubicin (Adriamycin) or idarubicin (Idamycin)
 14. Monitor pulmonary status when administering bleomycin sulfate (Blenoxane)
 15. Avoid the use of aspirin, anticoagulants, and thrombolytic agents with plicamycin (Mithracin)

IV. Antimetabolite Medications (Box 50–3)

A. Description
 1. Halt the synthesis of cell protein
 2. Replace normal proteins required for DNA synthesis
 3. Cell cycle phase-specific and affect the S phase
B. Side Effects
 1. Anorexia
 2. Nausea
 3. Vomiting
 4. Diarrhea
 5. Alopecia
 6. Stomatitis
 7. Depression of bone marrow
 8. Cytarabine HCl (ara-C; Cytosar-U) may cause alopecia, stomatitis, hyperuricemia, and hepatotoxicity
 9. 5-Fluorouracil (5-FU; Adrucil) may cause alopecia, stomatitis, diarrhea, phototoxicity reactions, and cerebellar dysfunction
 10. 6-Mercaptopurine (Purinethol) may cause hyperuricemia and hepatotoxicity
 11. Methotrexate (Folex) may cause alopecia, stomatitis, hyperuricemia, photosensitivity,

BOX 50–3. Antimetabolite Medications

FOLIC ACID ANTAGONIST

Methotrexate (Folex)

PYRIMIDINE ANALOGS

Cytarabine HCl (ara-C; Cytosar-U)
Floxuridine (FUDR)
5-Fluorouracil (5-FU; Adrucil)
Procarbazine HCl (Matulane)

PURINE ANALOGS

6-Mercaptopurine (Purinethol)
Thioguanine

MISCELLANEOUS RIBONUCLEOTIDE REDUCTASE INHIBITORS

Hydroxyurea (Hydrea)
Trimetrexate glucuronate (NeuTrexin)

ANTIMICROTUBULE

Enzyme inhibitor
Paclitaxel (Taxol)
Pentostatin (Nipent)

PODOPHYLLOTOXIN DERIVATIVE

Etoposide (VePesid, VP-16)
Teniposide (Vumon, VM-26)

OTHER ANTIMETABOLITE MEDICATIONS

Cladribine (Leustatin)
Fludarabine (Fludara)

hepatotoxicity, and hematological, GI, and skin toxicity

C. Implementation
  1. Monitor vital signs
  2. Monitor temperature for signs of infection
  3. Assess CBC, WBC, uric acid, and platelet count
  4. Hold medication if WBC count is less than 4000 cells/μL or platelet count is less than 75,000 cells/μL and notify physician
  5. Monitor renal function studies
  6. Monitor for cerebellar dysfunction
  7. Assess for photosensitivity
  8. Administer antiemetics 30 to 60 minutes before medication as prescribed
  9. Monitor IV site for extravasation
  10. Encourage fluid intake of 2 to 3 liters a day
  11. Encourage good oral hygiene
  12. Instruct client to monitor for signs of infection or bleeding
  13. Instruct client how to avoid infections and bleeding
  14. When administering 5-fluorouracil (5-FU; Adrucil), assess for signs of cerebellar dysfunction, such as dizziness, weakness, and ataxia, and assess for stomatitis and diarrhea, which may necessitate medication discontinuation
  15. When administering methotrexate (Folex) in large doses, administer leucovorin (folinic acid or citrovorum factor) as prescribed to prevent fatal toxicity (known as leucovorin rescue)
  16. When administering 5-fluorouracil (5-FU, Adrucil) or methotrexate (Folex), instruct client to use sunscreen and wear protective clothing to prevent photosensitivity reactions

V. Vinca Alkaloids (Box 50–4)

A. Description
  1. Prevent mitosis causing cell death
  2. Mitotic inhibitor that prevents cell division
  3. Cell cycle phase-specific and act on the M phase

B. Side Effects
  1. Leukopenia
  2. Neurotoxicity with vincristine sulfate (Oncovin), manifested as numbness and tingling in the finger and toes
  3. Ptosis
  4. Hoarseness
  5. Motor instability
  6. Anorexia
  7. Nausea
  8. Vomiting
  9. Constipation
  10. Peripheral neuropathy
  11. Alopecia
  12. Stomatitis
  13. Hyperuricemia
  14. Phlebitis at IV site

C. Implementation
  1. Monitor vital signs
  2. Monitor WBC, CBC, uric acid, and platelet counts
  3. Monitor for hoarseness
  4. Assess eyes for ptosis
  5. Assess motor stability and initiate safety precautions as necessary
  6. Monitor for neurotoxicity with vincristine-sulfate (Oncovin), manifested as numbness and tingling in the finger and toes

VI. Hormonal Medications and Enzymes (Box 50–5)

A. Description
  1. Suppress the immune system and block normal hormones in hormone-sensitive tumors

BOX 50–4. Vinca Alkaloids

MEDICATIONS

Vinblastine sulfate (Velban)
Vincristine sulfate (Oncovin)
Vinorelbine (Navelbine)

BOX 50–5. Hormonal Medications and Enzymes

ANDROGENS

Progesterone (Gesterol 50)
Testolactone (Teslac)

HORMONAL ANTAGONISTS, ENZYMES

Aminoglutethimide (Cytadren)
Asparaginase (Elspar)
Diethylstilbestrol (DES; Stilphostrol)
Flutamide (Eulexin)
Goserelin acetate (Zoladex)
Leuprolide acetate (Lupron)
Megestrol acetate (Megace)
Mitotane (Lysodren)
Tamoxifen citrate (Nolvadex)

2. Change the hormonal balance and slow the growth rates of certain tumors
B. Side Effects
1. Anorexia
2. Nausea
3. Vomiting
4. Leukopenia
5. Impaired pancreatic function with asparaginase (Elspar)
6. Gynecomastia
7. Breast swelling
8. Hot flashes
9. Weight gain
10. Hemorrhagic cystitis, hypouricemia, and hypercholesterolemia, with mitotane (Lysodren)
11. Hypertension
12. Thromboembolitic disorders
13. Edema
14. Sex characteristic alterations
15. Electrolyte imbalances
16. Tamoxifen citrate (Nolvadex) may cause edema and hypercalcemia
17. Diethylstilbestrol (DES; Stilphostrol) may cause impotence and gynecomastia in men
18. Tamoxifen citrate (Nolvadex) decreases the effects of estrogen
19. Diethylstilbestrol (DES; Stilphostrol) may alter effects of insulin, oral anticoagulants, and oral hypoglycemic agents
C. Implementation
1. Monitor vital signs
2. Assess medications client is currently taking
3. Monitor serum calcium levels with androgens
4. Monitor for signs of alterations in sexual characteristics
5. Monitor pancreatic function with asparaginase (Elspar)
6. Encourage 2 to 3 liters of fluids per day
7. Monitor uric acid and cholesterol levels
8. Monitor for signs of hemorrhagic cystitis

PRACTICE QUESTIONS

1. The client with breast cancer is being treated with cyclophosphamide (Cytoxan). The nurse understands that this medication is:
   1 Cell cycle phase-specific, affecting cells only during a certain phase of the cell reproductive cycle
   2 Cell cycle phase-nonspecific, affecting cells in any phase of the reproductive cell cycle
   3 Cell cycle phase-specific, affecting the S phase of the reproductive cell cycle
   4 Cell cycle phase-specific, affecting the M phase of the reproductive cell cycle

2. The client with bladder cancer is receiving cisplatin (Platinol) and vincristine (Oncovin). The nurse understands that the purpose of administering both of these medications is to:
   1 Prevent gastrointestinal side effects
   2 Prevent alopecia
   3 Decrease the destruction of cells
   4 Decrease medication resistance and reduce medication toxicity

3. The nurse is monitoring the laboratory values of a client receiving an antineoplastic medication intravenously. The nurse initiates bleeding precautions when which of the following laboratory results is noted?
   1 A WBC of 3000/μL
   2 A platelet count of 70,000 cells/μL
   3 A clotting time of 10 minutes
   4 An ammonia level of 20 μg/dL

4. The nurse is monitoring the intravenous infusion of an antineoplastic medication. During the infusion, the client complains of pain at the insertion site. On inspection of the site, the nurse notes redness and swelling and sees that the infusion of the medication has slowed in rate. The most appropriate nursing action is to:
   1 Elevate the extremity of the IV site and slow the infusion
   2 Apply ice and maintain the infusion rate as prescribed
   3 Administer pain medication to reduce the discomfort
   4 Discontinue the infusion and notify the physician

5. The client with leukemia is receiving busulfan (Myleran). Allopurinol (Zyloprim) is prescribed for the client. The purpose of the allopurinol is to:
   1 Prevent gouty arthritis
   2 Prevent hyperuricemia
   3 Prevent stomatitis
   4 Prevent diarrhea

6. The nurse is providing instructions to a client with breast cancer. Cyclophosphamide (Cytoxan) had been prescribed for the client. Which of the

following would the nurse plan to include in the discharge instructions?
1 Take the medication with food
2 Increase fluid intake to 2000 to 3000 mL daily
3 Decrease sodium intake while taking the medication
4 Increase potassium intake while taking the medication

7. The client with non-Hodgkin's lymphoma is receiving daunorubicin (Cerubidine). Which of the following assessment signs indicate to the nurse that the client is experiencing a toxic effect related to the medication?
1 Nausea and vomiting
2 Fever
3 Rales on auscultation of the lungs
4 Diarrhea

8. The client with testicular cancer is receiving plicamycin (Mithracin). Which of the following physician's orders would the nurse question?
1 Warfarin (Coumadin)
2 Allopurinol (Zyloprim)
3 Acetaminophen (Tylenol)
4 Ondansetron (Zofran)

9. The client with squamous cell carcinoma of the larynx is receiving bleomycin sulfate (Blenoxane) by IV. Which of the following diagnostic studies does the nurse anticipate will be prescribed for this client?
1 Pulmonary function studies
2 Electrocardiogram
3 Cervical radiographs
4 Echocardiogram

10. Cytarabine HCL (Cytosar-U) is prescribed for the client with acute lymphocytic leukemia. The nurse understands that this medication is classified as an antimetabolite and is a:
1 Cell cycle-nonspecific medication
2 Cell cycle-specific medication affecting the M phase
3 Cell cycle-specific medication affecting the S phase
4 Medication that affects cells in any phase of the reproductive cell cycle

11. The clinic nurse prepares a teaching plan for the client receiving an antineoplastic medication. Which of the following does the nurse include in the plan of care?
1 Take aspirin (acetylsalicylic acid, ASA) as needed for headache
2 Drink beverages containing alcohol in moderate amounts
3 Consult with the physician before receiving immunizations
4 Be sure to receive the flu and pneumonia vaccine

12. The client with lung cancer is receiving a high dose of methotrexate (Folex). Leucovorin (citrovorum factor, folic acid) is also prescribed. The nurse understands that the purpose of administering the leucovorin is to:
1 Preserve normal cells
2 Promote DNA synthesis
3 Promote medication excretion
4 Promote the synthesis of nucleic acids

13. The client with ovarian cancer is being treated with vincristine (Oncovin). Which of the following indicates a side effect specific to this medication?
1 Diarrhea
2 Numbness and tingling in the fingers and toes
3 Chest pain
4 Hair loss

14. Asparaginase (Elspar), an antineoplastic agent, is contraindicated in which of the following conditions?
1 Myocardial infarction
2 Chronic obstructive pulmonary disease
3 Diabetes mellitus
4 Pancreatitis

15. Tamoxifen citrate (Nolvadex) is prescribed for the client with metastatic breast carcinoma. The primary action of this medication is to:
1 Increase DNA and RNA synthesis
2 Compete with estradiol for binding to estrogen in tissues containing high concentrations of receptors
3 Increase estrogen concentration and estrogen response
4 Promote the biosynthesis of nucleic acids

16. The client with metastatic breast cancer is receiving tamoxifen citrate (Nolvadex). Which of the following laboratory values would the nurse specifically monitor while the client is taking this medication?
1 Potassium level
2 Glucose level
3 Calcium level
4 Prothrombin time

17. Megestrol acetate (Megace), an antineoplastic medication, is prescribed for the client with metastatic endometrial carcinoma. This medication would be used with caution if the client had a history of:
1 Asthma
2 Myocardial infarction
3 Thrombophlebitis
4 Gout

18. A female client with carcinoma of the breast is admitted to the hospital for treatment with IV vincristine sulfate (Oncovin). The client tells the nurse that she has been told by her friends that

she is going to lose all of her hair. The most appropriate nursing response is which of the following?

1 "You will not lose your hair."
2 "Your friends are correct."
3 "Hair loss may occur, but it will grow back just as it is now."
4 "Hair loss may occur, and it will grow back, but it may have a different color or texture."

19. The clinic nurse prepares instructions for a client who developed stomatitis following the administration of a course of antineoplastic medications. Which of the following instructions is most appropriate to include in the plan of care?

1 To rinse the mouth with baking soda or saline
2 To avoid foods and fluids for the next 24 hours
3 To swab the mouth daily with lemon and glycerin pads
4 To brush teeth and use waxed dental floss three times a day

20. The client with acute myelocytic leukemia is being treated with busulfan (Myleran). Which of the following laboratory values would the nurse specifically monitor during treatment with this medication?

1 Blood glucose
2 Uric acid level
3 Potassium level
4 Clotting time

ANSWERS

1. **2**

Rationale: Cyclophosphamide is an antineoplastic medication of the alkylating classification. Medications in this classification affect all phases of the reproductive cell cycle. Cell phase-specific medications affect cells only during a certain phase of the reproductive cycle. Antimetabolite medications are cell cycle phase-specific and affect the S phase. Vinca alkaloids are cell cycle phase-specific and act on the M phase.

Test-Taking Strategy: Knowledge regarding the classification of this medication and the specific action of alkylating agents is required to answer the question. Use the process of elimination to answer the question, noting that option 2, the correct option, is different from the others. Option 2 addresses the action as cell cycle phase-nonspecific, whereas options 1, 3, and 4 address a cell cycle phase-specific action. If you had difficulty with this question, take time now to review the action of alkylating medications!

Level of Cognitive Ability: Analysis
Phase of Nursing Process: Analysis
Client Needs: Physiological Integrity
Content Area: Pharmacology

Reference

LeFever Kee, J., & Hayes, E. (1997). *Pharmacology: A nursing process approach* (2nd ed.). Philadelphia: W. B. Saunders, p. 410.

2. **4**

Rationale: Cisplatin is an alkylating-like medication, and vincristine is a vinca alkaloid. Alkylating medications are cell cycle phase-nonspecific. Vinca alkaloids are cell cycle phase-specific and act on the M phase. Single agent medication therapy is seldom used. Combinations of medications are used to enhance tumoricidal effects. Use of combination medications decreases medication resistance, shortens and intensifies the therapeutic effects of medications, increases destruction of cancer cells, and reduces medication toxicity.

Test-Taking Strategy: Knowledge of the rationale of combination medication therapy is required to answer the question. Use the process of elimination to answer the question. Eliminate option 3 first as the least likely option. Eliminate options 1 and 2. It may be possible, with some specific inter-

ventions, to reduce GI effects and alopecia, but it is unlikely that these occurrences can be prevented.

Level of Cognitive Ability: Analysis
Phase of Nursing Process: Analysis
Client Needs: Physiological Integrity
Content Area: Pharmacology

Reference

LeFever Kee, J., & Hayes, E. (1997). *Pharmacology: A nursing process approach* (2nd ed.). Philadelphia: W. B. Saunders, p. 409.

3. **2**

Rationale: Bleeding precautions need to be initiated when the platelet count drops. Bleeding precautions include avoiding all trauma, such as rectal temperatures or injections. The normal platelet count is 150,000 to 450,000 cells/μL. The normal WBC is 5000 to 10,000/μL. When the WBC count drops, neutropenic precautions need to be implemented. The normal clotting time is 8 to 15 minutes. The normal ammonia value is 15 to 45 μg/dL.

Test-Taking Strategy: Knowledge regarding normal laboratory values and the significance of the specific laboratory tests is required to answer the question. Options 3 and 4 identify normal laboratory values. To select between the last two options, correlate a low platelet count with the need for bleeding precautions, and a low WBC count with the need for neutropenic precaution. Learn this now! You are likely to find a question related to this concept on NCLEX-RN!

Level of Cognitive Ability: Application
Phase of Nursing Process: Implementation
Client Needs: Physiological Integrity
Content Area: Pharmacology

Reference

LeFever Kee, J., & Hayes, E. (1997). *Pharmacology: A nursing process approach* (2nd ed.). Philadelphia: W. B. Saunders, p. 413.

4. **4**

Rationale: When antineoplastic medications are administered by IV, great care must be taken to prevent the medication from escaping into the tissues surrounding the injection site, because pain, tissue damage, and necrosis can result. The nurse monitors for signs of extravasation, such as redness or swelling at the insertion site, a decreased infusion rate, inability to obtain a return of blood, and pain or resistance during the injection of medication. If extravasation occurs, discontinue the infusion but leave the needle or catheter in place. The physician needs to be notified.

Test-Taking Strategy: Use the process of elimination to answer the question. Eliminate options 1 and 2 first. Antineoplastic medications must be administered at the prescribed rate; therefore, you would not slow the rate. Based on the information in the question, you would not be able to maintain the prescribed rate. Administering pain medication to reduce discomfort at an IV site is not an appropriate action. Further investigation of the cause of the discomfort is required. This leaves option 4 as the correct nursing action.

Level of Cognitive Ability: Application
Phase of Nursing Process: Implementation
Client Needs: Physiological Integrity
Content Area: Pharmacology

Reference
Clark, J., Queener, S., & Karb V. (1997). *Pharmacologic basis of nursing practice* (5th ed.). St. Louis: Mosby–Year Book, p. 601.

5. **2**

Rationale: Busulfan is an alkylating medication used in the treatment of acute myelocytic leukemia and in the palliative treatment of chronic myelogenous leukemia. Hyperuricemia can result from the use of this medication, as it may produce uric acid nephropathy, renal stones, and acute renal failure. Allopurinol, an antigout medication, is used with chemotherapy to prevent or treat hyperuricemia secondary to blood dyscrasias caused by cancer chemotherapy. It may be used in mouthwash following fluorouracil (Adrucil) therapy to prevent stomatitis. Allopurinol is not used to prevent diarrhea.

Test-Taking Strategy: Knowledge of the side effects associated with busulfan and the purpose of administering allopurinol during the administration of antineoplastic medication is required to answer this question. Take time now to review both of these medications if you had difficulty with this question. You are likely to find a similar question on NCLEX-RN!

Level of Cognitive Ability: Analysis
Phase of Nursing Process: Analysis
Client Needs: Physiological Integrity
Content Area: Pharmacology

Reference
Hodgson, B., & Kizior, R. (1999). *Saunders nursing drug handbook 1999.* Philadelphia: W. B. Saunders, pp. 24, 132.

6. **2**

Rationale: Hemorrhagic cystitis is a toxic effect that can occur with the use of cyclophosphamide. The client needs to be instructed to drink copious amounts of fluid during the administration of this medication. Clients should also monitor urine output for hematuria. The medication should be taken on an empty stomach, unless GI upset occurs. Hyperkalemia can result from the use of the medication; therefore, the client would not be encouraged to increase potassium intake. The client would not be instructed to alter the sodium intake.

Test-Taking Strategy: Knowledge of the toxic effects of cyclophosphamide will assist you to answer this question correctly. If you correlated cyclophosphamide with hemor-

rhagic cystitis, then, by the process of elimination, option 2 would be selected. If you had difficulty with this question, take time now to review the toxic effects associated with this medication!

Level of Cognitive Ability: Application
Phase of Nursing Process: Planning
Client Needs: Health Promotion and Maintenance
Content Area: Pharmacology

Reference
Hodgson, B., & Kizior, R. (1999). *Saunders nursing drug handbook 1999.* Philadelphia: W. B. Saunders, pp. 270–272.

7. **3**

Rationale: Cardiotoxicity, noted as acute or transient abnormal ECG findings and/or cardiomyopathy manifested as congestive heart failure (CHF), is a toxic effect of daunorubicin. Bone marrow depression is also a toxic effect. Nausea and vomiting is a frequent side effect associated with the medication that begins a few hours after administration and lasts 24 to 48 hours. Fever is a frequent side effect, and diarrhea can occur occasionally.

Test-Taking Strategy: The ability to distinguish between side effects and toxic effects is required to answer the question. Use the process of elimination, keeping in mind that the question is asking for a toxic effect. This concept should direct you to the option addressing a sign of CHF. Additionally, the correct option presents the most serious concern. If you had difficulty with this question, take time now to review the toxic effects associated with daunorubicin!

Level of Cognitive Ability: Analysis
Phase of Nursing Process: Assessment
Client Needs: Physiological Integrity
Content Area: Pharmacology

Reference
Hodgson, B., & Kizior, R. (1999). *Saunders nursing drug handbook 1999.* Philadelphia: W. B. Saunders, p. 286.

8. **1**

Rationale: Plicamycin is an antitumor antibiotic. Because plicamycin affects bleeding time, the use of aspirin, anticoagulants, and thrombolytic agents should be avoided. Warfarin is an anticoagulant, and the risk of hemorrhage is increased if administered during plicamycin therapy. Allopurinol, an antigout medication, may be used with cancer chemotherapy to prevent or treat hyperuricemia secondary to blood dyscrasias. Acetaminophen may be used to treat mild discomfort. Ondansetron is an antiemetic used to prevent or treat nausea and vomiting during chemotherapy.

Test-Taking Strategy: Knowledge regarding the classifications of the medications identified in the options would assist in answering the question. With this knowledge, use the process of elimination to answer the question. If you are unfamiliar with these medications, take time now to review their classifications and purposes. Additionally, review the medication interactions associated with plicamycin!

Level of Cognitive Ability: Analysis
Phase of Nursing Process: Implementation
Client Needs: Safe, Effective Care Environment
Content Area: Pharmacology

Reference
Hodgson, B., & Kizior, R. (1999). *Saunders nursing drug handbook 1999.* Philadelphia: W. B. Saunders, p. 838.

9. **1**

Rationale: Bleomycin sulfate is an antineoplastic medication that can cause interstitial pneumonitis that can progress to pulmonary fibrosis. Pulmonary function studies, along with hematological, hepatic, and renal function tests, need to be monitored. The nurse needs to monitor lung sounds for dyspnea and rales that indicate pulmonary toxicity. The medication must be discontinued immediately if pulmonary toxicity occurs.

Test-Taking Strategy: Knowledge of the toxic effects of bleomycin sulfate is required to answer this question. Eliminate options 2 and 4 first as they are both cardiac related and therefore similar in nature. From this point, prioritize and select option 1 since it relates to airway. If you had difficulty with this question, take time now to review the toxic effects of this medication!

Level of Cognitive Ability: Analysis
Phase of Nursing Process: Analysis
Client Needs: Physiological Integrity
Content Area: Pharmacology

Reference

Hodgson, B., & Kizior, R. (1999). *Saunders nursing drug handbook 1999.* Philadelphia: W. B. Saunders, pp. 120–122.

10. **3**

Rationale: Cytarabine is an antimetabolite. Antimetabolites are classified as cell cycle-specific and affect the S phase (DNA synthesis and metabolism) of the reproductive cell cycle. Alkylating medications affect all phases of the cell reproductive cycle. Vinca alkaloids are cell cycle phase-specific and act on the M phase of the cell reproductive cycle.

Test-Taking Strategy: Eliminate options 1 and 4 first as they are similar. From this point, knowledge regarding the action of an antimetabolite is required to answer the question. Take time now to review this action if you had difficulty with this question!

Level of Cognitive Ability: Analysis
Phase of Nursing Process: Analysis
Client Needs: Physiological Integrity
Content Area: Pharmacology

Reference

LeFever Kee, J., & Hayes, E. (1997). *Pharmacology: A nursing process approach* (2nd ed.). Philadelphia: W. B. Saunders, p. 414.

11. **3**

Rationale: Since antineoplastic medications lower the body's resistance, clients must be informed not to receive immunizations without a physician's approval. Clients also need to avoid contact with individuals who have recently taken oral polio vaccine. Aspirin and aspirin-containing products need to be avoided to minimize the risk of bleeding. Alcohol needs to be avoided to minimize the risk of toxicity.

Test-Taking Strategy: Knowledge of the contraindications and cautions associated with the administration of antineoplastic medications is required to answer this question. Use the process of elimination, remembering that antineoplastic medications lower the body's resistance. Take time now to review the client-teaching points about these medications, if you had difficulty with this question!

Level of Cognitive Ability: Application
Phase of Nursing Process: Planning
Client Needs: Health Promotion and Maintenance
Content Area: Pharmacology

References

Hodgson, B., & Kizior, R. (1999). *Saunders nursing drug handbook 1999.* Philadelphia: W. B. Saunders, p. 430.
Pinnell, N. (1996). *Nursing pharmacology.* Philadelphia: W. B. Saunders, p. 946

12. **1**

Rationale: High concentrations of methotrexate cause harm and damage to normal cells. To save normal cells, leucovorin is given. This is known as leucovorin rescue. Leucovorin bypasses the metabolic block caused by methotrexate, thereby permitting normal cells to synthesize. It should be noted that leucovorin rescue is potentially hazardous. Failure to administer leucovorin in the right dose at the right time can be fatal.

Test-Taking Strategy: Knowledge of the action of leucovorin and the purpose of administering this medication with methotrexate is required to answer this question. Eliminate options 2 and 4 first as they are similar. Nucleic acids include RNA and DNA. Eliminate option 3 because increased fluids and diuretics are normally administered to promote medication excretion. This leaves option 1 as the correct answer. If you had difficulty with this question, take time now to review leucovorin rescue!

Level of Cognitive Ability: Analysis
Phase of Nursing Process: Analysis
Client Needs: Physiological Integrity
Content Area: Pharmacology

Reference

Lehne, R. (1998). *Pharmacology for nursing care* (3rd ed.). Philadelphia: W. B. Saunders, p. 1027.

13. **2**

Rationale: A side effect specific to vincristine is peripheral neuropathy, which occurs in nearly every client. This can be manifested as numbness and tingling in the fingers and toes. Depression of the Achilles tendon reflex may be the first clinical sign indicating peripheral neuropathy. Constipation rather than diarrhea is most likely to occur with this medication, although diarrhea may occur occasionally. Hair loss occurs with nearly all the antineoplastic medications. Chest pain is unrelated to this medication.

Test-Taking Strategy: Knowledge of the side effects associated with this medication is required to answer this question. Eliminate options 1 and 4 first as these side effects are associated with many of the antineoplastic agents. Note that the question asks for the side effect "specific" to this medication. Correlate peripheral neuropathy with vincristine!

Level of Cognitive Ability: Analysis
Phase of Nursing Process: Assessment
Client Needs: Physiological Integrity
Content Area: Pharmacology

Reference

Hodgson, B., & Kizior, R. (1999). *Saunders nursing drug handbook 1999.* Philadelphia: W. B. Saunders, pp. 1053–1054.

14. 4

Rationale: Asparaginase is contraindicated if hypersensitivity exists, in pancreatitis, or if the client has a history of pancreatitis. The medication impairs pancreatic function, so pancreatic function tests should be performed before therapy begins and when a week or more has elapsed between the administration of the doses. The client needs to be monitored for signs of pancreatitis, which include nausea, vomiting, and abdominal pain.

Test-Taking Strategy: Knowledge of the contraindications associated with asparaginase is required to answer this question. Take time now to review this medication if you had difficulty answering this question!

Level of Cognitive Ability: Analysis
Phase of Nursing Process: Assessment
Client Needs: Physiological Integrity
Content Area: Pharmacology

Reference
Hodgson, B., & Kizior, R. (1999). *Saunders nursing drug handbook 1999.* Philadelphia: W. B. Saunders, pp. 72–74.

15. 2

Rationale: Tamoxifen is an antineoplastic medication that competes with estradiol for binding to estrogen in tissues containing high concentrations of receptors. It is used in the treatment of metastatic breast carcinoma in women and men. It is also effective in delaying the recurrence of cancer following mastectomy. It reduces DNA synthesis and estrogen response.

Test-Taking Strategy: Eliminate options 1 and 4 first as they are similar. Nucleic acids include DNA and RNA. From this point, select option 2, because it is unlikely that treatment of metastatic breast carcinoma would focus on increasing estrogen concentration and estrogen response. If you had difficulty with this question, take time now to review the action of this medication!

Level of Cognitive Ability: Analysis
Phase of Nursing Process: Analysis
Client Needs: Physiological Integrity
Content Area: Pharmacology

Reference
Hodgson, B., & Kizior, R. (1999). *Saunders nursing drug handbook 1999.* Philadelphia: W. B. Saunders, p. 961.

16. 3

Rationale: Tamoxifen may increase calcium, cholesterol, and triglyceride levels. Prior to the initiation of therapy, a CBC, platelet count, and serum calcium levels should be assessed. These blood levels should be monitored periodically during therapy. The nurse should assess for hypercalcemia while the client is taking this medication. Signs of hypercalcemia include increased urine volume, excessive thirst, nausea, vomiting, constipation, hypotonicity of muscles, and deep bone or flank pain.

Test-Taking Strategy: Knowledge of the laboratory values that are affected while the client is taking this medication is required to answer this question. Take time now to review this important medication if you had difficulty answering this question!

Level of Cognitive Ability: Analysis
Phase of Nursing Process: Assessment
Client Needs: Physiological Integrity
Content Area: Pharmacology

Reference
Hodgson, B., & Kizior, R. (1999). *Saunders nursing drug handbook 1999.* Philadelphia: W. B. Saunders, p. 962.

17. 3

Rationale: Megestrol acetate suppresses the release of luteinizing hormone from the anterior pituitary by inhibiting pituitary function and regressing tumor size. It is used with caution if the client has a history of thrombophlebitis.

Test-Taking Strategy: Knowledge of the contraindications associated with the administration of this medication is required to answer this question. Take time now to review this important medication if you had difficulty answering this question!

Level of Cognitive Ability: Analysis
Phase of Nursing Process: Assessment
Client Needs: Physiological Integrity
Content Area: Pharmacology

Reference
Hodgson, B., & Kizior, R. (1999). *Saunders nursing drug handbook 1999.* Philadelphia: W. B. Saunders, p. 634.

18. 4

Rationale: Alopecia, hair loss, can occur following the administration of many antineoplastic medications. Alopecia is reversible, but new hair growth may have a different color and texture.

Test-Taking Strategy: Use knowledge of the side effects of antineoplastic medications and therapeutic communication techniques to answer this question. Eliminate options 1 and 2 first. Option 1 is incorrect, and option 2 is a nontherapeutic response. Take time now to review content related to hair loss and antineoplastic medications, if you had difficulty with this question!

Level of Cognitive Ability: Application
Phase of Nursing Process: Implementation
Client Needs: Psychosocial Integrity
Content Area: Pharmacology

Reference
Hodgson, B., & Kizior, R. (1999). *Saunders nursing drug handbook 1999.* Philadelphia: W. B. Saunders, p. 1054.

19. 1

Rationale: Stomatitis, ulceration in the mouth, can occur as a result of the administration of antineoplastic medications. The client should be instructed to examine the mouth daily and to report any signs of ulceration. If stomatitis occurs, instruct the client to rinse the mouth with baking soda or saline. Food and fluid are important and should not be restricted. If chewing and swallowing are painful, the client may switch to a liquid diet that includes milkshakes and ice cream. Instruct the client to avoid spicy foods and foods with hard crusts or edges. The client should avoid toothbrushing and flossing when stomatitis is severe. Lemon and glycerin swabs may cause pain and further irritation.

Test-Taking Strategy: Knowing that stomatitis involves ulcerations in the mucous membrane of the mouth will assist you in the process of eliminating the incorrect options. Eliminate option 2 first because foods and fluids would not be restricted in a client who received antineoplastic medication. Eliminate option 3 because lemon can be irritating to ulcerated lesions. Eliminate option 4 because a toothbrush and floss will also irritate ulcerations and may cause bleeding. If you had difficulty with this question, take time now to review the client-teaching points related to stomatitis!

Level of Cognitive Ability: Application
Phase of Nursing Process: Implementation
Client Needs: Physiological Integrity
Content Area: Pharmacology

Reference
LeFever Kee, J., & Hayes, E. (1997). *Pharmacology: A nursing process approach* (2nd ed.). Philadelphia: W. B. Saunders, p. 417.

20. **2**

Rationale: Busulfan can cause an increase in the uric acid level. Hyperuricemia can produce uric acid nephropathy, renal stones, and acute renal failure.

Test-Taking Strategy: Knowledge of the adverse effects of this medication is required to answer this question. If you had difficulty with this question, take time now to review the effects of busulfan!

Level of Cognitive Ability: Analysis
Phase of Nursing Process: Assessment
Client Needs: Physiological Integrity
Content Area: Pharmacology

Reference
Hodgson, B., & Kizior, R. (1999). *Saunders nursing drug handbook 1999.* Philadelphia: W. B. Saunders, pp. 133–134.

BIBLIOGRAPHY

Clark, J., Queener, S., & Karb V. (1997). *Pharmacologic basis of nursing practice* (5th ed.). St. Louis: Mosby–Year Book.

Hodgson, B., & Kizior, R. (1999). *Saunders nursing drug handbook 1999.* Philadelphia: W. B. Saunders.

LeFever Kee, J., & Hayes, E. (1997). *Pharmacology: A nursing process approach* (2nd ed.). Philadelphia: W. B. Saunders

Lehne, R. (1998). *Pharmacology for nursing care* (3rd ed.). Philadelphia: W. B. Saunders.

Pinnell, N. (1996). *Nursing pharmacology.* Philadelphia: W. B. Saunders.

UNIT XI

The Adult Client with an Endocrine Disorder

PYRAMID TERMS

Addisonian Crisis—A life-threatening disorder caused by adrenal hormone insufficiency. It is precipitated by infection, trauma, stress, or surgery. Death can occur from shock, vascular collapse, or hyperkalemia.

Addison's Disease—Hyposecretion of adrenal cortex hormones (glucocorticoids and mineralocorticoids) from the adrenal gland, resulting in deficiency of the steroid hormones. The condition is fatal if left untreated.

Adrenalectomy—The surgical removal of an adrenal gland. Lifelong steroid replacement is necessary with a bilateral adrenalectomy. Temporary steroid replacement, up to 2 years, is necessary for a unilateral adrenalectomy.

Chvostek's Sign—A spasm of the facial muscles elicited by tapping the facial nerve in the region of the parotid gland. It is noted in hypocalcemia.

Cushing's Syndrome—A condition resulting from the hypersecretion of glucocorticoids from the adrenal cortex.

Dawn Phenomenon—Results from a nocturnal release of growth hormone secretion that may cause blood glucose elevations at about 5 to 6 A.M. Treatment includes administering an evening dose of intermediate-acting insulin at 10 P.M.

Diabetic Ketoacidosis (DKA)—A complication of diabetes mellitus that develops when a severe insulin deficiency occurs. DKA is a life-threatening condition. Hyperglycemia that progresses to ketoacidosis occurs. Seen in clients with insulin-dependent diabetes mellitus (IDDM), undiagnosed diabetics, and persons who stop prescribed treatment for diabetes. It develops over a period of several hours to days.

Diabetes Insipidus—The hyposecretion of antidiuretic hormone (ADH) and a deficiency of vasopressin. Results in failure of tubular reabsorption of water in the kidneys.

Diabetes Mellitus—A chronic and potentially disabling disease characterized by elevated blood sugar levels. A chronic disorder of glucose intolerance and impaired carbohydrate, protein, and lipid metabolism because of a deficiency of insulin. A deficiency of insulin results in hyperglycemia.

Graves' Disease (Hyperthyroidism)—Known as thyrotoxicosis. A hyperthyroid state resulting from a hypersecretion of thyroid hormone.

Hyperglycemia—Elevated blood glucose level.

Hyperosmolar Hyperglycemic Nonketotic Coma (HHNC)—Extreme hyperglycemia without acidosis. Usually occurs in noninsulin-dependent diabetics when diabetes is uncontrolled or undiagnosed, or during stress or infection. The major difference between HHNC and DKA is the lack of ketone production with HHNC. Onset is usually slow, taking from hours to days.

Hypoglycemia (Insulin Reaction)—Described as a blood glucose level below 50 to 60 mg/dL. Occurs as a result of too much insulin, not enough food, or excessive activity.

Hypophysectomy—The removal of the pituitary gland.

Myxedema (Hypothyroidism)—A hypothyroid state resulting from a hyposecretion of thyroid hormone. The condition occurs in adulthood.

Myxedema Coma—A rare but serious disorder that results from a persistent low thyroid production. It can be precipitated by acute illness, rapid withdrawal of thyroid medication, anesthesia and surgery, hypothermia, and the use of sedatives and narcotics.

Somogyi's Phenomenon—A rebound phenomenon occurring in diabetes mellitus. Overtreatment with insulin induces hypoglycemia, which initiates the release of epinephrine, ACTH, glucagon, and growth hormone. Lipolysis, glyconeogenesis, and glycogenolysis result in rebound hyperglycemia and ketosis. Occurs during the initial period of serum glucose control; develops at peak insulin times and during the night.

Thyroidectomy—Removal of the thyroid gland. Performed in conditions in which persistent hyperthryoidism exists.

Thyroid Storm—An acute and fatal thyroid condition that occurs from manipulation of the thyroid gland during surgery and the release of thyroid hormone into the blood stream. It can also occur from severe infection and stress.

Trousseau's Sign—A sign found in hypocalcemia in which carpal spasm can be elicited by compressing the upper arm and causing ischemia to the nerves distally.

PYRAMID TO SUCCESS

The endocrine system is made up of organs or glands that secrete hormones and release these hormones directly into the circulation. The endocrine system can be easily understood if you remember that basically one of two situations can occur; that is, either hyposecretion or hypersecretion of hormones from the organ or gland. When an excess of the hormone occurs, treatment is aimed at blocking the hormone release through medication or surgery. When a deficit of the hormone exists, treatment is aimed at replacement therapy. Pyramid points focus on diabetes mellitus; the prevention and treatment of complications and insulin therapy, hypoglycemic and hyperglycemic reactions, and diabetic ketoacidosis; Addison's disease and addisonian crisis; Cushing's syndrome; thyroid disorders; thyroid storm; and care to the client following thyroidectomy or adrenalectomy.

NURSING PROCESS

ASSESSMENT

Appetite changes
Growth imbalances
Weight gain or loss
Fluid and electrolyte imbalances
Gastrointestinal (GI) disturbances
Headache
Hypotension or hypertension
Hyperglycemia or hypoglycemia
Cardiac dysrhythmias
Abnormal skin pigmentation
Skin turgor
Signs of impaired healing

Fever and diaphoresis
Generalized weakness
Sensitivity to cold or heat
Exophthalmos
Visual disturbances
Hirsutism
Polyuria, polydipsia, and polyphagia
Mental status changes and emotional disturbances
Personality changes and mood swings
Menstrual changes
Impotence

ANALYSIS: Altered Nutrition

PLANNING	IMPLEMENTATION	EVALUATION
The client will verbalize the prescribed diet plan. The client will maintain glucose levels to as near normal as possible.	Instruct client in prescribed diet therapy. Instruct client and family how to shop and select items required to maintain prescribed dietary therapies.	The client maintains appropriate body weight. Blood glucose levels remain within the expected range.

ANALYSIS: Fluid Deficit or Excess

PLANNING	IMPLEMENTATION	EVALUATION
The client's fluid imbalance will return to normal.	Monitor fluid and electrolyte balance closely. Administer replacement therapy as prescribed.	Maintenance of normal fluid balance is achieved as evidenced by balanced intake and output (I&O), stable vital signs, stable weight, and normal laboratory values.

ANALYSIS: Altered Tissue Perfusion

PLANNING	IMPLEMENTATION	EVALUATION
The client will identify factors that increase the risk for altered tissue perfusion.	Assess neurological status. Monitor client for alterations in neurovascular and cardiovascular status.	Adequate tissue perfusion is maintained.

ANALYSIS: Alteration in Comfort

PLANNING	IMPLEMENTATION	EVALUATION
The client verbalizes the need for pain relief measures.	Encourage client to verbalize measures that reduce pain.	The client remains comfortable.

ANALYSIS: Infection

PLANNING	IMPLEMENTATION	EVALUATION
The client remains free of infection.	Instruct client regarding measures to prevent infection. Instruct client in signs and symptoms of infection.	The client remains free of signs of infection.

ANALYSIS: Impaired Skin Integrity

PLANNING	IMPLEMENTATION	EVALUATION
The client will maintain intact skin.	Assess skin integrity. Instruct client in measures to maintain skin integrity.	The client complies with treatment measures to prevent complications related to skin integrity.

ANALYSIS: Sensory Perceptual Alterations

PLANNING	IMPLEMENTATION	EVALUATION
The client will maintain an appropriate sensory and perceptual status.	Assess vision and hearing abilities. Instruct client to obtain vision examinations every 6 to 12 months as prescribed.	Client remains free of sensory or perceptual disturbances.

ANALYSIS: Altered Thought Processes

PLANNING	IMPLEMENTATION	EVALUATION
The client will remain free of injury. The client verbalizes changes in feelings and mood.	Orient client to environment. Encourage client to discuss feelings related to personality changes. Discuss the causes of the changes that occur in personality. Promote a positive and calm environment.	The client is free of injury. The client is oriented to person, place and time. The client describes altered feelings.

ANALYSIS: Body Image Disturbances

PLANNING	IMPLEMENTATION	EVALUATION
The client will experience an improvement in body image.	Encourage client to discuss feelings related to body image.	The client states that body image improves.

ANALYSIS: Sexual Dysfunction

PLANNING	IMPLEMENTATION	EVALUATION
The client achieves a personal desired level of sexual functioning.	Identify problems that the client is experiencing related to sexual functioning. Encourage the client to express the effect that sexual dysfunction has had on the sexual partner.	The client participates in sexual activity as desired.

ANALYSIS: Knowledge Deficit

PLANNING	IMPLEMENTATION	EVALUATION
The client verbalizes the treatments prescribed. The client verbalizes the importance of the prescribed therapies. The client correctly demonstrates how to administer medications and injections.	Instruct client regarding the prescribed treatment plan. Instruct client on the disease process and the rationale for the prescribed plan. Instruct the client in measures to prevent complications. Instruct the client in the signs and symptoms of complications related to the disorder. Instruct client in preventive measures of complications. Instruct client and family regarding medications and the administration of injections.	The client complies with the prescribed treatment plan. The client obtains and carries or wears a Medic-Alert bracelet. The client notifies the physician when appropriate.

CLIENT NEEDS

SAFE, EFFECTIVE CARE ENVIRONMENT

Advocacy related to client's decisions
Informed consent related to diagnostic tests and procedures
Confidentiality related to client condition
Accident prevention in the client with altered mental status
Asepsis
Handling hazardous and infectious materials

HEALTH PROMOTION AND MAINTENANCE

Describing expected body image changes
Disease prevention related to potential complications
Health screening related to diabetes
Instructions regarding the prescribed treatment plan
Instructions regarding the effect of diet therapy, exercise, and the administration of insulin to the diabetic client
Addressing lifestyle choices

PSYCHOSOCIAL INTEGRITY

Coping mechanisms related to the endocrine disturbance
Sensory or perceptual alterations related to the disorder
Unexpected body image disturbances
Role changes and support systems

PHYSIOLOGICAL INTEGRITY

Basic care and comfort measures
Expected effects of medication administration
Laboratory values of diagnostic tests
Identifying potential complications
Providing care in emergencies

BIBLIOGRAPHY

Black, J., & Matassarin-Jacobs, E. (1997). *Medical-surgical nursing: Clinical management for continuity of care* (5th ed.). Philadelphia: W. B. Saunders.

Monahan, F., & Neighbors, M. (1998). *Medical-surgical nursing: Foundations for clinical practice* (2nd ed.). Philadelphia: W. B. Saunders.

National Council of State Boards of Nursing (eds.) (1997). *Test plan for the National Council Licensure Examination for Registered Nurses. Chicago:* Author.

O'Toole, M. (ed.) (1997). *Miller-Keane encyclopedia & dictionary of medicine, nursing, & allied health* (6th ed.). Philadelphia: W. B. Saunders.

CHAPTER 51

Endocrine System

. . . .

I. Anatomy and Physiology of Endocrine Glands (Box 51–1)

A. Functions
1. Maintenance and regulation of vital functions
2. Response to stress and injury
3. Growth and development
4. Energy metabolism
5. Reproduction
6. Fluid, electrolyte, and acid-base balance

B. Pituitary gland (Box 51–2)
1. The master gland
2. Located at the base of the brain
3. Influenced by the hypothalamus
4. Directly affects function of other endocrine glands
5. Promotes growth of body tissue
6. Influences water absorption by the kidney
7. Controls sexual development and function

C. Adrenal gland
1. Rests upon each kidney
2. Regulates sodium and electrolyte balance
3. Affects carbohydrate, fat, and protein metabolism
4. Influences the development of sexual characteristics
5. Sustains the "flight or fight" response
6. Adrenal cortex
   a. The inner core of the adrenal gland
   b. Synthesizes glucocorticoids and mineralocorticoids and secretes small amounts of sex hormones (androgens, estrogens) (Box 51–3)
7. Adrenal medulla
   a. The outer shell of the adrenal gland
   b. Works as part of the sympathetic nervous system
   c. Produces epinephrine and norepinephrine

D. Thyroid gland
1. Located in the anterior part of the neck
2. Controls the rate of body metabolism and growth
3. Produces thyroxine (T_4), triiodothyronine (T_3), and thyrocalcitonin

E. Parathyroid gland
1. Located near the thyroid
2. Controls calcium and phosphorus metabolism
3. Produces parathyroid hormone (PTH)

F. Pancreas
1. Located posterior to the liver
2. Influences carbohydrate metabolism
3. Indirectly influences fat and protein metabolism
4. Produces insulin and glucagon

G. Ovaries and testes
1. Ovaries
   a. Located in the pelvic cavity
   b. Produce estrogen and progesterone
2. Testes
   a. Located in the scrotum
   b. Control the development of the secondary sex characteristics
   c. Produce testosterone

BOX 51–2. Pituitary Gland

ANTERIOR LOBE PRODUCTION

ACTH (adrenocorticotropic hormone)
TSH (thyroid-stimulating hormone)
STH (somatotropic growth-stimulating hormone)
FSH (follicle-stimulating hormone)
LH (lutcinizing hormone)
PRL (prolactin)
GH (growth hormone)
MSH (melanocyte-stimulating hormone)

POSTERIOR LOBE PRODUCTION

ADH (vasopressin, antidiuretic hormone)
Oxytocin

Box 51–1. Endocrine Glands

Pituitary	Parathyroid	Ovaries
Adrenal	Pancreas	Testes
Thyroid		

BOX 51–3. Glucocorticoids

CORTISOL, CORTISONE, CORTICOSTERONE

Responsible for glucose metabolism, protein metabolism, fluid and electrolyte balance, suppression of the inflammatory response to injury, the protective immune response to invasion by infectious agents, and resistance to stress

MINERALOCORTICOIDS

ALDOSTERONE

Regulates electrolyte balance by promoting sodium retention and potassium excretion

---

II. Diagnostic Tests

A. Radioactive iodine (RAI) uptake
   1. A thyroid function test that measures the absorption of the iodine isotope to determine how the thyroid gland is functioning
   2. The amount of radioactivity is measured 2, 6, and 24 hours after ingestion of the capsule
   3. Normal value is 5% to 35% in 24 hours
   4. Elevated values are indicative of **hyperthyroidism, thyrotoxicosis**, decreased iodine intake or increased iodine excretion
   5. Decreased values indicate a low T_4, the use of antithyroid medications, thyroiditis, myxedema, or **hypothyroidism**
B. T_3 and T_4 resin uptake test
   1. Blood tests for the diagnosis of thyroid disorders
   2. T_3 and T_4 regulate thyroid-stimulating hormone
   3. Normal values
      a. T_3: 25% to 35%
      b. T_4: 3.8% to 11.4%
   4. The T_3 is elevated in **hyperthyroidism** and T_3 toxicosis, decreases with the aging process, and may be decreased in hypothyroidism
   5. The T_4 is elevated in **hyperthyroidism** and decreased in **hypothyroidism**
C. Thyroid-stimulating hormone (TSH)
   1. Blood test used to differentiate the diagnosis of primary **hypothyroidism**
   2. Normal value is 0 to 6 μU/mL
   3. Elevated values indicate primary **hypothyroidism**
   4. Decreased values indicate **hyperthyroidism** or secondary **hypothyroidism**
D. Thyroid scan
   1. Performed to identify nodules or growths in the thyroid gland
   2. A radioisotope of iodine or technetium is administered prior to the scanning of the thyroid gland
   3. Reassure the client that the level of radioactive medication is not dangerous to self and others
   4. Determine whether the client has received radiographic contrast agents within the past 3 months, as these may invalidate the scan
   5. Check with the physician regarding discontinuing medications containing iodine for 14 days prior to the test and the need to discontinue thyroid medication 4 to 6 weeks before the test
   6. Instruct the client to maintain an NPO status after midnight on the day prior to the test; if iodine is used, the client will fast for an additional 45 minutes after ingestion of the oral isotope and the scan will be performed in 24 hours
   7. If technetium is used, it is administered IV 30 minutes before the scan
E. Needle aspiration of thyroid tissue
   1. Aspiration of thyroid tissue for cytological examination
   2. No special client preparation
   3. Light pressure is applied to the aspiration site after the procedure
F. Glucose tolerance test (GTT)
   1. Aids in the diagnosis of **diabetes mellitus**
   2. If the glucose levels peak at higher than normal at 1 and 2 hours after injection or ingestion of glucose, and are slower than normal to return to fasting levels, then **diabetes mellitus** is confirmed
   3. Instruct client to eat a high carbohydrate (200 to 300 g) diet for 3 days before the test
   4. Instruct client to avoid alcohol, coffee, and smoking for 36 hours before testing
   5. Instruct client to fast for 10 to 16 hours prior to the test
   6. Instruct client to avoid strenuous exercise for 8 hours before and after the test
   7. Instruct diabetic client to withhold morning insulin or oral hypoglycemic medication
   8. Instruct client that test will take 3 to 5 hours, requires IV or oral administration of glucose, and multiple blood samples
G. Glycosylated hemoglobin (HbA_{1c})
   1. HbA_{1c} is blood glucose bound to hemoglobin
   2. HbA_{1c} is a reflection of how well blood glucose levels have been controlled for up to the prior 4 months
   3. Hyperglycemia in diabetics is usually a cause of an increase in HbA_{1c}
   4. Values are expressed as percentage of total hemoglobin
      a. Nondiabetic: 5.5% to 8.5%
      b. Diabetic with good control: 7.5% to 11.4%
      c. Diabetic with moderate control: 11.5% to 15%
      d. Diabetic with poor control: greater than 15%
   5. Fasting is not required

BOX 51–4. Risk Factors for Endocrine Disorders

Hereditary	Environmental
Congenital	Secondary to other
Trauma	disorders

> **BOX 51–5. Pituitary Disorders**
>
> **ANTERIOR PITUITARY**
> Acromegaly
> Giantism
> Dwarfism
>
> **POSTERIOR PITUITARY**
> Diabetes insipidus
> SIADH (syndrome of inappropriate antidiuretic hormone)

III. Disorders of Pituitary Gland (Box 51–5)

A. Acromegaly
   1. Description: The hypersecretion of growth hormone (GH) by the anterior pituitary gland. Acromegaly occurs in middle age, after the closure of the epiphyses of the long bones
   2. Assessment
       a. Large hands and feet
       b. Visual problems
       c. Headache
       d. **Hyperglycemia**
       e. Hypercalcemia
       f. Deepened voice
       g. Thickening and protrusion of the jaw
       h. Increased hair growth
       i. Joint pain
       j. Diaphoresis
       k. Oily, rough skin
       l. Menstrual disturbances
       m. Impotence
   3. Implementation
       a. Provide emotional support to client
       b. Encourage client to express feelings related to altered body image
       c. Provide frequent skin care
       d. Provide pharmacological and nonpharmacological interventions for joint pain
       e. Prepare client for radiation of the pituitary gland if prescribed
       f. Prepare client for **hypophysectomy** if planned

B. Giantism
   1. Description
       a. The hypersecretion of GH by the anterior pituitary gland
       b. Giantism occurs in childhood before the closure of the epiphyses of the long bones
   2. Assessment
       a. Overgrowth of long bones
       b. Increased height in early adulthood
       c. Deterioration of mental and physical status
   3. Implementation
       a. Provide emotional support to client and family
       b. Encourage client and family to express feelings related to altered body image

   c. Prepare client for radiation of the pituitary gland if prescribed
   d. Prepare client for **hypophysectomy** if planned

C. **Hypophysectomy**
   1. Description
       a. The removal of the pituitary gland
       b. Complications include increased intracranial pressure, bleeding, rhinorrhea, and meningitis
   2. Postoperative implementation
       a. Initiate postoperative care similar to craniotomy care
       b. Monitor vital signs
       c. Assess level of consciousness
       d. Assess neurological status
       e. Monitor for increased ICP
       f. Monitor for bleeding
       g. Elevate the head of the bed
       h. Monitor for adrenal insufficiency
       i. Administer corticosteroids as prescribed on time
       j. Monitor fluids and electrolyte values
       k. Monitor for temporary **diabetes insipidus** due to antidiuretic hormone (ADH) disturbances
       l. Avoid water intoxication
       m. Instruct client to avoid sneezing, coughing, and blowing nose
       n. Instruct client in the administration of prescribed medications

D. Dwarfism
   1. Description
       a. The hyposecretion of GH by the anterior pituitary gland
       b. Occurs in childhood
   2. Assessment
       a. Retarded physical growth
       b. Premature aging
       c. Low intellectual development
       d. Dry skin
       e. Poor development of secondary sex characteristics
   3. Implementation
       a. Provide emotional support to client and family
       b. Encourage client and family to express feelings related to altered body image
       c. Prepare to administer hGH (human growth hormone)

E. **Diabetes insipidus**
   1. Description
       a. The hyposecretion of ADH and a deficiency of vasopressin
       b. Results in failure of tubular reabsorption of water in the kidneys
   2. Assessment
       a. Polyuria of 4 to 24 L per day
       b. Polydipsia
       c. Dehydration
       d. Decreased skin turgor, dry mucous membranes

e. Inability to concentrate urine
f. A low urinary specific gravity of 1.006 or less
g. Fatigue
h. Muscle pain and weakness
i. Headache
j. Postural hypotension
k. Tachycardia
3. Implementation
a. Monitor vital signs, neurological and cardiovascular status
b. Monitor electrolyte values
c. Administer vasopressin tannate (Pitressin Tannate) or DDAVP (desmopressin acetate) as prescribed
d. Monitor intake and output (I&O), weights, specific gravity of urine
e. Instruct client to avoid foods or liquids with a diuretic type of action
f. Maintain the intake of adequate fluids
g. Instruct client in the administration of medications as prescribed
h. Instruct client to wear a Medic-Alert bracelet
F. Syndrome of inappropriate antidiuretic hormone (SIADH) secretion
1. Description
a. A disorder of the posterior pituitary gland in which a continued release of ADH occurs
b. Results in water intoxication
2. Assessment
a. Changes in level of consciousness (LOC)
b. Mental status changes
c. Weight gain
d. Hypertension
e. Signs of fluid volume overload
f. Tachycardia
g. Anorexia
h. Nausea and vomiting
i. Hyponatremia
3. Implementation
a. Monitor vital signs
b. Monitor neurological status
c. Monitor cardiac status
d. Protect the client from injury
e. Monitor I&O
f. Obtain daily weights
g. Restrict water intake as prescribed
h. Monitor fluid and electrolyte balance
i. Administer diuretics and IV fluids as prescribed

IV. Disorders of Adrenal Glands (Box 51-6)

A. **Addison's disease**
1. Description
a. Hyposecretion of adrenal cortex hormones (glucocorticoids and mineralocorticoids)
b. The condition is fatal if left untreated
2. Assessment
a. Weakness

BOX 51-6. Disorders of Adrenal Glands

ADRENAL CORTEX
Addison's disease
Cushing's syndrome
Aldosteronism (Conn's syndrome)

ADRENAL MEDULLA
Pheochromocytoma

b. GI disturbances
c. Weight loss
d. Emotional disturbances
e. Bronze pigmentation of skin
f. Electrolyte imbalances
g. Hypotension
h. Hyponatremia
i. **Hypoglycemia**
j. Hyperkalemia
k. Elevated blood urea nitrogen (BUN)
3. Implementation
a. Monitor vital signs
b. Monitor weight and I&O
c. Maintain fluid and electrolyte balance
d. Monitor for infection
e. Instruct client in a high-protein, high-carbohydrate diet
f. Instruct client in the avoidance of stress
g. Instruct client to avoid individuals with an infection
h. Instruct client in the need for lifelong corticosteroids
i. Instruct client to avoid over-the-counter medications
j. Instruct client to avoid strenuous exercise
k. Instruct client to wear a Medic-Alert bracelet
l. Observe for **addisonian crisis** secondary to stress, infection, trauma, surgery
B. **Addisonian crisis**
1. Description
a. A life-threatening disorder caused by acute adrenal insufficiency
b. It is precipitated by infection, trauma, stress, or surgery
c. Can cause hyponatremia, hyperkalemia, hypoglycemia, and shock
2. Assessment
a. Severe headache
b. Severe abdominal, leg, and lower back pain
c. Generalized weakness
d. Irritability and confusion
e. Severe hypotension
f. Shock
3. Implementation
a. Monitor vital signs
b. Monitor neurological status, noting irritability and confusion
c. Monitor I&O

d. Administer IV fluids as prescribed to restore electrolyte balance

e. Administer adrenocorticosteroids as prescribed on time schedule

f. Protect client from infection

g. Maintain bed rest and provide a quiet environment

C. **Cushing's syndrome**

1. Description

a. A condition resulting from the hypersecretion of glucocorticoids from the adrenal cortex

b. Can result from the prolonged administration of corticosteroids

2. Assessment

a. Obesity with thin extremities

b. Moonface

c. Buffalo hump

d. Fragile skin that easily bruises

e. Hirsutism (masculine characteristics in female)

f. Mood swings

g. Muscular weakness

h. Signs of infection

i. Signs of osteoporosis

j. Hypertension

k. Hypokalemia

l. **Hyperglycemia**

m. Glycosuria

n. Elevated white blood cells (WBC)

o. Sodium and water retention

3. Implementation

a. Monitor I&O

b. Monitor weight

c. Monitor for urinary glucose

d. Provide good skin care

e. Allow client to discuss feelings related to body appearance

f. High-protein, low-calorie diet with potassium supplements

g. Prepare client for **adrenalectomy** if prescribed

h. Prepare client for radiation if prescribed

i. Administer hormone replacement therapy as prescribed

j. Administer steroids as prescribed if **adrenalectomy** was performed

k. Administer chemotherapeutic agents as prescribed

l. Instruct client in the administration of medications as prescribed

m. Instruct client to avoid infection, stress, and accidents

n. Instruct client in measures for adequate nutrition and rest

D. Aldosteronism (Conn's syndrome)

1. Description

a. A hypersecretion of aldosterone from the adrenal cortex of the adrenal gland

b. Due to an adrenal lesion that is usually benign

2. Assessment

a. Generalized weakness

b. Increased thirst, nocturia, and polyuria

c. Edema

d. Weight gain

e. Headache

f. Hypertension

g. Positive **Chvostek's sign**

h. Increased urinary aldosterone

i. Hypokalemia

j. Hypernatremia

k. Metabolic alkalosis

3. Implementation

a. Monitor vital signs

b. Monitor weight

c. Monitor I&O

d. Assess muscular strength

e. Monitor for positive **Chvostek's sign**

f. Monitor electrolytes

g. Maintain sodium restriction as prescribed

h. Administer potassium supplements as prescribed

i. Administer antihypertensives and spironolactone (Aldactone) as prescribed

j. Prepare client for surgical removal of tumor if prescribed

E. Pheochromocytoma

1. Description

a. A catecholamine-producing tumor usually found in the adrenal gland but also may be found in the abdomen

b. It causes hypersecretion of the hormones of the adrenal medulla and secretion of excessive amounts of epinephrine and norepinephrine

c. It is typically a benign tumor but can be malignant

d. Surgical excision of the adrenal gland is the primary treatment

e. Symptomatic treatment is initiated if surgical excision is not possible; however, the complications associated with pheochromocytoma include hypertensive retinopathy and nephropathy, myocarditis, congestive heart failure (CHF), increased platelet aggregation, and cerebrovascular accident (CVA)

f. Death can occur from shock, CVA, renal failure, dysrhythmias, and dissecting aortic aneurysm

2. Assessment

a. Hypertension and headaches

b. Hypermetabolism

c. Diaphoresis

d. Palpitation and tachycardia

e. Apprehension

f. Emotional instability

g. **Hyperglycemia** and glycosuria

h. Pain in the chest or abdomen with nausea and vomiting

i. Weight loss

j. Fatigue and exhaustion

3. Implementation
   a. Monitor vital signs
   b. Monitor cardiovascular, neurological, and renal status
   c. Monitor for hypertensive attacks as hypertension can precipitate a CVA or sudden blindness
   d. Keep phentolamine (Regitine) at the bedside for hypertensive crisis
   e. Prepare to administer an alpha-adrenergic blocking agent, phenoxybenzamine (Dibenzyline), as prescribed to control blood pressure
   f. Be alert to stimuli that can precipitate a paroxysm, such as increased abdominal pressure, micturition, and vigorous abdominal palpation
   g. Avoid opiates preoperatively as they can precipitate a hypertensive crisis
   h. Monitor urine for glucose and acetone
   i. Promote rest and a nonstressful environment
   j. Provide a diet high in calories, vitamins, and minerals
   k. Prohibit caffeine-containing beverages and food

F. **Adrenalectomy**
   1. Description
      a. The surgical removal of an adrenal gland
      b. Lifelong steroid replacement is necessary with a bilateral **adrenalectomy**
      c. Temporary steroid replacement, up to 2 years, is necessary for a unilateral **adrenalectomy**
      d. Catecholamine levels drop as a result of surgery, which can result in cardiovascular collapse, hypotension, and shock, and the client needs to be monitored closely
      e. Hemorrhage can also occur owing to the high vascularity of the adrenal glands
   2. Preoperative implementation
      a. Prepare client for surgical procedure
      b. Monitor electrolytes and correct electrolyte imbalances
      c. Assess for dysrhythmias
      d. Monitor for **hyperglycemia**
      e. Protect client from infections
      f. Administer steroids as prescribed
   3. Postoperative implementation
      a. Monitor vital signs
      b. Monitor I&O, and if urinary output is less that 30 mL per hour, notify the physician, as this may be indicative of impending shock and renal failure
      c. Monitor daily weights
      d. Monitor electrolytes
      e. Monitor for signs of shock and hemorrhage, particularly during the first 24 to 48 hours
      f. Assess dressing
      g. Monitor for paralytic ileus, as manifested by abdominal distention and pain, nausea,

vomiting, and diminished or absent bowel sounds, as paralytic ileus can develop from internal bleeding
   h. Administer IV fluids as prescribed to maintain blood volume
   i. Administer pain medication as prescribed, remembering that meperidine (Demerol) can cause hypotension
   j. Administer steroid replacement as prescribed
   k. Instruct client in the importance of steroid therapy following surgery

V. Disorders of the Thyroid Gland (Box 51–7)

A. Cretinism
   1. Description: A severe thyroid hypofunction that results in hyposecretion of thyroid hormones in the fetus or soon after birth
   2. Assessment
      a. Severe physical and mental retardation
      b. Dry skin
      c. Coarse, dry, brittle hair
      d. Slow teething
      e. Large tongue
      f. Poor appetite
      g. Constipation
      h. Yellowish coloration to skin
      i. Pot belly with umbilical hernia
      j. Sensitivity to cold
   3. Implementation
      a. Provide emotional support
      b. Provide warmth and skin care
      c. Prevent injury
      d. Prevent constipation
      e. Encourage parents to discuss feelings regarding the disorder
      f. Administer hormone replacement of desiccated thyroid, thyroxine (Synthroid), or triiodothyronine (Cytomel) as prescribed
      g. Instruct parents regarding the administration of medication

B. **Myxedema (hypothyroidism)**
   1. Description
      a. A hypothyroid state resulting from a hyposecretion of thyroid hormone
      b. The condition occurs in adulthood
   2. Assessment
      a. Slowed rate of body metabolism
      b. Lethargy and fatigue
      c. Intolerance to cold
      d. Weight gain
      e. Dry skin and hair
      f. Loss of body hair
      g. Bradycardia
      h. Constipation

BOX 51–7. Disorders of the Thyroid Gland	
Cretinism	Graves' disease (thyrotoxicosis,
Myxedema	hyperthyroidism)

i. Generalized puffiness and nonpitting edema
j. Forgetfulness and loss of memory
k. Menstrual disturbances
l. Cardiac disorders

3. Implementation
   a. Monitor vital signs
   b. Monitor for cardiac complications
   c. Administer and monitor thyroid replacement of desiccated thyroid, thyroxine (Synthroid), or triiodothyronine (Cytomel) as prescribed
   d. Instruct client in low-calorie, low-cholesterol, low-saturated fat diet
   e. Assess client for anorexia and fecal impaction
   f. Provide roughage and fluids to prevent constipation
   g. Provide a warm environment for the client
   h. Avoid sedatives and narcotics due to intolerance
   i. Monitor for overdose of thyroid medications, characterized by tachycardia, restlessness, nervousness, and insomnia

◆ C. **Myxedema coma**
1. Description
   a. A rare but serious disorder that results from a persistent, low thyroid production
   b. It can be precipitated by acute illness, rapid withdrawal of thyroid medication, anesthesia and surgery, hypothermia, and the use of sedatives and narcotics

2. Assessment
   a. Hypotension
   b. Hypothermia
   c. Bradycardia
   d. Mental depression
   e. Mood swings
   f. Hyponatremia
   g. **Hypoglycemia**
   h. Coma

3. Implementation
   a. Maintain a patent airway
   b. Monitor vital signs and LOC
   c. Assess client's temperature frequently
   d. Assess blood pressure
   e. Administer IV fluids as prescribed
   f. Monitor electrolytes and glucose level
   g. Administer IV glucose as prescribed
   h. Keep client warm
   i. Monitor for changes in mental status
   j. Administer levothyroxine sodium IV as prescribed
   k. Administer corticosteroids as prescribed
   l. Avoid the use of sedatives and hypnotics

◆ D. **Graves' disease (hyperthyroidism)**
1. Description
   a. A hyperthyroid state resulting from a hypersecretion of thyroid hormone
   b. Also known as thyrotoxicosis

2. Assessment
   a. Increased rate of body metabolism

b. Enlarged thyroid gland (goiter)
c. Cardiac dysrhythmias, such as tachycardia and palpitations
d. Protruding eyeballs (exophthalmos)
e. Hypertension
f. Heat intolerance
g. Diaphoresis
h. Weight loss
i. Smooth, soft skin and hair
j. Nervousness and fine tremors of hands
k. Personality changes
l. Irritability and agitation
m. Mood swings

3. Implementation
   a. Provide adequate rest
   b. Administer sedatives as prescribed
   c. Provide cool and quiet environment
   d. Obtain daily weights
   e. Provide a high-calorie diet
   f. Avoid stimulants
   g. Provide psychosocial support
   h. Administer antithyroid medications, methimazole (Tapazole), or propylthiouracil, which blocks thyroid synthesis, as prescribed
   i. Administer iodine preparations, Lugol's solution, saturated solution of potassium iodide (SSKI), which inhibits the release of thyroid hormone, as prescribed
   j. Administer propranolol (Inderal) for tachycardia as prescribed
   k. Prepare the client for radioiodine therapy as prescribed to destroy thyroid cells
   l. Prepare client for **thyroidectomy** if prescribed

E. **Thyroid storm**
1. Description
   a. An acute and fatal thyroid condition that occurs from manipulation of the thyroid gland during surgery and the release of thyroid hormone into the blood stream
   b. It can also occur from severe infection and stress

2. Assessment
   a. Fever
   b. Diaphoresis
   c. Dehydration
   d. Tachycardia
   e. Congestive heart failure and pulmonary edema
   f. Nausea, vomiting, and diarrhea
   g. systolic hypertension
   h. Tremors
   i. Irritability, agitation, and restlessness
   j. Delirium and coma

3. Implementation
   a. Monitor vital signs
   b. Decrease temperature, avoiding the use of salicylates as they increase free thyroid hormone levels
   c. Avoid palpating the thyroid gland
   d. Monitor I&O

e. Monitor fluid and electrolyte balance
f. Monitor for dehydration and overhydration
g. Monitor pulmonary and cardiac status
h. Administer iodine preparations, Lugol's solution, or saturated solution of potassium iodide (SSKI), which inhibits the release of thyroid hormone, as prescribed
i. Administer propranolol (Inderal) for tachycardia and to reverse toxic manifestations of **thyroid storm** as prescribed
j. Administer glucocorticoids as prescribed to allay stress effects
k. Administer cardiac medications as prescribed to decrease heart activity

F. **Thyroidectomy**
1. Description
   a. Removal of the thyroid gland
   b. Performed when persistent hyperthyroidism exists
2. Preoperative implementation
   a. Obtain vital signs
   b. Obtain weight
   c. Assess electrolyte levels
   d. Assess for **hyperglycemia** and glycosuria
   e. Assess level of consciousness
   f. Assess for signs of **thyroid storm**
   g. Administer antithyroid medications as prescribed to deplete iodine and hormones
   h. Administer iodine as prescribed to decrease vascularity of the thyroid gland
3. Postoperative implementation
   a. Monitor for respiratory distress
   b. Have tracheotomy set, oxygen, and suction at the bedside
   c. Maintain semi-Fowler's position
   d. Monitor for signs of bleeding
   e. Check dressing anteriorly and at the back of the neck
   f. Limit client talking, and assess level of hoarseness
   g. Monitor for laryngeal nerve damage, as evidenced by respiratory obstruction, dysphonia, high- pitched voice, stridor, dysphagia, and restlessness
   h. Monitor for signs of tetany, which can be due to trauma to the parathyroid gland (Box 51–8)
   i. Prepare to administer calcium gluconate as prescribed for tetany

---

BOX 51–8. Signs of Tetany

Positive Chvostek's sign
Positive Trousseau's sign
Numbness of extremities and spasm of glottis
Irritability
Wheezing and dyspnea
Visual disturbances
Muscle and abdominal cramps

VI. Disorders of the Parathyroid Gland

A. Hypoparathyroidism
1. Description
   a. A condition caused by hyposecretion of parathyroid hormone by the parathyroid gland
   b. Occurs following **thyroidectomy** from removal of parathyroid tissue
2. Assessment
   a. Hypocalcemia and elevated phosphorus levels
   b. Numbness and tingling of extremities
   c. Cramping
   d. Signs of tetany, such as muscular spasms, irritability, seizures, positive **Trousseau's sign**, positive **Chvostek's sign**, laryngospasm, and cardiac dysrhythmias
   e. Signs of hypocalcemia, such as weakness and tingling of the extremities, painful muscle spasms, dysrhythmias, irritability and anxiety
   f. Increased neuromuscular irritability
   g. Confusion
   h. Visual problems
   i. Depression
3. Implementation
   a. Monitor vital signs
   b. Monitor cardiac status
   c. Monitor for tetany
   d. Initiate seizure precautions
   e. Place a tracheotomy set, oxygen, and suctioning at the bedside
   f. Provide a high-calcium, low-phosphorus diet
   g. Provide a quiet environment with no stimulus
   h. Administer aluminum hydroxide as prescribed to decrease phosphate levels
   i. Administer parathyroid hormone as prescribed
   j. Prepare to administer IV calcium gluconate for hypocalcemia
   k. Instruct client in the administration of calcium carbonate (OsCal) and vitamin D (Calciferol) as prescribed

B. Hyperparathyroidism
1. Description: A condition caused by hypersecretion of parathyroid hormone by the parathyroid gland
2. Assessment
   a. Bone deformities
   b. Fractures
   c. Calcium deposits in organs
   d. Gastric ulcers
   e. Nausea, vomiting, anorexia, constipation
   f. Personality changes
   g. Polydipsia and polyuria
   h. Elevated calcium and low phosphorus levels
3. Implementation
   a. Monitor cardiac function

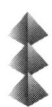

b. Monitor renal status
c. Monitor I&O
d. Provide hydration
e. Monitor fluid and electrolyte balance
f. Monitor calcium and phosphorus levels
g. Administer furosemide (Lasix) as prescribed to lower calcium levels
h. Administer IV saline as prescribed to lower calcium levels
i. Notify the physician immediately if a precipitous drop in the calcium level occurs
j. Assess client for tingling and numbness in the muscles, which is caused by a sudden drop in calcium levels
k. Administer phosphates as prescribed, which interfere with calcium absorption
l. Administer calcitonin (Calcimar) as prescribed to decrease skeletal calcium release and increase renal clearance of calcium
m. Administer cytotoxic antibiotics as prescribed to lower calcium levels, and monitor client closely for thrombocytopenia and renal and hepatic toxicity
n. Prepare client for parathyroidectomy as prescribed

C. Parathyroidectomy
1. Description: Removal of one or more of the parathyroid glands
2. Preoperative implementation
a. Monitor electrolytes, calcium, phosphate, and magnesium levels
b. Assure that calcium levels are decreased to near-normal
c. Inform the client that talking may be painful for the first day or two postoperative
3. Postoperative implementation
a. Monitor for respiratory distress
b. Place a tracheotomy set, oxygen, and suctioning at the bedside
c. Monitor vital signs
d. Position client in semi-Fowler's
e. Assess neck dressing for bleeding—1 to 5 mL of serosanguineous drainage is expected
f. Monitor for hypocalcemic crisis, as

evidenced by tingling and twitching in the extremities and face
g. Assess for positive **Trousseau's** and **Chvostek's signs**, which signal the potential of tetany
h. Monitor for laryngeal nerve damage
i. Monitor for changes in voice pattern and hoarseness
j. Instruct client in the administration of calcium and vitamin D as prescribed

VII. Disorders of the Pancreas
A. **Diabetes mellitus** (Table 51–1)
1. Description
a. A chronic and potentially disabling disease characterized by elevated blood sugar levels
b. A chronic disorder of impaired glucose intolerance and carbohydrate, protein, and lipid metabolism because of a deficiency of insulin
c. A deficiency of insulin results in **hyperglycemia**
d. Macrovascular complications include coronary disease, cardiomyopathy, hypertension, cerebrovascular disease, peripheral vascular disease, and infection
e. Microvascular complications include retinopathy, nephropathy, and neuropathy.
2. Assessment
a. Polyuria
b. Polydipsia
c. Polyphagia
d. **Hyperglycemia**
e. Weight loss
f. Blurred vision
g. Slow wound healing
h. Weakness
i. Paresthesias
j. Signs of inadequate circulation to the feet
k. Vaginal infections
3. Diet
a. Total amount of calories is individualized, based on the client's current or desired weight
b. Weight control centers on a diet high in complex carbohydrates and low in fat; behavior modification; and evaluation of eating habits
c. As prescribed by the physician, the client may be advised to follow the food exchange from the American Diabetic Association diet or the dietary guidelines for Americans (Food Guide Pyramid) issued by the U.S. Departments of Agriculture and Health Services
d. Incorporate diet into individual client needs, lifestyle, and cultural and socioeconomic patterns
4. Exercise
a. Decreases cholesterol and triglyceride levels

Table 51–1. **Major Types of Diabetes**

Type 1—(Insulin-Dependent Diabetes Mellitus) (IDDM)
Usually abrupt in onset
Clients require insulin injections
Occurs primarily in childhood or adolescence but can occur at any age

Type 2—(Noninsulin-Dependent Diabetes Mellitus) (NIDDM)
Generally slow in onset
Onset after the age of 30 years
Ability to produce some insulin, with a favorable response to oral hypoglycemic agents

b. Decreases blood pressure

c. Helps the body burn excess sugar

d. Improves circulation

e. Encourages weight loss

f. Decreases the body's need for oral hypoglycemic agents or insulin

g. Instruct client in dietary adjustments when exercising

h. Instruct client to monitor blood glucose prior to exercising

i. If the exercise is of short duration and of low to moderate intensity, and if the blood glucose is less than 100 mg/dL, increase food intake by 10 to 15 g of carbohydrate per hour (1 fruit or 1 starch/bread exchange) of exercise

j. If the exercise is of moderate intensity, and if the blood glucose is less than 100 mg/dL, increase food intake by 25 to 50 g of carbohydrate before exercise, then 10 to 15 g per hour (1 fruit or 1 starch/bread exchange) of exercise

k. If the exercise is strenuous, and if the blood glucose is less than 100 mg/dL, increase food intake by 50 g of carbohydrate (1 meat sandwich with a milk and fruit exchange), and monitor blood glucose carefully

l. If the exercise is strenuous, and if the blood glucose is between 100 and 180 mg/dL, increase food intake by 25 to 50 g of carbohydrate (1/2 meat sandwich with a milk and fruit exchange), and monitor blood glucose carefully

m. If the blood sugar is 180 to 300 mg/dL or above, instruct client not to exercise until the blood glucose is under better control

5. Oral hypoglycemic medications

a. Prescribed for clients with **diabetes mellitus** Type 2

b. Assess the client's knowledge of diabetes and the use of oral antidiabetic agents

c. Assess vital signs and blood sugar levels

d. Assess the medications that the client is currently taking

e. Aspirin, alcohol, sulfonamides, oral contraceptives, and MAO inhibitors increase the hypoglycemic effect

f. Glucocorticoids, thiazide diuretics, and estrogen increase blood sugar levels

g. Instruct the client how to recognize symptoms of **hypoglycemia** and **hyperglycemia**

h. Instruct client to avoid over-the-counter medications unless prescribed by the physician

i. Instruct client not to ingest alcohol with sulfonylureas

j. Inform the client that insulin may be needed during stress, surgery, or infection

k. Instruct the client in the necessity of compliance with prescribed medication

l. Advise client to obtain a Medic-Alert bracelet

6. Insulin

a. Used in the treatment of Type 1 diabetes mellitus and in Type 2 diabetes mellitus when diet and weight control therapy have failed to maintain satisfactory blood glucose levels

b. Regular insulin is used in emergency treatment of ketoacidosis

c. Aspirin, alcohol, oral anticoagulants, oral hypoglycemics, beta-blockers, tricyclic antidepressants, tetracycline, and MAO inhibitors increase the hypoglycemic effect when taking insulin

d. Glucocorticoids, thiazide diuretics, thyroid agents, oral contraceptives, and estrogen increase blood sugar levels

e. Illness, infection, and stress increase the need for insulin, and insulin should not be withheld during illness, infection, or stress, as **hyperglycemia** and ketoacidosis can result

f. Instruct the client to recognize symptoms of **hypoglycemia** and **hyperglycemia**

g. The peak action time of insulin is very important because of the possibility of hypoglycemic reactions occurring during that time

B. Complications of insulin therapy

1. **Dawn phenomenon**

a. Results from a nocturnal release of growth hormone secretion that may cause blood glucose elevations at about 5 to 6 A.M.

b. Treatment includes administering an evening dose of intermediate-acting insulin at 10 P.M.

2. **Somogyi's phenomenon**

a. A rebound phenomenon occurring in **diabetes mellitus**

b. Overtreatment with insulin induces **hypoglycemia**, which initiates the release of epinephrine, adrenocorticotropic hormone (ACTH), glucagon, and growth hormone

c. Lipolysis, glyconeogenesis, and glycogenolysis result in rebound **hyperglycemia** and ketosis

d. Occurs during the initial period of serum glucose control; develops at peak insulin times and during the night

e. Treatment includes adjusting the insulin dose, the evening diet and bedtime snack, and the exercise program to prevent **hypoglycemia**

C. Continuous subcutaneous infusion of insulin

1. Administered by an externally worn pump containing a syringe and reservoir, with regular insulin connected to the client by an infusion set

2. Continuous infusion of a basal dose of insulin with meal-associated increases in insulin

seems to be more effective than a multiple injection protocol in providing metabolic control

3. Buffered insulin is used to prevent the precipitation of insulin crystals within the catheter

4. Instruct the client to adjust the amount of insulin received by regulating the pump settings on the basis of blood glucose monitoring

5. To prevent infections, the needle insertion site is cleaned every 48 hours, and needle placement is changed every 3 days

6. The cessation of insulin administration quickly results in **hyperglycemia**, leading to ketoacidosis, and the client is instructed to perform regular urine tests for the presence of ketones

D. Insulin pumps
1. Implanted in the peritoneal cavity where insulin can be absorbed in a more physiological manner
2. Buffered insulin is used
3. Mechanical problems associated with the pump, the catheter, and the insulin delivery exist

E. Blood glucose monitoring
1. Provides the client with current blood glucose levels
2. Results provide the client with information to maintain good glycemic control
3. More accurate than urine testing
4. Requires clients to prick themselves several times a day as prescribed
5. Must be used with caution for clients with diabetic retinopathy and neuropathy
6. Instruct client in the proper procedure for obtaining the blood glucose level
7. Inform client that the procedure must be done precisely to obtain accurate results
8. Stress the importance of following the manufacturer's instructions
9. Stress the importance of handwashing before and after performing the procedure, to prevent infection
10. Instruct client to calibrate the monitor as instructed by the manufacturer
11. Instruct client to check the expiration date on the test strips
12. Instruct client that if blood glucose results do not seem reasonable, reread the instructions, reassess technique, check the expiration date of the test strips, and perform the procedure again to verify results

F. Urine testing
1. Instruct client in the procedure for testing urine for ketones and glucose
2. Teach client that the second voided urine specimen is most accurate
3. The presence of ketones may indicate impending ketoacidosis
4. Urine glucose testing is not recommended as a

means of monitoring for clients taking insulin, as it is a less reliable indicator compared with blood glucose monitoring

VIII. Acute Complications of Diabetes Mellitus

A. **Hypoglycemia (insulin reaction)**
1. Description
   a. Described as a blood glucose level below 50 to 60 mg/dL
   b. Occurs as a result of too much insulin, not enough food, or excessive activity
2. Assessment
   a. Cool, clammy skin
   b. Diaphoresis
   c. Irritable, nervous, weepy
   d. Difficulty concentrating, speaking, focusing, coordinating
   e. Shaky feeling, tremors, and dizziness
   f. Hunger
   g. Headache
   h. Shallow respirations
   i. Tachycardia
   j. Blood glucose below 50 mg/dL
   k. Negative ketones
   l. Late signs: Hyperreflexia, dilated pupils, convulsions, shock, coma
3. Implementation
   a. Monitor vital signs and blood glucose
   b. Monitor neurological status
   c. Provide carbohydrate food items
4. Mild **hypoglycemia**
   a. A capillary blood glucose level of 40 to 60 mg/dL
   b. Provide 10 to 15 g of carbohydrate (Box 51–9) and repeat the treatment in 10 to 15 minutes if symptoms do not subside; instruct client to eat additional food or the next scheduled meal in 15 to 30 minutes
5. Moderate **hypoglycemia**
   a. A capillary blood glucose level of 20 to 40 mg/dL
   b. Provide 15 to 30 g of carbohydrate and repeat the treatment in 10 to 15 minutes if symptoms do not subside
   c. Instruct client to eat additional food such as low-fat milk or cheese, after 15 to 30 minutes
6. Severe **hypoglycemia**
   a. The client who is unconscious or experiencing seizures
   b. Administer IM or SC glucagon or 50% dextrose IV as prescribed

BOX 51–9. Food Items Providing 10 to 15 Grams of Carbohydrate	
2–3 glucose tablets	6–10 hard candies
½ cup orange or grape juice	4 cubes sugar
½ cup regular soft drink	6 saltines
8 oz skim milk	3 graham crackers

c. Administer a second dose if the client remains unconscious

d. Provide a small meal when the client wakes up and is no longer nauseated

e. Instruct family on the administration of glucagon

B. **Hyperglycemia**

1. Description: Described as an elevated blood glucose level

2. Assessment
   a. Gradual onset
   b. Lethargy dulled sensorium, and confusion
   c. Thirst
   d. Weakness
   e. Nausea, vomiting, and abdominal pain
   f. Flushed
   g. Signs of dehydration
   h. Dry, crusty mucous membranes
   i. Deep, rapid respirations and weak pulse
   j. Fruity, acetone breath
   k. Paresthesia and diminished reflexes
   l. Acidosis, coma
   m. Blood glucose of 250 mg/dL or more
   n. Ketones high
   o. Polyuria (early) to oliguria (late)

3. Implementation
   a. Instruct client to monitor for signs of hyperglycemia
   b. Instruct client to notify physician when blood sugar results are greater than 250 mg/dL, when ketonuria is present for more than 24 hours, when unable to take food or fluids, and when illness persists for more than 2 days

C. **Diabetic ketoacidosis (DKA)**

1. Description
   a. A complication of **diabetes mellitus** that develops when a severe insulin deficiency occurs
   b. **DKA** is a life-threatening condition
   c. Hyperglycemia occurs that progresses to metabolic acidosis
   d. Seen primarily in clients with Type 1 diabetes mellitus, undiagnosed diabetics, and persons who stop prescribed treatment for diabetes
   e. It develops over a period over several hours to days

2. Assessment
   a. Fatigue and weakness
   b. Headache
   c. Sunken eyeballs
   d. Dry mucous membranes
   e. Thirst
   f. Kussmaul's respirations
   g. Polyuria
   h. Fruity odor to breath
   i. Warm, flushed skin
   j. Nausea, vomiting, abdominal pain
   k. Tachycardia
   l. Drowsiness, stupor
   m. Urinary glucose and ketones

n. Potassium imbalances

o. Late signs include oliguria, anuria, and hypotension

3. Implementation
   a. Restore circulating volume and protect against cerebral, coronary, or renal hypoperfusion
   b. Correct **hyperglycemia** with IV Regular insulin administration as prescribed
   c. Monitor vital signs, urine outputs, and mental status closely
   d. Correct dehydration with rapid IV infusions of 0.9% or 0.45% normal saline as prescribed
   e. Correct acidosis if pH is less than 7.10
   f. Correct electrolyte imbalance
   g. Administer oxygen as prescribed
   h. Monitor blood glucose closely
   i. Monitor client closely for signs of fluid overload
   j. Monitor potassium closely, because when the client receives insulin to lower the blood sugar level, the serum potassium will decrease as the acidosis improves, and potassium replacement may be required
   k. Treat cause of **hyperglycemia**

4. Insulin IV administration
   a. Use Regular insulin only
   b. A dose of 5 to 10 units of Regular insulin by IV bolus may be prescribed before the continuous infusion
   c. Mix the prescribed dose of Regular insulin in 0.9% or 0.45% normal saline as prescribed
   d. Prime the IV tubing with IV solution before adding insulin, because insulin adheres to IV tubing
   e. Always place the insulin drip on an IV pump
   f. Monitor the blood glucose closely, and monitor the client for signs of **hypoglycemia**
   g. The IV insulin is usually discontinued and 5% dextrose in 0.45% normal saline is administered when the blood sugar reaches 250 mg/dL
   h. A dose of SC Regular insulin may be prescribed 20 to 30 minutes before the continuous infusion is stopped

5. Administering IV fluids
   a. Administer normal saline as prescribed to restore circulating volume and protect against organ hyperperfusion
   b. IV dextrose is added as prescribed when the blood sugar reaches 250 mg/dL
   c. Monitor potassium levels, glucose levels, and urinary output and for signs of increased intracranial pressure
   d. If the blood glucose falls too far and too fast before the brain has time to equilibrate, water is pulled from the blood to the cerebrospinal fluid (CFS) and the

brain, causing cerebral edema and increased intracranial pressure (ICP)

 e. The potassium level will fall rapidly within the first hour of treatment as fluids and insulin are replaced

 f. IV potassium may be added to the IV when the potassium level falls to normal level and urinary output is normal

D. **Hyperosmolar hyperglycemic nonketotic coma (HHNC)**

 1. Description

  a. Extreme **hyperglycemia** without acidosis

  b. Usually occurs in noninsulin-dependent diabetics when diabetes is uncontrolled or undiagnosed, or during stress or infection

  c. The major difference between **HHNC** and **DKA** is the lack of production of ketones with **HHNC**

  d. Onset is usually slow, taking from hours to days

 2. Assessment

  a. Polyuria, polydipsia, polyphagia

  b. Glycosuria

  c. Dehydration

  d. Abdominal discomfort

  e. Hyperventilation

  f. Alterations in LOC

  g. Hypotension

  h. Blood glucose is extremely high, from 800 up to 2400 mg/dL

  i. Absent ketones

  j. Shock and coma

 3. Implementation

  a. The most critical element is the choice and rate of fluid replacement

  b. The initial objective for fluid replacement is to raise the circulating blood volume

  c. Monitor vital signs, urine output, and mental status closely

  d. Monitor fluid and electrolyte levels closely

  e. Monitor potassium levels and glucose levels and for signs of increased intracranial pressure

  f. Correct hydration with IV fluids of 0.9% or 0.45% normal saline as prescribed

  g. Administer IV potassium replacement as prescribed

  h. Administer IV Regular insulin to correct the **hyperglycemia** as prescribed

IX. Chronic Complications of Diabetes Mellitus

A. Diabetic retinopathy

 1. Description

  a. A chronic and progressive noninflammatory impairment of the retinal circulation that eventually causes hemorrhage

  b. Permanent vision changes and blindness can occur

  c. The client has difficulty with carrying out the daily tasks of glucose testing and insulin injections

 2. Assessment

  a. A change in vision due to ruptured vessels

  b. Blurred vision due to macular edema

  c. Sudden loss of vision due to retinal detachment

  d. Cataracts due to lens opacity

 3. Implementation

  a. Maintain safety

  b. Early prevention by the control of hypertension and blood sugar levels

  c. Photocoagulation (laser therapy) to remove hemorrhagic tissue to decrease scarring

  d. Vitrectomy to remove vitreous hemorrhages and thus decrease tension on the retina, preventing detachment

  e. Cataract removal with lens implant

B. Diabetic nephropathy

 1. Description: A progressive decrease in kidney function as a result of the diabetes

 2. Assessment

  a. Microalbuminuria

  b. Thirst

  c. Fatigue

  d. Anemia

  e. Weight loss

  f. Signs of malnutrition

  g. Frequent urinary tract infections

  h. Signs of a neurogenic bladder

 3. Implementation

  a. Early prevention by the control of hypertension and blood sugar levels

  b. Assess vital signs

  c. Monitor I&O

  d. Monitor BUN and creatinine, and for albuminuria

  e. Restrict dietary protein, sodium, and potassium as prescribed

  f. Avoid nephrotoxic medications

  g. Prepare client for dialysis procedures as prescribed

  h. Prepare client for kidney transplants as prescribed

  i. Prepare client for pancreas transplants as prescribed

C. Diabetic neuropathy

 1. Description

  a. General deterioration of the nervous system as a result of the diabetes disease process

  b. Complications include foot injuries resulting from trauma and diabetic ulcers, frequently requiring amputation

 2. Assessment

  a. Paresthesias

  b. Decreased or absent reflexes

  c. Decreased sensation to vibration or light touch

  d. Pain, aching, and burning in the lower extremities

  e. Poor peripheral pulses

f. Skin breakdown and signs of infection
g. Weakness or loss of sensation in cranial nerves III, IV, V, or VI
h. Dizziness and postural hypotension
i. Nausea and vomiting
j. Diarrhea or constipation
k. Incontinence
l. Dyspareunia
m. Impotence
n. Hypoglycemic unawareness
3. Implementation
a. Early prevention by the control of hypertension and blood sugar levels
b. Careful foot care to prevent trauma (Box 51–10)
c. Apply topical capsaicin (Axsain, Zostrix) for temporary relief of neuralgia
d. Administer antidepressants as prescribed for pain relief
e. Initiate bladder-training programs
f. Instruct in the use of estrogen-containing lubricants for women with dyspareunia
g. Prepare the male client with impotence for penile injections or implantable devices as prescribed
h. Prepare for surgical decompression for

BOX 51–10. Preventive Foot Care

- Teach client meticulous skin care and proper foot care
- Instruct client to inspect feet daily
- Monitor feet for redness, swelling, or break in skin integrity
- Instruct client to wash feet with lukewarm water and dry thoroughly
- Do not soak feet
- Do not treat corns, blisters, or ingrown toenails
- Do not cross legs or wear tight garments that may constrict blood flow
- Apply moisturizing lotion to the feet but not between the toes
- Prevent moisture from accumulating between toes
- Wear loose socks and well-fitting shoes, and instruct client not to go barefoot
- Notify physician if redness or a break in the skin occurs
- Instruct client to avoid thermal injuries from hot water, heating pads, and baths
- Change into clean cotton socks daily
- Wear socks to keep feet warm
- Avoid tight-fitting garments and shoes
- Do not wear the same pair of shoes two days in a row
- Wear leather shoes
- Do not wear open-toed shoes or shoes with a strap that goes between the toes
- Check shoes for cracks or tears in the lining and for foreign objects before putting them on
- Break in new shoes gradually
- Cut toenails straight across, and smooth nails with an emery board
- Do not smoke

---

compression lesions related to the cranial nerves, as prescribed

X. Operative Care for the Diabetic Client

A. Preoperative care
1. Discontinue sulfonylurea medications, as prescribed 36 to 72 hours before surgery
2. Monitor blood glucose
3. Administer IV fluids as prescribed
4. Administer insulin as prescribed
5. In stable clients undergoing minor procedures, hold the prescribed morning dose of insulin or oral agent if the client is fasting; monitor blood glucose levels and notify physician of results, since a supplemental short-acting insulin may be prescribed preoperatively
B. Postoperative care
1. Administer glucose and insulin infusions as prescribed until the client can tolerate oral feedings
2. Administer supplemental short-acting insulin as prescribed, based on blood glucose results
3. Monitor blood glucose levels closely if the diabetic is receiving total parenteral nutrition (TPN)
4. When the client is tolerating food, ensure that the client receives an adequate amount of carbohydrates daily to prevent **hypoglycemia** and ketosis
C. Whole pancreas transplants
1. The goal of pancreatic transplantation is to halt or reverse the complications of diabetes
2. The pancreas is transplanted into the peritoneal cavity, with drainage of exocrine secretions into the urinary bladder
3. Monitor urinary amylase, since a decrease indicates the need to treat the client for rejection
4. **Hyperglycemia** is a late sign of rejection and indicates irreversible graft failure
5. Immunosuppressive therapy is prescribed to prevent and treat rejection
6. Inform client of the potential for future insulin injections which may be necessary to treat hyperglycemia caused by immunosuppressive medications

PRACTICE QUESTIONS

1. The nurse is caring for a client scheduled for a transsphenoidal hypophysectomy. The preoperative teaching plan includes which of the following most important statements?
   1 "Your hair will need to be shaved"
   2 "Deep breathing and coughing will be needed after surgery"
   3 "Toothbrushing will not be permitted for at least 2 weeks following surgery"
   4 "You will receive spinal anesthesia"

2. Following hypophysectomy, the client complains of being very thirsty and having to urinate frequently. The initial nursing action is to:
   1 Document the complaints
   2 Increase fluid intake
   3 Assess urine specific gravity
   4 Assess for urinary glucose

3. The nurse is caring for a client following hypophysectomy. The nurse notices clear nasal drainage from the client's nostril. The initial nursing action is to:
   1 Continue to observe drainage
   2 Test the drainage for glucose
   3 Lower the head of the bed
   4 Obtain a culture of the drainage

4. Following several diagnostic tests, a client is diagnosed with diabetes insipidus. Which of the following symptoms is indicative of this disorder?
   1 Diarrhea
   2 Polydipsia
   3 Weight gain
   4 Fatigue

5. The nurse caring for a client with Addison's disease would expect to note which of the following?
   1 Obesity
   2 Edema
   3 Hypotension
   4 Hirsutism

6. The client with Cushing's syndrome verbalizes concern to the nurse regarding the appearance of the buffalo hump that has developed. Which of the following statements by the nurse is most appropriate?
   1 "This is permanent, but looks are deceiving and not that important"
   2 "Don't be concerned, this problem can be covered with clothing"
   3 "Try not to worry about it, there are other things to be concerned about"
   4 "Usually these physical changes slowly improve following treatment"

7. The nurse develops a plan of care for a client with Graves' disease. Which of the following would the nurse include in the plan of care?
   1 Provide small meals
   2 Provide client with extra blankets
   3 Provide a high-fiber diet
   4 Provide a restful environment

8. The nurse is caring for a client following thyroidectomy. The nurse notes that calcium gluconate is prescribed for the client. The nurse determines that this medication has been prescribed to:
   1 Treat thyroid storm
   2 Prevent cardiac irritability
   3 Stimulate release of parathyroid hormone
   4 Treat hypocalcemic tetany

9. The nurse is performing an assessment on the client following a thyroidectomy. The nurse notes that the client has developed hoarseness and a weak voice. Which of the following nursing actions is appropriate?
   1 Notify the physician immediately
   2 Reassure the client that this is usually a temporary condition
   3 Check for signs of bleeding
   4 Administer calcium gluconate

10. A client is admitted to the emergency department, and a diagnosis of myxedema coma is made. Which of the following nursing actions does the nurse prepare to carry out initially?
    1 Warm the client
    2 Replace fluids
    3 Maintain an airway
    4 Administer thyroid hormone

11. The nurse is reviewing the physician's orders for a client with hypothyroidism. Which of the following medications, if prescribed for the client, does the nurse question and verify?
    1 Docusate sodium (Colace)
    2 Morphine sulfate
    3 Levothyroxine (Synthroid)
    4 Atenolol (Tenormin)

12. The client is taking NPH insulin daily every morning. The nurse instructs the client that the most likely time for a hypoglycemic reaction to occur is:
    1 2 to 4 hours after administration
    2 6 to 12 hours after administration
    3 12 to 16 hours after administration
    4 18 to 24 hours after administration

13. The client with Type 1 diabetes is to begin an exercise program, and the nurse is providing instructions to the client regarding the program. Which of the following should the nurse include in the teaching plan?
    1 Exercise is best performed during peak times of insulin
    2 Administer insulin after exercising
    3 Take a blood glucose test before exercising
    4 Try to exercise prior to meal time

14. The nurse is preparing a teaching plan for the diabetic client regarding proper foot care. Which of the following instructions should be included in the plan?
    1 Soak feet in hot water
    2 Apply a lanolin lotion to dry feet
    3 Always have a podiatrist cut your toenails, never cut them yourself
    4 Avoid using soap on the feet

15. A client is brought to the emergency department in an unresponsive state, and a diagnosis of hyperglycemic hyperosmolar nonketotic (HHNK)

syndrome is made. The nurse prepares to immediately administer which of the following?
1 100 units of NPH insulin
2 Oxygen via nasal cannula
3 IV replacement of bicarbonate
4 IV infusion of normal saline

16. The nurse provides dietary instructions to a diabetic client regarding the prescribed diabetic diet. Which statement, if made by the client, indicates a need for further teaching?
1 "I need to drink diet soft drinks"
2 "I'll eat a balanced meal plan"
3 "I need to buy special dietetic foods"
4 "I'll snack on fruit instead of cake"

17. An external insulin pump is prescribed for the client with diabetes. The client asks the nurse about the functioning of the pump. The nurse bases the response on the information that the pump:
1 Gives a small, continuous dose of Regular insulin subcutaneously, and the client can bolus self with additional dosage from the pump prior to each meal
2 Is timed to release programmed doses of Regular or NPH insulin into the blood stream at specific intervals
3 Is surgically attached to the pancreas and infuses Regular insulin into the pancreas, which in turn releases the insulin into the blood stream
4 Continuously infuses small amounts of NPH insulin into the blood stream while regularly monitoring blood glucose levels

18. The newly diagnosed client with diabetes mellitus has been stabilized with insulin injections daily. The nurse prepares a discharge teaching plan regarding the insulin. The teaching plan reinforces which of the following concepts?
1 Increase the amount of insulin prior to unusual exercise
2 Acetone in the urine will signify a need for less insulin
3 Always keep insulin vials refrigerated
4 Systematically rotate insulin injection sites

19. A client with a diagnosis of diabetic ketoacidosis (DKA) is being treated in the emergency department. Which of the following findings does the nurse expect to note as confirming this diagnosis?
1 Elevated blood sugar and low plasma bicarbonate
2 Decreased urine output
3 Increased respirations and an increase in pH
4 Coma

20. The client received 20 units of NPH insulin subcutaneously at 8:00 A.M. The nurse should assess the client for a hypoglycemic reaction at:

1 10:00 A.M.
2 11:00 A.M.
3 5:00 P.M.
4 11:00 P.M.

21. The nurse teaches a diabetic client about differentiating between hypoglycemia and ketoacidosis. The client demonstrates an understanding of the teaching by stating that glucose will be taken if which of the following symptoms develops?
1 Fruity breath odor
2 Shakiness
3 Blurred vision
4 Polyuria

22. A diabetic client demonstrates acute anxiety when first admitted for the treatment of hyperglycemia. The most appropriate intervention to decrease the clients' anxiety is to:
1 Administer a sedative
2 Make sure the client knows all the correct medical terms to understand what is happening
3 Ignore the signs and symptoms of anxiety so that they will soon disappear
4 Convey empathy, trust, and respect toward the client

23. The nurse provides instructions to a newly diagnosed Type 1 diabetic client. The nurse evaluates accurate understanding of measures to prevent DKA when the client says:
1 "I will stop taking my insulin if I'm too sick to eat"
2 "I will decrease my insulin dose during times of illness"
3 "I will notify my physician if my blood glucose level is greater than 250 mg/dL"
4 "I will adjust my insulin dose according to the level of glucose in my urine"

24. The client is admitted with a diagnosis of DKA. The initial serum glucose level was 950 mg/dL. IV insulin was started, along with rehydration with IV normal saline. The serum glucose level is now 240 mg/dL. The nurse next prepares to administer which of the following?
1 IV fluids containing 5% glucose
2 NPH insulin subcutaneously
3 An ampule of 50% glucose
4 Phenytoin (Dilantin) for prevention of seizures

25. A diabetic client is being discharged following treatment for hyperglycemic hyperosmolar non-ketotic (HHNK) syndrome precipitated by acute illness. The client tells the nurse, "I will call the doctor next time I can't eat for more than a day or so." Which of the following statements reflects the most appropriate analysis of this client's level of knowledge?

1 The client needs immediate education prior to discharge

2 The client's statement is accurate, but knowledge should be evaluated further

3 The client's statement is inaccurate and the client should be scheduled for outpatient diabetic counseling

4 The client requires follow-up teaching regarding the administration of insulin

26. The physician has prescribed propylthiouracil (PTU) for a client with hyperthyroidism. The nurse develops a plan of care for the client. A priority nursing assessment to be included in the plan regarding this medication is:

    1 Assess for signs and symptoms of hypothyroidism

    2 Assess the client for signs and symptoms of hyperglycemia

    3 Assess the client for relief of pain

    4 Assess the client for signs of renal toxicity

27. The nurse develops a plan of care for a client with hyperparathyroidism receiving calcitonin (Calcimar). Which of the following outcome criteria has the highest priority regarding this medication?

    1 Absence of side effects

    2 Achievement of normal serum calcium levels

    3 Relief of pain

    4 Verbalization of appropriate medication knowledge

28. The physician prescribes levothyroxine (Synthroid), 0.15 mg PO daily, for the client with hypothyroidism. The nurse will prepare to administer this medication:

    1 Three times a day in equal doses of 0.5 mg each to ensure consistent serum drug levels

    2 In the morning to prevent sleeplessness

    3 Only when the client complains of fatigue and cold intolerance

    4 At various times of the day to prevent tolerance from occurring

29. The nurse is monitoring a client receiving chlorpropamide (Diabinese). Which of the following is not a therapeutic outcome for this client?

    1 A decrease in polyuria

    2 A fasting blood sugar (FBS) of 110

    3 A decrease in polyphagia

    4 A glycosylated hemoglobin of 12%

30. The nurse is monitoring a client with diabetes insipidus. Desmopressin (DDAVP) has been prescribed for the client. Which of the following outcomes reflects a therapeutic effect of this medication?

    1 Serum osmolality greater than 320 mOsm/kg

    2 Increased blood pressure

    3 Decreased urine output

    4 Urine osmolality less than 100 mOsm/kg

31. The nurse is monitoring a newly diagnosed diabetic client for signs of complications. Which of the following, if exhibited in the client, indicates hyperglycemia and warrants physician notification?

    1 Hypertension

    2 Diaphoresis

    3 Polyuria

    4 Increased pulse rate

32. The nurse is preparing a care plan for a diabetic client with hyperglycemia. The priority nursing diagnosis is:

    1 High risk for fluid volume deficit

    2 Knowledge deficit: Disease process and treatment

    3 Altered nutrition: Less than body requirements

    4 Ineffective family coping: Compromised

33. The home health nurse visits a client with a diagnosis of Type 1 diabetes. The client reports a history of vomiting and diarrhea. No food nor medication has been consumed for 36 hours. Which of the following statements by the client indicates a need for further teaching?

    1 "I need to stop my insulin."

    2 "I need to increase my fluid intake."

    3 "I need to call my doctor."

    4 "I need to monitor my blood glucose every 4 to 6 hours."

34. The nurse is teaching a client with diabetes mellitus recovering from DKA to develop a plan to prevent a recurrence. Which of the following is most important to include in the plan of care?

    1 Eat 6 small meals per day

    2 Receive appropriate follow-up health care

    3 Monitor blood glucose levels frequently

    4 Test urine for ketone levels

35. The nurse is caring for a client admitted to the emergency department with DKA. In the acute phase, the priority nursing action is to prepare to:

    1 Administer IV Regular insulin

    2 Administer IV 5% dextrose

    3 Correct acidosis

    4 Apply an electrocardiographic monitor

36. A client with Type 2 diabetes mellitus has a blood sugar over 600 mg/dL and is complaining of polydipsia, polyuria, weight loss, and weakness. The nurse reviews the physician's documentation and expects to note which of the following diagnoses?

    1 Diabetic ketoacidosis

    2 Hypoglycemia

    3 Hyperglycemic hyperosmolar nonketotic (HHNK) syndrome

    4 Pheochromocytoma

37. The family of a bedridden client with Type 2 diabetes mellitus calls the nurse to report the

following symptoms: blood glucose 400 (by fingerstick), polydipsia, and increased lethargy. In determining a possible diagnosis, the most important question to the family is which of the following?

1 "Has there been any change in tube feeding?"
2 "Have there been any ketones in the urine?"
3 "Has there been any fever?"
4 "Have you increased the amount of fluids provided?"

38. The nurse performs a physical assessment on a client with Type 2 diabetes mellitus. Findings include a fasting blood sugar of 180 mg/dL, temperature of 101°F, pulse of 88, respirations of 22, blood pressure of 140/84. Which of the data is of most concern to the nurse?

1 Pulse
2 Blood pressure
3 Respiration
4 Temperature

39. The nurse is interviewing a client with Type 2 diabetes mellitus. Which statement by the client indicates an understanding of the medications?

1 "I am taking oral insulin instead of shots."
2 "The medications I'm taking help release the insulin I already make."
3 "By taking these medications I am able to eat more."
4 "When I become ill I need to increase the number of pills I take."

40. The client with Type 1 is having trouble remembering the types, duration, and onset of action of insulin. The client's family members have not been supportive. The nurse's best response is:

1 "You can't always depend on your family to help."
2 "Let me go over the types of insulin with you again."
3 "It's not really necessary for you to remember this."
4 "What is it you don't understand?"

41. A nurse is doing discharge teaching with a client who has Cushing's syndrome. Which of the following statements by the client indicates that instructions related to dietary management were understood?

1 "I am fortunate that I do not need to follow any special diet."
2 "I will need to limit the amount of protein in my diet."
3 "I am fortunate that I can eat all the salty foods I enjoy."
4 "I can eat foods that have a lot of potassium in them."

42. The nurse is preparing to administer an IV insulin injection. The vial of Regular insulin has been refrigerated. Upon inspection of the vial, the nurse finds the medication frozen. The nurse should:

1 Wait for the insulin to thaw at room temperature
2 Check the temperature settings of the refrigerator
3 Discard the insulin and obtain another vial
4 Roll the vial between the hands until the medication becomes liquid

43. A client with Type 1 calls the nurse to report recurrent episodes of hypoglycemia. Which of the following statements by the client indicates an inadequate understanding of NPH insulin and exercise?

1 "The best time for me to exercise is every afternoon."
2 "The best time for me to exercise is after lunch."
3 "The best time for me to exercise is after breakfast."
4 "The best time for me to exercise is before bedtime."

44. The nurse is completing an assessment on an elderly client who is being admitted for a diagnostic workup for primary hyperparathyroidism. Which client complaint is characteristic of this disorder?

1 Diarrhea
2 Polyuria
3 Polyphagia
4 Weight gain

45. The nurse is caring for a postoperative parathyroidectomy client. Which client complaint indicates that a serious life-threatening complication may be developing, requiring immediate notification of the physician?

1 Difficulty in voiding
2 Abdominal cramps
3 Laryngeal stridor
4 Mild to moderate incisional pain

46. The nurse is preparing to discharge a client who has had a parathyroidectomy. Part of the discharge instructions includes medication administration for oral calcium supplements that the client will need daily. Which statement by the nurse is appropriate regarding oral calcium supplement therapy?

1 Store the tablets in the refrigerator to maintain potency
2 Check the pulse daily; if it is below 60 beats per minute, do not take the tablets
3 Take the tablets with food or following a meal
4 Avoid sunlight as it can cause skin color change

47. A nurse is assessing a newly diagnosed diabetic client's learning readiness. Which client behavior

indicates to the nurse that the client is not ready to learn?

1 The client complains of fatigue whenever the nurse plans a teaching session
2 The client asks if the spouse can attend the classes also
3 The client asks for written materials about diabetes before class
4 The client asks appropriate questions about what will be taught

48. The nurse notes that the Type 1 diabetic has lipodystrophy on both upper thighs. The nurse would appropriately inquire whether the client:
    1 Cleanses the skin with alcohol before each injection
    2 Rotates sites for injection
    3 Aspirates for blood prior to injection into the subcutaneous tissue
    4 Administers the insulin at a 45° angle

49. The nurse is caring for a Type 1 client. Which of the following client complaints would alert the nurse to a possible hypoglycemic reaction?
    1 Hot, dry skin
    2 Muscle cramps
    3 Anorexia
    4 Tremors

50. A young Type 1 male diabetic client tells the nurse that he might lose his job because he has been having frequent hypoglycemic reactions. His boss thinks that he is drunk during these episodes, and that he has been drinking on the job. Which action by the nurse would best assist this client to meet his needs?
    1 Contact the local employment office to help him find another job
    2 Ask the client if he indeed has been drinking at work
    3 Examine factors with the client that may be causing frequent hypoglycemic episodes
    4 Ask the client what he does to treat his hypoglycemia

51. The nurse needs to maintain food and fluid intake to minimize the risk of dehydration in a frail, elderly diabetic client with gastroenteritis. An appropriate intervention for the nurse to perform is:
    1 Offer water only, until the client is able to tolerate solid foods
    2 Withhold all fluids until vomiting has ceased for at least 4 hours
    3 Encourage the client to take 8 to 12 ounces of fluid every hour while awake
    4 Maintain a clear liquid diet for at least 5 days before advancing to allow inflammation of the bowel to dissipate

52. A client who is currently taking levothyroxine (Synthroid) complains of cold intolerance, constipation, dry skin, weight gain, and puffy eyes. Based on these findings, the nurse anticipates which of the following prescriptions?
    1 Increase Synthroid dosage after checking the T4 level
    2 Decrease Synthroid dosage after checking the T_4 level
    3 Discontinue Synthroid—the client is having an adverse reaction
    4 No change in medication; these are common side effects that will diminish with time

53. A client with diabetes mellitus visits the health care clinic. The client's diabetes mellitus had previously been well controlled with glyburide (DiaBeta), 5 mg PO QD, but recently the fasting blood glucose has been running 180 to 200 mg/dL. Which of the following medications, if added to the client's regimen, may contribute to the hyperglycemia?
    1 Prednisone (Deltasone)
    2 Atenolol (Tenormin)
    3 Phenelzine (Nardil)
    4 Allopurinol (Zyloprim)

54. The nurse is caring for a client with diabetes insipidus who is receiving vasopressin (Pitressin). Which of the following is not a therapeutic effect of this medication?
    1 Increased GI tract smooth muscle tone and contractions
    2 Decreased urine output
    3 Increased reabsorption of water by the renal tubules
    4 Vasodilation of vascular vessels

55. The client is diagnosed with pheochromocytoma. The nurse prepares a nursing care plan for the client, and in the planning the nurse understands that pheochromocytoma is a condition:
    1 That causes profound hypotension
    2 That causes the release of excessive amounts of catecholamines
    3 That is not a curable condition and is treated symptomatically
    4 That is manifested by severe hypoglycemia

56. The nurse is performing an admission assessment on a client admitted with a diagnosis of pheochromocytoma. The nurse assesses for the major symptom associated with pheochromocytoma when:
    1 Testing the client's urine for glucose
    2 Taking the client's weight
    3 Palpating the skin for its temperature
    4 Taking the client's blood pressure

57. The nurse collects urine specimens for catecholamine testing from the client with suspected pheochromocytoma. The results of the catecholamine test are reported as 20 µg/dL urine. The nurse analyzes these results as:

1 Normal

2 Lower than normal, ruling out pheochromocytoma

3 Higher than normal, indicating pheochromocytoma

4 Insignificant and unrelated to pheochromocytoma

58. The physician orders a 24-hour urine collection for VMA (vanillylmandelic acid). The community health nurse visits the client at home and instructs the client in the procedure for the collection of the urine. Which of the following statements, if made by the client, indicates a need for further instruction?

1 "I will start the collection in 2 days. Starting now, I cannot eat or drink any tea, chocolate, vanilla, or fruit until the test is completed."

2 "When I start the collection, I will urinate and discard that specimen."

3 "I will pour the urine in the collection bottle each time I urinate and refrigerate the urine."

4 "I can take medication if I need to during the collection."

59. The nurse is caring for a client with pheochromocytoma. The client is scheduled for adrenalectomy. In the preoperative period, the priority nursing action is to monitor:

1 Vital signs

2 Urine for glucose and acetone

3 I&O

4 BUN laboratory values

60. The nurse is caring for a client with pheochromocytoma. As part of the nursing care plan, the nurse monitors for hypertensive crisis. In the event that hypertensive crisis occurs, the nurse anticipates that the most likely medication to be prescribed would be:

1 Propranolol (Inderal)

2 Phentolamine mesylate (Regitine)

3 Phenoxybenzamine hydrochloride (Dibenzyline)

4 Prazosin hydrochloride (Minipress)

61. The nurse is caring for a client with pheochromocytoma. The client asks for a snack and something warm to drink. The most appropriate choice for this client to meet nutritional needs is which of the following?

1 Graham crackers and warm milk

2 Toast with peanut butter and cocoa

3 Crackers with cheese and tea

4 Vanilla wafers and coffee with cream and sugar

62. Which of the following assessment data indicates a potential complication associated with pheochromocytoma?

1 A urinary output of 50 mL per hour

2 Rales heard on auscultation

3 A BUN of 20 mg/dL

4 A coagulation time of 5 minutes

63. The client with pheochromocytoma is scheduled for surgery and says to the nurse, "I'm not sure that surgery is the best thing to do." The most appropriate response by the nurse is which of the following?

1 "You have concerns about the surgical treatment for your condition?"

2 "There is no reason to worry. Your doctor is a wonderful surgeon."

3 "You are very ill. Your physician has made the correct decision."

4 "I think you are making the right decision to have the surgery."

64. The community health nurse visits a client at home. Prednisone (Deltasone), 10 mg PO daily, has been prescribed for the client. The nurse teaches the client about the medication. Which of the following statements, if made by the client, indicates that further teaching is necessary?

1 "I need to take the medication every day at the same time."

2 "I can take aspirin or my antihistamine if I need it."

3 "If I gain more than 5 pounds a week, I will call my doctor."

4 "I need to avoid coffee, tea, cola, and chocolate in my diet."

65. The nurse is caring for a client following thyroidectomy and is monitoring for signs of thyroid storm. Which of the following is a manifestation associated with this disorder?

1 Low-grade temperature

2 Bradycardia

3 Hypotension

4 Constipation

66. The nurse is providing instructions to the client with Addison's disease regarding diet therapy. Which of the following diets would most likely be prescribed for this client?

1 Low sodium

2 High sodium

3 Low protein

4 Low carbohydrate

67. The nursing instructor asks the student to describe the pathophysiology that occurs in Cushing's disease. Which of the following statements by the student indicates an accurate understanding of this disorder?

1 "It is characterized by an oversecretion of glucocorticoid hormones."

2 "It is characterized by an undersecretion of glucocorticoid hormones."

3 "It is characterized by an oversecretion of insulin."

4 "It is characterized by an undersecretion of corticotropic hormones."

ANSWERS

1. **3**

Rationale: Based on the location of the surgical procedure, spinal anesthesia would not be used. Additionally, the hair would not be shaved. Although coughing and deep breathing are important, specific to this procedure is avoiding toothbrushing to prevent disruption of the surgical site.

Test-Taking Strategy: Consider the anatomical location and the surgical procedure itself to eliminate options 1 and 4. Although you may be tempted to select option 2, read carefully. Because of the anatomical location of the surgery, option 3 is most important. Review this surgical procedure now, if you had difficulty with this question!

Level of Cognitive Ability: Application
Phase of Nursing Process: Implementation
Client Needs: Physiological Integrity
Content Area: Adult Health/Endocrine

Reference
Black, J., & Matassarin-Jacobs, E. (1997). *Medical-surgical nursing: Clinical management for continuity of care* (5th ed.). Philadelphia: W. B. Saunders. p. 2064.

2. **3**

Rationale: Following hypophysectomy, diabetes insipidus can occur temporarily because of antidiuretic hormone deficiency. This deficiency is related to surgical manipulation. The nurse should assess specific gravity and notify the physician if the results are less than 1.005.

Test-Taking Strategy: Knowledge that diabetes insipidus is a complication of this type of surgery will assist in eliminating option 4. Note the key word "initial." Knowledge of the nursing assessment measures in diabetes insipidus will easily direct you to option 3.

Level of Cognitive Ability: Application
Phase of Nursing Process: Implementation
Client Needs: Physiological Integrity
Content Area: Adult Health/Endocrine

Reference
Black, J., & Matassarin-Jacobs, E. (1997). *Medical-surgical nursing: Clinical management for continuity of care* (5th ed.). Philadelphia: W. B. Saunders. p. 2064.

3. **2**

Rationale: Following hypophysectomy, the client should be monitored for rhinorrhea, which could indicate a CSF leak. If this occurs, the drainage should be collected and tested for the presence of CSF. The head of the bed should not be lowered to prevent increased intracranial pressure. Clear nasal drainage would not indicate the need for a culture. Continuing to observe the drainage without taking action could result in a serious complication.

Test-Taking Strategy: Note the key word "initial." This indicates that an action is required. Option 3 can be easily eliminated. Option 4 can be easily eliminated because the drainage is clear. Because an action is required, eliminate option 1. Review the complications following hypophysectomy if you had difficulty with this question!

Level of Cognitive Ability: Application
Phase of Nursing Process: Implementation
Client Needs: Physiological Integrity
Content Area: Adult Health/Endocrine

Reference
Black, J., & Matassarin-Jacobs, E. (1997). *Medical-surgical nursing: Clinical management for continuity of care* (5th ed.). Philadelphia: W. B. Saunders. p. 2064.

4. **2**

Rationale: Polydipsia and polyuria are classic symptoms of diabetes insipidus. The urine is pale in color, and the specific gravity is low. Anorexia and weight loss occur.

Test-Taking Strategy: Eliminate option 4 first because this symptom is rather vague and occurs in many conditions. Knowledge of the manifestations of diabetes insipidus will assist in eliminating options 1 and 3. If you had difficulty with this question, review the clinical manifestations associated with diabetes insipidus!

Level of Cognitive Ability: Analysis
Phase of Nursing Process: Assessment
Client Needs: Physiological Integrity
Content Area: Adult Health/Endocrine

Reference
Monahan, F., & Neighbors, M. (1998). *Medical-surgical nursing: Foundations for clinical practice* (2nd ed.). Philadelphia: W. B. Saunders. pp. 1274–1275.

5. **3**

Rationale: Common manifestations of Addison's disease include postural hypotension from fluid loss, syncope, muscle weakness, anorexia, nausea and vomiting, abdominal cramps, weight loss, depression, and irritability.

Test-Taking Strategy: Knowledge regarding the clinical manifestations associated with Addison's disease is required to answer this question. If you had difficulty with this question, be sure to review this very important endocrine disorder!

Level of Cognitive Ability: Analysis
Phase of Nursing Process: Assessment
Client Needs: Physiological Integrity
Content Area: Adult Health/Endocrine

Reference
Monahan, F., & Neighbors, M. (1998). *Medical-surgical nursing: Foundations for clinical practice* (2nd ed.). Philadelphia: W. B. Saunders. p. 1278.

6. **4**

Rationale: The client with Cushing's syndrome should be reassured that most physical changes resolve with treatment. Options 1, 2, and 3 are not therapeutic responses.

Test-Taking Strategy: Use knowledge regarding the physical changes that occur in Cushing's syndrome to answer this question. If you are unfamiliar with this disorder, you can easily eliminate options 1, 2, and 3 because these statements are not therapeutic responses to a client!

Level of Cognitive Ability: Application
Phase of Nursing Process: Implementation
Client Needs: Psychosocial Integrity
Content Area: Adult Health/Endocrine

Reference
Monahan, F., & Neighbors, M. (1998). *Medical-surgical nursing: Foundations for clinical practice* (2nd ed.). Philadelphia: W. B. Saunders. p. 1289.

7. **4**

Rationale: Because of the hypermetabolic state, the client with Graves' disease needs to be provided with an environment that is restful both physically and mentally. Six full meals a day that are well balanced and high in calories are required because of the accelerated metabolic rate. Foods that increase peristalsis, such as high-fiber foods, need to be avoided. These clients suffer from heat intolerance and require a cool environment.

Test-Taking Strategy: The key concept to bear in mind when answering this question is that clients with Graves' disease experience an accelerated metabolic rate. This concept should assist you in eliminating options 1, 2, and 3.

Level of Cognitive Ability: Application
Phase of Nursing Process: Planning
Client Needs: Physiological Integrity
Content Area: Adult Health/Endocrine

Reference

Black, J., & Matassarin-Jacobs, E. (1997). *Medical-surgical nursing: Clinical management for continuity of care* (5th ed.). Philadelphia: W. B. Saunders. p. 2020.

8. **4**

Rationale: Hypocalcemia can develop after thyroidectomy if the parathyroid glands are accidentally removed during surgery. Manifestations develop 1 to 7 days after surgery. If the client develops numbness and tingling around the mouth, fingertips, or toes; muscle spasms; or twitching, the physician is notified immediately. Calcium gluconate should be kept at the bedside.

Test-Taking Strategy: Noting the name of the medication (calcium gluconate) should easily direct you to option 4. Calcium would be given if hypocalcemic tetany occurs.

Level of Cognitive Ability: Analysis
Phase of Nursing Process: Analysis
Client Needs: Physiological Integrity
Content Area: Pharmacology

Reference

Black, J., & Matassarin-Jacobs, E. (1997). *Medical-surgical nursing: Clinical management for continuity of care* (5th ed.). Philadelphia: W. B. Saunders. p. 2023.

9. **2**

Rationale: Weakness and hoarseness of the voice can occur because of trauma or damage of the laryngeal nerve. If this develops, the client should be reassured that the problem will subside in a few days. Unnecessary talking should be discouraged. It is not necessary to notify the physician. These signs do not indicate bleeding or the need to administer calcium gluconate.

Test-Taking Strategy: Knowledge regarding the complications following thyroidectomy will easily direct you to option 2. Options 3 and 4 can easily be eliminated because they are unrelated to the signs presented in the question. No data are presented requiring physician notification.

Level of Cognitive Ability: Analysis
Phase of Nursing Process: Assessment
Client Needs: Physiological Integrity
Content Area: Adult Health/Endocrine

Reference

Black, J., & Matassarin-Jacobs, E. (1997). *Medical-surgical nursing: Clinical management for continuity of care* (5th ed.). Philadelphia: W. B. Saunders. p. 2023.

10. **3**

Rationale: The initial nursing action would be to maintain a patent airway. Oxygen would be administered, followed by fluid replacement, keeping the client warm, monitoring vital signs, and administering thyroid hormones IV.

Test-Taking Strategy: Note the key phrase "carry out initially." All the options are appropriate interventions, but utilize the ABCs in selecting the correct option.

Level of Cognitive Ability: Application
Phase of Nursing Process: Implementation
Client Needs: Physiological Integrity
Content Area: Adult Health/Endocrine

Reference

Black, J., & Matassarin-Jacobs, E. (1997). *Medical-surgical nursing: Clinical management for continuity of care* (5th ed.). Philadelphia: W. B. Saunders. p. 2009.

11. **2**

Rationale: The client with hypothyroidism experiences fatigue, lethargy, and increased somnolence. The decreased metabolism and oxygen consumption are manifested by a slow heart rate, decreased cardiac output, and decreased blood pressure. Synthroid, a thyroid hormone, is a component of therapy. Stool softeners such as Colace are prescribed to promote defecation. Morphine would further depress bodily functions. Atenolol is used with caution in clients with hyperthyroidism.

Test-Taking Strategy: Keeping in mind that a decreased metabolic rate occurs in the client with hypothyroidism will easily direct you to option 2 as the medication that would be avoided in this condition. Review the pathophysiology associated with hypothyroidism now, if you had difficulty with this question!

Level of Cognitive Ability: Analysis
Phase of Nursing Process: Analysis
Client Needs: Physiological Integrity
Content Area: Pharmacology

Reference

Monahan, F., & Neighbors, M. (1998). *Medical-surgical nursing: Foundations for clinical practice* (2nd ed.). Philadelphia: W. B. Saunders. p. 1301.

12. **2**

Rationale: NPH is an intermediate-acting insulin. The onset of action is 1 to 2 hours, it peaks in 6 to 12 hours, and its duration of action is 18 to 24 hours. Hypoglycemic reactions most likely occur during peak time.

Test-Taking Strategy: Knowledge regarding the onset, peak, and duration of action for NPH insulin is required to answer this question. Be sure to learn these characteristics of NPH insulin. You are likely to find a question regarding NPH and Regular insulin on NCLEX-RN!

Level of Cognitive Ability: Application
Phase of Nursing Process: Implementation
Client Needs: Health Promotion and Maintenance
Content Area: Pharmacology

Reference

Lehne, R. (1998). *Pharmacology for nursing care* (3rd ed.). Philadelphia: W. B. Saunders. p. 580.

13. 3

Rationale: A blood glucose test performed before exercising lets the client know whether to eat a snack first. Exercising during the peak times of insulin or prior to mealtime places the client at risk for hypoglycemia. Insulin should be administered as prescribed.

Test-Taking Strategy: The issue of the question relates to the occurrence of a hypoglycemic reaction. Utilize the process of elimination, keeping in mind this issue and the action of insulin. You should easily be able to eliminate options 1, 2, and 4.

Level of Cognitive Ability: Application
Phase of Nursing Process: Implementation
Client Needs: Health Promotion and Maintenance
Content Area: Adult Health/Endocrine

Reference
Monahan, F., & Neighbors, M. (1998). *Medical-surgical nursing: Foundations for clinical practice* (2nd ed.). Philadelphia: W. B. Saunders. p. 1234.

14. 2

Rationale: The client should be instructed not to soak the feet and should avoid hot water to prevent burns. The client may cut toenails straight and even with the toe itself, and would consult a podiatrist if the toenails were thick, hard to cut, or vision was poor. The client should be instructed to wash the feet daily using a mild soap.

Test-Taking Strategy: Eliminate option 3 first because of the word "always." Options 1 and 4 can be easily eliminated, leaving option 2 as the correct choice. Review diabetic foot care instructions now, if you had difficulty with this question!

Level of Cognitive Ability: Application
Phase of Nursing Process: Planning
Client Needs: Health Promotion and Maintenance
Content Area: Adult Health/Endocrine

Reference
Monahan, F., & Neighbors, M. (1998). *Medical-surgical nursing: Foundations for clinical practice* (2nd ed.). Philadelphia: W. B. Saunders. p. 1252.

15. 4

Rationale: The primary goal of treatment is to rehydrate the client to restore fluid volume and to correct electrolyte deficiency. IV fluid replacement is similar to that administered in DKA and begins with IV infusion of normal saline. Regular, not NPH, insulin would be administered. The use of sodium bicarbonate to correct acidosis is avoided because it can precipitate a further drop in serum potassium levels. Oxygen is not necessarily required to treat HHNC.

Test-Taking Strategy: Knowledge regarding the treatment for HHNC is required to answer this question. If you can recall the treatment for DKA, you will easily be able to answer this question. Treatment for HHNC is similar to the treatment for DKA.

Level of Cognitive Ability: Application
Phase of Nursing Process: Implementation
Client Needs: Physiological Integrity
Content Area: Adult Health/Endocrine

Reference
Monahan, F., & Neighbors, M. (1998). *Medical-surgical nursing: Foundations for clinical practice* (2nd ed.). Philadelphia: W. B. Saunders. pp. 1249–1250.

16. 3

Rationale: It is important to emphasize to the client and family that they are not eating a diabetic diet but rather a balanced meal plan. Adherence to nutrition principles is an important component of diabetic management, and an individualized meal plan should be developed for the client.

Test-Taking Strategy: Careful reading of this question and the options will easily direct you to the correct answer. Note the key phrase "indicates a need for further teaching." By the process of elimination, you will easily be directed to option 3.

Level of Cognitive Ability: Analysis
Phase of Nursing Process: Evaluation
Client Needs: Health Promotion and Maintenance
Content Area: Adult Health/Endocrine

Reference
Black, J., & Matassarin-Jacobs, E. (1997). *Medical-surgical nursing: Clinical management for continuity of care* (5th ed.). Philadelphia: W. B. Saunders. p. 1975.

17. 1

Rationale: An insulin pump provides a small, continuous dose of Regular insulin SC throughout the day and night, and the client can bolus self with additional dosage from the pump prior to each meal as needed. Regular insulin is used in an insulin pump. An external pump is not surgically attached to the pancreas.

Test-Taking Strategy: Knowledge that Regular insulin is used in an insulin pump will assist in eliminating options 2 and 4. Careful reading of the question noting the word "external" will assist in eliminating option 3. Review the use of the insulin pump now, if you are unfamiliar with it!

Level of Cognitive Ability: Analysis
Phase of Nursing Process: Analysis
Client Needs: Health Promotion and Maintenance
Content Area: Adult Health/Endocrine

Reference
Monahan, F., & Neighbors, M. (1998). *Medical-surgical nursing: Foundations for clinical practice* (2nd ed.). Philadelphia: W. B. Saunders. pp. 1238–1239.

18. 4

Rationale: Insulin dosages should not be adjusted and should not be increased prior to unusual exercise. If acetone is found in the urine, it may possibly indicate the need for additional insulin. To minimize the discomfort associated with insulin injections, insulin should be administered at room temperature. Injection sites should be systematically rotated from one area to another. The client should be instructed to give injections in one area, about an inch apart, until the whole area has been used, then change to another site. This prevents dramatic changes in daily insulin absorption.

Test-Taking Strategy: Eliminate option 3 first because of the word "always." Knowledge regarding insulin administration and the significance of acetone in the urine will assist in eliminating options 1 and 2. If you had difficulty with this question, take time now to review insulin management!

Level of Cognitive Ability: Application
Phase of Nursing Process: Implementation
Client Needs: Health Promotion and Maintenance
Content Area: Pharmacology

Reference
Black, J., & Matassarin-Jacobs, E. (1997). *Medical-surgical nursing: Clinical management for continuity of care* (5th ed.). Philadelphia: W. B. Saunders. p. 1979.

19. 1

Rationale: In DKA, the arterial pH is less than 7.35, plasma bicarbonate is less than 15 mEq/L, the blood glucose level is higher than 250 mg/dL, and ketones are present in the blood and urine. The client would be experiencing polyuria, and Kussmaul's respirations would be present. Coma may occur if DKA is not treated, but coma would not confirm the diagnosis.

Test-Taking Strategy: Note the key word "confirm" in the stem of the question. Eliminate option 4 because coma can exist in many conditions. Eliminate option 3 because in acidosis the pH would be low. Remember that polyuria exists in DKA. This leaves option 1 as the correct choice.

Level of Cognitive Ability: Analysis
Phase of Nursing Process: Analysis
Client Needs: Physiological Integrity
Content Area: Adult Health/Endocrine

Reference
Monahan, F., & Neighbors, M. (1998). *Medical-surgical nursing: Foundations for clinical practice* (2nd ed.). Philadelphia: W. B. Saunders. pp. 1249, 1251.

20. 3

Rationale: NPH is an intermediate-acting insulin. The onset of action is 1 to 2 hours, it peaks in 6 to 12 hours, and its duration of action is 18 to 24 hours. Hypoglycemic reactions most likely occur during peak time.

Test-Taking Strategy: Knowledge regarding the onset, peak, and duration of action for NPH insulin is required to answer this question. Knowing that peak action is between 6 and 12 hours will easily direct you to option 3. Be sure to learn these characteristics of NPH insulin. You are likely to find a question regarding NPH and Regular insulin on NCLEX-RN!

Level of Cognitive Ability: Analysis
Phase of Nursing Process: Assessment
Client Needs: Physiological Integrity
Content Area: Pharmacology

Reference
Lehne, R. (1998). *Pharmacology for nursing care* (3rd ed.). Philadelphia: W. B. Saunders. p. 580.

21. 2

Rationale: Shakiness is a sign of hypoglycemia and would indicate the need for food, glucose, or glycogen. A fruity breath odor, blurred vision, and polyuria are signs of hyperglycemia.

Test-Taking Strategy: Knowledge regarding the signs and symptoms of hypoglycemia and hyperglycemia is required to answer this question. If you are unfamiliar with these signs, be sure to learn them. You are likely to find a question regarding these signs and the treatment required on NCLEX-RN!

Level of Cognitive Ability: Analysis
Phase of Nursing Process: Evaluation
Client Needs: Health Promotion and Maintenance
Content Area: Adult Health/Endocrine

Reference
Monahan, F., & Neighbors, M. (1998). *Medical-surgical nursing: Foundations for clinical practice* (2nd ed.). Philadelphia: W. B. Saunders. p. 1251.

22. 4

Rationale: The most appropriate intervention is to address the client's feelings related to the anxiety. Administering a sedative is not the most appropriate intervention. The nurse should not ignore the client's anxious feelings. A client will not relate to medical terms, particularly when anxiety exists.

Test-Taking Strategy: Utilize therapeutic communication techniques to answer the question. Remember that the client's feelings come first. Keeping this in mind will easily direct you to option 4.

Level of Cognitive Ability: Application
Phase of Nursing Process: Implementation
Client Needs: Psychosocial Integrity
Content Area: Adult Health/Endocrine

Reference
Leahy, J., & Kizilay, P. (1998). *Foundations of nursing practice: A nursing process approach*. Philadelphia: W. B. Saunders. p. 223.

23. 3

Rationale: During illness, the client should monitor blood glucose levels and should notify the physician if the level is over 250 mg/dL. Insulin should never be stopped. In fact, insulin may need to be increased. Doses should not be adjusted without the physician's advice.

Test-Taking Strategy: Note that options 1, 2, and 4 all relate to adjustment of insulin doses. Therefore, eliminate these options. Review diabetic management during illness now, if you had difficulty with this question!

Level of Cognitive Ability: Analysis
Phase of Nursing Process: Evaluation
Client Needs: Health Promotion and Maintenance
Content Area: Adult Health/Endocrine

Reference
Monahan F., & Neighbors, M. (1998). *Medical-surgical nursing: Foundations for clinical practice* (2nd ed.). Philadelphia: W. B. Saunders. pp. 1240–1241.

24. 1

Rationale: During management of DKA, when the blood glucose level falls to 300 mg/dL, the infusion rate is reduced and 5% dextrose is added to maintain a blood glucose level of about 250 mg/dL, or until the client recovers from ketosis. NPH insulin is not used to treat DKA. Fifty percent glucose is used to treat hypoglycemia. Dilantin is not a normal treatment measure in DKA.

Test-Taking Strategy: Eliminate option 2 first, knowing that Regular insulin is used in the management of DKA. Eliminate option 3 next, knowing that this is the treatment for hypoglycemia. Note the key phrase "the serum glucose level is now 240 mg/dL." This should indicate that the IV solution of 5% dextrose is the next step in management of care.

Level of Cognitive Ability: Application
Phase of Nursing Process: Implementation
Client Needs: Physiological Integrity
Content Area: Adult Health/Endocrine

Reference
Monahan, F., & Neighbors, M. (1998). *Medical-surgical nursing: Foundations for clinical practice* (2nd ed.). Philadelphia: W. B. Saunders. pp. 1249–1250.

25. 1

Rationale: If the client becomes ill and cannot retain fluids or food for a period of 4 hours, the physician should be notified. The client's statement in this question indicates a need for immediate education to prevent HHNC, a life-threatening emergency situation.

Test-Taking Strategy: Knowledge regarding the causes of HHNC will assist in answering the question. Eliminate option 2 first because the client's statement is inaccurate. Eliminate option 3 next because the client requires immediate education. Eliminate option 4 because HHNC most commonly occurs with Type 2 diabetes mellitus. Review diabetic management during times of illness now, if you had difficulty with this question!

Level of Cognitive Ability: Analysis
Phase of Nursing Process: Analysis
Client Needs: Health Promotion and Maintenance
Content Area: Adult Health/Endocrine

Reference
Monahan, F., & Neighbors, M. (1998). *Medical-surgical nursing: Foundations for clinical practice* (2nd ed.). Philadelphia: W. B. Saunders. pp. 1240–1241.

26. 1

Rationale: Excessive dosing with PTU may convert the client from a hyperthyroid state to a hypothyroid state. If this occurs, the dosage should be reduced. Temporary administration of thyroid hormone may be required. PTU is not used for pain and does not cause hyperglycemia or renal toxicity.

Test-Taking Strategy: Noting that PTU is used to treat hyperthyroidism should easily direct you to option 1. If you had difficulty with this question, take time now to review this important medication!

Level of Cognitive Ability: Application
Phase of Nursing Process: Planning
Client Needs: Physiological Integrity
Content Area: Adult Health/Endocrine

Reference
Lehne, R. (1998). *Pharmacology for nursing care* (3rd ed.). Philadelphia: W. B. Saunders. pp. 602–603.

27. 2

Rationale: Calcitonin can lower plasma calcium levels in clients with hypercalcemia secondary to hyperparathyroidism. The therapeutic effect in this client situation would be a reduction in serum calcium levels. Calcitonin is a very safe medication. It is the medication of choice for rapid relief of pain associated with Paget's disease.

Test-Taking Strategy: Reading the question carefully, noting the client diagnosis, will assist in directing you to option 2. Additionally, note the relationship between the name of the medication and the word "calcium" in option 2. If you are unfamiliar with this medication, take time now to review!

Level of Cognitive Ability: Analysis
Phase of Nursing Process: Evaluation
Client Needs: Health Promotion and Maintenance
Content Area: Adult Health/Endocrine

Reference
Lehne, R. (1998). *Pharmacology for nursing care* (3rd ed.). Philadelphia: W. B. Saunders. pp. 820, 828.

28. 2

Rationale: Synthroid is a synthetic thyroid hormone that increases cellular metabolism. It should be given in the morning in a single dose to prevent sleeplessness. It should be given at the same time each day to maintain drug level.

Test-Taking Strategy: Options 1 and 3 can be eliminated because it is not the nurse's decision to change or alter a physician's order. When choosing between options 2 and 4, option 2 has more validity based on common nursing sense, even if you do not know the action of Synthroid.

Level of Cognitive Ability: Application
Phase of Nursing Process: Implementation
Client Needs: Physiological Integrity
Content Area: Adult Health/Endocrine

Reference
Hodgson, B., & Kizior, R. (1998). *Saunders nursing drug handbook 1998*. Philadelphia: W. B. Saunders. pp. 589–590.

29. 4

Rationale: Diabinese is an oral hypoglycemic agent given to reduce serum glucose and the signs and symptoms of hyperglycemia. Therefore, a decrease in both polyuria and polyphagia, and symptoms of hyperglycemia, would denote a beneficial response to Diabinese. Laboratory values are also used to assess the client's response to treatment. An FBS of 110 mg/dL is within normal limits. However, a glycosylated hemoglobin of 12% indicates that diabetes is not well controlled.

Test-Taking Strategy: Note the key word "not" in the stem of the question. Knowledge of Diabinese as an oral hypoglycemic agent tells you to look for an option that would denote hyperglycemia (lack of response to medication). Options 1 and 3 are similar, a clue that they are both either true or false and therefore could not be the one option to select. Knowledge of the normal blood glucose level will easily direct you to option 4.

Level of Cognitive Ability: Analysis
Phase of Nursing Process: Evaluation
Client Needs: Physiological Integrity
Content Area: Adult Health/Endocrine

Reference
Lehne, R. (1998). *Pharmacology for nursing care* (3rd ed.). Philadelphia: W. B. Saunders. pp. 594–595.

30. 3

Rationale: DDAVP is a synthetic form of antidiuretic hormone. It causes increased reabsorption of water with a resultant decrease in urine output. Therapeutic response to DDAVP would demonstrate a decrease in serum osmolality as more fluid is retained, and an increase in urine osmolality as less fluid is excreted. Increased blood pressure is a side effect rather than a therapeutic effect of DDAVP.

Test-Taking Strategy: Knowledge of the medication action of DDAVP is necessary to select the correct option. This knowledge easily allows you to select option 3. The key word in the stem "therapeutic" directs you to eliminate option 2, as this is a side effect rather than an intended therapeutic effect. Review this important medication now, if you had difficulty with this question!

Level of Cognitive Ability: Analysis
Phase of Nursing Process: Evaluation
Client Needs: Physiological Integrity
Content Area: Adult Health / Endocrine

Reference
Hodgson, B., & Kizior, R. (1998). *Saunders nursing drug handbook 1998*. Philadelphia: W. B. Saunders. pp. 293–295.

31. **3**

Rationale: Regular monitoring may detect hyperglycemia early enough to prevent serious complications. Classic symptoms of hyperglycemia include polydipsia, polyuria, and polyphagia.

Test-Taking Strategy: Knowledge regarding the signs and symptoms of hyperglycemia is required to answer this question. Remember the 3 Ps: polyuria, polydipsia, polyphagia. Learn the signs of hyperglycemia now, if you had difficulty with this question!

Level of Cognitive Ability: Application
Phase of Nursing Process: Assessment
Client Needs: Physiological Integrity
Content Area: Adult Health/Endocrine

Reference
Monahan, F., & Neighbors, M. (1998). *Medical-surgical nursing: Foundations for clinical practice* (2nd ed.). Philadelphia: W. B. Saunders. p. 1251.

32. **1**

Rationale: Increased blood glucose will cause the kidneys to excrete the glucose in the urine. This glucose is accompanied by fluids and electrolytes, causing an osmotic diuresis leading to dehydration. This fluid loss must be replaced when it becomes severe.

Test-Taking Strategy: Use Maslow's Hierarchy of Needs to answer this question. Option 1 indicates a physiological response to the hyperglycemia, which should be a priority. Options 2, 3, and 4 are nursing diagnoses that may need to be addressed after providing for the high-priority physiological needs.

Level of Cognitive Ability: Application
Phase of Nursing Process: Planning
Client Needs: Physiological Integrity
Content Area: Adult Health/Endocrine

Reference
Monahan, F., & Neighbors, M. (1998). *Medical-surgical nursing: Foundations for clinical practice* (2nd ed.). Philadelphia: W. B. Saunders. pp. 1250–1251.

33. **1**

Rationale: When a diabetic client is unable to eat normally due to illness, the client should still take the prescribed insulin or oral medication. Additional fluids should be consumed, and a call placed to health care providers. The client should monitor the blood glucose levels every 4 to 6 hours.

Test-Taking Strategy: Knowledge regarding the principles related to sick day care in the diabetic is required to answer this question. Remembering that clients need to take their insulin will easily direct you to option 1. Review these principles now, if you had difficulty with this question!

Level of Cognitive Ability: Analysis
Phase of Nursing Process: Evaluation
Client Needs: Health Promotion and Maintenance
Content Area: Adult Health/Endocrine

Reference
Burrell, L., Gerlach, M., & Pless, B. (1997). *Adult nursing: Acute and community care* (2nd ed.). Stamford, CT: Appleton & Lange. pp. 1154, 1189.

34. **3**

Rationale: Client education following DKA should emphasize the need for home glucose monitoring two to four times per day. It is also important to instruct the client to notify the health care provider when illness occurs. The presence of urine ketones indicates that DKA has already occurred. The client should eat well-balanced meals with snacks as prescribed.

Test-Taking Strategy: Treatment of DKA focuses on maintenance of appropriate blood sugars, therefore this knowledge is necessary to provide the client with correct instructions. Option 1 is not an accurate component of diabetic care. Option 2 will not prevent DKA, and option 4 does not prevent DKA but actually confirms the diagnosis.

Level of Cognitive Ability: Application
Phase of Nursing Process: Implementation
Client Needs: Health Promotion and Maintenance
Content Area: Adult Health/Endocrine

Reference
Monahan, F., & Neighbors, M. (1998). *Medical-surgical nursing: Foundations for clinical practice* (2nd ed.). Philadelphia: W. B. Saunders. pp. 1242–1243.

35. **1**

Rationale: Lack (absolute or relative) of insulin is the primary cause leading to DKA. Treatment consists of insulin administration, IV fluids (normal saline initially), and potassium replacement, followed by correcting acidosis.

Test-Taking Strategy: Note the key word "priority." Remember that in DKA, the initial treatment is Regular insulin. Normal saline is administered initially, therefore option 2 is incorrect. Options 3 and 4 may be components of the treatment plan but are not the priority.

Level of Cognitive Ability: Application
Phase of Nursing Process: Implementation
Client Needs: Physiological Integrity
Content Area: Adult Health/Endocrine

Reference
Burrell, L., Gerlach, M., & Pless, B. (1997). *Adult nursing: Acute and community care* (2nd ed.). Stamford, CT: Appleton & Lange. pp. 1167–1169.

36. **3**

Rationale: HHNK is seen primarily in Type 2 diabetes mellitus with a "relative deficiency" of insulin. The onset of symptoms may be gradual. The symptoms may include polyuria, polydipsia, dehydration, mental status alterations, weight loss, and weakness.

Test-Taking Strategy: The key phrase is the "Type 2 diabetes mellitus with a blood sugar over 600." You can easily eliminate option 4 and then option 2. Recalling that HHNK most commonly occurs in Type 2 diabetes mellitus will easily direct you to option 3.

Level of Cognitive Ability: Analysis
Phase of Nursing Process: Analysis
Client Needs: Physiological Integrity
Content Area: Adult Health/Endocrine

Reference
Burrell, L., Gerlach, M., & Pless, B. (1997). *Adult nursing: Acute and community care* (2nd ed.). Stamford, CT: Appleton & Lange. pp. 1166–1168.

37. 2

Rationale: HHNK is differentiated from DKA by the absence of excessive ketone bodies. Options 1, 3, and 4 will not assist in determining a potential diagnosis.

Test-Taking Strategy: Note the signs and symptoms presented in the question. Options 1 and 3 can be eliminated first because they are unrelated to these signs and symptoms. From the remaining options, option 2 is most specific in assisting to determine the client's diagnosis. Review the differences between DKA and HHNK coma if you had difficulty with this question!

Level of Cognitive Ability: Analysis
Phase of Nursing Process: Assessment
Client Needs: Physiological Integrity
Content Area: Adult Health/Endocrine

Reference
Burrell, L., Gerlach, M., & Pless, B. (1997). *Adult nursing: Acute and community care* (2nd ed.). Stamford, CT: Appleton & Lange. p. 1166.

38. 4

Rationale: Elevated temperature may be indicative of infection. Infection is a leading cause of HHNK or DKA.

Test-Taking Strategy: Basic knowledge of the normal values of vital signs will easily direct you to the correct option. The client's temperature is the only abnormal value. Remember that an elevated temperature can indicate an infectious process, which may lead to diabetic complications.

Level of Cognitive Ability: Analysis
Phase of Nursing Process: Analysis
Client Needs: Physiological Integrity
Content Area: Adult Health/Endocrine

Reference
Burrell, L., Gerlach, M., & Pless, B. (1997). *Adult nursing: Acute and community care* (2nd ed.). Stamford, CT: Appleton & Lange. p. 1174.

39. 2

Rationale: Clients with Type 2 diabetes have decreased or impaired insulin secretion. Oral hypoglycemic agents are given to these clients to facilitate glucose utilization. Insulin injections may be given during times of stress-induced hyperglycemia. Oral insulin is not available due to the breakdown of the insulin by digestion.

Test-Taking Strategy: Be careful and read the options completely to prevent any confusion. You must be able to determine the specific treatment for Type 2 diabetes mellitus and analyze the client's response regarding medication. Option 1 is incorrect because there is no "oral insulin"; options 3 and 4 are not accepted treatment of diabetes.

Level of Cognitive Ability: Analysis
Phase of Nursing Process: Evaluation
Client Needs: Physiological Integrity
Content Area: Adult Health/Endocrine

Reference
Monahan, F., & Neighbors, M. (1998). *Medical-surgical nursing: Foundations for clinical practice* (2nd ed.). Philadelphia: W. B. Saunders. p. 1227.

40. 2

Rationale: Reinforcement of knowledge and behaviors is vital to the success of the client's self-care. Knowledge and understanding of insulin are essential in maintaining optimum health.

Test-Taking Strategy: Remember to be therapeutic in your interaction with the client. By analyzing the responses, you find option 1 may devalue a client's family, option 3 places the issue on "hold," and option 4 requests an explanation by the client. Option 2 is the correct option because it validates/clarifies previous information.

Level of Cognitive Ability: Analysis
Phase of Nursing Process: Analysis
Client Needs: Psychosocial Integrity
Content Area: Adult Health/Endocrine

Reference
Leahy, J., & Kizilay, P. (1998). *Foundations of nursing practice: A nursing process approach*. Philadelphia: W. B. Saunders. pp. 222–225.

41. 4

Rationale: A diet low in calories, carbohydrates, and sodium but ample in protein and potassium content is encouraged for a client with Cushing's syndrome. Such a diet promotes weight loss, reduction of edema and hypertension, controls hypokalemia, and rebuilding of wasted tissue. The client with Cushing's syndrome who also is experiencing diabetes mellitus or gastric ulcers needs further modifications in diet.

Test-Taking Strategy: To measure whether teaching was understood or not, you must first recall the effect that Cushing's syndrome has on the body, particularly in relation to metabolic processes. Option 1 is the only option that says no change is necessary. Using the process of elimination, this option could probably be eliminated. Protein is usually limited in renal disorders. Excess sodium is not healthy in general, so, by using the process of elimination, you should be directed to option 4.

Level of Cognitive Ability: Analysis
Phase of Nursing Process: Evaluation
Client Needs: Health Promotion and Maintenance
Content Area: Adult Health/Endocrine

Reference
Luckmann, J. (1997). *Saunders manual of nursing care*. Philadelphia: W. B. Saunders p. 1405.

42. 3

Rationale: Insulin preparations are stable at room temperature for up to 1 month without significant loss of activity. Insulin should not be frozen.

Test-Taking Strategy: Eliminate options 1 and 4 because they are similar. From the remaining options, option 3 is most directly related to client safety. Therefore select this option. Review insulin storage principles now, if you had difficulty with this question!

Level of Cognitive Ability: Application
Phase of Nursing Process: Implementation
Client Needs: Physiological Integrity
Content Area: Adult Health/Endocrine

Reference
Lehne, R. (1998). *Pharmacology for nursing care* (3rd ed.). Philadelphia: W. B. Saunders. p. 583.

43. **1**

Rationale: Hypoglycemia reaction may occur in response to increased exercise. Clients should avoid exercise during the peak time of insulin. NPH insulin peaks at 6 to 12 hours, therefore afternoon exercise will occur during the peak of the medication. The client should be educated to adjust the exercise schedule.

Test-Taking Strategy: Knowledge that the client should not exercise within 1 hour of an insulin injection or at the peak time of insulin action is required to answer this question. Remember these important points and you will easily be able to answer questions similar to this one!

Level of Cognitive Ability: Analysis
Phase of Nursing Process: Evaluation
Client Needs: Physiological Integrity
Content Area: Adult Health/Endocrine

Reference

Ignatavicius, D., Workman, M., & Mishler, M. (1995). *Medical-surgical nursing: A nursing process approach* (2nd ed.). Philadelphia: W. B. Saunders. p. 1893.

44. **2**

Rationale: Hypercalcemia is the hallmark of hyperparathyroidism. Elevated serum calcium levels produce osmotic diuresis, thus option 2 is the correct answer. This diuresis leads to dehydration, therefore option 4 can be eliminated. Both options 1 and 3 are gastrointestinal symptoms but are not associated with the common GI symptoms typical of hyperparathyroidism (i.e., nausea, vomiting, anorexia, constipation).

Test-Taking Strategy: Knowledge of the symptoms associated with hypercalcemia, the hallmark of hyperparathyroidism, is required to answer this question. If you were unsure of these symptoms, note that options 1, 3, and 4 are all GI symptoms, whereas option 2 is the only renal symptom.

Level of Cognitive Ability: Application
Phase of Nursing Process: Assessment
Client Needs: Physiological Integrity
Content Area: Adult Health/Endocrine

Reference

Black, J., & Matassarin-Jacobs, E. (1997). *Medical-surgical nursing: Clinical management for continuity of care* (5th ed.). Philadelphia: W. B. Saunders. p. 2031.

45. **3**

Rationale: During the postoperative period, the nurse carefully observes the client for signs of hemorrhage, which causes swelling and compression of adjacent tissue. Laryngeal stridor is a harsh, high-pitched sound heard on inspiration and expiration, caused by compression of the trachea leading to respiratory distress. It is an acute emergency situation that requires immediate attention to avoid complete obstruction of the airway.

Test-Taking Strategy: Consider the anatomical location of the surgical procedure and use the ABCs to select the correct option. Options 1, 2, and 4 are usual postoperative problems that are not life-threatening. Option 3 addresses airway!

Level of Cognitive Ability: Analysis
Phase of Nursing Process: Assessment
Client Needs: Physiological Integrity
Content Area: Adult Health/Endocrine

Reference

Black, J., & Matassarin-Jacobs, E. (1997). *Medical-surgical nursing: Clinical management for continuity of care* (5th ed.). Philadelphia: W. B. Saunders. p. 2035.

46. **3**

Rationale: Oral calcium supplements need to be given with food in the stomach to enhance its absorption as well as decrease gastrointestinal irritation. All other options are inappropriate and unrelated to oral calcium therapy.

Test-Taking Strategy: Knowledge of the specifics about this medication is required to answer this question. Eliminate those choices that seem unusual. Checking for a pulse is usually done for cardiac medications. Avoidance of sunlight and refrigeration of tablets are required for some medications but are not as common an intervention as option 3. Review this medication now, if you had difficulty with this question!

Level of Cognitive Ability: Application
Phase of Nursing Process: Implementation
Client Needs: Health Promotion and Maintenance
Content Area: Adult Health/Endocrine

Reference

Hodgson, B., & Kizior, R. (1998). *Saunders nursing drug handbook 1998*. Philadelphia: W. B. Saunders. p. 139.

47. **1**

Rationale: Physical symptoms can interfere with an individual's ability to learn and can also indicate to the teacher that the learner lacks motivation to learn if the symptoms repeatedly recur when teaching is initiated.

Test-Taking Strategy: Options 2, 3, and 4 identify the client as actively seeking information. Option 1 suggests avoidance on the part of the client.

Level of Cognitive Ability: Analysis
Phase of Nursing Process: Assessment
Client Needs: Psychosocial Integrity
Content Area: Adult Health/Endocrine

Reference

Potter, P., & Perry, A. (1997). *Fundamentals of nursing: Concepts, process, and practice* (4th ed.). St. Louis: Mosby–Year Book. pp. 269–270.

48. **2**

Rationale: Lipodystrophy (hypertrophy of subcutaneous tissue at the injection site) occurs in some diabetic clients when injection sites are used repeatedly. Thus, clients are instructed to adhere to a rotating injection site plan to avoid tissue changes. Cleansing with alcohol, aspiration, and the angle of insulin administration do not produce tissue damage.

Test-Taking Strategy: Knowledge of the definition of lipodystrophy will easily direct you to the correct option. If you are unfamiliar with this complication, take time now to review this important component in diabetic teaching!

Level of Cognitive Ability: Application
Phase of Nursing Process: Assessment
Client Needs: Physiological Integrity
Content Area: Adult Health/Endocrine

Reference

Ignatavicius, D., Workman, M., & Mishler, M. (1995). *Medical-surgical nursing: A nursing process approach* (2nd ed.). Philadelphia: W. B. Saunders. p. 1882.

49. 4

Rationale: Decreased blood glucose levels produce adrenergic (autonomic) manifestations, which are classically manifested as nervousness, irritability, and tremors. Option 1 is more likely to occur with hyperglycemia. Options 2 and 3 are unrelated to the signs of hypoglycemia.

Test-Taking Strategy: Knowledge regarding the signs associated with a hypoglycemic reaction is required to answer the question. If you had difficulty with this question, take time now to review this important complication!

Level of Cognitive Ability: Analysis
Phase of Nursing Process: Assessment
Client Needs: Physiological Integrity
Content Area: Adult Health/Endocrine

Reference
Black, J., & Matassarin-Jacobs, E. (1997). *Medical-surgical nursing: Clinical management for continuity of care* (5th ed.). Philadelphia: W. B. Saunders. p. 1988.

50. 3

Rationale: Hypoglycemic reactions present adrenergic symptoms of tremor, shakiness, and nervousness that are similar to alcohol intoxication. The best strategy to deal with this client's psychosocial need is to decrease the episodes of hypoglycemia by first identifying and then eliminating those factors that precipitate this event. Frequent hypoglycemic reactions can have an impact on the client's self-esteem, as well as physiological integrity.

Test-Taking Strategy: This is a complex question because it involves a biophysical problem that is having an impact on the client's psychosocial functioning. Always remember that the nurse's role is to assist the client to adapt to the illness. Option 1 presumes that the problem is unavoidable, and thus the client is at fault. Option 2 is absolutely nontherapeutic because it presumes that the client may be drinking, and option 4 is avoidance of the psychosocial aspects of the client's problem.

Level of Cognitive Ability: Analysis
Phase of Nursing Process: Analysis
Client Needs: Psychosocial Integrity
Content Area: Adult Health/Endocrine

Reference
Black, J., & Matassarin-Jacobs, E. (1997). *Medical-surgical nursing: Clinical management for continuity of care* (5th ed.). Philadelphia: W. B. Saunders. pp. 1988, 1990.

51. 3

Rationale: Offer liquids containing both glucose and electrolytes. Small amounts of fluid may be tolerated even when vomiting is present. Advance diet as tolerated, including a minimum of 100 to 150 g of carbohydrates daily.

Test-Taking Strategy: Eliminate options 1 and 2 because of the words "only" and "all." The time frame in option 4 seems unreasonable; therefore, select option 3. Review care to the diabetic client during illness now, if you had difficulty with this question!

Level of Cognitive Ability: Application
Phase of Nursing Process: Implementation
Client Needs: Physiological Integrity
Content Area: Adult Health/Endocrine

Reference
Ignatavicius, D., Workman, M., & Mishler, M. (1995). *Medical-surgical nursing: A nursing process approach* (2nd ed.). Philadelphia: W. B. Saunders. p. 1888.

52. 1

Rationale: Manifestations of hypothyroid syndrome include cold intolerance, constipation, loss of initiative, thick and dry skin, a notably puffy appearance of the skin around the eyes, slowed intellectual function including retarded speech and apathy, and low metabolic rate. Synthroid is used to correct hypothyroid syndrome. This dosage would appear to be subtherapeutic.

Test-Taking Strategy: Note the key phrase "currently taking Synthroid." Knowledge that the signs presented in the question relate to the manifestations associated with hypothyroidism will easily direct you to option 1. The dosage needs to be increased.

Level of Cognitive Ability: Analysis
Phase of Nursing Process: Analysis
Client Needs: Physiological Integrity
Content Area: Adult Health/Endocrine

Reference
Hodgson, B., & Kizior, R. (1998). *Saunders nursing drug handbook 1998.* Philadelphia: W. B. Saunders. pp. 589–590.

53. 1

Rationale: Options 2, a beta-blocker, and 3, an MAO inhibitor, have their own intrinsic hypoglycemic activity. Option 4 decreases urinary excretion of sulfonylurea agents, causing increased levels of the oral agents that can lead to hypoglycemia. Prednisone may decrease the effect of oral hypoglycemics, insulin, diuretics, and potassium supplements.

Test-Taking Strategy: This question requires that you know the medication classifications of the options and correlate that with their potential hypoglycemic or hyperglycemic effect. Review these medications now, if you are unfamiliar with them!

Level of Cognitive Ability: Analysis
Phase of Nursing Process: Analysis
Client Needs: Physiological Integrity
Content Area: Adult Health/Endocrine

Reference
Hodgson, B., & Kizior, R. (1998). *Saunders nursing drug handbook 1998.* Philadelphia: W. B. Saunders. p. 856.

54. 4

Rationale: Vasopressin, an antidiuretic hormone, causes vasoconstriction with reduced blood flow in coronary, peripheral, cerebral, and pulmonary vessels. Options 1, 2, and 3 are therapeutic effects of the medication.

Test-Taking Strategy: Note the key word "not" in the stem of the question. Eliminate options 2 and 3 because they are similar. Knowledge regarding the therapeutic effects of this medication is required to answer this question. If you had difficulty with this question, take time now to review this important medication!

Level of Cognitive Ability: Analysis
Phase of Nursing Process: Analysis
Client Needs: Physiological Integrity
Content Area: Adult Health/Endocrine

Reference
Hodgson, B., & Kizior, R. (1998). *Saunders nursing drug handbook 1998.* Philadelphia: W. B. Saunders. p. 1064.

55. **2**

Rationale: Pheochromocytoma is a catecholamine-producing tumor and causes secretion of excessive amounts of epinephrine and norepinephrine. Hypertension is the principal manifestation, and the client has episodes of high blood pressure accompanied by pounding headaches. The excessive release of catecholamine also results in excessive conversion of glycogen into glucose in the liver. Consequently, hyperglycemia and glucosuria occur during attacks. Pheochromocytoma is curable. The primary treatment is surgical removal of one or both of the adrenal glands, depending on whether the tumor is unilateral or bilateral.

Test-Taking Strategy: In both options 1 and 4, a similarity exists in the sense of hypotension and hypoglycemia. There is only one correct answer. If a similarity exists in the answers, then neither one is likely to be the answer. The word "not" in 3 is an absolute term, and it is best to avoid selecting statements that include absolute terminology.

Level of Cognitive Ability: Analysis
Phase of Nursing Process: Planning
Client Needs: Physiological Integrity
Content Area: Adult Health/Endocrine

Reference
Black, J., & Matassarin-Jacobs, E. (1997). *Medical-surgical nursing: Clinical management for continuity of care* (5th ed.). Philadelphia: W. B. Saunders. pp. 2057–2058.

56. **4**

Rationale: Hypertension is the major symptom associated with pheochromocytoma. The blood pressure status would be assessed by taking the client's blood pressure. Glycosuria, weight loss, and diaphoresis are also clinical manifestations of pheochromocytoma, yet hypertension is the major symptom.

Test-Taking Strategy: Utilize the principles associated with prioritizing when answering this question. Remember your ABCs: Airway, Breathing, and Circulation. A method of assessing circulation is to take the blood pressure.

Level of Cognitive Ability: Application
Phase of Nursing Process: Assessment
Client Needs: Physiological Integrity
Content Area: Adult Health/Endocrine

Reference
Luckmann, J. (1997). *Saunders manual of nursing care.* Philadelphia: W. B. Saunders. p. 1411.

57. **3**

Rationale: Assays of catecholamines are performed on single-voided urine specimens, 2- to 4-hour specimens, and 24-hour urine specimens. The normal range of urinary catecholamines is up to 14 µg/dL of urine, with higher levels occurring in pheochromocytoma.

Test-Taking Strategy: Knowing that pheochromocytoma is a catecholamine-producing tumor, you would expect that the results of such a test would indicate higher than normal amounts of catecholamine. Additionally, the question addresses that the client is suspected of having pheochromocytoma. If you need to select an answer and you are not quite sure, select the response that has similarity to a thought in the question. In this case, suspected pheochromocytoma is similar to indicating pheochromocytoma found in option 3.

Level of Cognitive Ability: Analysis
Phase of Nursing Process: Analysis
Client Needs: Physiological Integrity
Content Area: Adult Health/Endocrine

Reference
Black, J., & Matassarin-Jacobs, E. (1997). *Medical-surgical nursing: Clinical management for continuity of care* (5th ed.). Philadelphia: W. B. Saunders. p. 2058.

58. **4**

Rationale: Since a 24-hour urine collection is a timed quantitative determination, it is essential that the client start the test with an empty bladder. Therefore, the client is instructed to void and discard the first urine, then note the time and start the test. The 24-hour urine specimen collection bottle must be kept on ice or refrigerated. In a VMA collection, the client is instructed to avoid tea, chocolate, vanilla, and all fruits for 2 days before urine collection begins. Also, clients are reminded not to take medications for 2 to 3 days before the test.

Test-Taking Strategy: The question asks you to select the response which indicates that the client needs further instruction. Be careful with these types of questions, and read them carefully or they can easily confuse you. Read each response, and eliminate those answers that are accurate statements made by the client. Look for the response that is an inaccurate statement, as this would reflect the need for further education. Knowledge regarding the procedure for 24-hour urine collections will assist you in answering this question correctly. Options 2 and 3 can be eliminated. Looking at the remaining options, remember that medications can affect the results of a test. If you need to make a choice, your best option to select would be an option such as 4.

Level of Cognitive Ability: Analysis
Phase of Nursing Process: Evaluation
Client Needs: Physiological Integrity
Content Area: Adult Health/Endocrine

Reference
Black, J., & Matassarin-Jacobs, E. (1997). *Medical-surgical nursing: Clinical management for continuity of care* (5th ed.). Philadelphia: W. B. Saunders. p. 2058.

59. **1**

Rationale: Hypertension is the hallmark of pheochromocytoma. Severe hypertension can precipitate a cerebrovascular accident or sudden blindness. Although all the responses are accurate nursing interventions for the client with pheochromocytoma, the priority nursing action is to monitor the vital signs, particularly the blood pressure.

Test-Taking Strategy: Utilize the principles associated with prioritizing when answering this question. Remember your ABCs: Airway, Breathing, and Circulation. Monitoring vital signs is the nursing action that would assess airway, breathing, and circulation. Also, you can use the strategy of selecting the response that is different. Options 2, 3, and 4 all refer to assessment of the renal system, whereas option 1 does not. In this situation, it is more likely that the response that is different is the correct response.

Level of Cognitive Ability: Application
Phase of Nursing Process: Implementation
Client Needs: Physiological integrity
Content Area: Adult/Health Endocrine

Reference
Black, J., & Matassarin-Jacobs, E. (1997). *Medical-surgical nursing: Clinical management for continuity of care* (5th ed.). Philadelphia: W. B. Saunders. p. 2058.

60. 2

Rationale: The most likely medication to be ordered in hypertensive crisis is phentolamine (Regitine). This medication is a short-acting alpha-adrenergic blocker and would be given by IV bolus or drip for a hypertensive crisis. Phenoxybenzamine hydrochloride (Dibenzyline) is an oral medication that produces long-acting alpha-adrenergic blockade. It is used in the management of pheochromocytoma and is most suitable for preoperative management of hypertension and prevention of hypertensive crisis. Prazosin hydrochloride (Minipress), an alpha-blocker, is used less frequently for the preoperative pheochromocytoma client because of its shorter duration of action. The physician never uses beta-receptor blocking agents in clients with suspected or confirmed pheochromocytoma until after alpha-adrenergic blockade has been initiated, because these medications may cause the blood pressure to rise. After alpha-adrenergic blockade, low doses of propranolol (Inderal) may be used to treat tachycardia and dysrhythmias.

Test-Taking Strategy: Knowledge of the actions and uses of these medications is required to assist you in answering this question. If you knew that phentolamine mesylate (Regitine) is a short-acting medication, then you would want to select this option. The question asks about hypertensive crisis, and such a situation requires immediate intervention. If you are unfamiliar with the medications addressed in this question, it would be important to review them.

Level of Cognitive Ability: Application
Phase of Nursing Process: Implementation
Client Needs: Physiological Integrity
Content Area: Adult/Health Endocrine

Reference
Black, J., & Matassarin-Jacobs, E. (1997). *Medical-surgical nursing: Clinical management for continuity of care* (5th ed.). Philadelphia: W. B. Saunders. p. 2058.

61. 1

Rationale: The client with pheochromocytoma needs to be provided with a diet high in vitamins, minerals, and calories. Of particular importance is that food or beverages that contain caffeine, such as coffee, tea, or colas, are prohibited. Cocoa, tea, and coffee are caffeine-containing products.

Test-Taking Strategy: Be careful with the selection of your answer when the answer contains the word "and." Remember that the entire option needs to be correct. Therefore, carefully read the content before and after the "and." Options 2, 3, and 4 are similar in that they all mention a drink that contains caffeine. Use the strategy of selection of the option that is different: option 1 is the different option that does not identify a caffeine-containing drink. Additionally, clients with pheochromocytoma are prohibited from eating or drinking any caffeine-containing products.

Level of Cognitive Ability: Application
Phase of Nursing Process: Implementation
Client Needs: Physiological Integrity
Content Area: Adult Health/Endocrine

Reference
Luckmann, J. (1997). *Saunders manual of nursing care* Philadelphia: W. B. Saunders. p. 1411.

62. 2

Rationale: The complications associated with pheochromocytoma include hypertensive retinopathy and nephropathy, myocarditis, CHF, increased platelet aggregation, and CVA. Death can occur from shock, CVA, renal failure, dysrhythmias, and dissecting aortic aneurysm. Rales heard on auscultation are indicative of CHF. A urinary output of 50 mL per hour is an appropriate output, and the nurse would become concerned if the output were below 30 mL per hour. A BUN of 20 mg/dL is a normal finding. Normal BUN is 11 to 23 mg/dL. A coagulation time of 5 minutes is normal. Normal coagulation time is 5 to 15 minutes.

Test-Taking Strategy: Utilize the principles associated with prioritizing when answering this question. Remember your ABCs: Airway, Breathing, and Circulation. Rales heard on auscultation in the lungs is associated with airway. Additionally, if you knew the normal hourly expectations associated with urinary output and the normal laboratory values for coagulation time and BUN, by the process of elimination you will determine that option 2 is the correct answer.

Level of Cognitive Ability: Analysis
Phase of Nursing Process: Assessment
Client Needs: Physiological Integrity
Content Area: Adult Health/Endocrine

Reference
Luckmann, J. (1997). *Saunders manual of nursing care* Philadelphia: W. B. Saunders. p. 1412.

63. 1

Rationale: Paraphrasing is restating the client's messages in the nurse's own words. Option 1 addresses the therapeutic communication technique of paraphrasing. The client is reaching out for understanding. In the nurse's response in option 2, the nurse is offering a false reassurance, and this type of response will block communication. Option 3 also represents a communication block in that it reflects a lack of the client's right to an opinion. In option 4, the nurse is expressing approval, which can be harmful to a nurse-client relationship.

Test-Taking Strategy: Remember that therapeutic communication techniques are the answers to your questions regarding responses to a client. Therapeutic communication techniques enhance communication. Always select the answers that will enhance communication. Avoid selecting responses that will block communication. Always address the client's concerns and feelings.

Level of Cognitive Ability: Application
Phase of Nursing Process: Implementation
Client Needs: Psychosocial Integrity
Content Area: Adult Health/Endocrine

Reference
Leahy, J., & Kizilay, P. (1998). *Foundations of nursing practice: A nursing process approach*. Philadelphia: W. B. Saunders. pp. 229–231.

64. **2**

Rationale: Aspirin and other over-the-counter medications should not be used unless the client consults with the physician. Abrupt discontinuation of corticosteroids can result in withdrawal syndrome, and the client needs to be instructed not to stop the medication. A slight weight gain with improved appetite is expected, but after the dosage is stabilized, a sudden slow but steady increase in weight of 5 pounds or more weekly should be reported to the physician. Caffeine-containing foods and fluids need to be avoided as they may contribute to steroid-ulcer development.

Test-Taking Strategy: Knowledge of the use of steroids is required to assist you in answering this question. However, a very important point to remember is that clients should not take other medications, especially over-the-counter medications, without first consulting their physicians.

Level of Cognitive Ability: Analysis
Phase of Nursing Process: Evaluation
Client Needs: Health Promotion and Maintenance
Content Area: Adult Health/Endocrine

Reference

Black, J., & Matassarin-Jacobs, E. (1997). *Medical-surgical nursing: Clinical management for continuity of care* (5th ed.). Philadelphia: W. B. Saunders. p. 2048.

65. **3**

Rationale: Clinical manifestations associated with thyroid storm include a fever as high as 106°, severe tachycardia, profuse diarrhea, extreme vasodilation, hypotension, atrial fibrillation, hyperreflexia, abdominal pain, diarrhea, and dehydration rapidly progressing to coma and cardiovascular collapse.

Test-Taking Strategy: Knowledge regarding the manifestations associated with thyroid storm is required to answer the question. This condition is a rare but potentially fatal hypermetabolic state. If you are unfamiliar with this disorder, take time now to review!

Level of Cognitive Ability: Analysis
Phase of Nursing Process: Assessment
Client Needs: Physiological Integrity
Content Area: Adult Health/Endocrine

Reference

Monahan, F., & Neighbors, M. (1998). *Medical-surgical nursing: Foundations for clinical practice* (2nd ed.). Philadelphia: W. B. Saunders. p. 1308.

66. **2**

Rationale: A high-sodium, high-complex carbohydrate, and high-protein diet will be prescribed for the client with Addison's disease. To prevent excess fluid and sodium loss, the client is instructed to maintain adequate salt intake of up to 8 g of sodium daily and to increase salt intake during hot weather, before strenuous exercise, and in response to fever, vomiting, or diarrhea.

Test-Taking Strategy: Knowledge regarding the pathophysiology associated with Addison's disease will assist in answering this question. If you were unfamiliar with this disorder, it is important to review now. You are likely to find questions related to this disorder on NCLEX-RN!

Level of Cognitive Ability: Analysis
Phase of Nursing Process: Analysis
Client Needs: Health Promotion and Maintenance
Content Area: Adult Health/Endocrine

Reference

Monahan, F., & Neighbors, M. (1998). *Medical-surgical nursing: Foundations for clinical practice* (2nd ed.). Philadelphia: W. B. Saunders. p. 1284.

67. **1**

Rationale: Cushing's syndrome is characterized by an oversecretion of glucocorticoid hormones. Addison's disease is characterized by the failure of the adrenal cortex to produce and secrete adrenocortical hormones. Options 3 and 4 are inaccurate regarding Cushing's syndrome.

Test-Taking Strategy: Option 3 can be easily eliminated, remembering that in C"u"shing's (up) syndrome, there is an oversecretion, and in A"dd"ison's (down) disease, there is an undersecretion. This may assist in answering questions similar to this one.

Level of Cognitive Ability: Analysis
Phase of Nursing Process: Evaluation
Client Needs: Physiological Integrity
Content Area: Adult Health/Endocrine

Reference

Monahan, F., & Neighbors, M. (1998). *Medical-surgical nursing: Foundations for clinical practice* (2nd ed.). Philadelphia: W. B. Saunders. p. 1285.

BIBLIOGRAPHY

Black, J., & Matassarin-Jacobs, E. (1997). *Medical-surgical nursing: Clinical management for continuity of care* (5th ed.). Philadelphia: W. B. Saunders.

Burrell, L., Gerlach, M., & Pless, B. (1997). *Adult nursing: Acute and community care* (2nd ed.). Stamford, CT: Appleton & Lange.

Chernecky, C., & Berger, B. (1997). *Laboratory tests and diagnostic procedures* (2nd ed.). Philadelphia: W. B. Saunders.

Hodgson, B., & Kizior, R. (1998). *Saunders nursing drug handbook 1998*. Philadelphia: W. B. Saunders.

Ignatavicius, D., Workman, M., & Mishler, M. (1995). *Medical-surgical nursing: A nursing process approach* (2nd ed.). Philadelphia: W. B. Saunders.

Lehne, R. (1998). *Pharmacology for nursing care* (3rd ed.). Philadelphia: W. B. Saunders.

Leahy, J., & Kizilay, P. (1998). *Foundations of nursing practice: A nursing process approach*. Philadelphia: W. B. Saunders.

Lewis, S., Collier, I., & Heitkemper, M. (1996). *Medical-surgical nursing: Assessment and management of clinical problems* (4th ed.). St. Louis: Mosby–Year Book.

Luckmann, J. (1997). *Saunders manual of nursing care*. Philadelphia: W. B. Saunders.

Lutz, C., & Przytulski, K. (1997). *Nutrition and diet therapy* (2nd ed.). Philadelphia: F. A. Davis.

Monahan, F., & Neighbors, M. (1998). *Medical-surgical nursing: Foundations for clinical practice* (2nd ed.). Philadelphia: W. B. Saunders.

O'Toole, M. (ed.) (1997). *Miller-Keane encyclopedia & dictionary of medicine, nursing, & allied health* (6th ed.). Philadelphia: W. B. Saunders.

Potter, P., & Perry, A. (1997). *Fundamentals of nursing: Concepts, process, and practice* (4th ed). St Louis: Mosby–Year Book.

Smeltzer, S., & Bare, B. (1996). *Brunner and Suddarth's textbook of medical-surgical nursing* (8th ed.). Philadelphia: Lippincott-Raven.

CHAPTER 52

Endocrine Medications

· ·

I. Pituitary Medications

A. Description
  1. Anterior pituitary gland: Secretes growth hormone (GH), thyroid-stimulating hormone (TSH), adrenocorticotropic hormone (ACTH), and gonadotropins (follicle-stimulating hormone, or FSH, and luteinizing hormone, or LH)
  2. Posterior pituitary gland: Secretes antidiuretic hormones (ADH, vasopressin) and oxytocin
B. Growth hormones (Box 52–1)
  1. Description
    a. Secreted by the anterior pituitary gland
    b. Interact with specific receptors to produce enzymatic actions that stimulate linear growth
    c. Used for pituitary dwarfism
  2. Side effects
    a. Pain at injection site
    b. Glucose intolerance
    c. **Hypothyroidism**
    d. Giantism in children with excessive doses
  3. Implementation
    a. Assess child's physical growth and compare growth with standards
    b. Recommend annual bone age determinations for children receiving growth hormones
    c. Monitor blood and urine glucose levels
    d. Teach client and family about the importance of follow-up regarding blood and urine glucose testing

◆ II. Antidiuretic Hormones (Box 52–2)

A. Description
  1. Enhance reabsorption of water in the kidneys, promoting an antidiuretic effect and regulating fluid balance
  2. Used in **diabetes insipidus**
B. Side effects
  1. Flushing
  2. Headache
  3. Nausea and abdominal cramps
  4. Water intoxication
  5. Hypertension with water intoxication
  6. Nasal congestion with nasal administration
C. Implementation
  1. Monitor weight
  2. Monitor intake and output (I&O) and urine osmolality
  3. Monitor electrolytes
  4. Restrict intake as necessary to prevent water intoxication
  5. Monitor for signs of water intoxication, such as drowsiness, listlessness, and headache
  6. Instruct client how to use the intranasal drug form
  7. Instruct client to report signs of water intoxication or symptoms of headache or shortness of breath

III. Thyroid Hormones (Box 52–3)

A. Description
  1. Control the metabolic rate of tissues and accelerate heat production and oxygen consumption
  2. To replace hormonal deficit in the treatment of **hypothyroidism, myxedema,** or cretinism
  3. Enhance the action of oral anticoagulants, sympathomimetics, and antidepressants and

---

BOX 52–1. Growth Hormones

Somatrem (Protropin)
Somatropin (Humatrope)

BOX 52–2. Antidiuretic Hormones

Desmopressin acetate (DDAVP)
Desmopressin (Stimate)
Lypressin (Diapid)
Vasopressin (Pitressin)

BOX 52–3. Thyroid Hormones

Levothyroxine sodium (Synthroid)
Liothyronine sodium (Cytomel)
Liotrix (Euthroid, Thyrolar)
Thyroglobulin (Proloid)
Thyroid (Armour Thyroid, Thyrar)

---

decrease the action of insulin, oral hypoglycemics, and digitalis preparations
   4. Phenytoin (Dilantin) and aspirin can enhance the action of thyroid hormone
B. Side effects
   1. Nausea and vomiting
   2. Cramps and diarrhea
   3. Weight loss
   4. Nervousness and tremors
   5. Headache
   6. Hypertension
   7. Tachycardia and dysrhythmias
   8. Sweating and heat intolerance
   9. Insomnia
C. Implementation
   1. Assess the client for history of medications currently being taken
   2. Monitor vital signs
   3. Monitor weight
   4. Monitor triiodothyronine (T_3), thyroxine (T_4), and thyroid stimulating hormone (TSH) levels
   5. Instruct client to take the medication at the same time each day, preferably in the morning without food
   6. Instruct client to monitor pulse rate
   7. Advise the client to report symptoms of **hyperthyroidism,** such as tachycardia, chest pain, palpitations, and excessive sweating
   8. Instruct client to avoid foods that can inhibit thyroid secretion, such as strawberries, peaches, pears, cabbage, turnips, spinach, kale, Brussels sprouts, cauliflower, radishes, and peas
   9. Advise the client to avoid over-the-counter medications
   10. Instruct client to wear a Medic-Alert bracelet

IV. Antithyroid Medications (Box 52–4)

A. Description
   1. Inhibit the synthesis of thyroid hormone
   2. Used for **hyperthyroidism** or **Graves' disease**
B. Side effects
   1. Nausea and vomiting

BOX 52–4. Antithyroid Medications

Iodine solution (Lugol solution, potassium iodide solution)
Methimazole (Tapazole)
Propylthiouracil (PTU)

---

   2. Diarrhea
   3. Hypersensitivity
   4. Rash
   5. Agranulocytosis
   6. **Hypothyroidism**
   7. Iodism characterized by vomiting, abdominal pain, brassy taste, rash, and sore salivary glands
C. Implementation
   1. Monitor vital signs
   2. Monitor T_3, T_4, and TSH levels
   3. Monitor weight
   4. Instruct client to take medication with meals to avoid gastrointestinal (GI) upset
   5. Instruct client how to take the pulse
   6. Inform client of side effects and when to notify the physician
   7. Advise client to contact physician if a fever or sore throat develops
   8. Instruct client in the signs of **hypothyroidism**
   9. Instruct client regarding the importance of drug compliance and that abruptly stopping the medication could cause thyroid crisis
   10. Assess for signs and symptoms of thyroid crisis **(thyroid storm),** which include fever, flushed skin, confusion and behavioral changes, tachycardia, dysrhythmias, and heart failure
   11. Advise client to consult physician before eating iodized salt and iodine-rich foods
   12. Instruct client to avoid aspirin and medications containing iodine

V. Parathyroid Medications (Table 52–1)

A. Description
   1. Parathyroid hormone regulates serum calcium levels
   2. Low serum levels of calcium stimulate parathyroid hormone release
   3. Hyperparathyroidism results in high serum calcium levels and bone demineralization, and medication is used to lower serum calcium levels
   4. Hypoparathyroidism results in low serum calcium levels, which increase neuromuscular

---

Table 52–1. Parathyroid Medications

For Hypoparathyroidism and Hypocalcemia

Calcifediol (Calderol)
Calcitriol (Rocaltrol)
Ergocalciferol (Drisdol)
Calcium carbonate (Os-Cal)
Calcium gluconate

For Hyperparathyroidism and Hypercalcemia

Calcitonin (human) (Cibacalcin)
Calcitonin (salmon) (Calcimar)
Etidronate (Didronel)

excitability, and the treatment includes calcium and vitamin D supplements
5. Parathyroid and antihypercalcemic agents may cause hypermagnesemia
6. Calcium salts administered with digitalis increases the risk of digitalis toxicity
7. Oral calcium salts reduce the absorption of tetracycline

B. Implementation
1. Monitor electrolyte and calcium levels
2. Assess for signs and symptoms of hypocalcemia and hypercalcemia
3. Assess for symptoms of tetany in hypocalcemia, such as twitching of the mouth, tingling and numbness of the fingers, carpopedal spasm, spasmodic contractions, and laryngeal spasm
4. Monitor for signs and symptoms of hypercalcemia, such as bone pain, anorexia, nausea, vomiting, thirst, constipation, lethargy, bradycardia, polyuria
5. Instruct client in the signs and symptoms in hypercalcemia and hypocalcemia
6. Instruct client to check over-the-counter medication labels for the possibility of calcium content
7. Instruct client receiving oral calcium to maintain an adequate intake of vitamin D, as vitamin D enhances absorption of calcium

VI. Adrenocorticotropic Hormones (Box 52–5)

A. Description
1. Stimulate the adrenal cortex to secrete cortisol
2. Produce an anti-inflammatory effect
3. Used to diagnose adrenocortical disorders
4. Used to treat acute multiple sclerosis

B. Side effects
1. Nausea and vomiting
2. Increased appetite
3. Mood swings
4. Petechiae
5. Water and sodium retention
6. Hypokalemia
7. Hypocalcemia

C. Implementation
1. Monitor vital signs
2. Monitor I&O
3. Monitor for signs of infection
4. Monitor weight
5. Monitor for edema
6. Monitor electrolyte and calcium levels
7. Avoid administering to client with adrenocortical hyperfunction

---

BOX 52–5. Adrenocorticotropic Hormones

Corticotropin (Acthar)
Corticotropin repository (Acthar gel)
Cosyntropin (Cortrosyn)

BOX 52–6. Use of Corticosteroids

Trauma
Surgery
Infections
Emotional upsets and anxiety
Autoimmune disorders
Inflammatory diseases
Allergic reactions
By organ transplant recipients to prevent rejection

---

8. Instruct client to decrease salt intake
9. Instruct client to report muscle weakness, edema, petechiae, ecchymosis, decrease in growth, decreased wound healing, and menstrual irregularities
10. Monitor for adverse effects when the medication is discontinued
11. Dose should be tapered and not stopped abruptly because adrenal hypofunction may result

VII. Corticosteroids

A. Description
1. Corticosteroids are normally secreted by the adrenal cortex
2. Produce metabolic effects
3. Suppress inflammation
4. Alter the normal immune response
5. Promote sodium and water retention and potassium excretion
6. Produce anti-inflammatory, antiallergic, and antistress effects (Box 52–6)

B. Contraindications and cautions
1. Contraindicated in hypersensitivity, psychosis, and fungal infections
2. Use with caution in **diabetes mellitus**
3. Dexamethasone decreases the effects of oral anticoagulants and oral antidiabetic agents
4. Corticosteroids increase the potency of drugs taken concurrently, such as aspirin and nonsteroidal anti-inflammatory drugs (NSAIDs), thus increasing the risk of GI bleeding and ulceration
5. Use of potassium-wasting diuretics increases potassium loss, resulting in hypokalemia
6. Barbiturates, phenytoin (Dilantin), and rifampin (Rifadin) decrease the effect of prednisone
7. The action of dexamethasone is decreased by the use of phenytoin (Dilantin), theophylline, rifampin (Rifadin), barbiturates, and antacids
8. NSAIDs, aspirin, and estrogen increase the effect of dexamethasone
9. Glucocorticoids should be used with extreme caution in clients with infections because they mask the signs and symptoms of an infection

---

BOX 52–7. Glucocorticoids

Betamethasone (Celestone)
Cortisone acetate (Cortone Acetate)
Dexamethasone (Decadron)
Hydrocortisone (Cortef, Hydrocortone)
Methylprednisolone (Depo-Medrol, Medrol, Solu-Medrol)
Prednisolone (Delta-Cortef, Prelone)
Prednisone
Triamcinolone (Aristocort, Kenalog, Kenacort)

C. Glucocorticoids (Box 52–7)
   1. Description: Used as a replacement for adrenocortical insufficiency
   2. Side effects
      a. **Hyperglycemia**
      b. Edema
      c. Sodium and water retention
      d. Hypokalemia
      e. Cause muscle wasting, osteoporosis, growth retardation in children, peptic ulcer, increased serum glucose levels, hypertension, convulsions, mood swings, cataracts, glaucoma, fragile skin, hirsutism, altered fat distribution
      f. Mask the signs and symptoms of infection
   3. Implementation
      a. Monitor vital signs
      b. Monitor serum electrolytes and blood sugar
      c. Monitor for hypokalemia and **hyperglycemia**
      d. Monitor weight
      e. Monitor for hypertension
      f. Monitor for edema
      g. Monitor urine output
      h. Assess medical history for glaucoma, cataracts, peptic ulcer, mental health disorders, or diabetes
      i. Instruct client that topical medication should be applied in a thin layer and to report any rashes, infection, or purpura
      j. Monitor the older client for signs and symptoms of increased osteoporosis
      k. Assess for changes in muscle strength
      l. Prepare a schedule for the client on short-term, tapered doses
      m. Instruct client to take at mealtime or with food
      n. Advise client to eat foods high in potassium
      o. Instruct the client to avoid individuals with respiratory infections
      p. Advise the client to inform all health care providers of taking the medication
      q. Instruct client to report signs and symptoms of a drug overdose or **Cushing's syndrome,** including a moon face, puffy eyelids, edema in the feet, increased bruising, dizziness, bleeding and menstrual irregularities

   r. Note that the client may need additional doses during periods of stress, such as surgery
   s. Instruct client not to stop medication abruptly, as abrupt withdrawal can result in severe adrenal insufficiency
   t. Advise client to consult with physician before receiving vaccinations
   u. Advice client to wear Medic-Alert bracelet
D. Mineralocorticoid (Box 52–8)
   1. Description
      a. Mineralocorticoid deficiency usually occurs with a glucocorticoid deficiency, frequently called corticosteroid deficiency
      b. Enhances reabsorption of sodium and chloride and promotes excretion of potassium and hydrogen from the renal tubules, thereby helping maintain fluid and electrolyte balance
      c. Used for replacement therapy in primary and secondary adrenal insufficiency in **Addison's disease**
   2. Side effects
      a. Sodium and water retention
      b. Hypokalemia
      c. Hypocalcemia
      d. Increased susceptibility to infection
      e. Delayed wound healing
      f. GI distress
      g. Diarrhea or constipation
      h. Increased appetite
      i. Weight gain
      j. Insomnia
      k. Mood swings
      l. Abdominal distention
   3. Implementation
      a. Monitor vital signs
      b. Monitor weight
      c. Monitor electrolytes and calcium and glucose level
      d. Monitor for signs of electrolyte imbalances
      e. Instruct client to take medication with food or milk
      f. Instruct client to consume a high potassium diet
      g. Instruct client not to stop the medication abruptly
      h. Instruct client to notify physician if signs of infection, muscle aches, sudden weight gain, or headaches occur
      i. Instruct client to avoid exposure to disease or trauma
      j. Instruct client not to take aspirin or any other medication without consulting the physician

---

BOX 52–8. Mineralocorticoid

Fludrocortisone acetate (Florinef Acetate)

k. Instruct client to wear a Medic-Alert bracelet

VIII. Androgens (Box 52–9)

A. Description
1. The androgens are steroids that stimulate the action of endogenous hormones
2. Used either to replace deficient hormones or to treat hormone-sensitive disorders
3. Used as replacement therapy for clients who have reduced endogenous androgen production
4. Prescribed as a palliative treatment for androgen-sensitive breast cancer or fibrocystic breast disease, and to treat endometriosis or advanced prostatic cancer
5. Can cause bleeding if the client is taking oral anticoagulants
6. Cause decreased serum glucose concentration, thereby reducing insulin requirements in the diabetic client

B. Side effects
1. Masculine secondary sexual characteristics
2. Body hair growth
3. Lowered voice
4. Muscle growth
5. Bladder irritation and urinary tract infections
6. Breast tenderness and impotence in men
7. Gynecomastia
8. Priapism
9. Menstrual irregularities
10. Edema
11. Nausea, vomiting, and diarrhea
12. Acne
13. Changes in libido
14. Hepatotoxicity
15. Sodium and water retention
16. Weight gain
17. Mood swings

C. Implementation
1. Monitor vital signs
2. Monitor for edema, weight gain, and skin changes
3. Assess heart and lung sounds
4. Assess mental status and neurological function

BOX 52–9. Androgens

Fluoxymesterone (Halotestin)
Methyltestosterone (Android, Oreton Methyl, Testred, Virilon)
Testosterone (Andronaq, Histerone)
Testosterone cypionate (Depotest, Depo-Testosterone)
Testosterone enanthate (Delatest)
Testosterone propionate (Testex)
Flutamide (Eulexin)
Leuprolide acetate (Lupron)

BOX 52–10. Estrogens

Diethylstilbestrol (DES, Stilphostrol)
Ethinyl estradiol (Estinyl)
Chlorotrianisene (Tace)
Conjugated estrogens (Premarin)

---

5. Assess for signs of depression
6. Assess for signs of liver dysfunction, including right upper quadrant abdominal pain, malaise, fever, jaundice, pruritus
7. Assess for the development of secondary sexual characteristics
8. Instruct client to take with meals or a snack
9. Instruct client to notify physician if priapism develops
10. Instruct client to notify physician if fluid retention occurs
11. Instruct women to use a nonhormonal contraceptive while on therapy

IX. Estrogens and Progestins

A. Description
1. Used to stimulate the endogenous hormones to restore hormonal balance and to treat hormone-sensitive tumors
2. Lactation suppressants decrease the serum prolactin level, thereby relieving postpartal breast engorgement
3. Fertility medications stimulate ovarian function by increasing levels of pituitary gonadotropins
4. Oxytocic medications enhance uterine motility by directly stimulating uterine and smooth muscle contractions
5. Labor suppressants relax uterine muscles and decrease uterine contractions

B. Estrogens (Box 52–10)
1. Estrogen preparations suppress tumor growth
2. Estrogen therapy is a palliative treatment used in men to decrease the progression of prostatic cancer and in postmenopausal women to decrease the progression of breast cancer

C. Progestins: Used for breast cancer, endometrial cancer, and renal cancer (Box 52–11)

D. Contraindications and cautions
1. Contraindicated in embolism, thrombophlebitis, undiagnosed breast

---

BOX 52–11. Progestins

Hydroxyprogesterone caproate (Duralutin)
Medroxyprogesterone acetate (Depo-Provera)
Megestrol acetate (Megace)

neoplasms, and history of cerebrovascular accident (CVA)
   2. Associated with an increased risk of endometrial cancer
E. Side effects
   1. Nausea, vomiting, and diarrhea
   2. Weight gain
   3. Edema and fluid retention
   4. Rash
   5. Headache
   6. Insomnia
   7. Hypertension
   8. Thromboembolitic disorders
F. Implementation
   1. Monitor vital signs
   2. Monitor for hypertension
   3. Assess for edema
   4. Monitor weight
   5. Advise client not to smoke
   6. Advise client to undergo routine breast and pelvic examinations

X. Gonadotropin-Releasing Hormones (Box 52–12)

A. Description
   1. Stimulate synthesis and release of LH and FSH from the anterior pituitary
   2. Used as palliative treatment for advanced prostatic cancer, to treat endometriosis, and to treat hypothalamic amenorrhea
B. Side effects
   1. Headache
   2. Nausea, vomiting, abdominal discomfort
   3. Lightheadedness
   4. Hot flashes
   5. Vaginitis
   6. Decreased libido
C. Implementation
   1. Instruct client to use contraceptive measures during therapy
   2. Monitor for side effects related to therapy
   3. Stress the importance of follow-up with the physician as scheduled

◆ XI. Diabetic Medications

◆ A. Insulin and oral hypoglycemic medications
   1. Description
      a. Insulin increases glucose transport into cells and promotes conversion of glucose

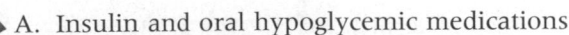

BOX 52–12. Gonadotropin-Releasing Hormones

Gonadorelin acetate (Lutrepulse)
Gonadorelin hydrochloride (Factrel)
Goserelin acetate (Zoladex)
Leuprolide acetate (Lupron)
Nafarelin acetate (Synarel)

---

to glycogen, decreasing serum glucose levels
      b. Oral hypoglycemic agents stimulate the pancreas to produce more insulin and increase the sensitivity of peripheral receptors to insulin, thereby decreasing serum glucose levels
      c. Used in **diabetes mellitus**
   2. Contraindications and concerns
      a. Insulin is contraindicated in clients with hypersensitivity
      b. Oral hypoglycemic agents are contraindicated in Type 1 insulin-dependent **diabetes mellitus** and in those individuals allergic to sulfonylureas
      c. Sulfonylureas can increase cardiac function and oxygen consumption and lead to cardiac dysrhythmias
      d. Use of antidiabetic medications with beta-adrenergic blocking agents mask signs and symptoms of **hypoglycemia**
      e. Use of antidiabetic medications with alcohol, steroids, salicylates, or MAO inhibitors may cause **hypoglycemia**
      f. Anticoagulants, chloramphenicol, and sulfonamides may cause **hypoglycemia**
      g. Use of insulin with corticosteroids, sympathomimetics, thiazide diuretics or thyroid preparations, oral contraceptives, and estrogen may cause **hyperglycemia**
   3. Implementation
      a. Monitor serum and urine glucose and ketone levels
      b. Monitor for signs of **hypoglycemia** and **hyperglycemia**
      c. Note that stress, fever, trauma, and infection may increase insulin requirements or necessitate switching from an oral hypoglycemic agent to insulin
      d. Note that IV glucose or glucagon may be necessary in severe hypoglycemic states
      e. Inform client that antidiabetic agents control but do not cure diabetes
      f. Emphasize the need for lifelong therapy
      g. Instruct client in the signs and symptoms of **hypoglycemia** and **hyperglycemia**
      h. Instruct client about diet and the use of the exchange system when planning meals
      i. Instruct client how to monitor serum and urine glucose levels
      j. Instruct client in the importance of regular exercise
      k. Instruct client about the importance of daily foot inspection
      l. Instruct client regarding alcohol intake
      m. Instruct client to notify physician if unable to eat
      n. Instruct client to carry sugar and to wear a Medic-Alert bracelet

Table 52–2. First- and Second-Generation Sulfonylureas and Nonsulfonylureas

Medication	Implementation
First-Generation Sulfonylureas	
Short-Acting	
Tolbutamide (Orinase)	Administer 30 minutes before meals to provide the best reduction in postprandial hyperglycemia
Intermediate-Acting	
Acetohexamide (Dymelor)	Stress eating habits and patterns as there is a high incidence of hypoglycemia in clients with renal impairment Monitor renal function
Tolazamide (Tolinase)	Administer with meals to avoid GI upset
Long-Acting	
Chlorpropamide (Diabinese)	Stress eating habits and patterns as the long half-life of the medication is associated with hypoglycemia
Second-Generation Sulfonylureas	
Glipizide (Glucotrol)	Administer 30 minutes before meals to provide the best reduction in postprandial hyperglycemia
Glyburide (DiaBeta, Micronase, Glynase)	Administer with meals to avoid GI upset Stress eating habits and patterns as the long half-life of the medication is associated with hypoglycemia
Glimepiride (Amaryl)	Administer with breakfast Contraindicated in clients with severe renal or hepatic impairment
Nonsulfonylureas	
Metformin (Glucophage)	Monitor renal function Should not be used in clients with renal impairment
Acarbose (Precose)	Intended for use in clients who do not achieve results with diet alone

 B. Oral hypoglycemic medications
1. Prescribed for clients with **diabetes mellitus** Type II
2. Sulfonylureas
   a. Classified as first- and second-generation sulfonylureas (Table 52–2)
   b. Stimulate the beta-cells to produce more insulin
3. Nonsulfonylureas
   a. Affect the hepatic and gastrointestinal production of glucose
   b. May be used in combination with a sulfonylurea
4. Implementation
   a. Assess the client's knowledge of diabetes and the use of oral antidiabetic agents
   b. Assess vital signs and blood sugar levels
   c. Assess the medications that the client is currently taking
   d. Instruct client to recognize symptoms of **hypoglycemia** and **hyperglycemia**
   e. Instruct client to avoid over-the-counter medications unless prescribed by the physician
   f. Instruct client not to ingest alcohol with sulfonylureas
   g. Inform the client that insulin may be needed during stress, surgery, or infection
   h. Instruct the client in the necessity of compliance with prescribed medication
   i. Advise client to obtain a Medic-Alert bracelet

C. Insulin (Table 52–3)
1. Primarily acts in the liver, muscle, and adipose tissue by attaching to receptors on cellular membranes and facilitating the passage of glucose, potassium, and magnesium
2. Prescribed for clients with **diabetes mellitus** Type I
3. Insulin injection sites
   a. Insulin injected into the abdomen may absorb more evenly and rapidly than other sites
   b. Insulin administered SC has a slower absorption rate than if administered IM
   c. Heat, massage, and exercise of the injected area can increase absorption rates
   d. Injection into scar tissue may delay absorption of insulin

Table 52–3. **Types of Insulin**

Type	Onset	Peak	Duration
Short-Acting Insulin			
Humulin (Regular)	0.5–1 hour	2–4 hours	5–7 hours
Lispro (Humalog)	5 minutes	0.5–1 hour	2–4 hours
Intermediate-Acting Insulin			
Humulin N (NPH)	1–2 hours	6–12 hours	18–24 hours
Humulin L (Lente)	1–2 hours	6–12 hours	18–24 hours
Long-Acting Insulin			
Humulin U Ultralente	4–6 hours	16–18 hours	20–36 hours
Premixed Insulin			
70% NPH and 30% Regular	0.5 hour	2–12 hours	18–24 hours

e. Insulin injection sites should be rotated to prevent hypertrophic lipodystrophy, a spongy swelling at or around the injection site, which can interfere with insulin absorption

f. Lipoatrophic lipodystrophy, a loss of fat at the injection site, is most often due to the use of animal insulins

g. Rotation within one anatomical site is preferred to rotation from one anatomical site to another

h. Administer the insulin in the same general area, rotating sites within that area, to predict the absorption rate

i. Injections should be 1.5 inches apart at a site area each day

4. Storing insulin: Vials of insulin not in use should be refrigerated

5. Administering insulin (Box 52–13)
a. To prevent dosage errors, be certain that there is a match of the insulin concentration with the calibration of units on the insulin syringe

b. Before use, roll, not shake, the insulin bottle to ensure that the insulin and ingredients are mixed well and to avoid bubbles, causing drawing an inaccurate dose

c. When mixing insulin, inject an amount of

BOX 52–13. Client Instructions for Insulin

- Instruct client and a family member in the administration of the insulin
- Instruct client to keep insulin in use at room temperature and refrigerate any extra supplies of insulin
- Instruct client to draw up Regular insulin prior to NPH insulin if a mix is prescribed
- Illness, infection, and stress increase the need for insulin, and insulin should not be withheld during illness, infection, or stress, because hyperglycemia and ketoacidosis can result
- Instruct the client how to recognize symptoms of hypoglycemia and hyperglycemia
- The peak action times of insulin is very important because of the possibility of hypoglycemic reactions occurring during that time
- Orange juice, sugar-sweetened beverages, or hard candy should be kept available and administered if a hypoglycemic reaction occurs
- Instruct client that hypoglycemic reactions are likely to occur during peak time and that orange juice, sugar-containing drinks, and hard candy may be used when a hypoglycemic reaction occurs
- Instruct family in administering glucagon by injection if the client has a hypoglycemic reaction and is unable to drink sugar-containing fluid
- Instruct client to avoid over-the-counter medications unless prescribed by the physician
- Instruct the client always to have a spare bottle of insulin available
- Avise the client to obtain a Medic-Alert bracelet indicating the type and daily insulin dosage

---

air equal to the insulin dose into the longer-acting insulin first

d. Always withdraw the shorter-acting insulin first

e. Be careful not to inject any shorter-acting insulin into the NPH bottle

f. Regular insulin may be mixed with any other type of insulin

g. Insulin zinc suspensions may be mixed only with each other and Regular insulin, not with other types of insulin

h. Administer a mixed dose of insulin within 5 minutes of preparation, for after this time the Regular insulin binds with the NPH insulin and its action is reduced

i. Administer insulin at a 45° to 90° angle and at a 45° to 60° angle in thin persons

j. REMEMBER: Regular insulin is the only type of insulin that can be administered by IV

D. Glucagon
1. A hormone secreted by the alpha-cells of the islets of Langerhans in the pancreas
2. Increases blood sugar by stimulating glycogenolysis in the liver
3. Can be administered SC, IM, or IV
4. Used to treat insulin-induced **hypoglycemia** when the client is semiconscious or unconscious and is unable to ingest liquids
5. The blood glucose level begins to increase within 5 to 20 minutes after administration

E. Diazoxide (Proglycem)
1. Increases blood sugar by inhibiting insulin release from the beta-cells and stimulating the release of epinephrine from the adrenal medulla
2. Used to treat chronic **hypoglycemia** caused by hyperinsulinism due to islet cell cancer or hyperplasia
3. It is not used for **hypoglycemic** reactions from insulin

PRACTICE QUESTIONS

1. Somatren (Protropin) is administered to a client with pituitary dwarfism. The expected therapeutic effect of this medication is to:
   1 Promote weight gain
   2 Stimulate linear growth
   3 Increase bone density
   4 Decrease the mobilization of fats

2. Somatropin (Humatrope), a growth hormone, is contraindicated in which of the following conditions?
   1 In a child with growth hormone deficiency
   2 In pituitary dwarfism
   3 In a 20-year-old with growth failure
   4 In a child with growth failure

3. Side effects associated with the administration of growth hormone replacement therapy include which of the following?

1 Hyperglycemia
2 Hyperthyroidism
3 Hypoglycemia
4 IIypocalciuria

4. Octreotide acetate (Sandostatin) is prescribed for the client with acromegaly. Side effects associated with the administration of this medication include which of the following?
   1 Constipation
   2 Polyuria
   3 Abdominal pain
   4 Hypotension

5. Desmopressin (DDAVP) is prescribed for the treatment of diabetes insipidus. The nurse administering the medication understands that the primary action of the medication is to:
   1 Decrease permeability in the kidneys to water
   2 Decrease water reabsorption
   3 Increase renal excretion of water
   4 Promote renal conservation of water

6. The nurse is monitoring a client receiving desmopressin (DDAVP). Which of the following indicates an adverse reaction to the medication?
   1 Increased urination
   2 Weight loss
   3 Drowsiness
   4 Insomnia

7. Vasopressin (Pitressin) is prescribed for the client with diabetes insipidus. The nurse is particularly cautious in monitoring the client with which of the following pre-existing conditions?
   1 Depression
   2 Endometriosis
   3 Coronary artery disease
   4 Pheochromocytoma

8. The client is diagnosed with hypothyroidism. Levothyroxine (Synthroid) is prescribed. The client is presently taking warfarin (Coumadin). The nurse anticipates which of the following medication prescriptions?
   1 An increased dosage of Coumadin
   2 A decreased dosage of Coumadin
   3 An increased dosage of Synthroid
   4 A decreased dosage of Synthroid

9. The nurse provides instructions to a client taking levothyroxine (Synthroid). The nurse evaluates effective client teaching if the client states to take the medication:
   1 With food
   2 On an empty stomach
   3 At bedtime
   4 At lunchtime

10. Thyroid replacement therapy is prescribed for the client diagnosed with hypothyroidism. The client asks the nurse when the medication will no longer be needed. The most appropriate nursing response is which of the following?
    1 "You will need to ask your physician."
    2 "Most clients require medication therapy for about 1 year."
    3 "It depends on the results of the laboratory values."
    4 "The medication will need to be continued for life."

11. The nurse provides medication instructions to a client taking levothyroxine (Synthroid). The nurse instructs the client to notify the physician if which of the following occurs?
    1 Cold intolerance
    2 Tremors
    3 Excessively dry skin
    4 Fatigue

12. An adult client with hypothyroidism is admitted to the hospital. On admission assessment, the nurse notes that the client is taking a maintenance dose of levothyroxine (Synthroid). The normal adult maintenance dose of this medication is:
    1 0.025 to 0.05 mg daily
    2 0.075 to 0.1 mg daily
    3 0.05 to 0.075 mg daily
    4 0.1 to 0.2 mg daily

13. The nurse performs an admission assessment on a client who visits the health care clinic for the first time. The client tells the nurse that propylthiouracil (PTU) is taken daily. The nurse suspects that the client has a history of:
    1 Cushing's syndrome
    2 Addison's disease
    3 Myxedema
    4 Graves' disease

14. A client is seen in the clinic for complaints of thirst, frequent urination, and headaches. Following diagnostic studies, diabetes insipidus is diagnosed. Lypressin (Diapid) is prescribed. The nurse instructs the client that the medication is prescribed to:
    1 Relieve the headaches
    2 Increase water reabsorption
    3 Decrease production of antidiuretic hormone
    4 Stimulate the production of aldosterone

15. The nurse is instructing a client regarding the administration of lypressin (Diapid). The nurse instructs the client that the medication will be taken by which of the following routes?
    1 Oral
    2 Subcutaneous
    3 Intranasal
    4 Intramuscular

16. Somatrem (Protropin) is prescribed for the client with pituitary dwarfism. The nurse explains that the expected outcome of the medication is:
    1 Growth that begins in 4 to 5 years
    2 An increase in height that will begin in adulthood
    3 An immediate increase in growth
    4 Growth spurts that occur every 2 years

17. The client is receiving somatropin (Humatrope). Which of the following laboratory studies is most significant to monitor during therapy with this medication?
    1 Amylase
    2 Lipase
    3 Blood urea nitrogen (BUN)
    4 Thyroid stimulating hormone (TSH)

18. A client arrives at the clinic complaining of fatigue, a lack of energy, constipation, and depression. Following diagnostic studies, hypothyroidism is diagnosed. Levothyroxine (Synthroid) is prescribed. The nurse instructs the client that the expected outcome of the medication is to:
    1 Increase energy levels
    2 Achieve normal thyroid hormone levels
    3 Increase blood glucose levels
    4 Alleviate depression

19. A client diagnosed with hypothyroidism is taking levothyroxine (Synthroid). The client returns to the clinic 1 week after beginning the medication and tells the nurse that the medication has not helped. The most appropriate nursing response to the client is based on which of the following?
    1 A higher dosage is required
    2 The medication may need to be changed
    3 Full therapeutic effect may take 1 to 3 weeks
    4 Full therapeutic effect may take up to 4 months

20. Propylthiouracil (PTU) is prescribed for the client with hyperthyroidism. The nurse provides instructions to the client regarding the medication. The nurse informs the client to notify the physician if which of the following signs occur?
    1 Drowsiness
    2 Sore throat
    3 Polyuria
    4 Dry mouth

21. The client is scheduled for subtotal thyroidectomy. Strong iodine solution (Lugol's solution) is prescribed. The therapeutic effect of this medication is to:
    1 Increase thyroid hormone production
    2 Suppress thyroid hormone production
    3 Replace thyroid hormone
    4 Prevent the oxidation of iodide

22. Strong iodine solution (Lugol's solution) is prescribed for the client with thyrotoxic crisis. The client calls the clinic nurse and complains of a brassy taste and burning sensations in the mouth. The most appropriate instruction to the client is which of the following?
    1 Continue with the medication
    2 Take half of the prescribed dose for the next 24 hours
    3 Stop the medication for the next 24 hours and then continue as prescribed
    4 Stop the medication and notify the physician

23. A client is admitted to the emergency room and an iodine overdose is suspected. Gastric lavage is initiated to remove the iodine from the stomach. In addition to treatment with gastric lavage, the nurse anticipates that which of the following will be administered?
    1 Calcium gluconate
    2 Vitamin K
    3 Mucomyst
    4 Sodium thiosulfate

24. Fludrocortisone (Florinef) is prescribed for the client with Addison's disease. The primary action of this medication is to:
    1 Enhance the reabsorption of sodium and chloride ions in the distal tubules of the kidney
    2 Promote the retention of potassium in the distal tubules of the kidney
    3 Promote the retention of hydrogen ions in the distal tubules of the kidney
    4 Promote the excretion of water in the distal tubules of the kidney

25. The nurse provides instructions to the client taking fludrocortisone (Florinef). The nurse instructs the client to notify the physician if which of the following occurs?
    1 Weight loss
    2 Nausea
    3 Swelling of the feet
    4 Fatigue

26. Calcium carbonate (Os-Cal) is prescribed for the client with hypocalcemia. The nurse will instruct the client to take the medication:
    1 With meals
    2 One hour after meals
    3 Before meals
    4 At bedtime

27. Calcifediol (Calderol) is prescribed for the client with hypoparathyroidism in the management of hypocalcemia. The client arrives at the clinic for a follow-up visit and complains of chronic constipation. Which of the following would not be a component of the teaching plan to alleviate the constipation?
    1 Increase daily fluid intake
    2 Add one half ounce of mineral oil to the daily diet
    3 Increase high-fiber foods
    4 Increase activity level as tolerated

28. Calcitriol (Rocaltrol) is prescribed for the client with hypocalcemia. The nurse provides dietary instructions to the client. Which of the following food items does the nurse instruct the client to avoid while taking this medication?
   1 Dark green leafy vegetables
   2 Milk
   3 Whole grain cereals
   4 Sardines

29. Etidronate (Didronel), an antihypercalcemic medication, is prescribed for the client. The nurse instructs the client to take the medication:
   1 Two hours before meals
   2 With meals
   3 With milk
   4 With an antacid

30. A daily dose of prednisone (Deltasone) is prescribed for the client. The nurse provides instructions to the client regarding administration of the medication. The nurse instructs the client that the best time to take this medication is:
   1 At bedtime
   2 At noon
   3 Early morning
   4 Anytime, at the same time, each day

31. Cortisone (Cortone) is prescribed for a client with adrenal insufficiency. The nurse provides instructions to the client regarding the medication. Which of the following statements, if made by the client, indicates a need for further instruction?
   1 "I will eat a good breakfast every day."
   2 "I will avoid people with colds."
   3 "I will limit my sodium intake."
   4 "I will stop the medication when I feel better."

32. Prednisone (Deltasone) is prescribed for a diabetic client who is taking NPH insulin daily. Which of the following prescriptions does the nurse anticipate during therapy with the prednisone?
   1 A decreased amount of daily NPH insulin
   2 An increased amount of daily NPH insulin
   3 An additional dose of prednisone daily
   4 Addition of an oral hypoglycemic medication daily

33. The hospitalized diabetic client received NPH insulin in the morning. When would the nurse expect the peak action of the insulin dose to occur?
   1 2 to 4 hours after administration
   2 6 to 12 hours after administration
   3 12 to 16 hours after administration
   4 18 to 24 hours after administration

34. The nurse is teaching the client how to mix Regular insulin and NPH insulin in the same syringe. Which of the following actions, if performed by the client, indicates the need for further teaching?
   1 Injects air into the NPH insulin vial first
   2 Injects the amount of air equal to the desired dose of insulin into the vial
   3 Withdraws the NPH insulin first
   4 Withdraws the Regular insulin first

35. The home care nurse visits a client recently diagnosed with diabetes mellitus. The client is taking NPH insulin daily. The client asks the nurse how to store the unopened vials of insulin. Which of the following instructions does the nurse provide to the client?
   1 Freeze the insulin
   2 Refrigerate the insulin
   3 Keep the insulin at room temperature
   4 Store the insulin in a dark, dry place

36. The home care nurse prefills syringes containing NPH and Regular insulin for the diabetic client who has difficulty with seeing and accurately preparing dosages. The client can administer the injection. Considering the stability of insulin, how many prefilled syringes can the nurse prepare for the client?
   1 Three-day supply
   2 Five-day supply
   3 Seven-day supply
   4 One-month supply

37. A diabetic client is self-administering NPH insulin from a vial that is kept at room temperature. The client asks the nurse about the length of time an unrefrigerated vial of insulin will maintain its potency. The most appropriate response is which of the following?
   1 Two weeks
   2 One month
   3 Two months
   4 Six months

38. Lispro insulin (Humalog), a rapid-acting form of insulin, is prescribed for the client. The client is instructed to administer the insulin prior to meals. The nurse instructs the client to administer the insulin:
   1 Immediately before eating
   2 30 minutes before eating
   3 45 minutes before eating
   4 60 minutes before eating

39. The emergency room nurse is caring for a client admitted with diabetic ketoacidosis. The physician prescribes IV insulin. The nurse plans to prepare which type of insulin for the client?
   1 NPH
   2 Regular
   3 Lente
   4 Ultralente

40. The nurse instructs a diabetic client regarding blood glucose monitoring and monitoring for signs of hypoglycemia. The nurse informs the client that hypoglycemia is a blood glucose level of:
   1 Less than 120 mg/dL
   2 Less than 100 mg/dL
   3 Less than 70 mg/dL
   4 Less than 50 mg/dL

41. The new diabetic client is instructed by the physician to obtain glucagon for emergency home use. The client asks the home care nurse about the purpose of the medication. The nurse instructs the client that the purpose of the medication is to treat:
   1 Hypoglycemia from insulin overdose
   2 Hyperglycemia from insufficient insulin
   3 Lipoatrophy from insulin injections
   4 Lipohypertrophy from inadequate insulin absorption

42. Tolbutamide (Orinase) is prescribed for the client with diabetes. The nurse instructs the client to avoid which of the following while taking this medication?
   1 Carbonated beverages
   2 Organ meats
   3 Alcohol
   4 Whole grain cereals

43. Metformin (Glucophage) is prescribed for the client with noninsulin-dependent diabetes mellitus. The most common side effect of the medication is:
   1 Hypoglycemia
   2 GI disturbances
   3 Weight gain
   4 Flushing and palpitations

44. The diabetic nurse specialist conducts a teaching session to a group of nursing students regarding sulfonylureas, oral hypoglycemic medications used for noninsulin-dependent diabetes mellitus. The primary action of these medications is described as which of the following?
   1 Decrease glucose production by the liver
   2 Inhibit carbohydrate digestion
   3 Promote insulin secretion by the pancreas
   4 Decrease insulin resistance

45. The diabetic client calls the clinic and tells the nurse that he/she has been nauseated during the night. The client asks the nurse if the morning insulin should be administered. Which of the following is the most appropriate nursing response?
   1 Omit the insulin
   2 Administer half the prescribed dose
   3 Administer the full dose as prescribed
   4 Wait until noon before making a decision

ANSWERS

1. 2

Rationale: Protropin is a growth stimulator used in the long-term treatment of growth failure due to endogenous growth hormone deficiency. It stimulates linear growth and increases the number and size of muscle cells and red cell mass. It affects carbohydrate metabolism by antagonizing the action of insulin, increases mobilization of fats, and increases cellular protein synthesis.

Test-Taking Strategy: Use the client diagnosis in the question to assist in the process of elimination in answering the question. Note the relationship between "dwarfism" in the question and "growth" in the correct option. Review the action of this medication now, if you had difficulty with this question!

Level of Cognitive Ability: Analysis
Phase of Nursing Process: Analysis
Client Needs: Physiological Integrity
Content Area: Pharmacology

Reference
Hodgson, B., & Kizior, R. (1998). *Saunders nursing drug handbook 1998.* Philadelphia: W. B. Saunders. p. 939.

2. 3

Rationale: Humatrope should not be administered during or after epiphyseal closure. Efficacy of therapy declines as the client grows older and is usually lost entirely by age 20 to 24 years.

Test-Taking Strategy: Note the similarity between options 1, 2, and 4. These options all relate to growth failure. Note the difference in option 3, as it identifies a particular age of a client. Review the contraindications associated with the administration of Humatrope now, if you had difficulty with this question!

Level of Cognitive Ability: Analysis
Phase of Nursing Process: Analysis
Client Needs: Physiological Integrity
Content Area: Pharmacology

Reference
Lehne, R. (1998). *Pharmacology for nursing care* (3rd ed.). Philadelphia: W. B. Saunders. p. 611.

3. 1

Rationale: Hyperglycemia can occur from the administration of growth hormone, particularly in clients with diabetes. Growth hormone therapy is associated with a decline in thyroid function. Hypercalciuria can occur, particularly during the first 2 to 3 months of therapy. Glucose and thyroid hormone levels should be monitored.

Test-Taking Strategy: Knowledge regarding the side effects associated with growth hormone replacement therapy is required to answer the question. Review these side effects now, if you are unfamiliar with them!

Level of Cognitive Ability: Analysis
Phase of Nursing Process: Analysis
Client Needs: Physiological Integrity
Content Area: Pharmacology

References
Lehne, R. (1998). *Pharmacology for nursing care* (3rd ed.). Philadelphia: W. B. Saunders. p. 611.
Hodgson, B., & Kizior, R. (1998). *Saunders nursing drug handbook 1998*. Philadelphia: W. B. Saunders. p. 939.

4. 3

Rationale: Sandostatin is used to reduce GH levels in clients with acromegaly. The most common side effects of Sandostatin include diarrhea, nausea, gallstone formation, and abdominal discomfort. Hypertension, although rare, may occur. Polyuria is not associated with this medication.

Test-Taking Strategy: Knowledge regarding the side effects associated with Sandostatin is required to answer the question. Review these side effects now, if you had difficulty with this question!

Level of Cognitive Ability: Analysis
Phase of Nursing Process: Assessment
Client Needs: Physiological Integrity
Content Area: Pharmacology

Reference
Hodgson, B., & Kizior, R. (1998). *Saunders nursing drug handbook 1998*. Philadelphia: W. B. Saunders. p. 764.

5. 4

Rationale: DDAVP promotes renal conservation of water. The hormone accomplishes this by acting on the collecting ducts of the kidney to increase their permeability to water, which results in increased water reabsorption.

Test-Taking Strategy: Utilize the diagnosis in the question to assist you in answering the question. Recalling the manifestations related to the loss of large volumes of urine in this disorder will assist in directing you to option 4. Review diabetes insipidus and the action of DDAVP now, if you had difficulty answering this question!

Level of Cognitive Ability: Analysis
Phase of Nursing Process: Analysis
Client Needs: Physiological Integrity
Content Area: Pharmacology

Reference
Lehne, R. (1998). *Pharmacology for nursing care* (3rd ed.). Philadelphia: W. B. Saunders. p. 612.

6. 3

Rationale: Water intoxication or hyponatremia is an adverse reaction to DDAVP. Early signs include drowsiness, listlessness, and headache. Decreased urination, rapid weight gain, confusion, seizures, and coma may also occur in overhydration.

Test-Taking Strategy: Knowledge that this medication is used in the treatment of diabetes insipidus will assist in eliminating options 1 and 2. Recalling the action of the medication will assist you in determining that water intoxication is an adverse reaction. This thought process will assist

in directing you to option 3. Review the adverse reactions related to this important medication now, if you had difficulty with this question!

Level of Cognitive Ability: Analysis
Phase of Nursing Process: Assessment
Client Needs: Physiological Integrity
Content Area: Pharmacology

Reference
Hodgson, B., & Kizior, R. (1998). *Saunders nursing drug handbook 1998*. Philadelphia: W. B. Saunders. p. 295.

7. 3

Rationale: Because of its powerful vasoconstrictor actions, vasopressin can cause adverse cardiovascular effects. By constricting arteries of the heart, vasopressin can cause angina pectoris and even myocardial infarction, especially if administered to clients with coronary artery disease. In addition, vasopressin may cause gangrene by decreasing blood flow in the periphery.

Test-Taking Strategy: Attempt to make a relationship between the name of the medication: "vaso" pressin, and coronary artery disease, the correct option. If you are unfamiliar with the cautions associated with the administration of this important medication, take time now to review!

Level of Cognitive Ability: Analysis
Phase of Nursing Process: Analysis
Client Needs: Physiological Integrity
Content Area: Pharmacology

Reference
Lehne, R. (1998). *Pharmacology for nursing care* (3rd ed.). Philadelphia: W. B. Saunders. p. 614.

8. 2

Rationale: Synthroid accelerates the degradation of vitamin K–dependent clotting factors. As a result, effects of Coumadin are enhanced. If thyroid hormone replacement therapy is instituted in a client who has been taking Coumadin, the dosage of Coumadin should be reduced.

Test-Taking Strategy: Knowledge regarding the medication interactions that can occur with Synthroid is required to answer the question. Review these interactions now, if you had difficulty with this question. Both Coumadin and Synthroid are very important medications to become familiar with!

Level of Cognitive Ability: Analysis
Phase of Nursing Process: Analysis
Client Needs: Physiological Integrity
Content Area: Pharmacology

Reference
Lehne, R. (1998). *Pharmacology for nursing care* (3rd ed.). Philadelphia: W. B. Saunders. p. 601.

9. 2

Rationale: Oral doses of Synthroid should be taken on an empty stomach to enhance absorption. Dosing is usually done in the morning before breakfast.

Test-Taking Strategy: Knowledge regarding the administration of Synthroid is required to answer the question. You are likely to find questions regarding this medication on NCLEX-RN. If you are unfamiliar with this medication, review it now!

Level of Cognitive Ability: Analysis
Phase of Nursing Process: Evaluation
Client Needs: Health Promotion and Maintenance
Content Area: Pharmacology

Reference

Lehne, R. (1998). *Pharmacology for nursing care* (3rd ed.). Philadelphia: W. B. Saunders. p. 601.

10. **4**

Rationale: For most hypothyroid clients, replacement therapy must be continued for life. Treatment provides symptomatic relief but does not produce a cure. The client should be told that although therapy will cause symptoms to improve, these improvements do not constitute a reason to interrupt or discontinue the medication.

Test-Taking Strategy: Knowledge regarding the physiology associated with hypothyroidism is required to answer the question. If you are unfamiliar with this disorder and the medication therapy associated with it, take time now to review!

Level of Cognitive Ability: Application
Phase of Nursing Process: Implementation
Client Needs: Health Promotion and Maintenance
Content Area: Pharmacology

Reference

Lehne, R. (1998). *Pharmacology for nursing care* (3rd ed.). Philadelphia: W. B. Saunders. p. 601.

11. **2**

Rationale: Excessive doses of Synthroid can produce signs and symptoms of hyperthyroidism (thyrotoxicosis). These include tachycardia, angina, tremor, nervousness, insomnia, hyperthermia, heat intolerance, and sweating. The client should be instructed to notify the physician if these occur. Options 1, 3, and 4 are signs of hypothyroidism.

Test-Taking Strategy: Utilize the process of elimination, recalling the symptoms associated with hypothyroidism, the purpose of administering Synthroid, and the effects of the medication. Options 1, 3, and 4 are symptoms related to hypothyroidism. Review the adverse effects of the medication now, if you are unfamiliar with it!

Level of Cognitive Ability: Application
Phase of Nursing Process: Implementation
Client Needs: Health Promotion and Maintenance
Content Area: Pharmacology

Reference

Lehne, R. (1998). *Pharmacology for nursing care* (3rd ed.). Philadelphia: W. B. Saunders. p. 601.

12. **4**

Rationale: The normal maintenance dose of Synthroid in an adult is 0.1 to 0.2 mg daily. Maintenance dose for infants 0 to 6 months of age is 0.025 to 0.05 mg daily; children 1 to 5 years, 0.075 to 0.1 mg daily; and children 6 to 12 months, 0.05 to 0.075 mg daily.

Test-Taking Strategy: Knowledge regarding the normal adult dosage of Synthroid is required to answer the question. Learn this dosage range now, if you had difficulty with this question!

Level of Cognitive Ability: Analysis
Phase of Nursing Process: Analysis
Client Needs: Physiological Integrity
Content Area: Pharmacology

Reference

Hodgson, B., & Kizior, R. (1998). *Saunders nursing drug handbook 1998.* Philadelphia: W. B. Saunders. pp. 589–590.

13. **4**

Rationale: PTU inhibits thyroid hormone synthesis and is used to treat hyperthyroidism or Graves' disease. Myxedema indicates hypothyroidism. Cushing's syndrome and Addison's disease are disorders related to adrenal function.

Test-Taking Strategy: Knowledge regarding the action of the medication and the treatment measures for Graves' disease is required to answer the question. If you are unfamiliar with either of these, review now!

Level of Cognitive Ability: Analysis
Phase of Nursing Process: Analysis
Client Needs: Physiological Integrity
Content Area: Pharmacology

Reference

Lehne, R. (1998). *Pharmacology for nursing care* (3rd ed.). Philadelphia: W. B. Saunders. p. 601.

14. **2**

Rationale: Lypressin is an antidiuretic hormone used in the treatment of diabetes insipidus. It promotes renal conservation of water by acting on the collecting ducts of the kidney to increase their permeability to water, which results in increased water reabsorption.

Test-Taking Strategy: Note the diagnosis identified in the question. Recalling the pathophysiology associated with the disorder will easily assist in the process of elimination and in directing you to the correct option. Review the action of lypressin now, if you had difficulty with this question!

Level of Cognitive Ability: Application
Phase of Nursing Process: Implementation
Client Needs: Physiological Integrity
Content Area: Pharmacology

Reference

Lehne, R. (1998). *Pharmacology for nursing care* (3rd ed.). Philadelphia: W. B. Saunders. p. 612.

15. **3**

Rationale: Lypressin is administered by the intranasal route. It is used for diabetes insipidus. The usual adult dosage is 1 to 2 sprays into each nostril four times daily.

Test-Taking Strategy: Knowledge that lypressin is administered by the nasal route is required to answer the question. If you are unfamiliar with this medication, take time now to review!

Level of Cognitive Ability: Application
Phase of Nursing Process: Implementation
Client Needs: Health Promotion and Maintenance
Content Area: Pharmacology

Reference

Lehne, R. (1998). *Pharmacology for nursing care* (3rd ed.). Philadelphia: W. B. Saunders. p. 613.

16. 3

Rationale: Protropin is a growth hormone used in the treatment of dwarfism. When treatment is started, height may be increased by as much as 6 inches. To monitor treatment, height and weight should be measured monthly.

Test-Taking Strategy: Utilize the process of elimination. Options 1, 2, and 4 are similar in that each identifies lengthy and specific time frames related to the expected outcome of the medication. Review the expected outcome of Protropin now, if you had difficulty with this question!

Level of Cognitive Ability: Analysis
Phase of Nursing Process: Evaluation
Client Needs: Physiological Integrity
Content Area: Pharmacology

Reference
Lehne, R. (1998). *Pharmacology for nursing care* (3rd ed.). Philadelphia: W. B. Saunders. p. 611.

17. 4

Rationale: An adverse reaction to Humatrope is hypothyroidism. Thyroid function is monitored throughout therapy. Options 1 and 2 would evaluate pancreatic function, and option 3 evaluates renal function.

Test-Taking Strategy: Knowledge that Humatrope is a growth hormone will assist in the process of elimination and direct you to option 4. Eliminate options 1 and 2 first because both evaluate pancreatic function and therefore are similar. Option 3 evaluates renal function. If you had difficulty with this question, take time now to review interventions associated with the administration of Humatrope!

Level of Cognitive Ability: Analysis
Phase of Nursing Process: Assessment
Client Needs: Physiological Integrity
Content Area: Pharmacology

Reference
Kuhn, M. (1998). *Pharmacotherapeutics: A nursing process approach* (4th ed.). Philadelphia: F. A. Davis. p. 625.

18. 2

Rationale: Laboratory determinations of serum TSH are an important means of evaluation. Successful therapy will cause elevated TSH levels to fall. These levels will begin their decline within hours of the onset of therapy and will continue to drop as plasma levels of thyroid hormone build up. If an adequate dosage is established, TSH levels will remain suppressed for the duration of the therapy.

Test-Taking Strategy: Note the key phrase "expected outcome." Relate the diagnosis hypo"thyroidism" with "thyroid" hormone levels in the correct option. If you had difficulty with this question, take time now to review the therapeutic effect of Synthroid!

Level of Cognitive Ability: Application
Phase of Nursing Process: Evaluation
Client Needs: Physiological Integrity
Content Area: Pharmacology

Reference
Lehne, R. (1998). *Pharmacology for nursing care* (3rd ed.). Philadelphia: W. B. Saunders. p. 601.

19. 3

Rationale: Synthroid is used in the treatment of hypothyroidism. Although therapy with Synthroid may begin with small doses that are gradually increased, the most appropriate response is to inform the client that a full therapeutic effect may take 1 to 3 weeks.

Test-Taking Strategy: Eliminate options 1 and 2 first because they are similar. Knowledge regarding the therapeutic action of Synthroid is required to select between options 3 and 4. If you had difficulty with this question, take time now to review the therapeutic effects of this medication!

Level of Cognitive Ability: Analysis
Phase of Nursing Process: Analysis
Client Needs: Physiological Integrity
Content Area: Pharmacology

Reference
Hodgson, B., & Kizior, R. (1998). *Saunders nursing drug handbook 1998*. Philadelphia: W. B. Saunders. p. 590.

20. 2

Rationale: An adverse effect of PTU is agranulocytosis. The client needs to be informed of the early signs of this adverse effect, which include fever or sore throat. Drowsiness is an occasional side effect of the medication. Polyuria and dry mouth are unrelated to this medication.

Test-Taking Strategy: Knowledge that agranulocytosis is an adverse effect of PTU is required to answer this question. If you are unfamiliar with this important medication, take time now to review!

Level of Cognitive Ability: Application
Phase of Nursing Process: Implementation
Client Needs: Health Promotion and Maintenance
Content Area: Pharmacology

Reference
Lehne, R. (1998). *Pharmacology for nursing care* (3rd ed.). Philadelphia: W. B. Saunders. p. 606.

21. 2

Rationale: Lugol's solution is administered to hyperthyroid individuals in preparation for thyroidectomy to suppress thyroid function. Initial effects develop within 24 hours; peak effects develop in 10 to 15 days. In most cases, plasma levels of thyroid hormone are reduced with PTU before initiating Lugol's solution therapy. Then, iodine solution along with PTU is administered for the last 10 days prior to surgery.

Test-Taking Strategy: Eliminate options 1 and 3 first because they are similar. From the remaining options, select option 2 because of its relationship to the issue of the question. If you had difficulty with this question, take time now to review the purpose of this medication!

Level of Cognitive Ability: Analysis
Phase of Nursing Process: Evaluation
Client Needs: Physiological Integrity
Content Area: Pharmacology

Reference
Lehne, R. (1998). *Pharmacology for nursing care* (3rd ed.). Philadelphia: W. B. Saunders. p. 604.

22. **4**

Rationale: Chronic ingestion of iodine can produce iodism. The client needs to be instructed about the symptoms of iodism, which include a brassy taste, burning sensations in the mouth, soreness of gums and teeth, frontal headache, coryza, salivation, and skin eruptions. The client needs to be instructed to notify the physician if these symptoms occur.

Test-Taking Strategy: Eliminate options 2 and 3 first because the nurse cannot legally alter medication prescriptions without a physician's order. Considering the client symptoms presented in the question, eliminate option 1 as a reasonable choice. Review the adverse effects of Lugol's solution now, if you had difficulty with this question!

Level of Cognitive Ability: Application
Phase of Nursing Process: Implementation
Client Needs: Physiological Integrity
Content Area: Pharmacology

Reference
Lehne, R. (1998). *Pharmacology for nursing care* (3rd ed.). Philadelphia: W. B. Saunders. pp. 604, 607.

23. **4**

Rationale: Lugol's solution can cause iodine toxicity. Iodine is corrosive, and overdose will injure the gastrointestinal tract. Symptoms include abdominal pain, vomiting, and diarrhea. Swelling of the glottis may result in asphyxiation. Treatment consists of gastric lavage to remove iodine from the stomach and administration of sodium thiosulfate to reduce iodine to iodide. Calcium gluconate is used for acute hypocalcemia. Mucomyst is the antidote for acetaminophen (Tylenol) overdose. Vitamin K is the antidote for warfarin (Coumadin).

Test-Taking Strategy: Knowledge of the specific antidotes for medication overdose is required to answer this question. You should be able to easily eliminate options 1, 2, and 3 because these medications should be familiar to you. If they are not familiar and you are unsure of these antidotes, be sure to learn them now!

Level of Cognitive Ability: Analysis
Phase of Nursing Process: Analysis
Client Needs: Physiological Integrity
Content Area: Pharmacology

Reference
Lehne, R. (1998). *Pharmacology for nursing care* (3rd ed.). Philadelphia: W. B. Saunders. p. 604.

24. **1**

Rationale: Florinef has mineralocorticoid activity and also has a modest glucocorticoid effect. It acts primarily on the kidneys' distal tubules, enhancing the reabsorption of sodium and chloride ions and the excretion of potassium and hydrogen ions. It promotes water retention.

Test-Taking Strategy: Knowledge regarding the action of Florinef is required to answer the question. If you are unfamiliar with this medication, try to recall the pathophysiology associated with Addison's disease to assist in answering the question. Review this medication action now, if you are unfamiliar with it!

Level of Cognitive Ability: Analysis
Phase of Nursing Process: Analysis
Client Needs: Physiological Integrity
Content Area: Pharmacology

Reference
Kuhn, M. (1998). *Pharmacotherapeutics: A nursing process approach* (4th ed.). Philadelphia: F. A. Davis. p. 632.

25. **3**

Rationale: Excessive doses of Florinef cause retention of sodium and water and excessive excretion of potassium, resulting in expansion of blood volume, hypertension, cardiac enlargement, edema, and hypokalemia. The client needs to be informed about the signs of salt and water retention, such as unusual weight gain or swelling of the feet or lower legs. If these signs occur, the physician needs to be notified.

Test-Taking Strategy: Recalling that Florinef can cause water retention will easily direct you to option 3. If you are unfamiliar with the adverse effects associated with this medication, review them now!

Level of Cognitive Ability: Application
Phase of Nursing Process: Implementation
Client Needs: Health Promotion and Maintenance
Content Area: Pharmacology

Reference
Lehne, R. (1998). *Pharmacology for nursing care* (3rd ed.). Philadelphia: W. B. Saunders. p. 623.

26. **2**

Rationale: The client should be instructed to take the medication exactly as prescribed, and it is best administered 1 to 1.5 hours after meals. The client should take the tablets with a full glass of water; however, it can be taken with milk.

Test-Taking Strategy: Knowledge regarding the administration of Os-Cal is required to answer the question. If you are unfamiliar with the administration of this medication, take time now to review!

Level of Cognitive Ability: Application
Phase of Nursing Process: Implementation
Client Needs: Health Promotion and Maintenance
Content Area: Pharmacology

Reference
Kuhn, M. (1998). *Pharmacotherapeutics: A nursing process approach* (4th ed.). Philadelphia: F. A. Davis. p. 684.

27. **2**

Rationale: Clients taking antihypocalcemic medications should be instructed to avoid the use of mineral oil as a laxative because it decreases vitamin D absorption, and vitamin D is needed to assist in the absorption of calcium. Options 1, 3, and 4 are basic measures to alleviate constipation.

Test-Taking Strategy: Note the key word "not" in the stem of the question. Use the process of elimination and eliminate options 1, 3, and 4 because they are general and basic teaching measures that will assist in alleviating constipation. If you had difficulty with this question, review these basic measures and review the contraindications associated with the administration of Calderol!

Level of Cognitive Ability: Application
Phase of Nursing Process: Implementation
Client Needs: Health Promotion and Maintenance
Content Area: Pharmacology

Reference
Kuhn, M. (1998). *Pharmacotherapeutics: A nursing process approach* (4th ed.). Philadelphia: F. A. Davis. p. 684.

28. 3

Rationale: The client taking an antihypocalcemic medication should be instructed to avoid eating too much spinach, rhubarb, bran, or whole grain cereals because they decrease calcium absorption. Good dietary sources of calcium are milk products, dark green leafy vegetables, clams, oysters, sardines, and orange juice with calcium.

Test-Taking Strategy: Note that the client diagnosis is "hypocalcemia." Note the key word "avoid" in the stem of the question. Use the process of elimination and knowledge regarding food items high in calcium to assist in selecting the correct option. This should assist in eliminating options 1, 2, and 4.

Level of Cognitive Ability: Application
Phase of Nursing Process: Implementation
Client Needs: Health Promotion and Maintenance
Content Area: Pharmacology

Reference
Kuhn, M. (1998). *Pharmacotherapeutics: A nursing process approach* (4th ed.). Philadelphia: F. A. Davis. p. 684.

29. 1

Rationale: Didronel should be taken on an empty stomach 2 hours before meals. It should not be taken within 2 hours of vitamins, or with mineral supplements, antacids, or medications high in calcium, magnesium, iron, or albumin.

Test-Taking Strategy: Eliminate options 2, 3, and 4 because they are similar. Note that each of these options suggests administering the medication with another substance. Option 1 is the only option that reflects administering the medication on an empty stomach. Review concepts related to the administration of this medication now, if you had difficulty with this question!

Level of Cognitive Ability: Application
Phase of Nursing Process: Implementation
Client Needs: Health Promotion and Maintenance
Content Area: Pharmacology

Reference
Hodgson, B., & Kizior, R. (1998). *Saunders nursing drug handbook 1998*. Philadelphia: W. B. Saunders. p. 393.

30. 3

Rationale: Glucocorticoids should be administered before 9 A.M., and the client should be instructed to do so. Administration at this time helps minimize adrenal insufficiency and mimics the burst of glucocorticoids released naturally by the adrenals each morning.

Test-Taking Strategy: Knowledge regarding the administration of glucocorticoids is required to answer this question. If you had difficulty with this question, take time now to review the concepts!

Level of Cognitive Ability: Application
Phase of Nursing Process: Implementation
Client Needs: Health Promotion and Maintenance
Content Area: Pharmacology

Reference
Lehne, R. (1998). *Pharmacology for nursing care* (3rd ed.). Philadelphia: W. B. Saunders. p. 717.

31. 4

Rationale: Glucocorticoids should not be abruptly discontinued to prevent acute adrenal insufficiency. They can cause sodium and water retention and the loss of potassium, and clients should be instructed to limit sodium intake and consume potassium-rich foods. These medications can increase the risk of infection, and the client should avoid contact with persons who are ill.

Test-Taking Strategy: Note the key phrase "indicates a need for further instruction." Use knowledge regarding the administration of glucocorticoids and the process of elimination to assist in answering the question. You should easily be able to eliminate options 1, 2, and 3, remembering that the client should not stop these medications, or in fact any medication, without physician approval.

Level of Cognitive Ability: Analysis
Phase of Nursing Process: Evaluation
Client Needs: Health Promotion and Maintenance
Content Area: Pharmacology

Reference
Lehne, R. (1998). *Pharmacology for nursing care* (3rd ed.). Philadelphia: W. B. Saunders. p. 718.

32. 2

Rationale: Glucocorticoids can elevate blood levels of glucose. Diabetic clients may need their dosage of insulin or oral hypoglycemic medications increased during glucocorticoid therapy.

Test-Taking Strategy: Remember that glucocorticoids can increase the level of the blood glucose. Keep this important concept in mind when answering these types of questions because you are likely to find questions similar to this one on NCLEX-RN!

Level of Cognitive Ability: Analysis
Phase of Nursing Process: Analysis
Client Needs: Physiological Integrity
Content Area: Pharmacology

Reference
Lehne, R. (1998). *Pharmacology for nursing care* (3rd ed.). Philadelphia: W. B. Saunders. p. 719.

33. 2

Rationale: NPH insulin is an intermediate-acting insulin. Its onset of action is 1 to 2 hours, it peaks in 6 to 12 hours, and its duration of action is 18 to 24 hours.

Test-Taking Strategy: Read the question carefully, noting that the question is asking about NPH insulin. Knowledge regarding the onset, peak, and duration of action is required to answer the question. Review these points regarding both NPH and Regular insulin now, if you are unfamiliar with these points, because you are likely to find questions related to these concepts on NCLEX-RN!

Level of Cognitive Ability: Analysis
Phase of Nursing Process: Analysis
Client Needs: Physiological Integrity
Content Area: Pharmacology

Reference
Lehne, R. (1998). *Pharmacology for nursing care* (3rd ed.). Philadelphia: W. B. Saunders. p. 580.

34. **3**

Rationale: When preparing a mixture of Regular insulin with another insulin preparation, the Regular insulin should be drawn into the syringe first. This sequence will avoid contaminating the vial of Regular insulin with insulin of another type.

Test-Taking Strategy: Knowledge regarding the appropriate method of preparing insulin for injection is required to answer the question. Remember "RN"; draw up the "R"egular insulin before the "N"PH insulin. You are likely to find a question related to this method of insulin preparation on NCLEX-RN!

Level of Cognitive Ability: Analysis
Phase of Nursing Process: Evaluation
Client Needs: Health Promotion and Maintenance
Content Area: Pharmacology

Reference
Lehne, R. (1998). *Pharmacology for nursing care* (3rd ed.). Philadelphia: W. B. Saunders. p. 583.

35. **2**

Rationale: Insulin in unopened vials should be stored under refrigeration until needed. Vials should not be frozen. When stored unopened under refrigeration, insulin can be used up to the expiration date on the vial.

Test-Taking Strategy: Note the key word "store" in the question. Remembering that insulin should not be frozen will assist in eliminating option 1. Options 3 and 4 are similar and should be eliminated. Review client teaching points related to insulin now, if you had difficulty with this question!

Level of Cognitive Ability: Application
Phase of Nursing Process: Implementation
Client Needs: Health Promotion and Maintenance
Content Area: Pharmacology

Reference
Lehne, R. (1998). *Pharmacology for nursing care* (3rd ed.). Philadelphia: W. B. Saunders. p. 583.

36. **3**

Rationale: Mixtures of insulin in prefilled syringes should be stored in a refrigerator where they will be stable for at least 1 week, and perhaps 2. The syringe should be stored vertically, with the needle pointing up to avoid clogging the needle. Prior to administration, the syringe should be agitated gently to resuspend the insulin.

Test-Taking Strategy: Knowledge regarding home care concepts and the diabetic client is required to answer the question. Review these concepts now, if you are unfamiliar with the principles related to prefilling insulin syringes!

Level of Cognitive Ability: Application
Phase of Nursing Process: Implementation
Client Needs: Health Promotion and Maintenance
Content Area: Pharmacology

Reference
Lehne, R. (1998). *Pharmacology for nursing care* (3rd ed.). Philadelphia: W. B. Saunders. p. 583.

37. **2**

Rationale: An insulin vial in current use can be kept at room temperature for up to 1 month without significant loss of activity. Direct sunlight and heat must be avoided.

Test-Taking Strategy: Note the key word "unrefrigerated" in the stem of the question. This word will assist in directing you to the correct option. However, if you are unfamiliar with the concepts related to insulin stability, review now!

Level of Cognitive Ability: Application
Phase of Nursing Process: Implementation
Client Needs: Health Promotion and Maintenance
Content Area: Pharmacology

Reference
Lehne, R. (1998). *Pharmacology for nursing care* (3rd ed.). Philadelphia: W. B. Saunders. p. 583.

38. **1**

Rationale: The effect of Lispro insulin begins within 5 minutes of SC injection and persists for 2 to 4 hours. Lispro insulin acts more rapidly that Regular insulin but has a shorter duration of action. Because of its rapid onset, it can be administered immediately before eating. In contrast, Regular insulin is generally administered 30 to 60 minutes before meals.

Test-Taking Strategy: Note the key phrase "rapid-acting." You should easily be able to eliminate options 3 and 4. From the remaining two options, remember that the question is asking about Lispro, not Regular, insulin. This should direct you to option 1.

Level of Cognitive Ability: Application
Phase of Nursing Process: Implementation
Client Needs: Health Promotion and Maintenance
Content Area: Pharmacology

Reference
Lehne, R. (1998). *Pharmacology for nursing care* (3rd ed.). Philadelphia: W. B. Saunders. p. 583.

39. **2**

Rationale: Only Regular insulin may be administered by IV. Also, it is the only type of insulin that may be administered by the IM route. Since Regular insulin forms a true solution, it is safe for IV use.

Test-Taking Strategy: Remember that Regular insulin is the only type of insulin that can be administered IV. If you were unable to answer this question, it is necessary that you review this content now!

Level of Cognitive Ability: Application
Phase of Nursing Process: Planning
Client Needs: Safe, Effective Care Environment
Content Area: Pharmacology

Reference
Lehne, R. (1998). *Pharmacology for nursing care* (3rd ed.). Philadelphia: W. B. Saunders. p. 582.

40. **4**

Rationale: The principal adverse effect of insulin therapy is hypoglycemia, a blood glucose level of less then 50 mg/dL.

Test-Taking Strategy: Recalling the normal blood glucose level will assist in eliminating options 1, 2, and 3. If you are unfamiliar with the normal blood glucose level or the concept of hypoglycemia, review now!

Level of Cognitive Ability: Application
Phase of Nursing Process: Implementation
Client Needs: Health Promotion and Maintenance
Content Area: Pharmacology

Reference
Lehne, R. (1998). *Pharmacology for nursing care* (3rd ed.). Philadelphia: W. B. Saunders. p. 593.

41. **1**

Rationale: Glucagon is used to treat hypoglycemia resulting from insulin overdose. The family of the client is instructed in how to administer the medication. In an unconscious client, arousal usually occurs within 20 minutes of glucagon injection. Once consciousness has been produced, oral carbohydrates should be given. Lipoatrophy and lipohypertrophy result from insulin injections.

Test-Taking Strategy: Noting the word "glucagon" will assist in determining that the medication contains some form of glucose. This relationship should easily direct you to option 1. If you are unfamiliar with this medication, review now!

Level of Cognitive Ability: Application
Phase of Nursing Process: Implementation
Client Needs: Health Promotion and Maintenance
Content Area: Pharmacology

Reference
Lehne, R. (1998). *Pharmacology for nursing care* (3rd ed.). Philadelphia: W. B. Saunders. p. 592.

42. **3**

Rationale: When alcohol is combined with tolbutamide, a disulfiram-like reaction may occur. This syndrome includes flushing, palpitations, and nausea. Alcohol can potentiate the hypoglycemic effects of tolbutamide. Clients must be warned about alcohol consumption while taking this medication.

Test-Taking Strategy: Utilize the process of elimination. Eliminate options 1, 2, and 4 as these food items are allowed in a diabetic diet. Remembering that alcohol can affect the action of many medications will assist in directing you to option 3. Review this medication now, if you had difficulty with this question!

Level of Cognitive Ability: Application
Phase of Nursing Process: Implementation
Client Needs: Health Promotion and Maintenance
Content Area: Pharmacology

Reference
Lehne, R. (1998). *Pharmacology for nursing care* (3rd ed.). Philadelphia: W. B. Saunders. p. 588.

43. **2**

Rationale: The most common side effect of Glucophage is GI disturbances including decreased appetite, nausea, and diarrhea. These generally subside over time. This medication does not cause weight gain; in fact, clients lose an average of 7 to 8 pounds because the medication causes nausea and decreased appetite.

Test-Taking Strategy: Knowledge regarding the side effects associated with Glucophage is required to answer this question. If you are unfamiliar with this medication, take time now to review!

Level of Cognitive Ability: Analysis
Phase of Nursing Process: Assessment
Client Needs: Physiological Integrity
Content Area: Pharmacology

Reference
Lehne, R. (1998). *Pharmacology for nursing care* (3rd ed.). Philadelphia: W. B. Saunders. p. 589.

44. **3**

Rationale: Sulfonylureas promote insulin secretion by the pancreas and may also increase tissue response to insulin. Alpha-glucosidase inhibitors inhibit carbohydrate digestion. Biguanides decrease glucose production by the liver. Thiazolidinediones decrease insulin resistance.

Test-Taking Strategy: Knowledge regarding the specific action of the sulfonylureas is required to answer this question. If you are not familiar with this important classification of medications, review now!

Level of Cognitive Ability: Analysis
Phase of Nursing Process: Analysis
Client Needs: Physiological Integrity
Content Area: Pharmacology

Reference
Lehne, R. (1998). *Pharmacology for nursing care* (3rd ed.). Philadelphia: W. B. Saunders. p. 587.

45. **3**

Rationale: When the diabetic client becomes ill, control is more difficult. Insulin is not omitted, and the client is encouraged to consume liquid carbohydrates if unable to eat regular meals. The client is instructed to notify the physician if vomiting or diarrhea occurs, or if the illness progresses past 2 days.

Test-Taking Strategy: You can easily eliminate options 1, 2, and 4 because it is not within the legal parameters of nursing responsibilities to adjust or alter medication dosages. If you had difficulty with this question, review the client teaching points related to the administration of insulin on "sick days"!

Level of Cognitive Ability: Application
Phase of Nursing Process: Implementation
Client Needs: Health Promotion and Maintenance
Content Area: Pharmacology

Reference
Kuhn, M. (1998). *Pharmacotherapeutics: A nursing process approach* (4th ed.). Philadelphia: F. A. Davis. p. 670.

BIBLIOGRAPHY

Black, J., & Matassarin-Jacobs, E. (1997). *Medical-surgical nursing: Clinical management for continuity of care* (5th ed.). Philadelphia: W. B. Saunders.

Hodgson, B., & Kizior, R. (1998). *Saunders nursing drug handbook 1998.* Philadelphia: W. B. Saunders

Kuhn, M. (1998). *Pharmacotherapeutics: A nursing process approach* (4th ed.). Philadelphia: F. A. Davis.

Leahy, J., & Kizilay, P. (1998). *Foundations of nursing practice: A nursing process approach.* Philadelphia: W. B. Saunders.

Lehne, R. (1998). *Pharmacology for nursing care* (3rd ed.). Philadelphia: W. B. Saunders.

Luckmann, J. (1997). *Saunders manual of nursing care.* Philadelphia: W. B. Saunders.

Monahan, F., & Neighbors, M. (1998). *Medical-surgical nursing: Foundations for clinical practice* (2nd ed.). Philadelphia: W. B. Saunders.

O'Toole, M. (1997). *Miller-Keane encyclopedia & dictionary of medicine, nursing, & allied health* (6th ed.). Philadelphia: W. B. Saunders.

UNIT XII

....

The Adult Client with a Gastrointestinal Disorder

PYRAMID TERMS

Ascites—The accumulation of fluid within the peritoneal cavity that results in venous congestion of the hepatic capillaries. This leads to plasma leaking directly from the liver surface and portal vein.

Asterixis—Also termed liver flap. A coarse tremor characterized by rapid, nonrhythmic extensions and flexions in the wrist and fingers.

Billroth I—Also called gastroduodenostomy. Partial gastrectomy with the remaining segment anastomosed to the duodenum.

Billroth II—Also called gastrojejunostomy. Partial gastrectomy with the remaining segment anastomosed to the jejunum.

Cholecystectomy—Removal of the gallbladder.

Cholecystitis—An inflammation of the gallbladder that may occur as an acute or a chronic process. Acute inflammation is associated with gallstones (cholelithiasis). Chronic cholecystitis results when inefficient bile emptying and gallbladder muscle wall disease cause a fibrotic and contracted gallbladder.

Choledochotomy—Incision into the common bile duct to remove the stone.

Cirrhosis—A chronic, progressive disease of the liver characterized by diffuse damage to cells with fibrosis and nodular regeneration. Repeated destruction of hepatic cells causes the formation of scar tissue.

Crohn's Disease—An inflammatory disease that can occur anywhere in the gastrointestinal (GI) tract but most often affects the terminal ileum and leads to thickening and scarring, a narrowed lumen, fistulas, ulcerations, and abscesses. It is characterized by remissions and exacerbations.

Cullen's Sign—Bluish discoloration of the abdomen and periumbilical area, seen in acute hemorrhagic pancreatitis.

Diverticulitis—Inflammation of one or more diverticuli. Results when a diverticulum perforates, with local abscess formation. A perforated diverticulum can progress to intra-abdominal perforation with generalized peritonitis.

Diverticulosis—Outpouching or herniations of the intestinal mucosa. They can occur in any part of the intestine but are most common in the sigmoid colon.

Dumping Syndrome—Rapid emptying of the gastric contents into the small intestine. Occurs following gastric resection.

Esophageal Varices—Dilated and tortuous veins in the submucosa of the esophagus. They are caused by portal hypertension, are often associated with liver cirrhosis, and are at high risk for rupture if portal circulation pressure rises.

Fetor Hepaticus—The fruity, musty breath odor associated with chronic liver disease.

Gastrectomy—Also called esophagojejunostomy. Removal of the stomach with attachment of the esophagus to the jejunum or duodenum.

Gastric Resection—Also called antrectomy. Involves removal of the lower half of the stomach and usually includes a vagotomy.

Hiatus Hernia—Also known as esophageal or diaphragmatic hernia. A portion of the stomach herniates through the diaphragm and into the thorax. It results from weakening of the muscles of the diaphragm and is aggravated by factors that increase abdominal pressure, such as pregnancy, ascites, obesity, tumors, and heavy lifting.

Kock Pouch—An intra-abdominal pouch is constructed from the terminal ileum. The pouch is connected to the stoma with a nipple-like valve constructed from a portion of the ileum. The stoma is flush with the skin.

Murphy's Sign—A sign of gallbladder disease, consisting of pain on taking a deep breath when the examiner's fingers are on the approximate location of the gallbladder.

Pancreatitis—An acute or chronic inflammation of the pancreas, with associated escape of pancreatic enzymes into surrounding tissue. Acute pancreatitis occurs suddenly as one attack or can be recurrent but resolves. Chronic pancreatitis is a continual inflammation and destruction of the pancreas, with scar tissue replacing pancreatic tissue.

Peristalsis—Wavelike rhythmic contractions that propel material through the GI tract.

Portal Hypertension—A persistent increase in pressure within the portal vein that develops as a result of obstruction to flow.

Pyloroplasty—Enlarging the pylorus to prevent or decrease pyloric obstruction, thereby enhancing gastric emptying.

Turner's Sign—A gray-blue discoloration of the flanks, seen in acute hemorrhagic pancreatitis.

Ulcerative Colitis—Ulcerative and inflammatory disease of the bowel that results in poor absorption of nutrients. Acute ulcerative colitis results in vascular congestion, hemorrhage, and edema and ulceration of the bowel mucosa. Chronic ulcerative colitis causes muscular hypertrophy, fat deposits, and fibrous tissue, with bowel thickening, shortening, and narrowing.

Vagotomy—Surgical division of the vagus nerve to eliminate the vagal impulses that stimulate hydrochloric acid secretion in the stomach.

PYRAMID TO SUCCESS

Pyramid points focus on diagnostic tests, nursing care related to the various gastric or intestinal tubes, gastric surgery, cirrhosis, hepatitis, pancreatitis, and colostomy care. Focus on preprocedure and postprocedure care of the client undergoing a GI diagnostic test. Remember that an informed consent is required for any invasive procedure. Focus on diet restrictions before and following the diagnostic test, and remember that the gag reflex or bowel sounds must return before allowing a client to consume food or fluids. Pyramid points include instructions to the client and family regarding the prevention of GI disorders and the complications associated with the disorder. Focus on teaching the client and family about diet and nutrition specific to the disorder, tube and wound care, preventing the transmission of infection, and care to a colostomy or ileostomy. Remember that body image disturbances can occur in clients with a GI disorder. Specific focus relates to the client with a diversion, such as an ileostomy or colostomy, to the social isolation issues that can occur, and coping strategies.

NURSING PROCESS

ASSESSMENT

Medical and family history
Socioeconomic status
Cultural and religious patterns
Vital signs
Respiratory pattern
Level of consciousness
Appearance as emaciated or obese
Dietary patterns
Nutritional and fluid intake
Weight changes
Nausea and vomiting

Condition of mouth, teeth, tongue, and gums
Swallowing ability and gag reflex
Skin color, turgor, and appearance
Abdominal assessment, including girth
Pain
Edema
Ascites
Bowel patterns
Bowel sounds and motility
Stool for the presence of blood, mucus, bile

ANALYSIS: Ineffective Breathing Pattern

PLANNING	IMPLEMENTATION	EVALUATION
The client will maintain a patent airway. The client demonstrates effective breathing patterns.	Monitor vital signs. Assess respiratory status. Encourage coughing and deep breathing and splinting procedures. Position client based on disorder for optimal breathing.	Client's airway remains patent. Lung sounds remain clear. Respiratory status remains within normal limits.

ANALYSIS: Alteration in Nutrition

PLANNING	IMPLEMENTATION	EVALUATION
The client will tolerate nutritional intake to meet body needs. The client describes components of a nutritionally adequate diet. The client verbalizes understanding of fluid and dietary restrictions.	Monitor food and fluid intake. Monitor for signs of dehydration, such as dry mucous membranes, poor skin turgor, decreased urination, and increased pulse. Monitor weight. Develop meal plan with client. Instruct client in requirements and restrictions as prescribed based on the GI disorder.	The client maintains adequate nutritional intake. The client maintains a stable weight. The client demonstrates the ability to select appropriate foods, based on restrictions or requirements.

ANALYSIS: Alteration in Elimination

PLANNING	IMPLEMENTATION	EVALUATION
The client passes stool of normal consistency for the disorder.	Perform abdominal assessment. Assess for and document the presence of bowel sounds and abdominal distention. Monitor stool patterns and consistency. Evaluate laboratory results of stool specimens.	The client verbalizes the presence of an optimal bowel pattern.

ANALYSIS: Impaired Skin Integrity

PLANNING	IMPLEMENTATION	EVALUATION
The client demonstrates an optimal skin care routine.	Monitor skin integrity. Instruct client in the care of the diversion, such as the colostomy/ileostomy if present. Establish a skin care routine and instruct client in measures to prevent skin breakdown.	Skin remains intact.

ANALYSIS: Pain

PLANNING	IMPLEMENTATION	EVALUATION
The client reports a decrease in reflux symptoms. The client demonstrates the use of nonpharmacological pain relief measures. The client verbalizes the need for pain medication and obtains relief from medication.	Monitor for pain. Demonstrate the use of nonpharmacological pain relief measures. Utilize comfort measures to assist in reducing pain. Administer pain medication as prescribed. Monitor for effectiveness of pain medication and document results.	The client utilizes pain relief techniques. The client remains free of pain.

ANALYSIS: Social Isolation

PLANNING

The client identifies personal strengths that may promote effective coping. The client identifies community resources and support systems that will assist in decreasing social isolation.

IMPLEMENTATION

Assist the client to identify personal strengths and methods of coping. Assist the client to identify behaviors that contribute to feelings of social isolation. Provide information on community resources that may decrease social isolation after discharge.

EVALUATION

The client utilizes support systems and community resources.

ANALYSIS: Altered Health Maintenance

PLANNING

The client verbalizes knowledge of preventive health measures.

IMPLEMENTATION

Instruct client in preventive health measures specific to needs, such as lifestyle, plan modifications, dietary changes, cessation of smoking, stress reduction and exercise. Instruct client and family regarding measures to prevent disease transmission. Consult with social service to plan for health maintenance needs at discharge.

EVALUATION

The client follows prescribed treatment. The client implements preventive health measures.

CLIENT NEEDS

SAFE, EFFECTIVE CARE ENVIRONMENT

Confidentiality issues related to GI disorder
Informed consent for treatments and surgical procedures
Consultation related to nutritional status
Referrals to home care and community services
Handling infectious drainage and secretions
Standard precautions
Preventing the transmission of disease

HEALTH PROMOTION AND MAINTENANCE

Health screening related to GI disorders
Health promotion programs related to GI disorders
Physical assessment techniques of the GI system
Teaching related to prescribed dietary and other treatment measures
Teaching related to colostomy or ileostomy care
Teaching related to preventing the transmission of disease

PSYCHOSOCIAL INTEGRITY

Coping mechanisms
Support systems
Body image changes related to colostomy or ileostomy

PHYSIOLOGICAL INTEGRITY

Nutrition and oral hydration
Personal hygiene
Elimination
Nonpharmacological and pharmacological comfort measures
Medication therapy specific to GI disorder
Total parenteral nutrition
Diagnostic tests related to GI system
Care of GI tubes
Monitoring for complications related to tests, procedures, and surgical interventions
Fluid and electrolyte imbalances
Infectious diseases of the GI tract

BIBLIOGRAPHY

Black, J., & Matassarin-Jacobs, E. (1997). *Medical-surgical nursing: Clinical management for continuity of care* (5th ed.). Philadelphia: W. B. Saunders.

Leahy, J., & Kizilay, P. (1998). *Foundations of nursing practice: A nursing process approach.* Philadelphia: W. B. Saunders.

National Council of State Boards of Nursing (eds.) (1977). *Test plan for the National Council Licensure Examination for Registered Nurses.* Chicago: Author.

O'Toole, M. (ed.) (1997). *Miller-Keane encyclopedia & dictionary of medicine, nursing, & allied health* (6th ed.). Philadelphia: W. B. Saunders.

CHAPTER 53

Gastrointestinal System

. . . .

I. Anatomy and Physiology

A. Functions of the gastrointestinal (GI) system
   1. Process food substances
   2. Absorb the products of digestion into the blood
   3. Excrete unabsorbed materials
   4. Provide an environment for microorganisms to synthesize nutrients, such as vitamin K
   5. For risk factors associated with the GI system, see Box 53–1
B. Mouth
   1. Contains the lips, cheeks, palate, tongue, teeth (mastication), salivary glands (lubrication), muscles, and maxillary bones
   2. Saliva contains the enzyme amylase (ptyalin) that aids in digestion
C. Esophagus
   1. A collapsible muscular tube, about 10 inches long
   2. Carries food from the pharynx to the stomach
D. Stomach: Contains the cardia, the fundus, the body, and the pylorus

   1. Mucous glands
      a. Located in mucosa
      b. Prevent autodigestion by providing an alkaline protective covering
   2. Cardiac opening: Prevents reflux into the esophagus
   3. Pyloric sphincter: Regulates the rate of stomach emptying into the small intestine
   4. Hydrochloric acid: Kills microorganisms, breaks food into small particles, and provides a chemical environment that is required by the gastric enzymes
   5. Pepsin: The chief coenzyme of gastric juice, which converts proteins into proteases and peptones
   6. Intrinsic factor: Necessary for the absorption of vitamin B_{12}
   7. Gastrin: Controls gastric acidity
E. Small intestine
   1. The small intestine terminates in the cecum
   2. Duodenum: Contains the openings of the bile and pancreatic ducts
   3. Jejunum: Approximately 8 feet long
   4. Ileum: Approximately 12 feet long
F. Intestinal juice enzymes
   1. Amylase digests starch to maltose
   2. Maltase reduces maltose to monosaccharide glucose
   3. Lactase splits lactose into galactose and glucose
   4. Sucrase reduces sucrose to fructose and glucose
   5. Nucleoses split nucleic acids to nucleotides
   6. Enterokinase activates trypsinogen to trypsin
G. Large intestine
   1. Approximately 5 feet long
   2. Absorbs water and eliminates wastes
   3. Manufacture of vitamins, including some B vitamins and vitamin K
   4. Colon
      a. Ascending
      b. Transverse
      c. Descending

BOX 53–1. Risk Factors Associated with the GI System

Family history of GI disorders
Chronic laxative use
Tobacco use
Chronic alcohol use
Chronic high stress levels
Allergic reactions to food or medications
Long-term GI conditions such as ulcerative colitis may predispose to colorectal cancer
Previous abdominal surgery or trauma may lead to adhesions
Neurological disorders can impair movement, particularly with chewing and swallowing
Cardiac, respiratory, and endocrine disorders may lead to constipation
Diabetes mellitus may predispose to oral candidal infections

---

d. Sigmoid
e. Rectum
5. Ileocecal valve: Prevents contents of large intestine from entering ileum
6. Anal sphincters: Guard the anal canal

H. Peritoneum
1. Lines the abdominal cavity
2. Forms the mesentery that supports the intestines and blood supply

I. Liver
1. The largest gland in the body, weighing 3 to 4 pounds
2. Contains Kupffer's cells, which remove bacteria in the portal venous blood
3. Removes excess glucose and amino acids from the portal blood
4. Synthesizes glucose, amino acids, and fats
5. Aids in the digestion of fats, carbohydrates, and proteins
6. Stores and filters blood (200 to 400 mL of blood stored)
7. Stores vitamins A, D, and B_{12} and iron
8. Secretes bile to emulsify fats (500 to 1000 mL of bile a day)
9. Hepatic ducts
   a. Deliver bile to the gallbladder via the cystic duct
   b. Deliver bile to the duodenum via the common bile duct
   c. The common bile duct opens into the duodenum, with the pancreatic duct at the ampulla of Vater
   d. The sphincter prevents the reflux of intestinal contents into the common bile duct and pancreatic duct

J. Gallbladder
1. Stores and concentrates bile
2. Contracts to force bile into the duodenum during the digestion of fats
3. The cystic duct joins the hepatic duct to form the common bile duct
4. The sphincter of Oddi guards the entrance into the duodenum
5. The presence of fatty materials in the duodenum stimulates the liberation of cholecystokinin, which causes contraction of the gallbladder and relaxation of the sphincter of Oddi

K. Pancreas
1. Exocrine gland
   a. Secretes sodium bicarbonate to neutralize the acidity of the stomach contents as they enter the duodenum
   b. Pancreatic juices contain enzymes for digesting carbohydrates, fats, and proteins
2. Endocrine gland
   a. Insulin secretion is produced by the islets of Langerhans
   b. Insulin is secreted into the blood stream
   c. Insulin is important for carbohydrate metabolism

II. Diagnostic Procedures

A. Upper GI (barium swallow)
1. Description: An examination of the upper GI tract under fluoroscopy after the client drinks barium sulfate
2. Preprocedure: Instruct the client to fast from foods and fluids overnight prior to the study
3. Postprocedure
   a. A laxative may be prescribed
   b. Instruct client to drink 6 to 8 glasses of water each day for 2 days to help pass the barium
   c. Monitor stools for the passage of barium (stools will appear chalky white)

B. Lower GI (barium enema)
1. Description
   a. A fluoroscopic and radiographic examination of the large intestine after rectal instillation of barium sulfate
   b. May be done with or without air
2. Preprocedure
   a. Laxatives on the day prior to and the morning of the test
   b. Liquid diet 1 day prior to and on the morning of the test
3. Postprocedure
   a. Increase fluid intake for 24 to 48 hours
   b. Administer mild laxatives to facilitate emptying of the barium
   c. Monitor stool for passage of barium
   d. Notify physician if a bowel movement does not occur within 2 days

C. Gastroscopy
1. Description: Insertion of an endoscopic instrument through the esophagus into the stomach and upper portion of the small intestine to visualize the mucosal lining
2. Preprocedure
   a. Obtain informed consent
   b. Remove dentures
   c. Administer sedative as required
   d. Obtain baseline vital signs
   e. Maintain NPO status for 12 hours prior to procedure
3. Postprocedure
   a. Assess vital signs and respiratory, cardiac, and neurological status
   b. Monitor for return of gag reflex
   c. Do not administer food or fluid until gag reflex returns
   d. Monitor for signs of bleeding, as evidenced by hypotension, pallor, and tachycardia
   e. Monitor for perforation as evidenced by pain, tachypnea, and rales

D. Sigmoidoscopy
1. Description: Endoscopic visualization of the sigmoid colon using a sigmoidoscope
2. Preprocedure
   a. Obtain informed consent
   b. A full liquid diet the evening before the test

c. Laxatives the evening before the test and an enema or suppository 1 hour prior to the test

3. Postprocedure

a. Assess for side effects related to sedative if administered

b. Normal activities and diet may be resumed

c. Notify physician if temperature is higher than 101°F, if breathing is difficult, or if stomach pain or bright red rectal bleeding occurs

E. Colonoscopy

1. Description: A fiberoptic endoscopic study in which the lining of the large intestine is visually examined

2. Preprocedure

a. Obtain informed consent

b. Clear liquid diet for 48 hours prior to the test

c. Bowel preparation with laxatives on the evening prior to the test and an enema on the day of the test

3. Postprocedure

a. Monitor vital signs

b. Monitor for side effects if sedation was administered

c. A normal diet may be resumed

d. Monitor for signs of colon perforation, as evidenced by abdominal pain or distention, malaise, fever, purulent rectal drainage, or lower GI bleeding

F. Gastric analysis

1. Description: The passage of a nasogastric (NG) tube into the stomach to aspirate gastric contents for analysis of acidity, appearance, and volume

2. Preprocedure

a. Fast for 12 hours prior to the test

b. Avoiding tobacco and chewing gum for 6 hours prior to the test

3. Postprocedure

a. May resume normal activities

b. Refrigerate gastric samples if not tested within 4 hours

G. Gallbladder series

1. Description: Oral cholecystography to study the dye-filled gallbladder by radiographic film

2. Preprocedure

a. A low-fat meal on the evening prior to the test and then fasting from midnight the day before the test

b. Administer six 0.5-g iopanoic acid (Telepaque) tablets 12 hours prior to the test

c. Tablets should be taken with a large amount of water at 5-minute intervals

d. Instruct client to go to the emergency department if a rash, itching or hives, or difficulty in breathing occurs after taking the tablets

3. Postprocedure

a. Inform the client that dysuria is common because the dye is excreted in the urine

b. A normal diet may be resumed; however, a fatty meal may enhance dye excretion

H. Liver biopsy

1. Description: A needle is inserted through the abdominal wall to the liver to obtain a tissue sample for biopsy and microscopic examination

2. Preprocedure

a. Obtained informed consent

b. Assess hematological laboratory results

c. Administer sedative as prescribed

d. NPO after midnight on the day prior to the test

e. Note that the client is placed in the supine or left lateral position during the procedure

3. Postprocedure

a. Assess vital signs frequently

b. Assess biopsy site for bleeding

c. Monitor for peritonitis

d. Maintain bed rest for 24 hours

e. Place client on the right side for 1 to 2 hours to decrease the risk of hemorrhage

I. Paracentesis

1. Description: Transabdominal removal of fluid from the peritoneal cavity for the analysis of electrolytes, red blood cells, white blood cells, bacterial and viral cultures, and cytology studies

2. Preprocedure

a. Obtain informed consent

b. Have the client void prior to the start of the procedure to empty the bladder and to move the bladder out of the way of the paracentesis needle

c. Measure abdominal girth, weight, and baseline vital signs

d. Note that the client is positioned sitting on the edge of the bed with the back supported and the feet resting on a stool, or lying prone during the procedure

3. Postprocedure

a. Monitor vital signs

b. Maintain bed rest

c. Apply a dry sterile dressing to the insertion site

d. Monitor insertion site for bleeding

e. Measure abdominal girth and weight

f. Monitor for hematuria due to bladder trauma

g. Instruct client to notify physician if the urine becomes bloody, pink, or red

J. Stool specimens

1. Description: Examination of stool for the presence of occult bleeding

2. Preprocedure: Instruct client to avoid aspirin, nonsteroidal anti-inflammatory drugs (NSAIDs), red meat, poultry, and fish 3 days prior to the collection

K. Liver and pancreas laboratory studies

1. Alkaline phosphatase

a. Released during liver damage or biliary obstruction

b. Normal value: 4.5 to 13 King-Armstrong U/dL

2. Prothrombin time (PT)
   a. Prolonged with liver damage
   b. Normal value: 9.6 to 18.0 sec
3. Serum ammonia
   a. Assesses the ability of the liver to deaminate protein by-products
   b. Normal value: 15 to 45 μg/dL
4. Liver enzymes (transaminase studies)
   a. Elevated with liver damage
   b. SGOT (serum glutamic-oxaloacetic transaminase): 10 to 50 IU/L
   c. SGPT (serum glutamate pyruvate transaminase): 5 to 35 IU/L
   d. LDH (lactate dehydrogenase): 70 to 200 IU/L
5. Cholesterol
   a. Increase can indicate **pancreatitis** or biliary obstruction
   b. Normal value: 120 to 200 mg/dL
6. Bilirubin
   a. Increase indicates liver damage or biliary obstruction
   b. Bilirubin direct: 0 to 0.3 mg/dL
   c. Bilirubin indirect: 0.1 to 1.0 mg/dL
   d. Bilirubin total: Less than 1.5 mg/dL
7. Amylase and lipase
   a. Elevations indicate **pancreatitis**
   b. Amylase: 50 to 180 Somogyi units/dL
   c. Lipase: 31 to 186 U/L

III. Assessment

A. Abdominal assessment
   1. Inspect skin for color, abnormalities, contour, and tautness and the abdomen for distention
   2. Auscultate for bowel sounds
   3. Percuss for air or solids
   4. Palpate for tenderness
B. Bowel sounds
   1. Auscultate bowel sounds before percussion and palpation
   2. Normal bowel sounds occur 5 to 34 times a minute or every 5 to 15 seconds
   3. Auscultate in all quadrants
   4. Listen at least 5 minutes in each quadrant before assuming sounds are absent

IV. Nasogastric Tubes

A. Description
   1. Short tubes used to intubate the stomach
   2. Inserted from nose to stomach
B. Types of tubes
   1. Levine
      a. Single-lumen NG tube
      b. Used to remove gastric contents via intermittent suction, or to provide tube feedings

2. Salem sump
   a. Double-lumen NG tube with an air vent
   b. Used for decompression with continuous suction
   c. Air vent is not to be clamped and is to be kept above the level of the stomach
   d. If leakage occurs through the air vent, instill 30 mL of air into the air vent and irrigate the main lumen with normal saline (NS)
C. Intubation procedures
   1. Place client in high Fowler's position
   2. Measure from tip of nose to earlobe to xiphoid process to determine the length of insertion and mark with tape
   3. Lubricate tube about 3 inches with a water-soluble jelly only, to prevent the development of pneumonia if the tube accidentally slips into the bronchus
   4. Instruct client to bend the head forward to close the epiglottis and open the esophagus
   5. Insert into nostril, advance backward and through the nasopharynx
   6. Have client take a sip of water and advance tube as client swallows
   7. Do not force tube
   8. If the client experiences any respiratory distress (coughing or choking) during insertion, pull back on the tube and wait until the distress subsides
   9. Advance until tape mark is reached; tape in place when correct placement is confirmed
   10. If feedings are prescribed, x-ray confirmation should be done prior to initiating feedings
   11. When GI tubes are attached to suction, it may be continuous or intermittent, with a pressure not exceeding 25 mmHg as prescribed by the physician
D. Assessing placement
   1. Note that the most reliable method to determine placement is by x-ray and should be performed after initial placement
   2. Assess tube placement every 4 hours and before administering feedings or medications
   3. Assess tube placement by aspirating gastric contents and measuring the pH, which should be 4 or less (pH values greater than 6 indicate intestinal placement)
   4. Inserting 5 to 10 mL of air into the NG tube and listening for the rush of air over the stomach with a stethoscope is an alternative method for assessing placement but is not as reliable as an x-ray or checking gastric pH
E. Assessing residual
   1. Check residual volumes every 4 hours, before each feeding, and before giving medications
   2. Aspirate all stomach contents (residual) and measure amount
   3. Reinstill residual feeding to prevent excessive fluid and electrolyte losses unless the residual volume appears abnormal
   4. Usually, if the residual is less than 100 to 150

mL, feeding, if prescribed, is administered; if residual is greater than 150 mL, hold the feeding

F. Irrigating
   1. Check patency of tube every 4 hours
   2. Assess placement before irrigating
   3. Gently instill 30 to 50 mL water or NS (depending on agency policy) with irrigation syringe
   4. Pull back on syringe plunger to withdraw the fluid to check patency; repeat if tube remains sluggish

G. Removal of an NG tube: instruct client to exhale, and remove tube with one very smooth continuous pull

V. GI Tube Feedings

A. Tubes
   1. Nasogastric: Nose to stomach
   2. Nasoduodenal/nasojejunal: Nose to duodenum or jejunum
   3. Gastrostomy: Stomach
   4. Jejunostomy: Jejunum

B. Types of administration
   1. Bolus
      a. Resembles normal meal feeding patterns
      b. Approximately 300 to 400 mL of formula is administered over a 30- to 60-minute period every 3 to 6 hours
   2. Continuous
      a. Administered continuously for 24 hours
      b. An infusion pump regulates the flow
   3. Cyclical
      a. Administered either in the daytime or nighttime for 8 to 16 hours
      b. An infusion pump regulates the flow
      c. Feedings at night allow for more freedom during the day

C. Administering feedings
   1. Position client in high Fowler's and on right side if comatose
   2. Warm feeding to room temperature to prevent diarrhea and cramps
   3. Aspirate all stomach contents (residual), measure amount, and return contents to stomach to prevent electrolyte imbalances
   4. Usually if the residual is less than 100 to 150 mL, feeding is administered; if the residual is greater than 150 mL, hold the feeding
   5. Assess tube placement by aspirating gastric contents and measuring the pH (should be 4 or less)
   6. Assess bowel sounds, hold feeding, and notify physician if bowel sounds are absent
   7. Use a feeding pump for continuous or cyclic feedings
   8. Flush tubing with water following feeding to maintain fluid balance and patency of tube
   9. For bolus feeding, leave client in a high Fowler's position for 30 minutes after feeding

   10. For a continuous feeding, keep client in a 30° Fowler's position at all times

D. Precautions
   1. Change feeding container and tubing every 24 hours
   2. Do not hang more solution than will be required for a 4-hour period to prevent bacterial growth
   3. Check expiration date on the formula prior to administering
   4. Shake formula well prior to inserting into container
   5. Always assess placement of tube prior to feeding
   6. Always assess bowel sounds and do not administer any feedings if bowel sounds are absent
   7. If an obstruction occurs, try flushing with water, saline, cranberry juice, gingerale, or cola, if not contraindicated, after checking placement
   8. Add a drop of blue food coloring to the feeding, particularly with clients who have endotracheal or tracheal tubes
   9. Suspect tracheoesophageal fistula when blue gastric contents appear in tracheal excretion and, if this occurs, notify physician immediately
   10. Administer feeding at prescribed rate, or via gravity flow (intermittent, bolus feedings) with a 60-mL syringe with the plunger removed
   11. Gently flush with 30 to 50 mL of water or NS (depending on agency policy) with irrigation syringe after feeding

VI. Medications Via NG or Gastrostomy Tube

A. Crush medications or use elixir forms of medications
B. Ensure that the medication ordered can be crushed or that the capsule can be opened
C. Dissolve in 5 to 10 mL of water
D. Check placement and residual prior to instilling medications
E. Draw up the medication into a catheter-tip syringe, clear excess air, and insert medication into the tube
F. Flush with 30 mL of water (depending on agency policy)
G. Clamp tube for 30 to 60 minutes (depending on medication and agency policy)

VII. Intestinal Tubes

A. Description
   1. Passed nasally into small intestine
   2. Used to decompress the bowel or to remove intestinal contents
   3. Designed to enter the small intestine through the pyloric sphincter because of the weight of a small bag of mercury at the end

B. Types of Tubes
1. Cantor
   a. Single-lumen tube with a reservoir for 5 to 10 mL of mercury located at its tip, below the level of the drainage holes
   b. Mercury is inserted before the tube is passed through the nose, making the procedure uncomfortable
2. Miller-Abbott tube
   a. Double-lumen tube
   b. One lumen is for the instillation of mercury once the tube is in the stomach, and the other for irrigation or drainage

◆ C. Implementation
1. Assess physician's orders and agency policy for advancement and removal of tube
2. Position on right side to allow the mercury weights within the tube to facilitate passage through the pylorus of the stomach and into the small intestine
3. Do not secure tube to face with tape until it has reached final placement in the intestines
4. Allow tube to advance over several hours
5. Radiography is performed to verify desired placement
6. Monitor drainage from the tube
7. If the tube becomes blocked, notify the physician; a small amount of air injected into the lumen may be prescribed to clear the tube
8. Assess the abdomen and measure abdominal girth
9. In removal, to avoid pulling on the intestines remove the intestinal tube about 6 inches every 10 minutes as prescribed, until it reaches the stomach; then, withdraw as you would an NG tube
10. Dispose of the mercury in the appropriate manner as per agency policy

VIII. Esophageal and Gastric Tubes

A. Description
1. Used to apply pressure against esophageal veins to control bleeding
2. Not used if the client has ulceration or necrosis of the esophagus or had previous esophageal surgery
◆ B. Sengstaken-Blakemore tube
1. Triple-lumen gastric tube with an inflatable esophageal balloon, an inflatable gastric balloon, and a gastric aspiration lumen
2. The gastric balloon applies pressure at the cardioesophageal junction to decrease blood flow to **esophageal varices** and directly compresses gastric varices; traction is applied to maintain the gastric balloon in place
3. The esophageal balloon directly compresses **esophageal varices**
4. If bleeding is not stopped with inflation of the gastric balloon, the esophageal balloon is inflated to 25 to 45 mmHg

5. An x-ray film of the upper abdomen and chest confirms placement
6. Gastric contents are aspirated by gastric lavage or intermittent suction via the gastric aspiration port
7. With the Sengstaken-Blakemore tube, a nasogastric tube is also inserted in the opposite nares to collect secretions that accumulate above the esophageal balloon
C. Minnesota tube
1. Four-lumen gastric tube
2. A modified Sengstaken-Blakemore tube with an additional lumen for aspirating esophagopharyngeal secretions
D. Implementation
1. Check patency and integrity of all balloons prior to insertion
2. Label each lumen
3. Place the client in an upright or Fowler's position for insertion
4. Prepare for radiography immediately after insertion to verify placement
5. Maintain head elevation once tube is in place
6. Double-clamp the balloon ports to prevent air leaks
7. Keep scissors at the bedside at all times
8. Monitor for respiratory distress and, if it occurs, cut tubes to deflate balloons
9. Release esophageal pressure as prescribed and per agency policy to prevent ulceration or necrosis of the esophagus
10. Monitor for increased bloody drainage, which may indicate persistent bleeding
11. Monitor for signs of esophageal rupture, which includes a drop in blood pressure, increased heart rate, back and upper abdominal pain
12. Esophageal rupture is an emergency and must be reported to the physician immediately

IX. Lavage Tubes

A. Description: Used to remove toxic substances from the stomach
B. Types of tubes
1. Lavacuator
   a. An orogastric tube with a large suction lumen and a smaller lavage/vent lumen that provides continuous suction
   b. Irrigation solution enters the lavage lumen while stomach contents are removed through the suction lumen
2. Ewald: Reusable single-lumen large tube used for rapid one-time irrigation and evacuation

X. Hiatus Hernia

A. Description
1. Also known as esophageal or diaphragmatic hernia

2. A portion of the stomach herniates through the diaphragm and into the thorax
3. It results from weakening of the muscles of the diaphragm and is aggravated by factors that increase abdominal pressure, such as pregnancy, **ascites**, obesity, tumors, and heavy lifting
4. Complications include ulceration, hemorrhage, regurgitation and aspiration of stomach contents, and incarceration of the stomach in the chest with possible necrosis, peritonitis, and mediastinitis

B. Assessment
1. Heartburn
2. Feeling of fullness
3. Discomfort or pain
4. Regurgitation or vomiting
5. Dysphagia
6. Bleeding

C. Implementation
1. Provide small, frequent meals and minimize the amount of liquids
2. Elevate the head of the bed while eating and for 30 minutes after eating
3. Administer antacids after meals and at bedtime as prescribed to relieve heartburn and to increase lower esophageal sphincter pressure
4. Administer histamine H₂-receptor antagonists as prescribed to control esophageal reflux
5. Avoid anticholinergics, which delay stomach emptying
6. Instruct client to avoid vigorous coughing
7. Instruct client to avoid constrictive clothing around the waist
8. Instruct client to avoid sharp, forward bending
9. Instruct client to avoid highly seasoned and fatty foods
10. Instruct client to avoid alcohol, smoking, caffeine, chocolate, and carbonated and acidic beverages
11. Instruct client to avoid nighttime snacking to ensure that the stomach is empty
12. Encourage weight reduction, since obesity increases intra-abdominal pressure

D. Surgical implementation
1. Indicated when the risk of complications such as aspiration exists and damage from chronic reflux is severe
2. Surgical approaches include reinforcement of the lower esophageal sphincter (LES) to restore sphincter competence and prevent reflux
3. Achieved by a procedure that involves wrapping of a portion of the stomach fundus around the distal esophagus to anchor it and reinforce the LES

XI. Esophageal Varices

A. Description

1. Dilated and tortuous veins in the submucosa of the esophagus
2. They are caused by **portal hypertension**, are often associated with liver **cirrhosis**, and are at high risk for rupture if portal circulation pressure rises
3. Bleeding varices is an emergency
4. The goal of treatment is to control bleeding, prevent complications, and prevent the recurrence of a bleed

B. Assessment
1. Hematemesis
2. Melena
3. Tarry stools
4. **Ascites**
5. Jaundice
6. Hepatomegaly and splenomegaly
7. Dilated abdominal veins
8. Hemorrhoids
9. Bleeding and shock

C. Implementation
1. Monitor vital signs
2. Elevate the head of the bed
3. Monitor for orthostatic hypotension
4. Monitor lung sounds and for the presence of respiratory distress
5. Administer oxygen as prescribed to prevent tissue hypoxia
6. Maintain NPO status
7. Monitor level of consciousness (LOC)
8. Monitor intake and output (I&O)
9. Administer IV fluids as prescribed to restore fluid volume and electrolyte imbalances
10. Monitor hemoglobin, hematocrit, and coagulation factors
11. Administer blood or clotting factors as prescribed
12. Assist in inserting a nasogastric tube or a balloon tamponade as prescribed
13. Assist with the administration of iced saline irrigations to achieve vasoconstriction of the varices
14. Prepare to assist with administering vasopressin (Pitressin) by IV or intra-arterial infusion as prescribed to induce vasoconstriction and reduce bleeding
15. Prepare to assist with administering nitroglycerin (Tridil) with the vasopressin to prevent vasoconstriction of coronary arteries
16. Instruct client to avoid activities that will initiate vasovagal responses
17. Prepare client for endoscopic procedures or surgical procedures as prescribed

D. Endoscopic injection (sclerotherapy)
1. Injection of a sclerosing agent into and around bleeding varices
2. Complications include chest pain, pleural effusion, aspiration pneumonia, esophageal stricture, and perforation of the esophagus

E. Endoscopic variceal ligation
1. Ligation of the varices with an elastic rubber band

2. Sloughing, followed by superficial ulceration, occurs in the area of ligation within 3 to 7 days

F. Surgical shunt procedures
1. Splenorenal: Involves splenectomy, with anastomosis of the splenic vein to the left renal vein
2. Portacaval: Shunting of the blood from the portal vein to the inferior vena cava
3. Mesocaval: Involves a side anastomosis of the superior mesenteric vein to the proximal end of the inferior vena cava
4. Transjugular intrahepatic portal/systemic
   a. Uses the normal vascular anatomy of the liver to create a shunt with the use of a metallic stent
   b. The shunt is between the portal and systemic venous system within the liver and is aimed at relieving **portal hypertension**

XII. Peptic Ulcer Disease

A. Description
1. An ulceration in the mucosal wall of the stomach, pylorus, or duodenum in portions that are accessible to gastric secretions
2. Erosion may extend through the muscle to the peritoneum
3. The most common peptic ulcers are gastric ulcers and duodenal ulcers

B. Gastric ulcers
1. Description
   a. Involves ulceration of the mucosal lining that extends to the submucosal layer of the stomach
   b. Predisposing factors include stress, smoking, the use of steroids, nonsteroidal anti-inflammatory drugs (NSAIDs), alcohol, a history of gastritis, family history of gastric ulcers, or infection with *Helicobacter pylori*
   c. Complications include hemorrhage, perforation, and pyloric obstruction
2. Assessment
   a. Gnawing, sharp pain in or left of the midepigastric region 1 to 2 hours after eating
   b. Nausea and vomiting
   c. Hematemesis
3. Implementation
   a. Monitor vital signs
   b. Monitor for bleeding
   c. Administer small, frequent bland feedings during the active phase
   d. Administer histamine H_2-receptor antagonists as prescribed to decrease the secretion of gastric acid
   e. Administer antacids as prescribed to neutralize gastric secretions
   f. Administer anticholinergics as prescribed to reduce gastric motility

g. Administer mucosal barrier protectants as prescribed 1 hour before each meal
h. Administer prostaglandins as prescribed for their protective and antisecretory actions
i. Instruct client to avoid alcohol
j. Instruct client to avoid caffeine and chocolate
k. Instruct client to avoid smoking
l. Instruct client to avoid aspirin or NSAIDs
m. Instruct client to obtain adequate rest and reduce stress

4. Implementation during active bleeding
   a. Monitor vital signs
   b. Assess for signs of dehydration, hypovolemic shock, sepsis, and respiratory insufficiency
   c. Monitor I&O
   d. Maintain NPO status and administer IV fluid replacement as prescribed
   e. Monitor hemoglobin and hematocrit
   f. Administer blood transfusion as prescribed
   g. Assist with insertion of an NG tube for decompression and for lavage access
   h. Assist with normal saline or tap water lavage at room temperature to reduce active bleeding
   i. Prepare to assist with administering vasopressin (Pitressin) by IV as prescribed to induce vasoconstriction and reduce bleeding

5. Estimating the amount of blood loss
   a. Less than 500 mL: Pulse rate begins to rise
   b. 500 to 1000 mL: Pulse increases to 100 to 110, blood pressure (BP) begins to decrease, urine output declines, and signs of shock are present
   c. 1000 to 2000 mL: Pulse increases beyond 110 to 120, and BP continues to decrease
   d. More than 2000 mL: Pulse increases beyond 120, and BP and urine output decline significantly

6. Surgical implementation
   a. Total **gastrectomy**: Also called esophagojejunostomy; removal of the stomach with attachment of the esophagus to the jejunum or duodenum
   b. **Vagotomy**: Surgical division of the vagus nerve to eliminate the vagal impulses that stimulate hydrochloric acid secretion in the stomach
   c. **Gastric resection**: Also called antrectomy; involves removal of the lower half of the stomach and usually includes a **vagotomy**
   d. **Billroth I**: Also called gastroduodenostomy; partial **gastrectomy**, with the remaining segment anastomosed to the duodenum
   e. **Billroth II**: Also called gastrojejunostomy; partial **gastrectomy**, with the remaining segment anastomosed to the jejunum
   f. **Pyloroplasty**: Enlarges the pylorus to

prevent or decrease pyloric obstruction, thereby enhancing gastric emptying

7. Postoperative implementation
   a. Monitor vital signs
   b. Position in Fowler's for comfort and to promote drainage
   c. Monitor I&O
   d. Administer fluids and electrolyte replacements IV as prescribed
   e. Assess bowel sounds
   f. Monitor NG suction as prescribed
   g. Do not irrigate the NG tube or remove it
   h. Assist physician with NG irrigation or removal of NG tube
   i. Maintain NPO status as prescribed for 1 to 3 days until **peristalsis** returns
   j. Progress the diet from NPO to sips of clear water to 6 small bland meals a day as prescribed when bowel sounds return
   k. Monitor for postoperative complications of hemorrhage, **dumping syndrome**, diarrhea, hypoglycemia, and vitamin B_{12} deficiency

XIII. Duodenal Ulcers

A. Description
   1. A break in the mucosa of the duodenum
   2. Risk factors and causes include alcohol intake, smoking, stress, caffeine, the use of aspirin, corticosteroids and NSAIDs, and infection with *Helicobacter pylori*
   3. The goals of treatment are to eliminate the cause, decrease gastric acidity, and prevent complications
   4. Complications include bleeding, perforation, gastric outlet obstruction, and intractable disease
B. Assessment
   1. Burning pain in the midepigastric area 2 to 4 hours after eating and during the night
   2. Pain that is often relieved by eating
   3. Melena
C. Implementation
   1. Monitor vital signs
   2. Perform abdominal assessment
   3. Instruct client in a bland diet with small frequent meals
   4. Provide for adequate rest
   5. Encourage the cessation of smoking
   6. Instruct client to avoid alcohol intake, caffeine, the use of aspirin, corticosteroids, and NSAIDs
   7. Administer antacids as prescribed to neutralize acid secretions
   8. Administer histamine H_2-receptor antagonists as prescribed to block the secretion of acid
D. Surgical implementation: Surgery is performed only if the ulcer is unresponsive to medications or if hemorrhage, obstruction, or perforation occurs

XIV. Dumping Syndrome

A. Description
   1. Rapid emptying of the gastric contents into the small intestine
   2. Occurs following **gastric resection**.
B. Assessment
   1. Symptoms occurring 30 minutes after eating
   2. Nausea and vomiting
   3. Abdominal cramping
   4. Feelings of fullness
   5. Diarrhea
   6. Palpitation
   7. Tachycardia
   8. Perspiration
   9. Weakness and dizziness
   10. Borborygmi
C. Implementation
   1. Instruct client to eat a high-protein, high-fat, low-carbohydrate diet
   2. Instruct client to eat small meals and to avoid fluids with meals
   3. Instruct client to avoid sugar and salt
   4. Instruct client to lie down after meals
   5. Instruct client to take sedatives and antispasmodic medications as prescribed to delay gastric emptying

XV. Vitamin B_{12} Deficiency

A. Description
   1. Results from either an inadequate intake of vitamin B_{12} or a lack of absorption of ingested vitamin B_{12} from the intestinal tract
   2. Pernicious anemia results from a deficiency of intrinsic factor, which is necessary for intestinal absorption of vitamin B_{12}
B. Assessment
   1. Severe pallor
   2. Fatigue
   3. Weight loss
   4. Smooth, beefy red tongue
   5. Slight jaundice
   6. Paresthesias of the hands and feet
   7. Disturbances with gait and balance
C. Implementation
   1. Increase dietary intake of food rich in vitamin B_{12} if the anemia is the result of a dietary deficiency (Box 53–2)
   2. Administer vitamin B_{12} injections as prescribed on a weekly basis initially and then monthly for maintenance (lifelong) if the anemia is the result of a deficiency of the intrinsic factor

BOX 53–2. Foods Rich in Vitamin B_{12}	
Liver	Green leafy vegetables
Organ meats	Citrus fruits
Dried beans	Brewer's yeast
Nuts	

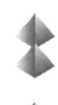

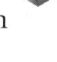

XVI. Gastric Cancer

A. Description
1. An abnormal, malignant growth in the abdomen
2. Risk factors include a diet high in starch and salt and low in fresh, green leafy vegetables and fresh fruit; smoking; alcohol; a history of gastric ulcers, and the presence of *Helicobacter pylori*
3. Complications include hemorrhage, obstruction, metastasis, and **dumping syndrome**
4. The goal of treatment is to remove the tumor and provide a nutritional program

B. Assessment
1. Anorexia
2. Nausea and vomiting
3. Indigestion and epigastric discomfort
4. A sensation of pressure
5. Dysphagia
6. Weight loss
7. Palpable mass
8. Fatigue
9. Anemia
10. **Ascites**

C. Implementation
1. Monitor vital signs
2. Assess nutritional status
3. Encourage small, bland, easily digestible meals, with vitamin and mineral supplements
4. Monitor weight
5. Administer pain medication as prescribed
6. Monitor hemoglobin and hematocrit and administer blood transfusion as prescribed
7. Provide emotional support
8. Prepare the client for chemotherapy or radiation therapy as prescribed
9. Prepare the client for surgical resection of the tumor as prescribed (Box 53–3)

D. Postoperative implementation
1. Monitor vital signs
2. Position in Fowler's for comfort and to promote drainage
3. Monitor I&O
4. Administer fluids and electrolyte replacements IV as prescribed
5. Assess bowel sounds
6. Monitor NG suction as prescribed
7. Do not irrigate or remove NG tube
8. Assist physician with NG irrigation or removal of NG tube
9. Maintain NPO status as prescribed for 1 to 3 days until **peristalsis** returns

---

BOX 53–3. Surgical Treatment for Gastric Cancer

Total gastrectomy	Billroth I
Vagotomy	Billroth II
Gastric resection	Pyloroplasty

---

10. Progress the diet from NPO to sips of clear water to 6 small bland meals a day as prescribed when bowel sounds return
11. Monitor for postoperative complications of hemorrhage, **dumping syndrome**, diarrhea, hypoglycemia, and vitamin B_{12} deficiency

XVII. Ulcerative Colitis

A. Description
1. Ulcerative and inflammatory disease of the bowel that results in poor absorption of nutrients
2. Commonly begins in the rectum and spreads upward toward the cecum
3. The colon becomes edematous and may develop bleeding lesions and ulcers
4. The ulcers may lead to perforation
5. Scar tissue develops and causes loss of elasticity and loss of ability to absorb nutrients
6. Characterized by various periods of remissions and exacerbations
7. Acute **ulcerative colitis** results in vascular congestion, hemorrhage, edema, and ulceration of the bowel mucosa
8. Chronic **ulcerative colitis** causes muscular hypertrophy, fat deposits, and fibrous tissue, with bowel thickening, shortening, and narrowing

B. Assessment
1. Anorexia
2. Weight loss
3. Malaise
4. Abdominal tenderness and cramping
5. Severe diarrhea that may contain blood and mucus
6. Dehydration and electrolyte imbalances
7. Anemia
8. Vitamin K deficiency

C. Implementation
1. Maintain NPO status and administer IVs and electrolytes as prescribed during the acute phase
2. Administer total parenteral nutrition (TPN) as prescribed during an acute phase
3. Restrict the client's activity, to reduce intestinal activity
4. Monitor bowel sounds
5. Monitor for abdominal tenderness and cramping
6. Monitor stools, noting color, consistency, and the presence or absence of blood
7. Monitor for perforation, peritonitis, and hemorrhage
8. Following the acute phase, the diet progresses from clear liquids to low residue as tolerated
9. Instruct client to consume a low-roughage, low-residue diet and to avoid such foods as whole wheat grains, nuts, raw fruits, and vegetables

10. Instruct client to avoid gas-forming foods and milk products
11. Instruct client to chew solid foods thoroughly
12. Instruct client to avoid caffeinated beverages, alcohol, and pepper
13. Encourage client to stop smoking
14. Administer antidiarrheal medications as prescribed
15. Administer antimicrobials, corticosteroids, and immunosuppressants as prescribed to prevent infection and reduce inflammation

D. Surgical implementation
1. Total proctocolectomy with permanent ileostomy
   a. Involves removal of the colon, rectum, and anus, with anal closure
   b. The end of the terminal ileum forms the stoma, which is located in the right lower quadrant
2. **Kock pouch** (ileostomy)
   a. An intra-abdominal pouch is constructed from the terminal ileum
   b. The pouch is connected to the stoma with a nipple-like valve constructed from a portion of the ileum
   c. The stoma is flush with the skin
3. Ileoanal reservoir
   a. A two-stage procedure that involves excision of the rectal mucosa, abdominal colectomy, construction of the reservoir to the anal canal, and a temporary loop ileostomy
   b. The ileostomy is closed in approximately 4 months after the capacity of the reservoir is increased
4. Preoperative colostomy/ileostomy
   a. Consult with the enterostomal therapist to assist in identifying optimal placement of the ostomy
   b. Instruct client to eat a low-residue diet for a day or two prior to surgery as prescribed
   c. Administer intestinal antiseptics and antibiotics as prescribed to cleanse the bowel and to decrease the bacterial content of the colon
   d. Administer laxatives and enemas as prescribed
5. Postoperative colostomy
   a. Place a petrolatum gauze over the stoma as prescribed to keep it moist, followed by a dry sterile dressing if a pouch system is not in place
   b. Place a pouch system on the stoma as soon as possible
   c. Monitor the stoma for size, unusual bleeding, or necrotic tissue
   d. Monitor for color changes in the stoma
   e. Note that the normal stoma color is red or pink, indicating high vascularity

f. Note that a pale pink stoma indicates low hemoglobin and hematocrit levels and a purple-black stoma indicates compromised circulation, requiring physician notification
g. Assess the functioning of the colostomy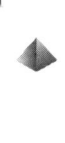
h. Expect that stool is liquid immediately postoperative but becomes more solid depending on the area of the colostomy: ascending colon—liquid stool; transverse colon—loose to semiformed; descending colon—close to normal
i. Monitor the pouch system for proper fit and signs of leakage
j. Empty pouch when one third full
k. Fecal matter should not be allowed to remain on skin
l. Administer analgesics and antibiotics as prescribed
m. Irrigate the perineal wound if present as prescribed and monitor for signs of infection
n. Instruct the client to avoid foods that cause excess gas formation and odor
o. Instruct client on stoma care and irrigations as prescribed (Box 53–4)
p. Instruct client that normal activities may be resumed when approved by the physician
6. Postoperative ileostomy
   a. Note that the healthy stoma is red
   b. Monitor for color change in the stoma to dark blue or black; if it occurs, it should be reported to the physician
   c. Note that normal stool is liquid
   d. Monitor for dehydration and electrolyte imbalance
   e. Do not give suppositories through the ileostomy

BOX 53–4. Colostomy Irrigation

DESCRIPTION

Instilling 500 to 1000 mL of tepid H_2O through the stoma and allowing H_2O and stool to drain into the collection bag

PROCEDURE

If ambulatory, position the client sitting on toilet
If on bed rest, position client on side
Hang the irrigation bag so that the bottom of the bag is at the level of the client's shoulder, or slightly higher
Insert the irrigation tube carefully without force
Begin the flow of irrigation
Clamp tubing if cramping occurs; release tubing as cramping subsides
Avoid frequent irrigations with H_2O, which can lead to loss of fluids and electrolytes
Perform irrigation around the same time each day
Perform irrigation preferably 1 hour after a meal

XVIII. Crohn's Disease (Regional Enteritis)

A. Description
1. An inflammatory disease that can occur anywhere in the GI tract but most often affects the terminal ileum and leads to thickening and scarring, a narrowed lumen, fistulas, ulcerations, and abscesses
2. It is characterized by remissions and exacerbations

B. Assessment
1. Fever
2. Cramplike pain after meals
3. Diarrhea semisolid and may contain mucus, pus, and blood
4. Abdominal distention
5. Anorexia, nausea, and vomiting
6. Weight loss
7. Anemia
8. Dehydration
9. Electrolyte imbalances

C. Implementation: Care is similar to that of the client with **ulcerative colitis**

XIX. Intestinal Tumors

A. Description
1. Malignant lesions that develop in the cells lining the bowel wall or develop as polyps in the colon or rectum
2. Complications include bowel perforation with peritonitis, abscess and/or fistula formation, frank hemorrhage, and complete intestinal obstruction
3. Metastasis occurs via the circulatory or lymphatic system or by direct extension to other areas in the colon or other organs

B. Assessment
1. Blood in stools
2. Abnormal stools
3. Anorexia
4. Vomiting
5. Weight loss
6. Malaise
7. Anemia
8. Ascending colon tumor—diarrhea
9. Descending colon tumor—constipation or some diarrhea, or flat, ribbon-shaped stool due to a partial obstruction
10. Rectal tumor—alternating constipation and diarrhea
11. Guarding or abdominal distention
12. Abdominal mass (a late sign)
13. Cachexia (a late sign)

C. Implementation
1. Monitor for signs of complications, which include bowel perforation with peritonitis, abscess and/or fistula formation, frank hemorrhage, and complete intestinal obstruction
2. Monitor for signs of intestinal perforation, including low BP, rapid weak pulse, distended abdomen, and elevated temperature

3. Monitor for signs of intestinal obstruction, which may include vomiting (may be fecal contents), pain, constipation, and abdominal distention
4. Note that an early sign of intestinal obstruction includes increased peristaltic activity, which produces an increase in bowel sounds, and as the obstruction progresses, hypoactive sounds

D. Nonsurgical implementation
1. Radiation preoperatively to facilitate surgical resection and postoperatively to decrease the risk of recurrence or to reduce pain, hemorrhage, bowel obstruction, or metastasis
2. Chemotherapy used postoperatively to assist in the control of symptoms and spread of the disease

E. Surgical implementation: Bowel resection and creation of colostomy or ileostomy

XX. Diverticulosis and Diverticulitis

A. Description
1. **Diverticulosis**
   a. Outpouching or herniations of the intestinal mucosa
   b. They can occur in any part of the intestine but are most common in the sigmoid colon
2. **Diverticulitis**
   a. Inflammation of one or more diverticuli
   b. Results when a diverticulum perforates, with local abscess formation
   c. A perforated diverticulum can progress to intra-abdominal perforation with generalized peritonitis

B. Assessment
1. Left lower quadrant abdominal pain that increases with coughing, straining, or lifting
2. Elevated temperature
3. Nausea and vomiting
4. Flatulence
5. Cramplike pain
6. Abdominal distention and tenderness
7. Palpable, tender rectal mass
8. Blood in stools

C. Implementation
1. Provide bed rest during the acute phase
2. Maintain NPO status or provide clear liquids during the acute phase as prescribed
3. Introduce a fiber-containing diet gradually, when the inflammation is resolved
4. Instruct client to refrain from lifting, straining, coughing, or bending to avoid increased intra-abdominal pressure
5. Administer antibiotics and pain medication as prescribed
6. Monitor for perforation, hemorrhage, fistulas, abscesses
7. Instruct client on the signs and symptoms of diverticular disease, such as fever, abdominal pain, and bloody stools
8. Instruct client to eat a diet high in cellulose,

such as wheat bran, whole grains, and cereals

9. Instruct client to eat fruits and vegetables with high fiber content and to avoid foods containing indigestible roughage or seeds

10. Instruct client to avoid gas-forming foods, hot and cold liquids, and alcohol

11. Instruct client to avoid enemas and laxatives other than bulk-forming products such as psyllium (Metamucil)

D. Surgical implementation
1. Colon resection with primary anastomosis
2. Temporary or permanent colostomy may be required for increased bowel inflammation

XXI. Hemorrhoids

A. Description
1. Dilated varicose veins of the anal canal
2. May be either internal, external, or prolapsed
3. Internal hemorrhoids lie above the anal sphincter and cannot be seen upon inspection of the perianal area
4. External hemorrhoids lie below the anal sphincter and can be seen on inspection
5. Prolapsed hemorrhoids can become thrombosed or inflamed
6. Hemorrhoids are caused from **portal hypertension**, straining, irritation, increased venous or abdominal pressure

B. Assessment
1. Bright red rectal bleeding
2. Pain associated with thrombosis
3. Rectal itching
4. Mucous rectal discharge

C. Implementation
1. Apply cold packs to the anal/rectal area, followed by sitz baths as prescribed
2. Apply witch hazel soaks and topical anesthetics as prescribed
3. Encourage a high-fiber diet and fluids to promote bowel movements without straining
4. Administer stool softeners as prescribed

D. Endoscopic procedures
1. Sclerotherapy
2. Endoscopic ligation

E. Surgical procedures
1. Cryosurgery
2. Hemorrhoidectomy

F. Postoperative implementation
1. Assist client to prone or side-lying position to prevent bleeding
2. Maintain ice packs over dressing as prescribed until the packing is removed by the physician
3. Monitor for urinary retention
4. Administer stool softeners as prescribed
5. Instruct client to increase fluids and fiber foods
6. Instruct client to limit sitting to short periods
7. Instruct the client in the use of sitz baths three to four times a day as prescribed

XXII. Appendicitis

A. Description
1. Inflammation of the appendix
2. When the appendix becomes inflamed or infected, rupture may occur within a matter of hours, leading to peritonitis and sepsis

B. Assessment
1. Pain in periumbilical area that descends to the right lower quadrant
2. Abdominal pain that is most intense at McBurney's point
3. Rebound tenderness and abdominal rigidity
4. Low-grade fever
5. Elevated white blood cell (WBC) count
6. Anorexia, nausea, and vomiting
7. Client in side-lying position, with abdominal guarding and legs flexed
8. Constipation or diarrhea

C. Peritonitis: Inflammation of the peritoneum
1. Increased fever and chills
2. Progressive abdominal distention and abdominal pain
3. Right guarding of abdomen
4. Tachycardia and tachypnea
5. Pallor
6. Restlessness

D. Appendectomy: Surgical removal of the appendix
1. Preoperative implementation
a. Maintain NPO status
b. Administer IV fluids to prevent dehydration
c. Monitor for changes in level of pain
d. Monitor for signs of ruptured appendix and peritonitis
e. Position right side-lying or low to semi-Fowler's position to promote comfort
f. Monitor bowel sounds
g. Apply ice packs to abdomen for 20 to 30 minutes every hour
h. Administer antibiotics as prescribed
i. Avoid application of heat to abdomen
j. Avoid laxatives or enemas
2. Postoperative implementation
a. Monitor temperature for signs of infection
b. Assess incision for signs of infection such as redness, swelling, and pain
c. Maintain NPO status until bowel function has returned
d. Advance diet gradually as tolerated when bowel sounds return
e. If rupture of the appendix has occurred, expect a Penrose drain to be inserted, or the incision may be left open to heal from the inside out
f. Expect that drainage from the Penrose drain may be profuse for the first 12 hours
g. Position client in right side-lying or low to semi-Fowler's position, with legs flexed, to facilitate drainage
h. Change dressing as prescribed
i. Record type and amount of drainage

    j. Perform wound irrigations if prescribed

    k. Maintain NG suction and patency of NG tube if present

    l. Administer antibiotics and analgesics as prescribed

XXIII. Cirrhosis (Box 53–5)

A. Description

    1. A chronic, progressive disease of the liver, characterized by diffuse damage to cells with fibrosis and nodular regeneration

    2. Repeated destruction of hepatic cells causes the formation of scar tissue

B. Complications

    1. **Portal hypertension**: A persistent increase in pressure within the portal vein that develops as a result of obstruction to flow

    2. **Ascites**

      a. The accumulation of fluid within the peritoneal cavity that results in venous congestion of the hepatic capillaries

      b. This leads to plasma leaking directly from the liver surface and portal vein

    3. Bleeding **esophageal varices**: Fragile, thin-walled, distended esophageal veins that become irritated and rupture

    4. Coagulation defects

      a. Decreased synthesis of bile fats in the liver prevent the absorption of fat-soluble vitamins

      b. Without vitamin K and clotting factors II, VII, IX, and X, the client is prone to bleeding

    5. Jaundice: Occurs because the liver is unable to metabolize bilirubin and because the edema, fibrosis, and scarring of the hepatic bile ducts interfere with normal bile and bilirubin secretion

    6. Portal systemic encephalopathy: End stage hepatic failure and **cirrhosis**, characterized by altered LOC, neurologic symptoms, impaired thinking, and neuromuscular disturbances

    7. Hepatorenal syndrome

      a. Progressive renal failure associated with hepatic failure

      b. Characterized by a sudden decrease in urinary output, elevated BUN and creatinine, decreased urine sodium excretion, and increased urine osmolarity

C. Assessment

    1. Anorexia and weight loss

    2. Early morning nausea and vomiting

    3. Dyspepsia

    4. Flatulence and changes in bowel habits

    5. Emaciation

    6. Fatigue

    7. Jaundice

    8. Abdominal pain or tenderness

    9. **Ascites**

    10. Peripheral edema

    11. Dry skin and rashes

    12. Petechiae or ecchymosis

    13. Spider angiomas on the nose, cheeks, upper thorax, and shoulders

    14. Hepatomegaly

    15. Protruding umbilicus

    16. Dilated abdominal veins

    17. Presence of blood in vomitus

    18. **Fetor hepaticus,** the fruity, musty breath odor of chronic liver disease

    19. Amenorrhea and testicular atrophy

    20. Gynecomastia

    21. Impotence

    22. **Asterixis** (liver flap): A coarse tremor characterized by rapid, nonrhythmic extensions and flexions in the wrist and fingers

    23. Delirium

D. Implementation

    1. Elevate head of bed to minimize shortness of breath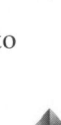

    2. Provide a low-sodium diet initially, restricting daily sodium to 200 to 500 mg and restricting daily protein to 50 to 60 g (to reduce excess protein breakdown by intestinal bacteria), as prescribed

    3. Provide supplemental vitamins with thiamine, folate, and multivitamins, as prescribed

    4. Initiate TPN as prescribed

    5. Restrict fluid intake to 1500 mL daily as prescribed

    6. Administer diuretics as prescribed

    7. Monitor I&O

    8. Monitor electrolyte balance

    9. Weigh client and measure abdominal girth daily

BOX 53–5. Types of Cirrhosis

LAENNEC'S CIRRHOSIS

Alcohol-induced, nutritional, or portal cirrhosis
Cellular necrosis causes eventual widespread scar tissue, with fibrotic infiltration of the liver

POSTNECROTIC CIRRHOSIS

Occurs after massive liver necrosis
Results as a complication of acute viral hepatitis or exposure to hepatotoxins
Scar tissue causes destruction of liver lobules and entire lobes

BILIARY CIRRHOSIS

Develops from chronic biliary obstruction, bile stasis, and inflammation resulting in severe obstructive jaundice

CARDIAC CIRRHOSIS

Associated with severe, right-sided congestive heart failure (CHF) and results in an enlarged, edematous, congested liver
The liver becomes anoxic, resulting in liver cell necrosis and fibrosis

10. Monitor LOC
11. Assess for precoma state (tremors, delirium)
12. Monitor for **asterixis**
13. Maintain gastric intubation to assess bleeding
14. Maintain esophagogastric balloon tamponade to control bleeding varices if prescribed
15. Administer blood products as prescribed
16. Monitor coagulation laboratory results
17. Administer vitamin K if prescribed
18. Avoid hepatotoxin intake
19. Instruct client to restrict alcohol
20. Administer low-sodium antacids as prescribed
21. Administer lactulose (Chronulac), which decreases the pH of the bowel, decreases production of ammonia by bacteria in the bowel, and facilitates the excretion of ammonia
22. Administer neomycin (Mycifradin) as prescribed to inhibit protein synthesis in bateria and decrease production of ammonia
23. Avoid medications such as narcotics, sedatives, and barbiturates
24. Prepare client for paracentesis to remove abdominal fluid
25. Prepare client for surgical shunting procedures if prescribed

XXIV. Cholecystitis

A. Description
1. An inflammation of the gallbladder that may occur as an acute or chronic process
2. Acute inflammation is associated with gallstones (cholelithiasis)
3. Chronic **cholecystitis** results when inefficient bile emptying and gallbladder muscle wall disease cause a fibrotic and contracted gallbladder
4. A calculous **cholecystitis** occurs in the absence of gallstones and is due to bacterial invasion via the lymphatic or vascular systems

B. Assessment
1. Nausea and vomiting
2. Indigestion
3. Belching
4. Flatulence
5. Epigastric pain that radiates to the scapula 2 to 4 hours after eating fatty foods and may persist for 4 to 6 hours
6. Pain localized in right upper quadrant
7. Guarding, rigidity, and rebound tenderness
8. Mass palpated in the right upper quadrant
9. **Murphy's sign** (cannot take a deep breath when examiner's fingers are passed below hepatic margin)
10. Elevated temperature
11. Tachycardia
12. Signs of dehydration

C. Biliary obstruction
1. Jaundice
2. Dark orange and foamy urine
3. Steatorrhea and clay-colored feces
4. Pruritus

D. Implementation
1. Maintain NPO status during nausea and vomiting episodes
2. Maintain nasogastric decompression as prescribed for severe vomiting
3. Administer analgesics as prescribed to relieve pain and reduce spasm (note: morphine or codeine may cause spasm of the sphincter of Oddi and increase pain)
4. Administer antispasmodics (anticholinergics) as prescribed to relax smooth muscle
5. Administer antiemetics as prescribed for nausea and vomiting
6. Instruct clients with chronic cholecystitis to eat more frequent low-fat meals in small amounts
7. Instruct client to avoid gas-forming foods
8. Prepare client for nonsurgical and surgical procedures as prescribed

E. Nonsurgical implementation
1. Dissolution therapy
   a. To remove cholesterol stones
   b. Chenodeoxycholic acid (Chenodiol) or ursodiol (Actigall) is administered PO to decrease size of stones or to dissolve small stones
   c. Direct contact with repeated injections and aspirations of a dissolution agent via percutaneous catheter may be performed
2. Extracorporeal shock wave lithotripsy
   a. Shock waves are administered that disintegrate stones in the biliary system
   b. Oral dissolution follows

F. Surgical implementation
1. **Cholecystectomy:** Removal of the gallbladder
2. **Choledochotomy:** Incision into the common bile duct to remove the stone

G. Postoperative implementation
1. Monitor for respiratory complications secondary to pain at incision site
2. Encourage coughing and deep breathing
3. Encourage early ambulation
4. Instruct client about splinting abdomen to prevent discomfort during coughing
5. Administer antiemetics as prescribed for nausea and vomiting
6. Administer analgesics as prescribed for pain relief
7. Maintain NPO status as prescribed for 24 to 48 hours
8. Maintain NG tube suction as prescribed
9. Advance diet from clear liquids to solids when prescribed and as tolerated by the client
10. Maintain T tube (Box 53–6)

XXV. Pancreatitis

A. Description
1. An acute or chronic inflammation of the

BOX 53–6. Care of a T Tube

DESCRIPTION

- Surgically inserted to decompress biliary tree and maintain patency of the bile duct

IMPLEMENTATION

- Position client in semi-Fowler's to facilitate drainage
- Monitor the amount, color, consistency, and odor of drainage
- Monitor for inflammation and protect the skin from irritation
- Collect and administer excess bile output to the client via NG tube or administer synthetic bile salts as prescribed
- Keep the drainage system below the level of the gallbaldder
- Report sudden increases in bile output to the physician
- Monitor for foul odor and purulent drainage and report to the physician
- Avoid irrigation, aspiration, or clamping of the T tube without a physician's order
- As prescribed, clamp tube before eating, and observe for abdominal discomfort and distention, nausea, chills, or fever
- Unclamp tube if nausea or vomiting occurs

---

pancreas with associated escape of pancreatic enzymes into surrounding tissue

2. Acute **pancreatitis** occurs suddenly as one attack or can be recurrent, but resolves
3. Chronic **pancreatitis** is a continual inflammation and destruction of the pancreas, with scar tissue replacing pancreatic tissue
4. Precipitating factors include trauma, the use of alcohol, biliary tract disease, viral or bacterial disease, hyperlipidemia, hypercalcemia, cholelithiasis, hyperparathyroidism, ischemic vascular disease, and peptic ulcer disease

B. Acute
  1. Assessment
     a. Abdominal pain, including a sudden onset midepigastric or left upper quadrant location with radiation to the back
     b. Pain that is aggravated by a fatty meal, alcohol, or lying in a recumbent position
     c. Abdominal tenderness and guarding
     d. Nausea and vomiting
     e. Weight loss
     f. **Cullen's sign** (discoloration of the abdomen and periumbilical area)
     g. **Turner's sign** (bluish discoloration of the flanks)
     h. Absent or decreased bowel sounds
     i. Elevated temperature
     j. Hypotension
     k. Tachycardia

  l. Elevated WBC, glucose, bilirubin, alkaline phosphatase, urinary amylase
  m. Elevated lipase and amylase
  n. Abnormally low calcium, sodium, and magnesium owing to dehydration

  2. Implementation
     a. Maintain NPO status and maintain hydration with IV fluids
     b. Administer TPN for severe nutritional depletion
     c. Provide small, frequent high-carbohydrate, high-protein and low-fat foods when prescribed and when tolerated by the client
     d. Administer supplemental preparations and vitamins and minerals to increase caloric intake if prescribed
     e. Maintain NG tube to decrease gastric distention and suppress pancreatic secretion
     f. Administer meperidine hydrochloride (Demerol) as prescribed for pain because it causes less incidence of smooth muscle spasm of the pancreatic ducts and sphincter of Oddi (note: avoid morphine or codeine, which may cause spasms)
     g. Administer antacids as prescribed to neutralize gastric secretions
     h. Administer histamine receptor–blocking medications as prescribed to decrease hydrochloric acid production so pancreatic enzymes are not activated
     i. Administer anticholinergics as prescribed to decrease vagal stimulation, decrease GI motility, and inhibit pancreatic enzyme secretion
     j. Instruct client in the importance of avoiding alcohol
     k. Instruct client in the importance of follow-up visits with the physician
     l. Instruct client to notify physician for acute abdominal pain, jaundice, clay-colored stools, and dark urine

C. Chronic
  1. Assessment
     a. Abdominal pain as continuous burning or gnawing, dullness with intense exacerbations
     b. Abdominal tenderness
     c. Left upper quadrant mass
     d. Steatorrhea and foul-smelling stools that may increase in volume as pancreatic insufficiency increases
     e. Weight loss
     f. Muscle wasting
     g. Jaundice
     h. Signs and symptoms of diabetes
  2. Implementation
     a. Administer meperidine hydrochloride (Demerol) as prescribed for pain because it causes less incidence of smooth muscle spasm of the pancreatic ducts and

sphincter of Oddi (note: avoid morphine or codeine, which may cause spasms)

b. Maintain NPO status to avoid pain caused by eating

c. Administer TPN for nutritional depletion as prescribed

d. Provide small, frequent high-carbohydrate, high-protein and low-fat diet when prescribed as tolerated by the client

e. Provide supplemental preparations and vitamins and minerals to increase caloric intake

f. Administer pancreatic enzymes as prescribed to aid in digestion and absorption of fat and protein

g. Administer insulin or oral hypoglycemic medications as prescribed to control diabetes

h. Instruct client to avoid alcohol, caffeinated beverages, rich fatty foods

i. Instruct client in the use of pancreatic enzyme medications

j. Instruct client in the treatment plan for glucose management

k. Instruct client to notify physician if increased steatorrhea occurs or if abdominal distention, cramping, or skin breakdown develops

l. Instruct client in the importance of follow-up visits

PRACTICE QUESTIONS

1. The nurse has inserted a nasogastric tube to the level of the oropharynx and has repositioned the client's head in a flexed-forward position. The client has been asked to begin swallowing. The nurse starts to advance the nasogastric tube slowly with each swallow. The client begins to cough, gag, and choke. Which of the following nursing actions is least likely to result in proper tube insertion and promote client relaxation?
   1 Continuing to advance the tube to the desired distance
   2 Pulling the tube back slightly
   3 Checking the back of the pharynx, using a tongue blade and flashlight
   4 Instructing the client to breathe slowly and take sips of water

2. The nurse is caring for a client receiving bolus feedings via a Levin type of nasogastric tube. As the nurse is finishing the feeding, the client asks for the bed to be positioned flat to sleep. Which of the following positions is the most appropriate choice for this client at this time?
   1 Head of bed flat, with client in the supine position for 30 minutes
   2 Head of bed elevated 30° to 45°, with client in the right lateral position for 60 minutes
   3 Head of bed elevated 45° to 60°, with client in the supine position for 30 minutes

   4 Head of bed in semi-Fowler's, with client in the left lateral position for 60 minutes

3. Prior to administering an intermittent tube feeding through an NG tube, the nurse assesses for gastric residual. The nurse aspirates the stomach contents and withdraws 40 mL of undigested formula. What is the rationale for assessing gastric residual prior to administering the tube feeding?
   1 To confirm proper nasogastric tube placement
   2 To observe the digestion of formula
   3 To assess fluid and electrolyte status
   4 To evaluate absorption of the last feeding

4. A client presents to the emergency department with upper GI bleeding and is in moderate distress. In planning priorities for care, which nursing action is the first priority for this client?
   1 Thorough investigation of precipitating events
   2 Insertion of a nasogastric tube and Hematest of emesis
   3 Complete abdominal physical examination
   4 Determination of vital signs

5. The nurse is caring for a client with possible cholelithiasis who is being prepared for a cholangiogram. The nurse teaches the client about the procedure. Which of the following client statements indicates that the client understands the purpose of a cholangiogram?
   1 "They are going to 'look at' my gallbladder and ducts."
   2 "This procedure will drain my gallbladder."
   3 "My gallbladder will be irrigated."
   4 "They will put medication in my gallbladder."

6. The nurse is caring for a client with acute pancreatitis and a history of alcoholism. Which of the following assessment data is a sign of paralytic ileus?
   1 Firm, nontender mass palpable at the lower right costal margin
   2 Severe, constant pain with rapid onset
   3 Inability to pass flatus
   4 Loss of anal sphincter control

7. The nurse inspects the color of the drainage from an NG tube on a postoperative client approximately 24 hours following a laparoscopic procedure. The previous shift reported the drainage as "dark red drainage since the surgery." Which of the following current assessment data indicates a potential complication requiring notification of the physician?
   1 Light yellowish-brown drainage
   2 Dark red drainage
   3 "Coffee ground" granules in the drainage
   4 Greenish-tinged drainage

8. After performing an initial abdominal assessment on a client with a diagnosis of cholelithiasis, the nurse reports that the bowel sounds are normal.

Which of the following best describes "normal bowel sounds"?
1 Waves of loud gurgles auscultated in all four quadrants
2 Very high-pitched loud rushes auscultated especially in one or two quadrants
3 Relatively high-pitched clicks or gurgles auscultated in all four quadrants
4 Low-pitched swishing auscultated in one or two quadrants

9. The nurse is preparing to discontinue a client's NG tube. The client is positioned properly and the tube has been flushed with 15 mL of air to clear secretions. The nurse must take a second precaution to prevent possible aspiration of gastric secretions during removal of the tube. Which of the following choices is the best instruction for the nurse to give the client to meet this goal?
1 "Take a deep breath when I tell you and breathe normally while I remove the tube."
2 "Take a deep breath when I tell you and bear down while I remove the tube."
3 "Take a deep breath when I tell you and slowly exhale while I remove the tube."
4 "Take a deep breath when I tell you and hold it while I remove the tube."

10. The nurse is caring for a client with an NG tube connected to continuous gastric suction. During the assessment, the nurse observes that the client is mouth breathing and has dry mucous membranes and that the breath has a foul odor. In planning care, which of the following nursing orders is the most appropriate choice to maintain the integrity of this client's oral mucosa?
1 Offer small sips of water frequently
2 Encourage client to suck on sour hard candy
3 Brush teeth frequently; use mouthwash and water
4 Use lemon-glycerin swabs to provide oral hygiene

11. A client with a small bowel obstruction asks the nurse to explain the purpose of the NG tube and continuous gastric suction. After the teaching is completed, the nurse evaluates the client's progress toward meeting the teaching goal by eliciting client feedback. Which of the following client responses indicates that the teaching goal was met? The client states: "The purpose of the continuous gastric suction is to:
1 Provide nourishment."
2 Relieve the bronchi of mucus."
3 Withdraw gastric contents for laboratory analysis."
4 Remove gas and fluids from the stomach and intestine."

12. The nurse is caring for a client with a resolved intestinal obstruction who has an NG tube in place. The client has tolerated the tube being clamped every 2 hours for 1 hour. The physician has now ordered the NG tube to be discontinued. To determine whether it is appropriate to discontinue the NG tube, the nurse should assess:
1 Proper NG tube placement
2 The client's serum electrolyte levels
3 Presence of bowel sounds in all four quadrants
4 The pH of the gastric aspirate

13. The nurse has administered approximately half of a high cleansing enema when the client complains of pain and cramping. Which of the following nursing actions is the most appropriate?
1 Raise the enema bag so that the solution can be completed quickly
2 Clamp the tubing for 30 seconds and restart the flow at a slower rate
3 Reassure the client and continue the flow
4 Discontinue the enema and notify the physician

14. The nurse is preparing to administer a high cleansing enema. The nurse positions the client in the:
1 Left lateral position with the right leg acutely flexed
2 Right Sims' position
3 Dorsal recumbent position
4 Right lateral position with the left leg acutely flexed

15. The nurse has aspirated 40 mL of undigested formula from the client's NG tube before administering an intermittent tube feeding. The nurse understands that before administering the tube feeding, the 40 mL of gastric aspirate should be:
1 Discarded properly and recorded as output on the client's I&O record
2 Poured into the NG tube through a syringe with the plunger removed
3 Mixed with the formula and poured into the NG tube through a syringe without a plunger
4 Diluted with water and injected into the NG tube by putting pressure on the plunger

16. The nurse observes that the client's NG tube has suddenly stopped draining. The tube is connected to suction, the machine is on and functioning, and all connections are snug. The tube is secured properly and does not appear to have been dislodged. After checking placement, the nurse gently flushes the tube with 30 mL of normal saline, but the tube still is not draining. The nurse analyzes this problem as:
1 Channels of gastric secretions may be bypassing the holes in the tube, and turning the client will promote stomach emptying
2 Thick gastric secretions may be blocking the tube, and removing this tube and reinserting a new tube will correct the problem
3 It is normal for an NG tube to stop draining, and no action is required

4 This is a potentially serious complication and the physician must be notified immediately

17. The home care nurse is providing instructions to the spouse of a client with gastroenteritis. The most appropriate instruction to prevent dehydration is to:
    1 Offer water only, until the client is able to tolerate solid foods
    2 Withhold all fluids until vomiting has ceased for at least 4 hours
    3 Encourage the client to take 8 to 12 ounces of fluid every hour while awake
    4 Maintain a clear liquid diet for at least 5 days before advancing, to allow inflammation of the bowel to subside

18. The nurse is participating in a health screening clinic and is preparing teaching materials about colorectal cancer. The nurse would plan to include which of the following in a list of risk factors for colorectal cancer?
    1 Age over 30 years
    2 High-fiber, low-fat diet
    3 Distant relative with colorectal cancer
    4 Personal history of ulcerative colitis or GI polyps

19. The hospitalized client with gastroesophageal reflux disease (GERD) is complaining of chest discomfort that feels like heartburn following a meal. After administering an ordered antacid, the nurse encourages the client to lie in which of the following positions?
    1 Supine with the head of the bed flat
    2 On the stomach, with the head flat
    3 On the left side, with the head of bed elevated 30°
    4 On the right side, with the head of the bed elevated 30°

20. The nurse is planning to teach the client with gastroesophageal reflux disease about substances that will increase the lower esophageal sphincter (LES) pressure. Which of the following items does the nurse include on this list?
    1 Fatty foods
    2 Nonfat milk
    3 Chocolate
    4 Coffee

21. The client has undergone esophagogastroduodenoscopy (EGD). The nurse places highest priority on which of the following items as part of the client's care plan?
    1 Assessing for return of the gag reflex
    2 Giving warm gargles for sore throat
    3 Monitoring temperature
    4 Monitoring complaints of heartburn

22. The nurse has taught the client about an upcoming endoscopic retrograde cholangiopancreatography (ERCP) procedure. The nurse evaluates that the client has not fully understood the information if the client makes which of the following statements?
    1 "I know I must sign the consent form."
    2 "I'm glad I don't have to lie still for this procedure."
    3 "I'm glad some medication will be given IV to relax me."
    4 "I hope the throat spray keeps me from gagging."

23. The client being seen in a physician's office has just been scheduled for a barium swallow (esophagography) the next day. The nurse writes down which of the following instructions for the client to follow before the test?
    1 Remove all metal and jewelry before the test
    2 Eat a regular supper and breakfast
    3 Continue to take all oral medications as scheduled
    4 Monitor own bowel movement pattern for constipation

24. The nurse is planning care for the client who has just returned to the nursing unit following an oral cholecystogram. The nurse would expect to be able to delete which of the following orders on the client's care plan?
    1 Monitor client's hydration status
    2 Assess for nausea and vomiting
    3 Maintain clear liquid status for 72 hours
    4 Monitor client for abdominal discomfort

25. The nurse is teaching the client about an upcoming colonoscopy procedure. The nurse includes in the instructions that the client will be placed in which of the following positions for the procedure?
    1 Left Sims'
    2 Right Sims'
    3 Knee-chest
    4 Lithotomy

26. The nurse has given postprocedure instructions to a client who underwent colonoscopy. The nurse evaluates that the client did not fully understand the directions if the client states that:
    1 Intake should be light at first, then progress to regular intake
    2 It is normal to feel gassy or bloated after the procedure
    3 The abdominal muscles may be tender from stretching during the procedure
    4 It is all right to drive after being home for an hour or so

27. The nurse is performing an abdominal assessment. The initial assessment would be which of the following?
    1 Auscultation
    2 Inspection
    3 Palpation
    4 Percussion

28. The nurse is scheduling diagnostic tests for a client. If all the following diagnostic tests are ordered, which would be performed last?
    1 Gallbladder series
    2 Barium enema
    3 Barium swallow
    4 Oral cholecystogram

29. The client is scheduled for an oral cholecystogram. The nurse plans to order what type of diet for the evening meal prior to the test?
    1 Low-protein
    2 High-carbohydrate
    3 Fat-free
    4 Liquid

30. The client is scheduled for an upper GI endoscopy. Which of the following assessments is essential to include in the plan of care following the procedure?
    1 Monitoring for rectal bleeding
    2 Assessment of pulses
    3 Monitoring urine output
    4 Assessment of the gag reflex

31. Polyethylene glycol-electrolyte solution (Go-LYTELY) is prescribed for the client scheduled for a colonoscopy. The client begins to experience diarrhea following administration of the solution. What action by the nurse is most appropriate?
    1 Cancel the examination
    2 Start an IV
    3 Administer an enema
    4 Explain that diarrhea is expected

32. The nurse is preparing to insert an NG tube into a client. What nursing measure will best facilitate easy insertion of the NG tube ?
    1 Placing the NG tube in warm water
    2 Removing the tube if any resistance to insertion is met
    3 Asking the client to swallow as the tube is being advanced
    4 Hyperextend the head to insert the tube

33. A nasogastric tube has been inserted into a client, and the physician prescribes that the tube be attached to intermittent suction. The nurse attaches the suction, noting that the pressure should not exceed:
    1 10 mmHg
    2 20 mmHg
    3 25 mmHg
    4 30 mmHg

34. The nurse is caring for a client with a diagnosis of chronic gastritis. The nurse anticipates that this client is at risk for which of the following vitamin deficiencies?
    1 Vitamin A
    2 Vitamin B_{12}
    3 Vitamin C
    4 Vitamin E

35. The nurse is reviewing the medication record of a client with acute gastritis. Which of the following medications, if noted on the client's record, would the nurse question?
    1 Digoxin (Lanoxin)
    2 Indomethacin (Indocin)
    3 Furosemide (Lasix)
    4 Propranolol hydrochloride (Inderal)

36. The nurse is assessing a client 24 hours following a cholecystectomy. The nurse notes that the T tube has drained 750 mL of green-brown drainage since surgery. Which of the following nursing interventions is most appropriate?
    1 Notify the physician
    2 Document the findings
    3 Irrigate the T tube
    4 Clamp the T tube

37. The nurse is monitoring a client with a diagnosis of peptic ulcer. Which of the following assessment findings most likely indicates perforation of the ulcer?
    1 Bradycardia
    2 Numbness in the legs
    3 Nausea and vomiting
    4 A rigid, boardlike abdomen

38. The nurse provides medication instructions to a client with peptic ulcer disease. Which statement, if made by the client, indicates the best understanding of the medication therapy?
    1 "The cimetidine (Tagamet) will cause me to produce less stomach acid."
    2 "Sucralfate (Carafate) will change the fluid in my stomach."
    3 "Antacids will coat my stomach."
    4 "Omeprazole (Prilosec) will coat the ulcer and help it heal."

39. The client with peptic ulcer disease is scheduled for a pyloroplasty. The client asks the nurse about the procedure. The nurse bases the response on which of the following?
    1 A pyloroplasty involves cutting the vagus nerve
    2 A pyloroplasty involves removing the distal portion of the stomach
    3 A pyloroplasty involves removal of the ulcer and a large portion of the cells that produce hydrochloric acid
    4 A pyloroplasty involves an incision and resuturing of the pylorus to relax the muscle and enlarge the opening from the stomach to the duodenum

40. The client is diagnosed with a GI bleed, and the bleeding has been controlled. Antacids are prescribed to be administered every hour. The nurse should plan on maintaining an approximate gastric pH of:
    1 3
    2 6
    3 9
    4 15

41. A client with a peptic ulcer is scheduled for a vagotomy. The client asks the nurse about the purpose of this procedure. The best nursing response is which of the following?
    1 "Decreases food absorption in the stomach."
    2 "Heals the gastric mucosa."
    3 "Halts stress reactions."
    4 "Reduces the stimulus to acid secretions."

42. The nurse is caring for a client following a Billroth II procedure. On review of the postoperative orders, which of the following, if prescribed, does the nurse question and verify?
    1 Irrigating the NG tube
    2 Coughing and deep-breathing exercises
    3 Leg exercises
    4 Early ambulation

43. The nurse is providing discharge instructions to a client following gastrectomy. Which of the following measures will the nurse instruct the client to follow to assist in preventing dumping syndrome?
    1 Eat high-carbohydrate foods
    2 Limit the fluids taken with meals
    3 Ambulate following a meal
    4 Sit in a high Fowler's position during meals

44. The nurse is monitoring a client for the early signs and symptoms of dumping syndrome. Which of the following symptoms indicates this occurrence?
    1 Abdominal cramping and pain
    2 Bradycardia and indigestion
    3 Sweating and pallor
    4 Double vision and chest pain

45. The nurse is preparing a discharge teaching plan for the client who had a herniorrhaphy. Which of the following does the nurse include in the plan of care?
    1 Restricting pain medication
    2 Maintaining bed rest
    3 Avoiding coughing
    4 Irrigating the drain

46. The nurse is instructing the client who had a herniorrhaphy how to reduce postoperative swelling following the procedure. Which of the following does the nurse suggest to the client to prevent swelling?

1 Heat to the abdomen
2 Elevation of the scrotum
3 Limiting fluids
4 A low-roughage diet

47. The nurse is caring for a hospitalized client with a diagnosis of ulcerative colitis. When assessing the client, which finding, if noted, would the nurse report to the physician?
    1 Bloody diarrhea
    2 Hypotension
    3 A hemoglobin level of 12 mg/dL
    4 Rebound tenderness

48. Diphenoxylate hydrochloride and atropine sulfate (Lomotil) is prescribed for the client with ulcerative colitis. Which of the following is a therapeutic effect of this medication?
    1 Elimination of peristalsis
    2 Reduced diarrhea
    3 Decreased cramping
    4 Improved intestinal tone

49. A client is diagnosed as having irritable bowel syndrome. Which of the following instructions does the nurse not include in the plan of care?
    1 Maintain a low-residue diet
    2 Provide fiber and bulk in the diet
    3 Eat regular meals
    4 Drink 8 to 10 cups of liquid each day

50. Sulfasalazine (Azulfidine) is prescribed for the client with a diagnosis of ulcerative colitis. The nurse prepares a teaching plan for the client. Which of the following is not included in the plan regarding this medication?
    1 Sensitivity to sunlight may occur
    2 Take Azulfidine with meals
    3 This medication should be taken as prescribed
    4 The medication will cause constipation

51. The nurse is caring for a client postoperatively following creation of a colostomy. Which of the following nursing diagnoses does the nurse include in the plan of care?
    1 Altered Nutrition; More Than Body Requirements
    2 Body Image Disturbance
    3 Fear Related to Poor Prognosis
    4 Sexual Dysfunction

52. The nurse is reviewing the record of a client with Crohn's disease. Which of the following stool characteristics does the nurse expect to note in this client?
    1 Bloody stools
    2 Diarrhea
    3 Constipation alternating with diarrhea
    4 Stool constantly oozing from the rectum

53. The nurse is performing a colostomy irrigation on a client. During the irrigation, the client begins to complain of abdominal cramps. Which of the following is the most appropriate nursing action?
    1 Notify the physician
    2 Increase the height of the irrigation
    3 Stop the irrigation temporarily
    4 Medicate for pain and resume irrigation

54. The nurse is teaching a client how to perform a colostomy irrigation. To enhance the effectiveness of the irrigation, what measure should the nurse instruct the client to do?
    1 Increase fluid intake
    2 Reduce the amount of irrigation solution
    3 Massage the abdomen gently
    4 Place heat on the abdomen

55. The nurse is reviewing the record of a client with a diagnosis of cirrhosis and notes that there is documentation of the presence of asterixis. To assess for the presence of this sign, the nurse does which of the following?
    1 Asks client to extend the arms
    2 Assesses for the presence of Homan's sign
    3 Instructs the client to lean forward
    4 Measures the abdominal girth

56. The client with cirrhosis has ascites and a fluid volume excess. Which measure will the nurse include in the plan of care for this client?
    1 Increase the amount of sodium in the diet
    2 Restrict the amount of fluids consumed
    3 Encourage ambulation frequently
    4 Administer magnesium antacids

57. The client with ascites is scheduled for a paracentesis. The nurse is assisting the physician in performing the procedure. Which of the following positions will the nurse assist the client to assume for this procedure?
    1 Supine
    2 Left side lying
    3 Right side lying
    4 Upright

58. The nurse is reviewing the laboratory results in a client with cirrhosis and notes that the ammonia level is elevated. Which of the following diets does the nurse anticipate would most likely be prescribed for this client?
    1 High-carbohydrate
    2 Moderate-fat
    3 High-protein
    4 Low-protein

59. Lactulose (Chronulac) is prescribed for a client with a diagnosis of hepatic encephalopathy. Which assessment finding indicates that the client is responding to this medication therapy as anticipated?
    1 The fecal pH is acidic

2 The client experiences diarrhea
3 The client is able to tolerate a full diet
4 Vomiting occurs

60. An ultrasound of the gallbladder is scheduled for the client with a suspected diagnosis of cholecystitis. The nurse explains to the client that this test:
    1 Requires the client to lie still for short intervals
    2 Requires that the client be NPO
    3 Requires the administration of oral tablets
    4 Is uncomfortable

61. The nurse is providing preoperative teaching to a client scheduled for a cholecystectomy. Which of the following interventions is of highest priority in the preoperative teaching plan?
    1 Teaching coughing and deep breathing exercises
    2 Teaching leg exercises
    3 Instructions regarding fluid restrictions
    4 Assessing the client's understanding of the surgical procedure

62. A Penrose drain is in place on the first postoperative day following a cholecystectomy. Serosanguineous drainage is noted on the dressing covering the drain. Which nursing intervention is most appropriate?
    1 Notify the physician
    2 Change the dressing
    3 Circle the amount on the dressing with a pen
    4 Continue to monitor the drainage

63. Cholestyramine resin (Questran Light) is prescribed for the client with an elevated serum cholesterol level. The nurse instructs the client to administer the medication:
    1 After meals
    2 Mixed with fruit juice
    3 Via a rectal suppository
    4 At least 3 hours before meals

64. The nurse is reviewing the physician's orders written for a client admitted with acute pancreatitis. Which physician order would the nurse question if noted on the client's chart?
    1 NPO status
    2 Insert NG tube
    3 An anticholinergic medication
    4 Morphine sulfate for pain

65. Pancrelipase (Viokase) is prescribed for a client with postgastrectomy syndrome. Which of the following assessment findings indicates a therapeutic effect of this medication?
    1 The client's appetite improves
    2 The client experiences a weight loss
    3 Vitamin B_{12} deficiency is controlled
    4 Stools are less fatty and decrease in frequency

66. The nurse is evaluating the plan of care for the client with peptic ulcer disease (PUD) with a nursing diagnosis of Pain. The nurse would determine that the client has not met the expected outcomes if the client states:
    1 That pain is relieved with histamine receptor antagonists
    2 That irritating foods have been eliminated from the diet
    3 That he may be awakened at 2 A.M. with heartburn
    4 Pain is absent before meals

67. The nurse is doing an admission assessment for the client with a history of duodenal ulcer. To determine whether the problem is currently active, the nurse assesses the client for which of the following most frequent symptoms of duodenal ulcer?
    1 Pain that is relieved by food intake
    2 Pain that radiates down the right arm
    3 Nausea and vomiting
    4 Weight loss

68. A client with peptic ulcer states that stress frequently causes exacerbation of the disease. The nurse interprets that which of the following items mentioned by the client is most likely responsible for the exacerbations?
    1 Sleeping 8 to 10 hours a night
    2 Eating 5 to 6 small meals per day
    3 Ability to work at home periodically
    4 Frequent need to work overtime on short notice

69. The client with peptic ulcer disease needs dietary modification to reduce episodes of epigastric pain. The nurse plans to teach the client that which of the following items, which the client enjoys, does not need to be limited or eliminated with this disease?
    1 Wine
    2 Baked chicken
    3 Coffee
    4 Fresh fruit

70. The medication history of a client with peptic ulcer disease reveals intermittent use of the following medications. The nurse teaches the client to avoid which of these medications altogether because of the irritating effects on the lining of the GI tract?
    1 Omeprazole (Prilosec)
    2 Ibuprofen (Motrin)
    3 Sucralfate (Carafate)
    4 Nizatidine (Axid)

71. The client with a history of gastric ulcer suddenly complains of a sharp, severe pain in the midepigastric area, which then spreads over the entire abdomen. The client's abdomen is rigid and boardlike to palpation, and the client obtains most comfort from lying in the knee-chest position. The nurse calls the physician immediately, suspecting that the client is experiencing which of the following complications of peptic ulcer disease?
    1 Perforation
    2 Obstruction
    3 Hemorrhage
    4 Intractability

72. The nurse instructs the ileostomy client to do which of the following as part of essential care of the stoma?
    1 Cleanse the peristomal skin meticulously
    2 Take in high-fiber foods such as nuts
    3 Massage the area below the stoma
    4 Limit fluid intake to prevent diarrhea

73. The client is admitted with dehydration following creation of an ileostomy. The nurse assesses that the client has lost 3 pounds of weight, has poor skin turgor, and has concentrated urine. The nurse interprets that the client's clinical picture correlates most closely with recent intake of which of the following medications, which is contraindicated for the ileostomy client?
    1 Ferrous sulfate (Feosol)
    2 Folate (folic acid)
    3 Phenolphthalein (Ex-Lax)
    4 Cyanocobalamin (vitamin B_{12})

74. The client with hiatal hernia chronically experiences heartburn following meals. The nurse plans to teach the client to avoid which of the following, which is contraindicated with hiatal hernia?
    1 Taking in small, frequent, bland meals
    2 Lying recumbent following meals
    3 Raising the head of bed on 6-inch blocks
    4 Taking histamine receptor–antagonist medication

75. The client who has undergone creation of a colostomy has a nursing diagnosis of Body Image Disturbance. The nurse evaluates that the client is making the most significant progress toward identified goals if the client:
    1 Watches the nurse empty the ostomy bag
    2 Looks at the ostomy site
    3 Reads the ostomy product literature
    4 Practices cutting the ostomy appliance

76. The nurse is assessing for stoma prolapse in a client with a recent colostomy. The nurse observes to see whether the stoma is:
    1 Sunken and hidden
    2 Dark and bluish in color
    3 Narrowed and flattened
    4 Protruding and swollen

77. The client has a new colostomy, created 2 days earlier. The client is beginning to pass malodorous flatus from the stoma. The nurse interprets that:
    1 This indicates inadequate preoperative bowel preparation

2 This is a normal, expected event

3 The client is experiencing early signs of ischemic bowel

4 The client should not have the NG tube removed

78. The client with a new colostomy is concerned about odor from stool in the ostomy drainage bag. The nurse should teach the client to include which of the following foods in the diet to reduce odor?
    1 Yogurt
    2 Broccoli
    3 Cucumbers
    4 Eggs

79. The nurse is giving dietary instructions for the client who has a new colostomy. The nurse encourages the client to eat foods representing which of the following diets for the first 4 to 6 weeks postoperatively?
    1 High-protein
    2 High-carbohydrate
    3 Low-calorie
    4 Low-residue

80. The nurse has given instructions to the client with an ileostomy about foods to eat to thicken the stool. The nurse evaluates that the client did not fully understand the instructions if the client stated that eating which of the following foods makes the stool less watery?
    1 Pasta
    2 Boiled rice
    3 Bran
    4 Low-fat cheese

81. The client has just had surgery to create an ileostomy. The nurse assesses the client in the immediate postoperative period for which of the following most frequent complications of this type of surgery?
    1 Intestinal obstruction
    2 Fluid and electrolyte imbalance
    3 Malabsorption of fat
    4 Folate deficiency

82. The nurse is doing preoperative teaching with the client who is about to undergo creation of a Kock pouch. The nurse interprets that the client has the best understanding of the nature of the surgery if the client makes which of the following statements?
    1 "I will need to drain the pouch regularly with a catheter."
    2 "I will need to wear a drainage bag for the rest of my life."
    3 "The drainage from this type of ostomy will be formed."
    4 "I will be able to pass stool by the rectum eventually."

83. The client with a newly created Kock pouch has an order to discontinue the continuous suction to the catheter placed in the pouch during surgery. The nurse anticipates that which of the following solutions will be ordered for periodic catheter irrigation once the suction has been removed?
    1 10 to 20 mL of normal saline
    2 50 to 60 mL of tap water
    3 30 to 40 mL of sterile water
    4 120 mL of normal saline

84. The nurse is caring for a client admitted to the hospital with a suspected diagnosis of acute appendicitis. Which of the following laboratory results does the nurse expect to note if the client does indeed have appendicitis?
    1 Leukopenia with a shift to the right
    2 Leukocytosis with a shift to the right
    3 Leukocytosis with a shift to the left
    4 Leukopenia with a shift to the left

85. The nurse is monitoring a client admitted to the hospital with a diagnosis of appendicitis. The client is scheduled for surgery in 2 hours. The client begins to complain of increased abdominal pain and begins to vomit. On assessment, the nurse notes that the abdomen is distended and bowel sounds are diminished. Which of the following is the most appropriate nursing intervention?
    1 Administer prescribed pain medication
    2 Notify the physician
    3 Call and ask the operating room team to perform the surgery as soon as possible
    4 Reposition the client and apply a heating pad on warm setting to the client's abdomen

86. The client has been admitted with a diagnosis of acute pancreatitis. The nurse would assess this client for pain that is:
    1 Severe and unrelenting, located in the epigastric area and radiating to the back
    2 Severe and unrelenting, located in the left lower quadrant and radiating to the groin
    3 Burning and aching, located in the epigastric area and radiating to the umbilicus
    4 Burning and aching, located in the left lower quadrant and radiating to the hip

87. The nurse is reviewing the laboratory test results of the client with acute pancreatitis who also has chronic alcoholism. The nurse interprets that which of the following results could represent a laboratory error?
    1 Elevated blood glucose
    2 Elevated serum lipase
    3 Elevated serum amylase
    4 Elevated magnesium level

88. The client with chronic pancreatitis needs information on dietary modification to manage the health problem. The nurse should plan as priority

instruction to teach the client to limit which of the following items in the diet?
1 Carbohydrate
2 Protein
3 Fat
4 Water-soluble vitamins

89. The client with acute pancreatitis is experiencing severe pain from the disorder. The nurse teaches the client to avoid which of the following positions that could aggravate the pain?
    1 Sitting up
    2 Lying flat
    3 Leaning forward
    4 Flexing the left leg

90. The nurse had taught the client with chronic pancreatitis about risk factor modification to reduce the incidence of recurrences. The nurse evaluates that the client has understood the information if the client states it will be necessary to control which of the following?
    1 Diabetes mellitus
    2 Alcohol intake
    3 Duodenal ulcer
    4 Crohn's disease

91. The nurse is evaluating the effect of dietary counseling on the client with cholecystitis. The nurse evaluates that the client understands the instructions given if the client stated that which of the following food items is acceptable in the diet?
    1 Baked scrod
    2 Sauces and gravies
    3 Fried chicken
    4 Fresh whipped cream

92. The nurse assesses the client experiencing an acute episode of cholecystitis for pain that is located in the right:
    1 Upper quadrant and radiates to the left scapula and shoulder
    2 Upper quadrant and radiates to the right scapula and shoulder
    3 Lower quadrant and radiates to the umbilicus
    4 Lower quadrant and radiates to the back

93. The client with cirrhosis is beginning to show signs of hepatic encephalopathy. The nurse plans a dietary consult to limit the amount of which of the following ingredients in the client's diet?
    1 Fat
    2 Carbohydrate
    3 Protein
    4 Minerals

94. The client with cirrhosis complicated by ascites is admitted to the hospital. The client experienced a 10-pound weight gain over the last week and a half. The client has edema of both feet and ankles. The abdomen is distended, taut, and shiny

with striae. The nurse selects which of the following as the most appropriate nursing diagnosis for this client?
1 Altered Nutrition: More Than Body Requirements
2 Impaired Gas Exchange
3 Risk for Impaired Skin Integrity
4 Fluid Volume Excess

95. The client with Crohn's disease has a nursing diagnosis of Pain. The nurse teaches the client to avoid which of the following in managing this problem?
    1 Lying supine with legs straight
    2 Applying heat to the abdomen
    3 Utilizing antispasmodic medication
    4 Utilizing relaxation techniques

96. The client with Crohn's disease has an order to begin taking antispasmodic medication. The nurse should time the medication so that each dose is taken:
    1 30 minutes before meals
    2 During meals
    3 60 minutes after meals
    4 Upon arising and at bedtime

97. The client with ulcerative colitis is diagnosed with a mild case of the disease. The nurse doing dietary teaching gives the client examples of foods to eat that represent which of the following therapeutic diets?
    1 High-fat with milk
    2 High-protein without milk
    3 Low-roughage without milk
    4 Low-roughage with milk

98. The client is admitted to the hospital for treatment of acute hepatitis B. Which activity order does the nurse expect to be prescribed?
    1 Bed rest
    2 Encourage ambulation
    3 Out of bed in a chair
    4 No activity restrictions

99. It has been determined that the client with hepatitis has contracted the infection from contaminated food. What type of hepatitis is this client most likely experiencing?
    1 Hepatitis A
    2 Hepatitis B
    3 Hepatitis C
    4 Hepatitis D

100. A client is suspected of having hepatitis. Which of the following diagnostic test results will assist in confirming this diagnosis?
     1 Decreased erythrocyte sedimentation rate
     2 Elevated serum bilirubin
     3 Elevated hemoglobin
     4 Elevated BUN

ANSWERS

1. 1

Rationale: As the NG tube is passed through the oropharynx, the gag reflex is stimulated, which may cause coughing, gagging, and/or choking. Instead of passing through to the esophagus, the NG tube may coil around itself in the oropharynx, or it may enter the larynx and obstruct the airway. The flexed position of the head closes off the upper airway to the trachea and opens the esophagus. Swallowing closes the epiglottis over the trachea and helps move the tube into the esophagus. Since the tube may enter the larynx and obstruct the airway, pulling the tube back slightly will remove it from the larynx; advancing the tube might position it in the trachea. Slow breathing helps the client relax to reduce the gag response. The tube may be advanced after the client relaxes.

Test-Taking Strategy: Note that you are asked to identify the nursing action that would be "least likely" to result in proper tube insertion and promote client relaxation. Options 2, 3, and 4 all aim at assessing and promoting relaxation, whereas option 1 could result in an unsafe malposition of the NG tube into the trachea. The tube may be advanced to the desired distance after the client relaxes.

Level of Cognitive Ability: Application
Phase of Nursing Process: Implementation
Client Needs: Physiological Integrity
Content Area: Adult Health/Gastrointestinal

Reference
Lammon, C., Foote, A., Leli, P., et al. (1995). *Clinical nursing skills.* Philadelphia: W. B. Saunders. pp. 418–421.

2. 2

Rationale: Aspiration is a possible complication associated with NG tube feeding. The head of the bed is elevated 30°–45° for at least 30 minutes following bolus tube feeding to prevent vomiting and aspiration. The right lateral position uses gravity to facilitate gastric retention to prevent vomiting. The flat supine position is to be avoided for the first 30 minutes after a tube feeding.

Test-Taking Strategy: There are three components to each answer: the level of elevation of the head, the client's position, and the duration. The entire option needs to be correct. Option 1 can be eliminated immediately because this position could result in aspiration. Options 2 and 4 are the same elevation, but the right lateral position is the correct position and 60 minutes is the correct duration. Option 3 is eliminated because of the supine position and the length of duration.

Level of Cognitive Ability: Application
Phase of Nursing Process: Implementation
Client Needs: Physiological Integrity
Content Area: Adult Health/Gastrointestinal

Reference
Lammon, C., Foote, A., Leli, P., et al. (1995). *Clinical nursing skills.* Philadelphia: W. B. Saunders. pp. 426–427.

3. 4

Rationale: All the stomach contents are aspirated and measured prior to administering a tube feeding. This procedure measures the gastric residual. The gastric residual is assessed in order to confirm whether undigested formula from a previous feeding remains and thereby evaluates absorption of the last feeding. It is important to assess gastric residual because administration of a tube feeding to a full stomach could result in overdistention, thus predisposing the client to regurgitation and possible aspiration.

Test-Taking Strategy: Note that the issue of the question is the purpose of assessing residual. Focusing on this issue should direct you to option 4. Review this procedure now, if you had difficulty with this question!

Level of Cognitive Ability: Analysis
Phase of Nursing Process: Assessment
Client Needs: Physiological Integrity
Content Area: Adult Health/Gastrointestinal

Reference
Lammon, C., Foote, A., Leli, P., et al. (1995). *Clinical nursing skills.* Philadelphia: W. B. Saunders. p. 427.

4. 4

Rationale: An initial nursing assessment should be performed while getting the client ready for initial treatment. The immediate determination of vital signs indicates whether the client is in shock from blood loss and also provides a baseline blood pressure and pulse by which to monitor the progress of treatment. Signs and symptoms of shock include low blood pressure; rapid, weak pulse; increased thirst; cold, clammy skin; and restlessness. Vital signs should be monitored every 10 to 15 minutes, and the physician should be informed of any significant changes. The client may not be able to provide subjective data until the immediate physical needs are met.

Test-Taking Strategy: Although all the choices are important components of a complete nursing assessment for this client, utilize principles of prioritization when answering this question. A client with an acute upper GI bleed is at risk for shock. Monitoring vital signs is the nursing action that will assess circulation, provide information about the client's circulating volume status, and alert the nurse to early stages of shock.

Level of Cognitive Ability: Application
Phase of Nursing Process: Planning
Client Needs: Physiological Integrity
Content Area: Adult Health/Gastrointestinal

Reference
Lewis, S., Collier, I., & Heitkemper, M. (1996). *Medical-surgical nursing: Assessment and management of clinical problems* (4th ed.). St. Louis: Mosby–Year Book. pp. 1235–1237.

5. 1

Rationale: An IV cholangiogram is for diagnostic purposes. It outlines both the gallbladder and the ducts, so gallstones that have moved into the ductal system can be detected. X-ray films are used to visualize the biliary duct system after IV injection of radiopaque dye.

Test-Taking Strategy: Knowledge of the pathophysiology of cholelithiasis and the purpose of the cholangiogram will help in answering this question. Eliminate options 2, 3, and 4 because they are similar. If you are unfamiliar with this procedure, take time now to review!

Level of Cognitive Ability: Analysis
Phase of Nursing Process: Evaluation
Client Needs: Physiological Integrity
Content Area: Adult Health/Gastrointestinal

Reference
Monahan, F., & Neighbors, M. (1998). *Medical-surgical nursing: Foundations for clinical practice* (2nd ed.). Philadelphia: W. B. Saunders. p. 972.

6. 3

Rationale: An inflammatory reaction such as acute pancreatitis can cause paralytic ileus, the most common form of nonmechanical obstruction. Inability to pass flatus is a clinical manifestation of paralytic ileus. Option 1 is the description of the physical finding of liver enlargement. The liver is usually enlarged in cases of cirrhosis or hepatitis. Although this client may have an enlarged liver, an enlarged liver is not a sign of paralytic ileus or intestinal obstruction. Pain is associated with paralytic ileus, but the pain usually presents as a more constant generalized discomfort. Pain that is severe, constant, and rapid in onset is more likely caused by strangulation of the bowel. Loss of sphincter control is not a sign of paralytic ileus.

Test-Taking Strategy: Knowledge of the clinical manifestations and abdominal physical assessment findings of paralytic ileus will assist you in answering this question. Noting the word "paralytic" will assist in directing you to option 3. Review these clinical manifestations now, if you had difficulty with this question!

Level of Cognitive Ability: Analysis
Phase of Nursing Process: Assessment
Client Needs: Physiological Integrity
Content Area: Adult Health/Gastrointestinal

Reference

Monahan, F., & Neighbors, M. (1998). *Medical-surgical nursing: Foundations for clinical practice* (2nd ed.). Philadelphia: W. B. Saunders. p. 1076.

7. 2

Rationale: For the first 12 hours following a laparoscopic procedure, the NG tube drainage may be dark brown to dark red. Later, the drainage should change to a light yellowish-brown color. The presence of bile may cause a greenish tinge. However, the physician should be notified at once of the possibility of hemorrhage if the dark red color continues or if bright red blood is observed. Because of the presence of small amounts of blood and the action of gastric secretions, "coffee-ground" granules may be seen in the NG tube drainage.

Test-Taking Strategy: Knowledge of the anticipated postoperative course following a laparoscopic procedure, including evolution of the color and character of NG drainage, is helpful in answering this question. Even though option 2 is not a change from the color of the drainage since surgery, after 12 hours it is an indicator of possible hemorrhage and the physician should be notified.

Level of Cognitive Ability: Analysis
Phase of Nursing Process: Analysis
Client Needs: Physiological Integrity
Content Area: Adult Health/Gastrointestinal

Reference

Lewis, S., Collier, I., & Heitkemper, M. (1996). *Medical-surgical nursing: Assessment and management of clinical problems* (4th ed.). St. Louis: Mosby–Year Book. p. 1217.

8. 3

Rationale: Although frequency and intensity of bowel sounds will vary depending on the phase of digestion, normal bowel sounds are relatively high-pitched clicks or gurgles. Loud gurgles (borborygmi) indicate hyperperistalsis. Bowel sounds will be more high-pitched and loud (hyperresonance) when the intestines are under tension, such as in intestinal obstruction. A swishing or buzzing sound represents turbulent blood flow associated with a bruit. No aortic bruits should be heard.

Test-Taking Strategy: A knowledge of normal auscultation findings for bowel sounds is helpful in answering this question. Normally, bowel sounds should be audible in all four quadrants; therefore, options 2 and 4 can be eliminated easily.

Level of Cognitive Ability: Application
Phase of Nursing Process: Assessment
Client Needs: Physiological Integrity
Content Area: Adult Health/Gastrointestinal

Reference

Lewis, S., Collier, I., & Heitkemper, M. (1996). *Medical-surgical nursing: Assessment and management of clinical problems* (4th ed.). St. Louis. Mosby–Year Book. pp. 1085, 1089.

9. 3

Rationale: The client should take a deep breath because the airway will be temporarily obstructed during the tube's removal. The client is then told to exhale slowly, and the tube is withdrawn during exhalation. Bearing down could inhibit the removal of the tube. Breathing normally could result in aspiration of gastric secretions during inhalation.

Test-Taking Strategy: Attempt to visualize the process of tube removal in answering this question. You should easily be directed to option 3 by thinking about the process of removal. Exhaling slowly will facilitate the process of removal. Review this procedure now, if you had difficulty with this question!

Level of Cognitive Ability: Application
Phase of Nursing Process: Implementation
Client Needs: Physiological Integrity
Content Area: Adult Health/Gastrointestinal

Reference

Monahan, F., & Neighbors, M. (1998). *Medical-surgical nursing: Foundations for clinical practice* (2nd ed.). Philadelphia: W. B. Saunders. p. 980.

10. 3

Rationale: After the NG tube is in place, mouth care is extremely important. With one naris occluded, the client tends to mouth breathe, drying the mucous membranes. Previous vomiting will leave a bad taste in the client's mouth, and a fecal odor may be present. Frequent, small sips of water would be contraindicated when the client is on gastric suction. The hard candy would increase the salivation but would not be useful in cleaning the oral cavity. Lemon glycerin swabs have a drying or irritating effect on the mucous membranes.

Test-Taking Strategy: The issue of this question is a specific nursing action. It is important to know that a client on gastric suction will be NPO, and swallowing water or other liquids would be prohibited The goal for this client is to maintain the integrity of the oral mucosa. Options 1, 2, and 4 are similar in that they provide moisture. Option 3 is the one that is different. It includes cleaning and providing moisture, and these are the two key elements to maintaining mucosal integrity.

Level of Cognitive Ability: Application
Phase of Nursing Process: Planning
Client Needs: Physiological Integrity
Content Area: Adult Health/Gastrointestinal

Reference

Lewis, S., Collier, I., & Heitkemper, M. (1996). *Medical-surgical nursing: Assessment and management of clinical problems* (4th ed.). St. Louis: Mosby–Year Book. p. 1239.

11. **4**

Rationale: Treatment of intestinal obstruction is directed toward decompression of the intestine by removal of gas and fluid. Nasogastric tubes may be used to decompress the bowel. Continuous gastric suction does not provide nourishment. Option 2 is the purpose for tracheal suctioning. Although gastric contents may be sent for laboratory analysis, it is not the main purpose for continuous gastric suction.

Test-Taking Strategy: Knowledge of the pathophysiology of small bowel obstruction and the use of continuous gastric suction will help you in answering this question. Although the question asks you to evaluate the client's understanding of the purpose of the NG continuous suctioning, you must know that the purpose is to remove air and fluid from the stomach and intestine.

Level of Cognitive Ability: Analysis
Phase of Nursing Process: Evaluation
Client Needs: Physiological Integrity
Content Area: Adult Health/Gastrointestinal

References

Lewis, S., Collier, I., & Heitkemper, M. (1996). *Medical-surgical nursing: Assessment and management of clinical problems* (4th ed.). St. Louis: Mosby–Year Book. p. 1237.

12. **3**

Rationale: Distention, vomiting, and abdominal pain are a few of the symptoms associated with intestinal obstruction. Nasogastric tubes may be used to empty the stomach and relieve distention and vomiting. They are also used to treat partial or complete small bowel obstruction. The nurse may evaluate peristaltic movements by auscultating the abdomen. Bowel sounds return to normal as the obstruction is relieved and normal bowel function is restored. Discontinuing the NG tube prior to normal bowel function may result in a return of the symptoms, necessitating reinsertion of the NG tube. Serum electrolyte levels, tube placement, and the pH of gastric aspirate are important assessments for the client with an NG tube in place but would not assist in determining the appropriateness of removing the NG tube.

Test-Taking Strategy: Knowing the pathophysiology for intestinal obstruction and the purpose of NG tubes as a therapy, you will know that the tube is left in until normal bowel function returns. Checking for the presence of bowel sounds is the assessment indicator for normal bowel function. It is not appropriate to discontinue the NG tube until bowel sounds are present. Assessing the pH of gastric aspirate is one method of assessing tube placement. Checking tube placement is necessary routinely and prior to instilling substances through the tube but not necessary prior to discontinuing the tube.

Level of Cognitive Ability: Application
Phase of Nursing Process: Assessment
Client Needs: Physiological Integrity
Content Area: Adult Health/Gastrointestinal

Reference

Lewis, S., Collier, I., & Heitkemper, M. (1996). *Medical-surgical nursing: Assessment and management of clinical problems* (4th ed.). St. Louis: Mosby–Year Book. pp. 1235–1239.

13. **2**

Rationale: The enema fluid should be administered slowly. If the client complains of fullness or pain, stop the flow for 30 seconds and restart at a slower rate. Slow enema administration and stopping the flow temporarily, if necessary, will decrease the likelihood of intestinal spasm and premature ejection of the solution. The higher the solution container is held above the rectum, the faster the flow and the greater the force in the rectum. Pain and cramping are usually due to intestinal spasm and will subside when the enema is stopped briefly, after which the enema may be resumed. There is no need to discontinue the enema and notify the physician at this time.

Test-Taking Strategy: Knowledge of the procedure for enema administration will assist you in answering this question. Noting the client's symptoms will assist in directing you to the correct option. Review this procedure now, if you had difficulty with this question!

Level of Cognitive Ability: Application
Phase of Nursing Process: Implementation
Client Needs: Physiological Integrity
Content Area: Adult Health/Gastrointestinal

Reference

Kozier, B., Erb, G., & Blais, K. (1998). *Fundamentals of nursing: Concepts, process, and practice* (5th ed.). Reading, MA: Addison-Wesley. pp. 1203, 1205.

14. **1**

Rationale: The sigmoid and descending colon are located on the left side. Therefore, the left lateral position uses gravity to facilitate the flow of solution into the sigmoid and descending colon. Acute flexion of the right leg allows for adequate exposure of the anus.

Test-Taking Strategy: Knowledge of anatomy of the rectum will assist in eliminating options 2 and 4. Attempt to visualize the remaining positions presented in options 1 and 3. By doing so, you should easily be able to eliminate option 3. Review this procedure now, if you had difficulty with this question!

Level of Cognitive Ability: Application
Phase of Nursing Process: Implementation
Client Needs: Physiological Integrity
Content Area: Adult Health/Gastrointestinal

Reference

Kozier, B., Erb, G., & Blais, K. (1998). *Fundamentals of nursing: Concepts, process, and practice* (5th ed.). Reading, MA: Addison-Wesley. p. 1204.

15. **2**

Rationale: After checking residual feeding contents, reinstill the gastric contents into the stomach by removing the syringe bulb or plunger and pouring the gastric contents via the syringe into the NG tube. Removal of the contents could disturb the client's electrolyte balance.

Test-Taking Strategy: Knowledge of the procedure for NG intermittent tube feeding will assist you in answering this question. The question is asking you what should be done with aspirated gastric residual. It does not need to be mixed with water, nor should it be discarded. Gastric contents should be reinstilled in order to maintain the client's electrolyte balance. The gastric contents should be poured into the NG tube through a syringe without a plunger and not injected by pushing on the plunger.

Level of Cognitive Ability: Application
Phase of Nursing Process: Implementation
Client Needs: Physiological Integrity
Content Area: Adult Health/Gastrointestinal

Reference

Kozier, B., Erb, G., & Blais, K. (1998). *Fundamentals of nursing: Concepts, process, and practice* (5th ed.). Reading, MA: Addison-Wesley. p. 1050.

16. 1

Rationale: The nurse must check the NG tube regularly to ensure that it is draining properly and is patent. Nasogastric tubes are used to decompress the stomach. The gastric distention will be relieved only if the tube drains properly. One cause of improper tube drainage is channels of gastric secretions forming along the walls of the stomach and bypassing the holes in the NG tube. Turning the client regularly helps collapse the channels and promotes gastric emptying. The tube has already been flushed, so it is unlikely that it is still blocked by thick secretions. Although this is a problem that requires attention, it is within the practice of nursing to maintain patency of the NG tube.

Test-Taking Strategy: The question addresses that the NG tube is not draining properly and asks for the nurse to analyze the problem. The stem includes some important data to note. Option 2 can be eliminated because the tube has just been flushed. Option 4 can be eliminated because there are still some nursing options available to re-establish NG tube patency. Option 3 can be eliminated because it is not acceptable to ignore the tube that has suddenly stopped draining.

Level of Cognitive Ability: Analysis
Phase of Nursing Process: Analysis
Client Needs: Physiological Integrity
Content Area: Adult Health/Gastrointestinal

Reference

Lewis, S., Collier, I., & Heitkemper, M. (1996). *Medical-surgical nursing: Assessment and management of clinical problems* (4th ed.). St. Louis: Mosby–Year Book. pp. 1237–1238.

17. 3

Rationale: The nurse should instruct the spouse to offer liquids containing both glucose and electrolytes. Small amounts of fluid may be tolerated even when vomiting is present. The diet should be advanced as tolerated.

Test-Taking Strategy: Identify words like "only" and "all" in options 1 and 2 and eliminate these options. Maintaining a clear liquid diet for at least 5 days is rather a lengthy time; therefore, eliminate this option also!

Level of Cognitive Ability: Application
Phase of Nursing Process: Implementation
Client Needs: Physiological integrity
Content Area: Adult Health/Gastrointestinal

Reference

Ignatavicius, D., Workman, M., & Mishler, M. (1995). *Medical-surgical nursing: A nursing process approach.* (2nd ed.) Philadelphia: W. B. Saunders. p. 1888.

18. 4

Rationale: Common risk factors for colorectal cancer include age over 40 years; first-degree relative with colorectal cancer; high-fat, low-fiber diet; and a history of bowel problems, such as ulcerative colitis or familial polyposis. Clients should be aware of risk factors as part of general health maintenance and primary disease prevention.

Test-Taking Strategy: Specific knowledge of risk factors related to colorectal cancer is needed to answer this question correctly. If needed, take a few moments to review this content area now!

Level of Cognitive Ability: Application
Phase of Nursing Process: Planning
Client Needs: Health Promotion and Maintenance
Content Area: Adult Health/Gastrointestinal

Reference

Monahan, F., & Neighbors, M. (1998). *Medical-surgical nursing: Foundations for clinical practice* (2nd ed.). Philadelphia: W. B. Saunders. p. 969.

19. 3

Rationale: The discomfort of reflux is aggravated by positions that compress the abdomen and the stomach. These include lying flat either on the back or stomach after a meal, or lying on the right side. The left side–lying position with head of the bed elevated is most likely to give relief to the client.

Test-Taking Strategy: To answer this question correctly, evaluate each of the positions described in terms of their ability to put pressure on the stomach and cause reflux. Using knowledge of anatomy and these basic nursing positions, you should be able to eliminate each of the incorrect options systematically!

Level of Cognitive Ability: Application
Phase of Nursing Process: Implementation
Client Needs: Physiological Integrity
Content Area: Adult Health/Gastrointestinal

Reference

Beare, P., & Myers, J. (1998). *Adult health nursing* (3rd ed.). St. Louis; Mosby–Year Book. p. 1485.

20. 2

Rationale: Foods that increase the LES pressure will decrease reflux, and lessen the symptoms of GERD. The food substance that will increase the LES pressure is nonfat milk. The other substances listed decrease the LES pressure, thus increasing reflux symptoms. Aggravating substances include chocolate, coffee, fatty foods, and alcohol.

Test-Taking Strategy: To answer this question accurately, it is necessary to understand the effect of various food substances on LES pressure and GERD. This will allow you to eliminate each of the incorrect options systematically. Review this now, if you had difficulty with this question!

Level of Cognitive Ability: Application
Phase of Nursing Process: Planning
Client Needs: Health Promotion and Maintenance
Content Area: Adult Health/Gastrointestinal

Reference

Beare, P., & Myers, J. (1998). *Adult health nursing* (3rd ed.). St. Louis: Mosby–Year Book. p. 1484.

21. 1

Rationale: The nurse places highest priority on assessing for return of the gag reflex and managing the client's airway. The client's vital signs are monitored also; a sudden, sharp increase in temperature could indicate perforation of the GI tract. This would be accompanied by other signs as well, such as pain. Monitoring for sore throat and heartburn are also important; the client's airway still takes priority however.

Test-Taking Strategy: Remember the ABCs: Airway, Breathing, and Circulation. Note also that the question contains the key words "highest priority." This tells you that more than one or all of the options may be partially or totally correct. Use the ABCs to set your priorities.

Level of Cognitive Ability: Application
Phase of Nursing Process: Planning
Client Needs: Physiological Integrity
Content Area: Adult Health/Gastrointestinal

Reference
Beare, P., & Myers, J. (1998). *Adult health nursing* (3rd ed.). St. Louis: Mosby–Year Book. p. 1465.

22. **2**

Rationale: The client does have to lie still for ERCP, which takes about an hour to perform. The client does also have to sign a consent form. IV sedation is given to relax the client, and an anesthetic spray is used to help keep the client from gagging as the endoscope is passed.

Test-Taking Strategy: Note the key words "has not fully understood." Invasive procedures require consent, so option 1 can be eliminated. Noting the name of the procedure and considering the anatomical location will assist in eliminating options 3 and 4. Review this procedure now, if you had difficulty with this question!

Level of Cognitive Ability: Analysis
Phase of Nursing Process: Evaluation
Client Needs: Physiological Integrity
Content Area: Adult Health/Gastrointestinal

Reference
Beare, P., & Myers, J. (1998). *Adult health nursing* (3rd ed.). St. Louis: Mosby–Year Book. p. 1472.

23. **1**

Rationale: A barium swallow, or esophagography, is an x-ray study that uses a substance called barium for contrast to highlight abnormalities in the GI tract. The client is told to remove all jewelry before the test, so it won't interfere with x-ray visualization of the field. The client should fast for 8 to 12 hours before the test, depending on physician instructions. Most oral medications are also withheld before the test. It is important after the procedure to monitor for constipation, which can occur as a result of the presence of barium in the GI tract.

Test-Taking Strategy: Note that the key words in the stem of the question are "barium swallow" and "before." This tells you that the correct answer is an item that the client needs to comply with before the test is done. Eliminate option 4 first, since it is a part of aftercare. Knowing that the procedure is a type of x-ray study that involves barium for contrast allows you to eliminate each of the incorrect options successfully.

Level of Cognitive Ability: Application
Phase of Nursing Process: Implementation
Client Needs: Safe, Effective Care Environment
Content Area: Adult Health/Gastrointestinal

Reference
Beare, P., & Myers, J. (1998). *Adult health nursing* (3rd ed.). St. Louis: Mosby–Year Book. p. 1465.

24. **3**

Rationale: The client should be able to resume the usual diet once the nurse is assured that the GI function is normal. It is not necessary to keep the client on clear liquids for 72 hours following the procedure. The nurse would monitor the client for complaints of GI discomfort and nausea and vomiting. The nurse would also assess the client's hydration status as part of routine care for the client undergoing a GI diagnostic test.

Test-Taking Strategy: Note that the key words in the stem of the question are "delete" and "following." This tells you that the correct option is one that would have been needed before the procedure but is no longer necessary. Utilize knowledge of concepts related to dietary preparations for GI studies to choose correctly.

Level of Cognitive Ability: Application
Phase of Nursing Process: Planning
Client Needs: Physiological Integrity
Content Area: Adult Health/Gastrointestinal

Reference
Monahan, F., & Neighbors, M. (1998). *Medical-surgical nursing: Foundations for clinical practice* (2nd ed.). Philadelphia: W. B. Saunders. p. 972.

25. **1**

Rationale: The client is placed in the left Sims' position for the procedure. This position takes the best advantage of the client's anatomy for ease in introducing the colonoscope. The other options are incorrect.

Test-Taking Strategy: Utilize concepts related to GI anatomy to answer this question. The answer is the same position utilized for giving the client an enema while lying down. When answering factual questions such as these, remember the guiding principles and attempt to visualize the procedure to help you select the correct option.

Level of Cognitive Ability: Application
Phase of Nursing Process: Implementation
Client Needs: Physiological Integrity
Content Area: Adult Health/Gastrointestinal

Reference
Monahan, F., & Neighbors, M. (1998). *Medical-surgical nursing: Foundations for clinical practice* (2nd ed.). Philadelphia: W. B. Saunders. p. 975.

26. **4**

Rationale: The client should not drive for several hours after discharge because the client would have received sedative medications during the procedure. Important decisions should also be delayed for at least 24 hours for the same reason. The client should resume intake slowly, and progress as tolerated. The client may experience gas or abdominal tenderness for a short while after the procedure, and this is normal.

Test-Taking Strategy: Note that the question contains the key words "did not fully understand." This tells you that the correct answer is an incorrect statement on the part of the client. Utilize knowledge of events during the procedure to choose the correct option. Knowledge that sedating medications are administered will direct you to option 4.

Level of Cognitive Ability: Analysis
Phase of Nursing Process: Evaluation
Client Needs: Health Promotion and Maintenance
Content Area: Adult Health/Gastrointestinal

Reference
Monahan, F., & Neighbors, M. (1998). *Medical-surgical nursing: Foundations for clinical practice* (2nd ed.). Philadelphia: W. B. Saunders. p. 976.

27. 2

Rationale: The appropriate technique for abdominal examination is inspection, auscultation, percussion, and palpation. Auscultation is performed after inspection to ensure that the motility of the bowel and bowel sounds are not altered. The sequence of maneuvers is inspect, auscultate, percuss, and palpate.

Test-Taking Strategy: Knowledge regarding the techniques used to assess the abdomen is required to answer the question. Remember that the sequence for abdominal assessment is different from the usual systematic approach. Review this technique now, if you had difficulty with this question!

Level of Cognitive Ability: Application
Phase of Nursing Process: Assessment
Client Needs: Health Promotion and Maintenance
Content Area: Adult Health/Gastrointestinal

Reference
Lammon, C., Foote, A., Leli, P., et al. (1995). *Clinical nursing skills.* Philadelphia: W. B. Saunders. pp. 727, 763.

28. 3

Rationale: A barium swallow should be done after a barium enema or gallbladder series to prevent the mixture used in the barium swallow from obstructing the view of other organs. It takes several days for swallowed barium to pass completely out of the GI tract.

Test-Taking Strategy: Eliminate options 1 and 4 first because a gallbladder series is the same procedure as an oral cholecystogram. In selecting from the remaining options, think about the use of barium and its effect in blocking the visualization of organs. This concept should easily direct you to option 3.

Level of Cognitive Ability: Application
Phase of Nursing Process: Implementation
Client Needs: Physiological Integrity
Content Area: Adult Health/Gastrointestinal

Reference
Monahan, F., & Neighbors, M. (1998). *Medical-surgical nursing: Foundations for clinical practice* (2nd ed.). Philadelphia: W. B. Saunders. pp. 970–971.

29. 3

Rationale: Normal dietary intake of fat should be maintained during the days preceding the test in order to empty bile from the gallbladder. A fat-free diet is ordered on the evening before the test. The fat-free supper prevents contraction of the gallbladder and allows accumulation of the contrast substance needed for x-ray visualization.

Test-Taking Strategy: Knowledge that an oral cholecystogram is an x-ray study of the gallbladder will assist in directing you to the correct option. Think about the function of the gallbladder to assist in selecting the correct option.

Level of Cognitive Ability: Application
Phase of Nursing Process: Planning
Client Needs: Physiological Integrity
Content Area: Adult Health/Gastrointestinal

Reference
Monahan, F., & Neighbors, M. (1998). *Medical-surgical nursing: Foundations for clinical practice* (2nd ed.). Philadelphia: W. B. Saunders. p. 972.

30. 4

Rationale: Following the procedure, the client remains NPO until the gag reflex returns, which is usually in 1 to 2 hours. Options 1, 2, and 3 are not specific assessments related to this procedure.

Test-Taking Strategy: Note the key words "upper GI endoscopy." The only option that relates to the anatomical location of this procedure is option 4. Review postprocedure care following endoscopy now, if you had difficulty with this question!

Level of Cognitive Ability: Application
Phase of Nursing Process: Planning
Client Needs: Physiological Integrity
Content Area: Adult Health/Gastrointestinal

Reference
Monahan, F., & Neighbors, M. (1998). *Medical-surgical nursing: Foundations for clinical practice* (2nd ed.). Philadelphia: W. B. Saunders. p. 973.

31. 4

Rationale: The solution GoLYTELY is a bowel evacuant used in preparation for colonoscopy to cleanse the bowel. It is expected to cause a mild diarrhea and will clear the bowel in 4 to 5 hours.

Test-Taking Strategy: Knowledge regarding the purpose of this medication will assist in eliminating option 3 and easily direct you to option 4. Options 1 and 2 are not within the scope of nursing practice and should be eliminated.

Level of Cognitive Ability: Application
Phase of Nursing Process: Implementation
Client Needs: Physiological Integrity
Content Area: Adult Health/Gastrointestinal

Reference
Hodgson, B., & Kizior, R. (1998). *Saunders nursing drug handbook 1998.* Philadelphia: W. B. Saunders. p. 841.

32. 3

Rationale: To best facilitate insertion, when the tube reaches the pharynx the client is encouraged to lower the head slightly, swallow, and if allowed take sips of water. The NG tube would be iced so that it is stiff, to ease insertion. Hyperextension of the head is done in preparation for insertion. If the tube enters the trachea, it must be withdrawn and repassed. Option 3 is the only option that would facilitate insertion.

Test-Taking Strategy: The issue of the question relates to facilitating easy insertion of the NG tube. Option 1 can be easily eliminated. From the remaining options, focusing on the issue will assist in eliminating options 2 and 4.

Level of Cognitive Ability: Application
Phase of Nursing Process: Planning
Client Needs: Physiological Integrity
Content Area: Adult Health/Gastrointestinal

Reference
Monahan, F., & Neighbors, M. (1998). *Medical-surgical nursing: Foundations for clinical practice* (2nd ed.). Philadelphia: W. B. Saunders. p. 978.

33. **3**

Rationale: When GI tubes are attached to suction, the suction may be continuous or intermittent, with a pressure not exceeding 25 mmHg. The specific pressure and the intervals are prescribed by the physician.

Test-Taking Strategy: Knowledge regarding the restrictions related to the amount of pressure with suction on a GI tube is required to answer this question. Learn this now, if you are unfamiliar with this procedure!

Level of Cognitive Ability: Analysis
Phase of Nursing Process: Implementation
Client Needs: Physiological Integrity
Content Area: Adult Health/Gastrointestinal

Reference

Monahan, F., & Neighbors, M. (1998). *Medical-surgical nursing: Foundations for clinical practice* (2nd ed.). Philadelphia: W. B. Saunders. p. 978.

34. **2**

Rationale: Deterioration and atrophy of the lining of the stomach lead to the loss of function of the parietal cells. When the acid secretion decreases, the source of the intrinsic factor is lost, which results in the inability to absorb vitamin B_{12}. This leads to the development of pernicious anemia.

Test-Taking Strategy: Knowledge regarding the pathophysiology related to the lining of the stomach is required to answer this question. If you are unfamiliar with vitamin B_{12} deficiency and its relationship to gastric disorders, review now!

Level of Cognitive Ability: Analysis
Phase of Nursing Process: Analysis
Client Needs: Physiological Integrity
Content Area: Adult Health/Gastrointestinal

Reference

Black, J., & Matassarin-Jacobs, E. (1997). *Medical-surgical nursing: Clinical management for continuity of care* (5th ed.). Philadelphia: W. B. Saunders. p. 1763.

35. **2**

Rationale: Indocin is an NSAID and can cause ulceration of the esophagus, stomach, duodenum, or small intestine. It is contraindicated in a client with GI disorders. Lasix is a loop diuretic. Digoxin is an antidysrhythmic. Inderal is a beta-adrenergic blocker. Lasix, digoxin, and Inderal are not contraindicated in clients with gastric disorders.

Test-Taking Strategy: Knowledge regarding the side effects associated with the medications identified in the options is required to answer this question. If you are unfamiliar with these medications, take time now to review them!

Level of Cognitive Ability: Analysis
Phase of Nursing Process: Implementation
Client Needs: Physiological Integrity
Content Area: Adult Health/Gastrointestinal

Reference

Hodgson, B., & Kizior, R. (1998). *Saunders nursing drug handbook 1998.* Philadelphia: W. B. Saunders. pp. 528–530, 324–326, 452–454, 877–880.

36. **2**

Rationale: Following cholecystectomy, drainage from the T tube is initially bloody and then turns green-brown and is measured as output. The amount of expected drainage will range from 500 to 1000 mL per day. The nurse would document the output.

Test-Taking Strategy: Knowledge regarding normal expectations following a cholecystectomy is required to answer this question. Options 3 and 4 can be eliminated because a T tube is not irrigated and would not be clamped with this amount of drainage. Review postoperative assessment findings following cholecystectomy now, if you had difficulty with this question!

Level of Cognitive Ability: Analysis
Phase of Nursing Process: Implementation
Client Needs: Physiological Integrity
Content Area: Adult Health/Gastrointestinal

Reference

Monahan, F., & Neighbors, M. (1998). *Medical-surgical nursing: Foundations for clinical practice* (2nd ed.). Philadelphia: W. B. Saunders. p. 1114.

37. **4**

Rationale: Perforation is a surgical emergency. It is characterized by sudden, sharp, intolerable severe pain beginning in the midepigastric area and spreading over the abdomen, which becomes rigid and boardlike. Nausea and vomiting may occur. Tachycardia may occur as hypovolemic shock develops. Numbness in the legs is not an associated finding.

Test-Taking Strategy: Note the key words "most likely" in the stem of the question. Option 2 can be easily eliminated. Eliminate option 1 next because tachycardia rather than bradycardia would develop if the client is bleeding. From the remaining two options, focusing on the key words will assist in directing you to option 4.

Level of Cognitive Ability: Analysis
Phase of Nursing Process: Assessment
Client Needs: Physiological Integrity
Content Area: Adult Health/Gastrointestinal

Reference

Monahan, F., & Neighbors, M. (1998). *Medical-surgical nursing: Foundations for clinical practice* (2nd ed.). Philadelphia: W. B. Saunders. p. 1029.

38. **1**

Rationale: Tagamet, a histamine H_2-receptor antagonist, will decrease the secretion of gastric acid. Carafate promotes healing by coating the ulcer. Antacids neutralize acid in the stomach. Prilosec inhibits gastric acid secretion.

Test-Taking Strategy: Knowledge regarding the actions of the medications used to treat peptic ulcers is required to answer this question. If you are unfamiliar with these medications or their actions, take time now to review them!

Level of Cognitive Ability: Analysis
Phase of Nursing Process: Evaluation
Client Needs: Health Promotion and Maintenance
Content Area: Adult Health/Gastrointestinal

Reference

Monahan, F., & Neighbors, M. (1998). *Medical-surgical nursing: Foundations for clinical practice* (2nd ed.). Philadelphia: W. B. Saunders. pp. 1027–1028.

39. 4

Rationale: Option 4 describes the procedure for a pyloroplasty. A vagotomy involves cutting the vagus nerve. A subtotal gastrectomy involves removing the distal portion of the stomach. A Billroth II procedure involves removal of the ulcer and a large portion of the cells that produce hydrochloric acid.

Test-Taking Strategy: Note the relationship between the words "pyloroplasty" and "pylorus" in the correct option. If you are unfamiliar with this procedure, take time now to review!

Level of Cognitive Ability: Analysis
Phase of Nursing Process: Analysis
Client Needs: Physiological Integrity
Content Area: Adult Health/Gastrointestinal

Reference
Monahan, F., & Neighbors, M. (1998). *Medical-surgical nursing: Foundations for clinical practice* (2nd ed.). Philadelphia: W. B. Saunders. p. 1028.

40. 2

Rationale: During the first few days after hemorrhage, gastric pH should be increased to between 5.5 and 7.0 and maintained at this level to control secretory activity. Ranitidine (Zantac) or cimetidine (Tagamet) may be prescribed in addition to antacids to accomplish this. The use of antacids complements the effectiveness of H_2-antagonists for maintaining the pH level of gastric secretions.

Test-Taking Strategy: Knowledge regarding treatment goals following a GI bleed will assist in answering this question. Remembering that gastric secretions are acidic will assist in eliminating option 1. Options 3 and 4 identify an alkaline pH. Therefore, option 2 is the best choice.

Level of Cognitive Ability: Application
Phase of Nursing Process: Planning
Client Needs: Physiological Integrity
Content Area: Adult Health/Gastrointestinal

Reference
Ignatavicius, D., Workman, M., & Mishler, M. (1995). *Medical-surgical nursing: A nursing process approach.* (2nd ed.) Philadelphia: W. B. Saunders. p. 1578.

41. 4

Rationale: A vagotomy, or cutting of the vagus nerve, is done to eliminate parasympathetic stimulation of gastric secretion. Options 1, 2, and 3 are incorrect descriptions of a vagotomy.

Test-Taking Strategy: Knowledge regarding the procedure and purpose of a vagotomy is required to answer this question. If you are unfamiliar with this procedure, take time now to review!

Level of Cognitive Ability: Application
Phase of Nursing Process: Implementation
Client Needs: Physiological Integrity
Content Area: Adult Health/Gastrointestinal

Reference
Monahan, F., & Neighbors, M. (1998). *Medical-surgical nursing: Foundations for clinical practice* (2nd ed.). Philadelphia: W. B. Saunders. p. 1028.

42. 1

Rationale: In a Billroth II resection, the proximal remnant of the stomach is anastamosed to the proximal jejunum. Patency of the NG tube is critical for preventing the retention of gastric secretions. The nurse, however, should never irrigate or reposition the gastric tube after gastric surgery unless specifically ordered to do so by the physician. In this situation, the nurse should clarify the order. Options 2, 3, and 4 are appropriate postoperative interventions.

Test-Taking Strategy: Eliminate options 2, 3, and 4 because they are general postoperative measures. Consider the anatomical location of the surgical procedure to assist in directing you to option 1. Review postoperative measures now, if you had difficulty with this question!

Level of Cognitive Ability: Analysis
Phase of Nursing Process: Implementation
Client Needs: Physiological Integrity
Content Area: Adult Health/Gastrointestinal

Reference
Ignatavicius, D., Workman, M., & Mishler, M. (1995). *Medical-surgical nursing: A nursing process approach.* (2nd ed.) Philadelphia: W. B. Saunders. p. 1581.

43. 2

Rationale: The client should be instructed to decrease the amount of fluid taken at meals. The client should also be instructed to avoid high-carbohydrate foods, including fluids such as fruit nectars; to assume a low Fowler's position during meals; to lie down for 30 minutes after eating to delay gastric emptying; and to take antispasmodics as prescribed.

Test-Taking Strategy: Eliminate options 3 and 4 first because these measures will promote gastric emptying. From the remaining options, select option 2 because this measure will delay gastric emptying. If you are unfamiliar with this syndrome, take time now to review the important client teaching points!

Level of Cognitive Ability: Application
Phase of Nursing Process: Implementation
Client Needs: Health Promotion and Maintenance
Content Area: Adult Health/Gastrointestinal

Reference
Monahan, F., & Neighbors, M. (1998). *Medical-surgical nursing: Foundations for clinical practice* (2nd ed.). Philadelphia: W. B. Saunders. p. 1000.

44. 3

Rationale: Early manifestations occur 5 to 30 minutes after eating. Symptoms include vertigo, tachycardia, syncope, sweating, pallor, palpitations, and the desire to lie down.

Test-Taking Strategy: Knowledge regarding the early manifestations associated with dumping syndrome is required to answer this question. If you are unfamiliar with these manifestations, review them now!

Level of Cognitive Ability: Analysis
Phase of Nursing Process: Assessment
Client Needs: Physiological Integrity
Content Area: Adult Health/Gastrointestinal

Reference
Ignatavicius, D., Workman, M., & Mishler, M. (1995). *Medical-surgical nursing: A nursing process approach* (2nd ed.). Philadelphia: W. B. Saunders. p. 1581.

45. 3

Rationale: Bed rest is not required following this surgical procedure. The client should take analgesics as needed and as prescribed. A drain is not placed in this procedure, although the client may be instructed in simple dressing changes. Coughing is avoided to prevent disruption of the tissue integrity, which can occur due to the location of this surgical procedure.

Test-Taking Strategy: General postoperative measures will assist in eliminating options 1 and 2. Consider the anatomical location of the surgery and the surgical procedure to assist in selecting option 3. Review postoperative measures now, if you had difficulty with this question!

Level of Cognitive Ability: Application
Phase of Nursing Process: Implementation
Client Needs: Health Promotion and Maintenance
Content Area: Adult Health/Gastrointestinal

Reference
Monahan, F., & Neighbors, M. (1998). *Medical-surgical nursing: Foundations for clinical practice* (2nd ed.). Philadelphia: W. B. Saunders. p. 1096.

46. 2

Rationale: Following herniorrhaphy, the client should be instructed to elevate the scrotum and apply ice packs while in bed to decrease pain and swelling. Instruct the client to apply a scrotal support when out of bed.

Test-Taking Strategy: The issue of the question is to prevent swelling. Basic knowledge regarding the effects of heat will assist in eliminating option 1. Options 3 and 4 can be eliminated next by focusing on the issue of the question. Review postoperative care following herniorrhaphy now, if you had difficulty with this question!

Level of Cognitive Ability: Application
Phase of Nursing Process: Implementation
Client Needs: Health Promotion and Maintenance
Content Area: Adult Health/Gastrointestinal

Reference
Monahan, F., & Neighbors, M. (1998). *Medical-surgical nursing: Foundations for clinical practice* (2nd ed.). Philadelphia: W. B. Saunders. p. 1096.

47. 4

Rationale: Rebound tenderness may be indicative of peritonitis. Bloody diarrhea is expected to occur in ulcerative colitis. Because of the blood loss, the client may be hypotensive, and the hemoglobin may be lower than normal. Signs of peritonitis must be reported to the physician.

Test-Taking Strategy: Consider the expected manifestations that would occur in ulcerative colitis. This should assist you in eliminating option 1. This manifestation would cause a lowered hemoglobin and hypotension; therefore, eliminate options 2 and 3. Review the normal assessment findings in ulcerative colitis now, if you had difficulty with this question!

Level of Cognitive Ability: Analysis
Phase of Nursing Process: Assessment
Client Needs: Physiological Integrity
Content Area: Adult Health/Gastrointestinal

Reference
Ignatavicius, D., Workman, M., & Mishler, M. (1995). *Medical-surgical nursing: A nursing process approach.* (2nd ed.) Philadelphia: W. B. Saunders. p. 1640.

48. 2

Rationale: Lomotil is an antidiarrheal product that decreases the frequency of stools, usually by reducing the volume of liquid in the stools. Options 1, 3, and 4 are not associated therapeutic effects of this medication.

Test-Taking Strategy: Think about the diagnosis presented in the question. Knowledge of the clinical manifestations that occur in this condition will easily direct you to option 2. If you had difficulty with this question, review the therapeutic effect of Lomotil now!

Level of Cognitive Ability: Analysis
Phase of Nursing Process: Evaluation
Client Needs: Physiological Integrity
Content Area: Adult Health/Gastrointestinal

Reference
Ignatavicius, D., Workman, M., & Mishler, M. (1995). *Medical-surgical nursing: A nursing process approach.* (2nd ed.) Philadelphia: W. B. Saunders. p. 1641.

49. 1

Rationale: The client with irritable bowel syndrome should be encouraged to include fiber and bulk in the diet to help produce bulky, soft stools and establish regular bowel habits. The client should ingest approximately 30 to 40 g of fiber each day. Eating regular meals, drinking 8 to 10 cups of liquids each day, and chewing food slowly promote normal bowel function.

Test-Taking Strategy: Note the key word "not" in the stem of the question. Also note that options 1 and 2 are opposite client instructions. This should indicate that one of these options is the correct one. Recalling that the goal is to establish regular bowel habits will assist in directing you to option 1.

Level of Cognitive Ability: Application
Phase of Nursing Process: Planning
Client Needs: Health Promotion and Maintenance
Content Area: Adult Health/Gastrointestinal

Reference
Ignatavicius, D., Workman, M., & Mishler, M. (1995). *Medical-surgical nursing: A nursing process approach* (2nd ed.). Philadelphia: W. B. Saunders. p. 1598.

50. 4

Rationale: Azulfidine is an anti-inflammatory sulfonamide. It can cause photosensitivity, and the client should be instructed to avoid sun and ultraviolet light. It should be administered with meals if possible to prolong intestinal passage. The client needs to take the medication as prescribed and continue for the full length of treatment even if symptoms are relieved. Constipation is not associated with this medication.

Test-Taking Strategy: Note the key word "not" in the stem of the question. Eliminate option 3 first because this is a general measure regarding medication therapy. Knowing that this medication is a sulfonamide will assist in eliminating options 1 and 2. Review client teaching points regarding this medication now, if you had difficulty with this question!

Level of Cognitive Ability: Application
Phase of Nursing Process: Planning
Client Needs: Health Promotion and Maintenance
Content Area: Adult Health/Gastrointestinal

Reference
Hodgson, B., & Kizior, R. (1998). *Saunders nursing drug handbook 1998*. Philadelphia: W. B. Saunders. pp. 953–955.

51. 2

Rationale: Risk for Body Image Disturbance relates to loss of bowel control, the presence of a stoma, the release of fecal material onto the abdomen, the passage of flatus, odor, and the need for an appliance. No data in the question support options 3 and 4. Risk for Altered Nutrition; Less Than Body Requirements is the more likely nursing diagnosis.

Test-Taking Strategy: Use the data presented in the question to assist in selecting the correct option. No data in the question support options 3 and 4. Reading option 1 carefully will assist in eliminating this option and direct you to option 2.

Level of Cognitive Ability: Analysis
Phase of Nursing Process: Planning
Client Needs: Psychosocial Integrity
Content Area: Adult Health/Gastrointestinal

Reference
Monahan, F., & Neighbors, M. (1998). *Medical-surgical nursing: Foundations for clinical practice* (2nd ed.). Philadelphia: W. B. Saunders. p. 1007.

52. 2

Rationale: Crohn's disease is characterized by nonbloody diarrhea of usually not more than 4 to 5 stools daily. Over time, the diarrheal episodes do increase in frequency, duration, and severity. Options 3 and 4 are not characteristics of Crohn's disease.

Test-Taking Strategy: Options 3 and 4 can be easily eliminated. From the remaining options, it is necessary to be familiar with the characteristics of Crohn's disease. If you are unfamiliar with this disorder, take time now to review!

Level of Cognitive Ability: Analysis
Phase of Nursing Process: Assessment
Client Needs: Physiological Integrity
Content Area: Adult Health/Gastrointestinal

Reference
Monahan, F., & Neighbors, M. (1998). *Medical-surgical nursing: Foundations for clinical practice* (2nd ed.). Philadelphia: W. B. Saunders. p. 1067.

53. 3

Rationale: If cramping occurs during colostomy irrigation, stop the irrigation flow temporarily and allow the client to rest. Cramping may occur from infusion that is too rapid or is causing too much pressure. Increasing the height of the irrigation will cause further discomfort. The physician does not need to be notified. Medicating the client for pain is not the most appropriate action.

Test-Taking Strategy: Focus on the issue of the question. This will assist in eliminating options 1, 2, and 4 and easily direct you to the correct option. If you had difficulty answering this question, take time now to review the procedure for colostomy irrigation!

Level of Cognitive Ability: Application
Phase of Nursing Process: Implementation
Client Needs: Physiological Integrity
Content Area: Adult Health/Gastrointestinal

Reference
Lammon, C., Foote, A., Leli, P., et al. (1995). *Clinical nursing skills*. Philadelphia: W. B. Saunders. p. 471.

54. 3

Rationale: To enhance effectiveness of the irrigation, instruct the client to change position, ambulate, massage the abdomen gently, and drink something warm. Options 1, 2, and 4 will not enhance the effectiveness of this procedure.

Test-Taking Strategy: Focus on the issue of the question, which is the measure that will enhance the effectiveness of the irrigation. This focus will assist in eliminating options 1, 2, and 4. If you are unfamiliar with this procedure, take time now to review!

Level of Cognitive Ability: Application
Phase of Nursing Process: Implementation
Client Needs: Health Promotion and Maintenance
Content Area: Adult Health/Gastrointestinal

Reference
Ignatavicius, D., Workman, M., & Mishler, M. (1995). *Medical-surgical nursing: A nursing process approach* (2nd ed.). Philadelphia: W. B. Saunders. p. 1609.

55. 1

Rationale: Asterixis is irregular, flapping movements of the fingers and wrists when the hands and arms are outstretched, with the palms down, wrists bent up, and fingers spread. It is the most common and reliable sign that hepatic encephalopathy is developing.

Test-Taking Strategy: Knowledge regarding the procedure for this important assessment is required to answer this question. If you are unfamiliar with this assessment procedure, be sure to review now!

Level of Cognitive Ability: Application
Phase of Nursing Process: Assessment
Client Needs: Physiological Integrity
Content Area: Adult Health/Gastrointestinal

Reference
Monahan, F., & Neighbors, M. (1998). *Medical-surgical nursing: Foundations for clinical practice* (2nd ed.). Philadelphia: W. B. Saunders. p. 1150.

56. 2

Rationale: Fluid volume excess, related to the accumulation of fluid in the peritoneal cavity and dependent areas of the body, can occur in the client with cirrhosis. Fluids should be restricted, including fluids given with medications and meals. Sodium restriction will also aid in reducing fluid volume excess. Options 3 and 4 will not assist in reducing fluid volume excess.

Test-Taking Strategy: Note that the issue is to reduce fluid excess. Options 3 and 4 can be eliminated first. Recalling that sodium will retain fluids will assist in eliminating option 1. Review care to the client with cirrhosis now, if you had difficulty with this question!

Level of Cognitive Ability: Application
Phase of Nursing Process: Implementation
Client Needs: Physiological Integrity
Content Area: Adult Health/Gastrointestinal

Reference
Monahan, F., & Neighbors, M. (1998). *Medical-surgical nursing: Foundations for clinical practice* (2nd ed.). Philadelphia: W. B. Saunders. p. 1190.

57. **4**

Rationale: An upright position allows the intestine to float away from the paracentesis site and helps prevent intestinal laceration during catheter insertion.

Test-Taking Strategy: Attempt to visualize this procedure in selecting the correct option. Knowing that fluid will be aspirated from the abdominal cavity will assist in directing you to option 4. If you had difficulty with this question, review this procedure now!

Level of Cognitive Ability: Application
Phase of Nursing Process: Implementation
Client Needs: Physiological Integrity
Content Area: Adult Health/Gastrointestinal

Reference
Lammon, C., Foote, A., Leli, P., et al. (1995). *Clinical nursing skills.* Philadelphia: W. B. Saunders. p. 157.

58. **4**

Rationale: Most of the ammonia in the body is found in the GI tract. Protein provided by the diet is transported to the liver by the portal vein. The liver breaks down protein, and this results in the formation of ammonia. A low-protein diet would be prescribed.

Test-Taking Strategy: Recall the physiology of the liver in answering this question. Note that the question stem states "most likely." You should be easily directed to option 4. Also note that options 3 and 4 are opposite, which should provide you with the clue that one of these options is correct.

Level of Cognitive Ability: Application
Phase of Nursing Process: Implementation
Client Needs: Physiological Integrity
Content Area: Adult Health/Gastrointestinal

Reference
Ignatavicius, D., Workman, M., & Mishler, M. (1995). *Medical-surgical nursing: A nursing process approach* (2nd ed.). Philadelphia: W. B. Saunders. p. 1668.

59. **1**

Rationale: Lactulose is an osmotic laxative. The desired effect is 2 to 3 soft stools per day with an acid fecal pH. Lactulose creates an acid environment in the bowel, resulting in a fall of the colon's pH from 7 to 5. This causes ammonia to leave the circulatory system and move into the colon. Diarrhea may indicate excessive administration of the medication. Options 3 and 4 do not determine that a desired effect has occurred.

Test-Taking Strategy: Knowledge regarding the purpose and action of this medication is required to answer this question. Review this important medication now, if you had difficulty with this question!

Level of Cognitive Ability: Analysis
Phase of Nursing Process: Evaluation
Client Needs: Physiological Integrity
Content Area: Adult Health/Gastrointestinal

Reference
Ignatavicius, D., Workman, M., & Mishler, M. (1995). *Medical-surgical nursing: A nursing process approach.* (2nd ed.) Philadelphia: W.B. Saunders. p. 1680.

60. **1**

Rationale: Ultrasound of the gallbladder is a noninvasive procedure and is frequently used for emergency diagnosis of acute cholecystitis. The client does not need to be NPO but may be instructed to avoid carbonated beverages for 48 hours before the test to help decrease intestinal gas. It is a painless test and does not require the administration of oral tablets as preparation.

Test-Taking Strategy: Attempt to vizualize this procedure in selecting the correct option. This should be relatively easy; however, if you are unfamiliar with this test take time now to review!

Level of Cognitive Ability: Application
Phase of Nursing Process: Implementation
Client Needs: Physiological Integrity
Content Area: Adult Health/Gastrointestinal

Reference
Monahan, F., & Neighbors, M. (1998). *Medical-surgical nursing: Foundations for clinical practice* (2nd ed.). Philadelphia: W. B. Saunders. p. 976.

61. **1**

Rationale: After cholecystectomy, breathing tends to be shallow because deep breathing is painful as a result of the location of the incision. Teaching the importance of perfoming coughing and deep breathing exercises is the priority.

Test-Taking Strategy: Utilize Maslow's Hierarchy of Needs theory to answer the question. Option 1 relates to airway. Additionally, recalling the anatomical location of the abdominal incision will assist in directing you to the correct option.

Level of Cognitive Ability: Application
Phase of Nursing Process: Planning
Client Needs: Physiological Integrity
Content Area: Adult Health/Gastrointestinal

Reference
Monahan, F., & Neighbors, M. (1998). *Medical-surgical nursing: Foundations for clinical practice* (2nd ed.). Philadelphia: W. B. Saunders. p. 1116.

62. **2**

Rationale: Serosanguineous drainage with a small amount of bile is expected from the Penrose drain for the first 24 hours. Drainage then decreases and the drain is removed, usually in 48 hours. The physician does not need to be notified. A sterile dressing covers the site and should be changed to prevent infection and skin excoriation..

Test-Taking Strategy: Eliminate options 3 and 4 first because they are similar. Knowledge of the normal expected findings following cholecystectomy will easily direct you to option 2.

Level of Cognitive Ability: Application
Phase of Nursing Process: Implementation
Client Needs: Physiological Integrity
Content Area: Adult Health/Gastrointestinal

Reference
Monahan, F., & Neighbors, M. (1998). *Medical-surgical nursing: Foundations for clinical practice* (2nd ed.). Philadelphia: W. B. Saunders. p. 1114.

63. **2**

Rationale: This medication binds with bile salts in the intestines to form a compound that is excreted in the feces. The client should be instructed to mix the medication with 3 to 6 oz of water, milk, fruit juice, or soup. It should be administered before meals. It is not administered via rectal suppository.

Test-Taking Strategy: Knowledge regarding the administration of this medication is required to answer this question. Knowledge that is it available in oral form will assist in eliminating option 3. Review this medication now, if you had difficulty with this question!

Level of Cognitive Ability: Application
Phase of Nursing Process: Implementation
Client Needs: Health Promotion and Maintenance
Content Area: Adult Health/Gastrointestinal

Reference
Hodgson, B., & Kizior, R. (1998). *Saunders nursing drug handbook 1998.* Philadelphia: W. B. Saunders. p. 216.

64. **4**

Rationale: Meperidine hydrochloride (Demerol) rather than morphine is the medication of choice because morphine can cause spasms in the sphincter of Oddi. Options 1, 2, and 3 are appropriate interventions for the client with acute pancreatitis.

Test-Taking Strategy: Note the key word "acute" in the question. Knowledge regarding the treatment measures for acute pancreatitis is required to answer this question. Review this content now. You are likely to find a question related to this content on NCLEX-RN!

Level of Cognitive Ability: Analysis
Phase of Nursing Process: Implementation
Client Needs: Physiological Integrity
Content Area: Adult Health/Gastrointestinal

Reference
Monahan, F., & Neighbors, M. (1998). *Medical-Surgical nursing: Foundations for clinical practice* (2nd ed.). Philadelphia: W. B. Saunders. p. 1118.

65. **4**

Rationale: Viokase aids in the digestion of protein, carbohydrate, and fat in the GI tract. It is used to treat steatorrhea associated with postgastrectomy syndrome for bowel resection. The nurse should record the number of stools per day and the stool consistency to monitor the effectiveness of this enzyme therapy. If it is effective, the stools should become less frequent and less fatty.

Test-Taking Strategy: Knowledge regarding the use and therapeutic effect of this medication is required to answer this question. If you are unfamiliar with this medication, take time now to review!

Level of Cognitive Ability: Analysis
Phase of Nursing Process: Evaluation
Client Needs: Physiological Integrity
Content Area: Adult Health/Gastrointestinal

Reference
Hodgson, B., & Kizior, R. (1998). *Saunders nursing drug handbook 1998.* Philadelphia: W. B. Saunders. p. 787.

66. **3**

Rationale: Expected outcomes for the client with PUD experiencing pain include elimination of irritating foods from the diet, ability to take prescribed medications that will reduce pain, reporting that pain is relieved or prevented with medication, and an ability to sleep through the night without pain. The client who continues to be awakened by pain requires further modification of medication therapy, which may include adjustment of timing of histamine receptor-antagonist, or an additional dose of antacid prior to the time when pain awakens the client.

Test-Taking Strategy: Note that the stem of the question contains the key words "expected outcomes" and "not met." This tells you that the correct answer is an option that indicates insufficient pain management. Utilize knowledge of medication therapy for PUD to eliminate each of the incorrect options systematically.

Level of Cognitive Ability: Analysis
Phase of Nursing Process: Evaluation
Client Needs: Physiological Integrity
Content Area: Adult Health/Gastrointestinal

Reference
Monahan, F., & Neighbors, M. (1998). *Medical-surgical nursing: Foundations for clinical practice* (2nd ed.). Philadelphia: W. B. Saunders. p. 1032.

67. **1**

Rationale: The most frequent symptom of duodenal ulcer is pain that is relieved by food intake. These clients generally describe the pain as a burning, heavy, sharp, or "hungry" pain that often localizes in the midepigastric area. The client with duodenal ulcer does not usually experience weight loss or nausea and vomiting. These symptoms are more typical in the client with a gastric ulcer.

Test-Taking Strategy: To answer this question accurately, it is necessary to be able to discriminate between symptoms of duodenal and gastric ulcers. This will allow you to eliminate options 3 and 4 first. You would choose option 1 over option 2 by knowing that pain does not radiate down the right arm, or by knowing that there is a pattern of relief of pain by food with duodenal ulcer.

Level of Cognitive Ability: Application
Phase of Nursing Process: Assessment
Client Needs: Physiological Integrity
Content Area: Adult Health/Gastrointestinal

Reference
Monahan, F., & Neighbors, M. (1998). *Medical-surgical nursing: Foundations for clinical practice* (2nd ed.). Philadelphia: W. B. Saunders. p. 1026.

68. **4**

Rationale: Psychological or emotional stressors that exacerbate peptic ulcer disease may be found either at home or in the workplace. The frequent need to work overtime on short notice is the option that is potentially most stressful, since it is the item that the client has least control over. An ability to work at home periodically is not necessarily stressful, because there is increased client control over timing of work and location. Adequate rest and proper dietary pattern (options 1 and 2) should alleviate symptoms, not worsen them.

Test-Taking Strategy: Begin to answer this question by eliminating options 1 and 2 because they are healthy living habits. Recall that psychological stress may be worsened in situations in which there is little client control. This would help you to choose option 4 over option 3 as the correct answer, given the wording of the question.

Level of Cognitive Ability: Analysis
Phase of Nursing Process: Analysis
Client Needs: Psychosocial Integrity
Content Area: Adult Health/Gastrointestinal

Reference
Monahan, F., & Neighbors, M. (1998). *Medical-surgical nursing: Foundations for clinical practice* (2nd ed.). Philadelphia: W. B. Saunders. p. 1027.

69. **2**

Rationale: Dietary modification for the client with PUD includes eliminating foods that are irritating to the client. Items that are generally eliminated or avoided are highly spiced foods, alcohol, caffeine, chocolate, and fresh fruits. Other foods may be taken according to the client's tolerance of that specific food.

Test-Taking Strategy: To answer this question accurately, it is necessary to understand which types of foods and beverages are irritating to the gastrointestinal mucosa. This will allow you to eliminate each of the incorrect options systematically. If this question was difficult, take a few moments to review this important content area now.

Level of Cognitive Ability: Application
Phase of Nursing Process: Planning
Client Needs: Health Promotion and Maintenance
Content Area: Adult Health/Gastrointestinal

Reference
Monahan, F., & Neighbors, M. (1998). *Medical-surgical nursing: Foundations for clinical practice* (2nd ed.). Philadelphia: W. B. Saunders. p. 1027.

70. **2**

Rationale: Ibuprofen is an NSAID, which is typically irritating to the lining of the GI tract and should be avoided by clients with a history of peptic ulcer disease. The other medications listed are frequently used in the treatment of PUD. Omeprazole is a proton-pump inhibitor, which blocks transport of hydrogen ions into the lumen of the GI tract. Sucralfate coats the surface of an ulcer to promote healing. Nizatidine is a histamine receptor-antagonist, which reduces the secretion of gastric acid.

Test-Taking Strategy: To answer this question accurately, it is necessary to know either the types of medications that are irritating to the GI tract, or to know which medications are used in the treatment of PUD. Knowledge in either of these areas will allow you to eliminate all of the incorrect choices easily.

Level of Cognitive Ability: Application
Phase of Nursing Process: Implementation
Client Needs: Health Promotion and Maintenance
Content Area: Adult Health/Gastrointestinal

References
Deglin, J., & Vallerand, A. (1997). *Davis's drug guide for nurses* (5th ed.). Philadelphia: F. A. Davis. pp. 593, 622.
Monahan, F., & Neighbors, M. (1998). *Medical-surgical nursing: Foundations for clinical practice* (2nd ed.). Philadelphia: W. B. Saunders. p. 1028.

71. **1**

Rationale: The signs and symptoms described in the stem are consistent with perforation of the ulcer, which then progresses to peritonitis if the perforation is large enough. The client with intestinal obstruction would most likely complain of abdominal pain, distention, and nausea and vomiting. The client with hemorrhage would be vomiting blood or coffee-ground material or would be expelling black, tarry, or bloody stools. Intractability is a term that refers to continued symptoms of a disease process, despite ongoing medical treatment.

Test-Taking Strategy: To answer this question correctly, it is necessary to be familiar with the signs and symptoms of each of the three complications of ulcer disease. If this question was difficult, take a few moments at this time to review this important content area.

Level of Cognitive Ability: Analysis
Phase of Nursing Process: Analysis
Client Needs: Physiological Integrity
Content Area: Adult Health/Gastrointestinal

Reference
Monahan, F., & Neighbors, M. (1998). *Medical-surgical nursing: Foundations for clinical practice* (2nd ed.). Philadelphia: W. B. Saunders. p. 1029.

72. **1**

Rationale: The peristomal skin must receive meticulous cleansing because the ileostomy drainage has more enzymes and is more caustic to the skin than colostomy drainage. Foods such as nuts and those with seeds will pass through the ileostomy. The client should be taught that these foods will remain undigested. The area below the ileostomy may be massaged if needed if the ileostomy becomes blocked by high-fiber foods. Fluid intake should be maintained to at least 6 to 8 glasses of water per day to prevent dehydration.

Test-Taking Strategy: Note that the question contains the key words "essential care" and "stoma." This tells you that the correct answer will be the option that deals with the stoma directly. This helps you eliminate each of the incorrect options easily.

Level of Cognitive Ability: Application
Phase of Nursing Process: Implementation
Client Needs: Health Promotion and Maintenance
Content Area: Adult Health/Gastrointestinal

Reference
Monahan, F., & Neighbors, M. (1998). *Medical-surgical nursing: Foundations for clinical practice* (2nd ed.). Philadelphia: W. B. Saunders. p. 1014.

73. **3**

Rationale: The client with an ileostomy is prone to dehydration due to the location of the ostomy and should not take laxatives. This will compound this potential risk for the client. Clients are at risk for deficiency of iron, folate, and cyanocobalamin and should receive these as supplements if necessary.

Test-Taking Strategy: To answer this question accurately, it is necessary to know that dehydration is an important risk for ileostomy clients, and to know what can trigger episodes of dehydration. This will allow you to eliminate each of the incorrect options systematically.

Level of Cognitive Ability: Analysis
Phase of Nursing Process: Analysis
Client Needs: Physiological Integrity
Content Area: Adult Health/Gastrointestinal

Reference
Monahan, F., & Neighbors, M. (1998). *Medical-surgical nursing: Foundations for clinical practice* (2nd ed.). Philadelphia: W. B. Saunders. p. 1013.

74. **2**

Rationale: Hiatal hernia is due to protrusion of a portion of the stomach above the diaphragm, where the esophagus usually is positioned. The client usually experiences pain due to reflux with ingestion of irritating foods, lying flat following meals or at night, and with large or fatty meals. Relief is obtained with intake of small, frequent, and bland meals; with use of histamine antagonists and antacids; and with elevation of the thorax following meals and during sleep.

Test-Taking Strategy: To answer this question accurately, it is necessary to know the aggravating factors for hiatal hernia and corrective actions. Note that the key word in the stem of the question is "contraindicated." This tells you that the correct answer will be the option that represents an aggravating factor for hiatal hernia discomfort.

Level of Cognitive Ability: Application
Phase of Nursing Process: Planning
Client Needs: Health Promotion and Maintenance
Content Area: Adult Health/Gastrointestinal

Reference
Monahan, F., & Neighbors, M. (1998). *Medical-surgical nursing; Foundations for clinical practice* (2nd ed.). Philadelphia: W. B. Saunders. p. 1044.

75. **4**

Rationale: The client is expected to have a Body Image Disturbance after colostomy. The client progresses through normal grieving stages to adjust to this change. The client demonstrates the greatest acceptance when participating in the actual colostomy care. Each of the incorrect options represents an interest in colostomy care but is a passive activity. The correct option shows the client participating in self-care.

Test-Taking Strategy: To answer this question accurately, it is necessary to be familiar with the nursing diagnosis of Body Image Disturbance and with behaviors that exemplify various stages of grieving. Note the key words in the question are "colostomy" and "most significant progress." This tells you that more than one or all of the options may be partially or totally correct, and that you will have to prioritize your answer.

Level of Cognitive Ability: Analysis
Phase of Nursing Process: Evaluation
Client Needs: Psychosocial Integrity
Content Area: Adult Health/Gastrointestinal

Reference
Monahan, F., & Neighbors, M. (1998). *Medical-surgical nursing: Foundations for clinical practice* (2nd ed.). Philadelphia: W. B. Saunders. p. 1010.

76. **4**

Rationale: A prolapsed stoma is one in which bowel protrudes through the stoma, with an elongated and swollen appearance. A stoma retraction is characterized by sinking of the stoma. Ischemia of the stoma would be associated with a dusky or bluish color. A stoma with a narrowed opening either at the level of the skin or fascia is said to be stenosed.

Test-Taking Strategy: Focus on the key word "prolapse." To answer this question correctly, it is necessary to be familiar with the different complications that can occur with ostomy formation. If this question was difficult, take a few moments now to review these important items!

Level of Cognitive Ability: Application
Phase of Nursing Process: Assessment
Client Needs: Physiological Integrity
Content Area: Adult Health/Gastrointestinal

Reference
Monahan, F., & Neighbors, M. (1998). *Medical-surgical nursing: Foundations for clinical practice* (2nd ed.). Philadelphia: W. B. Saunders. p. 1005.

77. **2**

Rationale: As peristalsis returns following creation of a colostomy, the client begins to pass malodorous flatus. This indicates returning bowel function and is an expected event. Within 72 hours of surgery, the client should begin passing stool via the colostomy. Options 1, 3, and 4 are incorrect.

Test-Taking Strategy: To answer this question accurately, it is necessary to know the normal progression of bowel activity following ostomy formation. This will allow you to eliminate each of the incorrect choices systematically.

Level of Cognitive Ability: Application
Phase of Nursing Process: Analysis
Client Needs: Physiological Integrity
Content Area: Adult Health/Gastrointestinal

Reference
Monahan, F., & Neighbors, M. (1998). *Medical-surgical nursing: Foundations for clinical practice* (2nd ed.). Philadelphia: W. B. Saunders. pp. 1004–1005.

78. **1**

Rationale: The client should be taught to include deodorizing foods in the diet, such as beet greens, parsley, buttermilk, and yogurt. Spinach also reduces odor but is a gas-forming food as well. Broccoli, cucumbers, and eggs are gas-forming foods.

Test-Taking Strategy: To answer this question correctly, it is necessary to know the effect of various foods on the GI tract of the client with an ostomy. If this question was difficult, take a few moments to review which foods cause odor or gas, and those that have a deodorizing effect.

Level of Cognitive Ability: Application
Phase of Nursing Process: Implementation
Client Needs: Health Promotion and Maintenance
Content Area: Adult Health/Gastrointestinal

Reference
Monahan, F., & Neighbors, M. (1998). *Medical-surgical nursing: Foundations for clinical practice* (2nd ed.). Philadelphia: W. B. Saunders. p. 1009.

79. **4**

Rationale: For the first 4 to 6 weeks following colostomy formation, the client should take in a low-residue diet. Following this period, the client should eat a high-carbohydrate, high-protein diet. The client is also instructed to add new foods, one at a time, to determine tolerance to that food.

Test-Taking Strategy: To answer this question accurately, it is necessary to understand the type of diet needed to establish a measure of bowel control following colostomy. If needed, take a few moments to review dietary considerations at this time.

Level of Cognitive Ability: Application
Phase of Nursing Process: Implementation
Client Needs: Physiological Integrity
Content Area: Adult Health/Gastrointestinal

Reference
Monahan, F., & Neighbors, M. (1998). *Medical-surgical nursing: Foundations for clinical practice* (2nd ed.). Philadelphia: W. B. Saunders. p. 1009.

80. **3**

Rationale: Foods that help thicken the stool of the client with an ileostomy include pasta, boiled rice, and low-fat cheese. Bran is high in dietary fiber and thus will increase output of watery stool by increasing propulsion through the bowel. Ileostomy output is liquid by nature. Addition or elimination of various foods can help thicken or loosen this liquid drainage.

Test-Taking Strategy: To answer this question accurately, it is necessary to know that high-fiber foods such as bran can aggravate watery stools. This will help you eliminate each of the incorrect options systematically. The wording of the question tells you that you are looking for an incorrect choice on the part of the client.

Level of Cognitive Ability: Analysis
Phase of Nursing Process: Evaluation
Client Needs: Health Promotion and Maintenance
Content Area: Adult Health/Gastrointestinal

Reference
Monahan, F., & Neighbors, M. (1998). *Medical-surgical nursing: Foundations for clinical practice* (2nd ed.). Philadelphia: W. B. Saunders. p. 1014.

81. **2**

Rationale: A major complication that occurs most frequently following ileostomy is fluid and electrolyte imbalance. The client requires constant monitoring of I & O to prevent this from occurring. Losses require replacement by IV until the client can tolerate a diet orally. Intestinal obstruction is a less frequent complication. Fat malabsorption and folate deficiency are complications that could occur later in the postoperative period.

Test-Taking Strategy: Note that the question contains the key words "ileostomy," "complications," and "immediate postoperative period." This tells you that the correct answer is one that occurs early in the postoperative course, and that occurs with relative frequency. Use your knowledge of this type of procedure to choose correctly.

Level of Cognitive Ability: Application
Phase of Nursing Process: Assessment
Client Needs: Physiological Integrity
Content Area: Adult Health/Gastrointestinal

Reference
Monahan, F., & Neighbors, M. (1998). *Medical-surgical nursing: Foundations for clinical practice* (2nd ed.). Philadelphia: W. B. Saunders. p. 1013.

82. **1**

Rationale: A Kock pouch is a continent ileostomy. As the ileostomy begins to function, the client drains it every 3 to 4 hours, then decreasing to about three times a day or as needed when full. The client does not need to wear a drainage bag but should wear an absorbent dressing to absorb mucous drainage from the stoma. Ileostomy drainage is liquid in nature. The client would be able to pass stool from the rectum only if an ileal-anal pouch or anastamosis was created. This type of operation is a two-stage procedure.

Test-Taking Strategy: To answer this question accurately, it is necessary to understand the different surgical procedures that are performed with ileostomy, and their consequences on the bowel habits of the client. If this question was difficult, take a few moments to review this material at this time!

Level of Cognitive Ability: Analysis
Phase of Nursing Process: Evaluation
Client Needs: Physiological Integrity
Content Area: Adult Health/Gastrointestinal

Reference
Monahan, F., & Neighbors, M. (1998). *Medical-surgical nursing: Foundations for clinical practice* (2nd ed.). Philadelphia: W. B. Saunders. pp. 1012–1013.

83. **1**

Rationale: To maintain catheter patency and drainage, the catheter is irrigated with 10 to 20 mL of normal saline. This prevents the pouch from overfilling, causing tension on the new suture lines. Water is not used because it is hypotonic. Small amounts are used to prevent rupture of suture lines in the newly created pouch.

Test-Taking Strategy: Begin to answer this question by eliminating options 2 and 4 first. These amounts are large and could cause harm to the suture lines. Choose option 1 over option 3 because it is a smaller volume, and because it is an isotonic solution.

Level of Cognitive Ability: Analysis
Phase of Nursing Process: Analysis
Client Needs: Physiological Integrity
Content Area: Adult Health/Gastrointestinal

Reference
Monahan, F., & Neighbors, M. (1998). *Medical-surgical nursing: Foundations for clinical practice* (2nd ed.). Philadelphia: W. B. Saunders. p. 1013.

84. **3**

Rationale: Laboratory findings do not establish the diagnosis of appendicitis, but there is often a moderate elevation of the WBC count (leukocytosis) to 10,000 to 18,000/mm³ with a "shift to the left" (an increased number of immature WBCs).

Test-Taking Strategy: Knowledge that an inflammatory process causes a rise in the WBC count will assist in eliminating options 1 and 4. If you are unfamiliar with the meaning of "shift to the left," take time now to review!

Level of Cognitive Ability: Analysis
Phase of Nursing Process: Analysis
Client Needs: Physiological Integrity
Content Area: Adult Health/Gastrointestinal

Reference
Ignatavicius, D., Workman, M., & Mishler, M. (1995). *Medical-surgical nursing: A nursing process approach* (2nd ed.). Philadelphia: W. B. Saunders. p. 1629.

85. **2**

Rationale: Based on the signs and symptoms presented in the question, the nurse should suspect peritonitis and the physician should be notified. Administering pain medication is not an appropriate intervention. Heat should never be applied to the abdomen of a client with suspected appendicitis. It is not within the scope of nursing practice to schedule the surgical time, although the physician would probably perform the surgery earlier than the prescheduled time.

Test-Taking Strategy: Focus on the signs and symptoms in the question and consider the complications that can occur with appendicitis. Options 3 and 4 can be easily eliminated. Noting that the signs presented in the question indicate a complication will assist in directing you to option 2.

Level of Cognitive Ability: Analysis
Phase of Nursing Process: Implementation
Client Needs: Physiological Integrity
Content Area: Adult Health/Gastrointestinal

Reference
Ignatavicius, D., Workman, M., & Mishler, M. (1995). *Medical-surgical nursing: A nursing process approach* (2nd ed.). Philadelphia: W. B. Saunders. p. 1630.

86. **1**

Rationale: The pain associated with acute pancreatitis is often severe and unrelenting, is located in the epigastric region, and radiates to the back. The other options are incorrect.

Test-Taking Strategy: To answer this question accurately, it is necessary to be familiar with the signs and symptoms of pancreatitis. Because the pain radiates to the back, it is a little easier to discriminate this pain in relation to other GI disorders. If needed, take a few moments to review the signs and symptoms of acute pancreatitis at this time.

Level of Cognitive Ability: Application
Phase of Nursing Process: Assessment
Client Needs: Physiological Integrity
Content Area: Adult Health/Gastrointestinal

Reference
Burrell, P., Gerlach, M., & Pless, B. (1997). *Adult nursing: Acute and community care* (2nd ed.). Stamford, CT: Appleton & Lange. p. 1545.

87. **4**

Rationale: The client with chronic alcoholism who is experiencing acute pancreatitis is expected to show elevations in serum blood glucose, lipase, and amylase. The client with alcoholism typically has low magnesium levels. A high reading does not match the clinical picture, and the result should be questioned.

Test-Taking Strategy: To answer this question correctly, it is necessary to be familiar with the expected trends in laboratory test results for pancreatitis. If needed, take a few moments to review these basic tests now!

Level of Cognitive Ability: Analysis
Phase of Nursing Process: Analysis
Client Needs: Physiological Integrity
Content Area: Adult Health/Gastrointestinal

Reference
Burrell, P., Gerlach, M., & Pless, B. (1997). *Adult nursing: Acute and community care* (2nd ed.). Stamford, CT: Appleton & Lange. p. 1546.

88. **3**

Rationale: The client should limit fat in the diet. The client should also take in small meals at each sitting. This will also reduce the amount of carbohydrate and protein that the client must digest at any one time. The client does not need to limit water-soluble vitamins in the diet.

Test-Taking Strategy: Note that the stem of the question contains the key words "priority instruction." This tells you that more than one or all of the options may be partially or totally correct. Use knowledge related to pancreatic function and the ability to prioritize to make your selection.

Level of Cognitive Ability: Application
Phase of Nursing Process: Planning
Client Needs: Health Promotion and Maintenance
Content Area: Adult Health/Gastrointestinal

Reference
Burrell, P., Gerlach, M., & Pless, B. (1997). *Adult nursing: Acute and community care* (2nd ed.). Stamford, CT: Appleton & Lange. p. 1548.

89. **2**

Rationale: Positions such as sitting up, leaning forward, and flexing the legs (especially the left leg) may alleviate some of the pain associated with pancreatitis. The pain is aggravated by lying supine or walking. This is because the pancreas is located retroperitoneally, and the edema and inflammation intensify the irritation of the posterior peritoneal wall with these positions.

Test-Taking Strategy: Use your critical thinking skills to visualize the pancreas and the potential effects from stretching associated with the various positions listed. This may help you eliminate the incorrect options. Remember also that options that are similar are not likely to be correct. This will help you to eliminate at least options 1 and 3.

Level of Cognitive Ability: Application
Phase of Nursing Process: Implementation
Client Needs: Physiological Integrity
Content Area: Adult Health/Gastrointestinal

Reference
Burrell, P., Gerlach, M., & Pless, B. (1997). *Adult nursing: Acute and community care* (2nd ed.). Stamford, CT: Appleton & Lange. p. 1545.

90. **2**

Rationale: Chronic pancreatitis is aggravated by continued alcohol intake. Each of the other responses is not correct.

Test-Taking Strategy: Remember that options that are similar are not likely to be correct. In this instance, two of the incorrect options (3 and 4) represent other disorders of the digestive system. You would choose option 2 over option 1 by recalling that diabetes mellitus is an endocrine disorder of the pancreas, whereas pancreatitis is an exocrine disorder.

Level of Cognitive Ability: Analysis
Phase of Nursing Process: Evaluation
Client Needs: Health Promotion and Maintenance
Content Area: Adult Health/Gastrointestinal

Reference

Burrell, P., Gerlach, M., & Pless, B. (1997). *Adult nursing: Acute and community care* (2nd ed.). Stamford, CT: Appleton & Lange. p. 1548.

91. 1

Rationale: The client with cholecystitis should decrease overall intake of dietary fat. Foods that generally should be avoided to achieve this end include sauces and gravies, fatty meats, fried foods, products made with cream, and heavy desserts. The correct answer is baked scrod, which is low in fat.

Test-Taking Strategy: To answer this question correctly, it is necessary to know that clients with cholecystitis should decrease fat intake. Utilize knowledge of basic nutrition to make the selection accordingly.

Level of Cognitive Ability: Analysis
Phase of Nursing Process: Evaluation
Client Needs: Health Promotion and Maintenance
Content Area: Adult Health/Gastrointestinal

Reference

Monahan, F., & Neighbors, M. (1998). *Medical-surgical nursing: Foundations for clinical practice* (2nd ed.). Philadelphia: W. B. Saunders. p. 1111.

92. 2

Rationale: During an acute "gallbladder attack," the client may complain of severe right upper quadrant pain that radiates to the right scapula and shoulder. This is governed by the pattern of dermatomes in the body. The other responses are incorrect.

Test-Taking Strategy: Knowledge of anatomical location of organs is needed to help answer this question. Begin by eliminating options 3 and 4 as anatomically incorrect. Choose option 2 over option 1 by knowing symptoms of acute cholecystitis.

Level of Cognitive Ability: Application
Phase of Nursing Process: Assessment
Client Needs: Physiological Integrity
Content Area: Adult Health/Gastrointestinal

Reference

Monahan, F., & Neighbors, M. (1998). *Medical-surgical nursing: Foundations for clinical practice* (2nd ed.). Philadelphia: W. B. Saunders. p. 1109.

93. 3

Rationale: Ammonia is yielded as a product of protein metabolism. Clients with hepatic encephalopathy have high serum ammonia levels, which is responsible for the encephalopathy symptoms. Limiting protein intake will curb the elevation in serum ammonia and prevent further deterioration of the client's mental status.

Test-Taking Strategy: To answer this question correctly, it is necessary to have an understanding of the relationships between cirrhosis, encephalopathy, and protein intake. If needed, take a few moments to review these key concepts at this time.

Level of Cognitive Ability: Application
Phase of Nursing Process: Planning
Client Needs: Health Promotion and Maintenance
Content Area: Adult Health/Gastrointestinal

Reference

Monahan, F., & Neighbors, M. (1998). *Medical-surgical nursing: Foundations for clinical practice* (2nd ed.). Philadelphia: W. B. Saunders. p. 1183.

94. 4

Rationale: The client with weight gain who also has cirrhosis complicated by ascites is most often retaining fluid. This is especially true when the client has not demonstrated an appreciable increase in food intake, or when the weight gain is massive in relation to the time frame given. This makes Fluid Volume Excess the most appropriate nursing diagnosis. The client does not have Altered Nutrition: More Than Body Requirements; in fact, this client is most likely malnourished as part of the overall clinical picture. No data are given to support Impaired Gas Exchange, although in some clients, upward pressure on the diaphragm from ascites does impair respiration. Risk for Impaired Skin Integrity assumes a lower priority than diagnoses that are actual.

Test-Taking Strategy: Note that the question contains the key words "most appropriate." This tells you that more than one or all of the options may be partially or totally correct. Begin to answer this question by eliminating option 3, since it is not an actual nursing diagnosis. Eliminate option 2 next because there are no supportive data. Choose correctly between the remaining two knowing that the weight gain is due to fluid retention.

Level of Cognitive Ability: Analysis
Phase of Nursing Process: Analysis
Client Needs: Physiological Integrity
Content Area: Adult Health/Gastrointestinal

Reference

Monahan, F., & Neighbors, M. (1998). *Medical-surgical nursing: Foundations for clinical practice* (2nd ed.). Philadelphia: W. B. Saunders. p. 1155.

95. 1

Rationale: Pain associated with Crohn's disease is alleviated by use of analgesics and antispasmodics. It is also reduced by having the client practice relaxation techniques, applying local heat to the abdomen, and lying with the legs flexed. Lying with the legs extended is not useful because it increases the muscle tension in the abdomen, which could aggravate inflamed intestinal tissues as the abdominal muscles are stretched.

Test-Taking Strategy: Utilize general knowledge of pain management strategies, application of heat, and client positioning to answer this question. If this question was difficult, take a few moments now to review the essential elements found in the various options.

Level of Cognitive Ability: Application
Phase of Nursing Process: Implementation
Client Needs: Physiological Integrity
Content Area: Adult Health/Gastrointestinal

Reference

Monahan, F., & Neighbors, M. (1998). *Medical-surgical nursing: Foundations for clinical practice* (2nd ed.). Philadelphia: W. B. Saunders. p. 1069.

96. **1**

Rationale: To be effective in decreasing bowel motility, antispasmodic medications should be administered 30 minutes before mealtimes. The other options are incorrect.

Test-Taking Strategy: Utilize concepts related to medication action to anticipate when the doses should be timed. Knowing that antispasmodics slow down gut motility, it can be reasoned that they should be taken before meals, an activity that normally stimulates increased GI motility.

Level of Cognitive Ability: Application
Phase of Nursing Process: Implementation
Client Needs: Physiological Integrity
Content Area: Adult Health/Gastrointestinal

Reference
Monahan, F., & Neighbors, M. (1998). *Medical-surgical nursing: Foundations for clinical practice* (2nd ed.). Philadelphia: W. B. Saunders. p. 1069.

97. **3**

Rationale: The client with a mild to moderate case of ulcerative colitis is often prescribed a diet that is low in roughage and that does not include milk. This will help reduce the frequency of diarrhea for this client.

Test-Taking Strategy: To answer this question correctly, it is necessary to know that the disorder is characterized by diarrhea. It is then necessary to know which types of diet reduce this symptom. Knowing that milk products aggravate diarrhea, eliminate options 1 and 4 first. Choose between the remaining two by deciding which is less irritating to the inflamed tissue of the colon.

Level of Cognitive Ability: Application
Phase of Nursing Process: Implementation
Client Needs: Health Promotion and Maintenance
Content Area: Adult Health/Gastrointestinal

Reference
Monahan, F., & Neighbors, M. (1998). *Medical-surgical nursing: Foundations for clinical practice* (2nd ed.). Philadelphia: W. B. Saunders. p. 1071.

98. **1**

Rationale: Fatigue is a normal response to hepatic cellular damage. During the acute stage, rest is an essential intervention to reduce the liver's metabolic demands and increase its blood supply. Options 2, 3, and 4 are incorrect.

Test-Taking Strategy: Note the key word "acute" in the question. Knowing that the liver will need to rest in order to heal will easily assist you to option 1. If you are unfamiliar with the care of a client with hepatitis, take time now to review!

Level of Cognitive Ability: Analysis
Phase of Nursing Process: Planning
Client Needs: Physiological Integrity
Content Area: Adult Health/Gastrointestinal

Reference
Monahan, F., & Neighbors, M. (1998). *Medical-surgical nursing: Foundations for clinical practice* (2nd ed.). Philadelphia: W. B. Saunders. p. 1177.

99. **1**

Rationale: Hepatitis A is transmitted by the fecal-oral route via contaminated food or infected food handlers. Hepatitis B, C, and D is most commonly transmitted via infected blood or body fluids.

Test-Taking Strategy: Knowledge regarding the modes of transmission of the various types of hepatitis is required to answer this question. If you are unfamiliar with this important content area, take time now to review!

Level of Cognitive Ability: Analysis
Phase of Nursing Process: Analysis
Client Needs: Safe, Effective Care Environment
Content Area: Adult Health/Gastrointestinal

Reference
Monahan, F., & Neighbors, M. (1998). *Medical-surgical nursing: Foundations for clinical practice* (2nd ed.). Philadelphia: W. B. Saunders. p. 1170.

100. **2**

Rationale: Laboratory indicators of hepatitis include elevated liver enzyme levels, elevated serum bilirubin levels, elevated erythrocyte sedimentation rates, and leukopenia. An elevated BUN may indicate renal dysfunction. A hemoglobin level is unrelated to this diagnosis.

Test-Taking Strategy: Eliminate option 4 because a BUN identifies renal rather than hepatic dysfunction. Thinking about the organ that is involved in hepatitis should assist in directing you to option 2, the liver function test.

Level of Cognitive Ability: Analysis
Phase of Nursing Process: Analysis
Client Needs: Physiological Integrity
Content Area: Adult Health/Gastrointestinal

Reference
Monahan, F., & Neighbors, M. (1998). *Medical-surgical nursing: Foundations for clinical practice* (2nd ed.). Philadelphia: W. B. Saunders. p. 1172.

BIBLIOGRAPHY

Beare, P., & Myers, J. (1998). *Adult health nursing* (3rd ed.). St. Louis: Mosby–Year Book.

Black, J., & Matassarin-Jacobs, E. (1997). *Medical-surgical nursing: Clinical management for continuity of care* (5th ed.). Philadelphia: W. B. Saunders.

Burrell, P., Gerlach, M., & Pless, B. (1997). *Adult nursing: Acute and community care* (2nd ed.). Stamford, CT: Appleton & Lange.

Chernecky, C., & Berger, B. (1997). *Laboratory tests and diagnostic procedures* (2nd ed.). Philadelphia: W. B. Saunders.

Hodgson, B., & Kizior, R. (1998). *Saunders nursing drug handbook 1998*. Philadelphia: W. B. Saunders.

Ignatavicius, D., Workman, M., & Mishler, M. (1995). *Medical-surgical nursing: A nursing process approach* (2nd ed.). Philadelphia: W. B. Saunders.

Kozier, B., Erb, G., & Blais, K. (1998). *Fundamentals of nursing: Concepts, process, and practice* (5th ed.). Reading, MA: Addison-Wesley.

Lammon, C., Foote, A., Leli, P., et al. (1995). *Clinical nursing skills*. Philadelphia: W. B. Saunders.

Leahy, J., & Kizilay, P. (1998). *Foundations of nursing practice: A nursing process approach*. Philadelphia: W. B. Saunders.

Lehne, R. (1998). *Pharmacology for nursing care* (3rd ed.). Philadelphia: W. B. Saunders.

Lewis, S., Collier, I., & Heitkemper, M. (1996). *Medical-surgical nursing: Assessment and management of clinical problems* (4th ed.). St. Louis: Mosby–Year Book.

Luckmann, J. (1997). *Saunders manual of nursing care*. Philadelphia: W. B. Saunders.

Lutz, C., & Pryztulski, K. (1997). *Nutrition and diet therapy* (2nd ed.). Philadelphia: F. A. Davis.

Mahan, L., & Escott-Stump, S. (1996). *Krause's food, nutrition and diet therapy* (9th ed.). Philadelphia: W. B. Saunders.

Monahan, F., & Neighbors, M. (1998). *Medical-surgical nursing: Foundations for clinical practice* (2nd ed.). Philadelphia: W. B. Saunders.

O'Toole, M. (ed.) (1997). *Miller-Keane encyclopedia & dictionary of medicine, nursing, & allied health* (6th ed.). Philadelphia: W. B. Saunders.

CHAPTER 54

Gastrointestinal Medications

I. Antacids

A. Description
1. React with gastric acid to produce neutral salts or salts of low acidity
2. Inactivate pepsin and enhance mucosal protection but do not coat the ulcer crater to protect it from the acid and pepsin
3. Used for peptic ulcer disease and gastroesophageal reflux disease
4. Should be taken on a regular schedule
5. Are usually administered seven times a day, 1 and 3 hours after each meal and at bedtime
6. To provide maximum benefit, treatment should elevate the gastric pH above 5
7. Antacid tablets should be chewed thoroughly and followed with a glass of water or milk
8. Liquid preparations should be shaken before dispensing
9. Interactions with other medications can be minimized by allowing 1 hour between antacid administration and the administration of other medications
10. Can interfere with the action of sucralfate (Carafate), and to minimize this interaction the medications should be administered 1 hour apart from each other

B. Magnesium hydroxide
1. Rapid-acting
2. Also referred to as milk of magnesia
3. Most prominent side effect is diarrhea
4. Usually administered in combination with aluminum hydroxide, an antacid that assists in preventing diarrhea
5. Contraindicated in clients with intestinal obstruction, appendicitis, or undiagnosed abdominal pain
6. In clients with renal impairment, magnesium can accumulate to high levels, causing signs of toxicity

C. Aluminum hydroxide (Amphojel, Alu-Cap, Dialume)
1. Slow-acting
2. Contains significant amounts of sodium
3. Used with caution for clients with hypertension and heart failure
4. Most common side effect is constipation
5. Can reduce the effects of tetracyclines, warfarin sodium (Coumadin), and digoxin (Lanoxin)
6. Can reduce phosphate absorption and thereby cause hypophosphatemia

D. Calcium carbonate (Tums)
1. Rapid-acting
2. Common side effect is constipation

E. Sodium bicarbonate
1. Rapid onset
2. Liberates carbon dioxide, increases intradominal pressure, and promotes flatulence
3. Used with caution in clients with hypertension and heart failure
4. Can cause systemic alkalosis in clients with renal impairment
5. Is useful for treating acidosis and elevating urinary pH to promote excretion of acidic medications following overdose

II. Histamine H₂ Inhibitors (Box 54–1)

A. Description
1. Suppress secretions of gastric acid
2. Alleviate symptoms of heartburn and assist in preventing complications of peptic ulcer disease

BOX 54–1. Histamine H₂ Inhibitors	
Cimetidine (Tagamet)	Nizatidine (Axid)
Famotidine (Pepcid)	Ranitidine (Zantac)

3. Prevent stress ulcers and reduce the recurrence of all ulcers
4. Promote healing in gastroesophageal reflux disease
5. Contraindicated in hypersensitivity
6. Used with caution in clients with impaired renal or hepatic function

B. Cimetidine (Tagamet)
1. Can be administered orally, intramuscularly, and IV
2. Food reduces the rate of absorption; if taken with meals, absorption will be slowed
3. By IV route, a 300-mg dose can be diluted in a total volume of 20 mL and injected slowly over 2 minutes, or it may diluted in 100 mL and infused over 15 to 20 minutes
4. Antacids can decrease the absorption of cimetidine
5. Cimetidine and antacids should be administered at least 1 hour apart from each other
6. Passes the blood-brain barrier, and central nervous system (CNS) side effects can occur
7. May cause mental confusion, agitation, psychosis, depression, anxiety, and disorientation
8. Dosage should be reduced in clients with renal impairment
9. IV administration can cause hypotension and dysrhythmias
10. If administered with warfarin sodium (Coumadin), phenytoin (Dilantin), theophylline, or lidocaine, the dosages of these medications should be reduced

C. Ranitidine (Zantac)
1. Can be administered orally, IM, or IV
2. Side effects are uncommon
3. It does not penetrate the blood-brain barrier as cimetidine does
4. Zantac is not affected by food
5. For IV injection, it should be diluted with a volume of 20 mL and administered slowly over 5 minutes or more, or diluted in 100 mL and administered over 15 to 20 minutes

D. Famotidine (Pepcid) and nizatidine (Axid)
1. Similar to Zantac and Tagamet
2. Does not need to be administered with food

III. Proton Pump Inhibitors (Box 54–2)

A. Suppress gastric acid secretion
B. Used with active ulcer disease, erosive esophagitis, and pathological hypersecretory conditions

---

BOX 54–3. Gastrointestinal Stimulants

Metoclopramide (Reglan)
Cisapride (Propulsid)

C. Contraindicated in hypersensitivity
D. Common side effects include headache, diarrhea, abdominal pain, and nausea

IV. Sucralfate (Carafate)

A. Creates a protective barrier against acid and pepsin
B. Administered orally; should be taken on an empty stomach
C. Administer at least 30 minutes apart from an antacid
D. May cause constipation
E. May impede absorption of warfarin sodium (Coumadin), phenytoin (Dilantin), theophylline, digoxin (Lanoxin), and some antibiotics and should be administered at least 2 hours apart from these medications

V. Misoprostol (Cytotec)

A. Used to prevent gastric ulcers caused by long-term therapy with nonsteroidal anti-inflammatory drugs (NSAIDs)
B. Suppresses secretion of gastric acid
C. Promotes secretion of bicarbonate and cytoprotective mucus
D. Maintains submucosal blood flow by promoting vasodilation
E. Administered with meals
F. Causes diarrhea and abdominal pain
G. Contraindicated for use in pregnancy

VI. Gastrointestinal Stimulants (Box 54–3)

A. Stimulate motility of the upper GI tract and increase the rate of gastric emptying without stimulating gastric, biliary, or pancreatic secretions
B. Used for gastroesophageal reflux
C. May cause restlessness, drowsiness, extrapyramidal reactions, dizziness, insomnia, headache
D. Contraindicated for clients with sensitivity
E. Contraindicated in clients with mechanical obstruction, perforation, or GI hemorrhage
F. Can precipitate hypertensive crisis in clients with pheochromocytoma

---

BOX 54–2. Proton Pump Inhibitors

Omeprazole (Prilosec)
Iansoprazole (Prevacid)

BOX 54–4. Bile Acid Sequestrants

Cholestyramine (Questran, Prevalite)
Colestipol (Colestid)

BOX 54–5. Medications for Cholelithiasis

Chenodiol (Chenix)
Monoctanoin (Moctanin)
Ursodiol (Actigall)

BOX 54–7. Bulk-Forming Laxatives

Methylcellulose (Citrucel)
Calcium polycarbophil (FiberCon)
Psyllium (Metamucil)

G. Safety in pregnancy is not established
H. Reglan can cause Parkinson-like reactions, and if this occurs the medication is discontinued
I. Propulsid may increase the absorption of cimetidine (Tagamet) and ranitidine (Zantac) when administered concurrently
J. Anticholinergics and narcotic analgesics antagonize the effects of Reglan
K. Alcohol, sedatives, cyclosporine (Sandimmune), and tranquilizers produce an additive effect

VII. Bile Acid Sequestrants (Box 54–4)

A. Description
  1. Used to treat pruritus associated with biliary disease
  2. Act by absorbing and combining with intestinal bile salts, which are then secreted in the feces, preventing intestinal reabsorption
  3. May be used in the treatment of hypercholesterolemia in adults

  4. Used cautiously in clients with bowel obstruction or severe constipation because of the adverse GI effects
  5. Taste and palatability are often reasons for noncompliance and can be improved by the use of flavored products or mixing the medication with various juices
  6. Stool softeners and other sources of fiber can be used to abate the GI side effects
B. Side effects
  1. Constipation
  2. Bloating
  3. Flatulence
  4. Nausea
  5. Fecal impaction and intestinal obstruction
  6. Exacerbation of hemorrhoids
  7. Hypoprothrombinemia
  8. Decreased vitamin absorption

VIII. Medications for Cholelithiasis (Box 54–5)

A. Chenodiol (Chenix)
  1. Decreases cholesterol production, lowering content of bile, thus facilitates dissolution of gallstones

  2. Can cause diarrhea and possible hepatotoxicity
  3. Baseline liver function studies should be performed
  4. Client should be instructed to contact physician if abdominal pain, sudden right upper quadrant pain, nausea, or vomiting occurs
B. Monoctanoin (Moctanin)
  1. Used when stones made of calcium are resistant to dissolution by oral chenodiol
  2. Administered through a T tube, nasal biliary catheter, or percutaneous transhepatic catheter
  3. Effective only when in contact with the stone
  4. Major side effects include diarrhea, nausea, and abdominal pain
C. Ursodiol (Actigall)
  1. A naturally occurring bile salt
  2. Suppresses hepatic synthesis and secretion of cholesterol and inhibits intestinal absorption of cholesterol
  3. Requires months of therapy for dissolution of a gallstone to occur
  4. Ultrasound images are obtained within 6 months to determine effectiveness of therapy
  5. Clients should be instructed to report nausea, vomiting, diarrhea, or rash to the physician

IX. Medications to Treat Hepatic Encephalopathy (Box 54–6)

A. Lactulose (Cephulac)
  1. Reduces ammonia levels
  2. Improves protein tolerance in clients with advanced hepatic **cirrhosis**
  3. Lowers the colonic pH from 7 to 5; this acidification pulls ammonia into the bowel to be excreted in the feces, thus lowering the ammonia level
  4. Administered orally in the form of a syrup
B. Neomycin (Mycifradin)
  1. Reduces the number of colonic bacteria that normally convert urea and amino acids into ammonia

---

BOX 54–6. Medications to Treat Hepatic Encephalopathy

Lactulose (Cephulac)
Neomycin (Mycifradin)

BOX 54–8. Saline Cathartics

Magnesium hydroxide (milk of magnesia, MOM)
Magnesium sulfate (Epsom salt)
Phospho-Soda

BOX 54–9. Stool Softeners

Docusate calcium (Surfak)
Docusate sodium (Colace)
Docusate with casanthranol (Peri-Colace)

---

2. Administered orally or via nasogastric (NG) tube
3. Used with caution in clients with kidney impairment

X. Laxatives

A. Bulk-forming laxatives (Box 54–7)
   1. Description
      a. Absorb water into feces and increase bulk to produce large and soft stools
      b. For short-term use
      c. Contraindicated in bowel obstruction
   2. Side effects
      a. GI disturbances
      b. Dehydration
      c. Electrolyte imbalance
      d. Dependency with chronic use
B. Stimulant cathartics
   1. Description: Stimulate motility of large intestine
   2. Bisacodyl (Dulcolax): Do not administer within 60 minutes of an antacid or milk
   3. Cascara (castor oil): Administer with juice; produces results in 2 to 6 hours
C. Saline cathartics (Box 54–8)
   1. Attract water into the large intestine to produce bulk
   2. Stimulate **peristalsis**
   3. Achieve results in 2 to 6 hours
D. Stool softeners (Box 54–9)
   1. Inhibit absorption of water so fecal mass remains large and soft
   2. Used to avoid straining
E. Lubricants
   1. Act to soften the feces
   2. Ease the strain of passing stool
   3. Lessen irritation to hemorrhoids
   4. Mineral oil
      a. Can cause lipid pneumonia if accidentally aspirated
      b. Interferes with absorption of fat-soluble vitamins A, D, E, and K
F. Opioids (Box 54–10)
   1. Decrease intestinal motility

BOX 54–10. Opioids

Codeine
Diphenoxylate hydrochloride with atropine (Lomotil)
Loperamide hydrochloride (Imodium)
Tincture of opium

BOX 54–11. Antispasmodics

Dicyclomine hydrochloride (Antispas)
Dicyclomine hydrochloride (Bentyl)

---

2. Decrease **peristalsis**
3. When poisons, infections, or bacterial toxins are the cause of diarrhea, opioids worsen the condition by delaying the elimination of toxins
4. Tincture of opium has an unpleasant taste and can be diluted with 15 to 30 mL of water for administration

XI. Antispasmodics (Box 54–11)

A. Description: Relax smooth muscle of GI tract
B. Side effects
   1. Constipation or diarrhea
   2. Rash
   3. Euphoria
   4. Dizziness
   5. Drowsiness
   6. Headache
   7. Nausea
   8. Weakness

PRACTICE QUESTIONS

1. The client has received a dose of dimenhydrinate (Dramamine). The nurse evaluates that the medication has been effective if the client states relief of:
   1 Headache
   2 Chills
   3 Nausea and vomiting
   4 Buzzing sound in the ears

2. The nurse in the preoperative holding unit administers a dose of scopolamine to a client. The nurse tells the client to expect which of the following side effects of the medication?
   1 Excessive urination
   2 Diaphoresis
   3 Dry mouth
   4 Pupillary constriction

3. The nurse is preparing to administer a dose of hydroxyzine (Vistaril) to a client by the intramuscular route. The nurse tells the client to expect:
   1 Pain at the injection site from the medication
   2 Relief from nausea within 5 minutes
   3 Excessive salivation as a side effect
   4 Increased alertness lasting generally 4 hours

4. The physician tells the nurse that a client can be given droperidol (Inapsine) for the relief of postoperative nausea. The nurse anticipates that the physician will order the medication by which of the following routes?

1 Oral
2 Intravenous
3 Subcutaneous
4 Intramuscular

5. The client is receiving propantheline (Pro-Banthine) as adjunctive treatment for peptic ulcer disease. The nurse should administer this medication:
   1 With meals
   2 Just after meals
   3 30 minutes before meals
   4 With antacids

6. The client is taking docusate (Colace). The nurse monitors which of the following to determine whether the client is having a therapeutic effect from this medication?
   1 Abdominal pain
   2 Hematest-negative stools
   3 Reduction in steatorrhea
   4 Regular bowel movements

7. The client is taking cascara sagrada and develops abdominal cramps. The nurse interprets that the client is most likely experiencing:
   1 A common side effect of this medication
   2 Partial bowel obstruction
   3 A case of influenza
   4 Peptic ulcer disease

8. The client taking bisacodyl (Dulcolax) wants to achieve rapid effect from the medication. The nurse then tells the client to take the medication:
   1 With a large meal
   2 On an empty stomach
   3 At bedtime
   4 With two glasses of juice

9. The client who is advised to take senna (Senokot) for the treatment of constipation asks the nurse how this medication works. The nurse would incorporate which of the following when formulating a response?
   1 It coats the bowel wall and makes it slippery
   2 It adds fiber and bulk to the stool
   3 It accumulates water and increases peristalsis
   4 It stimulates the vagus nerve to improve bowel tone

10. The client has a PRN order for loperamide (Imodium). The nurse should plan to administer this medication if the client has:
    1 Hematest-positive nasogastric tube drainage
    2 Abdominal pain
    3 Constipation
    4 An episode of diarrhea

11. The nurse has given instructions to the client who just received a prescription for diphenoxylate with atropine (Lomotil). The nurse evaluates that the client understands the use of the medication and its properties if the client states to:

1. Stay within the prescribed dose because it can be habit-forming
2. Take the medication with a bulk-forming laxative
3. Expect increased salivation while taking the medication
4. Anticipate side effects of nervous system excitability

12. The client has been started on psyllium (Metamucil). The nurse would teach this client to take this medication with:
    1 Gelatin, applesauce, or pudding
    2 A full glass of liquid, followed by a second
    3 A multivitamin and mineral supplement
    4 A dose of antacid

13. The client with diabetic gastroparesis has been given a prescription for metoclopramide (Reglan) four times a day. The nurse teaches the client to take the medication:
    1 30 minutes before meals and at bedtime
    2 With each meal and at bedtime
    3 One hour after each meal and at bedtime
    4 Every 6 hours spaced evenly around the clock

14. The nurse teaches the client taking metoclopramide (Reglan) to discontinue the medication immediately and call the physician if which of the following side effects occurs with long-term use?
    1 Anxiety or irritability
    2 Dry mouth not minimized by use of sugar-free hard candy
    3 Excessive excitability
    4 Uncontrolled rhythmic movements of the face or limbs

15. The client has just taken a dose of trimethobenzamide (Tigan). The nurse plans to monitor this client for relief of:
    1 Nausea and vomiting
    2 Abdominal pain
    3 Heartburn
    4 Constipation

16. The client has a PRN order for ondansetron (Zofran). The nurse would administer this medication to the postoperative client for relief of:
    1 Urinary retention
    2 Incisional pain
    3 Nausea and vomiting
    4 Paralytic ileus

17. The client has an order to take magnesium citrate to prevent constipation following a barium study of the upper GI tract. The nurse plans to administer this medication:
    1 With a full glass of water
    2 With fruit juice only
    3 On ice
    4 At room temperature

18. The nurse is administering a dose of prochlorperazine (Compazine) to a client for nausea and

vomiting. The nurse would assess the client for which of the following frequent side effects of this medication?

1 Diarrhea
2 Drooling
3 Excessive lacrimation
4 Blurred vision

19. The client has begun medication therapy with pancrelipase (Pancrease). The nurse evaluates that the medication is having the optimal intended benefit if which of the following effects is observed?

1 Reduction of steatorrhea
2 Absence of abdominal pain
3 Relief of heartburn
4 Weight loss

20. The client asks the nurse why the medication cisapride (Propulsid) has been prescribed. The nurse incorporates which of the following thoughts in a reply?

1 It is being used to relieve nighttime heartburn from gastroesophageal reflux
2 It is used to prevent nausea and vomiting
3 It can help heal GI hemorrhage sites more quickly
4 It may reverse a bowel obstruction, thus avoiding surgery

21. The nurse is giving the client directions for proper use of aluminum hydroxide tablets (Alu-Caps). The nurse tells the client to:

1 Chew the tablets thoroughly and follow with 4 ounces of water
2 Swallow whole with a full glass of water
3 Take the tablet at the same time as other medications
4 Take each dose with a laxative to prevent constipation

22. The client with a history of duodenal ulcer is taking calcium carbonate chewable tablets. The nurse evaluates that the client is experiencing optimal effects of the medication if:

1 Muscle twitching stops
2 Heartburn is relieved
3 Serum calcium levels rise
4 Serum phosphorus levels decrease

23. The hospitalized client asks the nurse for sodium bicarbonate to relieve heartburn following a meal. The nurse interprets that this client could not receive this medication if the client is currently being treated for which of the following conditions?

1 Urinary calculi
2 Chronic bronchitis
3 Metabolic alkalosis
4 Respiratory acidosis

24. The client is complaining of gas pains following surgery and requests medication. The nurse se-

lects which of the following medications from the PRN medication list to give to the client?

1 Magnesium hydroxide (milk of magnesia)
2 Droperidol (Inapsine)
3 Acetaminophen (Tylenol)
4 Simethicone (Mylicon)

25. The elderly client has recently been started on cimetidine (Tagamet). The nurse would plan to monitor the client for which of the following most frequent central nervous system side effects of this medication?

1 Confusion
2 Dizziness
3 Tremors
4 Hallucinations

26. The client with a gastric ulcer has an order for sucralfate, 1 g by mouth QID. The nurse schedules the medication for which of the following times?

1 With meals and at bedtime
2 One hour before meals and at bedtime
3 Every 6 hours around the clock
4 One hour after meals and at bedtime

27. The client who chronically uses nonsteroidal anti-inflammatory drugs (NSAIDs) has been taking misoprostol (Cytotec). The nurse evaluates that the medication is having the intended therapeutic effect if the client did not experience which of the following symptoms?

1 Decreased platelet count
2 Decreased white blood cell count
3 Epigastric pain
4 Diarrhea

28. The physician has written an order for ranitidine (Zantac), 300 mg once daily. The nurse schedules the medication for which of the following times?

1 Before breakfast
2 After lunch
3 With supper
4 At bedtime

29. The client is taking lansoprazole (Prevacid) for the chronic management of Zollinger-Ellison syndrome. The nurse advises the client to take which of the following products if needed for headache?

1 Acetaminophen (Tylenol)
2 Ibuprofen (Motrin)
3 Naproxen (Aleve)
4 Acetylsalicylic acid (aspirin)

30. The client has been taking omeprazole (Prilosec) for 4 weeks. The ambulatory care nurse evaluates that the client is receiving the optimal intended effect of the medication if the client reports absence of which of the following symptoms?

1 Constipation
2 Heartburn
3 Diarrhea
4 Flatulence

ANSWERS

1. **3**

Rationale: Dimenhydrinate is used to treat and prevent the symptoms of dizziness, vertigo, nausea, and vomiting that accompany motion sickness. The other options are incorrect.

Test-Taking Strategy: To answer this question accurately, it is necessary to be familiar with this medication and its uses. If the medication is unfamiliar to you, take a moment or two to review it briefly.

Level of Cognitive Ability: Analysis
Phase of Nursing Process: Evaluation
Client Needs: Physiological Integrity
Content Area: Pharmacology

Reference
Lehne, R. (1998). *Pharmacology for nursing care* (3rd ed.). Philadelphia: W. B. Saunders. p. 798.

2. **3**

Rationale: Scopolamine is an anticholinergic medication that causes the frequent side effects of dry mouth, urinary retention, decreased sweating, and dilation of the pupils. The other options are completely incorrect.

Test-Taking Strategy: To answer this question accurately, it is necessary to be familiar with this medication and its uses. If the medication is unfamiliar to you, take a moment or two to review it briefly.

Level of Cognitive Ability: Application
Phase of Nursing Process: Implementation
Client Needs: Physiological Integrity
Content Area: Pharmacology

Reference
Lehne, R. (1998). *Pharmacology for nursing care* (3rd ed.). Philadelphia: W. B. Saunders. p. 798.

3. **1**

Rationale: Hydroxyzine is an antiemetic and sedative/hypnotic. It is often used in conjunction with narcotic analgesics for added effect. Medications administered by the IM route generally take 20 to 30 minutes to become effective. Hydroxyzine causes dry mouth and drowsiness as side effects.

Test-Taking Strategy: Begin to answer this question by eliminating option 2, since IM medications do not work that rapidly. Use medication knowledge to choose correctly among the remaining three options.

Level of Cognitive Ability: Application
Phase of Nursing Process: Implementation
Client Needs: Physiological Integrity
Content Area: Pharmacology

Reference
Hodgson, B., & Kizior, R. (1998). *Saunders nursing drug handbook 1998.* Philadelphia: W. B. Saunders. p. 508.

4. **2**

Rationale: Droperidol may be administered by the IM or IV route. The IV route is the route used when relief of nausea is needed. The IM route may be used when the medication is used as an adjunct to anesthesia.

Test-Taking Strategy: To answer this question accurately, it is necessary to be familiar with this medication and its uses. If the medication is unfamiliar to you, take a moment or two to review it briefly.

Level of Cognitive Ability: Analysis
Phase of Nursing Process: Analysis
Client Needs: Physiological Integrity
Content Area: Pharmacology

Reference
Deglin, J., & Vallerand, A. (1997). *Davis's drug guide for nurses* (5th ed.). Philadelphia: F. A. Davis. pp. 420–421.

5. **3**

Rationale: Propantheline is an antimuscarinic anticholinergic medication that decreases GI secretions. It should be administered 30 minutes prior to meals. The other options are incorrect.

Test-Taking Strategy: To answer this question accurately, it is necessary to be familiar with this medication and its uses. Option 4 could be eliminated immediately since most medications cannot be administered with antacids due to interactive effects. If the medication is unfamiliar to you, take time now to review!

Level of Cognitive Ability: Application
Phase of Nursing Process: Implementation
Client Needs: Physiological Integrity
Content Area: Pharmacology

Reference
Deglin, J., & Vallerand, A. (1997). *Davis's drug guide for nurses* (5th ed.). Philadelphia: F. A. Davis. pp. 1023–1024.

6. **4**

Rationale: Docusate is a stool softener that promotes absorption of water into the stool, producing a softer consistency of stool. The intended effect is relief or prevention of constipation. The medication does not relieve abdominal pain, stop GI bleeding, or decrease the amount of fat in the stools.

Test-Taking Strategy: To answer this question accurately, it is necessary to be familiar with this medication and its uses. If you answered incorrectly, take a few minutes to review this commonly used medication at this time.

Level of Cognitive Ability: Application
Phase of Nursing Process: Assessment
Client Needs: Health Promotion and Maintenance
Content Area: Pharmacology

Reference
Hodgson, B., & Kizior, R. (1998). *Saunders nursing drug handbook 1998.* Philadelphia: W. B. Saunders. pp. 344–345.

7. **1**

Rationale: Cascara sagrada is a laxative that causes nausea and abdominal cramps as the most frequent side effects. Other health problems are not determined based on a single symptom.

Test-Taking Strategy: Remember that options that are similar are not likely to be correct. This will allow you to eliminate the two GI disorders (options 2 and 4). Choose option 1 over option 3 knowing that laxatives can cause abdominal cramping.

Level of Cognitive Ability: Analysis
Phase of Nursing Process: Analysis
Client Needs: Physiological Integrity
Content Area: Pharmacology

Reference
Hodgson, B., & Kizior, R. (1998). *Saunders nursing drug handbook 1998.* Philadelphia: W. B. Saunders. pp. 157–158.

8. **2**

Rationale: Most rapid results from Dulcolax occur when it is taken on an empty stomach. It will not have a rapid effect if taken with a large meal. If it is taken at bedtime, the client will have a bowel movement in the morning. Taking the medication with two glasses of juice will not add to its effect.

Test-Taking Strategy: General knowledge related to laxatives is needed to answer this question accurately. If needed, take a few moments to briefly review this commonly administered category of medications at this time.

Level of Cognitive Ability: Application
Phase of Nursing Process: Implementation
Client Needs: Health Promotion and Maintenance
Content Area: Pharmacology

Reference
Deglin, J., & Vallerand, A. (1997). *Davis's drug guide for nurses* (5th ed.). Philadelphia: F. A. Davis. pp. 155–156.

9. **3**

Rationale: Senna works by changing the transport of water and electrolytes in the large intestine, which causes accumulation of water in the mass of stool and increased peristalsis. The other options are incorrect.

Test-Taking Strategy: To answer this question accurately, it is necessary to be familiar with this medication and its actions. If you answered incorrectly, take a few minutes to review this commonly used medication at this time.

Level of Cognitive Ability: Analysis
Phase of Nursing Process: Analysis
Client Needs: Health Promotion and Maintenance
Content Area: Pharmacology

Reference
Deglin, J., & Vallerand, A. (1997). *Davis's drug guide for nurses* (5th ed.). Philadelphia: F. A. Davis. p. 1081.

10. **4**

Rationale: Loperamide is an antidiarrheal agent. It is commonly administered after loose stools. It is used in the management of acute diarrhea, and also in chronic diarrhea such as with inflammatory bowel disease. It can also be used to reduce the volume of drainage from an ileostomy.

Test-Taking Strategy: Specific information about this medication is needed to answer this question correctly. If needed, take a few moments to review this medication now.

Level of Cognitive Ability: Application
Phase of Nursing Process: Planning
Client Needs: Physiological Integrity
Content Area: Pharmacology

Reference
Lehne, R. (1998). *Pharmacology for nursing care* (3rd ed.). Philadelphia: W. B. Saunders. p. 799.

11. **1**

Rationale: The client should not exceed the recommended dose because it may be habit-forming. The medication is an antidiarrheal and therefore should not be taken with a laxative. Side effects of the medication include dry mouth and drowsiness.

Test-Taking Strategy: To answer this question accurately, it is necessary to be familiar with this medication and its habit-forming properties. Familiarity with atropine as an ingredient may help you eliminate options 3 and 4 immediately. Take a moment to review this medication if the question was difficult for you.

Level of Cognitive Ability: Analysis
Phase of Nursing Process: Evaluation
Client Needs: Physiological Integrity
Content Area: Pharmacology

Reference
Deglin, J., & Vallerand, A. (1997). *Davis's drug guide for nurses* (5th ed.). Philadelphia: F. A. Davis. pp. 384–385.

12. **2**

Rationale: Metamucil is a bulk-forming laxative. It should be taken with a full glass of water or juice, followed by another glass of liquid. This will help prevent impaction of the medication in the stomach or small intestine. The other options are incorrect.

Test-Taking Strategy: Use knowledge of this common medication to eliminate each of the incorrect options systematically. Option 4 should be eliminated first because most medications are not taken with antacids. Eliminate options 1 and 3 next because they have no physiological benefit for medication effect.

Level of Cognitive Ability: Application
Phase of Nursing Process: Implementation
Client Needs: Physiological Integrity
Content Area: Pharmacology

Reference
Hodgson, B., & Kizior, R. (1998). *Saunders nursing drug handbook 1998.* Philadelphia: W. B. Saunders. p. 886.

13. **1**

Rationale: The client should be taught to take this medication 30 minutes before meals and at bedtime. This allows the medication time to begin working before the client takes in food, which requires digestion and movement. The other options are incorrect.

Test-Taking Strategy: Remember that for an option to be correct, all its parts must be correct. Eliminate option 4 first as incorrect because is it the least plausible. Choose from among the remaining three options by reasoning that if the medication is used to treat gastroparesis, it must be taken before meals to enhance digestion.

Level of Cognitive Ability: Application
Phase of Nursing Process: Implementation
Client Needs: Physiological Integrity
Content Area: Pharmacology

Reference
Hodgson, B., & Kizior, R. (1998). *Saunders nursing drug handbook 1998.* Philadelphia: W. B. Saunders. p. 671.

14. 4

Rationale: If the client experiences tardive dyskinesia (rhythmic movements of the face or limbs), the client should stop the medication and call the physician. These side effects may be irreversible. Excitability is not a side effect of this medication. Anxiety, irritability, and dry mouth are side effects that are not so harmful to the client.

Test-Taking Strategy: To answer this question correctly, it is necessary to know that the medication can cause tardive dyskinesia, and to know what the signs and symptoms are. If needed, take a few moments to review the side effects of this medication now.

Level of Cognitive Ability: Application
Phase of Nursing Process: Implementation
Client Needs: Health Promotion and Maintenance
Content Area: Pharmacology

Reference
Hodgson, B., & Kizior, R. (1998). *Saunders nursing drug handbook 1998.* Philadelphia: W. B. Saunders. p. 672.

15. 1

Rationale: Tigan is an antiemetic agent that is used in the treatment of nausea and vomiting. All the other options are incorrect.

Test-Taking Strategy: To answer this question accurately, it is necessary to know the classification of this medication. This will allow you to eliminate each of the incorrect options systematically.

Level of Cognitive Ability: Application
Phase of Nursing Process: Planning
Client Needs: Physiological Integrity
Content Area: Pharmacology

Reference
Lehne, R. (1998). *Pharmacology for nursing care* (3rd ed.). Philadelphia: W. B. Saunders. p. 766.

16. 3

Rationale: Ondansetron is an antiemetic used in the treatment of postoperative nausea and vomiting, as well as nausea and vomiting associated with chemotherapy. All the other options are incorrect.

Test-Taking Strategy: To answer this question accurately, it is necessary to know the classification of this medication. This will allow you to eliminate each of the incorrect options systematically.

Level of Cognitive Ability: Application
Phase of Nursing Process: Implementation
Client Needs: Physiological Integrity
Content Area: Pharmacology

Reference
Lehne, R. (1998). *Pharmacology for nursing care* (3rd ed.). Philadelphia: W. B. Saunders. p. 794.

17. 3

Rationale: Magnesium citrate is available as an oral solution. It is used commonly as a laxative following certain studies of the GI tract. It should be served on ice and should not be allowed to stand for prolonged periods. This would reduce the carbonation and make the solution even less palatable.

Test-Taking Strategy: Eliminate options 1 and 2 first knowing that magnesium citrate is itself a liquid. To discriminate between the last two options, it is necessary to know it should be given cold to enhance palatability.

Level of Cognitive Ability: Application
Phase of Nursing Process: Planning
Client Needs: Physiological Integrity
Content Area: Pharmacology

Reference
Lehne, R. (1998). *Pharmacology for nursing care* (3rd ed.). Philadelphia: W. B. Saunders. pp. 792–793.

18. 4

Rationale: The nurse would assess the client for blurred vision as a frequent side effect of prochlorperazine. Other frequent side effects of this phenothiazine-type antiemetic and antipsychotic are dry eyes, dry mouth, and constipation.

Test-Taking Strategy: To answer this question accurately, it is necessary to know the common side effects of phenothiazines. This would allow you to eliminate each of the incorrect options systematically.

Level of Cognitive Ability: Application
Phase of Nursing Process: Assessment
Client Needs: Physiological Integrity
Content Area: Pharmacology

Reference
Hodgson, B., & Kizior, R. (1998). *Saunders nursing drug handbook 1998.* Philadelphia: W. B. Saunders. p. 867.

19. 1

Rationale: Pancrease is a pancreatic enzyme used as a digestive aid in clients with pancreatitis. The medication should reduce the amount of fatty stools (steatorrhea). Another intended effect could be improved nutritional status. It is not used to treat abdominal pain or heartburn. It could result in weight gain but should not result in weight loss if it is aiding in digestion.

Test-Taking Strategy: The name of the medication gives an indication of its possible uses. Use knowledge of physiology of the pancreas to assist in directing you to the correct option!

Level of Cognitive Ability: Analysis
Phase of Nursing Process: Evaluation
Client Needs: Physiological Integrity
Content Area: Pharmacology

Reference
Hodgson, B., & Kizior, R. (1998). *Saunders nursing drug handbook 1998.* Philadelphia: W. B. Saunders. pp. 786–787.

20. 1

Rationale: Cisapride is a GI prokinetic agent that is often given to treat nighttime heartburn associated with gastroesophageal reflux disease. It is not used as an antiemetic. It is contraindicated in conditions in which increased GI motility could cause harm, such as with GI hemorrhage, bowel perforation, or mechanical bowel obstruction.

Test-Taking Strategy: Familiarity with this medication is needed to answer this question correctly. If needed, take a few moments to review this medication at this time.

Level of Cognitive Ability: Analysis
Phase of Nursing Process: Analysis
Client Needs: Physiological Integrity
Content Area: Pharmacology

Reference
Hodgson, B., & Kizior, R. (1998). *Saunders nursing drug handbook 1998.* Philadelphia: W. B. Saunders. pp. 225–226.

21. **1**

Rationale: Aluminum hydroxide tablets should be chewed thoroughly before swallowing. This prevents them from entering the small intestine undissolved. They should not be swallowed whole. Antacids should be taken at least 2 hours apart from other medications to prevent interactive effects. Constipation is a side effect of use of aluminum products, but it is not correct for the client to take a laxative with each dose. This promotes laxative abuse; the client should first try other means to prevent constipation.

Test-Taking Strategy: Eliminate option 4 first since it does not promote healthy bowel function. Next eliminate option 3 using general knowledge of antacid interactive effects. Discriminate between the final two options using principles of digestion and medication use.

Level of Cognitive Ability: Application
Phase of Nursing Process: Implementation
Client Needs: Physiological Integrity
Content Area: Pharmacology

Reference
Hodgson, B., & Kizior, R. (1998). *Saunders nursing drug handbook 1998.* Philadelphia: W. B. Saunders. pp. 34–35.

22. **2**

Rationale: Calcium carbonate is used as an antacid for the relief of heartburn and indigestion. It can also be used as a calcium supplement (option 3), or to bind phosphorus in the GI tract with renal failure (option 4). Option 1 is incorrect, although proper calcium levels are needed for proper neurological function.

Test-Taking Strategy: The key words in the stem are "duodenal ulcer" and "optimal effects." This tells you that more than one option may be correct, and that you must discriminate the correct therapeutic effect. Knowledge of concepts related to duodenal ulcer will allow you to eliminate each of the incorrect options easily.

Level of Cognitive Ability: Analysis
Phase of Nursing Process: Evaluation
Client Needs: Health Promotion and Maintenance
Content Area: Pharmacology

Reference
Deglin, J., & Vallerand, A. (1997). *Davis's drug guide for nurses* (5th ed.). Philadelphia: F. A. Davis. pp. 208, 210.

23. **3**

Rationale: Sodium bicarbonate is an electrolyte modifier and antacid. It would further aggravate metabolic alkalosis, which is a difficult acid-base disturbance to correct. The other options are incorrect.

Test-Taking Strategy: Utilize knowledge of acid-base concepts to answer this question. Eliminate options 2 and 4 because respiratory acidosis can result from bronchitis. You would then eliminate option 1 as irrelevant.

Level of Cognitive Ability: Analysis
Phase of Nursing Process: Analysis
Client Needs: Physiological Integrity
Content Area: Pharmacology

Reference
Hodgson, B., & Kizior, R. (1998). *Saunders nursing drug handbook 1998.* Philadelphia: W. B. Saunders. p. 932.

24. **4**

Rationale: Simethicone is an antiflatulent used in the relief of pain due to excessive gas in the GI tract. MOM is an antacid and laxative. Droperidol is used to treat postoperative nausea and vomiting. Acetaminophen is a non-narcotic analgesic.

Test-Taking Strategy: The key words in this question are "gas pains." Knowledge of the classifications to which each of the medications belong is needed to answer this question. If it was difficult, take a brief moment to review this drug.

Level of Cognitive Ability: Analysis
Phase of Nursing Process: Analysis
Client Needs: Physiological Integrity
Content Area: Pharmacology

Reference
Deglin J., & Vallerand, A. (1997). *Davis's drug guide for nurses* (5th ed.). Philadelphia: F. A. Davis. p. 1086.

25. **1**

Rationale: Elderly clients are especially susceptible to CNS side effects of cimetidine. The most frequent of these is confusion. Less common CNS side effects include headache, dizziness, drowsiness, and hallucinations.

Test-Taking Strategy: Note that the stem of the question contains the key words "most frequent." This modifier tells you that more than one or all of the options may be partially or totally correct. Use your knowledge of elderly clients and medications to choose correctly.

Level of Cognitive Ability: Application
Phase of Nursing Process: Planning
Client Needs: Physiological Integrity
Content Area: Pharmacology

Reference
Lehne, R. (1998). *Pharmacology for nursing care* (3rd ed.). Philadelphia: W. B. Saunders. p. 779.

26. **2**

Rationale: The medication should be scheduled for administration 1 hour before meals and at bedtime. The drug is timed to allow it to form a protective coating over the ulcer before food intake stimulates gastric acid production and mechanical irritation. All the other options are incorrect.

Test-Taking Strategy: Specific knowledge of this medication and its timing is needed to answer this question. If needed, take a few moments to review this drug at this time.

Level of Cognitive Ability: Application
Phase of Nursing Process: Implementation
Client Needs: Physiological Integrity
Content Area: Pharmacology

Reference
Hodgson, B., & Kizior, R. (1998). *Saunders nursing drug handbook 1998.* Philadelphia: W. B. Saunders. p. 951.

27. **3**

Rationale: The client who chronically uses NSAIDs is prone to gastric mucosal injury. Misoprostol is specifically given to prevent this occurrence. Diarrhea can be a side effect of the medication but is not an intended effect. Options 1 and 2 are completely incorrect.

Test-Taking Strategy: The key words in this question are "intended therapeutic effect" and "did not experience." This tells you that the medication is being given to prevent the occurrence of specific symptoms. Knowledge of the drug's use is needed to discriminate correctly among the options.

Level of Cognitive Ability: Analysis
Phase of Nursing Process: Evaluation
Client Needs: Health Promotion and Maintenance
Content Area: Pharmacology

Reference
Hodgson, B., & Kizior, R. (1998). *Saunders nursing drug handbook 1998.* Philadelphia: W. B. Saunders. p. 693.

28. **4**

Rationale: A single daily dose of ranitidine is scheduled to be given at bedtime. This allows for prolonged effect and the greatest protection of gastric mucosa. All the other options are incorrect.

Test-Taking Strategy: Specific knowledge of the timing of this medication is needed to answer this question. If needed, take a few moments to review this medication at this time.

Level of Cognitive Ability: Application
Phase of Nursing Process: Implementation
Client Needs: Physiological Integrity
Content Area: Pharmacology

Reference
Hodgson, B., & Kizior, R. (1998). *Saunders nursing drug handbook 1998.* Philadelphia: W. B. Saunders. p. 901.

29. **1**

Rationale: Zollinger-Ellison syndrome is a hypersecretory condition of the stomach. The client should avoid taking medications that are irritating to the stomach lining. Irritants would include aspirin and NSAIDs (naprosyn and ibuprofen). The client should be advised to take Tylenol for headache.

Test-Taking Strategy: Remember that options that are similar are not likely to be correct. With this in mind, eliminate options 2 and 3 first. Choose Tylenol over aspirin because it is least irritating to the stomach.

Level of Cognitive Ability: Application
Phase of Nursing Process: Implementation
Client Needs: Physiological Integrity
Content Area: Pharmacology

Reference
Hodgson, B., & Kizior, R. (1998). *Saunders nursing drug handbook 1998.* Philadelphia: W. B. Saunders. pp. 577–579.

30. **2**

Rationale: Omeprazole is a gastric pump inhibitor and is classified as an antiulcer agent. The intended effect of the drug is relief of pain from gastric irritation, often referred to as heartburn by clients.

Test-Taking Strategy: Specific knowledge of this medication and its uses is needed to answer this question. If needed, take a few moments to review this medication at this time.

Level of Cognitive Ability: Analysis
Phase of Nursing Process: Evaluation
Client Needs: Health Promotion and Maintenance
Content Area: Pharmacology

Reference
Hodgson, B., & Kizior, R. (1998). *Saunders nursing drug handbook 1998.* Philadelphia: W. B. Saunders. pp. 771–772.

BIBLIOGRAPHY

Black, J., & Matassarin-Jacobs, E. (1997). *Medical-surgical nursing: Clinical management for continuity of care* (5th ed.). Philadelphia: W. B. Saunders.

Chernecky, C., & Berger, B. (1997). *Laboratory tests and diagnostic procedures* (2nd ed.). Philadelphia: W. B. Saunders.

Clark, J., Queener, S., & Karb, V. (1997). *Pharmacologic basis of nursing practice* (5th ed.). St. Louis: Mosby–Year Book.

Deglin, J., & Vallerand, A. (1997). *Davis's drug guide for nurses* (5th ed.). Philadelphia: F. A. Davis.

Hodgson, B., & Kizior, R. (1998). *Saunders nursing drug handbook 1998.* Philadelphia: W. B. Saunders.

Ignatavicius, D., Workman, M., & Mishler, M. (1995). *Medical-surgical nursing: A nursing process approach* (2nd ed.). Philadelphia: W. B. Saunders.

Kuhn, M. (1998). *Pharmacotherapeutics: A nursing process approach* (4th ed.). Philadelphia: F. A. Davis.

Lehne, R. (1998). *Pharmacology for nursing care* (3rd ed.). Philadelphia: W. B. Saunders.

Luckmann, J. (1997). *Saunders manual of nursing care.* Philadelphia: W. B. Saunders.

Monahan, F., & Neighbors, M. (1998). *Medical-surgical nursing: Foundations for clinical practice* (2nd ed.). Philadelphia: W. B. Saunders.

O'Toole, M. (ed.) (1997). *Miller-Keane encyclopedia & dictionary of medicine, nursing, & allied health* (6th ed.). Philadelphia: W. B. Saunders.

CHAPTER 55

Client with Hepatitis

NURSING PROCESS

ASSESSMENT

Psychosocial Data
Known exposure to a person with hepatitis
Exposure to possible contamination of food or water
Recent ingestion of shellfish
Received a recent blood transfusion
Receiving hemodialysis
Sexual activity with multiple sex partners
IV drug user
Received recent ear piercing or tattooing
Living accommodations
Employment history related to exposure to blood or blood products
Recent travel to foreign country

Subjective Data
Fatigue
Weakness
Muscle pain
Joint pain
Headache
Pruritus
Nausea
Vomiting
Loss of appetite late in the day
Changes in taste
Intolerance to noxious odors

Objective Data
Fever
Jaundice
Clay-colored stools
Dark urine
Right upper quadrant tenderness
Skin rashes
Irritability

ANALYSIS: Altered Nutrition

PLANNING
The client maintains the prescribed daily calorie requirement.

IMPLEMENTATION
Assess the client's food likes and dislikes. Provide a diet high in carbohydrates and calories. Provide moderate to low amounts of fat and protein in the diet. Provide small frequent meals with increased amounts of clear liquids for anorexia. Offer high-calorie snacks. Provide supplemental vitamins and feedings. Increase fluid intake. Maintain a calorie count. Perform and offer mouth care. Remove noxious odors from the client's environment.

EVALUATION
The client maintains optimal intake of nutrients and calories to promote healing. The client complies with increased nutritional intake and has a full return of appetite. The client experiences a decreased incidence of nausea and vomiting.

ANALYSIS: Potential for Injury

PLANNING	IMPLEMENTATION	EVALUATION
The client verbalizes the need for precautions. The client verbalizes the need to avoid hepatotoxic substances.	Standard precautions at all times. Avoid the administration of prochlorperazine maleate (Compazine) for nausea because of its potential hepatotoxic effects. Monitor bilirubin level. Monitor serum ammonia and BUN levels.	Universal precautions are maintained. The client avoids hepatotoxic substances. Laboratory values return to normal.

ANALYSIS: Pain

PLANNING	IMPLEMENTATION	EVALUATION
The client identifies measures to control pain.	Assess level of pain. Administer analgesics as prescribed, avoiding hepatotoxic medications. Instruct client to avoid medications unless they are prescribed by the physician.	The client reports the absence of pain.

ANALYSIS: Activity Intolerance

PLANNING	IMPLEMENTATION	EVALUATION
The client describes the importance of adequate rest periods. The client alternates rest periods with activity.	Reinforce the importance of bed rest in the initial stage. Provide bed rest for 1 to 2 weeks, gradually increasing activity. Provide several periods of rest during the day. Plan care so client does not become fatigued.	The client verbalizes need for long-term rest. The client adheres to physical and activity limitation. The client gradually increases activity to the level experienced before illness.

ANALYSIS: Risk for Impaired Skin Integrity

PLANNING	IMPLEMENTATION	EVALUATION
The client monitors skin for breakdown. The client verbalizes discomfort related to itching.	Assess skin integrity, particularly during the period of bed rest. Instruct client to monitor skin integrity. Assess for rash and itching. Provide comfort measures as prescribed.	Skin remains intact. The client reports relief of discomfort.

ANALYSIS: Social Isolation

PLANNING	IMPLEMENTATION	EVALUATION
The client verbalizes appropriate diversional activities.	Encourage diversional activities on the basis of the client's interests. Encourage family members to visit for short periods.	The client participates in appropriate diversional activities.

ANALYSIS: Knowledge Deficit

PLANNING
The client verbalizes the treatment plan and the need for follow-up care.

IMPLEMENTATION
Instruct client to avoid fried and fatty foods, which can increase nausea. Instruct client in the importance of abstaining from alcohol. Instruct client and family in appropriate home care measures. Instruct client in the importance of follow-up care.

EVALUATION
The client complies with seeking medical help for routine follow-up and laboratory analysis.

I. Hepatitis

A. Description
  1. An inflammation of the liver caused by a virus, bacteria, or exposure to medications or hepatotoxins
  2. The goals of treatment include resting the inflamed liver to reduce metabolic demands and increasing the blood supply, thus promoting cellular regeneration and preventing complications

II. Viral Hepatitis

A. Types of Viral Hepatitis
  1. Hepatitis A (HAV), infectious hepatitis
  2. Hepatitis B (HBV)
  3. Hepatitis C (non-A, non-B)
  4. Hepatitis D (delta agent hepatitis)
  5. Hepatitis E (enterically transmitted non-A, non-B hepatitis)
B. Stages of Viral Hepatitis (Box 55–1)
C. Assessment
  1. Preicteric stage
    a. Fatigue
    b. Malaise
    c. Headache
    d. Lethargy
    e. Increased temperature
    f. Anorexia
    g. Nausea and vomiting
    h. Abdominal tenderness
    i. Diarrhea or constipation
    j. Weight loss
    k. Dark urine
    l. Joint pain
    m. Elevated AST, ALT, and bilirubin
  2. Icteric stage
    a. Tea-colored urine
    b. Clay-colored stools
    c. Jaundice
    d. Pruritus
    e. Enlarged and tender liver
  3. Posticteric stage
    a. Jaundice disappears
    b. Fatigue and malaise continues
    c. Appetite improves
    d. Stool and urine color returns to normal
    e. Liver remains enlarged

    f. Absence of clay-colored stools is an indication of resolution
D. Laboratory Assessment
  1. ALT (alanine aminotransferase)
    a. Elevated to more than 1000 mU/mL and may rise to as high as 4000 mU/mL
    b. Normal adult blood value: 6 to 24 U/L depending on age
  2. AST (aspartate aminotransferase)
    a. May rise to 1000 to 2000 mU/mL
    b. Normal adult blood value: 8 to 26 U/L depending on age with highest normal value in the newborn
  3. Alkaline phosphate levels
    a. May be normal or mildly elevated
    b. Normal: 30 to 90 IU/L or 4.5 to 13 King-Armstrong units/dL depending on age
  4. Serum total bilirubin levels
    a. Elevated to greater than 2.5 mg/dL
    b. Normal: 0.3 to 1.0 mg/dL (less than 1.5 mg/dL)
    c. Elevated levels of bilirubin in the urine

III. Hepatitis A (HAV), Infectious Hepatitis

A. Description
  1. Commonly seen during the fall and winter
  2. Is most prevalent in areas of poverty and areas with poor sanitation
  3. Increased risk
    a. Contact with infected materials
    b. Handling contaminated feces
    c. Eating or drinking contaminated water, milk, or food
    d. Eating raw fish from contaminated water
B. Transmission
  1. Fecal-oral route
  2. Person-to-person contact
  3. Parenteral
  4. Contaminated uncooked shellfish, fruits, and vegetables
  5. Contaminated water and milk
  6. Poorly washed utensils
C. Incubation and Infectious Periods
  1. Incubation period is 2–6 weeks
  2. Infectious period is 2 to 3 weeks prior to, and 1 week after, developing jaundice

BOX 55–1. Stages of Viral Hepatitis

PREICTERIC STAGE

The first stage of hepatitis preceding the appearance of jaundice

ICTERIC STAGE

The second stage of hepatitis, which includes the appearance of jaundice and associated symptoms such as elevated bilirubin levels, dark or tea-colored urine, and clay-colored stools

POSTICTERIC STAGE

The convalescent stage in which the jaundice decreases and the color of the urine and stool return to normal

D. Testing
   1. Infection is established by the presence of hepatitis A virus (HAV) antibodies (anti-HAV) in the blood
   2. IgM and IgG are normally present in the blood, and increased levels indicate infection and inflammation
   3. Ongoing inflammation of the liver is evidenced by the presence of elevated immunoglobulin M (IgM) antibodies, which persist in the blood for 4–6 weeks
   4. Previous infection is indicated by the presence of elevated immunoglobulin G (IgG) antibodies
E. Complication: Fulminant Hepatitis
F. Prevention
   1. Good handwashing
   2. Stool and needle precautions
   3. Treatment of municipal water supplies
   4. Serologic screening of food handlers
   5. Passive immunization
      a. Pre- and postexposure prophylaxis of immune globulin (IG)
      b. Immune globulin (IG) is not administered postexposure if clinical manifestations have developed
      c. Clients who live in or visit high-risk areas can be protected for up to 3 months following the administration of immune globulin (IG)
      d. The earlier in the incubation period that the immune globulin is given, the greater the protection
   6. Havrix
      a. Vaccine containing the inactivated virus of hepatitis A
      b. May replace gamma globulin for travelers
      c. A single dose is administered intramuscularly (IM)
      d. For maximum antibody titer, a booster is recommended 6–12 months after initial injection

IV. **Hepatitis B (HBV)**

A. Description
   1. Formerly called serum hepatitis
   2. Is nonseasonal in nature
   3. Prevalence increases in areas of overpopulation and poor hygiene
   4. Increased-risk individuals
      a. Those who receive multiple blood transfusions
      b. Health care providers in contact with blood and blood products
      c. Hemodialysis clients
      d. Sexually active individuals with multiple partners
      e. Morticians
      f. Those undergoing tattooing
      g. Parenteral drug abusers
   5. Sequelae of chronic hepatitis B infection may include chronic liver disease, **cirrhosis**, and primary liver cancer
B. Transmission
   1. Blood or body fluid contact
   2. Infected blood and blood products
   3. Infected saliva or semen
   4. Contaminated needles and equipment
   5. Oral or sexual contact
   6. Parenteral
   7. Perinatal period
   8. Blood or body fluid contact at birth
C. Incubation Period: 6–24 weeks
D. Testing
   1. Infection is established by the presence of hepatitis B antigen-antibody systems in the blood
   2. Presence of hepatitis B surface antigens (HBsAG) is the serologic marker to establish the diagnosis of hepatitis B
   3. The client is considered infectious if these antigens are present in the blood
   4. If the serologic marker (HBsAG) is present after 6 months, it indicates a carrier state or chronic hepatitis
   5. Normally the serologic marker (HBsAG) level declines and disappears after the acute hepatitis B episode
   6. The presence of antibodies to HBsAG (anti-HBS) indicates recovery and immunity to hepatitis B
   7. Hepatitis B early antigen (HBeAG) is detected in the blood about 1 week after the appearance of HBsAG and its presence determines the infective state of the client
E. Complications
   1. Fulminant hepatitis
   2. Chronic liver disease
   3. **Cirrhosis**
   4. Primary hepatocellular carcinoma
F. Prevention
   1. Good handwashing
   2. Screening blood donors
   3. Testing of all pregnant women

4. Needle precautions
5. Instructing clients to avoid sharing personal items
6. Avoiding intimate sexual contact if hepatitis B surface antigen (HBsAG) is positive
7. Engerix-B, Recombivax HB: hepatitis B vaccine involving three doses, an initial dose, a dose at 1 month, and a dose at 6 months
8. Hepatitis B immune globulin: may be given for postexposure prophylaxis when there has been percutaneous exposure to blood that contains HBsAg

V. Hepatitis C (Non-A, Non-B)

A. Description
   1. Occurs year-round
   2. Is common among drug abusers and is the major cause of post-transfusion hepatitis
   3. Risk factors are similar to HBV since hepatitis C is also parenterally transmitted
   4. Hepatitis C has been treated with interferon-alpha, which boosts the body's immune system
   5. Increased-risk individuals
      a. Parenteral drug abusers
      b. Dialysis clients
B. Transmission
   1. Same as HBV
   2. Infected blood and blood products
   3. Infected saliva or semen
   4. Contaminated needles and equipment
   5. Personal contact
   6. Possibly by fecal-oral route
   7. Parenteral
C. Incubation Period: 5–10 weeks
D. Testing: there is not an acceptable reliable serological screening test to detect hepatitis C
E. Complications
   1. Chronic liver disease
   2. Cirrhosis
   3. Primary hepatocellular carcinoma
F. Prevention
   1. Good handwashing
   2. Stool and needle precautions
   3. Screen blood donors

VI. Hepatitis D (delta agent hepatitis, HDV)

A. Description
   1. Common in the Mediterranean and Middle Eastern areas
   2. Seen with hepatitis B and may cause infection only in the presence of active HBV infection
   3. Coinfection with the delta agent intensifies the acute symptoms of hepatitis B
   4. Transmission and risk of infection are the same as in HBV, via contact with blood and blood products
   5. Prevention of HBV infection also prevents HDV infection, since HDV is dependent on HBV for replication

B. Transmission
   1. Infected saliva or semen
   2. Parenteral
   3. Contaminated needles and equipment
   4. Oral or sexual contact
   5. Blood and blood products among persons already infected with HBV
   6. Perinatal period
   7. Via blood or body fluid contact at birth
C. Incubation Period: 7–8 weeks
D. Testing
   1. Confirmed by the identification of intrahepatic delta antigen or a rise in the hepatitis D virus antibodies (anti-HD) titer
   2. Circulating hepatitis D antigen (HD Ag) is diagnostic of acute disease
E. Complications
   1. Chronic liver disease
   2. Fulminant hepatitis
F. Prevention: because hepatitis D must coexist with hepatitis B, the precautions that help prevent hepatitis B are also useful in preventing delta hepatitis

VII. Hepatitis E (Enterically Transmitted Non-A, Non-B Hepatitis)

A. Description
   1. A waterborne virus
   2. Prevalent in areas where sewage disposal is inadequate or where communal bathing in contaminated rivers is practiced
   3. Risk of infection is the same as HAV
   4. Presents as a mild disease except in infected women in the third trimester of pregnancy, with whom the mortality rate is high
   5. Increased risk
      a. With travel to countries that have a high incidence of hepatitis E such as India, Burma (Myanmar), Afghanistan, Algeria, and Mexico
      b. Eating or drinking food or water contaminated with the virus
B. Transmission
   1. Same as HAV
   2. Fecal-oral route
   3. Person-to-person contact
   4. Eating contaminated uncooked shellfish, fruits, and vegetables
   5. Drinking contaminated water and milk
   6. Poorly washed utensils
   7. Parenteral
C. Incubation Period: 2–9 weeks
D. Testing: no available serological markers for hepatitis E
E. Complications
   1. High mortality rate in pregnant women
   2. Fetal demise
F. Prevention
   1. Good handwashing
   2. Good personal hygiene

BOX 55–2. Client and Family Education for Hepatitis

- Frequent handwashing
- Do not share bathrooms unless the client strictly adheres to personal hygiene measures
- Individual washcloths, towels, drinking and eating utensils, as well as toothbrushes and razors, must be labeled and identified
- The client must not prepare food for other family members
- The client should avoid alcohol and over-the-counter medications, particularly acetaminophen (Tylenol) and sedatives, because these medications are hepatotoxic
- The client should increase activity gradually to prevent fatigue
- The client should consume small, frequent, high-carbohydrate, low-fat foods
- The client is not to donate blood
- The client may maintain normal contact with people as long as proper personal hygiene is maintained
- The client is to avoid sexual activity until hepatitis B surface antigen (HBsAg) results are negative
- Close personal contact such as kissing should be discouraged until HBsAg test results are negative
- If the client has hepatitis A and B, the family members should have immunoglobulin injections or vaccinations
- The client needs to carry a MedicAlert card noting the date of hepatitis onset
- The client needs to inform other health professionals, such as medical or dental personnel, of the onset of hepatitis
- The client needs to keep follow-up appointments with the health care provider

3. Treatment of water supplies
4. Good sanitation measures

◆ **VIII. Instruction for Home Care for the Client and Family** (Box 55–2)

PRACTICE QUESTIONS

1. A client is admitted to the hospital with acute viral hepatitis. Which of the following signs or symptoms would the nurse expect based upon this diagnosis?
   1 Spider angiomas
   2 Fatigue
   3 Pale urine
   4 Weight gain

2. The client with viral hepatitis, in discussing with the nurse the need to avoid alcohol, states, "I'm not sure I can do that." The nurse should respond by saying:
   1 "Everything will be all right."
   2 "I think you should talk more with the doctor about this."

   3 "I don't believe that."
   4 "I'm not sure that I understand. Would you please explain?"

3. Of the following infection control methods, which would be most appropriate to include in the plan of care to prevent hepatitis B in a client considered to be at high risk for exposure?
   1 Correct handwashing technique
   2 Hepatitis B (HBV) vaccine
   3 Proper personal hygiene
   4 Use of immune globulin

4. An infant is born to a mother with hepatitis B. Which of the following prophylaxis measures is indicated?
   1 Immune globulin (IG) given as soon as possible after delivery
   2 Hepatitis B immune globulin (HBIG) within 14 days after birth
   3 Hepatitis B immune globulin (HBIG) and hepatitis B vaccine within 12 hours of birth
   4 Hepatitis B vaccine within 24 hours of birth

5. The nurse is caring for a client that is a hepatitis B carrier. Which statement made by the client indicates the best understanding of how to prevent transmission of the disease?
   1 "I should be vaccinated as soon as possible."
   2 "I never will share towels with anyone else."
   3 "It is all right to kiss my wife."
   4 "My wife should get the vaccine."

6. A client has been in the hospital for several days with a diagnosis of viral hepatitis. To detect any difficulty with coping with this disease, the nurse should ask which of the following questions?
   1 "Are you losing weight?"
   2 "Do you rest sometime during the day?"
   3 "Have you enjoyed having visitors?"
   4 "Do you have a fever?"

7. To detect the development of a chronic carrier state in a client with hepatitis, the nurse assesses the client's serum for:
   1 Antibody to surface antigen (anti-HBs)
   2 Hepatitis B surface antigen (HBsAg)
   3 HBV-DNA
   4 Prolonged prothrombin time

8. The client with hepatitis is scheduled for a liver biopsy. Which of these nursing measures is included in the plan of care to assess for the possible development of bile peritonitis following a liver biopsy?
   1 Monitoring for bloody diarrhea
   2 Assessing for rebound tenderness
   3 Assessing for increased flatulence
   4 Monitoring for abdominal pain

9. The client is admitted to the hospital with viral hepatitis, complaining of "no appetite" and "los-

ing my taste for food." In order to provide adequate nutrition, the nurse teaches the client to:
1 Eat a good supper when anorexia is not as severe
2 Eat less often, preferably only three large meals daily
3 Drink lots of fluids, especially carbonated beverages
4 Select foods high in fat

10. The nurse is caring for a developmentally disabled client with hepatitis A who resides at a group home. Which of the following outcomes indicates that the most important goal has been achieved?
1 Avoids transmitting the virus to others in the group home
2 Gains at least 0.5 to 1 pound per week until at ideal weight
3 Progressively increases activity with planned rest periods
4 Resumes normal bowel elimination patterns

11. A client has developed hepatitis A after eating contaminated oysters. Which of the following signs and symptoms are expected?
1 Dark stools
2 Left upper quadrant discomfort
3 Malaise
4 Weight gain

12. An African-American client has a diagnosis of acute viral hepatitis. Which of the following specific areas should the nurse assess for jaundice in this client?
1 Flexor surfaces of the extremities
2 Hard palate of the mouth
3 Nailbeds
4 Skin

13. In planning care for a client with viral hepatitis who states, "I am so yellow," the nurse should include measures such as:
1 Assisting the client in expressing feelings
2 Doing most ADLs for the client
3 Providing information to the client only when the client requests it
4 Restricting visitors until the jaundice subsides

14. After a liver biopsy, the client should be instructed to:
1 Avoid alcohol for 8 hours
2 Save all stools to be checked for blood
3 Lie flat for 24 hours
4 Lie on the right side for 2 hours

15. A sexually active 20-year-old client has developed viral hepatitis. Which of the following statements made by the client indicates a need for further teaching?
1 "A condom should be used for sexual intercourse."

2 "I can never drink alcohol again."
3 "I won't go back to work right away."
4 "My close friends should get the vaccine."

16. After a business trip to an underdeveloped country 3 weeks ago, a client is diagnosed with hepatitis A. In completing the assessment, the nurse might expect which of the following statements to be most likely associated with the client's contracting the disease?
1 "I went hunting last fall and was swarmed by mosquitoes."
2 "Three months ago, I ate oysters while in Africa."
3 "I drank lemonade from a roadside stand while on this trip."
4 "My business partner is a hepatitis carrier."

17. A client is admitted to the hospital with severe jaundice and is having diagnostic testing. With no complaints of fatigue, the client is encouraged to ambulate in the hall to maintain muscle strength. The client paces around the room, but will not enter the hallway. Which of the following problems most likely is the reason for the client's reluctance to walk in the hall?
1 Fear of catching another disease
2 Not wanting to overexert and get overly tired
3 Feeling self-conscious about self-image
4 Unfamiliarity with the hospital

18. After giving an IM injection to a client with hepatitis B, the nurse accidentally pricks a finger with the needle. Which of the following prophylactic measures would prevent the development of hepatitis B in the nurse from this needlestick?
1 Hepatitis B immune globulin and hepatitis B vaccine
2 Hepatitis B immune globulin
3 Immune globulin
4 Hepatitis B vaccine

19. A client with viral hepatitis has no appetite, and food makes the client nauseated. Which of the following nursing interventions are appropriate?
1 Explain that high-fat diets are usually better tolerated
2 Encourage foods high in protein
3 Explain that the majority of calories need to be consumed in the evening hours
4 Monitor for fluid and electrolyte imbalance

20. Which of the following outcomes would the nurse expect to find in the client who has developed no complications from viral hepatitis?
1 Decreased absorption of vitamin K in intestine
2 Increasing prothrombin time values
3 Presence of asterixis
4 Decrease in AST (aspartate aminotransferase)

ANSWERS

1. 2

Rationale: Common signs of acute viral hepatitis include weight loss, dark urine, and fatigue. The client is anorexic possibly from a toxin produced by the diseased liver and finds food distasteful. The urine darkens because of excess bilirubin excreted by the kidneys. Fatigue occurs during all phases of hepatitis. Spider angiomas (small, dilated blood vessels) are commonly seen in cirrhosis of the liver.

Test-Taking Strategy: Knowledge of the signs and symptoms of viral hepatitis is needed to answer this question. If you know the function of the liver, then by the process of elimination you will be able to select the correct response. Lethargy is a classic symptom associated with hepatitis. If you had difficulty with this question, take time now to review content associated with hepatitis!

Level of Cognitive Ability: Application
Phase of Nursing Process: Assessment
Client Needs: Physiological Integrity
Content Area: Adult Health/Gastrointestinal

Reference
Lewis, S., Collier, I., & Heitkemper, M. (1996). *Medical-surgical nursing: Assessment and management of clinical problems* (4th ed.). St. Louis: Mosby–Year Book. p. 1261.

2. 4

Rationale: Striving to explain that which is vague or clarifying the meaning of what has been said increases the understanding for both the client and the nurse. Giving false reassurance devalues the client's feelings. Telling the client what to do implies that the nurse knows what is best and discourages independent thinking. Refusing to consider the client's ideas may cause the client to discontinue interaction with the nurse for fear of further rejection. Placing the client's feelings on hold by referring the client to the doctor for further information is a block to communication.

Test-Taking Strategy: Use therapeutic communication techniques in answering this question. The use of communication blocks indicates an incorrect answer. Such blocks used are giving false reassurance in option 1, giving advice and placing the client's feelings on hold in option 2, and showing approval or disapproval in option 3. Remember to always focus on the client's feelings first.

Level of Cognitive Ability: Application
Phase of Nursing Process: Implementation
Client Needs: Psychosocial Integrity
Content Area: Adult Health/Gastrointestinal

Reference
Townsend, M. (1996). *Psychiatric mental health nursing concepts of care* (2nd ed.). Philadelphia: F. A. Davis. p. 109.

3. 2

Rationale: Immunization is the most effective method of preventing HBV infection. Another general measure is handwashing. Immune globulin may be given for postexposure prophylaxis. Personal hygiene, such as handwashing after bowel movements and before eating also helps prevent the transmission of hepatitis.

Test-Taking Strategy: Note the key words "most appropriate" and "prevent." Knowledge regarding the most effective preventative measure will easily direct you to option 2. Review prevention measures in hepatitis B now, if you had difficulty with this question!

Level of Cognitive Ability: Application
Phase of Nursing Process: Planning
Client Needs: Safe, Effective Care Environment
Content Area: Adult Health/Gastrointestinal

Reference
Lewis, S., Collier, I., & Heitkemper, M. (1996). *Medical-surgical nursing: Assessment and management of clinical problems* (4th ed.). St. Louis: Mosby–Year Book. p. 1268.

4. 3

Rationale: HBIG and the vaccine are given to infants with perinatal exposure to prevent hepatitis and achieve lifelong prophylaxis and are administered within 12 hours of birth. Immune globulin (IG) is given to prevent hepatitis A.

Test-Taking Strategy: Knowledge of the different types of pre- and postexposure prophylaxis for hepatitis A and B is needed to answer this question. Noting the key words "mother with hepatitis B" will assist in directing you to option 3. If you had difficulty with this question, take time now to review content associated with hepatitis immunization!

Level of Cognitive Ability: Analysis
Phase of Nursing Process: Analysis
Client Needs: Physiological Integrity
Content Area: Adult Health/Gastrointestinal

Reference
LeMone, P., & Burke, K. (1996). *Medical-surgical nursing: Critical thinking in client care.* Reading, MA: Addison-Wesley. p. 513.

5. 4

Rationale: The vaccine is recommended for both sexual and household contacts of HBV carriers. Hepatitis B can be transmitted through intimate contact, such as kissing or sexual intercourse. The vaccine is used for prevention and is not given to carriers.

Test-Taking Strategy: Note that the question addresses a client who is a hepatitis B carrier. Noting the issue of the question, to prevent transmission, will easily direct you to option 4.

Level of Cognitive Ability: Analysis
Phase of Nursing Process: Evaluation
Client Needs: Health Promotion and Maintenance
Content Area: Adult Health/Gastrointestinal

Reference
LeMone, P., & Burke, K. (1996). *Medical-surgical nursing: Critical thinking in client care.* Reading, MA: Addison-Wesley. p. 511.

6. 3

Rationale: Clients with hepatitis may experience anxiety due to an anticipated change in lifestyle or fear of prognosis. They may also have a disturbance in body image related to the stigma of having a communicable disease or change in appearance. Option 3 relates to the client's possible feelings of not wanting to be seen by others due to appearance. Remember that the client with hepatitis is jaundiced.

Test-Taking Strategy: Knowledge of the psychosocial problems related to hepatitis is helpful in answering this question. Recalling the altered body image that occurs in hepatitis as a result of jaundice will easily direct you to option 3.

Level of Cognitive Ability: Application
Phase of Nursing Process: Assessment
Client Needs: Psychosocial Integrity
Content Area: Adult Health/Gastrointestinal

Reference

Lewis, S., Collier, I., & Heitkemper, M. (1996). *Medical-surgical nursing: Assessment and management of clinical problems* (4th ed.). St. Louis: Mosby–Year Book. p. 1267.

7. 2

Rationale: The Hepatitis B surface antigen (HBsAg) is positive in chronic carriers. Anti-HBs (antibody to surface antigen) is a marker for the response to the vaccine and it indicates immunity to hepatitis B. HBV-DNA indicates viral replication. A prolonged prothrombin time is caused by decreased absorption of vitamin K in the intestine with decreased production of prothrombin by the liver.

Test-Taking Strategy: Knowledge of the serologic tests for viral hepatitis is needed to answer this question. If you had difficulty with this question, take time now to review these serological tests!

Level of Cognitive Ability: Analysis
Phase of Nursing Process: Analysis
Client Needs: Physiological Integrity
Content Area: Adult Health/Gastrointestinal

Reference

Lewis, S., Collier, I., & Heitkemper, M. (1996). *Medical-surgical nursing: Assessment and management of clinical problems* (4th ed.). St. Louis: Mosby–Year Book. p. 1263.

8. 4

Rationale: Abdominal pain is the most common symptom of peritonitis. Although tenderness over the involved area is a universal sign, rebound tenderness is associated with appendicitis. Bloody diarrhea is a major symptom of ulcerative colitis. Increased flatulence commonly occurs with irritable bowel syndrome.

Test-Taking Strategy: Look for the specific issue of the question that can include a specific nursing action or a complication. The question asks for the assessment finding that indicates peritonitis. The best response is abdominal pain. Review the assessment findings associated with peritonitis now if you had difficulty with this question!

Level of Cognitive Ability: Application
Phase of Nursing Process: Planning
Client Needs: Physiological Integrity
Content Area: Adult Health/Gastrointestinal

Reference

Lewis, S., Collier, I., & Heitkemper, M. (1996). *Medical-surgical nursing: Assessment and management of clinical problems* (4th ed.). St. Louis: Mosby–Year Book. p. 1221.

9. 3

Rationale: Although no special diet is required in the treatment of viral hepatitis, it is generally recommended that clients have a diet with low fat content since fat may be poorly tolerated because of decreased bile production. Small, frequent meals are preferable and may even prevent nausea. Frequently, appetite is better in the morning, so it is easier to eat a good breakfast. Carbonated beverages are used to counteract anorexia. An adequate fluid intake of 2500–3000 mL/day is also important.

Test-Taking Strategy: Knowledge of nutritional needs during hepatitis is helpful in answering this question. In this question, it is asking about adequate nutrition for a client with anorexia. This key issue should easily direct you to option 3.

Level of Cognitive Ability: Application
Phase of Nursing Process: Implementation
Client Needs: Physiological integrity
Content Area: Adult Health/Gastrointestinal

Reference

Lewis, S., Collier, I., & Heitkemper, M. (1996). *Medical-surgical nursing: Assessment and management of clinical problems* (4th ed.). St. Louis: Mosby–Year Book. p. 1264.

10. 1

Rationale: All of the options are expected outcomes of care for this client. However, one of the most important goals when caring for clients with acute viral hepatitis is preventing the spread of infection.

Test-Taking Strategy: Note the relationship between "group home" in the question and in the correct option. Options 2, 3, and 4 are client specific. Option 1 is addressing prevention of transmission of the disease.

Level of Cognitive Ability: Analysis
Phase of Nursing Process: Evaluation
Client Needs: Health Promotion and Maintenance
Content Area: Adult Health/Gastrointestinal

Reference

LeMone, P., & Burke, K. (1996). *Medical-surgical nursing: Critical thinking in client care*. Reading, MA: Addison-Wesley. pp. 513, 515.

11. 3

Rationale: Hepatitis causes gastrointestinal symptoms such as anorexia, nausea, right upper quadrant discomfort, and weight loss. Fatigue and malaise are common. Stools will be light or clay colored if conjugated bilirubin is unable to flow out of the liver because of inflammation or obstruction of the bile ducts.

Test-Taking Strategy: Knowledge regarding the anatomical location and functions of the liver will easily direct you to option 3. If you had difficulty answering this question, review the signs and symptoms of hepatitis now!

Level of Cognitive Ability: Analysis
Phase of Nursing Process: Assessment
Client Needs: Physiological integrity
Content Area: Adult Health/Gastrointestinal

Reference

Lewis, S., Collier, I., & Heitkemper, M. (1996). *Medical-surgical nursing: Assessment and management of clinical problems* (4th ed.). St. Louis: Mosby–Year Book. p. 1261.

12. 2

Rationale: Jaundice occurs in the skin and mucous membranes. In light-skinned persons, it is first seen in the sclera of the eyes and later in the skin. In dark-skinned persons, jaundice is observed in the inner canthus of the eyes and hard palate of the mouth. Pallor is detected in the nailbeds, and flushing that occurs with increased body temperature may be noted in the flexor surfaces of the extremities.

Test-Taking Strategy: If you know that jaundice is not observed in the skin of a dark-skinned client, you can eliminate options 1 and 4. Knowing that pallor is assessed in the nailbeds will assist in directing you to option 2. Review assessment techniques now, if you had difficulty with this question!

Level of Cognitive Ability: Analysis
Phase of Nursing Process: Assessment
Client Needs: Physiological integrity
Content Area: Adult Health/Gastrointestinal

Reference
Lewis, S., Collier, I., & Heitkemper, M. (1996). *Medical-surgical nursing: Assessment and management of clinical problems* (4th ed.). St. Louis: Mosby–Year Book. p. 1269.

13. **1**

Rationale: To assist the client in adapting to changes in appearance, it is important for the nurse to encourage participation in self-care to foster independence and self-esteem. The client should be encouraged to ask questions in order to clarify misconceptions, learn ways to prevent the spread of hepatitis to reduce fear, and make decisions. The client's feelings should be explored to discover how the client feels about the disease process and appearance so appropriate interventions can be planned.

Test-Taking Strategy: Use the process of elimination in answering the question. In order to promote coping and psychosocial adaptation, identify the use of therapeutic communication tools. Option 1 is the only option that addresses the client's feelings. Always focus on the client's feelings first.

Level of Cognitive Ability: Application
Phase of Nursing Process: Planning
Client Needs: Psychosocial Integrity
Content Area: Adult Health/Gastrointestinal

Reference
Lewis, S., Collier, I., & Heitkemper, M. (1996). *Medical-surgical nursing: Assessment and management of clinical problems* (4th ed.). St. Louis: Mosby–Year Book. p. 1267.

14. **4**

Rationale: In order to splint the puncture site, the client is kept on the right side for a minimum of 2 hours. The client should lie flat for 12–14 hours. Complications of the procedures include peritonitis, shock, or pneumothorax. No instructions are given regarding alcohol and this procedure.

Test-Taking Strategy: Knowledge of care of a client undergoing a liver biopsy is needed to answer this question. Use your knowledge of the anatomy of the body to assist you in selecting the correct option. This should easily direct you to option 4. Review postprocedure care following liver biopsy now, if you had difficulty with this question!

Level of Cognitive Ability: Application
Phase of Nursing Process: Implementation
Client Needs: Physiological Integrity
Content Area: Adult Health/Gastrointestinal

Reference
Lewis, S., Collier, I., & Heitkemper, M. (1996). *Medical-surgical nursing: Assessment and management of clinical problems* (4th ed.). St. Louis: Mosby–Year Book. p. 1094.

15. **2**

Rationale: To prevent transmission of hepatitis, a condom is advised during sexual intercourse as well as vaccination of the partner and close contacts. Alcohol should be avoided for 1 year since it is detoxified in the liver and may interfere with recovery. Rest is especially important until laboratory studies show that the liver function has returned to normal. The client's activity is increased gradually.

Test-Taking Strategy: Note the absolute term "never" in option 2. This should assist in directing you to this option. Review client teaching points now, if you had difficulty with this question!

Level of Cognitive Ability: Analysis
Phase of Nursing Process: Evaluation
Client Needs: Physiological Integrity
Content Area: Adult Health/Gastrointestinal

Reference
Lewis, S., Collier, I., & Heitkemper, M. (1996). *Medical-surgical nursing: Assessment and management of clinical problems* (4th ed.). St. Louis: Mosby–Year Book. p. 1269.

16. **3**

Rationale: Hepatitis A is transmitted through the fecal-oral route by ingestion of food or liquid infected with the virus. It occurs in poor hygiene, crowded living conditions, or poor sanitation. Sources of transmission are contaminated food, water, or shellfish. The greatest risk of transmission occurs before clinical symptoms appear. The average incubation period for hepatitis A is 28 days and for hepatitis B, 2–4 months.

Test-Taking Strategy: Knowledge of the mode of transmission, incubation period, and carrier state of hepatitis A and B is needed to answer this question. Key words you should look for and focus your attention on in this question include "most likely" and "3 weeks ago." These key words should direct you to option 3. Take time now to review modes of transmission and incubation periods of hepatitis A and B if you had difficulty with this question!

Level of Cognitive Ability: Analysis
Phase of Nursing Process: Assessment
Client Needs: Physiological Integrity
Content Area: Adult Health/Gastrointestinal

Reference
Lewis, S., Collier, I., & Heitkemper, M. (1996). *Medical-surgical nursing: Assessment and management of clinical problems* (4th ed.). St. Louis: Mosby–Year Book, p. 1259.

17. **3**

Rationale: Clients frequently have a body image disturbance because of a change in appearance. This can be manifested in negative verbal or nonverbal behavior.

Test-Taking Strategy: Note the key words "severe jaundice." This should easily direct you to option 3. Review psychosocial issues related to the client with hepatitis now, if you had difficulty with this question!

Level of Cognitive Ability: Analysis
Phase of Nursing Process: Analysis
Client Needs: Psychosocial Integrity
Content Area: Adult Health/Gastrointestinal

Reference
Lewis, S., Collier, I., & Heitkemper, M. (1996). *Medical-surgical nursing: Assessment and management of clinical problems* (4th ed.). St. Louis: Mosby–Year Book. p. 1267.

18. **2**

Rationale: Immune globulin is given prophylactically for hepatitis A. Hepatitis B immune globulin is indicated for persons exposed to the hepatitis B virus. Vaccination is very effective in preventing hepatitis B long term in health care workers. Both the vaccine and hepatitis B immune globulin may be given at the same time.

Test-Taking Strategy: Knowledge of the postexposure prophylaxis of hepatitis A and B is needed to answer this question. The stem of this question specifically asks how to prevent hepatitis B after "this needlestick." These key words should easily direct you to option 2. Review postexposure prophylaxis now, if you had difficulty with this question!

Level of Cognitive Ability: Analysis
Phase of Nursing Process: Analysis
Client Needs: Health Promotion and Maintenance
Content Area: Adult Health/Gastrointestinal

Reference

Lewis, S., Collier, I., & Heitkemper, M. (1996). *Medical-surgical nursing: Assessment and management of clinical problems* (4th ed.). St. Louis: Mosby–Year Book. p. 1269.

19. **4**

Rationale: If nausea persists, the client will need to be assessed for fluid and electrolyte imbalances. It is important to explain to the client that the majority of calories should be eaten in the morning hours, since nausea occurs in the afternoon and evening. Clients should select a diet high in calories since energy is required for healing, and adequate carbohydrates can spare the protein. Changes in bilirubin interfere with fat absorption, so low-fat diets are better tolerated.

Test-Taking Strategy: Knowledge of the nutritional aspects of care for clients with acute hepatitis is helpful in answering this question. This knowledge will assist in eliminating options 1, 2, and 3. Review these concepts now if you had difficulty answering this question!

Level of Cognitive Ability: Application
Phase of Nursing Process: Implementation
Client Needs: Physiological Integrity
Content Area: Adult Health/Gastrointestinal

Reference

LeMone, P., & Burke, K. (1996). *Medical-surgical nursing: Critical thinking in client care.* Reading, MA: Addison-Wesley. p. 514.

20. **4**

Rationale: Complications from viral hepatitis include bleeding tendencies with increasing prothrombin time values as well as greatly abnormal liver function tests. Clients can also develop encephalopathy. A characteristic symptom of encephalopathy is asterixis. Serum transaminase levels (AST or SGOT) decrease and vitamin K becomes absorbed as liver cells heal and regenerate.

Test-Taking Strategy: Knowledge of the diagnostic findings along with complications of viral hepatitis is needed to answer this question. Identify the specific subject content of the question, which in this question is "complications from viral hepatitis." Review laboratory values now if you had difficulty with this question!

Level of Cognitive Ability: Analysis
Phase of Nursing Process: Evaluation
Client Needs: Physiological Integrity
Content Area: Adult Health/Gastrointestinal

Reference

Lewis, S., Collier, I., & Heitkemper, M. (1996). *Medical-surgical nursing: Assessment and management of clinical problems* (4th ed.). St. Louis: Mosby–Year Book. p. 1263.

BIBLIOGRAPHY

Black, J. M., & Matassarin-Jacobs, E. (1997). *Medical-surgical nursing: Clinical management for continuity of care* (5th ed.). Philadelphia: W. B. Saunders.

Chernecky, C., & Berger, B. (1997). *Laboratory tests and diagnostic procedures* (2nd ed.). Philadelphia: W. B. Saunders.

Ignatavicius, D., Workman, M., & Mishler, M. (1995). *Medical-surgical nursing: A nursing process approach* (2nd ed.). Philadelphia: W. B. Saunders.

LeMone, P., & Burke, K. (1996). *Medical-surgical nursing: Critical thinking in client care.* Reading, MA: Addison-Wesley.

Lehne, R. (1998). *Pharmacology for nursing care* (3rd ed.). Philadelphia: W. B. Saunders.

Lewis, S., Collier, I., & Heitkemper, M. (1996). *Medical-surgical nursing: Assessment and management of clinical problems* (4th ed.). St. Louis: Mosby–Year Book.

Luckmann, J. (1997). *Saunders manual of nursing care.* Philadelphia: W. B. Saunders.

O'Toole, M. (ed.). (1997). *Miller-Keane encyclopedia & dictionary of medicine, nursing, & allied health* (6th ed.). Philadelphia: W. B. Saunders.

Townsend, M. (1996). *Psychiatric mental health nursing concepts of care* (2nd ed.). Philadelphia: F. A. Davis.

UNIT XIII

....

The Adult Client with a Respiratory Disorder

PYRAMID TERMS

Bacille Calmette-Guérin (BCG) Vaccine—A vaccine containing attenuated tubercle bacilli that may be given to people in foreign countries or to those traveling to foreign countries, to produce increased resistance to TB.

Chest Tubes—Placed in the pleural space to remove air or fluid from the chest and thus restore negative pressure to re-expand the lung.

Chronic Airflow Limitation (CAL), Chronic Obstructive Lung Disease (COLD), Chronic Obstructive Pulmonary Disease (COPD)—A group of diseases that includes emphysema, asthma, bronchiectasis, and bronchitis. Characterized by progressive airflow limitations into and out of the lungs, elevated airway resistance, irreversible lung distention, and arterial blood gas imbalance. Can lead to pulmonary insufficiency, pulmonary hypertension, and cor pulmonale. In emphysema, the stimulus to breathe is a low PO_2 instead of increased PCO_2.

Emphysema—A chronic pulmonary disease marked by a narrowing of the small airways and the trapping of air, with destructive changes in their walls. Also known as chronic obstructive pulmonary disease (COPD).

Endotracheal Tube—A large-bore catheter inserted into the trachea through either the nose or the mouth. Used to maintain a patent airway and indicated when the client needs mechanical venti

lation. The tube isolates the airway, provides access for suctioning secretions from the large airways of the pulmonary tree, and allows delivery of specific concentrations of oxygen up to 100%.

Mantoux Test—The most reliable determinant of infection with tuberculosis (TB). A small amount (0.1 mL) of intermediate-strength purified protein derivative (PPD) containing 5 tuberculin units is given intradermally in the forearm. An area of induration measuring 10 mm or more in diameter 48 to 72 hours after injection indicates that the individual has been exposed to TB

Mechanical Ventilation—The use of a ventilator if the client is unable to ventilate enough to maintain proper levels of oxygen and carbon dioxide in the blood. Types of ventilators include negative pressure or positive pressure ventilators. Various ventilator modes are adjusted to the client's individual needs.

Multidrug-Resistant Strain (MDR-TB)—A multidrug-resistant strain (MDR-TB) of TB can occur as a result of improper or noncompliant use of treatment programs and the development of mutations in the tubercle bacilli.

Mycobacterium tuberculosis—The causative organism (bacillus) of tuberculosis. An aerobic bacterium that is a nonmotile, nonsporulating, acid-fast rod that secretes niacin.

Pneumothorax—The accumulation of atmospheric air in the pleural space, which results in a rise in intrathoracic pressure and reduced vital capacity. The loss of negative intrapleural pressure results in collapse of the lung. A spontaneous pneumothorax occurs with the rupture of a bleb. An open pneumothorax occurs when an opening through the chest wall allows the entrance of positive atmospheric pressure into the pleural space. A tension pneumothorax can occur from a blunt chest injury or from mechanical ventilation with positive end-expiratory pressure when there is a build-up of positive pressure in the pleural space. Diagnosis of pneumothorax is made by chest x-ray film.

Suctioning—A sterile procedure that involves the removal of respiratory secretions that accumulate in the tracheal bronchial airway when the client is unable to expectorate. Performed to maintain a patent airway.

Tracheostomy—An artificial opening into the trachea created to establish an airway. It may be temporary or permanent. Provides a patent airway by bypassing complete upper airway obstruction, as from pharyngeal tumors or laryngeal edema, by facilitating the removal of secretions, or by preventing aspiration of gastric contents. Also used to allow for long-term mechanical ventilation.

Tuberculosis—A highly communicable disease caused by *Mycobacterium tuberculosis*. It is transmitted by the airborne route via droplet infection.

PYRAMID TO SUCCESS

The Pyramid to Success focuses on respiratory acid-base imbalances and reading arterial blood gas results; infectious diseases, particularly acquired immunodeficiency syndrome (AIDS) and tuberculosis; and respiratory care in relation to oxygen delivery systems, endotracheal and tracheostomy tubes, and mechanical ventilation. Focuses on the care of the client with chest tubes and the expected and unexpected assessment findings. Pyramid points also focus on the client with pneumonia, respiratory failure, chronic obstructive pulmonary disease, and pneumothorax. The pyramid to success includes the care to the client with tuberculosis, especially with regard to the importance of the medication regimen, providing adequate nutrition and adequate rest to promote the healing process, and the prevention of the progression of the disease. Focuses on assisting the client to cope with the social isolation issues that exist during the period of illness and on teaching the client and family the critical measures of screening and of preventing respiratory disease and the transmission of disease.

NURSING PROCESS

ASSESSMENT

Risk factors related to respiratory disorders
Exposure to respiratory irritants, infectious disease, or TB
Medical and social history
Fatigue and lethargy
Anorexia and weight loss
Chills or fever
Cough
Dyspnea
Sputum production

Hemoptysis
Adventitious sounds
Changes in pattern of respirations
Chest tightness and a dull, aching chest pain that may accompany the cough
Voice changes
Presence of night sweats
Skin color changes
Changes in mentation

ANALYSIS: Ineffective Airway Clearance

PLANNING	IMPLEMENTATION	EVALUATION
Client consumes adequate fluids. Client expectorates sputum. Client performs respiratory treatments as prescribed.	Monitor vital signs. Auscultate lung sounds to evaluate air movement. Monitor sputum production noting color, amount, consistency, and odor. Provide adequate fluids and hydration to prevent retention of thick secretions. Position client for comfort and ease of respiration. Instruct client in the use of incentive spirometry and breathing exercises. Suction PRN.	Airway remains patent.

ANALYSIS: Ineffective Breathing Patterns

PLANNING	IMPLEMENTATION	EVALUATION
The client exhibits normal breathing patterns.	Monitor vital signs. Monitor respirations and breathing patterns. Monitor for signs of altered respirations. Monitor for changes in skin color, altered mentation, cyanosis.	Respirations remain normal in rate and depth.

ANALYSIS: Impaired Gas Exchange (Cerebral and Cardiovascular Tissue Perfusion)

PLANNING	IMPLEMENTATION	EVALUATION
The client exhibits signs of adequate gas exchange.	Monitor respiratory status, noting skin color. Monitor for changes in mental status. Monitor for cardiac dysrhythmias. Monitor peripheral vascular status. Administer oxygen as prescribed. Provide several periods of rest during the day.	Airway remains patent and the client does not exhibit signs of cyanosis.

ANALYSIS: Potential for Infection

PLANNING	IMPLEMENTATION	EVALUATION
Client identifies signs of infection. The client verbalizes actions to prevent the transmission of the disease.	Monitor temperature. Monitor for signs of infection. Monitor sputum culture and sensitivity results and chest x-ray results. Provide respiratory isolation during the infectious stage of respiratory disease until treatment is well established. Instruct the client to cover the mouth and nose when coughing, sneezing, and laughing. Instruct client how to properly dispose of used tissues. Educate the client, family, and close contacts about transmission and prevention. Perform Mantoux test on all known contacts of the client with tuberculosis.	Temperature remains within normal limits. Client complies with the treatment regimen. Demonstrates behaviors that will prevent the transmission of the disease.

ANALYSIS: Knowledge Deficit

PLANNING	IMPLEMENTATION	EVALUATION
The client describes the treatment plan. The client describes the importance of adequate rest periods. The client alternates rest periods with activity. The client verbalizes the need for follow up care.	Instruct client regarding prescribed treatment plan and the importance of compliance. Instruct client in the importance of adequate rest and activity. Instruct client in breathing techniques. Instruct client regarding administration of prescribed medications. Instruct client/family in prescribed respiratory treatments, care to tracheostomy site if present, and suctioning techniques. Identify support systems. Mobilize home care and community resources as appropriate. Instruct client in the importance of follow-up care and sputum culture testing if prescribed.	Client complies with treatment plan. Client demonstrates performance of prescribed respiratory treatments. Client complies with seeking medical help for routine follow-up and laboratory analysis. Client utilizes appropriate community resources.

ANALYSIS: Altered Nutrition

PLANNING	IMPLEMENTATION	EVALUATION
The client complies with increased nutritional intake. The client maintains prescribed daily calorie requirements.	Perform and offer mouth care. Assess the client's food likes and dislikes. Provide foods rich in iron, protein, and vitamin C; Increase fluid intake. Monitor body weight. Plan meal and snack times after rest periods.	Client maintains body weight through adequate nutritional intake. Maintains the optimal intake of nutrients and calories to promote tissue healing and to prevent infection.

ANALYSIS: Social Isolation

PLANNING	IMPLEMENTATION	EVALUATION
The client verbalizes appropriate diversional activities. Client identifies support system.	Encourage diversional activities on the basis of the client's interests. Encourage family members to visit during hospitalization for short periods, maintaining respiratory precautions if prescribed.	Client participates in appropriate diversional activities. Client utilizes support systems.

CLIENT NEEDS

SAFE, EFFECTIVE CARE ENVIRONMENT

Client rights
Confidentiality related to the respiratory disorder
Informed consent related to diagnostic and surgical procedures
Consultations and referrals related to respiratory disorder
Handling infectious materials such as sputum or body fluids
Respiratory precautions
Standard precautions
Asepsis when caring for wounds, tracheostomy sites, and mechanical ventilation and when performing suctioning

HEALTH PROMOTION AND MAINTENANCE

Respiratory assessment techniques
Prevention of respiratory disorders and infectious diseases
Health promotion programs
Health screening related to risks for respiratory disorders or AIDS
Instructions related to the prevention or transmission of infection
Instructions related to medication administration
Instructions related to breathing exercises and respiratory therapy and care
Instructions related to adequate fluid and nutritional intake
Instructions related to care to tracheostomy site and suctioning if appropriate
Instructions related to need for follow-up care

PSYCHOSOCIAL INTEGRITY

Religious and spiritual influences
Coping mechanisms
Grief and loss
Situational role changes
Body image changes related to tracheostomy if performed
Support systems
Community resources

PSYCHOSOCIAL INTEGRITY

Assistive devices related to laryngectomy client
Comfort interventions
Nutrition and oral hygiene
Personal hygiene and rest and sleep
Medication administration
Alterations in body systems
Acid-base imbalances
Infectious diseases
Respiratory care
Reading arterial blood gas results
Oxygen delivery systems
Endotracheal and tracheostomy tubes
Mechanical ventilation
Chest tubes
Pneumonia
Respiratory failure
Chronic obstructive pulmonary disease
Pneumothorax
Tuberculosis
Acquired immunodeficiency syndrome (AIDS)

BIBLIOGRAPHY

Black, J. & Matassarin-Jacobs, E. (1997). *Medical-surgical nursing: Clinical management for continuity of care* (5th ed.). Philadelphia: W. B. Saunders.

Luckmann, J. (1997). *Saunders manual of nursing care.* Philadelphia: W. B. Saunders.

National Council of State Boards of Nursing. (1997). *Plan for the National Licensure Examination for Registered Nurses.* Chicago: Author.

CHAPTER 56

The Respiratory System

I. Anatomy and Physiology

A. Primary functions
  1. Provides oxygen for metabolism in the tissues
  2. Removes carbon dioxide, the waste product of metabolism
B. Secondary functions
  1. Facilitates sense of smell
  2. Produces speech
  3. Maintains acid-base balance
  4. Maintains body water levels
  5. Maintains heat balance
C. Upper respiratory tract
  1. Nose: Humidifies, warms, and filters inspired air
  2. Sinuses
    a. Air-filled cavities within the hollow bones that surround the nasal passages
    b. Provide resonance during speech
  3. Pharynx
    a. Located behind the oral and nasal cavities
    b. Divided into the nasopharynx, oropharynx and laryngopharynx
    c. Passageway for both the respiratory and digestive tracts
  4. Larynx
    a. Located above the trachea and just below the pharynx at the root of the tongue
    b. Commonly called the voice box
    c. Contains two pairs of vocal cords, the false and true cords
    d. The opening between the true vocal cords is the glottis
    e. The glottis plays an important role in coughing, which is the most fundamental defense mechanism of the lungs
  5. Epiglottis
    a. Leaf-shaped elastic structure that is attached along one end to the top of the larynx
    b. It prevents food from entering the tracheobronchial tree by closing over the glottis during swallowing

D. Lower respiratory tract
  1. Trachea
    a. Located in front of the esophagus
    b. Branches into the right and left main stem bronchi at the carina
  2. Main stem bronchi
    a. Begin at the carina
    b. The right bronchus is slightly wider, shorter, and more vertical than the left bronchus
    c. The main stem bronchi divide into five secondary or lobar bronchi that enter each of the five lobes of the lung
    d. The bronchi are lined with cilia, which propel mucus up and away from the lower airway to the trachea where it can be expectorated or swallowed
  3. Bronchioles
    a. Branch from the secondary bronchi and subdivide into the small terminal and respiratory bronchioles
    b. They contain no cartilage and depend on the elastic recoil of the lung for patency
    c. The terminal bronchioles contain no cilia and do not participate in gas exchange
  4. Alveolar ducts and alveoli
    a. Acinus (pl: acini) is a term used to indicate all structures distal to the terminal bronchiole
    b. Alveolar ducts branch from the respiratory bronchioles
    c. Alveolar sacs, which arise from the ducts, contain clusters of alveoli, which are the basic units of gas exchange
    d. Cells in the walls of the alveoli secrete surfactant, a phospholipid protein that reduces the surface tension in the alveoli
    e. Without surfactant, the alveoli would collapse
  5. Lungs
    a. Located in the pleural cavity in the thorax
    b. Extend from just above the clavicles to the diaphragm, the major muscle of inspiration

c. The right lung, which is larger than the left, is divided into three lobes, the upper, middle, and lower

d. The left lung, which is somewhat narrower that the right lung to accommodate the heart, is divided into two lobes

e. Innervation of the respiratory structures is accomplished by the phrenic nerve, vagus nerve, and thoracic nerves

f. The parietal pleura lines the inside of the thoracic cavity, including the upper surface of the diaphragm

g. The visceral pleura covers the pulmonary surfaces

h. A thin fluid layer that is produced by the cells lining the pleura lubricates the visceral pleura and parietal pleura, allowing them to glide smoothly and painlessly during respiration

i. Blood flow through the lungs occurs via the pulmonary system and the bronchial system

6. Accessory muscles of respiration: Includes the scalene muscles, which elevate the first two ribs; the sternocleidomastoid muscles, which raise the sternum; and the trapezius and pectoralis muscles, which fix the shoulders

7. The respiratory process

a. The diaphragm descends into the abdominal cavity during inspiration, causing negative pressure in the lungs

b. The negative pressure draws air from the area of greater pressure, the atmosphere, into the area of lesser pressure, the lungs

c. In the lungs, air passes through the terminal bronchioles into the alveoli to oxygenate the body tissues

d. At the end of inspiration, the diaphragm and intercostal muscles relax and the lungs recoil

e. As the lungs recoil, pressure within the lungs becomes greater than atmospheric pressure, causing the air, which now contains the cellular waste products of carbon dioxide and water, to move from the alveoli in the lungs to the atmosphere

f. Expiration is a passive process (Box 56-1)

II. Diagnostic Tests

A. Chest x-ray (CXR) film (radiograph)

1. Description: Provides information regarding the anatomic location and appearance of the lungs

2. Preprocedure

a. Remove all jewelry and other metal objects from chest area

b. Assess ability to inhale and hold breath

c. Question women regarding pregnancy or the possibility of pregnancy

---

BOX 56-1. Risk Factors for Respiratory Disease

Smoking
Use of chewing tobacco
Allergies
Frequent respiratory illnesses
Chest injury
Surgery
Exposure to chemicals and environmental pollutants
Crowded living conditions
Family history of infectious disease
Geographic residence and travel to foreign countries

---

3. Postprocedure: Assist client to dress

B. Sputum specimen

1. Description: A specimen obtained by expectoration or tracheal **suctioning** to assist in the identification of organisms or abnormal cells (see Box 56-4)

2. Preprocedure

a. Determine specific purpose of collection and check with institutional policy for appropriate collection of specimen

b. Obtain an early morning sterile specimen from **suctioning** or expectoration after a respiratory treatment, if a treatment is prescribed

c. Obtain 15 mL of sputum

d. Instruct client to rinse mouth with water prior to collection; instruct client to take several deep breaths and then cough deeply to obtain sputum

e. Always collect specimen before starting antibiotics

3. Postprocedure

a. If culture of sputum is prescribed, transport specimen to laboratory immediately

b. Assist client with mouth care

C. Bronchoscopy

1. Description: Direct visual examination of the larynx, trachea, and bronchi with a fiberoptic bronchoscope

2. Preprocedure

a. Obtain informed consent

b. NPO from midnight prior to the procedure

c. Obtain vital signs

d. Monitor coagulation studies

e. Remove dentures or eyeglasses

f. Prepare suction equipment

g. Administer medication for sedation as prescribed

h. Have emergency resuscitation equipment readily available

3. Postprocedure

a. Monitor vital signs

b. Maintain semi-Fowler's position

c. Assess gag reflex

d. Maintain NPO status until gag reflex returns

e. Have an emesis basin readily available for client to expectorate saliva

f. Monitor for bloody sputum

g. Monitor respiratory status, particularly if sedation was administered

h. Monitor for complications, such as bronchospasm, bacteremia, bronchial perforation indicated by facial or neck crepitus, dysrhythmias, fever, hemorrhage, hypoxemia, and **pneumothorax**

i. Notify physician if fever or difficulty in breathing occurs following the procedure

D. Pulmonary angiography

1. Description: An invasive fluoroscopic procedure following injection of iodine or radiopaque or contrast material through a catheter inserted through the antecubital or femoral vein into the pulmonary artery or one of its branches

2. Preprocedure

a. Obtain informed consent

b. Assess for allergies to iodine, seafood, other radiopaque dyes

c. Maintain NPO status for 8 hours prior to the procedure

d. Monitor vital signs

e. Monitor coagulation studies

f. Establish an IV access

g. Administer sedation as prescribed

h. Instruct clients that they must lie still during the procedure

i. Instruct clients that they may feel an urge to cough or experience flushing, nausea, or a salty taste following injection of the dye

j. Have emergency resuscitation equipment available

3. Postprocedure

a. Monitor vital signs

b. Avoid taking blood pressures in the extremity used for injection for 24 hours

c. Monitor peripheral neurovascular status

d. Assess insertion site for bleeding

e. Monitor for delayed reaction to the dye

E. Thoracentesis

1. Description: Removal of fluid or air from the pleural space via a transthoracic aspiration

2. Preprocedure

a. Obtain consent

b. Obtain baseline vital signs

c. Prepare client for ultrasound or chest radiograph if prescribed prior to procedure

d. Assess coagulation studies

e. Note that client is positioned sitting upright, with arms and head supported by a table at the bedside during the procedure

f. If the client cannot sit up, the client is placed lying in bed on the unaffected side with the head of the bed elevated 45°

g. Inform client not to cough, breath deeply, or move during the procedure

3. Postprocedure

a. Monitor vital signs

b. Monitor respiratory status

c. Apply a pressure dressing and assess puncture site for bleeding and crepitus

d. Monitor for signs of **pneumothorax,** air embolism, and pulmonary edema

F. Pulmonary function tests (PFTs)

1. Description: Include a number of different tests used to evaluate lung mechanics, gas exchange, and acid-base disturbance through spirometric measurements, lung volumes, and arterial blood gases (see Box 56–3)

2. Preprocedure

a. Determine whether an analgesic that may depress the respiratory function is being administered

b. Consult with physician regarding holding bronchodilators prior to testing

c. Instruct client to void prior to procedure and to wear loose clothing

d. Remove dentures

e. Instruct client to refrain from smoking or eating a heavy meal for 4 to 6 hours prior to the test

3. Postprocedure: Resume normal diet and any bronchodilators and respiratory treatments that were held prior to procedure

G. Lung biopsy

1. Description

a. A percutaneous lung biopsy is performed to obtain tissue for analysis by culture or cytologic examination

b. A needle biopsy is done to identify pulmonary lesions, changes in lung tissue, and the cause of pleural effusion

2. Preprocedure

a. Obtain informed consent

b. Maintain NPO status prior to the procedure

c. Inform the client that a local anesthetic will be used but that a sensation of pressure during needle insertion and aspiration may be felt

d. Administer analgesics and sedatives as prescribed

3. Postprocedure

a. Monitor vital signs

b. Apply a dressing to the biopsy site and monitor for drainage or bleeding

c. Monitor for signs of respiratory distress, and notify physician if they occur

d. Monitor for signs of **pneumothorax** and air emboli, and notify physician if they occur

c. Prepare client for chest x-ray film if prescribed

H. Ventilation perfusion lung scan
   1. Description
      a. In the perfusion scan, blood flow to the lungs is evaluated
      b. The ventilation scan determines the patency of the pulmonary airways and detects abnormalities in ventilation
      c. A radionuclide may be injected for the procedure
   2. Preprocedure
      a. Obtain informed consent
      b. Assess for allergies to dye, iodine, or seafood
      c. Remove jewelry from the chest area
      d. Review breathing methods that may be required during testing
      e. Establish an IV access
      f. Administer sedation if prescribed
      g. Have emergency resuscitation equipment available
   3. Postprocedure
      a. Monitor client for reaction to the radionuclide
      b. For 24 hours following the procedure, rubber gloves that are worn when urine is being discarded should be washed with soap and water before removing; then, wash the hands after the gloves are removed
      c. Instruct client to wash hands carefully with soap and water for 24 hours following the procedure

I. Bronchography
   1. Description
      a. A liquid contrast medium is instilled into the trachea, followed by chest x-ray films of the bronchial tree
      b. It is performed to diagnose abnormalities of the bronchi, such as narrowing, dilation, and obstruction
   2. Preprocedure
      a. Obtain informed consent
      b. Assess for allergies to iodine, seafood, and contrast media (dye)
      c. Maintain NPO status for several hours prior to the test to prevent postprocedure aspiration
      d. Administer sedation as prescribed
   3. Postprocedure
      a. Assess vital signs
      b. Assess for dyspnea or bleeding
      c. Encourage coughing and deep breathing
      d. Maintain NPO status until gag reflex returns
      e. Encourage fluid intake when gag reflex returns

J. Skin tests
   1. Description: An intradermal injection used to assist in diagnosing various infectious diseases
   2. Preprocedure: Determine hypersensitivity or previous reactions to skin tests

   3. Procedure
      a. Use a test site that is free of excessive body hair, dermatitis, and blemishes
      b. Apply at upper one third of inner surface of left arm
      c. Circle and mark injection test site
      d. Document date, time, and test site
   4. Postprocedure
      a. Advise client not to scratch the test site, to prevent infection and abscess formation
      b. Instruct client to avoid washing the test site
      c. Interpret reaction at injection site 24 to 72 hours after administration of the test antigen
      d. Assess test site for the amount of induration (hard swelling) in millimeters and the presence of erythema and vesiculation (small blister-like elevations)

K. Arterial blood gases (ABGS)
   1. Description: Measures the dissolved oxygen and carbon dioxide in the arterial blood and reveals the acid-base state and how well the oxygen is being carried to the body (Box 56–2)
   2. Preprocedure
      a. Perform Allen's test on both wrists prior to drawing radial artery specimens
      b. Have client rest for 30 minutes prior to specimen collection
      c. Avoid **suctioning** prior to drawing blood gases
      d. Do not turn off oxygen unless blood gases are ordered to be drawn at room air
   3. Postprocedure
      a. Place specimen on ice
      b. Note client's temperature on laboratory form
      c. Note O_2 and type of ventilation client is receiving on the laboratory form
      d. Apply pressure to puncture site for 5 to 10 minutes and longer if the client is on anticoagulant therapy or has a bleeding disorder
      e. Transport the specimen to the laboratory within 15 minutes

III. Pulse Oximetry

A. Description
   1. A noninvasive test that registers the oxygen saturation of the client's hemoglobin

---

BOX 56–2. Normal ABG Values

pH—7.35–7.45
PCO_2—35–45 mmHg
HCO_3—22–27 mEq/L
PO_2—80–100 mmHg
O_2 saturation—96% to 100%
Oxyhemoglobin dissociation curve—No shift

BOX 56–3. Client Instructions for Incentive Spirometry

Use lips to form seal around mouthpiece
Inspire deeply
Hold inspiration for a few seconds
Forcefully exhale
Avoid use of spirometry at meal times as it may produce nausea

---

2. This arterial oxygen saturation (SaO_2) is recorded as a percentage
3. The normal value is 95% to 100%
4. After a hypoxic client uses up the readily available oxygen (measured as the arterial oxygen pressure, PaO_2, on arterial blood gas testing), the reserve oxygen, that oxygen attached to the hemoglobin (SaO_2), is drawn on to provide oxygen to the tissues
5. A pulse oximeter reading can alert the nurse to hypoxemia before clinical signs occur

B. Procedure
1. A sensor is placed on the client's finger, toe, nose, earlobe, or forehead to measure oxygen saturation, which is then displayed on a monitor
2. Maintain transducer at heart level
3. Do not select an extremity with an impediment to blood flow
4. Results lower than 91% necessitate immediate treatment
5. If the SaO_2 is below 85%, the body's tissues have a difficult time becoming oxygenated; an SaO_2 of less than 70% is life-threatening

IV. Chest Physiotherapy (CPT)

A. Description: Percussion and vibration over the thorax to loosen secretions in the affected area of the lungs
B. Implementation
1. A layer of material (gown or pajamas) is placed between the nurse's hands and the client's skin

---

BOX 56–4. Suctioning

Aseptic technique
Hyperoxygenate by Ambu bag, increasing O_2 flow rate, or by deep breaths
Lubricate catheter with sterile water
Tracheal suctioning—insert catheter 4 inches
Nasotracheal suctioning—insert catheter to induce cough reflex
Do not apply suction while inserting catheter
Apply suction intermittently for 10 to 15 seconds; rotate catheter and withdraw
Hyperoxygenate and encourage deep breaths

---

2. Best time is in the morning upon rising, 1 hour before meals, or 2 to 3 hours after meals
3. Stop if pain occurs
4. Dispose of sputum properly
5. Provide mouth care after procedure
C. Contraindications
1. When bronchospasm is increased by its use
2. History of pathological fractures
3. Rib fractures
4. Chest incisions

V. Postural Drainage

A. Description
1. Use of gravity to drain secretions from segments of the lungs
2. May be combined with CPT
B. Implementation
1. Position client properly (lung segment to be drained is uppermost)
2. Best time is in the morning upon arising, 1 hour before meals, or 2 to 3 hours after meals
3. Stop if cyanosis or exhaustion occurs
4. Maintain position 5 to 20 minutes after procedure
5. Dispose of sputum properly
6. Provide mouth care after the procedure
C. Contraindications
1. Unstable vital signs
2. Increased intracranial pressure

VI. Intermittent Positive Pressure Breathing (IPPB)

A. Description: Delivery of aerosolized medications to the respiratory tree by positive pressure
B. Adverse Effects
1. Dizziness
2. Headache
3. Anxiety
4. Cardiac dysrhythmias
5. **Pneumothorax**

VII. Oxygen

A. Implementation
1. Assess color and vital signs prior to and during treatment
2. Place a "NO SMOKING, OXYGEN IN USE" sign at client's bedside
3. Assess for presence of chronic lung problems
4. Humidify the oxygen
B. Nasal cannula (nasal prongs) (Box 56–5)
1. Description
a. Used at flow rates of 1 to 6 L/minute, providing approximate oxygen concentrations of 24% (at 1 L/minute) to 44% (at 6 L/minute)
b. Flow rates higher than 6 L/minute do not significantly increase oxygenation,

BOX 56–5. FIO₂ Delivered Via Nasal Cannula

24% at 1 L/minute	36% at 4 L/minute
28% at 2 L/minute	40% at 5 L/minute
32% at 3 L/minute	44% at 6 L/minute

because the anatomic reserve, or dead space (oral and nasal cavities), is full

  c. Used for the client with chronic airflow limitation (**CAL, COPD**) and for long-term oxygen use; however, the **CAL** client who retains carbon dioxide should never receive oxygen at a rate higher than 2 to 3 L/minute unless on a mechanical ventilator, because of the potential for apnea or respiratory arrest

  d. Effective oxygen concentration can be delivered to both nose breathers and mouth breathers with the use of a nasal cannula

  2. Implementation
  a. Place the nasal prongs in the nostrils, with the openings facing the client
  b. Add humidification as prescribed when a flow rate higher than 2 L/minute is prescribed
  c. Check the water level and change the humidifier as needed
  d. Assess the client for changes in respiratory rate or depth
  e. Assess mucosa, as high flow rates have a drying effect and increase mucosal irritation
  f. Assess skin integrity, as the oxygen tubing can irritate the skin
  g. Provide water-soluble jelly to the nares PRN

C. Simple face mask (Box 56–6)
  1. Description
  a. A face mask is used to deliver oxygen concentrations of 40% to 60% for short-term oxygen therapy or in an emergency
  b. A minimal flow rate of 5 L/minute is needed to prevent the rebreathing of exhaled air
  2. Implementation
  a. Be sure mask fits securely over nose and mouth since a poorly fitting mask reduces the FIO₂ delivered
  b. Assess skin and provide skin care to the

area covered by the mask, as pressure and moisture under the bag may cause skin breakdown

  c. Monitor the client closely for risk of aspiration, because the mask limits the client's ability to clear the mouth, especially if vomiting occurs
  d. Provide emotional support to decrease anxiety to the client who feels claustrophobic
  e. Consult with physician regarding switching the client from a mask to a nasal cannula during eating

D. Partial rebreather mask (Box 56–7)
  1. Description
  a. A partial rebreather mask consists of a mask with a reservoir bag that provides an oxygen concentration of 70% to 90%, with flow rates of 6 to 15 L/minute
  b. The client rebreathes one third of the exhaled tidal volume, which is high in oxygen, thus providing a high FIO₂
  2. Implementation
  a. Make sure that the reservoir does not twist or kink, which results in a deflated bag
  b. Adjust the flow rate to keep the reservoir bag inflated two thirds full during inspiration, as deflation results in decreased oxygen delivered and rebreathing of exhaled air

E. Nonrebreather Mask
  1. Description
  a. A nonrebreather mask provides the highest concentration of the low-flow systems and can deliver an FIO₂ greater than 90%, depending on the client's ventilatory pattern
  b. It is most frequently used in the client with deteriorating respiratory status who might require intubation
  c. The nonrebreather mask has a one-way valve between the mask and the reservoir and two flaps over the exhalation ports
  d. The valve allows the client to draw his or her entire oxygen from the reservoir bag
  e. The flaps prevent room air from entering through the exhalation ports
  f. During exhalation, air leaves through these exhalation ports while the one-way valve prevents exhaled air from re-entering the reservoir bag

BOX 56–6. FIO₂ Delivered Via Simple Face Mask

Flow rate must be set to at least 5 L/minute to flush the mask of carbon dioxide
40% at 5 L/min
45%–50% at 6 L/min
55%–60% at 8 L/min

BOX 56–7. FIO₂ Delivered Via Partial Rebreather Mask

A flow rate high enough to maintain the bag two thirds full during inspiration is needed; 70% to 90% FIO₂ is delivered at 6–15 L/minute

2. FIO_2 delivered: 60% to 100% FIO_2 at a liter flow that maintains the bag two thirds full
3. Implementation
   a. Remove mucus or saliva from the mask
   b. Assess the client closely
   c. Ensure that the valve and flaps are intact and functional during each breath
   d. Valves should open during exhalation and close during inhalation
   e. Suffocation can occur if the reservoir bag kinks or if the oxygen source disconnects
F. High-flow oxygen delivery systems
   1. A high-flow system provides oxygen concentrations of 24% to 100% at 8 to 15 L/minute
   2. High-flow systems include the Venturi mask, aerosol mask, face tent, **tracheostomy** collar, and T-piece
   3. These devices, when properly fitted, deliver a consistent and accurate oxygen concentration that meets the client's inspiratory effort
G. Venturi mask
   1. Description
      a. The Venturi mask delivers the most accurate oxygen concentration
      b. Its operation is based on a mechanism that pulls in a specific proportional amount of room air for each liter flow of oxygen
      c. An adapter is located between the bottom of the mask and the oxygen source; the adapter contains holes of different sizes that allow only specific amounts of air to mix with the oxygen
      d. The adapter allows selection of the amount of oxygen desired
   2. FIO_2 delivered: 24% to 55% FIO_2 with flow rates of 4 to 10 L/minute
   3. Implementation
      a. Monitor closely to ensure an accurate flow rate for specific FIO_2
      b. Keep the orifice for the Venturi adapter open and uncovered to assure adequate oxygen delivery
      c. Assure that mask fits snugly and tubing is free of kinks, as the FIO_2 is altered if kinking occurs or if the mask fits poorly
      d. Assess the client for dry mucous membranes since humidity or aerosol can be added to the system
H. Face tent, aerosol mask, **tracheostomy** collar, and T-piece
   1. Face tent
      a. Fits over the client's chin, with the top extending halfway across the face
      b. The oxygen concentration varies, but the face tent is useful instead of a tight-fitting mask for the client who has facial trauma and burns
   2. Aerosol mask: Used for the client who requires high humidity after extubation or

upper airway surgery or for the client who has thick secretions
   3. **Tracheostomy** collar and T-piece
      a. The **tracheostomy** collar can be used to deliver high humidity and the desired oxygen to the client with a **tracheostomy**
      b. A special adapter called the T-piece can be used to deliver any desired FIO_2 to the client with a **tracheostomy,** laryngectomy, or **endotracheal tube**
   4. FIO_2 delivered: 24% to 100% FIO_2 with flow rates at least 10 L/minute
   5. Implementation
      a. Change delivery system to a nasal cannula during mealtimes
      b. Assess that aerosol mist escapes from the vents of the delivery system during inspiration and expiration
      c. Empty condensation from the tubing to prevent the client from being lavaged with water and to promote an adequate flow rate
      d. Ensure that there is sufficient water in the canister, and change the aerosol water container as needed
      e. Keep the exhalation port on the T-piece open and uncovered (if the port is occluded, the client can suffocate)
      f. Position the T-piece so that it does not pull on the **tracheostomy** or **endotracheal tube** and cause erosion of skin at the **tracheostomy** insertion site
      g. Make sure the humidifier creates enough mist; a mist should be seen during inspiration and expiration

VIII. Endotracheal (ET) Tubes

A. Description
   1. Used to maintain a patent airway.
   2. Indicated when the client needs **mechanical ventilation**
   3. If the client requires an artificial airway for longer than 10 to 14 days, a **tracheostomy** may be created to avoid mucosal and vocal cord damage that can be caused by the **endotracheal tube**
   4. The cuff (located at the distal end of the tube), when inflated, produces a seal between the trachea and the cuff to prevent aspiration and insure delivery of a set tidal volume when **mechanical ventilation** is used; an inflated cuff also prevents air from passing to the vocal cords, nose, or mouth
   5. The pilot balloon permits air to be inserted into the cuff, prevents air from escaping, and is used as a guideline for determining the presence or absence of air in the cuff
   6. The universal adapter enables attachment of the tube to **mechanical ventilation** tubing or other types of oxygen delivery systems

B. Orotracheal
1. Allows use of a larger-diameter tube and reduces the work of breathing
2. Indicated when the client has a nasal obstruction or a predisposition to epistaxis
3. Uncomfortable and can be manipulated by the tongue, causing airway obstruction; an oral airway may be needed to keep the client from biting on the tube

C. Nasotracheal
1. Smaller-sized tube increases resistance and increases client's work of breathing
2. Discouraged in clients with bleeding disorders
3. More comfortable for the client, and client is unable to manipulate with tongue

D. Implementation
1. Placement confirmed by chest x-ray film (correct placement is 1 to 2 cm above carina)
2. Placement assessed by auscultating both sides of the chest while manually ventilating with a resuscitation (Ambu) bag
3. If breath sounds and chest wall movement are absent on the left side, the tube may be in the right main stem bronchus
4. Auscultation over the stomach is performed to rule out esophageal intubation
5. If the tube is in the stomach, louder breath sounds will be heard over the stomach than over the chest, and abdominal distention will be present
6. Secure the tube immediately after intubation with adhesive tape
7. Monitor position of tube at lip or nose
8. Monitor skin and mucous membranes
9. Suction only when needed
10. The oral tube needs to be moved to the opposite side of the mouth daily to prevent pressure and necrosis of the lip and mouth area, prevent nerve damage, and facilitate inspection and cleaning of the mouth; moving the tube to the opposite side of the mouth should be done by two health care providers
11. Prevent pulling or tugging on the tube to prevent dislodgment; suction, coughing, and speaking attempts by the client place extra stress on the tube and can cause dislodgment
12. Keep a resuscitation (Ambu) bag at bedside at all times
13. Assess pilot balloon to ensure cuff is inflated; maintain cuff inflation, which creates a seal and allows complete mechanical control of respiration
14. Monitor cuff pressures at least every 8 hours, which should not exceed 20 mmHg

E. Minimal leak technique
1. Inflate cuff until a seal is established
2. No harsh sound should be heard through a stethoscope placed over the trachea when the client breathes in, but a slight leak on peak inspiration is present

3. Client cannot make vocal sounds, and no air is felt coming out of client's mouth

F. Minimal occluding volume
1. Provides an adequate seal in the trachea at the lowest possible cuff pressure
2. Same procedure as minimal leak technique, without an air leak

G. Extubation
1. Hyperoxygenate the client and suction the **ET tube** and the oral cavity
2. Place client in semi-Fowler's position
3. The cuff is deflated; the client is instructed to take a deep breath and the tube is withdrawn
4. Instruct client to cough and deep breath to assist in removing accumulated secretions in the throat
5. Apply oxygen therapy as prescribed
6. Monitor respiratory status for signs of obstruction, and notify the physician if they occur
7. Inform client that hoarseness or a sore throat is normal and tell client to limit talking if it occurs

IX. Tracheostomy

A. Description
1. A tracheotomy is a surgical incision into the trachea for the purpose of establishing an airway
2. A **tracheostomy** is the stoma or opening that results from the tracheotomy (Table 56–1).
3. The **tracheostomy** can be temporary or permanent

B. Implementation
1. Assess respirations and bilateral breath sounds
2. Monitor ABGs and pulse oximetry
3. Encourage coughing and deep breathing
4. Maintain a semi- to high-Fowler's position
5. Monitor for bleeding, difficulty in breathing, absence of breath sounds, and crepitus, which are indications of hemorrhage, **pneumothorax,** and subcutaneous **emphysema**
6. Provide respiratory treatments as prescribed
7. Suction PRN; hyperoxygenate the client before **suctioning**
8. If client is allowed to eat, sit client up for meals, and assure that the cuff is inflated (if the tube is not capped) for meals and for 1 hour after meals
9. Monitor cuff pressures as prescribed
10. Assess the stoma and secretions for blood or purulent drainage
11. Follow physician's orders and agency policy for cleaning the **tracheostomy** site and inner cannula; usually one-half strength hydrogen peroxide is used
12. Administer humidified oxygen as prescribed, as the normal humidification process is bypassed in a client with a **tracheostomy**

BOX 56–8. Complications of a Tracheostomy

Tube obstruction
Tube dislodgment
Pneumothorax
Subcutaneous emphysema
Bleeding
Infection
Tracheomalacia
Tracheal stenosis
Tracheoesophageal fistula
Trachea–innominate artery fistula

13. Obtain assistance in changing **tracheostomy** ties; cut and remove old ties holding the **tracheostomy** in place after placing new ties
14. Keep a resuscitation (Ambu) bag, obturator, clamps, and a tracheotomy set at the bedside (Box 56–8)

C. Tube obstruction
   1. Assessment
      a. Difficulty in breathing
      b. Noisy respirations
      c. Difficulty in inserting the suction catheter
      d. Thick, dry secretions
      e. Unexplained peak pressures if on a mechanical ventilator
   2. Implementation
      a. Assist the client to cough and deep breathe
      b. Provide humidification and **suctioning**
      c. Clean the inner cannula regularly
      d. Instill saline into the **tracheostomy** tube as prescribed to loosen secretions
D. Tube dislodgment
   1. Prevention
      a. Secure the tube in place

Table 56–1. Types of Tracheostomy Tubes

Type	Description
Double-Lumen Tube	The double-lumen tube has three major parts: • *Outer cannula*—fits into the stoma and keeps the airway open. The face plate indicates the size and type of tube and has small holes on both sides for securing the tube with tracheostomy ties. • *Inner cannula*—fits snugly into the outer cannula and locks into place. Provides the universal adapter for use with the ventilator and other respiratory therapy equipment. Some may be removed, cleaned, and reused; others are disposable. • *Obturator*—is a stylet with a blunt end, used to facilitate direction of the tube when inserting or changing a tracheostomy tube. It is removed immediately after tube placement and is always kept with the client and at the bedside in case of accidental decannulation.
Single-Lumen Tube	The single-lumen tube is a long tube used for clients with long or extra thick necks. Often called a "bull neck trach" because of the long distance from the skin to the trachea or the longer length of the trachea in large people. More intensive nursing care is required with this tube because there is no inner cannula to ensure a patent lumen.
Cuffed Tube	A cuff, when inflated, seals the airway. Used with mechanical ventilation, in preventing aspiration of oral or gastric secretions, or for tube feeding. A pilot balloon attached to the outside of the tube may indicate the presence or absence of air in the cuff.
Cuffless Tube	The cuffless tube is a plastic, silicone-like (Silastic), or metal tube, usually double-lumen. Used for long-term airway management in those clients who require a tracheostomy and can protect themselves from aspiration and who do not require mechanical ventilation. Many people can speak with this tube in place.
Fenestrated Tube	The fenestrated tube has a pre-cut opening (fenestration) in the upper posterior wall of the outer cannula. It is used to wean the client from a tracheostomy by ensuring that the client can tolerate breathing through his or her natural airway before the entire tube is removed. This tube allows the client to speak.
Cuffed Fenestrated Tube	The cuffed fenestrated tube facilitates mechanical ventilation and speech. It is often used for clients with spinal cord paralysis or neuromuscular disease who do not require ventilation all the time. When not on the ventilator, the client can have the cuff deflated and the tube capped for speech. A cuffed fenestrated tube is never used in weaning from a tracheostomy because the cuff, even fully deflated, may partially obstruct the airway.
Metal Tracheostomy Tube	The metal tracheostomy tube is used for permanent tracheostomy. It is a cuffless double-lumen tube and can be cleaned and reused indefinitely. A special adapter attaches a manual resuscitation bag. Popular types are the Jackson and Holinger tubes.
Talking Tracheostomy Tube	The talking tracheostomy tube provides a means of communication for the client who is using a ventilator on a long-term basis. An extra air channel allows air to flow up through the vocal cords so that the client can speak with the cuff inflated. The air can cause drying of the vocal cords from constant dry airflow. Examples are the Pitt Trach Speaking Tube (National Catheter Corporation) and Communitrach (Implant Technologies, Inc.).

From Ignatavicius, D., Workman, M., & Mishler, M. (1995). *Medical-surgical nursing; A nursing process approach.* Philadelphia: W. B. Saunders. p. 660.

b. Minimize manipulation and traction on the tube

c. Assure that client does not pull on the tube

d. Ensure that a **tracheostomy** tube of the same type and size is at the client's bedside

2. Implementation

a. Extend the client's neck and open the tissues of the stoma to secure the airway

b. Maintain ventilation by bag and mask

c. Use tracheal dilator (curved clamp) to hold the stoma open

d. Assess airflow and bilateral breath sounds

e. If unable to secure an airway, call the resuscitation team and anesthesiologist

f. Be familiar with institutional policy regarding replacement of a **tracheostomy** tube as a nursing procedure

g. Prepare to insert **tracheostomy** tube; place obturator into **tracheostomy** tube, replace the tube and remove the obturator

h. See Table 56–2 for other **tracheostomy** complications

◆ **X. Chest Tube** Drainage System (Fig. 56–1)

A. Description

1. Returns negative pressure to the intrapleural space

2. Used to remove abnormal accumulations of air and fluids from the pleural space

B. Collection chamber

1. Where the **chest tube** from the client connects to the system

2. Drainage from the tube collects in a series of calibrated columns in this chamber

◆ C. Water seal chamber

1. Establishes 2 cm of water pressure

2. If positive pressure is greater than 2 cm, air or fluid is expelled into the drainage system

3. Allows for air to move from the pleural space into the drainage system but not back into the chest

4. Water oscillates (moves up as the client inhales and moves down as the client exhales)

5. Constant bubbling indicates an air leak from the lung or bronchus

◆ D. Suction control chamber

1. Provides the suction, which can be controlled to provide negative pressure to the chest

2. This chamber is filled with various levels of water to achieve the desired level of suction; without this control, lung tissue could be sucked into the **chest tube**

3. Bubbling in this chamber indicates that there is suction, and it does not indicate that air is escaping from the pleural space

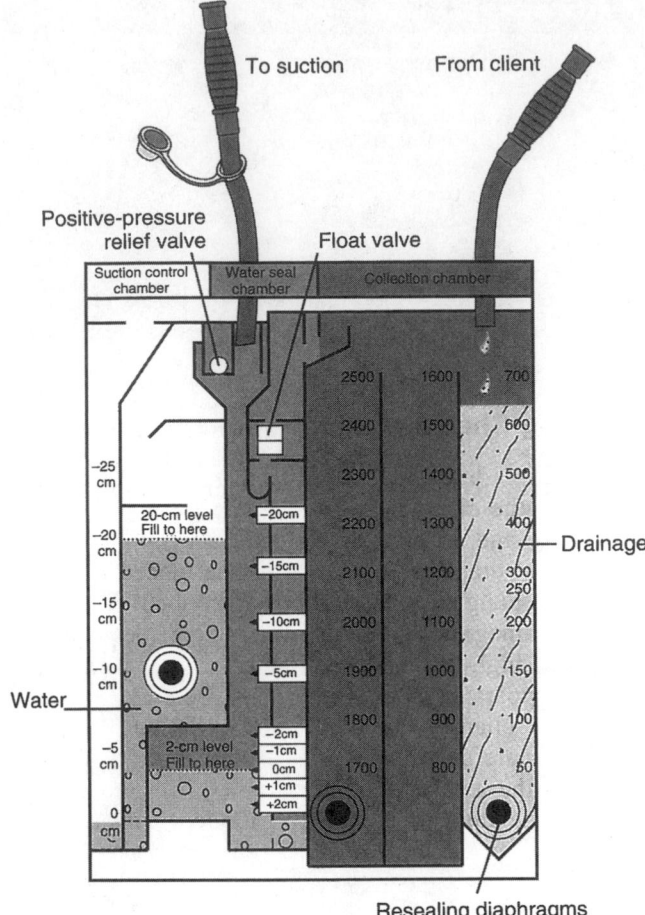

FIGURE 56–1. A commonly used disposable chest drainage system that combines the three bottles into a single device. (Courtesy of Deknatel, Fall River, MA.)

E. Implementation

1. An occlusive sterile dressing is maintained at the insertion site

2. A chest x-ray film assesses the position of the tube and determines whether the lung has re-expanded

3. Assess respiratory status and auscultate for lung sounds

4. Monitor for signs of extended pneumothorax or hemothorax

5. Keep the drainage system below the level of the chest and free of kinks, dependent loops, or other obstructions

6. Assure that all connections are secure

7. Monitor drainage, as it should not exceed 200 mL per hour for 2 consecutive hours

8. Monitor for fluctuation of the fluid level in the water seal chamber

9. Fluctuation in the water seal chamber stops if the tube is obstructed, if a dependent loop exists, if suction is not working properly, or if the lung has re-expanded

10. If the client has a known **pneumothorax,** intermittent bubbling in the water seal

Table 56–2. **Complications of Tracheostomy**

Complications and Description	Signs and Symptoms	Management	Prevention
Tracheomalacia: Constant pressure exerted by the cuff causes tracheal dilation and erosion of cartilage.	An increased amount of air is required in the cuff to maintain the seal. A larger tracheostomy tube is required to prevent an air leak at the stoma. Food particles are seen in tracheal secretions. The client does not receive tidal volume on the ventilator.	No special management is needed unless bleeding occurs.	Use an uncuffed tube as soon as possible. Monitor cuff pressure and air volumes closely and detect changes.
Tracheal stenosis: Narrowed tracheal lumen is due to scar formation from irritation of tracheal mucosa by the cuff.	Stenosis is usually seen after the cuff is deflated or the tracheostomy tube is removed. The client has increased coughing, inability to expectorate secretions, or difficulty in breathing or talking.	Tracheal dilation or surgical intervention is used.	Prevent pulling of and traction on the tracheostomy tube. Properly secure the tube in the midline position. Maintain proper cuff pressure. Minimize oronasal intubation time.
Tracheoesophageal fistula (TEF): Excessive cuff pressure causes erosion of the posterior wall of the trachea. A hole is created between the trachea and the anterior esophagus. The client at highest risk also has a nasogastric tube present.	Similar to tracheomalacia: • Food particles are seen in tracheal secretions. • Increased air in cuff is needed to achieve a seal. • The client has increased coughing and choking while eating. • The client does not receive the set tidal volume on the ventilator.	Oxygen is given manually by mask to the client to prevent hypoxemia. A small, soft feeding tube is used instead of a nasogastric tube for tube feedings. A gastrostomy or jejunostomy may be performed. The client with an NG tube is monitored closely, and assessment is done for tracheoesophageal fistula and aspiration.	Maintain cuff pressure. Monitor the amount of air needed for inflation and detect changes. Progress to deflated cuff or cuffless tube as soon as possible.
Trachea-innominate artery fistula: A malpositioned tube causes its distal tip to push against the lateral wall of the tracheostomy. Continued pressure causes necrosis and erosion of the innominate artery. **This is a medical emergency.**	The tracheostomy tube pulsates in synchrony with the heart beat. There is exsanguination from the stoma. This is a life-threatening complication.	The tracheostomy tube is removed immediately. Direct pressure is applied to the innominate artery at the stoma site. Emergency surgery is done for repair.	Correct the tube size, length, and midline position. Prevent pulling or tugging on the tracheostomy tube. Immediately notify the physician of pulsating tube.

From Ignatavicius, D., Workman, M., & Mishler, M. (1995). *Medical-surgical nursing; A nursing process approach.* Philadelphia: W. B. Saunders. p. 659.

chamber is expected as air is drained from the chest, but constant bubbling is indicative of an air leak in the system
11. Encourage coughing and deep breathing
12. Change client position frequently to promote drainage and ventilation
13. Do not milk a **chest tube** unless specifically directed to by a physician and if the agency policy allows
14. Keep a clamp and a sterile occlusive dressing at the bedside at all times
15. Mark the **chest tube** drainage in the collection chamber at 1- to 4-hour intervals, using a piece of tape
16. Notify the physician if there is constant bubbling in the water seal chamber or if drainage becomes bright red or increases suddenly

17. If the drainage system is broken or interrupted, clamp the tube or place the end of the tube in a bottle of sterile saline held below the level of the chest, and immediately replace the system (determine agency policy for clamping **chest tubes**)
18. If the **chest tube** is accidentally removed, immediately cover the opening in the chest with an occlusive petrolatum gauze dressing
19. When the **chest tube** is removed, the client is asked to perform the Valsalva maneuver; an airtight dressing is taped in place after removal of the **chest tube**

XI. Mechanical Ventilation

A. Types
    1. Pressure-cycled ventilator

a. Pushes air into the lungs until an airway pressure is reached

b. Used for short periods, such as in the postanesthesia care unit and for respiratory therapy

2. Time-cycled ventilator

a. Pushes air into the lungs until a preset time has elapsed

b. Primarily used in pediatric and neonatal clients

3. Volume-cycled ventilator

a. Pushes air into the lungs until a preset volume is delivered

b. A constant tidal volume is delivered regardless of the changing compliance of the lungs and chest wall, or the airway resistance in the client or ventilator

4. Microprocessor ventilator

a. A computer or microprocessor is built into the ventilator to allow continuous monitoring of ventilatory functions, alarms, and client parameters

b. Is more responsive to clients who have severe lung disease or require prolonged weaning

B. Modes of ventilation

1. Controlled

a. ·The client receives a set tidal volume at a set rate

b. Used for clients who cannot initiate respiratory effort

c. The least used mode; if the client attempts to initiate a breath, the efforts are blocked by the ventilator

2. Assist-control (AC) ventilator

a. Most commonly used mode

b. Tidal volume and ventilatory rate are preset on the ventilator

c. The ventilator takes over the work of breathing for the client

d. The ventilator is programmed to respond to the client's inspiratory effort if the client does initiate a breath

e. The ventilator delivers the preset tidal volume when the client initiates a breath, while allowing the client to control the rate of breathing

f. If the client's spontaneous ventilatory rate increases, the ventilator continues to deliver a preset tidal volume with each breath, which may cause hyperventilation and respiratory alkalosis

3. Synchronized intermittent mandatory ventilation (SIMV)

a. Similar to AC in that the tidal volume and ventilatory rate are preset on the ventilator; SIMV allows clients to breath spontaneously at their own rate and tidal volume between the ventilator breaths

b. Can be used in a primary ventilatory mode or in a weaning mode

c. When SIMV is used in a weaning mode, the number of SIMV breaths is gradually decreased, and the client gradually resumes spontaneous breathing

C. Ventilator controls and settings

1. Tidal volume: The volume of air that the client receives with each breath

2. Rate: Number of ventilator breaths delivered per minute

3. Fraction of inspired oxygen (FIO_2): The oxygen concentration delivered to the client, which is determined by the client's condition and the arterial blood gases

4. Sighs

a. Volumes of air that are 1.5 to 2 times the set tidal volume, delivered 6 to 10 times per hour

b. May be used to prevent atelectasis

5. Peak airway inspiratory pressure (PIP)

a. Pressure needed by the ventilator to deliver a set tidal volume at a given compliance

b. Monitoring PIP reflects changes in compliance of the lungs and resistance in the ventilator or client

6. Continuous positive airway pressure (CPAP)

a. Application of positive airway pressure throughout the entire respiratory cycle for spontaneously breathing clients

b. Keeps the alveoli open during inspiration and prevents alveolar collapse

c. Used primarily as a weaning modality

d. During CPAP, no ventilator breaths are delivered, but the ventilator delivers oxygen and provides monitoring and an alarm system

e. The respiratory pattern is determined by the client's efforts

7. Positive end-expiratory pressure (PEEP)

a. Positive pressure exerted during the expiratory phase of ventilation

b. Improves oxygenation by enhancing gas exchange and preventing atelectasis

c. The need for PEEP indicates a severe gas exchange disturbance

8. Implementation

a. Assess the client first and the ventilator second

b. Assess vital signs, lung sounds, respiratory status, and breathing patterns

c. Monitor skin color, particularly in the lips and nail beds

d. Monitor chest for bilateral expansion

e. Obtain pulse oximetry reading

f. Monitor ABG results

g. Assess the need for **suctioning** and observe type, color, and amount of secretions

h. Assess ventilator settings

i. Assess level of water in humidifier and temperature of the humidification system, as extremes in temperature can cause damage to the mucosa airway

j. Assure that the alarms are set

k. If a cause of an alarm cannot be determined, ventilate the client manually with a resuscitation bag until the problem is corrected

l. Empty ventilator tubings when moisture collects

m. Turn client at least every 2 hours or get client out of bed as prescribed to prevent complications of immobility

n. Have resuscitation equipment available at the bedside

D. Causes of alarms

1. High-pressure alarm

a. Increased secretions in the airway

b. Wheezing or bronchospasm causing decreased airway size, **pneumothorax**

c. Displacement of the **ET tube**

d. Obstructed **ET tube** due to water or a kink in the tubing

e. Client coughs, gags, or bites on the oral **ET tube**

f. Client is anxious or fights the ventilator

2. Low-pressure alarm

a. Disconnection or leak in the ventilator system or in the client's airway cuff

b. The client stops spontaneous breathing

E. Complications

1. Hypotension caused by the application of positive pressure, which increases intrathoracic pressure and inhibits blood return to the heart

2. Respiratory complications such as **pneumothorax** or subcutaneous **emphysema** due to positive pressure

3. Gastrointestinal alterations such as stress ulcers

4. Malnutrition

5. Infections

6. Muscular deconditioning

7. Ventilator dependence or inability to wean

F. Weaning: The process of going from ventilator dependence to spontaneous breathing

1. SIMV

a. The client breathes between the ventilator's preset breaths per minute rate

b. The SIMV rate is gradually decreased until the client is breathing on his or her own without the use of the ventilator

2. T-piece

a. The client is taken off the ventilator and the ventilator is replaced with a T-piece or CPAP, which delivers humidified oxygen

b. The client is taken off the ventilator for short periods initially and allowed to breathe spontaneously

c. Weaning progresses as the client is able to tolerate progressively longer periods off the ventilator

3. Pressure support (PS)

a. A predetermined pressure on the ventilator assists the client in the respiratory effort

b. As weaning continues, the amount of pressure is gradually decreased

c. With PS, pressure may be maintained while gradually decreasing the ventilator's preset breaths per minute

XII. Chest Injuries

A. Rib fracture

1. Description

a. Results from direct blunt chest trauma and causes a potential for intrathoracic injury, such as **pneumothorax** or pulmonary contusion

b. Pain with movement and chest splinting result in impaired ventilation and inadequate clearance of secretions

2. Assessment

a. Pain at injury site that increases with inspiration

b. Tenderness at site

c. Shallow respirations

d. Client splints chest

e. Fractures noted on chest x-ray film

3. Implementation

a. Note that ribs usually unite spontaneously

b. Place client in high Fowler's position

c. Administer pain medication as prescribed to maintain adequate ventilatory status

d. Monitor for increased respiratory distress

e. Instruct client to self-splint with hands and arms

f. Prepare the client for an intercostal nerve block as prescribed if the pain is severe

B. Flail chest

1. Description

a. A blunt chest trauma associated with accidents, which may result in hemothorax and rib fractures

b. The loose segment of the chest wall becomes paradoxical to the expansion and contraction of the rest of the chest wall

2. Assessment

a. Paradoxical respirations (the inward movement of the thorax during inspiration with outward movement during expiration)

b. Severe pain in chest

c. Dyspnea

d. Cyanosis

e. Tachycardia

f. Hypotension

g. Shallow respirations

h. Tachypnea

i. Diminished breath sounds

3. Implementation

a. Place client in high Fowler's position

b. Administer humidified oxygen as prescribed

c. Monitor for increased respiratory distress

d. Encourage coughing and deep breathing

e. Administer pain medication as prescribed
f. Maintain bed rest and limit activity to reduce O$_2$ demands
g. Prepare for intubation with **mechanical ventilation,** with positive end-expiratory pressure for severe flail chest associated with respiratory failure and shock

C. Pulmonary contusion
  1. Description
     a. Characterized by interstitial hemorrhage associated with intra-alveolar hemorrhage, resulting in decreased pulmonary compliance
     b. The major complication is adult respiratory distress syndrome (ARDS)
  2. Assessment
     a. Dyspnea
     b. Hypoxemia
     c. Increased bronchial secretions
     d. Hemoptysis
     e. Restlessness
     f. Decreased breath sounds
     g. Rales and wheezes
  3. Implementation
     a. Maintain airway and ventilation
     b. Position client in high Fowler's
     c. Administer oxygen as prescribed
     d. Monitor for increased respiratory distress
     e. Maintain bed rest and limit activity to reduce O$_2$ demands
     f. Prepare for **mechanical ventilation** with positive end-expiratory pressure if required

D. **Pneumothorax**
  1. Description
     a. The accumulation of atmospheric air in the pleural space, which results in a rise in intrathoracic pressure and reduced vital capacity
     b. The loss of negative intrapleural pressure results in collapse of the lung
     c. A spontaneous **pneumothorax** occurs with the rupture of a bleb
     d. An open **pneumothorax** occurs when an opening through the chest wall allows the entrance of positive atmospheric pressure into the pleural space
     e. A tension **pneumothorax** can occur from a blunt chest injury or from **mechanical ventilation** with positive end-expiratory pressure when there is a build up of positive pressure in the pleural space
     f. Diagnosis of **pneumothorax** is made by chest x-ray film
  2. Assessment
     a. Dyspnea
     b. Tachycardia
     c. Tachypnea
     d. Sharp chest pain
     e. Absent breath sounds on affected side
     f. Decreased chest expansion unilaterally

g. Cyanosis
h. Hypotension
i. Subcutaneous **emphysema**
j. Sucking sound with open chest wound
k. Tracheal deviation to the unaffected side with tension **pneumothorax**
  3. Implementation
     a. Apply pressure dressing over open chest wound
     b. Administer oxygen as prescribed
     c. Position client in high Fowler's
     d. Prepare for **chest tube** placement with underwater seal drainage until the lung has fully expanded
     e. Monitor **chest tube** drainage system
     f. Monitor for subcutaneous **emphysema**

XIII. Respiratory Failure

A. Description
  1. Occurs when the client cannot eliminate carbon dioxide from the alveoli
  2. The carbon dioxide retention results in hypoxemia
  3. Oxygen reaches the alveoli but cannot be absorbed or used properly
  4. The lungs can move air sufficiently but cannot oxygenate the pulmonary blood properly
  5. Respiratory failure occurs as a result of a mechanical abnormality of the lungs or chest wall, a defect in the respiratory control center in the brain, or an impairment in the function of the respiratory muscles
  6. The PaCO$_2$ level is greater than 45 mmHg
B. Assessment
  1. Dyspnea
  2. Headache
  3. Confusion
  4. Restlessness
  5. Tachycardia
  6. Cyanosis
  7. Dysrhythmias
  8. Decreased level of consciousness
  9. Alterations in respirations and breath sounds
C. Implementation
  1. Identify and treat the cause of respiratory failure
  2. Administer oxygen to maintain the PaO$_2$ level above 60 mmHg
  3. Position the client in high Fowler's
  4. Encourage deep breathing
  5. Administer bronchodilators as prescribed
  6. Prepare the client for **mechanical ventilation** if supplemental oxygen cannot maintain acceptable PaO$_2$ levels

XIV. Adult Respiratory Distress Syndrome (ARDS)

A. Description
  1. A form of acute respiratory failure caused by

a diffuse lung injury, leading to extravascular lung fluid
2. The major site of injury is the alveolar capillary membrane
3. The interstitial edema causes compression and obliteration of the terminal airways and leads to reduced lung volume and compliance
4. The ABGs identity respiratory acidosis and hypoxemia that does not respond to an increased percentage of oxygen
5. The chest x-ray film shows interstitial edema
6. Some of the causes include sepsis, fluid overload, shock, trauma, neurological injuries, burns, disseminated intravascular coagulation (DIC), drug ingestion, and inhalation of toxic substances

B. Assessment
1. Tachypnea
2. Dyspnea
3. Decreased breath sounds
4. Deteriorating blood gas levels
5. Hypoxemia despite high concentrations of delivered oxygen
6. Decreased pulmonary compliance
7. Pulmonary infiltrates

C. Implementation
1. Identify and treat cause of the ARDS
2. Administer oxygen as prescribed
3. Position client in high Fowler's
4. Restrict fluid intake as prescribed
5. Provide respiratory treatments as prescribed
6. Administer diuretics, anticoagulants, or steroids as prescribed
7. Prepare the client for intubation and **mechanical ventilation,** using positive end-expiratory pressure (PEEP)

XV. Chronic Obstructive Pulmonary Disease (COPD)

A. Description
1. Also known as **chronic obstructive lung disease (COLD) and chronic airflow limitation (CAL)**
2. A group of diseases that includes **emphysema,** asthma, bronchiectasis, and bronchitis
3. Characterized by progressive airflow limitations into and out of the lungs, elevated airway resistance, irreversible lung distention, and arterial blood gas imbalance
4. **COPD** leads to pulmonary insufficiency, pulmonary hypertension, and cor pulmonale
5. In **emphysema,** the stimulus to breathe is a low PO_2 instead of increased PCO_2

B. Assessment
1. Cough
2. Exertional dyspnea
3. Wheezing and crackles

4. Sputum production
5. Weight loss
6. Barrel chest **(emphysema)**
7. Use of accessory muscles
8. Cyanosis
9. Clubbing of fingers
10. Orthopnea
11. Cardiac dysrhythmias
12. Congestion and hyperinflation of lungs on chest x-ray film
13. ABGs indicate respiratory acidosis and hypoxemia
14. PFTs demonstrate decreased vital capacity

C. Implementation
1. Monitor vital signs
2. Administer oxygen as prescribed at 2 to 3 L/minute
3. Monitor pulse oximetry
4. Provide respiratory treatments and chest physical therapy
5. Reposition client for breathing comfort and to mobilize secretions
6. Instruct client in diaphragmatic or abdominal and pursed-lip breathing techniques
7. Record the color, amount, and consistency of sputum
8. Suction client if necessary to clear airway and prevent infection
9. Monitor weight
10. Encourage small, frequent meals to prevent dyspnea
11. Encourage fluids up to 3000 mL/day to keep secretions thin, unless contraindicated
12. Position in high Fowler's and leaning forward to aid in breathing
13. Provide a high-calorie, high-protein diet with dietary supplements
14. Allow activity as tolerated
15. Administer bronchodilators as prescribed and instruct client in the use of both oral and inhalant medications
16. Administer steroids as prescribed to reduce inflammation
17. Administer mucolytics as prescribed to thin secretions
18. Administer antibiotics for infection if prescribed

D. Client education
1. Stop smoking
2. Recognize the signs and symptoms of respiratory infection and hypoxia
3. Adhere to activity limitations, alternating rest periods with activity
4. Avoid exposure to individuals with infections and avoid crowds
5. Demonstrate pursed-lip and diaphragmatic or abdominal breathing
6. Instruct in the use of medications and inhalers
7. Instruct in the use of oxygen therapy
8. Instruct client in nutritional requirements

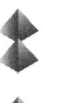

9. Avoid eating gas-producing foods, spicy foods, and extremely hot or cold foods
10. Instruct in the importance of receiving the influenza vaccine as recommended
11. When dusting, use a wet cloth
12. Avoid powerful odors
13. Avoid extremes in temperature
14. Avoid fireplaces, pets, and feather pillows

XVI. Pneumonia

A. Description
   1. An infection of the pulmonary tissue, including the interstitial spaces, alveoli, and bronchioles
   2. The edema associated with inflammation stiffens the lung, decreases compliance in vital capacity, and causes hypoxemia
   3. Can be community-acquired or hospital-acquired
   4. The chest x-ray film shows diffuse patches throughout the lungs or consolidated in a lobe
   5. A sputum culture identifies the organism
   6. The white blood cells (WBCs) and erythrocyte sedimentation rate (ESR) are elevated
B. Assessment
   1. Chills
   2. Elevated temperature
   3. Pleuritic pain
   4. Rales, rhonchi, and wheezes
   5. Use of accessory muscles
   6. Cyanosis
   7. Mental status changes
   8. Sputum production
      a. Rusty, green, or bloody (pneumococcal pneumonia)
      b. Yellow-green (bronchopneumonia)
C. Implementation
   1. Administer oxygen as prescribed
   2. Monitor respiratory status
   3. Monitor for labored respirations, cyanosis, cold and clammy skin
   4. Encourage coughing and deep breathing and use of incentive spirometer
   5. Position in semi-Fowler's to facilitate breathing and lung expansion
   6. Change position frequently and ambulate as tolerated to mobilize secretions
   7. Provide chest physical therapy
   8. Perform nasotracheal **suctioning** if client is unable to clear secretions
   9. Monitor pulse oximetry
   10. Monitor and record color, consistency, and amount of sputum
   11. Provide a high-calorie, high-protein diet, with small frequent meals
   12. Encourage fluids to 3 liters a day to liquefy secretions, unless contraindicated
   13. Provide a balance of rest and activity, increasing activity gradually

14. Administer antibiotics as prescribed
15. Administer antipyretics, bronchodilators, cough suppressants, mucolytic agents, and expectorants as prescribed
16. Prevent the spread of infection by handwashing and the proper disposal of secretions
D. Client education
   1. The importance of rest, proper nutrition, and adequate fluid intake
   2. Avoid chilling and exposure to other individuals with respiratory infections or viruses
   3. Instruct regarding medications and the use of inhalants as prescribed
   4. Instruct to notify physician if chills, fever, dsypnea, hemoptysis, or increased fatigue occur
   5. Instruct in the importance of receiving the influenza vaccine as recommended

XVII. Pleural Effusion

A. Description
   1. The collection of fluid in the pleural space
   2. Any condition that interferes with either secretion or drainage of this fluid will lead to pleural effusion
B. Assessment
   1. Pleuritic pain that is sharp and increases with inspiration
   2. Dyspnea on exertion
   3. Dry, nonproductive cough caused by bronchial irritation or mediastinal shift
   4. Malaise
   5. Tachycardia
   6. Elevated temperature
   7. Decreased breath sounds
   8. CXR film shows pleural effusion and a mediastinal shift away from the fluid
C. Implementation
   1. Identify and treat underlying cause
   2. Monitor vital signs
   3. Monitor breath sounds
   4. Position client in high Fowler's
   5. Encourage coughing and deep breathing
   6. Prepare client for thoracentesis
   7. If pleural effusion is recurrent, prepare client for pleurectomy or pleurodesis
D. Pleurectomy
   1. Consists of surgically stripping the parietal pleura away from the visceral pleura
   2. This produces an intense inflammatory reaction that promotes adhesion formation between the two layers during healing
E. Pleurodesis
   1. Involves the instillation of a sclerosing substance into the pleural space via a thorocotomy tube
   2. This creates an inflammatory response that scleroses tissues together

XVIII. Empyema

A. Description
1. The collection of pus within the pleural cavity
2. The fluid is thick, opaque, and foul-smelling
3. The most common cause is pulmonary infection and lung abscess caused by thoracic surgery or chest trauma, in which bacteria are introduced directly into the pleural space
4. Treatment focuses on emptying the empyema cavity, re-expanding the lung, and controlling the infection

B. Assessment
1. Recent febrile illnesses or trauma
2. Chest pain
3. Cough
4. Dyspnea
5. Anorexia and weight loss
6. Malaise
7. Elevated temperature and chills
8. Night sweats
9. Diminished chest wall movement on the affected side
10. Pleural exudate on CXR

C. Implementation
1. Monitor vital signs
2. Monitor breath sounds
3. Position client in semi- or high Fowler's
4. Encourage coughing and deep breathing
5. Administer antibiotics as prescribed
6. Instruct client to splint chest as necessary
7. Assist with **chest tube** insertion to promote drainage and lung expansion
8. If marked pleural thickening occurs, prepare client for decortication, if prescribed; this is a surgical procedure that involves removal of the restrictive mass of fibrin and inflammatory cells

XIX. Pleurisy

A. Description
1. Inflammation of the visceral and parietal membranes
2. These membranes rub together during respiration and cause pain
3. May be caused by pulmonary infarction or pneumonia
4. It usually occurs on one side of the chest, usually in the lower lateral portions in the chest wall

B. Assessment
1. Knife-like pain that is aggravated on deep breathing and coughing
2. Dyspnea
3. Pleural friction rub heard on auscultation
4. Apprehension

C. Implementation
1. Monitor vital signs
2. Monitor lung sounds
3. Identify and treat cause
4. Administer analgesics as prescribed
5. Apply hot or cold applications as prescribed
6. Encourage coughing and deep breathing
7. Instruct client to lie on affected side to splint chest

XX. Pulmonary Embolism

A. Description
1. Occurs when a thrombus that forms in a deep vein detaches and travels to the right side of the heart and then lodges in a branch of the pulmonary artery
2. Clients prone to pulmonary embolism are those at risk for deep vein thrombosis, including prolonged immobilization, surgery, obesity, pregnancy, congestive heart failure (CHF), advanced age, and prior history of thromboembolism
3. Fat emboli can occur as a complication following a fracture of a flat long bone
4. Treatment is aimed at preventing venous stasis and includes range-of-motion exercises and early ambulation following surgery, the use of antiembolism or pneumatic compression stockings, and preventing pressure under the popliteal space

B. Assessment
1. Dyspnea accompanied by anginal and pleuritic pain, exacerbated by inspiration
2. Cough
3. Blood-tinged sputum
4. Tachycardia
5. Chest pain
6. Tachypnea
7. Hypotension
8. Shallow respirations
9. Rales on auscultation
10. Low-grade fever
11. Distended neck veins
12. Cyanosis
13. Positive Homan's sign with deep vein thrombosis

C. Implementation
1. Monitor vital signs
2. Monitor lung sounds
3. Assess for positive Homan's sign
4. Administer oxygen as prescribed
5. Position client in high Fowler's
6. Maintain bed rest and active and passive range-of-motion exercises as prescribed
7. Encourage use of incentive spirometry as prescribed
8. Monitor pulse oximetry
9. Prepare for intubation and **mechanical ventilation** for severe hypoxemia
10. Administer anticoagulation with IV heparin (bolus), followed by continuous infusion during acute phase
11. Administer warfarin (Coumadin) orally when heparin drip is discontinued
12. Monitor prothrombin time (PT) and partial thromboplastin time (PTT) levels closely

13. Prepare client for embolectomy, vein ligation, or insertion of an umbrella filter as prescribed

XXI. Lung Cancer

A. Description
1. Malignant tumor of the lung that may be primary or metastatic
2. The lungs are a common target for metastasis from other organs
3. Bronchogenic carcinoma spreads through direct extension and lymphatic dissemination
4. The four major types of lung cancer include small cell (oat cell), epidermal (squamous cell), adenocarcinoma, and large cell anaplastic carcinoma
5. Diagnosis is made by a chest x-ray film that will show a lesion or mass, and bronchoscopy and sputum studies that will demonstrate a positive cytology for cancer cells
6. Causes include cigarette smoking, exposure to environmental pollutants, and exposure to occupational pollutants
B. Assessment
1. Cough
2. Dyspnea
3. Hoarseness
4. Hemoptysis
5. Chest pain
6. Weight loss
7. Weakness
8. Anorexia
C. Implementation
1. Monitor vital signs
2. Assess breathing patterns and for signs of respiratory impairment
3. Assess breath sounds
4. Assess for tracheal deviation
5. Administer analgesics as prescribed for pain management
6. Position client upright for ease in breathing
7. Administer oxygen as prescribed and humidification to moisten and loosen secretions
8. Monitor pulse oximetry
9. Provide respiratory treatments as prescribed
10. Administer bronchodilators and steroids as prescribed to decrease bronchospasm, inflammation, and edema
11. Provide a high-protein, high-calorie diet
12. Provide activity as tolerated and active and passive range-of-motion exercises
13. Monitor for bleeding, infection, and electrolyte imbalance
14. Provide rest periods
D. Nonsurgical implementation
1. Radiation therapy for localized intrathoracic lung cancers
2. Chemotherapy to promote tumor regression
3. Immunotherapy with tumor extracts, irradiated whole tumor cells, or cells killed by other methods
4. Immunotherapy directed at enhancing an effective immune response
E. Surgical implementation
1. Laser therapy: To relieve endobronchial obstruction
2. Thoracotomy with pneumonectomy: Surgical removal of a lung for bronchiogenic carcinoma
3. Thoracotomy with lobectomy: Surgical removal of one lobe of the lung for tumors confined to a single lobe
4. Thoracotomy with segmental resection: Surgical removal of a lobe segment for clients unable to tolerate lobectomy or pneumonectomy
5. Preoperative
   a. Explain the potential postoperative need for **chest tubes**
   b. Note that a **chest tube** is not inserted for a pneumonectomy, and the serum fluid that accumulates in the empty thoracic cavity eventually consolidates, preventing shifts of the mediastinum, heart, and remaining lung
6. Postoperative
   a. Monitor vital signs
   b. Assess cardiac and respiratory status
   c. Maintain **chest tube** drainage system, which will drain air or blood or both that accumulates in the pleural space
   d. Monitor for the absence and presence of lung sounds
   e. Assess **chest tube** insertion site for subcutaneous air and drainage
   f. Administer oxygen as prescribed
   g. Monitor pulse oximetry
   h. Provide activity as tolerated
   i. Encourage active performance of range-of-motion exercises to the operative shoulder as prescribed
   j. Maintain client position based on procedure performed
7. Pneumonectomy
   a. Avoid complete lateral positioning because the mediastinum is no longer held in place on both sides by lung tissue
   b. Extreme turning may cause mediastinum shift and compression of the remaining lung
8. Segmental (wedge) resection: Elevate the head of the bed 30° to 45° and avoid positioning client on operative side

XXII. Laryngeal Cancer

A. Description
1. A malignant tumor of the larynx
2. Laryngeal cancer presents as malignant ulcerations with underlying filtration
3. Metastasis to the lung is common
4. Diagnosis is made by laryngoscopy and

biopsy showing a positive cytology for cancer cells

    5. Causes include cigarette smoking, alcohol abuse, exposure to environmental pollutants, exposure to radiation, and voice strain

B. Assessment

    1. Persistent hoarseness
    2. Persistent sore throat
    3. Painless neck mass
    4. A feeling of a lump in the throat
    5. Burning sensation in the throat
    6. Dysphagia
    7. Change in voice quality
    8. Dyspnea
    9. Hemoptysis
    10. Weakness
    11. Weight loss
    12. Foul breath

C. Implementation

    1. Place in Fowler's position to promote optimal air exchange
    2. Administer oxygen as prescribed
    3. Provide respiratory treatments as prescribed
    4. Monitor respiratory status
    5. Monitor for signs of aspiration of food and fluid
    6. Provide activity as tolerated
    7. Provide a high-calorie, high-vitamin, high-protein diet
    8. Provide nutritional support via total parenteral nutrition (TPN), nasogastric (NG) tube feedings, and gastrostomy as prescribed
    9. Administer analgesic as prescribed

D. Nonsurgical implementation

    1. Radiation therapy if the cancer is limited to a small area in one vocal cord
    2. Chemotherapy, which may be done in combination with radiation and surgery

E. Surgical implementation

    1. Small tumor excision, or total laryngectomy: Performed for infiltrate tumors that involve vocal cord paralysis and for tumors that do not respond to radiation therapy
    2. Radical neck dissection
      a. Involves a laryngectomy and **tracheostomy**
      b. Performed when lymph node involvement is present
    3. Preoperative
      a. Establish methods of communication for the client
      b. Encourage the client to express feelings about changes in body image and loss of voice
      c. Describe the rehabilitation program and information about the tracheotomy and **suctioning**
    4. Postoperative
      a. Monitor vital signs
      b. Assess respiratory status
      c. Position client in high Fowler's
      d. Monitor airway patency and provide

frequent **suctioning** to remove bloody secretions

      e. Maintain mechanical ventilator support or a **tracheostomy** collar with humidification as prescribed
      f. Maintain surgical drains in the neck area if present
      g. Observe for hemorrhage and edema in the neck
      h. Administer oxygen via high-humidity **tracheostomy** mask as prescribed
      i. Monitor pulse oximetry
      j. Assess the color, amount, and consistency of sputum
      k. Monitor IV fluids or TPN until nutrition is administered via an NG, gastrostomy, or jejunostomy tube
      l. Assess gag and cough reflex and ability to swallow
      m. Provide oral hygiene
      n. Provide stoma and laryngectomy care
      o. Increase intake in fluids when prescribed
      p. Increase activity, as tolerated
      q. Provide consultation with speech and language pathologist as prescribed
      r. Prepare the client for rehabilitation and speech therapy through the use of an artificial larynx, followed by esophageal speech
      s. Reinforce method of communication established preoperatively

F. Client education

    1. Teach clean **suctioning** technique
    2. Instruct client how to clean incision and provide stoma care
    3. Protect neck from injury
    4. Avoid swimming, showering, and using aerosol sprays
    5. Demonstrate ways to prevent debris from entering the stoma
    6. Instruct client to wear a stoma guard to shield the stoma
    7. Advise client to wear loose-fitting, high-collar clothing to hide the stoma
    8. Advise client to increase humidity in the home
    9. Instruct in range-of-motion exercises for arms, shoulders, and neck daily
    10. Avoid exposure to people with infections
    11. Alternate rest periods with activity
    12. Increase fluid intake to 3000 mL/day
    13. Advise client to obtain a MedicAlert bracelet

XXIII. Carbon Monoxide Poisoning

A. Description

    1. Carbon monoxide is a colorless, odorless, and tasteless gas that has an affinity for hemoglobin 200 times greater than that of oxygen
    2. Oxygen molecules are displaced and carbon monoxide reversibly binds to hemoglobin to

form carboxyhemoglobin; tissue hypoxia occurs

B. Assessment
  1. Carbon monoxide levels of 5% to 10%: Impaired visual acuity
  2. Carbon monoxide levels of 11% to 20%: Flushing
  3. Carbon monoxide levels of 21% to 30%: Nausea and impaired dexterity
  4. Carbon monoxide levels of 31% to 40%: Vomiting, dizziness, and syncope
  5. Carbon monoxide levels of 41% to 50%: Tachypnea and, tachycardia
  6. Carbon monoxide level greater than 50%: Coma and death

C. Implementation
  1. Remove victim from exposure
  2. Administer oxygen
  3. Assess need for Basic Life Support
  4. Monitor vital signs
  5. Monitor carbon monoxide levels

XXIV. Histoplasmosis

A. Description
  1. A pulmonary fungal infection caused by spores of *Histoplasma capsulatum*
  2. Transmission occurs by the inhalation of spores, which are commonly located in contaminated soil
  3. Spores are also usually found in bird droppings

B. Assessment
  1. Dyspnea
  2. Chills
  3. Chest pain
  4. Elevated temperature
  5. Pulmonary infiltrates on CXR film
  6. Elevated WBCs
  7. Positive skin test
  8. Positive agglutination test
  9. Splenomegaly
  10. Hepatomegaly

C. Implementation
  1. Administer oxygen as prescribed
  2. Administer antiemetics, antihistamines, antipyretics, and steroids as prescribed
  3. Administer fungicidal medications as prescribed
  4. Encourage coughing and deep breathing
  5. Position client in semi-Fowler's
  6. Monitor vital signs
  7. Monitor breath sounds
  8. Monitor for nephrotoxicity from fungicidal medications
  9. Instruct client to spray area with water before sweeping barn and chicken coops

XV. Sarcoidosis

A. Description
  1. Epithelioid cell tubercles in lung

2. Cause is unknown
3. High titer of Epstein-Barr virus may be identified
4. Incidence is highest in blacks and young adults

B. Assessment
  1. Night sweats
  2. Fever
  3. Weight loss
  4. Cough
  5. Skin nodules
  6. Polyarthritis
  7. Kveim test: Sarcoid node antigen is injected intradermally and causes local nodular lesion in approximately 1 month

C. Implementation
  1. Corticosteroids to control symptoms
  2. Monitor temperature
  3. Increase fluid intake
  4. Frequent periods of rest
  5. Small, nutritious meals

XXVI. Occupational Lung Disease—Silicosis

A. Description
  1. Known as asbestosis and coal workers' pneumoconiosis
  2. Fibrotic disease of lungs caused by inhalation of inorganic dusts over long periods
  3. Common in miners and sandblasters
  4. Tuberculosis (TB) is a frequent complication

B. Assessment
  1. Frequent respiratory infections
  2. Blood-streaked sputum
  3. Cough
  4. CXR film: Nodular lesions of lungs

C. Implementation
  1. Antitussive for cough
  2. Medication for TB
  3. Eliminate toxic substances
  4. Oxygen
  5. Encourage coughing and deep breathing

XXVII. Acquired Immune Deficiency Syndrome 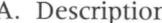 (AIDS)

A. Description
  1. An infectious disease characterized by severe deficits in cellular function
  2. Manifested clinically by opportunistic infection, unusual neoplasms, or both
  3. Etiology: Human immunodeficiency virus (HIV)
  4. The disease has a long incubation period, sometimes up to 10 years or more
  5. Manifestations may not appear until late in the infection

B. Aids-related complex (ARC)
  1. Similar to AIDS
  2. Two or more symptoms or two or more laboratory findings characteristic of immunodeficiency

Table 56–3. AIDS Medications

Action	Side Effects
Zidovudine (AZT, Retrovir)	
Inhibits HIV replication by suppressing synthesis of viral DNA Delays onset of symptoms Reduces severity of symptoms	Bone marrow depression; anemia; GI symptoms: anorexia, nausea, vomiting, diarrhea, abdominal pain; CNS symptoms: headache, confusion, anxiety, insomnia, nervousness, seizures; rash; muscle pain; changes in nail pigmentation
Didanosine (Videx)	
Blocks synthesis of viral DNA Reduces severity of symptoms	Pancreatitis: Increased amylase and triglycerides, decreased calcium, nausea, vomiting, abdominal pain; diarrhea; peripheral neuropathy; leukopenia; fever; rash and pruritus; headache; insomnia; hyperuricemia
Zalcitabine (Hivid)	
Inhibits viral DNA synthesis	Peripheral neuropathy, causing sharp, shooting pain and severe burning; pancreatitis can occur but is uncommon
Ganciclovir (Cytovene)	
Inhibits replication of DNA	Bone marrow depression—granulocytopenia and thrombocytopenia; fever; rash; anemia; liver dysfunction; confusion
Foscarnet (Foscavir)	
Provides selective inhibition on binding site on virus-specific DNA	Nephrotoxity; electrolyte imbalances; fever; anemia; nausea, vomiting, diarrhea; headache
Pentamidine (Pentam 300, NebuPent)	
Disrupts synthesis of DNA, RNA, phospholipids, and proteins	Hypotension; hypoglycemia or hyperglycemia; necrosis at injection site

3. Client is not as ill as the AIDS client
4. May lead to AIDS

C. High-risk groups
   1. Male homosexuals or bisexuals
   2. Intravenous drug abusers
   3. Persons receiving blood transfusions (hemophiliacs, surgical clients)
   4. Those individuals with frequent exposure to blood and body fluids
   5. Heterosexual contact with high-risk individuals
   6. Babies born to infected mothers

D. Assessment
   1. Malaise, weight loss
   2. Lymphadenopathy of at least 3 months
   3. Leukopenia
   4. Diarrhea
   5. Fatigue
   6. Night sweats
   7. Presence of opportunistic infections

8. *Pneumocystis carinii* pneumonia (major source of mortality)
9. Kaposi's sarcoma: Purplish/red lesions on internal organs and skin
10. Fungal infections
11. Candidiasis
12. Cytomegalovirus (CMV)

E. Implementation (Table 56–3)
   1. Respiratory support
   2. Pulmonary treatments
   3. Oxygen
   4. Maintain fluid and electrolyte balance
   5. Prevent spread of infection
   6. Blood and body fluids precautions
   7. Skin care
   8. High-nutrition and low-residue meals

PRACTICE QUESTIONS

1. The nurse is monitoring the chest tube drainage system in a client with a chest tube. The nurse notes intermittent bubbling in the water seal compartment. Which of the following is the most appropriate action?
   1 Change the chest tube drainage system
   2 Document the findings
   3 Check for an airleak
   4 Notify the physician

2. The nurse is planning care for a client scheduled for insertion of a tracheostomy. What equipment should the nurse plan to have at the bedside when the client returns from surgery?
   1 Oral airway
   2 Epinephrine
   3 Obturator
   4 Tracheostomy set with the next larger size

3. The nursing instructor is observing a nursing student suctioning a client through a tracheostomy tube. Which of the following observations, if made by the nursing instructor, indicates an inappropriate action?
   1 Hyperventilating the client with 100% oxygen prior to suctioning
   2 Instilling 3 to 5 mL of normal saline in the tracheotomy tube to loosen secretions
   3 Suctioning the client every hour
   4 Applying suction only during withdrawal of the catheter

4. The nurse is changing the tracheotomy ties on a client with a tracheotomy. The nurse is assessing the security of the ties. What method is used to assure that the ties are not too tightly placed?
   1 The nurse places 2 fingers between the tie and the neck
   2 The tracheotomy tube can be pulled slightly away from the neck
   3 The ties leave no marks on the neck
   4 The nurse uses a 12-inch tie that is affixed with Velcro tightly

5. The nurse is caring for a client with an endotracheal tube attached to a ventilator. The high-pressure alarm sounds on the ventilator. Which of the following is the most appropriate nursing intervention?
   1 Assess for a disconnection
   2 Evaluate the cuff for a leak
   3 Notify the respiratory therapist
   4 Suction the client

6. The nurse is preparing to obtain a sputum specimen from the client. Which of the following nursing actions will facilitate obtaining the specimen?
   1 Limiting fluids
   2 Having the client take three deep breaths
   3 Ask the client to spit into the collection container
   4 Ask the client to obtain the specimen after eating

7. The nurse is caring for a client following a bronchoscopy and biopsy. Which of the following signs, if noted in the client, should be reported immediately to the physician?
   1 Blood-streaked sputum
   2 Dry cough
   3 Hematuria
   4 Laryngeal stridor

8. The nurse is suctioning an adult client via a tracheostomy tube. When suctioning, the nurse must limit the suctioning to a maximum of:
   1 5 seconds
   2 15 seconds
   3 30 seconds
   4 1 minute

9. The nurse is suctioning a client through an endotracheal tube. During the suctioning procedure the nurse notes cardiac irregularities on the monitor. Which of the following is the most appropriate nursing intervention?
   1 Continue to suction
   2 Assure that the suction is limited to 15 seconds
   3 Stop the procedure and reoxygenate the client
   4 Notify the physician immediately

10. The nurse is preparing for removal of an endotracheal tube from a client. In preparing to assist the physician in this procedure, which of the following initial nursing actions is most appropriate?
    1 Suction the ET tube
    2 Deflate the cuff
    3 Turn the ventilator to the off position
    4 Obtain a code cart and place it at the bedside

11. The nurse is preparing to care for a client who will be weaned from a tracheostomy tube. The nurse is planning to use a tracheostomy plug and plans to insert it into the opening in the outer cannula. Which of the following nursing interventions is required prior to plugging the tube?
    1 Suction the client
    2 Deflate the cuff
    3 Assure that the client is able to swallow
    4 Assure that the client is able to speak

12. The nurse is caring for a client with a chest tube drainage system. The nurse notes a fluctuating water level on inspiration and expiration in the submerged tube in the water seal chamber of the chest tube system. Which nursing action is most appropriate?
    1 No action is necessary
    2 Encourage coughing and deep breathing
    3 Suction the client
    4 Increase the suction

13. The nurse is caring for a client with a chest tube drainage system. The nurse notes constant bubbling in the water seal chamber. Which of the following nursing actions is most appropriate?
    1 Reposition the client
    2 Change the chest tube drainage system
    3 Notify the physician
    4 This is a normal expected finding; no action is necessary

14. An unconscious client is admitted to the emergency department. Arterial blood gas level measurement reveals a pH of 7.30, a low bicarbonate level, a normal carbon dioxide level, and a normal oxygen level. An elevated potassium level is also present. These laboratory values indicate the presence of:
    1 Metabolic acidosis
    2 Respiratory acidosis
    3 Combined respiratory and metabolic acidosis
    4 Overcompensated respiratory acidosis

15. The emergency department nurse is assessing a client who sustained a blunt injury to the chest wall. Which of the following signs indicate the presence of a pneumothorax?
    1 A sucking sound at the site of injury
    2 Diminished breath sounds
    3 A low respiratory rate
    4 The presence of a barrel chest

16. The nurse is caring for a client hospitalized with acute exacerbation of chronic obstructive pulmonary disease. Which of the following does the nurse expect to note in assessing this client?
    1 Increased oxygen saturation with exercise
    2 A shortened expiratory phase of respiration
    3 A hyperinflated chest on the x-ray film
    4 A widened diaphragm noted on the chest x-ray film

17. An oxygen delivery system is prescribed for the client with chronic airflow limitation in order to deliver a precise oxygen concentration. Which of

the following types of oxygen delivery systems does the nurse anticipate to be prescribed?
1 Venturi mask
2 Aerosol mask
3 Face tent
4 Tracheostomy collar

18. Theophylline (Theo-Dur) tablets are prescribed for the client with chronic airflow limitation. The nurse instructs the client about the medication. Which of the following nursing statements is not a component of the teaching plan?
1 "Take the medication on an empty stomach."
2 "Take the medication with food."
3 "Continue to take the medication even if you are feeling better."
4 "Periodic blood levels will need to be obtained."

19. The nurse is instructing the hospitalized client with a diagnosis of emphysema about measures that will enhance the effectiveness of breathing during dyspneic periods. Which of the following positions will the nurse instruct the client to assume?
1 Side-lying in bed
2 Sitting in a recliner chair
3 Sitting up in bed
4 Sitting on the side of the bed, leaning on an overbed table

20. The community nurse is conducting an educational session to community members regarding tuberculosis. The first symptom associated with tuberculosis is:
1 Bloody, productive cough
2 A morning cough with expectoration of mucoid sputum
3 Chest pain
4 Dyspnea

21. The nurse performs an admission assessment on a client with a diagnosis of tuberculosis. The nurse reviews the results of which of the following diagnostic tests that will confirm this diagnosis?
1 Bronchoscopy
2 Chest x-ray film
3 Sputum culture
4 Tuberculin skin test

22. The nursing instructor asks the nursing student to describe the route of transmission of tuberculosis. The nursing instructor evaluates that the student understands this route of transmission if the student states that TB is transmitted by:
1 The airborne route
2 Blood and body fluids
3 Fomites
4 Hand-to-mouth

23. The nurse is caring for a client with emphysema. The client is receiving oxygen. The nurse assesses

the oxygen flow rate to assure that it does not exceed:
1 1 liter per minute
2 1 to 3 liters per minute
3 6 liters per minute
4 10 to 12 liters per minute

24. Which of the following arterial blood gases indicates metabolic alkalosis?
1 pH of 7.34, PCO_2 of 50, HCO_3 of 32, PO_2 of 70
2 pH of 7.46, PCO_2 of 30, HCO_3 of 26, PO_2 of 80
3 pH of 7.38, PCO_2 of 45, HCO_3 of 32, PO_2 of 50
4 pH of 7.47, PCO_2 of 40, HCO_3 of 36, PO_2 of 78

25. The nurse reviews the arterial blood gas values of a client. The results indicate respiratory acidosis. Which of the following values indicate that this acid-base imbalance exists?
1 pH of 7.48
2 PCO_2 of 32
3 pH of 7.30
4 HCO_3 of 20

26. The nurse instructs the client to use the pursed-lip method of breathing. The client asks the nurse about the purpose of this type of breathing. The primary purpose of pursed-lip breathing is to:
1 Promote oxygen intake
2 Strengthen the diaphragm
3 Strengthen the intercostal muscles
4 Promote carbon dioxide elimination

27. The client is intubated with an endotracheal tube by the anesthesiologist. What is the responsibility of the nurse in regard to checking for tube placement immediately following tube insertion?
1 It is not the responsibility of the nurse to check for tube placement
2 Arrange for a daily CXR
3 Auscultate the lungs for the presence of bilateral breath sounds
4 Instill air into the endotracheal tube and listen for it being forced into the lungs

28. The low-pressure alarm sounds on the ventilator. The nurse assesses the client and then attempts to determine the cause of the alarm. The nurse is unsuccessful in determining the cause of the alarm. Which of the following initial actions will the nurse take?
1 Check the client's vital signs
2 Ventilate the client manually
3 Administer oxygen
4 Start CPR

29. The client has requested and undergone testing for human immunodeficiency virus. The client now asks what will be done next, since the results of 2 enzyme-linked immunosorbent assay

(ELISA) tests have been positive. The nurse's response is based on the understanding that:
1 The client will probably have a bone marrow biopsy done
2 A Western blot assay will be done to confirm these findings
3 A CD4 cell count will be done to measure T-helper lymphocytes
4 The client will be definitively diagnosed as HIV-positive at this point

30. The nurse is caring for the client with acquired immunodeficiency syndrome (AIDS). The nurse detects early infection with *Pneumocystis carinii* by assessing the client for which of the following clinical manifestations?
1 Dyspnea on exertion
2 Dyspnea at rest
3 Fever
4 Cough

31. The nurse reviews the arterial blood gas values and notes a pH of 7.50, PCO_2 of 30, and HCO_3 of 25. The nurse interprets these values as indicating:
1 Respiratory acidosis uncompensated
2 Respiratory alkalosis uncompensated
3 Metabolic acidosis uncompensated
4 Metabolic acidosis partially compensated

32. Aminophylline is administered to a client with acute bronchitis. The primary action of this medication is to:
1 Promote expectoration
2 Suppress the cough
3 Relax smooth muscles of the bronchial airway
4 Prevent infection

33. The nurse evaluates the blood theophylline level of a client receiving theophylline IV. The nurse determines that a therapeutic blood level exists if which of the following is noted in the laboratory report?
1 1 to 5 μg/mL
2 5 to 15 μg/mL
3 20 to 25 μg/mL
4 25 to 30 μg/mL

34. The nurse is caring for a client with adult respiratory distress syndrome (ARDS). Which of the following does the nurse expect to note in the client?
1 Decreased respiratory rate
2 Pallor
3 Low arterial PaO_2
4 An elevated arterial PaO_2

35. The client is receiving isoetharine hydrochloride (Bronkosol) using a nebulizer. Which of the following is a side effect of this medication?
1 Constipation
2 Diarrhea
3 Bradycardia
4 Tachycardia

36. Isoniazid (INH) and rifampin (Rifadin) have been prescribed for the client with tuberculosis. The nurse reviews the medical record of the client. Which of the following, if noted in the client's record, would require physician notification?
1 Heart disease
2 Allergy to penicillin
3 Hepatitis B
4 Rheumatic fever

37. The client with tuberculosis is being treated with isoniazid (INH) and rifampin (Rifadin). The nurse is preparing instructions for the client regarding these medications. Which of the following statements would be included in the plan of care?
1 "You must discontinue the medication if GI irritation occurs."
2 "You must take the medication with meals."
3 "The entire year-long course of the medication needs to be completed."
4 "Fluids must be increased while taking this medication to prevent renal failure."

38. The client exposed to tuberculosis is taking isoniazid (INH) and develops signs and symptoms of the disease. The client is instructed to add rifampin (Rifadin) to the medication regimen. The nurse explains to the client that the purpose of adding this second medication is:
1 Because rifampin offsets side effects of INH
2 To be certain resistant organisms are eliminated
3 Because these medications potentiate each other
4 Because INH offsets side effects of rifampin

39. The nurse is caring for a client who is on strict bed rest. The nurse develops a plan of care and goals related to the prevention of deep vein thrombosis and pulmonary emboli. Which of the following nursing actions is most helpful to prevent these disorders from developing?
1 Applying a heating pad to the lower extremities
2 Active range-of-motion exercises
3 Placing a pillow under the knees
4 Restricting fluids

40. A client is suspected of having a pulmonary embolus (PE). Which of the following is not a common clinical manifestation of PE?
1 Decreased respirations
2 Tachypnea
3 Dyspnea
4 Chest pain

41. The nurse is teaching a client about the use of a respiratory inhaler. Which of the following is not a component of the teaching plan?
1 Remove the cap and shake the inhaler well before use

2 Press the canister down with your finger as you breath in

3 Inhale the mist and quickly exhale

4 Wait 1 minute between puffs if more than 1 puff has been prescribed

42. The nurse is assigned to care for a client following a left pneumonectomy. The nurse avoids positioning this client:
    1 On the side
    2 Semi-Fowler's
    3 Low Fowler's
    4 With the head of the bed elevated 40°

43. The nurse is preparing a care plan for the client who will be returning from surgery following a right wedge resection. In the postoperative period, the nurse avoids positioning this client:
    1 In low Fowler's position
    2 In semi-Fowler's position
    3 On the left side
    4 On the right side

44. The nurse is performing nasotracheal suctioning of a client. The nurse interprets that the client is adequately tolerating the procedure if which of the following observations is made?
    1 Secretions are becoming bloody
    2 Heart rate decreases from 78 to 54
    3 Coughing occurs with suctioning
    4 Skin color becomes cyanotic

45. The client with a newly inserted tracheostomy has Risk for Impaired Gas Exchange. The nurse assesses for which of the following items as the best indication of adequate ongoing respiratory status?
    1 Moderate amounts of tracheobronchial secretions
    2 Small to moderate amounts of frank blood suctioned from the tube
    3 Respiratory rate of 18 per minute
    4 Oxygen saturation of 91%

46. The nurse is monitoring the respiratory status of a client following insertion of a tracheostomy. The nurse understands that oxygen saturation measurements obtained by pulse oximetry may be inaccurate if the client has which of the following coexisting problems?
    1 Hypotension
    2 Fever
    3 Respiratory failure
    4 Epilepsy

47. The nurse is monitoring the function of a client's chest tube. The chest tube is attached to a Pleurevac drainage system. The nurse notes that the fluid in the water seal chamber rises with inspiration and falls with expiration. The nurse interprets that:
    1 The client has residual pneumothorax

2 The system is patent

3 Suction should be added to the system

4 There is a leak in the system

48. The client has a chest tube attached to a Pleurevac drainage system. As part of routine nursing care, the nurse assures that:
    1 The connection between the chest tube and the drainage system is taped, and that an occlusive dressing is maintained at the insertion site
    2 The amount of drainage into the chest tube is noted and recorded every 24 hours in the client's record
    3 The suction control chamber has sterile water added every shift, and that the system is kept below waist level
    4 The water seal chamber has continuous bubbling, and that assessment for crepitus is done once a shift

49. The client is returned to the nursing unit following thoracic surgery with chest tubes in place. During the first few hours postoperatively, the nurse assesses for drainage and expects to note that it is:
    1 Serous
    2 Serosanguineous
    3 Bloody
    4 Bloody with frequent small clots

50. A female client is scheduled to have a chest x-ray film. Which of the following questions is of most importance to the nurse assessing this client?
    1 "Is there any possibility that you could be pregnant?"
    2 "Are you wearing any metal chains or jewelry?"
    3 "Can you hold your breath easily?"
    4 "Are you able to hold your arms above your head?"

51. The client has just returned to the nursing unit following bronchoscopy. The nurse implements which of the following nursing interventions for this client?
    1 Forcing fluids for the next 24 hours
    2 Assuring return of the cough reflex before offering food or fluids
    3 Administering atropine intravenously
    4 Administering small doses of midazolam (Versed)

52. The nurse is caring for the client after pulmonary angiography with catheter insertion via the left groin. The nurse assesses for allergic reaction to the contrast medium by noting the presence of:
    1 Hematoma in the left groin
    2 Discomfort in the left groin
    3 Stridor
    4 Hypothermia

53. The client has an order to have a radial arterial blood gas analysis performed. Prior to drawing the sample, the nurse occludes the:
    1 Brachial and radial artery, then releases them and observes the circulation to the hand
    2 Radial and ulnar arteries, releases one, evaluates the color of the hand, and repeats the process with the other artery
    3 Radial artery and observes for color changes in the affected hand
    4 Ulnar artery and observes for color changes in the affected hand

54. The nurse is assessing the respiratory status of the client who has suffered a fractured rib. Which of the following observations, if made by the nurse, is not related to the rib fracture?
    1 Pain, especially with inspiration
    2 Slow, deep respirations
    3 Splinting or guarding the chest
    4 Bruising over the fracture area

55. An elderly client hospitalized with a rib fracture asks why the nurse is not strapping the ribs. Which of the following responses by the nurse is the most appropriate?
    1 "That isn't done anymore because people would often develop pneumonia from the constricting effect on the lungs."
    2 "That might help you breathe better, but this facility does not carry them in the stockroom. When you get home, you can purchase one at the medical supply store."
    3 "Those are only useful if the ribs are fractured in several places at once."
    4 "That's a good idea. I'll ask the physician for an order for one this afternoon."

56. The client with chest injury has suffered flail chest. The nurse assesses the client for which of the following as the most distinctive sign of flail chest?
    1 Cyanosis
    2 Hypotension
    3 Dyspnea, especially on exhalation
    4 Paradoxical chest movement

57. The client who has just suffered a large flail chest is experiencing severe pain and dyspnea. The client's central venous pressure is rising, and the arterial blood pressure is falling. The nurse interprets that the client is experiencing:
    1 Mediastinal flutter
    2 Mediastinal shift
    3 Hypovolemic shock
    4 Fat embolism

58. The client has been admitted with chest trauma after a motor vehicle accident and has undergone subsequent intubation. The nurse checks the client when the ventilator's high-pressure alarm sounds and notes that the client has absence of breath sounds in the right upper lobe of the lung. The nurse immediately assesses for other signs of:
    1 Displaced endotracheal tube
    2 Adult respiratory distress syndrome
    3 Pulmonary embolism
    4 Right pneumothorax

59. A client with no history of respiratory disease is admitted with respiratory failure. The nurse assesses the arterial blood gas reports for which of the following results that are consistent with this disorder?
    1 PaO_2 58 mmHg, $PaCO_2$ 32 mmHg
    2 PaO_2 60 mmHg, $PaCO_2$ 45 mmHg
    3 PaO_2 49 mmHg, $PaCO_2$ 52 mmHg
    4 PaO_2 73 mmHg, $PaCO_2$ 62 mmHg

60. The nurse is teaching the client with chronic respiratory failure how to use a metered-dose inhaler correctly. The nurse instructs the client to:
    1 Inhale through the nose
    2 Inhale quickly
    3 Take two inhalations during one breath
    4 Hold the breath after inhalation

61. The nurse is assessing the client with multiple trauma who is at risk for developing adult ARDS. The nurse assesses for which of the following as the earliest sign of ARDS?
    1 Inspiratory crackles
    2 Bilateral wheezing
    3 Intercostal retractions
    4 Increased respiratory rate

62. The nurse is taking pulmonary artery catheter measurements of the client with ARDS. The pulmonary capillary wedge pressure reading is 12 mmHg. The nurse interprets that this reading is:
    1 High and expected
    2 Low and unexpected
    3 Normal and expected
    4 Uncertain and unexpected

63. The nurse is assessing the client with CAL and notes that the client has a barrel chest. The nurse interprets that this client has which of the following forms of CAL?
    1 Chronic obstructive bronchitis
    2 Emphysema
    3 Bronchial asthma
    4 Both bronchial asthma and bronchitis

64. The client diagnosed with pleurisy is being started on medication therapy with indomethacin (Indocin). The nurse teaches the client that this medication is a:
    1 Topical anesthetic that alleviates surface pain
    2 Mild narcotic analgesic to allow the client to deep-breathe
    3 Corticosteroid to decrease the inflammatory response at the site
    4 Nonsteroidal anti-inflammatory drug (NSAID)

to allow more effective coughing and deep breathing

65. The client has experienced pulmonary embolism. The nurse assesses for which one of the following symptoms, which is most commonly reported?
    1 Dyspnea noted when deep breaths are taken
    2 Hot, flushed feeling
    3 Chest pain that occurs suddenly
    4 Sudden chills and fever

66. The nurse is caring for the client who is suspected of having lung cancer. The nurse assesses the client for which of the following most frequent early symptom of lung cancer?
    1 Hemoptysis
    2 Cough
    3 Hoarseness
    4 Pleuritic pain

67. The nurse is caring for the postoperative pneumonectomy client. The nurse assesses the client for which of the following adverse signs and symptoms indicating acute pulmonary edema?
    1 Respiratory rate of 20
    2 Pain with deep breathing
    3 Bilateral lung crackles
    4 Increased chest tube drainage

68. The nurse is caring for the client who has had a pulmonary resection. The nurse would avoid which of the following as the least effective method of splinting the client's incision for coughing and deep breathing?
    1 Apply firm, even pressure to the site after a deep breath and before a cough
    2 Apply firm pressure with the hands before the client takes a deep breath to cough
    3 Have the client hold a pillow firmly against the incision during a cough
    4 Put support under the incision and push down on the shoulder during a cough

69. The nurse is caring for the client who has just returned from the postanesthesia care unit after radical neck dissection. The nurse assesses the portable wound suction for which of the following types of drainage expected in the immediate postoperative period?
    1 Serosanguineous
    2 Grossly bloody
    3 Serous
    4 Serous with sputum

70. The client has had a radical neck dissection and begins to hemorrhage at the incision site. Which of the following actions by the nurse is contraindicated?
    1 Lowering the head of the bed to a flat position
    2 Applying manual pressure over the site
    3 Monitoring the client's airway
    4 Calling the physician immediately

71. The nurse is admitting a client to the emergency department with suspected carbon monoxide poisoning. The nurse assesses that which of the following manifestations is the least reliable for determining the oxygenation status of the client?
    1 Complaints of headache
    2 Muscular weakness
    3 Palpitations
    4 Skin color

72. A client is admitted to the nursing unit experiencing confusion and tremors. An initial arterial blood gas report indicates that the $PaCO_2$ level is 72 mmHg, while the PaO_2 level is 64 mmHg. The nurse interprets that the client is experiencing:
    1 Carbon monoxide poisoning
    2 Carbon dioxide narcosis
    3 Respiratory alkalosis
    4 Metabolic acidosis

73. The client with carbon dioxide narcosis has a potassium level of 6.2 mEq/L. The nurse interprets that this result is:
    1 Unexpected, and indicates a concurrent history of renal insufficiency
    2 Unexpected, and indicates a deficit of hydrogen ions in the blood stream
    3 Expected, and indicates the result of massive hemolysis
    4 Expected, and indicates that acidosis has driven hydrogen ions into the cell, forcing potassium out

74. The client is admitted with carbon dioxide narcosis. In addition to respiratory failure, the nurse plans to monitor the client for which of the following complications of this disorder?
    1 Paralytic ileus
    2 Hypernatremia
    3 Increased intracranial pressure
    4 Hyperglycemia

75. The nurse is evaluating the respiratory status of the client with carbon dioxide narcosis who is being mechanically ventilated. Upon evaluation of a set of arterial blood gas reports, the nurse notes that the client's carbon dioxide level has dropped significantly. The nurse then evaluates the client for which of the following adverse effects of this rapid change?
    1 Tachypnea
    2 Hyponatremia
    3 Seizure activity
    4 Confusion

76. The client with AIDS has become infected with histoplasmosis. The nurse assesses the client for which of the following signs and symptoms?
    1 Weight gain
    2 Dyspnea
    3 Hypothermia
    4 Headache

77. A client has been admitted to the nursing unit with pulmonary sarcoidosis. The nurse assesses the client for which of the following signs indicating a complication of the disorder?
    1 Bilateral lung crackles
    2 Flat neck veins
    3 Elevated central venous pressure (CVP)
    4 Shrunken liver

78. The nurse is caring for the client with exacerbation of sarcoidosis. The nurse teaches the client about adverse effects of medication therapy, which include:
    1 Weight loss
    2 Hyperglycemia
    3 Hyperkalemia
    4 Pruritus

79. The nurse is giving discharge instructions to the client with pulmonary sarcoidosis. The nurse evaluates that the client understands the information if the client reports which of the following early signs of exacerbation?
    1 Fever
    2 Weight loss
    3 Fatigue
    4 Shortness of breath

80. The nurse is taking the nursing history of a client with silicosis. The nurse assesses whether the client wears which of the following items during periods of exposure to silica particles?
    1 Mask
    2 Gown
    3 Gloves
    4 Eye protection

81. The client tells the nurse that the physician has stated a diagnosis of uncomplicated or simple silicosis. The client asks the nurse exactly what this means. In formulating a response, the nurse incorporates the knowledge that:
    1 There is evidence of silica in the blood stream, but no clinical symptoms
    2 The client has normal pulmonary function studies but has shortness of breath
    3 The client has mild ventilation restriction and has fibrosis on chest X-ray film
    4 There is massive pulmonary fibrosis on CXR but no extrapulmonary symptoms

82. The client has been taking benzonatate (Tessalon Perles) as prescribed. The nurse evaluates that the medication is having the intended effect if the client experiences:
    1 Decreased anxiety level
    2 Increased comfort level
    3 Reduction in nausea and vomiting
    4 Decreased frequency and intensity of cough

83. The client has been taking pyrazinamide for 1 month. The client asks the nurse if the therapy is due to be terminated soon. The nurse evaluates that the medication probably will be continued based on a positive finding on which of the following reports?
    1. Blood culture
    2 Sputum culture
    3 Urine culture
    4 Wound culture

84. The nursing diagnosis is Impaired Gas Exchange, related to decreased ventilation and mucous plugs. Which of the following provides the data needed to evaluate the expected outcome for this diagnosis?
    1 Client demonstrated effective coughing techniques
    2 ABGs = pH, 7.4; PO_2, 65; PCO_2, 40
    3 Venous oxygen saturation = 95%
    4 Respiratory rate = 20 breaths per minute

85. The nurse has an order to begin administering Foscarnet (Foscavir) to the client with cytomegalovirus retinitis and AIDS. The nurse assesses the latest results of which of the following laboratory studies prior to administering the dose?
    1 Serum albumin
    2 Serum creatinine
    3 CD4 cell count
    4 Lymphocyte count

86. The client with AIDS and *Pneumocystis carinii* infection has been receiving pentamidine (Pentam 300) IV. The client develops a fever of 101°. The nurse does further assessment of the client, knowing that this sign most likely indicates:
    1 The dose of the medication is too low
    2 The client is experiencing toxic effects of the medication
    3 The client has developed inadequacy of thermoregulation
    4 This is a result of another infection, caused by leukopenic effects of the medication

87. The client with AIDS has been started on therapy with zidovudine (AZT, Retrovir). The nurse carefully assesses which of the following laboratory results during treatment with this medication?
    1 Complete blood count
    2 Blood urea nitrogen
    3 Blood culture
    4 Blood glucose level

88. The nurse is reviewing the results of serum laboratory studies drawn on a client with AIDS who is receiving didanosine (Videx). The nurse interprets that the client may very well have the medication discontinued by the physician because of which of the following significantly elevated results?
    1 Serum cholesterol
    2 Serum amylase
    3 Blood glucose
    4 Serum protein

89. The nurse is preparing to administer a first dose of zalcitabine (Hivid) to a client. The nurse plans to include in medication instructions the need to have serial monitoring of which of the following tests to determine the effectiveness of therapy?
    1 Enzyme-linked immunosorbent assay (ELISA)
    2 Western blot
    3 CD4 cell count
    4 CBC with differential

90. The client with AIDS has a concurrent diagnosis of histoplasmosis. The nurse notes during physical assessment that the client has enlarged lymph nodes. The nurse interprets that:
    1 The client has disseminated histoplasmosis infection
    2 This is a side effect of the medications given to treat AIDS
    3 This indicates that the histoplasmosis is resolving
    4 The client probably has yet another infection that is developing

91. The nurse is caring for the client with AIDS who is experiencing night fever and night sweats. Which of the following nursing interventions is the least helpful in managing this symptom?
    1 Keep a change of bed linens nearby in case they are needed
    2 Administer an antipyretic after the client spikes the fever
    3 Make sure the pillow has a plastic cover
    4 Keep liquid at the bedside

92. The nurse is assessing a client with AIDS for early infection with *Pneumocystis carinii*. Which of the following clinical manifestations would the nurse note?
    1 Dyspnea on exertion
    2 Dyspnea at rest
    3 Fever
    4 Nonproductive cough

93. The client exposed to human immunodeficiency virus (HIV) approximately 3 months ago has seroconverted to HIV-positive status. The nurse antic-ipates that the client will experience which of the following at this time?
    1 Oral lesions
    2 Purplish skin lesions
    3 Chronic cough
    4 No signs and symptoms

94. The client with AIDS has raised, dark purplish-colored lesions on the trunk of the body. The nurse anticipates that which of the following procedures will be done to confirm whether these lesions are due to Kaposi's sarcoma?
    1 ELISA
    2 Western blot
    3 Skin biopsy
    4 Lung biopsy

95. The nurse participating in a health fair is setting up a booth on prevention of HIV transmission. A poster is planned that will list sexual behaviors in one of two columns, rated "safe" and "not safe." Which of the following behaviors would the nurse place in the "not safe" column?
    1 Use of latex condoms
    2 Use of "natural skin" condoms
    3 Abstinence
    4 Mutual monogamy

96. The client with AIDS is experiencing nausea and vomiting. The nurse makes which of the following dietary alterations for this client to enhance nutritional intake?
    1 Avoid dairy products and red meat
    2 Plan large, nutritious meals
    3 Add spices to food for added flavor
    4 Serve foods while they are very warm

97. The client with AIDS has diarrhea from lactose intolerance and a respiratory infection from *Pneumocystis carinii*. In evaluating the plan of care for the nursing diagnosis Impaired Gas Exchange, which of the following is not considered by the nurse to be a positive outcome criteria for this client?
    1 Is free of complaints of shortness of breath
    2 Expectorates secretions easily
    3 Has clear breath sounds
    4 Limits fluid intake

ANSWERS

1. **2**

Rationale: Bubbling in the water seal compartment is caused by air passing out of the pleural space into the fluid in the chamber. Intermittent bubbling is normal. It indicates that the system is accomplishing one of its purposes, that is, removing air from the pleural space. Continuous bubbling during both inspiration and expiration indicates that an air leak exists. If this occurs, it must be corrected.

Test-Taking Strategy: Knowledge regarding the functioning of chest tube drainage systems is required to answer this question. Carefully note the situation presented in the question to assist in determining the correct option. If you are unfamiliar with chest tube drainage systems, review now. You will surely see a question related to these tubes on NCLEX-RN!
Level of Cognitive Ability: Analysis
Phase of Nursing Process: Implementation
Client Needs: Physiological Integrity
Content Area: Adult Health/Respiratory

Reference:
Black, J., & Matassarin-Jacobs, E. (1997). *Medical-surgical nursing: Clinical management for continuity of care* (5th ed.). Philadelphia: W. B. Saunders. p. 1164.

2. 3

Rationale: A replacement tube of the same size and an obturator are kept at the bedside at all times in case the tracheostomy tube is dislodged. Additionally, a curved hemostat that could be used to hold the trachea open if dislodgment occurs should also be kept at the bedside. An oral airway and epinephrine would not be needed.

Test-Taking Strategy: Eliminate option 4 first because a tracheostomy set of the next larger size would not be appropriate for the client. Next eliminate option 2 because it is unrelated to the issue of the question. From the remaining options, recall that the airway has been altered because of the tracheostomy, so an oral airway would not be necessary. Remember that a replacement tube and an obturator should be kept at the bedside of a client with a tracheostomy, along with a curved hemostat, at all times.

Level of Cognitive Ability: Application
Phase of Nursing Process: Planning
Client Needs: Safe, Effective Care Environment
Content Area: Adult Health/Respiratory

Reference:
Monahan, F., & Neighbors, M. (1998). *Medical-surgical nursing: Foundations for clinical practice* (2nd ed.). Philadelphia: W. B. Saunders. p. 566.

3. 3

Rationale: The client should be suctioned as needed. Unnecessary suctioning needs to be avoided because it can increase secretions and cause mechanical trauma to the tissue. The client should be hyperoxygenated with 100% oxygen prior to suctioning, and if tracheal secretions are thick and not easily removed, directly instill 3 to 5 mL of sterile normal saline into the trachea to try to reduce the viscosity of the secretions and stimulate coughing. Suction is not applied during insertion of the catheter, and intermittent suction and a twirling motion of the catheter are utilized during withdrawal.

Test-Taking Strategy: Note the key word "inappropriate" in the question. Then carefully read each option, attempting to visualize the procedure. Note the key words in option 3: "every hour." This should help direct you to select this option. The client should be suctioned as needed, not on a preset scheduled time unless specifically required and indicated by the physician.

Level of Cognitive Ability: Analysis
Phase of Nursing Process: Evaluation
Client Needs: Safe, Effective Care Environment
Content Area: Adult Health/Respiratory

References:
Monahan, F., & Neighbors, M. (1998). *Medical-surgical nursing: Foundations for clinical practice* (2nd ed.). Philadelphia: W. B. Saunders. p. 566.
Black, J., & Matassarin-Jacobs, E. (1997). *Medical-surgical nursing: Clinical management for continuity of care* (5th ed.). Philadelphia: W. B. Saunders. p. 1072.

4. 1

Rationale: Following the changing of the tracheostomy tube, the nurse needs to assure that the ties are not too tight. The nurse should assess this by assuring that there is room for 2 fingers to slide comfortably under the ties.

Test-Taking Strategy: Utilize the process of elimination, noting the issue of the question. Option 4 can be eliminated because of the word "tightly." Next eliminate options 2 and 3 because these are not appropriate methods for assessing tightness of the ties. If you had difficulty with this question, take time now to review care of a tracheostomy!

Level of Cognitive Ability: Analysis
Phase of Nursing Process: Implementation
Client Needs: Physiological Integrity
Content Area: Adult Health/Respiratory

Reference:
Black, J., & Matassarin-Jacobs, E. (1997). *Medical-surgical nursing: Clinical management for continuity of care* (5th ed.). Philadelphia: W. B. Saunders. p. 1073.

5. 4

Rationale: When the high-pressure alarm sounds on a ventilator, it is most likely due to an obstruction. The obstruction can be caused by the client biting on the tube, kinking of the tubing, or mucus plugging that requires suctioning. It is also important to assess the tubing for the presence of any water and determine whether the client is out of rhythm with breathing with the ventilator.

Test-Taking Strategy: Note the key words "high-pressure alarm" in the question. Recalling that the high-pressure alarm indicates a possible obstruction will assist in directing you to the correct option. Review nursing interventions related to care of a client on a ventilator now, if you had difficulty with this question!

Level of Cognitive Ability: Analysis
Phase of Nursing Process: Implementation
Client Needs: Physiological Integrity
Content Area: Adult Health/Respiratory

Reference:
Black, J., & Matassarin-Jacobs, E. (1997). *Medical-surgical nursing: Clinical management for continuity of care* (5th ed.). Philadelphia: W. B. Saunders. p. 1186

6. 2

Rationale: To obtain a sputum specimen, the client should brush the teeth to reduce contamination, then cough into a sputum specimen container. The client should be encouraged to cough and not spit, so as to obtain sputum. Sputum can be thinned by fluids or by a respiratory treatment such as inhalation of nebulized saline or water. The optimal time to obtain a specimen is upon arising in the morning.

Test-Taking Strategy: Read each option carefully, utilizing the process of elimination. Option 1 can be eliminated first because general principles indicate that fluids assist in loosening or thinning secretions. Eliminate option 3 because of the word "spit." Spit is very different from saliva. Next eliminate option 4 because of the words "after eating."

Level of Cognitive Ability: Application
Phase of Nursing Process: Implementation
Client Needs: Physiological Integrity
Content Area: Adult Health/Respiratory

References:
Black, J., & Matassarin-Jacobs, E. (1997). *Medical-surgical nursing: Clinical management for continuity of care* (5th ed.). Philadelphia: W. B. Saunders. p. 1063.
Lammon, C., Foote, A., Leli, P., et al. (1995). *Clinical nursing skills.* Philadelphia: W. B. Saunders. p. 143.

7. 4

Rationale: If a biopsy was performed during a bronchoscopy, blood-streaked sputum is expected for several hours. Frank blood indicates hemorrhage. A dry cough may be expected. The client should be assessed for signs of complications, which would include cyanosis, dyspnea, stridor, hemoptysis, hypotension, tachycardia, and dysrhythmias. Hematuria is unrelated to this procedure.

Test-Taking Strategy: Eliminate option 3 first because it is unrelated to the procedure. Next eliminate option 2 because a dry cough may be expected. Noting that a biopsy has been performed will assist in eliminating option 1, as pink-tinged sputum would be expected. Note that option 4, the correct option, relates to airway. If you had difficulty with this question, review postprocedure care following bronchoscopy with biopsy!

Level of Cognitive Ability: Analysis
Phase of Nursing Process: Assessment
Client Needs: Physiological Integrity
Content Area: Adult Health/Respiratory

Reference:
Monahan, F., & Neighbors, M. (1998). *Medical-surgical nursing: Foundations for clinical practice* (2nd ed.). Philadelphia: W. B. Saunders. p. 549.

8. 2

Rationale: Hypoxemia can be caused by prolonged suctioning from stimulation of the pacemaker cells within the heart. A vasovagal response may occur, causing bradycardia. Limit the suctioning pass to 15 seconds and preoxygenate the client prior to suctioning.

Test-Taking Strategy: Knowledge regarding the procedure for suctioning is required to answer this question. Recall that during suctioning the client's airway is blocked; therefore, you should be able to eliminate options 3 and 4 easily. From the remaining two options, eliminate option 1 because of the very short time frame. It does not seem reasonable that 5 seconds would achieve removal of secretions. Review the procedure for suctioning now, if you had difficulty with this question!

Level of Cognitive Ability: Application
Phase of Nursing Process: Implementation
Client Needs: Physiological Integrity
Content Area: Adult Health/Respiratory

Reference:
Black, J., & Matassarin-Jacobs, E. (1997). *Medical-surgical nursing: Clinical management for continuity of care* (5th ed.). Philadelphia: W. B. Saunders. p. 1175.

9. 3

Rationale: During suctioning, the nurse should monitor the client closely for side effects, including hypoxemia, cardiac irregularities due to vagal stimulation, mucosal trauma, hypotension, and paroxysmal coughing. If side effects develop, especially cardiac irregularities, stop the procedure and reoxygenate the client.

Test-Taking Strategy: Utilize the process of elimination, recalling that suction can cause cardiac irregularities. This principle should easily direct you to option 3. If you had difficulty with this question, review the complications and interventions associated with suctioning procedure!

Level of Cognitive Ability: Application
Phase of Nursing Process: Implementation
Client Needs: Physiological Integrity
Content Area: Adult Health/Respiratory

Reference:
Black, J., & Matassarin-Jacobs, E. (1997). *Medical-surgical nursing: Clinical management for continuity of care* (5th ed.). Philadelphia: W. B. Saunders. p. 1176.

10. 1

Rationale: Once the client has been weaned successfully and has achieved an acceptable level of consciousness to sustain spontaneous respiration, an ET tube may be removed. The ET tube is suctioned first, then the cuff is deflated and the tube is removed. There is no reason to have a code cart placed at the bedside as this may cause alarm and concern in the client. Additionally, resuscitative equipment should have already been at the client's bedside.

Test-Taking Strategy: Note the key word "initial" in the stem of the question. Use Maslow's Hierarchy of Needs theory. Remember, airway is the first priority!

Level of Cognitive Ability: Application
Phase of Nursing Process: Implementation
Client Needs: Physiological Integrity
Content Area: Adult Health/Respiratory

Reference:
Black, J., & Matassarin-Jacobs, E. (1997). *Medical-surgical nursing: Clinical management for continuity of care* (5th ed.). Philadelphia: W. B. Saunders. p. 1184.

11. 2

Rationale: Plugging a tracheostomy tube is usually done by inserting the tracheostomy plug (decannulation stopper) into the opening of the outer cannula. This closes off the tracheostomy, and airflow and respiration occur normally through the nose and mouth. When plugging a cuffed tracheostomy tube, the cuff must be deflated. If it remains inflated, ventilation cannot occur and respiratory arrest could result.

Test-Taking Strategy: Note the key word "required" in the question. This should assist in directing you to the option that addresses a priority physiological need. Utilize the process of elimination and you should easily be directed to option 2, as an inflated cuff would cause airway obstruction.

Level of Cognitive Ability: Application
Phase of Nursing Process: Implementation
Client Needs: Physiological Integrity
Content Area: Adult Health/Respiratory

Reference:
Black, J., & Matassarin-Jacobs, E. (1997). *Medical-surgical nursing: Clinical management for continuity of care* (5th ed.). Philadelphia: W. B. Saunders. p. 1071.

12. 1

Rationale: With normal breathing, the water level rises with inspiration and falls with expiration. The opposite, falls with inspiration and rises with expiration, occurs when the client is on positive pressure mechanical ventilation. This is an expected normal occurrence in a chest tube drainage system; therefore, no action is necessary.

Test-Taking Strategy: Knowledge regarding the normal expected findings in monitoring a chest tube drainage system is required to answer this question. Knowing that the water level is expected to fluctuate will assist in directing you easily to option 1. Review chest tube drainage systems now, if you had difficulty with this question!

Level of Cognitive Ability: Analysis
Phase of Nursing Process: Implementation
Client Needs: Physiological Integrity
Content Area: Adult Health/Respiratory

Reference:
Monahan, F., & Neighbors, M. (1998). *Medical-surgical nursing: Foundations for clinical practice* (2nd ed.). Philadelphia: W. B. Saunders. p. 578.

13. **3**

Rationale: Constant bubbling in the water seal chamber may indicate a leak in the system. From the options provided, the most appropriate is to notify the physician.

Test-Taking Strategy: Note the key words "constant bubbling in the water seal chamber." Knowing that this is an unexpected occurrence and that it may indicate a potential complication with the chest tube drainage system will assist in directing you to option 3. If you had difficulty with this question or are unfamiliar with the care of the chest tube drainage system, take time now to review!

Level of Cognitive Ability: Analysis
Phase of Nursing Process: Implementation
Client Needs: Physiological Integrity
Content Area: Adult Health/Respiratory

Reference:
Black, J., & Matassarin-Jacobs, E. (1997). *Medical-surgical nursing: Clinical management for continuity of care* (5th ed.). Philadelphia: W. B. Saunders. p. 1164.

14. **1**

Rationale: In a metabolic acidotic condition, the pH is low, indicating the acidosis. Additionally, a low bicarbonate level along with a low pH indicates a metabolic state.

Test-Taking Strategy: This question requires the skill of evaluating the results of a blood gas determination. Remember to look at the pH first. This pH of 7.30 indicates an acidosis. Next look at the CO_2 level, which in this situation is normal; therefore, a respiratory condition does not exist. This will assist in eliminating options 2, 3, and 4. Noting that the bicarbonate level is low, as is the pH, should assist in directing you to option 1, a metabolic condition.

Level of Cognitive Ability: Analysis
Phase of Nursing Process: Evaluation
Client Needs: Physiological Integrity
Content Area: Adult Health/Respiratory

Reference:
Monahan, F., & Neighbors, M. (1998). *Medical-surgical nursing: Foundations for clinical practice* (2nd ed.). Philadelphia: W. B. Saunders. p. 544.

15. **2**

Rationale: This client has sustained a blunt or a closed-chest injury. Basic symptoms of a closed pneumothorax are shortness of breath and chest pain. A larger pneumothorax may present with tachypnea, cyanosis, diminished breath sounds, and subcutaneous emphysema. There may also be hyperresonance on the affected side.

Test-Taking Strategy: Note the key word "blunt" in the question. This will assist in elimination of option 1, a suck-ing chest wound injury. Knowing that increased respirations will occur in a respiratory injury will assist in eliminating option 3. Option 4 can be eliminated because a barrel chest is a characteristic finding in a client with COPD.

Level of Cognitive Ability: Analysis
Phase of Nursing Process: Assessment
Client Needs: Physiological Integrity
Content Area: Adult Health/Respiratory

Reference:
Monahan, F., & Neighbors, M. (1998). *Medical-surgical nursing: Foundations for clinical practice* (2nd ed.). Philadelphia: W. B. Saunders. pp. 692–693.

16. **3**

Rationale: Clinical manifestations of COPD include hypoxemia, hypercapnia, dyspnea on exertion and at rest, oxygen desaturation with exercise, use of accessory muscles of respiration, and a prolonged expiratory phase of respiration. CXR will reveal a hyperinflated chest and a flattened diaphragm if the disease is advanced.

Test-Taking Strategy: Utilize the process of elimination, reading each option carefully. Eliminate option 1 because oxygen desaturation rather than saturation would occur. Next eliminate option 2 because in the client with COPD, a prolonged expiratory phase would be noted. From the remaining options, reading carefully will assist in directing you to option 3, the correct option. If you are unfamiliar with the manifestations associated with COPD, take time now to review!

Level of Cognitive Ability: Analysis
Phase of Nursing Process: Assessement
Client Needs: Physiological Integrity
Content Area: Adult Health/Respiratory

Reference:
Monahan, F., & Neighbors, M. (1998). *Medical-surgical nursing: Foundations for clinical practice* (2nd ed.). Philadelphia: W. B. Saunders. p. 668.

17. **1**

Rationale: The Venturi mask delivers the most accurate oxygen concentration. It is the best oxygen delivery system for the client with CAL because it delivers a precise oxygen concentration. The face tent, aerosol mask, and tracheostomy collar are also high-flow oxygen delivery systems but are most often used to administer high humidity.

Test-Taking Strategy: Note the key words "precise oxygen concentration." Knowledge regarding the various types of oxygen delivery systems will assist in answering this question. Eliminate options 2, 3, and 4 because they are similar in that they are used to provide high humidity.

Level of Cognitive Ability: Analysis
Phase of Nursing Process: Planning
Client Needs: Physiological Integrity
Content Area: Adult Health/Respiratory

Reference:
Ignatavicius, D., Workman, M., & Mishler, M. (1995). *Medical-surgical nursing: A nursing process approach* (2nd ed.). Philadelphia: W. B. Saunders. p. 694.

18. **1**

Rationale: The medication should be administered with food, such as milk and crackers, to prevent GI irritation. Options 2, 3, and 4 are appropriate instructions regarding the use of this medication.

Test-Taking Strategy: Noting that options 2 and 3 are opposite in terms of administering the medication should alert you that one of these options is the correct answer. Knowledge regarding the administration of this medication is required to answer correctly. If you are unfamiliar with this important medication, take time now to review!

Level of Cognitive Ability: Application
Phase of Nursing Process: Implementation
Client Needs: Health Promotion and Maintenance
Content Area: Pharmacology

Reference:
Ignatavicius, D., Workman, M., & Mishler, M. (1995). *Medical-surgical nursing: A nursing process approach* (2nd ed.). Philadelphia: W. B. Saunders. p 701.

19. **4**

Rationale: Positions that will assist the client with breathing include sitting up and leaning on an overbed table, sitting up and resting elbows on the knees, or standing and leaning against the wall.

Test-Taking Strategy: Eliminate options 2 and 3 first because they are similar. Next eliminate option 1 because this position will not enhance breathing. If you had difficulty with this question, take time now to review the positions that will decrease the work of breathing in a client with emphysema!

Level of Cognitive Ability: Application
Phase of Nursing Process: Implementation
Client Needs: Physiological Integrity
Content Area: Adult Health/Respiratory

Reference:
Ignatavicius, D., Workman, M., & Mishler, M. (1995). *Medical-surgical nursing: A nursing process approach* (2nd ed.). Philadelphia: W. B. Saunders. p 689.

20. **2**

Rationale: The first pulmonary symptom includes a slight morning cough with the expectoration of mucoid sputum. Options 1, 3, and 4 are late symptoms and signify cavitation and extensive lung involvement.

Test-Taking Strategy: Note the key word "first" in the stem of the question. This should easily direct you to option 2. If you are unfamiliar with the signs associated with TB, take time now to review this important disease!

Level of Cognitive Ability: Analyses
Phase of Nursing Process: Assessment
Client Needs: Health Promotion and Maintenance
Content Area: Adult Health/Respiratory

Reference:
Monahan, F., & Neighbors, M. (1998). *Medical-surgical nursing: Foundations for clinical practice* (2nd ed.). Philadelphia: W. B. Saunders. p. 651.

21. **3**

Rationale: Definitive diagnosis of TB is confirmed through culture and isolation of *Mycobacterium tuberculosis*. A presumptive diagnosis is made on the basis of a tuberculin skin test, a sputum smear that is positive for acid fast bacteria, a chest x-ray film, and histologic evidence of graunulomatous disease on biopsy.

Test-Taking Strategy: Note the key word "confirm" in the stem of the question. Confirmation is made by identifying *Mycobacterium tuberculosis*. If you had difficulty with this question, take time now to review diagnostic procedures related to TB!

Level of Cognitive Ability: Analysis
Phase of Nursing Process: Analysis
Client Needs: Physiological Integrity
Content Area: Adult Health/Respiratory

Reference:
Monahan, F., & Neighbors, M. (1998). *Medical-surgical nursing: Foundations for clinical practice* (2nd ed.). Philadelphia: W. B. Saunders. p. 652.

22. **1**

Rationale: Tuberculosis is an infectious disease caused by the bacillus *Mycobacterium tuberculosis* and spread primarily by the airborne route. Options 2, 3, and 4 are incorrect.

Test-Taking Strategy: Knowledge that TB is a respiratory disease should easily direct you to option 1. If you had difficulty with this question, take time now to review the transmission of this important disease!

Level of Cognitive Ability: Analysis
Phase of Nursing Process: Evaluation
Client Needs: Safe, Effective Care Environment
Content Area: Adult Health/Respiratory

Reference:
Monahan, F., & Neighbors, M. (1998). *Medical-surgical nursing: Foundations for clinical practice* (2nd ed.). Philadelphia: W. B. Saunders. p. 650.

23. **2**

Rationale: One to three liters of oxygen by nasal cannula may be required to raise the PaO_2 to 60 to 80 mmHg. However, oxygen is used cautiously and should not exceed 3 L. Because of the long-standing hypercapnia, the respiratory drive is triggered by low oxygen levels rather than by increased carbon dioxide levels, as is the case in a normal respiratory system.

Test-Taking Strategy: Knowledge regarding the physiology associated with emphysema is required to answer this question. If you are unfamiliar with this important concept, take time now to review!

Level of Cognitive Ability: Analysis
Phase of Nursing Process: Assessment
Client Needs: Physiological Integrity
Content Area: Adult Health/Respiratory

Reference:
Black, J., & Matassarin-Jacobs, E. (1997). *Medical-surgical nursing: Clinical management for continuity of care* (5th ed.). Philadelphia: W. B. Saunders. p. 1117.

24. **4**

Rationale: In a metabolic alkalosis, the pH is elevated along with the bicarbonate level. Option 4 is the only option that reflects these values.

Test-Taking Strategy: Remember that when an alkalotic condition exists, the pH will be elevated. This will assist in eliminating options 1 and 3. Next, recall that in a metabolic condition, the HCO_3 will move in the same direction as the pH. The only option that represents these conditions is option 4. Review the process of blood gas analysis now, if you had difficulty with this question!

Level of Cognitive Ability: Analysis
Phase of Nursing Process: Analysis
Client Needs: Physiological Integrity
Content Area: Adult Health/Respiratory

Reference:
Monahan, F., & Neighbors, M. (1998). *Medical-surgical nursing: Foundations for clinical practice* (2nd ed.). Philadelphia: W. B. Saunders. p. 544.

25. 3

Rationale: In respiratory acidosis, the pH will be lower than normal and the Pco_2 will be elevated. The normal pH is 7.35 to 7.45. The normal Pco_2 is 35 to 45 mmHg. The only option that reflects these conditions is option 3.

Test-Taking Strategy: Remember that when an acidotic condition exists, the pH will be low. Next, recall that in a respiratory acidotic condition, the Pco_2 will move in the opposite direction from the pH. The only option that represents these conditions is option 3. Review the process of blood gas analysis now, if you had difficulty with this question!

Level of Cognitive Ability: Analysis
Phase of Nursing Process: Analysis
Client Needs: Physiological Integrity
Content Area: Adult Health/Respiratory

Reference:
Monahan, F., & Neighbors, M. (1998). *Medical-surgical nursing: Foundations for clinical practice* (2nd ed.). Philadelphia: W. B. Saunders. p. 544.

26. 4

Rationale: Pursed-lip breathing facilitates maximal expiration for clients with obstructive lung disease. This type of breathing allows better expiration by increasing airway pressure that keeps air passages open during exhalation. Options 1, 2, and 3 are not the purposes of this type of breathing.

Test-Taking Strategy: Attempt to visualize the use of this procedure to assist you in answering correctly. Knowledge regarding the respiratory conditions in which this type of breathing is helpful will also assist in directing you to option 4. Review the purpose of this procedure now, if you had difficulty with this question!

Level of Cognitive Ability: Analysis
Phase of Nursing Process: Analysis
Client Needs: Physiological Integrity
Content Area: Adult Health/Respiratory

Reference:
Lammon, C., Foote, A., Leli, P., et al. (1995). *Clinical nursing skills.* Philadelphia: W. B. Saunders. p. 523.

27. 3

Rationale: Immediately after an ET tube is inserted, tube placement is verified by both auscultation and CXR. Auscultating the lungs would be the immediate action. It is the responsibility of the nurse to auscultate for air movement. Option 4 is an inappropriate action.

Test-Taking Strategy: Note the key word "immediate" in the stem of the question. Although a nurse will prepare the client for a chest x-ray film, the immediate action is to auscultate for air movement. Options 1 and 4 can be easily eliminated. Review the procedure for checking ET placement following insertion now, if you had difficulty with this question!

Level of Cognitive Ability: Application
Phase of Nursing Process: Implementation
Client Needs: Physiological Integrity
Content Area: Adult Health/Respiratory

Reference:
Black, J., & Matassarin-Jacobs, E. (1997). *Medical-surgical nursing: Clinical management for continuity of care* (5th ed.). Philadelphia: W. B. Saunders. p. 1173.

28. 2

Rationale: If at any time an alarm is sounding and the nurse cannot quickly ascertain the problem, the client is disconnected from the ventilator and manual resuscitation is used to support respirations until the problem can be corrected. There is no reason to begin CPR. Checking vital signs is not the initial action. Although oxygen is helpful, it will not provide ventilation to the client.

Test-Taking Strategy: Read the question carefully and note that the issue relates to adequate ventilation of the client. Focusing on this issue will easily direct you to option 2. If you are unfamiliar with management of ventilators and alarms, take time now to review!

Level of Cognitive Ability: Application
Phase of Nursing Process: Implementation
Client Needs: Physiological Integrity
Content Area: Adult Health/Respiratory

Reference:
Black, J., & Matassarin-Jacobs, E. (1997). *Medical-surgical nursing: Clinical management for continuity of care* (5th ed.). Philadelphia: W. B. Saunders. p. 1186.

29. 2

Rationale: If the results of two ELISA tests are positive, the Western blot is done to confirm the findings. If the result of the Western blot is positive, then the client is considered to be positive for HIV and infected with the HIV virus.

Test-Taking Strategy: Knowledge of the procedural steps in diagnosing HIV is needed to answer this question. Review these now if they are unfamiliar to you. This is a subject of great concern to clients, and you would want to have the appropriate information to share. The increasing incidence of HIV infection as a major health problem also makes it a reasonably popular area for testing.

Level of Cognitive Ability: Analysis
Phase of Nursing Process: Analysis
Client Needs: Physiological Integrity
Content Area: Adult Health/Respiratory

Reference:
Black, J., & Matassarin-Jacobs, E. (1997). *Medical-surgical nursing: Clinical management for continuity of care* (5th ed.). Philadelphia: W. B. Saunders. p. 611.

30. 4

Rationale: The client with *Pneumocystis carinil* infection usually has a cough as the first symptom, which begins as nonproductive, then progresses to productive. Later signs include fever, dyspnea on exertion, and finally dyspnea at rest.

Test-Taking Strategy: The key word in the stem of this question is "early." While all these symptoms may appear at some point in the client with *Pneumocystis carinii* infection knowing that the cough appears first helps you eliminate each of the other responses.

Level of Cognitive Ability: Application
Phase of Nursing Process: Assessment
Client Needs: Physiological Integrity
Content Area: Adult Health/Respiratory

Reference:
Black, J., and Matassarin-Jacobs, E. (1997). *Medical-surgical nursing: Clinical management for continuity of care* (5th ed.). Philadelphia: W. B. Saunders. p. 629.

31. **2**

Rationale: In respiratory alkalosis, the pH will be higher than normal and the PCO_2 will be low. The normal pH is 7.35 to 7.45. The normal PCO_2 is 35 to 45 mmHg. The only option that reflects these conditions is option 2.

Test-Taking Strategy: Remember that when an alkalotic condition exists, the pH will be high. Next, recall that in a respiratory alkalotic condition, the PCO_2 will move in the opposite direction as the pH. The only option that represents these conditions is option 2. Compensation can be identified if the pH is within normal limits. Review the process of blood gas analysis now, if you had difficulty with this question!

Level of Cognitive Ability: Analysis
Phase of Nursing Process: Analysis
Client Needs: Physiological Integrity
Content Area: Adult Health/Respiratory

Reference:
Monahan, F., & Neighbors, M. (1998). *Medical-surgical nursing: Foundations for clinical practice* (2nd ed.). Philadelphia: W. B. Saunders. p. 544.

32. **3**

Rationale: Aminophylline is a bronchodilator that directly relaxes the smooth muscles of the bronchial airway. Options 1, 2, and 4 are not direct actions of this medication.

Test-Taking Strategy: Knowledge regarding the classification of this medication will assist in directing you to the correct option. Although bronchial dilation may assist in promoting expectoration, this is not the primary action of this medication. Take time now to review this important medication, if you had difficulty with this question!

Level of Cognitive Ability: Analysis
Phase of Nursing Process: Analysis
Client Needs: Physiological Integrity
Content Area: Pharmacology

Reference
Hodgson, B., & Kizior, R. (1999). Saunders nursing drug handbook 1999. Philadelphia: W. B. Saunders. pp. 44–47

33. **2**

Rationale: Safe and effective therapy requires periodic measurement of theophylline blood levels. Levels between 5 and 15 μg/mL are appropriate. Adverse effects occur at levels above 20 μg/mL. Options 3 and 4 represent toxic levels. Option 1 indicates that the client may require an increased dose of medication.

Test-Taking Strategy: Knowledge regarding the therapeutic blood levels for theophylline is required to answer this question. If you had difficulty with this question, it is important to learn this level now!

Level of Cognitive Ability: Analysis
Phase of Nursing Process: Analysis
Client Needs: Physiological Integrity
Content Area: Pharmacology

Reference
Lehne, R. (1998). *Pharmacology for nursing care* (3rd ed.). Philadelphia: W. B. Saunders. p. 755.

34. **3**

Rationale: The earliest clinical sign of ARDS is an increased respiratory rate. Breathing becomes labored, and the client may exhibit air hunger, retractions, and cyanosis. Blood gas analysis reveals increasing hypoxemia, with a PaO_2 of less than 60 mmHg.

Test-Taking Strategy: Knowledge regarding the clinical manifestations related to ARDS is required to answer this question. Note, however, that options 3 and 4 relate to the same issue but present opposite conditions. This may provide you with the clue that one of these options is the correct one. Considering the diagnosis of the client, the best choice is option 3!

Level of Cognitive Ability: Analysis
Phase of Nursing Process: Assessment
Client Needs: Physiological Integrity
Content Area: Adult Health/Respiratory

Reference
Black, J., & Matassarin-Jacobs, E. (1997). *Medical-surgical nursing: Clinical management for continuity of care* (5th ed.). Philadelphia: W. B. Saunders. p. 1171.

35. **4**

Rationale: Side effects that can occur from the use of this medication include tremors, nausea, nervousness, palpitations, tachycardia, peripheral vasodilation, and dryness of the mouth or throat.

Test-Taking Strategy: Knowledge that this medication causes sympathomimetic stimulation will easily direct you to option 4. If you are unfamiliar with the side effects related to this medication, take time now to review!

Level of Cognitive Ability: Analysis
Phase of Nursing Process: Assessment
Client Needs: Physiological Integrity
Content Area: Pharmacology

Reference
Hodgson, B., & Kizior, R. (1999). *Saunders nursing drug handbook 1999.* Philadelphia: W. B. Saunders. pp. 548–550.

36. **3**

Rationale: Both isoniazid and rifampin are contraindicated in clients with acute liver disease or history of hepatic injury. Option 3 is the only option that addresses hepatic dysfunction.

Test-Taking Strategy: Eliminate options 1 and 4 first because they both relate to cardiac disorders. From the remaining two options, it is necessary to know that these medications may cause hepatotoxicity.

Level of Cognitive Ability: Application
Phase of Nursing Process: Implementation
Client Needs: Physiological Integrity
Content Area: Pharmacology

Reference
Hodgson, B., & Kizior, R. (1999). *Saunders nursing drug handbook 1999.* Philadelphia: W. B. Saunders. pp. 550–552, 906–908.

37. 3

Rationale: The client needs to be instructed that the entire year-long course of the medication needs to be completed. It is preferable to take the medication 1 hour before or 2 hours after meals. If GI irritation occurs, the medication should not be discontinued, and in this situation a small amount of food may be taken to reduce the irritation. It is not necessary to increase fluids during this medication therapy.

Test-Taking Strategy: Use the process of elimination to answer the question. Note that options 1, 2, and 4 contain the absolute terms "must." Review the client teaching points related to these medications now, if you had difficulty with this question!

Level of Cognitive Ability: Application
Phase of Nursing Process: Planning
Client Needs: Health Promotion and Maintenance
Content Area: Pharmacology

Reference

Hodgson, B., & Kizior, R. (1999). *Saunders nursing drug handbook 1999.* Philadelphia: W. B. Saunders. pp. 550–552, 906–908.

38. 2

Rationale: Clients with diagnoses of active TB are usually started on more than one medication to be certain the resistant organisms are eliminated. The dosage of some medications may initially be large because the bacilli are difficult to kill. Options 1, 3, and 4 are inaccurate.

Test-Taking Strategy: Knowledge regarding the medication therapy for the treatment of TB is required to answer this question. If you are unfamiliar with this important therapy, take time now to review!

Level of Cognitive Ability: Application
Phase of Nursing Process: Implementation
Client Needs: Health Promotion and Maintenance
Content Area: Pharmacology

Reference

Black, J., & Matassarin-Jacobs, E. (1997). *Medical-surgical nursing: Clinical management for continuity of care* (5th ed.). Philadelphia: W. B. Saunders. p. 1143.

39. 2

Rationale: Persons at greatest risk for pulmonary emboli are immobilized clients. Basic preventive measures include early ambulation, leg elevation, active leg exercises, elastic stockings, and intermittent pneumatic calf compression. Keeping the client well-hydrated is essential because dehydration predisposes to clotting. A pillow under the knees may cause venous stasis. Heat should not be applied without a physician's prescription.

Test-Taking Strategy: Knowledge regarding preventive measures related to preventing deep venous thrombosis (DVT) and pulmonary emboli is required to answer this question. Use basic principles related to care of the immobile client to assist in answering this question. If you are unfamiliar with these basic measures, it is important that you review now!

Level of Cognitive Ability: Application
Phase of Nursing Process: Implementation
Client Needs: Physiological Integrity
Content Area: Adult Health/Respiratory

Reference

Monahan, F., & Neighbors, M. (1998). *Medical-surgical nursing; Foundations for clinical practice* (2nd ed.). Philadelphia: W. B. Saunders. p. 682.

40. 1

Rationale: The most common clinical manifestations of PE are tachypnea, dyspnea, and chest pain.

Test-Taking Strategy: Note the key word "not" in the stem of the question. Knowledge regarding the most common clinical manifestations of PE is required to answer this question. Note, however, that options 1 and 2 address a similar issue but opposite effects. This may provide you with the clue that one of these options is the correct one. You would expect an increased respiratory rate in PE; therefore, select option 1.

Level of Cognitive Ability: Analysis
Phase of Nursing Process: Assessment
Client Needs: Physiological Integrity
Content Area: Adult Health/Respiratory

Reference

Black, J., & Matassarin-Jacobs, E. (1997). *Medical-surgical nursing: Clinical management for continuity of care* (5th ed.). Philadelphia: W. B. Saunders. p. 1127.

41. 3

Rationale: Clients should be instructed that they should hold their breaths at least 5 to 10 seconds before exhaling the mist. Options 1, 2, and 4 are accurate instructions regarding the use of the inhaler.

Test-Taking Strategy: Knowledge regarding the use of the inhaler is required to answer this question. If you are unfamiliar with the client teaching points related to the use of an inhaler, take time now to review!

Level of Cognitive Ability: Application
Phase of Nursing Process: Implementation
Client Needs: Health Promotion and Maintenance
Content Area: Adult Health/Respiratory

Reference

Black, J., & Matassarin-Jacobs, E. (1997). *Medical-surgical nursing: Clinical management for continuity of care* (5th ed.). Philadelphia: W. B. Saunders. p. 1112.

42. 1

Rationale: Complete lateral positioning should be avoided following pneumonectomy. Because the mediastinum is no longer held in place on both sides by lung tissue, extreme turning may cause mediastinal shift and compression of the remaining lung.

Test-Taking Strategy: Eliminate options 2, 3, and 4 because they are similar. Additionally, option 4 describes semi-Fowler's position. If you had difficulty with this question, take time now to review care to the client following pneumonectomy!

Level of Cognitive Ability: Application
Phase of Nursing Process: Implementation
Client Needs: Physiological Integrity
Content Area: Adult Health/Respiratory

Reference

Black, J., & Matassarin-Jacobs, E. (1997). *Medical-surgical nursing: Clinical management for continuity of care* (5th ed.). Philadelphia: W. B. Saunders. p. 1161.

43. 4

Rationale: Following a wedge resection, the client should not be placed on the operative side. Lying on the operative side hinders expansion of remaining lung tissue and may accentuate perfusion of poorly ventilated tissue, thus further impeding normal gas exchange.

Test-Taking Strategy: Eliminate options 1 and 2 first because they are similar. From the remaining options, it is necessary to know that the client should not be positioned on the operative side. Attempt to visualize this surgical procedure to assist in answering the question. If you had difficulty with this question, take time now to review!

Level of Cognitive Ability: Application
Phase of Nursing Process: Implementation
Client Needs: Physiological Integrity
Content Area: Adult Health/Respiratory

Reference
Black, J., & Matassarin-Jacobs, E. (1997). *Medical-surgical nursing: Clinical management for continuity of care* (5th ed.). Philadelphia: W. B. Saunders. p. 1161.

44. 3

Rationale: The nurse monitors for adverse effects of suctioning, which include cyanosis, excessively rapid or slow heart rate, or sudden development of bloody secretions. If they occur, the nurse stops suctioning and reports these signs to the physician immediately. Coughing is a normal response to suctioning for the client with an intact cough reflex and does not indicate that the client cannot tolerate the procedure.

Test-Taking Strategy: The wording of the question asks you to select an option that would be a normal or expected finding while suctioning a client. Cyanosis and bradycardia are abnormal findings, and are eliminated first. Of the two remaining choices, the use of the word "becoming" in association with bloody secretions tells you that this has not been an ongoing problem, making this an incorrect option also. Since the cough reflex is normally present, and suction triggers coughing, this is the preferable one of the two remaining options.

Level of Cognitive Ability: Analysis
Phase of Nursing Process: Analysis
Client Needs: Physiological Integrity
Content Area: Adult Health/Respiratory

Reference
Taylor, C., Lillis, C., & LeMone, P. (1997). *Fundamentals of nursing: The art and science of nursing care* (3rd ed.). Philadelphia: Lippincott-Raven. p. 1348.

45. 3

Rationale: Impaired gas exchange could occur following tracheostomy from excessive secretions, bleeding into the trachea, restricted lung expansion due to immobility, or concurrent respiratory conditions. An oxygen saturation of 91% is less than optimal. The respiratory rate of 18 is well within the normal range of 14 to 20 breaths per minute.

Test-Taking Strategy: The question asks for the "best" indication of normal respiratory status. An oxygen saturation of 91% is suboptimal and is eliminated first. Bloody secretions (option 2) are also abnormal, although secretions may be blood-tinged for a few days after tracheostomy insertion. While tracheobronchial secretions may be expected, they are not the "best indication" of respiratory adequacy, making the respiratory rate of 18 the correct answer.

Level of Cognitive Ability: Application
Phase of Nursing Process: Assessment
Client Needs: Physiological Integrity
Content Area: Adult Health/Respiratory

Reference
Black, J., & Matassarin-Jacobs, E. (1997). *Medical-surgical nursing: Clinical management for continuity of care* (5th ed.). Philadelphia: W. B. Saunders. p. 1074.

46. 1

Rationale: Hypotension, shock, or the use of peripheral vasoconstricting medications may result in inaccurate pulse oximetry readings from impaired peripheral perfusion. Fever and epilepsy would not affect the accuracy of measurement. Respiratory failure also would not affect the accuracy of measurement, although the readings may be abnormally low in this condition.

Test-Taking Strategy: Recall that pulse oximetry measures oxygen saturation in blood flowing through the blood vessels in the periphery of the body. Inaccurate measurement may result from any factor that impairs blood flow through the periphery. Evaluating each of the options from this viewpoint helps you select hypotension as the answer. Epilepsy and fever do not affect the readings adversely. To discriminate between the respiratory failure option and hypotension, look again at the stem. The question asks which item gives an inaccurate reading, not a low reading!

Level of Cognitive Ability: Analysis
Phase of Nursing Process: Analysis
Client Needs: Physiological Integrity
Content Area: Adult Health/Respiratory

Reference
Black, J., & Matassarin-Jacobs, E. (1997). *Medical-surgical nursing: Clinical management for continuity of care* (5th ed.). Philadelphia: W. B. Saunders. p. 1074.

47. 2

Rationale: When the chest tube is patent, the water in the water seal chamber rises with inspiration and falls with expiration. This is referred to as tidaling and indicates proper function of the system.

Test-Taking Strategy: Knowing that there is negative pressure (pulling pressure) with inspiration, it is natural that the fluid level in the water seal chamber would rise on inspiration. It is also a natural consequence that with exhalation the opposite would be true. This makes options 3 and 4 totally incorrect. You would choose option 2 over option 1 because the stem makes no mention of bubbling in the water seal chamber. This would occur if the client had pneumothorax, even though the fluid would still rise and fall. Review the important assessment measures required in the care of a client with a chest tube now, if you had difficulty with this question!

Level of Cognitive Ability: Analysis
Phase of Nursing Process: Analysis
Client Needs: Physiological Integrity
Content Area: Adult Health/Respiratory

Reference
Black, J., & Matassarin-Jacobs, E. (1997). *Medical-surgical nursing: Clinical management for continuity of care* (5th ed.). Philadelphia: W. B. Saunders. p. 1163.

48. 1

Rationale: The nurse assures that all system connections are securely taped to prevent accidental disconnection, and that an occlusive dressing is maintained at the chest tube insertion site. Drainage is noted and recorded every hour in the first 24 hours after insertion and every 8 hours thereafter. The system is kept below the level of the waist. Assessment for crepitus is done once every 8 hours. Sterile water is added to the suction control chamber only as needed to replace evaporation losses. Continuous bubbling in the water seal chamber indicates an air leak in the system and requires immediate investigation and correction.

Test-Taking Strategy: Note that each option has two parts. For the option to be correct, both parts of the answer must be correct. Knowing this, eliminate options 3 and 4 first. Water needs to be added only as needed, and there should not be continuous bubbling in the water seal. Knowing that chest tube assessment is done every 8 hours at least helps you choose option 1 over option 2. Review the important assessment measures required in the care of a client with a chest tube now, if you had difficulty with this question!

Level of Cognitive Ability: Application
Phase of Nursing Process: Implementation
Client Needs: Physiological Integrity
Content Area: Adult Health/Respiratory

Reference
Black, J., & Matassarin-Jacobs, E. (1997). *Medical-surgical nursing: Clinical management for continuity of care* (5th ed.). Philadelphia: W. B. Saunders. pp. 1163–1165.

49. **3**

Rationale: In the first few hours after surgery, the drainage from the chest tube is bloody. After several hours, it becomes serosanguineous. The client should not experience significant clotting. Proper chest tube function should allow for drainage of blood before it has the chance to clot in the chest or the tubing.

Test-Taking Strategy: Recall that following thoracic surgery there may be considerable capillary oozing for some hours in the postoperative period. This would lead you to choose the bloody drainage over serous or serosanguineous. Knowing that patent chest tubes do not allow blood to collect in the pleural space eliminates the option of blood with clots. Review the important assessment measures required in the care of a client with a chest tube now, if you had difficulty with this question!

Level of Cognitive Ability: Application
Phase of Nursing Process: Assessment
Client Needs: Physiological Integrity
Content Area: Adult Health/Respiratory

Reference
Black, J., & Matassarin-Jacobs, E. (1997). *Medical-surgical nursing: Clinical management for continuity of care* (5th ed.). Philadelphia: W. B. Saunders. p. 1163.

50. **1**

Rationale: The most important item to ask about is the client's pregnancy status, because pregnant women should not be exposed to radiation. Clients are also asked to remove any chains or metal objects that could interfere with obtaining an adequate film. A chest x-ray film is most often taken at full inspiration, which gives optimal lung expansion. If a lateral view of the chest is ordered, the client is asked to raise the arms above the head. Most films are done in posterioanterior (PA) view.

Test-Taking Strategy: This question asks which is the "most important" question to the nurse. This implies that more than one or all of the options are correct. Eliminate options 3 and 4 first, because they can be determined by the radiologic technologist. Option 1 is a higher priority than option

2 because of potential negative teratogenic consequences to the fetus.

Level of Cognitive Ability: Analysis
Phase of Nursing Process: Assessment
Client Needs: Physiological Integrity
Content Area: Adult Health/Respiratory

Reference
Black, J., & Matassarin-Jacobs, E. (1997). *Medical-surgical nursing: Clinical management for continuity of care* (5th ed.). Philadelphia: W. B. Saunders. pp. 1059–1060.

51. **2**

Rationale: Following bronchoscopy, the nurse keeps the client on NPO status until the cough reflex returns. This is because the preoperative sedation and the local anesthesia impair swallowing and the protective laryngeal reflexes for a number of hours. Forcing fluids is unnecessary since there is no use of contrast dye that would need flushing from the system. Atropine and midazolam would be administered before the procedure, not after.

Test-Taking Strategy: The critical concept being tested with this question is that the client has lost the protective cough, gag, and swallow reflexes during this procedure. Knowledge of this implication helps you choose option 2 as the only possible answer. Review nursing care measures following bronchoscopy now, if you had difficulty with this question!

Level of Cognitive Ability: Application
Phase of Nursing Process: Implementation
Client Needs: Safe, Effective Care Environment
Content Area: Adult Health/Respiratory

Reference
Smeltzer, S., & Bare, B. (1996). *Brunner and Suddarth's textbook of medical-surgical nursing* (8th ed.). Philadelphia: Lippincott-Raven. p. 455.

52. **3**

Rationale: Signs of allergic reaction to the contrast dye include early signs such as localized itching and edema, which are then followed by more severe symptoms such as respiratory distress, stridor, and decreased blood pressure.

Test-Taking Strategy: Hypothermia is an unrelated event and is eliminated first. Discomfort is expected and is eliminated next. Hematoma formation is a complication of the procedure but does not indicate allergic reaction and is therefore eliminated. The remaining option is stridor, which is a sign of severe allergic reaction and possible anaphylaxis. Review the signs of an allergic reaction to the contrast medium now, if you had difficulty with this question!

Level of Cognitive Ability: Application
Phase of Nursing Process: Assessment
Client Needs: Physiological Integrity
Content Area: Adult Health/Respiratory

Reference
Black, J., & Matassarin-Jacobs, E. (1997). *Medical-surgical nursing: Clinical management for continuity of care* (5th ed.). Philadelphia: W. B. Saunders. pp. 638, 1062.

53. **2**

Rationale: Prior to drawing blood for an arterial blood gas determination, the nurse assesses the collateral circulation to the hand with Allen's test. This involves compressing both the radial and ulnar arteries and asking the client to close and open the fist. This should cause the hand to become pale. The nurse then releases pressure on one artery and observes whether circulation is quickly restored. The process is then repeated, releasing the other artery. The blood sample may be safely taken if there is adequate collateral circulation.

Test-Taking Strategy: To answer this question correctly, you must first know that collateral circulation to the hand must be assured before drawing arterial blood gas samples. Once this concept is in mind, you must then know the proper technique to answer the question correctly. If you are unfamiliar with this practice, take a moment to review it now!

Level of Cognitive Ability: Application
Phase of Nursing Process: Assessment
Client Needs: Physiological Integrity
Content Area: Adult Health / Respiratory

Reference
Black, J., & Matassarin-Jacobs, E. (1997). *Medical-Surgical nursing: Clinical management for continuity of care* (5th ed.). Philadelphia: W. B. Saunders. p. 1057.

54. **2**

Rationale: Rib fractures are a common injury, especially in elderly people, and result from a blunt injury or a fall. Typical signs and symptoms include pain and tenderness that are localized at the fracture site and are exacerbated by inspiration and palpation; shallow respirations; splinting or guarding the chest protectively to minimize chest movement; and possible bruising at the fracture site.

Test-Taking Strategy: Knowing that fractured ribs can cause pain and bruising helps you eliminate options 1 and 4 first. To discriminate between options 2 and 3, knowing that pain causes shallow, guarded respirations helps you choose option 2 as the unrelated finding. Review the assessment findings in rib fractures now, if you had difficulty with this question!

Level of Cognitive Ability: Analysis
Phase of Nursing Process: Assessment
Client Needs: Physiological Integrity
Content Area: Adult Health / Respiratory

Reference
Black, J., & Matassarin-Jacobs, E. (1997). *Medical-surgical nursing: Clinical management for continuity of care* (5th ed.). Philadelphia: W. B. Saunders. p. 2526.

55. **1**

Rationale: Strapping the ribs is an outmoded therapy. Its use had a constricting effect on the ribs and deep breathing, and it can actually increase the risk of atelectasis and pneumonia.

Test-Taking Strategy: This question can be answered by logically thinking through the physiological effects of restricting lung mobility. This will help eliminate each of the incorrect responses. Review interventions for rib fractures now, if you had difficulty with this question!

Level of Cognitive Ability: Application
Phase of Nursing Process: Implementation
Client Needs: Physiological Integrity
Content Area: Adult Health / Respiratory

Reference
Black, J., & Matassarin-Jacobs, E. (1997) *Medical-surgical nursing: Clinical management for continuity of care* (5th ed.). Philadelphia: W. B. Saunders. p. 2526.

56. **4**

Rationale: Flail chest results from fracture of two or more ribs in at least two places each. This results in a "floating" section of ribs. Because this section is unattached to the rest of the bony rib cage, this segment results in paradoxical chest movement. This means that the force of inspiration pulls the fractured segment inward, while the rest of the chest expands. Likewise, during exhalation the segment balloons outward while the rest of the chest moves inward. This is a tell-tale sign of flail chest.

Test-Taking Strategy: The key to answering this question is the use of the words "most distinctive" in the stem. Cyanosis and hypotension occur with many different disorders and are therefore eliminated first. Of the two remaining, you would choose paradoxical chest movement over dyspnea on exhalation by remembering that a flail chest has broken rib segments that move independently of the rest of the rib cage.

Level of Cognitive Ability: Application
Phase of Nursing Process: Assessment
Client Needs: Physiological Integrity
Content Area: Adult Health / Respiratory

Reference
Black, J., & Matassarin-Jacobs, E. (1997). *Medical-surgical nursing: Clinical management for continuity of care* (5th ed.). Philadelphia: W. B. Saunders. p. 2527.

57. **1**

Rationale: The client with severe flail chest will have significant paradoxical chest movement. This causes the mediastinal structures to swing back and forth with respiration. This movement can affect hemodynamics. Specifically, the client's central venous pressure rises, the filling of the right side of the heart is impaired, and the arterial blood pressure falls. This is referred to as mediastinal flutter.

Test-Taking Strategy: This is a difficult question. Since the stem makes no mention of hemorrhage or bleeding, hypovolemic shock is ruled out first. Knowing that these signs and symptoms are not compatible with fat embolism helps you eliminate that option next. Of the two remaining options, knowing that mediastinal shift is a result of tension pneumothorax helps you choose mediastinal flutter as the correct answer.

Level of Cognitive Ability: Analysis
Phase of Nursing Process: Analysis
Client Needs: Physiological Integrity
Content Area: Adult Health / Respiratory

Reference
Black, J., & Matassarin-Jacobs, E. (1997). *Medical-surgical nursing: Clinical management for continuity of care* (5th ed.). Philadelphia: W. B. Saunders. p. 2527.

58. **4**

Rationale: Pneumothorax is characterized by restlessness, tachycardia, dyspnea, pain with respiration, asymmetrical chest expansion, and diminished or absent breath sounds on the affected side. Pneumothorax can cause increased airway pressure because of resistance to lung inflation. ARDS and pulmonary embolism are not characterized by absent breath sounds. An endotracheal tube that is inserted too far can cause absent breath sounds, but the lack of breath sounds would most likely be on the left side because of the degree of curvature of the right and left main stem bronchus.

Test-Taking Strategy: Begin to answer this question by recalling that the high-pressure alarm on the ventilator sounds when there is increased tension and pressure within the intubated client's airways. The least likely causes with the wording of the question are ARDS and pulmonary embolism, so these are eliminated first. Either of the two remaining options could cause increased airway pressure. Knowing that a displaced tube usually enters the right main stem bronchus (and aerates the right lung only), you conclude that it cannot be a displaced endotracheal tube. The client has absent breath sounds in that lung. This leaves right pneumothorax as the only possible choice; absent breath sounds on the right is consistent with this complication. Review the manifestations associated with pneumothorax now, if you had difficulty with this question!

Level of Cognitive Ability: Application
Phase of Nursing Process: Assessment
Client Needs: Physiological Integrity
Content Area: Adult Health / Respiratory

Reference

Black, J., & Matassarin-Jacobs, E. (1997). *Medical-surgical nursing: Clinical management for continuity of care* (5th ed.). Philadelphia: W. B. Saunders. p. 2524.

59. **3**

Rationale: Respiratory failure is described as a PaO_2 of 50 mmHg or less and a $PaCO_2$ of 50 mmHg or greater in a client with no history of respiratory disease. In a client with a history of respiratory disorder with hypercapnia, elevations of 5 mm or more from the client's baseline are considered diagnostic.

Test-Taking Strategy: Knowing that the carbon dioxide level in respiratory failure is above 50 mmHg helps you eliminate options 1 and 2 first. You would choose option 3 over option 4 because the arterial oxygen level in respiratory failure is less than 50 mmHg. Review the blood gas findings in a client with respiratory failure now, if you had difficulty with this question!

Level of Cognitive Ability: Application
Phase of Nursing Process: Assessment
Client Needs: Physiological Integrity
Content Area: Adult Health/Respiratory

Reference

Black, J., & Matassarin-Jacobs, E. (1997). *Medical-surgical nursing: Clinical management for continuity of care* (5th ed.). Philadelphia: W. B. Saunders. p. 1169.

60. **4**

Rationale: Instructions for using a metered-dose inhaler include to shake the canister; hold it right side up; inhale slowly and evenly through the mouth; deliver one spray per breath; and hold the breath after inhalation.

Test-Taking Strategy: This question is straightforward and tests a fundamental concept of medication administration using inhalers. If you made an incorrect choice, review the key principles of this medication therapy now!

Level of Cognitive Ability: Application
Phase of Nursing Process: Implementation
Client Needs: Physiological Integrity
Content Area: Adult Health/Respiratory

Reference

Taylor, C., Lillis, C., & LeMone, P. (1997). *Fundamentals of nursing: The art and science of nursing care* (3rd ed.). Philadelphia: Lippincott-Raven. p. 1335.

61. **4**

Rationale: The earliest detectable sign of ARDS is an increased respiratory rate, which can begin anywhere from 1 to 96 hours after the initial insult to the body. This is followed by increasing dyspnea, air hunger, retraction of accessory muscles, and cyanosis. Breath sounds may be clear or may consist of fine inspiratory crackles or diffuse coarse crackles.

Test-Taking Strategy: Note that the question is asking for the "earliest" sign. Eliminate option 3 first, since muscle retraction is a later sign of respiratory distress. Of the three remaining, adventitious breath sounds (options 1 and 2) would occur later than an increased respiratory rate, which makes option 4 the correct answer. Review the early signs of ARDS now, if you had difficulty with this question!

Level of Cognitive Ability: Application
Phase of Nursing Process: Assessment
Client Needs: Physiological Integrity
Content Area: Adult Health/Respiratory

Reference

Ignatavicius, D., Workman, M., & Mishler, M. (1995). *Medical-surgical nursing: A nursing process approach* (2nd ed.). Philadelphia: W. B. Saunders. p. 753.

62. **3**

Rationale: The normal pulmonary capillary wedge pressure (PCWP) is 8 to 13 mmHg, and the client is considered to have high readings if they exceed 18 to 20 mmHg. The client with ARDS has a normal PCWP, which is an expected finding, since the edema is in the interstitium of the lung and is noncardiac in origin.

Test-Taking Strategy: To answer this question correctly, it is necessary to know that the PCWP is normal. This makes sense, knowing that fluid accumulates in the interstitium of the lung and not in the vascular bed. Thus, your answer could only be option 3, that the reading is normal and expected. Learn the normal PCWP reading now, if you are unfamiliar with it!

Level of Cognitive Ability: Analysis
Phase of Nursing Process: Analysis
Client Needs: Physiological Integrity
Content Area: Adult Health/Respiratory

Reference

Black, J., & Matassarin-Jacobs, E. (1997). *Medical-surgical nursing: Clinical management for continuity of care* (5th ed.). Philadelphia: W. B. Saunders. p. 1233.

63. **2**

Rationale: The client with emphysema has hyperinflation of the alveoli and flattening of the diaphragm. These lead to an increased anteroposterior diameter, which is referred to as barrel chest. The client also has dyspnea with prolonged expiration and lungs hyperresonant to percussion.

Test-Taking Strategy: To answer this question correctly, it is necessary to understand that the barrel chest is a result of long-term hyperinflation of the lungs and air trapping. By knowing that emphysema is the only type of CAL in which this occurs, you are able to eliminate each of the other incorrect options. Review the characteristics of emphysema now, if you had difficulty with this question!

Level of Cognitive Ability: Analysis
Phase of Nursing Process: Analysis
Client Needs: Physiological Integrity
Content Area: Adult Health/Respiratory

Reference

Black, J., & Matassarin-Jacobs, E. (1997). *Medical-surgical nursing: Clinical management for continuity of care* (5th ed.). Philadelphia: W. B. Saunders. pp. 1114–1115.

64. **4**

Rationale: Indomethacin is a nonsteroidal anti-inflammatory drug that has an analgesic effect and allows the client to cough and deep-breathe more effectively.

Test-Taking Strategy: Knowing that the medication needed to treat this condition would be an anti-inflammatory helps you eliminate options 1 and 2. In order to discriminate between options 3 and 4, you should recall that indomethacin is an NSAID. This medication is also used to treat inflammation of the epicardium in the pericardial sac, which is called pericarditis. If you are unfamiliar with this medication, take time now to review its uses and actions!

Level of Cognitive Ability: Application
Phase of Nursing Process: Implementation
Client Needs: Physiological Integrity
Content Area: Pharmacology

Reference

Smeltzer, S., & Bare, B. (1996). *Brunner and Suddarth's textbook of medical-surgical nursing* (8th ed.). Philadelphia: Lippincott-Raven. p. 502.

65. **3**

Rationale: The most common initial symptom in pulmonary embolism is chest pain that is sudden in onset. The next most commonly reported symptom is dyspnea, which is accompanied by an increased respiratory rate. Other typical symptoms of pulmonary embolism include cough, tachycardia, fever, diaphoresis, cough, anxiety, and possibly syncope.

Test-Taking Strategy: Since pulmonary embolism does not result from either an infectious process or an allergic reaction, options 2 and 4 are eliminated first. To discriminate between options 1 and 3, look at them closely. Option 1 states dyspnea when deep breaths are taken. Although dyspnea commonly occurs with pulmonary embolism, dyspnea is not associated only with deep breathing. Therefore, option 3 is correct, and option 1 is eliminated. Review the signs of pulmonary embolism now, if you had difficulty with this question!

Level of Cognitive Ability: Application
Phase of Nursing Process: Assessment
Client Needs: Physiological Integrity
Content Area: Adult Health/Respiratory

Reference

Smeltzer, S., & Bare, B. (1996). *Brunner and Suddarth's textbook of medical-surgical nursing* (8th ed.). Philadelphia: Lippincott-Raven. p. 526.

66. **2**

Rationale: Cough is the most frequent symptom of lung cancer, which begins as nonproductive and hacking and progresses to productive. In the smoker who already has a cough, a change in the character and frequency of cough usually occurs. Wheezing and blood-streaked sputum are later signs. Pain is a very late sign and is usually pleuritic in nature.

Test-Taking Strategy: Begin to answer this question by eliminating pain and hemoptysis, because it is reasonable that these would be later signs. To discriminate between

cough and hoarseness, think about location. Hoarseness would indicate that the affected tissue is the upper airway, whereas cough would indicate lower airway. Since the question is asking about lung cancer, which is lower airway, the answer must be cough. Review the common early signs of lung cancer now, if you had difficulty with this question!

Level of Cognitive Ability: Application
Phase of Nursing Process: Assessment
Client Needs: Physiological Integrity
Content Area: Adult Health/Respiratory

Reference

Monahan, F., & Neighbors, M. (1998). *Medical-surgical nursing: Foundations for clinical practice* (2nd ed.). Philadelphia: W. B. Saunders. p. 696.

67. **3**

Rationale: The client developing pulmonary edema after pneumonectomy demonstrates dyspnea, cough, frothy sputum, crackles, and possibly cyanosis. A respiratory rate of 20 is within normal limits. Pain with deep breathing is expected and managed with analgesics. The client with pneumonectomy does not have a chest tube.

Test-Taking Strategy: Increased chest drainage indicates hemorrhage, not pulmonary edema, and is eliminated first. Additionally, the client with pneumonectomy does not have a chest tube. A respiratory rate of 20 is normal, and pain with deep breathing is expected in the immediate postoperative period, so these may be eliminated next. Bilateral crackles in lung fields indicate pulmonary edema and the correct choice. Review the signs of pulmonary edema now, if you had difficulty with this question!

Level of Cognitive Ability: Application
Phase of Nursing Process: Assessment
Client Needs: Physiological Integrity
Content Area: Adult Health/Respiratory

Reference

Black, J., & Matassarin-Jacobs, E. (1997). *Medical-surgical nursing: Clinical management for continuity of care* (5th ed.). Philadelphia: W. B. Saunders. p. 1159.

68. **2**

Rationale: The nurse avoids putting pressure on the chest during inspiration, as it interferes with lung expansion. Acceptable methods of splinting include the use of the hands, a pillow, or a towel or drawsheet during a forced expiratory cough.

Test-Taking Strategy: The wording of the question guides you to look for an incorrect response. Option 3 is obviously correct and is eliminated. Option 4 is not as widely used but is a technique that supports the area above and below an incision. Since this option is also correct, it is eliminated next. Options 1 and 2 seem to oppose each other. To choose correctly, you would need to know that applying pressure to the chest before the breath interferes with lung expansion and is not as helpful to the client overall. This would force you to choose option 2 as the answer to the question according to the way it is worded.

Level of Cognitive Ability: Application
Phase of Nursing Process: Implementation
Client Needs: Physiological Integrity
Content Area: Adult Health/Respiratory

Reference
Black, J., & Matassarin-Jacobs, E. (1997). *Medical-surgical nursing: Clinical management for continuity of care* (5th ed.). Philadelphia: W. B. Saunders. p. 1157.

69. **1**

Rationale: Immediately following radical neck dissection, the client will have a wound drain in the neck attached to portable suction, which drains serosanguineous drainage. In the first 24 hours after surgery, the drainage may total 30 to 120 mL.

Test-Taking Strategy: Note the key word "immediate" in the stem of the question. Since the wound suction tube does not sit in the airway, option 4 is quickly eliminated. Since serous drainage has no blood, this is not likely in the immediate postoperative period, and this option is also eliminated as a choice. Knowing that grossly bloody drainage indicates bleeding or hemorrhage, you would choose option 1 (serosanguineous drainage) as the correct answer. Review normal expected assessment findings following radical neck dissection now, if you had difficulty with this question!

Level of Cognitive Ability: Application
Phase of Nursing Process: Assessment
Client Needs: Physiological Integrity
Content Area: Adult Health/Respiratory

Reference
Smeltzer, S., & Bare, B. (1996). *Brunner and Suddarth's textbook of medical-surgical nursing* (8th ed.). Philadelphia: Lippincott-Raven. p. 845.

70. **1**

Rationale: If the client begins to hemorrhage from the surgical site following radical neck dissection, the nurse elevates the head of the bed to maintain airway patency and prevent aspiration. The nurse applies pressure over the bleeding site and calls the physician immediately.

Test-Taking Strategy: This question is very straightforward. Options 2 and 3 are obviously indicated and are eliminated immediately as possible options. Calling the physician is also indicated immediately, while lowering the head of bed does not help with airway maintenance. Thus, option 1 is the contraindicated action and is the answer to the question.

Level of Cognitive Ability: Application
Phase of Nursing Process: Implementation
Client Needs: Physiological Integrity
Content Area: Adult Health/Respiratory

Reference
Smeltzer, S., & Bare, B. (1996). *Brunner and Suddarth's textbook of medical-surgical nursing* (8th ed.). Philadelphia: Lippincott-Raven. p. 845.

71. **4**

Rationale: Skin color is the least reliable sign for determining the oxygenation status of the client with carbon monoxide poisoning. It may range from pink to cherry red, or pale to cyanotic. Other signs that result from the lack of oxygen include dizziness, headache, muscular weakness, palpitations, and mental confusion that can progress rapidly to coma.

Test-Taking Strategy: Without specific knowledge of this condition, this question may be difficult to answer. Since palpitations could accompany tachycardia (which is expected with hypoxia), you may deduce that this sign is reliable and eliminate it from the list of possible choices. Since headache is a CNS symptom and the CNS relies heavily on a ready oxygen supply, this one may be eliminated also, since this should be a reliable sign. Muscular weakness is an example of the effects of hypoxia at the tissue level and therefore should be considered reliable also. By the process of elimination, skin color is the unreliable sign, since it may vary considerably. Review the clinical manifestations associated with carbon monoxide poisoning now, if you had difficulty with this question!

Level of Cognitive Ability: Analysis
Phase of Nursing Process: Assessment
Client Needs: Physiological Integrity
Content Area: Adult Health/Respiratory

Reference
Smeltzer, S., & Bare, B. (1996). *Brunner and Suddarth's textbook of medical-surgical nursing* (8th ed.). Philadelphia: Lippincott-Raven. pp. 2024–2025.

72. **2**

Rationale: Carbon dioxide narcosis is a condition that results from extreme hypercapnia, with carbon dioxide levels in excess of 70 mmHg. The client experiences symptoms such as confusion and tremors, which may progress to convulsions and possibly coma.

Test-Taking Strategy: To answer this question, you need to be able to interpret arterial blood gases at a fundamental level. Knowing that the client has a highly elevated carbon dioxide level, you may deduce that the client is expected to be in respiratory acidosis. Knowing this, you would eliminate options 3 and 4 quickly. To differentiate between options 1 and 2, knowing that there is a difference between carbon monoxide and carbon dioxide helps you easily choose option 2. Additionally, noting that the CO_2 level is elevated will easily direct you to the correct option, CO_2 narcosis!

Level of Cognitive Ability: Analysis
Phase of Nursing Process: Assessment
Client Needs: Physiological Integrity
Content Area: Adult Health/Respiratory

Reference
Smeltzer, S., & Bare, B. (1996). *Brunner and Suddarth's textbook of medical-surgical nursing* (8th ed.). Philadelphia: Lippincott-Raven. p. 234.

73. **4**

Rationale: With the severe respiratory acidosis that occurs in carbon dioxide narcosis, compensatory mechanisms fail. As hydrogen ion concentrations continue to rise, they are driven into the cell, forcing intracellular potassium out. This is an expected finding in this situation.

Test-Taking Strategy: To answer this question, an understanding of the effects of acidosis on the body is required. With build-up of carbon dioxide, the body attempts to eliminate hydrogen ions from the circulation, since they are another source of body acid. The blood buffer system tries to buffer them as the first line of defense. With a rapid build-up of carbon dioxide, this is insufficient, and the body needs to find another way to lose hydrogen ions. Since the renal system doesn't "kick in" for almost 24 hours, the hydrogen ions are driven into the cells, and potassium comes out. (Hydrogen and potassium are both cations.) With these concepts in mind, hyperkalemia is an expected finding, which eliminates options 1 and 2. Since this disorder has nothing to do with hemolysis, the only correct choice is option 4!

Level of Cognitive Ability: Analysis
Phase of Nursing Process: Analysis
Client Needs: Physiological Integrity
Content Area: Adult Health/Respiratory

Reference
Smeltzer, S., & Bare, B. (1996). *Brunner and Suddarth's textbook of medical-surgical nursing* (8th ed.). Philadelphia: Lippincott-Raven. p. 234.

74. **3**

Rationale: Carbon dioxide acts as a vasodilator to cerebral blood vessels. With sufficient rise in carbon dioxide, the client may suffer increased intracranial pressure, which is initially reflected as papilledema and dilated conjunctival blood vessels.

Test-Taking Strategy: Begin to answer this question by eliminating options 2 and 4 as the least plausible of the options. Knowing that carbon dioxide vasodilates the cerebral blood vessels guides you to choose option 3 as the correct answer, since the cerebral circulation is one of the three components that contributes to the net intracranial pressure. Review the complications associated with carbon dioxide narcosis now, if you had difficulty with this question!

Level of Cognitive Ability: Application
Phase of Nursing Process: Planning
Client Needs: Physiological Integrity
Content Area: Adult Health/Respiratory

Reference
Smeltzer, S., & Bare, B. (1996). *Brunner and Suddarth's textbook of medical-surgical nursing* (8th ed.). Philadelphia: Lippincott-Raven. p. 235.

75. **3**

Rationale: With a rapid drop in carbon dioxide levels, the kidneys are unable to excrete bicarbonate ions at the same pace. The client can experience rebound metabolic alkalosis, with resulting seizure activity. The nurse evaluates the client's status carefully during this period.

Test-Taking Strategy: To answer this question accurately, an understanding of how the body maintains acid-base balance is needed. With a drop in carbon dioxide, the body also needs to drop bicarbonate levels correspondingly. Otherwise, the body is in a state of metabolic alkalosis. However, it is difficult for the body to do this, because bicarbonate must be eliminated by the kidneys, which do not "kick in" to restore acid-base balance for 24 hours or so. Because of this, rapid declines in carbon dioxide levels often do result in metabolic alkalosis, putting the client at risk for seizure activity. This is a difficult question to answer unless you understand these concepts. If needed, review the basic acid-base abnormalities and their manifestations!

Level of Cognitive Ability: Analysis
Phase of Nursing Process: Evaluation
Client Needs: Physiological Integrity
Content Area: Adult Health/Respiratory

Reference
Smeltzer, S., & Bare, B. (1996). *Brunner and Suddarth's textbook of medical-surgical nursing* (8th ed.). Philadelphia: Lippincott-Raven. p. 235.

76. **2**

Rationale: Histoplasmosis is an opportunistic fungal infection that can occur in the client with AIDS. The infection begins as a respiratory infection and can progress to disseminated infection. Typical signs and symptoms include fever, dyspnea, cough, and weight loss. There may be enlargement of the client's lymph nodes, liver, and spleen as well.

Test-Taking Strategy: This question can be most easily answered if you know that histoplasmosis begins as a respiratory infection and can progress to a generalized infection. Knowing that histoplasmosis is an infectious process helps you eliminate option 3. Since the client has AIDS as well as another infection, weight gain is an unlikely symptom and can be eliminated next. Knowing that histoplasmosis begins as a respiratory infection helps you choose dyspnea over headache as the final discriminating factor. Review the signs of histoplasmosis now, if you had difficulty with this question!

Level of Cognitive Ability: Application
Phase of Nursing Process: Assessment
Client Needs: Physiological Integrity
Content Area: Adult Health/Respiratory

Reference
Ignatavicius, D., Workman, M., & Mishler, M. (1995). *Medical-surgical nursing: A nursing process approach* (2nd ed.). Philadelphia: W. B. Saunders. p. 506.

77. **3**

Rationale: Pulmonary sarcoidosis can lead to cor pulmonale (or right-sided heart failure), which is characterized by distended neck veins, elevated CVP, engorged liver, and peripheral edema. Bilateral crackles would indicate left-sided heart failure, not right-sided heart failure.

Test-Taking Strategy: To answer this question accurately, it is necessary to know that sarcoidosis is a restrictive lung disease. A complication of restrictive lung disease is cor pulmonale, since the right side of the heart has to work hard on a continuous basis to overcome pulmonary resistance. Knowing this, you would eliminate options 2 and 4, as they are the opposite of the symptoms expected with right-sided heart failure. You would choose option 3 over option 1 by knowing how to discriminate between left- and right-sided heart failure. Review the complications of pulmonary sarcoidosis and the signs of right- and left-sided heart failure now, if you had difficulty with this question!

Level of Cognitive Ability: Application
Phase of Nursing Process: Assessment
Client Needs: Physiological Integrity
Content Area: Adult Health/Respiratory

Reference
Ignatavicius, D., Workman, M., & Mishler, M. (1995). *Medical-surgical nursing: A nursing process approach* (2nd ed.). Philadelphia: W. B. Saunders. p. 724.

78. **2**

Rationale: The usual treatment for exacerbations of sarcoidosis includes systemic corticosteroids. Side effects of this therapy include weight gain, changes in mood, and hyperglycemia. Hyperkalemia and pruritus are unrelated findings.

Test-Taking Strategy: To answer this question successfully, it is necessary to know that sarcoidosis is a restrictive lung disease, with exacerbations that are treated with corticosteroids. Knowing that corticosteroids cause hyperglycemia, you can eliminate each of the incorrect options in turn. Review the medication therapy used in the treatment of sarcoidosis now, if you had difficulty with this question!

Level of Cognitive Ability: Application
Phase of Nursing Process: Implementation
Client Needs: Physiological Integrity
Content Area: Adult Health/Respiratory

Reference

Black, J., & Matassarin-Jacobs, E. (1997). *Medical-surgical nursing: Clinical management for continuity of care* (5th ed.). Philadelphia: W. B. Saunders. p. 1150.

79. 4

Rationale: Dry cough and dyspnea are typical signs and symptoms of pulmonary sarcoidosis. Others include chest pain, hemoptysis, and pneumothorax. Systemic signs and symptoms include weakness and fatigue, malaise, fever, and weight loss.

Test-Taking Strategy: Note the key word "early" in the stem of the question. Since sarcoidosis is a pulmonary problem, you would eliminate options 1 and 2 first. You would choose option 4 over option 3 since the shortness of breath (and impaired ventilation) appears first and would cause the fatigue as a secondary symptom.

Level of Cognitive Ability: Analysis
Phase of Nursing Process: Evaluation
Client Needs: Health Promotion and Maintenance
Content Area: Adult Health/Respiratory

Reference

Black, J., & Matassarin-Jacobs, E. (1997). *Medical-surgical nursing: Clinical management for continuity of care* (5th ed.). Philadelphia: W. B. Saunders. p. 1150.

80. 1

Rationale: Silicosis results from chronic, excessive inhalation of particles of free crystalline silica dust. The client should wear a mask to limit inhalation of this substance, which can cause restrictive lung disease after years of exposure.

Test-Taking Strategy: To answer this question, it is necessary to know that exposure to silica dust causes the illness. The dust is inhaled into the respiratory tract. Knowing this, each of the incorrect options can be readily eliminated. If you had difficulty with this question, take time now to review the protective measures associated with silicosis!

Level of Cognitive Ability: Application
Phase of Nursing Process: Assessment
Client Needs: Safe, Effective Care Environment
Content Area: Adult Health/Respiratory

Reference

Ignatavicius, D., Workman, M., & Mishler, M. (1995). *Medical-surgical nursing: A nursing process approach* (2nd ed.). Philadelphia: W. B. Saunders. p. 725.

81. 3

Rationale: The client with simple silicosis may be asymptomatic or have mild ventilatory restriction and has evidence of fibrosis on CXR. Pulmonary function studies reveal some decreases in vital capacity and total lung volume. There is no evidence of massive fibrosis at this stage. This disease is restricted to the respiratory system only.

Test-Taking Strategy: Option 4 has the least amount of "fit" with a disorder that is described as simple or uncomplicated,

and therefore is eliminated as a possible answer first. Since silicosis is a pulmonary disease, option 1 is also eliminated. Option 2 doesn't make sense; it would be difficult for one to have shortness of breath but yet have normal pulmonary function tests. By elimination, the answer is option 3. Review the pathophysiology associated with simple silicosis now, if you had difficulty with this question!

Level of Cognitive Ability: Analysis
Phase of Nursing Process: Analysis
Client Needs: Physiological Integrity
Content Area: Adult Health/Respiratory

Reference

Ignatavicius, D., Workman, M., & Mishler, M. (1995). *Medical-surgical nursing: A nursing process approach* (2nd ed.). Philadelphia: W. B. Saunders. pp. 725–726.

82. 4

Rationale: Benzonatate is a locally acting antitussive. Its effectiveness is measured by the degree to which it decreases the intensity and frequency of cough, without eliminating the cough reflex.

Test-Taking Strategy: This is a basic question testing knowledge of the purpose and effects of this medication. If the question was difficult and you are unfamiliar with this medication, take time now to review!

Level of Cognitive Ability: Analysis
Phase of Nursing Process: Evaluation
Client Needs: Physiological Integrity
Content Area: Pharmacology

Reference

Hodgson, B., & Kizior, R. (1999). *Saunders nursing drug handbook 1999.* Philadelphia: W. B. Saunders. pp. 101–102.

83. 2

Rationale: Pyrazinamide is an antitubercular medication that is given in conjunction with other antitubercular medications. Its use might not be discontinued if sputum cultures continue to be positive.

Test-Taking Strategy: This question tests basic knowledge of the purpose and action of this medication. Knowing that this medication is an antitubercular medication helps you eliminate each of the incorrect options in turn. If this question was difficult, take a few moments to review this medication, in particular, and possibly other antitubercular medications as well!

Level of Cognitive Ability: Analysis
Phase of Nursing Process: Evaluation
Client Needs: Physiological Integrity
Content Area: Pharmacology

Reference

Hodgson, B., & Kizior, R. (1999). *Saunders nursing drug handbook 1999.* Philadelphia: W. B. Saunders. pp. 887–888.

84. 2

Rationale: Adequate gas exchange can be demonstrated only when both PO_2 and PCO_2 levels are known. The other responses do not indicate gas exchange. Remember that oxygen saturation index is a measure of the percent of oxygen attached to the available hemoglobin and does not indicate the arterial PO_2 level.

Test-Taking Strategy: This question requires that you use your knowledge to analyze the options that are available.

Focus on the issue of decreased ventilation and the data that would evaluate ventilation status. You should easily be directed to option 2.

Level of Cognitive Ability: Analysis
Phase of Nursing Process: Evaluation
Client Needs: Physiological Integrity
Content Area: Adult Health/Respiratory

Reference
Polaski, A., & Tatro, S. (1996). *Luckmann's core principles and practice of medical-surgical nursing.* Philadelphia: W. B. Saunders. p. 580.

85. 2

Rationale: Foscarnet is very toxic to the kidneys. Serum creatinine is monitored prior to therapy, two to three times per week during induction therapy, and at least weekly during maintenance therapy. It also may cause decreased levels of calcium, magnesium, phosphorus, and potassium in the blood stream. Thus, these levels are also measured with the same frequency.

Test-Taking Strategy: It is necessary to know the toxicities and important side effects of this medication to discriminate among the various options correctly. If needed, take a few moments to review this medication now.

Level of Cognitive Ability: Application
Phase of Nursing Process: Assessment
Client Needs: Physiological Integrity
Content Area: Adult Health/Respiratory

Reference
Deglin, J., & Vallerand A. (1997). *Davis's drug guide for nurses* (5th ed.). Philadelphia: F. A. Davis. pp. 522–523.

86. 4

Rationale: Frequent side effects of this medication include leukopenia, thrombocytopenia, and anemia. The client should be routinely assessed for signs and symptoms of infection. The client should also have ongoing monitoring of a number of parameters owing to the nature and side effects of the medication, including blood glucose, BUN, serum creatinine, CBC, liver function studies, and serum calcium and magnesium levels.

Test-Taking Strategy: Options 2 and 3 are the least plausible, given the information in the stem, and are eliminated first. To discriminate between the last two, you need to know that the medication has leukopenic side effects to choose correctly.

Level of Cognitive Ability: Analysis
Phase of Nursing Process: Analysis
Client Needs: Physiological Integrity
Content Area: Pharmacology

Reference
Deglin, J., & Vallerand, A. (1997). *Davis's drug guide for nurses* (5th ed.). Philadelphia: F. A. Davis. pp. 931–933.

87. 1

Rationale: A common side effect of this medication therapy is granulocytopenia and anemia. The nurse carefully monitors CBC results for these changes. With early HIV infection or in the client who is asymptomatic, CBC levels are monitored monthly for 3 months, then every 3 months thereafter. In clients with advanced disease, they are monitored every 2 weeks for the first 2 months, and then once a month if the medication is tolerated well.

Test-Taking Strategy: It is necessary to know the toxicities and important side effects of this medication to discriminate among the various options correctly. If needed, take a few moments to review this medication now.

Level of Cognitive Ability: Application
Phase of Nursing Process: Assessment
Client Needs: Physiological Integrity
Content Area: Pharmacology

Reference
Deglin, J., & Vallerand, A. (1997). *Davis's drug guide for nurses* (5th ed.). Philadelphia: F. A. Davis. pp. 1235–1236.

88. 2

Rationale: A serum amylase level that is increased 1.5 to 2 times normal may signify pancreatitis in the AIDS client, which is potentially fatal. The medication may have to be discontinued. The medication is also hepatotoxic and can result in liver failure.

Test-Taking Strategy: It is necessary to know the toxicities and important side effects of this medication to discriminate among the various options correctly. If needed, take a few moments to review this medication now.

Level of Cognitive Ability: Analysis
Phase of Nursing Process: Analysis
Client Needs: Physiological Integrity
Content Area: Pharmacology

Reference
Deglin, J., & Vallerand, A. (1997). *Davis's drug guide for nurses* (5th ed.). Philadelphia: F. A. Davis. pp. 358–360.

89. 3

Rationale: This medication slows the progression of HIV disease by improving the CD4 cell count. The ELISA and Western blot tests are done to diagnose AIDS initially. A CBC with differential may be done as part of an ongoing monitoring of the status of the client with AIDS, and to detect adverse effects of other medications.

Test-Taking Strategy: It is necessary to know the purpose and action of this medication to discriminate among the various options correctly. If needed, take a few moments to review this medication now.

Level of Cognitive Ability: Application
Phase of Nursing Process: Planning
Client Needs: Physiological Integrity
Content Area: Pharmacology

Reference
Deglin, J., & Vallerand, A. (1997). *Davis's drug guide for nurses* (5th ed.). Philadelphia: F. A. Davis. pp. 1232–1233.

90. 1

Rationale: Histoplasmosis usually starts as a respiratory infection in the client with AIDS. It then becomes a disseminated infection, with enlargement of lymph nodes, spleen, and liver.

Test-Taking Strategy: Knowing that lymph nodes may enlarge with generalized infection helps you narrow the plausible choices to options 1 and 4. Since the stem contains no information that indicates that option 4 is true, option 1 is the correct choice by elimination.

Level of Cognitive Ability: Analysis
Phase of Nursing Process: Analysis
Client Needs: Physiological Integrity
Content Area: Adult Health/Respiratory

Reference
Ignatavicius, D., Workman, M., & Mishler, M. (1995). *Medical-surgical nursing: A nursing process approach* (2nd ed.). Philadelphia: W. B. Saunders. p. 506.

91. **2**

Rationale: For clients with AIDS who experience night fever and night sweats, it is useful to offer the client an antipyretic of choice prior to going to sleep. It is also helpful to keep a change of bed linens and night clothes nearby for use. The pillow should have a plastic cover, and a towel may be placed over the pillowcase if there is profuse diaphoresis. The client should have liquids at the bedside to drink.

Test-Taking Strategy: The wording of the question guides you to look for a response that is not the best or most correct action. Options 1 and 3 are helpful from an environmental viewpoint, so they are eliminated first as answers to this question. Knowing that liquids will help prevent dehydration causes you to eliminate this option next. This leaves option 2 as the answer. Since night fever and sweats occur serially, it is most helpful to give the antipyretic before sleep as a prophylactic measure.

Level of Cognitive Ability: Application
Phase of Nursing Process: Implementation
Client Needs: Physiological Integrity
Content Area: Adult Health/Respiratory

Reference
Black, J., & Matassarin-Jacobs, E. (1997). *Medical-surgical nursing: Clinical management for continuity of care* (5th ed.). Philadelphia: W. B. Saunders. p. 632.

92. **4**

Rationale: The client with *Pneumocystis carinii* infection usually has a cough as the first symptom, which begins as nonproductive, then progresses to productive. Later signs include fever, dyspnea on exertion, and finally dyspnea at rest.

Test-Taking Strategy: The key word in the stem of this question is "early." While all these symptoms may appear at some point in the client with *Pneumocystis carinii* infection, knowing that the cough appears first helps you eliminate each of the other responses.

Level of Cognitive Ability: Application
Phase of Nursing Process: Assessment
Client Needs: Physiological Integrity
Content Area: Adult Health/Respiratory

Reference
Black, J., & Matassarin-Jacobs, E. (1997). *Medical-surgical nursing: Clinical management for continuity of care* (5th ed.). Philadelphia: W. B. Saunders. p. 629.

93. **4**

Rationale: The client in stage 1 (Seroconversion) acute HIV infection has laboratory documentation of HIV-positive status but is asymptomatic. Following introduction of the infection and seroconversion in stage 1, the client may remain asymptomatic for a period of 6 months to in excess of 11 years (stage 2: Chronic asymptomatic status). The client's T4 cell count is normal during these two stages. The client will begin to show symptoms in stage 3: Symptomatic stage, when the T4 cell count drops below 500/mm^3. At this time, the client experiences opportunistic infections, including oral lesions (thrush) and skin lesions (Kaposi's sarcoma). The client may also experience signs of respiratory infection in stage 3.

Test-Taking Strategy: The wording of the question tells you that there are clearly three incorrect options. Utilize knowledge of concepts related to seroconversion to help you eliminate each of the incorrect options.

Level of Cognitive Ability: Application
Phase of Nursing Process: Assessment
Client Needs: Physiological Integrity
Content Area: Adult Health/Respiratory

Reference
Burrell, P., Gerlach, M., & Pless, B. (1997). *Adult nursing: Acute and community care* (2nd ed.). Stamford, CT: Appleton & Lange. p. 183.

94. **3**

Rationale: The skin biopsy is the procedure of choice to diagnose Kaposi's sarcoma, which frequently complicates the clinical picture of the client with AIDS. Lung biopsy would confirm *Pneumocystis carinii* infection. The ELISA and Western blot are tests to diagnose HIV status.

Test-Taking Strategy: Begin to answer this question by eliminating options 1 and 2, which are used to diagnose whether or not the client is HIV-positive. Knowledge of the meaning of Kaposi's sarcoma, or attention to the words "lesions" and "trunk," will help you choose correctly between the remaining two options.

Level of Cognitive Ability: Analysis
Phase of Nursing Process: Analysis
Client Needs: Physiological Integrity
Content Area: Adult Health/Respiratory

Reference
Burrell, P., Gerlach, M., & Pless, B. (1997). *Adult nursing: Acute and community care* (2nd ed.). Stamford, CT: Appleton & Lange. p. 184.

95. **2**

Rationale: Abstinence is the safest way to avoid HIV infection. The next most reliable method is participation in a mutually monogamous relationship. The use of latex condoms is considered safe, because the latex prevents the transmission of the HIV virus as long as the condom is used properly and remains in place. The use of "natural skin" condoms is not considered safe because the pores in the condom are large enough for the virus to pass through.

Test-Taking Strategy: Utilize knowledge of transmission of sexually transmitted diseases and universal precautions to answer this question. The wording of the question tells you that there is one option that is dissimilar from the others, which in this case is the correct answer to the question.

Level of Cognitive Ability: Application
Phase of Nursing Process: Planning
Client Needs: Health Promotion and Maintenance
Content Area: Adult Health/Respiratory

References
Burrell, P., Gerlach, M., & Pless, B. (1997). *Adult nursing: Acute and community care* (2nd ed.). Stamford, CT: Appleton & Lange. p. 181.
Lewis, S., Collier, I., and Heitkemper, M. (1996). *Medical-surgical nursing: Assessment and management of clinical problems* (4th ed.). St. Louis: Mosby–Year Book p. 245.

96. 1

Rationale: The AIDS client with nausea and vomiting should avoid fatty products such as dairy products and red meat. Meals should be small and frequent to lessen the chance of vomiting. Spices and odorous foods should be avoided since they aggravate nausea. Foods are best tolerated either cold or at room temperature.

Test-Taking Strategy: Utilize knowledge of the effects of AIDS on the GI tract and general principles for treating nausea and vomiting to answer this question. Doing so will guide you to eliminate each of the incorrect options systematically.

Level of Cognitive Ability: Application
Phase of Nursing Process: Implementation
Client Needs: Health Promotion and Maintenance
Content Area: Adult Health/Respiratory

Reference

Lewis, S., Collier, I., & Heitkemper, M. (1996). *Medical-surgical nursing: Assessment and management of clinical problems* (4th ed.). St. Louis: Mosby–Year Book. p. 247.

97. 4

Rationale: The status of the client with a diagnosis of Impaired Gas Exchange would be evaluated against the standard outcome criteria for this nursing diagnosis. These would include that the client states that breathing is easier, coughs up secretions effectively, and has clear breath sounds. The client should not limit fluid intake, because fluids are needed to decrease the viscosity of secretions for expectoration. The client with diarrhea also should not limit fluid intake because of the risk of dehydration.

Test-Taking Strategy: Note that the stem of the question contains the key word "not." This tells you that the answer to the question is an incorrect goal for the client. Use knowledge related to airway management and fluid balance to choose correctly.

Level of Cognitive Ability: Analysis
Phase of Nursing Process: Evaluation
Client Needs: Physiological Integrity
Content Area: Adult Health/Respiratory

Reference

Lewis, S., Collier, I., & Heitkemper, M. (1996). *Medical-surgical nursing: Assessment and management of clinical problems* (4th ed.). St. Louis: Mosby–Year Book. p. 253.

BIBLIOGRAPHY

Black, J., & Matassarin-Jacobs, E. (1997). *Medical-surgical nursing: Clinical management for continuity of care* (5th ed.). Philadelphia: W. B. Saunders.

Burrell, P., Gerlach, M., & Pless, B. (1997). *Adult nursing: Acute and community care* (2nd ed.). Stamford, CT: Appleton & Lange.

Deglin, J., and Vallerand, A. (1997). *Davis's drug guide for nurses* (5th ed.). Philadelphia: F. A. Davis

Hodgson, B., & Kizior, R. (1999). *Saunders nursing drug handbook 1999.* Philadelphia: W. B. Saunders.

Ignatavicius, D., Workman, M., and Mishler, M. (1995). *Medical-surgical nursing: A nursing process approach* (2nd ed.). Philadelphia: W. B. Saunders.

Lammon, C., Foote, A., Leli, P., et al. (1995). *Clinical nursing skills.* Philadelphia: W. B. Saunders.

Leahy, J., & Kizilay, P. (1998). *Foundations of nursing practice: A nursing process approach.* Philadelphia: W. B. Saunders.

Lehne, R. (1998). *Pharmacology for nursing care* (3rd ed.). Philadelphia: W. B. Saunders.

Lewis, S., Collier, I., & Heitkemper, M. (1996). *Medical-surgical nursing: Assessment and management of clinical problems* (4th ed.). St. Louis: Mosby–Year Book.

Luckmann, J. (1997). *Saunders manual of nursing care.* Philadelphia: W. B. Saunders.

Mahan, L., & Escott-Stump, S. (1996). *Krause's food, nutrition, and diet therapy* (9th ed.). Philadelphia: W. B. Saunders.

Monahan, F., & Neighbors, M. (1998). *Medical-surgical nursing: Foundations for clinical practice* (2nd ed.). Philadelphia: W. B. Saunders.

O'Toole, M. (ed.) (1997). *Miller-Keane encyclopedia & dictionary of medicine, nursing, & allied health* (6th ed.). Philadelphia: W. B. Saunders.

Polaski, A., & Tatro, S. (1996). *Luckmann's core principles and practice of medical-surgical nursing.* Philadelphia: W. B. Saunders.

Smeltzer, S., & Bare, B. (1996). *Brunner and Suddarth's textbook of medical-surgical nursing* (8th ed.). Philadelphia: Lippincott-Raven.

Taylor, C., Lillis, C., & LeMone, P. (1997). *Fundamentals of nursing: The art and science of nursing care* (3rd ed.). Philadelphia: Lippincott-Raven.

CHAPTER 57

Client with Tuberculosis

I. Tuberculosis

A. Description
1. A highly communicable disease caused by *Mycobacterium tuberculosis*
2. *Mycobacterium tuberculosis* is a nonmotile, nonsporulating, acid-fast rod that secrets niacin, and when the bacillus reaches a susceptible site, it multiplies freely
3. Because *Mycobacterium tuberculosis* is an aerobic bacterium, it primarily affects the pulmonary system, especially the upper lobes where the oxygen content is greatest, but can also affect other areas of the body such as the brain, intestines, peritoneum, kidney, joints, and liver
4. An exudative-type response causes a nonspecific pneumonitis and the development of granulomas in the lung tissue
5. **Tuberculosis (TB)** has an insidious onset, and many clients are not aware of symptoms until the disease is well advanced
6. **Multidrug-resistant tuberculosis (MDR-TB)** can exist as a result of improper or noncompliant use of treatment programs and the development of mutations in the tubercle bacilli
7. The goal of treatment is to prevent transmission, control symptoms, and prevent progression of the disease

B. Risk factors
1. Alcoholism
2. Intravenous drug use
3. Malnutrition
4. Infection
5. The elderly
6. The homeless
7. Refugees
8. Minority groups
9. Individuals from a lower socioeconomic group
10. Children younger than 5 years of age
11. Individuals living in crowded areas, such as long-term care facilities, prisons, and mental health facilities
12. Individuals in constant, frequent contact with an untreated or undiagnosed individual
13. Individuals with immune dysfunction, HIV, or who are immunosuppressed from medication therapy
14. Drinking unpasteurized milk if cow is infected with bovine **TB**

C. Transmission
1. Via aerosolization or airborne route by droplet infection
2. When an infected individual coughs, laughs, sneezes, or sings, droplet nuclei containing **TB** bacteria enter the air and may be inhaled by others
3. Identification of those individuals in close contact with the infected individual is important so that they can be tested and treated as necessary
4. When contacts have been identified, these people are assessed with a tuberculin test and chest x-ray to determine infection with **TB**
5. After the infected individual has received **TB** medication for 2 to 3 weeks, the risk of transmission is greatly reduced

D. Disease Progression
1. Droplets enter the lungs and the bacteria form a tubercle lesion
2. The body's defense systems may encapsulate the tubercle, leaving a scar
3. If encapsulation does not occur, bacteria may enter the lymph system, travel to the lymph nodes, and cause an inflammatory response called granulomatous inflammation
4. Other bacilli are attacked and primary lesions (primary infection) form
5. The primary lesions may become dormant,

but can be reactivated and become a secondary infection when reexposed to the bacterium

6. In an active phase, **TB** can cause necrosis and cavitation in the lesions, leading to rupture and the spread of necrotic tissue and damage to various parts of the body

II. Diagnostic Findings

A. Client History
   1. Past exposure to **TB**
   2. Client's country of origin and travel to foreign countries in which there is a high incidence of **TB**
   3. Recent history of influenza, pneumonia, febrile illness, cough, and foul-smelling sputum production
   4. Previous tests for **TB** and what the results were
   5. Recent **bacille Calmette-Guérin (BCG) vaccine** (a vaccine containing attenuated tubercle bacilli that may be given in foreign countries or if traveling to foreign countries to produce increased resistance to **TB**)
   6. An individual who has received **BCG** will have a positive skin test and should be evaluated for **TB** with a chest x-ray

B. Clinical Manifestations
   1. May be asymptomatic in primary infection
   2. Fatigue
   3. Lethargy
   4. Anorexia
   5. Weight loss
   6. Low-grade fever
   7. Chills
   8. Night sweats
   9. Persistent cough and the production of mucoid and mucopurulent sputum, which is occasionally streaked with blood
   10. Chest tightness and a dull, aching chest pain may accompany the cough

C. Chest Assessment
   1. A physical examination of the chest does not provide conclusive evidence of **TB**
   2. Chest x-ray is not definitive but the presence of multinodular infiltrates with calcification in the upper lobes suggests **TB**
   3. If the disease is active, caseation and inflammation may be seen on the chest x-ray
   4. Advanced disease
      a. Dullness with percussion over involved parenchymal areas, bronchial breath sounds, rhonchi and/or crackles
      b. Partial obstruction of a bronchus, caused by endobronchial disease or compression by lymph nodes, may produce localized wheezing and dyspnea

D. Sputum Cultures
   1. Sputum specimens are obtained for an acid-fast smear
   2. A sputum culture identifying *Mycobacterium tuberculosis* confirms the diagnosis
   3. After medications are started, sputum samples are obtained again to determine the effectiveness of therapy
   4. Most clients have negative cultures after 3 months of compliance to medication therapy

E. **Mantoux Test**
   1. The most reliable determinant of infection with **TB**
   2. A positive reaction does not mean that active disease is present but indicates exposure to **TB** or the presence of inactive (dormant) disease
   3. Once the test result is positive, it will be positive in any future tests
   4. A small amount (0.1 mL) of standard-strength purified protein derivative (PPD) containing 5 tuberculin units is administered intradermally in the forearm
   5. An area of induration measuring 10 mm or more in diameter, 48–72 hours after injection, indicates the individual has been exposed to **TB**
   6. For individuals with HIV infection or who are immunosuppressed, a reaction of 5 mm or greater is considered positive
   7. Once an individual's skin test is positive, a chest x-ray is necessary to rule out active **TB** or to detect old, healed lesions

III. Implementation

A. The Hospitalized Client
   1. The client with active **TB** is placed in respiratory isolation precautions in a well-ventilated room
   2. The room should have at least six exchanges of fresh air per hour and should be ventilated to the outside environment if possible
   3. The nurse wears a particulate respirator (a special individually fitted mask) when caring for the client and a gown when there is a possibility of contamination of clothing
   4. Hands are always thoroughly washed before and after caring for the client
   5. If the client needs to leave the room for a test or procedure, the client is required to wear a mask
   6. Isolation is discontinued when the client is no longer considered infectious
   7. After the infected individual has received **TB** medication for 2–3 weeks, the risk of transmission is greatly reduced
   8. When the results of two sputum cultures are negative, the client is no longer considered infectious

B. The Client at Home
   1. Provide the client and family with information about **TB** and allay concerns about the contagious aspect of the infection

2. Instruct the client to follow the medication regimen exactly as prescribed and always to have a supply of the medication on hand
3. Advise the client of the side effects of the medication and ways of minimizing them to ensure compliance
4. Reassure the client that after 2–3 weeks of medication therapy, it is unlikely that the client will infect anyone
5. Inform the client that activities should be resumed gradually
6. Instruct the client about the need for adequate nutrition and a well-balanced diet to promote healing and to prevent recurrence of infection
7. Instruct client to increase foods rich in iron, protein, and vitamin C
8. Inform the client and family that respiratory isolation is not necessary because family members have already been exposed
9. Instruct the client to cover mouth and nose when coughing or sneezing and to confine used tissues to plastic bags
10. Instruct the client and family about thorough handwashing
11. Inform the client that examination of the sputum is needed every 2–4 weeks once medication therapy is initiated
12. Inform the client that when the results of two sputum cultures are negative, the client is no longer considered infectious and can usually return to his or her former employment
13. Advise the client to avoid excessive exposure to silicone or dust because these substances can cause further lung damage
14. Instruct the client regarding the importance of compliance to treatment, follow-up care and sputum cultures as prescribed

IV. Medications

A. Description
1. The most effective method for treating the disease and preventing transmission
2. Treatment of identified lesions depends on whether the individual has active disease or has been exposed to the disease
3. Treatment is difficult because the bacterium has a waxy substance on the capsule, which makes penetration and destruction difficult
4. The use of a multiple medication regimen destroys organisms as quickly as possible and minimizes the emergence of medication-resistant organisms
5. Active **TB** is treated with a combination of medications to which the organism is susceptible
6. Individuals with active **TB** are treated for 6–9 months; however, clients with HIV infection will be treated for a longer period of time

7. After the infected individual has received medication for 2–3 weeks, the risk of transmission is greatly reduced
8. Most clients have negative sputum cultures after 3 months with compliance to medication therapy
9. Individuals who have been exposed to active **TB** are treated with preventive isoniazid (INH) for 9–12 months

B. First-Line or Second-Line Medications
1. First-line medications provide the most effective antituberculosis activity
2. Second-line medications are used in combination with first-line medications but are more toxic
3. Current infecting organisms are proving resistant to standard first-line medications and the resistant organisms develop because individuals with the disease fail to complete the course of treatment; surviving bacteria adapt to the drug and become resistant
4. Multidrug therapies are instituted because of the resistant bacteria

C. **Multidrug-Resistant Tuberculosis (MDR-TB)**
1. Occurs when a client receiving two medications (first-line and second-line medications) discontinues one of the medications without the physician's knowledge
2. The client briefly experiences some response from the single medication, but then large numbers of resistant organisms begin to grow
3. The client, infectious again, transmits the drug-resistant organism to other individuals
4. As this event is repeated, an organism develops that is resistant to many of the first-line tuberculosis medications

V. First-Line Medications (Table 57–1)

A. Isoniazid (INH)
1. Description
   a. Bactericidal
   b. Inhibits synthesis of mycolic acids and acts to kill actively growing organisms in the extracellular environment
   c. Inhibits growth of dormant organisms in

Table 57–1. First-Line and Second-Line Medications

First-Line	Second-Line
Isoniazid (INH)	Capreomycin sulfate (Capastat Sulfate)
Rifampin (Rifadin)	Kanamycin sulfate (Kantrex)
Ethambutol HCl (Myambutol)	Ethionamide (Trecator-SC)
Streptomycin	Aminosalicylate sodium (Sodium para-aminosalicylic acid [PAS])
Pyrazinamide	Cycloserine (Seromycin)

the macrophages and caseating granulomas

d. Active only during cell division

e. Used in combination with other antitubercular medications

2. Contraindications and cautions

a. Contraindicated in clients with hypersensitivity or with acute liver disease

b. Use with caution in clients with chronic liver disease, alcoholism, or renal impairment

c. Use with caution in clients taking niacin, nicotinic acid (Nicobid)

d. Use with caution in clients taking hepatotoxic medications as the risk for hepatotoxicity increases

e. Alcohol increases the risk of hepatotoxicity

f. Isoniazid (INH) may increase the risk of toxicity of carbamazepine (Tegretol) and phenytoin (Dilantin)

g. Isoniazid (INH) may decrease ketoconazole (Nizoral) concentrations

3. Side effects

a. Peripheral neuritis

b. Neurotoxicity

c. Irritation at injection site with IM administration

d. Nausea and vomiting

e. Dry mouth

f. Pyridoxine (vitamin B_6) deficiency

g. Dizziness

h. Hyperglycemia

i. Increased liver function tests

j. Hepatotoxicity

k. Hepatitis

l. Hypersensitivity reactions

4. Implementation

a. Assess for hypersensitivity

b. Assess for hepatic dysfunction

c. Assess for sensitivity to niacin, nicotinic acid (Nicobid)

d. Monitor liver function tests

e. Monitor for signs of hepatitis as anorexia, nausea, vomiting, weakness, fatigue, dark urine, or jaundice, and if these symptoms occur, hold medication and notify physician

f. Monitor for tingling, numbness, or burning of the extremities

g. Assess mental status

h. Monitor for visual changes and notify the physician if they occur

i. Assess for dizziness and initiate safety precautions

j. Monitor complete blood count (CBC) and blood glucose results

k. Administer 1 hour before or 2 hours after a meal as food may delay absorption

l. Administer at least 1 hour before

antacids, especially those antacids that contain aluminum

5. Client education

a. Instruct client not to skip doses and to take medication for the full length of the prescribed therapy

b. Instruct client not to take any other medication without consulting the physician

c. Advise client of the importance of follow-up physician visits, vision testing, and lab tests

d. Instruct client to avoid alcohol

e. Advise client to take medication on an empty stomach with 8 oz of water 1 hour before or 2 hours after meals and to avoid taking antacids with the medication

f. Instruct client to avoid tyramine-containing foods as they may cause a reaction as red and itching skin, a pounding heartbeat, lightheadedness, a hot or clammy feeling, or a headache, and if this does occur, to notify the physician

g. Instruct client in the signs of neurotoxicity, hepatitis, and hepatotoxicity

h. Instruct client to notify physician if signs of neurotoxicity, hepatitis and hepatotoxicity, or visual changes occur

B. Rifampin (Rifadin)

1. Description

a. Inhibits bacterial RNA synthesis

b. Binds to DNA-dependent RNA polymerase

c. Blocks RNA transcription

d. Used in conjunction with at least one other antitubercular medication

2. Contraindications and cautions

a. Contraindicated in clients with hypersensitivity

b. Use with caution in clients with hepatic dysfunction or alcoholism

c. Use of alcohol or hepatotoxic medications may increase the risk of hepatotoxicity

d. Decreases the effects of several medications including oral anticoagulants, oral hypoglycemics, chloramphenicol (Chloromycetin), digoxin (Lanoxin), disopyramide phosphate (Norpace), mexiletine (Mexitil), quinidine polygalacturonate (Cardioquin), tocainide HCl (Tonocard), fluconazole (Diflucan), methadone HCl (Dolophine), phenytoin (Dilantin), and verapamil HCl (Calan)

3. Side effects

a. Heartburn

b. Nausea

c. Vomiting

d. Diarrhea

e. Hypersensitivity reaction including fever,

chills, shivering, headache, muscle and bone pain, and dyspnea
   f. Increased liver function tests
   g. Hepatotoxicity and hepatitis
   h. Increased uric acid levels
   i. Blood dyscrasias
   j. Colitis
4. Implementation
   a. Assess for hypersensitivity
   b. Evaluate CBC, uric acid, and liver function tests
   c. Assess for signs of hepatitis and if they occur, hold medication and notify the physician
   d. Monitor stools and for signs of colitis
   e. Monitor mental status
   f. Assess for visual changes
5. Client education
   a. Instruct client not to skip doses and to take medication for the full length of the prescribed therapy
   b. Instruct client not to take any other medication without consulting the physician
   c. Advise client of the importance of follow-up physician visits and lab tests
   d. Instruct client to avoid alcohol
   e. Advise client to take medication on an empty stomach with 8 oz of water 1 hour before or 2 hours after meals and to avoid taking antacids with the medication
   f. Instruct the client that urine, feces, sweat, and tears will be red-orange in color and that soft contact lenses can become permanently discolored
   g. Instruct client to notify physician if yellow eyes or skin develops or if weakness, fatigue, nausea, vomiting, sore throat, fever, or unusual bleeding occurs

C. Ethambutol (Myambutol)
   1. Description
      a. Bacteriostatic
      b. Interferes with cell metabolism and multiplication by inhibiting one or more metabolites in susceptible bacteria
      c. Inhibits bacterial RNA synthesis
      d. Active only during cell division
      e. It is slow acting and must be used in combination with other bactericidal agents
   2. Contraindications and cautions
      a. Contraindicated in clients with hypersensitivity, optic neuritis, and in children under 13 years of age
      b. Use with caution in clients with renal dysfunction, gout, ocular defects, diabetic retinopathy, cataracts, and ocular inflammatory conditions
      c. Use with caution in the client taking neurotoxic medications as the risk for neurotoxicity increases

   3. Side effects
      a. Anorexia
      b. Nausea
      c. Vomiting
      d. Dizziness
      e. Malaise
      f. Mental confusion
      g. Joint pain
      h. Dermatitis
      i. Optic neuritis
      j. Peripheral neuritis
      k. Thrombocytopenia
      l. Increased uric acid levels
      m. Anaphylactoid reaction
   4. Implementation
      a. Assess for hypersensitivity
      b. Evaluate results of CBC and renal and liver function tests
      c. Obtain baseline visual acuity and color discrimination, especially to the color green
      d. Monitor for visual changes as altered color perception and decreased visual acuity, and if changes occur, discontinue medication and notify the physician
      e. Administer once every 24 hours and administer with food to decrease gastrointestinal (GI) upset
      f. Monitor uric acid concentrations and assess for painful or swollen joints or signs of gout
      g. Monitor intake and output (I&O) and for adequate renal function
      h. Assess mental status
      i. Monitor for dizziness and initiate safety precautions
      j. Assess for peripheral neuritis (numbness, tingling, or burning of the extremities) and if it occurs, notify the physician
   5. Client education
      a. Inform clients that they can prevent nausea related to the medications by taking the daily dose at bedtime or take prescribed antinausea medications as prescribed
      b. Instruct client not to skip doses and to take medication for the full length of the prescribed therapy
      c. Instruct client not to take any other medication without consulting the physician
      d. Advise client of the importance of follow-up physician visits, vision testing, and lab tests
      e. Instruct client to notify physician immediately if any visual problems occur, a rash, swelling and pain in the joints, or numbness, tingling, or burning in the hands or feet
D. Streptomycin
   1. Description
      a. An aminoglycoside antibiotic that is used

in conjunction with at least one other antitubercular medication

b. Bactericidal because of receptor binding action, interfering with protein synthesis in susceptible microorganisms

2. Contraindications and cautions

 a. Contraindicated in clients with hypersensitivity, myasthenia gravis, parkinsonism, or eighth cranial nerve damage

 b. Use with caution in the elderly, in neonates because of renal insufficiency and immaturity, and in young infants as it may cause central nervous system (CNS) depression

 c. The risk of toxicity increases when taken with other aminoglycosides, or nephrotoxic- or ototoxic-producing medications

3. Side effects (Box 57–1)

 a. Hypersensitivity

 b. Loss of vision

 c. Neuromuscular blockade

 d. Increased liver and renal function tests

 e. Signs of peripheral neuritis such as burning of the face or mouth

4. Implementation

 a. Assess for hypersensitivity

 b. Monitor liver and renal function tests

 c. Obtain baseline audiometric test and repeat every 1 to 2 months as the medication impairs the eighth cranial nerve

 d. Monitor for ototoxic, neurotoxic, and nephrotoxic reactions

 e. Assess hearing acuity

 f. Monitor for visual changes

 g. Assess hydration status and maintain adequate hydration during therapy

 h. Monitor I&O

 i. Assess urinalysis

 j. Monitor for superinfections

 k. Monitor for signs of peripheral neuritis

5. Client education

 a. Instruct client not to skip doses and to take medication for the full length of the prescribed therapy

---

BOX 57–1. Toxic Effects of Streptomycin

Nephrotoxicity	**Neurotoxicity**
Changes in urine output	Muscle twitching
Increased thirst	Tingling
Decreased appetite	Numbness
Nausea/vomiting	Changes in vision
Proteinuria	
Vestibular Ototoxicity	**Auditory Ototoxicity**
Dizziness	Ringing in the ears
Vertigo	Loss of hearing
	A full feeling in the ears

---

b. Instruct client not to take any other medication without consulting the physician

c. Advise client of the importance of follow-up physician visits and lab tests

d. Instruct client to notify physician if hearing loss, changes in vision, or urinary problems occur

E. Pyrazinamide

1. Description

 a. Exact mechanism of action is unknown

 b. May be bacteriostatic or bactericidal depending on its concentration at infection site and susceptibility of infecting bacteria

 c. Used in conjunction with at least one other antitubercular medication after failure or ineffectiveness of the primary medication occurs

2. Contraindications and cautions

 a. Contraindicated in clients with hypersensitivity

 b. Use with caution in clients with diabetes mellitus, renal impairment, gout, and in children

 c. May decrease the effects of allopurinol (Zyloprim), colchicine, probenecid (Benemid), sulfinpyrazone (Anturane)

 d. Cross-sensitivity is possible with isoniazid (INH), ethionamide (Trecator-SC), or niacin, nicotinic acid (Nicobid)

3. Side effects

 a. Increases liver function and uric acid levels

 b. Arthralgia

 c. Myalgia

 d. Photosensitivity

 e. Hepatotoxicity

 f. Thrombocytopenia

4. Implementation

 a. Assess for hypersensitivity

 b. Evaluate CBC, liver function tests, and uric acid levels

 c. Observe for hepatotoxic effects and if they occur, hold medication and notify the physician

 d. Assess for painful or swollen joints

 e. Evaluate blood glucose and diabetic status as diabetes may be difficult to control while on medication

5. Client education

 a. Instruct client to take the medication with food to reduce GI distress

 b. Instruct client to avoid sunlight or ultraviolet light until photosensitivity is determined

 c. Instruct client to notify the physician if any side effects occur

 d. Instruct client not to skip doses and to take medication for the full length of the prescribed therapy

 e. Instruct client not to take any other

medication without consulting the physician

f. Advise client of the importance of follow-up physician visits and lab tests

VI. Second-Line Medications (see Table 57–1)

A. Capreomycin Sulfate (Capastat Sulfate)
1. Description
   a. Mechanism of action is unknown
   b. Used to treat **MDR-TB** when significant resistance to other medications is expected
   c. Must be given by IM route
2. Contraindications and cautions
   a. The risk of nephrotoxicity, ototoxicity, and neuromuscular blockade is increased with the use of aminoglycosides or loop diuretics
   b. Use with caution in clients with renal insufficiency, acoustic nerve impairment, hepatic disorder, myasthenia gravis, and parkinsonism
   c. Do not administer to client receiving streptomycin
3. Side effects
   a. Nephrotoxicity
   b. Ototoxicity
   c. Neuromuscular blockade
4. Implementation
   a. Perform baseline audiometric testing
   b. Assess renal and hepatic electrolyte levels before administration
   c. Monitor I&O
   d. Reconstituted medication may be stored for 48 hours at room temperature
   e. Administer deep IM in a large muscle mass
   f. Rotate injection sites
   g. Observe injection site for redness, excessive bleeding, and inflammation
5. Client education
   a. Instruct client not to perform tasks that require mental alertness
   b. Instruct client to report any hearing loss, balance disturbances, respiratory difficulty, weakness, or signs of hypersensitivity reactions
B. Kanamycin (Kantrex)
1. Description
   a. An aminoglycoside antibiotic that is used in conjunction with at least one other antitubercular medication
   b. Bactericidal because of receptor binding action, interfering with protein synthesis in susceptible microorganisms
2. Contraindications and cautions
   a. Contraindicated in clients with hypersensitivity, neuromuscular disorders, or eighth cranial nerve damage
   b. Use with caution in the elderly, in neonates because of renal insufficiency

and immaturity, and in young infants as it may cause CNS depression
   c. The risk of toxicity increases when taken with other aminoglycosides or nephrotoxic- or ototoxic-producing medications
3. Side effects
   a. Hypersensitivity
   b. Pain and irritation at injection site
   c. Nephrotoxicity as evidenced by increased blood urea nitrogen (BUN) and serum creatinine
   d. Ototoxicity as evidenced by tinnitus, dizziness, ringing/roaring in the ears, and reduced hearing
   e. Neurotoxicity as evidenced by headache, dizziness, lethargy, tremors, and visual disturbances
   f. Superinfections
4. Implementation
   a. Assess for hypersensitivity
   b. Monitor liver and renal function tests
   c. Obtain baseline audiometric test and repeat every 1 to 2 months as the medication impairs the eighth cranial nerve
   d. Monitor for ototoxic, neurotoxic, and nephrotoxic reactions
   e. Assess hearing acuity
   f. Monitor for visual changes
   g. Assess hydration status and maintain adequate hydration during therapy
   h. Monitor I&O
   i. Assess urinalysis
   j. Monitor for superinfections
5. Client education
   a. Instruct client not to skip doses and to take medication for the full length of the prescribed therapy
   b. Instruct client not to take any other medication without consulting the physician
   c. Advise client of the importance of follow-up physician visits and lab tests
   d. Instruct client to notify physician if hearing loss, changes in vision, or urinary problems occur
C. Ethionamide (Trecator-SC)
1. Description
   a. Mechanism of action is unknown
   b. Used to treat **MDR-TB** when significant resistance to other medications is expected
2. Contraindications and cautions
   a. Contraindicated in clients with hypersensitivity
   b. Use with caution in clients with diabetes mellitus or renal dysfunction
3. Side effects
   a. Anorexia
   b. Nausea
   c. Vomiting

d. Metallic taste in the mouth
e. Orthostatic hypotension
f. Jaundice
g. Mental changes
h. Peripheral neuritis
i. Rash

4. Implementation
   a. Assess liver and renal function tests
   b. Monitor glucose levels in the diabetic client
   c. Administer pyridoxine (vitamin B$_6$) as prescribed to reduce the risk of neurotoxicity

5. Client education
   a. Instruct client to take medication with food or meals to minimize GI irritation
   b. Instruct client to change positions slowly
   c. Instruct client to report signs of a rash, which can progress to exfoliative dermatitis if the medication is not discontinued
   d. Instruct client to avoid alcohol
   e. Instruct client to report signs of jaundice
   f. Instruct client to report side effects of the medication if they occur

D. Aminosalicylate Sodium (sodium para-aminosalicylic acid [PAS])
   1. Description
      a. Inhibits folic acid metabolism in mycobacteria
      b. Used to treat **MDR-TB** when significant resistance to other medications is expected
   2. Contraindications and cautions
      a. Contraindicated with hypersensitivity to aminosalicylates, salicylates, or compounds containing para-aminophenyl group
      b. Aminobenzoates block the absorption of aminosalicylate sodium (sodium para-aminosalicylic acid [PAS])
   3. Side effects
      a. Bitter taste in the mouth
      b. GI tract irritation
      c. Allergic reactions
      d. Exfoliative dermatitis
      e. Blood dyscrasias
      f. Crystalluria
      g. Changes in thyroid function
   4. Implementation
      a. Assess for hypersensitivity
      b. Offer clear water to rinse mouth; chewing gum or hard candy to alleviate the bitter taste
      c. Encourage fluid intake to prevent crystalluria
      d. Monitor I&O
   5. Client education
      a. Instruct client to discard the medication if a purplish brown discoloration occurs
      b. Instruct client to take medication with food or antacid

c. Inform client that urine may turn red on contact with hypochlorite bleach if the bleach was used to clean a toilet
d. Instruct the client not to take aspirin or over-the-counter medications without the physician's approval
e. Inform diabetic client that a false-positive result can occur in glucose monitoring
f. Instruct client to report signs of blood dyscrasia as sore throat or mouth, malaise, fatigue, bruising, or bleeding

E. Cycloserine (Seromycin)
   1. Description
      a. Interferes with cell wall biosynthesis
      b. Used to treat **MDR-TB** when significant resistance to other medications is expected
   2. Contraindications and cautions
      a. Use of alcohol or ethionamide (Trecator-SC) increases the risk of seizures
      b. Use with caution in clients with epilepsy, depression, severe anxiety, psychosis, renal insufficiency, or the client that uses alcohol
   3. Side effects
      a. Hypersensitivity
      b. CNS reactions
      c. Neurotoxicity
      d. Seizures
      e. Congestive heart failure (CHF)
      f. Headache
      g. Vertigo
      h. Altered level of consciousness (LOC)
      i. Anxiety
      j. Confusion
      k. Depression
      l. Irritability
      m. Nervousness
      n. Mood changes
      o. Thoughts of suicide
   4. Implementation
      a. Monitor LOC
      b. Monitor for changes in mental status and thought processes
      c. Monitor renal and hepatic function tests
      d. Monitor serum drug level to avoid the risk of neurotoxicity; peak concentrations, measured 2 hours after dosing, should be 25 to 35 µg/mL
   5. Client education
      a. Instruct the client to take the medication after meals to prevent GI upset
      b. Instruct the client to avoid alcohol
      c. Instruct the client to report signs of a rash or signs of CNS toxicity
      d. Instruct client to avoid driving or performing tasks that require alertness until the reaction to the medication has been determined
      e. Advise client of the need for weekly serum drug levels

PRACTICE QUESTIONS

1. The nurse working on a medical respiratory nursing unit is caring for several clients with respiratory disorders. The nurse assesses which of the following clients on the nursing unit as being at the least risk for infection with tuberculosis?
   1 A woman newly immigrated from Korea
   2 An uninsured man who is homeless
   3 An elderly woman admitted from a long-term care facility
   4 A man who is an inspector for the U.S. Postal Service

2. The client has an order to receive purified protein derivative (PPD), 0.1 mL intradermally. The nurse administers the medication utilizing a tuberculin syringe with a:
   1 26-gauge, ⅝-inch needle inserted almost parallel to the skin with bevel side up
   2 26-gauge, ⅝-inch needle inserted at a 45-degree angle with bevel side down
   3 20-gauge, 1-inch needle inserted almost parallel to the skin with bevel side up
   4 20-gauge, 1-inch needle inserted at a 30-degree angle with bevel side down

3. The nurse is reading the PPD skin test for a client with no documented health problems. The site has no induration and a 1-mm area of ecchymosis. The nurse interprets that the result is:
   1 Positive
   2 Negative
   3 Uncertain
   4 Borderline

4. The client who is HIV-positive has had a Mantoux skin test. The results show a 7-mm area of induration. The nurse evaluates that this result is:
   1 Negative
   2 Borderline
   3 Uncertain
   4 Positive

5. The nurse reads the client's Mantoux skin test as positive. The nurse notes that previous tests were negative. The client becomes upset and asks the nurse what this means. The nurse's response is based on the understanding that the client has:
   1 No evidence of tuberculosis
   2 Systemic tuberculosis
   3 Pulmonary tuberculosis
   4 Exposure to tuberculosis

6. The nurse is caring for the client who had a PPD skin test implanted 48 hours ago upon admission to the nursing unit. The nurse reads the result as positive. Which of the following actions by the nurse has the highest priority?
   1 Call the physician
   2 Call the radiology department for a chest x-ray
   3 Document the finding in the client's record
   4 Call the employee health service department

7. The nurse is caring for the client with tuberculosis who is fearful of the disease and anxious about prognosis. In planning nursing care, the nurse incorporates which of the following as the best strategy to assist the client in coping with the illness?
   1 Encourage the client to visit with the pastoral care department chaplain
   2 Ask family members if they wish a psychiatric consult
   3 Provide reassurance that continued compliance with medication therapy is the most proactive way to cope with the disease
   4 Allow the client to deal with the disease in an individual fashion

8. The nurse has instructed the client diagnosed with tuberculosis about how to prevent the spread of infection after discharge. The nurse evaluates that the client needs further reinforcement of information if the client makes which of the following statements?
   1 "It's very important to wash my hands after I touch my mask, tissues, or body fluids."
   2 "I should cough into tissues and throw them away carefully."
   3 "It's important to cover my mouth if I laugh, sneeze, or cough."
   4 "I should use disposable plates, forks, and knives."

9. The nurse is caring for the client diagnosed with tuberculosis. Which of the following assessments, if made by the nurse, are not consistent with the usual clinical presentation of tuberculosis?
   1 Nonproductive or productive cough
   2 Anorexia and weight loss
   3 Chills and night sweats
   4 High-grade fever

10. The client is being discharged to home after 2 weeks with a diagnosis of tuberculosis (TB), and is worried about the possibility of infecting family and others. The nurse interprets that the client would get the most reassurance from which of the following accurate statements?
   1 The family does not need therapy, and the client will not be contagious after 1 month of medication therapy
   2 The family does not need therapy, and the client will not be contagious after 6 consecutive weeks of medication therapy
   3 The family will receive prophylactic therapy, and the client will not be contagious after 1 continuous week of medication therapy
   4 The family will be treated prophylactically, and the client will not be contagious after 2–3 consecutive weeks of medication therapy

11. The client diagnosed with tuberculosis is distressed over the loss of physical stamina and fatigue. The nurse plans to teach the client that:
    1 This is a short-lived problem, which should be gone within 1 week of medication therapy
    2 This is an unexpected finding with TB, but it should resolve within a month or so
    3 This is expected, and the client should very gradually increase activity as tolerated
    4 This is expected, and will last for at least a year

12. The nurse is teaching the client with tuberculosis (TB) about dietary elements that should be increased in the diet. The nurse suggests that the client increase intake of:
    1 Meats and citrus fruits
    2 Grains and broccoli
    3 Eggs and spinach
    4 Potatoes and fish

13. The nurse has conducted discharge teaching with the client who was diagnosed with tuberculosis. The client has been on medication for a week and a half. The nurse evaluates that the client has understood the information if the client makes which of the following statements?
    1 "I need to continue medication therapy for 2 months."
    2 "I should not be contagious after 2 to 3 weeks of medication therapy."
    3 "I can't shop at the mall for the next 6 months."
    4 "I can return to work if a sputum culture comes back negative."

14. The nurse is assessing the client with the typical clinical manifestations of tuberculosis (TB). The nurse expects the client to report having symptoms of fatigue and cough that have been present for:
    1 A day or two
    2 Almost a week
    3 One to two weeks
    4 Several weeks to months

15. The client with tuberculosis asks the nurse about precautions to take after discharge to prevent infection of others. The nurse develops a response to the client's question based on the understanding that:
    1 The client should maintain enteric precautions only
    2 The disease is transmitted by droplet nuclei
    3 Clothing and sheets should be bleached after each use
    4 Deep-pile carpet should be removed from the home

16. The nurse is preparing to give a bed bath to the immobilized client with tuberculosis (TB). The nurse should wear which of the following items when performing this care?
    1 Particulate respirator, gown, and gloves
    2 Particulate respirator and protective eyewear
    3 Surgical mask and gloves
    4 Surgical mask, gown, and protective eyewear

17. The client is being started on preventive treatment for tuberculosis (TB). The nurse teaches the client that the standard medication therapy consists of:
    1 Cycloserine (Seromycin) 1 g/day in divided doses for 6 to 12 months
    2 Rifampin (Rifadin) 600 mg/day for 3 to 6 months
    3 Isoniazid (INH) 300 mg/day for 6 to 12 months
    4 Capreomycin sulfate (Capastat Sulfate) 1 g/day for 2 to 4 months

18. The client with tuberculosis, whose status is being monitored in an ambulatory care clinic, asks the nurse when it is permissible to return to work. The nurse replies that the client may resume employment when:
    1 Two sputum cultures are negative
    2 Five sputum cultures are negative
    3 A sputum culture and a chest x-ray are negative
    4 A sputum culture and a PPD test are negative

19. The client with tuberculosis is being started on antituberculosis therapy with isoniazid (INH). The nurse assesses that which of the following baseline studies have been completed before giving the client the first dose?
    1 Coagulation times
    2 Electrolytes
    3 Serum creatinine
    4 Liver enzymes

20. The client being seen in an ambulatory clinic with a primary tuberculosis infection is fearful that the infection will progress to active disease. The client asks the nurse about the likelihood of this occurrence. The nurse responds to the client based on the understanding that the percent of clients who develop the disease after primary infection is only:
    1 1% to 2%
    2 2% to 5%
    3 5% to 15%
    4 25% to 50%

21. The nurse is admitting a client to the nursing unit who is suspected of having tuberculosis. The nurse plans to admit the client to a room that has:
    1 Ultraviolet light and three air exchanges per hour
    2 Ten air exchanges per hour and venting to the outside
    3 Venting to the outside and ultraviolet light
    4 Venting to the outside, six air exchanges per hour, and ultraviolet light

22. The client with HIV who has contracted tuberculosis asks the nurse how long the medication therapy lasts. The nurse responds that the duration of therapy would most likely be for at least:
    1 Six total months, and at least one month after cultures convert to negative
    2 Six total months, and at least 3 months after cultures convert to negative
    3 Nine total months, and at least 3 months after cultures convert to negative
    4 Nine total months, and at least 6 months after cultures convert to negative

23. The nurse has given the client with tuberculosis instructions for proper handling and disposal of respiratory secretions. The nurse evaluates that the client understands the instructions if the client verbalizes to:
    1 Wash hands at least four times a day
    2 Turn the head to the side if coughing or sneezing
    3 Discard used tissues in a plastic bag
    4 Brush the teeth and rinse the mouth once a day

24. The client with active tuberculosis (TB) demonstrates less than expected interest in learning about the prescribed medication therapy. The nurse assesses that this client may ultimately need:
    1 More medication instructions
    2 Involvement of the family in teaching
    3 Reinforcement by the physician
    4 Directly observed therapy

25. The nurse in an ambulatory clinic is preparing to administer a PPD skin test to a client who may have been exposed to an individual with TB. The client reports having had the bacille Calmette-Guérin (BCG) vaccine before moving to the United States from a foreign country. The nurse interprets that:
    1 The client's PPD will be negative, and will require sputum culture to diagnose
    2 The client's PPD will be positive, and will require chest x-ray for evaluation
    3 The client has no risk of acquiring TB, and needs no further workup
    4 The client is at more risk of acquiring TB, and needs immediate medication therapy

26. The client has been taking isoniazid (INH) for a month and a half. The client complains to the nurse about numbness, paresthesias, and tingling in the extremities. The nurse interprets that the client is experiencing:
    1 Small–blood vessel spasm
    2 Impaired peripheral circulation
    3 Hypercalcemia
    4 Peripheral neuritis

27. The client is to begin a 6-month course of therapy with isoniazid (INH). The nurse plans to teach the client to:
    1 Use alcohol in small amounts only
    2 Report yellow eyes or skin immediately
    3 Increase intake of Swiss or aged cheeses
    4 Avoid vitamin supplements during therapy

28. The client has been started on long-term therapy with rifampin (Rifadin). The nurse teaches the client that the medication:
    1 Should be double-dosed if one dose is forgotten
    2 May be discontinued independently if symptoms are gone in 3 months
    3 Causes orange discoloration of sweat, tears, urine, and feces
    4 Should always be taken with food or antacids

29. The nurse has given the client taking ethambutol HCl (Myambutol) information about the medication. The nurse evaluates that the client understands the instructions if the client states to immediately report:
    1 Distressing GI side effects
    2 Impaired sense of hearing
    3 Orange-red discoloration of body secretions
    4 Difficulty discriminating the color red from green

30. Cycloserine (Seromycin) is added to the medication regimen for a client with tuberculosis. Which of the following would the clinic nurse include in the client teaching plan regarding this medication?
    1 To take the medication before meals
    2 To return to the clinic weekly for serum drug levels
    3 It is not necessary to call the physician if a skin rash occurs
    4 It is not necessary to restrict alcohol intake with this medication

ANSWERS

1. **4**

Rationale: People at high risk for acquiring tuberculosis include immigrants from Asia, Africa, Latin America, and Oceania; medically underserved populations (ethnic minorities, homeless); those with HIV or other immunosuppressive disorders; residents in group settings (long-term care, correctional facilities); and health care workers.

Test-Taking Strategy: The question asks for the client at least risk. Begin to answer this question by eliminating options 1 and 2, since immigrants and the medically underserved are more frequently affected by the disease. To discriminate between the last two, the postal inspector, option 4, may or may not come in contact with many people, depending on job description. The client from the long-term care facility, however, lives in a group setting where a large number of people share a common environment 24 hours a day. This makes option 4 the correct answer, as the postal worker is at less overall risk than any of the others in the question.

Level of Cognitive Ability: Application
Phase of Nursing Process: Assessment
Client Needs: Health Promotion and Maintenance
Content Area: Adult Health/Respiratory

Reference

Black, J., & Matassarin-Jacobs, E. (1997). *Medical-surgical nursing: Clinical management for continuity of care* (5th ed.). Philadelphia: W. B. Saunders. p. 1140.

2. **1**

Rationale: A Mantoux skin test is administered by giving 0.1 mL of purified protein derivative (PPD) intradermally. This involves drawing the medication into a tuberculin syringe with a 25- to 27-gauge, ⅝-inch needle. The injection is given by inserting the needle as close as possible to a parallel position with the skin, and with the needle bevel facing up. This results in formation of a wheal when administered correctly.

Test-Taking Strategy: This question tests basic knowledge of intradermal injection technique. Remember that a tuberculin syringe is small and measures small amounts of medication dosages. Use the process of elimination to eliminate options 3 and 4 first, as these two options indicate larger syringes and needles. Remembering that the bevel side is up during administration of PPD will assist in directing you to the correct option from the remaining choices. If this question was difficult for you, take a few moments to review the basics of this injection technique!

Level of Cognitive Ability: Application
Phase of Nursing Process: Implementation
Client Needs: Physiological Integrity
Content Area: Adult Health/Respiratory

Reference

Taylor, C., Lillis, C., & LeMone, P. (1997). *Fundamentals of nursing: The art and science of nursing care* (3rd ed.). Philadelphia: Lippincott-Raven. pp. 825–826.

3. **2**

Rationale: A positive PPD reading has induration measuring 10 mm or more, and is considered abnormal. A small area of ecchymosis is insignificant and is probably related to injection technique.

Test-Taking Strategy: To answer this question accurately, it is necessary to know that induration is necessary for a positive response. Since the client in this question has no induration, the result can only be negative. Take time to review PPD skin testing results if you had difficulty with this question!

Level of Cognitive Ability: Analysis
Phase of Nursing Process: Analysis
Client Needs: Physiological Integrity
Content Area: Adult Health/Respiratory

Reference

Black, J., & Matassarin-Jacobs, E. (1997). *Medical-surgical nursing: Clinical management for continuity of care* (5th ed.). Philadelphia: W. B. Saunders. p. 720.

4. **4**

Rationale: The client with HIV is considered to have positive results on Mantoux skin testing with an area of 5 mm of induration or greater. The client without HIV is positive with induration greater than 10 mm. The client with HIV is immunosuppressed, making a smaller area of induration positive for this type of client. It is also possible for the client infected with HIV to have false-negative readings because of the immunosuppression factor.

Test-Taking Strategy: Use the process of elimination to answer the question. Begin by eliminating options 2 and 3 as they are similar. Remembering that the client with HIV is immunosuppressed will assist in directing you to option 4, the correct option. Take time now to review results of TB skin testing if you had difficulty with this question!

Level of Cognitive Ability: Analysis
Phase of Nursing Process: Evaluation
Client Needs: Physiological Integrity
Content Area: Adult Health/Respiratory

Reference

Ignatavicius, D., Workman, M., & Mishler, M. (1995). *Medical-surgical nursing: A nursing process approach* (2nd ed.). Philadelphia: W. B. Saunders. p. 720.

5. **4**

Rationale: A client who tests positive on a Mantoux skin test either has been exposed to tuberculosis or has inactive (dormant) tuberculosis. The client must then undergo chest x-ray and sputum culture to confirm the diagnosis.

Test-Taking Strategy: It is necessary to be familiar with the concept and possible results of Mantoux skin testing to be able to answer this question correctly. Use the process of elimination to eliminate options 2 and 3 first, as they are similar, both indicating the presence of TB. In selecting between options 1 and 4, review the case of the question, noting that the Mantoux skin test is positive. From this information, it is best to eliminate option 1. Because of the imformation of this item, be sure to review this area now if the question was difficult for you!

Level of Cognitive Ability: Analysis
Phase of Nursing Process: Analysis
Client Needs: Psychosocial Integrity
Content Area: Adult Health/Respiratory

Reference

Black, J., & Matassarin-Jacobs, E. (1997). *Medical-surgical nursing: Clinical management for continuity of care* (5th ed.). Philadelphia: W. B. Saunders. p. 1142.

6. **1**

Rationale: The nurse who obtains a positive PPD reading calls the physician immediately. The physician would order a chest x-ray to rule out whether the client has clinically active TB or old, healed lesions. Sputum culture would be done next as indicated to confirm the diagnosis of active TB. The client can be placed on TB precautions prophylactically until a final diagnosis is made.

Test-Taking Strategy: The question asks for the highest-priority action, which implies that one or all of the responses may be correct. Since the nurse may not order diagnostic tests, eliminate option 2 first. Likewise, option 4 can be eliminated, since calling employee health service is of no benefit to the client. To discriminate between the last two options, notifying the physician should have a higher priority than the documentation, even though they may both be done in the same narrow time period. Note that the question asks for the highest priority, not the first nursing action.

Level of Cognitive Ability: Application
Phase of Nursing Process: Implementation
Client Needs: Safe, Effective Care Environment
Content Area: Adult Health/Respiratory

Reference
Ignatavicius, D., Workman, M., & Mishler, M. (1995). *Medical-surgical nursing: A nursing process approach* (2nd ed.). Philadelphia: W. B. Saunders. p. 720.

7. **3**

Rationale: A primary role of the nurse in working with the client with tuberculosis is to teach the client about medication therapy. The anxious client may not absorb information optimally. The nurse continues to reinforce teaching using a variety of methods (repetition, teaching aids), and teaches the family about the medications as well. The most effective way of coping with the disease is to learn about the therapy that will eradicate it. This gives the client a measure of power over the situation and outcome.

Test-Taking Strategy: The question asks for the best strategy for coping with anxiety about the disease and its prognosis. This implies that more than one or all responses are partially or completely true. Options 2 and 4 are the least useful of the four choices, and may be eliminated first. Option 2 does not involve the client, and option 4 gives no active assistance to the client. The two remaining alternatives are both viable, but option 3 is the better of the two choices. TB is a controllable disease, and not necessarily a fatal one, which may help to discriminate between these plausible options.

Level of Cognitive Ability: Application
Phase of Nursing Process: Planning
Client Needs: Psychosocial Integrity
Content Area: Adult Health/Respiratory

Reference
Ignatavicius, D., Workman, M., & Mishler, M. (1995). *Medical-surgical nursing: A nursing process approach* (2nd ed.). Philadelphia: W. B. Saunders. p. 720.

8. **4**

Rationale: Since tuberculosis is transmitted by droplet, it cannot be carried on clothing, eating utensils, or other possessions. It is important to perform proper handwashing after contact with body substances, tissues, or face masks. The client should cover the mouth with a tissue with laughing, coughing, or sneezing, and dispose of tissues carefully. The client may also need to wear a tight-fitting mask as advised by the physician.

Test-Taking Strategy: Use the process of elimination to answer the question. Options 2 and 3 are obvious correct actions on the part of the client, and are therefore eliminated according to the way this question is worded. To discriminate between the last two options, you need to recall that TB is an airborne disease, so the organisms cannot be carried on inanimate objects. Using this knowledge, you would choose option 4 as the answer to the question as it is stated. Review client teaching points related to the prevention of the spread of TB now if you had difficulty with this question!

Level of Cognitive Ability: Analysis
Phase of Nursing Process: Evaluation
Client Needs: Health Promotion and Maintenance
Content Area: Adult Health/Respiratory

Reference
Black, J., & Matassarin-Jacobs, E. (1997). *Medical-surgical nursing: Clinical management for continuity of care* (5th ed.). Philadelphia: W. B. Saunders. p. 1146.

9. **4**

Rationale: The client with tuberculosis usually experiences cough (either productive or nonproductive), fatigue, anorexia, weight loss, dyspnea, hemoptysis, chest discomfort or pain, chills and sweats (which may occur at night), and a low-grade fever.

Test-Taking Strategy: Knowledge of the usual signs and symptoms of TB is needed to answer this question correctly. Options 1 and 2 may be eliminated first, since they are symptoms that are common in the client with TB. To discriminate between the last two, you need to know either that the client may get night sweats, or that the fever is low grade. Take time now to review the clinical manifestations associated with TB if you had difficulty with this question!

Level of Cognitive Ability: Application
Phase of Nursing Process: Assessment
Client Needs: Physiological Integrity
Content Area: Adult Health/Respiratory

Reference
Black, J., & Matassarin-Jacobs, E. (1997). *Medical-surgical nursing: Clinical management for continuity of care* (5th ed.). Philadelphia: W. B. Saunders. p. 1141.

10. **4**

Rationale: Family members or others who have been in close association with a client diagnosed with TB are placed on prophylactic therapy with isoniazid for 6 to 12 months. The client is usually not communicable after taking medication for 2 to 3 consecutive weeks. However, the client must take the full course of therapy (for 6 months or longer) to prevent reinfection or drug-resistant TB.

Test-Taking Strategy: Each of the options for this question has two parts. Remember that in order for the option to be correct, both of the parts must also be correct. Knowing that the family requires prophylactic therapy allows you to eliminate options 1 and 2. In order to discriminate between options 3 and 4, you need to recall that the client is not contagious after 2–3 weeks of therapy. Take time now to review the concepts related to the prevention of the spread of TB if you had difficulty with this question!

Level of Cognitive Ability: Analysis
Phase of Nursing Process: Analysis
Client Needs: Psychosocial Integrity
Content Area: Adult Health/Respiratory

Reference
Black, J., & Matassarin-Jacobs, E. (1997). *Medical-surgical nursing: Clinical management for continuity of care* (5th ed.). Philadelphia: W. B. Saunders. p. 1143.

11. **3**

Rationale: The client with TB has significant fatigue and loss of physical stamina. This can be very frightening for the client. The nurse teaches the client that this will resolve as the therapy progresses, and that the client should gradually increase activity as energy levels permit.

Test-Taking Strategy: A helpful concept to remember in answering this question is that fatigue due to respiratory problems may not resolve easily, and is an expected occurrence, due to tissue hypoxia. Knowing this, you can eliminate options 1 and 2 first. Discriminate between options 3 and 4 in this way: since the client is on medication therapy for 6 to 9 months, or even up to 12 months, it is not reasonable that the fatigue would last for "at least a year." Thus, option 3 is more plausible than option 4, and is the correct response.

Level of Cognitive Ability: Application
Phase of Nursing Process: Planning
Client Needs: Health Promotion and Maintenance
Content Area: Adult Health/Respiratory

Reference
Ignatavicius, D., Workman, M., & Mishler, M. (1995). *Medical-surgical nursing: A nursing process approach* (2nd ed.). Philadelphia: W. B. Saunders. pp. 721–722.

12. **1**

Rationale: The nurse teaches the client with TB to increase intake of protein, iron, and vitamin C. Foods rich in vitamin C include citrus fruits, berries, melons, pineapple, broccoli, cabbage, green peppers, tomatoes, potatoes, chard, kale, asparagus, and turnip greens. Food sources that are rich in iron include liver and other meats, from which 10% to 30% of available iron is absorbed. Less than 10% of iron is absorbed from eggs, and less than 5% is absorbed from grains and vegetables.

Test-Taking Strategy: This question is difficult. To answer it correctly, you must recall that the diet in tuberculosis should be high in protein, vitamin C, and calories. It is then necessary to know which types of foods contain these various nutrients. If you had difficulty with this question, take a few moments to review these nutritional concepts briefly now!

Level of Cognitive Ability: Application
Phase of Nursing Process: Implementation
Client Needs: Health Promotion and Maintenance
Content Area: Adult Health/Respiratory

References
Ignatavicius, D., Workman, M., & Mishler, M. (1995). *Medical-surgical nursing: A nursing process approach* (2nd ed.). Philadelphia: W. B. Saunders. p. 720.
Lutz, C., & Przytulski, K. (1997). *Nutrition and diet therapy* (2nd ed.). Philadelphia: F. A. Davis. pp. 107, 135.

13. **2**

Rationale: The client is continued on medication therapy for 6 to 12 months, depending on the situation. The client is generally considered to be not contagious after 2 to 3 weeks of medication therapy. The client is instructed to wear a mask if there will be exposure to crowds until the medication is effective in preventing transmission. The client is allowed to return to employment when the results of two sputum cultures are negative.

Test-Taking Strategy: This question is worded to make you look for a correct statement. Knowing that the medication therapy lasts for at least 6 months helps you to eliminate option 1 first. Knowing that two sputum cultures must be negative helps you to eliminate option 4 next. To discriminate between the remaining choices, knowing that the client is not contagious after 2–3 weeks of therapy helps you to choose option 2 and discard option 3, since they basically

oppose each other. If you had difficulty with this question, take time now to review the infectious period of TB!

Level of Cognitive Ability: Analysis
Phase of Nursing Process: Evaluation
Client Needs: Physiological Integrity
Content Area: Adult Health/Respiratory

Reference
Ignatavicius, D., Workman, M., & Mishler, M. (1995). *Medical-surgical nursing: A nursing process approach* (2nd ed.). Philadelphia: W. B. Saunders. p. 720.

14. **4**

Rationale: The client with tuberculosis may report symptoms that have been present for weeks or even months. The symptoms may include fatigue, lethargy, chest pain, anorexia and weight loss, night sweats, low-grade fever, cough with mucoid, or blood-streaked sputum. It may be the production of blood-tinged sputum that finally forces some clients to seek care.

Test-Taking Strategy: To answer this question, it is necessary to be familiar with the usual clinical manifestations of TB. Even without specific knowledge, you may be able to determine the correct answer by knowing that TB is an insidious health problem, which is hard to eradicate. It makes sense that if clients reported it early, it would not be the increasingly prominent health problem that it is.

Level of Cognitive Ability: Analysis
Phase of Nursing Process: Assessment
Client Needs: Physiological Integrity
Content Area: Adult Health/Respiratory

Reference
Ignatavicius, D., Workman, M., & Mishler, M. (1995). *Medical-surgical nursing: A nursing process approach* (2nd ed.). Philadelphia: W. B. Saunders. p. 719.

15. **2**

Rationale: Tuberculosis is spread by droplet nuclei, or the airborne route. The disease is not carried on objects such as clothing, eating utensils, linens, or furniture. Bleaching clothing and linens is unnecessary, although the client and family members should use good handwashing technique. It is unnecessary to remove carpeting from the home.

Test-Taking Strategy: Knowing that TB is not carried on inanimate objects helps you to eliminate options 3 and 4 first. To discriminate between options 1 and 2, you must be able to recall that the disease is transmitted by the airborne route. If you had difficulty with this question, take time now to review the transmission mode of TB!

Level of Cognitive Ability: Analysis
Phase of Nursing Process: Analysis
Client Needs: Safe, Effective Care Environment
Content Area: Adult Health/Respiratory

Reference
Black, J., & Matassarin-Jacobs, E. (1997). *Medical-surgical nursing: Clinical management for continuity of care* (5th ed.). Philadelphia: W. B. Saunders. p. 1146.

16. **1**

Rationale: The nurse who is in contact with a client with TB should wear an individually fitted particulate respirator. The nurse would also wear gloves as per universal precautions. The nurse wears a gown when there is a possibility that the clothing could become contaminated, such as when giving a bed bath.

Test-Taking Strategy: Knowing that the nurse should wear a particulate respirator helps you to eliminate options 3 and 4 first. Knowledge of basic universal precautions forces you to choose option 1 over option 2. In this nursing situation, option 1 is the best option!

Level of Cognitive Ability: Application
Phase of Nursing Process: Planning
Client Needs: Safe, Effective Care Environment
Content Area: Adult Health/Respiratory

Reference
Ignatavicius, D., Workman, M., & Mishler, M. (1995). *Medical-surgical nursing: A nursing process approach* (2nd ed.). Philadelphia: W. B. Saunders. p. 720.

17. **3**

Rationale: The most widely used first-line agent against tuberculosis is isoniazid (INH), which is given in doses up to 300 mg/day for 6 to 12 months. This is the medication that is used for preventive treatment. For the treatment of acute infection, it is given with other first-line agents such as rifampin, ethambutol HCl, streptomycin, and pyrazinamide. These medications are given in combination, with a specific timetable for each medication, and overall therapy lasts for a total of 6 to 12 months. Second-line agents include capreomycin, kanamycin, ethionamide, para-aminosalicylic acid, and cycloserine.

Test-Taking Strategy: The key phrase in the stem of this question is "preventive treatment." Knowing that a first-line agent is used as preventive treatment helps you to eliminate options 1 and 4. Knowing that isoniazid (INH) is the most commonly used medication helps you to choose it over rifampin. If you had difficulty with this question, take time now to review first-line and second-line medications!

Level of Cognitive Ability: Application
Phase of Nursing Process: Implementation
Client Needs: Physiological Integrity
Content Area: Adult Health/Respiratory

Reference
Black, J., & Matassarin-Jacobs, E. (1997). *Medical-surgical nursing: Clinical management for continuity of care* (5th ed.). Philadelphia: W. B. Saunders. pp. 1143–1145.

18. **1**

Rationale: The client must have sputum cultures performed every 2 to 4 weeks after initiation of antituberculosis medication therapy. The client may return to work when the results of two sputum cultures are negative, because the client is considered noninfectious at that point.

Test-Taking Strategy: Use the process of elimination to answer the question. Knowing that a positive PPD never reverts to negative helps you to automatically eliminate option 4 as a possible answer. To discriminate among the other three choices, it is necessary to know that two negative sputum cultures are required. If this question was difficult, review these key points now!

Level of Cognitive Ability: Application
Phase of Nursing Process: Implementation
Client Needs: Health Promotion and Maintenance
Content Area: Adult Health/Respiratory

Reference
Ignatavicius, D., Workman, M., & Mishler, M. (1995). *Medical-surgical nursing: A nursing process approach* (2nd ed.). Philadelphia: W. B. Saunders. p. 720.

19. **4**

Rationale: Isoniazid (INH) therapy can cause an elevation of hepatic enzymes and hepatitis. Therefore, liver enzymes are monitored when therapy is initiated and during the first 3 months of therapy. They may be monitored longer in the client who is over age 50 or abuses alcohol.

Test-Taking Strategy: In order to answer this question correctly, it is necessary to know that this medication can be toxic to the liver. Take time now to review the adverse effects of the various anti-TB medications if this is an area that is unfamiliar to you!

Level of Cognitive Ability: Analysis
Phase of Nursing Process: Assessment
Client Needs: Physiological Integrity
Content Area: Adult Health/Respiratory

Reference
Black, J., & Matassarin-Jacobs, E. (1997). *Medical-surgical nursing: Clinical management for continuity of care* (5th ed.). Philadelphia: W. B. Saunders. p. 1144.

20. **3**

Rationale: A minority of persons (5%–15%) with primary tuberculosis infection actually progress to active disease. The nurse also can reassure the client that preventive medication therapy will be initiated.

Test-Taking Strategy: This is a difficult question if you are unfamiliar with content associated with primary tuberculosis infection. Specific knowledge is needed to answer this question. TB is a health problem that is resurfacing in the nation, and may be a popular area for testing on NCLEX-RN. It would be helpful to review information in this area if you had difficulty with this question!

Level of Cognitive Ability: Analysis
Phase of Nursing Process: Analysis
Client Needs: Psychosocial Integrity
Content Area: Adult Health/Respiratory

References
Black, J., & Matassarin-Jacobs, E. (1997). *Medical-surgical nursing: Clinical management for continuity of care* (5th ed.). Philadelphia: W. B. Saunders. pp. 1142–1143.
Ignatavicius, D., Workman, M., & Mishler, M. (1995). *Medical-surgical nursing: A nursing process approach* (2nd ed.). Philadelphia: W. B. Saunders. p. 718.

21. **4**

Rationale: The client is admitted to a private room that has at least six air exchanges per hour, and which has negative pressure in relation to surrounding areas. The room should be vented to the outside and should have ultraviolet lights installed.

Test-Taking Strategy: Begin to answer this question by recalling the specific requirements of physical facilities that are used in the care of clients with TB. Knowing that the air must vent to the outside helps to eliminate option 1. Knowing that ultraviolet light is useful in killing these organisms helps you to eliminate option 2. To discriminate between the last two options, it is necessary to know that there must be an airflow system that allows for at least six air exchanges per hour. If you had difficulty with this question, take time now to review the care to the hospitalized client with TB!

Level of Cognitive Ability: Application
Phase of Nursing Process: Planning
Client Needs: Safe, Effective Care Environment
Content Area: Adult Health/Respiratory

Reference
Black, J., & Matassarin-Jacobs, E. (1997). *Medical-surgical nursing: Clinical management for continuity of care* (5th ed.). Philadelphia: W. B. Saunders. p. 1143.

22. **4**

Rationale: The client with tuberculosis who is coinfected with HIV requires that antituberculosis therapy last longer than usual. The current guideline is for a total of 9 months, and at least 6 months after sputum cultures convert to negative.

Test-Taking Strategy: This question asks specific but important formation. Knowing that the client with HIV requires longer baseline antituberculosis therapy helps you to eliminate options 1 and 2 first. To discriminate between the last two, it is necessary to recall that sputum cultures must be negative for 6 months before terminating medication therapy, due to the immunosuppressed status of the client. If you had difficulty with this question, take time now to review medication therapy for tuberculosis in the immunosuppressed client!

Level of Cognitive Ability: Application
Phase of Nursing Process: Implementation
Client Needs: Physiological Integrity
Content Area: Adult Health/Respiratory

Reference
Ignatavicius, D., Workman, M., & Mishler, M. (1995). *Medical-surgical nursing: A nursing process approach* (2nd ed.). Philadelphia: W. B. Saunders. p. 721.

23. **3**

Rationale: The client with tuberculosis should wash the hands carefully after each contact with respiratory secretions. The client should cover the mouth and nose when laughing, sneezing, or coughing. Used tissues are discarded in a plastic bag. Oral care is done as for any other client.

Test-Taking Strategy: Note that the question specifically asks for information about handling and disposal of secretions. The only options that address this topic directly are options 2 and 3, so options 1 and 4 are eliminated. Since turning the head to the side for coughing and sneezing does not specifically address the handling of secretions, eliminate that option. Disposal of tissues in a plastic bag is correct, and is therefore chosen as the more correct response.

Level of Cognitive Ability: Analysis
Phase of Nursing Process: Evaluation
Client Needs: Health Promotion and Maintenance
Content Area: Adult Health/Respiratory

Reference
Ignatavicius, D., Workman, M., & Mishler, M. (1995). *Medical-surgical nursing: A nursing process approach* (2nd ed.). Philadelphia: W. B. Saunders. p. 720.

24. **4**

Rationale: TB is a highly communicable disease that is reportable to the local public health departments. Each of these agencies has regulations that may be enforced to ensure compliance with TB therapy. The client may be required to have directly observed therapy to reduce the risk to the general public. This involves having a responsible person actually observe the client taking the medication each day.

Test-Taking Strategy: Note the word "ultimately" in the stem. This implies an action that would be taken as a last resort. Knowing that TB is a highly communicable, reportable disease, you would eliminate options 1, 2, and

then 3 as a final action. This leaves directly observed therapy, which is closely overseen and enforced through the public health department.

Level of Cognitive Ability: Analysis
Phase of Nursing Process: Assessment
Client Needs: Psychosocial Integrity
Content Area: Adult Health/Respiratory

Reference
Black, J., & Matassarin-Jacobs, E. (1997). *Medical-surgical nursing: Clinical management for continuity of care* (5th ed.). Philadelphia: W. B. Saunders. pp. 1145–1146.

25. **2**

Rationale: The bacille Calmette-Guérin (BCG) vaccine is routinely given in many foreign countries to enhance resistance to TB. The vaccine uses attenuated tubercle bacilli, so the client will always test positive on PPD skin testing. This client needs to be evaluated for TB with a chest x-ray.

Test-Taking Strategy: Knowledge of this specific vaccine is necessary to answer this question correctly. If you are unfamiliar with it, take a few moments now to review it briefly. It has important implications for clients who have received it, in terms of monitoring TB exposure.

Level of Cognitive Ability: Analysis
Phase of Nursing Process: Analysis
Client Needs: Physiological Integrity
Content Area: Adult Health/Respiratory

Reference
Ignatavicius, D., Workman, M., & Mishler, M. (1995). *Medical-surgical nursing: A nursing process approach* (2nd ed.). Philadelphia: W. B. Saunders. p. 719.

26. **4**

Rationale: A common side effect of INH is peripheral neuritis. This is manifested by numbness, tingling, and paresthesias in the extremities. This side effect can be minimized with pyridoxine (vitamin B_6) intake.

Test-Taking Strategy: Options 1 and 2 would not yield the symptoms presented in the stem, but instead would be manifested by pallor and coolness. Thus, these two may be eliminated first. To discriminate between the last two, you should know either that peripheral neuritis is a side effect of the medication or that these signs and symptoms do not correlate with hypercalcemia. Take time now to review the side effects associated with INH if you had difficulty with this question!

Level of Cognitive Ability: Analysis
Phase of Nursing Process: Analysis
Client Needs: Physiological Integrity
Content Area: Adult Health/Respiratory

Reference
Hodgson, B., & Kizior, R. (1999). *Saunders' nursing drug handbook 1999.* Philadelphia: W. B. Saunders. p. 551.

27. **2**

Rationale: INH is hepatotoxic, and therefore the client is taught to report signs and symptoms of hepatitis immediately (which includes yellow skin and sclera). For the same reason, alcohol should be avoided during therapy. The client should avoid intake of Swiss cheese, fish such as tuna, and foods containing tyramine because they may cause a reaction characterized by redness and itching of the skin, flushing, sweating, fast heartbeat, headache, or lightheadedness. The client can avoid developing peripheral neuritis by increasing intake of pyridoxine (vitamin B_6) during the course of INH therapy.

Test-Taking Strategy: Use the process of elimination to answer the question. Since alcohol intake is prohibited with many medications, option 1 should be eliminated first. Since the client receiving this medication typically is supplemented with vitamin B₆, option 4 is incorrect and is eliminated next. Knowing that the medication is hepatotoxic allows you to choose option 2 over option 3. If you had difficulty with this question, take time now to review this important medication!

Level of Cognitive Ability: Application
Phase of Nursing Process: Planning
Client Needs: Health Promotion and Maintenance
Content Area: Adult Health/Respiratory

Reference

Deglin, J., & Vallerand, A. (1997). *Davis's drug guide for nurses* (5th ed.). Philadelphia: F. A. Davis. p. 664.

28. **3**

Rationale: Rifampin should be taken exactly as directed. Doses should not be doubled or skipped. The client should not stop therapy until directed to do so by a physician. The medication should be administered on an empty stomach unless it causes GI upset, and then it may be taken with food. Antacids, if prescribed, should be taken at least 1 hour before the medication. Rifampin causes orange-red discoloration to body secretions, and will permanently stain soft contact lenses.

Test-Taking Strategy: Options 1 and 2 are examples of poor medication advice in general, and are eliminated first. Knowing that this medication causes discoloration of body secretions helps you to choose option 3 over option 4. You may also choose option 3 by noting the word "always" in option 4. It is not often that a distracter containing such an absolute descriptor is correct. If you had difficulty with this question, take time now to review the side effects associated with this medication!

Level of Cognitive Ability: Application
Phase of Nursing Process: Implementation
Client Needs: Physiological Integrity
Content Area: Adult Health/Respiratory

Reference

Pinnell, N. (1996). *Nursing pharmacology.* Philadelphia: W. B. Saunders. pp. 771–772.

29. **4**

Rationale: Ethambutol HCl causes optic neuritis, which decreases visual acuity and the ability to discriminate between the colors red and green. This poses a potential safety haz-

ard when driving a motor vehicle. The client is taught to report this symptom immediately. The client is also taught to take the medication with food if GI upset occurs. Impaired hearing results from antitubercular therapy with streptomycin. Orange-red discoloration of secretions occurs with rifampin (Rifadin).

Test-Taking Strategy: Option 1 is the least likely symptom to report; rather, it should be managed by taking the medication with food. Thus, this option may be eliminated first. To discriminate among the other options, it is necessary to know that this medication causes optic neuritis, and causing difficulty with red-green discrimination. If this question was difficult, take a moment to review antitubercular medications, since the incorrect options for this question are typical side effects of other antitubercular medications!

Level of Cognitive Ability: Analysis
Phase of Nursing Process: Evaluation
Client Needs: Health Promotion and Maintenance
Content Area: Adult Health/Respiratory

Reference

Pinnell, N. (1996). *Nursing pharmacology.* Philadelphia: W. B. Saunders. p. 770.

30. **2**

Rationale: Cycloserine (Seromycin) is an antitubercular medication that requires weekly serum drug level determinations to monitor for the potential of neurotoxicity. Serum drug levels less than 30 mg/mL reduce the incidence of neurotoxicity. The medication needs to be taken after meals to prevent GI irritation. The client needs to be instructed to notify the physician if a skin rash or early signs of CNS toxicity are noted. Alcohol needs to be avoided as it increases the risk of seizure activity.

Test-Taking Strategy: Knowledge regarding the medication is helpful to answer the question. Use the process of elimination to answer the question. Eliminate options 3 and 4 first, as they are the least likely correct options. From this point, knowing that the medication level needs to be monitored will assist you in selecting the correct option. If you had difficulty with this question, take time now to review this medication!

Level of Cognitive Ability: Analysis
Phase of Nursing Process: Planning
Client Needs: Health Promotion and Maintenance
Content Area: Adult Health/Respiratory

Reference

Pinnell, N. (1996). *Nursing pharmacology.* Philadelphia: W. B. Saunders. p. 775.

BIBLIOGRAPHY

Black, J., & Matassarin-Jacobs, E. (1997). *Medical-surgical nursing: Clinical management for continuity of care* (5th ed.). Philadelphia: W. B. Saunders.

Chernecky, C., & Berger, B. (1997). *Laboratory tests and diagnostic procedures* (2nd ed.). Philadelphia: W. B. Saunders.

Deglin, J., & Vallerand, A. (1997). *Davis's drug guide for nurses* (5th ed.). Philadelphia: F. A. Davis.

Hodgson, B., & Kizior, R. (1999). *Saunders nursing drug handbook 1999.* Philadelphia: W. B. Saunders.

Ignatavicius, D., Workman, M., & Mishler, M. (1995). *Medical-surgical nursing: A nursing process approach* (2nd ed.). Philadelphia: W. B. Saunders.

Kuhn, M. (1998). *Pharmacotherapeutics: A nursing process approach* (4th ed.). Philadelphia: F. A. Davis.

Lammon, C., Foote, A., Leli, P., et al. (1995). *Clinical nursing skills.* Philadelphia: W. B. Saunders.

Lehne, R. (1998). *Pharmacology for nursing care* (3rd ed.). Philadelphia: W. B. Saunders.

Luckmann, J. (1997). *Saunders manual of nursing care.* Philadelphia: W. B. Saunders.

Lutz, C., & Przytulski, K. (1997). *Nutrition and diet therapy* (2nd ed.). Philadelphia: F. A. Davis.

O'Toole, M. (ed.). (1997). *Miller-Keane encyclopedia & dictionary of medicine, nursing, & allied health* (6th ed.). Philadelphia: W. B. Saunders.

Pinnell, N. (1996). *Nursing pharmacology.* Philadelphia: W. B. Saunders.

CHAPTER 58

Respiratory Medications

I. Sympathomimetic Bronchodilators
(Box 58-1)

A. Description
1. Dilates the airways of the respiratory tree, thereby making air exchange and respiration easier for the client
2. Relaxes the smooth muscle of the bronchi
3. Used to treat allergic rhinitis and sinusitis, acute bronchospasm, acute and chronic asthma, bronchitis, **chronic obstructive pulmonary disease**, and **emphysema**
4. Contraindicated in individuals with hypersensitivity, peptic ulcer disease, severe cardiac disease and cardiac dysrhythmias, hyperthyroidism, and uncontrolled seizure disorders
5. Used cautiously with clients with hypertension and diabetes mellitus
6. Use with caution in clients with narrow-angle glaucoma

B. Side Effects
1. Tachycardia
2. Dizziness
3. May increase blood glucose levels
4. Headaches
5. Nausea and vomiting
6. Tremors
7. Nervousness
8. Palpitations
9. Muscle cramping in extremities
10. Mouth dryness and throat irritation with inhalers
11. Tolerance and paradoxic bronchoconstriction with inhalers

C. Implementation
1. Assess vital signs
2. Monitor for cardiac dysrhythmias
3. Assess for wheezing, decreased breath sounds, and sputum production
4. Monitor for confusion and restlessness
5. Provide adequate hydration
6. Administer oral medications after meals to decrease gastrointestinal (GI) upset
7. Instruct client in the side effects of bronchodilators
8. Instruct client how to monitor pulse and to report any abnormalities to the physician
9. Instruct client how to use inhaler or nebulizer and how to monitor the amount of medication remaining in an inhaler canister
10. Instruct client to avoid over-the-counter medications
11. Instruct client to avoid smoking
12. Instruct diabetic client to monitor blood glucose levels
13. Instruct clients with asthma to wear Medic-Alert bracelets

II. Methylxanthine-Derivative Bronchodilators
(Box 58-2)

A. Description
1. Relaxes smooth muscle and decreases bronchospasm

BOX 58-1. Sympathomimetics

ADRENERGIC BRONCHODILATORS

Ephedrine sulfate (Ephedol)
Epinephrine (Adrenalin)
Albuterol (Proventil, Ventolin)
Bitolterol mesylate (Tornalate)
Isoetharine HCl (Bronkosol)
Isoproterenol (Isuprel)
Metaproterenol sulfate (Alupent, Metaprel)
Pirbuterol acetate (Maxair)
Salmeterol (Serevent)
Terbutaline sulfate (Brethine, Bricanyl)

ANTICHOLINERGIC

Ipratropium bromide (Atrovent)

BOX 58–2. Methylxanthine (Xanthine) Derivatives

Aminophylline (Truphylline)
Theophylline
Theophylline (Aerolate, Slo-phyllin, Theolair)
Theophylline (Theo-Dur, Slo-Bid, Theo-24,
  Uni-Dur, Uniphyl)
Oxtriphylline (Choledyl)

---

2. Stimulates the CNS and respiration, dilates coronary and pulmonary vessels, and causes diuresis
3. Used to treat asthma
4. Contraindicated in individuals with hypersensitivity, peptic ulcer disease, severe cardiac disease and cardiac dysrhythmias, hyperthyroidism and uncontrolled seizure disorders
5. Used cautiously with clients with hypertension and diabetes mellitus
6. Theophylline increases the risk of digitalis toxicity, decreases the effects of lithium, and decreases theophylline levels when administered with phenytoin (Dilantin)
7. If theophylline and a beta-adrenergic agonist are given together, cardiac dysrhythmias may result
8. Beta blockers, cimetidine (Tagamet), and erythromycin increase the effects of theophylline
9. Barbiturate and carbamazepine (Tegretol) decrease the effects of theophylline

B. Side Effects
1. Anorexia, nausea, vomiting
2. Gastric irritation
3. Dizziness
4. Palpitations
5. Tachycardia
6. Dysrhythmias
7. Hypotension
8. Headache
9. CNS stimulation
10. Muscle tremors
11. Seizures
12. Restlessness, irritability, and insomnia
13. Flushing
14. Rash
15. Hyperglycemia
16. Decreased clotting time

C. Implementation
1. Monitor vital signs
2. Assess for cardiac dysrhythmias
3. Monitor for decreased breath sounds, wheezing, cough, and sputum production
4. Monitor for confusion and restlessness
5. Administer with food to avoid GI distress
6. Instruct client not to crush enteric-coated or sustained-release tablets or capsules
7. Instruct client to increase fluid intake
8. Instruct client to avoid caffeine products such as coffee, tea, cola, and chocolate

9. Administer medication at regular intervals around the clock to maintain a sustained therapeutic level
10. Advise client not to take over-the-counter medications
11. Instruct client to monitor pulse rate and to report any abnormalities to the physician
12. Monitor for a therapeutic serum theophylline level of 10–20 µg/mL
13. Note that toxicity is likely to occur when the serum level is greater than 20 µg/mL
14. IV aminophylline or theophylline preparations should be administered slowly and always via an infusion pump

III. Glucocorticoids (Steroids) (Box 58–3)

A. Description
1. Anti-inflammatory
2. Reduces edema of the airways
B. Side Effects
1. Anorexia or increased appetite
2. GI irritation
3. Impaired immune response
4. Throat irritation, hoarseness, dry mouth, and coughing with the use of inhalers
5. Fungal infections with the use of inhalers
6. Fluid retention
7. Puffy eyelids
8. Edema in the lower extremities
9. Weight gain
10. Moon face
11. Thinning of the skin and bruising
12. Mood swings
13. Hyperglycemia
14. Hypokalemia
C. Implementation
1. Monitor vital signs
2. Monitor for edema
3. Monitor weight
4. Administer oral medications with food, milk, or antacids
5. Monitor glucose and electrolyte levels
6. Instruct client in the use of medication
7. Instruct client to avoid exposure to infections
8. Instruct client to avoid sodium in the diet
9. Instruct client in eating foods high in potassium
10. Instruct client to avoid missing, changing, or withdrawing the medication abruptly
11. Instruct client to wear a Medic-Alert bracelet

BOX 58–3. Glucocorticoids (Steroids)

Beclomethasone (Vanceril, Beclovent)
Triamcinolone (Amcort, Aristocort, Azmacort)
Fluticasone (Flonase, Flovent)
Dexamethasone (Decadron)
Hydrocortisone (Cortef)
Prednisone (Deltasone)

BOX 58–4. Mast-Cell Stabilizer
Cromolyn sodium (Intal)

IV. Mast-Cell Stabilizer (Box 58–4)

A. Description
1. An antiasthmatic, antiallergic, and a mast-cell stabilizer that inhibits mast-cell release after exposure to antigens
2. Cromolyn sodium (Intal) is not an antihistamine but is used for the treatment of allergic rhinitis, bronchial asthma, and exercised-induced bronchospasm
3. Cromolyn sodium is contraindicated in clients with known hypersensitivity
4. Oral cromolyn sodium is used with caution in clients with impaired hepatic or renal function

B. Side effects
1. Cough or bronchospasm following inhalation
2. Nasal sting or sneezing following inhalation
3. Bad taste in the mouth

C. Implementation
1. Monitor vital signs
2. Monitor respirations and assess lung sounds for rhonchi, wheezing, and rales
3. Instruct client to drink a few sips of water before and after inhalation to prevent cough and bad taste in the mouth
4. Administer oral capsules at least 30 minutes before meals
5. Instruct client not to discontinue medication abruptly because a rebound asthmatic attack can occur

V. Leukotriene Receptor Antagonist (Box 58–5)

A. Description
1. Used in the prophylaxis and chronic treatment of bronchial asthma
2. Not used for acute asthma episodes
3. Inhibits bronchoconstriction caused by specific antigens
4. Reduces airway edema and smooth muscle constriction
5. Contraindicated with hypersensitivity and in breast-feeding mothers
6. Used with caution in clients with impaired hepatic function
7. Coadministration of inhaled corticosteroids increases the risk of upper respiratory infection

BOX 58–5. Leukotriene Receptor Antagonist
Zafirlukast (Accolate)

B. Side Effects
1. Headache
2. Nausea
3. Vomiting
4. Dyspepsia
5. Diarrhea
6. Generalized pain
7. Myalgia
8. Fever
9. Dizziness

C. Implementation
1. Assess liver function laboratory values
2. Monitor vital signs
3. Assess lung sounds for rhonchi, wheezing, and rales
4. Monitor for cyanosis
5. Instruct client to take medication 1 hour before or 2 hours after meals
6. Instruct client to increase fluid intake
7. Instruct client not to discontinue medication and to take as prescribed even during symptom-free periods

VI. Antihistamines (Box 58–6)

A. Description
1. Called histamine antagonists or H_1 blockers and these medications compete with histamine for receptor sites, thus preventing a histamine response
2. When the H_1 receptor is stimulated, the extravascular smooth muscles including those lining the nasal cavity are constricted
3. Decrease nasopharyngeal secretions by blocking the H_1 receptor and decrease nasal itching that causes sneezing
4. Used for the common cold, rhinitis, nausea and vomiting, motion sickness, urticaria, and as a sleep aid

BOX 58–6. Antihistamines
Chlorpheniramine maleate (Chlor-Trimeton)
Diphenhydramine (Benadryl)
Promethazine HCl (Phenergan)
Trimeprazine tartrate (Temaril)
Hydroxyzine (Atarax, Vistaril)
Terfenadine (Seldane)
Clemastine fumarate (Tavist)
Tripelennamine HCl (Pelamine)
Azatadine maleate (Optimine)
Cyproheptadine HCl (Periactin)
Brompheniramine maleate (Dimetane)
Dexchlorpheniramine maleate (Polaramine)
Triprolidine and pseudoephedrine (Actifed)
Triprolidine HCl (Alleract)
Astemizole (Hismanal)
Cetirizine (Zyrtec)
Loratadine (Claritin)
Methdilazine HCl (Tacaryl)

BOX 58–7. Nasal and Systemic Decongestants

Ephedrine
Naphazoline HCl (Allerest)
Oxymetazoline HCl (Afrin)
Phenylephrine HCl (Neo-Synephrine)
Phenylpropanolamine HCl (Dimetapp)
Pseudoephedrine (Sudafed)
Tetrahydrozoline HCl (Tyzine)
Xylometazoline HCl (Otrivin)

5. Diphenhydramine (Benadryl) has anticholinergic effects and should be avoided in clients with narrow-angle glaucoma
6. Can cause CNS depression if taken with alcohol, narcotics, hypnotics, or barbiturates
7. Used with caution in clients with chronic obstructive pulmonary disease (COPD) because of their drying effect

B. Side Effects
1. Drowsiness
2. Dizziness
3. Fatigue
4. Urinary retention
5. Blurred vision
6. Wheezing
7. Constipation
8. Dry mouth
9. GI irritation
10. Hypotension
11. Hearing disturbances
12. Photosensitivity
13. Nervousness and irritability
14. Nightmares
15. Confusion

C. Implementation
1. Monitor vital signs
2. Monitor for signs of urinary dysfunction
3. Administer with food or milk
4. Avoid subcutaneous (SC) injection and administer intramuscular (IM) in a large muscle if parenteral route is prescribed
5. Instruct client to avoid hazardous activities
6. Instruct client to avoid alcohol and other CNS depressants
7. Instruct client taking medication for motion sickness to take the medication 30 minutes before the event, and then before meals and at bedtime during the event
8. Instruct client to take hard candy or ice chips for dry mouth

VII. Nasal and Systemic Decongestants
(Box 58–7)

A. Description
1. Stimulates the alpha-adrenergic receptors, thus producing vasoconstriction of the capillaries within the nasal mucosa
2. Shrinks nasal mucosal membranes and reduces fluid secretion

3. Used for allergic rhinitis, hay fever, and acute coryza (profuse nasal discharge)
4. Contraindicated or used with extreme caution in clients with hypertension, cardiac disease, hyperthyroidism, and diabetes mellitus
5. Nasal decongestants can cause tolerance and rebound nasal congestion (vasodilation), caused by irritation of the nasal mucosa, and should not be used for more than 48 hours

B. Side Effects
1. Frequent use of decongestants, especially nasal sprays or drops, can result in tolerance and rebound nasal congestion (vasodilation), caused by irritation of the nasal mucosa
2. Nervousness
3. Restlessness
4. Hypertension
5. Hyperglycemia

C. Implementation
1. Assess client for existing medical disorders
2. Monitor for cardiac dysrhythmias
3. Monitor blood glucose levels
4. Instruct client to avoid caffeine in large amounts because it can increase restlessness and palpitations
5. Instruct client in the importance of limiting the use of nasal sprays and drops

VIII. Mucolytic Medications (Expectorants)
(Box 58–8)

A. Description
1. Loosen bronchial secretions so that they can be eliminated with coughing
2. Used for dry unproductive cough and to stimulate bronchial secretions
3. Guaifenesin and dextromethorphan (Robitussin-DM) are both an antitussive and expectorant
4. Mucolytic agents with dextromethorphan should not be used with clients with COPD because they suppress the cough
5. Acetylcysteine (Mucomyst) can increase airway resistance and should not be used in clients with asthma

B. Side Effects
1. GI irritation
2. Skin rash
3. Oropharyngeal irritation

BOX 58–8. Mucolytic Agents (Expectorants)

Guaifenesin (glyceryl guaiacolate) (Glycotuss, Humibid, Robitussin)
Iodinated glycerol (Iophen)
Potassium iodide (SSKI)
Acetylcysteine (Mucomyst)
Guaifenesin and dextromethorphan (Robitussin-DM)

C. Implementation
1. Instruct client to take medication with a full glass of water to loosen mucus
2. Instruct client to drink the diluted liquid form of saturated solution of potassium iodide (SSKI) through a straw to avoid discoloration of tooth enamel
3. Avoid the administration of potassium iodide if hyperkalemia is present
4. Instruct client to maintain an adequate fluid intake
5. Encourage client to cough and deep-breathe
6. Acetylcysteine sodium (Mucomyst), administered by nebulization, should not be mixed with another medication
7. Acetylcysteine sodium (Mucomyst), if administered with a bronchodilator. The bronchodilator should be administered 5 minutes before the Mucomyst
8. Monitor for side effects of acetylcysteine (Mucomyst) such as nausea and vomiting, stomatitis, and runny nose

IX. Antitussives (Box 58–9)

A. Description
1. Act on the cough control center in the medulla to suppress the cough reflex
2. Used for a cough that is nonproductive and irritating
B. Side Effects
1. Drowsiness
2. GI irritation
3. Nausea
4. Dizziness
5. Sedation
6. Dry mouth
7. Constipation
8. Respiratory depression
C. Implementation
1. Instruct client that if the cough lasts longer than 1 week and a fever or rash occurs, the physician should be notified
2. Encourage client to take adequate fluids with the medication
3. Encourage client to sleep with the head of the bed elevated

---

BOX 58–9. Antitussives

NARCOTICS
Codeine
Guaifenesin and codeine (Cheracol Cough, Robitussin A-C)
Hydrocodone bitartrate (Hycodan)

NONNARCOTICS
Benzonatate (Tessalon)
Diphenhydramine HCl (Benadryl)
Promethazine with dextromethorphan

BOX 58–10. Narcotic Antagonist

Naloxone HCl (Narcan)

---

4. Instruct client to avoid hazardous activities
5. Note that drug dependency can occur
6. Avoid administration in the client with a head injury or postoperative cranial surgery
7. Avoid administering to clients using narcotics, sedative hypnotics, barbiturates, or antidepressants, as CNS depression can occur
8. Instruct client to avoid the use of alcohol

X. Narcotic Antagonist (Box 58–10)

A. Description
1. Reverses respiratory depression in narcotic overdose
2. Avoid use in non-narcotic respiratory depression
B. Side Effects
1. CNS depression
2. Nausea
3. Vomiting
4. Tremors
5. Sweating
6. Increased blood pressure
7. Tachycardia
C. Implementation
1. Assess vital signs especially respirations
2. Have oxygen and resuscitative equipment available during administration

XI. Instructing the Client to Use an Inhaler

A. Shake inhaler well before using
B. Remove cap from inhaler
C. Breathe deeply in and out through the mouth
D. Insert the mouthpiece into the mouth or in front of the open mouth holding the inhaler upright
E. If a spacer is used, attach the spacer to the inhaler and place the end of the spacer in the mouth, passing the teeth and above the tongue
F. With the index finger on top of the canister, depress the top while inhaling slowly
G. Remove inhaler and hold breath for as long as possible, then exhale slowly
H. Wait 1–2 minutes before the next dose
I. If two different inhalers are prescribed, and one of the medications contains a steroid, administer the bronchodilator first and the steroid second
J. Wait 5 minutes following the bronchodilator before inhaling the steroid
K. Clean the mouthpiece following use

PRACTICE QUESTIONS

1. The nurse is preparing to administer albuterol (Proventil) to a client. The nurse assesses which of the following parameters before and during therapy?
   1 Urine output and blood urea nitrogen (BUN)
   2 Nausea and vomiting
   3 Lung sounds and presence of dyspnea
   4 Headache and level of consciousness

2. The home care nurse has observed the client self-administer a dose of metaproterenol sulfate (Alupent) via metered-dose inhaler. Within a short time, the client begins to wheeze loudly. The nurse interprets that this is due to:
   1 Insufficient dosage of the medication, which needs to be increased
   2 Probable interaction of this medication with an over-the-counter cold remedy
   3 Tolerance to the medication, indicating a need for a stronger type of bronchodilator
   4 Paradoxical bronchospasm, which must be reported to the physician

3. The nurse is administering a dose of isoproterenol HCl (Isuprel) to a client. The nurse plans to monitor for which of the following side effects of this medication?
   1 Increased pulse and blood pressure
   2 Drowsiness
   3 Hyperglycemia
   4 Hypokalemia

4. The nurse has an order to give the client metaproterenol sulfate (Alupent) two puffs and beclomethasone (Vanceril) two puffs by metered-dose inhaler. The nurse administers the medication by giving the:
   1 Beclomethasone first and then the metaproterenol
   2 Metaproterenol first and then the beclomethasone
   3 Alternating a single puff of each, beginning with the beclomethasone
   4 Alternating a single puff of each, beginning with the metaproterenol

5. The client with an exacerbation of chronic obstructive pulmonary disease (COPD) has been on oral glucocorticoids and is currently being weaned to triamcinolone (Azmacort) by inhalation. The nurse evaluates that the client understands the potential adverse effects to watch for during this medication change if the client states to report:
   1 Blurred vision, headache, and insomnia
   2 Chills, fever, generalized rash
   3 Anorexia, nausea, weakness, and fatigue
   4 Vomiting and diarrhea, increased thirst

6. The client receiving theophylline (Theo-Dur) is due to have a theophylline level drawn. The nurse questions the client to ensure that the client has not ingested which of the following substances prior to the sample being drawn?
   1 Sedatives
   2 Narcotics
   3 Glucose
   4 Caffeine

7. The nurse receives a report of the serum theophylline level of a client taking theophylline (Theo-Dur). The result is 20 mcg/mL. The nurse interprets that this result is:
   1 Below the therapeutic range
   2 In the middle of the therapeutic range
   3 At the top of the therapeutic range
   4 In excess of the therapeutic range

8. The client has begun therapy with oxtriphylline (Choledyl). The nurse plans to teach the client to limit the intake of which of the following while taking this medication?
   1 Oysters, lobster, and shrimp
   2 Coffee, cola, and chocolate
   3 Cottage cheese, cream cheese, and dairy creamers
   4 Grapefruit, oranges, and pineapple

9. The nurse has administered a dose of salmeterol (Serevent) to a client. The client develops a generalized rash and urticaria, and the eyelids begin to swell. The nurse should:
   1 Call the physician immediately
   2 Encourage the client to quickly drink oral fluids
   3 Apply a lanolin-based cream to the rash
   4 Assess the client's vision with a Snellen chart

10. The client with an order to take theophylline (Slo-Bid) daily has been given medication instructions by the nurse. The nurse evaluates that the client needs further information on the medication if the client states to:
    1 Avoid changing brands of the medication without physician approval
    2 Avoid over-the-counter (OTC) cough and cold medications unless approved by the physician
    3 Drink at least 2 liters of fluid per day
    4 Take the daily dose at bedtime

11. The client is taking brompheniramine maleate (Dimetane). The nurse assesses for which of the following side effects of this medication?
    1 Excitability
    2 Drowsiness
    3 Excess salivation
    4 Diarrhea

12. The client taking brompheniramine maleate (Dimetane) is scheduled for allergy skin testing, and tells the nurse in the physician's office that a dose was taken this morning. The nurse interprets that:
    1 A lower dose of allergen should be injected
    2 A higher dose of allergen should be injected
    3 The client should have the skin test read a day later than usual
    4 The client should reschedule the appointment

13. The client is receiving acetylcysteine (Mucomyst) by nebulizer. The nurse should have which of the following items available for possible use after giving this medication?
    1 Suction equipment
    2 Nasogastric tube
    3 Intubation tray
    4 Ambu bag

14. The nurse has an order to administer acetylcysteine (Mucomyst) to a client admitted with acetaminophen (Tylenol) overdose. Before giving this medication, the nurse would ensure that:
    1 The client knows how to use a nebulizer
    2 That the antidote to acetylcysteine is readily available
    3 The stomach is empty from emesis or lavage
    4 The solution is given full strength

15. The client has an order to take guaifenesin (Humibid). The nurse evaluates that the client understands the most effective use of this medication if the client states to:
    1 Take the tablet with a full glass of water
    2 Take an extra dose if the cough is accompanied by fever
    3 Beware of irritability as a side effect
    4 Crush the sustained-release tablet if immediate relief is needed

16. The postoperative client has received a dose of naloxone HCl (Narcan) for respiratory depression shortly after transfer to the nursing unit from the postanesthesia care unit. Following administration of the medication, the nurse assesses the client for:
    1 Pupillary changes
    2 Sudden episodes of vomiting
    3 Sudden increase in pain
    4 Scattered lung wheezes

17. The client with suspected narcotic overdose has received a dose of naloxone HCl (Narcan). The client subsequently becomes restless, starts to vomit, and complains of abdominal cramping. The blood pressure increases from 110/72 mm Hg to 160/86 mm Hg. The nurse provides emotional support and reassurance while administering care to the client, knowing that:
    1 These effects will only last a few moments
    2 These are signs of opioid withdrawal

3 The client may otherwise sign out against medical advice
    4 The client may next become suicidal

18. The nurse is preparing to administer a dose of naloxone HCl (Narcan) intravenously to a client with intravenous narcotic overdose. The nurse plans to have which of the following available as supportive equipment in case it is needed?
    1 Nasogastric tube
    2 Paracentesis tray
    3 Central line insertion tray
    4 Resuscitation equipment

19. The nurse is teaching the client about the effects of diphenhydramine HCl (Benadryl), which has been ordered as a cough suppressant. The nurse does not include which of the following items in the instructions?
    1 Avoid driving or other activities requiring mental alertness while taking this medication
    2 Use sugarless gum, candy, or oral rinses to decrease dry mouth
    3 Avoid using alcohol while taking this medication
    4 Administer on an empty stomach

20. The client has been prescribed a cough formula containing codeine. The nurse has given the client instructions for its use. The nurse evaluates that the client understands the instructions if the client verbalizes to self-assess for:
    1 Excitability
    2 Constipation
    3 Rapid pulse
    4 Excessive urination

21. The nurse is caring for the client who has been taking hydrocodone bitartrate (Hycodan) for the past 3 months. The nurse assesses the client for which of the following side effects of this medication?
    1 Psychological and physical dependence
    2 Tachycardia and hypertension
    3 Diarrhea and abdominal cramping
    4 Increased respiratory rate and bronchospasm

22. Cromolyn sodium (Intal) is prescribed for the client with allergic asthma. The nurse understands that this medication acts to:
    1 Inhibit the release of mediators from mast cells after exposure to an antigen
    2 Promotes the migration of eosinophils into the inflammatory site
    3 Increases the number of eosinophils
    4 Dilates the bronchi

23. Cromolyn sodium (Intal) inhaler is prescribed for the client with allergic asthma. The nurse provides instructions regarding the side effects of this medication. Which of the following undesirable side effects is associated with this medication?

1 Constipation
2 Hypotension
3 Insomnia
4 Bronchospasm

24. Terbutaline sulfate (Brethine) is prescribed for the client with bronchitis. This medication should be used with caution if which of the following existing medical conditions were present in the client?
    1 Hypothyroidism
    2 Polycystic disease

3 Osteoarthritis
4 Diabetes mellitus

25. Zafirlukast (Accolate) is prescribed for the client with bronchial asthma. Which of the following laboratory tests does the nurse expect to be prescribed before the administration of this medication?
    1 Platelet count
    2 Complete blood cell count
    3 Liver function tests
    4 Neutrophil count

ANSWERS

1. **3**

Rationale: Albuterol is a bronchodilator of the adrenergic type. The nurse assesses respiratory pattern, lung sounds, pulse, and blood pressure prior to and during therapy. The color, character, and amount of sputum are also noted.

Test-Taking Strategy: This questions tests fundamental knowledge about this medication. Knowing that this medication is a bronchodilator allows you to eliminate each of the incorrect options systematically. Use the ABCs, Airway, Breathing, and Circulation, to answer the question. Option 3 is the only option that addresses Airway!

Level of Cognitive Ability: Application
Phase of Nursing Process: Assessment
Client Needs: Physiological Integrity
Content Area: Pharmacology

Reference
Deglin, J., & Vallerand, A. (1997). *Davis's drug guide for nurses* (5th ed.). Philadelphia: F. A. Davis. p. 173.

2. **4**

Rationale: The client taking adrenergic bronchodilators may experience paradoxical bronchospasm, which is evident by the client's wheezing. This can occur with excessive use of inhalers. Further medication should be withheld, and the physician should be notified.

Test-Taking Strategy: Eliminate option 1 first, since the client began wheezing after the medication was administered, and not before. Option 3 may be eliminated next, since tolerance does not generally occur. To discriminate between options 2 and 4, knowing that wheezing is associated with bronchospasm may help you choose option 4.

Level of Cognitive Ability: Analysis
Phase of Nursing Process: Analysis
Client Needs: Physiological Integrity
Content Area: Pharmacology

Reference
Hodgson, B., & Kizior, R. (1999). *Saunders nursing drug handbook 1999.* Philadelphia: W. B. Saunders. pp. 648–650.

3. **1**

Rationale: Isoproterenol is an adrenergic bronchodilator. Side effects can include tachycardia, hypertension, chest pain, dysrhythmias, nervousness, restlessness, and head-

ache, among others. The nurse monitors for these effects during therapy.

Test-Taking Strategy: To answer this question accurately, it is necessary to understand that this medication is an adrenergic agent. Thus, it causes bronchodilation but also increases pulse and blood pressure due to its cardiovascular effects. With this in mind, you can eliminate each of the incorrect options easily. Remembering that tachycardia is a side effect should assist in selecting the option that identifies an increased pulse, option 1.

Level of Cognitive Ability: Application
Phase of Nursing Process: Planning
Client Needs: Physiological Integrity
Content Area: Pharmacology

Reference
Hodgson, B., & Kizior, R. (1999). *Saunders nursing drug handbook 1999.* Philadelphia: W. B. Saunders. p. 554.

4. **2**

Rationale: Metaproterenol sulfate is an adrenergic type of bronchodilator. Beclomethasone is a glucocorticoid. Bronchodilators are always administered before glucocorticoids, when both are to be given on the same time schedule. This allows for widening of the air passages by the bronchodilator, which then makes the glucocorticoid more effective.

Test-Taking Strategy: To answer this question correctly, it is necessary to know two different things. First you must know that a bronchodilator is always given before a glucocorticoid. This would allow you to eliminate options 3 and 4, since you would not alternate the medications. To discriminate between options 1 and 2, it is necessary to know that metaproterenol is a bronchodilator, while beclomethasone is a glucocorticoid. Learn this now, as you will likely find a question related to this concept on NCLEX-RN!

Level of Cognitive Ability: Application
Phase of Nursing Process: Implementation
Client Needs: Physiological Integrity
Content Area: Pharmacology

Reference
Pinnell, N. (1996). *Nursing pharmacology.* Philadelphia: W. B. Saunders. p. 565.

5. **3**

Rationale: The client being changed from oral to inhalation glucocorticoids could experience signs of adrenal insufficiency. The nurse teaches the client to report anorexia, nausea, weakness, and fatigue. Other signs that can be detected, which are objective in nature, include hypotension and hypoglycemia.

Test-Taking Strategy: To answer this question accurately, it is necessary to know that tapering could result in adrenal insufficiency, and then you must know what those typical signs and symptoms are. Since option 4 seems most compatible with dehydration, eliminate that option first. Option 1 implies CNS involvement, so that may be eliminated next. To discriminate between the remaining options, you would choose option 3 as more plausible than option 2, which seems to resemble a hypersensitivity reaction.

Level of Cognitive Ability: Analysis
Phase of Nursing Process: Evaluation
Client Needs: Physiological Integrity
Content Area: Pharmacology

Reference
Deglin, J., & Vallerand, A. (1997). *Davis's drug guide for nurses* (5th ed.). Philadelphia: F. A. Davis. p. 540.

6. **4**

Rationale: Theophylline is a xanthine bronchodilator. Before drawing a serum level of the medication, the client should avoid taking in foods or beverages that contain xanthine, such as colas, coffee, or chocolate. Thus, the client is told to avoid caffeine intake before the test.

Test-Taking Strategy: Specific knowledge is required to answer this question. Since this is a medication commonly used for respiratory disorders, and monitoring laboratory values associated with its administration is very important, take time now to review if this question was difficult!

Level of Cognitive Ability: Application
Phase of Nursing Process: Assessment
Client Needs: Physiological Integrity
Content Area: Pharmacology

Reference
Deglin, J., & Vallerand, A. (1997). *Davis's drug guide for nurses* (5th ed.). Philadelphia: F. A. Davis. pp. 182, 184.

7. **3**

Rationale: The normal therapeutic range for theophylline levels is 10–20 mcg/mL. A level above 20 mcg/mL is considered toxic. The value of 20 mcg/mL places the client at the top of the therapeutic range.

Test-Taking Strategy: Specific knowledge is required to answer this question. Since this is a common medication, take a few moments now to review this briefly if this question was difficult. This is an example of a helpful value to memorize. You are likely to see a question related to this laboratory value on NCLEX-RN!

Level of Cognitive Ability: Analysis
Phase of Nursing Process: Analysis
Client Needs: Physiological Integrity
Content Area: Pharmacology

Reference
Pinnell, N. (1996). *Nursing pharmacology.* Philadelphia: W. B. Saunders. p. 563.

8. **2**

Rationale: Oxtriphylline (Choledyl) is a xanthine bronchodilator. The nurse teaches the client to limit the intake of xanthine-containing foods while taking this medication. These include coffee, cola, and chocolate.

Test-Taking Strategy: To answer this question correctly, it is necessary to understand that oxtriphylline is a xanthine bronchodilator, and to know that intake of excessive amounts of foods naturally high in xanthines should be curtailed. With this in mind, you would eliminate each of the incorrect options in turn, because shellfish (option 1), dairy products (option 3), and citrus and other fruits (option 4) are unrelated. Take time now to review the foods naturally high in xanthines if you had difficulty with this question!

Level of Cognitive Ability: Application
Phase of Nursing Process: Planning
Client Needs: Health Promotion and Maintenance
Content Area: Pharmacology

Reference
Deglin, J., & Vallerand, A. (1997). *Davis's drug guide for nurses* (5th ed.). Philadelphia: F. A. Davis. pp. 178, 184.

9. **1**

Rationale: Hypersensitivity reaction can occur in clients taking ephedrine, epinephrine, isoproterenol, or salmeterol. Signs and symptoms include rash, urticaria, and swelling of the face, lips, or eyelids. The nurse should call the physician immediately if any of these occur. All of the other responses are completely incorrect.

Test-Taking Strategy: Specific medication knowledge is not even necessarily needed to answer this question. Recognizing that the signs and symptoms listed in the stem are typical of hypersensitivity reaction allows you to eliminate options 3 and 4 first. To discriminate between options 1 and 2, you would need to know that the client needs treatment with an antihistamine or epinephrine, not oral fluids.

Level of Cognitive Ability: Application
Phase of Nursing Process: Implementation
Client Needs: Physiological Integrity
Content Area: Pharmacology

Reference
Hodgson, B., & Kizior, R. (1999). *Saunders nursing drug handbook 1999.* Philadelphia: W. B. Saunders. p. 917.

10. **4**

Rationale: The client taking a single daily dose of theophylline, a xanthine bronchodilator, should take the medication early in the morning. This enables the client to have maximal benefit from the medication during daytime activities. Additionally, this medication causes insomnia. The client should take in at least 2 liters of fluid per day to decrease viscosity of secretions. The client should check with the physician before changing brands of the medication, as there may be different levels of bioavailability. The client also checks with the physician before taking OTC cough, cold, or other respiratory preparations with theophylline because they could have interactive effects, increasing the side effects of theophylline and causing dysrhythmias.

Test Taking Strategy: Note the key words "needs further information." General principles related to medication therapy will assist in eliminating options 1 and 2. Additionally, recalling that option 3 is an important measure to thin secretions will direct you to option 4 as the answer to this question as it is stated.

Level of Cognitive Ability: Analysis
Phase of Nursing Process: Evaluation
Client Needs: Health Promotion and Maintenance
Content Area: Pharmacology

Reference
Lehne, R. (1998). *Pharmacology for nursing care* (3rd ed.). Philadelphia: W. B. Saunders. pp. 755–756.

11. **2**

Rationale: A frequent side effect of brompheniramine maleate (Dimetane), an antihistamine, is drowsiness or sedation. Others include blurred vision, hypertension (and sometimes hypotension), dry mouth, constipation, urinary retention, and sweating.

Test-Taking Strategy: This is an example of a classic question related to antihistamine use, which typically causes drowsiness in users. To answer this question correctly, it is necessary to know that this medication is an antihistamine. Knowledge of the· effects of antihistamines lets you eliminate each of the incorrect options quickly. Take time now to review the side effects of antihistamines if you had difficulty with this question!

Level of Cognitive Ability: Application
Phase of Nursing Process: Assessment
Client Needs: Physiological Integrity
Content Area: Pharmacology

Reference
Kee, J. LeFever, & Hayes, E. (1997). *Pharmacology: A nursing process approach* (2nd ed.). Philadelphia: W. B. Saunders. pp. 445–447.

12. **4**

Rationale: Brompheniramine maleate is an antihistamine, which provides relief of symptoms caused by allergy. Antihistamines should be discontinued for at least 3 days (72 hours) before allergy skin testing to avoid false-negative readings. This client should have the appointment rescheduled for 3 days after discontinuing the medication.

Test-Taking Strategy: To answer this question correctly, it is necessary to know that this medication is an antihistamine. It is also necessary to know that antihistamines reduce the allergic response by virtue of their action. With this in mind, option 1 is eliminated first, since it makes no sense. Options 2 and 3 are also discarded, because the medication would still interfere with the test results.

Level of Cognitive Ability: Analysis
Phase of Nursing Process: Analysis
Client Needs: Physiological Integrity
Content Area: Pharmacology

Reference
Deglin, J., & Vallerand, A. (1997). *Davis's drug guide for nurses* (5th ed.). Philadelphia: F. A. Davis. pp. 166–167.

13. **1**

Rationale: Acetylcysteine can be given orally or by nasogastric tube to treat acetaminophen overdose, or it may be given by inhalation for use as a mucolytic. The nurse administering this medication as a mucolytic should have suction equipment available, in case the client cannot manage to clear the increased volume of liquefied secretions.

Test-Taking Strategy: To answer this question, it is necessary to know that Mucomyst may be given for either acetaminophen overdose or as a mucolytic agent. It is also necessary to know that the inhalation route is used only for mucolytic effects. With this in mind, options 3 and 4 may be eliminated, since the client does not need resuscitation. Option 2 is eliminated also, since this may be used in the client with acetaminophen overdose. If you had difficulty with this question, take time now to review the purpose of this medication and the related nursing interventions!

Level of Cognitive Ability: Application
Phase of Nursing Process: Planning
Client Needs: Physiological Integrity
Content Area: Pharmacology

Reference
Deglin, J., & Vallerand, A. (1997). *Davis's drug guide for nurses* (5th ed.). Philadelphia: F. A. Davis. pp. 7–9.

14. **3**

Rationale: Acetylcysteine can be given orally or by nasogastric tube to treat acetaminophen overdose, or it may be given by inhalation for use as a mucolytic. Before giving the medication as an antidote to acetaminophen, the nurse ensures that the client's stomach is empty through emesis or gastric lavage. The solution is diluted in cola, water, or juice to make the solution more palatable. It is then administered orally or by nasogastric tube.

Test-Taking Strategy: Begin to answer this question by eliminating options 1 and 2. This medication is not given by the inhalation route to treat acetaminophen overdose, and acetylcysteine *is* the antidote (to acetaminophen). To discriminate between the last two options, it is necessary to know either of two things. First, knowing that the solution must be diluted forces you to choose option 3 as correct. Second, knowing that the stomach must be emptied for maximal effect of the antidote also forces you to choose option 3 as correct.

Level of Cognitive Ability: Analysis
Phase of Nursing Process: Planning
Client Needs: Physiological Integrity
Content Area: Pharmacology

Reference
Deglin, J., & Vallerand, A. (1997). *Davis's drug guide for nurses* (5th ed.). Philadelphia: F. A. Davis. pp. 7–9.

15. **1**

Rationale: Guaifenesin (Humibid) is an expectorant. It should be taken with a full glass of water to decrease viscosity of secretions. Sustained-release preparations should not be broken open, crushed, or chewed. The medication may occasionally cause dizziness, headache, or drowsiness as side effects. The client should contact the physician if the cough lasts longer than 1 week, or is accompanied by fever, rash, sore throat, or persistent headache.

Test-Taking Strategy: Begin to answer this question by eliminating option 4 first. Sustained-relief preparations are not crushed or broken. Option 2 is eliminated next because fever indicates infection, and an "extra dose" of an expectorant is not helpful in treating infection. To discriminate between the last two options, knowing that increased fluids helps to liquefy secretions for more effective coughing allows you to choose option 1 as correct. If you had difficulty with this question, take time now to review this medication!

Level of Cognitive Ability: Analysis
Phase of Nursing Process: Evaluation
Client Needs: Health Promotion and Maintenance
Content Area: Pharmacology

Reference
Hodgson, B., & Kizior, R. (1999). *Saunders nursing drug handbook 1999.* Philadelphia: W. B. Saunders. p. 482.

16. 3

Rationale: Naloxone HCl is an antidote to opioids, and it may also be given to the postoperative client to treat respiratory depression. When given to the postoperative client for respiratory depression, it may also reverse the effects of analgesics. Therefore, the nurse must assess the client for a sudden increase in the level of pain experienced.

Test-Taking Strategy: To answer this question correctly, it is necessary to know that this medication is an antidote to narcotic analgesics, and that it would likely cause sudden pain in the postoperative client, or return of pain in clients who receive narcotic analgesics. All of the other options are incorrect and are eliminated. If you had difficulty with this question, take time now to review this medication!

Level of Cognitive Ability: Application
Phase of Nursing Process: Assessment
Client Needs: Physiological Integrity
Content Area: Pharmacology

Reference

Deglin, J., & Vallerand, A. (1997). *Davis's drug guide for nurses* (5th ed.). Philadelphia: F. A. Davis. p. 841.

17. 2

Rationale: Signs of opioid withdrawal include increased temperature and blood pressure, abdominal cramping, vomiting, and restlessness. They can occur anywhere from a few minutes to a few hours after administration of naloxone HCl, depending on the opioid involved, the degree of dependence, and the dose of naloxone.

Test-Taking Strategy: Eliminate option 1 first as the least plausible, since these types of symptoms identified in the question are not likely to disappear in a few moments. Option 4 is eliminated next, because there is no supporting information in the stem. To discriminate between the remaining two, knowing that the client with narcotic overdose may well have a history of prior chronic use, would cause you to choose option 2 over option 3.

Level of Cognitive Ability: Analysis
Phase of Nursing Process: Analysis
Client Needs: Psychosocial Integrity
Content Area: Pharmacology

Reference

Hodgson, B., & Kizior, R. (1999). *Saunders nursing drug handbook 1999.* Philadelphia: W. B. Saunders. pp. 719–720.

18. 4

Rationale: The nurse administering naloxone HCl for suspected narcotic overdose should have resuscitation equipment readily available to support naloxone therapy if it is needed. Other adjuncts that may be needed include oxygen, mechanical ventilator, and vasopressors.

Test-Taking Strategy: The key to answering this question is "intravenous narcotic overdose." Knowing the effects of these medications, you would want to have other resuscitation equipment available. The option that best meets this criterion is option 4. Option 4 is also the most global response.

Level of Cognitive Ability: Application
Phase of Nursing Process: Planning
Client Needs: Physiological Integrity
Content Area: Pharmacology

Reference

Deglin, J., & Vallerand, A. (1997). *Davis's drug guide for nurses* (5th ed.). Philadelphia: F. A. Davis. p. 841.

19. 4

Rationale: Diphenhydramine (Benadryl) has several uses, including antihistamine, antitussive, antidyskinetic, and sedative/hypnotic. Instructions for use include to take with food or milk to decrease GI upset, and to use oral rinses or sugarless gum or hard candy to minimize dry mouth. Since the medication causes drowsiness, the client should avoid use of alcohol or CNS depressants, operating a car, or engaging in other activities requiring mental acuity during use.

Test-Taking Strategy: The wording of the question guides you to look for an incorrect response. Knowing that the medication has a sedative effect helps to eliminate options 1 and 3 first. Knowing that the medication causes dry mouth helps you choose option 4 as the answer to the question, according to the way the question is stated. If you had difficulty with this question, take time now to review client education related to this medication!

Level of Cognitive Ability: Application
Phase of Nursing Process: Implementation
Client Needs: Physiological Integrity
Content Area: Pharmacology

Reference

Deglin, J., & Vallerand, A. (1997). *Davis's drug guide for nurses* (5th ed.). Philadelphia: F. A. Davis. p. 383.

20. 2

Rationale: The client is taught about side effects that could occur with use of codeine. The most common side effects include drowsiness, confusion, hypotension, nausea and vomiting, and constipation. Others include bradycardia, respiratory depression, and urinary retention.

Test-Taking Strategy: This question tests the concept that narcotic analgesics cause constipation as a side effect. Knowing that the medication causes drowsiness helps you to eliminate option 1 first. Knowing that the medication causes decreased pulse helps you to eliminate option 3 next. Finally, knowing that constipation and urinary retention go together as effects helps you to choose option 2 over option 4.

Level of Cognitive Ability: Analysis
Phase of Nursing Process: Evaluation
Client Needs: Physiological Integrity
Content Area: Pharmacology

Reference

Kee, J. LeFever, & Hayes, E. (1997). *Pharmacology: A nursing process approach* (2nd ed.). Philadelphia: W. B. Saunders. p. 236.

21. 1

Rationale: Hydrocodone bitartrate is an opioid analgesic, Schedule III, which also has antitussive properties. Side effects of this medication include physical and psychological dependence, bradycardia and hypotension, respiratory depression, nausea, vomiting, constipation, sedation, and confusion.

Test-Taking Strategy: Use the process of elimination to answer this question. This question tests the concept of hydrocodone as an opioid analgesic, which causes physical and psychological dependence. If this question was problematic, review information on the implications of opioid use and the side effects of this medication now!

Level of Cognitive Ability: Application
Phase of Nursing Process: Assessment
Client Needs: Physiological Integrity
Content Area: Pharmacology

Reference

Hodgson, B., & Kizior, R. (1999). *Saunders nursing drug handbook 1999.* Philadelphia: W. B. Saunders. p. 497.

22. **1**

Rationale: Cromolyn sodium (Intal) is an antiasthmatic, antiallergic and a mast-cell stabilizer that inhibits release of mediators from mast cells after exposure to an antigen. It can also interrupt the migration of eosinophils into the inflammatory site and decrease the number of eosinophils. These actions decrease airway hyperresponsiveness in some clients with asthma. It has no bronchodilating action.

Test-Taking Strategy: Knowledge regarding the action of this medication is required to answer this question. Eliminate options 2 and 3 first as they are similar responses. To select between the remaining options, it is certainly helpful to know that cromolyn sodium (Intal) has no bronchodilating action. Also, note the relationship between the words "antigen" in the correct option and "allergic" in the question. Take time now to review the action of this medication if you had difficulty with this question!

Level of Cognitive Ability: Analysis
Phase of Nursing Process: Analysis
Client Needs: Physiological Integrity
Content Area: Pharmacology

Reference

Pinnell, N. (1996). *Nursing pharmacology.* Philadelphia: W. B. Saunders. p. 566.

23. **4**

Rationale: The most common undesired clinical responses associated with inhalation therapy of cromolyn sodium (Intal) are bronchospasm, cough, nasal congestion, throat irritation, and wheezing. Clients receiving this medication orally may experience pruritus, nausea, diarrhea, and myalgia.

Test-Taking Strategy: Use the process of elimination to answer this question. Note that the stem of the question asks for the "undesirable" side effect. This should assist in directing you to option 4. Additionally, utilize the ABCs, Airway, Breathing, and Circulation, to select the correct option. Option 4 addresses Airway!

Level of Cognitive Ability: Analysis
Phase of Nursing Process: Assessment
Client Needs: Physiological Integrity
Content Area: Pharmacology

Reference

Pinnell, N. (1996). *Nursing pharmacology.* Philadelphia: W. B. Saunders. p. 566.

24. **4**

Rationale: Terbutaline sulfate (Brethine) is contraindicated in clients with hypersensitivity to sympathomimetics. It should be used with caution in clients with impaired cardiac function, diabetes mellitus, hypertension, hyperthyroidism, and clients with a history of seizures. The medication may increase blood glucose levels.

Test-Taking Strategy: This is a difficult question, and knowledge regarding this medication is required to answer correctly. Take time now to review the contraindications associated with this medication if you had difficulty with this question!

Level of Cognitive Ability: Analysis
Phase of Nursing Process: Analysis
Client Needs: Physiological Integrity
Content Area: Pharmacology

Reference

Hodgson, B., & Kizior, R. (1999). *Saunders nursing drug handbook 1999.* Philadelphia: W. B. Saunders. pp. 969–970.

25. **3**

Rationale: Zafirlukast (Accolate) is a leukotriene receptor antagonist that is used in the prophylaxis and chronic treatment of bronchial asthma. It is used with caution in clients with impaired hepatic function. Liver function laboratory values should be obtained as a baseline and should be monitored during administration of the medication.

Test-Taking Strategy: Knowledge regarding this medication is required to answer the question. Use the process of elimination, eliminating options 2 and 4 first, as a complete blood count would include a neutrophil count. From this point, you would need to know that this medication would affect hepatic function. If you had difficulty with this question, take time now to review this medication!

Level of Cognitive Ability: Analysis
Phase of Nursing Process: Analysis
Client Needs: Physiological Integrity
Content Area: Pharmacology

Reference

Hodgson, B., & Kizior, R. (1999). *Saunders nursing drug handbook 1999.* Philadelphia: W. B. Saunders. pp. 1064–1065.

BIBLIOGRAPHY

Deglin, J., & Vallerand, A. (1997). *Davis's drug guide for nurses* (5th ed.). Philadelphia: F. A. Davis.

Hodgson, B., & Kizior, R. (1999). *Saunders nursing drug handbook 1999.* Philadelphia: W. B. Saunders.

Kee, J. LeFever, & Hayes, E. (1997). *Pharmacology: A nursing process approach* (2nd ed.). Philadelphia: W. B. Saunders.

Kuhn, M. (1998). *Pharmacotherapeutics: A nursing process approach* (4th ed.). Philadelphia: F. A. Davis.

Lehne, R. (1998). *Pharmacology for nursing care* (3rd ed.). Philadelphia: W. B. Saunders.

Pinnell, N. (1996). *Nursing pharmacology.* Philadelphia: W. B. Saunders.

UNIT XIV

....

The Adult Client with a Cardiovascular Disorder

PYRAMID TERMS

Afterload—The force against which the heart has to pump to eject blood from the ventricle. Factors and conditions that would impede blood flow increase left ventricular afterload.

Arterial Anastomoses—Ensures that when one of the blood-supplying arteries is damaged, flow is maintained from the other arteries. Blood flow to the hands, feet, brain, and other organs is protected by arterial anastomoses.

Arterial Pressure—The pressure of the blood against the arterial walls. It can be measured indirectly by sphygmomanometer or directly by arterial catheter. Readings are expressed as systolic over diastolic. Arterial pressure increases when the cardiac output (CO), peripheral resistance, or blood volume increases.

Automaticity—The ability of cardiac cells to initiate an impulse spontaneously and repetitively without external neurohormonal control. The pacemaker cells have the highest rate of automaticity of all cardiac cells.

Baroreceptors—Also called pressoreceptors, baroreceptors are located in the walls of the aortic arch and carotid sinuses. Baroreceptors are specialized nerve endings that are affected by changes in the arterial blood pressure. Increases in arterial pressure stimulate baroreceptors, and the heart rate and arterial pressure decrease. Decreases in arterial pressure lead to a lessened stimulation of the baroreceptors and vasoconstriction occurs, as does an increase in heart rate.

Blood Pressure (BP)—Measures the force exerted by the blood against the walls of the blood vessels. If the BP falls too low, blood flow to the tissues, heart, brain, and other organs becomes inadequate. If the BP becomes too high, the risk of vessel rupture and damage increases.

Capillary Pressure or Hydrostatic Pressure—The pressure exerted by the blood against the capillary wall. Normal capillary pressure is 25 to 30 mmHg at the arterial end of the capillaries, and 10 to 15 mmHg at the venous end.

Cardiac Output—The total volume of blood pumped through the heart in 1 minute. The normal cardiac output is 4 to 8 liters per minute. Cardiac output = stroke volume × heart rate.

Chemoreceptors—Located in the aortic arch and carotid bodies. Hypoxemia stimulates chemoreceptors, which then transmit impulses to the central nervous system.

Conductivity—The ability of the heart muscle fibers to propagate electrical impulses along and across cell membranes.

Contractility—Refers to the inherent ability of the myocardium to alter contractile force and velocity. Sympathetic stimulation increases myocardial contractility, thus increases stroke volume. Conditions that decrease myocardial contractility reduce stroke volume.

Diastole—The phase of the cardiac cycle in which the heart relaxes between contractions. It represents the period of time when the two ventricles are dilated by the blood flowing into them.

Diastolic Pressure—The force of the blood exerted against the artery walls when the heart relaxes or fills. Normal diastolic pressure is 60 to 90 mmHg.

Excitability—The ability of cardiac muscle cells to depolarize in response to a stimulus. Excitability is influenced by hormones, electrolytes, nutrition, oxygen supply, medication, infections, and nerve characteristics.

Frank-Starling Law—States that the more the heart fills within reasonable limits during diastole, the greater the force of contraction during systole and the greater the stroke volume. The exception to the law is during heart failure, when increasing blood volume into the ventricle decreases stroke volume. If the left ventricle fills to such an extent that it overdistends the myocardium, cardiac output begins to decrease and the heart begins to fail.

Hepatojugular Reflex—Position the client with the head of the bed elevated 45° and locate the internal jugular vein. Compress the upper right abdomen for 30 to 40 seconds. Sudden distention of the neck veins after abdominal compression is usually indicative of right-sided heart failure.

Mean Arterial Pressure (MAP)—Is equivalent to one third of the pulse pressure plus the diastolic blood pressure. MAP is used in hemodynamic monitoring.

Paradoxical Blood Pressure—An exaggerated decrease in systolic pressure by more than 10 mmHg during the inspiratory phase of the respiratory cycle. Normal value is 3 to 10 mmHg.

Postural (Orthostatic) Hypotension—A blood pressure fall of more than 10 to 15 mmHg of the systolic pressure or a fall of more than 10 mmHg of the diastolic pressure and a 10% to 20% increase in heart rate. Occurs when the client's blood pressure is not adequately maintained when moving from a lying to a sitting or standing position.

Preload—The volume of blood stretching the left ventricle at the end of diastole. Preload is determined by the total circulating blood volume and is increased by an increase in venous return to the heart.

Pulse Pressure—The difference between the systolic pressure and diastolic pressure. Normal pulse pressure is 30 to 40 mmHg.

Refractoriness—The heart's inability to respond to a new stimulus while still in a state of contraction from an earlier stimulus. Refractoriness prevents uncontrolled rapid cardiac contractions and helps preserve the heart rhythm.

Stretch Receptors—Located in the vena cava and the right atrium. Respond to pressure changes that affect circulatory blood volume. When the blood pressure decreases because of hypovolemia, a sympathetic response occurs, causing an increased heart rate and blood vessel constriction. When the blood pressure increases because of hypervolemia, an opposite effect occurs.

Stroke Volume—The amount of blood ejected from the left ventricle with each contraction. The normal stroke volume is 70 to 130 mL per heart beat. The stroke volume can be affected by preload, afterload, contractility, and the Frank-Starling law.

Systole—The phase of contraction of the heart, especially of the ventricles, during which blood is forced into the aorta and pulmonary artery.

Systolic Pressure—The maximum pressure of blood exerted against the artery walls when the heart contracts. Normal systolic pressure is 100 to 140 mmHg.

Venous Pressure—The force exerted by the blood against the vein walls. Normal venous pressures are highest in the extremities (5 to 14 cm of H_2O in the arm), and lowest closest to the heart (6 to 8 cm of H_2O in the inferior vena cava).

PYRAMID TO SUCCESS

Pyramid points focus on assessment data related to cardiovascular risks, health screening and promotion, complications of the various cardiovascular disorders, emergency implementation measures, and client education. Focus on the assessment findings in angina, myocardial infarction (MI), congestive heart failure (CHF) and pulmonary edema, pericarditis, dysrhythmias, pacemakers, aneurysms, hypertension, and arterial and vascular disorders. Focus on the care of the client following diagnostic treatments and surgical procedures. Note appropriate and therapeutic client positions, particularly with arterial and venous disorders of the extremities. Focus on treatments and medications prescribed for the various cardiovascular disorders and client teaching related to prescribed treatment plans. Be familiar with the components related to cardiac rehabilitation.

NURSING PROCESS

ASSESSMENT

Demographic data, including age, sex, and cultural background

Medical and family history

Lifestyle habits, dietary and activity patterns

Characteristics of chest pain

Dyspnea—exertional, paroxysmal, and nocturnal, and orthopnea

Altered level of consciousness, syncope or fainting

Palpitations and dysrhythmias

Abnormal heart sounds or lung sounds, including rales or crackles

Respiratory distress, cough, or blood-tinged sputum

An increase or decrease in heart rate, blood pressure, or respirations

Jugular vein distention (JVD)

Weight gain and edema

Fatigue and weakness

Extremity pain

Skin color and temperature changes

Capillary filling time and peripheral pulses

Cardiac enzymes, electrocardiography (ECG), and laboratory and diagnostic tests

Psychosocial assessment

ANALYSIS: Alteration in Comfort

PLANNING	IMPLEMENTATION	EVALUATION
The client verbalizes chest discomfort. The client describes measures to relieve chest discomfort, including medication and activity restrictions.	Assess characteristics of pain. Determine precipitants of pain. Identify measures that relieve the pain. Administer nitroglycerin or pain medication as prescribed. Document the effectiveness of the medication.	The client obtains relief of chest discomfort.

ANALYSIS: Altered Cardiopulmonary, Cerebral, and Peripheral Tissue Perfusion

---

PLANNING	IMPLEMENTATION	EVALUATION
The client maintains adequate cardiac output.	Assess vital signs and hemodynamic parameters. Auscultate lung sounds. Monitor for dysrhythmias. Administer oxygen as prescribed. Monitor for the presence of cyanosis. Monitor for fluid overload and the presence of edema; Assess weight. Assess level of consciousness. Assess extremities for color, temperature, and sensation. Instruct client in measures to avoid circulatory compromise.	The client maintains hemodynamic stability.

ANALYSIS: Denial

PLANNING	IMPLEMENTATION	EVALUATION
Client describes barriers to compliance with treatment plan and identifies methods to modify barriers.	Assess client's understanding of illness. Assist client to explore denial. Engage client in anxiety, fears, symptoms, and impact of illness. Initiate follow-up, support services, and resources for the client.	The client acknowledges cardiovascular symptoms.

ANALYSIS: Knowledge Deficit

PLANNING

The client describes the required diet, medications, activity, and limitations. The client verbalizes reportable signs and symptoms of activity worsening the condition. The client verbalizes the significance of symptoms. The client reports significant symptoms.

IMPLEMENTATION

Instruct client in the correct procedure for taking nitroglycerin and other prescribed medications. Instruct client in diet and prescriptions. Instruct client regarding signs and symptoms requiring notifying health care provider. Initiate home care and community support.

EVALUATION

Client verbalizes accurate information regarding medications, diet, and the modification of risk factors associated with cardiovascular disorders. Client remains asymptomatic and implements appropriate treatments to alter the atherosclerotic progression. The client utilizes resources in the community.

CLIENT NEEDS

SAFE, EFFECTIVE CARE ENVIRONMENT

Informed consent related to treatments and procedures
Cardiovascular consultations and referrals
Standard precautions

HEALTH PROMOTION AND MAINTENANCE

Prevention of cardiovascular disease
Health screening and health promotion programs
Alterations in lifestyle
Cardiovascular assessment
Teaching related to diet therapy, exercise, and the administration of medications
Mobilization of appropriate community resources
Cardiac rehabilitation

PSYCHOSOCIAL INTEGRITY

Fear, anxiety, and denial
Accepting lifestyle changes
Body image changes
Coping mechanisms
Support systems

PHYSIOLOGICAL INTEGRITY

Nonpharmacological and pharmacological comfort interventions
Assisting with basic care measures
Activity limitations and rest and sleep
Administration of IV medications
Monitoring for therapeutic effects of IV medications
Monitoring cardiac enzymes and laboratory values related to the cardiovascular system
Monitoring for complications related to cardiovascular disorders
Interventions required in emergencies

BIBLIOGRAPHY

Black, J., & Matassarin-Jacobs, E. (1997). *Medical-surgical nursing: Clinical management for continuity of care* (5th ed.). Philadelphia: W.B. Saunders.

Leahy, J., & Kizilay, P. (1998). *Foundations of nursing practice: A nursing process approach.* Philadelphia: W.B. Saunders.

Monahan, F., & Neighbors, M. (1998). *Medical-surgical nursing: Foundations for clinical practice* (2nd ed.). Philadelphia: W.B. Saunders.

National Council of State Boards of Nursing. (1997). Plan for the National Licensure Examination for *Registered Nurses.* Chicago: Author.

O'Toole, M. (ed.). (1997). *Miller-Keane encyclopedia & dictionary of medicine, nursing & allied health* (6th ed.). Philadelphia: W.B. Saunders.

CHAPTER 59

Cardiovascular Disorders

. . . .

I. Anatomy and Physiology

A. Heart and heart layers
1. The heart is located in the left side of the mediastinum
2. The epicardium covers the outer surface of the heart
3. The myocardium is the middle layer and is the actual contracting muscle of the heart
4. The endocardium is the innermost layer and lines the inner chambers and the heart valves

B. Pericardium
1. The pericardium encases and protects the heart from trauma and infection
2. The parietal pericardium is the tough, fibrous outer membrane that is attached anteriorly to the lower half of the sternum, posteriorly to the thoracic vertebrae, and inferiorly to the diaphragm
3. The visceral pericardium is the thin inner layer that closely adheres to the heart
4. The pericardial space is between the parietal and visceral layers; it holds 5 to 20 mL of pericardial fluid, which lubricates the pericardial surfaces and cushions the heart

C. Heart chambers
1. The right atrium receives deoxygenated blood from the body via the superior and inferior venae cavae
2. The right ventricle receives blood from the right atrium and pumps it to the lungs via the pulmonary artery
3. The left atrium receives oxygenated blood from the lungs via four pulmonary veins
4. The left ventricle is the largest and most muscular chamber; it receives oxygenated blood from the lungs via the left atrium and pumps blood into the systemic circulation via the aorta

D. Heart valves
1. The atrioventricular valves lie between the atria and ventricles
2. The atrioventricular valves close at the beginning of ventricular contraction and prevent blood from flowing back into the atria from the ventricles; these valves open when the ventricle relaxes
3. The bicuspid or mitral valve is located on the left side of the heart
4. The tricuspid valve is located on the right side of the heart
5. The pulmonic semilunar valve lies between the right ventricle and the pulmonary artery
6. The aortic semilunar valve lies between the left ventricle and the aorta
7. The semilunar valves prevent blood from flowing back into the ventricles during relaxation; they open during ventricular contraction and close when the ventricles begin to relax

E. Atrioventricular (AV) node
1. The AV node is located in the lower aspect of the atrial septum
2. The AV node receives electrical impulses from the sinoatrial (SA) node

F. The bundle of His (AV bundle)
1. The bundle of His fuses with the AV node to form another pacemaker site
2. It branches into the right bundle branch (RBB), which branches down the right side of the interventricular septum, and the left bundle branch (LBB), which extends into the left ventricle
3. The right and left bundle branches terminate into Purkinje's fibers
4. If the SA node fails, the bundle of His can initiate and sustain a heart rate at 40 to 60 beats per minute

G. Purkinje's fibers
1. A diffuse network of conducting strands located beneath the ventricular endocardium

2. These fibers spread the wave of depolarization through the ventricles

H. Coronary arteries
1. The coronary arteries supply the capillaries of the myocardium with blood
2. The right coronary artery (RCA) supplies the right atrium and ventricle, the inferior portion of the left ventricle, the posterior septal wall, and the SA and AV nodes
3. The left coronary artery (LCA) consists of two major branches, the left anterior descending (LAD) and the circumflex arteries
4. The LAD artery supplies blood to the anterior wall of the left ventricle, the anterior ventricular septum, and the apex of the left ventricle
5. The circumflex artery supplies blood to the left atrium and the lateral and posterior surfaces of the left ventricle

I. Sinoatrial (SA) node
1. The SA node or pacemaker initiates each heart beat
2. Its location is at the junction of the superior vena cava and the right atrium
3. It generates electrical impulses at approximately 60 to 100 times per minute and is controlled by the sympathetic and parasympathetic systems

J. Heart sounds
1. The first heart sound (S_1) is heard as the AV valves close
2. The second heart sound (S_2) is heard when the semilunar valves close
3. A third heart sound (S_3) may be heard if ventricular wall compliance is decreased and structures in the ventricular wall vibrate; this can occur in such conditions as congestive heart failure (CHF) or valvular regurgitation; however, an S_3 heart sound may be a normal finding in individuals younger than 30 years of age
4. A fourth heart sound (S_4) may be heard on atrial **systole** if resistance to ventricular filling is present; this is not a normal finding, and the causes include cardiac hypertrophy, disease, or injury to the ventricular wall

K. Heart rate
1. The faster the heart rate, the less time the heart has for filling and the **cardiac output** decreases
2. An increase in heart rate increases oxygen consumption
3. The normal heart rate is 60 to 100 beats per minute
4. Sinus tachycardia is a rate of more than 100 beats per minute
5. Sinus bradycardia is a rate of less than 60 beats per minute

L. Autonomic nervous system
1. Stimulation of sympathetic nerve fibers releases the neurotransmitter norepinephrine, producing an increased heart rate, increased conduction speed through the AV node, increased atrial and ventricular **contractility,** and peripheral vasoconstriction; stimulation occurs when a decrease in pressure is detected
2. Stimulation of the parasympathetic nerve fibers releases the neurotransmitter acetylcholine, which decreases the heart rate and lessens atrial and ventricular **contractility** and **conductivity;** stimulation occurs when an increase in pressure is detected

M. Blood pressure control
1. **Baroreceptors,** also called pressoreceptors, are located in the walls of the aortic arch and carotid sinuses
2. **Baroreceptors** are specialized nerve endings that are affected by changes in the arterial **blood pressure**
3. Increases in **arterial pressure** stimulate **baroreceptors** and the heart rate, and **arterial pressure** decreases
4. Decreases in **arterial pressure** lead to a lessened stimulation of the **baroreceptors,** and vasoconstriction occurs, as does an increase in heart rate
5. **Stretch receptors,** located in the vena cava and the right atrium, respond to pressure changes that affect circulatory blood volume
6. When the **blood pressure** decreases because of hypovolemia, a sympathetic response occurs, causing an increased heart rate and blood vessel constriction; when the **blood pressure** increases because of hypervolemia, an opposite effect occurs
7. The antidiuretic hormone (ADH) influences **blood pressure** indirectly by regulating vascular volume
8. Increases in blood volume result in decreased ADH release, increasing diuresis, and decreasing blood volume and thus **blood pressure**
9. Decreases in blood volume result in increased ADH release; this promotes an increase in blood volume and thus **blood pressure**
10. Renin, a potent vasoconstrictor, causes the **blood pressure** to increase
11. Renin converts angiotensinogen to angiotensin I; angiotensin I is then converted to angiotensin II in the lungs
12. Angiotensin II stimulates the release of aldosterone, which promotes water and sodium retention by the kidneys; this action increases blood volume and **blood pressure**

N. The vascular system
1. The arteries are vessels through which the blood passes away from the heart to various parts of the body; they convey blood with high concentrations of oxygen from the left side of the heart to the tissues

2. The arterioles control the blood flow into the capillaries
3. The capillaries allow the exchange of fluid and nutrients between the blood and the interstitial spaces
4. Venules receive blood from the capillary bed and move blood into the veins
5. Veins transport deoxygenated blood from the tissues back toward the heart and lungs for oxygenation
6. Valves help return blood to the heart against the force of gravity
7. The lymphatic system drains the tissues and returns the tissue fluid to the blood

II. Diagnostic Tests and Procedures

A. Cardiac enzymes
1. CK-MB (isoenzyme specific to myocardial cells)
   a. An elevation in value indicates myocardial damage
   b. An elevation occurs within 4 to 6 hours and peaks 18 to 24 hours following the acute ischemic attack
   c. Normal value in conventional units is 0 to 7 U/L
2. LDH (lactic acid dehydrogenase)
   a. Elevations in LDH occur within 48 hours following myocardial infarction
   b. When the serum concentration of LDH 1 is higher than the LDH 2, the pattern is indicated as "flipped," signifying myocardial necrosis
   c. Normal value in conventional units is 70 to 200 IU/L
B. CBC (complete blood [cell] count)
1. The red blood cell (RBC) count decreases in rheumatic heart disease and infective endocarditis and increases in conditions characterized by inadequate tissue oxygenation
2. The white blood cell count increases in infectious and inflammatory diseases of the heart and following myocardial infarction, because large numbers of WBCs are required to dispose of the necrotic tissue resulting from the infarction
3. An elevated hematocrit can result from vascular volume depletion
4. A decrease in hematocrit and hemoglobin can indicate anemia and produce heart murmurs
5. The normal RBC count is 4.0 to 5.5 million/μL in women and 4.5 to 6.2 million/μL in men
6. The normal WBC count is 4500 to 11,000/mm^3
7. The normal hemoglobin count is 12.0 to 15.0 g/dL in women and 14.0 to 16.5 g/dL in men

8. The normal hematocrit count is 35% to 47% in women and 42% to 52% in men
C. Blood coagulation factors
1. An increase in coagulation factors can occur during and after a myocardial infarction, which places the client at greater risk of thrombophlebitis and extension of clots in the coronary artery
2. The normal bleeding time is 2.75 to 8.0 minutes
3. The normal coagulation time is 8 to 15 minutes
4. The normal PTT (partial thromboplastin time) is 20 to 36 seconds
5. The normal PT (prothrombin time) is 9.6 to 11.8 seconds (male); 9.5 to 11.3 seconds (female)
6. International Normalized Ratio (INR) of 2.0 to 3.0 for standard Coumadin therapy
7. INR of 3.0 to 4.5 for high-dose Coumadin therapy
D. Serum lipids
1. The lipid profile measures serum cholesterol, triglycerides, and lipoprotein levels
2. The lipid profile is used to assess the risk of developing coronary artery disease
3. The normal serum total lipids is 400 to 800 mg/dL
4. The normal serum triglycerides will range from 10 to 190 mg/dL depending on sex and age
5. The desirable range for serum cholesterol is less than 200 mg/dL, with the LDL cholesterol at 60 to 80 mg/dL and the HDL cholesterol at 30 to 80 mg/dL, depending on age
E. Electrolytes
1. Potassium level
   a. Hypokalemia causes increased cardiac electrical instability, ventricular dysrhythmias, and increased risk of digitalis toxicity
   b. In hypokalemia, the electrocardiogram (ECG) shows flattening and inversion of the T wave, the appearance of a U wave, and sagging of the ST segment
   c. Hyperkalemia causes **asystole** and ventricular dysrhythmias
   d. The normal serum potassium level is 3.5 to 5.1 mEq/L
2. Sodium level
   a. The serum sodium level decreases with the use of diuretics
   b. The serum sodium level decreases in congestive heart failure, indicating water excess
   c. The normal serum sodium level is 135 to 145 mEq/L
F. Calcium level
1. Hypocalcemia can cause ventricular dysrhythmias, prolonged QT intervals, and cardiac arrest
2. Hypercalcemia can cause a shortened QT

interval, AV block, tachycardia or bradycardia, digitalis hypersensitivity, and cardiac arrest
3. The normal serum calcium level is 8.6 to 10.2 mg/dL, or 4.5 to 5.5 mEq/L

G. Phosphorus level
   1. Phosphorus levels should be interpreted with calcium levels because the kidneys retain or excrete one electrolyte in an inverse relationship to the other
   2. The normal serum phosphorus level is 2.4 to 4.5 mg/dL or 1.8 to 2.6 mEq/L

H. Magnesium level
   1. A low magnesium level can cause ventricular tachycardia and fibrillation
   2. A high magnesium level can cause muscle weakness, hypotension, bradycardia, and a prolonged PR interval and wide QRS complex
   3. The normal serum magnesium level is 1.8 to 2.6 mg/dL or 1.5 to 2.3 mEq/L

I. Blood urea nitrogen (BUN)
   1. The BUN is elevated in heart disorders such as congestive heart failure and cardiogenic shock that adversely affects renal circulation
   2. The normal serum urea nitrogen level is 5 to 20 mg/dL

J. Blood glucose
   1. An acute cardiac episode can elevate the blood glucose level
   2. The normal serum glucose level is 70 to 105 mg/dL

K. Chest x-ray film
   1. Description
      a. Done to determine the size, silhouette, and position of the heart
      b. Specific pathological changes are difficult to determine via x-ray, but anatomic changes can be seen
   2. Implementation
      a. Prepare client for x-ray film, explaining purpose and procedure
      b. Remove jewelry

◄ L. ECG (electrocardiogram) (Box 59–1)
   1. Description: A common noninvasive diagnostic test that evaluates the heart's function by recording electrical activity
   2. Implementation
      a. Determine the client's ability to lie still and advise the client to lie still, breathe normally, and refrain from talking during the test
      b. Reassure client that an electrical shock will not occur
      c. Document any cardiac medications the client is taking

M. Holter monitoring
   1. Description
      a. A noninvasive test in which the client wears a Holter monitor and an ECG tracing is recorded continuously over a period of 24 or more hours

---

BOX 59–1. Electrocardiogram (ECG) Basics

- An ECG reflects the electrical activity of cardiac cells and records electrical activity at a speed of 25 mm/second
- An ECG strip consists of horizontal squares representing seconds, and vertical squares representing voltage
- Each small square represents 0.04 second
- Each large square represents 0.20 second
- The P wave represents atrial depolarization
- The PR interval represents the time it takes an impulse to travel from the atria through the AV node, bundle of His, and bundle branches to the Purkinje fibers
- Normal PR interval duration ranges from 0.12 to 0.2 second
- The PR interval is measured from the beginning of the P wave to the end of the PR segment
- The QRS complex represents ventricular depolarization
- Normal QRS complex duration ranges from 0.04 to 0.1 second
- The Q wave appears as the first negative deflection in the QRS complex and reflects initial ventricular septal depolarization
- The R wave is the first positive deflection in the QRS complex
- The S wave appears as the second negative deflection in the QRS complex
- The J point marks the end of the QRS complex and the beginning of the ST segment
- The QRS duration is measured from the end of the PR segment to the J point
- The ST segment represents part of ventricular repolarization
- The T wave represents ventricular repolarization and ventricular diastole
- The U wave may follow the T wave
- A prominent U wave may indicate an electrolyte abnormality such as hypokalemia
- The QT interval represents ventricular refractory time, or the total time required for ventricular depolarization and repolarization
- The QT interval is measured from the beginning of the QRS complex to the end of the T wave
- The QT interval normally lasts 0.32 to 0.4 second but varies with the client's heart rate, age, and sex

---

      b. It identifies dysrhythmias if they occur and evaluates the effectiveness of antidysrhythmics or pacemaker therapy
   2. Implementation: Instruct the client to resume normal daily activities and to maintain a diary documenting activities and any symptoms that may develop

N. Echocardiogram
   1. Description
      a. A noninvasive procedure, based on the principles of ultrasound
      b. It evaluates structural and functional changes in the heart
   2. Implementation: Determine the client's ability to lie still and advise the client to lie

still, breathe normally, and refrain from talking during the test

O. Exercise testing (stress)
 1. Description
  a. A noninvasive test that studies the heart during activity and detects and evaluates coronary artery disease
  b. Treadmill testing is the most commonly used mode of stress testing
  c. Stress testing may be used in conjunction with myocardial radionuclide testing, at which point the procedure becomes invasive because a radionuclide must be injected
  d. A consent form is required if a radionuclide is injected
 2. Preprocedure implementation
  a. Obtain consent if required
  b. Ensure the client has adequate rest the night before the procedure
  c. Instruct client to eat a light meal 1 to 2 hours before the procedure
  d. Instruct client to avoid smoking, alcohol, and caffeine prior to the procedure
  e. Ask the physician about taking prescribed medication on the day of the procedure
  f. Instruct the client to wear nonconstrictive, comfortable clothing and supportive shoes
 3. Postprocedure implementation
  a. Instruct the client to notify the physician if any chest pain, dizziness, or shortness of breath occurs
  b. Instruct the client to avoid taking a hot bath or shower for at least 1 to 2 hours

P. Digital substraction angiography
 1. Description
  a. Combines x-ray techniques and a computerized subtraction technique with fluoroscopy for visualization of the cardiovascular system
  b. A contrast medium (dye) is injected
 2. Preprocedure implementation
  a. Assess client for allergy to contrast medium (dye), iodine, or seafood
  b. Obtain consent
 3. Postprocedure implementation
  a. Monitor vital signs
  b. Assess injection site for bleeding or discomfort

Q. Nuclear cardiology
 1. Description
  a. The use of radionuclide techniques and scanning in cardiovascular assessment
  b. The most common tests include technetium pyrophosphate scanning, thallium imaging, and multigated cardiac blood pool imaging multigated angiogram [scan], or (MUGA)
 2. Preprocedure implementation
  a. Obtain consent
  b. Inform the client that a small amount of

radioisotope will be injected, and that the radiation exposure and risks are minimal
 3. Postprocedure implementation
  a. Assess vital signs
  b. Assess injection site for bleeding or discomfort
  c. Inform the client that fatigue may be experienced

R. Cardiac catheterization
 1. Description
  a. Involves insertion of a catheter into the heart and surrounding vessels
  b. Obtains information about the structure and performance of the heart valves and circulatory system
 2. Preprocedure implementation
  a. Obtain a consent form
  b. Assess for allergies to seafood, iodine, or radiopaque dyes
  c. Withhold solid food for 6 to 8 hours and liquids for 4 hours to prevent vomiting and aspiration during the procedure
  d. Document client's height and weight, as this information will be needed to determine the amount of dye to be administered
  e. Document baseline vital signs, and note the quality and presence of peripheral pulses for postprocedure comparison
  f. Inform client that a local anesthetic will be administered prior to catheter insertion
  g. Inform clients that they may feel fatigued because they must lie still and quiet on a relatively hard table for up to 2 hours
  h. Inform clients that they may feel a fluttery feeling as the catheter passes through the heart, a flushed, warm feeling when the dye is injected, a desire to cough, and palpitations caused by heart irritability
  i. Prepare insertion site by shaving and cleaning with an antiseptic solution if prescribed
  j. Administer preprocedure medications if prescribed
  k. Insert an IV if prescribed
 3. Postprocedure implementation
  a. Monitor vital signs (VS) and cardiac rhythm for dysrhythmias every 30 minutes for 2 hours initially
  b. Assess for chest pain, and if dysrhythmias or chest pain occurs, notify the physician
  c. Monitor peripheral pulses and the color, warmth, and sensation of the extremity distal to the insertion site every 30 minutes for 2 hours initially
  d. Notify the physician if the client complains of numbness and tingling, if the extremity becomes cool, pale or cyanotic, or if sudden loss of peripheral pulses occurs

e. Monitor the pressure dressing for bleeding or hematoma formation

f. Apply a sandbag to the insertion site to provide additional pressure if required

g. Monitor for bleeding; if bleeding occurs, apply pressure immediately and notify the physician

h. Monitor for hematoma, and if a hematoma develops, notify the physician

i. Keep extremity extended for 4 to 6 hours, keeping the leg straight to prevent arterial occlusion

j. Maintain strict bed rest for 6 to 12 hours; however, the client may turn from side to side; do not elevate the head of the bed more than 15°

k. If the antecubital vessel was used, immobilize the arm on an armboard

l. Encourage fluids, if not contraindicated, to promote renal excretion of the dye

m. Monitor for nausea, vomiting, and rash or other signs of hypersensitivity to the dye

S. Central venous pressure (CVP)

1. Description

a. The CVP is the pressure within the superior vena cava and reflects the pressure under which blood is returned to the superior vena cava and right atrium

b. CVP is measured with a central venous line in the superior vena cava or by a balloon flotation catheter in the pulmonary artery

c. Normal CVP pressure is 2 to 12 mmHg

d. An increase in the CVP measurement indicates an increase in blood volume due to sodium and water retention, excessive IV fluids, alterations in fluid balance, or renal failure

e. A decrease in the CVP measurement indicates a decrease in circulating blood volume and may be due to hemorrhage or severe vasodilation, with pooling of blood in the extremities, limited venous return, and fluid imbalances

2. Measuring CVP

a. The right atrium is located at the midaxillary line at the fourth intercostal space, and the zero point on the transducer needs to be at the level of the right atrium

b. The client needs to be supine, with the head of the bed at 45°

c. The client needs to be relaxed: note that activity that increases intrathoracic pressure, such as coughing or straining, will cause false increases in the readings

d. If the client is on a ventilator, the reading should be taken at the point of end-expiration

e. To maintain patency of the line, a constant small amount of fluid is delivered under pressure

III. Therapeutic Management

A. Percutaneous transluminal coronary angioplasty (PTCA)

1. Description

a. One or more arteries are dilated with a balloon catheter to open the vessel lumen and improve arterial blood flow

b. Clients can experience reocclusion after the procedure, and the procedure may need to be repeated

c. Complications can include arterial dissection or rupture, immobilization of plaque fragments, spasm, and acute myocardial infarction (MI)

d. Firm commitment is needed on the client's part to stop smoking, lose weight, alter exercise patterns, and stop any behaviors that lead to progression of artery occlusion

2. Preprocedure implementation

a. Maintain NPO status after midnight

b. Prepare the groin area with antiseptic soap and shave per institutional procedure and as prescribed

c. Assess baseline vital signs and peripheral pulses

3. Postprocedure implementation

a. Monitor vital signs closely

b. Assess distal pulses in both extremities

c. Maintain bed rest as prescribed, keeping the limb straight for 6 to 8 hours

d. Administer anticoagulants and antiplatelets as prescribed to prevent thrombus formation

e. Monitor IV nitroglycerin if prescribed to prevent coronary spasm

f. Instruct client in the administration of nitrates, calcium channel blockers, antiplatelets, and anticoagulants as prescribed

g. Instruct client to take daily aspirin permanently if prescribed

h. Assist client with planning lifestyle modifications

B. Laser-assisted angioplasty

1. Description

a. A laser probe is advanced through a cannula similar to that used for PTCA

b. Used for clients with small occlusions in the distal superficial femoral, proximal popliteal, and common iliac arteries

c. Heat from the laser vaporizes the plaque to open the occluded artery

2. Preprocedure and postprocedure care

a. Similar to that of the PTCA

b. Monitor for complications of coronary dissection, acute occlusion, perforation, embolism, and MI

C. Coronary artery stents

1. Description

a. Used instead of PTCA to eliminate the risk of acute coronary vessel closure and to improve long-term patency of the vessel

b. A balloon catheter bearing the stent is inserted into the coronary artery and positioned at the site of occlusion

c. When placed in the coronary artery, the stent reopens the blocked artery

2. Postprocedure implementation

a. Acute thrombosis is a major concern following the procedure, and the client is placed on antiplatelet and anticoagulation therapy for several months following the procedure

b. Monitor for complications of the procedure, such as stent migration or occlusion, coronary artery dissection, and bleeding due to anticoagulation

D. Atherectomy

1. Description

a. Removes plaque from an artery by the use of a cutting chamber on the inserted catheter or a rotating blade that pulverizes the plaque

b. Used to improve blood flow to ischemic limbs in individuals with peripheral arterial disease

2. Postprocedure implementation: Monitor for complications of perforation, embolus, and restenosis

E. Transmyocardial revascularization

1. Used for clients with widespread atherosclerosis involving vessels that are too small and numerous for replacement or balloon catheterization

2. Uses a high-powered laser that creates 15 to 30 holes (channels) in the heart

3. Blood enters these small channels to provide the affected region of the heart with oxygenated blood

4. Performed through a small chest incision

5. The opening on the heart's surface heals over; however, the main channels remain and perfuse the myocardium

F. Arterial revascularization

1. Description

a. Performed to increase arterial blood flow to the affected limb

b. Inflow procedures involve bypassing arterial occlusion above the superficial femoral arteries

c. Outflow procedures involve surgical bypassing of arterial occlusions at or below the superficial femoral arteries

d. Graft material is sutured above and below the occlusion to facilitate blood flow around the occlusion

2. Preoperative implementation

a. Assess baseline vital signs and peripheral pulses

b. Insert IV and urinary catheter as prescribed

c. Maintain central venous catheter and/or arterial line if inserted

3. Postoperative implementation

a. Assess vital signs

b. Monitor **blood pressure** and notify the physician if changes occur

c. Monitor for hypotension, which may indicate hypovolemia

d. Monitor for hypertension, which may place stress on the graft and facilitate clot formation

e. Maintain bed rest for 24 hours as prescribed

f. Instruct client to keep affected extremity straight, limit movement, and avoid bending the knee and hip

g. Monitor for warmth, redness, and edema, which are often expected outcomes as a result of increased blood flow

h. Monitor for graft occlusion, which often occurs within the first 24 hours

i. Assess peripheral pulses and for changes in color and temperature of the extremity

j. Monitor for a sharp increase in pain, as pain is frequently the first indicator of postoperative graft occlusion

k. If signs of graft occlusion occur, notify physician immediately

l. Encourage coughing and deep breathing and the use of incentive spirometry

m. Maintain NPO status and progression to clear liquids as prescribed

n. Use strict aseptic technique when in contact with the incision

o. Assess incision for drainage, warmth, or swelling

p. Monitor for excessive bleeding (a small amount of bloody drainage is expected)

q. Monitor the area over the graft for hardness, tenderness, and warmth, which may indicate infection; if this occurs, notify the physician immediately

r. Instruct client about proper foot care and measures to prevent ulcer formation

s. Instruct client to take medications as prescribed

t. Instruct client how to care for incision

u. Assist client in modifying lifestyle to prevent further plaque formation

G. Coronary artery bypass graft (CABG)

1. Description

a. The occluded coronary arteries are bypassed with the client's own venous or arterial blood vessels

b. The saphenous vein or internal mammary artery is used to bypass lesions in the coronary arteries

c. Performed when the client does not respond to medical management of CAD or when disease progression is evident

2. Preoperative implementation

a. Familiarize the client and family with the cardiac surgical critical care unit

b. Instruct client how to splint chest incision, cough and deep breathe, and perform arm and leg exercises
c. Instruct the client to inform the nurse of any postoperative pain, as pain medication will be available
d. Inform the client to expect a sternal incision, possibly a leg incision, one or two chest tubes, a Foley catheter, and several IV fluid catheters
e. Inform the client that an endotracheal tube will be in place and connected to a ventilator for 6 to 24 hours
f. Advise the client that he or she should breathe with the ventilator and not fight it
g. Inform family that the client will not be able to talk while the endotracheal tube is in place
h. Encourage client and family to discuss anxieties and fears related to surgery
i. Note that prescribed medications are to be discontinued preoperatively (diuretics 2 to 3 days prior to surgery, digitalis 12 hours prior to surgery, and aspirin and anticoagulants 1 week prior to surgery)
j. Administer medications as prescribed, which may include potassium chloride, antihypertensives, antidysrhythmics, and antibiotics

3. Cardiac surgical unit
a. Maintain mechanical ventilation for 6 to 24 hours as prescribed
b. Monitor heart rate and rhythm, pulmonary artery and **arterial pressures,** and neurological status
c. Monitor mediastinal tubes and water seal drainage system and report drainage exceeding 100 to 150 mL per hour
d. Ground epicardial pacer wires
e. Assess fluid and electrolyte balance
f. Restrict fluids as prescribed to 1500 to 2000 mL because the client usually has edema
g. Monitor for hypotension, which can cause collapse of a vein graft
h. Monitor for hypertension, as increased pressure promotes leakage from the suture line and may cause bleeding
i. Monitor temperature and initiate rewarming procedures using warm or thermal blankets if the temperature drops below 96.8°F; rewarm client no faster than 1.8°F per hour to prevent shivering, and discontinue rewarming when the temperature approaches 98.6°F
j. Administer potassium IV as prescribed to maintain potassium level between 4 and 5 mEq/L to prevent dysrhythmias
k. Monitor for signs of cardiac tamponade, which will include sudden cessation of previously heavily draining mediastinal

drainage, jugular vein distention with clear lung sounds, and pulsus paradoxus
l. Monitor pain, differentiating sternotomy pain from anginal pain, which would indicate graft failure

4. Transfer from the Special Care Unit
a. Monitor vital signs, level of consciousness, and peripheral perfusion
b. Monitor for dysrhythmias
c. Auscultate lungs and assess respiratory status
d. Encourage client to spit, cough, and deep breathe and to use the incentive spirometer to raise secretions and prevent atelectasis
e. Monitor temperature and WBC count, which, if elevated after 3 to 4 days, indicates infection
f. Provide adequate fluids and hydration as prescribed to liquefy secretions
g. Assess suture line and chest tube insertion sites for redness, purulent discharge, and signs of infection
h. Assess sternal suture line for instability, which may indicate an infection
i. Guide the client in a gradual resumption of activity
j. Assess client for tachycardia, **orthostatic hypotension,** and fatigue before, during, and after activity
k. Discontinue activities if **BP** drops more than 10 to 20 mmHg or pulse increases more than 10 beats per minute
l. Monitor episodes of pain closely
m. See Box 59–2 for home care instructions

BOX 59–2. Home Care Instructions Following Cardiac Surgery

- Instruct client on how to progress with activities at home
- Inform client to limit pushing or pulling activities for 6 weeks following discharge
- Instruct client about incisional care and to record signs of redness, swelling, or drainage
- Inform client that sternotomy heals in about 6 to 8 weeks
- Instruct client to avoid crossing legs, to wear elastic hose as prescribed until edema subsides, and to elevate surgical limb when sitting in a chair
- Instruct client in the use of prescribed medications
- Instruct client in dietary measures, including the avoidance of saturated fats and cholesterol and the use of salt
- Instruct client that sexual intercourse can be resumed on the advice of the physician after exercise tolerance is assessed; if clients can walk 1 block or climb 2 flights of stairs without symptoms, they can safely resume sexual activity

> **BOX 59–3. Six-Second Strip Method to Determine Heart Rate**
>
> - Can be used to determine heart rate for both regular and irregular rhythms
> - To determine atrial rate, count the number of PP intervals in 6 seconds and multiply by 10 to obtain a full minute rate
> - To determine ventricular rate, count the number of RR intervals in 6 seconds and multiply by 10 to obtain a full minute rate
> - For accuracy, timing should begin on the P wave or the QRS complex and end exactly at 30 large blocks later

H. Heart transplant
  1. A donor heart from an individual with a comparable body weight and ABO compatibility is transplanted into a recipient in less than 6 hours of procurement
  2. The surgeon removes the diseased heart, leaving the posterior portion of the atria, which serve as an anchor for the new heart
  3. Because a remnant of the client's atria remains, two unrelated P waves are noted on the ECG
  4. The transplanted heart is denervated and unresponsive to vagal stimulation; because the heart is denervated, clients do not experience angina
  5. Symptoms of heart rejection include hypotension, dysrhythmias, weakness, fatigue, and dizziness
  6. Endomyocardial biopsies are performed at regularly scheduled intervals and whenever rejection is suspected
  7. Clients require immunosuppressive therapy for the rest of their lives
  8. The heart rate approximates 100 beats per minute and responds slowly with increases in heart rate, **contractility,** and **cardiac output** to exercise and stress

IV. Cardiac Dysrhythmias

A. Normal sinus rhythm (Fig. 59–1)
  1. Rhythm originates from the SA node
  2. Atrial and ventricular rhythms are regular
  3. Atrial and ventricular rates are 60 to 100 beats per minute (Fig. 59–2; Box 59–3)

B. Sinus bradycardia
  1. Description: Atrial and ventricular rates are below 60 beats per minute
  2. Implementation
     a. Attempt to determine cause; if a medication is suspected as causing the bradycardia, hold the medication and notify the physician
     b. Administer oxygen as prescribed
     c. Administer atropine sulfate as prescribed to increase the heart rate to 60 beats per minute
     d. Application of a noninvasive pacemaker may be prescribed initially, if the atropine sulfate does not increase the heart rate sufficiently
     e. Avoid additional doses of atropine sulfate as they will induce tachycardia
     f. Monitor for hypotension and administer IV fluids as prescribed
     g. Depending on the cause of the bradycardia, the client may need a permanent pacemaker

C. Sinus tachycardia
  1. Description: Atrial and ventricular rates are 100 to 180 beats per minute
  2. Implementation
     a. Identify the cause of the tachycardia
     b. Decrease the heart rate to normal by treating the cause

D. Atrial fibrillation (Fig. 59–3)
  1. Description
     a. Multiple rapid impulses from many foci at a rate of 350 to 600 times per minute depolarize in the atria in a totally disorganized manner
     b. The atria quiver, which can lead to the formation of thrombi
     c. P wave is absent
  2. Implementation
     a. Administer oxygen
     b. Administer anticoagulants as prescribed because of the risk of emboli
     c. Administer cardiac medications as prescribed
     d. Prepare the client for cardioversion as prescribed
     e. Instruct client in the use of medications as prescribed to control the dysrhythmia

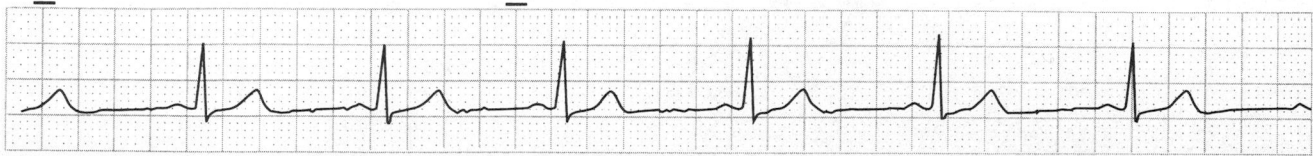

FIGURE 59–1. Normal sinus rhythm. (From Paul, S., & Hebra, J. [1998]. *The nurse's guide to cardiac rhythm interpretation.* Philadelphia: B. Saunders. p. 60.)

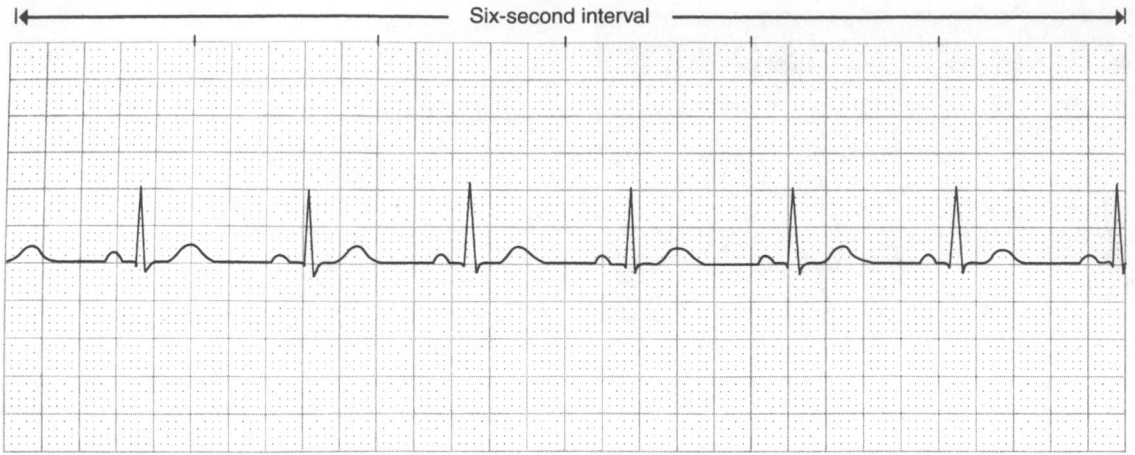

FIGURE 59–2. Six-second method for calculating heart rate: Seven QRS complexes in a 6-second interval is equal to a heart rate of 70 beats per minute. (From Paul, S., & Hebra, J. [1998]. *The nurse's guide to cardiac rhythm interpretation.* Philadelphia: W. B. Saunders. p. 34.)

E. Premature ventricular contractions (PVCs) (Box 59–4)
1. Description
   a. Also called ventricular premature beats (VPBs)
   b. Early ventricular complexes result from increased irritability of the ventricles
   c. PVCs frequently occur in repetitive rhythms, such as bigeminy, trigeminy, and quadrigeminy
   d. The QRS complexes may be unifocal or multifocal
2. Implementation
   a. Notify physician if PVCs are noted
   b. Identify the cause and treat based on the cause
   c. Evaluate electrolytes, particularly the potassium level, as hypokalemia can cause PVCs
   d. Administer oxygen as prescribed
   e. Administer lidocaine as prescribed
   f. Notify physician if the client complains of chest pain and if PVCs increase in frequency, are multifocal, are R on T, or occur in runs of ventricular tachycardia (Fig. 59–4)

F. Ventricular tachycardia (VT) (Fig. 59–4)
1. Description
   a. Occurs when there is a repetitive firing of an irritable ventricular ectopic focus at a rate of 140 to 250 beats or more per minute
   b. May present as a paroxysm of 3 self-limiting beats or more, or may be a sustained rhythm
   c. Can cause cardiac arrest
2. Stable client with sustained VT
   a. Administer oxygen as prescribed
   b. Administer lidocaine bolus and infusion as prescribed
   c. Administer procainamide (Pronestyl) bolus and infusion as prescribed
   d. Administer bretylium (Bretylol) bolus and infusion as prescribed
   e. Administer magnesium sulfate infusion as prescribed
3. Unstable client with VT
   a. Administer oxygen and antidysrhythmic therapy as prescribed
   b. Prepare for synchronized cardioversion if unstable
   c. Attempt cough cardiopulmonary resuscitation (CPR) by asking the client to cough hard every 1 to 3 seconds
4. Pulseless client: Defibrillation and CPR

G. Ventricular fibrillation (Fig. 59–5)
1. Description
   a. Impulses from many irritable foci fire in a totally disorganized manner
   b. Chaotic rapid rhythm in which the ventricles quiver
   c. Rapidly fatal if not successfully terminated within 3 to 5 minutes

---

BOX 59–4. Premature Ventricular Contractions (PVCs)

Bigeminy. PVC every other heart beat

Trigeminy. PVC every third heart beat

Quadrigeminy. PVC every fourth heart beat

Couplet or Pair. Two sequential PVCs

Unifocal. Uniform upward or downward deflection, arising from the same ectopic foci

Multifocal. Different shapes, with the impulse generation from different sites

R on T Phenomenon. PVC falls on preceding beats' T wave, which is considered a vunerable period; may precipitate ventricular fibrillation

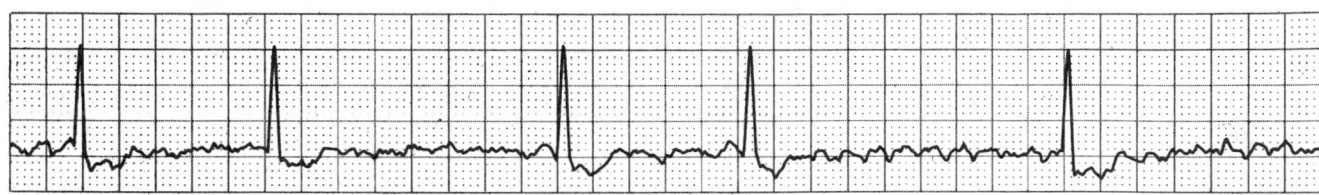

FIGURE 59–3. Atrial fibrillation. Note the chaotic undulations of the atria and irregular response of the ventricles. (From Paul, S., & Hebra, J. [1998]. *The nurse's guide to cardiac rhythm interpretation.* Philadelphia: W. B. Saunders. p. 87.)

    d. Client lacks a pulse, **blood pressure,** respirations, and heart sounds

  2. Implementation
    a. Defibrillate immediately
    b. Initiate CPR
    c. Administer oxygen as prescribed
    d. Administer epinephrine (Adrenalin) and antidysrhythmic therapy with lidocaine as prescribed
    e. Administer procainamide (Pronestyl) bolus and infusion as prescribed
    f. Administer bretylium (Bretylol) bolus and infusion as prescribed
    g. Administer magnesium sulfate infusion as prescribed

V. Management of Dysrhythmias

A. Vagal maneuvers
  1. Description: Induce vagal stimulation of the cardiac conduction system and used to terminate supraventricular tachydysrhythmias
  2. Carotid sinus massage
    a. The physician instructs the client to turn the head away from the side to be massaged
    b. The physician massages over the carotid artery for 6 to 8 seconds until there is a change in cardiac rhythm
    c. Observe the cardiac monitor for a change in rhythm
    d. Record an ECG rhythm strip before, during, and after the procedure
    e. Have a defibrillator and resuscitative equipment available
    f. Monitor vital signs, cardiac rhythm, and level of consciousness (LOC) following the procedure
  3. Valsalva maneuvers
    a. The physician instructs the client to bear down or induces a gag reflex in the client, both of which stimulate a vagal reflex
    b. Monitor the heart rate, rhythm, and **BP**
    c. Observe the cardiac monitor for a change in rhythm
    d. Record an ECG rhythm strip before, during, and after the procedure
    e. Provide an emesis basin if the gag reflex is stimulated, and initiate precautions to prevent aspiration
    f. Have a defibrillator and resuscitative equipment available

B. Cardioversion
  1. Description
    a. Synchronized countershock to convert an undesirable rhythm to a stable rhythm

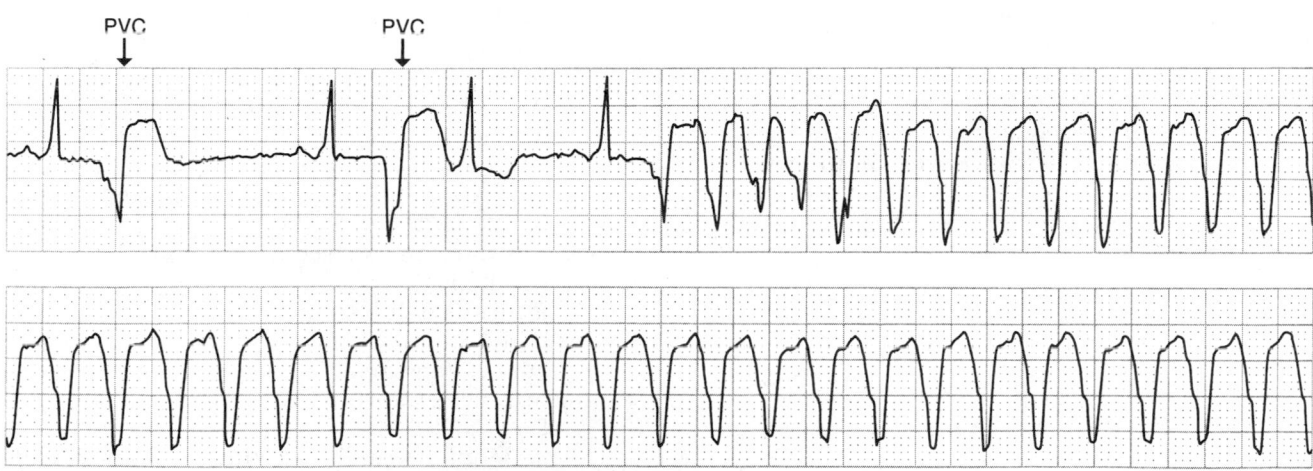

FIGURE 59–4. Ventricular tachycardia. Note the PVCs prior to the onset of the tachycardia (second and fourth beats on the strip). The PVC that initiates the tachycardia has the identical morphology (shape) of the first PVC. (From Paul, S., & Hebra, J. [1998]. *The nurse's guide to cardiac rhythm interpretation.* Philadelphia: W. B. Saunders. p. 138.)

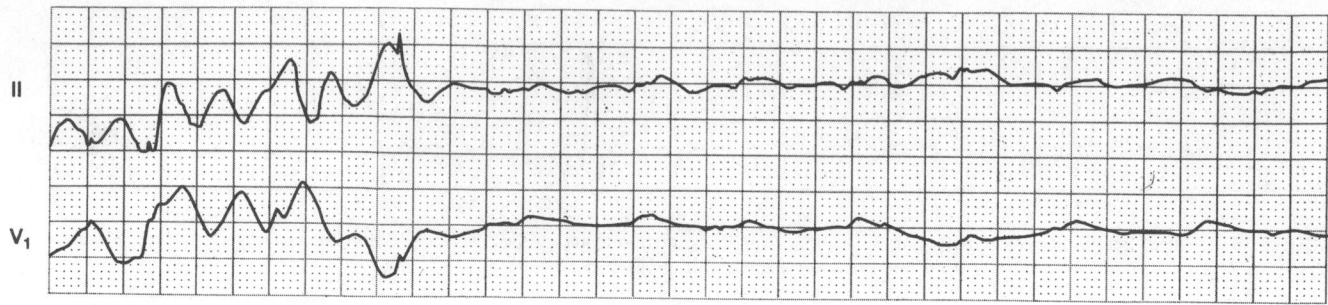

FIGURE 59–5. Coarse ventricular fibrillation degenerating into fine ventricular fibrillation. (From Paul, S., & Hebra, J. [1998]. *The nurse's guide to cardiac rhythm interpretation.* Philadelphia: W. B. Saunders. p. 144.)

b. An elective procedure done by the physician

c. A lower wattage of energy is used than with defibrillation

d. Defibrillator is synchronized to the client's R wave to avoid discharging the shock during the vunerable period (T wave)

e. If defibrillator were not synchronized, it would discharge on the T wave and cause ventricular fibrillation (VF)

2. Preprocedure implementation
   a. Obtain consent
   b. Administer sedation as prescribed
   c. Hold digoxin (Lanoxin) 48 hours preprocedure as prescribed to prevent postcardioversion ventricular irritability

3. During the Procedure
   a. Ensure skin is clean and dry in the area where the electrode paddles will be placed
   b. Oxygen is stopped during the procedure to avoid hazard of fire
   c. Be sure no one is touching the bed or the client when delivering the countershock

4. Postprocedure implementation
   a. Maintain airway patency
   b. Administer oxygen as prescribed
   c. Assess vital signs
   d. Assess LOC
   e. Monitor cardiac rhythm
   f. Monitor for indications of successful response, such as conversion to sinus rhythm, strong peripheral pulses, and an adequate **BP**

C. Defibrillation
   1. Description
      a. An asynchronous countershock used to terminate pulseless ventricular tachycardia (VT) or VF
      b. Three rapid consecutive shocks are delivered, with the first at an energy of 200 joules
      c. If unsuccessful, the shock is repeated at 200 to 300 joules
      d. The third and subsequent shock will be at 360 joules

2. During the procedure
   a. Oxygen is stopped during the procedure to avoid hazard of fire
   b. Be sure no one is touching the bed or the client when delivering the countershock

D. Use of paddle electrodes
   1. Apply conductive pads
   2. Place one paddle over pad on upper right chest to the right of sternum, and the other on the lower left chest with the center in the midaxillary line
   3. Apply firm pressure with the paddles
   4. Be sure no one is touching the bed or the client when delivering the countershock

E. Automatic external defibrillator (AED)
   1. Used by laypersons and emergency medical technicians for prehospital cardiac arrest
   2. Place client on a firm, dry surface
   3. Stop CPR
   4. Ensure that no one is touching the client to avoid motion artifact during rhythm analysis
   5. Place electrode paddles in correct position on the client's chest
   6. Press analyzer button, and when rhythm is analyzed, which may take 30 seconds, the machine will advise whether a shock is necessary
   7. Shocks are recommended for pulseless VF only
   8. If shock is recommended, the shock is delivered at an energy of 200 joules for the first one
   9. If unsuccessful, the shock is repeated at 200 to 300 joules
   10. The third and subsequent shock will be at 360 joules
   11. If unsuccessful, CPR is continued for 1 minute, and then another series of 3 shocks are delivered, each at 360 joules of energy

F. Implantable cardioverter defibrillator (ICD)
   1. Description
      a. Monitors cardiac rhythm and detects and terminates episodes of VT and VF
      b. It senses VT or VF and delivers 25 to 30 joules, up to four times if necessary
      c. Used in clients with a history of VF or in

unstable VT that is unresponsive to medications
  d. Electrodes are placed in the right atrium and ventricle and apical pericardium
  e. The generator is implanted in the abdomen
  2. Client education
  a. Basic functioning of the ICD
  b. How to perform cough CPR
  c. How to take pulse and to take pulse daily and maintain a diary of pulse rates
  d. Wear loose-fitting clothing
  e. Avoid contact sports and strenuous activities
  f. Report any fever, redness, swelling, or drainage from the insertion site
  g. Report symptoms of fainting, nausea, weakness, blackouts, and rapid pulse rates to the physician
  h. During shock discharge, the client may feel faint or short of breath
  i. Instruct client to sit or lie down if a shock is felt, and to notify the physician
  j. Instruct client and family how to access the emergency medical system
  k. Encourage family to learn CPR
  l. Advise client to maintain a diary of any shocks that are delivered, including the date, preceding activity, the number of shocks, and if the shocks were successful
  m. Instruct client to avoid electromagnetic fields directly over the ICD because they can inactivate the device
  n. Instruct client to move away from the magnetic field immediately if beeping tones are heard, and notify the physician
  o. Keep pacemaker ID in wallet and obtain and wear a Medic-Alert bracelet
  p. Inform all health care providers that an ICD is inserted

VI. Pacemakers (Box 59–5)

A. Description: A temporary or permanent device that provides electrical stimulation and maintains the heart rate when the client's intrinsic pacemaker fails to provide a perfusing rhythm

B. Settings
  1. Synchronous or demand pacemaker: Senses the client's rhythm and paces only if the client's intrinsic rate falls below the set pacemaker rate
  2. Asynchronous or fixed rate pacemaker: Paces at a preset rate regardless of the client's intrinsic rhythm
  3. Overdrive pacing: To suppress the underlying rhythm in tachydysrhythmias so that the sinus node will regain control of the heart

C. Spikes
  1. When a pacing stimulus is delivered to the heart, a spike (straight vertical line) is seen on the monitor or ECG strip
  2. Also referred to as "capture," meaning that

BOX 59–5. Pacemakers: Client Education

- Instruct client about the pacemaker, including the programmed rate
- Instruct client in the signs of battery failure and when to notify the physician
- Instruct client to report any fever, redness, swelling, or drainage from the insertion site
- Report signs of dizziness, weakness, or fatigue; swelling of the ankles or legs; chest pain; or shortness of breath
- Keep pacemaker ID in wallet and obtain and wear a Medic-Alert bracelet
- Instruct client how to take pulse, to take the pulse daily, and maintain a diary of pulse rates
- Wear loose-fitting clothing
- Avoid contact sports
- Inform all health care providers that a pacemaker is inserted
- Instruct clients to inform airport security that they have a pacemaker as the pacemaker may set off the security detector
- Instruct the client that most electrical appliances can be used without any interference with the functioning of the pacemaker; however, advise the client not to operate electrical appliances directly over the pacemaker site
- Avoid transmitter towers and antitheft devices in stores
- Instruct the client that if any unusual feelings occur when near any electrical devices, to move 5 to 10 feet away and check the pulse
- Emphasize the importance of follow-up with the physician

---

the pacemaker successfully depolarized or captured the chamber
  3. The spike should be followed by a P wave indicating atrial depolarization, or a QRS complex indicating ventricular depolarization
  4. If the electrode is in the ventricle, the spike is in front of the QRS complex; if the electrode is in the atria, the spike is before the P wave
  5. If the electrode is in both the atria and ventricle, the spike is before both QRS complex and P waves

D. Temporary pacemakers
  1. Noninvasive temporary pacing (NTP)
  a. Used as an emergency measure or when a client is transported and the risk of bradydysrhythmia exists in the client
  b. A large electrode patch is placed on the chest and back
  c. Wash skin with soap and water prior to applying electrodes
  d. Do not shave the hair or apply alcohol or tinctures to the skin
  e. The posterior electrode is placed between the spine and left scapula behind the heart, avoiding placement over bone
  f. The anterior electrode is placed between V2 and V5 position over the heart

g. Do not place the anterior electrode over female breast tissue; rather, displace breast tissue and place the electrode under the breast

h. Do not assess the pulse or take the **BP** on the left side, because the results will not be accurate due to the muscle twitching and electrical current

i. Ensure that electrodes are in good contact with the skin

j. If loss of "capture" occurs, assess the skin contact of the electrodes and increase the current until capture is regained

2. Transvenous invasive temporary pacing

a. Pacing lead wire is placed through the antecubital, femoral, jugular, or subclavian vein into the right atrium for atrial pacing, or the right ventricle, and positioned in contact with the endocardium

b. Monitor cardiac rhythm continuously

c. Monitor vital signs

d. Monitor pacemaker insertion site

e. Restrict client movement to prevent lead wire displacement

3. Epicardial invasive temporary pacing: Applied by a transthoracic approach, and the lead wires are loosely threaded on the epicardial surface of the heart after open heart surgery

4. Reducing the risk of microshock

a. Use only inspected and approved equipment

b. Insulate exposed portions of wires with plastic or rubber material (fingers of rubber gloves) when wires are not attached to the pulse generator, and cover with nonconductive tape

c. Ground all electrical equipment, using a three-pronged plug

d. Wear gloves when handling exposed wires

e. Keep dressings dry

E. Permanent pacemakers

1. Pulse generator is internal and surgically implanted in a subcutaneous pocket under the clavicle or abdominal wall

2. The leads are passed transvenously via the cephalic or subclavian vein to the endocardium on the right side of the heart

3. May be single-chambered, in which the lead wire is placed in the chamber to be paced, or may be dual-chambered, with lead wires placed in the atrium and right ventricle

4. It is programmed when inserted and can be reprogrammed if necessary by noninvasive transmission from an external programmer to the implanted generator

5. Pacemakers are powered by a lithium battery that has an average life span of 10 years, or are nuclear powered with a life span of 20

years or longer, or are designed to be recharged externally

VII. Coronary Artery Disease

A. Description

1. A narrowing or obstruction of the coronary arteries due to atherosclerosis, an accumulation in the arteries of fatty plaques made of lipids

2. Causes a decreased perfusion of myocardial tissue and inadequate myocardial oxygen supply

3. Leads to hypertension, angina, dysrhythmias, myocardial infarction, congestive heart failure, and death

4. Collateral circulation, more than one artery supplying a muscle with blood, is normally present in the coronary arteries, especially in older persons

5. The development of collateral circulation takes time and happens when chronic ischemia occurs to meet the metabolic demands; therefore, an occlusion of a coronary artery in a young individual is more likely to be lethal than in an older individual

6. Symptoms occur when the coronary artery is occluded to the point of inadequate blood supply to the muscle, causing ischemia

7. Coronary artery narrowing is significant if the lumen diameter of the left main artery is reduced at least 50%, or if any major branch is reduced at least 75%

8. The goal of treatment is to alter the atherosclerotic progression

B. Assessment

1. Findings may be normal during asymptomatic periods

2. Chest pain

3. Palpitations

4. Dyspnea

5. Syncope

6. Cough or hemoptysis

7. Excessive fatigue

C. Diagnostic studies

1. ECG

a. When blood flow is reduced and ischemia occurs, ST segment depression or T wave inversion is noted; the ST segment returns to normal when the blood flow returns

b. With infarction, cell injury results in ST segment elevation followed by T wave inversion

2. Cardiac catheterization

a. Provides the most definitive source for diagnosis

b. Would show the presence of atherosclerotic lesions

3. Blood lipid levels

a. May be elevated

b. Cholesterol-lowering medications may be prescribed to reduce the development of atherosclerotic plaques

D. Implementation

1. Instruct client regarding the purpose of diagnostic medical and surgical procedures and the expected preprocedure and postprocedure activities
2. Assist client to identify risk factors that can be modified
3. Assist client to set goals that will promote changes in lifestyle to reduce the impact of risk factors
4. Assist client to identify barriers to compliance with the therapeutic plan and to identify methods to overcome barriers
5. Instruct client regarding a low-calorie, low-sodium, low-cholesterol, and low-fat diet with an increase in dietary fiber
6. Stress to client that dietary changes are not temporary and must be maintained for life; instruct client regarding prescribed medications
7. Provide community resources to client regarding exercise, smoking reduction, and stress reduction

E. Surgical procedures

1. Percutaneous transluminal coronary angioplasty (PTCA) to compress the plaque against the walls of the artery and dilate the vessel
2. Laser angioplasty to vaporize the plaque
3. Atherectomy to remove the plaque from the artery
4. Vascular stent to prevent the artery from closing and prevent restenosis
5. Coronary artery bypass graft to improve blood flow to the myocardial tissues that are at risk for ischemia or infarction due to the occluded artery

F. Medications

1. Nitrates to dilate the coronary arteries and to decrease **preload** and **afterload**
2. Calcium channel blockers to dilate coronary arteries and reduce vasospasm
3. Cholesterol-lowering medications may be prescribed to reduce the development of atherosclerotic plaques
4. Beta-blockers to reduce **blood pressure** in those individuals who are hypertensive

VIII. Angina

A. Description

1. Chest pain resulting from myocardial ischemia caused by inadequate myocardial blood and oxygen supply
2. Caused by an imbalance between oxygen supply and demand
3. Causes include obstruction of coronary blood flow due to atherosclerosis, coronary artery

spasm, and conditions increasing myocardial oxygen consumption

4. The goal of treatment is to provide relief of an acute attack, correct the imbalance between myocardial oxygen supply and demand, prevent the progression of the disease and further attacks to reduce the risk of MI

B. Patterns of angina

1. Stable angina
   a. Also called exertional angina
   b. Occurs with such activities as exertion or emotional stress, and the pain is relieved with rest or nitroglycerin
   c. It usually has a stable pattern of onset, duration, severity, and relieving factors
2. Unstable angina
   a. Also called preinfarction angina
   b. Occurs with an unpredictable degree of exertion or emotion and increase in occurrence, duration, and severity over time
   c. Pain may not be relieved with nitroglycerin
3. Variant angina
   a. Also called Prinzmetal's or vasoplastic angina
   b. Results from coronary artery spasm and is similar to classic angina but lasts longer
   c. It may occur at rest
   d. Attacks may be associated with elevation of the ST segment on the ECG
4. Intractable angina: A chronic, incapacitating angina that is unresponsive to interventions
5. Preinfarction angina
   a. Associated with acute coronary insufficiency
   b. Angina that lasts longer than 15 minutes
   c. A symptom of worsening cardiac ischemia
6. Postinfarction angina: Occurs after an MI, when residual ischemia may cause episodes of angina

C. Assessment

1. Pain
   a. Can develop slowly or quickly
   b. Usually described as mild or moderate pain
   c. Substernal, crushing, squeezing pain
   d. May radiate to the shoulders, arms, jaw, neck, back
   e. Usually lasts less than 5 minutes; however, can last up to 15 to 20 minutes
   f. Relieved by nitroglycerin or rest
2. Dyspnea
3. Pallor
4. Sweating
5. Palpitations and tachycardia
6. Dizziness and faintness
7. Hypertension
8. Digestive disturbances

D. Diagnostic studies

1. ECG: Normal during rest, with ST depression

or elevation and/or T wave inversion during an episode of pain
2. Stress test: Chest pain or changes in the ECG or vital signs during testing may indicate ischemia
3. Cardiac enzymes: Normal findings in angina
4. Cardiac catheterization: Provides a definitive diagnosis by yielding information about the patency of the coronary arteries

E. Implementation
1. Immediate management
   a. Assess pain
   b. Provide bed rest
   c. Administer oxygen at 3-L nasal cannula as prescribed
   d. Administer nitroglycerin as prescribed to dilate the coronary arteries, reduce the oxygen requirements of the myocardium, and relieve the chest pain
   e. Obtain a 12-lead ECG
   f. Provide continuous cardiac monitoring
2. Following acute episode
   a. Instruct client regarding purpose of diagnostic medical and surgical procedures and the probable preprocedure and postprocedure expectations
   b. Assist client to identify angina-precipitating events
   c. Instruct client to stop activity and rest if chest pain occurs and to take nitroglycerin as prescribed
   d. Instruct client to seek medical attention if the pain persists
   e. Instruct client regarding prescribed medications
   f. Provide diet instruction to client, stressing that dietary changes are not temporary and must be maintained for life
   g. Assist client to identify risk factors that can be modified
   h. Assist client to set goals that will promote changes in lifestyle to reduce the impact of risk factors
   i. Assist client to identify barriers to compliance with the therapeutic plan and to identify methods to overcome barriers
   j. Provide community resources to client regarding exercise, smoking cessation, and stress reduction

F. Surgical procedures
1. Percutaneous transluminal coronary angioplasty (PTCA) to assess the condition of the coronary arteries and to compress the plaque, if present, against the walls of the artery and dilate the vessel
2. Laser angioplasty to vaporize the plaque if present
3. Atherectomy to remove the plaque, if present, from the artery
4. Vascular stent to prevent the artery from closing and prevent restenosis

5. Coronary artery bypass graft to improve blood flow to the myocardial tissue that is at risk for ischemia or infarction due to the occluded artery

G. Medications
1. Vasodilators to maintain coronary artery vasodilation and promote a greater flow of blood and oxygen to the heart
2. Calcium channel blockers to dilate coronary arteries and reduce vasospasm
3. Beta-blockers to reduce the oxygen requirements of the heart and reduce **blood pressure** in those individuals who are hypertensive
4. Antiplatelet therapy to inhibit platelet aggregation and reduce the risk of developing an acute MI

IX. Myocardial Infarction (MI)

A. Description
1. Occurs when myocardial tissue is abruptly and severely deprived of oxygen
2. Ischemia can lead to necrosis of myocardial tissue if blood flow is not restored
3. Infarction does not occur instantly but evolves over several hours
4. Obvious physical changes do not occur in the heart until 6 hours after the infarction, when the infarcted area appears blue and swollen
5. After 48 hours, the infarct turns gray with yellow streaks as neutrophils invade the tissue
6. By 8 to 10 days after infarction, granulation tissue forms
7. Over 2 to 3 months, the necrotic area develops into a scar; scar tissue permanently changes the size and shape of the entire left ventricle

B. Location of MI
1. Obstruction of the left anterior descending (LAD) artery results in anterior or septal MI or both
2. Obstruction of the circumflex artery results in posterior wall MI or lateral wall MI
3. Obstruction of the right coronary artery results in inferior wall MI

C. Risk factors
1. Atherosclerosis
2. CAD
3. Elevated cholesterol levels
4. Smoking
5. Hypertension
6. Obesity
7. Physical inactivity
8. Impaired glucose tolerance
9. Stress

D. Diagnostic studies
1. Total CK levels
   a. Rise within 3 hours after the onset of chest pain

b. Peak within 24 hours after damage and death of cardiac tissue

2. CK-MB isoenzyme
   a. Peak elevation occurs 12 to 24 hours after the onset of chest pain
   b. Levels return to normal 48 to 72 hours later

3. LDH levels
   a. Rise within 12 to 24 hours after MI
   b. Peak between 40 and 72 hours and fall to normal in 7 days
   c. Serum levels of LDH_1 isoenzyme rise higher than serum levels of LDH_2

4. WBC count: An elevated white blood cell count of 10,000 to 20,000 cells/mm³ appears on the second day post-MI and lasts up to a week

5. ECG
   a. ST segment elevation, T wave inversion, abnormal Q wave
   b. Hours to days after the MI, ST and T wave changes will return to normal, but the Q wave usually remains permanently abnormal

6. Diagnostic tests following the acute stage
   a. Exercise tolerance test or stress test may be prescribed to assess for ECG changes and ischemia and to evaluate for medical therapy or to identify clients who may need invasive therapy
   b. Thallium scans may be prescribed to assess for ischemia or necrotic muscle tissue
   c. MUGA scans: May be used to evaluate left ventricular function
   d. Cardiac catheterization: Performed to determine the extent and location of obstructions of the coronary arteries

E. Assessment
1. Pain
   a. Crushing substernal pain
   b. Radiates to the jaw, back, and left arm
   c. Occurs without cause, primarily early in the morning
   d. Is unrelieved by rest or nitroglycerin, and relieved only by opioids
   e. Pain lasts 30 minutes or more
2. Nausea and vomiting
3. Diaphoresis
4. Dyspnea
5. Dysrhythmias
6. Feelings of fear and anxiety
7. Pallor, cyanosis, coolness of extremities

F. Complications of MI
1. Dysrhythmias
2. Heart failure
3. Pulmonary edema
4. Cardiogenic shock
5. Thrombophlebitis
6. Pericarditis
7. Mitral valve insufficiency
8. Postinfarction angina
9. Ventricular rupture
10. Dressler's syndrome (a combination of pericarditis, pericardial effusion, and pleural effusion, which can occur several weeks to months following an MI)

G. Implementation, acute stage
1. Obtain a description of the chest discomfort
2. Assess vital signs
3. Assess cardiovascular status and maintain cardiac monitoring
4. Obtain a 12-lead ECG
5. Administer nitroglycerin as prescribed
6. Administer morphine sulfate as prescribed to relieve chest discomfort that is unresponsive to nitroglycerin
7. Administer oxygen at 2 to 4 L by nasal cannula as prescribed
8. Place client in semi-Fowler's position to enhance comfort and tissue oxygenation
9. Establish an IV access route
10. Administer IV nitroglycerin and antidysrhythmics as prescribed
11. Monitor thrombolytic therapy, which may be prescribed within the first 6 hours of the coronary event
12. Monitor for signs of bleeding if the client is receiving thrombolytics
13. Monitor laboratory values as prescribed
14. Administer beta-blockers to slow the heart rate and increase myocardial perfusion while reducing the force of myocardial contraction, as prescribed
15. Monitor for complications related to MI
16. Monitor for cardiac dysrhythmias, since tachycardia and PVCs frequently occur in the first few hours after MI
17. Assess distal peripheral pulses and skin temperature as poor **cardiac output** may be identified by cool, diaphoretic skin and diminished or absent pulses
18. Monitor intake and output (I&O)
19. Assess respiratory rate and breath sounds for signs of heart failure, as indicated by the presence of crackles or wheezes or dependent edema
20. Monitor **blood pressure** closely after the administration of medications, and if the **BP** is less than 100 systolic or is 25 mmHg lower than the previous reading, lower the head of the bed and notify the physician
21. Provide reassurance to client and family

H. Implementation following acute episode
1. Maintain bed rest for the first 24 to 36 hours
2. Use a bedside commode if prescribed; male client may be allowed to stand to void
3. Provide range of motion exercises to prevent thrombus formation and maintain muscle strength
4. Progress to dangling at the side of the bed or out of bed to the chair for 30 minutes three times a day as prescribed
5. Progress to ambulation in the client's room

and to the bathroom, then in the hallway, three times a day
6. Monitor for complications
7. Encourage client to verbalize feelings regarding the MI
I. Cardiac rehabilitation: Process of actively assisting the client with cardiac disease to achieve and maintain a vital and productive life within the limitations of the heart disease

◆ X. Heart Failure

A. Description
  1. The inability of the heart to maintain adequate circulation to meet the metabolic needs of the body, due to an impaired pumping capability
  2. **Cardiac output** is diminished, and peripheral tissue is not adequately perfused
  3. Congestion of the lungs and periphery may occur
B. Classification
  1. Acute: Occurs suddenly
  2. Chronic: Develops over time; however, a client with chronic heart failure can develop an acute episode
C. Types of heart failure
  1. Right-sided heart failure/left-sided heart failure
    a. Because the two ventricles of the heart represent two separate pumping systems, it is possible for one to fail alone for a short period
    b. Most heart failure begins with left ventricular failure and progresses to failure of both ventricles
    c. Acute pulmonary edema, a medical emergency, results from left ventricular failure
    d. If pulmonary edema is not treated, death will occur from suffocation as the client literally drowns in self-fluids
  2. Forward failure/backward failure
    a. In forward failure, an inadequate output of the affected ventricle causes decreased perfusion to vital organs
    b. In backward failure, blood backs up behind the affected ventricle, causing increased pressure in the atrium behind the affected ventricle
  3. Low output/high output
    a. In low-output failure, not enough **cardiac output** is available to meet the demands of the body
    b. High-output failure occurs when a condition causes the heart to work harder to meet the demands of the body
  4. Systolic failure/diastolic failure
    a. Systolic failure leads to problems with contraction and the ejection of blood
    b. Diastolic failure leads to problems with the heart relaxing and filling with blood

D. Compensatory mechanisms
  1. Act to restore **cardiac output** to near-normal levels
  2. Initially, these mechanisms increase **cardiac output;** however, they eventually have a damaging effect on pump action
  3. Contribute to an increase in myocardial oxygen consumption, and when this occurs, myocardial reserve is exhausted and clinical manifestations of heart failure develop
  4. Include increased heart rate, improved **stroke volume,** arterial vasoconstriction, sodium and water retention, and myocardial hypertrophy
E. Assessment
  1. Right-sided heart failure
    a. Signs of right-sided failure will be evident in the systemic circulation
    b. Pitting, dependent edema in feet, legs, sacrum, back, buttocks
    c. Ascites from portal hypertension
    d. Tenderness of right upper quadrant, organomegaly
    e. Distended neck veins
    f. Pulsus alternans (regular alternation of weak and strong beats noted in the pulse)
    g. Abdominal pain, bloating
    h. Anorexia, nausea
    i. Fatigue
    j. Weight gain
    k. Nocturnal diuresis
  2. Left-sided heart failure
    a. Signs of left-sided failure will be evident in the pulmonary system
    b. Cough, which may become productive, with frothy sputum
    c. Dyspnea upon exertion
    d. Orthopnea
    e. Paroxysmal nocturnal dyspnea
    f. Presence of rales or crackles on auscultation
    g. Tachycardia
    h. Pulsus alternans
    i. Fatigue
    j. Pallor
    k. Cyanosis
    l. Confusion and disorientation
    m. Signs of cerebral anoxia
  3. Acute pulmonary edema
    a. Severe dyspnea and orthopnea
    b. Pallor
    c. Tachycardia
    d. Expectoration of large amounts of blood-tinged, frothy sputum
    e. Wheezing and rales
    f. Bubbling respirations
    g. Acute anxiety, apprehension, restlessness
    h. Profuse sweating
    i. Cold, clammy skin
    j. Cyanosis
    k. Nasal flaring
    l. Use of accessory breathing muscles

m. Tachypnea

n. Hypocapnia evidenced by muscle cramps, weakness, dizziness, and paresthesia

F. Immediate management

1. Place client in high Fowler's position, with legs dependent, to reduce pulmonary congestion and relieve edema

2. Administer oxygen in high concentrations by mask or cannula as prescribed by the physician to improve gas exchange and pulmonary function

3. Prepare for intubation and ventilator support if required; monitor lung sounds for rales and decreased breath sounds

4. Suction as needed to maintain a patent airway

5. Assess LOC

6. Provide reassurance to the client

7. Monitor vital signs closely, noting tachycardia or pulsus alternans

8. Monitor for hypotension due to decreased tissue perfusion, or hypertension due to anxiety or history of hypertension

9. Monitor heart rate on a cardiac monitor for dysrhythmias

10. Assess for edema in dependent areas and in the sacral, lumbar, and posterior thigh region in the client in bed

11. Insert Foley catheter as prescribed and monitor urine output closely following administration of diuretic

12. Monitor I&O

13. Avoid the administration of unnecessary IV fluids

14. Administer morphine as prescribed to provide sedation and vasodilation, and monitor for respiratory depression or hypotension after administration

15. Administer diuretics as prescribed to reduce **preload,** enhance renal excretion of sodium and water, reduce circulating blood volume, and reduce pulmonary congestion

16. Administer digitalis as prescribed to increase ventricular **contractility** and improve **cardiac output**

17. Administer bronchodilators as prescribed for severe bronchospasm or bronchoconstriction

18. Administer additional inotropic medications such as dopamine, dobutamine, or amrinone, as prescribed, to facilitate myocardial **contractility** and enhance **stroke volume**

19. Administer vasodilators as prescribed to reduce **afterload,** increase the capacity of the systemic venous bed, and decrease venous return to the heart

20. Monitor weight to determine a response to treatment

21. Assess for hepatomegaly and ascites, and measure and record abdominal girth

22. Monitor peripheral pulses

23. Analyze blood gas results and evaluate electrolyte values for imbalances

24. Monitor potassium level closely, which may decrease due to the diuretic, and administer potassium supplements as prescribed to prevent digitalis toxicity

G. Following the acute episode

1. Encourage client to verbalize feelings about the necessary lifestyle changes that are required as a result of the heart failure

2. Assist the client to identify precipitating risk factors of heart failure and methods of eliminating these risk factors

3. Instruct the client in the prescribed medication regimen, which may include digoxin (Lanoxin), a diuretic, and vasodilators

4. Advise the client to notify the physician if side effects occur from the medications

5. Advise the client to avoid over-the-counter medications

6. Instruct the client to contact the physician if unable to take medications due to illness

7. Instruct the client to avoid large amounts of caffeine, found in coffee, tea, cocoa, chocolate, and some carbonated beverages

8. Instruct the client about the prescribed low-sodium, low-fat and low-cholesterol diet

9. Provide the client with a list of potassium-rich foods, since diuretics will cause hypokalemia (except for potassium-sparing diuretics)

10. Instruct the client regarding fluid restriction if prescribed, advising the client to spread the fluid out throughout the day and to suck on hard candy to reduce thirst

11. Instruct the client to space periods of activity and rest

12. Advise client to avoid isometric activities, which increase pressure in the heart

13. Instruct client to monitor weight

14. Instruct the client to report signs of fluid retention, such as edema or weight gain

XI. Cardiogenic Shock

A. Description

1. Failure of the heart to pump adequately, thereby reducing **cardiac output** and compromising tissue perfusion

2. Necrosis of more than 40% of the left ventricle occurs, usually as a result of occlusions of major coronary vessels

3. The goal of treatment is to relieve pain and decrease myocardial oxygen requirements through **preload,** and possibly **afterload,** reduction

B. Assessment

1. Hypotension

2. **Blood pressure** less than 90, or 30 mmHg less than the client's baseline

3. Urine output of less than 30 mL/hour

4. Cold, clammy skin
5. Poor peripheral pulses
6. Tachycardia
7. Pulmonary congestion
8. Tachypnea
9. Disorientation, restlessness, and confusion
10. Continuing chest discomfort

C. Implementation
1. Administer IV morphine as prescribed to decrease pulmonary congestion and relieve pain
2. Administer oxygen as prescribed
3. Prepare for intubation and mechanical ventilation
4. Administer diuretics and nitrates as prescribed while monitoring **blood pressure** constantly
5. Administer vasopressors and positive inotropics as prescribed to maintain organ perfusion
6. Prepare the client for insertion of intra-aortic balloon pump (IABP), which facilitates emptying of the left ventricle and improves **cardiac output,** if prescribed
7. Prepare the client for immediate reperfusion procedures, such as PTCA or CABG
8. Monitor arterial blood gas (ABG) levels and prepare to treat imbalances
9. Monitor urinary output
10. Assist with insertion of Swan-Ganz catheter to assess heart failure
11. Evaluate distal pulses and maintain transducer at level of right atrium if client has a Swan-Ganz catheter in place

XII. Inflammatory Diseases of the Heart

A. Pericarditis
1. Description
    a. An acute or chronic inflammation of the pericardium
    b. Chronic pericarditis, a chronic inflammatory thickening of the pericardium, constricts the heart causing compression
    c. The pericardial sac becomes inflamed
    d. Can result in loss of pericardial elasticity or an accumulation of fluid within the sac
    e. Heart failure or cardiac tamponade may result
2. Assessment
    a. Precordial pain in the anterior chest that radiates to the left side of the neck, shoulder, or back
    b. Pain that is aggravated by breathing (particularly inspiration), coughing, and swallowing
    c. Pain is worse when in the supine position and may be relieved by leaning forward
    d. Pericardial friction rub (scratchy, high-pitched sound) heard on auscultation,

produced by the rubbing of the inflamed pericardial layers
    e. Fever and chills
    f. Fatigue and malaise
    g. Elevated WBC count
    h. ECG changes
    i. Signs of right-sided heart failure in clients with chronic constrictive pericarditis
3. Implementation
    a. Assess the nature of the pain
    b. Position client side-lying, high Fowler's, or upright and leaning forward
    c. Administer analgesics, nonsteroidal anti-inflammatory drugs (NSAIDs), or steroids as prescribed for pain
    d. Avoid the administration of aspirin and anticoagulants because they increase the risk of tamponade
    e. Auscultate for a pericardial friction rub
    f. Evaluate blood culture report
    g. Administer antibiotics for bacterial infection as prescribed
    h. Administer diuretics and digoxin (Lanoxin) as prescribed to the client with chronic constrictive pericarditis
    i. Monitor for signs of cardiac tamponade, including pulsus paradoxus, jugular vein distention with clear lung sounds, muffled heart sounds, and decreased **cardiac output**
    j. Notify physician if signs of cardiac tamponade occur

B. Myocarditis
1. Description: An acute or chronic inflammation of the myocardium due to pericarditis, systemic infection, or allergic response
2. Assessment
    a. Fever
    b. Pericardial friction rub
    c. A gallop rhythm
    d. A murmur that sounds like fluid passing an obstruction
    e. Pulsus alternans
    f. Signs of heart failure
    g. Fatigue
    h. Dyspnea
    i. Tachycardia
    j. Chest pain
3. Implementation
    a. Assist client to a position of comfort, such as sitting up and leaning forward
    b. Administer analgesics, salicylates, NSAIDs as prescribed, to reduce fever and pain
    c. Administer oxygen as prescribed
    d. Provide adequate rest periods
    e. Limit activities to avoid overexertion and to decrease the workload of the heart
    f. Administer digoxin (Lanoxin) as prescribed, and monitor for signs of digoxin toxicity
    g. Administer antidysrhythmics as prescribed

h. Administer antibiotics as prescribed to treat causative organism

i. Monitor for complications, which can include thrombus, CHF, or cardiomyopathy

C. **Endocarditis**

1. Description

a. An inflammation of the inner lining of the heart and valves

b. Occurs primarily in clients who are IV drug abusers, have had valve replacements, or have mitral valve prolapse or other structural defects

c. Ports of entry for the infecting organism include the oral cavity (especially if the client had a dental procedure in the previous 3 to 6 months), cutaneous invasion, infections, or invasive procedures or surgery

2. Assessment

a. Fever

b. Anorexia

c. Weight loss

d. Fatigue

e. Cardiac murmurs

f. Heart failure

g. Embolic complications from vegetation fragments traveling through the circulation

h. Petechiae

i. Splinter hemorrhages in the nail beds

j. Osler's nodes (reddish and tender lesions) on the pads of the fingers, hands, and toes

k. Janeway's lesions (nontender hemorrhagic lesions) on the fingers, toes, nose, or earlobes

l. Splenomegaly

m. Clubbing of the fingers

3. Implementation

a. Provide adequate rest balanced with activity to prevent thrombus formation

b. Maintain antiembolism stockings

c. Monitor cardiovascular status

d. Monitor for signs of heart failure

e. Monitor for signs of emboli

f. Monitor for splenic emboli as evidenced by sudden abdominal pain radiating to the left shoulder, and the presence of rebound abdominal tenderness on palpation

g. Monitor for renal emboli as evidenced by flank pain radiating to the groin, hematuria, and pyuria

h. Monitor for confusion, aphasia, or dysphagia, which may be indicative of CNS emboli

i. Monitor for pulmonary emboli, as evidenced by pleuritic chest pain, dyspnea, and cough

j. Assess skin, mucous membranes, and conjunctiva for petechiae

k. Assess nail beds for splinter hemorrhages

l. Assess for Osler's nodes on the pads of the fingers, hands, and toes

m. Assess for Janeway's lesions on the fingers, toes, nose, or earlobes

n. Assess for clubbing of the fingers

o. Evaluate blood culture results

p. Administer IV antibiotic as prescribed

q. Plan and arrange for discharge, providing resources required for the continued administration of IV antibiotics

4. Client education

a. Instruct client regarding the signs and symptoms of complications and to notify the physician if they occur

b. Inform client about the importance of good oral hygiene

c. Instruct client to brush teeth twice daily with a soft toothbrush, followed by oral rinses

d. Instruct client to avoid irrigation devices, electric toothbrushes, and flossing, because these activities can cause the gums to bleed, allowing the entrance of bacteria into the mucous membranes and blood stream

e. Advise clients of the importance of prophylactic antibiotics prior to any invasive procedure and the importance of informing all health care professionals of their disease history

XIII. Cardiac Tamponade

A. Description

1. A pericardial effusion occurs when the space between the parietal and visceral layers of the pericardium fills with fluid

2. Pericardial effusion places the client at risk for cardiac tamponade, an accumulation of fluid in the pericardial cavity

3. Tamponade restricts ventricular filling, and **cardiac output** drops

4. Acute tamponade occurs when small volumes (20 to 50 mL) of fluid accumulate in the pericardium

B. Assessment

1. Pulsus paradoxus

2. Increased CVP

3. Jugular venous distention with clear lungs

4. Distant, muffled heart sounds

5. Decreased **cardiac output**

C. Implementation

1. Client will be placed in a critical care unit for hemodynamic monitoring

2. Administer IV fluids as prescribed to manage decreased **cardiac output**

3. Prepare client for chest x-ray film or echocardiogram

4. Prepare the client for pericardiocentesis to withdraw pericardial fluid if prescribed

5. Monitor for recurrence of tamponade following pericardiocentesis
6. If the client experiences recurrent tamponade or recurrent effusions, or develops adhesions from chronic pericarditis, a portion (pericardial window) or all of the pericardium (pericardiectomy) may be removed to allow adequate ventricular filling and contraction

XIV. Valvular Heart Disease

A. Description
   1. Occurs when the heart valves cannot fully open (stenosis) or close completely (insufficiency or regurgitation)
   2. Prevents efficient blood flow through the heart
B. Types
   1. Mitral stenosis: Valvular tissue thickens and narrows valve opening
   2. Mitral insufficiency/regurgitation: Valve is incompetent and prevents complete valve closure
   3. Mitral valve prolapse: Valve leaflets protrude into the left atrium during **systole**
   4. Aortic stenosis: Valvular tissue thickens and narrows the valve opening
   5. Aortic insufficiency: Valve is incompetent and prevents complete valve closure
C. Repair procedures
   1. Balloon valvuloplasty
      a. An invasive, nonsurgical procedure
      b. The passage of a balloon catheter from the femoral vein through the atrial septum to the mitral valve, or through the femoral artery to the aortic valve
      c. The balloon is inflated to enlarge the orifice
      d. Institute precautions for arterial puncture if appropriate
      e. Monitor for bleeding from the catheter insertion site
      f. Monitor for signs of systemic emboli
      g. Monitor for signs of a regurgitant valve by monitoring cardiac rhythm, heart sounds, and **cardiac output**
   2. Mitral annuloplasty: Tightening and suturing the malfunctioning valve annulus to eliminate or markedly reduce regurgitation
   3. Commissurotomy/valvotomy
      a. Accomplished with cardiopulmonary bypass during open heart surgery
      b. The valve is visualized, thrombi are removed from the atria, fused leaflets are incised, and calcium is debrided from the leaflets, thus widening the orifice
D. Valve replacement procedures (Box 59–6)
   1. Mechanical prosthetic valves
      a. Prosthetic valves are very durable but can fail
      b. Thromboembolism is a problem following

> ### BOX 59–6. Client Instruction Following Valve Replacement
>
> - Instruct client that adequate rest is important and that fatigue is usual
> - Instruct client in the need for anticoagulant therapy if a mechanical prosthetic valve was inserted
> - Instruct client in the hazards related to anticoagulant therapy, and to notify the physician if bleeding or excessive bruising occurs
> - Inform client about the importance of good oral hygiene to reduce the risk of infective endocarditis
> - Instruct client to brush teeth twice daily with a soft toothbrush, followed by oral rinses
> - Instruct client to avoid irrigation devices, electric toothbrushes, and flossing, because these activities can cause the gums to bleed, allowing the entrance of bacteria into the mucous membranes and blood stream
> - Instruct the client to monitor the incision and to report any drainage or redness
> - Inform client to avoid any dental procedures for 6 months
> - Inform client that heavy lifting (greater than 10 pounds) is to be avoided and to exercise caution when in an automobile to prevent injury to the sternal incision
> - Inform client with a prosthetic valve that a soft, audible clicking sound may be heard
> - Advise clients of the importance of prophylactic antibiotics prior to any invasive procedure and the importance of informing all health care professionals of the valvular disease history
> - Advise client to obtain and wear a Medic-Alert bracelet

the valve replacement, and anticoagulant therapy is required over a lifetime
   2. Bioprosthetic valves
      a. Biological grafts are xenografts (valves from other species): porcine valves (pig), bovine valves (cow); or homografts (human cadavers)
      b. Little risk of clot formation; therefore, long-term anticoagulation is not indicated
   3. Preoperative implementation: Consult with physician regarding discontinuing anticoagulants 72 hours prior to surgery
   4. Postoperative implementation
      a. Monitor closely for signs of bleeding
      b. Monitor **cardiac output** and for signs of heart pump failure
      c. Administer digoxin (Lanoxin) as prescribed to maintain **cardiac output** and prevent atrial fibrillation
E. Mitral stenosis
   1. Assessment
      a. Asymptomatic initially
      b. Symptoms occur when the orifice is reduced by 50%
      c. Dyspnea
      d. Orthopnea

e. Paroxysmal nocturnal dyspnea

f. Dry cough

g. Rumbling apical diastolic murmur

h. Right-sided heart failure

i. Hepatomegaly

j. Neck vein distention

k. Pitting peripheral edema

l. Hemoptysis and pulmonary edema as pulmonary hypertension and congestion progress

m. Development of atrial fibrillation, indicating that the client may decompensate (notify physician immediately)

2. Implementation

a. Administer prescribed treatment for CHF

b. Administer oxygen as prescribed

c. Provide a low-sodium diet

d. Administer diuretics and digoxin (Lanoxin) as prescribed

e. Administer antibiotics as prescribed if infective endocarditis is present

f. Administer antidysrhythmics and anticoagulants for atrial fibrillation as prescribed

g. Prepare client for commissurotomy or valve replacement as indicated

F. Mitral valve prolapse

1. Assessment

a. Fatigue

b. Atypical chest pain

c. Palpitations

d. Dizziness and syncope

e. Tachycardia

f. Systolic click

2. Implementation

a. Administer propranolol (Inderal) for dyspnea and chest pain as prescribed

b. Administer prophylactic antibiotics as prescribed

G. Mitral insufficiency

1. Assessment

a. Dyspnea

b. Orthopnea

c. Fatigue

d. Dizziness

e. Palpitations

f. Signs of right-sided heart failure

g. Atrial fibrillation

h. Neck vein distention

i. Pitting peripheral edema

j. High-pitched systolic murmur

2. Implementation

a. Administer prescribed treatment for CHF

b. Administer oxygen as prescribed

c. Provide a low-sodium diet

d. Administer diuretics and digoxin (Lanoxin) as prescribed

e. Administer antibiotics as prescribed if infective endocarditis is present

f. Administer antidysrhythmics and anticoagulants for atrial fibrillation as prescribed

g. Prepare client for commissurotomy or valve replacement as indicated

H. Aortic stenosis

1. Assessment

a. Dyspnea on exertion

b. Angina

c. Syncope on exertion

d. Fatigue

e. Orthopnea

f. Paroxysmal nocturnal dyspnea

g. Harsh systolic crescendo-decrescendo murmur

2. Implementation

a. Administer prescribed treatment for CHF

b. Administer oxygen as prescribed

c. Provide a low-sodium diet

d. Administer diuretics and digoxin (Lanoxin) as prescribed

e. Administer antibiotics as prescribed if infective endocarditis is present

f. Prepare client for valve replacement as indicated

I. Aortic insufficiency

1. Assessment

a. Dyspnea

b. Orthopnea

c. Paroxysmal nocturnal dyspnea

d. Fatigue

e. Angina

f. Tachycardia

g. Blowing decrescendo diastolic murmur

2. Implementation

a. Administer prescribed treatment for CHF

b. Administer oxygen as prescribed

c. Provide a low-sodium diet

d. Administer diuretics and digoxin (Lanoxin) as prescribed

e. Administer antibiotics as prescribed if infective endocarditis is present

f. Prepare client for valve replacement as indicated

J. Tricuspid stenosis

1. Assessment

a. Easily fatigued

b. Effort intolerance

c. Complaint of fluttering sensations in neck (obstructed venous flow)

d. Cyanosis

e. Signs of right-sided heart failure

f. Symptoms of decreased **cardiac output**

g. Ascites

h. Hepatomegaly

i. Peripheral edema

j. Rumbling diastolic murmur

k. Jugular vein distention with clear lung fields

2. Implementation

a. Administer prescribed treatment for CHF

b. Administer oxygen as prescribed

c. Provide a low-sodium diet

d. Administer diuretics and digoxin (Lanoxin) as prescribed

e. Administer antibiotics as prescribed if infective endocarditis is present

f. Prepare client for valve replacement as indicated

K. Tricuspid insufficiency
1. Assessment
   a. Asymptomatic in mild situations
   b. Signs of right-sided heart failure
   c. Ascites
   d. Hepatomegaly
   e. Pleural effusion
   f. Peripheral edema
   g. Systolic murmur heard at left sternal border, 4th intercostal space
2. Implementation
   a. Administer prescribed treatment for CHF
   b. Administer oxygen as prescribed
   c. Provide a low-sodium diet
   d. Administer diuretics and digoxin (Lanoxin) as prescribed
   e. Administer antibiotics as prescribed if infective endocarditis is present
   f. Prepare client for valve replacement as indicated

L. Pulmonary stenosis
1. Assessment
   a. Asymptomatic in mild condition
   b. Dyspnea
   c. Fatigue
   d. Syncope
   e. Signs of right-sided heart failure
   f. Ascites
   g. Hepatomegaly
   h. Peripheral edema
   i. Systolic thrill heard at left sternal border
2. Implementation
   a. Administer prescribed treatment for CHF
   b. Administer oxygen as prescribed
   c. Provide a low-sodium diet
   d. Administer diuretics and digoxin (Lanoxin) as prescribed
   e. Administer antibiotics as prescribed if infective endocarditis is present
   f. Prepare client for pulmonary valve commissurotomy as indicated

M. Pulmonary insufficiency
1. Assessment
   a. Asymptomatic in mild condition
   b. Dyspnea
   c. Fatigue
   d. Syncope
   e. Signs of right-sided heart failure
   f. Ascites
   g. Hepatomegaly
   h. Peripheral edema
   i. Systolic thrill heard at left sternal border
2. Implementation
   a. Administer prescribed treatment for CHF
   b. Administer oxygen as prescribed
   c. Provide a low-sodium diet

d. Administer diuretics and digoxin (Lanoxin) as prescribed

XV. Cardiomyopathy

A. Description
1. A subacute or chronic disorder of the heart muscle
2. Treatment is palliative, not curative, and clients need to deal with numerous lifestyle changes and a shortened life span

B. Dilated cardiomyopathy (DCM)
1. Description
   a. Most common type
   b. Heart ejects less than 40% of the blood in the left ventricle (normal is 70%) and reduced **cardiac output** leads to heart failure
2. Assessment
   a. Symptoms of left ventricular heart failure
   b. Weakness and fatigue
   c. Activity intolerance
   d. Chest pain
   e. Dysrhythmias
   f. Eventually signs of right-sided heart failure
3. Implementation
   a. Symptomatic treatment of heart failure
   b. Diuretics, cardiac glycosides, and vasodilators to increase **cardiac output**
   c. Antidysrhythmics to control dysrhythmias
   d. Instruct client to report any signs of dizziness or fainting, which may indicate a dysrhythmia
   e. Instruct client to avoid ingestion of alcohol because of its cardiac depressant effect
   f. Heart transplant

C. Hypertrophic cardiomyopathy (HCM)
1. Description
   a. Characterized by massive ventricular hypertrophy leading to hypercontraction of the left ventricle and rigid ventricular walls
   b. Causes obstruction in left ventricular outflow
2. Assessment
   a. Exertional dyspnea
   b. Syncope
   c. Chest pain that occurs at rest, is prolonged, has no relation to exertion, and is not relieved by nitrates
   d. Dysrhythmias
3. Implementation
   a. Symptomatic treatment of symptoms, similar to the care of a client with MI
   b. Conversion of atrial fibrillation if it occurs
   c. Instruct client to report any signs of dizziness or fainting, which may indicate a dysrhythmia
   d. Instruct client to avoid ingestion of

alcohol because of its cardiac depressant effect

  e. Beta-blockers and calcium antagonists to decrease the outflow obstruction and decrease heart rate

  f. Vasodilators and cardiac glycosides are contraindicated because vasodilating and positive inotropic effects augment the obstruction

  g. Ventriculomyotomy or muscle resection with mitral valve replacement

D. Restrictive cardiomyopathy

  1. Description: Characterized by restriction of filling of the ventricles

  2. Assessment

    a. Exertional dyspnea

    b. Weakness

  3. Implementation

    a. Symptomatic treatment of heart failure

    b. Exercise restriction

    c. Diuretics, cardiac glycosides, and vasodilators to increase **cardiac output**

    d. Antidysrhythmics to control dysrhythmias

    e. Instruct client to report any signs of dizziness or fainting, which may indicate a dysrhythmia

    f. Instruct client to avoid ingestion of alcohol because of its cardiac depressant effect

XVI. Vascular Disorders

A. Venous thrombosis

  1. Description

    a. Thrombus can be associated with an inflammatory process

    b. When a thrombus develops, inflammation occurs, thickening the vein wall and leading to embolization

  2. Types

    a. Thrombophlebitis: A thrombus associated with inflammation

    b. Phlebothrombus: A thrombus without inflammation

    c. Phlebitis: Vein inflammation associated with invasive procedures such as IVs

    d. Deep vein thrombophlebitis (DVT): More serious than a superficial thrombophlebitis because of the risk for pulmonary embolism

  3. Risk factors for thrombus formation

    a. Venous stasis from varicose veins, CHF, immobility

    b. Hypercoagulability disorders

    c. Injury to the venous wall from IV injections, fractures, trauma

    d. Following surgery, particularly hip surgery and open prostate surgery

    e. Pregnancy

    f. Ulcerative colitis

    g. Use of oral contraceptives

B. Phlebitis

  1. Assessment

    a. Red, warm area radiating up an extremity

    b. Pain and soreness

    c. Swelling

  2. Implementation

    a. Apply warm, moist soaks as prescribed to dilate the vein and promote circulation

    b. Assess temperature of soak prior to applying

    c. Assess for signs of complications, such as tissue necrosis, infection, or pulmonary embolus

C. Deep vein thrombophlebitis (DVT) (Box 59–7)

  1. Assessment

    a. Calf or groin tenderness or pain, with or without swelling

    b. Positive Homan's sign

    c. Warm skin that is tender to the touch

  2. Implementation

    a. Provide bed rest

    b. Elevate the affected extremity above the level of the heart as prescribed

    c. Avoid using the knee gatch or a pillow under the knees

    d. Do not massage the extremity

    e. Provide thigh-high compression or antiembolism stockings as prescribed to reduce venous stasis and to assist in the venous return of blood to the heart

    f. Administer intermittent or continuous warm, moist compresses as prescribed

    g. Palpate the site gently, monitoring for warmth and edema

    h. Measure and record the circumferences of the thighs and calves

---

BOX 59–7. Instructions for Client with Deep Vein Thrombosis

- Educate the client regarding the hazards of anticoagulation therapy
- Instruct the client to recognize the signs and symptoms of bleeding
- Instruct client to avoid prolonged sitting or standing, constrictive clothing, or crossing legs when seated
- Instruct client to elevate legs for 10–20 minutes every few hours each day
- Plan a progressive walking program with the client as prescribed
- Instruct client how to inspect legs for edema and how to measure the circumference of legs
- Instruct the client about the antiembolism stockings as prescribed
- Advise the client to avoid smoking
- Advise the client to avoid any medications unless they are prescribed by the physician
- Emphasize the importance of follow-up physician visits and laboratory studies
- Advise client to obtain and wear a Medic-Alert bracelet

i. Monitor for shortness of breath and chest pain as these may be indicative of pulmonary emboli

j. Administer thrombolytic therapy (t-PA, tissue-type plasminogen activator) as prescribed, which must be initiated within 5 days after the onset of symptoms

k. Administer heparin therapy as prescribed to prevent enlargement of the existing clot and prevent the formation of new clots

l. Monitor activated partial thromboplastin time (APTT) during heparin therapy

m. Administer warfarin (Coumadin) as prescribed when the symptoms of DVT have resolved

n. Monitor PT and INR (International Normalized Ratio) during warfarin (Coumadin) therapy

o. Monitor for the hazards and side effects associated with anticoagulant therapy

p. Administer analgesics as prescribed to reduce pain

q. Administer diuretics as prescribed to reduce lower extremity edema

D. Venous insufficiency
   1. Description
      a. Occurs as a result of prolonged venous hypertension, which stretches the veins and damages the valves
      b. The resultant edema and venous stasis cause venous stasis ulcers, swelling, and cellulitis
      c. Treatment focuses on decreasing edema and promoting venous return from the affected extremity
      d. Treatment for venous stasis ulcers focuses on healing the ulcer and preventing stasis and ulcer recurrence
   2. Assessment
      a. Stasis dermatitis or discoloration along the ankles extending up to the calf
      b. Edema
      c. The presence of ulcer formation
   3. Implementation
      a. Instruct client to wear elastic or compression stockings during the day and evening as prescribed
      b. Instruct client to don elastic stockings upon awakening, before getting out of bed
      c. Advise client to don a clean pair of elastic stockings each day and that it will probably be necessary to wear the stockings for the remainder of life
      d. Instruct client to avoid prolonged sitting or standing, constrictive clothing, or crossing legs when seated
      e. Instruct client to elevate legs for 10 to 20 minutes every few hours each day
      f. Instruct client to elevate legs above the level of the heart when in bed

g. Instruct the client in the use of an intermittent sequential pneumatic compression system if prescribed; instruct the client to apply the compression system twice daily for 1 hour in the morning and evening

h. Advise client with an open ulcer that the compression system is applied over a dressing

4. Wound care
   a. Provide care to the wound as prescribed by the physician
   b. Assess client's ability to care for the wound, and initiate home care resources as necessary
   c. If an Unna boot (a dressing constructed of gauze moistened with zinc oxide) is prescribed, it will be changed by the physician weekly
   d. The wound is cleansed with normal saline prior to application of the Unna boot; povidone-iodine (Betadine) and hydrogen peroxide are not used because they destroy granulation tissue
   e. The Unna boot is covered with an elastic wrap, which hardens to promote venous return and prevent stasis
   f. Monitor for signs of arterial occlusion from an Unna boot that may be too tight
   g. Keep tape off the client's skin
5. Medications
   a. Apply topical agents to wound as prescribed to debride the ulcer, eliminate necrotic tissue, and promote healing
   b. When applying topical agents, apply an oil-based agent such as petroleum jelly (Vaseline) on surrounding skin because debriding agents can injure healthy tissue
   c. Administer antibiotics as prescribed if infection or cellulitis occurs

E. Varicose veins
   1. Description
      a. Distended, protruding veins that appear darkened and tortuous
      b. Vein walls weaken and dilate, and valves become incompetent
   2. Assessment
      a. Pain in the legs, with dull aching after standing
      b. A feeling of fullness in the legs
      c. Ankle edema
   3. Trendelenburg test
      a. Place client in supine position with legs elevated
      b. When client sits up, if varicosities are present veins fill from the proximal end; veins normally fill from the distal end
   4. Implementation
      a. Assist with Trendelenburg test by placing client in supine position with legs elevated

b. Emphasize the importance of antiembolism stockings as prescribed

c. Instruct client to elevate legs as much as possible

d. Instruct client to avoid constrictive clothing and pressure on the legs

e. Prepare client for sclerotherapy or vein stripping as prescribed

5. Sclerotherapy

a. A solution is injected into the vein, followed by the application of a pressure dressing

b. An incision and drainage of the trapped blood in the sclerosed vein is performed 14 to 21 days after the injection, followed by the application of a pressure dressing for 12 to 18 hours

6. Vein stripping

a. Varicose veins are removed if they are larger than 4 mm in diameter or if they are in clusters

b. Preoperatively assist the physician with vein marking

c. Evaluate pulses as a baseline for comparison postoperatively

d. Maintain elastic (Ace) bandages on client's legs postoperatively

e. Monitor the groin and leg for bleeding through the elastic bandages

f. Monitor extremity for edema, warmth, color, and pulses

g. Elevate legs above level of heart postoperatively

h. Encourage range of motion exercises of the legs

i. Instruct client to avoid leg dangling or chair sitting

j. Instruct client to elevate legs when sitting

k. Emphasize the importance of wearing elastic stockings after bandage removal

XVII. Arterial Disorders

A. Peripheral arterial disease (PAD)

1. Description

a. A chronic disorder in which partial or total arterial occlusion deprives the lower extremities of oxygen and nutrients

b. Tissue damage occurs below the arterial occlusion

c. Atherosclerosis is the most common cause of PAD

2. Assessment

a. Intermittent claudication

b. Rest pain characterized by numbness, burning, or aching in the distal portion of the lower extremities that awakens the client at night and is relieved by placing the extremity in a dependent position

c. Lower back or buttock discomfort

d. Loss of hair and dry, scaly skin on lower extremities

e. Thickened toenails

f. Cold and gray-blue or darkened color of skin in lower extremities

g. Elevational pallor and dependent rubor in lower extremities

h. Decreased or absent peripheral pulses

i. Signs of arterial ulcer formation characterized as painful and occurring on or between the toes, or on the upper aspect of the foot

j. **Blood pressure** measurements at the thigh, calf, and ankle are lower than the brachial pressure (normally **BP** readings in the thigh and calf are higher than those in the upper extremities)

3. Implementation

a. Assess pain

b. Monitor the extremities for color, motion and sensation, and pulses

c. Obtain **blood pressure** measurements

d. Assess for signs of ulcer formation or signs of gangrene

e. Assist in developing an individualized exercise program that is initiated gradually and slowly increased

f. Encourage prescribed exercise that will improve arterial flow through the development of collateral circulation

g. Instruct client to walk to the point of claudication, stop and rest, then walk a little farther

h. As swelling in the extremities prevents arterial blood flow, instruct client to elevate the feet at rest but to refrain from elevating them above the level of the heart, as extreme elevation slows arterial blood flow to the feet

i. In severe cases of PAD, clients with edema may sleep with the affected limb hanging from the bed, or they may sit upright in a chair for comfort

j. Instruct all clients with PAD to avoid crossing their legs, which interferes with blood flow

k. Instruct client to avoid exposure to cold (causes vasoconstriction) to the extremities and to wear socks or insulated shoes for warmth at all times

l. Instruct client never to apply direct heat to the limb as with a heating pad or hot water, because the decreased sensitivity in the limb will cause burning

m. Instruct client to inspect skin on extremities daily and to report any signs of skin breakdown

n. Instruct client to avoid tobacco and caffeine because of their vasoconstrictive effects

o. Instruct client in the use of hemorrheologic and antiplatelet medications as prescribed

p. Inform client of the importance of taking

all medications prescribed by the physician

4. Procedures to improve arterial blood flow
   a. Percutaneous transluminal angioplasty
   b. Laser-assisted angioplasty
   c. Arthrectomy
   d. Bypass surgery

B. Raynaud's disease
   1. Description
      a. Vasospasms of the arterioles and arteries of the upper and lower extremities
      b. Vasospasm causes constriction of the cutaneous vessels
      c. Attacks are intermittent and occur with exposure to cold or stress
      d. Affects primarily fingers, toes, ears, and cheeks
   2. Assessment
      a. Blanching of the extremity, followed by cyanosis during vasoconstriction
      b. Reddened tissue when the vasospasm is relieved
      c. Numbness, tingling, swelling, and a cold temperature of the affected body part
   3. Implementation
      a. Monitor pulses
      b. Administer vasodilators as prescribed
      c. Instruct client regarding medication therapy
      d. Assist client to identify and avoid precipitating factors, such as cold and stress
      e. Instruct client to avoid smoking
      f. Instruct client to wear warm clothing, socks, and gloves in cold weather
      g. Advise client to avoid injuries to fingers and hands

C. Buerger's disease
   1. Description
      a. Also known as thromboangiitis obliterans
      b. An occlusive disease of the median and small arteries and veins
      c. The distal upper and lower limbs are most commonly affected
   2. Assessment
      a. Intermittent claudication (pain in the muscles resulting from an inadequate blood supply)
      b. Ischemic pain occurring in the digits while at rest
      c. Aching pain that is more severe at night
      d. Cool, numb, or tingling sensation
      e. Diminished pulses in the distal extremities
      f. Extremities are cool and red in the dependent position
      g. Development of ulcerations in extremities
   3. Implementation
      a. Instruct client to stop smoking
      b. Monitor pulses
      c. Instruct client to avoid injury to upper and lower extremities
      d. Administer vasodilators as prescribed

e. Instruct client regarding medication therapy

XVIII. Aortic Aneurysms

A. Description
   1. Abnormal dilation of the arterial wall, caused by localized weakness and stretching in the medial layer or wall of an artery
   2. The aneurysm can be located anywhere along the abdominal aorta
   3. The goal of treatment is to limit the progression of the disease by modifying risk factors, controlling the **BP** to prevent strain on the aneurysm, recognizing symptoms early, and preventing rupture

B. Types
   1. Fusiform: Diffuse dilation that involves the entire circumference of the arterial segment
   2. Saccular: Distinct localized outpouching of the artery wall
   3. Dissecting: Created when blood separates the layers of the artery wall, forming a cavity between them
   4. False (pseudoaneurysm)
      a. Results from development of a sac around a hematoma
      b. Maintains communication with artery lumen, the wall of which has ruptured

C. Assessment
   1. Thoracic aneurysm
      a. Pain extending to neck, shoulders, lower back, or abdomen
      b. Syncope
      c. Dyspnea
      d. Increased pulse
      e. Cyanosis
      f. Weakness
   2. Abdominal aneurysm
      a. Prominent, pulsating mass in abdomen, at or above umbilicus
      b. Systolic bruit over aorta
      c. Tenderness on deep palpation
      d. Abdominal or lower back pain
   3. Rupturing aneurysm
      a. Severe abdominal or back pain
      b. Lumbar pain radiating to flank and groin
      c. Hypotension
      d. Increased pulse rate
      e. Signs of shock
   4. Diagnostic tests
      a. Done to confirm the presence of an aneurysm
      b. Done to confirm the size and location of the aneurysm
      c. Include abdominal ultrasound, CT scan, and arteriography
   5. Implementation
      a. Monitor vital signs
      b. Assess risk factors for arterial disease process

c. Obtain information regarding back or abdominal pain
d. Question the client regarding the sensation of palpation in the abdomen
e. Inspect skin for presence of vascular disease or breakdown
f. Check peripheral circulation, including pulses, temperature, and color
g. Observe for signs of rupture
h. Note any tenderness over the abdomen
i. Monitor for abdominal distention

6. Nonsurgical implementation
   a. Modify risk factors
   b. Instruct the client regarding the procedure for monitoring **BP**
   c. Instruct the client of the importance of regular physician visits to follow the size of the aneurysm
   d. Instruct the client to notify physician immediately if severe back or abdominal pain, fullness or soreness over the umbilicus, sudden development of discoloration in the extremities, or a persistent elevation of **blood pressure** occurs
   e. Instruct the client with a thoracic aneurysm to report immediately the occurrence of chest or back pain, shortness of breath, difficulty in swallowing, or hoarseness

D. Pharmacological implementation
   1. Administer antihypertensives to maintain **BP** within normal limits and prevent strain on the aneurysm
   2. Instruct client in the purpose of the medications
   3. Instruct client about the side effects and schedule of the medication

E. Abdominal aneurysm resection
   1. Description: Surgical resection or excision of the aneurysm; the excised section is replaced with a graft that is sewn end to end
   2. Preoperative implementation
      a. Assess all peripheral pulses as a baseline for postoperative comparison
      b. Instruct client on coughing and deep breathing exercises
      c. Administer bowel preparation as prescribed
   3. Postoperative implementation
      a. Monitor vital signs
      b. Monitor peripheral pulses distal to the graft site
      c. Monitor for signs of graft occlusion, including changes in pulses, cool to cold extremities below the graft, white or blue extremities or flanks, severe pain, or abdominal distention
      d. Limit elevation of the head of the bed to 45° to prevent flexion of the graft
      e. Monitor for hypovolemia and renal

failure because of the large amount of blood loss during surgery
   f. Monitor urine output hourly, and if it is less than 50 mL per hour, notify physician
   g. Monitor serum creatinine and BUN daily
   h. Monitor respiratory status and auscultate breath sounds to identify respiratory complications
   i. Encourage turning, coughing, and deep breathing while splinting the incision
   j. Ambulate as prescribed
   k. Maintain nasogastric tube to low suction until bowel sounds return
   l. Assess for bowel sounds and report their return to the physician
   m. Monitor for pain and administer medication as prescribed
   n. Assess incision site for bleeding or signs of infection
   o. Prepare client for discharge by providing instructions regarding pain management, wound care and activity restrictions
   p. Instruct client not to lift objects heavier than 15 to 20 pounds for 6 to 12 weeks
   q. Advise client to avoid activities requiring pushing, pulling, or straining
   r. Instruct client not to drive a vehicle until the activity is approved by the physician

F. Thoracic aneurysm repair
   1. Description
      a. A thoracotomy or median sternotomy approach is used to enter the thoracic cavity
      b. The aneurysm is exposed and excised, and a graft or prosthesis is sewn onto the aorta
      c. Total cardiopulmonary bypass is necessary for excision of aneurysms in the ascending aorta
      d. Partial cardiopulmonary bypass is used for clients with an aneurysm in the descending aorta
   2. Postoperative implementation
      a. Monitor vital signs
      b. Monitor for such signs of hemorrhage as a drop in **blood pressure** and increased pulse rate and respirations, and report to physician immediately
      c. Monitor chest tubes for an increase in chest drainage, which may indicate bleeding or separation at the graft site
      d. Assess sensation and motion of all extremities; if deficits occur, which can be due to a lack of blood supply during surgery, notify physician
      e. Monitor respiratory status and auscultate breath sounds to identify respiratory complications
      f. Encourage turning, coughing, and deep breathing, splinting the incision
      g. Monitor cardiac status for dysrhythmias

h. Monitor for pain and administer medication as prescribed

i. Assess incision site for bleeding or signs of infection

j. Prepare client for discharge by providing instructions regarding pain management, wound care, and activity restrictions

k. Instruct client not to lift objects heavier than 15 to 20 pounds for 6 to 12 weeks

l. Advise client to avoid activities requiring pushing, pulling, or straining

m. Instruct client not to drive a vehicle until the activity is approved by the physician

XIX. Embolectomy

A. Description
   1. Removal of an embolus from an artery, using a catheter
   2. A patch graft may be required to close the artery

B. Preoperative implementation
   1. Obtain a baseline vascular assessment
   2. Administer anticoagulants as prescribed
   3. Administer thrombolytics as prescribed
   4. Place a bed cradle on the bed
   5. Avoid bumping or jarring the bed
   6. Maintain extremity in slightly dependent position

C. Postoperative implementation
   1. Assess cardiac, respiratory, and neurological status
   2. Monitor affected extremity for color, temperature, and pulse
   3. Assess sensory and motor function of affected extremity
   4. Monitor for signs and symptoms of new thrombi or emboli
   5. Administer oxygen as prescribed
   6. Monitor pulse oximetry
   7. Monitor for complications caused by reperfusion of the artery, such as spasms and swelling of skeletal muscles
   8. Monitor for signs of swollen skeletal muscles, such as edema, pain on passive movement, poor capillary refill, numbness, and muscle tension
   9. Maintain bed rest initially, with client in semi-Fowler's position
   10. Maintain a bed cradle on the bed
   11. Check incision site for bleeding or hematoma
   12. Administer anticoagulants or antithrombolytics as prescribed
   13. Monitor laboratory values related to anticoagulant therapy
   14. Instruct client to recognize the signs and symptoms of infection and edema
   15. Instruct client to avoid prolonged sitting or crossing legs when sitting
   16. Instruct client to elevate legs when sitting
   17. Instruct client to wear antiembolism stockings as prescribed and how to remove and reapply the stockings
   18. Instruct client to ambulate daily
   19. Instruct client about anticoagulant therapy and the hazards associated with anticoagulants

XX. Vena Caval Filter and Ligation of Inferior Vena Cava

A. Vena caval filter: Insertion of an intracaval filter (umbrella), which partially occludes the inferior vena cava and traps emboli, to prevent pulmonary emboli

B. Ligation: Suturing and placement of clips on the inferior vena cava to prevent pulmonary emboli

C. Preoperative implementation: If the client has been taking an anticoagulant, consult with physician regarding discontinuation of the medication to prevent hemorrhage

D. Postoperative implementation
   1. Monitor vital signs
   2. Assess cardiac and respiratory status
   3. Administer oxygen as prescribed
   4. Monitor pulse oximetry
   5. Maintain semi-Fowler's position
   6. Avoid hip flexion
   7. Provide activity as prescribed
   8. Check the insertion site for bleeding and hematoma
   9. Assess for peripheral edema
   10. Maintain antiembolism stockings as prescribed
   11. Monitor laboratory values related to anticoagulant therapy
   12. Instruct client to recognize the signs and symptoms of infection and edema
   13. Instruct client to avoid prolonged sitting or crossing legs when sitting
   14. Instruct client to elevate legs when sitting
   15. Instruct client to wear antiembolism stockings as prescribed and how to remove and reapply the stockings
   16. Instruct client to ambulate daily
   17. Instruct client about anticoagulant therapy and the hazards associated with anticoagulants

XXI. Hypertension

A. Description (Table 59–1)
   1. Persistent elevation of the systolic **blood pressure** above 140 mmHg and the diastolic **blood pressure** above 90 mmHg
   2. Most significant predictor of developing coronary artery disease
   3. Major risk factor for coronary, cerebral, renal, and peripheral vascular disease
   4. The disease is initially asymptomatic
   5. The goals of treatment include to reduce **blood pressure** and to prevent or lessen the extent of organ damage

Table 59–1. Hypertension

Organ Involvement	Complications
Eyes	Visual changes
Brain	Cerebrovascular accident (CVA)
Cardiovascular system	CHF, hypertensive crisis
Kidneys	Renal failure

CHF, congestive heart failure.

6. Nonpharmalogical approaches, such as lifestyle changes, may be initially prescribed; if the **BP** cannot be decreased after a reasonable time period (1 to 3 months), then the client may require pharmacological treatment

B. Primary or essential hypertension
1. No known etiology
2. Risk factors
a. Aging
b. Family history
c. Black race with higher prevalence in men
d. Obesity
e. Smoking
f. Stress

C. Secondary hypertension
1. Treatment depends on the cause and the organs involved
2. Occurs as a result of other disorders or conditions
3. Precipitating disorders or conditions
a. Cardiovascular disorders
b. Renal disorders
c. Endocrine system disorders
d. Pregnancy
e. Medications

D. Assessment
1. May be asymptomatic
2. Headache
3. Visual disturbances
4. Dizziness
5. Chest pain
6. Tinnitus
7. Flushed face
8. Epistaxis

E. Implementation
1. Goals
a. To reduce **blood pressure**
b. To prevent or lessen the extent of organ damage
2. Question client regarding signs and symptoms indicative of hypertension
3. Obtain **BP** two or more times on both arms with the client supine and standing
4. Compare **BP** with prior documentation
5. Determine family history
6. Identify current medication therapy
7. Obtain weight
8. Evaluate dietary patterns and sodium intake of client
9. Assess for visual changes or retinal damage
10. Assess for cardiovascular changes such as

distended neck veins, increased heart rate, dysrhythmias
11. Evaluate chest x-ray film for heart enlargement
12. Assess neurological system
13. Evaluate renal function
14. Evaluate results of diagnostic and laboratory studies

F. Nonpharmalogical implementation
1. Weight reduction if necessary, or maintenance of ideal weight
2. Dietary sodium restriction to 2 g daily as prescribed
3. Moderate intake of alcohol and caffeine-containing products
4. Initiation of a regular exercise program
5. Avoidance of smoking
6. Relaxation techniques and biofeedback therapy
7. Elimination of unnecessary medications that may contribute to the hypertension

G. Stepped-care approach
1. Description
a. If a pharmacological approach to treating hypertension is required, a single medication is prescribed and monitored for its effectiveness (Box 59–8)
b. Medications are added to the treatment regimen until the **BP** is controlled
2. Step 1: a single medication is prescribed, which may be a diuretic, beta-blocker, calcium channel blocker, or ACE inhibitor
3. Step 2:
a. Step 1 therapy is evaluated after 1 to 3 months
b. If the response is not adequate, compliance is evaluated
c. The medication may be increased or a new medication prescribed, or a second medication is added to the treatment plan
4. Step 3:
a. Compliance is evaluated
b. Further evaluation of Step 2
c. If a therapeutic response is not adequate, a second medication is substituted or a third medication is added to the treatment plan
5. Step 4:
a. Compliance is evaluated
b. Careful assessment is done of factors limiting the antihypertensive response
c. A third or fourth medication may be added to the treatment plan

H. See Box 59–9 for client education

BOX 59–8. Antihypertensive Medications

Diuretics	Vasodilators
ACE inhibitors	Beta-blockers
Calcium channel blockers	Sympatholytics

BOX 59–9. Client Education for Hypertension

- Educate the client to prevent noncompliance with the treatment plan
- Describe the disease process, explaining that symptoms usually do not develop until organs have suffered damage
- Initiate and assist the client in planning a regular exercise program, avoiding heavy weight-lifting and isometric exercises
- Emphasize the importance of beginning the exercise program gradually
- Encourage the client to express feelings about daily stress
- Assist the client to identify ways to reduce stress
- Teach relaxation techniques
- Instruct the client how to incorporate relaxation techniques into the daily living pattern
- Instruct the client and family in the technique for monitoring blood pressure
- Instruct the client to maintain a diary of blood pressure readings
- Emphasize the importance of lifelong medication and the need for follow-up treatment
- Emphasize the importance of medications, and instruct the client not to stop the medication without consulting with the physician
- Instruct the client and family on the dietary restrictions, which may include sodium, fat, calories, and cholesterol
- Instruct the client how to shop for and prepare low-sodium meals
- Provide a list of products that contain sodium
- Instruct client to read labels of products to determine sodium content, focusing on substances listed as sodium, NaCl, and MSG
- Instruct client to bake, roast, or boil foods, avoid salt in preparation of foods, and avoid salt at the table
- Instruct client that fresh foods are best to consume and to avoid canned foods
- Instruct the client about the action, side effects, and scheduling of medications
- Advise the client to contact the physician and not to stop the medication if uncomfortable side effects occur
- Instruct the client to avoid over-the-counter medication
- Stress the importance of follow-up care

XXII. Hypertensive Crisis

A. Description
   1. Any clinical condition requiring immediate reduction in **blood pressure**
   2. An acute and life-threatening condition
   3. The accelerated hypertension requires emergency treatment since target organ damage (brain, heart, retina of the eye) can occur quickly
   4. Death can be caused by stroke, renal failure, or cardiac disease

B. Assessment
   1. A **diastolic pressure** above 120 mmHg

   2. Headache
   3. Drowsiness
   4. Confusion
   5. Changes in neurological status
   6. Tachycardia and tachypnea
   7. Dyspnea
   8. Cyanosis
   9. Seizures

C. Implementation
   1. Maintain a patent airway
   2. Administer IV antihypertensive medications as prescribed, which may include nitroprusside (Nipride), diazoxide (Hyperstat), or trimethaphan (Arfonad)
   3. Monitor vital signs, assessing **BP** every 5 minutes
   4. Assess for hypotension during the administration of antihypertensives
   5. Place client in supine position if hypotension occurs
   6. Have emergency medications and resuscitation equipment readily available
   7. Maintain bed rest, with the head of the bed at 45°
   8. Monitor IV therapy, assessing for fluid overload
   9. Monitor I&O
   10. Insert Foley catheter as prescribed
   11. Monitor urinary output; if oliguria or anuria occurs, notify physician

PRACTICE QUESTIONS

1. A client with angina pectoris has a 12-lead ECG taken during an episode of chest pain. The nurse examines the tracing for which ECG change caused by myocardial ischemia?
   1 Prolonged PR interval
   2 Widened QRS complex
   3 ST segment elevation or depression
   4 Tall, peaked T waves

2. A client is scheduled for a cardiac catheterization using a radiopaque dye. Which of the following assessments is most critical before the procedure?
   1 Intake and output prior to procedure
   2 Baseline peripheral pulse rates
   3 Height and weight
   4 Allergy to iodine or shellfish

3. The client is scheduled for a dipyridamole (Persantine) thallium 201 scan. The nurse assesses to make sure that the client has not had which of the following prior to the procedure?
   1 Milk products
   2 Caffeine
   3 Excess sugar
   4 Fatty meal

4. A client with no history of cardiovascular disease presents to the ambulatory clinic with flulike symptoms. The client suddenly complains of chest pain. Which of the following questions best helps the nurse discriminate pain due to a noncardiac problem?
   1 "Have you ever had this pain before?"
   2 "Can you describe the pain to me?"
   3 "Does the pain get worse when you breathe in?"
   4 "Can you rate the pain on a scale of 1 to 10, with 10 being the worst?"

5. A client is admitted to the emergency department with chest pain and myocardial infarction is being ruled out. Vital signs: at 11:00 A.M.: P 92, RR 24, BP 140/88; 11:15 A.M., P 96, RR 26, BP 128/82; 11:30 A.M., P 104, RR 28, BP 104/68; 11:45 A.M., P 118, RR 32, BP 88/58. The nurse alerts the physician, as these changes are most consistent with:
   1 Cardiogenic shock
   2 Cardiac tamponade
   3 Pulmonary embolism
   4 Dissecting thoracic aortic aneurysm

6. The client with myocardial infarction has been transferred from the coronary care unit to the general medical unit with cardiac monitoring via telemetry. The nurse plans to allow for which of the following client activities?
   1 Strict bed rest for 24 hours after transfer
   2 Bathroom privileges and self-care activities
   3 Unsupervised hallway ambulation with distances under 200 feet
   4 Ad lib activities since the client is monitored

7. The nurse notes bilateral 2+ edema in the lower extremities of a client with myocardial infarction admitted 2 days ago. The nurse plans to do which of the following next?
   1 Review the intake and output records for the last 2 days
   2 Change the time of diuretic administration from morning to evening
   3 Request a sodium restriction of 1 g/day from the physician
   4 Order daily weights starting on the following morning

8. The nurse is conducting a health history with a client with a primary diagnosis of heart failure. Which of the following disorders reported by the client does not play a role in exacerbating the heart failure?
   1 Recent upper respiratory infection
   2 Nutritional anemia
   3 Peptic ulcer disease
   4 Atrial fibrillation

9. The nurse is admitting a client with heart failure who was sent directly to the hospital from the physician's office. The nurse plans on having which of the following medications readily available for use?
   1 Diltiazem (Cardizem)
   2 Digoxin (Lanoxin)
   3 Propranolol (Inderal)
   4 Metoprolol (Lopressor)

10. The client with myocardial infarction suddenly becomes tachycardic, shows signs of air hunger, and begins coughing up frothy, pink-tinged sputum. The nurse listens to breath sounds, expecting to hear bilateral:
    1 Rhonchi
    2 Crackles in bases
    3 Rales to the apices
    4 Wheezes

11. A nurse caring for a client in one room is told by another nurse that a second client has developed florid pulmonary edema. Upon entering the second client's room, the nurse expects the client to be:
    1 Slightly anxious
    2 Mildly anxious
    3 Moderately anxious
    4 Extremely anxious

12. The client with sudden pulmonary edema has been on diuretic therapy. The client has an order for additional furosemide (Lasix) in the amount of 40 mg IV push. Knowing that the client will also be started on digoxin, the nurse checks the client's most recent:
    1 Digoxin level
    2 Sodium level
    3 Potassium level
    4 Creatinine level

13. The client with myocardial infarction is going into cardiogenic shock. Because of myocardial ischemia, the nurse carefully assesses the client for:
    1 Ventricular dysrhythmias
    2 Bradycardia
    3 Rising diastolic blood pressure
    4 Falling central venous pressure

14. The client in cardiogenic shock has a multilumen pulmonary artery catheter in place. The nurse interprets that the client is most unstable if which of the following cardiac output (CO) and pulmonary capillary wedge pressure (PCWP) readings are obtained?
    1 CO 5 L/minute, PCWP low
    2 CO 4 L/minute, PCWP high
    3 CO 3 L/minute, PCWP high
    4 CO 2 L/minute, PCWP low

15. The client in cardiogenic shock had insertion of an intra-aortic balloon pump 24 hours ago via the left femoral approach. The nurse notes that

the left foot is cool and mottled, and the left pedal pulse is weak. The nurse would:

1 Document the data, as this is expected due to catheter size
2 Re-evaluate the neurovascular status in another hour
3 Increase the rate of intravenous nitroglycerin that is infusing
4 Call the physician immediately

16. The nurse assesses the sternotomy incision of a client on the third postoperative day after cardiac surgery. The incision shows some slight "puffiness" along the edges, is nonreddened, with no apparent drainage. Temperature is 99° oral. WBC count is 7500/mm³. The nurse interprets that the incision line:

1 Is slightly edematous but shows no active signs of infection
2 Shows no sign of infection although the WBC count is elevated
3 Shows early signs of infection although the temperature is near normal
4 Shows early signs of infection, supported by an elevated WBC count

17. The client who is 24 hours postcardiac surgery has a urine output averaging 20 mL/hr for 2 hours. The client received a single bolus of 500 mL of intravenous fluid. Urine output for the subsequent hour was 25 mL. Daily laboratory results indicate the BUN is 45 mg/dL and the serum creatinine is 2.2 mg/dL. The nurse interprets that the client is at risk for:

1 Hypovolemia
2 Urinary tract infection
3 Glomerulonephritis
4 Acute renal failure

18. The nurse is preparing to ambulate the client on the third postoperative day following cardiac surgery. The nurse plans to do which of the following to enable the client to tolerate the ambulation best?

1 Encourage the client to cough and deep breathe
2 Premedicate the client with an analgesic
3 Provide the client with a walker
4 Remove telemetry equipment

19. The nurse is assessing a client's ECG rhythm strip. The P waves and QRS complexes are regular. The PR interval is 0.16 second and QRS complexes measure 0.06 second. The overall heart rate is 64. The nurse assesses the cardiac rhythm as:

1 Normal sinus rhythm
2 Sinus bradycardia
3 Sick sinus syndrome
4 First-degree heart block

20. The client is wearing a continuous cardiac monitor, which begins to sound its alarm. The nurse sees no ECG complexes on the screen. The first action of the nurse is to:

1 Check the client status and lead placement
2 Press the recorder button on the ECG console
3 Call the physician
4 Call a code blue

21. The client's ECG strip shows atrial and ventricular rates of 80 complexes per minute. The PR interval is 0.14 second, the QRS complex measures 0.08 second, and the PP interval is slightly irregular. The nurse interprets that this rhythm is:

1 Normal sinus rhythm
2 Sinus bradycardia
3 Sinus tachycardia
4 Sinus dysrhythmia

22. The nurse notices frequent artifacts on the ECG monitor of the client whose leads are connected by cable to a console at the bedside. The nurse examines the client to determine the cause. Which of the following items is not responsible for the artifact?

1 Frequent movement of the client
2 Tightly secured cable connections
3 Leads applied over hairy areas
4 Leads applied to the limbs

23. The nurse is watching the cardiac monitor and notices that the rhythm suddenly changes. There are no P waves, the QRS complexes are wide, and the ventricular rate is regular but over 100. The nurse assesses that the client is experiencing:

1 Premature ventricular contractions
2 Ventricular tachycardia
3 Ventricular fibrillation
4 Sinus tachycardia

24. A client has frequent bursts of ventricular tachycardia on the cardiac monitor. The nurse is most concerned with this dysrhythmia because:

1 It is uncomfortable for the client, giving a sense of impending doom
2 It produces a low cardiac output that quickly leads to cerebral and myocardial ischemia
3 It is almost impossible to convert to a normal rhythm
4 It can develop into ventricular fibrillation at any time

25. The nurse is viewing the cardiac monitor in a client's room and notes that the client has just gone into ventricular tachycardia, and is awake and alert with good color. The nurse prepares to do which of the following?

1 Immediately defibrillate
2 Prepare for pacemaker insertion
3 Administer lidocaine intravenously
4 Administer epinephrine intravenously

26. The nurse is caring for a client with unstable ventricular tachycardia. The nurse instructs the client to do which of the following if prescribed during an episode of VT?
    1 Breathe deeply, regularly, and easily
    2 Inhale deeply and cough hard every 1 to 3 seconds
    3 Lie down flat in bed
    4 Remove any metal jewelry

27. The client is having frequent premature ventricular contractions (PVCs). The nurse places priority on assessment of which of the following items?
    1 Blood pressure and peripheral perfusion
    2 Sensation of palpitations
    3 Causative factors such as caffeine
    4 Precipitating factors such as infection

28. The client has developed atrial fibrillation, with a ventricular rate of 150 per minute. The nurse assesses the client for:
    1 Hypotension and dizziness
    2 Nausea and vomiting
    3 Hypertension and headache
    4 Flat neck veins

29. The nurse is watching the cardiac monitor, and a client's rhythm suddenly changes. There are no P waves; instead there are wavy lines. The QRS complexes measure 0.08 second, but they are very irregular, with a rate of 120 beats per minute. The nurse interprets that this rhythm is:
    1 Sinus tachycardia
    2 Atrial fibrillation
    3 Ventricular tachycardia
    4 Ventricular fibrillation

30. The client with rapid-rate atrial fibrillation asks the nurse why the physician is going to perform carotid massage. The nurse responds that this procedure may stimulate the:
    1 Vagus nerve to slow the heart rate
    2 Vagus nerve to increase the heart rate, overdriving the rhythm
    3 Diaphragmatic nerve to slow the heart rate
    4 Diaphragmatic nerve to overdrive the rhythm

31. The nurse notes that a client with sinus rhythm has a PVC that falls on the T wave of the preceding beat. The client's rhythm suddenly changes to one with no P waves nor definable QRS complexes. Instead, there are coarse wavy lines of varying amplitude. The nurse assesses this rhythm to be:
    1 Ventricular tachycardia
    2 Ventricular fibrillation
    3 Atrial fibrillation
    4 Asystole

32. The nurse is caring for a monitored client alone in a room at the end of the hall. The client has a short burst of ventricular tachycardia followed by ventricular fibrillation. The client immediately loses consciousness. The nurse:
    1 Calls for help and initiates cardiopulmonary resuscitation
    2 Starts oxygen by cannula at 10 L/minute and lowers the head of the bed
    3 Goes to the nurses' station quickly and calls a code
    4 Runs to get a defibrillator from an adjacent nursing unit

33. The nurse is preparing to defibrillate the client in ventricular fibrillation. The nurse places the paddles on the client's chest, and before defibrillating the client assesses that:
    1 The client has received lidocaine HCl (Xylocaine), 100 mg IV
    2 The rhythm is actually VF
    3 The machine has been set to the "synchronize" mode
    4 The client has been intubated

34. The client in ventricular fibrillation is about to be defibrillated. The nurse knows that in order to convert this rhythm effectively, the machine should be set at which of the following energy levels for the first delivery?
    1 50 joules
    2 100 joules
    3 200 joules
    4 360 joules

35. The nurse evaluates that defibrillation of a client was most successful if which of the following observations were made?
    1 Nonarousable, sinus rhythm, BP 88/60
    2 Arousable, sinus rhythm, BP 116/72
    3 Nonarousable, supraventricular tachycardia, BP 122/60
    4 Arousable, marked bradycardia, BP 86/54

36. The nurse is evaluating the client's response to cardioversion. Which of the following observations is of highest priority to the nurse?
    1 Oxygen flow rate
    2 Status of airway
    3 Blood pressure
    4 Level of consciousness

37. An automatic external defibrillator is available to treat the client who goes into cardiac arrest. The nurse assesses the cardiac rhythm by:
    1 Applying standard ECG monitoring leads to the client and observing the rhythm
    2 Holding the defibrillator paddles firmly against the chest
    3 Applying the adhesive patch electrodes to the skin and moving away from the client
    4 Connecting standard ECG electrodes to a transtelephonic monitoring device

38. The nurse assesses that which of the following clients is the least likely to have implantation of an internal automatic implantable cardioverter-defibrillator (AICD)?
    1 A client with three episodes of cardiac arrest unrelated to myocardial infarction
    2 A client with ventricular dysrhythmias despite medication therapy
    3 A client with an episode of cardiac arrest related to myocardial infarction
    4 A client with syncopal episodes related to ventricular tachycardia

39. The nurse is caring for a client who has just had implantation of an automatic implantable cardioverter-defibrillator. The nurse immediately determines which of the following items based on priority?
    1 Activation status of the device, heart rate cutoff, and number of shocks it is programmed to deliver
    2 Presence of a MedicAlert card for the client to carry
    3 Anxiety level of the client and family
    4 Knowledge of restrictions of postdischarge physical activity

40. The nurse is caring for the client immediately after insertion of a permanent demand pacemaker via the right subclavian vein. The nurse takes care not to dislodge the pacing catheter by:
    1 Limiting movement and abduction of the right arm
    2 Limiting movement and abduction of the left arm
    3 Assisting the client to get out of bed and ambulate with a walker
    4 Assisting the client to perform range-of-motion exercises to the right arm

41. The client diagnosed with thrombophlebitis 1 day ago suddenly complains of chest pain and shortness of breath and is visibly anxious. The nurse immediately assesses the client for other signs and symptoms of:
    1 Myocardial infarction
    2 Pneumonia
    3 Pulmonary embolism
    4 Pulmonary edema

42. A client seeks treatment in the physician's office for unsightly varicose veins, and sclerotherapy is recommended. Before leaving the examining room, the client says to the nurse, "Can you tell me again how this sclerotherapy is done?" In formulating a response, the nurse incorporates the knowledge that sclerotherapy consists of:
    1 Injecting an agent into the vein to damage the vein wall and close the vein off
    2 Tying off the vein at the upper end to prevent stasis from occurring

    3 Tying off the vein at the lower end to prevent stasis from occurring
    4 Surgical removal of the varicosity

43. The client is having a follow-up physician office visit after vein ligation and stripping. The client describes a sensation of "pins and needles" in the affected leg. Based on evaluation of this comment, the nurse:
    1 Reassures the client that this is only temporary
    2 Advises the client to take acetaminophen (Tylenol) until it is gone
    3 States that warm packs should help
    4 Reports the complaint to the physician

44. A 24-year-old man seeks medical attention for complaints of claudication in the arch of the foot. The nurse also notes superficial thrombophlebitis of the lower leg. The nurse next assesses the client for:
    1 Familial tendency toward peripheral vascular disease
    2 Smoking history
    3 Recent exposure to allergens
    4 History of recent insect bites

45. The nurse has given instructions to the client with Raynaud's disease about self-management of the disease process. The nurse evaluates that the client needs further reinforcement if the client states that:
    1 Smoking cessation is very important
    2 Sources of caffeine should be eliminated from the diet
    3 Taking nifedipine (Procardia) as prescribed will decrease vessel spasm
    4 Moving to a warmer climate should help

46. The nurse is caring for the client who had percutaneous insertion of an inferior vena cava filter and was on heparin therapy prior to surgery. The nurse inspects the surgical site for signs of:
    1 Thrombosis and infection
    2 Bleeding and infection
    3 Bleeding and wound dehiscence
    4 Wound dehiscence and evisceration

47. The nurse is assessing the blood pressure of a client diagnosed with primary hypertension. The nurse ensures accurate measurement by avoiding which of the following?
    1 Seating the client with arm bared, supported, and at heart level
    2 Measuring the blood pressure after the client is seated quietly for 5 minutes
    3 Using a cuff with a rubber bladder that encircles at least 80% of the limb
    4 Taking the blood pressure within 30 minutes following nicotine or caffeine ingestion

48. The client with hypertension tells the nurse that the client has been classified as having Stage 1 hypertension, and asks the nurse what this means. In formulating a response, the nurse knows that the parameters of Stage 1 hypertension are:
    1 Systolic BP (SBP) 130–139 mmHg and diastolic BP (DBP) 85–89 mmHg
    2 SBP 140–159 mmHg and DBP 90–99 mmHg
    3 SBP 160–179 mmHg and DBP 100–109 mmHg
    4 SBP 180–209 mmHg and DBP 110–119 mmHg

49. Intravenous heparin therapy is ordered for a client. While implementing this order, the nurse ensures that which of the following medications is available on the nursing unit?
    1 Vitamin K (AquaMEPHYTON)
    2 Aminocaproic acid (Amicar)
    3 Potassium chloride (KCl injection)
    4 Protamine sulfate (protamine injection)

50. The client is at risk for pulmonary embolism and is on anticoagulant therapy with warfarin (Coumadin). The client's prothrombin time is 20 seconds, with a control of 11 seconds. The nurse assesses that this result is:
    1 The same as the client's own baseline level
    2 Lower than the needed therapeutic level
    3 Within the therapeutic range
    4 Higher than the therapeutic range

51. The client who has been receiving heparin therapy is also started on warfarin (Coumadin). The client asks the nurse why both medications are being administered. In formulating a response, the nurse incorporates the understanding that warfarin:
    1 Stimulates breakdown of specific clotting factors by the liver, and it takes 2 to 3 days for this to exert an anticoagulant effect
    2 Inhibits synthesis of specific clotting factors in the liver, and it takes 3 to 4 days for this medication to exert an anticoagulant effect
    3 Stimulates production of the body's own thrombolytic substances, but it takes 2 to 4 days for this to begin
    4 Has the same mechanism of action as heparin, and the cross-over time is needed for the serum level of warfarin to be therapeutic

52. The nurse has an order to begin administering warfarin sodium (Coumadin) to a client. While implementing this order, the nurse ensures that which of the following medications is available on the nursing unit as the antidote for Coumadin?
    1 Vitamin K (AquaMEPHYTON)
    2 Aminocaproic acid (Amicar)
    3 Potassium chloride (KCl injection)
    4 Protamine sulfate (protamine injection)

53. A client is admitted to the hospital with acute myocardial infarction and is started on tissue plasminogen activator (t-PA, Activase) by infusion. Of the following parameters, which one would the nurse determine requires the least frequent assessment to detect complications with this therapy?
    1 Oxygen saturation
    2 Neurological signs
    3 Blood pressure and pulse
    4 Complaints of abdominal and back pain

54. The client is admitted with pulmonary thromboembolism and is to be treated with streptokinase (Streptase). The nurse reports which of the following assessments to the physician before this therapy is initiated?
    1 Adventitious breath sounds
    2 Respiratory rate of 28 per minute
    3 Temperature of 99.4°F oral
    4 Blood pressure of 198/110

55. The client is admitted with myocardial infarction and is given alteplase (Activase). Following this infusion, the nurse plans to administer which of the following medications as ordered for the client?
    1 Acetylsalicylic acid (aspirin) by mouth daily
    2 Heparin sodium (heparin) continuously by IV infusion
    3 Dipyridamole (Persantine) by mouth four times daily
    4 Warfarin (Coumadin) by mouth according to prothrombin time results

56. The client is receiving thrombolytic therapy with a continuous infusion of streptokinase. The client suddenly becomes extremely anxious and complains of itching. The nurse hears stridor and, upon examination of the client, notes generalized urticaria and hypotension. The nurse should:
    1 Administer oxygen and protamine sulfate
    2 Cut the infusion rate in half and sit the client up in bed
    3 Stop the infusion and call the physician
    4 Administer diphenhydramine (Benadryl) and continue the infusion

57. The client is admitted with an arterial ischemic leg ulcer. The nurse assesses that the ulcer:
    1 Has a pink base
    2 Is superficial, with uneven edges
    3 Has little granulation tissue
    4 Has brown pigmentation surrounding it

58. The nurse is assessing the neurovascular status of the client who returned to the surgical nursing unit 4 hours ago after undergoing aortoiliac bypass graft. The affected leg is warm, and the nurse notes redness and edema. The pedal pulse

is palpable and unchanged from admission. The nurse interprets that the neurovascular status is:
1 Normal, due to increased blood flow through the leg
2 Slightly deteriorating and should be monitored for another hour
3 Moderately impaired, and the surgeon should be called
4 Adequate from an arterial approach, but venous complications are arising

59. A client is admitted with possible rheumatic endocarditis. The nurse assess the client for signs and symptoms of concurrent:
1 Viral infection
2 Yeast infection
3 Staphylococcal infection
4 Streptococcal infection

60. The nurse is evaluating the condition of a client after pericardiocentesis for cardiac tamponade. Which of the following observations indicates that the procedure is not entirely effective?
1 Rising central venous pressure
2 Rising blood pressure
3 Client expressions of relief
4 Clearly audible heart sounds

61. The nurse is assessing the client with an abdominal aortic aneurysm. Which of the following assessment findings by the nurse is probably unrelated to the AAA?
1 Pulsatile abdominal mass
2 Hyperactive bowel sounds in the area
3 Systolic bruit over the area of the mass
4 Subjective sensation of "heart-beating" in the abdomen

62. The client with an abdominal aortic aneurysm is not a candidate for surgery because the aneurysm is not yet large enough. The client is fearful that the aneurysm will rupture, causing death. The nurse plans to assist the client in coping with this fear by emphasizing what the client can do for self-monitoring. Which of the following items is unnecessary for the nurse to include in discussions with the client?
1 Antibiotic prophylaxis before invasive procedures
2 Importance of follow-up CT scans
3 Management of hypertension
4 Reporting abdominal or back pain

63. The nurse is caring for a client who had resection of an abdominal aortic aneurysm yesterday. The client has an IV with an hourly rate of 150 mL/hour, unchanged for the last 10 hours. The client's urine output for the last 3 hours was 90 mL, 50 mL, and 28 mL (28 mL most recent). The client's BUN is 35 mg/dL, and serum creatinine is 1.8 mg/dL, drawn this morning. Which

of the following actions should the nurse take next?
1 Put the IV on a pump so the infusion rate is sure to stay stable
2 Check to see if the client had a serum albumin level drawn
3 Check the urine specific gravity
4 Call the physician

64. The client is admitted with a venous stasis leg ulcer. The nurse assesses that the ulcer:
1 Has a pale base
2 Is deep, with even edges
3 Has little granulation tissue
4 Has brown pigmentation surrounding it

65. The client has an Unna boot applied for treatment of venous stasis leg ulcer. The home care nurse notes that the client's toes are mottled and cool, and the client verbalizes some numbness and tingling of the foot. The nurse interprets that the boot:
1 Is controlling leg edema
2 Has been applied too tightly
3 Is impairing venous return
4 Has not yet dried

66. The nurse is planning care for an ambulatory client with a venous stasis leg ulcer. The nurse anticipates that which type of dressing will be used in the care of this client?
1 Damp to dry isotonic saline dressings
2 One-half strength Betadine dressings
3 Dry sterile dressings
4 Zinc oxide dressings (Unna boot)

67. The home care nurse is making a routine visit to the client receiving digoxin (Lanoxin) in the treatment of heart failure. The nurse assesses the client for:
1 Thrombocytopenia and weight gain
2 Anorexia, nausea, and yellow vision
3 Diarrhea and hypotension
4 Fatigue and muscle-twitching

68. The home care nurse has given instructions to the client who is beginning therapy with digoxin (Lanoxin). The nurse evaluates that the client needs reinforcement if the client made which of the following statements?
1 "I should call the doctor if my daily pulse rate is under 60 or over 100."
2 "If I miss a dose, I should just take two the next day."
3 "I shouldn't change brands without asking the doctor first."
4 "The pills should be kept in their original container, so they don't get mixed up with my other medicines."

69. The client with angina complains that the anginal pain is prolonged and severe and occurs at

the same time each day, most often in the morning. On further assessment, the nurse notes that the pain occurs in the absence of precipitating factors. This type of anginal pain is best described as:

1 Stable angina
2 Unstable angina
3 Variant angina
4 Nonanginal pain

70. The client is taking hydrochlorothiazide (Hydro-DIURIL, HCTZ) without taking any form of electrolyte supplement. The nurse encourages intake of which of the following foods?

1 Canned pears
2 Oranges
3 Cranberry juice
4 Applesauce

71. The client taking hydrochlorothiazide has been started on triamterene (Dyrenium) as well. The client asks the nurse why both medications are required. The nurse formulates a response based on the understanding that:

1 Dyrenium is a potassium-sparing diuretic, whereas HCTZ is a potassium-losing diuretic
2 HCTZ is a potassium-sparing diuretic, whereas Dyrenium is a potassium-losing diuretic
3 Both are weak potassium-losing diuretics
4 Both are weak potassium-sparing diuretics

72. The diabetic client who has been controlled with daily insulin has been placed on atenolol (Tenormin) for control of angina pectoris. Owing to the effects of the medication, the nurse assesses that which of the following signs or symptoms is the most reliable indicator of hypoglycemia?

1 Tachycardia
2 Sweating
3 Low blood glucose level
4 Anxiety

73. The hypertensive client who has been taking metoprolol (Lopressor) has been ordered to decrease the dose of the medication. The client asks the nurse why this must be done over a period of 1 to 2 weeks. In formulating a response, the nurse incorporates the understanding that abrupt withdrawal could:

1 Give the client insomnia
2 Cause enhanced side effects of other prescribed medications
3 Result in hypoglycemia
4 Precipitate rebound hypertension

74. The nurse is beginning an infusion of sodium nitroprusside (Nipride) for the client with hypertensive crisis. The nurse does not plan to do which of the following when beginning this therapy?

1 Monitor blood pressure initially every 30 seconds, then every 5 minutes when stable
2 Draw a thiocyanate level
3 Wrap the container in aluminum foil
4 Observe the solution for a faint brown tinge

75. The nurse is administering medications to a client newly admitted to the nursing unit with a history of cardiac disease. The client has an order for propranolol (Inderal), 20 mg PO, and albuterol (Proventil, Ventolin), 2 puffs by inhalation. The nurse should:

1 Administer the propranolol first, followed by the albuterol
2 Administer the albuterol first, followed by the propranolol
3 Let the client decide which to take first, according to preference
4 Call the physician to verify the order

76. A client taking enalapril (Vasotec) has tachycardia, complains of intestinal pain, and has muscle irritability and paresthesias. The ECG shows tall, narrow T waves. The nurse interprets that these manifestations are consistent with:

1 Hypomagnesemia
2 Hypercalcemia
3 Hypokalemia
4 Hyperkalemia

77. The client who has begun taking fosinopril (Monopril) is very distressed, telling the nurse that the client cannot taste food normally since beginning the medication 2 weeks ago. The nurse provides the best support to the client by:

1 Requesting that the physician change the order to another brand of ACE inhibitor
2 Reassuring the client that this is expected, and generally disappears in 2 to 3 months
3 Telling the client to take the medication with food
4 Suggesting that the client taper the dose until taste returns to normal

78. The nurse is caring for the client with a history of mild heart failure who is receiving diltiazem (Cardizem) for hypertension. The nurse assesses the client for:

1 Tachycardia and rebound hypertension
2 Wheezing and shortness of breath
3 Bradycardia, weight gain, and peripheral edema
4 Chest pain and tachycardia

79. The client receiving nifedipine (Procardia) for angina complains of feeling listless, with generalized weakness and no energy. To support the client most effectively, the nurse must understand that these symptoms:

1 Are unrelated to taking the medication
2 Are an expected effect of the medication
3 Indicate a toxic reaction to the medication
4 Indicate underdosing of the medication

80. The nurse is planning to administer amlodipine (Norvasc) to a client. The nurse plans to do which of the following before giving the medication?
    1 Check blood pressure and pulse
    2 Check respiratory rate
    3 Check lung sounds and heart rate
    4 Check level of consciousness and blood pressure

81. The nurse has an order to give verapamil (Isoptin, Calan), 5 mg intravenously, to a client. The nurse implements this order correctly by giving the medication:
    1 Over 5 minutes, with a pulse oximeter in place
    2 Over 2 minutes, with a pulse oximeter in place
    3 Over 5 minutes, with the client on a cardiac monitor
    4 Over 2 minutes, with the client on a cardiac monitor

82. The client taking nitroglycerin sublingually for control of episodes of chest pain says to the nurse that perhaps the medication shouldn't be used unless absolutely necessary for pain. On further assessment, the nurse determines that the client knows the reasons for taking the medication, and that the client can afford to pay for the medication. The nurse should next explore with the client any concerns about:
    1 Status of the heart disease
    2 Potential myocardial infarction
    3 Developing tolerance to the medication
    4 Inconvenience of the medication schedule

83. The client has been prescribed a transdermal nitroglycerin system (Nitrodisc, Nitro-Dur) for the management of angina pectoris. The client asks the nurse why the patch must be removed at bedtime each night. In formulating a reply, the nurse incorporates the understanding that:
    1 Lack of pain relief (tolerance) occurs when the patch is worn continuously for 24 hours
    2 Hypotension occurs frequently at night unless the patch is removed
    3 The system is too irritating to the skin to be worn for 24 hours
    4 The patch usually falls off from friction with the bedclothes anyway

84. The nurse has an order to administer a dose of nitroglycerin ointment (Nitro-Bid, Nitrostat) to a client. The nurse avoids doing which of the following in preparing the medication for administration?
    1 Using the manufacturer's papers
    2 Using the fingers to spread the ointment
    3 Applying the dose in an even layer
    4 Washing off the previous application

85. The nurse is giving the client instructions about the use of a transdermal nitroglycerin system (Nitro-Dur, Transderm-Nitro). The nurse does not include which of the following points?
    1 Apply patch with very light pressure to avoid rapid absorption
    2 Units are waterproof, so bathing and showering are allowed
    3 Do not change brands, as the dosages may not be equivalent
    4 Do not cut or trim patch to adjust dosage

86. The nurse has just administered a dose of hydralazine (Apresoline) intravenously to the client. The nurse initially assesses the:
    1 Cardiac rhythm continuously
    2 Oxygen saturation continuously
    3 Blood pressure every 5 minutes, then every 15 minutes
    4 Respiratory rate every 15 minutes, then every 30 minutes

87. A hypertensive client with target organ renal damage has been prescribed minoxidil (Loniten). The client asks the nurse why the physician has also prescribed propranolol (Inderal) for concurrent use. The nurse's response is based on the understanding that propranolol:
    1 Is used to get better control of hypertension than with minoxidil alone
    2 Prevents reflex tachycardia that is caused by the minoxidil
    3 Exerts a protective effect on the kidney
    4 Prevents fluid retention and weight gain

88. The nurse is preparing to administer lidocaine hydrochloride, 100 mg IV bolus, to a client. The nurse plans to make sure which of the following is in use when the medication is given?
    1 ECG monitor
    2 Noninvasive blood pressure cuff
    3 Intra-arterial line
    4 Pulmonary artery multilumen catheter

89. The client has begun antihypertensive therapy with prazosin (Minipress). Knowing the side effects that could affect the client's psychosocial well-being, the nurse does anticipatory counseling about the possibility of:
    1 Anxiety and confusion
    2 Anxiety and pain
    3 Paranoia
    4 Decreased libido and impotence

90. The nurse has given medication instructions to the client receiving disopyramide (Norpace). The nurse evaluates that the client needs clarification of the information if the client stated to:
    1 Change position slowly
    2 Avoid extreme heat
    3 Keep facial tissues nearby for excessive salivation
    4 Use caution with driving

91. The client has begun taking quinidine gluconate (Duraquin, Quinaglute). The nurse assesses for which of the following most frequent side effects of this medication?
    1 Constipation and dehydration
    2 Diarrhea, nausea, and cramping
    3 Tachycardia and hypertension
    4 Bleeding tendencies

92. The nurse is caring for a client receiving propafenone (Rythmol). The nurse would be especially cautious in administration of this medication if the client also has a history of:
    1 Tension headaches
    2 COPD
    3 Diverticulosis
    4 Congestive heart failure

93. The client is beginning amiodarone (Cordarone) therapy while in the hospital. To minimize gastrointestinal side effects, the nurse provides the client with:
    1 Antidiarrheal agents
    2 Antacids
    3 Increased fiber and fluids
    4 Soft diet

94. The client being seen in the physician's office has been prescribed colestipol hydrochloride (Colestid). The nurse assesses to see if which of the following baseline studies has been ordered before initiating therapy with this medication?
    1 Triglycerides and chylomicrons
    2 Triglycerides and very low density lipoproteins
    3 Serum cholesterol and chylomicrons
    4 Serum cholesterol and triglycerides

95. The nurse has an order to administer colestipol hydrochloride (Colestid) to a client. The nurse would verify the order if the client had a history of:
    1 Constipation
    2 Diarrhea
    3 Iodine allergy
    4 Sulfa allergy

96. The home care nurse is giving instructions to the client receiving colestipol hydrochloride (Colestid). The nurse advises the client to increase intake of:
    1 Carbohydrates
    2 Fats
    3 Fiber and fluids
    4 Protein

97. The nurse has begun a continuous infusion of dopamine (Intropin) intravenously. The nurse assesses for which untoward effect of this therapy?
    1 Falling pulmonary wedge pressure
    2 Falling central venous pressure
    3 Bradycardia
    4 Tachycardia

98. The nurse has begun an order for a continuous dobutamine (Dobutrex) infusion. The nurse would interpret that the infusion is most effective if which of the following hemodynamic measurements was obtained?
    1 Pulmonary capillary wedge pressure (PCWP) of 30 mmHg
    2 Pulmonary capillary wedge pressure of 25 mmHg
    3 Cardiac output (CO) of 4.8 L/min
    4 Cardiac output of 3.2 L/min

99. The nurse is administering epinephrine (Adrenalin) by continuous IV infusion to the cardiac client. During administration the nurse should continuously monitor:
    1 ECG and blood pressure
    2 ECG and respiratory rate
    3 Respiratory rate and blood pressure
    4 Heart rate and urine output

100. The nurse is administering norepinephrine bitartrate (Levophed) to a client by intravenous infusion. The nurse ensures that which of the following medications is available and drawn up in case of IV infiltration?
    1 Metaraminol (Aramine)
    2 Dopamine (Isoptin)
    3 Epinephrine (Adrenalin)
    4 Phentolamine (Regitine)

101. The client is receiving a continuous infusion of isoproterenol (Isuprel). The client begins to complain of chest pain. The nurse should:
    1 Continue to monitor status and vital signs
    2 Call the physician
    3 Cut the infusion rate in half
    4 Recalculate the standard adult dosage range

102. The client has just returned to the postoperative open heart unit. Which laboratory value deserves the nurse's immediate attention?
    1 Serum creatinine of 0.8 mEq/L
    2 Hemoglobin of 14.2 g/dL
    3 Serum potassium of 2.0 mEq/L
    4 Magnesium of 1.6 mEq/L

103. The client experiencing pulmonary edema is anxious and fearful. The client states, "I know I'm dying." The nurse utilizes therapeutic communication in responding to the client's statement. Which of the following findings indicates that the nurse's technique was effective in decreasing the client's anxiety?
    1 HR 100, RR 24, skin color pale pink
    2 HR 140, RR 36, flushed appearance
    3 HR 88, RR 42, cyanosis of extremities
    4 HR 52, RR 38, dyspneic

104. The nurse is performing an assessment on the client admitted with cardiogenic shock. The nurse expects to note signs and symptoms related to:
    1 Decreased intravascular volume
    2 Vasodilation of the vascular space
    3 Increased urinary output
    4 Left ventricular failure ·

105. The nurse measures hourly urinary output of the adult client in cardiogenic shock. The client's urinary output for the past hour was 15 mL/hr. The nurse analyzes these results as:
    1 Normal range
    2 Insignificant and not indicating a decrease in cardiac output
    3 Higher than normal, indicating adequate renal perfusion
    4 Lower than normal, indicating a decrease in renal perfusion

106. The nurse is performing an initial postoperative assessment on the client admitted with quadruple coronary artery bypass surgery. The nurse assesses for potential alteration in cardiac output by:
    1 Checking pupil reactivity to light
    2 Monitoring the client's temperature every 4 hours
    3 Documenting chest tube drainage every hour
    4 Palpating peripheral pulses every hour

107. The client had an aortic valve replacement 2 days ago. This morning the client says to the nurse, "I don't feel any better than I did before surgery." The most appropriate response by the nurse is:

    1 "It's only the second day post-op. Cheer up."
    2 "This is a normal frustration, it'll get better."
    3 "You are concerned that you don't feel any better after surgery."
    4 "You will feel better in a week or two."

108. The nurse is caring for a client with cardiogenic shock. As a part of the nursing care plan, the nurse monitors for decreased tissue perfusion. If the nurse assesses a decrease in peripheral perfusion, the nurse anticipates that the most likely medication to be prescribed would be:
    1 Amrinone (Inocor)
    2 Sodium nitroprusside (Nipride)
    3 Dexamethasone (Decadron)
    4 Nitroglycerin (Tridil)

109. The nurse caring for the conscious intubated client in cardiogenic shock identifies symptoms of anxiety in the client. The intervention that would best enhance emotional support is to:
    1 Medicate the client with antianxiety medication every 4 hours
    2 Monitor the ventilator settings every 2 hours
    3 Provide Magic Slate or pen/paper for communication of fears
    4 Ask the hospital chaplain to visit the client

110. A client has undergone aortic valve replacement. To avoid the most frequent complication of this type of surgery, the nurse places priority of care on which of the following postoperative activities?
    1 Coughing and deep breathing after extubation
    2 Testing nasogastric drainage for acidity
    3 Observing cardiac rate and rhythm
    4 Monitoring the character of chest tube drainage

ANSWERS

1. **3**

Rationale: An ECG taken with pain captures ischemic changes, which include ST segment elevation or depression. A prolonged PR interval indicates first-degree heart block. A widened QRS complex indicates delay in intraventricular conduction, such as bundle branch block. Tall, peaked T waves may indicate hyperkalemia.

Test-Taking Strategy: Recalling that myocardial ischemia causes cellular derangements that alter the processes of depolarization will easily direct you to option 3.

Level of Cognitive Ability: Analysis
Phase of Nursing Process: Analysis
Client Needs: Physiological Integrity
Content Area: Adult Health/Cardiovascular

Reference
Black, J., & Matassarin-Jacobs, E. (1997). *Medical-surgical nursing: Clinical management for continuity of care* (5th ed.). Philadelphia: W. B. Saunders. p. 1254.

2. **4**

Rationale: This procedure requires a signed consent, as it involves injection of a radiopaque dye into the blood vessel. The risk of allergic reaction and possible anaphylaxis is serious and must be assessed before the procedure.

Test-Taking Strategy: The question asks you for the "most critical" assessment, implying that several options may be plausible. Using the concept of criticality, eliminate options 1 and 3. The remaining options compete for priority, but the risk of anaphylaxis makes option 4 the correct choice. Review preprocedure interventions for a cardiac catheterization now, if you had difficulty with this question!

Level of Cognitive Ability: Analysis
Phase of Nursing Process: Assessment
Client Needs: Physiological Integrity
Content Area: Adult Health/Cardiovascular

Reference
Ignatavicius, D., Workman, M., & Mishler, M. (1995). *Medical-surgical nursing: A nursing process approach* (2nd ed.). Philadelphia: W. B. Saunders. p. 801.

3. **2**

Rationale: This test is an alternative to the exercise thallium 201 scan. The dipyridamole (Persantine) dilates the coronary arteries as exercise would. Before the procedure, any form of caffeine should be withheld, as well as aminophylline or theophylline. Aminophylline is the antagonist to dipyridamole.

Test-Taking Strategy: The question is looking for an incorrect item, evidenced by the word "not" in the stem. Factors that put a strain on the heart, such as nicotine and caffeine, can interfere with cardiac diagnostic test results. Look for items such as these in similarly worded questions.

Level of Cognitive Ability: Analysis
Phase of Nursing Process: Assessment
Client Needs: Physiological Integrity
Content Area: Adult Health/Cardiovascular

Reference
Black, J., & Matassarin-Jacobs, E. (1997). *Medical-surgical nursing: Clinical management for continuity of care* (5th ed.). Philadelphia: W. B. Saunders. p. 1230.

4. **3**

Rationale: Chest pain is assessed using the standard pain assessment parameters (e.g., characteristics, location, intensity, duration, precipitating and alleviating factors, and associated symptoms). Options 1, 2, and 4 may or may not help discriminate the origin of pain. Pain of pleuropulmonary origin usually worsens on inspiration.

Test-Taking Strategy: This question is looking for a method of discriminating among causes of pain. The three incorrect responses, although appropriate to use in practice, are general assessment questions only. Option 3 will discriminate between a cardiac and noncardiac cause of pain.

Level of Cognitive Ability: Analysis
Phase of Nursing Process: Assessment
Client Needs: Physiological Integrity
Content Area: Adult Health/Cardiovascular

Reference
Ignatavicius, D., Workman, M., & Mishler, M. (1995). *Medical-surgical nursing: A nursing process approach* (2nd ed.). Philadelphia: W. B. Saunders. pp. 788–789.

5. **1**

Rationale: Cardiogenic shock occurs with severe damage (greater than 40%) to the left ventricle. Classic signs include hypotension, rapid pulse that becomes weaker, decreased urine output, and cool, clammy skin. Respiratory rate increases as the body develops metabolic acidosis from shock. Cardiac tamponade is accompanied by distant, muffled heart sounds and prominent neck vessels. Pulmonary embolism presents suddenly with severe dyspnea accompanying the chest pain. Dissecting aortic aneurysms are usually accompanied by back pain.

Test-Taking Strategy: Recall that early serious complications of MI include dysrhythmias, cardiogenic shock, and sudden death. When given a question such as this one, look for the obvious. There is no extraneous information in the stem that would guide you to another conclusion. Review the complications of MI now, if you had difficulty with this question!

Level of Cognitive Ability: Analysis
Phase of Nursing Process: Analysis
Client Needs: Physiological Integrity
Content Area: Adult Health/Cardiovascular

Reference
Smeltzer, S., & Bare, B. (1996). *Brunner and Suddarth's textbook of medical-surgical nursing* (8th ed.). Philadelphia: Lippincott-Raven. p. 672.

6. **2**

Rationale: Upon transfer from CCU, the client is allowed self-care activities and bathroom privileges. Supervised ambulation in the hall for brief distances is encouraged, with distances gradually increased (50, 100, 200 feet).

Test-Taking Strategy: Eliminate options 3 and 4 first since they are excessive, given that the client has just transferred from the CCU. Option 1 is not viable since the client would be doing less activity than in the CCU prior to transfer. Review activity prescriptions for the client with an MI now, if you had difficulty with this question!

Level of Cognitive Ability: Application
Phase of Nursing Process: Planning
Client Needs: Physiological Integrity
Content Area: Adult Health/Cardiovascular

Reference
Black, J., & Matassarin-Jacobs, E. (1997). *Medical-surgical nursing: Clinical management for continuity of care* (5th ed.). Philadelphia: W. B. Saunders. p. 1264.

7. **1**

Rationale: Edema, the accumulation of excess fluid in the interstitial spaces, can be measured by intake greater than output and by a sudden increase in weight. Diuretics should be given in the morning whenever possible to avoid nocturia. Strict sodium restrictions are reserved for clients with severe symptoms.

Test-Taking Strategy: The question asks what the nurse should do next. Options 2 and 3 can be eliminated immediately. Options 1 and 4 are both correct choices, but option 1 can give the nurse immediate information about fluid balance.

Level of Cognitive Ability: Application
Phase of Nursing Process: Planning
Client Needs: Physiological Integrity
Content Area: Adult Health/Cardiovascular

Reference
Ignatavicius, D., Workman, M., & Mishler, M. (1995). *Medical-surgical nursing: A nursing process approach* (2nd ed.). Philadelphia: W. B. Saunders. p. 790.

8. **3**

Rationale: Heart failure is precipitated or exacerbated by physical or emotional stress, dysrhythmias, infections, anemia, thyroid disorders, pregnancy, Paget's disease, nutritional deficiencies (thiamine, alcoholism), pulmonary disease, and hypervolemia.

Test-Taking Strategy: The question asks for an item that is not related to the heart failure. Since heart failure is exacerbated by factors that increase the workload of the heart, options 1, 2, and 4 can be eliminated systematically. Review the precipitating factors associated with heart failure now, if you had difficulty with this question!

Level of Cognitive Ability: Analysis
Phase of Nursing Process: Analysis
Client Needs: Physiological Integrity
Content Area: Adult Health/Cardiovascular

Reference

Black, J., & Matassarin-Jacobs, E. (1997). *Medical-surgical nursing: Clinical management for continuity of care* (5th ed.). Philadelphia: W. B. Saunders. p. 1278.

9. **2**

Rationale: Digoxin exerts a positive inotropic effect on the heart while slowing the overall rate through a variety of mechanisms. It is the medication of choice to treat heart failure. Diltiazem (calcium channel blocker), propranolol, and metoprolol (beta-adrenergic blockers) have a negative inotropic effect and would worsen the failing heart.

Test-Taking Strategy: Medication knowledge is necessary to answer this question. Review them if necessary at this time. Similarities exist between options 3 and 4, which allows them to be eliminated first.

Level of Cognitive Ability: Application
Phase of Nursing Process: Planning
Client Needs: Physiological Integrity
Content Area: Pharmacology

Reference

Black, J., & Matassarin-Jacobs, E. (1997). *Medical-surgical nursing: Clinical management for continuity of care* (5th ed.). Philadelphia: W. B. Saunders p. 1283.

10. **3**

Rationale: Pulmonary edema is characterized by extreme breathlessness, dyspnea, air hunger, and production of frothy, pink-tinged sputum. Auscultation of the lungs reveals rales to the apices. Wheezes, rhonchi, and crackles in the bases are not associated with pulmonary edema.

Test-Taking Strategy: Fluid produces sounds that are called rales or crackles, which eliminates options 1 and 4. Option 2 is less plausible than option 3 because bibasilar crackles do not produce such extreme symptoms as are noted in pulmonary edema. If you had difficulty with this question, take time now to review the manifestations found in pulmonary edema!

Level of Cognitive Ability: Analysis
Phase of Nursing Process: Assessment
Client Needs: Physiological Integrity
Content Area: Adult Health/Cardiovascular

Reference

Luckmann, J. (1997). *Saunders manual of nursing care.* Philadelphia: W. B. Saunders. p. 1072.

11. **4**

Rationale: Pulmonary edema causes the client to be extremely agitated and anxious. The client may complain of a sense of drowning, suffocation, or smothering.

Test-Taking Strategy: The adjective "florid" in the stem implies a severe problem. The client with respiratory distress from any cause becomes extremely anxious, eliminating other options systematically.

Level of Cognitive Ability: Analysis
Phase of Nursing Process: Assessment
Client Needs: Psychosocial Integrity
Content Area: Adult Health/Cardiovascular

Reference

Luckmann, J. (1997). *Saunders manual of nursing care.* Philadelphia: W. B. Saunders. p. 1072.

12. **3**

Rationale: The serum potassium level is measured in clients receiving both digoxin and furosemide. Heightened digoxin effect is observed in the client with hypokalemia. Hypokalemia also predisposes the cardiac client to ventricular dysrhythmias.

Test-Taking Strategy: Option 1 can be eliminated because the client will just be beginning digoxin therapy. The question gives no indication of renal insufficiency, which helps eliminate option 4. Furosemide therapy can cause both hyponatremia and hypokalemia, but the risk of hypokalemia has more severe consequences in this situation.

Level of Cognitive Ability: Analysis
Phase of Nursing Process: Assessment
Client Needs: Physiological Integrity
Content Area: Adult Health/Cardiovascular

Reference

Smeltzer. S., & Bare, B. (1996). *Brunner and Suddarth's textbook of medical-surgical nursing* (8th ed.). Philadelphia: Lippincott-Raven. p. 660.

13. **1**

Rationale: Classic signs of cardiogenic shock as they relate to this question include low blood pressure and tachycardia. The CVP would rise as the backward effects of the left ventricular failure became apparent. Dysrhythmias commonly occur as a result of decreased oxygenation to the myocardium.

Test-Taking Strategy: The question is testing the concept of the effect of ischemia on the myocardial cells. Ischemia makes the myocardium irritable, producing dysrhythmias. Knowledge of the classic signs of shock help you systematically eliminate the other responses, which are incorrect. Review the clinical manifestations associated with cardiogenic shock now, if you had difficulty with this question!

Level of Cognitive Ability: Analysis
Phase of Nursing Process: Assessment
Client Needs: Physiological Integrity
Content Area: Adult Health/Cardiovascular

Reference

Smeltzer, S., & Bare, B. (1996). *Brunner and Suddarth's textbook of medical-surgical nursing* (8th ed.). Philadelphia: Lippincott-Raven. p. 672.

14. **3**

Rationale: The normal CO is 4 to 8 liters per minute. With cardiogenic shock, the cardiac output falls below normal, due to failure of the heart as a pump. The PCWP, on the other hand, rises, because it is a reflection of the left ventricular end-diastolic pressure (LVEDP), which rises with pump failure.

Test-Taking Strategy: Knowing that the normal cardiac output is 4 to 8 L/minute helps you eliminate options 1 and 2 quickly. If you are unsure how to discriminate between the last two options, think about what the pressure would do in the lungs behind a failing heart. This would help you select option 3 over option 4. Review these concepts now, if you had difficulty with this question!

Level of Cognitive Ability: Analysis
Phase of Nursing Process: Analysis
Client Needs: Physiological Integrity
Content Area: Adult Health/Cardiovascular

Reference
Luckmann, J. (1997). *Saunders manual of nursing care.* Philadelphia: W. B. Saunders. p. 998.

15. **4**

Rationale: The nursing interventions for the client with an intra-aortic balloon pump are the same as for any cardiovascular surgery client. The peripheral circulation to the affected limb is monitored for signs of occlusion, such as coolness, mottling, pain, tingling, and decreased or absent distal pulse. Adverse changes are reported immediately.

Test-Taking Strategy: This question tells you that an artificial obstruction has been introduced into the femoral vessel, and adverse circulatory signs are later noted. Use concepts related to care after cardiac catheterization. The physician must be notified!

Level of Cognitive Ability: Application
Phase of Nursing Process: Implementation
Client Needs: Physiological Integrity
Content Area: Adult Health/Cardiovascular

Reference
Luckmann, J. (1997). *Saunders manual of nursing care.* Philadelphia: W. B. Saunders. p. 1082.

16. **1**

Rationale: Sternotomy incision sites are assessed for signs and symptoms of infection, such as redness, swelling, induration, and "bogginess," or "stepping." An elevated temperature and WBC count after 3 to 4 days usually indicate infection.

Test-Taking Strategy: Rule out options 2 and 4 because the WBC count is normal. The lack of drainage, redness, or "bogginess" helps you choose option 1 over 4.

Level of Cognitive Ability: Analysis
Phase of Nursing Process: Analysis
Client Needs: Physiological Integrity
Content Area: Adult Health/Cardiovascular

Reference
Ignatavicius, D., Workman, M., & Mishler, M. (1995). *Medical-surgical nursing: A nursing process approach* (2nd ed.). Philadelphia: W. B. Saunders. p. 1013.

17. **4**

Rationale: The client who undergoes cardiac surgery is at risk for renal injury from poor perfusion, hemolysis, low cardiac output, or vasopressor drug therapy. Renal insult is signaled by decreased urine output and increased BUN and creatinine. The client may need medications such as dopamine to increase renal perfusion and could possibly need peritoneal dialysis or hemodialysis.

Test-Taking Strategy: The stem gives no evidence of any infection, so eliminate options 2 and 3 first. Hypovolemia is ruled out next because of the high BUN and creatinine values, and the poor response to fluid challenge. Review laboratory values and postcardiac surgery complications now, if you had difficulty with this question!

Level of Cognitive Ability: Analysis
Phase of Nursing Process: Analysis
Client Needs: Physiological Integrity
Content Area: Adult Health/Cardiovascular

Reference
Smeltzer, S., & Bare, B. (1996). *Brunner and Suddarth's textbook of medical-surgical nursing* (8th ed.). Philadelphia: Lippincott-Raven. p. 714.

18. **2**

Rationale: The nurse should encourage regular use of pain medication for the first 48 to 72 hours after cardiac surgery, because analgesia will promote rest, decrease myocardial oxygen consumption due to pain, and allow better participation in activities such as coughing, deep breathing, and ambulation.

Test-Taking Strategy: The question asks for the best action of the nurse to help a client tolerate ambulation. Coughing and deep breathing will not actively help endurance, so eliminate that first, as well as removal of telemetry equipment, which is contraindicated unless ordered. Options 2 and 3 are both helpful, but 2 is better, for the reasons just stated.

Level of Cognitive Ability: Application
Phase of Nursing Process: Planning
Client Needs: Physiological Integrity
Content Area: Adult Health/Cardiovascular

Reference
Smeltzer, S., & Bare, B. (1996). *Brunner and Suddarth's textbook of medical-surgical nursing* (8th ed.). Philadelphia: Lippincott-Raven. p. 714.

19. **1**

Rationale: Normal sinus rhythm is defined as a regular rhythm with an overall rate of 60 to 100 beats/minute. The PR and QRS measurements are normal, measuring 0.12 to 0.20 second and 0.04 to 0.10 second, respectively.

Test-Taking Strategy: A baseline knowledge of normal ECG measurements can help you decipher these questions fairly readily. Take the time to review these now if needed!

Level of Cognitive Ability: Analysis
Phase of Nursing Process: Assessment
Client Needs: Physiological Integrity
Content Area: Adult Health/Cardiovascular

Reference
Black, J., & Matassarin-Jacobs, E. (1997). *Medical-surgical nursing: Clinical management for continuity of care* (5th ed.). Philadelphia: W. B. Saunders. p. 1296.

20. **1**

Rationale: Sudden loss of ECG complexes indicates either ventricular asystole or possibly electrode displacement. Accurate assessment of the client and equipment is necessary to determine the cause and provide an appropriate response.

Test-Taking Strategy: Options 3 and 4 are incorrect because you are calling for assistance when you don't know what the problem is. Option 2 may sound reasonable, but the ECG monitor automatically starts recording when an alarm sounds. Option 1 is the best option because you should always assess the client directly before taking any action!

Level of Cognitive Ability: Application
Phase of Nursing Process: Implementation
Client Needs: Physiological Integrity
Content Area: Adult Health/Cardiovascular

Reference
Black, J., & Matassarin-Jacobs, E. (1997). *Medical-surgical nursing: Clinical management for continuity of care* (5th ed.). Philadelphia: W. B. Saunders. p. 1310.

21. **4**

Rationale: Sinus dysrhythmia has all the characteristics of normal sinus rhythm, except there is an irregular PP interval. This is due to phasic changes in the rate of firing of the SA node and may occur as a result of vagal tone alterations. It does not affect the cardiac output.

Test-Taking Strategy: Eliminate option 1 as the rate is irregular. Sinus tachycardia and sinus bradycardia are both rate-related dysrhythmias, but they are also regular rhythms. This leaves sinus dysrhythmia as the only choice.

Level of Cognitive Ability: Analysis
Phase of Nursing Process: Analysis
Client Needs: Physiological Integrity
Content Area: Adult Health/Cardiovascular

Reference

Black, J., & Matassarin-Jacobs, E. (1997). *Medical-surgical nursing: Clinical management for continuity of care* (5th ed.). Philadelphia: W. B. Saunders. p. 1299.

22. **2**

Rationale: Motion artifact, or "noise," can be caused by frequent client movement, electrode placement on limbs, and insufficient adhesion to the skin, such as placing electrodes over hairy areas of the skin. Electrode placement over bony prominences should also be avoided. Signal interference can also occur with electrode removal and cable disconnection.

Test-Taking Strategy: This one may be fairly easy even without much ECG knowledge. The question is actually seeking a response that promotes transmission of a good ECG signal, which guides you easily to the correct answer!

Level of Cognitive Ability: Analysis
Phase of Nursing Process: Analysis
Client Needs: Physiological Integrity
Content Area: Adult Health/Cardiovascular

Reference

Ignatavicius, D., Workman, M., & Mishler, M. (1995). *Medical-surgical nursing: A nursing process approach* (2nd ed.). Philadelphia: W. B. Saunders. pp. 821–822.

23. **2**

Rationale: Ventricular tachycardia is characterized by absence of P waves, wide QRS complex (usually greater than 0.14 second), and a rate between 100 and 250 impulses per minute. The rhythm is usually fairly regular.

Test-Taking Strategy: Eliminate option 4 first since there are no P waves. PVCs are isolated ectopic beats superimposed on an underlying rhythm, so that is eliminated next. There are no true QRS complexes with ventricular fibrillation, which limits your choice to ventricular tachycardia.

Level of Cognitive Ability: Analysis
Phase of Nursing Process: Assessment
Client Needs: Physiological Integrity
Content Area: Adult Health/Cardiovascular

Reference

Ignatavicius, D., Workman, M., & Mishler, M. (1995). *Medical-surgical nursing: A nursing process approach* (2nd ed.). Philadelphia: W. B. Saunders. p. 851.

24. **4**

Rationale: VT is a life-threatening dysrhythmia that results from an irritable ectopic focus that takes over as pacemaker for the heart. The low cardiac output that results can quickly lead to cerebral and myocardial ischemia. Clients frequently experience a feeling of impending death. VT is treated with antidysrhythmic medications or magnesium sulfate if the patient has a low magnesium level, cardioversion (client awake), or defibrillation (loss of consciousness). VT can deteriorate into ventricular fibrillation at any time.

Test-Taking Strategy: Note the key phrase "most concerned." Option 3 is false and is eliminated first. Of the three remaining choices, option 1 is eliminated next on the basis of acuity. Options 2 and 4 are both of significant concern, but option 4 takes precedence, because ventricular fibrillation is more life-threatening.

Level of Cognitive Ability: Analysis
Phase of Nursing Process: Analysis
Client Needs: Physiological Integrity
Content Area: Adult Health/Cardiovascular

Reference

Black, J., & Matassarin-Jacobs, E. (1997). *Medical-surgical nursing: Clinical management for continuity of care* (5th ed.). Philadelphia: W. B. Saunders. p. 1305.

25. **3**

Rationale: First-line treatment of ventricular tachycardia in a client who is hemodynamically stable is the use of antidysrhythmics, such as lidocaine, procainamide, and bretylium. Cardioversion may also be needed to correct the rhythm. Defibrillation is used only when there is loss of consciousness. Epinephrine would stimulate an already excitable ventricle and is contraindicated.

Test-Taking Strategy: Pacemakers are used most often to treat bradycardias and heart block, so this option can be eliminated fairly easily. Knowing that epinephrine is a sympathomimetic eliminates option 4. The stem tells you that the client is awake and alert, which serves as a warning that, of the two remaining options, defibrillation may not be the correct choice.

Level of Cognitive Ability: Application
Phase of Nursing Process: Planning
Client Needs: Physiological Integrity
Content Area: Adult Health/Cardiovascular

Reference

Black, J., & Matassarin-Jacobs, E. (1997). *Medical-surgical nursing: Clinical management for continuity of care* (5th ed.). Philadelphia: W. B. Saunders. p. 1305.

26. **2**

Rationale: Cough CPR is sometimes used in the client with unstable VT. The nurse tells the client to use cough CPR, if prescribed, by inhaling deeply and coughing forcefully every 1 to 3 seconds. It may either terminate the dysrhythmia or sustain the cerebral and coronary circulation for a short time until other measures can be implemented.

Test-Taking Strategy: The question is worded so there is only one correct choice. You should easily be able to eliminate options 1, 3, and 4. Review the concept of cough CPR if you are not familiar with it!

Level of Cognitive Ability: Application
Phase of Nursing Process: Implementation
Client Needs: Physiological Integrity
Content Area: Adult Health/Cardiovascular

Reference

Ignatavicius, D., Workman, M., & Mishler, M. (1995). *Medical-surgical nursing: A nursing process approach* (2nd ed.). Philadelphia: W. B. Saunders. p. 851.

27. 1

Rationale: PVCs can cause hemodynamic compromise. The shortened ventricular filling time with the ectopic beat leads to decreased stroke volume and, if frequent enough, to decreased cardiac output. The client may be asymptomatic or may feel palpitations. They can be caused by cardiac disorders, or by any number of physiological stressors, such as infection, illness, surgery, trauma, as well as intake of caffeine, nicotine, or alcohol.

Test-Taking Strategy: The question asks for "priority of assessment," implying more than one correct response. In this case, all responses are correct. Remembering the "ABCs" (airway, breathing, circulation) will help you answer this question quickly and easily!

Level of Cognitive Ability: Application
Phase of Nursing Process: Assessment
Client Needs: Physiological Integrity
Content Area: Adult Health/Cardiovascular

Reference
Ignatavicius, D., Workman, M., & Mishler, M. (1995). *Medical-surgical nursing: A nursing process approach* (2nd ed.). Philadelphia: W. B. Saunders. pp. 848–849.

28. 1

Rationale: The client with uncontrolled atrial fibrillation with a ventricular rate over 100 beats/minute is at risk for low cardiac output due to loss of atrial kick. The nurse assesses the client for palpitations, chest pain or discomfort, hypotension, pulse deficit, fatigue, weakness, dizziness, syncope, shortness of breath, and distended neck veins.

Test-Taking Strategy: Flat neck veins are normal or indicate hypovolemia, so option 4 is eliminated. Nausea and vomiting (option 2) are associated with vagus nerve activity, which doesn't match a tachycardic state. Of the remaining choices, the correct response can be chosen by thinking of the consequences of falling cardiac output (e.g., hypotension and dizziness, not hypertension).

Level of Cognitive Ability: Application
Phase of Nursing Process: Assessment
Client Needs: Physiological Integrity
Content Area: Adult Health/Cardiovascular

Reference
Ignatavicius, D., Workman, M., & Mishler, M. (1995). *Medical-surgical nursing: A nursing process approach* (2nd ed.). Philadelphia: W. B. Saunders. p. 841.

29. 2

Rationale: Atrial fibrillation is characterized by a loss of P waves; an undulating, wavy baseline; QRS duration that is often within normal limits; and a very irregular ventricular rate, which can range from 60 to 100 beats per minute (when controlled with medications) to a rate of 100 to 160 (when uncontrolled).

Test-Taking Strategy: The loss of P waves rules out sinus tachycardia as the correct choice. The QRS complex measures 0.08 second, which rules out either of the ventricular dysrhythmias. Atrial fibrillation is a common dysrhythmia that needs chronic management, so it is worth being familiar with. Review now, if you had difficulty with this question!

Level of Cognitive Ability: Analysis
Phase of Nursing Process: Analysis
Client Needs: Physiological Integrity
Content Area: Adult Health/Cardiovascular

Reference
Ignatavicius, D., Workman, M., & Mishler, M. (1995). *Medical-surgical nursing: A nursing process approach* (2nd ed.). Philadelphia: W. B. Saunders. p. 841.

30. 1

Rationale: Carotid sinus massage is one of the maneuvers used for vagal stimulation to decrease a rapid heart rate and possibly terminate a tachydysrhythmia. The others are the Valsalva maneuvers of inducing the gag reflex and asking the client to strain or bear down. Medication therapy is often needed as an adjunct to keep the rate down or to maintain the normal rhythm.

Test-Taking Strategy: Knowledge of anatomy and physiology alone may be sufficient to guide you through this question. A rapid-rate dysrhythmia would need to be slowed, which is the function of the vagus nerve. The diaphragmatic nerve affects respiration. If you are unfamiliar with the functions of these nerves, take time now to review!

Level of Cognitive Ability: Application
Phase of Nursing Process: Implementation
Client Needs: Physiological Integrity
Content Area: Adult Health/Cardiovascular

Reference
Ignatavicius, D., Workman, M., & Mishler, M. (1995). *Medical-surgical nursing: A nursing process approach* (2nd ed.). Philadelphia: W. B. Saunders. p. 864.

31. 2

Rationale: Ventricular fibrillation is characterized by irregular, chaotic undulations of varying amplitudes. There is no measurable rate, no visible P waves or QRS complexes. It results from electrical chaos in the ventricles.

Test-Taking Strategy: The lack of visible QRS complexes eliminates atrial fibrillation and ventricular tachycardia. Asystole is lack of any electrical activity of the heart, which leaves ventricular fibrillation as the correct option, by the process of elimination.

Level of Cognitive Ability: Analysis
Phase of Nursing Process: Assessment
Client Needs: Physiological Integrity
Content Area: Adult Health/Cardiovascular

Reference
Ignatavicius, D., Workman, M., & Mishler, M. (1995). *Medical-surgical nursing: A nursing process approach* (2nd ed.). Philadelphia: W. B. Saunders. p. 852.

32. 1

Rationale: When VF occurs, the nurse remains with the client and initiates CPR until a defibrillator is available and attached to the client.

Test-Taking Strategy: Eliminate options 3 and 4 first because you would never leave the client alone. Of the remaining two, lowering the head of the bed is appropriate (for resuscitation), but the oxygen by cannula at 10 liters is incorrect. Option 1 is the correct option!

Level of Cognitive Ability: Application
Phase of Nursing Process: Implementation
Client Needs: Physiological Integrity
Content Area: Adult Health/Cardiovascular

Reference
Black, J., & Matassarin-Jacobs, E. (1997). *Medical-surgical nursing: Clinical management for continuity of care* (5th ed.). Philadelphia: W. B. Saunders. p. 1305.

33. **2**

Rationale: Until the defibrillator is attached and charged, the client is resuscitated using CPR. Once the defibrillator is attached, the ECG is checked to verify that the rhythm is VF or pulseless ventricular tachycardia. Leads are also checked for any loose connections. A nitroglycerin patch, if present, is removed.

Test-Taking Strategy: The client does not have to be intubated in order to be defibrillated, so that option is incorrect. Lidocaine may be given subsequently but is not required before defibrillation, so that option is also discarded. The machine is not set to the synchronous mode, because there is no underlying rhythm to synchronize with. Thus, the only remaining option is to verify the actual rhythm before defibrillating.

Level of Cognitive Ability: Analysis
Phase of Nursing Process: Assessment
Client Needs: Physiological Integrity
Content Area: Adult Health/Cardiovascular

Reference
Black, J., & Matassarin-Jacobs, E. (1997). *Medical-surgical nursing: Clinical management for continuity of care* (5th ed.). Philadelphia: W. B. Saunders. p. 1311.

34. **3**

Rationale: The client may be defibrillated up to three times in succession if not successful. The energy levels used are 200, 300, and 360 joules for the first, second, and third attempts, respectively.

Test-Taking Strategy: This is a difficult question to answer unless you are familiar with the settings. As a general rule, though, remember that lower levels of energy are used for cardioversion. Higher levels are used in defibrillation. Review these procedures now, if you had difficulty with this question!

Level of Cognitive Ability: Analysis
Phase of Nursing Process: Analysis
Client Needs: Physiological Integrity
Content Area: Adult Health/Cardiovascular

Reference
Black, J., & Matassarin-Jacobs, E. (1997). *Medical-surgical nursing: Clinical management for continuity of care* (5th ed.). Philadelphia: W. B. Saunders. p. 1311.

35. **2**

Rationale: After defibrillation, the client requires continuous monitoring of ECG rhythm, hemodynamic status, and neurologic status. Respiratory acidosis and metabolic acidosis develop during ventricular fibrillation from lack of respiration and cardiac output. These can cause cerebral as well as cardiopulmonary complications. Arousable status, adequate BP, and a sinus rhythm indicate successful response to defibrillation.

Test-Taking Strategy: Note the key phrase "most successful" in the question. The options are arranged with three parameters: cardiac rhythm, BP, and neurologic status. Eliminate options 1 and 3 first, since the client is nonarousable. Of the remaining two, the correct answer contains the better rhythm (sinus rhythm) and better BP.

Level of Cognitive Ability: Analysis
Phase of Nursing Process: Evaluation
Client Needs: Physiological Integrity
Content Area: Adult Health/Cardiovascular

Reference
Black, J., & Matassarin-Jacobs, E. (1997). *Medical-surgical nursing: Clinical management for continuity of care* (5th ed.). Philadelphia: W. B. Saunders. p. 1311.

36. **2**

Rationale: Nursing responsibilities after cardioversion include maintenance of a patent airway, oxygen administration, assessment of vital signs and level of consciousness, and dysrhythmia detection.

Test-Taking Strategy: There is more than one correct answer, as evidence by the phrase "highest priority" in the stem. This question is easy, though, since it follows the ABCs of life support. Airway comes first!

Level of Cognitive Ability: Analysis
Phase of Nursing Process: Evaluation
Client Needs: Physiological Integrity
Content Area: Adult Health/Cardiovascular

Reference
Smeltzer, S., & Bare, B. (1996). *Brunner and Suddarth's textbook of medical-surgical nursing* (8th ed.). Philadelphia: Lippincott-Raven. p. 874.

37. **3**

Rationale: The nurse or rescuer puts two large adhesive patch electrodes on the client's chest in the usual defibrillator position. The nurse stops CPR and orders anyone near the client to move away and not touch the client. The defibrillator then analyzes the rhythm, which may take up to 30 seconds. The machine then indicates if it is necessary to defibrillate.

Test-Taking Strategy: If you are not familiar with this piece of equipment, look first at the word "automatic" in the name. This implies that a person is not as involved in the process as with a conventional defibrillator and may help you eliminate option 2. Since standard ECG monitoring leads do not play an active role once a resuscitation is underway (options 1 and 4), you can eliminate these other two similar, but incorrect, responses. Option 4 is especially "tricky" because automatic external defibrillation can be done transtelephonically, but it is done through the use of patch electrodes that interact via telephone lines to a base station, which controls any actual defibrillation.

Level of Cognitive Ability: Application
Phase of Nursing Process: Assessment
Client Needs: Physiological Integrity
Content Area: Adult Health/Cardiovascular

Reference
Ignatavicius, D., Workman, M., & Mishler, M. (1995). *Medical-surgical nursing: A nursing process approach* (2nd ed.). Philadelphia: W. B. Saunders. p. 879.

38. **3**

Rationale: An AICD detects and delivers an electric shock to terminate life-threatening episodes of ventricular tachycardia and ventricular fibrillation. These devices are implanted in clients who are considered high risk, including those who have survived sudden cardiac death that is unrelated to myocardial infarction, those who are refractory to medication therapy, and those who have syncopal episodes related to ventricular tachycardia.

Test-Taking Strategy: The question asks you to identify the client "least likely" to have implantation of the device. Ventricular dysrhythmias that induce syncope or occur while the client is on medication are likely to be true indications for the AICD, and so you eliminate those first. The last two choices are similar, but the main difference is whether or not the cardiac arrest was related to myocardial infarction. Of these two, the one most likely to be responsive to AICD would be the client without MI, since those dysrhythmias are spontaneous. Thus, the least likely client is the one whose dysrhythmias were primarily due to insult from MI. Review the indications for the use of an AICD now, if you had difficulty with this question!

Level of Cognitive Ability: Analysis
Phase of Nursing Process: Assessment
Client Needs: Physiological Integrity
Content Area: Adult Health/Cardiovascular

Reference
Ignatavicius, D., Workman, M., & Mishler, M. (1995). *Medical-surgical nursing: A nursing process approach* (2nd ed.). Philadelphia: W. B. Saunders. p. 881.

39. **1**

Rationale: The nurse caring for the client after insertion of an AICD needs to determine device settings, similar to after permanent pacemaker insertion. Specifically, the nurse needs to know whether it is activated, the heart rate cutoff above which it will fire, and number of shocks it is programmed to deliver. The nurse assesses the physiological and psychological status of the client postoperatively and provides postoperative care that is similar to that given after cardiac surgery.

Test-Taking Strategy: This question is worded to elicit a priority item that must be determined by the nurse post-AICD insertion. Thus, several of the options may be somewhat correct (as in fact, all of them are). However, the priority of care postprocedure is the physiological status of the client, including device status. Options 2 and 4 are important prior to discharge, and option 3 (anxiety) is the second priority after physiological safety.

Level of Cognitive Ability: Application
Phase of Nursing Process: Assessment
Client Needs: Physiological Integrity
Content Area: Adult Health/Cardiovascular

Reference
Ignatavicius, D., Workman, M., & Mishler, M. (1995). *Medical-surgical nursing: A nursing process approach* (2nd ed.). Philadelphia: W. B. Saunders. pp. 882–883.

40. **1**

Rationale: In the first several hours after insertion of either a permanent or temporary pacemaker, the most common complication is pacing electrode dislodgment. The nurse helps prevent this complication by limiting the client's activities.

Test-Taking Strategy: The stem of the question tells you that the pacemaker was inserted on the right side. Therefore, to prevent pacing electrode dislodgment, motion must be limited on that side. Options 3 and 4 involve movement of the right arm. Limiting the movement of the left arm (option 2) is of no benefit to the client. Thus, option 1 is the clear choice.

Level of Cognitive Ability: Application
Phase of Nursing Process: Implementation
Client Needs: Physiological Integrity
Content Area: Adult Health/Cardiovascular

Reference
Smeltzer, S., and Bare, B. (1996). *Brunner and Suddarth's textbook of medical-surgical nursing* (8th ed.). Philadelphia: Lippincott-Raven. p. 632.

41. **3**

Rationale: Pulmonary embolism is a life-threatening complication of deep vein thrombosis and thrombophlebitis. Chest pain is the most common symptom; it is sudden in onset and may be aggravated by breathing. Other signs and symptoms include dyspnea, cough, diaphoresis, and apprehension.

Test-Taking Strategy: This question tests your ability to analyze signs and symptoms of pulmonary embolism in a client at risk. Each of the incorrect options should be ruled out because myocardial infarction and pulmonary edema are cardiac-related problems and are therefore similar, and pneumonia is an infectious process. Review these concepts if needed. You are likely to find questions related to pulmonary embolism on NCLEX-RN!

Level of Cognitive Ability: Application
Phase of Nursing Process: Assessment
Client Needs: Physiological Integrity
Content Area: Adult Health/Cardiovascular

Reference
Black, J., & Matassarin-Jacobs, E. (1997). *Medical-surgical nursing: Clinical management for continuity of care* (5th ed.). Philadelphia: W. B. Saunders. p. 1435.

42. **1**

Rationale: Sclerotherapy is the injection of a sclerosing agent into a varicosity. The agent damages the vessel and causes aseptic thrombosis, which results in vein closure. With no blood flow through the vessel, there is no distention. The surgical procedure for varicose veins is vein ligation and stripping. This procedure involves tying off the varicose vein and large tributaries, and then removal of the vein with the use of hook and wires via multiple small incisions in the leg.

Test-Taking Strategy: If you are uncertain of the response to this question, look at the word "sclerotherapy." A vessel that is sclerosed is blocked. This may help you select the correct option. At the very least, you should be able to eliminate options 2 and 3 readily, because neither of these makes sense using principles of blood flow and gravity. Also, they are very similar and so are likely to be incorrect. Review this procedure now, if you had difficulty with this question!

Level of Cognitive Ability: Analysis
Phase of Nursing Process: Analysis
Client Needs: Physiological Integrity
Content Area: Adult Health/Cardiovascular

Reference
Black, J., & Matassarin-Jacobs, E. (1997). *Medical-surgical nursing: Clinical management for continuity of care* (5th ed.). Philadelphia: W. B. Saunders. p. 1439.

43. **4**

Rationale: Hypersensitivity, or a sensation of "pins and needles," in the surgical limb may indicate temporary or permanent nerve injury following surgery. The saphenous vein and the saphenous nerve run close together in the distal third of the leg. Since complications from this surgery are relatively rare, this symptom should be reported.

Test-Taking Strategy: Pins and needles sensations usually indicate nerve irritation or damage. Knowing this, options 2 and 3 can be eliminated as the least likely correct choices. Reassuring the client about something being "only temporary" is not often a good choice, unless this is known to be absolutely true. By the process of elimination, then, the physician should be notified.

Level of Cognitive Ability: Application
Phase of Nursing Process: Implementation
Client Needs: Physiological Integrity
Content Area: Adult Health/Cardiovascular

Reference

Black, J., & Matassarin-Jacobs, E. (1997). *Medical-surgical nursing: Clinical management for continuity of care* (5th ed.). Philadelphia: W. B. Saunders. p. 1439.

44. **2**

Rationale: The mixture of arterial and venous manifestations (claudication and phlebitis, respectively) in the young male client suggests thromboangiitis obliterans (Buerger's disease). This is a relatively uncommon disorder, characterized by inflammation and thrombosis of smaller arteries and veins. This disorder is typically found in young adult men who smoke. The cause is unknown but is suspected to have an autoimmune component.

Test-Taking Strategy: A basic knowledge of this disorder is really needed to answer this question rapidly and accurately. You can first eliminate options 3 and 4 because they would most likely cause local skin reactions. The question asks which item you should assess "next." It is often better to assess a modifiable factor before a nonmodifiable one. This may help you prioritize your answer.

Level of Cognitive Ability: Analysis
Phase of Nursing Process: Assessment
Client Needs: Physiological Integrity
Content Area: Adult Health/Cardiovascular

Reference

Ignatavicius, D., Workman, M., & Mishler, M. (1995). *Medical-surgical nursing: A nursing process approach* (2nd ed.). Philadelphia: W. B. Saunders. p. 952.

45. **4**

Rationale: The disorder responds favorably to removal of nicotine and caffeine. Medications such as calcium channel blockers may inhibit vessel spasm and prevent symptoms. Avoiding exposure to cold through a variety of means is very important. However, moving to a warmer climate may not necessarily be beneficial because the symptoms could still occur with the use of air conditioning and during periods of cooler weather.

Test-Taking Strategy: Note the key phrase "needs further reinforcement." All the options look good on first reading. However, when you analyze each of them, you realize that relocation is the least favorable of all the choices from the viewpoints of practicality and encountering new environmental concerns.

Level of Cognitive Ability: Analysis
Phase of Nursing Process: Evaluation
Client Needs: Health Promotion and Maintenance
Content Area: Adult Health/Cardiovascular

Reference

Lewis, S., Collier, I., & Heitkemper, M. (1996). *Medical-surgical nursing: Assessment and management of clinical problems* (4th ed.). St. Louis: Mosby–Year Book. p. 1053

46. **2**

Rationale: After IVC filter insertion, the nurse inspects the surgical site for bleeding and signs and symptoms of infection. Otherwise, care is the same as for any other postoperative client.

Test-Taking Strategy: Since these devices are inserted percutaneously through a deep vein, options 3 and 4 are not possible, as there is no abdominal incision. The client has been on anticoagulant therapy before surgery due to high risk of pulmonary embolism, which makes option 2 the option to choose.

Level of Cognitive Ability: Application
Phase of Nursing Process: Implementation
Client Needs: Physiological Integrity
Content Area: Adult Health/Cardiovascular

Reference

Ignatavicius, D., Workman, M., & Mishler, M. (1995). *Medical-surgical nursing: A nursing process approach* (2nd ed.). Philadelphia: W. B. Saunders p. 958.

47. **4**

Rationale: Blood pressure should be measured with the client seated with the arm bared, positioned with support, and at heart level. The client should sit with legs on floor, feet uncrossed, and not speak during the recording. The client should not have smoked tobacco or ingested caffeine in the 30 minutes preceding the measurement. The client should rest quietly for 5 minutes before the reading is taken. The cuff bladder should encircle at least 80% of the limb being measured. Gauges other than a mercury sphygmomanometer should be calibrated every 6 months to ensure accuracy. Finally, two or more readings should be averaged.

Test-Taking Strategy: Since blood pressure measurement is a finely honed skill, this should be fairly easy to answer. If you get a mental block, however, remember in questions worded such as these, variables that interfere with accuracy (such as caffeine and nicotine in this instance) are likely to be the correct choice.

Level of Cognitive Ability: Application
Phase of Nursing Process: Assessment
Client Needs: Physiological Integrity
Content Area: Adult Health/Cardiovascular

Reference

Black, J., & Matassarin-Jacobs, E. (1997). *Medical-surgical nursing: Clinical management for continuity of care* (5th ed.). Philadelphia: W. B. Saunders. p. 1399.

48. **2**

Rationale: The 1992 Joint National Committee on Detection, Evaluation, and Treatment of High Blood Pressure developed the following categories of hypertension for adults 18 years and older: High normal = SBP 130–139 mmHg and DBP 85–89 mmHg; Stage 1 (mild) = SBP 140–159 and DBP 90–99; Stage 2 (moderate) = SBP 160–179 and DBP 100–109; Stage 3 (severe) = SBP 180–209 and DBP 110–119; Stage 4 (very severe) = 210 or more and DBP 120 or more.

Test-Taking Strategy: If you can remember that hypertension is defined as BP of 140/90 or greater, you are off to a reasonable start to answer this question. Stage 1 by name implies a low degree of abnormality. These two thoughts would be sufficient for you to select the correct answer.

Level of Cognitive Ability: Analysis
Phase of Nursing Process: Analysis
Client Needs: Physiological Integrity
Content Area: Adult Health/Cardiovascular

Reference

Black, J., & Matassarin-Jacobs, E. (1997). *Medical-surgical nursing: Clinical management for continuity of care* (5th ed.). Philadelphia: W. B. Saunders. p. 1391.

49. **4**

Rationale: The antidote to heparin is protamine sulfate, and it should be readily available for use if excessive bleeding or hemorrhage should occur.

Test-Taking Strategy: This is an example of an item that must be memorized. It is a critical concept, and is a likely area for testing. Take the time to learn this now if needed!

Level of Cognitive Ability: Application
Phase of Nursing Process: Implementation
Client Needs: Physiological Integrity
Content Area: Pharmacology

Reference

Hodgson, B., & Kizior, R. (1998). *Saunders nursing drug handbook 1998*. Philadelphia: W. B. Saunders. p. 1098

50. **3**

Rationale: The therapeutic range for prothrombin time (PT) is 1.5 to 2 times the control for clients at high risk for thrombus. Based on the client's control value, the therapeutic range for this individual would be 16.5 to 22 seconds.

Test-Taking Strategy: A key to answering this question as stated is in the control value. If you know that the purpose of anticoagulant therapy is to prolong clotting times, then you can immediately eliminate options 1 and 2. Since the PT value in the stem is not even double the control, option 3 is your best choice.

Level of Cognitive Ability: Analysis
Phase of Nursing Process: Assessment
Client Needs: Physiological Integrity
Content Area: Pharmacology

Reference

Hodgson, B., & Kizior, R. (1998). *Saunders nursing drug handbook 1998*. Philadelphia: W. B. Saunders. pp. 1062–1064.

51. **2**

Rationale: Warfarin works in the liver. It inhibits synthesis of four vitamin K–dependent clotting factors (X, IX, VII, and II), but it takes 3 to 4 days before the therapeutic effect of warfarin is exhibited.

Test-Taking Strategy: Heparin and Coumadin do not act in the same way, so eliminate option 4 first. Warfarin is an anticoagulant, not a thrombolytic, so option 3 is incorrect. Recalling that the liver synthesizes clotting factors helps you choose option 2 over option 1.

Level of Cognitive Ability: Analysis
Phase of Nursing Process: Analysis
Client Needs: Health Promotion and Maintenance
Content Area: Pharmacology

Reference

Ignatavicius, D., Workman, M., & Mishler, M. (1995). *Medical-surgical nursing: A nursing process approach* (2nd ed.). Philadelphia: W. B. Saunders. p. 957.

52. **1**

Rationale: The antidote to coumadin is Vitamin K, and it should be readily available for use if excessive bleeding or hemorrhage should occur.

Test-Taking Strategy: This is an example of an item that must be memorized. It is a critical concept and is a likely area for testing. Take the time to learn this now if needed!

Level of Cognitive Ability: Application
Phase of Nursing Process: Implementation
Client Needs: Physiological Integrity
Content Area: Pharmacology

Reference

Hodgson, B., & Kizior, R. (1998). *Saunders nursing drug handbook 1998*. Philadelphia: W. B. Saunders. pp. 1062–1064.

53. **1**

Rationale: Thrombolytic agents dissolve existing clots, and bleeding can occur anywhere in the body. The nurse monitors for any obvious signs of bleeding and also for occult signs of bleeding, which would include hemoglobin and hematocrit levels, blood pressure and pulse, neurological signs, assessment of abdominal and back pain, and presence of blood in the urine or stool.

Test-Taking Strategy: Since bleeding is the prime complication of thrombolytic therapy, the nurse assesses for these signs and symptoms. The key phrase is "least frequent measurement," and therefore you are looking for an option that is not related to bleeding. A change in neurological signs could indicate cerebral bleeding; abdominal and back pain could indicate abdominal bleeding; change in blood pressure and pulse could be general indicators of hemorrhage. Oxygen saturation is not an indicator of bleeding in the respiratory tract; more likely, you would see hemoptysis. Therefore, this is the answer to the question.

Level of Cognitive Ability: Application
Phase of Nursing Process: Assessment
Client Needs: Physiological Integrity
Content Area: Pharmacology

Reference

Ignatavicius, D., Workman, M., & Mishler, M. (1995). *Medical-surgical nursing: A nursing process approach* (2nd ed.). Philadelphia: W. B. Saunders. p. 996.

54. **4**

Rationale: Thrombolytic therapy is contraindicated in a number of pre-existing conditions in which there is a risk of uncontrolled bleeding, similar to the case in anticoagulant therapy. It is also contraindicated in severe, uncontrolled hypertension because of the risk of cerebral hemorrhage.

Test-Taking Strategy: This question is straightforward in approach. Options 1, 2, and 3 may be present in the client with pulmonary thromboembolism and are not necessarily something that warrants reporting before this therapy is initiated. The correct response is the dangerously high BP, which could prove fatal to the client if untreated before this therapy is initiated.

Level of Cognitive Ability: Application
Phase of Nursing Process: Implementation
Client Needs: Physiological Integrity
Content Area: Pharmacology

Reference

Hodgson, B., & Kizior, R. (1998). *Saunders nursing drug handbook 1998*. Philadelphia: W. B. Saunders. pp. 946–948.

55. 2

Rationale: Once the thrombolytic therapy infusion is complete, a heparin drip is started without a loading dose. This is initiated when the thrombin time has decreased to less than twice the control value, which usually occurs within 4 hours of the time the infusion ended.

Test-Taking Strategy: To answer this question, you need to know that recurrent thrombosis can occur after thrombolytic therapy is complete, unless anticoagulation is started to prevent this. Do a quick review of this therapy now, if needed!

Level of Cognitive Ability: Application
Phase of Nursing Process: Planning
Client Needs: Physiological Integrity
Content Area: Pharmacology

Reference
Hodgson, B., & Kizior, R. (1998). *Saunders nursing drug handbook 1998.* Philadelphia: W. B. Saunders. p. 31.

56. 3

Rationale: The client is experiencing an anaphylactic reaction to streptokinase, which is allergenic. The infusion should be discontinued, and the client should receive treatment with epinephrine, antihistamines, and corticosteroids.

Test-Taking Strategy: This question is testing whether you know that allergic reaction and possible anaphylaxis are risks associated with streptokinase therapy. If you know this, or if you can recognize the signs and symptoms of anaphylaxis, you could probably answer this question correctly. With similar questions, when there is a severe allergic reaction, the substance (whatever it is) should be stopped, and life-saving treatment should begin!

Level of Cognitive Ability: Application
Phase of Nursing Process: Implementation
Client Needs: Physiological Integrity
Content Area: Pharmacology

Reference
Black, J., & Matassarin-Jacobs, E. (1997). *Medical-surgical nursing: Clinical management for continuity of care* (5th ed.). Philadelphia: W. B. Saunders. p. 513.

57. 3

Rationale: Arterial leg ulcers tend to be deep and pale, with uneven edges and little granulation tissue. The client usually has rest pain, and the ulcer site is painful. Surrounding skin has coloration consistent with peripheral arterial disease.

Test-Taking Strategy: This question is asking you to discriminate between signs and symptoms of arterial and venous leg ulcers. Since arterial ulcers are caused by marked reduction in blood flow and tissue malnutrition, you can eliminate options 1 and 2. Brown discoloration (option 4) indicates clogging of peripheral tissue with waste products of metabolism and indicates a venous problem. The answer is option 3, which is also consistent with tissue malnutrition.

Level of Cognitive Ability: Application
Phase of Nursing Process: Assessment
Client Needs: Physiological Integrity
Content Area: Adult Health/Cardiovascular

Reference
Ignatavicius, D., Workman, M., & Mishler, M. (1995). *Medical-surgical nursing: A nursing process approach* (2nd ed.). Philadelphia: W. B. Saunders. p. 940.

58. 1

Rationale: An expected outcome of surgery is warmth, redness, and edema in the surgical extremity, due to increased blood flow.

Test-Taking Strategy: Option 3 can be easily eliminated because the pedal pulse is unchanged. Venous complications from immobilization due to surgery would not be apparent within 4 hours, so eliminate that one next. To help you choose between options 1 and 2, think about the effects of sudden reperfusion in an ischemic limb. There would be redness from new blood flow, and edema from the sudden change in pressure in the blood vessels. Thus option 1 is better than option 2.

Level of Cognitive Ability: Analysis
Phase of Nursing Process: Analysis
Client Needs: Physiological Integrity
Content Area: Adult Health/Cardiovascular

Reference
Ignatavicius, D., Workman, M., & Mishler, M. (1995). *Medical-surgical nursing: A nursing process approach* (2nd ed.). Philadelphia: W. B. Saunders. p. 944.

59. 4

Rationale: Rheumatic endocarditis is a major indicator of rheumatic fever, which is a complication of infection with group A beta-hemolytic streptococci. It is frequently triggered by streptococcal pharyngitis.

Test-Taking Strategy: Streptococcal infections are largely responsible for rheumatic heart disease. Remembering this concept should help you navigate questions in this area!

Level of Cognitive Ability: Analysis
Phase of Nursing Process: Assessment
Client Needs: Physiological Integrity
Content Area: Adult Health/Cardiovascular

Reference
Ignatavicius, D., Workman, M., & Mishler, M. (1995). *Medical-surgical nursing: A nursing process approach* (2nd ed.). Philadelphia: W. B. Saunders. p. 917.

60. 1

Rationale: Following pericardiocentesis, a rise in blood pressure and a fall in CVP is expected. The client usually expresses immediate relief. Heart sounds are no longer muffled or distant.

Test-Taking Strategy: Note the key word "not." Successful therapy is measured by the disappearance of the original signs and symptoms of cardiac tamponade. The wording of the question makes you look for a sign consistent with continued tamponade, which would be option 1.

Level of Cognitive Ability: Analysis
Phase of Nursing Process: Evaluation
Client Needs: Physiological Integrity
Content Area: Adult Health/Cardiovascular

Reference
Smeltzer, S., & Bare, B. (1996). *Brunner and Suddarth's textbook of medical-surgical nursing* (8th ed.). Philadelphia: Lippincott-Raven. p. 674.

61. 2

Rationale: Only about 40% of clients with AAA exhibit symptoms. Those who do may describe a feeling of the "heart beating" in the abdomen when supine, or being able to feel the mass throbbing. A pulsatile mass may be palpated in the middle and upper abdomen. A systolic bruit may be auscultated over the mass. If the mass has thrombi attached, larger vessels could become occluded; smaller vessels suffer emboli, such as "blue toe syndrome" with digital obstruction.

Test-Taking Strategy: Note the key word "unrelated." Each of the incorrect options has a circulatory component. The correct option deals with an unrelated body system, even though it is an abdominal assessment!

Level of Cognitive Ability: Analysis
Phase of Nursing Process: Assessment
Client Needs: Physiological Integrity
Content Area: Adult Health/Cardiovascular

Reference
Smeltzer, S., & Bare, B. (1996). *Brunner and Suddarth's textbook of medical-surgical nursing* (8th ed.). Philadelphia: Lippincott-Raven. p. 739.

62. **1**

Rationale: Psychosocial care of the client with medical management of an AAA includes listening to the client's concerns, and reinforcing the rationales for ongoing medical surveillance. This includes periodic CT scans to monitor the size of the aneurysm and careful adherence to medication and diet therapy for hypertension. The client is instructed to report any sensation of abdominal fullness or complaints of abdominal or back pain to the physician without delay.

Test-Taking Strategy: This question is worded to make you look for an option that is not part of routine management for the client with unrepaired AAA. Options 2 and 4 can be eliminated quickly, as they are obviously good actions. If you have any difficulty with the last two, remember that increased blood pressure (option 3) could cause strain and rupture, which leaves option 1 as the correct answer.

Level of Cognitive Ability: Application
Phase of Nursing Process: Planning
Client Needs: Psychosocial Integrity
Content Area: Adult Health/Cardiovascular

Reference
Ignatavicius, D., Workman, M., & Mishler, M. (1995). *Medical-surgical nursing: A nursing process approach* (2nd ed.). Philadelphia: W. B. Saunders. p. 951.

63. **4**

Rationale: Following AAA resection or repair, the nurse monitors the client for signs of renal failure. This can occur because there is often much blood loss during the surgery, and, depending on aneurysm location, the renal arteries may be hypoperfused for a short period during surgery. The nurse monitors hourly intake and output and notes the results of daily BUN and creatinine levels. Urine output of less than 50 mL/hour is reported to the physician.

Test-Taking Strategy: In this question, there is an elevation in BUN and creatinine levels, as well as a significant drop in hourly urine output. Eliminate options 1 and 2 first. Option 3 may be useful information, but the elevated BUN and creatinine levels support your choice of option 4 as the best answer.

Level of Cognitive Ability: Analysis
Phase of Nursing Process: Implementation
Client Needs: Physiological Integrity
Content Area: Adult Health/Cardiovascular

Reference
Ignatavicius, D., Workman, M., & Mishler, M. (1995). *Medical-surgical nursing: A nursing process approach* (2nd ed.). Philadelphia: W. B. Saunders. p. 950.

64. **4**

Rationale: Venous leg ulcers, also called stasis ulcers, tend to be more superficial than arterial ulcers, and the ulcer bed is pink. The edges of the ulcer are uneven, and there is evidence of granulation tissue. There is a brown pigmentation to the skin, from accumulation of metabolic waste products due to venous stasis. The client also exhibits peripheral edema.

Test-Taking Strategy: This question is asking you to discriminate between signs and symptoms of arterial and venous leg ulcers. Knowing that the information in options 1, 2, and 3 is due to tissue malnutrition (and is thus an arterial problem), you can easily pick the correct choice.

Level of Cognitive Ability: Application
Phase of Nursing Process: Assessment
Client Needs: Physiological Integrity
Content Area: Adult Health/Cardiovascular

Reference
Ignatavicius, D., Workman, M., & Mishler, M. (1995). *Medical-surgical nursing: A nursing process approach* (2nd ed.). Philadelphia: W. B. Saunders. p. 940.

65. **2**

Rationale: An Unna boot that is applied too tightly can cause signs of arterial occlusion. The nurse assesses the circulation to the foot and teaches the client to do the same.

Test-Taking Strategy: The symptoms described in the stem are signs of arterial compromise. Option 2 is the only choice that is consistent with this circumstance. Whenever you have a question with this much information presented, it is there for a purpose; read it carefully and think about the message it is telling you.

Level of Cognitive Ability: Analysis
Phase of Nursing Process: Analysis
Client Needs: Physiological Integrity
Content Area: Adult Health/Cardiovascular

Reference
Ignatavicius, D., Workman, M., & Mishler, M. (1995). *Medical-surgical nursing: A nursing process approach* (2nd ed.). Philadelphia: W. B. Saunders. p. 960.

66. **4**

Rationale: Therapy for venous stasis ulcers consists of oxygen-permeable polyethylene film (Op Site) or oxygen-impermeable hydrocolloid dressing (DuoDerm). Opinions vary as to whether oxygen-permeable or oxygen-impermeable is better. For the ambulatory client, the physician may apply a gauze dressing moistened with zinc oxide to the leg, which hardens like a cast (Unna boot). This dressing then prevents venous stasis and provides a sterile environment for the wound. The dressing is changed on a weekly basis. Betadine is not used; it is a strong agent that could cause further damage to friable tissues. Dry sterile dressings do not keep the wound moist. Damp-to-dry dressings are not as effective.

Test-Taking Strategy: This question is a classic example of your ability to discriminate among the uses of different types of dressings. Review the purposes of each of them now if needed!

Level of Cognitive Ability: Analysis
Phase of Nursing Process: Planning
Client Needs: Physiological Integrity
Content Area: Adult Health/Cardiovascular

Reference

Ignatavicius, D., Workman, M., & Mishler, M. (1995). *Medical-surgical nursing: a nursing process approach* (2nd ed.). Philadelphia: W. B. Saunders. p. 960.

67. **2**

Rationale: The first signs and symptoms of digoxin toxicity in adults include abdominal pain, nausea, vomiting, visual disturbances (blurred, yellow or green vision, halos around lights), bradycardia, and other dysrhythmias.

Test-Taking Strategy: Medication side effects and toxicities are a difficult area to learn, simply because there are so many medications, and so many side effects. This one is a classic, though; take the time to learn this if you have the need!

Level of Cognitive Ability: Application
Phase of Nursing Process: Assessment
Client Needs: Physiological Integrity
Content Area: Pharmacology

Reference

Hodgson, B., & Kizior, R. (1999). *Saunders nursing drug handbook 1999.* Philadelphia: W. B. Saunders. pp. 324–326.

68. **2**

Rationale: Client teaching includes taking the dose exactly as prescribed each day. If more than 12 hours goes by, the client should omit that dose until the next scheduled one, and not double-dose. A daily pulse check is imperative, and the client should know parameters for which the physician should be called. Clients are advised not to mix digoxin in pill boxes with other medications as they may be similar in appearance. The physician should be consulted before changing brands, because the bioavailability of the medication may be different.

Test-Taking Strategy: This question is worded to make you look for an incorrect statement. Option 2 is a "red flag," not just for this medication, but many others as well. It is not good practice to "double-dose" any prescribed medications!

Level of Cognitive Ability: Analysis
Phase of Nursing Process: Evaluation
Client Needs: Health Promotion and Maintenance
Content Area: Pharmacology

Reference

Hodgson, B., & Kizior, R. (1998). *Saunders nursing drug handbook 1998.* Philadelphia: W. B. Saunders. pp. 324–326.

69. **3**

Rationale: Stable angina is induced by exercise and relieved by rest or nitroglycerin tablets. Unstable angina occurs at lower and lower levels of activity or at rest, is less predictable, and is often a precursor of myocardial infarction. Variant angina, or Prinzmetal's angina, is prolonged and severe and occurs at the same time each day, most often in the morning.

Test-Taking Strategy: Eliminate option 4 first. Evaluate the data presented in the question to determine the correct option. If you had difficulty with this question, review the characteristics of the various types of angina!

Level of Cognitive Ability: Analysis
Phase of Nursing Process: Assessment
Client Needs: Physiological Integrity
Content Area: Adult Health/Cardiovascular

Reference

Monahan, F., & Neighbors, M. (1998). *Medical-surgical nursing: Foundations for clinical practice* (2nd ed.). Philadelphia: W. B. Saunders. p. 286.

70. **2**

Rationale: HCTZ is a potassium-losing diuretic, and clients are at risk for hypokalemia. Potassium is found in many foods, especially unprocessed foods, many vegetables, fruits, and fresh meats. Since potassium is very water-soluble, foods that are prepared in water are often lower in potassium than the same foods cooked another way (e.g., boiled vs. baked potato). Clients who need potassium added to the diet are encouraged to eat these foods. Many salt substitutes are also high in potassium.

Test-Taking Strategy: Evaluating food choices in terms of their water content and according to how highly processed they are may be a helpful approach for some questions related to potassium. In this question, you will see that each of the incorrect options is processed to some degree and has a high water content.

Level of Cognitive Ability: Application
Phase of Nursing Process: Implementation
Client Needs: Physiological Integrity
Content Area: Adult Health/Cardiovascular

Reference

Lutz, C., & Przytulski, K. (1997). *Nutrition and diet therapy* (2nd ed.). Philadelphia: F. A. Davis. pp. 390–391.

71. **1**

Rationale: Distal tubule and potassium-sparing diuretics include amiloride (Midamor), spironolactone (Aldactone), and triamterene (Dyrenium). They are weak diuretics that are of particular use when combined with potassium-losing diuretics. This is especially useful when medication and dietary supplements of potassium are not appropriate.

Test-Taking Strategy: From the construct of this question, the options are visually divided into two sets: options 1 and 2, and options 3 and 4. Neither 3 nor 4 makes sense, so eliminate these first. Of the remaining two, it is especially helpful to remember that HCTZ (a common diuretic) is potassium-losing. This will help you answer correctly, using the process of elimination!

Level of Cognitive Ability: Analysis
Phase of Nursing Process: Analysis
Client Needs: Physiological Integrity
Content Area: Pharmacology

Reference

Hodgson, B., & Kizior, R. (1998). *Saunders nursing drug handbook 1998.* Philadelphia: W. B. Saunders. pp. 494–496, 1021–1022.

72. **3**

Rationale: Beta-adrenergic blocking agents, such as atenolol, inhibit the appearance of warning signs and symptoms of acute hypoglycemia, which include anxiety, increased heart rate, and sweating. Therefore, the client receiving this medication should adhere to the therapeutic regimen, and monitor blood glucose levels carefully.

Test-Taking Strategy: Note the use of the words "most reliable" in the stem. This indicates that more than one response could be partially or completely correct. Each of the options is, in fact, a sign or symptom of hypoglycemia. Knowledge of the masking effects of beta-adrenergic blocking agents helps you choose the blood glucose level as the most reliable indicator.

Level of Cognitive Ability: Analysis
Phase of Nursing Process: Assessment
Client Needs: Physiological Integrity
Content Area: Pharmacology

Reference
Hodgson, B., & Kizior, R. (1999). *Saunders nursing drug handbook 1999.* Philadelphia: W. B. Saunders. pp. 78–81.

73. 4

Rationale: Beta-adrenergic blocking agents should be tapered slowly. This will avoid abrupt withdrawal syndrome, characterized by headache, malaise, palpitations, tremors, sweating, rebound hypertension, dysrhythmias, and possibly myocardial infarction (in clients with cardiac disorders, including angina pectoris).

Test-Taking Strategy: This question is fairly straightforward. To answer it correctly, you need to know that all beta-adrenergic blocking agents should be tapered slowly to prevent the effects just noted, as well as a return of the symptoms for which the medication was prescribed. The stem guides you in the right direction by telling you that the client was taking this medication for hypertension. Remember, read the stem carefully. All information is there for a reason!

Level of Cognitive Ability: Analysis
Phase of Nursing Process: Analysis
Client Needs: Physiological Integrity
Content Area: Pharmacology

Reference
Hodgson, B., & Kizior, R. (1999). *Saunders nursing drug handbook 1999.* Philadelphia: W. B. Saunders. pp. 674–677.

74. 2

Rationale: Sodium nitroprusside is a powerful direct-acting vasodilator that significantly decreases arterial blood pressure. It does this by relaxing arterial and venous smooth muscle. It acts almost immediately after infusion and is often used to manage hypertensive crisis, as well as being used in combination with other medications, such as positive inotropes, to improve cardiac output. With initiation of the continuous IV therapy, the blood pressure should be monitored every 30 seconds to avoid rapid hypotension. Once BP is stable, it can be checked every 5 minutes. The solution has a faint brown tinge when mixed, and a fresh bag is constituted every 24 hours. It must be protected from light, using aluminum foil or some other opaque material. The medication is metabolized to cyanide by erythrocytes, and then to thiocyanate by the liver. For this reason, thiocyanate levels are measured after 72 hours of continuous therapy.

Test-Taking Strategy: You need to be familiar with this medication to answer this question quickly and accurately. However, look at option 2. Blood levels of a substance are usually checked once therapy has been initiated and ongoing for a period of time. This may help you choose this option over the others as incorrect, since this question specifies the action as occurring at the initiation of therapy!

Level of Cognitive Ability: Application
Phase of Nursing Process: Planning
Client Needs: Physiological Integrity
Content Area: Pharmacology

Reference
Hodgson, B., & Kizior, R. (1999). *Saunders nursing drug handbook 1999.* Philadelphia: W. B. Saunders. pp. 754–755.

75. 4

Rationale: Propranolol is a noncardioselective beta-adrenergic blocking agent. It blocks stimulation of beta$_1$- (myocardial) and beta$_2$- (pulmonary, vascular, and uterine) receptor sites. Albuterol is a sympathomimetic bronchodilator with relatively high beta$_2$-selectivity. The effects of the albuterol could be blocked by the action of propranolol. The nurse should verify the order with the physician.

Test-Taking Strategy: To answer this question successfully, you must know the basic actions of each of these medications, and know that propranolol is a noncardioselective beta-blocker. Since they oppose each other, they should be used cautiously together. The only option that indicates use of caution by the nurse is the option that verifies the order for the concurrent use of these two medications.

Level of Cognitive Ability: Application
Phase of Nursing Process: Implementation
Client Needs: Physiological Integrity
Content Area: Pharmacology

Reference
Hodgson, B., & Kizior, R. (1999). *Saunders nursing drug handbook 1999.* Philadelphia: W. B. Saunders. pp. 877–880.

76. 4

Rationale: Clients taking ACE inhibitors are at risk of developing hyperkalemia due to depressed aldosterone levels. Electrolyte levels are drawn periodically for the client receiving these medications.

Test-Taking Strategy: The key to answering this question lies in knowing that ACE inhibitors can cause hyperkalemia, and what the signs and symptoms of hyperkalemia are. Take a moment to review these now if needed!

Level of Cognitive Ability: Analysis
Phase of Nursing Process: Analysis
Client Needs: Physiological Integrity
Content Area: Pharmacology

Reference
Hodgson, B., & Kizior, R. (1999). *Saunders nursing drug handbook 1999.* Philadelphia: W. B. Saunders. pp. 361–363.

77. 2

Rationale: ACE inhibitors, such as fosinopril, cause temporary impairment of taste (dysgeusia). The nurse can tell the client that this effect usually disappears in 2 to 3 months even with continued therapy and can provide nutritional counseling if appropriate to avoid weight loss.

Test-Taking Strategy: Eliminate option 4 first as a poor nursing action. The nurse does not encourage ad lib dosage changes on any prescribed medication. Taking the drug with food is not going to change the taste of the food, so that can be eliminated next. Of the remaining two, you need to know that this effect occurs with all medications in the ACE inhibitor group. Thus, you are left with the correct option, which is supporting the client through teaching.

Level of Cognitive Ability: Application
Phase of Nursing Process: Implementation
Client Needs: Psychosocial Integrity
Content Area: Pharmacology

Reference

Hodgson, B., & Kizior, R. (1999). *Saunders nursing drug handbook 1999.* Philadelphia: W. B. Saunders. pp. 449–450.

78. 3

Rationale: Calcium channel blocking agents, such as diltiazem, are used cautiously in clients with conditions that could be worsened by the medication, such as aortic stenosis, bradycardia, heart failure, acute myocardial infarction, and hypotension. The nurse would assess for signs and symptoms that indicate worsening of these underlying disorders. In this question, the nurse assesses for signs and symptoms indicating heart failure.

Test-Taking Strategy: To answer this question, you must know that diltiazem is a calcium channel blocker, and that these medications decrease the rate and force of cardiac contraction. This helps you eliminate options 1 and 4, because bradycardia is expected. Option 2 is eliminated because these signs could indicate bronchoconstriction, which does not occur with calcium channel blockers but rather with some beta-adrenergic blockers.

Level of Cognitive Ability: Application
Phase of Nursing Process: Assessment
Client Needs: Physiological Integrity
Content Area: Pharmacology

Reference

Hodgson, B., & Kizior, R. (1999). *Saunders nursing drug handbook 1999.* Philadelphia: W. B. Saunders. pp. 327–329.

79. 2

Rationale: The client receiving a calcium channel blocking agent such as nifedipine (Procardia) may develop weakness and lethargy as an expected effect of the medication. The nurse may formulate a nursing diagnosis of "Activity Intolerance," and develop a plan of care to help the client adjust to the medication.

Test-Taking Strategy: To answer this question, you need to know that nifedipine is a calcium channel blocking agent, and that this medication decreases the rate and force of cardiac contraction, lowering the oxygen demand and also the cardiac output. By thinking through this process, you can reach the conclusion that decreased energy would then be an expected effect of the medication.

Level of Cognitive Ability: Analysis
Phase of Nursing Process: Analysis
Client Needs: Psychosocial Integrity
Content Area: Pharmacology

Reference

Hodgson, B., & Kizior, R. (1999). *Saunders nursing drug handbook 1999.* Philadelphia: W. B. Saunders. pp. 744–745.

80. 1

Rationale: Prior to administering a calcium channel blocking agent, the nurse should check the blood pressure and heart rate, which could both decrease in response to the action of this medication.

Test-Taking Strategy: To answer this question, you must know that amlodipine is a calcium channel blocker, and that this group of medications decrease the rate and force

of cardiac contraction. This in turn lowers the pulse rate and blood pressure. Option 2 can be eliminated rapidly because it is irrelevant. With options 3 and 4, note that only half the option is correct. When answering questions such as these, with two items per response, both the items must be correct for that option to be correct.

Level of Cognitive Ability: Application
Phase of Nursing Process: Planning
Client Needs: Physiological Integrity
Content Area: Pharmacology

Reference

Hodgson, B., & Kizior, R. (1999). *Saunders nursing drug handbook 1999.* Philadelphia: W. B. Saunders. pp. 51–52.

81. 4

Rationale: A single dose of verapamil given intravenously is administered over 2 minutes (or over 3 minutes with the elderly), with the client on a cardiac monitor. The solution should be clear, with no discoloration. Verapamil is a calcium channel blocking agent, with powerful antidysrhythmic action as well.

Test-Taking Strategy: Knowing that verapamil is a calcium channel blocker, you can eliminate options 1 and 2, since a pulse oximeter would be of no value. This particular medication is given slowly over 2 minutes; 5 minutes would be excessively slow.

Level of Cognitive Ability: Application
Phase of Nursing Process: Implementation
Client Needs: Physiological Integrity
Content Area: Pharmacology

Reference

Hodgson, B., & Kizior, R. (1999). *Saunders nursing drug handbook 1999.* Philadelphia: W. B. Saunders. pp. 1047–1049.

82. 3

Rationale: Tolerance to nitrates can develop over time. Some clients confuse tolerance with addiction. The nurse needs to explore the client's concerns and offer accurate information and support to help the client adapt to the illness and prescribed therapy.

Test-Taking Strategy: The stem tells you that the client is hesitant about taking the medication and that the nurse has ruled out lack of knowledge or financial barriers. Options 1 and 2 can be eliminated first because they are not reasons to stop taking the medication. Since the schedule is PRN for chest pain, there can be no inconvenience (option 4). Thus, you are left with the psychosocial concerns of the client to explore.

Level of Cognitive Ability: Application
Phase of Nursing Process: Assessment
Client Needs: Psychosocial Integrity
Content Area: Pharmacology

Reference

Lehne, R. (1998). *Pharmacology for nursing care* (3rd ed.). Philadelphia: W. B. Saunders. pp. 465–469.

83. 1

Rationale: Clients have developed tolerance when wearing a transdermal system or using nitropaste continuously for 24 hours. This is manifested by lack of pain relief from the medication. This can be avoided by having the client wear the nitrate for 12 hours, leaving 12 hours "nitrate free."

Test-Taking Strategy: Option 4 should be eliminated first as the least plausible of all the options. Hypotension (option 2) is least likely to occur at night when the client is supine. Of the two remaining options, option 1 is more plausible than option 3; the product would not be very marketable if it were too irritating.

Level of Cognitive Ability: Analysis
Phase of Nursing Process: Analysis
Client Needs: Physiological Integrity
Content Area: Pharmacology

Reference
Lehne, R. (1998). *Pharmacology for nursing care* (3rd ed.). Philadelphia: W. B. Saunders. pp. 465–469.

84. **2**

Rationale: The ointment is readily absorbed through the skin, so using the fingers will result in the nurse becoming hypotensive. Proper administration of nitroglycerin ointment involves the use of the dose-measuring applicator paper supplied by the manufacturer, applying it in a thin, uniform, even layer, and applying it to a nonhairy area of the chest, abdomen, anterior thigh, or forearm. The previous dose is removed before applying, and sites are rotated to avoid inflammation.

Test-Taking Strategy: This question tests fundamental principles of medication administration for nitroglycerin ointment. Review these principles now if needed!

Level of Cognitive Ability: Application
Phase of Nursing Process: Planning
Client Needs: Safe, Effective Care Environment
Content Area: Pharmacology

Reference
Hodgson, B., & Kizior, R. (1999). *Saunders nursing drug handbook 1999.* Philadelphia: W. B. Saunders. pp. 750–753.

85. **1**

Rationale: Transdermal patches can be applied to a hairless site using firm pressure to ensure good contact with skin, especially at the edges. The units are waterproof but should not be trimmed to adjust the dose, because that will interfere with the absorption rate. Brands should not be switched back and forth because they may not be equivalent in dose. If the unit becomes loose or falls off, it should be replaced.

Test-Taking Strategy: Note the key word "not" in the stem. Each of the other options listed is a standard administration technique. If you are unfamiliar with these applications, take a moment to review them now!

Level of Cognitive Ability: Application
Phase of Nursing Process: Implementation
Client Needs: Health Promotion and Maintenance
Content Area: Pharmacology

Reference
Lehne, R. (1998). *Pharmacology for nursing care* (3rd ed.). Philadelphia: W. B. Saunders. pp. 465–469.

86. **3**

Rationale: Hydralazine is a powerful vasodilator that exerts its action on the smooth muscle walls of arterioles. After a parenteral dose, blood pressure is checked every 5 minutes until stable, and every 15 minutes thereafter.

Test-Taking Strategy: If you know that hydralazine is an antihypertensive medication, you should be able easily to select the correct answer to this question. The important parameter to follow would be blood pressure!

Level of Cognitive Ability: Application
Phase of Nursing Process: Assessment
Client Needs: Physiological Integrity
Content Area: Pharmacology

Reference
Hodgson, B., & Kizior, R. (1999). *Saunders nursing drug handbook 1999.* Philadelphia: W. B. Saunders. pp. 493–494.

87. **2**

Rationale: Minoxidil is a direct-acting peripheral vasodilator and acts on arterioles, with little effect on veins. It is used in severe hypertension with target organ damage, such as the kidneys. It causes reflex tachycardia, so a beta-adrenergic blocking agent must be prescribed for use at the same time. A diuretic is also needed to correct sodium and water retention that will occur.

Test-Taking Strategy: To answer this question, you must know that minoxidil is a vasodilator and that propranolol is a beta-adrenergic blocker. Option 1 is incorrect because minoxidil is not a first-line agent to use against hypertension. Propranolol exerts no protective effect on the kidney, so is eliminated next. Knowing that beta-blockers can cause fluid retention, this option is also discarded, leaving the reflex tachycardia by the process of elimination!

Level of Cognitive Ability: Analysis
Phase of Nursing Process: Analysis
Client Needs: Physiological Integrity
Content Area: Pharmacology

Reference
Hodgson, B., & Kizior, R. (1999). *Saunders nursing drug handbook 1999.* Philadelphia: W. B. Saunders. pp. 689–691.

88. **1**

Rationale: Lidocaine is a Group 1B antidysrhythmic and requires the use of a continuous ECG monitor when used. It is used in the acute treatment of ventricular dysrhythmias.

Test-Taking Strategy: You need to know that lidocaine is an antidysrhythmic to answer this question correctly. Since this is a first-line agent for ventricular dysrhythmias, it is worth reviewing quickly now, if you have the need!

Level of Cognitive Ability: Application
Phase of Nursing Process: Planning
Client Needs: Physiological Integrity
Content Area: Pharmacology

Reference
Hodgson, B., & Kizior, R. (1999). *Saunders nursing drug handbook 1999.* Philadelphia: W. B. Saunders. pp. 591–594.

89. **4**

Rationale: Minipress is classified as a competitive antagonist that produces selective blockade of alpha$_1$-adrenergic receptors. Fatigue, decreased libido, and impotence may result. For the total well-being of the client, medication instructions should address this aspect of therapy.

Test-Taking Strategy: This side effect may occur with other alpha-adrenergic blockers as well. This may be helpful to remember if questions arise on psychosocial aspects of care with these medications!

Level of Cognitive Ability: Application
Phase of Nursing Process: Implementation
Client Needs: Psychosocial Integrity
Content Area: Pharmacology

Reference
Lehne, R. (1998). *Pharmacology for nursing care* (3rd ed.). Philadelphia: W. B. Saunders. p. 166.

90. **3**

Rationale: Disopyramide is a Group 1A antidysrhythmic used in the treatment of atrial and ventricular tachydysrhythmias. It has fewer side effects than others in that group, but it does exert an anticholinergic effect. For that reason, clients should be cautioned about dry mouth and advised to keep sugarless hard candy or gum nearby, or take frequent oral rinses. Because of reduced perspiration, clients may develop heat intolerance and should avoid extremely warm weather. The possibility of dizziness and blurred vision indicates the use of caution when driving. Another possible side effect includes hypotension, so clients should change position slowly if this occurs.

Test-Taking Strategy: If you know that this medication is an antidysrhythmic, you can anticipate that it will have cardiovascular effects. This might help you eliminate options 1 and 2, since these options are cardiovascular in nature. You would need to know that this medication has an anticholinergic effect to discriminate between options 3 and 4!

Level of Cognitive Ability: Analysis
Phase of Nursing Process: Evaluation
Client Needs: Health Promotion and Maintenance
Content Area: Pharmacology

Reference
Hodgson, B., & Kizior, R. (1999). *Saunders nursing drug handbook 1999*. Philadelphia: W. B. Saunders. pp. 337–339.

91. **2**

Rationale: Quinidine is a Group 1A antidysrhythmic, which decreases myocardial excitability and slows the velocity of conduction through the heart. The most common side effects relate to the GI system and include diarrhea, cramping, nausea, and anorexia. Hypotension, tachycardia, and dysrhythmias are less frequent side effects that relate to the cardiovascular system.

Test-Taking Strategy: Note the key phrase "most frequent side effects." If you know that quinidine is an antidysrhythmic, you may be able to eliminate option 3 as an unlikely combination. Options 1 and 2 seem to oppose each other, so it is likely that one of these is correct. In fact, quinidine causes the distressing GI side effects noted earlier.

Level of Cognitive Ability: Application
Phase of Nursing Process: Assessment
Client Needs: Physiological Integrity
Content Area: Pharmacology

Reference
Hodgson, B., & Kizior, R. (1999). *Saunders nursing drug handbook 1999*. Philadelphia: W. B. Saunders. pp. 894–896.

92. **4**

Rationale: Propafenone is a group 1-C antidysrhythmic, which means that it has some beta-adrenergic blocking and calcium channel blocking activity. Thus, it should be used cautiously in clients with a history of heart failure because of its negative inotropic effects. It is indicated for control of life-threatening ventricular dysrhythmias, such as ventricular tachycardia. It potentiates the action of digoxin (35% to 85% increase) and warfarin (up to 25% increase), so these medications are adjusted as necessary.

Test-Taking Strategy: To answer this question, you need to know that this medication is an antidysrhythmic with the aforementioned properties. This would help you eliminate each of the other incorrect options. Looking at this particular question, the correct answer is also the only one that is connected to the cardiovascular system!

Level of Cognitive Ability: Analysis
Phase of Nursing Process: Analysis
Client Needs: Physiological Integrity
Content Area: Pharmacology

Reference
Hodgson, B., & Kizior, R. (1999). *Saunders nursing drug handbook 1999*. Philadelphia: W. B. Saunders. pp. 872–874.

93. **3**

Rationale: Gastrointestinal side effects occur in up to 25% of clients taking amiodarone. The nurse can minimize these effects by providing a diet high in fiber and by increasing fluids, unless contraindicated. This will minimize the risk of constipation.

Test-Taking Strategy: You can begin by eliminating a soft diet, as the client does not demonstrate difficulty in chewing or swallowing. Since GI side effects are generally of two types, irritation/diarrhea or constipation, examine the remaining options. Antacids and antidiarrheals are similar in that they represent treatment of irritation, whereas the only other response is for constipation. In this case, you should select the response that is different from the other two similar ones!

Level of Cognitive Ability: Application
Phase of Nursing Process: Implementation
Client Needs: Physiological Integrity
Content Area: Pharmacology

Reference
Hodgson, B., & Kizior, R. (1999). *Saunders nursing drug handbook 1999*. Philadelphia: W. B. Saunders. pp. 47–49.

94. **4**

Rationale: Colestipol is a bile acid sequestrant used to lower blood cholesterol. Serum cholesterol and triglyceride levels should be noted as a baseline before initiating therapy and should be monitored intermittently afterward to determine the effects of therapy.

Test-Taking Strategy: Knowing that colestipol lowers blood cholesterol levels helps narrow the realistic choices to options 3 and 4. Since chylomicrons are not a well-known source of difficulty, you may choose the correct option using principles of logic.

Level of Cognitive Ability: Application
Phase of Nursing Process: Assessment
Client Needs: Physiological Integrity
Content Area: Pharmacology

Reference
Hodgson, B., & Kizior, R. (1999). *Saunders nursing drug handbook 1999*. Philadelphia: W. B. Saunders. pp. 253, 1116.

95. **1**

Rationale: Colestipol is a nonabsorbable anion-exchange resin, and it is also called a bile-sequestering agent. It inhibits reabsorption of cholesterol-rich bile acids in the gut. The nurse uses caution in administering this medication to a client with a history of constipation because it could cause fecal impaction.

Test-Taking Strategy: This question is visually divided into two sets of options, one dealing with allergies and one dealing with GI effects. If you know that this medication lowers cholesterol in this manner, you can eliminate options 3 and 4. You would choose option 1 over option 2 because it is available as a powder or in a chewable bar, which makes constipation the more realistic problem.

Level of Cognitive Ability: Analysis
Phase of Nursing Process: Analysis
Client Needs: Physiological Integrity
Content Area: Pharmacology

Reference
Hodgson, B., & Kizior, R. (1999). *Saunders nursing drug handbook 1999.* Philadelphia: W. B. Saunders. pp. 253, 1116.

96. **3**

Rationale: Colestipol hydrochloride is a bile acid sequestrant useful in lowering serum cholesterol levels. The medication causes constipation in 10% to 50% of clients, with possible fecal impaction. Because of this, clients are advised to monitor their elimination patterns carefully, increase intake of fiber and fluids, and take stool softeners or possibly laxatives if needed.

Test-Taking Strategy: If you look at the way this question is written, you will notice that each of the incorrect options represents a major type of food (e.g., CHO, fat, protein). In this question, the correct answer is the one that is different from the others, that is, fiber and fluids.

Level of Cognitive Ability: Application
Phase of Nursing Process: Implementation
Client Needs: Health Promotion and Maintenance
Content Area: Pharmacology

Reference
Hodgson, B., & Kizior, R. (1999). *Saunders nursing drug handbook 1999.* Philadelphia: W. B. Saunders. pp. 253, 1116.

97. **4**

Rationale: Dopamine is a positive inotropic agent and vasopressor that is used to improve cardiac output, blood pressure, and urine output. The physician should be notified if the client experiences tachycardia, reduced urine output without hypotension, dysrhythmias, and decreasing pulse pressure. The dose should be reduced or stopped temporarily.

Test-Taking Strategy: The options are divided visually into hemodynamic measurements and effect on heart rate. Usually if there is a cardiac problem, hemodynamic measurements are high (not low), so falling values for CVP and PCWP would be considered a good effect. Because the medication is a beta-adrenergic stimulant, you may reason that the untoward effect you are looking for would be tachycardia.

Level of Cognitive Ability: Application
Phase of Nursing Process: Assessment
Client Needs: Physiological Integrity
Content Area: Pharmacology

Reference
Hodgson, B., & Kizior, R. (1999). *Saunders nursing drug handbook 1999.* Philadelphia: W. B. Saunders. pp. 345–348.

98. **3**

Rationale: Dobutamine is a beta-adrenergic stimulant that has a positive inotropic effect on the heart. It improves cardiac output without significantly increasing the heart rate. The best effects of this medication would be seen with a normal cardiac output (4 to 8 L/minute) and normal PCWP readings (8 to 15 mmHg).

Test-Taking Strategy: To answer this question correctly, you must know the normal ranges for CO and PCWP and that dobutamine is a positive inotropic agent. In doing so, you will select the correct answer, since each of the values in the incorrect options is too high (PCWP) or low (CO).

Level of Cognitive Ability: Analysis
Phase of Nursing Process: Analysis
Client Needs: Physiological Integrity
Content Area: Pharmacology

Reference
Black, J., & Matassarin-Jacobs, E. (1997). *Medical-surgical nursing: Clinical management for continuity of care* (5th ed.). Philadelphia: W. B. Saunders. pp. 1234, 1236.

99. **1**

Rationale: Epinephrine acts in a variety of ways to increase cardiac output, cardiac rate, and peripheral vascular resistance. Thus, it increases heart rate and blood pressure and so can be used to treat bradycardia and hypotension. It has a number of noncardiac uses as well.

Test-Taking Strategy: To answer this question, it is helpful to remember that this substance helps mediate the sympathetic nervous system's "fight or flight" response. The stem tells you that the client has a cardiac problem, which should guide you to look for heart rate (ECG) and blood pressure as the correct parameters to monitor.

Level of Cognitive Ability: Application
Phase of Nursing Process: Implementation
Client Needs: Physiological Integrity
Content Area: Pharmacology

Reference
Black, J., & Matassarin-Jacobs, E. (1997). *Medical-surgical nursing: Clinical management for continuity of care* (5th ed.). Philadelphia: W. B. Saunders. pp. 366–369, 112, 1130, 1189.

100. **4**

Rationale: Phentolamine will vasodilate the small blood vessels in the area of infiltration. Norepinephrine is a powerful vasoconstrictor and could cause tissue necrosis and sloughing if infiltration occurs.

Test-Taking Strategy: To answer this question, it is helpful to know that norepinephrine is a vasoconstrictor. This would allow you to conclude logically that a vasodilator would be needed in case of infiltration. Each of the other incorrect options exerts vasopressor action, which would compound the tissue damage!

Level of Cognitive Ability: Application
Phase of Nursing Process: Implementation
Client Needs: Physiological Integrity
Content Area: Pharmacology

Reference

Hodgson, B., & Kizior, R. (1998). *Saunders nursing drug handbook 1998*. Philadelphia: W. B. Saunders. pp. 756–758, 819–820.

101. 2

Rationale: Isoproterenol is a sympathomimetic that, when used for cardiovascular benefit, can be given to treat cardiac standstill, dysrhythmias, and sometimes shock. Blood pressure, ECG, respiratory rate, and urine output should be monitored during infusion. If chest pain, dysrhythmias, heart rate greater than 110, or hypertension occurs, the physician should be notified.

Test-Taking Strategy: This question requires that you know that isoproterenol is a sympathomimetic. Because of the stimulating effects on the heart, it also increases myocardial oxygen demand and could result in chest pain. None of the other options is a safe nursing action.

Level of Cognitive Ability: Application
Phase of Nursing Process: Implementation
Client Needs: Physiological Integrity
Content Area: Pharmacology

Reference

Hodgson, B., & Kizior, R. (1999). *Saunders nursing drug handbook 1999*. Philadelphia: W. B. Saunders. pp. 552–555.

102. 3

Rationale: A serum potassium level of 2.0 is hypokalemia, which can increase the client's risk of a dysrhythmia. Hypokalemia can result in ventricular ectopic rhythms or bradydysrhythmias. To prevent potential lethal dysrhythmias, serum potassium levels are maintained between 4.0 and 5.0 mEq/L.

Test-Taking Strategy: This question requires knowledge of normal ranges of the laboratory values. The creatinine level, magnesium level, and hemoglobin levels are all within normal range. Review these laboratory values now, if you had difficulty with this question!

Level of Cognitive Ability: Analysis
Phase of Nursing Process: Analysis
Client Needs: Physiological Integrity
Content Area: Adult Health/Cardiovascular

Reference

Ignatavicius, D., Workman, M., & Mishler, M. (1995) *Medical-surgical nursing: A nursing process approach.* (2nd ed.) Philadelphia: W. B. Saunders. p. 1009.

103. 1

Rationale: Physiological responses to anxiety increase the demands on the heart and further contribute to the client's symptoms of pulmonary edema. These clinical manifestations of a decrease in anxiety would be the client's HR and RR nearing norm for the client, and maximal perfusion to organs/peripheral extremities.

Test-Taking Strategy: Knowledge of the physiological impact of anxiety and pulmonary edema on the body is required to answer this question. Anxiety in the client experiencing pulmonary edema further increases the workload on a failing heart and increases dyspnea and hypoxia. Option 1 is the normal finding indicating effective response!

Level of Cognitive Ability: Analysis
Phase of Nursing Process: Evaluation
Client Needs: Psychosocial Integrity
Content Area: Adult Health/Cardiovascular

Reference

Burrell, L., Gerlach, M., & Pless, B. (1997). *Adult nursing: Acute and community care* (2nd ed.). Stamford, CT: Appleton & Lange. p. 423.

104. 4

Rationale: Cardiogenic shock occurs when the heart can no longer pump blood efficiently to all parts of the body. Cardiac output is decreased. The major cause of cardiogenic shock is extensive myocardial necrosis secondary to a myocardial infarction (MI).

Test-Taking Strategy: A knowledge of different classifications of shock is needed to answer this question. Option 2 describes distributive shock. Option 1 is defining hypovolemic shock. Option 3 is incorrect in all shock classifications as the nurse would expect to see a decrease in urinary output.

Level of Cognitive Ability: Analysis
Phase of Nursing Process: Assessment
Client Needs: Physiological Integrity
Content Area: Adult Health/Cardiovascular

Reference

Lewis, S., Collier, I., & Heitkemper, M. (1996) *Medical-surgical nursing: Assessment and management of clinical problems* (4th ed.). St. Louis: Mosby–Year Book. p. 126.

105. 4

Rationale: Urine output of less than 0.5 mL/kg or less than 20 mL/hour may indicate inadequate perfusion of the kidneys.

Test-Taking Strategy: A knowledge of normal urinary output for the adult will easily direct you to the correct option. Urinary output of less than 20 mL/hr indicates a decrease in perfusion to the kidneys. In this case, the decrease in perfusion to the kidneys is result of the client's experiencing cardiogenic shock, secondary to left ventricular failure.

Level of Cognitive Ability: Analysis
Phase of Nursing Process: Analysis
Client Needs: Physiological Integrity
Content Area: Adult Health/Cardiovascular

Reference

Lewis, S., Collier, I., & Heitkemper, M. (1996) *Medical-surgical nursing: Assessment and management of clinical problems* (4th ed.). St. Louis: Mosby–Year Book. p. 138.

106. 4

Rationale: A decrease in cardiac output is a complication that may occur in the post-open heart surgical client. The nurse would assess closely for the finding of decreased cardiac output by palpation of peripheral pulses and monitoring hourly urinary output and hemodynamic parameters that indicate adequate organ/tissue perfusion.

Test-Taking Strategy: Options 1, 2, and 3 do not directly measure outcomes of cardiac output. A decrease in cardiac output would result in decreased peripheral perfusion, which would result in a decrease in peripheral pulses in strength and quality!

Level of Cognitive Ability: Analysis
Phase of Nursing Process: Assessment
Client Needs: Physiological Integrity
Content Area: Adult Health/Cardiovascular

Reference

Monahan, F., & Neighbors, M. (1998). *Medical-surgical nursing: Foundations for clinical practice* (2nd ed.). Philadelphia: W. B. Saunders. p. 225.

107. 3

Rationale: Paraphrasing is restating the client's message in the nurse's own words. Option 3 utilizes the therapeutic communication technique of paraphrasing. The client is frustrated and is searching for understanding.

Test-Taking Strategy: Therapeutic communication techniques are the answers to your questions regarding responses to a client. Therapeutic communication techniques enhance communication. Always select responses that will enhance communication. Option 1 belittles the client's concerns/feelings. Options 2 and 4 offer false reassurance by the nurse.

Level of Cognitive Ability: Application
Phase of Nursing Process: Implementation
Client Needs: Psychosocial Integrity
Content Area: Adult Health/Cardiovascular

Reference

Leahy, J., & Kizilay, P. (1998). *Foundations of nursing practice: A nursing process approach.* Philadelphia: W. B. Saunders. pp. 227–231.

108. 1

Rationale: Amrinone produces an inotropic action increasing cardiac output. If you increase cardiac output, then the peripheral perfusion is increased. Amrinone directly relaxes vascular smooth muscle, decreasing preload and afterload. Sodium nitroprusside acts as a potent vasodilator on veins and arteries. This medication may decrease cardiac output. Dexamethasone is used in anaphylactic shock and inhibits the inflammatory process. Nitroglycerin primarily acts as a venous vasodilator causing a decrease in cardiac output.

Test-Taking Strategy: Knowledge of the actions and uses of these medications is required to assist in answering this question. Amrinone is a positive inotropic medication that will increase cardiac output and increase peripheral perfusion. If you are unfamiliar with the medications addressed in this question, it would be important to review them!

Level of Cognitive Ability: Analysis
Phase of Nursing Process: Analysis
Client Needs: Physiological Integrity
Content Area: Pharmacology

References

Lewis, S., Collier, I., & Heitkemper, M. (1996). *Medical-surgical nursing: Assessment and management of clinical problems* (4th ed.). St. Louis: Mosby–Year Book, p. 133.

109. 3

Rationale: For the nurse to support the client, the nurse must first establish a means of communication. The client must be able to express the source of the anxiety. Once the client has identified the cause of anxiety, the nurse can direct care for resolution.

Test-Taking Strategy: Prior to planning care for the client experiencing anxiety, the client must be able to communicate the origin of the anxiety. Option 1 may be instituted but does not identify the cause of the anxiety. This offers only temporary relief, not resolution. Option 2 deals with respiratory care of the client, not emotional support. Option 4 may or may not be appropriate, depending on the cause of anxiety.

Level of Cognitive Ability: Application
Phase of Nursing Process: Planning
Client Needs: Psychosocial Integrity
Content Area: Adult Health/Cardiovascular

Reference

Lewis, S., Collier, I., & Heitkemper, M. (1996) *Medical-surgical nursing: Assessment and management of clinical problems* (4th ed.). St. Louis: Mosby–year Book. p. 139.

110. 4

Rationale: The client with aortic valve replacement receives care similar to that of the client undergoing coronary artery bypass surgery. One difference, however, is that valve replacement clients are at greater risk for postoperative hemorrhage. Because of this, the nurse is especially diligent in monitoring bleeding.

Test-Taking Strategy: This question may look difficult on the surface. Since the procedure is similar to coronary bypass surgery, the risk of respiratory complications or ulcer development should be no greater than usual. This eliminates options 1 and 2. Options 3 and 4 compete for your attention. Option 3 would presume dysrhythmias, whereas option 4 presumes hemorrhage. Knowing that the aortic valve is subject to great changes in pressure with each heartbeat (left ventricular systole and diastole), it makes sense that hemorrhage is the more likely option.

Level of Cognitive Ability: Application
Phase of Nursing Process: Implementation
Client Needs: Physiological Integrity
Content Area: Adult Health/Cardiovascular

Reference

Ignatavicius, D., Workman, M., & Mishler, M. (1995). *Medical-surgical nursing: A nursing process approach* (2nd ed.). Philadelphia: W. B. Saunders. p. 909

BIBLIOGRAPHY

Black, J., & Matassarin-Jacobs, E. (1997). *Medical-surgical nursing: Clinical management for continuity of care* (5th ed.). Philadelphia: W. B. Saunders.

Burrell, L., Gerlach, M., & Pless, B. (1997). *Adult nursing: Acute and community care* (2nd ed.). Stamford, CT: Appleton & Lange.

Chernecky, C., & Berger, B. (1997). *Laboratory tests and diagnostic procedures* (2nd ed.). Philadelphia: W. B. Saunders.

Hodgson, B., & Kizior, R. (1999). *Saunders nursing drug handbook 1999.* Philadelphia: W. B. Saunders.

Ignatavicius, D., Workman, M., & Mishler, M. (1995). *Medical-surgical nursing: A nursing process approach* (2nd ed.). Philadelphia: W. B. Saunders.

Leahy, J., & Kizilay, P. (1998). *Foundations of nursing practice: A nursing process approach.* Philadelphia: W. B. Saunders.

Lehne, R. (1998). *Pharmacology for nursing care* (3rd ed.). Philadelphia: W. B. Saunders.

Lewis, S., Collier, I., & Heitkemper, M. (1996). *Medical-surgical nursing: Assessment and management of clinical problems* (4th ed.). St. Louis: Mosby–Year Book.

Luckmann, J. (1997). *Saunders manual of nursing care.* Philadelphia: W. B. Saunders.

Lutz, C., & Przytulski, K. (1997). *Nutrition and diet therapy* (2nd ed.). Philadelphia: F. A. Davis.

Monahan, F., & Neighbors, M. (1998). *Medical-surgical nursing: Foundations for clinical practice* (2nd ed.). Philadelphia: W. B. Saunders.

O'Toole, M. (ed.) (1997). *Miller-Keane encyclopedia & dictionary of medicine, nursing, & allied health* (6th ed.). Philadelphia: W. B. Saunders.

Paul, S., & Hebra, J. (1998). *The nurse's guide to cardiac rhythm interpretation.* Philadelphia: W. B. Saunders.

Smeltzer, S., & Bare, B. (1996). *Brunner and Suddarth's textbook of medical-surgical nursing* (8th ed.). Philadelphia: Lippincott-Raven.

CHAPTER 60

Cardiovascular Medications

....

I. Anticoagulants (Box 60–1)

A. Description
1. Prevents the extension and formation of clots by inhibiting factors in the clotting cascade and decreasing blood coagulability
2. Used for thrombosis, pulmonary embolism, and myocardial infarction (MI)
3. Contraindicated with active bleeding, except for disseminated intravascular coagulation (DIC), bleeding disorders or blood dyscrasias, ulcers, liver and kidney disease, and spinal cord or brain injuries

B. Side effects (Box 60–2)
1. Hemorrhage
2. Hematuria
3. Epistaxis
4. Ecchymosis
5. Bleeding gums
6. Thrombocytopenia
7. Hypotension

C. Heparin sodium (Liquaemin Sodium)
1. Description
   a. Prevents thrombin from converting fibrinogen to fibrin
   b. Prevents thromboembolism
   c. The therapeutic dose does not dissolve clots, but prevents new thrombus formation
2. Blood levels
   a. Normal activated partial thromboplastin time (APTT) is 20 to 36 seconds
   b. Maintain the APTT at 1.5 to 2.5 times normal
   c. At therapeutic levels, heparin will increase the APTT by a factor of 1.5 to 2, making the APTT 60 to 80 seconds
   d. APTT therapy should be measured every 4 to 6 hours during initial therapy, then on a daily basis
   e. If the APTT is too long, greater than 80 seconds, the dosage should be lowered
   f. If the APTT is too short, less than 60 seconds, the dosage should be increased
   g. Normal clotting time is 8 to 15 minutes
   h. Maintain clotting time at 15 to 20 minutes
3. Implementation
   a. Monitor clotting time and APTT
   b. Monitor platelet count
   c. Observe for bleeding gums, bruises, nosebleeds, hematuria, hematemesis, occult blood in the stool, and petechiae
   d. When administering heparin subcutaneously, inject into the abdomen using a small needle at a 90-degree angle and do not aspirate or rub the injection site
   e. Antidote: protamine sulfate

D. Warfarin sodium (Coumadin)
1. Description
   a. Decreases prothrombin activity and prevents the use of vitamin K by the liver

---

BOX 60–1. Anticoagulants

Heparin sodium (Liquaemin Sodium)
Warfarin sodium (Coumadin)

BOX 60–2. Substances to Avoid with Anticoagulants

Green leafy vegetables and foods high in vitamin K
Salicylates
Steroids
Nonsteroidal anti-inflammatory drugs (NSAIDs)
Sulfonamides
Phenytoin (Dilantin)
Cimetidine (Tagamet)
Allopurinol (Zyloprim)
Oral hypoglycemic agents

b. Used for long-term anticoagulation
c. Prolongs clotting time and is monitored by the prothrombin (PT) time
d. Used mainly to prevent thromboembolitic conditions such as thrombophlebitis, pulmonary embolism and embolism formation caused by atrial fibrillation, thrombosis, MI, or heart valve damage
e. Usually given for 2 to 3 months after an MI to decrease the incidence of deep vein thrombosis and thromboembolism

2. Blood levels
   a. Average PT is 9.5 to 11.8 seconds
   b. Warfarin prolongs the PT
3. INR (international normalized ratio)
   a. The normal INR is 1.3 to 2.0
   b. The PT ratio is the ratio of the client's PT to a control PT
   c. The INR is determined by multiplying the observed PT ratio by a correction factor specific to a particular thromboplastin preparation used in the testing
   d. The treatment goal is to raise the INR to an appropriate value
   e. An INR of 2 to 3 is appropriate for most clients, although for some clients, the target INR is 3.0 to 4.5
   f. If the INR is below the recommended range, warfarin should be increased
   g. If the INR is above the recommended range, warfarin should be reduced
4. Implementation
   a. Monitor the PT and INR
   b. Avoid the administration of salicylates
   c. Observe for bleeding gums, bruises, nosebleeds, tarry stools, hematuria, hematemesis, and petechiae
   d. Teach the client to use a soft toothbrush and electric razor
   e. Antidote: vitamin K, phytonadione (AquaMEPHYTON)

II. Thrombolytic Medications (Box 60–3)

A. Description
1. Activates plasminogen, leading to its conversion to plasma, a substance that degrades clots and dissolves formed blood clots
2. Plasminogen generates plasmin (the enzyme that dissolves clots)
3. Used early in the course of myocardial infarct, (within 4 to 6 hours of the onset of the infarct), to restore blood flow, limit myocardial damage, preserve left ventricular function, and prevent death

B. Contraindications
1. Active internal bleeding
2. History of cerebrovascular accident (CVA)
3. Intracranial problems
4. Intracranial surgery or trauma within the previous 2 months

---

BOX 60–3. Thrombolytic Medications

Alteplase (Activase, t-PA, Tissue Plasminogen Activator)
Clot specific and activates only fibrin bound plasminogen and promotes the conversion of plasminogen to plasmin.

Anistreplase (Eminase)
Clot specific and activates only fibrin bound plasminogen and promotes the conversion of plasminogen to plasmin.

Streptokinase (Kabikinase, Streptase)
Acts systemically and converts plasminogen to plasmin

Urokinase (Abbokinase)
Acts systemically and converts plasminogen to plasmin

---

5. History of thoracic, pelvic, or abdominal surgery in the previous 10 days
6. History of hepatic or renal disease
7. Uncontrolled hypertension
8. Recently required, prolonged cardiopulmonary resuscitation (CPR)

C. Side Effects
1. Bleeding
2. Dysrhythmias
3. Fever
4. Allergic reactions

D. Implementation
1. Obtain thrombin time (TT), APTT, PT, fibrinogen level, hematocrit, and platelet count
2. Monitor vital signs
3. Assess pulses
4. Monitor for bleeding
5. Monitor all excretions for occult blood
6. Monitor for neurological changes such as slurred speech, lethargy, confusion, and hemiparesis
7. Monitor for hypotension and tachycardia
8. Avoid injections
9. Apply direct pressure over a puncture site for 20 to 30 minutes
10. Handle the client as little as possible when moving
11. Instruct the client to use electric razor
12. Instruct the client to brush teeth gently
13. Discontinue medication if bleeding develops and call the physician
14. Antidote
    a. Aminocaproic acid (Amicar)
    b. Used only in acute, life-threatening conditions

III. Antiplatelet Medications (Box 60–4)

A. Description
1. Inhibits the aggregation of platelets in the

BOX 60–4. Antiplatelet Medications

Aspirin (acetylsalicylic acid, ASA)
Dipyridamole (Persantine)
Ticlopidine HCl (Ticlid)
Sulfinpyrazone (Anturane)

---

clotting process, thereby prolonging the
bleeding time
2. May be used in conjunction with
anticoagulants
3. Used in the prophylaxis of long-term
complications following MI, coronary
revascularization, and cerebral vascular
accidents
4. Sulfinpyrazone (Anturane) is also used for
treating gout and may be used in
atrioventricular (AV) shunts for hemodialysis
to prevent clotting
5. Contraindicated in bleeding disorders and
known sensitivity
B. Side Effects
1. Gastrointestinal (GI) bleeding
2. Bruising
3. Hematuria
4. Tarry stools
C. Implementation
1. Determine sensitivity prior to administration
2. Monitor vital signs
3. Instruct the client to take medication with
food if GI upset occurs
4. Monitor bleeding time
5. Monitor for side effects related to bleeding
6. Instruct the client in the use of the
medication
7. Instruct the client to monitor for side effects
related to bleeding

IV. Positive Inotropic/Cardiotonic Medication
(Box 60–5)

A. Description
1. Stimulates myocardial **contractility** and
produces a positive inotropic effect
2. The increase in myocardial **contractility**

**BOX 60–5. Positive Inotropic/
Cardiotonic Medications**

AMRINONE LACTATE (INOCOR)

Used for short-term management of congestive heart
failure in those who have not responded adequately to cardiac glycosides, diuretics, and vasodilators

MILRINONE LACTATE (PRIMACOR)

Used for short-term management of congestive heart
failure or may be given before heart transplantation

---

increases cardiac, peripheral, and kidney
function by increasing **cardiac output**,
decreasing **preload**, improving blood flow to
the periphery and kidneys, decreasing
edema, and increasing fluid excretion; as a
result, fluid retention in the lungs and
extremities is decreased
B. Side Effects
1. Dysrhythmias
2. Hypotension
3. Thrombocytopenia
C. Toxic/Adverse Reactions
1. Hepatotoxicity manifested by elevated liver
enzymes
2. Hypersensitivity manifested by wheezing,
shortness of breath, pruritus, urticaria,
clammy skin, and flushing
D. Implementation
1. For intravenous (IV) administration
a. Do not dilute with dextrose-containing
solutions
b. For continuous IV, administer using an
infusion pump
c. Stop infusion if client's **blood pressure**
drops or dysrhythmias occur
2. Monitor apical pulse and **blood pressure**
3. Monitor for hypersensitivity
4. Assess lung sounds for wheezing and rales
5. Monitor for edema
6. Monitor for relief of congestive heart failure
as noted by reduction in edema, lessening of
dyspnea, orthopnea, and fatigue
7. Monitor electrolytes, liver enzymes, platelet
count, and renal function studies: may
decrease potassium and increase liver
enzymes
E. Milrinone Lactate (Primacor)
1. Side effects
a. Headache
b. Hypotension
c. Angina
2. Toxic/adverse reactions: dysrhythmias
3. Implementation
a. For IV injection of loading dose,
administer slowly over 10 minutes
b. For continuous IV, administer using an
infusion pump
c. Monitor apical pulse and **blood pressure**
d. Stop infusion if client's **blood pressure**
drops or dysrhythmias occur
e. Assess lung sounds for wheezing and
rales
f. Monitor for edema
g. Monitor for relief of congestive heart
failure as noted by reduction in edema,
lessening of dyspnea, orthopnea, and
fatigue

V. Cardiac Glycosides (Box 60–6)

A. Description
1. Inhibits sodium potassium pump, thus
increases intracellular calcium, which causes

BOX 60–6. Cardiac Glycosides

Digoxin (Lanoxicaps, Lanoxin)
Digitoxin (Crystodigin)

---

the heart muscle fibers to contract more efficiently

2. Produces a positive inotropic action, which increases the force of myocardial contractions
3. Produces a negative chronotropic action that depresses the sinoatrial (SA) node, reduces conduction of the impulse through the AV node, and slows the heart rate
4. Produces a negative dromotropic action that decreases the conduction of the heart cells
5. The increase in myocardial **contractility** increases cardiac, peripheral, and kidney function by increasing **cardiac output**, decreasing **preload**, improving blood flow to the periphery and kidneys, decreasing edema, and increasing fluid excretion, as a result, fluid retention in the lungs and extremities is decreased
6. Used for congestive heart failure, atrial tachycardia, atrial fibrillation, and atrial flutter
7. Contraindicated in ventricular dysrhythmias and second- or third-degree heart block
8. Use with caution in clients with renal disease, hypothyroidism, and hypokalemia

B. Side Effects
1. Anorexia
2. Nausea
3. Vomiting
4. Headache
5. Blurred vision
6. Yellow-green halos
7. Diplopia
8. Photophobia
9. Drowsiness
10. Bradycardia
11. Fatigue
12. Weakness

C. Implementation
1. Monitor for toxicity as evidenced by anorexia, nausea, vomiting, visual disturbances, confusion, bradycardia, heart block, premature ventricular contractions (PVCs), and tachydysrhythmias
2. Monitor serum digoxin level, electrolyte levels, and renal function tests
3. Therapeutic digoxin range is 0.5 to 2.0 ng/mL, and levels above 2.0 mg/mL are toxic
4. An increased risk of toxicity exists in clients with hypercalcemia, hypokalemia, hypomagnesemia, or hypothyroidism
5. Monitor potassium level, and if hypokalemia occurs (potassium below 3.5 mEq/L), notify the physician

---

BOX 60–7. Classifications of Diuretics

Thiazide diuretics
Loop diuretics
Osmotic diuretics
Potassium-sparing diuretics
Carbonic anhydrase inhibitors

---

6. Instruct the client to avoid over-the-counter medications
7. Monitor the client taking a potassium-wasting diuretic or cortisone medication closely for hypokalemia because the hypokalemia can cause digoxin toxicity
8. Note that elderly clients are more sensitive to toxicity
9. Advise the client to eat foods high in potassium such as fresh and dried fruits, fruit juices, vegetables, and potatoes
10. Monitor the apical pulse
11. If the apical pulse rate is below 60, medication should be held and the physician notified
12. Teach the client how to measure the pulse
13. Teach the client to notify the physician if the pulse rate is below 60 or above 100
14. Teach the client signs and symptoms of toxicity
15. Antidote: digoxin immune Fab (Digibind) used in extreme toxicity

VI. Antihypertensive Medications (Box 60–7)

A. Thiazide Diuretics (Box 60–8)
  1. Description
     a. Increase sodium and water excretion by inhibiting sodium reabsorption in the distal tubule of the kidney
     b. Used for hypertension and peripheral edema

BOX 60–8. Thiazide and Thiazide-like Diuretics

THIAZIDE DIURETICS

Hydrochlorothiazide (Esidrix, Oretic, HydroDIURIL)
Chlorothiazide (Diuril)
Bendroflumethiazide (Naturetin)
Benzthiazide (Aquatag, Hydrex)
Hydroflumethiazide (Saluron, Diucardin)
Methyclothiazide (Aquatensen, Enduron)
Polythiazide (Renese-R)
Thichlormethiazide (Metahydrin, Naqua)

THIAZIDE-LIKE DIURETICS

Chlorthalidone (Hygroton)
Indapamide (Lozol)
Metolazone (Zaroxolyn)
Quinethazone (Hydromox)

c. Used in clients with normal renal function
d. Not effective for immediate diuresis
e. Contraindicated in renal failure
f. Use with caution in the client taking lithium because lithium toxicity can occur
g. Use with caution in clients taking digoxin, corticosteroids, and antidiabetic medications

2. Side effects
   a. Hypercalcemia
   b. Hyperglycemia
   c. Hypokalemia
   d. Hyperuricemia
   e. Hyponatremia
   f. Hypovolemia
   g. Hypotension
   h. Headaches
   i. Nausea
   j. Vomiting
   k. Constipation
   l. Rashes
   m. Photosensitivity
   n. Blood dyscrasias

3. Implementation
   a. Monitor vital signs
   b. Monitor weight
   c. Monitor urine output
   d. Monitor electrolytes, glucose, and uric acid levels
   e. Check the peripheral extremities for edema
   f. Instruct the client to take medication in the morning to avoid nocturia and sleep interruption
   g. Instruct the client how to record blood pressure
   h. Instruct the client to eat foods rich in potassium
   i. Instruct the client how to take potassium supplements if prescribed
   j. Instruct the client to take medication with food to avoid GI upset
   k. Instruct the client to change positions slowly to prevent **orthostatic hypotension**
   l. Instruct the client to use sunscreen when in direct sunlight
   m. Instruct the diabetic client to have blood glucose checked periodically

B. Loop Diuretics (Box 60–9)
   1. Description
      a. Inhibit sodium and chloride reabsorption from the loop of Henle and the distal tubule

BOX 60–9. Loop Diuretics	
Furosemide (Lasix)	Ethacrynic acid (Edecrine)
Bumetanide (Bumex)	Torsemide (Demadex)

b. They have little effect on the blood glucose; however, they cause marked depletion of water and electrolytes, increased uric acid levels, and cause the excretion of calcium
c. Are more potent than the thiazide diuretics, causing rapid diuresis, thus decreasing vascular fluid volume, **cardiac output**, and **blood pressure**
d. Used for hypertension, edema associated with congestive heart failure (CHF), hypercalcemia, and renal disease
e. Use with caution in clients taking digoxin or lithium
f. Use with caution in clients on aminoglycosides, anticoagulants, corticosteroids, and amphotericin B

2. Side effects
   a. Hypokalemia
   b. Hyponatremia
   c. Hypocalcemia
   d. Hypomagnesemia
   e. Hypochloremia
   f. Thrombocytopenia
   g. Hyperuricemia
   h. **Orthostatic hypotension**
   i. Skin disturbances
   j. Ototoxicity and deafness
   k. Thiamine deficiency
   l. Dehydration

3. Implementation
   a. Monitor vital signs
   b. Monitor weight
   c. Monitor urine output
   d. Monitor electrolytes, calcium, and uric acid levels
   e. Check the peripheral extremities for edema
   f. Monitor for signs of digitalis or lithium toxicity if the client is on these medications
   g. Instruct the client to take medication in the morning to avoid nocturia and sleep interruption
   h. Instruct the client how to record **blood pressure**
   i. Instruct clients to eat foods rich in potassium
   j. Instruct clients how to take potassium supplements if prescribed
   k. Instruct the client to take medication with food to avoid GI upset
   l. Instruct the client to change positions slowly to prevent **orthostatic hypotension**
   m. Administer IV furosemide (Lasix) slowly, as hearing loss can occur if injected rapidly

C. Osmotic Diuretics (Box 60–10)
   1. Description
      a. Increase osmotic pressure of the

BOX 60–10. Osmotic Diuretics

Mannitol (Osmitrol)
Urea (Ureaphil)

glomerular filtrate, inhibiting reabsorption of water and electrolytes
   b. Used for oliguria and to prevent renal failure
   c. Used to decrease intracranial pressure
   d. Used to decrease intraocular pressure in narrow-angle glaucoma
   e. Mannitol is used with chemotherapy to induce diuresis
 2. Side effects
   a. Fluid and electrolyte imbalances
   b. Pulmonary edema from the rapid shifts of fluid
   c. Nausea and vomiting
   d. Tachycardia from the rapid fluid loss
   e. Dehydration
 3. Implementation
   a. Monitor vital signs
   b. Monitor weight
   c. Monitor urine output
   d. Monitor electrolyte levels
   e. Monitor lungs and heart sounds for signs of pulmonary edema
   f. Monitor for signs of dehydration
   g. Monitor neurological status
   h. Assess for signs of decreasing intracranial pressure if appropriate
   i. Change the client's position slowly to prevent **orthostatic hypotension**
   j. Monitor for crystallization in the vial of mannitol before administering the medication, and if crystallization is noted, do not administer the medication
D. Carbonic Anhydrase Inhibitors (Box 60–11)
 1. Description
   a. Block the action of the enzyme carbonic anhydrase needed to maintain the acid-base balance
   b. Inhibition of this enzyme, carbonic anhydrase, causes increased sodium, potassium, and bicarbonate excretion
   c. Metabolic acidosis can occur with prolonged use
   d. Used to decrease intraocular pressure in open-angle (chronic) glaucoma, to produce diuresis, manage epilepsy, treat high-altitude sickness

BOX 60–11. Carbonic Anhydrase Inhibitors

Acetazolamide sodium (Diamox)
Dichlorphenamide (Daranide)
Methazolamide (Neptazane)

   e. Used to treat metabolic alkalosis
   f. Contraindicated in narrow-angle or acute glaucoma
 2. Side effects
   a. Hyperglycemia
   b. Hypokalemia
   c. Hyperuricemia
   d. Hypercalcemia
   e. Fluid and electrolyte imbalance
   f. Anorexia
   g. Nausea
   h. Vomiting
   i. **Orthostatic hypotension**
   j. Renal calculi
   k. Hemolytic anemia
 3. Implementation
   a. Monitor vital signs
   b. Monitor weight
   c. Monitor urine output
   d. Monitor electrolytes, glucose, calcium, and uric acid levels
   e. Monitor mental status
   f. Instruct clients to monitor for signs of renal calculi
E. Potassium-Sparing Diuretics (Box 60–12)
 1. Description
   a. Act on the distal tubule to promote sodium and water excretion and potassium retention
   b. Used for edema and hypertension, to increase urine output, to treat fluid retention and overload associated with CHF, hepatic cirrhosis, or nephrotic syndrome, and for diuretic-induced hypokalemia
   c. Contraindicated in severe kidney or hepatic disease or in severe hyperkalemia
   d. Use with caution in clients with diabetes
   e. Use with caution in clients taking antihypertensives and lithium
   f. Use with caution in clients taking angiotensin converting enzyme (ACE) inhibitors, as hyperkalemia can result
   g. Use with caution in clients taking potassium supplements
 2. Side effects
   a. Hyperkalemia
   b. Nausea

BOX 60–12. Potassium-Sparing Diuretics

Spironolactone (Aldactone)
Amiloride HCl (Midamor)
Triamterene (Dyrenium)
Amiloride HCl and hydrochlorothiazide (Moduretic)
Spironolactone and hydrochlorothiazide (Aldactazide)
Triamterene and hydrochlorothiazide (Dyazide, Maxzide)

    c. Vomiting
    d. Diarrhea
    e. Rash
    f. Dizziness
    g. Headache
    h. Weakness
    i. Dry mouth
    j. Photosensitivity
    k. Anemia
    l. Thrombocytopenia
  3. Implementation
    a. Monitor vital signs
    b. Monitor urine output
    c. Monitor for signs and symptoms of hyperkalemia such as nausea, diarrhea, abdominal cramps, tachycardia followed by bradycardia, peaked narrow T wave on the electrocardiogram (ECG), or oliguria
    d. Monitor for a potassium level greater than 5.3 mEq/L, which indicates hyperkalemia
    e. Instruct the client to avoid foods high in potassium
    f. Instruct the client to avoid exposure to direct sunlight
    g. Instruct the client to monitor for signs of hyperkalemia
    h. Instruct the client to avoid salt substitutes because they contain potassium
    i. Instruct the client to take with or after meals to decrease GI irritation

VII. Peripherally Acting Alpha-Adrenergic Blockers (Box 60–13)

A. Description
  1. Decrease sympathetic vasoconstriction by reducing the effects of norepinephrine at peripheral nerve endings, resulting in vasodilation and decreased **blood pressure**
  2. Used to maintain renal blood flow
  3. Used to treat hypertension
B. Side Effects
  1. **Orthostatic hypotension**
  2. Reflex tachycardia
  3. Sodium and water retention
  4. GI disturbances
  5. Nausea

BOX 60–13. Peripherally Acting Alpha-Adrenergic Blockers

    Doxazosin mesylate (Cardura)
    Prazosin (Minipress)
    Terazosin (Hytrin)
    Guanadrel sulfate (Hylorel)
    Guanethidine (Ismelin)
    Reserpine (Serpasil)
    Phenoxybenzamine (Dibenzyline)
    Phentolamine (Regitine)
    Tolazoline (Priscoline)

BOX 60–14. Centrally Acting Sympatholytics

    Clonidine HCl (Catapres)
    Methyldopa (Aldomet)
    Guanabenz acetate (Wytensin)
    Guanfacine (Tenex)

---

  6. Drowsiness
  7. Nasal congestion
  8. Edema
  9. Weight gain
  10. Reserpine (Serpasil) can cause depression, GI irritation, and impotence
C. Implementation
  1. Monitor vital signs
  2. Monitor for fluid retention and edema
  3. Instruct the client to change positions slowly to prevent **orthostatic hypotension**
  4. Instruct the client how to monitor **blood pressure**
  5. Instruct the client to monitor for edema
  6. Instruct the client to decrease salt intake
  7. Instruct the client to avoid over-the-counter medications

VIII. Centrally Acting Sympatholytics (Adrenergic Blockers) (Box 60–14)

A. Description
  1. Stimulate alpha receptors in the central nervous system (CNS) to inhibit vasoconstriction, thus reducing peripheral resistance
  2. Used to treat hypertension
  3. Contraindicated in impaired liver function
B. Side effects
  1. Sodium and water retention
  2. Drowsiness
  3. Dry mouth
  4. Dizziness
  5. Bradycardia
  6. Edema
  7. Impotence
  8. Hypotension
  9. Depression
C. Implementation
  1. Monitor vital signs
  2. Instruct clients not to discontinue medication, as abrupt withdrawal can cause severe rebound hypertension
  3. Monitor liver function tests

IX. ACE Inhibitors (Box 60–15)

A. Description
  1. Prevent peripheral vasoconstriction by blocking conversion of angiotensin I to angiotensin II
  2. Used to treat hypertension

BOX 60–15. ACE Inhibitors

Captopril (Capoten)
Enalapril maleate (Vasotec)
Benazepril (Lotensin)
Fosinopril (Monopril)
Lisinopril (Prinivil, Zestril)
Quinapril HCl (Accupril)
Ramipril (Altace)

3. Avoid use with potassium supplements and potassium-sparing diuretics
B. Side effects
1. Nausea
2. Vomiting
3. Diarrhea
4. Persistent cough
5. Hypotension
6. Hyperkalemia
7. Tachycardia
8. Headache
9. Dizziness
10. Fatigue
11. Insomnia
12. Hypoglycemic reaction in diabetics
13. Bruising, petechiae, bleeding
14. Diminished taste
C. Implementation
1. Monitor vital signs
2. Monitor protein, albumin, blood urea nitrogen (BUN), creatinine, white blood cells (WBC), potassium levels
3. Monitor for hypoglycemic reaction in diabetics
4. Instruct the client to take captopril (Capoten) 20 minutes to 1 hour before a meal
5. Monitor for bruising, petechiae, or bleeding with captopril
6. Instruct the client not to discontinue captopril, as rebound hypertension can occur
7. Instruct clients not to take over-the-counter medications
8. Instruct clients how to take **blood pressure**
9. Instruct clients that if dizziness occurs and persists to notify the physician
10. Inform clients that the taste of food may be diminished during the first month of therapy

X. Antianginal Medications (Box 60–16)

A. Nitrates
1. Description
a. Produce vasodilation
b. Decrease **preload** and **afterload** and reduce myocardial oxygen consumption
c. Contraindicated in clients with marked hypotension, increased intracranial pressure (ICP), or severe anemia
d. Use with caution with severe renal or hepatic disease

e. Avoid abrupt withdrawal of long-acting preparations to prevent the rebound effect of severe pain from myocardial ischemia
2. Side effects
a. Headache
b. **Orthostatic hypotension**
c. Dizziness
d. Weakness
e. Faintness
f. Nausea
g. Vomiting
h. Flushing or pallor
i. Confusion
j. Rash
k. Dry mouth
l. Reflex tachycardia
m. Paradoxical bradycardia
3. Sublingual medications
a. Monitor vital signs
b. Offer sips of water before giving, as dryness may inhibit medication absorption
c. Instruct the client to place under the tongue and leave until fully dissolved
d. Instruct the client not to swallow the medication
e. Instruct the client to take 1 tablet for pain, and repeat every 5 minutes for a total of three doses
f. Instruct the client to seek medical help immediately if pain is not relieved in 15 minutes, following the three doses
g. Inform the client that a stinging or biting sensation may indicate that the tablet is fresh
h. Instruct to store medication in a dark, tightly closed bottle
i. Instruct the client to check expiration date on the medication bottle, as expiration may occur within 6 months of obtaining medication
j. Instruct the client to take acetaminophen (Tylenol) for a headache
4. Translingual medications
a. Instruct clients to direct spray against the oral mucosa
b. Instruct clients to avoid inhaling the spray
5. Sustained-release medications: instruct clients to swallow and not to chew or crush the medication

BOX 60–16. Antianginal Medications

Nitroglycerin (Nitro-Bid, Nitrostat, Transderm-Nitro Patch)
Isosorbide mononitrate (Imdur)
Isosorbide dinitrate (Isordil, Sorbitrate)
Erythrityl tetranitrate (Cardilate)
Pentaerythritol tetranitrate (Peritrate)
Amyl nitrite

6. Transmucosal-buccal medications
   a. Instruct the client to place between the upper lip and gum or in the buccal area between the cheek and gum
   b. Inform the client that the medication will adhere to the oral mucosa and slowly dissolve
7. Transdermal patch
   a. Instruct the client to apply the patch to a hairless area, using a new patch and different site each day
   b. As prescribed, instruct the client to remove the patch after 12 to 14 hours, allowing 10 to 12 "patch-free" hours each day to prevent tolerance
   c. Do not apply the patch on the chest in the area of defibrillator-cardioverter paddle placement, as skin burns can result
8. Topical ointments
   a. Instruct the client to remove ointment on the skin from the previous dose
   b. Instruct the client to squeeze a ribbon of ointment of the prescribed length onto the applicator paper
   c. Instruct the client to spread the ointment over a 6- $\times$ 6-inch area using the chest, back, abdomen, upper arm, or anterior thigh (avoiding hairy areas), and cover with a plastic wrap
   d. Instruct the client to rotate sites and to avoid touching the ointment when applying
   e. Do not apply ointment on the chest in the area of defibrillator-cardioverter paddle placement, as skin burns can result

XI. Beta-Adrenergic Blockers (Box 60–17)

A. Description
   1. Inhibit response to beta-adrenergic stimulation, thus decreasing **cardiac output**
   2. Block the release of the catecholamines, epinephrine, and norepinephrine, thus decreasing the heart rate and **blood pressure**
   3. Decrease the workload of the heart and decrease oxygen demands
   4. Used for angina dysrhythmias, hypertension, migraine headaches, prevention of MI, and glaucoma
   5. Contraindicated in clients with asthma, bradycardia, CHF, severe renal or hepatic disease, hyperthyroidism, and CVA
   6. Use with caution in clients with diabetes, as it may mask symptoms of hypoglycemia
   7. Use with caution in clients on antihypertensives
B. Side Effects
   1. Decreased pulse rate
   2. Bradycardia

BOX 60–17. Beta-Adrenergic Blockers

Propranolol HCl (Inderal)
Metoprolol Tartrate (Lopressor)
Acebutolol (Sectral)
Atenolol (Tenormin)
Betaxolol (Kerlone)
Bisoprolol fumarate (Zebeta)
Nadolol (Corgard)
Penbutolol (Levatol)
Pindolol (Visken)
Timolol maleate (Blocadren)
Carteolol HCl (Cartrol)
Labetalol HCl (Normodyne, Trandate)
Carvedilol (Coreg)
Esmolol HCl (Brevibloc)
Levbunolol HCl (Betagan)
Metipranolol HCl (OptiPranolol)
Sotalol (Betapace)

---

3. Bronchospasm
4. Hypotension
5. Fatigue
6. Weakness
7. Nausea
8. Vomiting
9. Dizziness
10. Hypoglycemia
11. Agranulocytosis
12. Behavioral or psychotic response
13. Depression
14. Nightmares

C. Implementation
   1. Monitor vital signs and ECG
   2. Monitor **blood pressure**
   3. Hold medication if pulse or **blood pressure** is not within agreed parameters
   4. Monitor for signs of CHF
   5. Assess for respiratory distress and for signs of wheezing and dyspnea
   6. Instruct the client to report dizziness, lightheadedness, or nasal congestion
   7. Instruct the client not to stop medication as rebound hypertension, rebound tachycardia, or an anginal attack can occur
   8. Advise clients on insulin that early signs of hypoglycemia such as tachycardia and nervousness can be masked by the beta blocker
   9. Instruct clients on insulin to monitor their blood sugar
   10. Instruct the client and family how to take a pulse and **blood pressure**
   11. Instruct clients to change positions slowly to prevent **orthostatic hypotension**
   12. Instruct clients to avoid over-the-counter cold medications and nasal decongestants

XII. Calcium Channel Blockers (Box 60–18)

A. Description
   1. Decrease cardiac **contractility** (negative

BOX 60–18. Calcium Channel Blockers

Diltiazem (Cardizem)   Amlodipine (Norvasc)
Nifedipine (Procardia)   Bepridil (Vascor)
Verapamil HCl (Calan)   Felodipine (Plendil)
Nicardipine (Cardene)   Isradipine (DynaCirc)

---

inotropic effect by relaxing smooth muscle)
and the workload of the heart, thus
decreasing the need for oxygen
2. Promote vasodilation of the coronary and
peripheral vessels
3. Used for angina, dysrhythmias, and
hypertension
4. Used with caution in clients with CHF,
bradycardia, or AV block
B. Side Effects
1. Bradycardia
2. Hypotension
3. Reflex tachycardia as a result of hypotension
4. Headache
5. Dizziness
6. Lightheadedness
7. Fatigue
8. Peripheral edema
9. Constipation
10. Flushing of the skin
11. Changes in liver and kidney function
C. Implementation
1. Monitor vital signs
2. Monitor for signs of CHF
3. Monitor liver enzymes
4. Monitor kidney function tests
5. Instruct the client not to discontinue
medication
6. Instruct the client how to take a pulse
7. Instruct clients to notify the physician if
dizziness or fainting occurs
8. Instruct clients not to crush or chew
sustained-release tablets

XIII. Peripheral Vasodilators (Box 60–19)

A. Description
1. Decrease peripheral resistance by exerting a
direct action on the arteries or on both the
arteries and veins
2. Increase blood flow to the extremities
3. Used in peripheral vascular disorders of
venous and arterial vessels
4. Most effective for disorders resulting from
vasospasm (Raynaud's disease)
5. These medications may decrease some of the
symptoms of cerebral vascular insufficiency
B. Side Effects
1. Lightheadedness
2. Dizziness
3. **Postural hypotension**
4. Tachycardia
5. Palpitation

BOX 60–19. Peripheral Vasodilators

Alpha-adrenergic Blocker
Tolazoline (Priscoline)

Beta-adrenergic Agonist
Isoxsuprine (Vasodilan)
Nylidrin (Arlidin)

Direct-acting Peripheral Vasodilators
Cyclandelate (Cyclan, Cyclospasmol)
Ergoloid mesylates (Hydergine)
Nicotinyl alcohol

Alpha Blocker
Prazosin HCl (Minipress)

Calcium Channel Blocker
Nifedipine (Procardia)

Hemorrheologic
Pentoxifylline (Trental)
Increases microcirculation and tissue perfusion

---

6. Flushing
7. GI distress
C. Implementation
1. Monitor vital signs, especially **blood
pressure** and heart rate
2. Monitor for **orthostatic hypotension** and
tachycardia
3. Monitor for signs of inadequate blood flow
to the extremities such as pallor, coldness of
the extremities, and pain
4. Instruct the client that it may take up to 3
months for a desired therapeutic response
5. Advise the client not to smoke because
smoking increases vasospasm
6. Instruct the client to avoid aspirin or aspirin-
like compounds unless approved by the
physician
7. Instruct the client to take the medication
with meals if GI disturbances occur
8. Instruct the client to avoid alcohol as it may
cause a hypotensive reaction
9. Encourage the client to change positions
slowly to avoid **orthostatic hypotension**

XIV. Direct-Acting Arteriolar Vasodilators
(Box 60–20)

A. Description
1. Relax the smooth muscles of the blood
vessels, mainly the arteries, causing
vasodilation

BOX 60–20. Direct-Acting Arteriolar Vasodilators

Diazoxide (Hyperstat)
Sodium nitroprusside (Nipride)
Hydralazine HCl (Apresoline)
Minoxidil (Loniten)

---

2. Promote an increase in blood flow to the brain and kidneys
3. With vasodilation, the **blood pressure** drops and sodium and water are retained, resulting in peripheral edema
4. Diuretics may be given to decrease the edema
5. Used in clients with moderate to severe hypertension
6. Used during acute hypertensive emergencies

B. Side Effects
1. Hypotension
2. Reflex tachycardia caused by vasodilation and the drop in **blood pressure**
3. Palpitations
4. Edema
5. Dizziness
6. Headaches
7. Nasal congestion
8. GI bleeding
9. Neurological symptoms
10. Confusion
11. Excess hair growth with minoxidil (Loniten)
12. With sodium nitroprusside (Nipride), cyanide toxicity, and thiocyanate toxicity can occur

C. Implementation
1. Monitor vital signs
2. Sodium nitroprusside
    a. Monitor cyanide and thiocyanate levels
    b. Protect from light because the medication decomposes
    c. When administering, solution must be wrapped in aluminum foil and is stable for 24 hours
    d. Discard if the medication is red or blue

XV. Antidysrhythmic Medications

A. Description: suppress dysrhythmias by inhibiting abnormal pathways of electrical conduction through the heart
B. Class I Antidysrhythmics
1. Fast (sodium) channel blockers I
    a. Moricizine HCl (Ethmozine)
    b. Disopyramide (Norpace)
    c. Procainamide (Pronestyl)
    d. Quinidine sulfate (Quinidex)
2. Fast (sodium) channel blockers II
    a. Lidocaine (Xylocaine)
    b. Mexiletine (Mexitil)
3. Fast (sodium) channel blockers III
    a. Flecainide acetate (Tambocor)
    b. Tocainide HCl (Tonocard)
4. Side Effects
    a. Hypotension
    b. Heart failure
    c. CHF
    d. Worsened or new dysrhythmias
    e. Nausea, vomiting, or diarrhea
C. Class II Antidysrhythmics
1. Beta-adrenergic blockers
    a. Acebutolol (Sectral)
    b. Propranolol HCl (Inderal)
    c. Sotalol (Betapace)
2. Side effects
    a. Dizziness
    b. Fatigue
    c. Hypotension
    d. Bradycardia
    e. CHF
    f. Dysrhythmias
    g. Heart block
    h. Bronchospasms
    i. GI distress
D. Class III Antidysrhythmics
1. Medications
    a. Adenosine (Adenocard)
    b. Amiodarone HCl (Cordarone)
    c. Bretylium tosylate (Bretylol)
2. Side effects
    a. Hypotension
    b. Bradycardia
    c. Nausea
    d. Vomiting
    e. Adenosine can cause dysrhythmias, dyspnea, facial flushing
    f. Amiodarone HCl may cause pulmonary fibrosis, photosensitivity, bluish skin discoloration, corneal deposits, peripheral neuropathy, tremor, poor coordination, abnormal gait, hypothyroidism
    g. Bretylium tosylate may cause vertigo, syncope, dizziness
E. Class IV Antidysrhythmics
1. Calcium channel blockers
    a. Verapamil HCl (Calan)
    b. Diltiazem (Cardizem)
2. Side effects
    a. Dizziness
    b. Hypotension
    c. Bradycardia
    d. Edema
    e. Constipation
F. Other Antidysrhythmics
1. Medications
    a. Phenytoin (Dilantin)
    b. Digoxin (Lanoxin)
    c. Atropine sulfate
    d. Atropine is used to treat sinus bradycardia
    e. Atropine is contraindicated in glaucoma, urinary retention, and ileus
2. Side effects: atropine can cause hallucinations, tachycardia, dry mouth, and constipation
G. Implementation for Antidysrhythmics
1. Monitor heart rate, respiratory rate, and **blood pressure (BP)**
2. Monitor ECG
3. Provide cardiac monitoring
4. Maintain therapeutic serum drug levels
5. Before administering lidocaine, always check the vial label to prevent administering a form that contains epinephrine or

preservatives, as these solutions are used for local anesthesia only

6. Do not administer with food as food may affect absorption
7. Mexiletine or tocainide may be administered with food or antacids to reduce GI distress
8. Always administer IV antidysrhythmics via an infusion pump
9. Monitor for signs of fluid retention, such as weight gain, peripheral edema, or shortness of breath
10. Advise the client to limit fluid and salt intake to minimize fluid retention
11. Monitor respiratory, thyroid, and neurological function
12. After administering bretylium tosylate, keep the client supine and monitor for hypotension
13. Instruct the client to change positions slowly to minimize **orthostatic hypotension**
14. Instruct the client taking amiodarone to use a sunscreen and protective clothing to prevent photosensitivity reactions
15. Encourage the client to increase fiber intake to prevent constipation
16. Assess for bradycardia when administering atropine in low doses or by slow infusion

XVI. Adrenergic Agonists (Box 60–21)

A. Dobutamine (Dobutrex)
 1. Increases myocardial force and **cardiac output** through stimulation of beta receptors
 2. Used in CHF and for clients undergoing cardiopulmonary bypass surgery
B. Dopamine HCl (Intropin)
 1. Increases **blood pressure** and **cardiac output** through positive inotropic action and increases renal blood flow through its action on alpha and beta receptors
 2. Used to treat mild renal failure caused by low **cardiac output**
C. Epinephrine (Adrenalin)
 1. Used for cardiac stimulation in cardiac arrest
 2. Used for bronchodilation in asthma or allergic reactions
 3. Produces mydriasis
 4. Produces local vasoconstriction when combined with local anesthetics and prolongs anesthetic action by decreasing blood flow to site

D. Isoproterenol HCl (Isuprel)
 1. Stimulates beta receptors
 2. Used for cardiac stimulation and bronchodilation
E. Norepinephrine bitartrate (Levophed)
 1. Stimulates the heart in cardiac arrest
 2. Vasoconstricts and increases the **blood pressure** in hypotension and shock
F. Side Effects
 1. Dysrhythmias
 2. Tachycardia
 3. Angina
 4. Restlessness
 5. Urgency or urinary incontinence
G. Implementation
 1. Monitor vital signs
 2. Monitor lung sounds
 3. Monitor urinary output
 4. Monitor ECG
 5. Administer medication through a large vein
 6. If extravasation occurs, infiltrate the site with normal saline and phentolamine (Regitine)

XVII. Antilipemic Medications

A. Description
 1. Reduce serum levels of cholesterol, triglycerides, or low-density lipoprotein (LDL)
 2. When cholesterol, triglycerides, and LDL are elevated, the client is at increased risk for coronary artery disease
 3. In many cases diet alone will not lower blood lipid levels; therefore, antilipemic medications will be prescribed
B. Bile Acid Sequestrants (Box 60–22)
 1. Description
  a. Binds with acids in the intestines
  b. Bile acid sequestrants should not be used as the only therapy in clients with elevated triglycerides, because they typically raise triglyceride levels
 2. Side effects
  a. Constipation
  b. Peptic ulcer
 3. Implementation
  a. Cholestyramine resin (Questran) comes in a gritty powder that must be mixed thoroughly in juice or water before administration
  b. Monitor the client for early signs of peptic ulcer such as nausea and abdominal discomfort followed by abdominal pain and distention

---

BOX 60–21. Adrenergic Agonists

Dobutamine (Dobutrex)
Dopamine HCl (Intropin)
Epinephrine (Adrenalin)
Isoproterenol HCl (Isuprel)
Norepinephrine bitartrate (Levophed)

BOX 60–22. Bile Acid Sequestrants

Cholestyramine resin (Questran)
Colestipol (Colestid)

BOX 60–23. HMG-CoA Reductase Inhibitors

Pravastatin (Pravachol)
Lovastatin (Mevacor)

---

c. Instruct clients that the medication must be taken with and followed by sufficient fluids
C. HMG-CoA Reductase Inhibitors (Box 60–23)
  1. Description
    a. Lovastatin (Mevacor) is highly protein-bound and should not be administered with anticoagulants
    b. Lovastatin should not be administered with gemfibrozil (Lopid)
    c. Administer lovastatin with caution to clients on immunosuppressive medications
  2. Side effects
    a. Nausea
    b. Diarrhea or constipation
    c. Abdominal pain or cramps
    d. Flatulence
    e. Dizziness
    f. Headache
    g. Blurred vision
    h. Rash
    i. Pruritus
    j. Elevated liver enzymes
    k. Causes GI disturbances, headaches, muscle cramps, and fatigue
  3. Implementation
    a. Monitor serum liver enzymes
    b. Instruct client to receive an annual eye exam because the medication causes cataract formation
    c. If lovastatin is not effective in lowering the lipid level after 3 months, it should be discontinued
D. Other Antilipemic Medications (Box 60–24)
  1. Description
    a. Gemfibrozil should not be taken with anticoagulants because they compete for protein sites, and if the client is on an anticoagulant, the anticoagulant dose should be reduced during antilipemic therapy and the INR monitored closely
    b. Do not administer gemfibrozil with lovastatin

BOX 60–24. Other Antilipemic Medications

Fenofibrate (Lipidil)
Clofibrate (Atromid-S)
Gemfibrozil (Lopid)
Nicotinic acid, niacin (Nicobid)
Probucol (Lorelco)
Simvastatin (Zocor)
Fluvastatin (Lescol)

---

    c. Clofibrate (Atromid-S) should not be used long term because of its side effects such as dysrhythmias, angina, thromboembolism, and gallstones
    d. Probucol (Lorelco) is contraindicated in clients with cardiac dysryhthmias
  2. Implementation
    a. Monitor vital signs
    b. Monitor liver enzyme levels
    c. Monitor serum cholesterol and triglyceride levels
    d. Instruct the client to restrict intake of fats, cholesterol, carbohydrates, and alcohol
    e. Instruct the client to stop smoking
    f. Instruct the client to follow an exercise program
    g. Instruct the client that it will take several weeks before the lipid level declines
    h. Instruct the client to have an annual eye examination and to report any changes in vision
    i. Instruct diabetic clients taking gemfibrozil to monitor blood glucose levels regularly
    j. Instruct the client to increase fluid intake
    k. Note that nicotinic acid, niacin, has numerous side effects that include GI disturbances, flushing of the skin, elevated liver enzymes, hyperglycemia, and hyperuricemia
    l. Instruct the client that aspirin may assist in reducing the side effects of nicotinic acid, niacin
    m. Instruct the client to take nicotinic acid, niacin, with meals to reduce GI discomfort

PRACTICE QUESTIONS

1. The nurse provides discharge instructions to the postoperative client taking warfarin sodium (Coumadin). Which statement, if made by the client, reflects the need for further teaching?
   1 "I will take Ecotrin for my headaches because it is coated."
   2 "I will be certain to limit my alcohol consumption."
   3 "I will take my pills every day at the same time."
   4 "I have already called my family to pick up a Medic-Alert bracelet."

2. The client has a serum potassium (K^+) of 3.0 and is complaining of anorexia. The physician orders a digoxin level to rule out digoxin toxicity. What is the therapeutic serum level for digoxin?
   1 3.5 ng/mL
   2 1.2 to 2.8 ng/mL
   3 3.0 ng/mL
   4 0.5 to 2.0 ng/mL

3. When administering a subcutaneous injection of heparin, the nurse should:
   1 Administer with a 23- to 25-gauge, 1-inch needle
   2 Aspirate before injection
   3 Apply heat after the injection
   4 Administer with a 25- to 27-gauge, ⅝-inch needle

4. The client is being treated with procainamide HCl (Pronestyl) for cardiac dysrhythmia. Following intravenous administration of the medication, the client complains of dizziness. What intervention should the nurse do first?
   1 Administer ordered nitroglycerin tablets
   2 Auscultate the client's apical pulse and obtain a blood pressure
   3 Measure heart rate and rhythm on the rhythm strip
   4 Obtain a 12-lead electrocardiogram (ECG) immediately

5. A 51-year-old client is admitted with a diagnosis of myocardial infarction. The client is started on streptokinase (Streptase) therapy. The nurse knows that teaching has been effective when the client's wife states that the purpose of the medication is:
   1 "To thin the blood."
   2 "To slow the clotting of the blood."
   3 "To dissolve any clots in the coronary arteries."
   4 "To prevent further clots from forming in the coronary arteries."

6. The client is being treated for moderate hypertension and has been taking diltiazem (Cardizem) for several months. The client is seen by the physician, and Prinzmetal's angina is diagnosed. What action of the medication will provide a therapeutic effect for this new diagnosis?
   1 Increases oxygen demands within the myocardium
   2 Prevents influx of calcium ions in vascular smooth muscle
   3 Leads to increase in calcium absorption in the vascular smooth muscle
   4 Increases the force of contraction of ventricular tissues

7. Which of the following assessment data indicate a potential serious complication associated with propranolol HCl (Inderal)?
   1 A baseline blood pressure of 150/80 mm Hg followed by a blood pressure of 138/72 mm Hg after two doses of the medication
   2 A baseline resting heart rate of 88 beats per minute (bpm) followed by a resting heart rate of 72 bpm after two doses of the medication
   3 The development of audible expiratory wheezes
   4 The development of complaints of insomnia

8. The client is admitted to the emergency department with an acute anterior wall myocardial infarction. The nurse discusses streptokinase therapy with the client. The spouse is concerned about the dangers of this treatment. Which of the following statements by the nurse is most appropriate?
   1. "Your loved one is very ill. The physician has made the best decision for you."
   2 "There is no reason to worry. We use this medication all the time."
   3 "I'm certain you made the correct decision to use this medication."
   4 "You have concerns about whether this treatment is the best option."

9. The physician prescribed digoxin (Lanoxin) 0.25 mg for a client with atrial fibrillation. The medication is available as 0.125-mg tablets. The nurse calculates that the client will receive 2 tablets of digoxin. When the nurse administers the medication, the client looks at the medication and states, "Every time I get chest pain, I will take one of these heart pills." After double-checking the dosage calculation the nurse decides to:
   1 Not administer the medication as prescribed and calculated
   2 Administer one-half tablet of the medication instead of the dosage calculated
   3 Administer the medication as prescribed and calculated, and monitor for untoward effects such as seizures
   4 Administer the medication as prescribed and calculated and proceed with further client teaching

10. The home health care nurse is visiting an elderly client. Furosemide (Lasix) is prescribed for the client. The nurse teaches the client about the medication. Which of the following statements, if made by the client, indicates the need for further teaching?
    1 "I will take my medication every morning with breakfast."
    2 "I will call my doctor if my ankles swell or my rings get tight."
    3 "I need to drink lots of coffee and tea to keep myself healthy."
    4 "I will sit up slowly before standing each morning."

11. The client has a closed-head injury with increased intracranial pressure (ICP). The ICP is being effectively managed by mannitol (Osmitrol) IV. The nurse is planning to administer this medication via IV pump. The nurse should administer this medication:
    1 By giving it rapidly over 5 minutes IV bolus
    2 Mixed in solution with the IV antibiotics
    3 Piggybacked into the packed red blood cells
    4 By giving it slowly over 30 to 60 minutes

12. The nurse is administering lidocaine (Xylocaine) IV. Which of the following indicates to the nurse that the client is experiencing toxicity?
    1 Blurred vision and nausea
    2 Heart rate of 70 bpm, blood pressure (BP) of 130/72
    3 Headache and a temperature of 100°F orally
    4 Urine output of 275 mL over the past 8 hours

13. Which of the following laboratory studies will the physician order to monitor the therapeutic effect of heparin?
    1 Prothrombin time (PT)
    2 Activated partial thromboplastin time (APTT)
    3 Hematocrit (HCT)
    4 Hemoglobin (Hgb)

14. The client has suffered an acute myocardial infarction and is receiving tissue plasminogen activator (t-PA). Which of the following is a priority nursing intervention?
    1 Have heparin available
    2 Monitor for renal failure
    3 Monitor for signs of bleeding
    4 Monitor psychosocial status

15. The home health nurse instructs the client about the use of a nitrate patch. Which of the following will the nurse include in the teaching plan to prevent client tolerance to nitrates?
    1 Do not remove the patches
    2 Have a 12-hour "no nitrate" time
    3 Have a 24-hour "no nitrate" time
    4 Keep nitrates on 24 hours, then off 24 hours

16. The client was admitted to the medical unit with nausea and bradycardia. The family handed the nurse a small white envelope labeled "heart pill." The envelope is sent to pharmacy and reveals digitoxin (Crystodigin). The family stated, "That doctor doesn't know how to take care of my family." The most therapeutic response by the nurse is:
    1 "You are concerned your loved one receives the best care."
    2 "You're right! I've never seen a doctor put pills in an envelope."
    3 "I think you're wrong. That physician has been in practice over 30 years."
    4 "Don't worry about this. I'll take care of everything."

17. Which of the following potential nursing diagnoses is appropriate for the client receiving dopamine (Intropin) therapy at 10 mcg/kg/minute?
    1 Increased cardiac output
    2 Fluid volume excess
    3 Impaired tissue perfusion
    4 Altered sensory perception

18. The nurse is planning to administer furosemide (Lasix) 40 mg IVP (IV push). In order to deliver this medication safely the nurse must:

    1 Pinch the IV tubing below the injection port and inject slowly over 1 to 2 minutes
    2 Pinch the tubing above the injection port and inject slowly over 1 to 2 minutes
    3 Give the medication rapidly over 10 seconds
    4 Give the medication slowly diluted in 100 mL of D5W

19. The nurse is planning to administer hydrochlorothiazide (HydroDIURIL) to the client. Which of the following are concerns related to the administration of this medication?
    1 Hyperkalemia, hypoglycemia, penicillin allergy
    2 Hypouricemia, hyperkalemia
    3 Hypokalemia, hyperglycemia, sulfa allergy
    4 Increased risk of osteoporosis

20. The home health care nurse is visiting a client with elevated triglycerides and a serum cholesterol of 398 mg/dL. The client is taking cholestyramine resin (Questran). Which of the following statements, if made by the client, indicates the need for further education?
    1 "Constipation and bloating might be a problem."
    2 "I'll continue to watch my diet and reduce my fats."
    3 "I'll continue my nicotinic acid from the health food store."
    4 "Walking a mile each day will help the whole process."

21. The client is experiencing impotence after taking guanfacine (Tenex). The client states, "I would sooner have a stroke than keep living with the side effects of this medication." The most appropriate response by the nurse is:
    1 "I can understand completely."
    2 "The doctor should change your prescription."
    3 "You wouldn't really want to have a stroke."
    4 "You are concerned about the side effects of your medication."

22. The client with congestive heart failure is on a 1-g sodium diet. Which of the following medications promotes sodium excretion while conserving potassium?
    1 Spironolactone (Aldactone)
    2 Furosemide (Lasix)
    3 Ethacrynic acid (Edecrin)
    4 Hydrochlorothiazide (HydroDIURIL)

23. A client with coronary artery disease complains of substernal chest pain. After assessing the client's heart rate and blood pressure, the nurse administers nitroglycerin 0.4 mg sublingually. After 5 minutes, the client states, "My chest still hurts." If the vital signs have remained stable, the nurse should:
    1 Wait another 10 minutes and then administer a second nitroglycerin tablet

2 Apply 10 L of oxygen via nasal cannula

3 Administer another nitroglycerin tablet

4 Call the resuscitation team immediately

24. The client has developed paroxysmal nocturnal dyspnea (PND). Which of the following medications might be prescribed by the physician?
    1 Lidocaine (Xylocaine)
    2 Propranolol (Inderal)
    3 Bumetanide (Bumex)
    4 Urokinase (Abbokinase)

25. The client arrives in the emergency department after complaining of unrelieved chest pain for 2 days. The pain has subsided slightly but never disappeared. When the nurse approaches the client with a nitroglycerin 0.4-mg sublingual tablet, the client states, "I don't need that. My dad takes that for his heart. There's nothing wrong with my heart." Which of the following best describes the client's response?
    1 Obsessive-compulsive
    2 Denial
    3 Phobic
    4 Angry

26. The nurse has admitted a new client to the medical unit. The client is taking enalapril (Vasotec), atenolol (Tenormin), and aspirin (ASA) daily. The client admits the medications were prescribed by different physicians. The client is being admitted with syncope. The admitting physician wrote in the client's order sheet "administer medications as taken at home." Which of the following is the most appropriate action for the nurse to take?
    1 Give the medications as ordered by the physician
    2 Send the client's medication bottles to the pharmacy for identification and then administer the medications as ordered
    3 Call the physician, describe the medications, and request order clarification
    4 Refuse to give any medications and wait until the physician makes rounds to clarify the orders

27. A 66-year-old client is seen in the clinic complaining of not feeling well. The client is taking several medications to control heart disease and hypertension. These medications include atenolol, digoxin, and chlorothiazide (Diuril). A tentative diagnosis of digoxin toxicity is made. Which assessment data support this diagnosis?
    1 Chest pain, hypotension, and paresthesias
    2 Constipation, dry mouth, and sleep disorder
    3 Double vision, loss of appetite, and nausea
    4 Dyspnea, edema, and palpitations

28. A 79-year-old client is being treated for acute congestive heart failure with IV bumetanide (Bumex). The vital signs are blood pressure 100/60 mm Hg, pulse 96, and respirations 24. Following the initial dose, which of the following is the priority assessment?
    1 Monitoring blood pressure
    2 Monitoring potassium level
    3 Monitoring urine output
    4 Monitoring weight loss

29. A client with a diagnosis of congestive heart failure is seen in the clinic. The client is being treated with a variety of medications including digoxin (Lanoxin) and furosemide (Lasix). Which of the following assessment findings leads the nurse to suspect that the client is hypokalemic?
    1 Diarrhea
    2 Intermittent intestinal colic
    3 Muscle weakness and leg cramps
    4 Tingling around the mouth

30. The client is being discharged with a prescription for propranolol HCl (Inderal). In developing a medication teaching plan, the nurse includes which of the following instructions?
    1 Gentle exercising will prevent orthostatic hypotension
    2 Hot baths and showers are advised to increase vasodilation
    3 Medication should be taken on an empty stomach to enhance absorption
    4 Medication should be withheld if pulse rate drops below 60 bpm

ANSWERS

1. **1**

Rationale: Ecotrin is an aspirin-containing product and should be avoided. Excessive alcohol consumption should be avoided when taking warfarin. Taking prescribed medication at the same time increases client compliance. The Medic-Alert bracelet provides health care personnel emergency information.

Test-Taking Strategy: Knowledge regarding anticoagulants is important. Interactions between alcohol, food, and other medications create problems with many medications. The client should not take any over-the-counter medications without first consulting a health care provider. Use the process of elimination in answering the question. Read the stem carefully and note that the stem asks for the client statement that reflects the need for further education.

Level of Cognitive Ability: Analysis
Phase of Nursing Process: Evaluation
Client Needs: Health Promotion and Maintenance
Content Area: Pharmacology

Reference
Hodgson, B., & Kizior, R. (1999). *Saunders nursing drug handbook 1999.* Philadelphia: W. B. Saunders, pp. 75–77.

2. 4

Rationale: Therapeutic levels for digitalis range from 0.5 to 2.0 ng/mL.

Test-Taking Strategy: Knowledge of normal serum levels for digoxin is important. It is important to be aware of the reason for concern. The client's potassium was low and this increases the likelihood of digoxin toxicity. If you had difficulty with this question, take time now to learn the therapeutic levels for digoxin!

Level of Cognitive Ability: Analysis
Phase of Nursing Process: Analysis
Client Needs: Physiological Integrity
Content Area: Pharmacology

Reference
Lehne, R. (1998). *Pharmacology for nursing care* (3rd ed.). Philadelphia: W. B. Saunders. p. 485.

3. 4

Rationale: For subcutaneous heparin, use a 25- to 27-gauge, ³/₈- to ⁵/₈-inch needle to prevent tissue trauma and inadvertent intramuscular injection. A 1-inch needle would inject the heparin into the muscle. The application of heat may vary the absorption of the heparin. Aspiration before injection is avoided with heparin.

Test-Taking Strategy: Knowledge of anatomy of muscle and subcutaneous layers of tissue is important. Principles of safe medication injection specifically for heparin are key. If you had difficulty with this question, take time now to review the principles related to heparin administration!

Level of Cognitive Ability: Application
Phase of Nursing Process: Implementation
Client Needs: Physiological Integrity
Content Area: Pharmacology

Reference
Lehne, R. (1998). *Pharmacology for nursing care* (3rd ed.). Philadelphia: W. B. Saunders. p. 537.

4. 2

Rationale: Signs of toxicity from procainamide HCl include confusion, dizziness, drowsiness, decreased urination, nausea, vomiting, and tachydysrhythmias. Toxicity can cause widened QRS and prolonged PR interval. If this occurs, therapy is discontinued. Dizziness is a sign of toxicity. Option 2 identifies the first action followed by option 3 then option 4. Option 1 is an inappropriate action.

Test-Taking Strategy: Always assess the client first, not the monitoring devices. Therefore, option 2 is a better option than option 3. Option 4 will be implemented, but assess the blood pressure and heart rate first.

Level of Cognitive Ability: Application
Phase of Nursing Process: Implementation
Client Needs: Physiological Integrity
Content Area: Pharmacology

Reference
Deglin, J., & Vallerand, A. (1996). *Davis's drug guide for nurses* (4th ed.). Philadelphia: F. A. Davis. p. 1007.

5. 3

Rationale: Streptokinase converts plasminogen in the blood to plasmin. Plasmin is an enzyme that digests or dissolves fibrin clots wherever they exist. Options 1, 2, and 4 describe mechanisms of action of heparin and warfarin.

Test-Taking Strategy: This question requires a knowledge of the difference in the mechanism of action between heparin and streptokinase. Remember that streptokinase dissolves clots.

Level of Cognitive Ability: Analysis
Phase of Nursing Process: Evaluation
Client Needs: Physiological Integrity
Content Area: Pharmacology

Reference
Lehne, R. (1998). *Pharmacology for nursing care* (3rd ed.). Philadelphia: W. B. Saunders. p. 544.

6. 2

Rationale: Diltiazem is a calcium channel blocker that inhibits calcium influx through the slow channels of the membrane of smooth muscle cells. Calcium channel blockers decrease myocardial oxygen demands and block calcium channels thereby decreasing the force of contraction of the ventricular tissue.

Test-Taking Strategy: Knowledge of normal anatomy and physiology of cardiac electrical and mechanical structures is helpful in answering this question. Knowledge of the mechanisms involved in Prinzmetal's angina (coronary artery spasm) is required to understand why calcium channel blockers would be prescribed. Review the action of calcium channel blockers now if you had difficulty with this question!

Level of Cognitive Ability: Analysis
Phase of Nursing Process: Analysis
Client Needs: Physiological Integrity
Content Area: Pharmacology

Reference
Hodgson, B., & Kizior, R. (1999). *Saunders nursing drug handbook 1999.* Philadelphia: W. B. Saunders. pp. 327–329.

7. 3

Rationale: Audible expiratory wheezes may indicate a serious adverse reaction, bronchospasm. Beta blockers may induce this reaction, particularly in clients with chronic obstructive pulmonary disease (COPD) or asthma. A normal decrease in blood pressure and heart rate is expected. Insomnia is a frequent mild side effect and should be monitored.

Test-Taking Strategy: Knowledge regarding the side effects and adverse effects of propranolol are required to answer this question. Use the process of elimination, eliminating options 1 and 2, as these are expected responses from the medication. Read the question carefully. The question asks about the serious complication associated with the medication. This key phrase should direct you to the correct option.

Level of Cognitive Ability: Analysis
Phase of Nursing Process: Assessment
Client Needs: Physiological Integrity
Content Area: Pharmacology

Reference
Hodgson, B, & Kizior, R. (1999). *Saunders nursing drug handbook 1999.* Philadelphia: W. B. Saunders. pp. 877–880.

8. 4

Rationale: Paraphrasing is restating the client's or family member's own words. Option 1 represents a communication block that denies the person's right to an opinion.

Option 2 is offering a false reassurance. In option 3 the nurse is expressing approval, which can be harmful to the client-nurse or family-nurse relationship.

Test-Taking Strategy: Select the option with the most non-judgmental therapeutic nursing communication. A working knowledge of blocks to communication and ways to facilitate communication is essential. Note the client of the question. Address the client's feelings first!

Level of Cognitive Ability: Application
Phase of Nursing Process: Implementation
Client Needs: Psychosocial Integrity
Content Area: Pharmacology

Reference
Leahy, J., & Kizilay, P. (1998). *Foundations of nursing practice: A nursing process approach.* Philadelphia: W. B. Saunders. pp. 226–229.

9. **4**

Rationale: It is appropriate to treat atrial fibrillation with the prescribed and calculated dose of digoxin as indicated in the question. The issue of the question is that the client verbalizes inaccurate and unsafe knowledge regarding this medication and the treatment for chest pain. This client needs further education regarding the safe administration of medications for episodes of chest pain.

Test-Taking Strategy: Knowledge regarding the use of this medication is required to answer this question. Perform the calculation first and determine that the dose that the nurse is to give, is a correct dose. From this point, eliminate options 1 and 2. Note the issue of the question, which is the need for client teaching. This should direct you to the correct option.

Level of Cognitive Ability: Analysis
Phase of Nursing Process: Implementation
Client Needs: Health Promotion and Maintenance
Content Area: Pharmacology

Reference
Pinnell, N. L. (1996). *Nursing pharmacology.* Philadelphia: W. B. Saunders. pp. 351–356.

10. **3**

Rationale: Tea and coffee are stimulants as well as mild diuretics. These are a poor choice for hydration. Taking the medication at the same time each day improves compliance. Since furosemide is a diuretic, morning is the best time to take the medication so as not to interrupt sleep. Notification of the health care provider is appropriate if edema is noticed in the hands, feet, or face or if the client is short of breath. Sitting up slowly prevents postural hypotension.

Test-Taking Strategy: Knowledge of diuretics and the effects on the elderly is key. Client teaching regarding proper hydration with water and fruit juice is important. Tea and coffee are stimulants, and diuretics can worsen dehydration. Additionally, coffee and tea are not healthy foods. This should alert you that this is the correct option for this question, as stated.

Level of Cognitive Ability: Analysis
Phase of Nursing Process: Evaluation
Client Needs: Health Promotion and Maintenance
Content Area: Pharmacology

Reference
Pinnell, N. L. (1996). *Nursing pharmacology.* Philadelphia: W. B. Saunders. pp. 447–449.

11. **4**

Rationale: Mannitol is an osmotic diuretic. When used to lower increased intracranial pressure, mannitol is given slowly, over 30 to 60 minutes, not rapidly and not via IV bolus. The nurse should observe for an increased urine output greater than 30 mL/hour via Foley catheter. Mannitol should not be mixed in solution with antibiotics, and nothing should be piggybacked with packed red blood cells.

Test-Taking Strategy: Use the process of elimination to answer this question. Options containing the word "rapidly" or "slowly" should be assessed carefully. Generally it is incorrect to choose "rapidly" when giving most medications IV. Medications should not be mixed in solution with antibiotics. Nothing can be piggybacked with blood products.

Level of Cognitive Ability: Application
Phase of Nursing Process: Planning
Client Needs: Physiological Integrity
Content Area: Pharmacology

Reference
Pinnell, N. L. (1996). *Nursing pharmacology.* Philadelphia: W. B. Saunders. p. 452.

12. **1**

Rationale: Blurred vision and nausea are common indicators of lidocaine toxicity. The heart rate and blood pressure noted in option 2 are normal. A headache and elevated temperature are important assessment signs but are not related to the lidocaine. Urine output is greater than the minimum amount of 30 mL/hour and therefore is adequate.

Test-Taking Strategy: Use the process of elimination to answer the question. Knowledge of how lidocaine affects the central nervous system is required. Note that options 2, 3, and 4 reveal normal or mild physiological changes. The question stem asks for the indicator of toxicity.

Level of Cognitive Ability: Analysis
Phase of Nursing Process: Assessment
Client Needs: Physiological Integrity
Content Area: Pharmacology

Reference
Pinnell, N. L. (1996). *Nursing pharmacology.* Philadelphia: W. B. Saunders. p. 365.

13. **2**

Rationale: The PT will assess for the therapeutic effect of warfarin and the APTT will assess the therapeutic effect of heparin. HCT and Hgb assess red blood cell concentrations. Baseline assessment including an APTT value should be completed, as well as ongoing daily APTT values while the client is on heparin. Heparin doses are determined based on these laboratory results.

Test-Taking Strategy: Eliminate options 3 and 4. These laboratory values are not specific to heparin therapy. Knowledge of the appropriate test for monitoring therapeutic values of both heparin and warfarin is required to answer this question. Learn them now. You are likely to see a question as such on NCLEX-RN!

Level of Cognitive Ability: Analysis
Phase of Nursing Process: Evaluation
Client Needs: Physiological Integrity
Content Area: Pharmacology

Reference
Lehne, R. (1998). *Pharmacology for nursing care* (3rd ed.). Philadelphia: W. B. Saunders. pp. 534–539.

14. 3

Rationale: Tissue plasminogen activator is a thrombolytic. Hemorrhage is a complication of any type of thrombolytic medication. Monitor the client carefully for bleeding. Monitoring for renal failure and the client's psychosocial status is important; however, it is not the most critical. Heparin is given following thrombolytic therapy, but the question is not asking for the associated medications.

Test-Taking Strategy: The question asks for the priority nursing intervention. Use the process of elimination. Eliminate option 1, remembering that assessment is a priority. Use the ABCs to answer this question. Additionally, bleeding is a priority!

Level of Cognitive Ability: Application
Phase of Nursing Process: Implementation
Client Needs: Physiological Integrity
Content Area: Pharmacology

Reference
Lehne, R. (1998). *Pharmacology for nursing care* (3rd ed.). Philadelphia: W. B. Saunders. p. 546.

15. 2

Rationale: To help prevent tolerance, clients need a 12-hour "no nitrate" time, sometimes referred to as a pharmacological vacation from the medication.

Test-Taking Strategy: Knowledge of the absorption and distribution of nitrates is critical. In addition to having a 12-hour "no nitrate" vacation, the client must rotate the nitrate patch or paste and wash the hands to prevent topical absorption through the fingers.

Level of Cognitive Ability: Application
Phase of Nursing Process: Implementation
Client Needs: Physiological Integrity
Content Area: Pharmacology

Reference
Lehne, R. (1998). *Pharmacology for nursing care* (3rd ed.). Philadelphia: W. B. Saunders. p. 468.

16. 1

Rationale: This is a therapeutic nonjudgmental response. The statement reflects the family's concern, but remains nonjudgmental.

Test-Taking Strategy: Reflection of the client's or family's concern is the most therapeutic. The second option creates doubt in the physician's practice without actually knowing the circumstances. Option 3 is argumentative and nontherapeutic. Option 4 dismisses the family's concerns and disempowers the family.

Level of Cognitive Ability: Application
Phase of Nursing Process: Implementation
Client Needs: Psychosocial Integrity
Content Area: Pharmacology

Reference
Leahy, J., & Kizilay, P. (1998). *Foundations of nursing practice: A nursing process approach.* Philadelphia: W. B. Saunders. pp. 226–229.

17. 3

Rationale: The client receiving dopamine therapy should be assessed for impaired tissue perfusion related to peripheral vasoconstriction. As the dosage of dopamine increases, vasoconstriction increases.

Test-Taking Strategy: Use ABCs and eliminate options 2 and 4. Knowledge of how dopamine works is imperative. Assessment of impaired tissue perfusion is key to understanding underdosing, overdosing, or extravasation of dopamine. Knowledge of the action of this medication will direct you to the correct option, option 3.

Level of Cognitive Ability: Analysis
Phase of Nursing Process: Analysis
Client Needs: Physiological Integrity
Content Area: Pharmacology

Reference
Hodgson, B. & Kizior, R. (1999). *Saunders nursing drug handbook 1999.* Philadelphia: W. B. Saunders. pp. 345–348.

18. 2

Rationale: The tubing should be pinched above the injection port so the medication does not go back up the tubing. Most IVP medications should be injected slowly. Large and rapid doses of furosemide can lead to hearing loss.

Test-Taking Strategy: Knowledge of loop diuretic administration is imperative. Most IV injections should be delivered slowly. Therefore, eliminate option 3. Visualize the administration of the medication through the IV tubing. Pinching the tubing below the injection port prevents the medication from reaching the client and instead forces it back up the tubing. It is not necessary to dilute Lasix in 100 mL D5W. Also, the client might not tolerate the additional fluid, especially considering the action and purpose of furosemide.

Level of Cognitive Ability: Application
Phase of Nursing Process: Planning
Client Needs: Physiological Integrity
Content Area: Pharmacology

Reference
Hodgson, B., & Kizior, R. (1999). *Saunders nursing drug handbook 1999.* Philadelphia: W. B. Saunders. pp. 452–454.

19. 3

Rationale: Thiazide diuretics like hydrochlorothiazide are sulfa-based medications, and a client with a sulfa allergy is at risk for an allergic reaction. Also, clients are at risk for hypokalemia, hyperglycemia, hypercalcemia, hyperlipidemia, and hyperuricemia. Thiazide diuretics have been useful in reducing the incidence of osteoporosis in postmenopausal women by normalizing parathyroid function and calcium absorption.

Test-Taking Strategy: Knowledge of thiazide diuretics carrying a sulfa ring is imperative. When a client declares a sulfa allergy, this information must be communicated to the pharmacist, physician, nurse, and other health care providers. Eliminate option 4 because it is incorrect. Eliminate option 1 because this medication is not a penicillin. Eliminate option 2 because most diuretics, except for the potassium-sparing diuretics, cause hypokalemia. Note that option 3 addresses hypokalemia.

Level of Cognitive Ability: Analysis
Phase of Nursing Process: Planning
Client Needs: Physiological Integrity
Content Area: Pharmacology

Reference
Hodgson, B., & Kizior, R. (1999). *Saunders nursing drug handbook 1999.* Philadelphia: W. B. Saunders. pp. 494–496.

20. 3

Rationale: Nicotinic acid, even over-the-counter forms, should be avoided because it may lead to liver abnormalities. All lipid-lowering medications can also cause liver abnormalities, so a combination of nicotinic acid and cholestyramine resin is to be avoided. Constipation and bloating are the two most common side effects. Both walking and the reduction of fats in the diet are therapeutic measures to reduce cholesterol and triglyceride levels.

Test-Taking Strategy: Knowledge of elevated cholesterol and lipid-lowering medications is imperative. The most common complaints requiring medication adjustment are gastrointestinal, including bloating and constipation. In addition, any activity leading to an increased incidence of liver damage should be avoided. This includes lifestyle choices such as drinking alcohol and taking over-the-counter medications. The client should be encouraged to modify fat intake and increase activity. Remember that over-the-counter medications should be avoided when a client is taking a prescription medication!

Level of Cognitive Ability: Analysis
Phase of Nursing Process: Evaluation
Client Needs: Health Promotion and Maintenance
Content Area: Pharmacology

Reference
Hodgson, B., & Kizior, R. (1999). *Saunders nursing drug handbook 1999.* Philadelphia: W. B. Saunders. pp. 215–217.

21. 4

Rationale: Reflection of the client's own comment lets the client know you are hearing concerns without judging. The nurse cannot understand what the client is experiencing. Option 3 is confrontative and unsupportive.

Test-Taking Strategy: Remember that therapeutic communication techniques are important when responding to the client. Select nonjudgmental responses that reflect the fact you are listening to the client's concerns.

Level of Cognitive Ability: Application
Phase of Nursing Process: Implementation
Client Needs: Psychosocial Integrity
Content Area: Pharmacology

Reference
Leahy, J., & Kizilay, P. (1998). *Foundations of nursing practice.* Philadelphia: W. B. Saunders. pp. 226–229.

22. 1

Rationale: Spironolactone is a potassium-sparing diuretic that promotes sodium excretion while conserving potassium. Options 2, 3, and 4 identify diuretics that do not conserve potassium.

Test-Taking Strategy: Knowledge that spironolactone is a potassium-sparing diuretic is required to answer this question. Take time now to review the potassium-sparing diuretics if you had difficulty with this question!

Level of Cognitive Ability: Analysis
Phase of Nursing Process: Analysis
Client Needs: Physiological Integrity
Content Area: Pharmacology

Reference
Pinnell, N. L. (1996). *Nursing pharmacology.* Philadelphia: W. B. Saunders. pp. 450–451.

23. 3

Rationale: Nitroglycerin tablets are usually ordered one every 5 minutes p.r.n. for chest pain for a total dose of three tablets. The client with known coronary artery disease should have low-flow oxygen, 1 to 3 L/minute via nasal cannula, prescribed on admission.

Test-Taking Strategy: Use the process of elimination. Waiting 10 minutes is inappropriate if the client is having chest pain. Oxygen at 10 L is an unsafe dose. There is no need to call the resuscitation team at this time. This leaves option 3 as the correct option!

Level of Cognitive Ability: Application
Phase of Nursing Process: Implementation
Client Needs: Physiological Integrity
Content Area: Pharmacology

Reference
Pinnell, N. L. (1996). *Nursing pharmacology.* Philadelphia: W. B. Saunders. pp. 337–339.

24. 3

Rationale: Bumetanide is a diuretic. The PND may be a result of increased venous return when lying in bed and the client needs diuresis. Propranolol is a beta blocker, lidocaine is an antidysrhythmic, and urokinase is a thrombolytic.

Test-Taking Strategy: Knowledge of each medication type and purpose is critical. A diuretic assists the client with PND by increasing urine output and reducing right heart preload. The heart will have less volume to deal with and will reduce pulmonary capillary congestion. Review the actions of the medications identified in the options now if you had difficulty with this question!

Level of Cognitive Ability: Analysis
Phase of Nursing Process: Analysis
Client Needs: Physiological Integrity
Content Area: Pharmacology

Reference
Pinnell, N. L. (1996). *Nursing pharmacology.* Philadelphia: W. B. Saunders. pp. 448–449.

25. 2

Rationale: Denial is the most common reaction when a client has a myocardial infarction or anginal pain.

Test-Taking Strategy: Use the process of elimination to answer the question. Denial is the most common reaction when a person has chest pain. No angry behavior was demonstrated. Phobias and obsessive-compulsive disorders are psychiatric diagnoses.

Level of Cognitive Ability: Analysis
Phase of Nursing Process: Analysis
Client Needs: Psychosocial Integrity
Content Area: Pharmacology

Reference
Black, J, & Matassarin-Jacobs, E. (1997). *Medical surgical nursing: Clinical management for continuity of care* (5th ed.). Philadelphia: W. B. Saunders. p. 1266.

26. 3

Rationale: The nurse is ultimately responsible for giving the correct medication. When medication orders are vague, the nurse must call the physician. Often the physician is unaware of medications prescribed by other physicians. Always verify unclear orders for medications with the physician before giving them. When similar medications are being taken by the client, ask which physicians ordered them or look at the original prescription bottles if available.

Test-Taking Strategy: Use the process of elimination. Options 1 and 2 are easily eliminated. Eliminate option 4 because it is not appropriate to wait to clarify an unclear physician's order!

Level of Cognitive Ability: Application
Phase of Nursing Process: Implementation
Client Needs: Safe, Effective Care Environment
Content Area: Pharmacology

Reference
Lehne, R. (1998). *Pharmacology of nursing care* (3rd ed.). Philadelphia: W. B. Saunders. p. 70.

27. **3**

Rationale: Double vision, loss of appetite, and nausea are early signs of digoxin toxicity. Additional signs of digoxin toxicity include bradycardia, difficulty reading, visual alterations such as green and yellow vision, seeing spots or halos, confusion, vomiting, diarrhea, decreased libido, and impotence.

Test-Taking Strategy: Knowledge regarding the signs of digoxin toxicity is required to answer the question. Remember gastrointestinal (GI) and visual disturbances. If you had difficulty with this question, take time now to review digoxin toxicity. You are likely to see questions related to this content on NCLEX-RN!

Level of Cognitive Ability: Application
Phase of Nursing Process: Assessment
Client Needs: Physiological Integrity
Content Area: Pharmacology

Reference
Hodgson, B., & Kizior, R. (1999). *Saunders nursing drug handbook 1999.* Philadelphia: W. B. Saunders. pp 324–326.

28. **1**

Rationale: Hypotension is a common side effect with this medication and an increased risk exists in an elderly client. Options 2, 3, and 4 will also require assessment but are not the priority.

Test-Taking Strategy: Focus on the key word "priority." Blood pressure is mentioned in the question and also in option 1. Remember the ABCs. Blood pressure reflects circulation!

Level of Cognitive Ability: Analysis
Phase of Nursing Process: Assessment
Client Needs: Physiological Integrity
Content Area: Pharmacology

Reference
Deglin, J., & Vallerand, A. (1996). *Davis's drug guide for nurses* (4th ed.). Philadelphia: F. A. Davis. p. 393.

29. **3**

Rationale: Clients on potassium-wasting diuretics are at high risk of hypokalemia. Clinical manifestations of hypokalemia include fatigue, anorexia, nausea, vomiting, muscle weakness, leg cramps, decreased bowel motility, paresthesias, and dysrhythmias.

Test-Taking Strategy: Use the process of elimination and knowledge regarding the signs of electrolyte imbalances to answer the question. Diarrhea and intestinal colic are signs of hyperkalemia. Tingling around the mouth is a sign of hypocalcemia. If you had difficulty with this question, take time now to review the signs of electrolyte imbalances!

Level of Cognitive Ability: Analysis
Phase of Nursing Process: Assessment
Client Needs: Physiological Integrity
Content Area: Pharmacology

Reference
Smeltzer, S., & Bare, B. (1996). *Brunner and Suddarth's textbook of medical-surgical nursing* (18th ed.). Philadelphia: Lippincott-Raven. p. 220.

30. **4**

Rationale: Most beta blockers may be administered with food or on an empty stomach but propranolol is best absorbed if taken with meals or directly after eating. Exercise will not affect orthostatic hypotension. Hot showers and baths are not advised. The client needs to be instructed how to take pulse rate and to notify the physician if the heart rate falls below 60 beats per minute.

Test-Taking Strategy: Use the process of elimination to answer the question. Remember that bradycardia can occur with propranolol. If you had difficulty with question, take time now to review this medication!

Level of Cognitive Ability: Application
Phase of Nursing Process: Planning
Client Needs: Health Promotion and Maintenance
Content Area: Pharmacology

Reference
Deglin, J., & Vallerand, A. (1996). *Davis's drug guide for nurses* (4th ed.). Philadelphia: F. A. Davis. p. 142.

BIBLIOGRAPHY

Black, J. M., & Matassarin-Jacobs, E. (1997). *Medical-surgical nursing: Clinical management for continuity of care* (5th ed.). Philadelphia: W. B. Saunders.

Clark, J. Queener, S., & Karb, V. (1997). *Pharmacologic basis of nursing practice* (5th ed.). St. Louis: Mosby–Year Book.

Deglin, J., & Vallerand, A. (1996). *Davis's drug guide for nurses* (4th ed.). Philadelphia: F. A. Davis.

Hodgson, B., & Kizior, R. (1999). *Saunders nursing drug handbook 1999.* Philadelphia: W. B. Saunders.

Kee, J., & Hayes, E. (1997). *Pharmacology: A nursing process approach* (2nd ed.). Philadelphia: W. B. Saunders.

Leahy, J., & Kizilay, P. (1998). *Foundation of nursing practice: A nursing process approach.* Philadelphia: W. B. Saunders.

Pinnell, N. L. (1996). *Nursing pharmacology.* Philadelphia: W. B. Saunders.

Smeltzer, S., & Bare, B. (1996). *Brunner and Suddarth's textbook of medical-surgical nursing* (18th ed.). Philadelphia: Lippincott-Raven.

UNIT XV

The Adult Client with a Renal System Disorder

PYRAMID TERMS

Acute Renal Failure (ARF)—The sudden loss of kidney function caused by renal cell damage from ischemia or toxic substances. ARF occurs abruptly and can be reversible. It leads to hypoperfusion, cell death, and decompensation in renal function. The prognosis is dependent on the cause and the condition of the client. Near-normal or normal kidney function may resume gradually.

Anuria—Urine output of less than 100 mL a day.

Arterial Steal Syndrome—Can develop following the insertion of an AV fistula when too much blood is diverted to the vein and arterial perfusion to the hand is compromised.

Azotemia—The retention of nitrogenous waste products in the blood.

Chronic Renal Failure (CRF)—The progressive loss and ongoing deterioration in kidney function that occurs slowly over a period of time. It occurs in four stages, is irreversible, and results in uremia or end-stage renal disease. Chronic renal failure requires dialysis or kidney transplant to maintain life.

Disequilibrium Syndrome—A rapid change in the composition of the extracellular fluid (ECF) that occurs during hemodialysis. Solutes are removed from the blood faster than from the cerebrospinal fluid (CSF) and brain. Fluid is pulled into the brain causing cerebral edema.

Hemodialysis—The process of cleansing the client's blood. The diffusion of dissolved particles from one fluid compartment into another across a semipermeable membrane. The client's blood flows through one fluid compartment and the dialysate is in another fluid compartment.

Internal Arteriovenous Fistula (AV Fistula)—Access of choice for chronic dialysis clients. Created surgically by which an artery in the arm is anastomosed to a vein. This creates an opening, or fistula, between a large artery and a large vein. The flow of arterial blood into the venous system causes the vein to become engorged (maturity). It requires 1 to 2 weeks to mature before it can be used. Maturity is necessary so that the engorged vein can be punctured for the dialysis procedure, using a large-bore needle.

Nephrolithiasis—Refers to the formation of kidney stones. Kidney stones are formed in the renal parenchyma.

Oliguria—Urine output of less than 400 mL a day.

Peritoneal Dialysis—The peritoneum is the dialyzing membrane (semipermeable membrane) and substitutes for kidney function during kidney failure. Works on the principles of diffusion and osmosis, and the dialysis occurs via the transfer of fluid and solute from the blood stream through the peritoneum.

Renal Failure—The loss of kidney function. The types of renal failure are ARF or CRF. The signs and symptoms of renal failure are caused by the retention of wastes, the retention of fluids, and the inability of the kidneys to regulate electrolytes.

Urolithiasis—Refers to the formation of urinary stones or calculi. Urinary calculi are formed in the ureter.

PYRAMID TO SUCCESS

Pyramid points focus on ARF and CRF, dialysis procedures such as hemodialysis and continuous ambulatory peritoneal dialysis (CAPD), urinary diversions, and postoperative care to the client following urinary or renal surgery. Focus on the major problems associated with renal failure and the rationale for the prescribed treatment modalities. Be familiar with the complications associated with hemodialysis and peritoneal dialysis, the specific assessment data related to complications, and the expected treatment. Focus on the care of a peritoneal catheter and hemodialysis access devices, the complications associated with these access devices, and the appropriate nursing interventions if a complication is suspected. Review preoperative and postoperative care related to renal transplantation and the assessment data indicating rejection. Be familiar with urinary diversions, care to the client following prostatectomy, and treatment measures for the client with urinary or renal calculi. Refer to Chapter 9 for additional nursing care measures.

NURSING PROCESS

ASSESSMENT

Medications client is presently taking
Associated medical conditions
Family history
Trauma and injury
Changes in pattern of urination, such as frequency, nocturia, hesitancy, urgency, dribbling, incontinence, and retention
Urine output, such as polyuria, oliguria, anuria
Changes in appearance of urine, such as dilute, concentrated, hematuria, and pyuria

Proteinuria
Burning pain
Dysuria
Fever and chills
Flank pain
Hypertension
Periorbital and peripheral edema
Weight changes
Level of consciousness (LOC)
Laboratory values

ANALYSIS: Altered Urinary Elimination

PLANNING	IMPLEMENTATION	EVALUATION
The client maintains adequate urinary output.	Obtain a client assessment, noting family history, history of trauma and injury, associated medical conditions, and current medication therapy. Assess vital signs. Assess urinary patterns. Assess characteristics of urine. Monitor intake and output (I&O). Maintain patency of urinary catheter and tubes if present. Prepare client for dialysis procedure if prescribed.	The client is free of urinary obstruction.

ANALYSIS: Pain

PLANNING	IMPLEMENTATION	EVALUATION
The client verbalizes the need to implement pain control measures. The client describes methods of promoting comfort.	Obtain data regarding the presence and characteristics of pain. Provide comfort measures to relieve discomfort. Administer pain medication as prescribed. Document effectiveness of pain relief measures.	Client obtains relief from pain and is comfortable.

ANALYSIS: Fluid Volume Deficit or Excess

PLANNING	IMPLEMENTATION	EVALUATION
The client consumes an amount of fluids as prescribed. Laboratory values remain within normal range.	Assess vital signs; Assess LOC. Assess lungs for rales and rhonchi. Assess for cardiac dysrhythmias. Monitor weight, noting changes or fluctuations. Monitor for periorbital or peripheral, edema. Monitor for signs of dehydration. Evaluate results of electrolyte and laboratory values. Monitor for acid-base imbalances.	An acceptable fluid balance is maintained. Laboratory values remain within a safe range. Risks of complications related to fluid imbalances are minimized.

ANALYSIS: Potential for Infection

PLANNING	IMPLEMENTATION	EVALUATION
The client verbalizes the signs and symptoms of infection.	Monitor for signs of infection. Monitor for fever or alterations in blood pressure. Monitor incision site for drainage and infection. Monitor dialysis access site for signs of infection. Instruct client to monitor for signs and symptoms of infection.	The client does not exhibit signs of infection. The client is free of previous infection.

ANALYSIS: Potential for Alteration in Skin Integrity

PLANNING	IMPLEMENTATION	EVALUATION
The client monitors skin integrity and implements measures to prevent alteration in skin integrity.	Monitor skin integrity. Monitor dressings, wound, and stoma sites. Change wound dressings as necessary. Initiate measures as prescribed to prevent skin breakdown. Instruct client in measures to prevent skin breakdown.	Skin integrity remains intact.

ANALYSIS: Potential for Injury

PLANNING	IMPLEMENTATION	EVALUATION
The client implements measures to prevent injury.	Monitor for risks related to potential for injury; Monitor LOC. Provide a safe, hazard-free environment. Note nephrotoxic medications that may be prescribed. Assess dialysis access device for patency. Maintain safe precautions when caring for dialysis access device. Monitor for complications associated with dialysis.	The client remains free from injury.

ANALYSIS: Knowledge Deficit

PLANNING

The client describes the prescribed diet and fluid intake plan. The client performs self-care and self-care activities and prescribed exercises. The client obtains adequate sleep and rest. The client demonstrates the ability to apply an external pouch, provide skin care, empty a pouch, and self-catheterize correctly if a urinary diversion is present. The client demonstrates care measures related to the dialysis access device. The client demonstrates the procedure for peritoneal dialysis, if prescribed. The client describes the correct procedure for the administration of prescribed medications. The client describes the plan for post-treatment follow-up, including knowledge regarding medications and the need for physician notification.

IMPLEMENTATION

Instruct client in adequate diet related to disorder. Instruct client in the need for increased fluids unless contraindicated. Instruct client to obtain adequate rest and to avoid fatigue. Encourage and instruct client to perform bladder-training exercises as appropriate. Instruct client with urinary diversion how to apply an external pouch, provide skin care, empty a pouch, and self-catheterize. Instruct client in home care dialysis procedures. The client demonstrates the appropriate procedure for peritoneal dialysis if prescribed. Instruct client in measures to reduce the risk of bleeding that may be associated with certain renal disorders. Instruct client in signs of complications and the need to notify the physician. Instruct client regarding the importance of medications and follow-up care.

EVALUATION

Complies with prescribed diet and fluid prescription. The client achieves a state that promotes healing and prevents further deterioration. The client explains preventive health actions related to diet modification and fluid intake. The client demonstrates the use of selected exercises related to bladder-training programs. The client demonstrates the appropriate procedure for caring for urinary diversion or a dialysis access device if present. The client demonstrates the appropriate procedure for peritoneal dialysis if prescribed. The client explains the correct procedure regarding the administration of medications. The client keeps follow-up appointments and seeks medical care if signs of complications arise.

ANALYSIS: Body Image Disturbances

PLANNING

The client participates in social interactions and avoids self-isolation.

IMPLEMENTATION

Encourage client to verbalize feelings related to altered body image. Assist client in identifying coping mechanisms. Mobilize support services and community services as necessary.

EVALUATION

Demonstrates effective coping mechanisms related to limitations to personal lifestyle. Utilizes community and support services.

CLIENT NEEDS

SAFE, EFFECTIVE CARE ENVIRONMENT

    Confidentiality related to renal disorder
    Informed consent related to diagnostic and surgical
        procedures
    Renal organ donation
    Consultations and referrals related to renal disorder
    Accident prevention related to complications associ-
        ated with disorder
    Asepsis related to wound care and dialysis access de-
        vices
    Standard precautions related to care of the client

HEALTH PROMOTION AND MAINTENANCE

    Instructions regarding the prevention of the recur-
        rence of a urinary or renal disorder

Urinary and renal assessment techniques
Instructions regarding prescribed treatments related
    to urinary or renal disorder
Instructions regarding postoperative management
Instructions regarding care to a urinary diversion,
    dialysis access device, and dialysis procedures

PSYCHOSOCIAL INTEGRITY

Religious and spiritual influences
Body image disturbances
Loss of function of a body part that occurs in clients
    with a renal disorder
Coping mechanisms
Support systems
Community resources

PHYSIOLOGICAL INTEGRITY

Elimination measures
Comfort interventions
Prescribed nutrition and fluid measures
Personal hygiene
Adequate rest and sleep
Medication administration
Diagnostic tests and laboratory results
Fluid and electrolyte and acid-base disorders
Care related to hemodialysis and peritoneal dialysis
Care related to dialysis access devices

Prevention of complications arising as a result of dialysis
Preoperative and postoperative care related to renal transplantation
Assessment data indicating rejection of renal transplant
Urinary diversions
Care to the client following prostatectomy
Treatment measures for the client with urinary or renal calculi

BIBLIOGRAPHY

Black, J., & Matassarin-Jacobs, E. (1997). *Medical-surgical nursing: Clinical management for continuity of care* (5th ed.). Philadelphia: W. B. Saunders.

Leahy, J., & Kizilay, P. (1998). *Foundations of nursing practice: A nursing process approach.* Philadelphia: W. B. Saunders.

Luckmann, J. (1997). *Saunders manual of nursing care.* Philadelphia: W. B. Saunders.

National Council of State Boards of Nursing. (1997). *Plan for the National Licensure Examination for Registered Nurses.* Chicago: Author.

O'Toole, M. (ed.). (1997). *Miller-Keane encyclopedia & dictionary of medicine, nursing & allied health* (6th ed.). Philadelphia: W. B. Saunders.

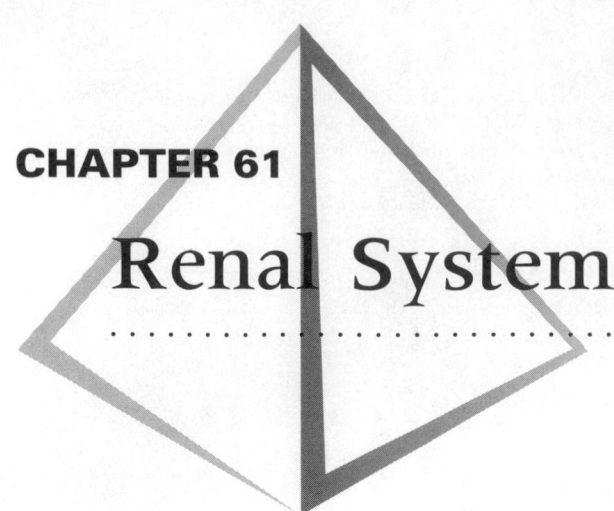

CHAPTER 61

Renal System

I. Anatomy and Physiology

A. Kidneys
1. There are two—each is attached to the abdominal wall at the level of the last thoracic and first three lumbar vertebrae
2. Enclosed in the renal capsule
3. The cortex is the outer layer of the renal capsule
4. The medulla is surrounded by the cortex
5. The nephron makes up the functional unit of the kidneys
6. Functions of kidneys
   a. Maintain homeostasis of the blood
   b. Excrete end-products of body metabolism
   c. Control fluid and electrolyte balance
   d. Excrete bacterial toxins, water-soluble drugs, and drug metabolites
   e. Secrete renin and erythropoietin, which play a role in the function of the parathyroid hormones and vitamin D
7. Nephron
   a. Functional renal unit
   b. Composed of glomerulus and tubules
8. Glomerulus
   a. Is encased in Bowman's capsule
   b. Filters the fluid out of blood
9. Tubules
   a. Include proximal, distal, and Henle's loop
   b. Fluid is converted to urine in the tubules and then the urine moves to the pelvis of the kidney
   c. The urine flows from the pelvis of the kidney through the ureter, and empties into the bladder

B. Bladder
1. The ureterovesical sphincter prevents reflux of urine from the bladder to the ureter
2. The total capacity of the bladder is 1 L

C. Prostate gland
1. Surrounds the male urethra
2. Contains a duct that opens into the prostatic portion of the urethra and secretes the alkaline portion of seminal fluid

D. Urine production
1. As fluid flows through the proximal tubules, water and solutes are reabsorbed
2. Water and solutes that are not reabsorbed become urine
3. The process of selective reabsorption determines the amount of water and solutes to be secreted

E. Homeostasis of water
1. The antidiuretic hormone (ADH) is primarily responsible for the reabsorption of water by kidneys
2. ADH is produced by the hypothalamus and secreted from the posterior lobe of the pituitary gland
3. Secretion of ADH is stimulated by dehydration or high sodium intake and by a fall in blood volume
4. ADH increases the permeability to water of the distal convoluted tubules and collecting duct
5. Water is drawn out of the tubules by osmosis into a high salt concentration of fluid in the medulla and its capillaries; water returns to the blood and concentrated urine remains in the tubule to be excreted
6. When clients lack ADH, they develop diabetes insipidus
7. Clients with diabetes insipidus produce very large amounts of dilute urine and without treatment have difficulty drinking sufficient water to survive

F. Homeostasis of sodium
1. When the amount of sodium increases, extra water is retained to preserve osmotic pressure
2. An increase in sodium and water produces an increase in the blood volume and blood pressure (BP)
3. When the BP increases, glomerular filtration increases, and extra water and salt are lost; blood volume is reduced and returns the BP to normal
4. Reabsorption of sodium in the distal convoluted tubules is controlled by the hormones of the renin-angiotensin system

5. Renin is secreted when the BP or concentration of fluid in the distal convoluted tubule is low
6. Renin is an enzyme that splits angiotensin I from angiotensinogen, which converts to angiotensin II as blood flows through the lung
7. Angiotensin II, a potent vasoconstrictor, stimulates the secretion of aldosterone
8. Aldosterone stimulates the distal convoluted tubules to reabsorb sodium and secrete potassium
9. The additional sodium increases water reabsorption and increases blood volume and BP, returning BP to normal; the stimulus for the secretion of renin is then removed

G. Homeostasis of potassium
1. Increases in potassium stimulate the secretion of aldosterone
2. Aldosterone stimulates the distal convoluted tubules to secrete potassium; this acts to return the potassium concentration to normal

H. Homeostasis of acidity (pH)
1. Blood pH is controlled by maintaining the concentration of buffer systems
2. Carbonic acid and sodium bicarbonate form the most important buffer for neutralizing acids in the plasma
3. The concentration of carbonic acid is controlled by the respiratory system
4. The concentration of sodium bicarbonate is controlled by the kidneys
5. Normal pH is 7.35 to 7.45, maintained by keeping the ratio of concentrations of sodium bicarbonate to carbon dioxide constant at 20:1
6. Strong acids are neutralized by sodium bicarbonate to produce carbonic acid and the sodium salts of the strong acid; this process quickly restores the ratio and thus blood pH
7. The carbonic acid produced dissociates into carbon dioxide and water; because the concentration of carbon dioxide is maintained at a constant level by the respiratory system, the excess carbonic acid is rapidly excreted
8. Sodium combined with the strong acid is actively reabsorbed in the distal convoluted tubules in exchange for hydrogen or potassium ions; the strong acid is neutralized by the secretion of ammonia and is excreted as ammonia or potassium salts

II. Diagnostic Tests (Box 61–2)

A. Urinalysis
1. Description: A urine test for evaluation of the renal system and for determining renal disease
2. Implementation
   a. Wash perineal area

BOX 61–1. Risk Factors Associated with Renal Disorders

Frequent urinary tract infections
High sodium diet
Contact sports
Trauma and injury
History of hypertension
Family history of renal disease
Medication use
Associated medical conditions

---

   b. Use a clean container
   c. Obtain 10 to 15 mL of the first morning sample
   d. Note that refrigerated samples may alter the specific gravity
   e. If the client is menstruating, indicate this on the laboratory requisition form

B. Specific gravity determination
1. Description: A urine test that measures the specific gravity of the urine
2. Implementation
   a. Obtain a freshly voided specimen
   b. Fill the specific gravity container one half to two thirds full
   c. Place the hydrometer (urinometer) in the urine and spin gently
   d. Read the scale at the level of the meniscus

C. Urine culture and sensitivity
1. Description: A urine test that identifies the presence of microorganisms and determines the specific antibiotics that will appropriately treat the existing microorganism
2. Implementation
   a. Clean perineal area and urinary meatus with bacteriostatic solution
   b. Collect midstream sample in a sterile container
   c. Send the collected specimen to the laboratory immediately
   d. Note that urine from clients who forced fluids may be too dilute to provide a positive culture
   e. Identify any sources of potential contaminants during the collection of the specimen, such as the hands, skin, clothing, hair, and vaginal or rectal secretions

---

BOX 61–2. Normal Renal Function Tests

BUN (blood urea nitrogen), 5–20 mg/dL
Serum creatinine, 0.6–1.3 mg/dL
Creatinine clearance, 100–120 mL/minute
Uric acid serum, 2.5–8.0 mg/dL
Uric acid urine, 250–750 mg/24 hours

D. Creatinine clearance test
   1. Description
      a. A blood and timed urine specimen that evaluates kidney function
      b. Blood is drawn at the start of the test and the morning of the day that the 24-hour urine specimen collection is complete
   2. Implementation
      a. Encourage adequate fluids before and during the test
      b. Instruct client as prescribed to avoid tea, coffee, and medications during testing
      c. If the client is taking ACTH, cortisone, or thyroxine, check with the physician regarding administration of these medications during testing
      d. Maintain the urine specimen on ice or refrigerate, and check with the laboratory regarding the addition of a preservative to the specimen during collection
E. VMA (vanillylmandelic acid) test
   1. Description
      a. A 24-hour urine collection to diagnose pheochromocytoma, a tumor of the adrenal gland
      b. The test identifies an assay of urinary catecholamines in the urine
   2. Implementation
      a. Instruct client to avoid foods such as caffeine, cocoa, vanilla, cheese, gelatin, licorice, and fruits for at least 2 days prior to beginning the urine collection and during the collection, and to avoid taking medications for 2 to 3 days prior to beginning the test as prescribed
      b. Instruct client to avoid stress and to maintain adequate food and fluids during the test
      c. Save all urine, label the container, add preservative, and place specimen on ice or refrigerate
      d. Check with the laboratory regarding medication restrictions
F. 17-Ketosteroids
   1. Description: A 24-hour urine collection to diagnose endocrine imbalances of adrenal glands, ovaries, and testes
   2. Implementation
      a. Encourage fluids and a normal diet during testing
      b. Add preservative and place specimen collection on ice or refrigerate
      c. Note that obesity and severe mental and physical stress may affect the test results
      d. Note that levels may increase during the third trimester of pregnancy
G. Uric acid test
   1. Description: A 24-hour urine collection to diagnose gout and kidney disease
   2. Implementation
      a. Encourage fluids and a regular diet during testing

b. Place specimen on ice or refrigerate, and check with the laboratory regarding the addition of a preservative
H. KUB (kidneys, ureters, and bladder) radiograph
   1. Description: An x-ray film that views the urinary system and adjacent structures; used to detect urinary calculi
   2. Implementation: There is no specific preparation
I. Intravenous pyelogram (IVP)
   1. Description
      a. The injection of a radiopaque dye that outlines the renal system
      b. Performed to identify abnormalities in the system
   2. Preprocedure implementation
      a. Obtain informed consent
      b. Assess the client for allergies to iodine, seafood, and radiopaque dyes
      c. Withhold food and fluids after midnight on the night before the test
      d. Administer laxatives as prescribed
      e. Inform the client about possible throat irritation, flushing of the face, warmth, or a salty taste that may be experienced during the test
   3. Postprocedure implementation
      a. Monitor vital signs
      b. Instruct the client to drink at least 1 L of fluids unless contraindicated
      c. Assess the venipuncture site for bleeding
      d. Monitor urinary output
J. Renal angiography
   1. Description: The injection of a radiopaque dye through a catheter for examination of the renal arterial supply
   2. Preprocedure implementation
      a. Obtain informed consent
      b. Assess the client for allergies to iodine, seafood, and radiopaque dyes
      c. Inform the client about a possible burning feeling or a feeling of heat along the vessel after the dye is injected
      d. Withhold food and fluids after midnight on the night before the test
      e. Instruct the client to void immediately before the procedure
      f. Administer enemas as prescribed
      g. Shave injection sites as prescribed
      h. Assess and mark the peripheral pulses
   3. Postprocedure implementation
      a. Assess vital signs and peripheral pulses
      b. Provide bed rest and use of a sandbag at insertion site for 4 to 8 hours
      c. Assess the color and temperature of the involved extremity
      d. Inspect the catheter insertion site for bleeding or swelling
      e. Force fluids unless contraindicated
      f. Monitor urinary output
K. Renal scan
   1. Description: An IV injection of a radioisotope for visual imaging of renal blood flow

2. Preprocedure implementation
   a. Obtain informed consent
   b. Assess for allergies
   c. Assist with administering radioisotope as necessary
   d. Instruct clients that they will be required to remain motionless
   e. Instruct clients that imaging may be repeated at various intervals before the test is complete
3. Postprocedure implementation
   a. Encourage fluids unless contraindicated
   b. Assess the client for signs of delayed allergic reaction, such as itching and hives
   c. Note that the radioactivity is eliminated in 24 hours
   d. Follow standard precautions when caring for incontinent clients and double-bag client linens per agency policy

L. Cystometrogram (CMG)
1. Description: A graphic recording of the pressures exerted at varying filling phases of the bladder
2. Preprocedure implementation: Inform the client of the voiding requirements during the procedure
3. Postprocedure implementation: Monitor client voiding after the procedure

M. Cystoscopy
1. Description: The bladder mucosa is examined for inflammation, calculi, or tumors by means of a cystoscope
2. Preprocedure implementation
   a. Obtain informed consent
   b. Withhold food and fluids after midnight on the night before the test
   c. Administer enemas and medications as prescribed
3. Postprocedure implementation
   a. Monitor vital signs
   b. Monitor for postural hypotension
   c. Force fluids as prescribed
   d. Monitor intake and output
   e. Encourage deep-breathing exercises to relieve bladder spasms
   f. Administer analgesics as prescribed
   g. Administer sitz baths for back and abdominal pain
   h. Note that leg cramps are common due to the lithotomy position maintained during the procedure
   i. Assess urine for color and consistency
   j. Note that pink-tinged or tea-colored urine is common
   k. Monitor for bright red urine or clots and notify physician if this occurs

N. Renal biopsy
1. Description: Insertion of a needle into the kidney to obtain a sample of tissue for examination
2. Preprocedure implementation
   a. Assess vital signs
   b. Assess baseline clotting studies
   c. Obtain informed consent
   d. Withhold food and fluids after midnight on the night before the test
3. Implementation during procedure: Position client prone with a pillow under the abdomen and shoulders
4. Postprocedure implementation
   a. Monitor vital signs
   b. Monitor hemoglobin and hematocrit
   c. Place client in the supine position on bed rest for 8 hours as prescribed
   d. Provide pressure to the biopsy site for 30 minutes
   e. Check the biopsy site for bleeding
   f. Force fluids from 1500 to 2000 mL as prescribed
   g. Instruct client to avoid heavy lifting and strenuous activity for 2 weeks

III. Renal Failure

A. Description
1. The loss of kidney function
2. The types of **renal failure** include **acute renal failure** or **chronic renal failure**
3. The signs and symptoms of **renal failure** are caused by the retention of wastes, the retention of fluids, and the inability of the kidneys to regulate electrolytes

B. **Acute renal failure (ARF)** (Box 61–3)
1. Description
   a. The sudden loss of kidney function caused by renal cell damage from ischemia or toxic substances
   b. **ARF** occurs abruptly and can be reversible
   c. It leads to hypoperfusion, cell death, and decompensation in renal function
   d. The prognosis is dependent on the cause and the condition of the client
   e. Near-normal or normal kidney function may resume gradually
2. Causes
   a. Infection
   b. Renal artery occlusion
   c. Obstruction
   d. Acute kidney disease
   e. Dehydration
   f. Diuretic therapy
   g. Ischemia from hypovolemia, heart failure, septic shock, and blood loss
   h. Toxic substances such as medications, particularly antibiotics
3. Oliguric phase (Table 61–1)

BOX 61–3. Phases of Acute Renal Failure

Oliguric	Recovery (Convalescent)
Diuretic	

Table 61-1. Phases of Acute Renal Failure

Oliguric Phase

Glomerular filtration rate decreased
Hyperkalemia
Sodium level normal or decreased
Fluid overload
Elevated BUN and creatinine

Diuretic Phase

Glomerular filtration rate begins to increase
Hypokalemia
Hyponatremia
Hypovolemia
Gradual decline in BUN and creatinine

Recovery Phase (Convalescent)

BUN is stable and normal
Complete recovery may take 1–2 years

---

a. Duration is 8 to 15 days, and the longer the duration, the less chance of recovery
b. Sudden drop in urine output; urine output less than 400 mL/day
c. Urine specific gravity of 1.010 to 1.016
d. Anorexia, nausea, and vomiting
e. Hypertension
f. Decreased skin turgor
g. Pruritus
h. Tingling of the extremities
i. Drowsiness progressing to disorientation to coma
j. Edema
k. Dysrhythmias
l. Signs of congestive heart failure (CHF) and pulmonary edema
m. Signs of pericarditis
n. Signs of acidosis
4. Diuretic phase
  a. Urine output rises slowly and then diuresis occurs (4–5 L/day)
  b. Excessive urine output indicates recovery of damaged nephrons
  c. Hypotension
  d. Tachycardia
  e. Improvement in level of consciousness (LOC)
5. Recovery phase (convalescent)
  a. A slow process; complete recovery may take 1 to 2 years
  b. Urine volume is normal
  c. Increase in strength
  d. Increase in LOC
  e. BUN is stable and normal
  f. Client can develop **chronic renal failure**
C. **Chronic renal failure (CRF)**
  1. Description
    a. The progressive loss and ongoing deterioration in kidney function that occurs slowly over a period of time
    b. It occurs in four stages, is irreversible, and

results in uremia or end-stage renal disease (Table 61–2)
  c. CRF requires dialysis or kidney transplant to maintain life
  d. Hypervolemia can occur owing to the inability of the kidneys to excrete sodium and water, or hypovolemia can occur owing to the inability of the kidneys to conserve sodium and water
2. Causes
  a. May follow ARF
  b. Renal artery occlusion
  c. Chronic urinary obstruction
  d. Recurrent infections
  e. Hypertension
  f. Metabolic disorders
  g. Diabetes mellitus
  h. Autoimmune disorders
3. Assessment
  a. Anorexia and nausea
  b. Headache
  c. Weakness and fatigue
  d. Hypertension
  e. Confusion and lethargy, followed by convulsions and coma
  f. Kussmaul respirations
  g. Diarrhea or constipation
  h. Muscle twitching and numbness of extremities
  i. Decreased urine output

Table 61-2. Stages of Chronic Renal Failure

First Stage

Characterized by diminished renal reserve
Polyuria
Nocturia
Polydipsia
Renal function tests abnormal

Second Stage

Characterized by renal insufficiency
Metabolic waste begins to accumulate
Increased BUN and creatinine

Third Stage

Characterized by renal failure
Hypertension
Edema
Poor urine output
Abnormal electrolyte values
Increased BUN and creatinine
Anemia
Metabolic acidosis

Fourth Stage

Characterized by uremia
Accumulation of nitrogenous waste products in blood
Increased urea, creatinine, and uric aid
Electrolyte imbalances
Anemia
Metabolic acidosis because of the inability of the kidney to excrete hydrogen ions
Urine concentration ability lost

j. Decreased urine specific gravity
k. Proteinuria
l. Anemia
m. **Azotemia**
n. Fluid overload and signs of heart failure
o. Uremic frost

D. Implementation
1. Monitor vital signs
2. Monitor urine and I&O (hourly in **ARF**)
3. Monitor weight, noting that an increase of 0.5 to 1 lb daily indicates fluid retention
4. Monitor BUN, creatinine, and electrolyte values
5. Monitor for acidosis and treat with sodium bicarbonate as prescribed
6. Assess urinalysis for protein, hematuria, casts, and specific gravity
7. Monitor LOC
8. Assess for signs of infection, since client may not demonstrate a temperature or an increased white blood cell (WBC) count
9. Assess for dysrhythmias, since a potassium level above 6 mEq/L will cause peaked T waves and a widened QRS complex
10. Monitor for fluid overload; assess lungs for rales and rhonchi
11. Monitor for edema
12. Administer prescribed diet of moderate protein to decrease the workload on the kidneys, high carbohydrate, and low potassium and phosphorus
13. Restrict sodium intake as prescribed based on the electrolyte level
14. Daily fluid allowances may be 400 to 1000 mL plus measured urinary output
15. Administer sodium polystyrene sulfonate (Kayexalate) to lower the potassium level as prescribed
16. Be alert to nephrotoxic medications, such as antibiotics, that may be prescribed
17. Prepare the client for dialysis if prescribed

E. Special problems in renal failure
1. Hypertension
   a. Failure of the kidneys to maintain homeostasis of the blood pressure
   b. Monitor vital signs
   c. Maintain fluid and sodium restrictions as prescribed
   d. Administer diuretics and antihypertensives as prescribed
   e. Administer propranolol (Inderal), a beta-adrenergic antagonist, as prescribed, which decreases renin release (renin causes vasoconstriction)
2. Hypervolemia
   a. Monitor vital signs
   b. Monitor I&O and weight
   c. Monitor for edema
   d. Monitor electrolytes
   e. Monitor for hypertension
   f. Monitor for CHF and pulmonary edema
   g. Administer diuretics as prescribed
   h. Instruct client to avoid foods with salt
   i. Instruct clients to avoid antacids or cold remedies containing sodium bicarbonate
3. Hypovolemia
   a. Monitor vital signs
   b. Monitor I&O
   c. Monitor electrolytes
   d. Monitor for hypotension
   e. Monitor for dehydration
   f. Provide replacement therapy based on electrolyte results
   g. Provide sodium supplements as prescribed depending on electrolyte value
4. Potassium retention
   a. Monitor vital signs and apical rate
   b. Monitor potassium level
   c. Monitor for dysrhythmias (peaked T waves and widened QRS complex) indicating hyperkalemia
   d. Provide a low-potassium diet
   e. Administer medication as prescribed to lower the potassium level
   f. Prepare the client for dialysis
5. Phosphorus retention
   a. Phosphorus rises and calcium drops, which leads to stimulation of parathyroid hormone, causing bone demineralization
   b. Treatment is aimed at lowering serum phosphorus levels
   c. Administer aluminum hydroxide preparations as prescribed (usually 1–5 g/day) that bind phosphorus in the intestine and allow the phosphorus to be eliminated
   d. Administer aluminum hydroxide preparations at meals and not with other medications because they bind medications in the intestinal tract
   e. Administer stool softeners and laxatives as prescribed to prevent constipation, because aluminum hydroxide preparations are constipating
6. Low calcium
   a. Occurs because of the high phosphorus level and because of the inability of the diseased kidney to activate vitamin D
   b. The absence of vitamin D causes poor absorption of calcium from the intestinal tract
   c. Monitor calcium level
   d. Administer calcium supplements as prescribed
   e. Administer activated vitamin D as prescribed
7. Metabolic acidosis
   a. The kidneys are unable to excrete hydrogen ions or manufacture bicarbonate, resulting in acidosis

b. Administer alkalizers such as sodium bicarbonate as prescribed
c. Note that clients with **CRF** adjust to low bicarbonate levels and do not become acutely ill

8. Anemia
a. A decreased rate of production of red blood cells (RBCs) occurs as a result of the diseased kidney and the decreased secretion of erythropoietin
b. Monitor hemoglobin and hematocrit
c. Administer epoetin alfa (Epogen) as prescribed to stimulate the production of RBCs
d. Administer folic acid (vitamin B$_9$) as prescribed instead of oral iron, since oral iron is not well absorbed by the GI tract in **CRF** and causes nausea and vomiting
e. Administer blood transfusions if prescribed, but blood transfusions are prescribed only when necessary because they decrease the stimulus to produce RBCs
f. Monitor bleeding
g. Instruct client to use a soft toothbrush
h. Administer stool softeners as prescribed
i. Avoid the administration of acetylsalicylic acid (aspirin) because the medication is excreted by the kidneys; if administered, high toxic levels will occur and prolong bleeding time

9. GI bleeding
a. Urea is broken down to ammonia by the intestinal bacteria, and ammonia is a mucosal irritant that causes ulceration and bleeding
b. Monitor hemoglobin and hematocrit
c. Monitor stools for occult blood

10. Infection and injury
a. Infection and injury need to be monitored and avoided because tissue breakdown causes increased potassium levels
b. Monitor for signs of infection
c. Avoid urinary catheters and provide strict asepsis during insertion and catheter care
d. Instruct client to avoid fatigue, which decreases body resistance
e. Instruct client to avoid persons with infections
f. Administer antibiotics as prescribed, monitoring for nephrotoxic effects

11. Pruritus
a. Urate crystals are excreted through the skin to rid the body of excess wastes
b. This deposit of crystals is called uremic frost and it is seen in advanced stages of **renal failure**
c. Monitor for skin breakdown, rash, and uremic frost
d. Provide good skin care and oral hygiene
e. Avoid the use of soaps
f. Administer antipruritics as prescribed

12. Muscle cramps
a. Occur in the extremities and hands and can be due to the low sodium level
b. Monitor electrolytes
c. Administer electrolyte replacements as prescribed
d. Administer heat and massage as prescribed

13. Ocular irritation
a. Calcium deposits in the conjunctiva cause burning and watering of the eyes
b. Administer medications to control the phosphate level as prescribed
c. Administer lubricating eye drops

14. Insomnia and fatigue
a. The diseased kidneys cause a build-up of wastes, causing fatigue in the client
b. Provide adequate rest periods
c. Administer mild CNS depressants as prescribed

15. Neurological changes
a. The build-up of active particles and fluids causes changes in the brain cells and leads to confusion and impairment in decision-making ability
b. Monitor for confusion and monitor LOC
c. Protect the client from injury
d. Provide a safe and hazard-free environment
e. Use side rails on bed as needed
f. Provide a calm and restful environment
g. Provide comfort measures and backrubs

16. Psychosocial problems: Monitor client for psychological problems such as depression, anxiety, suicidal behavior, denial, dependence/independence conflict, changes in body image

IV. Hemodialysis

A. Description
1. The diffusion of dissolved particles from one fluid compartment into another across a semipermeable membrane
2. The client's blood flows through one fluid compartment and the dialysate is in another fluid compartment

B. Functions of **hemodialysis**
1. Cleanses the blood of accumulated waste products
2. Removes the by-products of protein metabolism, such as urea, creatinine, and uric acid
3. Removes excessive fluids
4. Maintains or restores the body's buffer system
5. Maintains or restores electrolyte levels

C. Principles of **hemodialysis**
1. The semipermeable membrane is made of a thin, porous cellophane
2. The pore size of the membrane allows small

particles to pass through, such as urea, creatinine, uric acid, and water molecules

3. Proteins, bacteria, and blood cells are too large to pass through the membrane

4. The client's blood flows into the dialyzer; the movement of substances occurs from the blood to the dialysate

5. Diffusion: The movements of particles from an area of greater concentration to one of lesser concentration

6. Osmosis: The movement of fluids across a semipermeable membrane from an area of lesser to an area of greater concentration

7. Ultrafiltration: The movement of fluid across a semipermeable membrane as a result of an artificially created pressure gradient

D. Dialysate bath
   1. Composed of water and major electrolytes
   2. The dialysate bath need not be sterile because bacteria are too large to pass through

E. Implementation
   1. Monitor vital signs
   2. Monitor laboratory values before, during, and after dialysis
   3. Assess client for fluid overload prior to the procedure
   4. Assess patency of the blood access device
   5. Weigh client before and after procedure to determine fluid loss
   6. Hold antihypertensives and sedatives prior to the procedure as prescribed
   7. Monitor for shock and hypovolemia during the procedure
   8. Provide adequate nutrition (client may eat prior to the procedure)

V. Complications of Hemodialysis (Box 61–4)

A. Disequilibrium syndrome
   1. Description
      a. A rapid change in the composition of the extracellular fluid (ECF) occurs during hemodialysis
      b. Solutes are removed from the blood faster than from the cerebrospinal fluid (CSF) and brain; fluid is pulled into the brain, causing cerebral edema
   2. Assessment

BOX 61–4. Complications of Hemodialysis

Hypotension and shock
Muscle cramping
Electrolyte changes
Sepsis
Loss of blood
Hepatitis
Disequilibrium syndrome
Dialysis encephalopathy

---

   a. Nausea
   b. Vomiting
   c. Headache
   d. Hypertension
   e. Restlessness and agitation
   f. Confusion
   g. Seizures
   3. Implementation
      a. Monitor for signs of **disequilibrium syndrome**
      b. Notify physician if signs of **disequilibrium syndrome** occur
      c. Prepare to dialyze the client for a shorter period at reduced blood flow rates to prevent occurrence

B. Dialysis encephalopathy
   1. Description: An aluminum toxicity that occurs as a result of aluminum in the H_2O sources used in the dialysate bath and the ingestion of aluminum-containing antacids (phosphate binders)
   2. Assessment
      a. Progressive neurological impairment
      b. Mental cloudiness
      c. Speech disturbances
      d. Dementia
      e. Muscle incoordination
      f. Bone pain
      g. Seizures
   3. Implementation
      a. Monitor for signs of dialysis encephalopathy
      b. Notify physician if signs of dialysis encephalopathy occur
      c. Administer aluminum-chelating agents as prescribed so that the aluminum is freed and dialyzed from the body

VI. Access for Hemodialysis

A. Subclavian and femoral catheter (Fig. 61–1)
   1. Description
      a. A subclavian (subclavian vein) or femoral (femoral vein) catheter may be inserted for short-term or temporary use in **ARF**
      b. May be used until a fistula or graft matures, or when the client has fistula or graft access failure due to infection or clotting
   2. Implementation
      a. Assess insertion site for hematoma, bleeding, dislodging, and infection
      b. Do not use these catheters for any other reason other than dialysis
   3. Subclavian vein catheter
      a. Is usually filled with 10,000 units of heparin and capped to maintain patency between dialysis treatments
      b. The catheter should not be uncapped
      c. The catheter may be left in place for up to 6 weeks if complications do not occur

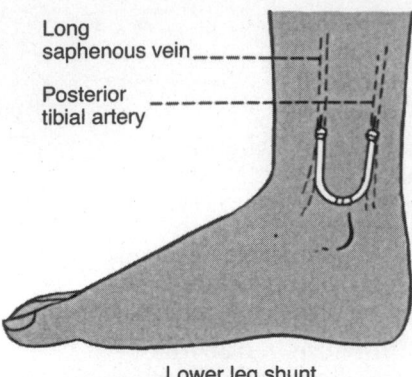
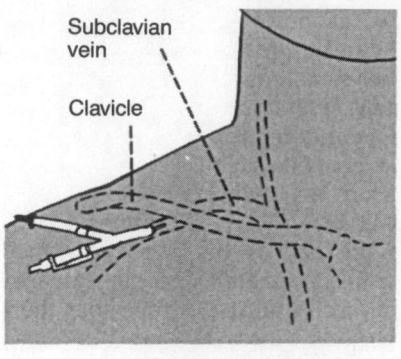
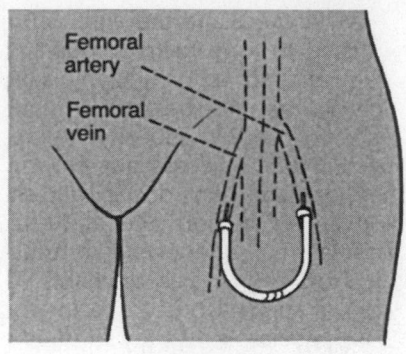

Long saphenous vein

Posterior tibial artery

Lower leg shunt

Subclavian vein

Clavicle

Subclavian cannula

Femoral artery

Femoral vein

Femoral catheter

FIGURE 61–1. Alternative access areas for hemodialysis: ankle, clavicle, and thigh. (From Black, J., & Matassarin-Jacobs, E. [1997]. *Medical-surgical nursing: Clinical management for continuity of care* [5th ed.]. Philadelphia: W. B. Saunders. p. 1514.)

4. Femoral vein catheter
   a. The client should not sit up at more than 45° or lean forward or the catheter may kink and occlude
   b. Assess extremity for circulation, temperature and pulses
   c. Prevent pulling or disconnecting of the catheter when giving care
   d. Maintain an IV of 250 mL of normal saline with 1250 units of heparin at 10 to 20 gtt/minute as prescribed to maintain the line
   e. Use an IV control pump with microdrip tubing if the heparin infusion is prescribed

B. External arteriovenous shunt (AV shunt) (Fig. 61–2)
   1. Description
      a. Access is formed by the surgical insertion of two Silastic cannulas into an artery and a vein in the forearm or leg, to form an external blood path
      b. The cannulas are connected to form a U shape; blood flows from the client's artery through the shunt into the vein
      c. A tube leading to the membrane compartment of the dialyzer is connected to the arterial cannula
      d. Blood fills the membrane compartment and flows back to the client by way of a tube connected to the venous cannula
      e. When dialysis is complete, the cannulas are clamped and reattached to form their U shape
   2. Advantages
      a. Can be used immediately following creation
      b. No venipuncture is necessary for dialysis
   3. Disadvantages
      a. External danger of disconnecting or dislodging
      b. Risk of hemorrhage, infection, or clotting
      c. Skin erosion around the catheter site can occur

4. Implementation
   a. Avoid wetting the shunt
   b. A dressing is completely wrapped around the shunt and kept dry and intact
   c. Cannula clamps need to be available at the client's bedside
   d. Do not measure a blood pressure, draw blood, place an IV, or administer injections in the shunt extremity
   e. Monitor for hemorrhage, infection, and clotting
   f. Monitor skin integrity around the insertion site
   g. Note that the shunt is patent if warm
   h. Auscultate and palpate for a bruit, although a bruit may not be heard and is not always felt with the shunt
   i. Notify physician immediately if signs of clotting, hemorrhage, or infection occur
5. Signs of clotting
   a. Fold back Ace wrap to expose Silastic tubing and assess for signs of clotting
   b. Fibrin-white flecks noted in the tubing
   c. The separation of serum and cells
   d. The absence of a previously heard bruit
   e. Coolness of the tubing or extremity
   f. Client complaints of a tingling sensation

C. Internal arteriovenous fistula (AV fistula) (Fig. 61–3)
   1. Description
      a. Access of choice for chronic dialysis clients
      b. Created surgically by anastamosing an artery in the arm to a vein; this creates an opening or fistula between a large artery and a large vein
      c. The flow of arterial blood into the venous system causes the veins to become engorged (maturity)
      d. Maturity takes about 1 to 2 weeks and is required before the fistula can be used, so that the engorged vein can be punctured with a large-bore needle for the dialysis procedure

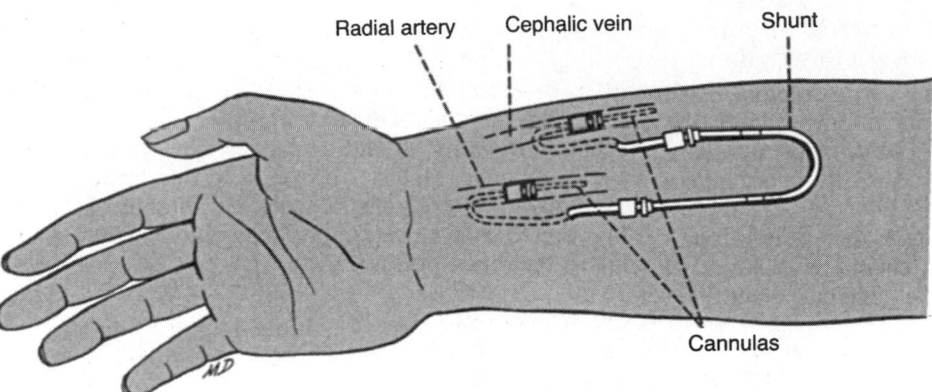

FIGURE 61–2. External arteriovenous shunt provides access to blood for hemodialysis. Arterial cannula is connected to a dialyzer, and blood returns through a venous cannula. When not connected to a hemodialyzer, the arterial cannula is connected to a venous cannula with a U-shaped shunt and secured carefully to the skin. (From Black, J., & Matassarin-Jacobs, E. [1997]. *Medical-surgical nursing: Clinical management for continuity of care* [5th ed.]. Philadelphia: W. B. Saunders. p. 1512.)

e. Subclavian or femoral catheters, peritoneal dialysis, or an external AV shunt can be used for dialysis while the fistula is maturing
2. Advantages
   a. Since the fistula is internal, there is less danger of clotting and bleeding
   b. The fistula can be used indefinitely
   c. Decreased incidence of infection
   d. No external dressing is required
   e. Allows freedom of movement
3. Disadvantages
   a. Cannot be used immediately after insertion
   b. Needle insertions are required for dialysis
   c. Infiltration of the needles during dialysis can occur and cause hematomas
   d. An aneurysm can form in the fistula
   e. **Arterial steal syndrome** can develop (too much blood is diverted to the vein and arterial perfusion to the hand is compromised)
   f. CHF can occur from the increased blood flow in the venous system

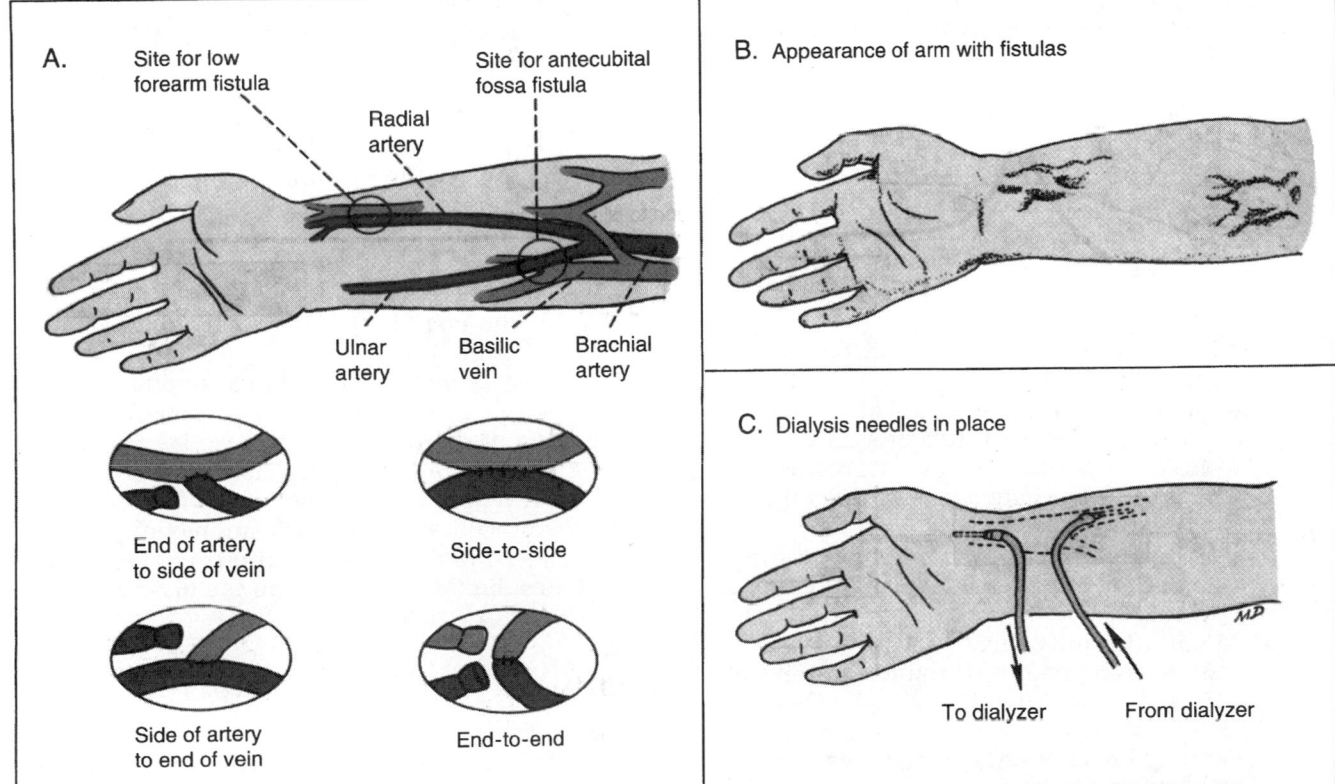

FIGURE 61–3. Internal arteriovenous fistula. Surgical creation of an arteriovenous anastomosis provides easy access to blood for hemodialysis. This method reduces the risk of infection and makes external shunts unnecessary except during hemodialysis. The internal fistula must be created 2 to 6 weeks before it can be used. Note that in this illustration, arteries, not veins, are toned. (From Black, J., & Matassarin-Jacobs, E. [1997]. *Medical-surgical nursing: Clinical management for continuity of care* [5th ed.]. Philadelphia: W. B. Saunders. p. 1513.)

D. Internal arteriovenous graft (AV graft)
   1. Description
      a. The internal graft is used primarily for chronic dialysis clients who do not have adequate blood vessels for the creation of a fistula
      b. An artificial graft made of Gore-Tex or a bovine (cow) carotid artery is used to create an artificial vein for blood flow
      c. The procedure involves the anastomosis of the graft to the artery, a tunneling under the skin, and anastomosis to a vein
      d. The graft can be used 2 weeks after insertion
      e. Complications of the graft include clotting, aneurysms, and infection
   2. Advantages
      a. Since the graft is internal, there is less danger of clotting and bleeding
      b. The graft can be used indefinitely
      c. Decreased incidence of infection
      d. No external dressing is required
      e. Allows freedom of movement
   3. Disadvantages
      a. Cannot be used immediately after insertion
      b. Needle insertions are required for dialysis
      c. Infiltration of the needles during dialysis can occur and cause hematomas
      d. An aneurysm can form in the fistula
      e. **Arterial steal syndrome** can develop (too much blood is diverted to the vein and arterial perfusion to the hand is compromised)
      f. CHF can occur from the increased blood flow in the venous system
E. Implementation for AV fistula and AV graft
   1. Do not measure a blood pressure, draw blood, place an IV, or administer injections in the fistula extremity
   2. Monitor for clotting
      a. Complaints of tingling or discomfort in the extremity
      b. Inability to palpate or auscultate a bruit or thrill over the fistula or graft
   3. Monitor for **arterial steal syndrome**
   4. Palpate or auscultate for bruit or thrill over the fistula or graft
   5. Palpate pulses below the fistula or graft and monitor for hand swelling as an indication of ischemia
   6. Monitor for infection
   7. Monitor lung and heart sounds for signs of CHF
   8. Notify physician immediately if signs of clotting, infection, or **arterial steal syndrome** occur

VII. Peritoneal Dialysis

A. Description
   1. The peritoneum is the dialyzing membrane (semipermeable membrane) and substitutes for kidney function during kidney failure
   2. Works on the principles of diffusion and osmosis, and the dialysis occurs via the transfer of fluid and solute from the blood stream through the peritoneum
   3. The peritoneal membrane is large and porous, allowing solutes and fluid to move via an osmotic gradient from an area of higher concentration in the body to lower concentration in the dialyzing fluid
   4. The peritoneal cavity is rich in capillaries; therefore, it provides a ready access to blood supply
B. Contraindications to peritoneal dialysis
   1. Peritonitis
   2. Recent abdominal surgery
   3. Abdominal adhesions
   4. Impending renal transplant
C. Dialysate solution
   1. Solution is sterile
   2. Electrolytes
      a. Sodium, 140 to 145 mEq
      b. Chloride, 101 to 110 mEq
      c. Calcium, 3.5 to 4.0 mEq
      d. Magnesium, 1.5 mEq
      e. Lactate/acetate (base), 43 to 45 mEq
   3. Osmolarity
      a. 1.5% = 365 mOsm
      b. 4.25% = 504 mOsm
   4. Glucose concentrations
      a. 1.5%
      b. 2.5%
      c. 4.25%
      d. The higher the glucose concentration, the greater the amount of fluid removed during an exchange
      e. Increasing the glucose concentration increases the concentration of active particles that cause osmosis and increases the rate of ultrafiltration and the amount of fluid removed
   5. Potassium: If hyperkalemia is not a problem, 4 mEq of potassium may be added to each bag of solution
   6. Heparin: Added to the dialysate solution to prevent clotting of the catheter
   7. Antibiotics: Prophylactic antibiotics may be added to the dialysate to prevent peritonitis
   8. Insulin: May be added to the dialysate for the diabetic client

VIII. Access for Peritoneal Dialysis (Fig. 61–4)

A. Description
   1. Surgical insertion of a siliconized rubber catheter into the abdominal cavity is required to allow infusion of dialysis fluid
   2. The preferred insertion site is 3 to 5 cm below the umbilicus as this area is relatively avascular and has less fascial resistance
   3. The catheters are tunneled under the skin to

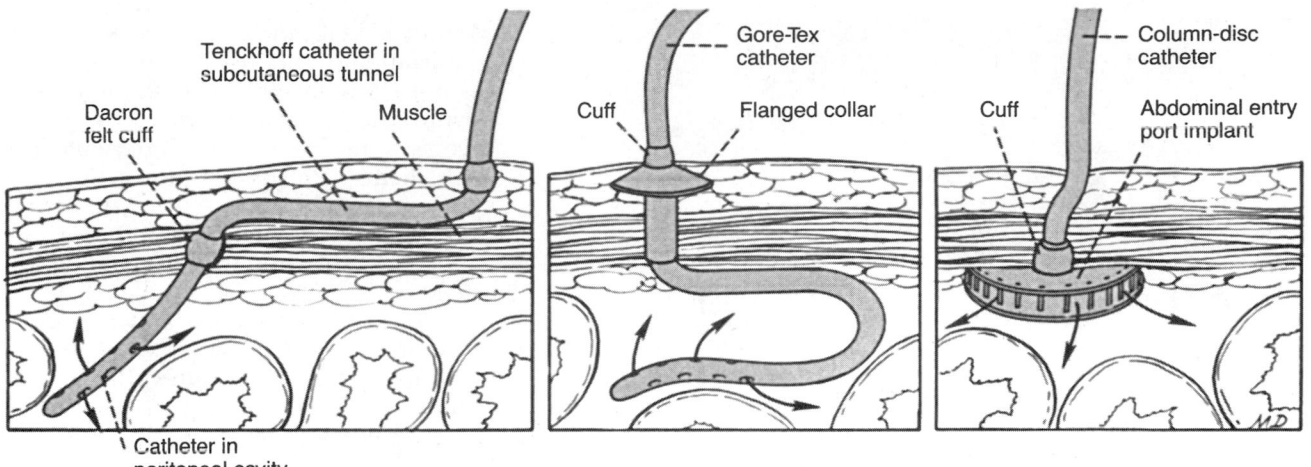

FIGURE 61–4. Three types of peritoneal dialysis catheters. The Tenckhoff catheter has two Dacron felt cuffs that hold the catheter in place and prevent dialysate leakage and bacterial invasion; the subcutaneous tunnel also helps prevent infection. The Gore-Tex catheter has a Dacron cuff above a flanged collar. The column-disc catheter has a cuff and a large abdominal entry port implant. (From Black, J., & Matassarin-Jacobs, E. [1997]. *Medical-surgical nursing: Clinical management for continuity of care* [5th ed.]. Philadelphia: W. B. Saunders. p. 1511.)

stabilize the catheter and reduce the risk of infection
4. Over a period of 1 to 2 weeks following insertion, there is an ingrowth of fibroblasts and blood vessels into the cuffs of the catheter, which fix the catheter in place and provide an extra barrier against dialysate leakage and bacterial invasion
B. Types of **peritoneal dialysis**
   1. Continuous ambulatory **peritoneal dialysis** (CAPD)
      a. Closely resembles renal function because it is a continuous process
      b. Does not require a machine for the procedure
      c. Promotes client independence
      d. The client performs self-dialysis 24 hours a day, 7 days a week
      e. Four dialysis cycles are administered in 24 hours, including an 8 hour dwell overnight
      f. One and a half to three liters of dialysate is instilled into the abdomen four times daily and allowed to dwell as prescribed
      g. The dialysis bag, attached to the catheter, is folded and carried in the client's clothing until time for outflow
      h. After dwell, the bag is placed lower than the insertion site so fluid drains by gravity flow
      i. When full, the bag is changed, new dialysate is instilled into the abdomen, and the process continues
   2. Automated **peritoneal dialysis** (APD) (Box 61–5)
      a. Similar to CAPD in that it is a continuous dialysis process
      b. Requires a peritoneal cycling machine

c. Can be done as intermittent peritoneal dialysis (IPD), continuous cycling peritoneal dialysis (CCPD), or nightly peritoneal dialysis (NPD)
C. Peritoneal dialysis infusion (Fig. 61–5)
   1. Description
      a. One infusion (inflow), dwell, and outflow is considered one exchange
      b. Uses an open system that presents a risk of infection
      c. Inflow: The infusion of 1 to 2 liters of dialysate is infused by gravity into the

---

BOX 61–5. Types of Automated Peritoneal Dialysis

CONTINUOUS CYCLING PERITONEAL DIALYSIS (CCPD)

Requires a peritoneal cycling machine
Consists of three cycles done at night and one cycle with an 8-hour dwell done in the morning
The peritoneal cavity is opened only for the on and off procedures, which reduces the risk of infection
The client does not need to do exchanges during the day

INTERMITTENT PERITONEAL DIALYSIS (IPD)

Requires a peritoneal cycling machine
Not a continuous dialysis procedure
Performed for 10 to 14 hours, three to four times a week

NIGHTLY PERITONEAL DIALYSIS (NPD)

Performed 8 to 12 hours each night with no daytime dwells

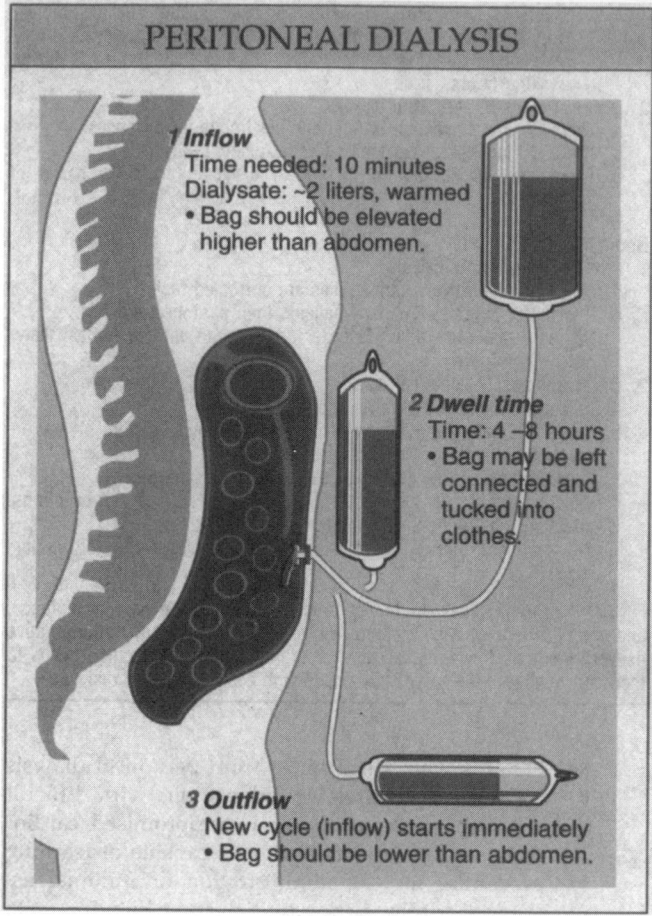

PERITONEAL DIALYSIS

1 Inflow
Time needed: 10 minutes
Dialysate: ~2 liters, warmed
• Bag should be elevated higher than abdomen.

2 Dwell time
Time: 4 –8 hours
• Bag may be left connected and tucked into clothes.

3 Outflow
New cycle (inflow) starts immediately
• Bag should be lower than abdomen.

FIGURE 61–5. Components of a long-term peritoneal dialysis system. (From Luckmann, J. [1997]. *Saunders manual of nursing care.* Philadelphia: W. B. Saunders. p. 1191.)

peritoneal space, which usually takes approximately 10 to 20 minutes.
  d. Dwell time: The amount of time that the dialysate solution remains in the peritoneal space; prescribed by the physician
  e. Outflow: Fluid drains out of body by gravity into the drainage bag
  2. Implementation before treatment
    a. Monitor vital signs
    b. Obtain weight
    c. Have client void if possible
    d. Assess electrolyte and glucose levels
  3. Implementation during treatment
    a. Monitor vital signs
    b. Monitor for signs of infection
    c. Monitor for respiratory distress, pain, or discomfort
    d. Monitor for signs of pulmonary edema
    e. Monitor for hypotension and hypertension
    f. Monitor for malaise, nausea, vomiting
    g. Assess catheter site dressing for wetness or bleeding

    h. Monitor dwell time as prescribed by the physician and initiate outflow
    i. Do not allow dwell time to extend beyond the physician's order as this increases the risk for hyperglycemia
    j. Turn client from side to side or have client sit upright if flow is slow to start
    k. Monitor outflow, which should be a continuous stream after the clamp is opened
    l. Monitor outflow for color and clarity
    m. Monitor I&O accurately
    n. If outflow is less than inflow, the difference is equal to the amount absorbed or retained by the client during dialysis and should be counted as intake

IX. Complications of Peritoneal Dialysis

A. Peritonitis
  1. Maintain meticulous sterile technique when hooking up or clamping off bags, and when caring for a catheter insertion site
  2. Follow institutional procedure for hooking up or clamping off bags, which may include scrubbing the connection sites with an antiseptic
  3. Monitor temperature closely
  4. Monitor for fever, cloudy outflow, and rebound abdominal tenderness
  5. If peritonitis is suspected, obtain a culture of the outflow to determine the infective organism
  6. Administer antibiotics as prescribed
B. Abdominal pain
  1. Pain during inflow is common during the first few exchanges, is caused by peritoneal irritation, and usually disappears after a week or two
  2. The cold temperature of dialysate aggravates the discomfort, and the dialysate should be warmed before use only with a special dialysate warmer pad
  3. Place a heating pad on the abdomen during the inflow to relieve discomfort
C. Insufficient outflow
  1. May be caused by catheter migration out of the peritoneal area; if this occurs, the catheter must be repositioned by the physician
  2. Insufficient outflow can also be caused by a full colon
  3. Maintain drainage bag below the client's abdomen
  4. Change client's outflow position by turning or ambulating
  5. Check for kinks in the tubing
  6. Encourage a high-fiber diet
  7. Administer stool softeners as prescribed
D. Leakage around the catheter site
  1. Over a period of 1 to 2 weeks following insertion of the catheter, an ingrowth of

fibroblasts and blood vessels into the cuffs of the catheter occurs, which fixes the catheter in place and provides an extra barrier against dialysate leakage and bacterial invasion

   2. It may take up to 2 weeks for the client to tolerate a full 2-L exchange without leaking around the catheter site

E. Characteristics of outflow
   1. During the first or initial exchanges, the outflow may be bloody; outflow should be clear and colorless thereafter
   2. A brown outflow indicates bowel perforation
   3. If the outflow is the same color as urine, this indicates bladder perforation
   4. Cloudy outflow indicates peritonitis

X. Uremic Syndrome

A. Description
   1. The accumulation of nitrogenous waste products in the blood due to the inability of the kidneys to filter out these waste products
   2. It may occur as a result of **acute** or **chronic renal failure**

B. Assessment
   1. **Oliguria**
   2. The presence of protein, red blood cells, and casts in the urine
   3. A urine specific gravity of 1.010
   4. Elevated levels of urea, uric acid, potassium, and magnesium in the urine
   5. Hypotension or hypertension
   6. Alterations in LOC
   7. Electrolyte imbalances
   8. Stomatitis
   9. Nausea or vomiting
   10. Diarrhea or constipation

C. Implementation
   1. Monitor vital signs
   2. Monitor electrolyte values
   3. Monitor I&O
   4. Provide diet low in protein unless the client is on **peritoneal dialysis**
   5. Limit sodium, nitrogen, potassium, and phosphate intake as prescribed

XI. Cystitis/Urinary Tract Infections (UTI)
(Box 61–6)

A. Description
   1. Inflammation of the bladder from infection or obstruction of the urethra
   2. The most common causative organisms are *Escherichia coli, Enterobacter, Pseudomonas,* and *Serratia*
   3. More common in women because women have a shorter urethra than men, and the location of the urethra in the women is close to the rectum
   4. Sexually active and pregnant women are most vulnerable to cystitis

B. Assessment

BOX 61–6. Causes of Cystitis

- Hormonal changes influencing alterations in vaginal flora
- Loss of bactericidal properties of prostatic secretions in men
- Sexual intercourse
- Poor-fitting diaphragms
- Use of spermicides
- Synthetic underwear and pantyhose
- Wet bathing suits
- Allergens or irritants, such as soaps, sprays, bubble bath, perfumed sanitary napkins
- Invasive urinary tract procedures
- Indwelling urethral catheters
- Bladder distention
- Urinary stasis
- Calculus

---

   1. Frequency and urgency
   2. Burning on urination
   3. Voiding in small amounts
   4. Inability to void
   5. Incomplete emptying of the bladder
   6. Lower abdominal discomfort or back discomfort
   7. Cloudy, dark, foul-smelling urine
   8. Hematuria
   9. Bladder spasms
   10. Malaise, chills, fever
   11. Nausea and vomiting

C. Implementation
   1. Obtain a urine specimen for culture and sensitivity to identify bacterial growth prior to administering prescribed antibiotics
   2. Instruct client to force fluids up to 3000 mL a day, especially if the client is taking a sulfonamide, because these medications can form crystals in concentrated urine
   3. Maintain acid urine pH (5.5) by an acid ash diet; instruct the client about foods to consume on an acid ash diet
   4. Use strict aseptic technique when inserting a urinary catheter
   5. Maintain closed urinary drainage systems for clients with indwelling catheters
   6. Provide meticulous perineal care for clients with indwelling catheters
   7. Administer medications as prescribed, which may include analgesics, antiseptics, antispasmodics, antibiotics, and antimicrobials
   8. Note that if the client is prescribed an aminoglycoside, a sulfonamide, or nitrofurantoin (Macrodantin), the actions of these medications are diminished by acidic urine
   9. Discourage caffeine products like coffee, tea, and cola
   10. Instruct the client to avoid alcohol
   11. Provide heat to the abdomen or sitz baths for complaints of discomfort

12. Instruct client to take medications as prescribed
13. Instruct client to take antibiotics on schedule and to take entire course of medication as prescribed, which may be a course of 10 to 14 days
14. Instruct client in the importance of follow-up urine culture following treatment
15. Preventive measures are listed in Box 61–7

XII. Urosepsis

A. Description
1. A gram-negative bacteremia originating in the urinary tract
2. The most common responsible organism is *Escherichia coli*
3. The most common cause is the presence of an indwelling catheter or an untreated UTI in a client who is medically compromised
4. The major problem is the ability of this bacterium to develop resistant strains
5. Urosepsis can lead to septic shock if not treated aggressively
B. Assessment: Fever is the most common and earliest manifestation
C. Implementation
1. Obtain a urine specimen for urine culture and sensitivity
2. Administer IV antibiotics as prescribed, usually until the client has been afebrile for 3 to 5 days
3. Administer oral antibiotics as prescribed after the 3- to 5-day afebrile period

XIII. Urethritis

A. Description
1. An inflammation of the urethra commonly associated with sexually transmitted diseases (STD), it also may be seen with cystitis
2. In men, it is most often caused by gonorrhea and chlamydial infection

---

BOX 61–7. Prevention of Cystitis

Teach the female client good perineal care and to wipe from front to back
Instruct client to avoid bubble baths and tub baths and avoid vaginal deodorants
Instruct client to void every 2 to 3 hours
Instruct client to void and drink a glass of water after intercourse
Instruct women to wear cotton pants and to avoid wearing panty hose with slacks, tight clothes, and sitting in a wet bathing suit
Teach pregnant women to void every 2 hours
Encourage menopausal women to use estrogen vaginal creams to restore pH
Instruct women to use water-soluble lubricants for coitus, especially after menopause

---

3. In women, it is most often caused by feminine hygiene sprays, perfumed toilet paper and sanitary napkins, spermicidal jellies, UTIs, and changes in the vaginal mucosal lining
B. Assessment
1. Men
a. Burning on urination
b. Frequency
c. Urgency
d. Nocturia
e. Difficulty in voiding
f. Discharge from the penis
2. Women
a. Frequency
b. Urgency
c. Nocturia
d. Painful urination
e. Difficulty in voiding
f. Lower abdominal discomfort
C. Implementation
1. Encourage fluids
2. Prepare client for testing to determine whether an STD is present
3. Administer antibiotics as prescribed
4. Instruct client in the use of sitz baths
5. If stricture occurs, prepare client for dilation of the urethra and instillation of an antiseptic solution
6. Instruct client to avoid intercourse until the symptoms subside or treatment of the STD is complete
7. Instruct women to avoid the use of perfumed toilet paper, sanitary napkins, and feminine hygiene sprays

XIV. Ureteritis and Pyelonephritis

A. Ureteritis
1. An inflammation of the ureter that is commonly associated with pyelonephritis
2. Chronic pyelonephritis causes the ureter to become fibrotic and narrowed by strictures
B. Pyelonephritis
1. An inflammation of the renal pelvis and the parenchyma, commonly caused by bacterial invasion
2. Acute pyelonephritis often occurs after bacterial contamination of the urethra or following an invasive procedure of the urinary tract
3. Chronic pyelonephritis most commonly occurs following chronic obstruction with reflux or chronic disorders
4. *Escherichia coli* is the most common bacterial causative organism
C. Acute pyelonephritis
1. Usually a short course that recurs as a relapse of a previous infection or as a new infection
2. Can progress to bacteremia or chronic pyelonephritis

3. Assessment
   a. Fever and chills
   b. Nausea
   c. Flank pain on the affected side
   d. Costovertebral angle (CVA) tenderness
   e. Headache
   f. Muscular pain
   g. Dysuria
   h. Frequency and urgency
   i. Cloudy, bloody, or foul-smelling urine
   j. Increased white blood cells in the urine

D. Chronic pyelonephritis
  1. A slow, progressive disease that is usually associated with recurrent acute attacks
  2. Causes contraction of the kidneys and dysfunctioning of the nephrons, which are replaced by scar tissue
  3. Can lead to **renal failure**
  4. Assessment
   a. Frequently diagnosed incidentally when a client is being evaluated for hypertension
   b. Poor urine-concentrating ability
   c. Pyuria
   d. **Azotemia**
   e. Proteinuria
   f. Anemia
   g. Acidosis

E. Implementation
  1. Monitor vital signs
  2. Monitor I&O
  3. Monitor weight
  4. Encourage fluids up to 3000 mL a day
  5. Encourage adequate rest
  6. Instruct client in high-calorie, low-protein diet
  7. Provide warm moist compresses to flank area
  8. Encourage client to take warm baths
  9. Administer analgesics, antipyretics, and antiemetics as prescribed
  10. Administer antibiotics as prescribed
  11. Administer urinary antiseptics as prescribed
  12. Monitor for signs of **renal failure**

XV. Glomerulonephritis

A. Description
  1. A term that includes a variety of disorders, most of which are caused by an immunological reaction
  2. It results in proliferative and inflammatory changes within the glomerular structure
  3. Destruction, inflammation, and sclerosis of the glomeruli of both kidneys occurs
  4. The inflammation of the glomeruli results from an antigen-antibody reaction produced from an infection elsewhere in the body
  5. Loss of kidney function develops

B. Causes
  1. Immunological diseases
  2. Streptococcal infection Group A beta-hemolytic

3. History of pharyngitis or tonsillitis 2 to 3 weeks prior to symptoms
4. Autoimmune diseases

C. Types
  1. Acute: Occurs 2 to 3 weeks after a streptococcal infection
  2. Chronic: Can occur after the acute phase or slowly over time

D. Complications
  1. Heart failure
  2. Hypertensive encephalopathy
  3. Pulmonary edema
  4. Renal failure

E. Assessment
  1. Gross hematuria
  2. Dark, smoky, cola-colored or red-brown urine
  3. Proteinuria that produces a persistent and excessive foam in the urine
  4. Urinary debris
  5. Mid to high specific gravity
  6. Low urinary pH
  7. **Oliguria** or **anuria**
  8. Headache
  9. Chills and fever
  10. Fatigue and weakness
  11. Anorexia, nausea, and vomiting
  12. Pallor
  13. Edema in the face, periorbital area, and feet, or generalized
  14. Shortness of breath, ascites, pleural effusion, and CHF
  15. Abdominal or flank pain
  16. Hypertension
  17. Reduced visual acuity
  18. Increased BUN and creatinine levels
  19. Increased antistreptolysin O titer (used to diagnosis disorders caused by streptococcal infections)

F. Implementation
  1. Monitor vital signs
  2. Monitor I&O and urine closely
  3. Monitor daily weight
  4. Monitor for edema
  5. Monitor for fluid overload, ascites, pulmonary edema, and CHF
  6. Restrict fluid intake as prescribed
  7. Provide a high-calorie and low-protein diet
  8. Restrict sodium intake as prescribed if edema is present
  9. Provide bed rest and limited activity
  10. Instruct client to obtain treatment for infections—specifically, sore throats and upper respiratory infections
  11. Administer diuretics, antihypertensives, and antibiotics as prescribed
  12. Monitor for signs of **renal failure,** cardiac failure, hypertensive encephalopathy
  13. Initiate seizure precautions as indicated and provide safety measures
  14. Instruct client to report signs of bloody urine, headache, or edema

XVI. Nephrotic Syndrome

A. Description: A set of clinical manifestations arising from protein wasting secondary to diffuse glomerular damage

B. Assessment
1. Proteinuria
2. Hypoalbuminemia
3. Edema
4. Hyperlipidemia
5. Waxy pallor to the skin
6. Anemia
7. Anorexia
8. Malaise
9. Irritability
10. Amenorrhea or abnormal menses
11. Hematuria may be present
12. Hypertension

C. Implementation
1. Monitor vital signs
2. Monitor I&O
3. Bed rest if severe edema is present
4. Normal to low-protein diet as prescribed, with adequate carbohydrate and calorie intake
5. Monitor daily weight
6. Provide a mild sodium restriction as prescribed
7. Monitor potassium level, as potassium may be restricted from the diet if the potassium level rises
8. Administer diuretics as prescribed
9. Administer steroids and cytotoxic medications as prescribed
10. Administer plasma volume expanders, such as albumin, plasma, and dextran, to raise the osmotic pressure
11. Administer anticoagulants as prescribed for those clients who develop renal vein thrombosis

XVII. Hydronephrosis

A. Description
1. Distention of the renal pelvis and calices, caused by an obstruction of normal urine flow
2. The urine becomes trapped proximal to the obstruction
3. The causes include calculus, tumors, scar tissue, or kinks in the ureter

B. Assessment
1. Hypertension
2. Headache
3. Flank pain
4. Electrolyte imbalances

C. Implementation
1. Monitor vital signs frequently
2. Monitor for fluid and electrolyte imbalances, including dehydration after the obstruction is relieved

3. Monitor for diuresis, which can lead to fluid depletion
4. Monitor daily weight
5. Monitor urine for specific gravity, albumin, and glucose
6. Administer fluid replacement as prescribed

XVIII. Genitourinary Tuberculosis

A. Description
1. Usually a late manifestation of tuberculosis, caused by the spread of *Mycobacterium tuberculosis* from the lungs through the blood stream
2. *Mycobacterium tuberculosis* is the cause of tuberculosis and is most often seen in the poor, the malnourished, those living in close housing, and in the immunosuppressed client

B. Assessment
1. Frequency and pain on urination
2. Bladder spasms
3. Fatigue
4. Weight loss
5. Tubercle bacilli in urine culture
6. Lesions noted on x-ray film
7. Tuberculosis nodules noted on the prostate

C. Implementation
1. Administer antitubercular medications as prescribed
2. Use precautions when handling urine specimens since the bacillus in the urine is infectious
3. Instruct the client to use precautions to prevent the spread of the disease
4. Instruct the client to use condoms during intercourse to prevent the spread of the disease

XIX. Polycystic Disease

A. Description
1. Cystic formation and hypertrophy of the kidneys which leads to cystic rupture, infection, the formation of scar tissue, and damaged nephrons
2. There is no known way to arrest the progress of the destructive cysts
3. The ultimate result of this disease is **renal failure**

B. Types
1. Infantile polycystic disease: An inherited autosomal recessive trait that results in the death of the infant within a few months after birth
2. Adult polycystic disease: Autosomal dominant trait that results in end-stage renal disease

C. Assessment
1. Flank, lumbar, or abdominal pain
2. Fever and chills
3. UTIs

4. Hematuria, proteinuria, pyuria
5. Calculi
6. Hypertension
7. Palpable abdominal masses and enlarged kidneys

D. Implementation
1. Monitor for gross hematuria, which indicates cyst rupture
2. Increase sodium and water because sodium loss rather than retention occurs
3. Provide bed rest if ruptured cysts and bleeding occur
4. Prepare client for percutaneous cyst puncture for relief of obstruction, or for draining an abscess
5. Prepare client for dialysis or renal transplantation
6. Encourage client to seek genetic counseling

XX. Urolithiasis and Nephrolithiasis

A. Description
1. Calculi or stones can form anywhere in the urinary tract; however, the most frequent site is the kidneys
2. The problems that can occur as a result of calculi are pain, obstruction, and tissue trauma with secondary hemorrhage and infection
3. A KUB film, intravenous pyelogram (IVP), computed tomography (CT) scan, and renal ultrasonography will determine the stone location
4. A stone analysis will be done after passage to determine the type of stone and assist in determining treatment
5. **Urolithiasis** refers to the formation of urinary stones; urinary calculi are formed in the ureter
6. **Nephrolithiasis** refers to the formation of kidney stones; kidney stones are formed in the renal parenchyma
7. When a calculus occludes the ureter and blocks the flow of urine, the ureter dilates; this is known as hydroureter
8. If the obstruction is not removed, urinary stasis results in infection, impairment of renal function on the side of the blockage, and resultant hydronephrosis and irreversible kidney damage

B. Causes
1. Family history of stone formation
2. Diet high in calcium, vitamin D, milk, protein, oxalate, purines, or alkali
3. A high intake of purine-rich foods
4. Obstruction and urinary stasis
5. Dehydration
6. Use of diuretics, which can cause volume depletion
7. UTIs and prolonged urinary catheterization
8. Immobilization
9. Hypercalcemia and hyperparathyroidism
10. Elevated uric acid level, as in gout

C. Assessment
1. Renal colic originates in the lumbar region and radiates around the side and down toward the testicle in men, and to the bladder in women
2. Ureteral colic radiates toward the genitalia and thigh
3. Sharp, severe pain of sudden onset
4. Dull, aching kidney(s)
5. Nausea and vomiting, pallor, and diaphoresis during acute pain
6. Urinary frequency with alternating retention
7. Signs of UTI
8. Low-grade fever
9. RBCs, WBCs, and bacteria in urinalysis
10. Hematuria

D. Implementation
1. Monitor vital signs
2. Monitor I&O
3. Assess for fever, chills, and infection
4. Monitor for nausea, vomiting, and diarrhea
5. Force fluids up to 3000 mL/day unless contraindicated to facilitate the passage of the stone and prevent infection
6. Strain all urine for the presence of stones
7. Send stones to the laboratory for analysis
8. Provide warm baths and heat to flank area
9. Administer analgesics at regularly scheduled intervals as prescribed to relieve pain
10. Assess client's response to pain medication
11. Administer IV fluids as prescribed to increase the flow of urine and facilitate the passage of the stone
12. Assist the client in performing relaxation techniques to assist in relieving pain
13. Instruct client in the diet specific to the stone composition
14. Maintain urinary pH depending on type of stone
15. Turn and reposition immobilized clients
16. Prepare client for surgical procedures if prescribed

E. Stone composition (Boxes 61–8 and 61–9)
1. Calcium phosphate stones
   a. Caused by supersaturation of urine with calcium and phosphate

---

BOX 61–8. Alkaline Ash Diet

OUTCOME

Increases the pH
Reduces the acidity of the urine

FOODS TO INCLUDE

Milk
Fruits, except cranberries, plums, and prunes
Rhubarb
Most vegetables
Small amounts of beef, halibut, veal, trout, and salmon allowed

---

BOX 61–9. Acid Ash Diet

OUTCOME

Decreases pH
Makes the urine more acid

FOODS TO INCLUDE

Cheese, eggs
Meat, fish, oysters, poultry
Bread, cereal, whole grains
Pastries
Cranberries, prunes, plums, tomatoes
Corn and legumes

FOODS TO AVOID

Carbonated beverages
Baking soda or powder
All vegetables except corn and legumes
Olives, pickles
Nuts, other than peanuts

---

    b. Diet includes acid ash foods, because calcium stones have an alkaline chemistry

    c. Dietary prescription may include decreased intake of foods high in calcium and phosphate to reduce urinary calcium content, and avoidance of excess vitamin D intake to prevent stones from forming

  2. Calcium oxalate stones

    a. Caused by supersaturation of urine with calcium and oxalate

    b. Diet includes acid ash foods, because calcium stones have an alkaline chemistry

    c. Dietary prescription may include decreasing intake of foods high in calcium

    d. Dietary prescription may include avoiding oxalate food sources to reduce urinary oxalate content and the formation of stones

    e. Oxalate-rich foods sources include tea, almonds, cashews, chocolate, cocoa, beans, spinach, and rhubarb

  3. Struvite stones

    a. Also called triple phosphate stones—composed of magnesium and ammonium phosphate

    b. Caused by urea splitting by bacteria

    c. Struvite stones tend to form in alkaline urine

    d. Diet includes acid ash foods

    e. Dietary prescription includes limiting high-phosphate foods, such as dairy products, red and organ meats, and whole grains, to reduce urinary phosphate content

  4. Uric acid stones

    a. Caused by excess dietary purine or gout

    b. Uric acid stones tend to form in acidic urine

    c. Dietary prescription may include alkaline ash foods and decreased intake of purine sources, such as organ meats, gravies, red wines, and sardines, to reduce urinary purine content

    d. Allopurinol (Zyloprim) may be prescribed to lower uric acid levels

  5. Cystine stones

    a. Caused by cystine crystal formation

    b. Cystine stones tend to form in acidic urine

    c. Diet includes alkaline ash foods

    d. Dietary prescription may also include a low intake of methionine, an essential amino acid that forms cystine, and the client would be instructed to avoid meat, milk, cheese, and eggs

    e. Dietary measures also focus on encouraging fluids up to 3 L a day, unless contraindicated, to help dilute the urine and prevent cystine crystals from forming

XXI. Surgical Management of Kidney Stones

A. Cystoscopy

  1. May be done for stones located in the bladder or lower ureter

  2. There is no incision

  3. One or two ureteral catheters are inserted past the stone

  4. The stone may be manipulated and dislodged by the procedure

  5. The catheters may mechanically guide the stones downward as they are removed

  6. Catheters are left in place for 24 hours to drain the urine trapped proximal to the stone and to dilate the ureter

  7. A continuous chemical irrigation may be prescribed to dissolve the stone

B. Extracorporeal shock wave lithotripsy (ESWL)

  1. Noninvasive mechanical procedure for breaking up stones that are located in the kidney or upper ureter so that they can pass spontaneously or be removed by other methods

  2. Fluoroscopy is utilized to visualize the stone

  3. There are no incisions or drains

  4. Ultrasonic waves are delivered through a bath of warm water to the areas of the stone to disintegrate it

  5. Stones are passed in the urine within a few days

  6. Preprocedure: NPO for 8 hours prior to procedure; a laxative may be prescribed

  7. Postprocedure

    a. Monitor vital signs

    b. Monitor I&O

    c. Monitor for bleeding

    d. Monitor for pain and signs of urinary obstruction

    e. Instruct client to increase fluid intake to wash out the stone fragments

f. Inform client that ambulation is important

C. Percutaneous lithotripsy
1. Performed for stones in the bladder, ureter, or kidneys
2. An invasive procedure in which a guide is inserted under fluoroscopy near the area of the stone
3. An ultrasonic wave is aimed at the stone to break it into fragments
4. May be performed via cystoscopy or nephroscopy
5. No incision is required for cystoscopy; however, a small flank incision is needed for nephrostomy
6. The client may possibly have an indwelling catheter
7. A nephrostomy tube may be placed to administer chemical irrigations to break up the stone; nephrostomy tube may remain in place for 1 to 5 days
8. Encourage client to drink 3000 to 4000 mL of fluid per day following the procedure
9. Monitor for and instruct client to monitor for complications of infection, hemorrhage, and extravasation of fluid into the retroperitoneal cavity

D. Ureterolithotomy
1. An open surgical procedure, performed if lithotripsy is not effective
2. Performed if the location of the stone is in the ureter
3. Incision into the ureter is made through a lower abdominal or flank incision to remove the stone
4. The client may have a Penrose drain, ureteral stent catheter, and indwelling bladder catheter

E. Pyelolithotomy
1. A flank incision into the kidney is made to remove stones from the renal pelvis
2. A large flank incision is required
3. The client will have a Penrose drain and indwelling catheter

F. Nephrolithotomy
1. Incision into the kidney is made to remove the stone
2. A large flank incision is required
3. The client may have a nephrostomy tube and an indwelling catheter

G. Partial or total nephrectomy
1. Performed if there is extensive kidney damage, renal infection, or severe obstruction and to prevent stone recurrence
2. Postoperative implementation
   a. The plan of care will be based on the incision location and the type of drainage tubes present
   b. Monitor incision, particularly if a Penrose drain is in place, as it will drain large amounts of urine
   c. Protect the skin from urinary drainage

d. Place an ostomy pouch over the Penrose drain to protect the skin if urinary drainage is excessive
e. Monitor the nephrostomy tube, which may be attached to a drainage bag for a free flow of urine
f. If urethral catheters are in place, do not irrigate
g. Monitor indwelling Foley catheter for drainage
h. Encourage fluid intake to ensure 2500 to 3000 mL or more of urine output per day
i. Monitor I&O closely
j. Determine composition of stone from laboratory analysis
k. Instruct client in dietary restrictions if required
l. Instruct clients about medications that may be needed for long-term to reduce the development of calculi
m. Medications prescribed for calcium stones may include phosphates, thiazide diuretics, and allopurinol (Zyloprim)
n. Pyridoxine or magnesium oxide may be prescribed for clients with oxalate stones
o. Allopurinol (Zyloprim) may be prescribed for oxalate and uric acid stones
p. Long-term antibiotics may be prescribed for struvite or cystine stones

XXII. Kidney Tumors

A. Description
1. May be benign or malignant, bilateral or unilateral
2. Common site of metastasis includes bone, lungs, liver, spleen, or other kidney
3. The exact cause of renal carcinoma is unknown

B. Assessment
1. Dull flank pain
2. Palpable renal mass
3. Painless gross hematuria

C. Radical nephrectomy
1. Description
   a. Removal of the entire kidney, adjacent adrenal gland, and renal artery and vein
   b. Radiation therapy and possibly chemotherapy may follow radical nephrectomy
2. Postoperative implementation
   a. Monitor vital signs
   b. Monitor abdomen for distention caused by bleeding
   c. Observe bed linens under the client for bleeding
   d. Monitor for hypotension, decreases in urinary output, and alterations in LOC, as indicating signs of hemorrhage
   e. Monitor for signs of adrenal insufficiency
   f. In clients with adrenal insufficiency, a large urinary output followed by

hypotension and subsequent **oliguria** occurs
  g. Administer IV fluids and packed RBCs as prescribed
  h. Monitor I&O and daily weight
  i. Monitor for a urinary output of 30 to 50 mL an hour to ensure adequate renal function
  j. Monitor urine for specific gravity
  k. Maintain semi-Fowler's position
  l. Monitor for signs of respiratory complications related to surgery
  m. Encourage coughing and deep-breathing exercises
  n. Monitor bowel sounds for paralytic ileus
  o. Apply antiembolism stockings as prescribed
  p. Do not irrigate or manipulate the nephrostomy tube if in place
  q. Administer pain medications as prescribed

XXIII. Bladder Trauma

A. Description
  1. Occurs following a blunt or penetrating injury to the lower abdomen
  2. Penetrating wounds occur as a result of a stabbing or a gunshot wound, or from other objects piercing the abdominal wall
  3. A fractured pelvis that causes bone fragments to puncture the bladder is the most common cause of bladder trauma
  4. A blunt trauma causes compression of the abdominal wall and the bladder
B. Assessment
  1. **Anuria**
  2. Hematuria
  3. Pain over costovertebral angle (CVA)
  4. Nausea and vomiting
C. Implementation
  1. Monitor vital signs
  2. Monitor for hematuria, hemorrhage, and signs of shock
  3. Promote bed rest
  4. Monitor pain level
  5. Prepare client for insertion of a suprapubic catheter to aid in urinary drainage if prescribed
  6. Prepare client for surgical repair of the laceration if prescribed

XXIV. Epididymitis

A. Description
  1. An acute or chronic inflammation of the epididymis that occurs as a result of a UTI, STD, prostatitis, or long-term use of a Foley catheter
  2. The infective organism passes upward through the urethra and ejaculatory duct, along the vas deferens to the epididymis

B. Assessment
  1. Scrotal pain
  2. Groin pain
  3. Swelling in scrotum and groin
  4. Pus and bacteria in the urine
  5. Fever and chills
  6. Abscess development
C. Implementation
  1. Encourage fluid intake
  2. Encourage bed rest with the scrotum elevated to prevent traction on the spermatic cord, to facilitate drainage, and to relieve pain
  3. Instruct client in the intermittent application of cold compresses to scrotum
  4. Instruct client in the use of sitz baths
  5. Instruct client in the administration of antibiotics for self and sexual partner if chlamydia infection or gonorrhea is the cause
  6. Instruct client to avoid lifting, straining, and sexual contact until the infection subsides

XXV. Prostatitis

A. Description
  1. An inflammation of the prostate gland that can be caused by an infectious agent (bacterial) or by tissue hyperplasia (abacterial)
  2. Bacterial prostatitis occurs as a result of the organism reaching the prostate via the urethra or blood stream
  3. Abacterial prostatitis usually occurs following a viral illness or a decrease in sexual activity
B. Assessment
  1. Bacterial
    a. Fever and chills
    b. Dysuria
    c. Urethral discharge
    d. Boggy, tender prostate
    e. Urethral discharge on palpation of prostate
    f. WBCs found in prostatic secretions
  2. Abacterial
    a. Backache
    b. Dysuria
    c. Perineal pain
    d. Frequency
    e. Hematuria may be present
    f. Irregularly enlarged, firm, and tender prostate
C. Implementation
  1. Encourage adequate fluid intake
  2. Instruct client in the use of sitz baths to promote comfort
  3. Administer antibiotics, analgesics, antispasmodics, and stool softeners as prescribed
  4. Inform client of activities to drain the prostate, such as intercourse, masturbation, and prostatic massage

5. Instruct client to avoid spicy foods, coffee, alcohol, prolonged auto rides, and sexual intercourse during an acute inflammation

XXVI. Benign Prostatic Hypertrophy (BPH)

A. Description
1. A slow enlargement of the prostate gland, with hypertrophy and hyperplasia of normal tissue
2. The enlargement causes narrowing of the urethra and results in partial or complete obstruction
3. The cause is unknown, and the disorder usually occurs in men older than 50 years

B. Assessment
1. Urgency, frequency, and hesitancy
2. Changes in size and force of urinary stream
3. Retention
4. Dribbling
5. Nocturia
6. Hematuria
7. Urinary stasis
8. Urinary tract infections

C. Implementation
1. Encourage fluids up to 2000 to 3000 mL per day unless contraindicated
2. Prepare for bladder drainage via urinary catheterization for distention
3. Avoid administering medications that cause urinary retention, such as the anticholinergics, antihistamines and decongestants
4. Administer finasteride (Proscar) as prescribed to shrink the prostate gland and improve urine flow
5. Prepare client for surgery as prescribed (Box 61–10)

XXVII. Kidney Transplantation

A. Description
1. Implantation of a human kidney from a compatible donor into a recipient
2. Performed for irreversible kidney failure
3. Immunosuppressive medications must be taken by the recipient for life

B. Living related donors
1. Most desirable source of kidneys for transplant is living related donors who match the client closely
2. Screened for ABO blood group, tissue-specific antigen, human leukocyte antigen (HLA) suitability, and mixed lymphocyte culture index (histocompatibility)

BOX 61–10. Surgical Interventions for BPH

Transurethral resection (TUR)
Retropubic prostatectomy
Suprapubic prostatectomy
Perineal prostatectomy

---

3. Donor must be in excellent health with two properly functioning kidneys
4. The emotional well-being of the donor is determined
5. Complete understanding of the donation process and outcome is necessary

C. Cadaver donors
1. Must meet criteria of brain death
2. Must be under 60 years of age
3. Must have normal renal function
4. No malignant disease outside of the central nervous system (CNS) can be present
5. No generalized infection can be present
6. No abdominal or renal trauma can be present
7. Normal BP must be present
8. Potential donor must have a negative hepatitis B antigen and negative HIV antibody
9. Continuous ventilation and heartbeat are maintained until the kidneys are surgically removed
10. Once the potential donor has demonstrated cerebral death, it is crucial to restore intravascular volume, wean from vasopressors, and establish diuresis

D. Warm ischemic time
1. The time elapsed between cessation of perfusion and cooling of the kidney, and the time required for anastomosis of the kidney
2. Maximal allowable warm ischemic time is 30 to 60 minutes
3. The kidney can be cooled, and then the maximum time for transplantation is increased to 24 to 48 hours

E. Preoperative implementation
1. Verify histocompatability tests of identical twin or family member
2. Administer immunosuppressive medications to recipient as prescribed for 2 days before the transplantation
3. Maintain protective isolation
4. Verify that **hemodialysis** of recipient was completed 24 hours before transplant
5. Ensure client is free of any infections
6. Assess renal function studies
7. Encourage discussion of feelings of both donor and recipient

F. Postoperative implementation
1. Kidney begins to function immediately, or it may be delayed a few days
2. **Hemodialysis** is performed until adequate kidney function is established
3. Monitor vital signs
4. Monitor I&O
5. Monitor urine output every hour
6. Monitor daily laboratory studies, urine for blood and specific gravity, daily weight, pulse oximetry, BUN, and creatinine levels
7. Maintain client in semi-Fowler's position
8. Monitor for patency of Foley catheter
9. Note that urine is pink and bloody initially

but gradually returns to normal within several days to weeks

10. Monitor for gross hematuria and clots, which are not expected, and notify the physician if they occur

11. Monitor three-way Foley irrigation if prescribed, to prevent blood clot formation

12. Note that the Foley should be removed as soon as possible to prevent infection

13. Maintain protective isolation precautions and monitor for infection

14. Monitor IV fluids closely and for fluid overload

15. Begin oral fluids in 12 to 24 hours as prescribed

16. Monitor for bowel sounds and initiate diet as prescribed when bowel sounds return

17. Maintain good oral hygiene, monitoring for stomatitis and bacterial and fungal infections

18. Encourage coughing and deep-breathing exercises

19. Maintain strict aseptic technique with wound care

20. Administer medications as prescribed, which may include antifungal medications, antibiotics, immunosuppressive agents, and corticosteroids

21. Assess for organ rejection (Box 61–11)

22. Promote live donor and recipient relationship

23. Monitor client and recipient for depression

G. Graft rejection: Except for identical twin donor and recipient, the major postoperative complication is graft rejection

1. Assessment
   a. Fever
   b. Malaise
   c. Elevated WBC count
   d. Graft tenderness
   e. Signs of deteriorating renal function
   f. Acute hypertension
   g. Anemia

2. Hyperacute rejection
   a. Occurs immediately after surgery to 48 hours postoperatively

b. Implementation: Removal of rejected kidney

3. Acute rejection
   a. Occurs within 6 weeks but can occur as late as 2 years
   b. Potentially reversible with increased immunosuppression
   c. Implementation: High doses of steroids; if steroids are ineffective, monoclonal antibodies may be administered

4. Chronic rejection
   a. Occurs slowly months to years after transplant
   b. Can be irreversible
   c. Mimics **CRF**
   d. Implementation: Immunosuppressive medications

PRACTICE QUESTIONS

1. The home care nurse is making home visits to an elderly client with urinary incontinence, who is very disturbed by the incontinent episodes. The nurse explores the client's home situation to determine environmental barriers to normal voiding. Which of the following items, if assessed by the nurse, may be contributing to the client's problem?
   1 Presence of hand railings in the bathroom
   2 Having one bathroom on each floor of the home
   3 Nightlight present in the hall between bedroom and bathroom
   4 Bathroom located on the second floor, bedroom on the first floor

2. The nurse has inserted an indwelling Foley catheter and inflates the balloon. The client immediately complains of pain. Which of the following represents the best plan by the nurse?
   1 Tell the client that the discomfort will pass
   2 Withdraw 1 ml from the balloon of the catheter
   3 Deflate the balloon and push it farther into the bladder
   4 Deflate the balloon and replace it with another catheter

3. The nurse has an order to obtain a specimen for analysis from a client with an indwelling urinary catheter. The nurse plans to avoid which of the following, which could contaminate the specimen?
   1 Obtaining the specimen from the urinary drainage bag
   2 Clamping the tubing of the drainage bag
   3 Aspirating a sample from the port on the drainage bag
   4 Wiping the port with an alcohol swab prior to inserting the syringe

BOX 61–11. Client Instructions Following Kidney Transplant

Instruct client to avoid prolonged periods of sitting
Instruct client to recognize the signs and symptoms of infection and rejection
Instruct client to avoid contact sports
Instruct client to avoid exposure to people with infections
Instruct client in the signs and symptoms of infection and to monitor for infection
Instruct client in the use of medications as prescribed and in the importance of maintenance of immunosuppressive therapy for life

4. The nurse is caring for the client who has had a renal biopsy. Which of the following interventions would the nurse avoid in the care of the client after this procedure?
   1 Forcing fluids to at least 3 L in the first 24 hours
   2 Administering PRN narcotics
   3 Testing serial urine samples with dipsticks for occult blood
   4 Ambulating the client in the room and hall for short distances

5. The elderly client with cystitis also has an indwelling urinary catheter. The nurse plans to ensure that the nursing assistant does not:
   1 Use soap and water to cleanse the perineal area
   2 Keep the drainage bag below the level of the bladder
   3 Utilize the drainage tubing port to obtain urine samples
   4 Let the drainage tubing rest under the leg

6. The nurse is assisting the client with cystitis with diet selection in an acid ash diet. The nurse encourages the client to eat which of the following foods that the client enjoys?
   1 Low-fat milk
   2 Baked haddock
   3 Garden peas
   4 Apples

7. The client with acute pyelonephritis who was started on antibiotic therapy 24 hours ago is still complaining of burning with urination. The nurse checks the physician's orders to see whether which of the following medications is prescribed?
   1 Phenazopyridine (Pyridium)
   2 Bethanechol chloride (Urecholine)
   3 Oxybutinin chloride (Ditropan)
   4 Propantheline bromide (Pro-Banthine)

8. The nurse is teaching the client with nephrotic syndrome about managing the disorder. The nurse instructs the client to adjust which of the following upward or downward according to the amount of edema?
   1 Water
   2 Salt intake
   3 Use of diuretics
   4 Activity level

9. The client with urolithiasis has a history of chronic urinary tract infections. The nurse concludes that this client most likely has which of the following types of urinary stones?
   1 Calcium oxalate
   2 Uric acid
   3 Struvite
   4 Cystine

10. The client who has a history of gout is also diagnosed with urolithiasis. The stones are determined to be of uric acid type. The nurse gives the client instructions in foods to limit, which include:
    1 Liver
    2 Apples
    3 Carrots
    4 Milk

11. The nurse is caring for the client just after ureterolithotomy and is monitoring the drainage from the ureteral catheter hourly. The catheter stops draining suddenly. The nurse eliminates which of the following items that cannot be responsible for this occurrence?
    1 Blood clots
    2 Ureteral edema
    3 Catheter displacement
    4 Chemical sediment

12. The nurse is receiving in transfer from the postanesthesia care unit a client who has had percutaneous ultrasonic lithotripsy for calculi in the renal pelvis. The nurse anticipates that the client's care will involve monitoring of which of the following?
    1 Suprapubic tube
    2 Ureteral stent
    3 Nephrostomy tube
    4 Jackson-Pratt drain

13. The nurse is caring for a client who has been diagnosed as having a kidney mass. The client asks the nurse the reason for renal biopsy when other tests such as CT scan and ultrasound are available. In formulating a response, the nurse incorporates the knowledge that renal biopsy:
    1 Helps differentiate between a solid mass and a fluid filled cyst
    2 Provides an outline of the renal vascular system
    3 Gives specific cytological information about the lesion
    4 Determines whether the mass is growing rapidly or slowly

14. The client with renal cell carcinoma of the left kidney is scheduled for nephrectomy. The right kidney appears normal at this time. The client is anxious about whether dialysis will ultimately be a necessity. The nurse plans to utilize which of the following information in discussions with the client?
    1 There is absolutely no chance of needing dialysis due to the nature of the surgery
    2 Dialysis could become likely, but it depends on how well the client complies with fluid restriction after surgery
    3 One kidney is adequate to meet the needs of the body as long as it has normal function

4 There is a strong likelihood that the client will need dialysis within 5 to 10 years

15. The client with renal cancer is to undergo preoperative renal artery embolization. The nurse reinforces the primary benefit of this procedure by explaining to the client that:
    1 This will prevent the risk of pulmonary embolism, by occluding the renal artery and its branches
    2 This will shrink the tumor, because its blood supply will be removed after placement of an absorbable gelatin sponge
    3 The procedure will reduce the time needed for surgery by at least half because it provides hemostasis
    4 This will cause the tumor to become tougher, and easier to resect with the scalpel in surgery

16. The client with renal cancer is being treated preoperatively with radiation therapy. The nurse evaluates that the client has an understanding of proper care of the skin over the treatment field if the client states to:
    1 Avoid skin exposure to direct sunlight and chlorinated water
    2 Use lanolin-based cream on the affected skin on a daily basis
    3 Remove the lines or ink marks after each treatment, using a gentle soap
    4 Use the hottest water possible to wash the treatment site twice daily

17. The nurse is urging the client to cough and deep breathe after nephrectomy. The client tells the nurse, "That's easy for you to say! You don't have to do this." The nurse interprets that the client's statement is most likely a result of:
    1 A stress response to the ordeal of surgery
    2 A latent fear of needing dialysis if the surgery is unsuccessful
    3 Effects of circulating metabolites that have not been excreted by the remaining kidney
    4 Pain that is intensified because the location of the incision is near the diaphragm

18. The nurse is administering a dose of fentanyl (Sublimaze) to the client via an epidural catheter after nephrectomy. Before administering the medication, the nurse plans to:
    1 Aspirate to ensure that there is a CSF return
    2 Ensure that naloxone (Narcan) is readily available
    3 Place the head of the bed flat
    4 Flush the catheter with 6 mL of sterile water

19. The client is being evaluated as a potential kidney donor for a family member. The client asks the nurse why there are separate teams of people evaluating them as donor and recipient. In formulating a response, the nurse understands that this is being done to:
    1 Save the client and recipient valuable preoperative time
    2 Avoid a conflict of interest by the team evaluating the recipient and donor
    3 Help reduce the cost of the preoperative workup
    4 Have a sufficient number of people reviewing the case, so no information is overlooked

20. The nurse is administering care to the client immediately following nephrectomy. The nurse administers IV fluids as ordered, considering that the hourly rate should be calculated based on:
    1 The number of milliliters of the previous hour's urine output
    2 One half of the previous hour's urine output
    3 A strict hourly rate of 100 mL
    4 A strict hourly rate of 150 mL

21. The client presents to the emergency department with complaints of low abdominal pain and hematuria. The client is afebrile. The nurse next assesses the client to determine a history of:
    1 Renal cancer in the client's family
    2 Blow or trauma to the bladder or abdomen
    3 Glomerulonephritis
    4 Pyelonephritis

22. The client is admitted to the emergency department following a motor vehicle accident while wearing a lap seatbelt. The client has hematuria and lower abdominal pain. To further determine whether the pain is due to bladder trauma, the nurse asks the client whether the pain is referred to which of the following areas?
    1 Shoulder
    2 Umbilicus
    3 Costovertebral angle
    4 Hip

23. The female client is admitted to the emergency department following a fall from a horse. The physician orders insertion of a Foley catheter. The nurse notes blood at the urinary meatus while preparing for the procedure. The nurse should:
    1 Use extra povidone-iodine solution in cleansing the meatus
    2 Use a smaller-sized catheter
    3 Administer pain medication before inserting the catheter
    4 Notify the physician

24. The client is admitted with a suspicion of bladder cancer. The nurse assesses the client for which of the following earliest manifestations of the disease?
    1 Hematuria with no pain

2 Painful urination and hematuria

3 Pyuria and palpable abdominal mass

4 Proteinuria and dysuria

25. The female client who has been receiving radiation therapy for bladder cancer tells the nurse that it feels as though she is voiding through the vagina. The nurse interprets that the client may be experiencing:

1 Extreme stress due to the diagnosis of cancer

2 Altered perineal sensation as a side effect of radiation therapy

3 The development of a vesicovaginal fistula

4 Rupture of the bladder

26. The client is receiving intravesical chemotherapy for cancer of the bladder. The nurse plans to do which of the following after the completion of each treatment?

1 Provide increased doses of narcotic analgesics

2 Keep the client NPO for 6 hours

3 Place the client on contact isolation for 24 hours

4 Encourage increased intake of oral fluids

27. The client is coming to the nursing unit for admission after receiving a radium implant for bladder cancer. The nurse takes which of the following priority actions in the care of this client?

1 Encourage the client to take frequent rest periods

2 Admit the client to a private room

3 Encourage the family to visit

4 Place the client in reverse isolation

28. The client is to undergo weekly intravesical chemotherapy for bladder cancer for the next 8 weeks. The nurse interprets that the client understands management of the urine as a biohazard if the client states to:

1 Disinfect the urine and toilet with bleach for 6 hours after a treatment

2 Have one bathroom strictly set aside for the client's use for the next 2 months

3 Purchase extra bottles of scented disinfectant for daily bathroom cleansing

4 Void into a bedpan and then empty the urine into the toilet

29. The nurse is preparing to teach the client who has just had a urinary diversion about ostomy care. The client has a nursing diagnosis of Body Image Disturbance. The nurse interprets that the client is making the best initial positive adaptation if the client does which of the following?

1 Asks to defer ostomy care to the spouse

2 Asks to wait one more day before beginning to learn ostomy care

3 States that ostomy care is the nurse's job while in the hospital

4 Agrees to look at the ostomy

30. The home health nurse is planning to make a home visit to a client who has had the creation of an ileal conduit. The nurse plans to include which of the following items about ostomy care in discussions with the client?

1 Cut an opening in the faceplate of the appliance that is slightly smaller than the stoma

2 Plan to do appliance changes in the late evening hours

3 Appliance odor from urine breakdown to ammonia can be minimized by limiting fluids

4 Cleanse the skin around the stoma, use gentle soap and water, rinse and dry well

31. The client who is to have cystectomy and formation of an ileal conduit asks the nurse why the bowel needs to be cleansed before surgery if the bladder is being removed. The nurse gives the best response using which of the following pieces of information?

1 A portion of the bowel will be used to create the urinary diversion

2 All clients undergo bowel prep with major surgery

3 This will reduce the chance of the surgeon nicking the bowel during surgery

4 This will decrease the chance of postoperative paralytic ileus

32. The male client has a tentative diagnosis of urethritis. The nurse assesses the client for which of the following manifestations of the disorder?

1 Hematuria and penile discharge

2 Hematuria and pyuria

3 Dysuria and proteinuria

4 Dysuria and penile discharge

33. The nurse is planning a teaching session with the female client diagnosed with urethritis due to infection with *Chlamydia*. The nurse plans to include which of the following points in the teaching session?

1 The most serious complication of this infection is sterility

2 The infection can be prevented by using spermicide to alter the pH in the perineal area

3 Medication therapy should be continued for 2 weeks without interruption

4 Sexual partners during the last 12 months should be notified and treated

34. The male client who is admitted for an unrelated medical problem is diagnosed with urethritis due to chlamydial infection. The nursing assistant assigned to the client asks the nurse what measures are necessary to prevent contraction of the infection during care. The nurse tells the assistant that:

1 Enteric precautions should be instituted for the client

2 Contact isolation should be initiated, since the disease is highly contagious

3 Universal precautions are quite sufficient, since the disease is transmitted sexually

4 Gloves and mask should be used when in the client's room

35. The client with chlamydial infection has received instructions on self-care and prevention of further infection. The nurse evaluates that the client needs further reinforcement if the client states to:

1 Reduce the chance of reinfection by limiting the number of sexual partners

2 Use latex condoms to prevent disease transmission

3 Return to the clinic as requested for follow-up culture in 1 week

4 Use doxycycline prophylactically to prevent symptoms of chlamydia infection

36. The nurse is assessing the client with epididymitis. The nurse anticipates which of the following findings on physical examination?

1 Fever, diarrhea, groin pain, and ecchymosis

2 Fever, nausea and vomiting, and painful scrotal edema

3 Diarrhea, groin pain, and scrotal edema

4 Nausea and vomiting and scrotal edema with ecchymosis

37. The client with epididymitis is upset about the extent of scrotal edema. Attempts to reassure the client that this is temporary have not been effective. The nurse formulates which of the following nursing diagnoses for this client in addressing this problem?

1 Anxiety, related to inability to reduce scrotal swelling

2 Acute Pain, related to fluid accumulation in scrotum

3 Fear, related to possibility of sterility secondary to scrotal swelling

4 Body Image Disturbance, related to change in appearance of scrotum

38. The client is in extreme pain from scrotal swelling that is caused by epididymitis. The nurse administers an IM narcotic analgesic in the left arm to relieve the pain. The nurse should plan to do which of the following actions next?

1 Tell the client to do range of motion exercises to the left arm to absorb the medication into the blood stream

2 Check the name bracelet of the client

3 Put the side rails up on the bed

4 Dim the lights in the room

39. The nurse is caring for the client with epididymitis. The nurse avoids using which of the following treatment modalities in care of the client?

1 Bed rest

2 Scrotal elevation

3 Sitz bath

4 Use of heating pad

40. The client has epididymitis as a complication of urinary tract infection. The nurse is giving the client instructions to prevent a recurrence. The nurse evaluates that the client needs further instruction if the client states to:

1 Drink increased amounts of fluids

2 Continue to take antibiotics until all symptoms are gone

3 Limit the force of the stream during voiding

4 Utilize condoms to eliminate risk from *Chlamydia* infection and gonorrhea

41. The client complains of fever, perineal pain, and urinary urgency, frequency, and dysuria. To assess whether the client's problem is related to prostatitis, the nurse looks at results of the prostate examination, which should reveal that the prostate gland is:

1 Tender, indurated, and warm to the touch

2 Boggy, swollen, and warm to the touch

3 Tender and edematous, with ecchymosis

4 Reddened, swollen, and boggy

42. The client with acute prostatitis has difficulty voiding, which is accompanied by pain. The client asks the nurse, "Can't you just put a catheter in so I won't be in this misery when I try to go?" The nurse's response is based on the understanding that catheterization:

1 Will prolong the course of the inflammation

2 Could result in obstruction from rebound edema once the catheter is removed

3 Is avoided whenever possible to avoid pushing organisms up into the bladder

4 Could puncture the prostate gland since it is so inflamed

43. The nurse is taking the history of a client who has had benign prostatic hyperplasia (BPH) in the past. To determine whether the client is currently experiencing difficulty, the nurse asks the client about the presence of which of the following early symptoms?

1 Urge incontinence

2 Nocturia

3 Decreased force of the stream of urine

4 Urinary retention

44. The client who has a cold is seen in the emergency department with inability to void. Since the client has a history of BPH, the nurse determines that the client should be questioned about use of which of the following medications?

1 Diuretics

2 Antibiotics

3 Antitussives

4 Decongestants

45. The client is diagnosed with BPH, and is scheduled for transrectal ultrasound and measurement of a prostate-specific antigen (PSA) level.

The client says to the nurse, "I can't remember—can you tell me again why I need these tests to be done?" The nurse would respond that the tests:

1. Help rule out the presence of malignancy
2. Predict the course of BPH
3. Pinpoint the likelihood of developing urinary obstruction
4. Give an indication of whether intermittent self-catheterization is needed.

46. The client is being admitted to the nursing unit following radical prostatectomy for cancer. The nurse anticipates that which of the following nursing diagnoses will most likely apply to the client in the immediate postoperative period?
   1. Fear, related to outcome of surgery
   2. Chronic Pain, related to the effects of cancer
   3. Body Image Disturbance, related to presence of suprapubic catheter
   4. Impaired Home Maintenance Management, related to insufficient help postdischarge

47. The client who has had a prostatectomy is complaining of pain due to bladder spasm. The nurse looks at the physician's order sheet to see whether which of the following medications is ordered to treat the problem?
   1. Belladonna and opium (B&O) suppository
   2. Meperidine (Demerol)
   3. Morphine sulfate
   4. Hydromorphone (Dilaudid)

48. The client who has had a prostatectomy has learned perineal exercises to gain control of the urinary sphincter. The nurse evaluates that the client needs further instruction if the client states to perform which of the following as part of these exercises?
   1. Tighten the muscles as if trying to prevent urination
   2. Contract the abdominal, gluteal, and perineal muscles
   3. Tighten the rectal sphincter while relaxing abdominal muscles
   4. Perform the Valsalva maneuver

49. The client has developed acute renal failure (ARF) as a complication of glomerulonephritis. The nurse assesses this client for which of the following expected manifestations?
   1. Hypertension
   2. Bradycardia
   3. Decreased cardiac output
   4. Decreased central venous pressure

50. The client newly diagnosed with chronic renal failure (CRF) has many learning needs about the disease. The nurse prepares a teaching plan for this client to help the client adapt to the disease. The nurse recognizes that which of the following items pertaining to the client's situa-

tion is least likely to interfere with the client's ability to learn?
   1. Anxiety
   2. Memory deficits
   3. Short attention span
   4. Presence of family

51. The client with CRF is at risk of developing dementia related to excessive absorption of aluminum. The nurse teaches the client that this is the reason that the client is being prescribed which of the following phosphate-binding agents?
   1. Alu-Cap
   2. Tums
   3. Amphojel
   4. Basaljel

52. The client diagnosed with CRF is scheduled to begin hemodialysis. The nurse assesses that which of the following neurological and psychosocial manifestations, if exhibited by this client, is unrelated to the chronic renal failure?
   1. Labile emotions
   2. Withdrawal
   3. Euphoria
   4. Depression

53. The client with CRF is on fluid restriction. The client is fatigued and therefore has a limited tolerance for activity. The client takes aluminum hydroxide gel (ALternaGEL) as a phosphate binder. Based on this information, the nurse determines that the client is most at risk for which of the following problems?
   1. Impaired Physical Mobility
   2. Activity Intolerance
   3. Fluid Volume Deficit
   4. Constipation

54. The client with renal failure has a medication order for epoetin alfa (Epogen). The nurse administers this medication:
   1. Subcutaneously
   2. Intramuscularly
   3. With a full glass of water
   4. Diluted in juice to enhance taste

55. The nurse is working with the client newly diagnosed with CRF to set up a schedule for hemodialysis. The client states, "This is impossible! How can I even think about leading a normal life again if this is what I'm going to have to do?" The nurse assesses that the client is exhibiting:
   1. Withdrawal
   2. Depression
   3. Anger
   4. Projection

56. The nurse is analyzing the posthemodialysis laboratory results of a client with CRF. The nurse interprets that the dialysis is having an expected

but nontherapeutic effect if the results indicate a decreased:
1 Phosphorus level
2 Creatinine level
3 Potassium level
4 RBC count

57. The hemodialysis client with an AV fistula in the left arm has a nursing diagnosis of Risk for Infection. The nurse formulates which of the following outcome goals as most appropriate for this nursing diagnosis?
1 The client's temperature remains less than 101°F
2 The client's WBC count remains within normal limits
3 The client washes hands at least once per day
4 The client states to avoid BP measurement in the left arm

58. The nurse is giving general instructions to the client receiving hemodialysis. Which of the following statements is most appropriate for the nurse to include?
1 Several types of medications should be withheld on the day of dialysis until after the procedure
2 Medications should be double dosed on the morning of hemodialysis to prevent loss
3 It's acceptable to exceed the fluid restriction on the day before hemodialysis
4 It's acceptable to cheat on the renal diet on the day before hemodialysis

59. The client newly diagnosed with CRF has recently begun hemodialysis. Knowing that the client is at risk for disequilibrium syndrome, the nurse assesses the client during dialysis for:
1 Hypertension, tachycardia, and fever
2 Hypotension, bradycardia, and hypothermia
3 Restlessness, irritability, and generalized weakness
4 Headache, deteriorating LOC, and seizures

60. The client with CRF has been on dialysis for 3 years. The client is receiving the usual combination of medications for the disease, including aluminum hydroxide as a phosphate-binding agent. The client now presents with mental cloudiness, dementia, and complaints of bone pain. The nurse interprets that these assessment data are compatible with:
1 Phosphate overdose
2 Aluminum intoxication
3 Advancing uremia
4 Folic acid deficiency

61. The client undergoing hemodialysis is at risk for bleeding from the heparin used during the hemodialysis treatment. The nurse plans to minimize this occurrence by periodically measuring which of the following laboratory tests?

1 Partial thromboplastin time (PTT)
2 Prothrombin time (PT)
3 Thrombin time (TT)
4 Bleeding time

62. A client with CRF has completed a hemodialysis treatment. The nurse uses which of the following standard indicators to evaluate the client's status postdialysis?
1 Potassium level and client weight
2 BUN and creatinine levels
3 Vital signs and BUN
4 Vital signs and client weight

63. The hemodialysis client with a left arm fistula is at risk for steal syndrome. The nurse assesses this client for which of the following manifestations?
1 Warmth, redness, and pain in the left hand
2 Pallor, diminished pulse, and pain in the left hand
3 Edema and purplish discoloration of the left arm
4 Aching pain, pallor, and edema of the left arm

64. The nurse is monitoring the fluid balance of an assigned client. The nurse evaluates that the client has proper fluid balance if which of the following 24-hour I&O totals is noted?
1 Intake 1500 mL, output 800 mL
2 Intake 3000 mL, output 2400 mL
3 Intake 2400 mL, output 2900 mL
4 Intake 1800 mL, output 1750 mL

65. The nurse is reviewing the medical record of a client with a diagnosis of pyelonephritis. Which of the following disorders, if noted on the client's record, would the nurse identify as a risk factor for this disorder?
1 Hypoglycemia
2 Coronary artery disease
3 Diabetes mellitus
4 Orthostatic hypotension

66. The nurse is reviewing the client's record and notes that the physician has documented that the client has a renal disorder. On review of the laboratory results, the nurse would most likely expect to note which of the following?
1 Elevated BUN
2 Decreased hemoglobin
3 Decreased RBC count
4 Decreased WBC count

67. The client is undergoing diagnostic tests to rule out a diagnosis of renal disease. The laboratory results indicate a ratio of BUN to creatinine as 15:1. This indicates:
1 A fluid volume deficit
2 Liver failure
3 A fluid volume excess
4 The ratio is within normal limits

68. A nursing assistant collects a urine specimen from a client and is planning to deliver the specimen to the laboratory after completing morning care to other assigned clients. The registered nurse instructs the nursing assistant to place the collected specimen in the refrigerator. The nursing assistant asks the registered nurse about the reason that the urine needs refrigeration. The registered nurse bases the response on the fact that when urine is allowed to stand unrefrigerated:
    1 The urine becomes more acidic
    2 Bacteria and WBCs decompose
    3 The urine clumps
    4 The pH decreases

69. The nurse is collecting a 24-hour urine specimen from the client. Which of the following is an inaccurate action when collecting the specimen?
    1 Asking the client to void, save the specimen, and note the start time
    2 Discarding the urine specimen at the start time
    3 Placing the specimen on ice or refrigerating it
    4 Asking the client to void at the end of the collection and adding this to the collection

70. Which of the following would the nurse include in the plan of care for a client following a renal scan?
    1 Place the client on radiation precautions for 18 hours
    2 Save all urine in a radiation-safe container for 18 hours
    3 Limit contact with the client for 20 minutes per hour
    4 No special precautions except to wear gloves if coming in contact with the client's urine

71. The client is scheduled for an intravenous pyelogram (IVP). Prior to the test, the priority nursing action is to:
    1 Administer an oral preparation of radiopaque dye
    2 Restrict fluids
    3 Determine a history of allergies
    4 Administer a sedative

72. The nurse instructs the client to obtain a clean-catch urine specimen for culture. Which of the following statements, if made by the client, indicates that the client understands the procedure for collecting the specimen?
    1 To empty the bladder into a container so that the full amount of urine can be determined
    2 That a urine specimen will be obtained from a catheter
    3 To cleanse labia using cleansing towels, void into toilet, and then void into sterile specimen container

4 To clean labia with toilet paper and void into sterile specimen container

73. The client is scheduled for an excretory urogram. Which of the following would the nurse anticipate to be prescribed as a component of preparation for this test?
    1 NPO after midnight
    2 Administration of a sedative prior to the test
    3 Administration of IV fluids
    4 Bowel preparation to remove fecal contents

74. Following a renal biopsy, the client complains of pain at the biopsy site that radiates to the front of the abdomen. The nurse interprets this complaint and further assesses the client for:
    1 Bleeding
    2 Infection
    3 Renal colic
    4 A normal expected pain

75. A client is admitted to the hospital and has a diagnosis of early stage of CRF. Which of the following does the nurse expect to note on assessment of the client?
    1 Polyuria
    2 Edema
    3 Oliguria
    4 Anuria

76. The nurse is reviewing the medication record of a client diagnosed with CRF. The nurse notes that the client is receiving aluminum hydroxide (Amphojel). The nurse determines that the purpose of this medication is to:
    1 Combine with phosphorus and help eliminate phosphates from the body
    2 Prevent ulcers
    3 Promote the elimination of potassium from the body
    4 Prevent constipation

77. The client with CRF, who is receiving an antihypertensive drug, is experiencing frequent hypotensive episodes. Which one of the following medications, if prescribed, would have the greatest tendency to cause hypotension?
    1 Propranolol (Inderal)
    2 Epoetin alfa (Epogen)
    3 Methyldopa (Aldomet)
    4 Calcium carbonate (OsCal)

78. The client with CRF returns to the nursing unit following a hemodialysis treatment. On assessment, the nurse notes that the client's temperature is 100.2°F. Which of the following is the most appropriate nursing action?
    1 Encourage fluids
    2 Notify the physician
    3 Monitor site of shunt for infection
    4 Continue to monitor vital signs

79. The registered nurse is instructing a new nursing graduate about hemodialysis. Which of the following statements, if made by the new nursing graduate, indicates an inaccurate understanding of the procedure for hemodialysis?
    1 Sterile dialysate must be used
    2 Warming the dialysate increases the efficiency of diffusion
    3 Heparin is administered during dialysis
    4 Dialysis removes excess waste products from the blood

80. The nurse is performing an assessment on a client who has returned from the dialysis unit following hemodialysis. The client is complaining of a headache and nausea and is extremely restless. Which of the following is the most appropriate nursing action?
    1 Notify the physician
    2 Monitor the client
    3 Elevate the head of the bed
    4 Medicate the client for nausea

81. The nurse is caring for a client diagnosed with ARF caused by severe hemorrhage following trauma. The client is in the oliguric phase. Which of the following laboratory results does the nurse not expect to note during this phase?
    1 An elevated BUN-creatinine ratio
    2 Low specific gravity of urine
    3 Casts in the urine
    4 Low urine sodium

82. The client is receiving diagnostic tests because of a suspected diagnosis of renal disease. Which of the following laboratory tests best evaluates the kidneys' ability to regulate fluid balance?
    1 Urine specific gravity
    2 BUN
    3 Creatinine
    4 Urinary protein

83. The nurse is caring for a client with ARF. When performing an assessment, the nurse expects to note which of the following breathing patterns?
    1 Decreased respirations
    2 Apneic
    3 Cheyne-Stokes
    4 Kussmaul's

84. The nurse is assisting a client on a low-potassium diet to select food items from the menu. Which of the following food items, if selected by the client, indicates an understanding of this dietary restriction?
    1 Cantaloupe
    2 Spinach
    3 Lima beans
    4 Strawberries

85. The nursing student is assigned to care for a client with a diagnosis of ARF, diuretic phase.

The nursing instructor asks the student about the primary goal of the treatment plan for this client. Which of the following statements, if made by the nursing student, indicates an adequate understanding of the treatment plan for this client?
    1 Prevent loss of electrolytes
    2 Reduce the urine specific gravity
    3 Promote the excretion of wastes
    4 Prevent fluid overload

86. The nurse instructs a client about continuous ambulatory peritoneal dialysis (CAPD). Which of the following statements, if made by the client, indicates an accurate understanding of CAPD?
    1 A portable hemodialysis machine is used so the client will be able to ambulate during the treatment
    2 A cycling machine is used so the risk for infection is minimized
    3 No machinery is involved, and the client can pursue usual activities
    4 The drainage system can be used once during the day and a cycling machine for three cycles at night

87. The nurse is reviewing the list of components of the peritoneal dialysis solution with the client. The client asks the nurse about the purpose of the glucose contained in the solution. The nurse bases the response on which of the following?
    1 To prevent excess glucose from being removed from the client
    2 To decrease the risk of peritonitis
    3 To prevent disequilibrium syndrome
    4 To increase osmotic pressure to produce ultrafiltration

88. Which of the following would be included in the nursing plan of care to prevent the major complication associated with peritoneal dialysis?
    1 Monitor the client's LOC
    2 Maintain strict aseptic technique
    3 Add heparin to the dialysate
    4 Change catheter site dressing daily

89. A hospitalized client is receiving peritoneal dialysis, and during the infusion of the dialysate the client complains of abdominal pain. Which of the following actions by the nurse is most appropriate?
    1 Slow the infusion
    2 Decrease the amount to be infused
    3 Explain that the pain will subside after the first few exchanges
    4 Stop the dialysis

90. The nurse is monitoring a client receiving peritoneal dialysis. The nurse notes that the client's outflow is less than the inflow. Which of the following nursing actions is most appropriate?

1 Monitor for hypertension
2 Reposition the client
3 Irrigate the catheter
4 Continue to monitor outflow

91. The nurse is instructing a diabetic client about peritoneal dialysis. The nurse instructs the client regarding the importance of maintaining the dwell time for the dialysis at the prescribed time because of the risk of:
    1 Infection
    2 Hyperglycemia
    3 Fluid overload
    4 Disequilibrium syndrome

92. The nurse is providing dietary instructions to a client receiving peritoneal dialysis. Which of the following dietary components would most likely be limited in this client's diet?
    1 Sodium
    2 Glucose
    3 Protein
    4 Potassium

93. Which of the following clients is most at risk for developing a candidal urinary tract infection?
    1 A man with diabetes insipidus
    2 An obese woman
    3 A paraplegic on intermittent catheterization
    4 A young woman on antibiotic therapy

94. The nurse is caring for an 88-year-old woman suspected of having a urinary tract infection (UTI). Which of the following symptoms, if noted in the client, would alert the nurse to the possibility of the presence of a UTI?
    1 Fever
    2 Frequency
    3 Confusion
    4 Urgency

95. The clinic nurse is providing instructions to a client receiving methenamine (Mandelamine) for treatment of a UTI. Which of the following would the nurse include in the instructions?
    1 Explain that the medication will turn the urine orange
    2 Increase daily fluid intake to more than 3 L
    3 Explain how to maintain an acid pH of urine
    4 Be sure to take this medication with food

96. The nurse is providing dietary instructions to a client with a diagnosis of acute glomerulonephritis. Which of the following dietary measures would be included in the instructions?
    1 Restrict fluid intake
    2 Restrict protein intake
    3 Increase intake of high-fiber foods
    4 Increase intake of potassium-rich foods

97. The client passes a urinary stone, and laboratory analysis of the stone indicates that it is composed of calcium oxalate. Based on this analysis, which of the following would the nurse include in the dietary instructions?
    1 Increase intake of wheat bran and tea
    2 Avoid intake of cranberries and citrus juices
    3 Avoid green leafy vegetables such as spinach
    4 Increase intake of dairy products

98. The client returns to the nursing unit following a pyelolithotomy for removal of a kidney stone. A Penrose drain is in place. Which of the following does the nurse include in the client's postoperative plan of care?
    1 Sterile irrigation of the Penrose drain
    2 Frequent dressing changes around the Penrose drain
    3 Weighing dressings
    4 Maintaining the client's position on the affected side

99. The nurse is caring for a client following a kidney transplant. The client develops oliguria. Which of the following does the nurse anticipate to be prescribed as the treatment for the oliguria?
    1 Forcing fluids
    2 Administration of diuretics
    3 Irrigation of the Foley catheter
    4 Restricting fluids

100. The nurse is performing an admission assessment on a client with a diagnosis of bladder cancer. Which of the following symptoms does the nurse most likely expect to note on assessment of this client?
    1 Hematuria
    2 Burning
    3 Urgency
    4 Frequency

101. A week after kidney transplantation, the client develops a fever of 101°F, the blood pressure is elevated, and the kidney is tender. The x-ray film results indicate that the transplanted kidney is enlarged. Based on these assessment findings, the nurse suspects which of the following?
    1 Acute rejection
    2 Chronic rejection
    3 Kidney infection
    4 Kidney obstruction

102. A cystectomy is performed on the client with a diagnosis of bladder cancer, and a Kock pouch is created for a urinary diversion. The nurse is preparing a discharge teaching plan and includes which of the following in the plan?
    1 External pouch and application care
    2 Technique of catheterization
    3 Proper administration of prophylactic antibiotics
    4 Dietary restrictions

103. The client with benign prostatic hypertrophy (BPH) undergoes a transurethral resection (TUR). Postoperatively, the client is receiving continuous bladder irrigations. The nurse assesses the client for signs of TUR syndrome. Which of the following assessment data indicates the onset of this syndrome?
    1 Bradycardia and confusion
    2 Tachycardia and diarrhea
    3 Decreased urinary output and bladder spasms
    4 Increased urinary output and anemia

104. The client is admitted to the hospital with a diagnosis of BPH, and a TUR is performed. Four hours after surgery, the nurse takes the client's vital signs and empties the urinary drainage bag. Which of the following assessment findings indicates the need to notify the physician?
    1 Red bloody urine
    2 Urinary output of 200 mL greater than intake
    3 Blood pressure of 100/50, pulse 130
    4 Pain related to bladder spasms

105. A client is diagnosed with polycystic kidney disease. Which of the following does the nurse not expect to be a component of the treatment plan?
    1 Sodium restriction
    2 Antihypertensive medications
    3 Increased water intake
    4 Genetic counseling

106. The nurse is caring for the client who has undergone renal angiography using the left femoral artery for access. The nurse evaluates that the client is experiencing a complication of the procedure if which of the following observations is made?
    1 Urine output of 50 mL/hour
    2 Absence of hematoma in the left groin
    3 Blood pressure of 110/74
    4 Pallor and coolness of the left leg

107. The client with acute glomerulonephritis is awaiting results of a urinalysis. The report reveals hematuria and proteinuria. The nurse interprets that these results are:
    1 Consistent with glomerulonephritis
    2 Inconsistent with glomerulonephritis
    3 Unclear, and no conclusion can be drawn
    4 Indicative of impending renal failure

108. The nurse is caring for the client with acute glomerulonephritis. The nurse instructs the nursing assistant to do which of the following in the care of the client?
    1 Monitor the temperature every 2 hours
    2 Remove the water pitcher from the bedside
    3 Ambulate the client frequently
    4 Encourage a diet high in protein

109. The nurse has given the client with polycystic disease information about management of the disorder and prevention and recognition of complications. The nurse evaluates that the client needs further instruction if the client states to report:
    1 Lowered blood pressure
    2 Onset of shortness of breath
    3 Fever
    4 Burning on urination

110. The client is having difficulty coughing and deep breathing because of pain after nephrectomy. Which of the following actions by the nurse is least helpful in promoting optimal respiratory function?
    1 Administering pain medication only before ambulation
    2 Encouraging use of incentive spirometer hourly
    3 Assisting the client to splint the incision during respiratory exercise
    4 Offering PRN pain medication every 4 hours when due

111. The client being discharged home following renal transplant has a nursing diagnosis of Risk for Infection, related to immunosuppressive therapy. The nurse evaluates that the client needs further instruction on measures to prevent and control infection if the client states to:
    1 Take an oral temperature daily
    2 Utilize good handwashing technique
    3 Take all scheduled medications exactly as prescribed
    4 Monitor urine character and output at least 1 day each week

112. The client with bladder injury has had surgical repair of the injured area and placement of a suprapubic catheter. The nurse plans to do which of the following to prevent complications of this procedure?
    1 Monitor urine output every shift
    2 Encourage a high intake of oral fluids
    3 Prevent kinking of the catheter tubing
    4 Measure specific gravity once a shift

113. The client with prostatitis secondary to kidney infection has received instructions on management of the condition at home and prevention of recurrence. The nurse evaluates that the client understood the instructions if the client verbalized to:
    1 Keep fluid intake to a minimum to decrease the need to void
    2 Exercise as much as possible to stimulate circulation
    3 Stop antibiotic therapy when pain subsides
    4 Use warm sitz baths and analgesics to increase comfort

114. The nurse is participating in a prostate screening

clinic. The nurse interprets that a client understands the educational information that was shared if the nurse overhears the client tell another participant that:

1 Increased intake of green leafy vegetables is helpful
2 A daily supplement of vitamin E will prevent BPH
3 An annual prostate examination after age 40 years is best for early detection
4 Cigarette smoking triples the chance of developing BPH

115. The client with crush injury to the right lower leg develops ARF. The nurse interprets that this type of renal failure is due to:

1 Prerenal causes
2 Renal causes
3 Postrenal causes
4 Extrarenal causes

116. The client with ARF has a serum potassium level of 5.8 mEq/L. The nurse plans to take which of the following as a priority action?

1 Allow an extra 500 mL of fluid intake to dilute the electrolyte concentration
2 Encourage increased vegetables in the diet
3 Place the client on a cardiac monitor
4 Check the sodium level

117. The nurse tests the urine of a client with ARF with a multitest reagent strip. The strip tests highly positive for proteinuria. The nurse analyzes that this result is consistent with which of the following types of renal failure?

1 Atypical renal failure
2 Prerenal failure
3 Intrinsic renal failure
4 Postrenal failure

118. The client with CRF who is scheduled for hemodialysis this morning is due to receive a daily dose of enalapril (Vasotec). The nurse should plan to administer this medication:

1 Just prior to dialysis
2 During dialysis
3 Upon return from dialysis
4 The day after dialysis

119. The client with CRF has an indwelling catheter for peritoneal dialysis in the abdomen. The client spills water on the dressing while bathing. The nurse should plan to immediately:

1 Reinforce the dressing
2 Change the dressing
3 Flush the peritoneal dialysis catheter
4 Scrub the catheter with povidone-iodine

120. The client with chronic renal failure is about to begin hemodialysis therapy. The client asks the nurse about the frequency and scheduling of hemodialysis treatments. The nurse's response is based on an understanding that the typical schedule is:

1 Five hours of treatment 2 days per week
2 Three to four hours of treatment 3 days per week
3 Two to three hours of treatment 5 days per week
4 Two hours of treatment 6 days per week

121. The nurse is about to begin hemodialysis. Which of the following measures would the nurse plan to avoid in the care of the client?

1 Putting on a mask and giving one to the client to wear during connection to the machine
2 Wearing full protective clothing such as goggles, mask, apron, and gloves
3 Covering the connection site with a bath blanket to enhance extremity warmth
4 Using sterile technique for needle insertion

122. The client being hemodialyzed becomes suddenly short of breath and complains of chest pain. The client is tachycardic, pale, and anxious. The nurse suspects air embolism. The nurse should:

1 Continue dialysis at a slower rate after checking the lines for air
2 Discontinue dialysis and notify the physician
3 Monitor vital signs every 15 minutes for the next hour
4 Bolus the client with 500 mL of normal saline to break up the air embolus

123. The nurse has completed client teaching with the hemodialysis client about self-monitoring between hemodialysis treatments. The nurse evaluates that the client best understands the information given if the client states to record on a daily basis:

1 Pulse, respiratory rate
2 I&O and weight
3 BUN and creatinine levels
4 Activity log

124. The client is scheduled for surgical creation of an internal arteriovenous (AV) fistula on the following day. The client says to the nurse, "I'll be so happy when the fistula is made tomorrow. This means I can have that other hemodialysis catheter pulled right out." The nurse interprets that the client:

1 Does not understand that the site needs to mature for 1 to 2 weeks before use
2 Has an accurate understanding of the procedure and aftercare
3 Does not realize how painful removal of the dialysis catheter will be
4 Is not aware that the alternate access site is left in place prophylactically for 2 months

125. The client with an AV shunt in place for hemo-

dialysis is at risk for bleeding. The nurse does which of the following as a priority action to prevent this complication from occurring?

1 Check the results of PTT tests as they are ordered

2 Observe the site once per shift

3 Check the shunt for presence of bruit and thrill

4 Ensure that small clamps are attached to the AV shunt dressing

ANSWERS

1. **4**

Rationale: Having a bathroom on the second floor and the bedroom on the first floor may pose a problem for the elderly client with incontinence. The need to negotiate the stairs and the distance both may interfere with reaching the bathroom in a timely fashion. It is more helpful to the incontinent client to have a bathroom on the same floor as the bedroom, or to have a rented commode. The presence of nightlights and hand railings is helpful to the client in reaching the bathroom quickly and safely.

Test-Taking Strategy: Begin to answer this question by eliminating option 1 as obviously helpful. Option 2 is also helpful and cannot be the answer to the question as stated. Since option 3 is more helpful than option 4, at least for nighttime voiding, option 4 must be the correct answer.

Level of Cognitive Ability: Analysis
Phase of Nursing Process: Assessment
Client Needs: Psychosocial Integrity
Content Area: Adult Health/Renal

Reference
Black, J., & Matassarin-Jacobs, E. (1997). *Medical-surgical nursing: Clinical management for continuity of care* (5th ed.). Philadelphia: W. B. Saunders. pp. 1550–1551.

2. **4**

Rationale: The appropriate procedure if the client complains of pain after insertion is to remove the catheter after deflating the balloon and replace it with another one. This is preferred to option 3, which could make the client more at risk for developing urinary tract infection, since the catheter would be advanced after part of it was resting against the client's external genitalia. Options 1 and 2 are totally incorrect.

Test-Taking Strategy: Options 1 and 2 are the least plausible, and should be eliminated first. You would be able to discriminate correctly between options 3 and 4 using principles of aseptic technique.

Level of Cognitive Ability: Application
Phase of Nursing Process: Planning
Client Needs: Safe, Effective Care Environment
Content Area: Adult Health/Renal

Reference
Taylor, C., Lillis, C., & LeMone, P. (1997). *Fundamentals of nursing: The art and science of nursing care* (3rd ed.). Philadelphia: Lippincott-Raven. p. 1237.

3. **1**

Rationale: A urine specimen is not taken from the urinary drainage bag. Urine undergoes chemical changes while in the bag, which do not necessarily reflect current client status. In addition, urine may become contaminated with bacteria from opening the system.

Test-Taking Strategy: This question tests a core principle of asepsis. If this question was difficult in any way, take a few moments now to review this key area of nursing practice.

Level of Cognitive Ability: Application
Phase of Nursing Process: Planning
Client Needs: Safe, Effective Care Environment
Content Area: Adult Health/Renal

Reference
Black, J., & Matassarin-Jacobs, E. (1997). *Medical-surgical nursing: Clinical management for continuity of care* (5th ed.). Philadelphia: W. B. Saunders. pp. 1555–1556.

4. **4**

Rationale: Following renal biopsy, the nurse ensures that the client remains in bed for at least 24 hours. Vital signs and puncture site assessments are done frequently during this time. Forcing fluids is done to reduce possible clot formation at the biopsy site. Serial urine samples are hematested with urine dipsticks to evaluate bleeding. Narcotic analgesics are often needed to manage the renal colic pain that some clients feel after this procedure.

Test-Taking Strategy: Begin to answer this question by recalling that pain and bleeding are potential concerns after this procedure. This would allow you to eliminate options 2 and 3 as possible responses. To discriminate between the last two options, you would need to recall that forcing fluids will reduce clotting at the site, whereas ambulation could initiate or enhance bleeding at the biopsy site.

Level of Cognitive Ability: Application
Phase of Nursing Process: Implementation
Client Needs: Physiological Integrity
Content Area: Adult Health/Renal

Reference
Black, J., & Matassarin-Jacobs, E. (1997). *Medical-surgical nursing: Clinical management for continuity of care* (5th ed.). Philadelphia: W. B. Saunders. p. 1569.

5. **4**

Rationale: Proper care of an indwelling catheter is especially important to prevent prolonged infection or reinfection in the client with cystitis. The nurse and all caregivers must use strict aseptic technique when emptying the drainage bag or obtaining urine specimens. The perineal area is cleansed thoroughly, using mild soap and water, at least twice a day and following a bowel movement (BM). The drainage bag is kept below the level of the bladder to prevent urine from being trapped in the bladder, and for the same reason, the drainage tubing is not placed under the client's leg. The tubing must drain freely at all times.

Test-Taking Strategy: The wording of the question guides you to look for an incorrect response. Eliminate option 1 first, since this is a basic standard of care for the client with an indwelling catheter. Option 3 is also consistent with principles of asepsis and is eliminated next. To discriminate between options 2 and 4, recall that option 2 promotes drainage, whereas option 4 could impede drainage. Thus the answer to the question is option 4, according to the wording of the question.

Level of Cognitive Ability: Application
Phase of Nursing Process: Planning
Client Needs: Safe, Effective Care Environment
Content Area: Adult Health/Renal

Reference
Black, J., & Matassarin-Jacobs, E. (1997). *Medical-surgical nursing: Clinical management for continuity of care* (5th ed.). Philadelphia: W. B. Saunders. p. 1573.

6. 2

Rationale: Foods that are allowed on an acid ash diet include meat, fish, shellfish, cheese, eggs, poultry, grains, cranberries, prunes, plums, corn, lentils, and foods with high amounts of chlorine, phosphorus, and sulfur. Foods not included are all milk and milk products; all other vegetables except corn and lentils; all fruits except cranberries, plums, and prunes; and foods containing high amounts of sodium, potassium, calcium, and magnesium.

Test-Taking Strategy: This question is difficult to answer without specific knowledge of the types of foods that may be included in the acid ash diet. Knowing that most fruits and vegetables are not included on the list may help you eliminate options 3 and 4. To discriminate between options 1 and 2, it is necessary to know that foods such as meat, fish, cheese, and eggs are included, whereas milk and milk products are not.

Level of Cognitive Ability: Application
Phase of Nursing Process: Implementation
Client Needs: Physiological Integrity
Content Area: Adult Health/Renal

Reference
Black, J., & Matassarin-Jacobs, E. (1997). *Medical-surgical nursing: Clinical management for continuity of care* (5th ed.). Philadelphia: W. B. Saunders. p. 1577.

7. 1

Rationale: The pain experienced with pyelonephritis usually resolves as antibiotic therapy becomes effective. However, clients may be treated for urinary tract pain with phenazopyridine, which is a urinary analgesic. Bethanechol chloride is a cholinergic agent used with neurogenic bladder or for urinary retention. Oxybutinin and propantheline bromide are antispasmodics that are used to treat bladder spasm.

Test-Taking Strategy: Specific knowledge of the classifications of these medications is necessary to answer this question correctly. If this question was difficult, take a few moments to review these medications now!

Level of Cognitive Ability: Application
Phase of Nursing Process: Analysis
Client Needs: Physiological Integrity
Content Area: Pharmacology

Reference
Black, J., & Matassarin-Jacobs, E. (1997). *Medical-surgical nursing: Clinical management for continuity of care* (5th ed.). Philadelphia: W. B. Saunders. pp. 1576, 1629.

8. 4

Rationale: The client with nephrotic syndrome usually has a standard limit set on sodium intake. Fluids are not restricted unless the client is also hyponatremic. Diuretics are ordered on a specific schedule, and doses are not titrated according to the level of edema. The client is taught to adjust the activity level according to the amount of edema. As edema decreases, activity can increase. Correspondingly, as edema increases, the client should increase rest periods and limit activity. Bed rest is recommended during periods of severe edema.

Test-Taking Strategy: Knowing that sodium restrictions, if ordered, are not modified upward or downward allows you to discard option 2 first as obviously incorrect. Likewise, knowing that diuretics are not titrated allows you to eliminate option 3 next. To discriminate between options 1 and 4, it is necessary to know that fluids may or may not be restricted (depending on serum sodium level), whereas activity level is adjusted downward as edema increases.

Level of Cognitive Ability: Application
Phase of Nursing Process: Implementation
Client Needs: Health Promotion and Maintenance
Content Area: Adult Health/Renal

Reference
Black, J., & Matassarin-Jacobs, E. (1997). *Medical-surgical nursing: Clinical management for continuity of care* (5th ed.). Philadelphia: W. B. Saunders. p. 1635.

9. 3

Rationale: Struvite stones are commonly referred to as infection stones, because they form in urine that is alkaline and rich in ammonia, such as with UTI. Calcium oxalate stones result from increased calcium intake or conditions that raise serum calcium concentrations. Uric acid stones occur in clients with gout. Cystine stones are rare and occur in clients with a genetic defect, which results in decreased renal absorption of the amino acid cystine.

Test-Taking Strategy: Begin to answer this question by eliminating option 4, since cystine stones are rare and are linked to a genetic disorder. Option 2 may be eliminated next. Uric acid stones may occur with gout, and the stem makes no mention of this problem. To discriminate between the last two options, you would need to know that calcium oxalate stones may occur with excess calcium intake or other specific disorders, whereas struvite stones commonly occur in the client who experiences UTI. This knowledge would guide you to choose option 3 over option 1 as the correct answer.

Level of Cognitive Ability: Analysis
Phase of Nursing Process: Analysis
Client Needs: Physiological Integrity
Content Area: Adult Health/Renal

Reference
Smeltzer, S., & Bare, B. (1996). *Brunner and Suddarth's textbook of medical-surgical nursing* (8th ed.). Philadelphia: Lippincott-Raven. p. 1207.

10. 1

Rationale: Foods containing high amounts of purines should be avoided in the client with uric acid stones. This includes limiting or avoiding organ meats, such as liver, brain, heart, kidney, and sweetbreads. Other foods to avoid include herring, sardines, anchovies, meat extracts, consommés, and gravies. Foods that are low in purines include all fruits, many vegetables, milk, cheese, eggs, refined cereals, sugars and sweets, coffee, tea, chocolate, and carbonated beverages.

Test-Taking Strategy: To answer this question, begin by examining the options and classifying the types of food sources they represent. Options 2 and 3 represent foods that are grown, whereas options 1 and 4 represent foods that derive from animal sources. Since purines are end-products of protein metabolism, you would eliminate options 2 and 3 first. To discriminate between options 1 and 4, you would need to know that organ meats such as liver provide a greater quantity of protein than does milk. With this in mind, you would choose option 1 over option 4.

Level of Cognitive Ability: Application
Phase of Nursing Process: Implementation
Client Needs: Health Promotion and Maintenance
Content Area: Adult Health/Renal

References
Lutz, C., & Przytulski, K. (1997). *Nutrition and diet therapy* (2nd ed.). Philadelphia: F. A. Davis. p. 400.
Smeltzer, S., & Bare, B. (1996). *Brunner and Suddarth's textbook of medical-surgical nursing* (8th ed.). Philadelphia: Lippincott-Raven. p. 1210.

11. **2**

Rationale: Following ureterolithotomy, a ureteral catheter is put in place. Urine flows freely through it for the first 2 to 3 days. As ureteral edema diminishes, urine leaks around the ureteral catheter and drains directly into the bladder. At this point, drainage through the ureteral catheter diminishes. Immediately after surgery, absence of drainage is usually caused by blockage from blood clots, mucus shreds, or chemical sediment.

Test-Taking Strategy: The wording of this question guides you to look for an option that is not responsible for the problem described. Eliminate options 1 and 4 first, since either of these items could easily cause blockage of the tube. To discriminate between options 2 and 3, knowing that dislodgment causes failure of drainage would enable you to eliminate this option also. This leaves ureteral edema as the correct answer. Since the stent keeps the ureter open, ureteral edema cannot stop the flow of urine.

Level of Cognitive Ability: Analysis
Phase of Nursing Process: Analysis
Client Needs: Physiological Integrity
Content Area: Adult Health/Renal

Reference
Black, J., & Matassarin-Jacobs, E. (1997). *Medical-surgical nursing: Clinical management for continuity of care* (5th ed.). Philadelphia: W. B. Saunders. p. 1598.

12. **3**

Rationale: A nephrostomy tube is put in place after percutaneous ultrasonic lithotripsy to treat calculi in the renal pelvis. The client may also have a Foley catheter to drain urine produced by the other kidney. The nurse monitors the drainage from each of these tubes and strains the urine to detect elimination of the calculus fragments.

Test-Taking Strategy: The stem of the question tells you that the calculi are in the renal pelvis. Thus you can eliminate the suprapubic tube and the Jackson-Pratt drain, since these drainage tubes would not be placed in the kidney. You would then choose option 3 over option 2 for the same reason.

Level of Cognitive Ability: Analysis
Phase of Nursing Process: Analysis
Client Needs: Physiological Integrity
Content Area: Adult Health/Renal

Reference
Black, J., & Matassarin-Jacobs, E. (1997). *Medical-surgical nursing: Clinical management for continuity of care* (5th ed.). Philadelphia: W. B. Saunders. p. 1668.

13. **3**

Rationale: Renal biopsy is a definitive test that gives specific information about whether the lesion is benign or malignant. An ultrasound discriminates between a fluid-filled cyst and a solid mass. Renal arteriography outlines the renal vascular system.

Test-Taking Strategy: Begin to answer this question by eliminating options 1 and 2 first. Basic knowledge of the purposes of biopsy helps you discard these quickly. To discriminate between options 3 and 4, remember that with biopsy the cells are examined under a microscope. This examination then yields specific information about the type of neoplastic cell. Although some types of cancer grow more quickly than others, it is not possible to determine this for any one individual by biopsy. Thus you would choose option 3 as the better answer.

Level of Cognitive Ability: Analysis
Phase of Nursing Process: Analysis
Client Needs: Physiological Integrity
Content Area: Adult Health/Renal

Reference
Black, J., & Matassarin-Jacobs, E. (1997). *Medical-surgical nursing: Clinical management for continuity of care* (5th ed.). Philadelphia: W. B. Saunders. p. 1671.

14. **3**

Rationale: Fears about having only one functioning kidney are common in clients who must undergo nephrectomy for renal cancer. These clients need emotional support and reassurance that the remaining kidney should be able to meet the body's metabolic needs fully, as long as it has normal function.

Test-Taking Strategy: Begin to answer this question by eliminating option 1. An option that contains the phrase "absolutely no chance" is not likely to be correct. Knowing that there is no need for fluid restriction with a functioning kidney guides you to eliminate option 2 next. To discriminate between the last two options, remember that an individual can donate a kidney without adverse consequences or the need for dialysis. Applying that knowledge to this question would guide you to choose option 3 over option 4.

Level of Cognitive Ability: Application
Phase of Nursing Process: Planning
Client Needs: Psychosocial Integrity
Content Area: Adult Health/Renal

Reference
Black, J., & Matassarin-Jacobs, E. (1997). *Medical-surgical nursing: Clinical management for continuity of care* (5th ed.). Philadelphia: W. B. Saunders. p. 1672.

15. **2**

Rationale: Renal artery embolization may be done instead of radiation therapy to shrink the kidney tumor, by cutting off its blood supply and vascularity. A secondary benefit is that it reduces the risk of hemorrhage during surgery. This procedure can be accomplished in a number of ways, including placement of an absorbable gelatin sponge (Gelfoam), barium, a balloon, metal coil, or other substances.

Test-Taking Strategy: Eliminate option 1 first, knowing that this option is not plausible with normal anatomy and physiology. Option 4 is discarded next as there is no basis for determining that this procedure would make a tumor "tougher." To discriminate between options 2 and 3, notice the phrase "by at least half" in option 3. Although renal artery embolization does help in hemostasis, it is not guaranteed to have this much of an effect on the operative time. This leaves option 2 as the correct answer. This procedure does help shrink the tumor by depriving it of its blood supply and nutrients.

Level of Cognitive Ability: Application
Phase of Nursing Process: Implementation
Client Needs: Physiological Integrity
Content Area: Adult Health/Renal

Reference
Black, J., & Matassarin-Jacobs, E. (1997). *Medical-surgical nursing: Clinical management for continuity of care* (5th ed.). Philadelphia: W. B. Saunders. p. 1672.

16. **1**

Rationale: The client undergoing radiation therapy should avoid washing the site until instructed to do so. The client should then wash the site, using mild soap and warm or cool water, and pat the area dry. No lotions, creams, alcohol, or deodorants should be placed on the skin over the treatment site. Lines or ink marks that are placed on the skin to guide the radiation therapy should be left in place. The affected skin should be protected from temperature extremes, direct sunlight, and chlorinated water (as from swimming pools).

Test-Taking Strategy: Begin to answer this question by eliminating options 2 and 4, since they are contraindicated in the care of this client. Knowing that markings used to guide therapy are to be left in place helps you choose option 1 over option 3.

Level of Cognitive Ability: Analysis
Phase of Nursing Process: Evaluation
Client Needs: Physiological Integrity
Content Area: Adult Health/Renal

Reference
Black, J., & Matassarin-Jacobs, E. (1997). *Medical-surgical nursing: Clinical management for continuity of care* (5th ed.). Philadelphia: W. B. Saunders. pp. 571, 1673.

17. **4**

Rationale: The client after nephrectomy may be in considerable pain. This is due to the size of the incision and its location near the diaphragm, which makes coughing and deep breathing so uncomfortable. For this reason, narcotics are used liberally and may be most effective when provided as patient-controlled analgesia or through epidural analgesia.

Test-Taking Strategy: The question asks for the "most likely" reason for the client's statement, which implies that more than one option may be partially correct. Begin to answer the question by eliminating options 2 and 3 as the least plausible options. Knowing that coughing and deep breathing intensify pain after many surgical procedures helps you choose option 4 over option 1.

Level of Cognitive Ability: Analysis
Phase of Nursing Process: Analysis
Client Needs: Physiological Integrity
Content Area: Adult Health/Renal

Reference
Black, J., & Matassarin-Jacobs, E. (1997). *Medical-surgical nursing: Clinical management for continuity of care* (5th ed.). Philadelphia: W. B. Saunders. pp. 1672–1673.

18. **2**

Rationale: Epidural analgesia is used for clients with high levels of expected postoperative pain. The nurse carefully checks the medication, notes the client's level of sedation, and makes sure that the head of bed is elevated 30° unless contraindicated. The nurse aspirates to make sure there is no cerebrospinal fluid (CSF) return. If CSF returns with aspiration, the catheter has migrated from the epidural space into the subarachnoid space. The catheter is not flushed with 6 mL of sterile water. Narcan should be readily available for use if respiratory depression should occur.

Test-Taking Strategy: Begin to answer this question by eliminating option 4 first. Flushing 6 mL of sterile water through an epidural catheter is the least plausible and most dangerous option. Option 1 is eliminated next, since CSF aspiration should not occur with an epidural catheter. To discriminate between the last two options, you would choose option 2 as the correct answer if you knew that the antidote to fentanyl is naloxone. Or, you would choose option 2 by elimination if you knew that the head of the bed should be elevated at least 30°.

Level of Cognitive Ability: Application
Phase of Nursing Process: Planning
Client Needs: Physiological Integrity
Content Area: Pharmacology

Reference
Black, J., & Matassarin-Jacobs, E. (1997). *Medical-surgical nursing: Clinical management for continuity of care* (5th ed.). Philadelphia: W. B. Saunders. pp. 383, 1673.

19. **2**

Rationale: Both the kidney donor and recipient need thorough medical and psychological evaluation prior to transplant surgery. There are separate teams to evaluate the donor and recipient to avoid a conflict of interest on the part of the team. The psychosocial issues in living-related organ donation may be very complex, and conversations with the donor are held in strict confidence to preserve family relations.

Test-Taking Strategy: Begin to answer this question by eliminating options 3 and 4, which are the least plausible. You would choose option 2 over option 1 utilizing knowledge of concepts regarding client advocacy. One group cannot advocate for both parties simultaneously.

Level of Cognitive Ability: Analysis
Phase of Nursing Process: Analysis
Client Needs: Psychosocial Integrity
Content Area: Adult Health/Renal

Reference
Black, J., & Matassarin-Jacobs, E. (1997). *Medical-surgical nursing: Clinical management for continuity of care* (5th ed.). Philadelphia: W. B. Saunders. p. 1661.

20. **1**

Rationale: Intravenous fluids are managed very carefully following renal transplant. Fluids are given according to a formula that takes into account the previous hour's urine output. The desired urine output is generally high.

Test-Taking Strategy: Begin to answer this question by eliminating options 3 and 4 first, knowing that the intravenous fluid rate is titrated according to the urine output immediately following nephrectomy. To choose correctly between options 1 and 2, it is necessary to know that the formula adds the previous hour's urine output to a base rate.

Level of Cognitive Ability: Application
Phase of Nursing Process: Implementation
Client Needs: Physiological Integrity
Content Area: Adult Health/Renal

Reference

Black, J., & Matassarin-Jacobs, E. (1997). *Medical-surgical nursing: Clinical management for continuity of care* (5th ed.). Philadelphia: W. B. Saunders. p. 1664.

21. **2**

Rationale: Bladder trauma or injury should be considered or suspected in the client with low abdominal pain and hematuria. Renal cancer would not cause pain that is felt in the low abdomen; rather, it would be in the flank area. Glomerulonephritis and pyelonephritis would be accompanied by fever and are thus not applicable to the client in this question.

Test-Taking Strategy: Begin to answer this question by eliminating options 3 and 4, knowing that any inflammatory disease or infection is accompanied by fever. Since this client is afebrile, these are not possible choices. Knowledge of anatomy and pain assessment would guide you to choose option 2 over option 1. Pain from renal cancer is a later finding and is localized in the flank area.

Level of Cognitive Ability: Application
Phase of Nursing Process: Assessment
Client Needs: Physiological Integrity
Content Area: Adult Health/Renal

Reference

Black, J., & Matassarin-Jacobs, E. (1997). *Medical-surgical nursing: Clinical management for continuity of care* (5th ed.). Philadelphia: W. B. Saunders. p. 1619.

22. **1**

Rationale: Bladder trauma or injury is characterized by lower abdominal pain that may radiate to one of the shoulders. Bladder injury pain does not radiate to the umbilicus, costovertebral angle, or hip.

Test-Taking Strategy: To answer this question successfully, recall concepts related to dermatomes of the body and pain characteristics of bladder trauma. This would allow you to eliminate each of the incorrect options in turn.

Level of Cognitive Ability: Analysis
Phase of Nursing Process: Analysis
Client Needs: Physiological Integrity
Content Area: Adult Health/Renal

Reference

Black, J., & Matassarin-Jacobs, E. (1997). *Medical-surgical nursing: Clinical management for continuity of care* (5th ed.). Philadelphia: W. B. Saunders. p. 1619.

23. **4**

Rationale: The presence of blood at the urinary meatus may indicate urethral trauma or disruption. The nurse notifies the physician, knowing that the client should not be catheterized until the cause of the bleeding is determined by diagnostic testing.

Test-Taking Strategy: This question is straightforward in wording and intent. Basic knowledge of catheter insertion allows you to eliminate each of the incorrect options readily. If this question was difficult, take a few moments now to review this content area briefly.

Level of Cognitive Ability: Application
Phase of Nursing Process: Implementation
Client Needs: Physiological Integrity
Content Area: Adult Health/Renal

Reference

Black, J., & Matassarin-Jacobs, E. (1997). *Medical-surgical nursing: Clinical management for continuity of care* (5th ed.). Philadelphia: W. B. Saunders. p. 1619.

24. **1**

Rationale: The most common initial manifestation of bladder cancer is hematuria that is not accompanied by pain. The hematuria is intermittent at first. Later symptoms include hematuria with dysuria and frequency due to bladder irritation. Pyuria and proteinuria are not part of the clinical picture. A mass is usually not palpable.

Test-Taking Strategy: Begin to answer this question by eliminating option 3 first. Since this is not an infectious process, the client should not have pyuria. Knowing that pain and discomfort are later signs helps you eliminate options 2 and 4 next. This leaves option 1 as correct. The client usually presents with intermittent hematuria, which is not accompanied by pain.

Level of Cognitive Ability: Application
Phase of Nursing Process: Assessment
Client Needs: Physiological Integrity
Content Area: Adult Health/Renal

Reference

Black, J., & Matassarin-Jacobs, E. (1997). *Medical-surgical nursing: Clinical management for continuity of care* (5th ed.). Philadelphia: W. B. Saunders. p. 1583.

25. **3**

Rationale: A complication of radiation therapy for bladder cancer is fistula formation. In women, this is frequently manifested as a vesicovaginal fistula, which is an opening between the bladder and the vagina. With this complication, the client senses that urine is flowing out of the vagina. In men, a colovesical fistula may develop, which is an opening between the bladder and the colon. This is manifested as voiding urine that contains fecal material.

Test-Taking Strategy: Begin to answer this question by eliminating options 1 and 4 first as the least plausible of all the options. Specific knowledge of the usual effects of radiation therapy allows you to choose option 3 over option 2 as the correct answer.

Level of Cognitive Ability: Analysis
Phase of Nursing Process: Analysis
Client Needs: Physiological Integrity
Content Area: Adult Health/Renal

Reference

Black, J., & Matassarin-Jacobs, E. (1997). *Medical-surgical nursing: Clinical management for continuity of care* (5th ed.). Philadelphia: W. B. Saunders. p. 1584.

26. **4**

Rationale: Following intravesical chemotherapy, the nurse increases fluids to help flush the medication out of the bladder after the period of retention. The chemotherapy agent and the urine are treated as biohazards, but the client does not need to be placed on contact isolation. The client does not have a need for narcotic analgesics as a result of the chemotherapy session.

Test-Taking Strategy: Eliminate option 1 first, knowing that the client does not have a need for higher doses of narcotics as a result of this treatment. Knowing that the urine is the only biohazard helps you eliminate option 3 next. The client needs only universal precautions following this procedure. To discriminate between options 2 and 4, note that option 2 would have the effect of decreasing urine flow, whereas option 4 would increase urine flow. Knowing that increased urine flow will flush the residual chemotherapeutic agent from the bladder allows you to choose option 4 as correct.

Level of Cognitive Ability: Application
Phase of Nursing Process: Planning
Client Needs: Physiological Integrity
Content Area: Adult Health/Renal

Reference
Black, J., & Matassarin-Jacobs, E. (1997). *Medical-surgical nursing: Clinical management for continuity of care* (5th ed.). Philadelphia: W. B. Saunders. p. 1585.

27. **2**

Rationale: The client who has a radiation implant is placed in a private room and has limited visitors. This reduces the exposure of others to the radiation. Frequent rest periods are a helpful general intervention but are not a priority for the client in this situation. Reverse isolation is unnecessary.

Test-Taking Strategy: Note that the wording of the question asks for a priority action on the part of the nurse. This implies that more than one option may be totally or partially correct. Begin to answer the question by eliminating option 4 first as an unnecessary action. Option 1 is helpful but is not considered a priority and may be eliminated next. To discriminate between options 2 and 3, it is necessary to know that other people should have limited exposure to clients with radium implants. This would allow you to choose option 2 over option 3.

Level of Cognitive Ability: Application
Phase of Nursing Process: Implementation
Client Needs: Safe, Effective Care Environment
Content Area: Adult Health/Renal

Reference
Black, J., & Matassarin-Jacobs, E. (1997). *Medical-surgical nursing: Clinical management for continuity of care* (5th ed.). Philadelphia: W. B. Saunders. p. 1585.

28. **1**

Rationale: After intravesical chemotherapy, the client treats the urine as a biohazard. This involves disinfecting the urine and the toilet with household bleach for 6 hours. Scented disinfectants are of no particular use. The client does not need to have a separate bathroom for personal use. There is no value in using a bedpan for voiding.

Test-Taking Strategy: Option 4 is the least plausible of all the options for this question and may be eliminated first. Since scented disinfectants have no obvious value, option 3 is eliminated next. Knowing that the urine needs special treatment for only 6 hours after each session allows you to choose option 1 over option 2. Option 2 is unnecessary and may be unrealistic for a number of clients.

Level of Cognitive Ability: Analysis
Phase of Nursing Process: Evaluation
Client Needs: Safe, Effective Care Environment
Content Area: Adult Health/Renal

Reference
Black, J., & Matassarin-Jacobs, E. (1997). *Medical-surgical nursing: Clinical management for continuity of care* (5th ed.). Philadelphia: W. B. Saunders. p. 1585.

29. **4**

Rationale: The most positive initial step in learning to care for an ostomy and to accept it as a part of the self is to be able to look at the ostomy. Once the client is able to look at the ostomy and touch it, learning about ostomy care can then proceed more successfully. Each of the other responses indicates a deferral or refusal on the part of the client, which makes it a less than optimal choice.

Test-Taking Strategy: The wording of the question tells you that you are looking for "the best initial" adaptation. Options 2 and 3 do not illustrate adaptation in any way and are eliminated first. Option 4 is an action on the part of the client, whereas option 1 is still a refusal to participate in any way in ostomy care. Thus you would choose option 4 as the answer, since it is the only option that illustrates an action on the part of the client.

Level of Cognitive Ability: Analysis
Phase of Nursing Process: Analysis
Client Needs: Psychosocial Integrity
Content Area: Adult Health/Renal

Reference
Black, J., & Matassarin-Jacobs, E. (1997). *Medical-surgical nursing: Clinical management for continuity of care* (5th ed.). Philadelphia: W. B. Saunders. p. 1589.

30. **4**

Rationale: The skin around the stoma is cleansed at each appliance change, using a gentle, nonresidue soap and water. The skin is rinsed and then dried thoroughly. The appliance should be changed early in the morning, because urine production is slowest from no fluid intake during sleep. The appliance is cut so that the opening is not more than 3 mm larger than the stoma. An opening smaller than the stoma will prevent application of the appliance. Fluids are encouraged to dilute the urine, decreasing the incidence of odor.

Test-Taking Strategy: Begin to answer this question by eliminating option 3. Fluid limitation will not limit ammonia odor; in fact; decreased fluids will increase the concentration of the urine, making it stronger. Option 1 is eliminated next, because an appliance cut in this way will be too small to fit over the stoma. It may be difficult to choose between options 2 and 4. To choose correctly, you would need to realize that option 4 is completely correct, or you would need to recall that urine flow is slowest in the early morning from decreased intake during the night. Either of these thought processes would lead you to choose the correct answer to this question.

Level of Cognitive Ability: Application
Phase of Nursing Process: Planning
Client Needs: Health Promotion and Maintenance
Content Area: Adult Health/Renal

Reference
Black, J., & Matassarin-Jacobs, E. (1997). *Medical-surgical nursing: Clinical management for continuity of care* (5th ed.). Philadelphia: W. B. Saunders. p. 1592.

31. **1**

Rationale: The client who will have formation of either an ileal conduit or a reservoir undergoes bowel preparation the night before surgery. This includes clear liquids, laxatives, enemas, and antibiotics. This is done primarily because a loop of bowel will be used to create the urinary diversion.

Test-Taking Strategy: Options 3 and 4 are most obviously incorrect and may be eliminated first. You would choose option 1 over option 2 by knowing that the bowel is used to create the diversion, or by realizing that the response given in option 2 is not helpful to the client.

Level of Cognitive Ability: Application
Phase of Nursing Process: Implementation
Client Needs: Physiological Integrity
Content Area: Adult Health/Renal

Reference

Black, J., & Matassarin-Jacobs, E. (1997). *Medical-surgical nursing: Clinical management for continuity of care* (5th ed.). Philadelphia: W. B. Saunders. p. 1588.

32. **4**

Rationale: Urethritis in the male client often results from chlamydial infection and is characterized by dysuria, which is accompanied by a clear to mucopurulent discharge. Because this disorder often coexists with gonorrhea, diagnostic tests are done for both; these include culture and rapid assays.

Test-Taking Strategy: Begin to answer this question by eliminating options 1 and 2. Urethritis is generally accompanied by dysuria in the male client, which is present only in options 3 and 4. Knowing that the problem originates in the urethra, not the kidney, you would then eliminate the option with proteinuria, which indicates a problem with kidney function. This leaves option 4 as the correct answer. The male client with urethritis has dysuria and discharge from the penis.

Level of Cognitive Ability: Application
Phase of Nursing Process: Assessment
Client Needs: Physiological Integrity
Content Area: Adult Health/Renal

Reference

Black, J., & Matassarin-Jacobs, E. (1997). *Medical-surgical nursing: Clinical management for continuity of care* (5th ed.). Philadelphia: W. B. Saunders. p. 2469.

33. **1**

Rationale: The most serious complication of chlamydial infection is sterility. The infection can be prevented by the use of latex condoms. It is treated with doxycycline for 7 days, or with azithromycin (Zithromax) as a single dose. All sexual partners during the 30 days before diagnosis should be notified, examined, and treated as necessary.

Test-Taking Strategy: Eliminate option 2 first as a possible answer, using principles of infection control. Knowing that most courses of antibiotic therapy extend from 7 to 10 days in general may help you eliminate option 3 next. To discriminate accurately between options 1 and 4, it is necessary to know either that sterility is a serious and permanent complication, or that partners within the last month should be notified and treated as needed.

Level of Cognitive Ability: Application
Phase of Nursing Process: Planning
Client Needs: Physiological Integrity
Content Area: Adult Health/Renal

Reference

Black, J., & Matassarin-Jacobs, E. (1997). *Medical-surgical nursing: Clinical management for continuity of care* (5th ed.). Philadelphia: W. B. Saunders. p. 2470.

34. **3**

Rationale: Chlamydial infection is a sexually transmitted disease and is frequently called nongonococcal urethritis in the male client. It requires no special precautions. Caregivers cannot acquire the disease during administration of care, and using universal precautions is the only necessary measure.

Test-Taking Strategy: This question is straightforward in nature. A basic knowledge of infection control and disease transmission guides you to select option 3 as correct. If this question was difficult for you, take a few moments to review transmission of this disorder and universal precautions.

Level of Cognitive Ability: Application
Phase of Nursing Process: Implementation
Client Needs: Safe, Effective Care Environment
Content Area: Adult Health/Renal

Reference

Black, J., & Matassarin-Jacobs, E. (1997). *Medical-surgical nursing: Clinical management for continuity of care* (5th ed.). Philadelphia: W. B. Saunders. p. 2470.

35. **4**

Rationale: Antibiotics are not taken prophylactically to prevent acquisition of urethritis from chlamydial infection. The risk of reinfection can be reduced by limiting the number of sexual partners and by the use of condoms. In some instances, follow-up culture is requested in 4 to 7 days to confirm a cure.

Test-Taking Strategy: The wording of the question guides you to look for an incorrect response. Options 1 and 2 are the most obviously correct and are therefore eliminated as possible answers to the question. Knowing the basic principles of antibiotic therapy allows you to choose option 4, since antibiotics are not used intermittently at will for prophylaxis of this infection.

Level of Cognitive Ability: Analysis
Phase of Nursing Process: Evaluation
Client Needs: Health Promotion and Maintenance
Content Area: Adult Health/Renal

Reference

Black, J., & Matassarin-Jacobs, E. (1997). *Medical-surgical nursing: Clinical management for continuity of care* (5th ed.). Philadelphia: W. B. Saunders. p. 2470.

36. **2**

Rationale: Typical signs and symptoms of epididymitis include scrotal pain and edema, which are often accompanied by fever, nausea and vomiting, and chills. It is most often caused by infection, although sometimes it can be caused by trauma. It needs to be correctly distinguished from testicular torsion.

Test-Taking Strategy: Any disorder that ends in "itis" results from inflammation or infection. Therefore, an expected finding would be elevated temperature. With this in mind, you may eliminate options 3 and 4, since they do not contain fever as part of the response. Knowing that ecchymosis results from bleeding, which is not part of this clinical picture, helps you choose option 2 over option 1 as the answer.

Level of Cognitive Ability: Application
Phase of Nursing Process: Assessment
Client Needs: Physiological Integrity
Content Area: Adult Health/Renal

Reference

Black, J., & Matassarin-Jacobs, E. (1997). *Medical-surgical nursing: Clinical management for continuity of care* (5th ed.). Philadelphia: W. B. Saunders. p. 2381.

37. **4**

Rationale: Body Image Disturbance can be diagnosed when the client has either a verbal or a nonverbal response to a change in the structure or the function of a body part. Anxiety is a nonspecific feeling of unease. The diagnosis of Fear can be used when the client has an identifiable concern, but sterility is not mentioned as a concern by the client. Acute Pain may apply, but it does not match the information in the stem.

Test-Taking Strategy: Begin to answer this question by eliminating options 2 and 3, because the stem makes no mention of either pain or a fear of sterility. Knowing that anxiety cannot be traced to a specific cause helps you choose option 4 over option 1 as the correct answer.

Level of Cognitive Ability: Analysis
Phase of Nursing Process: Analysis
Client Needs: Psychosocial Integrity
Content Area: Adult Health/Renal

Reference

Cox, H., Hinz, M., Lubno, M., et al. (1997). *Clinical applications of nursing diagnosis: Adult, child, women's, psychiatric, gerontic and home health considerations* (3rd ed.). Philadelphia: F. A. Davis. pp. 453, 496, 506, 514.

38. **3**

Rationale: The client who receives a narcotic analgesic should immediately have the side rails raised on the bed, to prevent injury once the medication has taken effect. Dimming the light in the room is the next most helpful action. The name bracelet should have been checked before administering the medication. It is unnecessary to do range of motion exercise of the site of injection.

Test-Taking Strategy: Begin to answer this question by eliminating option 2, since this should have been done before administering the medication. Option 1 is not necessary and may be eliminated next. To discriminate between options 3 and 4, note that the question asks you for the action to be taken "next." With this in mind, you would choose option 3 over option 4. Although option 4 is a correct answer, it would be done upon leaving the room. As part of protecting the client's safety after administration of a narcotic analgesic, you would put the side rails up first.

Level of Cognitive Ability: Application
Phase of Nursing Process: Planning
Client Needs: Safe, Effective Care Environment
Content Area: Adult Health/Renal

Reference

Black, J., & Matassarin-Jacobs, E. (1997). *Medical-surgical nursing: Clinical management for continuity of care* (5th ed.). Philadelphia: W. B. Saunders. p. 2381.

39. **4**

Rationale: Common interventions used in the treatment of epididymitis include bed rest, elevation of the scrotum with a Bellevue bridge, ice packs, sitz baths, analgesics, and antibiotics. A heating pad would not be used because direct application of heat could increase blood flow to the area and increase the swelling.

Test-Taking Strategy: Begin to answer this question by eliminating options 1 and 2, since they are obviously the most helpful in the care of the client. In examining options 3 and 4, note that they both address the application of heat to the client. A sitz bath uses a milder temperature, and the heat is moist and soothing. Knowing that direct heat may increase inflammation with tissue that is already at risk would guide you to choose option 4 as the item to avoid.

Level of Cognitive Ability: Application
Phase of Nursing Process: Implementation
Client Needs: Physiological Integrity
Content Area: Adult Health/Renal

Reference

Black, J., & Matassarin-Jacobs, E. (1997). *Medical-surgical nursing: Clinical management for continuity of care* (5th ed.). Philadelphia: W. B. Saunders. p. 2381.

40. **2**

Rationale: The client who experiences epididymitis from urinary tract infection should increase intake of fluids to flush the urinary system. Since organisms can be forced into the vas deferens and epididymis from strain or pressure during voiding, the client may limit the force of the stream. Condom use can help prevent urethritis and epididymitis from STDs. Antibiotics are always taken until the full course of therapy is completed.

Test-Taking Strategy: The wording of the question guides you to look for an incorrect response. Since option 1 is consistent with good practices in the prevention of UTI, this option may be eliminated first. To eliminate options 3 and 4, it is necessary to know that the force of stream should be limited to prevent backflow into the epididymis, and that condoms are helpful in preventing this disorder from occurring as a complication of an STD. Remember that antibiotics are not stopped when symptoms subside but must be taken until the full course of therapy is completed.

Level of Cognitive Ability: Analysis
Phase of Nursing Process: Evaluation
Client Needs: Health Promotion and Maintenance
Content Area: Adult Health/Renal

Reference

Black, J., & Matassarin-Jacobs, E. (1997). *Medical-surgical nursing: Clinical management for continuity of care* (5th ed.). Philadelphia: W. B. Saunders. p. 2381.

41. **1**

Rationale: The client with prostatitis has a prostate gland that is swollen and tender, but which is also warm to the touch, firm, and indurated. Systemic symptoms include fever with chills, perineal and low back pain, and signs of urinary tract infection (which often accompany the disorder).

Test-Taking Strategy: Begin to answer this question by reasoning that inflammation of the prostate gland would cause the area to be tender. This would allow you to eliminate options 2 and 4. Knowing that inflammation is accompanied by local warmth, you could choose option 1 over option 3 as the correct answer. Or, you could also choose option 1 as correct knowing that ecchymosis is consistent with bleeding, but not inflammation.

Level of Cognitive Ability: Application
Phase of Nursing Process: Assessment
Client Needs: Physiological Integrity
Content Area: Adult Health/Renal

Reference

Black, J., & Matassarin-Jacobs, E. (1997). *Medical-surgical nursing: Clinical management for continuity of care* (5th ed.). Philadelphia: W. B. Saunders. p. 2372.

42. 3

Rationale: Occasionally, the client with acute prostatitis needs urinary catheterization if the client cannot void at all. Otherwise, catheterization is avoided to prevent introducing bacteria into the bladder by pushing them up the urethra. Catheterization does not prolong the course of the inflammation, nor does it cause rebound edema when it is discontinued. There is no reported risk of prostate gland puncture from this procedure, although it may be painful.

Test-Taking Strategy: Option 4 is the least plausible of all the choices and is eliminated first. Option 1 is also not very plausible and may be eliminated next. In comparing the remaining two responses, knowledge of transmission of infection would guide you to choose option 3 over option 2.

Level of Cognitive Ability: Analysis
Phase of Nursing Process: Analysis
Client Needs: Physiological Integrity
Content Area: Adult Health/Renal

Reference

Black, J., & Matassarin-Jacobs, E. (1997). *Medical-surgical nursing: Clinical management for continuity of care* (5th ed.). Philadelphia: W. B. Saunders. p. 2372.

43. 3

Rationale: Decreased force in the stream of urine is an early sign of BPH. The stream later becomes weak and dribbling. The client may then develop hematuria, frequency, urgency, urge incontinence, and nocturia. If untreated, complete obstruction and urinary retention can occur.

Test-Taking Strategy: Note that the question asks for an early symptom. If you know that BPH can lead to urinary obstruction, you can then work backward from the most severe symptom to the least, which should also be the earliest. Option 4 is obviously the most severe of symptoms and therefore is eliminated first. Options 1 and 2 are also more severe than option 3, which guides you to select option 3 as the answer to the question.

Level of Cognitive Ability: Application
Phase of Nursing Process: Assessment
Client Needs: Physiological Integrity
Content Area: Adult Health/Renal

Reference

Black, J., & Matassarin-Jacobs, E. (1997). Medical-surgical nursing: Clinical management for continuity of care (5th ed.). Philadelphia: W. B. Saunders. p. 2352.

44. 4

Rationale: In the client with BPH, episodes of urinary retention can be triggered by certain medications, such as decongestants, anticholinergics, and antidepressants. The client should be questioned about use of these medications if presenting with urinary retention. Retention can also be precipitated by other factors, such as drinking alcoholic beverages, infection, bed rest, and becoming chilled.

Test-Taking Strategy: The question is basically asking you about medications that could exacerbate or contribute to urinary retention in the client with BPH. Diuretics should help voiding, and therefore option 1 is readily eliminated. Antibiotics should have no effect at all, and thus option 2 is eliminated as well. To discriminate between options 3 and 4, it is necessary to know that medications that contain anticholinergics may cause urinary retention. This would guide you to choose option 4 over option 3 as the correct answer. Antitussives have no effect on urinary retention.

Level of Cognitive Ability: Analysis
Phase of Nursing Process: Analysis
Client Needs: Physiological Integrity
Content Area: Adult Health/Renal

Reference

Black, J., & Matassarin-Jacobs, E. (1997). *Medical-surgical nursing: Clinical management for continuity of care* (5th ed.). Philadelphia: W. B. Saunders. p. 2352.

45. 1

Rationale: A transrectal ultrasound and PSA level help rule out the possibility of prostate cancer. They do not predict the course of BPH nor the development of complications such as urinary obstruction. These tests have nothing to do with determining the need for self-catheterization.

Test-Taking Strategy: Begin to answer this question by eliminating options 2 and 3. Diagnostic tests do not predict the course of a disease nor the likelihood of developing complications (such as obstruction). In a similar vein, diagnostic tests will not determine whether self-catheterization is needed. Therefore, this option is eliminated as well. This leaves option 1 as the correct answer. You would also choose this option just by knowing that biopsy is done to rule out malignancy.

Level of Cognitive Ability: Application
Phase of Nursing Process: Implementation
Client Needs: Physiological Integrity
Content Area: Adult Health/Renal

Reference

Black, J., & Matassarin-Jacobs, E. (1997). *Medical-surgical nursing: Clinical management for continuity of care* (5th ed.). Philadelphia: W. B. Saunders. p. 2352.

46. 1

Rationale: In the immediate postoperative period, the client who has had surgery for cancer may experience Fear, related to the uncertain outcome of surgery. Postoperative pain is classified as acute, not chronic. The client may experience Body Image Disturbance, but it would more likely be related to anticipated change in sexual function, not the presence of the suprapubic catheter. The priority focus in the immediate postoperative period is not on diagnoses that apply to hospital discharge.

Test-Taking Strategy: Begin to answer this question by eliminating option 4 as the least appropriate in the time frame immediately following surgery. There is insufficient evidence in the stem of the question to support a nursing diagnosis of Chronic Pain, so option 2 is eliminated next. To discriminate between options 1 and 3, knowing that the suprapubic catheter is temporary may guide you to eliminate option 3 as the answer. Using a different line of reasoning, knowing that the client is concerned about prognosis upon awakening from surgery for cancer guides you to select option 1 as the correct answer.

Level of Cognitive Ability: Analysis
Phase of Nursing Process: Analysis
Client Needs: Psychosocial Integrity
Content Area: Adult Health/Renal

References

Black, J., & Matassarin-Jacobs, E. (1997). *Medical-surgical nursing: Clinical management for continuity of care* (5th ed.). Philadelphia: W. B. Saunders. p. 2360.
Cox, H., Hinz, M., Lubno, M., et al. (1997). *Clinical applications of nursing diagnosis: Adult, child, women's, psychiatric, gerontic and home health considerations* (3rd ed.). Philadelphia: F. A. Davis. pp. 506, 514.

47. **1**

Rationale: Bladder spasm following prostatectomy is treated with antispasmodic medications, such as B&O suppository or propantheline bromide (ProBanthine). Narcotic analgesics such as meperidine, morphine, and hydromorphone are usually not effective in treating pain caused by spasm.

Test-Taking Strategy: This question is straightforward in its analysis, even without knowing the specific answer to the question. Remember that options that are similar are not likely to be correct. Since options 2, 3, and 4 are all narcotic analgesics, the answer would most likely be option 1, the B&O suppository.

Level of Cognitive Ability: Application
Phase of Nursing Process: Analysis
Client Needs: Physiological Integrity
Content Area: Pharmacology

Reference

Black, J., & Matassarin-Jacobs, E. (1997). *Medical-surgical nursing: Clinical management for continuity of care* (5th ed.). Philadelphia: W. B. Saunders. p. 2361.

48. **4**

Rationale: The Valsalva maneuver is avoided following prostatectomy, because it increases the risk of bleeding in the postoperative period. An acceptable exercise is tightening the abdominal, gluteal, and perineal muscles, as if trying to prevent urination. Another acceptable exercise is tightening the rectal sphincter while relaxing the abdominal muscles; this prevents the Valsalva maneuver from occurring.

Test-Taking Strategy: Notice that the types of movement in the exercises described in options 1, 2, and 3 are all muscle-tightening types. On the other hand, the Valsalva maneuver in option 4 involves a bearing down or pushing type of movement. Knowing that options 1, 2, and 3 are similar will direct you to choose the Valsalva maneuver (option 4) as the item to avoid.

Level of Cognitive Ability: Analysis
Phase of Nursing Process: Evaluation
Client Needs: Health Promotion and Maintenance
Content Area: Adult Health/Renal

Reference

Black, J., & Matassarin-Jacobs, E. (1997). *Medical-surgical nursing: Clinical management for continuity of care* (5th ed.). Philadelphia: W. B. Saunders. p. 2363.

49. **1**

Rationale: ARF caused by glomerulonephritis is classified as intrinsic or intrarenal failure. This form of ARF is commonly manifested by hypertension, tachycardia, oliguria, lethargy, edema, and other signs of fluid overload. ARF from prerenal causes is characterized by decreased blood pressure or a recent history of the same, tachycardia, and decreased cardiac output and central venous pressure. Bradycardia is not part of the clinical picture for any form of renal failure.

Test-Taking Strategy: Begin to answer this question by recalling that renal failure is accompanied by fluid overload. This would guide you to eliminate option 4 first. Since fluid overload is accompanied by tachycardia (since the heart works harder to pump the volume), option 2 may be eliminated next. You would then choose option 1 over option 3 by knowing that hypertension accompanies ARF due to intrarenal causes, whereas decreased cardiac output accompanies ARF due to prerenal causes.

Level of Cognitive Ability: Application
Phase of Nursing Process: Assessment
Client Needs: Physiological Integrity
Content Area: Adult Health/Renal

Reference

Ignatavicius, D., Workman, M., & Mishler, M. (1995). *Medical-surgical nursing: A nursing process approach* (2nd ed.). Philadelphia: W. B. Saunders. pp. 2150–2151.

50. **4**

Rationale: The client with CRF may have several barriers to learning. Anxiety about the disease and its ramifications may frequently interfere with learning. Physiological effects of the disease process also impair the client's mental functioning. Specifically, the client may exhibit a short attention span and have memory deficits. This usually improves once hemodialysis has begun. The presence of family is helpful, since the family needs to understand the disease and treatment and may help reinforce information with the client after the formal teaching session is over.

Test-Taking Strategy: This question asks for the least interfering variable. Knowing that anxiety commonly interferes with learning, you would eliminate option 1 first. Options 2 and 3 are similar, in that they reflect neurological impairment. In this case, they are due to physiological effects of the disease on the nervous system. Recall that similar options are not likely to be correct. This would leave option 4 as the correct answer. The presence of family does not automatically interfere with learning; in fact, they may be quite helpful.

Level of Cognitive Ability: Analysis
Phase of Nursing Process: Analysis
Client Needs: Psychosocial Integrity
Content Area: Adult Health/Renal

Reference

Black, J., & Matassarin-Jacobs, E. (1997). *Medical-surgical nursing: Clinical management for continuity of care* (5th ed.). Philadelphia: W. B. Saunders. p. 1657.

51. **2**

Rationale: Phosphate-binding agents that contain aluminum include Alu-Cap, Basaljel, and Amphojel. These products are made from aluminum hydroxide. Tums are made from calcium carbonate and also bind phosphorus. Tums are being used more frequently in order to avoid the occurrence of dementia related to high intake of aluminum.

Phosphate-binding agents are needed by the client in renal failure because the kidneys cannot eliminate phosphorus.

Test-Taking Strategy: Option 1 may be eliminated rapidly since the name of the medication gives a clue as to its ingredients. Otherwise, specific knowledge of the types of antacids is needed to answer this question accurately. If needed, take a few moments now to review these two types of antacids and their use in renal failure.

Level of Cognitive Ability: Application
Phase of Nursing Process: Implementation
Client Needs: Physiological Integrity
Content Area: Pharmacology

Reference
Black, J., & Matassarin-Jacobs, E. (1997). *Medical-surgical nursing: Clinical management for continuity of care* (5th ed.). Philadelphia: W. B. Saunders. p. 1654.

52. 3

Rationale: The client with chronic renal failure often experiences a variety of psychosocial changes. These are related to uremia as well as the stress experienced by the client, who has a chronic disease that is life-threatening. These clients may have labile emotions and personality changes and may exhibit withdrawal, depression, or agitation. Delusions and psychosis can also occur. Euphoria is not part of the clinical picture for the client in renal failure.

Test-Taking Strategy: Options that are similar in nature are not likely to be correct. This would guide you to eliminate options 2 and 4 immediately. To discriminate between options 1 and 3, it is necessary to know that labile emotions are also characteristic of the disease and may be related to psychosocial factors as well as uremia.

Level of Cognitive Ability: Analysis
Phase of Nursing Process: Assessment
Client Needs: Psychosocial Integrity
Content Area: Adult Health/Renal

Reference
Black, J., & Matassarin-Jacobs, E. (1997). *Medical-surgical nursing: Clinical management for continuity of care* (5th ed.). Philadelphia: W. B. Saunders. pp. 1646–1647.

53. 4

Rationale: The client with renal failure is almost certain to have a problem with constipation due to factors such as fluid restriction, fatigue that limits exercise, and dietary restrictions on most high-fiber foods (which have high potassium content). In addition, phosphate-binding antacids such as ALternaGEL cause constipation as a side effect.

Test-Taking Strategy: Look for the response that is the most global; that is, look for the one that takes into account all the data presented in the stem. This would allow you to eliminate each of the incorrect responses, since each of them addresses only one piece of data supplied in the stem of the question.

Level of Cognitive Ability: Analysis
Phase of Nursing Process: Analysis
Client Needs: Physiological Integrity
Content Area: Adult Health/Renal

Reference
Black, J., & Matassarin-Jacobs, E. (1997). *Medical-surgical nursing: Clinical management for continuity of care* (5th ed.). Philadelphia: W. B. Saunders. p. 1656.

54. 1

Rationale: Epoetin alfa is erythropoietin that has been manufactured through the use of recombinant DNA technology. It is used to treat anemia in the client with chronic renal failure. The medication may be administered subcutaneously or intravenously.

Test-Taking Strategy: Specific knowledge of epoetin alfa is necessary to answer this question. If the medication or its methods of administration are unfamiliar to you, take a few moments to review this medication.

Level of Cognitive Ability: Application
Phase of Nursing Process: Implementation
Client Needs: Physiological Integrity
Content Area: Pharmacology

Reference
Black, J., & Matassarin-Jacobs, E. (1997). *Medical-surgical nursing: Clinical management for continuity of care* (5th ed.). Philadelphia: W. B. Saunders p. 1654.

55. 3

Rationale: Psychosocial reactions to chronic renal failure and hemodialysis are varied and may include anger. Other reactions include personality changes, emotional lability, withdrawal, and depression. The individual client's response may vary depending on the client's personality and support systems. The client in this question is exhibiting anger. The client has not projected blame on the nurse, nor does the client statement reflect withdrawal or depression.

Test-Taking Strategy: A knowledge of basic communication theory helps you answer this question. This would help you eliminate each of the incorrect options systematically.

Level of Cognitive Ability: Analysis
Phase of Nursing Process: Assessment
Client Needs: Psychosocial Integrity
Content Area: Adult Health/Renal

Reference
Black, J., & Matassarin-Jacobs, E. (1997). *Medical-surgical nursing: Clinical management for continuity of care* (5th ed.). Philadelphia: W. B. Saunders. pp. 1646–1647.

56. 4

Rationale: Hemodialysis typically lowers the amounts of fluid, sodium, potassium, urea, nitrogen, creatinine, uric acid, magnesium, and phosphate levels in the blood. Hemodialysis also enhances anemia, because RBCs are lost in dialysis from blood sampling and anticoagulation during the procedure, and from residual blood that is left in the dialyzer. While all these results are expected, only the lowered RBC count is nontherapeutic and enhances the anemia already caused by the disease process.

Test-Taking Strategy: Look for the key words in the question. They are "expected" and "nontherapeutic." Knowing that all the values are expected guides you then to focus on which of the results is nontherapeutic. An adequate understanding of dialysis would then guide you to eliminate each of the incorrect options.

Level of Cognitive Ability: Analysis
Phase of Nursing Process: Analysis
Client Needs: Physiological Integrity
Content Area: Adult Health/Renal

Reference
Black, J., & Matassarin-Jacobs, E. (1997). *Medical-surgical nursing: Clinical management for continuity of care* (5th ed.). Philadelphia: W. B. Saunders. pp. 1644, 1653.

57. **2**

Rationale: General indicators that the client is not experiencing infection include temperature and WBC count within normal limits. The client should also use proper handwashing technique as a general preventive measure. Handwashing once per day is insufficient and is therefore incorrect. It is true that the client should avoid blood pressure measurement in the affected arm; however, this would relate more closely to the nursing diagnosis Risk for Injury.

Test-Taking Strategy: Determine what the question is asking. The answer to this question will be the best indicator that the client is infection-free. Since option 4 is unrelated to infection, this is eliminated immediately. Since options 1 and 3 are less than optimal, they are also eliminated, leaving option 2 as the correct answer.

Level of Cognitive Ability: Application
Phase of Nursing Process: Planning
Client Needs: Physiological Integrity
Content Area: Adult Health/Renal

Reference
Black, J., & Matassarin-Jacobs, E. (1997). *Medical-surgical nursing: Clinical management for continuity of care* (5th ed.). Philadelphia: W. B. Saunders. p. 1658.

58. **1**

Rationale: Many medications are dialyzable, which means they are extracted from the blood-stream during dialysis. Therefore, many medications may be withheld on the day of dialysis until after the procedure. It is not typical for medications to be "double-dosed," since there is no way to be certain how much of each drug is cleared by dialysis. Clients receiving hemodialysis are not routinely taught that it is acceptable to disregard dietary and fluid restrictions.

Test-Taking Strategy: Note that the responses to this question are dichotomized into two groups. Knowing that clients are not taught to "cheat" on therapeutic diet or fluid orders helps you eliminate options 3 and 4. To discriminate between options 1 and 2, it is necessary to know that hemodialysis decreases serum drug levels, and that medications generally should not be given predialysis.

Level of Cognitive Ability: Application
Phase of Nursing Process: Implementation
Client Needs: Physiological Integrity
Content Area: Adult Health/Renal

Reference
Black, J., & Matassarin-Jacobs, E. (1997). *Medical-surgical nursing: Clinical management for continuity of care* (5th ed.). Philadelphia: W. B. Saunders. p. 1653.

59. **4**

Rationale: Disequilibrium syndrome is characterized by headache, mental confusion, decreasing level of consciousness, nausea, vomiting, twitching, and possible seizure activity. It is caused by rapid removal of solutes from the body during hemodialysis. At the same time, the blood-brain barrier interferes with the efficient removal of wastes from brain tissue. As a result, water goes into cerebral cells because of the osmotic gradient, causing brain swelling and onset of symptoms. It most often occurs in clients who are new to dialysis and is prevented by dialyzing for shorter times or at reduced blood flow rates.

Test-Taking Strategy: Familiarity with the causes and symptoms of disequilibrium syndrome is necessary to answer this question correctly. If this question was difficult, take a few moments to review this syndrome.

Level of Cognitive Ability: Application
Phase of Nursing Process: Assessment
Client Needs: Physiological Integrity
Content Area: Adult Health/Renal

Reference
Black, J., & Matassarin-Jacobs, E. (1997). *Medical-surgical nursing: Clinical management for continuity of care* (5th ed.). Philadelphia: W. B. Saunders. p. 1654.

60. **2**

Rationale: Aluminum intoxication may occur when there is accumulation of aluminum, an ingredient in many phosphate-binding antacids. It results in mental cloudiness, dementia, and bone pain from infiltration of the bone with aluminum. This condition was formerly known as dialysis dementia. It may be treated with aluminum-chelating agents, which make aluminum available to be dialyzed from the body. It can be prevented by avoiding or limiting the use of phosphate-binding agents that contain aluminum.

Test-Taking Strategy: To answer this question correctly, it is necessary to understand the potential implications of long-term use of aluminum-containing phosphate-binding agents by the hemodialysis client. If this question was difficult, take a few moments to review this information now.

Level of Cognitive Ability: Analysis
Phase of Nursing Process: Analysis
Client Needs: Physiological Integrity
Content Area: Adult Health/Renal

Reference
Black, J., & Matassarin-Jacobs, E. (1997). *Medical-surgical nursing: Clinical management for continuity of care* (5th ed.). Philadelphia: W. B. Saunders. p. 1654.

61. **1**

Rationale: Heparin is the anticoagulant used most often during hemodialysis. The hemodialysis nurse monitors the extent of anticoagulation by measuring the PTT, which is the appropriate test to measure heparin effect. The PT is used to monitor the effect of warfarin (Coumadin) therapy. Thrombin and bleeding times are not used to measure the effect of heparin therapy, although they are useful in the diagnosis of other clotting abnormalities.

Test-Taking Strategy: Specific knowledge about the effects of heparin therapy on blood coagulation studies is needed to answer this question. If needed, take a few moments to review this material now.

Level of Cognitive Ability: Application
Phase of Nursing Process: Planning
Client Needs: Physiological Integrity
Content Area: Adult Health/Renal

Reference
Black, J., & Matassarin-Jacobs, E. (1997). *Medical-surgical nursing: Clinical management for continuity of care* (5th ed.). Philadelphia: W. B. Saunders. p. 1653.

62. 4

Rationale: Following dialysis, the client's vital signs are monitored to determine whether the client is remaining hemodynamically stable. Weight is measured and compared with the client's "dry weight" to determine the effectiveness of fluid extraction. Laboratory studies are done as per protocol but are not necessarily done after the hemodialysis treatment has been ended.

Test-Taking Strategy: Note that the question asks about measures to determine the client's status postdialysis. Knowing that hemodialysis disturbs the client's hemodynamics, you would narrow your choices to options 3 and 4, which contain vital signs measurements. To discriminate between the last two, it is necessary to know that the client's weight is an important indicator of the effectiveness of fluid removal and also has an effect on hemodynamics.

Level of Cognitive Ability: Application
Phase of Nursing Process: Evaluation
Client Needs: Physiological Integrity
Content Area: Adult Health/Renal

Reference
Luckmann, J. (1997). *Saunders manual of nursing care.* Philadelphia: W. B. Saunders. pp. 1194–1195.

63. 2

Rationale: Steal syndrome results from vascular insufficiency after creation of a fistula. The client exhibits pallor and diminished pulse distal to the fistula and complains of pain distal to the fistula, which is due to tissue ischemia. Warmth, redness, and pain would more likely characterize a problem with infection. The patterns described in options 3 and 4 are not associated with steal syndrome.

Test-Taking Strategy: Knowledge of steal syndrome and its signs and symptoms is needed to answer this question correctly. If needed, take a few moments now to review this material.

Level of Cognitive Ability: Application
Phase of Nursing Process: Assessment
Client Needs: Physiological Integrity
Content Area: Adult Health/Renal

Reference
Luckmann, J. (1997). *Saunders manual of nursing care.* Philadelphia: W. B. Saunders. p. 1195.

64. 4

Rationale: For the client taking a normal diet, the normal fluid intake is approximately 1200 to 1800 mL of measurable fluids per day. The client's output in the same period should be about the same and not include insensible losses, which are extra. This is offset by the fluid in solid foods, which also is not measured.

Test-Taking Strategy: This question tests a fundamental concept and is straightforward in wording. Knowing that intake should approximately equal output helps you eliminate each of the incorrect choices. If this question was difficult, take a few moments to review this core principle.

Level of Cognitive Ability: Analysis
Phase of Nursing Process: Evaluation
Client Needs: Physiological Integrity
Content Area: Adult Health/Renal

Reference
Black, J., & Matassarin-Jacobs, E. (1997). *Medical-surgical nursing: Clinical management for continuity of care* (5th ed.). Philadelphia: W. B. Saunders. p. 1554.

65. 3

Rationale: Risk factors associated with pyelonephritis include diabetes mellitus, hypertension, chronic renal calculi, chronic cystitis, structural abnormalities of the urinary tract, presence of urinary stones, and indwelling catheter or frequent urinary catheterization.

Test-Taking Strategy: Eliminate options 1 and 4 first as least likely to be associated as risk factors. From the remaining options, remember that diabetes mellitus can cause renal complications. This will assist in directing you to the correct option.

Level of Cognitive Ability: Analysis
Phase of Nursing Process: Analysis
Client Needs: Physiological Integrity
Content Area: Adult Health/Renal

Reference
Black, J., & Matassarin-Jacobs, E. (1997). *Medical-surgical nursing: Clinical management for continuity of care* (5th ed.). Philadelphia: W. B. Saunders. p. 1628.

66. 1

Rationale: The BUN is the most frequently used laboratory test to determine renal function. The BUN starts to rise when the glomerular filtration rate falls below 40% to 60%. A decreased hemoglobin and RBC count may be noted if bleeding from the urinary tract occurs or if erythropoietic function by the kidney is impaired. An increased WBC count is most likely to be noted in renal disease.

Test-Taking Strategy: Note the key words "most likely expect to note" in the stem of the question. Eliminate option 4 first. Although options 2 and 3 may be noted in some renal disorders, option 1 is the most likely laboratory finding. Review significant laboratory tests now, if you had difficulty with this question!

Level of Cognitive Ability: Analysis
Phase of Nursing Process: Analysis
Client Needs: Physiological Integrity
Content Area: Adult Health/Renal

Reference
Black, J., & Matassarin-Jacobs, E. (1997). *Medical-surgical nursing: Clinical management for continuity of care* (5th ed.). Philadelphia: W. B. Saunders. p. 1562.

67. 4

Rationale: The ratio of BUN to creatinine is approximately 10:1 to 15:1. A value lower than 10:1 would indicate diminished urea concentration. A value greater than 15:1 would indicate inadequate renal function.

Test-Taking Strategy: Knowledge regarding the normal ratio of BUN to creatinine is required to answer the question. Learn the normal values and the importance of this test now, if you had difficulty with this question!

Level of Cognitive Ability: Analysis
Phase of Nursing Process: Analysis
Client Needs: Physiological Integrity
Content Area: Adult Health/Renal

Reference
Chernecky, C., & Berger, B. (1997). *Laboratory tests and diagnostic procedures* (2nd ed.). Philadelphia: W. B. Saunders. p. 261.

68. 2

Rationale: Refrigeration preserves the elements of urine, but the delay can cause crystals to precipitate. If the specimen stands at room temperature, the warmth causes bacteria and WBCs to decompose. When urine is allowed to stand unrefrigerated, the urea breaks down to ammonia and becomes more alkaline. The pH decreases in an acidic condition and increases in an alkaline environment.

Test-Taking Strategy: Careful reading will assist you to eliminate option 3 easily. Eliminate options 1 and 4 next because they are similar. pH decreases in acidic conditions. This leaves option 2 as the likely option.

Level of Cognitive Ability: Analysis
Phase of Nursing Process: Analysis
Client Needs: Safe, Effective Care Environment
Content Area: Adult Health/Renal

Reference
McMorrow, M.E., & Malarkey, L. (1998). *Laboratory and diagnostic tests: A pocket guide.* Philadelphia: W. B. Saunders. p. 329.

69. 1

Rationale: Since the 24-hour urine is a timed quantitative determination, it is essential to start the test with an empty bladder. The urine collection should be refrigerated or placed on ice to prevent changes in urine. Fifteen minutes prior to the end of the collection time, the client should be asked to void, and this specimen is added to the collection.

Test-Taking Strategy: Note that options 1 and 2 are addressing the same issue and are different in regards to this procedure. This would lead you to think that one of these options is the correct option. Try to think about the purpose of this timed test and eliminate option 2 because it would make sense that this test should be started when the client has an empty bladder. Review this procedure now, if you had difficulty with this question!

Level of Cognitive Ability: Application
Phase of Nursing Process: Implementation
Client Needs: Safe, Effective Care Environment
Content Area: Adult Health/Renal

Reference
Lammon, C., Foote, A., Leli, P., et al. (1995). *Clinical nursing skills.* Philadelphia: W. B. Saunders. pp. 133–134.

70. 4

Rationale: There are no specific precautions following a renal scan. If the client is able, urination into a commode is acceptable without risk from the small amount of radioactive material to be excreted. The nurse wears gloves to maintain body secretion precautions.

Test-Taking Strategy: Knowledge regarding the renal scan is required to answer this question. Knowing that there is generally no danger from the small amount of radioactive material used in this procedure will easily direct you to option 4. Review this procedure now, if you had difficulty with this question!

Level of Cognitive Ability: Application
Phase of Nursing Process: Planning
Client Needs: Safe, Effective Care Environment
Content Area: Adult Health/Renal

Reference
Ignatavicius, D., Workman, M., & Mishler, M. (1995). *Medical-surgical nursing: A nursing process approach* (2nd ed.). Philadelphia: W. B. Saunders. p. 2039.

71. 3

Rationale: The iodine-based dye used during the IVP can cause allergic reactions such as itching, hives, rash, tight feeling in the throat, shortness of breath, and bronchospasm. Assessing for allergies is the priority.

Test-Taking Strategy: Note the key word "priority" in the stem of the question. Utilize the nursing process as a guide. Option 1, 2, and 4 address implementation. Option 3 is the only option that addresses assessment.

Level of Cognitive Ability: Application
Phase of Nursing Process: Implementation
Client Needs: Physiological Integrity
Content Area: Adult Health/Renal

Reference
Chernecky, C., & Berger, B. (1997). *Laboratory tests and diagnostic procedures* (2nd ed.). Philadelphia: W. B. Saunders. p. 643.

72. 3

Rationale: Urine specimens for cultures should be obtained using proper cleansing and voiding techniques to avoid contamination from external sources. The use of paper towels will contaminate the specimen. The procedure described in option 1 would not provide a clean specimen. It is not necessary to obtain the specimen via catheter.

Test-Taking Strategy: Note the key words "clean catch." These words should assist in eliminating options 1 and 4 and easily direct you to option 3. If you had difficulty with this question, take time now to review the procedure for this type of urine collection!

Level of Cognitive Ability: Analysis
Phase of Nursing Process: Evaluation
Client Needs: Safe, Effective Care Environment
Content Area: Adult Health/Renal

Reference
Lammon, C., Foote, A., Leli, P., et al. (1995). *Clinical nursing skills.* Philadelphia: W. B. Saunders, pp. 123–125.

73. 4

Rationale: An excretory urogram is an invasive test that uses contrast radiopaque dye to assess the ability of the kidneys to excrete dye in the urine. Bowel preparation is necessary to permit adequate visualization of the kidneys, ureters, and bladder.

Test-Taking Strategy: Knowledge regarding this procedure is required to answer this question. The name of the procedure may provide you with the clue that visualization of the renal system is necessary. This information should easily direct you to option 4. Review test preparation for this procedure now, if you had difficulty with this question!

Level of Cognitive Ability: Analysis
Phase of Nursing Process: Planning
Client Needs: Physiological Integrity
Content Area: Adult Health/Renal

Reference
Chernecky, C., & Berger, B. (1997). *Laboratory tests and diagnostic procedures* (2nd ed.). Philadelphia: W. B. Saunders. p. 643.

74. 1

Rationale: If pain originates at the biopsy site and begins to radiate to the flank area and around the front of the abdomen, bleeding should be suspected. Hypotension, a decreasing hematocrit, and gross or microscopic hematuria would also indicate bleeding. Signs of infection would not appear immediately following a biopsy. Pain of this nature is not normal. There are no data to support the presence of renal colic.

Test-Taking Strategy: You can easily eliminate options 3 and 4. Recalling that signs of infection may not appear immediately following biopsy will assist in directing you to option 1.

Level of Cognitive Ability: Analysis
Phase of Nursing Process: Assessment
Client Needs: Physiological Integrity
Content Area: Adult Health/Renal

Reference
Black, J., & Matassarin-Jacobs, E. (1997). *Medical-surgical nursing: Clinical management for continuity of care* (5th ed.). Philadelphia: W. B. Saunders. p. 1569.

75. 1

Rationale: Polyuria occurs early in CRF and if untreated can cause severe dehydration. Polyuria progresses to anuria, and the client loses all normal functions of the kidney. Oliguria and anuria are not early signs and edema occurs in the later stages of renal failure.

Test-Taking Strategy: Note the key word "early" in the question. Eliminate options 3 and 4 because they are similar. From the remaining options select option 1 because this option relates to early renal function and is the correct answer to this question. Review the early and later signs of CRF now, if you had difficulty with this question!

Level of Cognitive Ability: Analysis
Phase of Nursing Process: Assessment
Client Needs: Physiological Integrity
Content Area: Adult Health/Renal

Reference
Black, J., & Matassarin-Jacobs, E. (1997). *Medical-surgical nursing: Clinical management for continuity of care* (5th ed.). Philadelphia: W. B. Saunders. p. 1644.

76. 1

Rationale: Amphojel binds with phosphate in the intestines to be excreted in the feces, thus lowering phosphorus levels. It can cause constipation, and it does not promote the elimination of potassium. It may be used in the treatment of hyperacidity associated with gastric ulcers, but this is not the purpose of its use in the client with renal failure.

Test-Taking Strategy: Knowledge regarding the purpose of this medication in CRF is required to answer this question. If you are unfamiliar with this medication, review now. You are likely to see a question regarding this medication on NCLEX-RN!

Level of Cognitive Ability: Analysis
Phase of Nursing Process: Analysis
Client Needs: Physiological Integrity
Content Area: Adult Health/Renal

Reference
Hodgson, B., & Kizior, R. (1998). *Saunders nursing drug handbook 1998.* Philadelphia: W. B. Saunders. p. 34.

77. 3

Rationale: Aldomet is metabolized by the kidneys and requires careful dosage adjustment according to the client's renal function to prevent hypotension. Epogen is an erythropoietin and is more likely to cause hypertension. Hypotension is a rare side effect of Inderal. Os-Cal is used in the treatment of calcium deficiency and does not cause hypotension when administered by the oral route. Parenteral administration of calcium may cause hypotension.

Test-Taking Strategy: Eliminate options 2 and 4 first because they are not used to control blood pressure. From the remaining options, knowledge that Aldomet is an antihypertensive medication will easily direct you to option 3. Review these important medications now, if you are unfamiliar with them!

Level of Cognitive Ability: Analysis
Phase of Nursing Process: Analysis
Client Needs: Physiological Integrity
Content Area: Pharmacology

Reference
Hodgson, B., & Kizior, R. (1998). *Saunders nursing drug handbook 1998.* Philadelphia: W. B. Saunders. pp. 141, 369–371, 879.

78. 4

Rationale: The client may have an elevated temperature following dialysis because the dialysis machine warms the blood slightly. If the temperature is elevated excessively and remains elevated, sepsis would be suspected, and a blood sample would be obtained as prescribed for culture and sensitivity determinations.

Test-Taking Strategy: Note the key words "most appropriate." Knowledge that an elevated temperature is expected following dialysis will assist in directing you to option 4. If you had difficulty with this question, review the normal expected findings following dialysis!

Level of Cognitive Ability: Application
Phase of Nursing Process: Implementation
Client Needs: Physiological Integrity
Content Area: Adult Health/Renal

Reference
Ignatavicius, D., Workman, M., & Mishler, M. (1995). *Medical-surgical nursing: A nursing process approach* (2nd ed.). Philadelphia: W. B. Saunders. p. 2137.

79. 1

Rationale: Dialysate is made from clear water and chemicals and is free from any metabolic waste products or medications. Bacteria and other microorganisms are too large to pass through the membrane; therefore, the dialysate does not need to be sterile. The dialysate is warmed to approximately 100°F to increase the efficiency of diffusion and to prevent a decrease in the client's blood temperature. Heparin inhibits the tendency of blood to clot when it comes in contact with foreign substances. Option 4 is the purpose of dialysis.

Test-Taking Strategy: Knowledge regarding the purpose of dialysis and the procedure will assist in eliminating options 2, 3, and 4. If you had difficulty with this question, review the components and characteristics of dialysate!

Level of Cognitive Ability: Analysis
Phase of Nursing Process: Evaluation
Client Needs: Safe, Effective Care Environment
Content Area: Adult Health/Renal

Reference
Ignatavicius, D., Workman, M., & Mishler, M. (1995). *Medical-surgical nursing: A nursing process approach* (2nd ed.). Philadelphia: W. B. Saunders. p. 2132.

80. 1

Rationale: Disequilibrium syndrome may be due to the rapid decrease in BUN levels during hemodialysis. These changes can cause cerebral edema, which leads to increased intracranial pressure. The client is exhibiting early signs of disequilibrium syndrome, and appropriate treatment with anticonvulsive medications and barbiturates may be necessary to prevent a life-threatening situation. The physician must be notified.

Test-Taking Strategy: Knowledge regarding the complications of hemodialysis and the signs and symptoms associated with the complications will assist in directing you to option 1. If you are unfamiliar with disequilibrium syndrome, review the signs and symptoms and the appropriate interventions required for this disorder.

Level of Cognitive Ability: Application
Phase of Nursing Process: Implementation
Client Needs: Physiological Integrity
Content Area: Adult Health/Renal

Reference
Ignatavicius, D., Workman, M., & Mishler, M. (1995). *Medical-surgical nursing: A nursing process approach* (2nd ed.). Philadelphia: W. B. Saunders. pp. 2137–2138.

81. 2

Rationale: The clinical signs of oliguric ARF are an elevated BUN and creatinine, urinary output of less than 400 mL for 24 hours, high specific gravity, low urinary sodium, traces of protein, and casts in the urine. In acute prerenal failure, which occurs as a result of impaired renal perfusion, specific gravity is high.

Test-Taking Strategy: Note the key words "not" and "oliguric" in the question. Knowing the clinical manifestations associated with this phase of ARF and that urine production falls below 400 mL/day will assist in directing you to option 2. If you are unfamiliar with the phases of ARF, review them now!

Level of Cognitive Ability: Analysis
Phase of Nursing Process: Analysis
Client Needs: Physiological Integrity
Content Area: Adult Health/Renal

References:
Black, J., & Matassarin-Jacobs, E. (1997). *Medical-surgical nursing: Clinical management for continuity of care* (5th ed.). Philadelphia: W. B. Saunders, p. 1638.
Luckmann, J. (1997). *Saunders manual of nursing care.* Philadelphia: W. B. Saunders. p. 1190.

82. 1

Rationale: Specific gravity evaluates the kidneys' ability to regulate fluid balance as well as the hydration status of the body. The BUN and creatinine more specifically evaluate renal function. A small amount of protein in the urine may be normal or proteinuria may be an indicator of renal pathology.

Test-Taking Strategy: Note the key words "regulate fluid balance." This should easily assist you in eliminating options 2, 3, and 4. If you are unfamiliar with the purposes of these tests and their relationship to renal function, review now!

Level of Cognitive Ability: Analysis
Phase of Nursing Process: Analysis
Client Needs: Physiological Integrity
Content Area: Adult Health/Renal

Reference
Chernecky, C., & Berger, B. (1997). *Laboratory tests and diagnostic procedures* (2nd ed.). Philadelphia: W. B. Saunders. pp. 846, 921, 1003.

83. 4

Rationale: Clinical manifestations associated with ARF occur as a result of the metabolic acidosis that occurs. The nurse would expect to note Kussmaul breathing as a result of the metabolic acidosis because the bodily response is to exhale excess carbon dioxide.

Test-Taking Strategy: Knowledge that the client with ARF experiences metabolic acidosis will easily direct you to option 4. Recalling that the client with diabetic ketoacidosis (metabolic acidosis) experiences Kussmaul breathing, will assist in answering this question.

Level of Cognitive Ability: Analysis
Phase of Nursing Process: Assessment
Client Needs: Physiological Integrity
Content Area: Adult Health/Renal

Reference
Luckmann, J. (1997). *Saunders manual of nursing care.* Philadelphia: W. B. Saunders. p. 1190.

84. 3

Rationale: Cantaloupe (¼ small), spinach (½ cup cooked), and strawberries (1¼ cups) are high-potassium foods and average 7 mEq per serving. Lima beans (⅓ cup) average 3 mEq per serving.

Test-Taking Strategy: Utilize the process of elimination, remembering that many fruits and green leafy vegetables are high in potassium. This may assist in directing you to option 3.

Level of Cognitive Ability: Analysis
Phase of Nursing Process: Evaluation
Client Needs: Health Promotion and Maintenance
Content Area: Adult Health/Renal

Reference
Black, J., & Matassarin-Jacobs, E. (1997). *Medical-surgical nursing: Clinical management for continuity of care* (5th ed.). Philadelphia: W. B. Saunders. p. 313.

85. 1

Rationale: In the diuretic phase, fluids and electrolytes are lost in the urine. As a result, the plan of care focuses on fluid and electrolyte replacement and monitoring.

Test-Taking Strategy: Noting that the issue of the question focuses on the diuretic phase should easily direct you to option 1.

Level of Cognitive Ability: Analysis
Phase of Nursing Process: Evaluation
Client Needs: Physiological Integrity
Content Area: Adult Health/Renal

Reference
Ignatavicius, D., Workman, M., & Mishler, M. (1995). *Medical-surgical nursing: A nursing process approach* (2nd ed.). Philadelphia: W. B. Saunders. p. 2152.

86. 3

Rationale: CAPD closely approximates normal renal function and the client will need to infuse and drain several times a day. No machinery is used, and CAPD is a manual procedure.

Test-Taking Strategy: Read the options carefully, noting that options 1, 2, and 4 address the use of a cycling machine. Option 3 is the option that is different and correctly describes the procedure for CAPD.

Level of Cognitive Ability: Analysis
Phase of Nursing Process: Evaluation
Client Needs: Health Promotion and Maintenance
Content Area: Adult Health/Renal

Reference
Monahan, F., & Neighbors, M. (1998). *Medical-surgical nursing: Foundations for clinical practice* (2nd ed.). Philadelphia: W. B. Saunders. pp. 1402–1403.

87. **4**

Rationale: Increasing the glucose concentration makes the solution increasingly more hypertonic. The more hypertonic the solution, the greater the osmotic pressure for ultrafiltration and thus the greater the amount of fluid removed from the client during an exchange.

Test-Taking Strategy: Knowledge regarding the principles related to ultrafiltration is required to answer this question. If you had difficulty with this question, take time now to review dialysate solutions for peritoneal dialysis!

Level of Cognitive Ability: Analysis
Phase of Nursing Process: Analysis
Client Needs: Physiological Integrity
Content Area: Adult Health/Renal

Reference
Ignatavicius, D., Workman, M., & Mishler, M. (1995). *Medical-surgical nursing: A nursing process approach* (2nd ed.). Philadelphia: W. B. Saunders. p. 2139.

88. **2**

Rationale: The major complication of peritoneal dialysis is peritonitis. Strict aseptic technique is required in caring for the client receiving this treatment. Although option 4 may assist in preventing infection, this option relates to an external site. Options 1 and 3 are unrelated to the major complication of peritoneal dialysis.

Test-Taking Strategy: Knowledge of the major complication of peritoneal dialysis will easily direct you to option 2. If you are unfamiliar with the complications associated with this procedure, review them now. You are likely to find a question related to this concept on NCLEX-RN!

Level of Cognitive Ability: Application
Phase of Nursing Process: Planning
Client Needs: Safe, Effective Care Environment
Content Area: Adult Health/Renal

Reference
Ignatavicius, D., Workman, M., & Mishler, M. (1995). *Medical-surgical nursing: A nursing process approach* (2nd ed.). Philadelphia: W. B. Saunders. p. 2140.

89. **3**

Rationale: Pain during the inflow of dialysate is common during the first few exchanges because of peritoneal irritation; however, it disappears after a week or two. The infusion amount should not be decreased, and the infusion should not be slowed or stopped.

Test-Taking Strategy: Eliminate options 2 and 4 first because this action is not within the scope of nursing practice. It is also inappropriate to slow the infusion. Review the complications associated with peritoneal dialysis and the

appropriate nursing actions now, if you had difficulty with this question!

Level of Cognitive Ability: Application
Phase of Nursing Process: Implementation
Client Needs: Physiological Integrity
Content Area: Adult Health/Renal

Reference
Ignatavicius, D., Workman, M., & Mishler, M. (1995). *Medical-surgical nursing: A nursing process approach* (2nd ed.). Philadelphia: W. B. Saunders. p. 2140.

90. **2**

Rationale: If outflow drainage is inadequate, the nurse attempts to stimulate outflow by changing the client's position. Turning the client to the other side or making sure that the client is in good body alignment may assist with outflow drainage. The catheter should not be irrigated. Although vital signs may be important, hypertension is not the concern. An intervention is required; therefore, to continue to monitor outflow is inappropriate at this time.

Test-Taking Strategy: Note that the issue of the question relates to inadequate outflow and the need for a nursing intervention. Option 3 should be eliminated first. Next eliminate option 1 because it is unrelated to the issue of the question. Eliminate option 4 because a nursing action is required to stimulate outflow. Review nursing interventions related to insufficient flow of dialysate now, if you had difficulty with this question!

Level of Cognitive Ability: Application
Phase of Nursing Process: Implementation
Client Needs: Physiological Integrity
Content Area: Adult Health/Renal

Reference
Ignatavicius, D., Workman, M., & Mishler, M. (1995). *Medical-surgical nursing: A nursing process approach* (2nd ed.). Philadelphia: W. B. Saunders. p. 2141.

91. **2**

Rationale: An extended dwell time increases the risk of hyperglycemia in diabetic clients as a result of absorption of glucose from the dialysate and electrolyte changes. Diabetic clients may require extra insulin.

Test-Taking Strategy: Note the key word "diabetic" in the question. This may assist you in making a relationship to option 2, a complication of both diabetes and an extended dwell time.

Level of Cognitive Ability: Application
Phase of Nursing Process: Implementation
Client Needs: Health Promotion and Maintenance
Content Area: Adult Health/Renal

Reference
Black, J., & Matassarin-Jacobs, E. (1997). *Medical-surgical nursing: Clinical management for continuity of care* (5th ed.). Philadelphia: W. B. Saunders. p. 1650.

92. **2**

Rationale: Clients with peritoneal dialysis have higher protein needs (about 1.2 to 1.5 g/kg of protein) because of greater protein losses. Clients are on more liberal fluid, sodium, and potassium allowances because the therapy is continuous and more of these products are removed. Weight gain is experienced by most clients receiving peritoneal dialysis as a result of absorbing 600 to 800 calories/day from the glucose dialysate. Dietary intake of calories and glucose may have to be modified to account for energy absorbed from dialysate.

Test-Taking Strategy: Note the key words "most likely be limited." Knowledge that glucose is a component of dialysate will assist in directing you to option 2.

Level of Cognitive Ability: Application
Phase of Nursing Process: Implementation
Client Needs: Health Promotion and Maintenance
Content Area: Adult Health/Renal

Reference
Mahan, L., & Escott-Stump, S. (1996). *Krause's food, nutrition and diet therapy* (9th ed.). Philadelphia: W. B. Saunders. p. 785.

93. 4

Rationale: Candidal infections, which are fungal, develop in persons who are on long-term antibiotic therapy because of the alteration of normal flora. It is also associated with clients who have blood dyscrasias, diabetes mellitus, cancer, immunosuppression, and a drug addiction.

Test-Taking Strategy: Knowledge regarding the causes of urinary tract infections is required to answer this question. Recalling that antibiotics alter normal flora and that women are more susceptible to cystitis will assist in directing you to option 4.

Level of Cognitive Ability: Analysis
Phase of Nursing Process: Analysis
Client Needs: Physiological Integrity
Content Area: Adult Health/Renal

Reference
Black, J., & Matassarin-Jacobs, E. (1997). *Medical-surgical nursing: Clinical management for continuity of care* (5th ed.). Philadelphia: W. B. Saunders. p. 1571.

94. 3

Rationale: In an elderly client, the only symptom of a UTI may be something as vague as increasing mental confusion or frequent unexplained falls. Frequency and urgency may commonly occur in an elderly client, and fever can be associated with a variety of conditions.

Test-Taking Strategy: Note the client's age in the question. Eliminate options 2 and 4 because they may commonly occur in an elderly client. Eliminate option 1 next because fever can be associated with a variety of conditions. Review clinical manifestations of UTI that occur in elderly people now, if you had difficulty with this question!

Level of Cognitive Ability: Analysis
Phase of Nursing Process: Assessment
Client Needs: Physiological Integrity
Content Area: Adult Health/Renal

Reference
Ignatavicius, D., Workman, M., & Mishler, M. (1995). *Medical-surgical nursing: A nursing process approach* (2nd ed.). Philadelphia: W. B. Saunders. p. 2047.

95. 3

Rationale: Mandelamine is bactericidal only in acidic urine. Under acidic conditions, the medication decomposes into ammonia and formaldehyde. The formaldehyde denatures bacterial proteins, causing death. For formaldehyde to be released, the urine must be acidic, with a pH of 5.5 or less. It is not necessary to take the medication with food unless gastric distress occurs. Ingestion of large amounts of fluid

(3 L.) will reduce antibacterial effects by diluting the medication and raising the urinary pH. Option 1 is incorrect.

Test-Taking Strategy: The question is addressing a specific medication. You may be tempted to select options 2 or 4; however, knowledge regarding this specific medication will direct you to option 3. Review this medication now, if you had difficulty with this question!

Level of Cognitive Ability: Application
Phase of Nursing Process: Implementation
Client Needs: Health Promotion and Maintenance
Content Area: Pharmacology

Reference
Lehne, R. (1998). *Pharmacology for nursing care* (3rd ed.). Philadelphia: W. B. Saunders. p. 904.

96. 2

Rationale: In acute glomerulonephritis, it is important to protect the kidneys while they are recovering their function. The diet is generally high calorie and low protein. This diet avoids protein catabolism and allows the kidneys to rest.

Test-Taking Strategy: Knowledge regarding the treatment measures in acute glomerulonephritis is required to answer this question. Recalling that protein would increase the workload of the kidneys will assist in directing you to option 2. Fluids are not restricted unless edema is present.

Level of Cognitive Ability: Application
Phase of Nursing Process: Implementation
Client Needs: Health Promotion and Maintenance
Content Area: Adult Health/Renal

Reference
Black, J., & Matassarin-Jacobs, E. (1997). *Medical-surgical nursing: Clinical management for continuity of care* (5th ed.). Philadelphia: W. B. Saunders. p. 1632.

97. 3

Rationale: Oxalate is found in dark green foods such as spinach. Other foods that raise the urinary oxalate level are rhubarb, strawberries, chocolate, wheat bran, nuts, beets, and tea.

Test-Taking Strategy: Knowledge regarding the foods that raise the urinary oxalate level will assist in answering this question. Remembering that green leafy foods are high in oxalate will assist in directing you to option 3. Review these foods now, if you had difficulty with this question!

Level of Cognitive Ability: Application
Phase of Nursing Process: Implementation
Client Needs: Health Promotion and Maintenance
Content Area: Adult Health/Renal

Reference
Mahan, L., & Escott-Stump, S. (1996). *Krause's food, nutrition and diet therapy* (9th ed.). Philadelphia: W. B. Saunders. p. 778.

98. 2

Rationale: Frequent dressing changes around the Penrose drain are required to protect the skin against breakdown from urinary drainage. If urinary drainage is excessive, an ostomy pouch may be placed over the drain to protect the skin. A Penrose drain is not irrigated. Weighting the dressings is not necessary. Placing the client on the affected side will prevent a free flow of urine through the drain.

Test-Taking Strategy: Identify the issue of the question, which relates to the Penrose drain. This should provide you with the clue that drainage is expected. Eliminate option 3 as the least likely answer. Eliminate option 1 because a Penrose drain is not irrigated. Visualize the effect that positioning on the affected side will have on the client. Review postoperative care now, if you had difficulty with this question!

Level of Cognitive Ability: Application
Phase of Nursing Process: Planning
Client Needs: Physiological Integrity
Content Area: Adult Health/Renal

Reference

Black, J., & Matassarin-Jacobs, E. (1997). *Medical-surgical nursing: Clinical management for continuity of care* (5th ed.). Philadelphia: W. B. Saunders. p. 1670.

99. **2**

Rationale: To increase urinary output, diuretics and osmotic agents such as mannitol are administered. The client should be monitored closely because fluid overload can cause hypertension, CHF, and pulmonary edema. Fluids would not be forced or restricted; irrigation of the Foley catheter will not assist in alleviating this occurrence.

Test-Taking Strategy: Knowledge regarding the definition of oliguria will easily direct you to option 2 as the treatment for this occurrence. If you are unfamiliar with the treatment of oliguria following kidney transplant, review now!

Level of Cognitive Ability: Analysis
Phase of Nursing Process: Analysis
Client Needs: Physiological Integrity
Content Area: Adult Health/Renal

Reference

Black, J., & Matassarin-Jacobs, E. (1997). *Medical-surgical nursing: Clinical management for continuity of care* (5th ed.). Philadelphia: W. B. Saunders. p. 1662.

100. **1**

Rationale: Gross, painless hematuria is most frequently the first manifestation of bladder cancer. As the disease progresses, the client may experience dysuria, frequency, and urgency.

Test-Taking Strategy: The issue of the question relates specifically to bladder cancer. Focusing on this issue should easily direct you to option 1. If you are unfamiliar with the specific manifestations associated with bladder cancer, review now!

Level of Cognitive Ability: Analysis
Phase of Nursing Process: Assessment
Client Needs: Physiological Integrity
Content Area: Adult Health/Renal

Reference

Black, J., & Matassarin-Jacobs, E. (1997). *Medical-surgical nursing: Clinical management for continuity of care* (5th ed.). Philadelphia: W. B. Saunders. p. 1583.

101. **1**

Rationale: Acute rejection usually occurs within 6 weeks after transplant. Clinical manifestations include fever, malaise, elevated WBC count, acute hypertension, graft tenderness, and manifestations of deteriorating renal function. Chronic rejection occurs over a period of months to years. Although kidney infection or obstruction can occur, the symptoms presented in the question do not specifically relate to these disorders.

Test-Taking Strategy: Note the key words "a week after kidney transplantation." These words should easily direct you to option 1, "acute" rejection. Review the signs of acute rejection now, if you had difficulty with this question!

Level of Cognitive Ability: Analysis
Phase of Nursing Process: Assessment
Client Needs: Physiological Integrity
Content Area: Adult Health/Renal

Reference

Black, J., & Matassarin-Jacobs, E. (1997). *Medical-surgical nursing: Clinical management for continuity of care* (5th ed.). Philadelphia: W. B. Saunders. p. 1662.

102. **2**

Rationale: Kock pouch is a continent internal ileal reservoir. The nurse instructs the client about the technique of catheterization. There is no external pouch. Antibiotics are not required unless an infection is present and one is prescribed by the physician. Dietary restrictions are not required.

Test-Taking Strategy: Knowledge regarding the physiology associated with a Kock pouch is required to answer this question. If you are unfamiliar with this urinary diversion procedure, take time now to review!

Level of Cognitive Ability: Application
Phase of Nursing Process: Implementation
Client Needs: Health Promotion and Maintenance
Content Area: Adult Health/Renal

Reference

Ignatavicius, D., Workman, M., & Mishler, M. (1995). *Medical-surgical nursing: A nursing process approach* (2nd ed.). Philadelphia: W. B. Saunders. pp. 2076–2077.

103. **1**

Rationale: TUR syndrome is caused by increased absorption of nonelectrolyte irrigating fluid used during surgery. The client may show signs of cerebral edema and increased intracranial pressure, such as increased BP, bradycardia, confusion, disorientation, muscle twitching, visual disturbances, and nausea and vomiting.

Test-Taking Strategy: Knowledge regarding TUR syndrome is required to answer this question. If you can recall that increased intracranial pressure is the concern, you can be easily directed to option 1. Review this disorder now, if you had difficulty with this question!

Level of Cognitive Ability: Analysis
Phase of Nursing Process: Assessment
Client Needs: Physiological Integrity
Content Area: Adult Health/Renal

Reference

Monahan, F., & Neighbors, M. (1998). *Medical-surgical nursing: Foundations for clinical practice* (2nd ed.). Philadelphia: W. B. Saunders. p. 1712.

104. **3**

Rationale: Frank bleeding, arterial or venous, may occur during the first day after surgery. Some hematuria is usual for several days after surgery. A urinary output of 200 mL greater than intake is adequate. Bladder spasms are expected to occur following surgery. A rapid pulse with a low BP is a potential sign of excessive blood loss. The physician should be notified.

Test-Taking Strategy: Knowledge regarding the normal expected findings following a TUR is required to answer this question. This knowledge will assist in eliminating options 1, 2, and 4. Reading each option carefully will direct you to option 3, as these vital signs are abnormal, indicating physician notification.

Level of Cognitive Ability: Application
Phase of Nursing Process: Implementation
Client Needs: Physiological Integrity
Content Area: Adult Health/Renal

Reference

Black, J., & Matassarin-Jacobs, E. (1997). *Medical-surgical nursing: Clinical management for continuity of care* (5th ed.). Philadelphia: W. B. Saunders. p. 2361.

105. **1**

Rationale: Individuals with polycystic kidney disease seem to waste rather than retain sodium. Thus, they need an increased sodium and water intake. Aggressive control of hypertension is essential. Genetic counseling is advisable because of the hereditary nature of the disease.

Test-Taking Strategy: Knowledge regarding the treatment for preserving kidney function in a client with polycystic kidney disease is required to answer this question. If you are unfamiliar with this disease, take time now to review!

Level of Cognitive Ability: Analysis
Phase of Nursing Process: Planning
Client Needs: Physiological Integrity
Content Area: Adult Health/Renal

Reference

Black, J., & Matassarin-Jacobs, E. (1997). *Medical-surgical nursing: Clinical management for continuity of care* (5th ed.). Philadelphia: W. B. Saunders. p. 1679.

106. **4**

Rationale: Potential complications after renal angiography include allergic reaction to the dye, renal damage from the dye, and a number of vascular complications, which include hemorrhage, thrombosis, or embolism. The nurse detects these complications by noting signs and symptoms of allergic reaction, decreased urine output, hematoma or hemorrhage at the insertion site, or decreased circulation to the affected leg.

Test-Taking Strategy: Begin to answer this question by eliminating options 1 and 3, since they are normal findings. Thus, they cannot be complications of this procedure. Since a hematoma is abnormal, then "absence of hematoma" is a normal finding, which eliminates this option also. Thus, you are left with option 4 as the answer to the question as stated. This is the only option that has any abnormal clinical findings.

Level of Cognitive Ability: Analysis
Phase of Nursing Process: Evaluation
Client Needs: Physiological Integrity
Content Area: Adult Health/Renal

Reference

Black, J., & Matassarin-Jacobs, E. (1997). *Medical-surgical nursing: Clinical management for continuity of care* (5th ed.). Philadelphia: W. B. Saunders. pp. 1564–1565.

107. **1**

Rationale: Gross hematuria and proteinuria are the cardinal signs of glomerulonephritis. The urine may be small in volume, dark or smoky in color from the hematuria, and foamy from the proteinuria. Concurrent serum studies would reveal elevated BUN, creatinine, C-reactive protein levels, and antistreptolysin O titer.

Test-Taking Strategy: Option 4 should be eliminated first, since these results do not indicate impending renal failure. Option 3 is not a likely answer, because there is no point is asking a question that has no definite answer. To choose correctly between options 1 and 2, it is necessary to know that these findings are consistent with glomerulonephritis.

Level of Cognitive Ability: Analysis
Phase of Nursing Process: Analysis
Client Needs: Physiological Integrity
Content Area: Adult Health/Renal

Reference

Black, J., & Matassarin-Jacobs, E. (1997). *Medical-surgical nursing: Clinical management for continuity of care* (5th ed.). Philadelphia: W. B. Saunders. p. 1631.

108. **2**

Rationale: The client with acute glomerulonephritis commonly experiences fluid volume excess and fatigue. Interventions include fluid restriction, as well as monitoring weight and I&O. The client is placed on bed rest or at least encouraged to rest. This is because there is a direct correlation between proteinuria and hematuria and increased activity levels. The diet is high in calories but low in protein. It is unnecessary to monitor the temperature as frequently as every 2 hours.

Test-Taking Strategy: The stem of the question gives you no information about the client's actual temperature, so option 1 may be eliminated first. Knowing that the client needs rest eliminates option 3. To choose correctly between the two remaining options, it is necessary to know either that fluids are restricted or that protein is limited. Knowledge of either concept would allow you to choose option 2 as correct.

Level of Cognitive Ability: Application
Phase of Nursing Process: Implementation
Client Needs: Safe, Effective Care Environment
Content Area: Adult Health/Renal

Reference

Black, J., & Matassarin-Jacobs, E. (1997). *Medical-surgical nursing: Clinical management for continuity of care* (5th ed.). Philadelphia: W. B. Saunders. p. 1632.

109. **1**

Rationale: The client with polycystic kidney disease should report any signs and symptoms of urinary tract infection so that treatment may begin promptly. The client should also report rises in blood pressure, as control of hypertension is essential. The client may experience heart failure as a result of hypertension, and thus any symptoms of heart failure, such as shortness of breath, are also reported.

Test-Taking Strategy: The wording of the question guides you to look for an incorrect response. Begin to answer this question by eliminating options 3 and 4 first, since signs of infection should be reported to the physician. To discriminate accurately between the remaining two options, it is necessary to know that the client with polycystic kidney disease is likely to be hypertensive. Since a complication of hypertension is heart failure, the nurse also teaches the client to report these signs and symptoms. With this in mind, you would know that shortness of breath should be reported. This leaves option 1, lowered blood pressure, as the correct answer. Lowered blood pressure is not a complication of polycystic kidney disease, and it is an expected effect of effective antihypertensive therapy. Thus, this does not need to be reported and is the answer to the question as stated.

Level of Cognitive Ability: Analysis
Phase of Nursing Process: Evaluation
Client Needs: Health Promotion and Maintenance
Content Area: Adult Health/Renal

Reference

Black, J., & Matassarin-Jacobs, E. (1997). *Medical-surgical nursing: Clinical management for continuity of care* (5th ed.). Philadelphia: W. B. Saunders. pp. 1678–1679.

110. **1**

Rationale: The client who has had a nephrectomy may have pain with coughing, deep breathing, and other respiratory exercise because of the location of the incision so close to the diaphragm. The nurse assists the client by using narcotic analgesics liberally, encouraging incentive spirometer use, and assisting the client to splint the incision during coughing. If the client takes pain medication only before ambulation, this may be insufficient and may not promote optimal respiratory function.

Test-Taking Strategy: By asking for the "least helpful" action in promoting respiratory function, the question is seeking the response that is the most incorrect. Options 2 and 3 are obviously helpful and are eliminated first. Since option 4 is more helpful than option 1, you would choose option 1 as the answer to the question as stated.

Level of Cognitive Ability: Application
Phase of Nursing Process: Implementation
Client Needs: Physiological Integrity
Content Area: Adult Health/Renal

Reference

Black, J., & Matassarin-Jacobs, E. (1997). *Medical-surgical nursing: Clinical management for continuity of care* (5th ed.). Philadelphia: W. B. Saunders. p. 1673.

111. **4**

Rationale: The client receiving immunosuppressive medication therapy must learn and utilize infection control methods for use at home. The client must learn proper hand-washing technique and should take the temperature daily to detect early infection. This is especially important since the client also takes corticosteroids, which mask signs and symptoms of infection. The client monitors own urine output and its characteristics on a daily basis. All medications should be taken exactly as ordered.

Test-Taking Strategy: The wording of this question guides you to look for an incorrect response on the part of the client. Options 1 and 2 are the most obviously correct and are therefore eliminated as possible choices. Since the client may be taking a combination of anti-infectives on a routine basis, along with immunosuppressive medication, it would be important to take scheduled medications on time. Thus, option 3 is correct and cannot be the answer to the question. This leaves option 4 as the answer. Knowing that the "once a week" frequency is insufficient makes this the answer to the question as stated.

Level of Cognitive Ability: Analysis
Phase of Nursing Process: Evaluation
Client Needs: Health Promotion and Maintenance
Content Area: Adult Health/Renal

Reference

Black, J., & Matassarin-Jacobs, E. (1997). *Medical-surgical nursing: Clinical management for continuity of care* (5th ed.). Philadelphia: W. B. Saunders. p. 1664.

112. **3**

Rationale: A complication after surgical repair of the bladder is disruption of sutures caused by tension on them from urine build-up. The nurse prevents this from happening by ensuring that the catheter is able to drain freely. This involves basic catheter care, including keeping the tubing free from kinks, keeping tubing below the level of the bladder, and monitoring the flow of urine frequently. Measurement of urine specific gravity and high oral fluid intake do not prevent complications of bladder surgery. Monitoring urine output every shift is insufficient to detect decreased flow from catheter kinking.

Test-Taking Strategy: Begin to answer this question by eliminating option 4 first. Specific gravity measurement is not a preventive action. Using the same reasoning, eliminate option 1 next, since once a shift measurement is not a preventive action, and it is also insufficient in frequency. To discriminate between the last two items, knowing that high oral fluid intake will not prevent complications from this procedure will allow you to choose option 3 as correct. Knowing that a key principle of catheter management is to prevent kinking of the tubing would also allow you to choose option 3 over option 2.

Level of Cognitive Ability: Application
Phase of Nursing Process: Planning
Client Needs: Physiological Integrity
Content Area: Adult Health/Renal

Reference

Black, J., & Matassarin-Jacobs, E. (1997). *Medical-surgical nursing: Clinical management for continuity of care* (5th ed.). Philadelphia: W. B. Saunders. p. 1619.

113. **4**

Rationale: Treatment of prostatitis includes medication with antibiotics, analgesics, and stool softeners. The client is also taught to rest, increase fluid intake; and use sitz baths for comfort. Antimicrobial therapy is always continued until the prescription is completely finished.

Test-Taking Strategy: Eliminate option 3 first since stopping medication therapy before the end of the course is contraindicated. Option 1 is also eliminated since fluid intake should be increased. To discriminate between the last two options correctly, it is necessary to understand that sitz baths provide comfort, or that rest is helpful in the healing process. Knowledge of either of these concepts would help you choose option 4 as the correct answer.

Level of Cognitive Ability: Analysis
Phase of Nursing Process: Evaluation
Client Needs: Health Promotion and Maintenance
Content Area: Adult Health/Renal

Reference

Black, J., & Matassarin-Jacobs, E. (1997). *Medical-surgical nursing: Clinical management for continuity of care* (5th ed.). Philadelphia: W. B. Saunders. p. 2372.

114. **3**

Rationale: Increasing age is the major risk factor for developing BPH. It is currently thought to be due to alteration in androgen levels, although the exact cause is still unknown. Increased intake of yellow vegetables and some elements of the Japanese diet may be helpful in reducing risk. Vitamin E and cigarette smoking have no known relationship with BPH. Early detection is the only method of prevention (and is actually secondary prevention). This is accomplished by annual prostate examination after the age of 40 years.

Test-Taking Strategy: This question tests knowledge of risk factors for development of BPH. Knowing that advancing age is the prime risk factor, you may systematically eliminate options 1, 2, and 4. Since the setting of the question is a prostate screening clinic, your attention is automatically drawn to detection, which would also guide you to choose option 3 as correct.

Level of Cognitive Ability: Analysis
Phase of Nursing Process: Evaluation
Client Needs: Health Promotion and Maintenance
Content Area: Adult Health/Renal

Reference

Black, J., & Matassarin-Jacobs, E. (1997). *Medical-surgical nursing: Clinical management for continuity of care* (5th ed.). Philadelphia: W. B. Saunders. p. 2350.

115. **2**

Rationale: Crush injuries may cause acute tubular necrosis, from the accumulation of large amounts of myoglobin and hemoglobin that are released from damaged muscle and blood cells. This type of renal failure is said to be due to renal causes; that is, conditions within the kidney itself. Prerenal causes are conditions that interfere with the perfusion of blood to the kidney. Postrenal causes include conditions that cause urinary obstruction distal to the kidney. It is necessary to determine the cause and type of renal failure, since this knowledge guides the interventions used in treatment to a certain extent.

Test-Taking Strategy: Knowledge of the categories of ARF is necessary to answer this question. Begin to answer this question by eliminating option 4 since it is not a category of ARF. Reflecting on the nature of the injury and its effect on the kidneys may help you eliminate each of the incorrect options.

Level of Cognitive Ability: Analysis
Phase of Nursing Process: Analysis
Client Need: Physiological Integrity
Content Area: Adult Health/Renal

Reference

Black, J., & Matassarin-Jacobs, E. (1997). *Medical-surgical nursing: Clinical management for continuity of care* (5th ed.). Philadelphia: W. B. Saunders. pp. 1636–1637.

116. **3**

Rationale: The client with hyperkalemia is at risk of developing cardiac dysrhythmias and cardiac arrest. Because of this, the client should be placed on a cardiac monitor. Fluid intake is not increased, since it contributes to fluid overload and would not significantly affect the serum potassium level. Vegetables are a natural source of potassium in the diet, and their use would not be increased. The nurse may also assess the sodium level, since it is another electrolyte that is commonly measured with the potassium level. However, this is not a priority action of the nurse.

Test-Taking Strategy: To answer this question successfully, it is necessary to know that the potassium level is high. It is also necessary to understand the critical effects of hyperkalemia on the heart. This knowledge will help you eliminate each of the incorrect options systematically.

Level of Cognitive Ability: Application
Phase of Nursing Process: Planning
Client Needs: Physiological Integrity
Content Area: Adult Health/Renal

Reference

Black, J., & Matassarin-Jacobs, E. (1997). *Medical-surgical nursing: Clinical management for continuity of care* (5th ed.). Philadelphia: W. B. Saunders. p. 1639.

117. **3**

Rationale: With intrinsic renal failure, there a fixed specific gravity, and the urine tests definitely positive for proteinuria. In prerenal failure, the specific gravity is high, and there is very little or no proteinuria. In postrenal failure, there is a fixed specific gravity and little or no proteinuria.

Test-Taking Strategy: Begin to answer this question by eliminating option 1 as a nonexistent entity. Knowing that proteinuria occurs due to leakage at the basement membrane of the glomerulus helps you choose option 3 over options 2 and 4 as the correct answer.

Level of Cognitive Ability: Analysis
Phase of Nursing Process: Analysis
Client Needs: Physiological Integrity
Content Area: Adult Health/Renal

Reference

Black, J., & Matassarin-Jacobs, E. (1997). *Medical-surgical nursing: Clinical management for continuity of care* (5th ed.). Philadelphia: W. B. Saunders. p. 1638.

118. **3**

Rationale: Antihypertensive medications such as enalapril are given to the client following hemodialysis. This prevents the client from becoming hypotensive during dialysis, and also from having the medication removed from the blood stream by dialysis. There is no rationale for waiting a full day to resume the medication. This would lead to ineffective control of the blood pressure.

Test-Taking Strategy: Begin to answer this question by thinking about the effects of an antihypertensive medication on the blood pressure when fluid is being removed from the body. Since hypotension is much more likely to occur in this circumstance, you would eliminate options 1 and 2 as possible answers. Most clients are hemodialyzed three times a week. If the medication was held for dialysis until the following day, the client would miss three of the seven doses that would usually be given in a week. This would lead to ineffective blood pressure control. Thus, option 4 is incorrect, leaving option 3 as correct. The medication is administered following return from hemodialysis.

Level of Cognitive Ability: Application
Phase of Nursing Process: Planning
Client Needs: Physiological Integrity
Content Area: Adult Health/Renal

Reference

Black, J., & Matassarin-Jacobs, E. (1997). *Medical-surgical nursing: Clinical management for continuity of care* (5th ed.). Philadelphia: W. B. Saunders. p. 1654.

119. **2**

Rationale: Clients with peritoneal dialysis catheters are at high risk for infection. A dressing that is wet is a conduit for bacteria to reach the catheter insertion site. The nurse ensures that the dressing is kept dry at all times. Reinforcing the dressing is not a safe practice to prevent infection in this circumstance. Flushing the catheter is not indicated. Scrubbing the catheter with povidone-iodine is done at the time of connection or disconnection of peritoneal dialysis.

Test-Taking Strategy: Determine what the question is asking. The stem states that the dressing is wet. The correct answer would focus on the dressing, not the catheter. Knowing that it is better to change a wet dressing than reinforce it, you would choose option 2 as the correct answer.

Level of Cognitive Ability: Application
Phase of Nursing Process: Planning
Client Needs: Safe, Effective Care Environment
Content Area: Adult Health/Renal

Reference
Black, J., & Matassarin-Jacobs, E. (1997). *Medical-surgical nursing: Clinical management for continuity of care* (5th ed.). Philadelphia: W. B. Saunders. p. 1658.

120. 2

Rationale: The typical schedule for hemodialysis is 3 to 4 hours of treatment 3 days per week. Individual adjustments may be made according to variables such as the size of the client, type of dialyzer, rate of blood flow, personal client preferences, and others.

Test-Taking Strategy: The question asks about a "typical" dialysis schedule. This is important baseline knowledge for the nurse to have. If needed, memorize this information now.

Level of Cognitive Ability: Analysis
Phase of Nursing Process: Analysis
Client Needs: Health Promotion and Maintenance
Content Area: Adult Health/Renal

Reference
Black, J., & Matassarin-Jacobs, E. (1997). *Medical-surgical nursing: Clinical management for continuity of care* (5th ed.). Philadelphia: W. B. Saunders. p. 1653.

121. 3

Rationale: Infection is a major concern in hemodialysis. For that reason, the use of sterile technique and the application of a face mask for both nurse and client are extremely important. It is also imperative that universal precautions be followed, which includes the use of goggles, mask, gloves, and apron. The connection site should not be covered; it should be visible so that the nurse can assess for bleeding, ischemia, and infection at the site during the hemodialysis procedure.

Test-Taking Strategy: The wording of the question guides you to look for an incorrect statement. Being able to recognize proper actions for infection control and universal precautions allows you to eliminate each of the incorrect responses systematically. You could also choose correctly if you know that the access site should remain visible to detect bleeding as well as signs of ischemia and infection.

Level of Cognitive Ability: Application
Phase of Nursing Process: Planning
Client Needs: Safe, Effective Care Environment
Content Area: Adult Health/Renal

Reference
Luckmann, J. (1997). *Saunders manual of nursing care.* Philadelphia: W. B. Saunders. p. 1194.

122. 2

Rationale: If the client experiences air embolus during hemodialysis, the nurse should terminate dialysis immediately, notify the physician, and administer oxygen as needed. All other actions are incorrect.

Test-Taking Strategy: To answer this question accurately, recall that air embolus is an emergency situation that affects the cardiopulmonary system suddenly and profoundly. With this in mind, all options except option 2 would be eliminated quickly.

Level of Cognitive Ability: Application
Phase of Nursing Process: Implementation
Client Needs: Physiological Integrity
Content Area: Adult Health/Renal

Reference
Luckmann, J. (1997). *Saunders manual of nursing care.* Philadelphia. W. B. Saunders. p. 1195.

123. 2

Rationale: The client on hemodialysis should monitor fluid status between hemodialysis treatments. This can be accomplished by recording I&O and measuring weight on a daily basis. Ideally, the hemodialysis client should not gain more than 0.5 kg of weight per day.

Test-Taking Strategy: To answer this question accurately, it is necessary to understand the pathophysiology of renal failure and the impact on the client's body functions. With this in mind, you would choose the option that relates to monitoring of fluid retention, which is option 2. Option 4 is not indicated. The client does not have the need or the ability to self-screen laboratory results. While it is helpful for the client to monitor own vital signs, it is not the best indicator of fluid status, which is the focus of the question.

Level of Cognitive Ability: Analysis
Phase of Nursing Process: Evaluation
Client Needs: Health Promotion and Maintenance
Content Area: Adult Health/Renal

Reference
Ignatavictus, D., Workman, M., & Mishler, M. (1995). *Medical-surgical nursing: A nursing process approach* (2nd ed.). Philadelphia: W. B. Saunders. p. 2126.

124. 1

Rationale: An AV fistula is the internal creation of an arterial to venous anastomosis. This causes engorgement of the vein, allowing both the artery and the vein to be easily cannulated for hemodialysis. Fistulas take 1 to 2 weeks to mature before they can be used for dialysis, so the current method of access must remain in place to be used during that time period. The statements in each of the other options are incorrect.

Test-Taking Strategy: To answer this question correctly, it is necessary to understand concepts related to the creation and use of internal AV fistulas. This is an important content area, so review this material briefly if needed.

Level of Cognitive Ability: Analysis
Phase of Nursing Process: Analysis
Client Need: Physiological Integrity
Content Area: Adult Health/Renal

Reference
Black, J., & Matassarin-Jacobs, E. (1997). *Medical-surgical nursing: Clinical management for continuity of care* (5th ed.). Philadelphia: W. B. Saunders. p. 1651.

125. 4

Rationale: An AV shunt is a less common form of access site but carries a risk for bleeding when it is used. This is because two ends of a cannula are tunneled subcutaneously into an artery and a vein, and the ends of the cannula are joined. If accidental disconnection occurs, the client could lose blood rapidly. For this reason, small clamps are attached to the dressing that covers the insertion site for use if needed. The shunt site should also be observed at least every 4 hours.

Test-Taking Strategy: Begin to answer this question by eliminating option 1, which is an assessment, not an action. Option 3 as worded addresses patency, not bleeding, and is therefore incorrect. The frequency of observation in option 2 is substandard and is eliminated. This leaves option 4, which is completely correct.

Level of Cognitive Ability: Application
Phase of Nursing Process: Implementation
Client Needs: Safe, Effective Care Environment
Content Area: Adult Health/Renal

Reference
Ignatavicius, D., Workman, M., & Mishler, M. (1995). *Medical-surgical nursing: A nursing process approach* (2nd ed.). Philadelphia: W. B. Saunders. pp. 2136–2137.

BIBLIOGRAPHY

Black, J., & Matassarin-Jacobs, E. (1997). *Medical-surgical nursing: Clinical management for continuity of care* (5th ed.). Philadelphia: W. B. Saunders.

Chernecky, C., & Berger, B. (1997). *Laboratory tests and diagnostic procedures* (2nd ed.). Philadelphia: W. B. Saunders.

Cox, H., Hinz, M., Lubno, M., et al. (1997). *Clinical applications of nursing diagnosis: Adult, child, women's, psychiatric, gerontic and home health considerations* (3rd ed.). Philadelphia: F. A. Davis.

Hodgson, B., & Kizior, R. (1998). *Saunders nursing drug handbook 1998.* Philadelphia: W. B. Saunders.

Ignatavicius, D., Workman, M., & Mishler, M. (1995). *Medical-surgical nursing: A nursing process approach* (2nd ed.). Philadelphia: W. B. Saunders.

Lammon, C., Foote, A., Leli, P., et al. (1995). *Clinical nursing skills.* Philadelphia: W. B. Saunders.

Leahy, J., & Kizilay, P. (1998). *Foundations of nursing practice: A nursing process approach.* Philadelphia: W. B. Saunders.

Lehne, R. (1998). *Pharmacology for nursing care* (3rd ed.). Philadelphia: W. B. Saunders.

Luckmann, J. (1997). *Saunders manual of nursing care.* Philadelphia: W. B. Saunders.

Lutz, C., & Przytulski, K. (1997). *Nutrition and diet therapy* (2nd ed.). Philadelphia: F. A. Davis.

Mahan, L., & Escott-Stump, S. (1996). *Krause's food, nutrition and diet therapy* (9th ed.). Philadelphia: W. B. Saunders.

McMorrow, M., & Malarkey, L. (1998). *Laboratory and diagnostic tests: A pocket guide.* Philadelphia: W. B. Saunders.

Monahan, F., & Neighbors, M. (1998). *Medical-surgical nursing: Foundations for clinical practice* (2nd ed.). Philadelphia: W. B. Saunders.

O'Toole, M. (ed.) (1997). *Miller-Keane encyclopedia & dictionary of medicine, nursing, & allied health* (6th ed.). Philadelphia: W. B. Saunders.

Smeltzer, S., & Bare, B. (1996). *Brunner and Suddarth's textbook of medical-surgical nursing* (8th ed.). Philadelphia: Lippincott-Raven.

Taylor, C., Lillis, C., & LeMone, P. (1997). *Fundamentals of nursing, The art and science of nursing care* (3rd ed.). Philadelphia: Lippincott-Raven.

CHAPTER 62

Renal Medications

....

I. Urinary Tract Antiseptics (Box 62–1)

A. Description
   1. Inhibit the growth of bacteria in the urine
   2. Act as disinfectants within the urinary tract
   3. Used to treat urinary tract infections
   4. These medications do not achieve effective antibacterial concentrations in blood or tissues and therefore cannot be used for infections at sites outside the urinary tract

B. Side effects and nursing considerations
   1. Nitrofurantoin
      a. Gastrointestinal effects such as anorexia, nausea, vomiting, and diarrhea
      b. Pulmonary reactions such as dyspnea, chest pain, chills, fever, cough, and alveolar infiltrates
      c. Hematological effects such as agranulocytosis, leukopenia, thrombocytopenia, and megaloblastic anemia
      d. Peripheral neuropathy such as muscle weakness, tingling sensations, and numbness
      e. Neurological effects such as headache, vertigo, drowsiness, and nystagmus
      f. Imparts a harmless brown color to the urine
      g. Pulmonary reactions resolve in 2 to 4 days following cessation of treatment
      h. Administration with milk or meals will minimize gastrointestinal (GI) distress
      i. Contraindicated in clients with renal impairment

j. Instruct client in expected side effects and those warranting notifying the physician
   2. Methenamine
      a. Relatively safe and well tolerated
      b. May cause gastric distress
      c. Chronic high-dose therapy can cause bladder irritation
      d. Can cause crystalluria and should not be used in clients with renal impairment
      e. Decomposition of medication generates ammonia, thus it should not be used for clients with liver dysfunction
      f. Requires acidic urine with pH of 5.5 or less
      g. Ingestion of large amounts of fluid will reduce antibacterial effects by diluting the medication and raising the urinary pH
      h. Should not be combined with sulfonamides because of the risk of crystalluria and urinary tract injury
      i. Clients taking this medication should not be given alkalinizing agents
   3. Nalidixic acid
      a. Gastrointestinal disturbances such as nausea, vomiting, and abdominal discomfort
      b. Rash
      c. Visual disturbances
      d. Photosensitivity reactions
      e. May produce intracranial hypertension in pediatric clients and should not be administered to children under age 3 months
      f. When used for more than 2 weeks, blood cell counts and liver function tests should be performed
      g. Can intensify the effects of oral anticoagulants
      h. Contraindicated in clients with a history of convulsive disorders
   4. Cinoxacin
      a. Side effects are similar to those of nalidixic acid
      b. Dosage should be reduced in clients with

BOX 62–1. Urinary Tract Antiseptics

Nitrofurantoin (Furadantin, Macrodantin, Macrobid)
Methenamine (Mandelamine, Hiprex, Urex)
Nalidixic acid (NegGram)
Cinoxacin (Cinobac)
Norfloxacin (Noroxin)

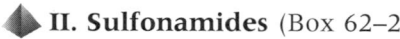

BOX 62–2. Sulfonamides

Sulfisoxazole (Gantrisin)
Sulfamethoxazole (Gantanol, Urobak)
Sulfadiazine
Sulfacytine (Renoquid)
Sulfamethizole (Thiosulfil Forte)
Trisulfapyrimidines (Triple Sulfa No. 2)

renal impairment; failure to do so could result in accumulation of medication to toxic levels

　5. Norfloxacin
　　a. Can cause fatigue, headache, nausea, constipation, rash, and elevated liver function tests
　　b. Encourage client to consume a high fluid intake
　　c. Advise client to take medication 1 hour before or 2 hours after meals because food may hamper absorption

II. Sulfonamides (Box 62–2)

A. Description
　1. Suppress bacterial growth by inhibiting synthesis of folic acid
　2. Active against a broad spectrum of microbes
B. Side effects and nursing considerations
　1. Hypersensitivity reactions such as rash, fever, and photosensitivity can occur
　2. Stevens-Johnson syndrome, the most severe hypersensitivity response, producing symptoms that include widespread lesions of the skin and mucous membranes, with fever, malaise, and toxemia
　3. Can cause hemolytic anemia and agranulocytosis, leukopenia, and thrombocytopenia
　4. Should be discontinued if any sort of rash is observed
　5. Instruct client to take medication on an empty stomach with a full glass of water
　6. Clients should be instructed to avoid prolonged exposure to sunlight, wear protective clothing, and apply a sunscreen to exposed skin
　7. Adults should maintain a daily urine output of 1200 mL by consuming 8 to 10 glasses of water each day to minimize the risk of renal damage from the medication
　8. Can intensify the effects of Coumadin, phenytoin (Dilantin), and oral hypoglycemics
　9. Administer with caution in clients with renal impairment
　10. Contraindicated in infants under age 2 months and in pregnant women or mothers who are breast-feeding
　11. Contraindicated if a hypersensitivity exists to sulfonamides, sulfonylureas, thiazide, or loop diuretics

III. Trimethoprim (Proloprim, Trimpex)

A. Description
　1. Active against a broad spectrum of microbes
　2. Suppresses bacterial synthesis of DNA, RNA, and proteins
B. Side effects and nursing considerations
　1. Itching and rash are the most frequent side effects
　2. GI reactions such as epigastric distress, nausea and vomiting, glossitis, and stomatitis occur occasionally
　3. Megaloblastic anemia, thrombocytopenia, and neutropenia may occur in individuals with pre-existing folic acid deficiency
　4. If early signs of bone marrow suppression occur such as sore throat, fever, or pallor, complete blood counts should be performed
　5. Contraindicated in women who are pregnant or are breast-feeding
　6. Contraindicated in clients with folate deficiency

IV. Trimethoprim-Sulfamethoxazole

A. Description
　1. A fixed-dose combination product (TMP-SMZ) that is a powerful broad-spectrum antimicrobial preparation
　2. Trade names include Bactrim, Cotrim, and Septra
B. Side effects and nursing considerations
　1. Nausea, vomiting, and rash are the most common side effects
　2. Can cause megaloblastic anemia in clients who are folate deficient
　3. Can cause central nervous system (CNS) effects such as headache, depression, and hallucinations
　4. Hyperkalemia can occur
　5. Toxicities may occur, such as hypersensitivity reactions, blood dyscrasias, and renal damage
　6. Contraindicated during pregnancy and lactation, for infants under age 2 months, in clients with a folate deficiency, and in clients with a history of hypersensitivity to sulfonamides and chemically related medications

V. Cholinergic (Box 62–3)

A. Description
　1. Used to treat nonobstructive urinary retention and neurogenic bladder
　2. Used to increase bladder tone and function

BOX 62–3. Cholinergic

Bethanechol chloride (Duvoid, Urecholine)

B. Side effects
1. Headache
2. Hypotension
3. Flushing and sweating
4. Increased salivation
5. Abdominal cramps
6. Nausea and vomiting
7. Diarrhea
8. Urinary urgency
9. Bronchoconstriction
C. Nursing considerations
1. Do not administer if client has urinary obstruction
2. Never administer by IM or IV route
3. Monitor intake and output (I&O)
4. Monitor for increased bladder tone and function
5. Administer on an empty stomach to decrease nausea and vomiting
6. Monitor for cholinergic overdose
7. Have atropine (antidote) readily available

VI. Antispasmodics

A. Description
1. Oxybutynin chloride (Ditropan) relaxes smooth muscles of the urinary tract
2. Propantheline bromide (Pro-Banthine) decreases bladder muscle spasms
B. Oxybutynin chloride (Ditropan)
1. Side effects
a. Leukopenia
b. Anxiety
c. Anorexia, nausea, vomiting
d. Palpitations
e. Sinus bradycardia
2. Nursing considerations
a. Do not administer to clients with known hypersensitivity, GI or genitourinary (GU) obstruction, glaucoma, severe colitis, or myasthenia gravis
b. Instruct client to avoid hazardous activities
C. Propantheline bromide (Pro-Banthine)
1. Side effects
a. Palpitations
b. Blurred vision
c. Confusion in elderly clients
d. Tachycardia
e. Constipation
f. Dry mouth
g. Urinary hesitancy and urgency
h. Decreased sweating
2. Nursing considerations
a. Monitor I&O
b. Provide gum or hard candy for dry mouth
c. Do not administer to clients with narrow angle glaucoma, obstructive uropathy, GI disease, or ulcerative colitis

---

BOX 62–4. Urinary Analgesic

Phenazopyridine HCl (Pyridium)

VII. Urinary Analgesic (Box 62–4)

A. Description
1. Used for pain from urinary tract irritation or infection
2. Administered with an antibiotic because it does not treat infection, it treats only pain
B. Side effects
1. Nausea
2. Headache
3. Vertigo
C. Nursing considerations
1. Instruct client that urine will turn red or orange
2. Contraindicated in renal or hepatic disease

VIII. Hematopoietic Growth Factor (Box 62–5)

A. Description
1. Used to stimulate red blood cell (RBC) production
2. Reverses anemia associated with **chronic renal failure**
3. Initial effects can be seen within 1 to 2 weeks, and the hematocrit reaches normal levels (30% to 33%) in 2 to 3 months
B. Side effect: Major side effect is hypertension
C. Nursing considerations
1. Monitor blood levels
2. Monitor vital signs, especially blood pressure for hypertension
3. The extent of hypertension is directly related to the rate of rise in the hematocrit
4. Contraindicated in clients with uncontrolled hypertension or hypersensitivity to mammalian cell–derived products or human albumin
5. Use with caution in clients with cancers of myeloid origin

IX. Preventing Organ Rejection (Box 62–6)

A. Description
1. Cyclosporine acts on T lymphocytes to suppress production of interleukin-2, gamma interferon, and other cytokines
2. Tacrolimus inhibits calcineurin and thereby prevents T cells from producing interleukin-2, gamma interferon, and other cytokines
3. Azathioprine (Imuran) suppresses cell-

BOX 62–5. Hematopoietic Growth Factor

Epoetin alfa (Epogen, Procrit)

BOX 62–6. Preventing Organ Rejection

IMMUNOSUPPRESSANTS

Cyclosporine (Sandimmune, Neoral)
Tacrolimus (Prograf)

CYTOTOXIC MEDICATIONS

Azathioprine (Imuran)
Mycophenolate mofetil (CellCept)

GLUCOCORTICOID

Prednisone (Deltasone)

ANTIBODIES

Muromonab-CD3 (Orthoclone OKT3)
Lymphocyte immune globulin, antithymocyte globulin (equine) (Atgam)

mediated and humoral immune responses by inhibiting the proliferation of B and T lymphocytes

4. Mycophenolate mofetil causes selective inhibition of B and T lymphocyte proliferation
5. Muromonab-CD3 blocks all T cell functions
6. Therapeutic effect of lymphocyte immune globulin results from a decrease in the number and activity of thymus-derived lymphocytes

B. Cyclosporine (Sandimmune, Neoral)
1. Used to prevent rejection of allogeneic kidney transplant
2. Prednisone is usually administered concurrently
3. Oral administration is preferred; IV administration is reserved for clients who cannot take the medication orally
4. Blood levels should be measured periodically
5. The most common adverse effects are nephrotoxicity, infection, hypertension, tremor, and hirsutism
6. Clients should be informed about the possibility of renal damage and liver damage and the need for periodic blood urea nitrogen (BUN), creatinine, and liver function tests
7. Clients should be instructed to monitor for early signs of infection and to report these signs immediately
8. Instruct client to dispense the oral liquid into a glass container using a specially calibrated pipette, mix well, and drink immediately; rinse the container with diluent and drink it to ensure ingestion of the complete dose; dry the outside of the pipette and return to its cover for storage
9. Instruct client to mix the concentrated medication solution with milk, chocolate milk, or orange juice just before administration
10. Assure client that hirsutism is reversible

11. Grapefruit juice can raise cyclosporine levels, thereby increasing the risk of toxicity
12. Phenytoin, phenobarbital, rifampin, and TMP-SMZ can decrease cyclosporine levels
13. Ketoconazole, erythromycin, and amphotericin B can elevate cyclosporine levels
14. Renal damage can be intensified by the concurrent use of other nephrotoxic medications
15. Contraindicated in the presence of hypersensitivity, pregnancy, and breast-feeding, recent inoculation with live virus vaccines, and recent contact with an active infection such as chickenpox or herpes zoster
16. Is embryotoxic, and women of child-bearing age should use a mechanical form of contraception and avoid oral contraceptives

C. Tacrolimus (Prograf)
1. Nephrotoxicity is the major concern
2. Other common reactions include neurotoxicity, GI effects, hypertension, hyperkalemia, and hyperglycemia
3. Increases the risk of infection and lymphomas
4. Concurrent use of glucocorticoids is recommended

D. Azathioprine (Imuran)
1. Used as an adjunct to cyclosporine and glucocorticoids to help suppress transplant rejection
2. Can cause neutropenia and thrombocytopenia from bone marrow suppression
3. Contraindicated in pregnancy and is associated with an increased incidence of neoplasms

E. Mycophenolate mofetil (CellCept)
1. Used in combination with cyclosporine and glucocorticoids
2. Major adverse effects include diarrhea, severe neutropenia, vomiting, and sepsis
3. Associated with an increased risk of infection and malignancies
4. Absorption is decreased by the use of magnesium and aluminum antacids and by cholestyramine (Questran, Prevalite)
5. Contraindicated in pregnancy

F. Muromonab-CD3 (Orthoclone OKT3)
1. Used to prevent acute allograft rejection of kidney transplants
2. Adverse reactions include fever, chills, dyspnea, chest pain, and nausea and vomiting

G. Lymphocyte immune globulin, antithymocyte globulin (equine) (Atgam)
1. Used to prevent rejection of renal transplants
2. Usually administered with glucocorticoids and azathioprine
3. Adverse reactions include chills, fever, leukopenia, and skin reactions

PRACTICE QUESTIONS

1. Cinoxacin (Cinobac) is prescribed for the client with a urinary tract infection. The clinic nurse is instructing the client regarding the administration of the medication. Which of the following is an appropriate instruction?
   1 Administer the medication 1 hour before meals
   2 Administer the medication with meals
   3 Administer the medication at bedtime
   4 Administer the medication in the morning prior to breakfast

2. Laboratory analysis of a urine specimen for culture and sensitivity reveals a gram-negative bacterial infection. The client is treated with nalidixic acid (NegGram). Which of the following existing disorders of the client alerts the nurse to question the prescription for this medication?
   1 Diabetes mellitus
   2 Seizure disorder
   3 Coronary artery disease
   4 Peptic ulcer disease

3. Norfloxacin (Noroxin) is prescribed for a client with *Pseudomonas* infection of the urinary tract. The nurse instructs the client to take the medication:
   1 With meals
   2 At bedtime
   3 Two hours after meals
   4 With a snack in the late afternoon

4. Nitrofurantoin (Macrodantin) is prescribed for the client with an acute urinary tract infection. Which of the following food items would the nurse instruct the client to avoid during the administration of this medication?
   1 Orange juice
   2 Cranberry juice
   3 Prune juice
   4 Rhubarb

5. Methenamine mandelate (Mandelamine) is prescribed for the client with a gram-positive urinary tract infection. Which of the following conditions, if noted in the client's record, alerts the nurse to question the order for this prescribed medication?
   1 Cirrhosis
   2 Diabetes mellitus
   3 Peripheral vascular disease
   4 Hypothyroidism

6. Co-trimoxazole (Bactrim) is prescribed to be administered by IV infusion to the client with a recurrent urinary tract infection. The nurse plans to administer this medication:
   1 Over 60 to 90 minutes
   2 Over a period of 30 minutes
   3 Piggybacked into the existing infusion of normal saline and potassium chloride

4 Piggybacked into the peripheral line containing total parenteral nutrition (TPN)

7. The client receiving nitrofurantoin calls the clinic complaining of side effects related to the medication. Which of the following side effects indicates the need to stop treatment with this medication?
   1 Anorexia
   2 Nausea
   3 Cough and chest pain
   4 Diarrhea

8. Nitrofurantoin is prescribed for an adult client for treatment of acute urinary tract infection. Which of the following is the appropriate adult dose?
   1 50 mg three to four times daily
   2 100 mg three times daily
   3 300 mg administered at bedtime
   4 1 g distributed evenly throughout the day

9. Methenamine (Mandelamine) is prescribed for the client with a chronic urinary tract infection. The mechanism of action of this medication is which of the following?
   1 Inhibits the replication of bacterial DNA
   2 Decomposes into ammonia and formaldehyde and denatures bacterial proteins
   3 Decreases bladder muscles and spasms
   4 Relaxes smooth muscles of the urinary tract

10. Nalidixic acid (NegGram) is prescribed for the client with a urinary tract infection. Reviewing the client's record, the nurse notes that the client is taking Coumadin on a daily basis. Which of the following prescriptions would the nurse anticipate because the client is on this oral anticoagulant?
    1 An increase in the anticoagulation dosage
    2 A reduction in the anticoagulation dosage
    3 The need to discontinue the Coumadin during therapy
    4 The need to administer an alternative medication to treat the urinary tract infection

11. Nalidixic acid is prescribed for the adult client with urinary tract infection. The normal adult dosage for this medication is:
    1 1 g four times daily for a period of 1 week
    2 500 mg daily administered at bedtime
    3 250 mg administered BID
    4 100 mg administered TID

12. Cinoxacin (Cinobac), a urinary antiseptic, is prescribed for the client. This medication would be used with caution in which of the following disorders?
    1 Hepatic disease
    2 Renal disease
    3 Diabetes insipidus
    4 Congestive heart failure

13. The nurse is providing discharge instructions to a client receiving sulfisoxazole (Gantrisin). Which of the following is included in the plan of care for instructions?
    1 Restrict fluid intake
    2 Maintain a high fluid intake
    3 Decrease the dosage when symptoms are improving to prevent an allergic response
    4 If the urine turns dark brown, call the physician immediately

14. Sulfamethoxazole (Gantanol) is prescribed for a client with a urinary tract infection. The client is a diabetic and is receiving tolbutamide (Orinase). Based on the administration of these two medications in combination, which of the following would the nurse anticipate may be prescribed?
    1 A decreased dosage of the tolbutamide
    2 An increased dosage of the tolbutamide
    3 A decreased dosage of the sulfamethoxazole
    4 An increased dosage of the sulfamethoxazole

15. Trimethoprim-sulfamethoxazole (Bactrim) is prescribed for the client. The nurse instructs the client to report which of the following symptoms if it developed during the course of this medication therapy?
    1 Headache
    2 Nausea
    3 Diarrhea
    4 Sore throat

16. Phenazopyridine (Pyridium) is prescribed for the client for symptomatic relief of pain resulting from a lower urinary tract infection. Which of the following would the nurse include in the teaching plan for the client?
    1 Take the medication prior to meals
    2 A reddish-orange discoloration of the urine may occur
    3 Discontinue the medication if a headache occurs
    4 Take the medication at bedtime

17. Bethanechol (Urecholine) is prescribed for the client with urinary retention. Which of the following disorders is a contraindication to the administration of this medication?
    1 Neurogenic atony
    2 Urinary strictures
    3 Gastroesophageal reflux
    4 Gastric atony

18. Bethanechol is prescribed for the client. The nurse instructs the client to take the medication:
    1 With meals
    2 Two hours after meals
    3 With a snack in the afternoon
    4 At bedtime with crackers and cheese

19. Bethanechol is prescribed for the client. The normal adult oral dosage of this medication ranges from:
    1 10 to 50 mg three to four times a day
    2 50 to 100 mg three to four times a day
    3 100 mg every 4 hours
    4 100 mg at bedtime

20. The nurse is administering 5 mg of bethanechol subcutaneously to a client with urinary retention. Which of the following would the nurse prepare to have readily available when administering this medication?
    1 Protamine sulfate
    2 Vitamin K
    3 Atropine
    4 Mucomyst

21. The nurse administering bethanechol is monitoring for acute toxicity associated with the medication. Which of the following is not a manifestation associated with overdose?
    1 Salivation
    2 Sweating
    3 Bradycardia
    4 Severe hypertension

22. Bethanechol is prescribed for the client with urinary retention. An injectable form of bethanechol is available for use. The nurse prepares to administer this medication by which of the following routes?
    1 Intravenously
    2 Intramuscularly
    3 Intradermally
    4 Subcutaneously

23. Oxybutynin (Ditropan) is prescribed for the client with neurogenic bladder. Which of the following indicates a possible toxic effect related to this medication?
    1 Bradycardia
    2 Pallor
    3 Restlessness
    4 Drowsiness

24. Propantheline bromide (Pro-Banthine) is prescribed for the client with bladder spasms. Which of the following disorders, if noted in the client's record, alerts the nurse to question the prescription for this medication?
    1 Glaucoma
    2 Hypothyroidism
    3 Myxedema
    4 Coronary artery disease

25. Following kidney transplant, cyclosporine (Sandimmune) is prescribed for the client. Which of the following laboratory results indicates an adverse effect from the use of this medication?
    1 Decreased white blood cell (WBC) count
    2 Decreased hemoglobin
    3 Elevated BUN
    4 Decreased creatinine

26. The nurse is providing dietary instructions to a client who has been prescribed cyclosporine. Which of the following food items would the nurse instruct the client to avoid?
    1 Orange juice
    2 Grapefruit juice
    3 Red meats
    4 Green leafy vegetables

27. Cyclosporine is prescribed for the client following a kidney transplant. The nurse would be most concerned if she noted that the client is presently taking which of the following prescribed medications?
    1 Digoxin (Lanoxin)
    2 Propranolol (Inderal)
    3 Phenytoin (Dilantin)
    4 Prednisone (Deltasone)

28. The nurse is caring for a client who will be receiving amphotericin B. The nurse notes that the client is also taking cyclosporine to prevent rejection of a kidney transplant performed 2 years ago. Which of the following prescriptions would the nurse anticipate to be prescribed for this client during the administration of these medications concurrently?
    1 An increased amount of amphotericin B
    2 A decreased amount of amphotericin B
    3 An increased amount of cyclosporine
    4 A decreased amount of cyclosporine

29. The nurse is preparing to administer a prescribed dose of cyclosporine by IV administration. Which of the following priority items would the nurse have available at the bedside during administration of this medication?
    1 Oral airway
    2 Epinephrine
    3 A code cart
    4 A suction catheter

30. Cyclosporine is prescribed to be administered by IV route. Which of the following indicates an inappropriate action in regard to preparing and administering this medication?
    1 Mixing 1 mL of concentrate in 10 mL of 0.9% sodium chloride and administering by bolus injection
    2 Mixing the solution and covering it with a paper bag
    3 Mixing 1 mL of concentrate in 50 mL of 0.9% sodium chloride
    4 Administering the medication over a period of 2 to 6 hours

31. The nurse provides instructions to the client prescribed to take cyclosporine oral solution. Which of the following instructions would the nurse provide to the client?
    1 Dilute the medication in a Styrofoam cup prior to administration

    2 Avoid diluting the concentrate for administration
    3 Mix the concentration with chocolate milk
    4 Mix the concentration with grapefruit juice

32. The nurse provides instructions regarding the administration of cyclosporine to a client. Which of the following statements, if made by the client, would indicate the need for further instruction?
    1 "I need to mix the concentrate well and drink it immediately."
    2 "After taking the medication, I need to rinse the container with diluent and drink it to ensure that I have taken the complete dose."
    3 "I will purchase a dropper from the pharmacist to calibrate the amount of medication that I need."
    4 "I will mix the concentrate with orange juice to improve the taste."

33. The nurse is monitoring a client receiving cyclosporine. Which of the following indicates to the nurse that the client is experiencing a side effect from this medication?
    1 Nausea
    2 Alopecia
    3 Tremor
    4 Hypotension

34. Tacrolimus (Prograf) is prescribed for a client for prevention of organ rejection following renal transplant. Which of the following would the nurse anticipate to be prescribed for this client during the administration of this medication?
    1 Prednisone (Deltasone)
    2 Erythromycin (E-Mycin)
    3 Fluconazole (Diflucan)
    4 Phenytoin (Dilantin)

35. Tacrolimus (Prograf) is prescribed for the client. Which of the following disorders, if noted on the client's record, indicates that the medication needs to be administered with caution?
    1 Diabetes insipidus
    2 Coronary artery disease
    3 Pancreatitis
    4 Ulcerative colitis

36. The nurse is reviewing the laboratory results of a client receiving tacrolimus. Which of the following indicates to the nurse that the client is experiencing an adverse effect of the medication?
    1 WBC of 6000/μL
    2 Blood glucose of 200 mg/dL
    3 Potassium level of 3.8 mEq/L
    4 Platelet count of 300,000 cells/μL

37. Muromonab-CD3 (Orthoclone OKT3) is prescribed for a client to manage allograft rejection following a renal transplant. The primary mechanism of action of this medication is that it:
    1 Binds to the CD3 site and blocks all T cell functions

2 Inhibits the proliferation of B lymphocytes
3 Cross-links DNA, causing cell injury and death
4 Suppresses B lymphocytes

38. The nurse is monitoring a client receiving Muromonab-CD3. Which of the following priority assessments is required in monitoring for adverse effects of the medication?
    1 Assessing pedal pulses
    2 Assessing lung sounds
    3 Assessing for positive bowel sounds
    4 Assessing for a positive Homan's sign

39. Mycophenolate mofetil (CellCept) is prescribed for a client as prophylaxis of organ rejection following allogeneic renal transplant. Which of the following instructions does the nurse provide to the client regarding administration of this medication?
    1 Administer following meals
    2 Open the capsule and mix with food for administration
    3 Contact the physician if a sore throat occurs
    4 Take the medication with a magnesium-type antacid

40. Azathioprine (Imuran) is prescribed for the client to suppress rejection of a renal transplant. The mechanism of action of this medication is that it:
    1 Inhibits the proliferation of B and T lymphocytes
    2 Cross-links DNA
    3 Blocks all T cell functions
    4 Decreases the activity of thymus-derived lymphocytes

41. Equine antithymocyte globulin (Atgam) is prescribed for the client for treatment of transplant rejection. Which of the following is the priority in planning the administration of this medication?
    1 Plan for a skin test dose to identify hypersensitivity
    2 Assess bowel sounds
    3 Premedicate the client with acetylsalicylic acid (aspirin)
    4 Assess the neurovascular status

42. The client with chronic renal failure is receiving epoetin alfa (erythropoietin). The nurse is evaluating the laboratory results. Which of the following results indicates a therapeutic effect of the medication?
    1 WBC count of 6000/μL
    2 Hematocrit count of 32%
    3 Platelet count of 400,000 cells/μL
    4 BUN of 15 mg/dL

43. Epoetin alfa has been prescribed for the client with chronic renal failure. The nurse will prepare to administer this medication by which of the following routes:
    1 PO
    2 IM

3 Intradermally
4 Subcutaneously

44. The nurse is monitoring the client receiving epoetin alfa for adverse effects of the medication. Which of the following indicates an adverse effect?
    1 Hypotension
    2 Hypertension
    3 Depression
    4 Bradycardia

45. The nurse is evaluating the laboratory studies of a client receiving epoetin alfa. The nurse expects to note a therapeutic effect of this medication:
    1 After 1 week of therapy
    2 Immediately
    3 3 days after therapy
    4 2 weeks after therapy

46. The nurse is instructing a client to administer epoetin alfa by the subcutaneous route. Which of the following indicates an accurate description of the instruction?
    1 Shake the bottle before use
    2 Keep the vial of medication at room temperature
    3 Use only 1 dose per vial
    4 Use alcohol to clean the top of the vial when reused

47. Aluminum hydroxide (Amphojel) is prescribed for the client with chronic renal failure. The nurse instructs the client to take this medication:
    1 On an empty stomach
    2 At bedtime
    3 With meals
    4 In the morning upon arising

48. A most common side effect associated with the administration of aluminum hydroxide is:
    1 Diarrhea
    2 Constipation
    3 Muscle weakness
    4 Headache

49. The client with hyperphosphatemia is receiving aluminum hydroxide. The usual adult dosage for this medication is:
    1 10 mL BID
    2 15 mL TID
    3 30 mL QD
    4 30 mL TID

50. The client with chronic renal failure is receiving ferrous sulfate (Feosol). Which of the following is a common side effect associated with this medication?
    1 Diarrhea
    2 Constipation
    3 Headache
    4 Weakness

ANSWERS

1. **2**

Rationale: Cinobac is a urinary antiseptic and is administered with meals to decrease GI side effects. The normal dosage is 1 g per day administered in two to four divided doses for a period of 7 to 14 days.

Test-Taking Strategy: Eliminate options 1 and 4 first because they are similar. To discriminate between the remaining options, knowledge that this medication is administered more than once daily will direct you to option 2.

Level of Cognitive Ability: Application
Phase of Nursing Process: Implementation
Client Needs: Health Promotion and Maintenance
Content Area: Pharmacology

Reference

Black, J., & Matassarin-Jacobs, E. (1997) *Medical-surgical nursing: Clinical management for continuity of care* (5th ed.). Philadelphia: W. B. Saunders. p. 1575.

2. **2**

Rationale: NegGram is used for acute and chronic UTIs, especially gram-negative bacterial infections. The medication is contraindicated in clients with a history of convulsions. It is used with caution in clients with liver or renal disorders.

Test-Taking Strategy: Knowledge regarding the contraindications associated with this medication is required to answer the question. Review this medication now, if you had difficulty with this question!

Level of Cognitive Ability: Analysis
Phase of Nursing Process: Analysis
Client Needs: Physiological Integrity
Content Area: Pharmacology

Reference

Black, J., & Matassarin-Jacobs, E. (1997). *Medical-surgical nursing: Clinical management for continuity of care* (5th ed.). Philadelphia: W. B. Saunders. p. 1575.

3. **3**

Rationale: Noroxin is administered 1 hour before or 2 hours after meals because food may hamper absorption. The normal dosage is 400 mg PO BID for 7 to 10 days for mild infections and for 10 to 21 days for severe infections.

Test-Taking Strategy: Eliminate options 1 and 4 first because they are similar. To discriminate between the remaining options, knowledge that this medication is administered more than once daily will direct you to option 3.

Level of Cognitive Ability: Application
Phase of Nursing Process: Implementation
Client Needs: Health Promotion and Maintenance
Content Area: Pharmacology

Reference

Black, J., & Matassarin-Jacobs, E. (1997). *Medical-surgical nursing: Clinical management for continuity of care* (5th ed.). Philadelphia: W. B. Saunders. p. 1575.

4. **4**

Rationale: When a client is receiving Macrodantin, the urinary pH must be maintained in an acid range. The client needs to be instructed to consume an acid ash diet. Rhubarb is a food item that will reduce the acidity of the urine, and it should be avoided when the client requires an acid ash urine.

Test-Taking Strategy: Note the key word "avoid" in the stem of the question. Knowledge that this medication requires that the urinary pH be maintained in an acid range will assist in directing you to option 4.

Level of Cognitive Ability: Application
Phase of Nursing Process: Implementation
Client Needs: Health Promotion and Maintenance
Content Area: Pharmacology

Reference

Black, J., & Matassarin-Jacobs, E. (1997). *Medical-surgical nursing: Clinical management for continuity of care* (5th ed.). Philadelphia: W. B. Saunders. p. 1575.

5. **1**

Rationale: Mandelamine is contraindicated in clients with renal or hepatic disease or clients with severe dehydration. The nurse would question the physician's prescription for this medication in the client with cirrhosis.

Test-Taking Strategy: Knowledge that this medication is contraindicated in hepatic disease will easily direct you to option 1. If you are unfamiliar with this medication, take time now to review!

Level of Cognitive Ability: Analysis
Phase of Nursing Process: Analysis
Client Needs: Physiological Integrity
Content Area: Pharmacology

Reference

Black, J., & Matassarin-Jacobs, E. (1997). *Medical-surgical nursing: Clinical management for continuity of care* (5th ed.). Philadelphia: W. B. Saunders. p. 1575.

6. **1**

Rationale: Bactrim may be administered by IV infusion but should not be mixed with any other medications or solutions. It is infused over a period of 60 to 90 minutes, and bolus infusions or rapid infusions must be avoided.

Test-Taking Strategy: Eliminate options 3 and 4 because they both address the issue of mixing the Bactrim with other solutions. From the remaining options, option 1 identifies the longer time frame and is the safe and correct choice!

Level of Cognitive Ability: Application
Phase of Nursing Process: Implementation
Client Needs: Safe, Effective Care Environment
Content Area: Pharmacology

Reference

Hodgson, B., & Kizior, R. (1999). *Saunders nursing drug handbook 1999.* Philadelphia: W. B. Saunders. p. 263.

7. **3**

Rationale: Gastrointestinal effects are the most frequent adverse reactions to this medication and can be minimized by administering the medication with milk or meals. Pulmonary reactions, manifested as dyspnea, chest pain, chills, fever, cough, and the presence of alveolar infiltrates on x-ray film, would indicate the need to stop the treatment. These symptoms would resolve in 2 to 4 days following discontinuation of this medication.

Test-Taking Strategy: Eliminate options 1, 2, and 4 because they are GI-related side effects. If you are unfamiliar with this medication, take time now to review it:

Level of Cognitive Ability: Analysis
Phase of Nursing Process: Analysis
Client Needs: Physiological Integrity
Content Area: Pharmacology

Reference
Lehne, R. (1998). *Pharmacology for nursing care* (3rd ed.). Philadelphia: W. B. Saunders. p. 903.

8. 1

Rationale: For treatment of acute UTI, the adult dosage is 50 mg three to four times a day. For prophylaxis of recurrent UTI, low doses are employed, such as 50 to 100 mg at bedtime for adults.

Test-Taking Strategy: Knowledge regarding the normal adult dosage of Macrodantin is required to answer this question. If you are unfamiliar with this medication, take time now to review!

Level of Cognitive Ability: Analysis
Phase of Nursing Process: Analysis
Client Needs: Physiological Integrity
Content Area: Pharmacology

Reference
Lehne, R. (1998). *Pharmacology for nursing care* (3rd ed.). Philadelphia: W. B. Saunders. p. 904

9. 2

Rationale: Methenamine, under acidic conditions, decomposes into ammonia and formaldehyde. The formaldehyde denatures bacterial proteins, causing death. Nalidixic acid (NegGram) is a medication that inhibits the replication of bacterial DNA. Antispasmodics relax smooth muscle of the urinary tract and decrease bladder muscle and spasms.

Test-Taking Strategy: Eliminate options 3 and 4 because they are similar. From the remaining options, it is necessary to know the action of this medication. If you had difficulty with this question, take time now to review it!

Level of Cognitive Ability: Analysis
Phase of Nursing Process: Analysis
Client Needs: Physiological Integrity
Content Area: Pharmacology

Reference
Lehne, R. (1998). *Pharmacology for nursing care* (3rd ed.). Philadelphia: W. B. Saunders. p. 904.

10. 2

Rationale: Nalidixic acid can intensify the effects of oral anticoagulants by displacing these agents from binding sites on plasma protein. When an oral anticoagulant is combined with nalidixic acid, a reduction in the anticoagulant dosage may be needed.

Test-Taking Strategy: Option 3 can be eliminated as the least likely choice. Next, eliminate option 1 as the next least likely prescription. From the remaining options, the most likely choice, based on the situation presented, would be option 2.

Level of Cognitive Ability: Analysis
Phase of Nursing Process: Analysis
Client Needs: Physiological Integrity
Content Area: Pharmacology

Reference
Lehne, R. (1998). *Pharmacology for nursing care* (3rd ed.). Philadelphia: W. B. Saunders. p. 905.

11. 1

Rationale: Nalidixic acid is dispensed in tablets of 250 mg, 500 mg, and 1 g, and in a suspension of 50 mg/mL for oral use. Adult dosage is 1 g four times a day for 1 week. It should not be administered to children less than 3 months of age because it may produce intracranial hypertension in pediatric clients.

Test-Taking Strategy: Knowledge regarding the normal adult dosage of nalidixic acid is required to answer this question. If you are unfamiliar with this medication, take time now to review!

Level of Cognitive Ability: Analysis
Phase of Nursing Process: Analysis
Client Needs: Physiological Integrity
Content Area: Pharmacology

Reference
Lehne, R. (1998). *Pharmacology for nursing care* (3rd ed.). Philadelphia: W. B. Saunders. p. 905.

12. 2

Rationale: Cinoxacin should be administered with caution in clients with renal impairment. The dosage should be reduced, and failure to do so could result in accumulation of cinoxacin to toxic levels.

Test-Taking Strategy: Knowledge that this medication is to be used with caution in clients with renal impairment will easily direct you to option 2. If you are unfamiliar with this medication, take time now to review!

Level of Cognitive Ability: Analysis
Phase of Nursing Process: Analysis
Client Needs: Physiological Integrity
Content Area: Pharmacology

Reference
Lehne, R. (1998). *Pharmacology for nursing care* (3rd ed.). Philadelphia: W. B. Saunders. p. 905.

13. 2

Rationale: Each dose of Gantrisin should be administered with a full glass of water, and the client should maintain a high fluid intake. The medication is more soluble in alkaline urine. The client should not be instructed to taper or discontinue the dose. Some forms of Gantrisin such as Azo Gantrisin causes urine to turn dark brown or red. This does not indicate the need to notify the physician.

Level of Cognitive Ability: Application
Phase of Nursing Process: Implementation
Client Needs: Health Promotion and Maintenance
Content Area: Pharmacology

Reference
Black, J., & Matassarin-Jacobs, E. (1997). *Medical-surgical nursing: Clinical management for continuity of care* (5th ed.). Philadelphia: W. B. Saunders. p. 1576.

14. 1

Rationale: Sulfonamides can intensify the effects of warfarin, phenytoin, and oral hypoglycemics such as tolbutamide. When combined with sulfonamides, these medications may require a reduction in dosage.

Test-Taking Strategy: Options 3 and 4 can be eliminated as the least likely choices. From the remaining options, the most likely choice, based on the situation presented, would be option 1.

Level of Cognitive Ability: Analysis
Phase of Nursing Process: Analysis
Client Needs: Physiological Integrity
Content Area: Pharmacology

Reference
Lehne, R. (1998). *Pharmacology for nursing care* (3rd ed.). Philadelphia: W. B. Saunders. p. 897.

15. 4

Rationale: Clients taking trimethoprim-sulfamethoxazole should be informed about early signs of blood disorders that can occur from this medication. These signs include sore throat, fever, or pallor, and the client should be instructed to notify the physician if these symptoms occur. The other options do not require physician notification.

Test-Taking Strategy: Knowledge that this medication can cause blood dyscrasias is required to answer the question. If you are unfamiliar with this medication, take time now to review!

Level of Cognitive Ability: Application
Phase of Nursing Process: Implementation
Client Needs: Health Promotion and Maintenance
Content Area: Pharmacology

Reference
Lehne, R. (1998). *Pharmacology for nursing care* (3rd ed.). Philadelphia: W. B. Saunders. p. 897.

16. 2

Rationale: The client should be instructed that a reddish-orange discoloration of urine may occur. The client should also be instructed that this discoloration can stain fabric. The medication should be taken after meals to reduce the possibility of GI upset. A headache is an occasional side effect of the medication and does not warrant discontinuation.

Test-Taking Strategy: Eliminate options 1 and 4 first because they are similar in that they both address time schedules for the administration of the medication. From the remaining options, eliminate option 3 because the nurse would not advise the client to discontinue this medication.

Level of Cognitive Ability: Application
Phase of Nursing Process: Implementation
Client Needs: Health Promotion and Maintenance
Content Area: Pharmacology

Reference
Hodgson, B., & Kizior, R. (1998). *Saunders nursing drug handbook 1998.* Philadelphia: W. B. Saunders. p. 813.

17. 2

Rationale: Urecholine can be hazardous to clients with urinary tract obstruction or weakness of the bladder wall. The medication has the ability to contract the bladder and thereby increase pressure within the urinary tract. Elevation of pressure within the urinary tract could rupture the bladder in clients with these conditions.

Test-Taking Strategy: Knowledge regarding the contraindications associated with this medication is required to answer this question. Noting that the medication is used for urinary retention may assist in directing you to option 2. Review this medication now, if you had difficulty with this question!

Level of Cognitive Ability: Application
Phase of Nursing Process: Implementation
Client Needs: Physiological Integrity
Content Area: Pharmacology

Reference
Lehne, R. (1998). *Pharmacology for nursing care* (3rd ed.). Philadelphia: W. B. Saunders. p. 122.

18. 2

Rationale: Administration of bethanechol with meals can cause nausea and vomiting in the client. To avoid this problem, oral doses should be administered 1 hour before meals or 2 hours after meals.

Test-Taking Strategy: Note that options 1, 3, and 4 are similar in that they all suggest administering the medication with a food item. Option 2 is the best selection.

Level of Cognitive Ability: Application
Phase of Nursing Process: Implementation
Client Needs: Health Promotion and Maintenance
Content Area: Pharmacology

Reference
Lehne, R. (1998). *Pharmacology for nursing care* (3rd ed.). Philadelphia: W. B. Saunders. p. 122.

19. 1

Rationale: The normal adult oral dosage of bethanechol ranges from 10 to 50 mg three to four times daily.

Test-Taking Strategy: Knowledge regarding the normal dosage of this medication is required to answer this question. Learn this dosage now, if you had difficulty with this question!

Level of Cognitive Ability: Analysis
Phase of Nursing Process: Analysis
Client Needs: Physiological Integrity
Content Area: Pharmacology

Reference
Lehne, R. (1998). *Pharmacology for nursing care* (3rd ed.). Philadelphia: W. B. Saunders. p. 122.

20. 3

Rationale: Cholinergic overdose can occur with bethanechol. The antidote is atropine administered SC or IV, which should be readily available for use should overdose occur. Protamine sulfate is the antidote for heparin. Vitamin K is the antidote for Coumadin. Mucomyst is the antidote for acetaminophen (Tylenol) overdose.

Test-Taking Strategy: Knowledge regarding the antidotes for certain medication overdoses is required to answer this question. If you could not answer this question, be sure to learn these antidotes now!

Level of Cognitive Ability: Application
Phase of Nursing Process: Planning
Client Needs: Physiological Integrity
Content Area: Pharmacology

Reference
Lehne, R. (1998). *Pharmacology for nursing care* (3rd ed.). Philadelphia: W. B. Saunders. p. 127.

21. 4

Rationale: Overdose produces manifestations of excessive muscarinic stimulation, such as salivation, sweating, involuntary urination and defecation, bradycardia, and severe hypotension. Treatment includes supportive measures and the administration of atropine SC or IV.

Test-Taking Strategy: Knowledge of the signs of cholinergic overdose is required to answer this question. If you are unfamiliar with these signs, learn them now. You are likely to find a question regarding this manifestation on NCLEX-RN!

Level of Cognitive Ability: Analysis
Phase of Nursing Process: Assessment
Client Needs: Physiological Integrity
Content Area: Pharmacology

Reference
Lehne, R. (1998). *Pharmacology for nursing care* (3rd ed.). Philadelphia: W. B. Saunders. p. 127.

22. 4

Rationale: The injectable form of bethanechol is intended for subcutaneous administration only. Bethanechol must never be injected IM or IV since the resulting high drug levels can cause severe toxicity, such as bloody diarrhea, bradycardia, profound hypotension, and cardiovascular collapse.

Test-Taking Strategy: Knowledge regarding the route of administration of this medication is required to answer this question. If you did not know the answer to this question, learn this administration route now!

Level of Cognitive Ability: Analysis
Phase of Nursing Process: Analysis
Client Needs: Physiological Integrity
Content Area: Pharmacology

Reference
Lehne, R. (1998). *Pharmacology for nursing care* (3rd ed.). Philadelphia: W. B. Saunders. pp. 122–123.

23. 3

Rationale: Overdosage produces CNS excitation, such as nervousness, restlessness, hallucinations, and irritability. Other signs of overdose include either hypotension or hypertension, confusion, tachycardia, flushed or red face, and signs of respiratory depression. Drowsiness is a frequent side effect of the medication but does not indicate overdosage.

Test-Taking Strategy: Knowledge regarding the manifestations related to overdose is required to answer this question. If you are unfamiliar with this medication, take time now to review!

Level of Cognitive Ability: Analysis
Phase of Nursing Process: Analysis
Client Needs: Physiological Integrity
Content Area: Pharmacology

Reference
Hodgson, B., & Kizior, R. (1999). *Saunders nursing drug handbook 1999.* Philadelphia: W. B. Saunders. p. 779.

24. 1

Rationale: Pro-Banthine is contraindicated in clients with narrow angle glaucoma, obstructive uropathy, GI disease, or ulcerative colitis. The medication decreases bladder muscle spasms.

Test-Taking Strategy: Eliminate options 2 and 3 because they are similar. From the remaining options, it is necessary to know the contraindications associated with the medication. Review these contraindications now, if you had difficulty with this question!

Level of Cognitive Ability: Analysis
Phase of Nursing Process: Analysis
Client Needs: Physiological Integrity
Content Area: Pharmacology

Reference
Ignatavicius, D., Workman, M., & Mishler, M. (1995). *Medical-surgical nursing: A nursing process approach* (2nd ed.). Philadelphia: W. B. Saunders. p. 2059.

25. 3

Rationale: Nephrotoxicity can occur from the use of Sandimmune. Nephrotoxicity is evaluated by monitoring for an elevated BUN and serum creatinine level. Sandimmune does not depress the bone marrow.

Test-Taking Strategy: Eliminate options 1 and 2 first because they are unrelated to renal function. Next, eliminate option 4 because the creatinine level would be elevated, not decreased. Option 3 is the only option that indicates an increased level of a renal function test.

Level of Cognitive Ability: Analysis
Phase of Nursing Process: Analysis
Client Needs: Physiological Integrity
Content Area: Pharmacology

Reference
Lehne, R. (1998). *Pharmacology for nursing care* (3rd ed.). Philadelphia: W. B. Saunders. p. 729.

26. 2

Rationale: A compound present in grapefruit juice inhibits metabolism of cyclosporine. As a result, consuming grapefruit juice can raise cyclosporine levels by 50% to 100%, thereby greatly increasing the risk of toxicity.

Test-Taking Strategy: Knowledge regarding substances that inhibit the metabolism of cyclosporine is required to answer this question. If you had difficulty with this question, review this very important medication now!

Level of Cognitive Ability: Application
Phase of Nursing Process: Implementation
Client Needs: Health Promotion and Maintenance
Content Area: Pharmacology

Reference
Lehne, R. (1998). *Pharmacology for nursing care* (3rd ed.). Philadelphia: W. B. Saunders. pp. 729–730.

27. 3

Rationale: Medications known to lower cyclosporine levels include Dilantin, phenobarbital, rifampin, and trimethoprim-sulfamethoxazole. Cyclosporine levels should be monitored and the dosage adjusted in clients taking these medications.

Test-Taking Strategy: Knowledge regarding the medications that lower cyclosporine levels is required to answer this question. If you are unfamiliar with these medications, take time now to review important points related to cyclosporine!

Level of Cognitive Ability: Analysis
Phase of Nursing Process: Analysis
Client Needs: Physiological Integrity
Content Area: Pharmacology

Reference
Lehne, R. (1998). *Pharmacology for nursing care* (3rd ed.). Philadelphia: W. B. Saunders. pp. 729–730.

28. 4

Rationale: Amphotericin B as well as erythromycin and ketoconazole can elevate cyclosporine levels. When either of these medications is combined with cyclosporine, the dosage of cyclosporine must be reduced to prevent accumulation to toxic levels.

Test-Taking Strategy: Knowledge regarding the medications that elevate cyclosporine levels is required to answer this question. If you are unfamiliar with these medications, take time now to review important points related to cyclosporine!

Level of Cognitive Ability: Analysis
Phase of Nursing Process: Analysis
Client Needs: Physiological Integrity
Content Area: Pharmacology

Reference

Lehne, R. (1998). *Pharmacology for nursing care* (3rd. ed.). Philadelphia: W. B. Saunders. pp. 729–730.

29. 2

Rationale: Because of the risk of anaphylaxis during the administration of cyclosporine IV, epinephrine and oxygen must be immediately available for use. An oral airway or a suction machine is not the priority item, and it is not necessary to have a code cart at the bedside.

Test-Taking Strategy: Knowledge that cyclosporine administered IV can cause anaphylaxis will assist in directing you to option 2. Options 1 and 4 can be eliminated first, followed by option 3. An oral airway and a suction catheter are components of a code cart. Focusing specifically on the issue of the question, the administration of cyclosporine IV, will direct you to option 2.

Level of Cognitive Ability: Application
Phase of Nursing Process: Planning
Client Needs: Physiological Integrity
Content Area: Pharmacology

Reference

Lehne, R. (1998). *Pharmacology for nursing care* (3rd ed.). Philadelphia: W. B. Saunders. p. 731.

30. 1

Rationale: When administering cyclosporine IV, 1 mL of concentrate is diluted in 20 to 100 mL of 0.9% sodium chloride or 5% dextrose. The initial dose is 5 to 6 mg/kg (1/3 the oral dose), administered over 2 to 6 hours. The solution should be protected from light.

Test-Taking Strategy: Note the key word "inappropriate" in the stem of the question. Read each option carefully, and if you are unsure of the procedure for administering cyclosporine IV, the best option to select is option 1. This option identifies administering the medication by IV bolus. Additionally, 10 mL is a small amount of diluent. Review this medication now, if you had difficulty with this question!

Level of Cognitive Ability: Application
Phase of Nursing Process: Implementation
Client Needs: Physiological Integrity
Content Area: Pharmacology

Reference

Lehne, R. (1998). *Pharmacology for nursing care* (3rd ed.). Philadelphia: W. B. Saunders. p. 713.

31. 3

Rationale: To improve palatability, the client should be taught to mix the concentrated drug solution with chocolate milk or orange juice just before administration. Grapefruit juice can raise cyclosporine levels. Instruct client to dispense the oral liquid into a glass container, using a specially calibrated pipette; mix well and drink immediately; rinse the container with diluent and drink it to ensure ingestion of the complete dose; dry the outside of the pipette and return it to its cover for storage.

Test-Taking Strategy: Knowledge regarding the administration of the oral concentrate is required to answer this question. If you are unfamiliar with this procedure, review now. You are likely to find questions related to this medication on NCLEX-RN!

Level of Cognitive Ability: Application
Phase of Nursing Process: Implementation
Client Needs: Health Promotion and Maintenance
Content Area: Pharmacology

Reference

Lehne, R. (1998). *Pharmacology for nursing care* (3rd ed.). Philadelphia: W. B. Saunders. p. 734.

32. 3

Rationale: The client needs to be instructed to dispense the oral liquid into a glass container using a specially calibrated pipette. The client should not use any other type of dropper to calibrate the amount of prescribed medication. Options 1, 2, and 4 are correct.

Test-Taking Strategy: Note the key words "indicate the need for further instruction." Knowledge regarding the administration of the oral concentrate is required to answer this question. If you are unfamiliar with this procedure, review now. You are likely to find questions related to this medication on NCLEX-RN!

Level of Cognitive Ability: Analysis
Phase of Nursing Process: Evaluation
Client Needs: Health Promotion and Maintenance
Content Area: Pharmacology

Reference

Lehne, R. (1998). *Pharmacology for nursing care* (3rd ed.). Philadelphia: W. B. Saunders. p. 734.

33. 3

Rationale: The most common adverse effects of cyclosporine are nephrotoxicity, infection, hypertension, tremor, and hirsutism. Of these, nephrotoxicity and infection are the most serious.

Test-Taking Strategy: Knowledge regarding the adverse effects associated with cyclosporine is required to answer this question. If you are unfamiliar with these effects, review now!

Level of Cognitive Ability: Analysis
Phase of Nursing Process: Assessment
Client Needs: Physiological Integrity
Content Area: Pharmacology

Reference

Lehne, R. (1998). *Pharmacology for nursing care* (3rd ed.). Philadelphia: W. B. Saunders. p. 729.

34. 1

Rationale: Prograf is an alternative medication to cyclosporine for prevention of organ rejection in clients receiving transplant. The medication is somewhat more effective than cyclosporine but also more toxic. Concurrent use of glucocorticoids is recommended during administration of this medication.

Test-Taking Strategy: Knowledge that glucocorticoids are administered concurrently with some medications used to prevent organ rejection will easily direct you to option 1. Review this medication now, if you are unfamiliar with it!

Level of Cognitive Ability: Analysis
Phase of Nursing Process: Analysis
Client Needs: Physiological Integrity
Content Area: Pharmacology

Reference
Lehne, R. (1998). *Pharmacology for nursing care* (3rd ed.). Philadelphia: W. B. Saunders. p. 731.

35. 3

Rationale: Tacrolimus is used with caution in immunosuppressed clients and in clients with renal or hepatic function impairment. It is contraindicated in clients with hypersensitivity to this medication or hypersensitivity to cyclosporine.

Test-Taking Strategy: Many medications affect renal and hepatic function. If you had to select an option and were unsure of the correct answer, select the option that addresses liver or hepatic function. Review the cautions and contraindications associated with the administration of this medication now, if you had difficulty with this question!

Level of Cognitive Ability: Analysis
Phase of Nursing Process: Analysis
Client Needs: Physiological Integrity
Content Area: Pharmacology

Reference
Hodgson, B., & Kizior, R. (1999). *Saunders nursing drug handbook 1999.* Philadelphia: W. B. Saunders. p. 959.

36. 2

Rationale: Nephrotoxicity is a major concern with this medication. Other common reactions include neurotoxicity evidenced by headache, tremor, and insomnia; GI effects such as diarrhea, nausea, and vomiting; hypertension; hyperkalemia; and hyperglycemia.

Test-Taking Strategy: Utilize the process of elimination, noting that options 1, 3, and 4 represent normal values. Option 2 is the only abnormal value reflecting an elevation. Option 2 is the correct option.

Level of Cognitive Ability: Analysis
Phase of Nursing Process: Analysis
Client Needs: Physiological Integrity
Content Area: Pharmacology

Reference
Lehne, R. (1998). *Pharmacology for nursing care* (3rd ed.). Philadelphia: W. B. Saunders. p. 731.

37. 1

Rationale: Orthoclone is a monoclonal antibody. Upon binding to the CD3 site, the antibody blocks all T cell function. Options 2, 3, and 4 are not actions of this medication.

Test-Taking Strategy: Knowledge regarding the action of this medication is required to answer this question. If you are unfamiliar with this medication, take time now to review!

Level of Cognitive Ability: Analysis
Phase of Nursing Process: Analysis
Client Needs: Physiological Integrity
Content Area: Pharmacology

Reference
Lehne, R. (1998). *Pharmacology for nursing care* (3rd ed.). Philadelphia: W. B. Saunders. p. 733.

38. 2

Rationale: Potentially fatal anaphylactic reactions can occur. Manifestations include pulmonary edema, cardiovascular collapse, and cardiac or respiratory arrest.

Test-Taking Strategy: Note the key word "priority" in the stem of the question. Use Maslow's Hierarchy of Needs theory to answer. Remember, airway is the first priority. Review this medication now, if you had difficulty with this question!

Level of Cognitive Ability: Analysis
Phase of Nursing Process: Assessment
Client Needs: Physiological Integrity
Content Area: Pharmacology

Reference
Lehne, R. (1998). *Pharmacology for nursing care* (3rd ed.). Philadelphia: W. B. Saunders. p. 733.

39. 3

Rationale: Mycophenolate mofetil should be administered on an empty stomach. The capsules should not be opened or crushed. The client should contact the physician if unusual bleeding or bruising, sore throat, mouth sores, abdominal pain, or fever occurs. Antacids containing magnesium and aluminum may decrease the absorption of the medication and therefore should not be taken with the medication. The medication is given in combination with corticosteroids and cyclosporine.

Test-Taking Strategy: Knowledge regarding the teaching points associated with the administration of this medication is required to answer this question. Review this medication now, if you had difficulty with it!

Level of Cognitive Ability: Application
Phase of Nursing Process: Implementation
Client Needs: Health Promotion and Maintenance
Content Area: Pharmacology

Reference
Hodgson, B., & Kizior, R. (1999). *Saunders nursing drug handbook 1999.* Philadelphia: W. B. Saunders. pp. 709–711.

40. 1

Rationale: Imuran suppresses cell-mediated and humoral immune responses by inhibiting the proliferation of B and T lymphocytes. It is generally used as an adjunct to cyclosporine and glucocorticoids to help suppress transplant rejection.

Test-Taking Strategy: Knowledge regarding the action of this medication is required to answer this question. If you are unfamiliar with this medication, take time now to review!

Level of Cognitive Ability: Analysis
Phase of Nursing Process: Assessment
Client Needs: Physiological Integrity
Content Area: Pharmacology

Reference
Lehne, R. (1998). *Pharmacology for nursing care* (3rd ed.). Philadelphia: W. B. Saunders. p. 732.

41. 1

Rationale: The nurse should plan for a skin test dose prior to IV administration of Atgam to identify hypersensitivity to the medication. Although options 2 and 4 may be implemented, the test dose is the priority nursing intervention. The client would not be premedicated with aspirin. Premedication with Tylenol and/or Benadryl may be prescribed to prevent reaction to the dose.

Test-Taking Strategy: Use Maslow's Hierarchy of Needs theory to answer the question. Option 1 addresses an intervention that could prevent a life-threatening situation.

Level of Cognitive Ability: Analysis
Phase of Nursing Process: Assessment
Client Needs: Physiological Integrity
Content Area: Pharmacology

Reference
Kuhn, M. (1998). *Pharmacotherapeutics: A nursing process approach* (4th ed.). Philadelphia: F. A. Davis. p. 925.

42. 2

Rationale: Epoetin alfa is used to reverse anemia associated with CRF. Therapeutic effect is seen when the hematocrit is between 30% and 33%.

Test-Taking Strategy: Relate the name of the medication "erythropoietin" to the potential action or effect. The only laboratory test that would reflect the effect of this medication is identified in option 2. Review the therapeutic effect of this medication now, if you had difficulty with this question!

Level of Cognitive Ability: Analysis
Phase of Nursing Process: Evaluation
Client Needs: Physiological Integrity
Content Area: Pharmacology

Reference
Lehne, R. (1998). *Pharmacology for nursing care* (3rd ed.). Philadelphia: W. B. Saunders. p. 567.

43. 4

Rationale: Epoetin alfa is administered parenterally by either the IV or SC route. Administration is by IV bolus for dialysis clients and by IV bolus or SC injection for nondialysis clients. It cannot be given orally because it is a glycoprotein and would be degraded in the gastrointestinal tract.

Test-Taking Strategy: Knowledge regarding the administration of this medication is required to answer this question. If you are unfamiliar with this important medication, take time now to review!

Level of Cognitive Ability: Application
Phase of Nursing Process: Planning
Client Needs: Physiological Integrity
Content Area: Pharmacology

Reference
Lehne, R. (1998). *Pharmacology for nursing care* (3rd ed.). Philadelphia: W. B. Saunders. p. 567.

44. 2

Rationale: Epoetin alfa is generally well tolerated. The most significant adverse effect is hypertension. Occasionally, a tachycardia may occur as a side effect. It may also cause an improved sense of well-being.

Test-Taking Strategy: Knowledge regarding the significant side effect associated with erythropoietin is required to answer this question. Review this important medication now, if you had difficulty with this question!

Level of Cognitive Ability: Analysis
Phase of Nursing Process: Assessment
Client Needs: Physiological Integrity
Content Area: Pharmacology

Reference
Lehne, R. (1998). *Pharmacology for nursing care* (3rd ed.). Philadelphia: W. B. Saunders. p. 567.

45. 4

Rationale: Epoetin alfa stimulates erythropoiesis. It takes 2 to 6 weeks after initiation of therapy before a clinically significant increase in hematocrit is observed. Therefore, this medication is not intended for clients who require immediate correction of severe anemia, and it is not a substitute for emergency transfusions.

Test-Taking Strategy: Knowledge that the medication stimulates erythropoiesis will assist in directing you to option 4. If you are unfamiliar with this medication and its therapeutic effects, review now!

Level of Cognitive Ability: Analysis
Phase of Nursing Process: Assessment
Client Needs: Physiological Integrity
Content Area: Pharmacology

Reference
Kuhn, M. (1998). *Pharmacotherapeutics: A nursing process approach* (4th ed.). Philadelphia: F. A. Davis. p 567.

46. 3

Rationale: The client should be instructed not to shake the bottle. The medication should be refrigerated at all times. All partially used vials should be discarded, and the client should use only 1 dose per vial and not re-enter the vial. Unused portions need to be discarded.

Test-Taking Strategy: Note the key words "accurate description." Note that options 3 and 4 are identifying opposite actions. This should provide you with the clue that one of these options may be the correct one. If you are not familiar with the teaching points related to this medication, review them now. You are likely to find questions related to this medication on NCLEX-RN!

Level of Cognitive Ability: Application
Phase of Nursing Process: Implementation
Client Needs: Health Promotion and Maintenance
Content Area: Pharmacology

Reference
Kuhn, M. (1998). *Pharmacotherapeutics: A nursing process approach* (4th ed.). Philadelphia: F. A. Davis. p. 569.

47. 3

Rationale: The client who is receiving Amphojel should take the medication with meals. The phosphate-binding effect is best when it is taken with food. If tablets are used, they should be chewed well before swallowing.

Test-Taking Strategy: Note that options 1, 2, and 4 are similar in that they all suggest administering the medication without a food item. Option 3 is the best selection.

Level of Cognitive Ability: Application
Phase of Nursing Process: Implementation
Client Needs: Health Promotion and Maintenance
Content Area: Pharmacology

Reference

Kuhn, M. (1998). *Pharmacotherapeutics: A nursing process approach* (4th ed.). Philadelphia: F. A. Davis. p. 574.

48. **2**

Rationale: Aluminum-containing antacids are constipating, and the client should be instructed to take a stool softener or additional bulk-type laxatives to relieve this uncomfortable side effect.

Test-Taking Strategy: Knowledge regarding the purpose and side effects associated with administration of this important medication is required to answer this question. If you are unfamiliar with this medication, take time now to review!

Level of Cognitive Ability: Analysis
Phase of Nursing Process: Analysis
Client Needs: Physiological Integrity
Content Area: Pharmacology

Reference

Kuhn, M. (1998). *Pharmacotherapeutics: A nursing process approach* (4th ed.). Philadelphia: F. A. Davis. p. 574.

49. **4**

Rationale: The usual adult dose of aluminum hydroxide is 30 to 60 mL or 1 to 3 capsules before each meal, or three times a day.

Test-Taking Strategy: Knowledge regarding the usual adult dosage for aluminum hydroxide is required to answer this question. If you are unfamiliar with this important medication, take time now to review!

Level of Cognitive Ability: Analysis
Phase of Nursing Process: Analysis
Client Needs: Physiological Integrity
Content Area: Pharmacology

Reference

Kuhn, M. (1998). *Pharmacotherapeutics: A nursing process approach* (4th ed.). Philadelphia: F. A. Davis. p. 567.

50. **2**

Rationale: Feosol is an iron supplement used to treat anemia. Constipation is a frequent and uncomfortable side effect associated with the administration of oral iron supplements. Stool softeners are often prescribed to prevent constipation.

Test-Taking Strategy: Recalling that oral iron can cause constipation will easily direct you to option 2. If you had difficulty with this question, take time now to review the side effects of Feosol.

Level of Cognitive Ability: Analysis
Phase of Nursing Process: Assessment
Client Needs: Physiological Integrity
Content Area: Pharmacology

Reference

Black, J., and Matassarin-Jacobs, E. (1997). *Medical-surgical nursing: Clinical management for continuity of care* (5th ed.). Philadelphia: W. B. Saunders. p. 2128.

BIBLIOGRAPHY

Black, J., and Matassarin-Jacobs, E. (1997). *Medical-surgical nursing: Clinical management for continuity of care* (5th ed.). Philadelphia: W. B. Saunders.

Hodgson, B., & Kizior, R. (1999). *Saunders nursing drug handbook 1999.* Philadelphia: W. B. Saunders.

Ignatavicius, D., Workman, M., & Mishler, M. (1995). *Medical-surgical nursing. A nursing process approach* (2nd ed.). Philadelphia: W. B. Saunders.

Kuhn, M. (1998). *Pharmacotherapeutics: A nursing process approach* (4th ed.). Philadelphia: F. A. Davis.

Lehne, R. (1998). *Pharmacology for nursing care* (3rd ed.). Philadelphia: W. B. Saunders.

UNIT XVI

....

The Adult Client with an Eye or Ear Disorder

PYRAMID TERMS

Accommodation—Process by which a clear visual image is maintained as the gaze is shifted from a distant to a near point.

Astigmatism—Corneal curvature; eye may be hyperopic or myopic.

Cataracts—An opacity of the lens that distorts the image projected onto the retina and which can progress to blindness.

Conductive Hearing Loss—When sound waves are blocked to the inner ear fibers because of external ear or middle ear disorders. Disorders can often be corrected with no damage to hearing, or minimal permanent hearing loss.

Cycloplegia—Refers to the paralysis of the ciliary muscles by medications that block muscarinic receptors. Cycloplegia causes blurred vision because the shape of the lens can no longer be adjusted to near vision.

Emmetropia—Term to describe ideal refraction of the eye.

Fenestration—Removal of the stapes with a small hole drilled in the footplate, and a prosthesis is connected between the incus and foot plate. Sounds cause the prosthesis to vibrate in the same manner as did the stapes.

Glaucoma—Increased intraocular pressure as a result of inadequate drainage of aqueous humor from the canal of Schlemm or overproduction of aqueous humor. The condition damages the optic nerve and can result in blindness.

Hyperopia—Farsightedness; objects converge to a point behind the retina. Vision beyond 20 feet is normal but near vision is poor. Correction is done by a convex lens.

Legally Blind—If the best visual acuity with corrective lenses in the better eye is 20/200 or less, or if visual acuity is less than 20 degrees of the visual field in the better eye.

Meniere's Syndrome—A syndrome also called endolymphatic hydrops, which refers to dilation of the endolymphatic system either by overproduction or decreased reabsorption of endolymphatic fluid. It is characterized by tinnitus, unilateral sensorineural hearing loss, and vertigo.

Miosis—Refers to a constricted pupil and is achieved primarily by stimulating the muscarinic receptors of the sphincter muscles.

Miotics—Medications that cause contraction of the pupil.

Mydriasis—Refers to a dilated pupil and is achieved by blocking the muscarinic receptors of the sphincter muscles or by stimulating the alpha receptors of the dilator muscles.

Mydriatics—Medications that dilate the pupil.

Myopia—Nearsightedness; rays coming from an object are focused in front of the retina. Near vision is normal but distant vision is defective. A biconcave lens is used for correction.

Otosclerosis—Disease of the labyrinthine capsule of the middle ear that results in a bony overgrowth of tissue surrounding the ossicles. Causes the development of irregular areas of new bone formation and causes fixation of the bones. Stapes fixation leads to conductive hearing loss.

Presbycusis—Common cause of sensorineural hearing loss associated with aging.

Refraction—Process of bending light rays so as to focus an image on the retina.

Retinal Detachment—Occurs when the layers of the retina separate because of the accumulation of fluid between them, or when both retinal layers elevate away from choroid as a result of a tumor. Partial separation becomes complete if untreated. When detachment becomes complete, blindness occurs.

Sensorineural Hearing Loss—A pathological process of the inner ear or of the sensory fibers that lead to the cerebral cortex. Is often permanent, and measures must be taken to reduce further damage or to attempt to amplify sound as a means of improving hearing to some degree.

PYRAMID TO SUCCESS

Pyramid points focus on nursing interventions for clients with an impairment in sight or hearing and on the nursing care related to disorders such as cataracts, glaucoma, and retinal detachment. Pyramid points also focus on emergency interventions for eye and ear disorders and injuries. Review nursing care related to organ donation for the donor and the recipient. Pyramid points also focus on client instructions related to medication administration, sensory perceptual alterations and safety issues, and available support systems.

NURSING PROCESS

ASSESSMENT

Risk factors related to eye or ear disorders
Visual impairment
Hearing impairment
Signs of infection
Risk for injury
Ability to care for self

ANALYSIS: Sensory and Perceptual Alterations

PLANNING	IMPLEMENTATION	EVALUATION
The client remains oriented to the environment.	Identify factors that contribute to sensory or perceptual alterations. Orient the client to the environment. Increase the amount of stimuli to achieve appropriate sensory input.	The client interacts appropriately with the environment. The client demonstrates the ability to compensate for sensory deficits by maximizing the use of unimpaired senses.

ANALYSIS: Potential for Infection

PLANNING	IMPLEMENTATION	EVALUATION
The client remains free of infection. The client identifies factors that increase the risk of infection.	Monitor vital signs. Monitor for signs of infection. Instruct the client regarding signs of infection and methods to avoid infection.	Vital signs remain normal; the client verbalizes the signs of infection. The client verbalizes methods to avoid infection.

ANALYSIS: Potential for Injury

PLANNING	IMPLEMENTATION	EVALUATION
The client remains free of injury.	Identify the risk for injury. Initiate safety precautions.	The client remains free of injury.

ANALYSIS: Self-Care Deficit

PLANNING	IMPLEMENTATION	EVALUATION
The client identifies limitations related to self-care.	Discuss limitations in self-care with the client. Encourage independence in self-care.	The client participates in self-care to the optimal level.

ANALYSIS: Fear Related to Visual or Hearing Loss

PLANNING	IMPLEMENTATION	EVALUATION
The client identifies behaviors that reduce fear.	Provide verbal and nonverbal reassurances that may assist in reducing fear. Encourage the client to verbalize feelings related to fear.	The client verbalizes comfort measures that reduce fear.

ANALYSIS: Social Isolation

PLANNING	IMPLEMENTATION	EVALUATION
The client identifies behaviors that may decrease social isolation.	Encourage the client to schedule time for social interaction.	The client identifies community resources that assist in decreasing social isolation.

ANALYSIS: Noncompliance

PLANNING	IMPLEMENTATION	EVALUATION
The client identifies the consequences of noncompliant behavior.	Identify probable causes of noncompliant behavior. Involve the client in identifying the importance of compliant behavior.	The client complies with the prescribed plan of care.

CLIENT NEEDS

SAFE, EFFECTIVE CARE ENVIRONMENT

Communication techniques for impaired vision and hearing

Client rights

Informed consent for invasive procedures

Organ donation

Accident prevention related to sensory impairments

Asepsis with procedures and treatments

Standard precautions

HEALTH PROMOTION AND MAINTENANCE

Aging process

Expected body image changes

The prevention and early detection of health problems and diseases related to the eye and the ear

Physical assessment of eye and ear disorders

Home care instructions following procedures related to the eye and ear

Instructions regarding the administration of eye and ear medications

Reinforcement regarding the importance of compliance to the prescribed therapy

PSYCHOSOCIAL INTEGRITY

The ability to cope with feelings of isolation and loss of independence

The threat to vision or hearing loss

Sensory perceptual alterations

Family support systems

Available community resources

PHYSIOLOGICAL INTEGRITY

Care to assistive devices such as glasses, contact lenses, and hearing aids

Self-care limitations

Pharmacological medications, actions, uses, side effects, and adverse effects

Complications related to procedures

Expected responses to therapy

Cataracts

Glaucoma

Retinal detachment

Initial treatment for eye and ear emergencies

Organ donation

Hearing or visual loss

BIBLIOGRAPHY

Black J., & Matassarin-Jacobs, E. (1997). *Medical-surgical nursing: Clinical management for continuity of care* (5th ed.). Philadelphia: W. B. Saunders.

National Council of State Boards of Nursing (1997). *Plan for the National Licensure Examination for Registered Nurses.* Chicago: Author.

CHAPTER 63

The Eye and the Ear

I. Anatomy and Physiology of the Eye

A. The Eye
   1. The eye is 1 inch in diameter
   2. It is located in the anterior portion of the orbit
   3. The orbit is the bony structure of the skull that surrounds the eye and offers protection to the eye
B. Layers of the Eye
   1. External layer
      a. The fibrous coat that supports the eye
      b. Contains the sclera, which is an opaque white tissue
      c. Contains the cornea, which is a dense transparent layer
   2. Middle layer
      a. The second layer of the eyeball
      b. Is vascular and heavily pigmented
      c. Consists of the choroid, the ciliary body, and the iris
      d. The choroid is the dark brown membrane located between the sclera and the retina
      e. The choroid lines most of the sclera and is attached to the retina, but can easily detach from the sclera
      f. The choroid contains many blood vessels and supplies nutrients to the retina
      g. The ciliary body connects the choroid with the iris and secretes aqueous humor that helps give the eye its shape
      h. The iris is the colored portion of the eye, is located in front of the lens, and has a central circular opening called the pupil
   3. Internal layer
      a. Consists of the retina
      b. The retina is a thin, delicate structure in which the fibers of the optic nerve are distributed
      c. The retina is bordered externally by the choroid and sclera and internally by the vitreous
      d. The retina contains blood vessels and photoreceptors called rods and cones

C. Vitreous Body
   1. Contains a gelatinous substance that occupies the vitreous chamber, which is the space between the lens and the retina
   2. It transmits light and gives shape to the posterior eye
D. Vitreous
   1. A jell-like substance that maintains the shape of the eye
   2. Provides additional physical support to the retina
E. Rods and Cones
   1. Rods are responsible for peripheral vision and function at reduced levels of illumination
   2. Cones function at bright levels of illumination and are responsible for color vision and central vision
F. Optic Disk
   1. A creamy pink to white depressed area in the retina
   2. The optic nerve enters and exits the eyeball at this area
   3. This area is called the blind spot because it contains only nerve fibers, lacks photoreceptor cells, and is insensitive to light
G. Macula Lutea
   1. A small, oval, yellowish pink area located lateral and temporal to the optic disk
   2. The central depressed part of the macula is the fovea centralis where most acute vision occurs
H. Aqueous Humor
   1. A clear watery fluid that fills the anterior and posterior chambers of the eye
   2. Produced by the ciliary processes and the fluid drains into the canal of Schlemm
   3. The anterior chamber lies between the cornea and the iris
   4. The posterior chamber lies between the iris and lens
I. Canal of Schlemm
   1. A passageway that extends completely around the eye

2. Permits fluid to drain out of the eye into the systemic circulation so a constant intraocular pressure is maintained

J. Lens
1. A transparent circular structure behind the iris and in front of vitreous body
2. Bends rays of light so that the light falls on the retina

K. Pupils
1. Control the amount of light that enters the eye and reaches the retina
2. Darkness produces dilation
3. Light produces constriction

L. Conjunctivae
1. The thin transparent mucous membranes
2. Line the posterior surface of each eyelid and is located over the sclera

M. Lacrimal Gland
1. Produces tears
2. Tears are drained throughout the punctum into the lacrimal duct and sac

N. Eye Muscles
1. Muscles do not work independently but in conjunction with the muscle that produces the opposite movement
2. Rectus muscles: exert their pull when the eye turns temporally
3. Oblique muscles: exert their pull when the eye turns nasally

O. Nerves
1. Cranial nerve III: oculomotor
2. Cranial nerve IV: trochlear
3. Cranial nerve VI: abducens
4. Cranial nerve II: optic nerve (nerve of sight)

P. Blood Vessels
1. Ophthalmic artery: major artery supplying the structures in the eye
2. Ophthalmic veins: venous drainage occurs through the veins

II. Anatomy and Physiology of the Ear

A. Functions
1. Hearing
2. Maintenance of balance

B. External Ear
1. Embedded in the temporal bone bilaterally at the level of the eyes
2. Extends from the auricle through the external canal to the tympanic membrane or eardrum
3. Includes the mastoid process, which is the bony ridge located over the temporal bone

C. Middle Ear
1. Consists of the medial side of the tympanic membrane
2. Contains three bony ossicles
   a. Malleus
   b. Incus
   c. Stapes
3. The tympanic membrane is a thick transparent sheet of tissue that provides a barrier between the external and the middle ear
4. The middle ear is protected from the inner ear by the round and the oval window membranes
5. The eustachian tube opens into the middle ear and allows for equalization of pressure on both sides of the tympanic membrane

D. Inner Ear
1. Contains the semicircular canals, the cochlea, and the distal end of the eighth cranial nerve
2. The semicircular canals contain fluid and hair cells connected to sensory nerve fibers of the vestibular portion of eighth cranial nerve
3. Maintains sense of balance or equilibrium
4. Cochlea: spiral-shaped organ of hearing
5. Organ of Corti: receptor and organ of hearing
6. Eighth cranial nerve
   a. Cochlear branch: transmits neuroimpulses from the cochlea to the brain where they are interpreted as sound
   b. Vestibular branch: maintains balance and equilibrium

E. Hearing and Equilibrium
1. The external ear conducts sound waves to the middle ear
2. The middle ear, also called the tympanic cavity, conducts sound vibrations to the inner ear
3. The middle ear is filled with air, which is kept at atmospheric pressure by the opening of the eustachian tube
4. The inner ear contains sensory receptors for sound and for equilibrium
5. The receptors in the inner ear transmit sound waves and changes in body position to the nerve impulses

III. Assessment of Vision

A. Acuity
1. Visual acuity tests measure the client's distance and near vision
2. Snellen chart
   a. A simple tool to record visual acuity
   b. The client stands 20 feet from the chart and covers one eye and uses the other eye to read the line that appears most clearly
   c. If the client is able to do this accurately, the client reads the next lower line
   d. This sequence is repeated until the client is unable to correctly identify more than half of the characters on the line
   e. The procedure is repeated for the other eye
   f. The findings are recorded as a comparison between what the client can read at 20 feet and the number of feet normally

required by an individual with normal vision to read the same line

g. A result of 20/50 means that the client is able to read at 20 feet from the chart what a healthy eye can read at 50 feet

h. Clients who wear corrective lenses other than for reading should have their vision tested with the lens in place

B. Confrontational Test

1. Performed to examine visual fields or peripheral vision

2. The examiner and the client sit facing each other

3. The client is asked to look directly into the eyes of the examiner throughout the test

4. The examiner covers the right eye while the client covers his or her left eye

5. The examiner moves a finger from a nonvisible area into the client's line of vision

6. Both examiner and client should see the object at approximately the same time

7. When the client sees the object coming into the line of vision, the client informs the examiner

8. The procedure is repeated on the opposite eye

9. The test assumes that the examiner has normal peripheral vision

C. Extraocular Muscle Function

1. Six cardinal positions of gaze

   a. Client's right (lateral position)

   b. Upward and right (temporal position)

   c. Down and right

   d. Client's left (lateral position)

   e. Upward and left (temporal position)

   f. Down and left

2. The client holds the head still and is asked to move the eyes and to follow a small object

3. The examiner notes for any parallel movements of the eye or for nystagmus, an involuntary rhythmic rapid twitching of the eyeballs

D. Color Vision

1. The standard tests for color vision involve picking numbers or letters out of a complex and colorful picture

2. Ishihara chart

   a. Consists of numbers that are composed of colored dots located within a circle of colored dots

   b. The client is asked to read the numbers on the chart

   c. Each eye is tested separately

   d. The test is sensitive for the diagnosis of red/green blindness but not effective for the detection of the discrimination of blue

E. Pupils

1. Round and of equal size

2. Increasing light causes pupillary constriction

3. Decreasing light causes pupillary dilation

4. Constriction of both pupils is a normal response to direct light

5. The client is asked to look straight ahead while the examiner quickly brings the beam of a flashlight in from the side and directs it onto the eye

6. The constriction of the eye is a direct response to the shining of a flashlight into that eye; constriction of the opposite eye is known as a consensual response

F. Sclera and Cornea

1. Normal sclera color is white

2. A yellow color to the sclera may indicate jaundice or systemic problems

3. In a dark-skinned person, the sclera may appear yellow; pigmented dots may be present

4. The cornea is transparent, smooth, shiny, and bright

5. Cloudy areas or specks on the cornea may be the result an accident or eye injury

G. Ophthalmoscopy

1. An instrument is used to examine the external structures and the interior of the eye

2. Darken the room so that the pupils will dilate

3. Hold the instrument with the right hand when examining the right eye and with the left hand when examining the left eye

4. Ask the client to look straight ahead at an object on the wall

5. Approach the client's eye from about 12 to 15 inches away and 15 degrees lateral to the client's line of vision

6. As the instrument is directed at the pupil, a red glare (red reflex) is seen in the pupil

7. The red reflex is the reflection of light on the vascular retina

8. Absence of the red reflex may indicate opacity of the lens

9. The retina, optic disk, optic vessels, fundus, and macula can be examined

IV. Diagnostic Tests for the Eye

A. Fluorescein Angiography

1. Description: detailed imaging and recording of ocular circulation by a series of photographs after the administration of a dye

2. Implementation preprocedure

   a. Assess client for allergies and previous reactions to dyes

   b. Obtain informed consent

   c. A mydriatic medication, which causes pupil dilation, is instilled in the eye 1 hour before the test

   d. The dye is injected into a vein of the client's arm

   e. Inform the client that the dye may cause the skin to appear yellow for several hours after the test and is gradually eliminated through the urine

   f. The client may experience nausea,

vomiting, sneezing, paresthesia of the tongue, or pain at the injection site

g. If hives appear, oral or intramuscular (IM) antihistamines as diphenhydramine (Benadryl) is administered as prescribed

3. Implementation postprocedure
   a. Encourage rest
   b. Encourage fluids to remove the dye from the client's system
   c. Remind the client that the yellow skin appearance will disappear
   d. Instruct the client that the urine will appear bright green until the dye is excreted
   e. Instruct the client to avoid direct sunlight for a few hours after the test
   f. Instruct the client that the photophobia will continue until pupil dilation returns to normal

B. Computed Tomography
   1. Description
      a. A beam of x-ray scans the skull and orbits of the eye
      b. A cross-sectional image is formed by the use of computer
      c. Contrast material is not usually administered
   2. Implementation
      a. No special client preparation or follow-up care is required
      b. Instruct the client that he or she will be positioned in a confined space and needs to keep the head still during procedure

C. Slit Lamp
   1. Description
      a. Allows examination of the anterior ocular structures under microscopic magnification
      b. The client leans on a chin rest to stabilize the head while a narrowed beam of light is aimed so it illuminates only a narrow segment of the eye
   2. Implementation
      a. Explain the procedure to the client
      b. Advise the client about the brightness of the light and the need to look forward at a point over the examiner's ear

D. Corneal Staining
   1. Description
      a. Instillation of a topical dye into the conjuctival sac to outline irregularities of the corneal surface that are not easily visible
      b. The eye is viewed through a blue filter, and a bright green color indicates areas of a nonintact corneal epithelium
   2. Implementation
      a. If the client wears contact lenses, they must be removed
      b. The client is instructed to blink after the dye has been applied to distribute the dye evenly across the cornea

E. Tonometry
   1. Description
      a. The test is primarily used to assess for an increase of intraocular pressure and potential **glaucoma**
      b. Normal ocular pressure is 10 to 21 mmHg
   2. Implementation
      a. Each eye may be anesthetized
      b. The client is asked to stare forward at a point above the examiner's ear
      c. A flattened cone is brought in contact with the cornea
      d. The amount of pressure needed to flatten the cornea is measured
      e. The client must be instructed to avoid rubbing the eye following the examination if the eye has been anesthetized and the potential for scratching the cornea exists

V. Assessment of the Ear

A. Otoscopic Exam
   1. The speculum is never blindly introduced into the external canal because of the risk of perforating the tympanic membrane
   2. Tilt the client's head slightly away and hold the otoscope upside down as if it were a large pen, as this permits the examiner's hand to lie against the client's head for support
   3. Pull the pinna up and back to straighten the external canal in an adult
   4. Visualize the external canal while slowly inserting the speculum
   5. The normal external canal is pink and intact without lesions and with various amounts of cerumen and fine little hairs
   6. Assess the tympanic membrane for intactness
   7. The normal tympanic membrane is intact and not perforated and should be free from lesions
   8. The tympanic membrane is transparent, opaque, pearly gray, and slightly concave

B. Auditory Assessment
   1. Sound is transmitted by air conduction and bone conduction
   2. Air conduction takes two to three times longer than bone conduction
   3. Hearing loss is categorized as **conductive, sensorineural,** and mixed **conductive** and **sensorineural**
   4. **Conductive hearing loss** is caused by any physical obstruction to the transmission of sound waves
   5. **Sensorineural hearing loss** is a result of a defect in the organ of hearing, in the eighth cranial nerve, or in the brain itself
   6. A mixed **conductive, sensorineural hearing loss** results in profound hearing loss

C. Voice Test
1. Ask the client to block one external canal
2. The examiner stands 1 to 2 feet away and quietly whispers a statement
3. The client is asked to repeat the whispered statement
4. Each ear is tested separately

D. Watch Test
1. A ticking watch to test for high frequency sounds
2. The examiner holds a ticking watch about 5 inches from each ear and asks the client if the ticking is heard

E. Tuning Fork Tests
1. Weber tuning fork test
   a. Place the vibrating tuning fork in the middle of the client's head at the midline of the forehead, or above the upper lip over the teeth
   b. Hold the fork by the stem only
   c. The client is asked whether the sound is heard equally in both ears or whether the sound is louder in one ear
   d. A normal test result is hearing the sound equally in both ears
   e. If the client hears the sound louder in one ear, the term lateralization is applied to the side hearing the loudest
   f. Such a finding may indicate that the client has a **conductive hearing loss** in the ear to which the sound is lateralized, or that there is a **sensorineural hearing loss** in the opposite ear
2. Rinne tuning fork test
   a. Compares the client's hearing by air conduction and bone conduction
   b. Air conduction is two to three times greater than bone conduction
   c. Place the vibrating tuning fork stem on the client's mastoid process and ask the client to indicate when he or she no longer hears the sound
   d. The examiner quickly brings the tuning fork in front of the pinna without touching the client and asks the client to indicate if he or she still hears the sound
   e. The client normally continues to hear the sound two times louder in front of the pinna; such results are a positive Rinne test
   f. The examiner records the duration of both phases, bone conduction followed by air conduction, and compares the times
   g. If the client is unable to hear the sound through the ear in front of the pinna, the client may have a **conductive hearing loss** on the side tested, because in this situation, the bone conduction is greater than the air conduction; such results are a negative Rinne test because air conduction is normally greater than bone conduction

h. The Rinne test is of no value in determining **sensorineural hearing loss**

F. Vestibular Assessment
1. Test for falling
   a. The examiner asks the client to stand with the feet together and arms hanging loosely at the sides and eyes closed
   b. The client normally remains erect with only slight swaying
   c. A significant sway or a fall is a positive Romberg sign
2. Test for past pointing
   a. The client sits in front of the examiner
   b. The client closes the eyes and extends the arms in front, pointing both index fingers at the examiner
   c. The examiner holds and touches his or her own extended index fingers under the extended index fingers of the client to give the client a point of reference
   d. The client is instructed to raise both arms and then lower them, attempting to return to the examiner's extended index fingers
   e. The normal test response is that the client can easily return to the point of reference
   f. Clients with vestibular function problems lack a normal sense of position and are unable to return their extended fingers to the point of reference; instead, they deviate either to the right or the left of the reference point
3. Gaze nystagmus evaluation
   a. Examine the client's eyes as they look straight ahead, 30 degrees to each side, upward and downward
   b. Any spontaneous nystagmus, a constant and involuntary cyclic movement of the eyeball in any direction, represents problems with the vestibular system
4. Hallpike maneuver
   a. Assesses for positional vertigo or induced dizziness
   b. The client assumes a supine position
   c. The head is rotated to one side for 1 minute
   d. A positive test results in nystagmus after 5 to 10 seconds

VI. Diagnostic Tests for the Ear

A. Tomography
1. Description
   a. May be performed with or without contrast enhancement
   b. Assesses the mastoid, middle ear, and inner ear structures
   c. Multiple x-rays of the head are done
   d. Especially helpful in the diagnosis of acoustic tumors
2. Implementation
   a. All jewelry is removed

b. Lead eye shields are used to cover the cornea to diminish the radiation dose to the eyes

c. The client must remain still in a supine position

d. No follow-up care is required

B. Audiometry

1. Description

a. Measures hearing acuity

b. Uses two types, pure tone audiometry and speech audiometry

c. Pure tone audiometry is used to identify problems with hearing, speech, music, and other sounds in the environment

d. In speech audiometry, the client's ability to hear spoken words is measured

e. After testing, audiogram patterns are depicted on a graph to determine the type and level of the hearing loss

2. Implementation

a. Inform the client regarding procedure

b. Instruct the client to identify the sounds as they are heard

C. Electronystagmography

1. Description

a. A vestibular test that evaluates spontaneous and induced eye movements known as nystagmus

b. Used to distinguish between normal nystagmus and either medication-induced nystagmus or nystagmus caused by a lesion in the central or peripheral vestibular pathway

c. Records changing electrical fields with the movement of the eye, as monitored by electrodes placed on the skin around the eye

2. Implementation

a. The client is instructed to take nothing by mouth 3 hours before testing

b. Unnecessary medications are omitted for 24 hours before testing

c. Instruct the client that this is a long and tiring procedure

d. The client should bring prescription eyeglasses to the exam

e. The client sits and is instructed to gaze at lights, focus on a moving pattern, focus on a moving point, and then sit with the eyes closed

f. While sitting in a chair, the client may be rotated to provide information about vestibular function

g. In addition, the client's ears are irrigated with both cool and warm water, which may cause nausea and vomiting

h. Following the procedure, the client begins taking clear fluids slowly and cautiously because nausea and vomiting may occur

i. Assistance with ambulation may also be necessary following the procedure

D. Caloric Test (Bithermal Test)

1. Description

a. Performed to evaluate the client who experiences dizziness

b. Nystagmus, nausea, vomiting, or ataxia may indicate a pathological condition of the labyrinth system, whereas a decreased response may indicate that the vestibular system is affected

2. Implementation

a. Warm water causes a greater response than cold water

b. Warm-water caloric testing precedes cool-water caloric testing

c. A 30-second irrigation with 120 to 200 mL of water at 44°C (111.2°F) is used first, followed by irrigation with water at 30°C (86°F)

d. The character and duration of the eye movements are measured

e. The client must assume a supine position with the eyes closed and head elevated to 30 degrees

f. Following the procedure, the client begins taking clear fluids slowly and cautiously because nausea and vomiting may occur

g. Assistance with ambulation may also be necessary following the procedure

VII. Disorders of the Eye

A. Risk Factors Related to Eye Disorders (Box 63–1)

B. **Legally Blind**

1. Description: If the best visual acuity with corrective lenses in the better eye is 20/200 or less, or if the widest diameter of the visual field in that eye is no greater than 20 degrees

2. Implementation

a. When speaking to the client who has limited sight or blindness, the nurse uses a normal tone of voice

b. Orient the client to the environment

c. Use a focal point and provide further orientation to the environment from that focal point

d. Allow the client to touch objects in the room

e. Use the clock placement of foods on the meal tray to orient the client

f. When ambulating, allow the client to grasp the nurse's arm at the elbow; the arm is kept close to the nurse's body so

BOX 63–1. **Risk Factors of Eye Disorders**	
Aging Process	Congenital
Trauma	Diabetes
Heredity	Medications

the client can detect the direction of movement

g. Instruct the client to remain one step behind the nurse when ambulating

h. Instruct the client in the use of the cane used for the blind, which is differentiated from other canes by its straight shape and white color with red tip

i. Instruct the client that the cane is held in the dominant hand several inches off the floor

j. Instruct the client that the cane sweeps the ground where the client's foot will be placed next, to determine the presence of obstacles

k. Alert the client when you are approaching

l. Provide radios, TVs, and clocks that give the time orally or provide Braille watches

m. Promote independence as much as is possible

C. **Cataracts**

1. Description

a. An opacity of the lens that distorts the image projected onto the retina and which can progress to blindness

b. Causes include the aging process (senile **cataracts**), inherited (congenital **cataracts**), injury (traumatic **cataracts**), and as a result of another eye disease (secondary **cataracts**)

c. Intervention is indicated when visual acuity has been reduced to a level that the client finds to be unacceptable or adversely affecting the lifestyle

2. Assessment

a. Opaque or cloudy white pupil

b. Gradual loss of vision

c. Blurred vision

d. Decreased color perception

e. Vision that is better in dim light with pupil dilation

f. Photophobia

g. Absence of the red reflex

3. Implementation

a. Surgical removal of the lens, one eye at a time

b. Extracapsular extraction: the lens is lifted out without removing the lens capsule; may be performed by phacoemulsification in which the lens is broken up by ultrasonic vibrations and extracted

c. Intracapsular extraction: the lens is removed within its capsule through a small incision

d. A partial iridectomy may be performed with the lens extraction to prevent acute secondary **glaucoma**

e. A lens implantation may be performed at the time of the surgical procedure

4. Preoperative Implementation

a. Instruct the client regarding measures postoperatively to decrease or prevent intraocular pressure

b. Administer preoperative eye medications including **mydriatics** and **cycloplegics** as prescribed

5. Postoperative Implementation

a. Elevate the head of the bed 30 to 45 degrees

b. Turn client to the back or nonoperated side

c. Maintain eye patch; orient client to the environment

d. Position the client's personal belongings to the nonoperated side

e. Use side rails for safety

f. Assist with ambulation

6. Client education (Box 63–2)

D. **Glaucoma**

1. Description

a. Increased intraocular pressure as a result of inadequate drainage of aqueous humor from canal of Schlemm or overproduction of aqueous humor

b. The condition damages the optic nerve and can result in blindness

2. Types

a. Acute closed-angle or narrow-angle **glaucoma:** results from obstruction to outflow to aqueous humor

---

BOX 63–2. Client Education Following Cataract Surgery

- Avoid eye straining
- Avoid rubbing or placing pressure on the eyes
- Avoid rapid movements, straining, sneezing, coughing, bending, vomiting, lifting objects over 5 pounds
- Instruct the client in measures to prevent constipation
- Instruct the client and significant other on dressing changes and prescribed eye drops and medications
- Wipe excess drainage or tearing with a sterile wet cotton ball from the inner to the outward canthus
- Instruct the client and significant other in the use of an eye shield at bedtime
- Instruct the client that if a lens implant is not performed, the eye cannot accommodate and glasses must be worn at all times
- Instruct clients that cataract glasses act as magnifying glasses and replace central vision only
- Instruct clients that cataract glasses magnify and objects will appear closer; therefore, they need to accommodate, judge distance, and climb stairs carefully
- Instruct the client that contact lenses will provide sharp visual acuity but that dexterity is needed to insert them
- Advise the client to contact the physician for any decrease in vision, severe eye pain, or increase in eye discharge

b. Chronic closed-angle **glaucoma**: follows an untreated attack of acute closed-angle **glaucoma**

c. Chronic open-angle **glaucoma**: results from overproduction or obstruction to the outflow of aqueous humor

d. Acute: a rapid onset of intraocular pressure greater than 50 to 70 mmHg

e. Chronic: a slow, progressive, gradual onset of intraocular pressure greater than 30 to 50 mmHg

3. Assessment
   a. Progressive loss of peripheral vision
   b. Elevated intraocular pressure (normal pressure is 10 to 21 mmHg)
   c. Vision worsening in the evening with difficulty in adjusting to dark rooms
   d. Blurred vision
   e. Halos around white lights
   f. Frontal headaches
   g. Eye pain
   h. Photophobia
   i. Lacrimation
   j. Progressive loss of central vision

4. Implementation for acute **glaucoma**
   a. Treat as a medical emergency
   b. Administer medications as prescribed to lower intraocular pressure
   c. Prepare the client for peripheral iridectomy, which allows aqueous humor to flow from the posterior to anterior chamber

5. Implementation for chronic **glaucoma**
   a. Instruct the client on the importance of medications (**miotics**) to constrict the pupils
   b. Instruct the client on the importance of medications (carbonic anhydrase inhibitors) to decrease the production of aqueous humor
   c. Instruct the client on the importance of medications (beta blockers) to decrease the production of aqueous humor and decrease intraocular pressure
   d. Instruct the client on the need for lifelong medication use
   e. Instruct the client to carry a MedicAlert tag
   f. Instruct the client to avoid anticholinergic medications
   g. Instruct the client to report eye pain, halos around the eyes, and changes in vision to the physician
   h. Instruct the client that when maximal medical therapy has failed to halt the progression of visual field loss and optic nerve damage, surgery will be recommended
   i. Prepare the client for trabeculoplasty as prescribed to facilitate aqueous humor drainage
   j. Prepare the client for trabeculectomy as

prescribed, which allows drainage of aqueous humor into the conjunctival spaces by the creation of an opening

E. Retinal Detachment
1. Description
   a. Occurs when the layers of the retina separate because of the accumulation of fluid between them, or when both retinal layers elevate away from choroid as a result of tumor
   b. Partial separation becomes complete if untreated
   c. When detachment becomes complete, blindness occurs

2. Assessment
   a. Flashes of light
   b. Floaters
   c. Increase in blurred vision
   d. Sense of a curtain being drawn
   e. Loss of a portion of the visual field

3. Immediate implementation
   a. Provide bed rest
   b. Cover both eyes with patches to prevent further detachment
   c. Position the client's head as prescribed
   d. Protect the client from injury
   e. Avoid jerky head movements
   f. Minimize eye stress
   g. Speak to the client before approaching
   h. Prepare the client for surgical procedures as prescribed

4. Surgical procedures
   a. Draining fluid from the subretinal space so that the retina can return to the normal position
   b. Sealing retinal breaks by cryosurgery, a cold probe applied to the sclera, to stimulate an inflammatory response leading to adhesions
   c. Diathermy, the use of electrode needle and heat through the sclera, to stimulate an inflammatory response
   d. Laser therapy, to stimulate an inflammatory response, to seal small retinal tears before the detachment occurs
   e. Scleral buckling, to hold the choroid and retina together with a splint, until scar tissue forms, closing the tear
   f. Insertion of gas or silicone oil to encourage attachment because these agents have a specific gravity less than vitreous or air, and can float against the retina

5. Postoperative implementation
   a. Maintain eyepatches bilaterally as prescribed
   b. Monitor for hemorrhage
   c. Prevent nausea and vomiting and monitor for restlessness, which can cause hemorrhage
   d. Monitor for sudden, sharp eye pain (notify the physician)

e. Encourage deep breathing but avoid coughing

f. Provide bed rest for 1 to 2 days as prescribed

g. Position client as prescribed

h. If gas has been inserted, position as prescribed on the abdomen and turn the head so the unaffected eye is down

i. Administer eye medications as prescribed

j. Assist the client with activities of daily living

k. Avoid sudden head movements or anything that increases intraocular pressure

l. Instruct the client to limit reading for 3 to 5 weeks

m. Instruct the client to avoid squinting, straining and constipation, lifting heavy objects, and bending from the waist

n. Instruct the client to wear dark glasses

o. Instruct the client to wear an eyepatch at night

p. Encourage follow-up care because of the danger of recurrence or occurrence in the other eye

F. Hyphema

1. Description

a. The presence of blood in the anterior chamber

b. Occurs as a result of an injury

c. The condition usually resolves in 5 to 7 days

2. Implementation

a. Encourage rest with client in semi-Fowler's position

b. Avoid sudden eye movements for 3 to 5 days to decrease the likelihood of bleeding

c. Administer **cycloplegic** eye drops as prescribed to place the eye at rest

d. Instruct the client in the use of eye shields or eyepatches as prescribed

e. Instruct the client to restrict reading and watching television

G. Contusions

1. Description

a. Bleeding into the soft tissue as a result of an injury

b. Causes a black eye, and the discoloration disappears in approximately 10 days

c. Visual acuity is usually not affected

d. Pain, photophobia, edema, and diplopia may occur

2. Implementation

a. Place ice on the eye immediately

b. Instruct the client to receive an eye examination

H. Foreign Bodies

1. Description: an object such as dust that enters the eye

2. Implementation

a. Have the client look upward, expose the lower lid, wet a cotton-tipped applicator with sterile normal saline, and gently twist the swab over the particle and remove it

b. If the particle cannot be seen, have the client look downward, place a cotton applicator horizontally on the outer surface of the upper eye lid, grasp the lashes, and pull the upper lid outward and over the cotton applicator; if particle is seen, gently twist swab over it to remove

I. Penetrating Objects

1. Description: an injury that occurs to the eye in which an object penetrates the eye

2. Implementation

a. Never remove the object because it may be holding ocular structures in place

b. The object must be removed by the physician

c. Cover the object with a cup

d. Do not allow the client to bend

e. Do not place pressure on the eye

f. Client is to be seen by a physician immediately

J. Chemical Burns

1. Description: an eye injury in which a caustic substance enters the eye

2. Implementation

a. Treatment should begin immediately

b. Flush the eyes at the site of injury with water for at least 15 to 20 minutes

c. At the scene of the accident, obtain a sample of the chemical involved

d. At the emergency room, the eye is irrigated with gentle solutions such as normal saline or an ophthalmic irrigation solution

e. The solution is directed across the cornea and toward the lateral canthus

f. Prepare for visual acuity assessment

g. Apply antibiotic ointment as prescribed

h. Cover the eye with a patch as prescribed

K. Enucleation and Exenteration

1. Description

a. Enucleation: removal of the entire eyeball

b. Exenteration: removal of the eyeball and surrounding tissues and bone

c. Performed for the removal of ocular tumors

d. After the eye is removed, a ball implant is inserted to provide a firm base for socket prosthesis and to facilitate the best cosmetic result

e. A prosthesis is fitted approximately 1 month after surgery

2. Preoperative implementation

a. Provide emotional support to the client

b. Encourage the client to verbalize feelings related to loss

3. Postoperative implementation

a. Monitor vital signs

b. Assess pressure patch or dressing
c. Report changes in vital signs or the presence of bright red drainage on the pressure patch or dressing

L. Organ Donation
1. Donor eyes
   a. Obtained from cadavers
   b. Must be enucleated soon after death because of rapid endothelial cell death
   c. Must be stored in a preserving solution
   d. Storage, handling, and coordination of donor tissue with surgeons is provided by a network of state eye bank associations across the country
2. Care to deceased client as a potential eye donor
   a. Raise the head of the bed 30 degrees
   b. Instill antibiotic eye drops such as neosporin or tobramycin as prescribed
   c. Close the eyes and apply a small ice pack to the closed eyes
   d. Contact the family and physician to discuss the option of eye donation
3. Preoperative care to the recipient
   a. Recipient may be told of the tissue availability only several hours to 1 day before the surgery
   b. Assist in alleviating client anxiety
   c. Assess eyes for signs of infection
   d. Report the presence of any redness, watery or purulent drainage, or edema around the eye to the physician
   e. Instill antibiotic drops into the eye as prescribed to reduce the number of microorganisms present
   f. Administer intravenous (IV) fluids and medications as prescribed
4. Postoperative care to the recipient
   a. The eye is covered with a pressure patch and protective shield that is left in place until the next day
   b. Do not remove or change the dressing without a physician's order
   c. Monitor vital signs
   d. Monitor the level of consciousness
   e. Assess the dressing
   f. Position the client on the nonoperative side to reduce intraocular pressure
   g. Orient the client frequently
   h. Monitor for complications of bleeding, wound leakage, infection, and graft rejection
   i. Instruct the client how to apply a patch and eye shield
   j. Instruct the client to wear the eye shield at night for 1 month and whenever around small children or pets
   k. Advise the client not to rub the eye
5. Graft rejection
   a. Can occur at any time
   b. Inform the client of the signs of rejection

c. Signs include redness, swelling, decreased vision, and pain (RSVP)
d. Treated with topical corticosteroids

VIII. Instillation of Eye Medications

A. Drops
1. Wash hands
2. Don gloves
3. Check the name, strength, and expiration date of the medication
4. Instruct the client to tilt the head backward, open the eyes, and look up
5. Pull the lower lid down against the cheekbone
6. Hold the bottle like a pencil with the tip downward
7. Holding the bottle, rest the wrist of the hand on the client's cheek
8. Squeeze the bottle gently to allow the drop to fall into the conjunctival sac
9. Instruct the client to close the eyes gently, not to squeeze them
10. Wait 3 to 5 minutes before instilling another drop to promote maximal absorption of the medication
11. Do not allow the medication bottle to come into contact with the eyeball

B. Ointments
1. Hold the ointment tube near but not touching the eye or eyelashes
2. Squeeze a thin ribbon of ointment along the lining of the sac from the inner to the outer canthus
3. Instruct the client to close the eyes gently and that vision may be blurred by the ointment

IX. Disorders of the Ear

A. Risk Factors Related to Ear Disorders (Box 63–3)
B. **Conductive Hearing Loss**
1. Description
   a. When sound waves are blocked to the inner ear fibers because of external ear or middle ear disorders
   b. Disorders can often be corrected with no damage to hearing, or minimal permanent hearing loss
2. Causes
   a. Any inflammatory process or obstruction of the external or middle ear
   b. Tumors
   c. **Otosclerosis**

BOX 63–3. Risk Factors of Ear Disorders	
Infection	Medications
Trauma	Tumors
Ototoxicity	Aging process

d. A build-up of scar tissue on the ossicles from previous middle ear surgery

C. **Sensorineural Hearing Loss**
1. Description
   a. A pathological process of the inner ear or of the sensory fibers that lead to the cerebral cortex
   b. Is often permanent and measures must be taken to reduce further damage or to attempt to amplify sound as a means of improving hearing to some degree
2. Causes
   a. Damage to the inner ear structures
   b. Damage to cranial nerve VIII
   c. Prolonged exposure to loud noise
   d. Medications
   e. Trauma
   f. Inherited disorders
   g. Metabolic and circulatory disorders
   h. Infections
   i. Surgery
   j. **Meniere's syndrome**
   k. Diabetes mellitus
   l. Myxedema

D. Mixed Hearing Loss
1. Also known as **conductive-sensorineural hearing loss**
2. Client has both **sensorineural** and **conductive hearing loss**

E. Signs of Hearing Loss and Facilitating Communication (Boxes 63–4 and 63–5)

F. Cochlear Implantation
1. Used for **sensorineural hearing loss**
2. A small computer converts sound waves into electrical impulses
3. Electrodes are placed by the internal ear with a computer device attached to the external ear
4. Electronic impulses directly stimulate nerve fibers

G. Hearing Aids
1. Used for the client with **conductive hearing loss**

2. Can help the client with **sensorineural** loss, although it is not as effective
3. A difficulty that exists is the amplification of background noise as well as voices
4. Client education (Box 63–6)

H. **Presbycusis**
1. Description

BOX 63–4. Signs of Hearing Loss

Frequently asking people to repeat statements
Straining to hear
Turning head or leaning forward to favor one ear
Shouting in conversation
Ringing in the ears
Failing to respond when not looking in the direction of the sound
Irritability
Answering questions incorrectly
Raising the volume of the television or radio
Avoiding large groups
Better understanding of speech when in small groups
Withdrawing from social interactions

BOX 63–5. Facilitating Communication

Using written words if the client is able to see, read, and write
Providing plenty of light in the room
Facing the client when speaking
Talking in a room without distracting noises
Moving close to the client and speaking slowly and clearly
Getting the attention of the client before you begin to speak
Keeping hands and other objects away from the mouth when talking to the client
Talking in lower tones because shouting is not helpful
Rephrasing sentences and repeating information
Validating with the client the understanding of statements made, by asking the client to repeat what was said
Reading lips
Encouraging the client to wear glasses when talking to someone to improve vision for lip reading
Using sign language, which combines speech with hand movements that signify letters, words, or phrases
Using telephone amplifiers
Installing flashing lights that are activated by ringing of the telephone or doorbell
Using specially trained dogs that help the client to be aware of sound and to alert the client of potential dangers

---

BOX 63–6. Client Education Regarding a Hearing Aid

- Encourage the client to start using the hearing aid slowly to develop an adjustment to the device
- Adjust the volume to the minimal hearing level to prevent feedback squeaking
- Teach the client to concentrate on the sounds that are to be heard and to filter out background noise
- Instruct the client to clean the ear mold with mild soap and water
- Avoid excessive wetting of hearing aid and try to keep the hearing aid dry
- Clean the ear cannula of the hearing aid with a toothpick or pipe cleaner
- Turn off the hearing aid and remove the battery when not in use
- Keep extra batteries on hand
- Keep hearing aid in a safe place
- Prevent hair sprays, oils, or other hair and face products to come in contact with the receiver of the hearing aid

a. Associated with aging

b. Leads to degeneration or atrophy of the ganglion cells in the cochlea and a loss of elasticity of the basilar membranes

c. Leads to compromise of the vascular supply to the inner ear with changes in several areas of the ear structure

2. Assessment

a. Hearing loss is gradual and bilateral

b. Clients state they have no problem with hearing, but they cannot understand what the words are

c. Clients think that the speaker is mumbling

I. External Otitis

1. Description

a. Infective inflammatory or allergic responses involving the structure of the external auditory canal or the auricles

b. An irritating or infective agent comes in contact with the epithelial layer of the external ear

c. This leads to either an allergic response or signs and symptoms of an infection

d. The skin becomes red, swollen, and tender to touch on movements

e. The extensive swelling of the canal can lead to **conductive hearing loss** because of obstruction

f. It is more common in children and is termed "swimmer's ear"

g. It occurs more often in hot, humid environments

h. Prevention includes the elimination of irritating or infecting agents

2. Assessment

a. Pain

b. Itching

c. Plugged feeling in the ear

d. Redness and edema

e. Exudate

f. Hearing loss

3. Implementation

a. Apply heat locally for 20 minutes three times a day as prescribed

b. Encourage bed rest to assist in reducing pain

c. Administer antibiotics or steroids as prescribed

d. Administer analgesics such as aspirin or acetaminophen (Tylenol) for the pain as prescribed

e. Instruct the client that the ears should be kept clean and dry

f. Instruct the client to use ear plugs for swimming

g. Instruct the client that cotton-tipped applicators should not be used to dry ears because their use can lead to trauma to the canal

h. Instruct the client that irritating agents such as hair products or headphones should be discontinued

J. Otitis Media

1. Description: infective inflammatory or allergic response involving the structure of the middle ear

2. Assessment

a. Pain

b. Pressure in the ear

c. Hearing loss

d. Tinnitus

e. Dizziness or vertigo

f. Fever

g. Headache

h. Malaise

i. Nausea and vomiting

j. Bulging tympanic membrane

k. Fluid behind the tympanic membrane

3. Implementation

a. Provide bed rest to limit head movements and prevent pain

b. Administer localized heat as prescribed

c. Administer antibiotics as prescribed

d. Administer analgesics as aspirin and acetaminophen as prescribed

e. Administer oral and nasal antihistamines and decongestants to decrease mucus production and decrease the levels of fluid in the middle ear

4. Myringotomy

a. Surgically performed perforation of the tympanic membrane

b. Allows drainage of middle ear fluids and thus alleviates pain

5. Needle aspiration: to remove fluid from the middle ear

6. Insertion of a grommet: placed through the tympanic membrane to allow continuous drainage of the middle ear

7. Postoperative Implementation

a. Administer antibiotic ear drops as prescribed

b. Administer systemic antibiotics for 10 to 14 days as prescribed

c. Provide a balanced diet with increased fluids

d. Provide adequate rest

8. Client education (Box 63–7)

K. Chronic Otitis Media

1. Description

a. A chronic infective, inflammatory, or allergic response involving the structure of the middle ear

b. Surgical treatment is necessary to restore hearing

c. The type of surgery can vary and includes either a simple reconstruction of the tympanic membrane, a myringoplasty, or replacement of the ossicles within the middle ear

d. A tympanoplasty, a reconstruction of the

BOX 63–7. Client Education Following Myringotomy

- Avoid strenuous activities
- Avoid rapid head movements, bouncing, or bending
- Avoid straining on bowel movement
- Avoid drinking through a straw
- Avoid traveling by air
- Avoid forceful coughing
- Avoid contact with persons with colds
- Instruct clients that if they need to blow their nose, blow one side at a time with mouth open
- Avoid washing hair, showering, or getting head wet for 1 week
- Instruct the client to keep ears dry for 6 weeks by keeping a ball of cotton coated with petroleum jelly in the ear and to change cotton ball daily
- Instruct the client to change ear dressing every 24 hours as prescribed
- Instruct the client to report excessive ear drainage to the physician

---

middle ear, may be attempted to improve **conductive hearing loss**

2. Preoperative Implementation
   a. Administer antibiotic drops as prescribed
   b. Clean the ear of debris as prescribed
   c. Irrigate the ear with a solution of equal parts of vinegar and sterile water as prescribed, to restore the normal pH of the ear
   d. Instruct the client to avoid persons with upper respiratory infections
   e. Instruct the client to obtain adequate rest, eat a balanced diet, and drink adequate fluids
   f. Instruct the client in deep breathing and coughing; forceful coughing, which increases pressure in middle ear, is avoided
3. Postoperative Implementation
   a. Inform the client that initial hearing after surgery is diminished because of the packing in the ear canal, and that hearing improvement will occur after the ear canal packing is removed
   b. Keep the dressing clean and dry
   c. Keep the client flat with the operative ear up for at least 12 hours
   d. Administer antibiotics as prescribed
   e. Instruct clients that they may return to work in approximately 3 weeks postoperatively as prescribed

L. **Mastoiditis**
   1. Description
      a. May be acute or chronic and results from untreated or inadequately treated chronic or acute otitis media
      b. The pain is not relieved by myringotomy
   2. Assessment

   a. Swelling behind the ear and pain with minimal movement of the head
   b. Cellulitis on the skin or external scalp over the mastoid process
   c. A reddened, dull, thick, immobile tympanic membrane with or without perforation
   d. Tender and enlarged postauricular lymph nodes
   e. Low-grade fever
   f. Malaise
   g. Anorexia
   3. Implementation
      a. Prepare the client for surgical removal of infected material
      b. Monitor for complications
      c. Simple or modified radical mastoidectomy with tympanoplasty is the most common treatment
      d. Once tissue that is infected is removed, tympanoplasty is performed to reconstruct the ossicles and the tympanic membranes in an attempt to restore normal hearing
   4. Complications
      a. Damage to the abducens and facial cranial nerves
      b. Damage exhibited by inability to look laterally (cranial nerve VI) and a drooping of the mouth on the affected side (cranial nerve VII)
      c. Meningitis
      d. Brain abscess
      e. Chronic purulent otitis media
      f. Wound infections
      g. Vertigo, if the infection spreads into the labyrinth
   5. Postoperative Implementation
      a. Monitor for dizziness
      b. Monitor for signs of meningitis as evidenced by a stiff neck and vomiting
      c. Prepare for a wound dressing change 24 hours postoperatively
      d. Monitor the surgical incision for edema, drainage, and redness
      e. Position the client flat with the operative side up
      f. Restrict the client to bed with bedside commode privileges for 24 hours as prescribed
      g. Assist the client with getting out of bed to prevent falling or injuries from dizziness
      h. With reconstruction of ossicles via graft, precautions are taken to prevent dislodging of the graft

M. **Otosclerosis**
   1. Description
      a. Disease of the labyrinthine capsule of the middle ear that results in a bony overgrowth of tissue surrounding the ossicles
      b. Causes the development of irregular areas

of new bone formation and causes the fixation of the bones

   c. Stapes fixation leads to a **conductive hearing loss**

   d. If the disease involves the inner ear, **sensorineural hearing loss** is present

   e. It is not uncommon to have bilateral involvement, although hearing loss may be worse in one ear

   f. The cause is unknown, although it is thought to have a familial tendency

   g. Nonsurgical intervention promotes the improvement of hearing through amplification

   h. Surgical intervention involves removal of the bony growth that is causing the hearing loss

   i. A partial stapedectomy or complete stapedectomy with prosthesis **(fenestration)** may be surgically performed

  2. Assessment

   a. Slowly progressing **conductive hearing loss**

   b. Bilateral hearing loss

   c. A ringing or roaring type of constant tinnitus

   d. Loud sounds heard in the ear when chewing

   e. Pinkish discoloration (Schwartze's sign) of the tympanic membrane, which indicates vascular changes within the ear

   f. Negative Rinne test

   g. Weber test shows lateralization of sound to the ear with the most **conductive hearing loss**

N. Fenestration

  1. Description

   a. Removal of the stapes with a small hole drilled in the footplate, and a prosthesis is connected between the incus and footplate

   b. Sounds cause the prosthesis to vibrate in the same manner as did the stapes

   c. Complications include complete hearing loss, prolonged vertigo, infection, or facial nerve damage

  2. Preoperative Implementation

   a. Instruct the client in measures to prevent middle ear or external ear infections

   b. Instruct the client to avoid excessive nose blowing

   c. Instruct the client not to clean the ear canal with any foreign object

   d. Instruct the client to remove hearing aid 2 weeks before surgery to ensure the integration of local tissue

  3. Postoperative Implementation

   a. Inform the client that hearing is initially worse after the surgical procedure because of swelling and that no

noticeable improvement in hearing may occur for as long as 6 weeks

   b. Inform the client that the Gelfoam ear packing interferes with hearing but is used to decrease bleeding

   c. Assist with ambulating during the first 1 to 2 days after surgery

   d. Provide side rails when the client is in bed

   e. Administer antibiotics, antivertiginous, and pain medications as prescribed

   f. Assess for facial nerve damage, weakness, changes in tactile sensation, changes in taste sensation, vertigo, nausea, and vomiting

   g. Instruct the client to move the head slowly when changing positions to prevent vertigo

   h. Instruct the client to avoid persons with upper respiratory tract infections

   i. Instruct the client to avoid showering and getting the head and wound wet

   j. Instruct the client to refrain from using small objects to clean the external ear canal

   k. Instruct the client to avoid rapid, extreme changes in pressure caused by quick head movements, sneezing, nose blowing, straining, and changes in altitude

   l. Instruct the client to avoid changes in middle ear pressure because they could dislodge the graft or prosthesis

O. Labyrinthitis

  1. Description: infection of the labyrinth that occurs as a complication of acute or chronic otitis media

  2. Assessment

   a. Hearing loss that may be permanent on the affected side

   b. Tinnitus

   c. Spontaneous nystagmus to the affected side

   d. Vertigo

   e. Nausea and vomiting

  3. Implementation

   a. Monitor for signs of meningitis, the most common complication, as evidenced by headache, stiff neck, and lethargy

   b. Administer systemic antibiotics as prescribed

   c. Advise the client to stay in bed in a darkened room

   d. Administer antiemetics and antivertiginous medications as prescribed

   e. Instruct the client that the vertigo subsides as the inflammation resolves

   f. Instruct the client that balance problems that persist may require gait training through physical therapy

P. Meniere's Syndrome

  1. Description

   a. A syndrome also called endolymphatic

hydrops, which refers to dilation of the endolymphatic system either by overproduction or decreased reabsorption of endolymphatic fluid
   b. It is characterized by tinnitus, unilateral **sensorineural hearing loss,** and vertigo
   c. Symptoms occur in attacks and last for several days and the client becomes totally incapacitated during the attacks
   d. Initial hearing loss is reversible, but as the frequency of attacks continues, hearing loss becomes permanent
   e. Repeated damage to the cochlea caused by increased fluid pressure leads to the permanent hearing loss
2. Causes
   a. Any factor that increases endolymphatic secretions in the labyrinth
   b. Viral and bacterial infections
   c. Allergic reactions
   d. Biochemical disturbances
   e. Vascular disturbance producing changes in the microcirculation in the labyrinth
3. Assessment
   a. Feelings of fullness in the ear
   b. Tinnitus, as a continuous low-pitched roar or humming sound, is present most of the time, but worsens just before and during severe attacks
   c. Hearing loss is worse during an attack
   d. Vertigo, as periods of whirling, which might cause the client to fall to the ground
   e. Vertigo, which is so intense that even while lying down, the client holds the bed or ground in an attempt to prevent the whirling
   f. Nausea and vomiting
   g. Nystagmus
   h. Severe headaches
4. Nonsurgical Implementation
   a. Prevent injury during vertigo attacks
   b. Provide bed rest in a quiet environment
   c. Provide assistance with walking
   d. Instruct the client to move the head slowly to prevent worsening of the vertigo
   e. Initiate salt and fluid restrictions as prescribed
   f. Instruct the client to stop smoking
   g. Administer nicotinic acid (Niacin) as prescribed for its vasodilatory effect
   h. Administer antihistamines as prescribed, which will reduce the production of histamine and the inflammation
   i. Administer antiemetics as prescribed
   j. Administer tranquilizers and sedatives as prescribed to calm the client and allow the client to rest, and to control vertigo, nausea, and vomiting
5. Surgical Implementation
   a. Performed when medical therapy is

ineffective and the functional level of the client has decreased significantly
   b. Endolymphatic drainage and insertion of a shunt may be performed early in the course of the disease to assist with the drainage of excess fluids
   c. A resection of the vestibular nerve or total removal of the labyrinth or a labyrinthectomy may be performed
6. Implementation postoperative
   a. Assess packing and dressing on the ear
   b. Speak to the client on the side of the unaffected ear
   c. Perform neurological assessments
   d. Maintain side rails
   e. Assist with ambulating
   f. Encourage the use of a bedside commode
   g. Administer antivertiginous and antiemetic medications as prescribed
Q. Acoustic Neuroma
   1. Description
      a. A benign tumor of the vestibular or acoustic nerve
      b. The tumor may cause damage to hearing and to facial movements and sensations
      c. Treatment includes surgical removal of the tumor via craniotomy
      d. Care is taken to preserve the function of the facial nerve
      e. The tumor rarely recurs after surgical removal
      f. Postoperative nursing care is similar to postoperative craniotomy care
   2. Assessment
      a. Symptoms usually begin with tinnitus and progress to gradual **sensorineural hearing loss**
      b. As the tumor enlarges, damage to adjacent cranial nerves occurs
R. Trauma
   1. Description
      a. The tympanic membrane has a limited stretching ability and gives way under high pressure
      b. Foreign objects placed in the external canal may exert pressure on the tympanic membrane and cause perforation
      c. If the object continues through the canal, the bony structure of the stapes, incus, and malleus may be damaged
      d. A blunt injury to the basal skull and ear can damage the middle ear structures through fractures extending to the middle ear
      e. Excessive nose blowing and rapid changes of pressure that occur with nonpressurized air flights can increase pressure in the middle ear
      f. Depending on the damage to the ossicles, hearing loss may or may not return
   2. Implementation

a. Tympanic membrane perforations usually heal within 24 hours

b. Surgical reconstruction of the ossicles and tympanic membrane through tympanoplasty or myringoplasty may be performed to improve hearing

S. Cerumen and Foreign Bodies

1. Description

a. Cerumen or wax is the most common cause of impacted canals

b. Foreign bodies can include vegetables, beads, pencil erasers, or insects

2. Assessment

a. Sensation of fullness in the ear with or without hearing loss

b. Pain, itching, or bleeding

3. Cerumen

a. Removal of wax by irrigation is a slow process

b. Irrigation is contraindicated in clients with a history of tympanic membrane perforation

c. To soften cerumen, add 3 drops of glycerin to the ear at bedtime, and 3 drops of hydrogen peroxide twice a day

d. After several days the ear is irrigated

e. 50 to 70 mL of solution is the maximal amount a client can tolerate during an irrigation sitting

4. Foreign bodies

a. With a foreign object of vegetable matter, irrigation is used with care because this material expands with hydration

b. Insects are killed before removal unless they can be coaxed out by flashlight or a humming noise

c. Mineral oil or alcohol is instilled to suffocate the insect, which is then removed using ear forceps

d. Use a small ear forceps to remove the object and avoid pushing the object farther into the canal and damaging the tympanic membrane

X. Ear Procedures

A. Irrigation

1. Warm tap water to body temperature

2. Fill a syringe with warm water

3. Place a basin under the ear to be irrigated as well as a towel around the client's neck to avoid getting the client wet

4. Use an otoscope to check the location of the impacted cerumen

5. Place the tip of the syringe at an angle so that the fluid pushes at one side of the impaction and not directly on the impaction; this helps to loosen the cerumen and avoids pushing it farther back in the canal

6. Watch fluid return for signs of cerumen plug removal

7. Continue to irrigate the ear with approximately 50 to 70 mL of fluid

8. If the cerumen does not drain out, wait about 10 minutes, then repeat the procedure

9. Monitor for signs of nausea; if nausea develops, stop the procedure

10. If cerumen cannot be removed by irrigation, glycerin drops as prescribed may be used three times a day for 2 days, and then the irrigation is repeated

B. Ear Drops

1. Tilt the client's head in the opposite direction of the affected ear and place drops in the ear

2. Insert a cotton ball into the ear canal to act as packing

PRACTICE QUESTIONS

1. The clinic nurse is testing the visual acuity of a client using a Snellen chart. Which of the following identifies the accurate procedure for this visual acuity test?

1 Both eyes are assessed together, followed by the assessment of the right and then the left eye

2 The right eye is tested, followed by the left eye; then both eyes are tested

3 The client is asked to stand at a distance of 40 feet from the chart and to read the largest line on the chart

4 The client is asked to stand at a distance of 40 feet from the chart and to read the line that can be read 200 feet away by an individual with unimpaired vision

2. The client's vision is tested with a Snellen chart. The results of the tests are documented as 20/60. The nurse interprets this as:

1 The client can read at a distance of 60 feet what a client with normal vision can read at 20 feet.

2 The client is legally blind.

3 The client's vision is normal.

4 The client can only read at a distance of 20 feet what a client with normal vision can read at 60 feet.

3. The clinic nurse notes that following several eye examinations, the physician has documented a diagnosis of legal blindness in the client's chart. Which of the following does the nurse expect to note as the result of the Snellen chart test?

1 20/20 vision

2 20/40 vision

3 20/60 vision

4 20/200 vision

4. The clinic nurse is evaluating the peripheral vision of a client by the confrontational method. Which of the following describes the accurate procedure?

1 The examiner and the client cover the same eyes and stare at each other's uncovered eye, and a small object is brought into the visual field

2 The examiner and the client cover the eyes directly opposite to each other and stare at each other's uncovered eye, and a small object is brought into the visual field

3 The client is asked to discriminate numbers from a chart composed of colored dots

4 The room is darkened and the client is asked to identify colored blocks and shapes when they appear in the visual field

5. Tonometry is performed on the client with a suspected diagnosis of glaucoma. The nurse analyzes the test results as documented in the client's chart, and understands that normal intraocular pressure is:
   1 2 to 7 mmHg
   2 10 to 21 mmHg
   3 22 to 30 mmHg
   4 31 to 35 mmHg

6. The nurse is developing a plan of care for the client scheduled for cataract surgery. Which of the following is the most appropriate nursing diagnosis?
   1 Self-care deficit
   2 Alteration in nutrition
   3 Sensory perceptual alterations
   4 Anxiety

7. The chief clinical manifestation that the nurse would expect to note in the early stages of cataract formation is:
   1 Eye pain
   2 Floating spots
   3 Blurred vision
   4 Diplopia

8. In preparation for cataract surgery, the nurse is to administer the prescribed eye drops. Which of the following types of eye drops will the nurse expect to be prescribed?
   1 An osmotic diuretic
   2 A miotic agent
   3 A mydriatic medication
   4 A thiazide diuretic

9. Postoperatively, the client who underwent cataract extraction should be positioned:
   1 On the operative side
   2 On the unoperative side
   3 Prone in a flat position
   4 Supine

10. During the early postoperative stage, the cataract extraction client complains of nausea and severe eye pain over the operative site. What is the initial nursing action in this situation?
    1 Call the physician

2 Administer the ordered pain medication and antiemetic

3 Reassure the client that this is normal

4 Turn the client on the operative side

11. The client is being discharged from the ambulatory care unit following cataract removal. The nurse provides instructions regarding home care. Which of the following, if stated by the client, indicates effective teaching?
    1 "I will take aspirin if I have any discomfort."
    2 "I will sleep on the side that I was operated on."
    3 "I will wear my eye shield at night and my glasses during the day."
    4 "I will not lift anything if it weighs more than 10 pounds."

12. The client is diagnosed with glaucoma. Which of the following assessment data gathered by the nurse indicates a risk factor associated with glaucoma?
    1 A history of migraine headaches
    2 Frequent urinary tract infections
    3 Cardiovascular disease
    4 Frequent upper respiratory tract infections

13. The client with glaucoma asks the nurse if complete vision will return. The most appropriate response is:
    1 "Although some vision has been lost and cannot be restored, further loss may be prevented by adhering to the treatment plan."
    2 "Your vision will return as soon as the medication begins to work."
    3 "Your vision will never return to normal."
    4 "Your vision loss is temporary and will return in about 3 to 4 weeks."

14. The nurse is developing a teaching plan for the client with glaucoma. Which of the following instructions does the nurse include in the plan of care?
    1 Decrease fluid intake to control the intraocular pressure
    2 Avoid overuse of the eyes
    3 Decrease the amount of salt in the diet
    4 Eye medications will need to be administered for the rest of the client's life

15. Which of the following assessment signs is associated with detachment of the retina?
    1 Pain in the affected eye
    2 Sudden and complete loss of vision
    3 A sense of a curtain falling across the field of vision
    4 A yellow discoloration of the sclera

16. Which of the following assessment signs indicates that bleeding has occurred as a result of retinal detachment?

1 Complaints of a burst of black spots or floaters
2 A sudden sharp pain in the eye
3 Total loss of vision
4 A reddened conjunctiva

17. The client with retinal detachment is admitted to the nursing unit in preparation for a scleral buckling procedure. Which of the following does the nurse anticipate to be prescribed?
    1 Bathroom privileges only
    2 Elevating the head of the bed to 45 degrees
    3 Placing an eyepatch over the client's affected eye
    4 Wearing dark glasses to read or watch TV

18. The client arrives in the emergency room following an automobile accident. The client's forehead hit the steering wheel and a hyphema is diagnosed. Which of the following does the nurse implement?
    1 Position the client flat on bed rest
    2 Place the client on bed rest in a semi-Fowler's position
    3 Place the client in a lateral position on the affected side
    4 Place the client in a lateral position on the unaffected side

19. The client sustains a contusion of the eyeball following a traumatic injury with a blunt object. Which of the following interventions should be initiated immediately?
    1 Notify the physician
    2 Irrigate the eye with cool water
    3 Apply ice to the affected eye
    4 Accompany the client to the emergency room

20. The client arrives in the emergency room with a penetrating eye injury from wood chips while cutting wood. The nurse assesses the eye and notes the piece of wood protruding from the eye. What is the initial nursing action?
    1 Remove the piece of wood using a sterile eye clamp
    2 Apply an eyepatch
    3 Assess visual acuity
    4 Irrigate the eye with sterile saline

21. The client sustains a chemical eye injury from a splash of battery acid. Emergency care includes which of the following?
    1 Assess visual acuity
    2 Irrigate the eye with sterile normal saline
    3 Swab the eye with antibiotic ointment
    4 Cover the eye with a pressure patch

22. The nurse is caring for a client following enucleation. The nurse notes the presence of bright red drainage on the dressing. Which of the following actions is appropriate?
    1 Notify the physician
    2 Continue to monitor vital signs

3 Document the finding
4 Mark the drainage on the dressing and monitor for any increase in bleeding

23. The nurse is performing an otoscopic examination on an adult client. Which of the following is the appropriate procedure?
    1 Pull the pinna up and back before inserting the speculum
    2 Pull the earlobe down and back before inserting the speculum
    3 Use the smallest speculum available to decrease the discomfort of the exam
    4 Tilt the client's head forward and down before inserting the speculum

24. The nurse is performing a voice test to assess hearing. Which of the following describes the accurate procedure?
    1 Stand 4 feet away from the client to ensure that the client can hear at this distance
    2 Quietly whisper a statement and ask the client to repeat it
    3 Whisper a statement with the examiner's back facing the client
    4 Whisper a statement while the client blocks both ears

25. During a hearing assessment, the nurse notes that the sound lateralizes to the client's left ear with the Weber test. The nurse analyses these results as:
    1 A normal finding
    2 A conductive hearing loss in the right ear
    3 A sensorineural or conductive loss
    4 The presence of nystagmus

26. The nurse is caring for a client who is hearing impaired. Which of the following approaches will facilitate communication?
    1 Speak frequently
    2 Speak loudly
    3 Speak directly into the impaired ear
    4 Speak in a normal tone

27. A client arrives at the emergency room with a foreign body in the left ear, which has been determined to be an insect. Which of the following interventions does the nurse anticipate to be prescribed initially?
    1 Irrigation of the ear
    2 Instillation of diluted alcohol
    3 Instillation of antibiotic ear drops
    4 Instillation of corticosteroid ointment

28. The nurse notes that the physician has documented a diagnosis of presbycusis on the client's chart. This condition is most accurately described as:
    1 A sensorineural loss that occurs with aging
    2 A conductive hearing loss that occurs with aging

3 Tinnitus that occurs with aging
4 Nystagmus that occurs with aging

29. The nurse has conducted discharge teaching for a client who had a fenestration procedure for the treatment of otosclerosis. Which of the following, if stated by the client, indicates that teaching was effective?
   1 "I should drink liquids through a straw for the next 2 to 3 weeks."
   2 "It is OK to take a shower and wash my hair."
   3 "I will take stool softeners as prescribed by my doctor."
   4 "I can resume my tennis lessons starting next week."

30. A client with Meniere's disease is experiencing severe vertigo. Which of the following instructions does the nurse give to the client to assist in controlling the vertigo?
   1 Increase fluid intake to 3000 mL a day
   2 Avoid sudden head movements
   3 Lie still and watch TV
   4 Increase sodium in the diet

31. Which of the following is most likely to be prescribed for the client with Meniere's disease?
   1 Low-cholesterol diet
   2 Low-sodium diet
   3 Low-carbohydrate diet
   4 Low-fat diet

32. The nurse is caring for a client following craniotomy for removal of an acoustic neuroma. Assessment of which of the following cranial nerves identifies a complication specifically associated with this surgery?
   1 Cranial nerve I, olfactory
   2 Cranial nerve III, oculomotor
   3 Cranial nerve IV, trochlear
   4 Cranial nerve VII, facial nerve

33. The nurse assesses the client with a blunt head injury sustained from a motor vehicle accident. Which of the following assessment signs indicates a basal skull fracture as a result of the injury?
   1 Purulent drainage from the auditory canal
   2 Bloody or clear drainage from the auditory canal
   3 Epistaxis
   4 Periorbital edema

34. Assessment findings in an otoscopic examination in a client with mastoiditis reveal which of the following?
   1 A pink-colored tympanic membrane
   2 A pearly colored tympanic membrane
   3 A red, dull, thick, and immobile tympanic membrane
   4 A transparent and clear tympanic membrane

35. The client is diagnosed with a disorder involving the inner ear. Which of the following is the most common client complaint associated with a disorder involving the inner ear?
   1 Hearing loss
   2 Pruritus
   3 Tinnitus
   4 Burning in the ear

ANSWERS

1. **2**

Rationale: Visual acuity is assessed in one eye at a time, then in both eyes together with the client comfortably seated. Begin with the right eye while the left eye is covered, then test the left eye with the right eye covered, followed by testing both eyes together. Visual acuity is measured with or without corrective lenses, and the client stands 20 feet from the chart.

Test-Taking Strategy: Use the process of elimination to answer this question. Remember that normal visual acuity as measured by a Snellen chart is 20/20 vision. This should assist you in eliminating options 3 and 4. It is best to test each eye separately first, then test both eyes together. This most accurately assesses visual acuity.

Level of Cognitive Ability: Analysis
Phase of Nursing Process: Assessment
Client Needs: Health Promotion and Maintenance
Content Area: Adult Health/Eye

Reference
Black, J., & Matassarin-Jacobs, E. (1997). *Medical-surgical nursing: Clinical management for continuity of care* (5th ed.). Philadelphia: W. B. Saunders. p. 945.

2. **4**

Rationale: Vision that is 20/20 is normal; that is, the client is able to read from 20 feet what a person with normal vision can read from 20 feet. A client with a visual acuity of 20/60 can only read at a distance of 20 feet what a person with normal vision can read at 60 feet.

Test-Taking Strategy: Understanding how to interpret the results of this visual acuity test is necessary to answer this question. If you had difficulty with this question, take time now to review!

Level of Cognitive Ability: Analysis
Phase of Nursing Process: Analysis
Client Needs: Health Promotion and Maintenance
Content Area: Adult Health/Eye

Reference
Black, J., & Matassarin-Jacobs, E. (1997). *Medical-surgical nursing: Clinical management for continuity of care* (5th ed.). Philadelphia: W. B. Saunders. p. 946.

3. **4**

Rationale: Legal blindness is defined as 20/200 or less with corrected vision (glasses or contact lenses), or less than 20 degrees of visual field in the better eye.

Test-Taking Strategy: Knowledge regarding the definition of legal blindness is required to answer this question. If you had difficulty with this question, take time now to review!

Level of Cognitive Ability: Analysis
Phase of Nursing Process: Analysis
Client Needs: Physiological Integrity
Content Area: Adult Health/Eye

Reference

Black, J., & Matassarin-Jacobs, E. (1997). *Medical-surgical nursing: Clinical management for continuity of care* (5th ed.). Philadelphia: W. B. Saunders. p. 946.

4. **2**

Rationale: The confrontational method assumes that the examiner has normal peripheral vision. The client sits facing the examiner approximately 2 feet away. The eyes of the client and the examiner should be at the same level. Both the examiner and the client cover the eyes directly opposite to each other and stare at each other's uncovered eye. A small object is brought from the peripheral visual field and tests the superior, temporal, inferior, and nasal fields. The client states when he or she sees the object.

Test-Taking Strategy: Knowledge regarding the procedure for assessing peripheral vision by the confrontational method is required to answer this question. Eliminate option 3 because this option describes the test for color vision. Option 4 does not describe a confrontational test. Try to visual the process of testing as you read through options 1 and 2. This may assist you in selecting the correct option. If you had difficulty with this question, take time now to review this assessment test!

Level of Cognitive Ability: Application
Phase of Nursing Process: Assessment
Client Needs: Health Promotion and Maintenance
Content Area: Adult Health/Eye

Reference

Black, J., & Matassarin-Jacobs, E. (1997). *Medical-surgical nursing: Clinical management for continuity of care* (5th ed.). Philadelphia: W. B. Saunders. p. 946.

5. **2**

Rationale: Tonometry is the method of measuring intraocular fluid pressure using a calibrated instrument that indents or flattens the corneal apex. Pressures between 10 and 21 mmHg are considered within the normal range.

Test-Taking Strategy: Knowledge regarding the normal intraocular pressure is required to answer this question. If you had difficulty with this question, take time now to learn this normal value!

Level of Cognitive Ability: Analysis
Phase of Nursing Process: Analysis
Client Needs: Physiological Integrity
Content Area: Adult Health/Eye

Reference

Black, J., & Matassarin-Jacobs, E. (1997). *Medical-surgical nursing: Clinical management for continuity of care* (5th ed.). Philadelphia: W. B. Saunders. p. 949.

6. **3**

Rationale: The most appropriate nursing diagnosis for the client scheduled for cataract surgery is sensory perceptual alterations (visual) related to lens extraction and replacement.

Test-Taking Strategy: Use the process of elimination to answer this question. When asked questions regarding nursing diagnosis, carefully review the information presented in the question before selecting an option. Use the information presented and avoid reading into the question. Remember that disorders of the eye or ear relate to sensory perceptual alterations. Option 3 is the correct option.

Level of Cognitive Ability: Analysis
Phase of Nursing Process: Planning
Client Needs: Psychosocial Integrity
Content Area: Adult Health/Eye

Reference

Black, J., & Matassarin-Jacobs, E. (1997). *Medical-surgical nursing: Clinical management for continuity of care* (5th ed.). Philadelphia: W. B. Saunders. p. 961.

7. **3**

Rationale: A gradual, painless blurring of central vision is the chief clinical manifestation of a cataract. Early symptoms include slightly blurred vision and a decrease in color perception.

Test-Taking Strategy: Remember the pathophysiology related to cataract development. As a cataract develops, the lens of the eye becomes opaque. This description will assist in directing you to the correct option. If you had difficulty with this question, take time now to review the assessment signs associated with cataract development!

Level of Cognitive Ability: Analysis
Phase of Nursing Process: Assessment
Client Needs: Physiological Integrity
Content Area: Adult Health/Eye

Reference

Ignatavicius, D., Workman, M., & Mishler, M. (1995). *Medical-surgical nursing: A nursing process approach* (2nd ed.). Philadelphia: W. B. Saunders. p. 1323.

8. **3**

Rationale: A mydriatic medication produces mydriasis or dilation of the pupil. Mydriatic medications are used preoperatively in the cataract client. These medications act by dilating the pupils. They also constrict blood vessels. An osmotic diuretic may be used to decrease intraocular pressure. A miotic medication constricts the pupil. A thiazide diuretic is not likely to be prescribed for a client with a cataract.

Test-Taking Strategy: Knowledge regarding the actions of the specific medications identified in the options is required to answer this question. Read the question carefully, noting that the client is being prepared for eye surgery. Dilation of the eye is necessary before cataract extraction.

Level of Cognitive Ability: Analysis
Phase of Nursing Process: Planning
Client Needs: Physiological Integrity
Content Area: Adult Health/Eye

Reference

Ignatavicius, D., Workman, M., & Mishler, M. (1995). *Medical-surgical nursing: A nursing process approach* (2nd ed.). Philadelphia: W. B. Saunders. p. 1328.

9. **2**

Rationale: Postoperatively, cataract extraction clients should be positioned on their backs in semi-Fowler's position or on the nonoperative side to prevent edema in the surgical site.

Test-Taking Strategy: Use the process of elimination to answer this question. Remember that edema to the surgical site can occur following the trauma of surgery. Think about the principles of gravity and the prevention of the accumulation of fluid around the surgical site. This will assist in directing you to the correct option. If you had difficulty with this question, take time now to review postoperative care of a client following cataract surgery!

Level of Cognitive Ability: Application
Phase of Nursing Process: Implementation
Client Needs: Physiological Integrity
Content Area: Adult Health/Eye

Reference

Ignatavicius, D., Workman, M., & Mishler, M. (1995). *Medical-surgical nursing: A nursing process approach* (2nd ed.). Philadelphia: W. B. Saunders. p. 1328.

10. **1**

Rationale: Severe pain or pain accompanied by nausea is an indicator of increased intraocular pressure and should be reported to the physician immediately.

Test-Taking Strategy: The key word in the question is "severe." From this point, use the process of elimination. Eliminate option 3 because this is not a normal condition. The client should not be turned to the operative side; therefore, eliminate option 4. Noting the key word in the question should direct you to eliminating option 2 and to selecting option 1 as the correct answer. If you had difficulty with this question, take time now to review the postoperative complications of cataract surgery requiring physician notification!

Level of Cognitive Ability: Application
Phase of Nursing Process: Implementation
Client Needs: Physiological Integrity
Content Area: Adult Health/Eye

Reference

Ignatavicius, D., Workman, M., & Mishler, M. (1995). *Medical-surgical nursing: A nursing process approach* (2nd ed.). Philadelphia: W. B. Saunders. p. 1329.

11. **3**

Rationale: The client is instructed to wear a metal or plastic shield to protect the eye from accidental injury and is instructed not to rub the eye. Glasses may be worn during the day. Aspirin or medications containing aspirin are not to be administered or taken by the client and the client is instructed to take acetaminophen (Tylenol) as needed for pain. The client is instructed not to sleep on the side of the body that was operated on. The client is not to lift more than 5 pounds.

Test-Taking Strategy: Use the process of elimination to answer this question. Read the stem of the question, carefully noting that the correct option indicates effective teaching. This will assist in directing you to the correct option. If you had difficulty with this question, take time now to review the discharge instructions for the client following cataract extraction!

Level of Cognitive Ability: Application
Phase of Nursing Process: Evaluation
Client Needs: Health Promotion and Maintenance
Content Area: Adult Health/Eye

Reference

Black, J., & Matassarin-Jacobs, E. (1997). *Medical-surgical nursing: Clinical management for continuity of care* (5th ed.). Philadelphia: W. B. Saunders. p. 961.

12. **3**

Rationale: Hypertension, cardiovascular disease, diabetes, and obesity are associated with the development of glaucoma. Smoking, ingestion of caffeine or large amounts alcohol, illicit drugs, corticosteroids, altered hormone levels, posture, and eye movements may cause varying transient increases in intraocular pressure.

Test-Taking Strategy: Use knowledge regarding the risk factors associated with glaucoma to answer this question. From this point, use the process of elimination to answer this question. If you had difficulty with this question, take time now to review the risk factors associated with this disorder!

Level of Cognitive Ability: Analysis
Phase of Nursing Process: Assessment
Client Needs: Health Promotion and Maintenance
Content Area: Adult Health/Eye

Reference

Black, J., & Matassarin-Jacobs, E. (1997). *Medical-surgical nursing: Clinical management for continuity of care* (5th ed.). Philadelphia: W. B. Saunders. p. 954.

13. **1**

Rationale: Vision loss to glaucoma is irreparable. Reassure the client that although some vision has been lost and cannot be restored, further loss may be prevented by adhering to the treatment plan.

Test-Taking Strategy: Knowledge regarding the effects of glaucoma on vision is required to answer this question. Read the options carefully. Eliminate option 3 because this option does not provide a reassuring response and will produce anxiety in the client as it is stated. Options 2 and 4 are similar and incorrect. Note that option 1 is more global in addressing the importance of compliance with the treatment plan.

Level of Cognitive Ability: Application
Phase of Nursing Process: Implementation
Client Needs: Psychosocial Integrity
Content Area: Adult Health/Eye

Reference

Black, J., & Matassarin-Jacobs, E. (1997). *Medical-surgical nursing: Clinical management for continuity of care* (5th ed.). Philadelphia: W. B. Saunders. pp. 955–956.

14. **4**

Rationale: The administration of eye drops is a critical component of the treatment plan for the client with glaucoma. The client needs to be instructed that medications will need to be taken for the rest of his or her life.

Test-Taking Strategy: Knowledge regarding the importance of eye medications is required to answer this question. Use process of elimination to answer the question. Limiting fluids and reducing salt will not decrease intraocular pressure. Knowing that medications are an integral component of the treatment plan will assist in directing you to the correct option. Review the treatment associated with the care of the client with glaucoma now if you had difficulty with this question!

Level of Cognitive Ability: Application
Phase of Nursing Process: Planning
Client Needs: Physiological Integrity
Content Area: Adult Health/Eye

Reference
Black, J., & Matassarin-Jacobs, E. (1997). *Medical-surgical nursing: Clinical management for continuity of care* (5th ed.). Philadelphia: W. B. Saunders. p. 956.

15. 3

Rationale: A characteristic clinical manifestation of retinal detachment described by clients is the feeling that a shadow or curtain is falling across the field of vision. There is no pain associated with detachment of the retina. A retinal detachment is an ophthalmic emergency.

Test-Taking Strategy: Knowledge regarding the clinical manifestations associated with retinal detachment is required to answer this question. Retinal detachment can occur suddenly and is an ophthalmic emergency. Review the clinical manifestations associated with this condition now if you had difficulty with this question!

Level of Cognitive Ability: Analysis
Phase of Nursing Process: Assessment
Client Needs: Physiological Integrity
Content Area: Adult Health/Eye

Reference
Black, J., & Matassarin-Jacobs, E. (1997). *Medical-surgical nursing: Clinical management for continuity of care* (5th ed.). Philadelphia: W. B. Saunders. p. 962.

16. 1

Rationale: Complaints of a sudden burst of black spots or floaters indicate that bleeding has occurred as a result of the detachment.

Test-Taking Strategy: Knowledge regarding the signs of hemorrhage associated with retinal detachment is required to answer this question. Hemorrhage is a serious complication associated with retinal detachment. Review the clinical manifestations associated with the complications of a detached retina now if you had difficulty with this question!

Level of Cognitive Ability: Analysis
Phase of Nursing Process: Assessment
Client Needs: Physiological Integrity
Content Area: Adult Health/Eye

Reference
Ignatavicius, D., Workman, M., & Mishler, M. (1995). *Medical-surgical nursing: A nursing process approach* (2nd ed.). Philadelphia: W. B. Saunders. p. 1139.

17. 3

Rationale: The nurse places an eyepatch over the client's affected eye to reduce eye movement. Some clients may need bilateral patching. Depending on the location and size of the retinal break, activity restrictions may be needed immediately. These restrictions are necessary to prevent further tearing or detachment and to promote drainage of any subretinal fluid. The nurse positions the client as prescribed by the physician.

Test-Taking Strategy: Use the process of elimination to answer the question. Eliminate options that suggest activity such as in options 1 and 4. Remember that the eye needs to be protected and rested. This should direct you to the correct option, option 3. If you had difficulty with this question, take time now to review care to the client with retinal detachment!

Level of Cognitive Ability: Analysis
Phase of Nursing Process: Analysis
Client Needs: Physiological Integrity
Content Area: Adult Health/Eye

Reference
Ignatavicius, D., Workman, M., & Mishler, M. (1995). *Medical-surgical nursing: A nursing process approach* (2nd ed.). Philadelphia: W. B. Saunders. p. 1339.

18. 2

Rationale: A hyphema is the presence of blood in the anterior chamber. It is produced when a force is sufficient to break the integrity of the blood vessels in the eye. It can be caused by direct injury such as a penetrating injury from a BB pellet, or indirectly such as from striking the forehead on a steering wheel during an accident. The client is treated by bed rest in a semi-Fowler's position to assist gravity in keeping the hyphema away from the optical center of the cornea.

Test-Taking Strategy: Use the process of elimination to answer this question. Placing the client flat will produce an increase in pressure at the injured site. Note that option 2 is the only option that identifies a position different from the other options. Take time now to review care to the client with hyphema if you had difficulty with this question!

Level of Cognitive Ability: Application
Phase of Nursing Process: Implementation
Client Needs: Physiological Integrity
Content Area: Adult Health/Eye

Reference
Ignatavicius, D., Workman, M., & Mishler, M. (1995). *Medical-surgical nursing: A nursing process approach* (2nd ed.). Philadelphia: W. B. Saunders. p. 1342.

19. 3

Rationale: Treatment for a contusion begins at the time of injury. Ice is applied immediately. The client should receive a thorough eye examination to rule out the presence of other eye injuries.

Test-Taking Strategy: Knowledge regarding the initial treatment following a contusion to the eye is required to answer this question. Use the process of elimination to answer this question. This will assist in directing you to the correct option. You are likely to see questions on NCLEX-RN regarding the initial treatment to various eye injuries. Review this content now if you had difficulty with this question!

Level of Cognitive Ability: Application
Phase of Nursing Process: Implementation
Client Needs: Physiological Integrity
Content Area: Adult Health/Eye

Reference
Ignatavicius, D., Workman, M., & Mishler, M. (1995). *Medical-surgical nursing: A nursing process approach* (2nd ed.). Philadelphia: W. B. Saunders. pp. 1342–1343.

20. 3

Rationale: If the laceration is the result of a penetrating injury, an object may be noted protruding from the eye. This object must never be removed except by the ophthalmologist because it may be holding ocular structures in place. Application of an eyepatch or irrigation of the eye may disrupt the foreign body and cause further tearing of the cornea.

Test-Taking Strategy: Use the process of elimination to answer this question. Note the key word "penetrating" in the question. This should indicate that a laceration has occurred and that interventions are directed at preventing further disruption of the integrity of the eye. The only option that is accurate in the options presented is to assess visual acuity. You are likely to see questions on NCLEX-RN regarding the initial treatment to various eye injuries. Review this content now if you had difficulty with this question!

Level of Cognitive Ability: Application
Phase of Nursing Process: Implementation
Client Needs: Physiological Integrity
Content Area: Adult Health/Eye

Reference

Ignatavicius, D., Workman, M., & Mishler, M. (1995). *Medical-surgical nursing: A nursing process approach* (2nd ed.). Philadelphia: W. B. Saunders. p. 1344.

21. 2

Rationale: Emergency care following a chemical burn to the eye includes irrigating the eye immediately with sterile normal saline or ocular irrigating solution. The irrigation should be maintained for at least 10 minutes. Following this emergency treatment visual acuity is assessed.

Test-Taking Strategy: Read the question carefully, noting the type of injury to the eye. From this point, use the process of elimination to answer the question. The question asks about emergency care; therefore, in this type of injury, it is necessary to irrigate the eye first! You are likely to see questions on NCLEX-RN regarding the initial treatment to various eye injuries. Review this content now if you had difficulty with this question!

Level of Cognitive Ability: Application
Phase of Nursing Process: Implementation
Client Needs: Physiological Integrity
Content Area: Adult Health/Eye

Reference

Ignatavicius, D., Workman, M., & Mishler, M. (1995). *Medical-surgical nursing: A nursing process approach* (2nd ed.). Philadelphia: W. B. Saunders. pp. 1344–1345.

22. 1

Rationale: If the nurse notes the presence of bright red drainage on the dressing, it must be reported to the physician because this can indicate hemorrhage.

Test-Taking Strategy: Note the key words "bright red" in the question. Bright red drainage indicates active bleeding. The physician needs to be notified if this type of drainage occurs. Review postoperative complications associated with an enucleation now if you had difficulty with this question!

Level of Cognitive Ability: Application
Phase of Nursing Process: Implementation
Client Needs: Physiological Integrity
Content Area: Adult Health/Eye

Reference

Black, J., & Matassarin-Jacobs, E. (1997). *Medical-surgical nursing: Clinical management for continuity of care* (5th ed.). Philadelphia: W. B. Saunders. p. 971.

23. 1

Rationale: The nurse tilts the client's head slightly away and holds the otoscope upside down as if it were a large pen. The pinna is pulled up and back and the nurse visualizes the external canal while slowly inserting the speculum.

Test-Taking Strategy: Use the process of elimination to answer the question. Note that the question addresses an adult client. Use the basic knowledge regarding the admin-

istration of ear medications in selecting the correct option. In the adult, the pinna is pulled up and back!

Level of Cognitive Ability: Application
Phase of Nursing Process: Assessment
Client Needs: Health Promotion and Maintenance
Content Area: Adult Health/Ear

Reference

Ignatavicius, D., Workman, M., & Mishler, M. (1995). *Medical-surgical nursing: A nursing process approach* (2nd ed.). Philadelphia: W. B. Saunders. pp. 1357–1358.

24. 2

Rationale: The examiner stands 1 to 2 feet away from the client and asks the client to block one external ear canal. The nurse quietly whispers a statement and asks the client to repeat it. Each ear is tested separately.

Test-Taking Strategy: Knowledge regarding the implementation of this examination is required to answer this question. Eliminate options 3 and 4 because they are not measures that would effectively assess hearing. Eliminate option 1, as distance hearing is not the issue of the question. This leaves option 2 as the correct option!

Level of Cognitive Ability: Application
Phase of Nursing Process: Assessment
Client Needs: Health Promotion and Maintenance
Content Area: Adult Health/Ear

Reference

Ignatavicius, D., Workman, M., & Mishler, M. (1995). *Medical-surgical nursing: A nursing process approach* (2nd ed.). Philadelphia: W. B. Saunders. p. 1359.

25. 3

Rationale: In the Weber tuning fork test, the nurse places the vibrating tuning fork in the middle of the client's head at the midline of the forehead, or above the upper lip over the teeth. Normally the sound is heard equally in both ears by bone conduction. If the client has a sensorineural hearing loss in one ear, the sound is heard in the other ear. If the client has a conductive hearing loss in one ear, the sound is heard in that ear.

Test-Taking Strategy: This is a difficult question. Knowledge regarding analyzing the results of the Weber tuning fork test is required to answer this question. If you had difficulty with this question, take time now to review this hearing test. Also, review the Rinne tuning fork test!

Level of Cognitive Ability: Analysis
Phase of Nursing Process: Analysis
Client Needs: Health Promotion and Maintenance
Content Area: Adult Health/Ear

Reference

Black, J., & Matassarin-Jacobs, E. (1997). *Medical-surgical nursing: Clinical management for continuity of care* (5th ed.). Philadelphia: W. B. Saunders. p. 989.

26. 4

Rationale: Speak in a normal tone to the client with impaired hearing and do not shout. Talk directly to the client while facing the client and speak clearly. If the client does not seem to understand what is said, express it differently. Moving closer to the client and toward the better ear may facilitate communication, but avoid talking directly into the impaired ear.

Test-Taking Strategy: Knowledge regarding effective communication techniques for the hearing impaired is required to answer this question. Use the process of elimination to answer this question. If you had difficulty with this question, take time now to review these techniques!

Level of Cognitive Ability: Application
Phase of Nursing Process: Implementation
Client Needs: Physiological Integrity
Content Area: Adult Health/Ear

Reference
Black, J., & Matassarin-Jacobs, E. (1997). *Medical-surgical nursing: Clinical management for continuity of care* (5th ed.). Philadelphia: W. B. Saunders. p. 1000.

27. **2**

Rationale: Insects are killed before removal unless they can be coaxed out by a flashlight or a humming noise. Mineral oil or diluted alcohol is instilled into the ear to suffocate the insect, which is then removed by using ear forceps. When the foreign object is vegetable matter, irrigation is not used because this material expands with hydration and the impaction becomes worse.

Test-Taking Strategy: Use the process of elimination and knowledge regarding care to the client with a foreign body in the ear to answer this question. If you had difficulty with this question, take time now to review the care required. You are likely to see questions on NCLEX-RN related to the initial care of ear injuries!

Level of Cognitive Ability: Analysis
Phase of Nursing Process: Implementation
Client Needs: Physiological Integrity
Content Area: Adult Health/Ear

Reference
Ignatavicius, D., Workman, M., & Mishler, M. (1995). *Medical-surgical nursing: A nursing process approach* (2nd ed.). Philadelphia: W. B. Saunders. p. 1370.

28. **1**

Rationale: Presbycusis is a type of hearing loss that occurs with aging. It is a gradual sensorineural loss caused by nerve degeneration in the inner ear or auditory nerve.

Test-Taking Strategy: Knowledge regarding the description of presbycusis is required to answer this question. If you are unfamiliar with this condition, take time now to review this age-related disorder!

Level of Cognitive Ability: Analysis
Phase of Nursing Process: Assessment
Client Needs: Physiological Integrity
Content Area: Adult Health/Ear

Reference
Black, J., & Matassarin-Jacobs, E. (1997). *Medical-surgical nursing: Clinical management for continuity of care* (5th ed.). Philadelphia: W. B. Saunders. p. 984.

29. **3**

Rationale: Following ear surgery, clients need to avoid straining when having a bowel movement. Clients need to be instructed to avoid drinking with a straw for 2 to 3 weeks, avoid air travel, and avoid coughing excessively. Clients need to avoid getting their head wet, washing their hair, and showering for 1 week. Clients need to avoid rapidly moving their head, bouncing, and bending over for 3 weeks.

Test-Taking Strategy: Note that the question asks for the client statement that indicates effective teaching. Consider the anatomical area of the client's condition and the surgical procedure in eliminating the incorrect options. If you had difficulty with this question, take time now to review client instructions following ear surgery!

Level of Cognitive Ability: Analysis
Phase of Nursing Process: Evaluation
Client Needs: Health Promotion and Maintenance
Content Area: Adult Health/Ear

Reference
Ignatavicius, D., Workman, M., & Mishler, M. (1995). *Medical-surgical nursing: A nursing process approach* (2nd ed.). Philadelphia: W. B. Saunders. p. 1373.

30. **2**

Rationale: The nurse instructs the client to make slow head movements and to avoid activities such as watching television to prevent worsening of the vertigo. Dietary changes such as salt and fluid restrictions that reduce the amount of endolymphatic fluid are sometimes prescribed. Clients are advised to stop smoking because of its vasoconstrictive effects.

Test-Taking Strategy: Identify the issue of the question. The issue is vertigo. Note the relationship between vertigo and the correct option, option 2, avoiding sudden head movements. If you had difficulty with this question, take time now to review measures that will reduce vertigo in the client with Meniere's disease!

Level of Cognitive Ability: Application
Phase of Nursing Process: Implementation
Client Needs: Health Promotion and Maintenance
Content Area: Adult Health/Ear

Reference
Ignatavicius, D., Workman, M., & Mishler, M. (1995). *Medical-surgical nursing: A nursing process approach* (2nd ed.). Philadelphia: W. B. Saunders. p. 1378.

31. **2**

Rationale: Dietary changes such as salt and fluid restrictions that reduce the amount of endolymphatic fluid are sometimes prescribed. Clients are advised to stop smoking because of its vasoconstrictive effects.

Test-Taking Strategy: Knowledge regarding the pathophysiology related to Meniere's disease is required to answer this question. From this point, using the process of elimination will direct you to the correct option. Review the pathophysiology related to this condition and the treatment now if you had difficulty with this question!

Level of Cognitive Ability: Analysis
Phase of Nursing Process: Analysis
Client Needs: Physiological Integrity
Content Area: Adult Health/Ear

Reference
Ignatavicius, D., Workman, M., & Mishler, M. (1995). *Medical-surgical nursing: A nursing process approach* (2nd ed.). Philadelphia: W. B. Saunders. p. 1378.

32. **4**

Rationale: Treatment for acoustic neuroma is surgical removal via a craniotomy. Extreme care is taken to preserve remaining hearing and the function of the facial nerve. Acoustic neuromas rarely occur following surgical removal.

Test-Taking Strategy: Use knowledge regarding the anatomical location of acoustic neuromas to answer this question. If you had difficulty with this question, take time now to review the complications associated with this surgical procedure!

Level of Cognitive Ability: Analysis
Phase of Nursing Process: Assessment
Client Needs: Physiological Integrity
Content Area: Adult Health/Ear

Reference

Ignatavicius, D., Workman, M., & Mishler, M. (1995). *Medical-surgical nursing: A nursing process approach* (2nd ed.). Philadelphia: W. B. Saunders. p. 1378.

33. **2**

Rationale: Bloody or clear watery drainage from the auditory canal indicates a cerebrospinal leak following trauma and suggests a basal skull fracture. This warrants immediate attention.

Test-Taking Strategy: Knowledge regarding the assessment signs associated with a basal skull fracture is required to answer this question. If you had difficulty with this question, take time now to review these assessment signs!

Level of Cognitive Ability: Analysis
Phase of Nursing Process: Assessment
Client Needs: Physiological Integrity
Content Area: Adult Health/Ear

Reference

Ignatavicius, D., Workman, M., & Mishler, M. (1995). *Medical-surgical nursing: A nursing process approach* (2nd ed.). Philadelphia: W. B. Saunders. p. 1271.

34. **3**

Rationale: Otoscopic examination in a client with mastoiditis reveals a red, dull, thick, and immobile tympanic membrane with or without perforation. Postauricular lymph nodes are tender and enlarged. Clients also have a low-grade fever, malaise, anorexia, swelling behind the ear, and pain with minimal movement of the head.

Test-Taking Strategy: Knowledge regarding the assessment findings associated with mastoiditis is required to answer this question. If you had difficulty with this question, take time now to review the assessment findings associated with this disorder!

Level of Cognitive Ability: Analysis
Phase of Nursing Process: Assessment
Client Needs: Physiological Integrity
Content Area: Adult Health/Ear

Reference

Ignatavicius, D., Workman, M., & Mishler, M. (1995). *Medical-surgical nursing: A nursing process approach* (2nd ed.). Philadelphia: W. B. Saunders. pp. 1371–1374.

35. **3**

Rationale: Tinnitus is the most common complaint of clients with otologic disorders, especially disorders involving the inner ear. Symptoms of tinnitus range from mild ringing in the ear, which can go unnoticed during the day, to a loud roaring in the ear, which can interfere with the client's thinking process and attention span.

Test-Taking Strategy: Knowledge regarding symptoms associated with inner ear disorders is required to answer this question. Use the process of elimination to select the correct option, and note that the question addresses a disorder of the inner ear!

Level of Cognitive Ability: Analysis
Phase of Nursing Process: Assessment
Client Needs: Physiological Integrity
Content Area: Adult Health/Ear

Reference

Ignatavicius, D., Workman, M., & Mishler, M. (1995). *Medical-surgical nursing: A nursing process approach* (2nd ed.). Philadelphia: W. B. Saunders. p. 1376.

BIBLIOGRAPHY

Black, J., & Matassarin-Jacobs, E. (1997). *Medical-surgical nursing: Clinical management for continuity of care* (5th ed.). Philadelphia: W. B. Saunders.

Clark, J., Queener, S., & Karb, V. (1997). *Pharmacologic basis for nursing practice* (5th ed.). St. Louis: Mosby–Year Book.

Hodgson, B., & Kizior, R. (1999). *Saunders nursing drug handbook 1999.* Philadelphia: W. B. Saunders.

Ignatavicius, D., Workman, M., & Mishler, M. (1995). *Medical-surgical nursing: A nursing process approach* (2nd ed.). Philadelphia: W. B. Saunders.

Kee, J., & Hayes, E. (1997). *Pharmacology: A nursing process approach* (2nd ed.). Philadelphia: W. B. Saunders.

Lammon, C. B., Foote, A. W., Leli, P. G., et al. (1995). *Clinical nursing skills.* Philadelphia: W. B. Saunders.

Lehne, R. (1998). *Pharmacology for nursing care* (3rd ed.). Philadelphia: W. B. Saunders.

Monahan, F., & Neighbors, M. (1998). *Medical-surgical nursing: Foundations for clinical practice* (2nd ed.). Philadelphia: W. B. Saunders.

Potter, P., & Perry, A. (1997). *Fundamentals of nursing: Concepts, process, & practice* (4th ed.). St. Louis: Mosby–Year Book.

CHAPTER 64

Ophthalmic and Otic Medications

I. Ophthalmic Medication Administration
(Box 64–1)

A. Guidelines for the Use of Eye Medications
1. Eye medications are usually in the form of drops or ointments
2. To prevent overflow of medication into the nasal and pharyngeal passages, thus reducing systemic absorption, instruct the client to occlude the nasolacrimal duct with one finger for 1 to 2 minutes after instilling the medication
3. When two or more eye medications are to be administered, wait at least 3 minutes between medications
4. Wash hands carefully before administering eye medications to avoid contaminating the eye or applicator
5. Wash hands after administering eye medications to rinse off any residue
6. Use a separate bottle or tube of medication for each client to avoid accidental cross contamination
7. Place the ordered dose of eye medication in the lower conjunctival sac, never directly onto the cornea
8. Avoid touching any part of the eye with the dropper or applicator
9. Administer drops or liquid preparations before ointments
10. Administer glucocorticoid preparations before other medications
11. Monitor the pulse of clients receiving beta blockers and instruct these clients to do the same

12. If the pulse is below 50 to 60 beats per minute (bpm) in an adult receiving a beta blocker, withhold the next dose of medication and notify the physician
13. Instruct the client how to instill medication correctly and supervise instillation until the client can do it safely
14. Instruct the client to read labels carefully to ensure administration of the correct medication and correct strength
15. Remind the client to keep these medications out of the reach of children
16. Instruct the client to avoid driving or operating hazardous equipment if vision is blurred
17. Inform clients that they may be unable to drive home after eye examinations when medications to dilate the pupil (**mydriatics**) or medications to paralyze the ciliary muscle (**cycloplegics**) are used
18. If photophobia occurs, instruct clients to wear sunglasses and avoid bright lights
19. Instruct clients to administer a missed dose as soon as remembered, unless the next dose is scheduled within 1 to 2 hours
20. Inform clients with **glaucoma** that the disorder cannot be cured, only controlled
21. Reinforce the importance of using medications to treat **glaucoma** as prescribed and not to discontinue these medications without consulting the physician
22. Inform the client that medications used to treat **glaucoma** may cause pain and blurred vision, especially when therapy is begun
23. Instruct clients to report the development of any eye irritation
24. Inform clients using eye gel to store the gel at room temperature or in the refrigerator but not to freeze it
25. Instruct the client to discard unused eye gel kept at room temperature after 8 weeks

---

BOX 64–1. Abbreviations

Left eye (OS)	Both eyes (OU)
Right eye (OD)	

26. Inform the client that soft contact lenses may absorb certain eye medications and that preservatives in eye medications may discolor the contact lenses
27. Advise clients wearing contact lenses to question the physician carefully about special precautions to observe
28. In infants, inform the parents that atropine eye drops may contribute to abdominal distention
29. Instruct parents to keep a record of the bowel movements of infants being administered atropine eye drops
30. Auscultate bowel sounds of infants and children receiving atropine eye drops

B. Instillation of Eye Medications
   1. Drops
      a. Wash hands
      b. Put gloves on
      c. Check the name, strength, and expiration date of the medication
      d. Instruct the client to tilt the head backward, open the eyes, and look up
      e. Pull the lower lid down against the cheekbone
      f. Hold the bottle like a pencil with the tip downward
      g. Holding the bottle, gently rest the wrist of the hand on the client's cheek
      h. Squeeze the bottle gently to allow the drop to fall into the conjunctival sac
      i. Instruct the client to close the eyes gently and not to squeeze the eyes shut
      j. Wait 3 to 5 minutes before instilling another drop to promote maximal absorption of the medication
      k. Do not allow the medication bottle to come in contact with the eyeball
   2. Ointments
      a. Hold the ointment tube near, but not touching, the eye or eyelashes
      b. Squeeze a thin ribbon of ointment along the lining of the sac from the inner to the outer canthus
      c. Instruct the client to close the eyes gently
      d. Instruct the client that vision may be blurred by the ointment

II. **Mydriatic/Cycloplegic and Anticholinergic Medications** (Box 64–2)

A. Description
   1. **Mydriatics** and **cycloplegics** dilate the pupils (**mydriasis**) and relax the ciliary muscles, causing blurred vision (**cycloplegia**)
   2. Anticholinergics block responses of the sphincter muscle in the ciliary body, producing **mydriasis** and **cycloplegia**
   3. Used preoperatively or for eye exams to produce **mydriasis**
   4. Contraindicated in clients with **glaucoma**

BOX 64–2. Mydriatic/Cycloplegic Eye Medications

Atropine sulfate (Isopto Atropine, Ocu-Tropine)
Scopolamine hydrobromide (Isopto Hyoscine)
Cyclopentolate HCl (Cyclogyl)
Homatropine hydrobromide (Isopto Homatropine)
Tropicamide (Mydriacyl)
Dipivefrin HCl (Propine)
Epinephrine HCl (Epifrin, Glaucon)
Epinephryl borate (Epinal, Eppy/N)
Phenylephrine HCl (AK-Dilate)

---

because of the risk of increased intraocular pressure
   5. **Mydriatics** are contraindicated in cardiac dysrhythmias and cerebral atherosclerosis and should be used with caution in the elderly and clients with prostatic hypertrophy, diabetes mellitus, or parkinsonism

B. Side Effects
   1. Tachycardia
   2. Photophobia
   3. Conjunctivitis
   4. Dermatitis

C. Atropine Toxicity
   1. Dry mouth
   2. Blurred vision
   3. Photophobia
   4. Tachycardia
   5. Fever
   6. Constipation
   7. Urinary retention
   8. Headache
   9. Brow pain
   10. Confusion
   11. Hallucinations
   12. Delirium
   13. Coma
   14. Worsening of narrow-angle **glaucoma**

D. Systemic Reactions of Anticholinergics
   1. Dry mouth
   2. Dry skin
   3. Fever
   4. Thirst
   5. Confusion
   6. Hyperactivity

E. Implementation
   1. Assess for allergic response
   2. Assess for risk of injury
   3. Assess for constipation and urinary retention
   4. Instruct the client that a burning sensation may occur on instillation
   5. Instruct the client not to drive or operate machinery for 24 hours after instillation of medication unless otherwise directed by the physician
   6. Instruct the client to wear sunglasses until the effects of the medication wear off
   7. Instruct the client to notify the physician if

blurring of vision, loss of sight, difficulty breathing, sweating, or flushing occurs

8. Instruct the client to report eye pain to the physician

III. Anti-Infective Eye Medications (Box 64–3)

A. Description: Kill or Inhibit the Growth of Bacteria, Fungi, and Viruses
B. Side Effects
   1. Superinfection
   2. Global irritation
C. Implementation
   1. Assess for risk of injury
   2. Instruct the client how to apply eye medications
   3. Instruct the client to continue treatment as prescribed
   4. Instruct the client to wash the hands thoroughly and frequently
   5. Advise the client that if improvement does not occur to notify the physician

IV. Anti-Inflammatory Eye Medications (Box 64–4)

A. Description
   1. Control inflammation, thereby reducing vision loss and scarring
   2. Used for uveitis, allergic conditions, and inflammation of the conjunctiva, cornea, and lids
B. Side Effects
   1. **Cataracts**
   2. Increased intraocular pressure
   3. Impaired healing
   4. Masking signs and symptoms of infection
C. Implementation
   1. Assess for risk of injury
   2. Instruct the client how to apply eye medications

BOX 64–3. Anti-Infective Eye Medications

ANTIBACTERIAL
Chloramphenicol (Chloromycetin, Chloroptic)
Ciprofloxacin HCl (Cipro)
Erythromycin (Ilotycin)
Gentamicin sulfate (Garamycin, Genoptic)
Norfloxacin (Chibroxin)
Tobramycin (Nebcin, Tobrex)
Silver nitrate 1%

ANTIFUNGAL
Natamycin (Natacyn ophthalmic)

ANTIVIRAL
Idoxuridine (Herplex Liquifilm)
Trifluridine (Viroptic)
Vidarabine (Vira-A ophthalmic)

BOX 64–4. Anti-Inflammatory Eye Medications

Dexamethasone (Maxidex)
Diclofenac sodium (Voltaren)
Flurbiprofen sodium (Ocufen)
Suprofen (Profenal)
Ketorolac tromethamine (Acular)
Medrysone (HMS, Liquifilm)
Prednisolone acetate (Predforte, Econopred)
Prednisolone sodium phosphate (AK-Pred, Inflamase)
Rimaxolone (Vexol)

---

3. Instruct the client to continue treatment as prescribed
4. Instruct the client to wash the hands thoroughly and frequently
5. Instruct the client that if improvement does not occur to notify the physician
6. Note that dexamethasone (Maxidex) should not be used for eye abrasions and wounds

V. Topical Anesthetics for the Eye (Box 64–5)

A. Description
   1. Produce corneal anesthesia
   2. Used for anesthesia for eye examinations, surgery, or to remove foreign bodies from the eye
B. Side Effects
   1. Temporary stinging or burning of the eye
   2. Temporary loss of corneal reflex
C. Implementation
   1. Assess for risk of injury
   2. Note that the medications should not be given to the client for home use and are not to be self-administered by the client
   3. Note that the blink reflex is temporarily lost and that the corneal epithelium needs to be protected
   4. Provide an eyepatch to protect the eye from injury until the corneal reflex returns

V. Eye Lubricants (Box 64–6)

A. Description
   1. Replace tears or add moisture to the eyes
   2. Moisten contact lenses or an artificial eye
   3. Protect the eyes during surgery or diagnostic procedures
   4. Used for keratitis, during anesthesia, or in a disorder that results in unconsciousness or decreased blinking

---

BOX 64–5. Topical Anesthetics for the Eye

Proparacaine HCl (Ophthaine, Ophthetic)
Tetracaine hydrochloride (Pontocaine)

BOX 64–6. Eye Lubricants

Hydroxypropyl methylcellulose (Lacril,
Isopto Plain)
Petroleum-based ointment (Artificial tears,
Liquifilm Tears)

B. Side Effects
   1. Burning on instillation
   2. Discomfort or pain on instillation
C. Implementation
   1. Inform the client that burning may occur on instillation
   2. Be alert to allergic responses to the preservatives in the lubricants

VII. Miotics (Box 64–7)

A. Description
   1. Reduce intraocular pressure by constricting the pupil and contracting the ciliary muscle, thereby increasing the blood flow to the retina and decreasing retinal damage and loss of vision
   2. Open the anterior chamber angle and increase the outflow of aqueous humor
   3. Miotic cholinergic medications reduce intraocular pressure by mimicking the action of acetylcholine
   4. Miotic acetylcholinesterase inhibitors reduce intraocular pressure by inhibiting the action of cholinesterase
   5. Used for chronic open-angle **glaucoma** or acute and chronic closed-angle **glaucoma**
   6. Used to achieve **miosis** during eye surgery
   7. Contraindicated in clients with **retinal detachment,** adhesions between the iris and lens, or in inflammatory diseases
   8. Use with caution in clients with asthma, hypertension, corneal abrasion, hyperthyroidism, coronary vascular disease, urinary tract obstruction, gastrointestinal (GI) obstruction, ulcer disease, parkinsonism, and bradycardia

---

BOX 64–7. Miotics

CHOLINERGICS

Acetylcholine chloride (Miochol)
Carbachol (Miostat)
Pilocarpine HCl (Isopto Carpine)
Pilocarpine nitrate (Ocusert Pilo-20, Pilo-40)
Echothiophate iodide (Phospholine Iodide)

CHOLINESTERASE MEDICATIONS

Physostigmine salicylate (Isopto Eserine)
Demecarium bromide (Humorsol)
Isoflurophate (Floropryl)

B. Side Effects
   1. Headache
   2. Eye pain
   3. Decreased vision in poor light
   4. **Myopia**
   5. Local irritation
   6. Systemic effects
      a. Flushing
      b. Diaphoresis
      c. GI upset
      d. Diarrhea
      e. Frequent urination
      f. Increased salivation
      g. Muscle weakness
      h. Respiratory difficulty
   7. Toxicity
      a. Vertigo
      b. Bradycardia
      c. Tremors
      d. Hypotension
      e. Syncope
      f. Cardiac dysrhythmias
      g. Seizures
C. Implementation
   1. Assess vital signs
   2. Assess for risk of injury
   3. Assess the client for the degree of diminished vision or blindness
   4. Monitor for side effects and toxic effects
   5. Monitor for postural hypotension and instruct the client to change positions slowly
   6. Assess breath sounds for rales and rhonchi as cholinergic medications can cause bronchospasms and increased bronchial secretions
   7. Maintain oral hygiene because of the increase in salivation
   8. Have atropine sulfate available as an antidote for pilocarpine
   9. Instruct the client or family regarding the correct administration of eye medications
   10. Instruct the client not to stop the medication suddenly
   11. Advise the client to avoid activities such as driving while vision is impaired
   12. Instruct clients with **glaucoma** to read labels on over-the-counter medications and to avoid atropine-like medications because atropine will increase intraocular pressure

VIII. Ocusert System

A. Description
   1. Ocusert is a thin eye wafer impregnated with time-release pilocarpine
   2. It is devised to overcome the frequent application of pilocarpine
   3. It is placed in the upper or lower cul-de-sac of the eye
   4. The pilocarpine is released over 1 week
   5. The disk is replaced every 7 days
   6. Drawbacks of its use include sudden leakage

of pilocarpine, migration of the system over the cornea, and unnoticed loss of the system

B. Implementation
1. Assess the client's ability to insert medication disk
2. Store the medication in the refrigerator
3. Instruct the client to discard damaged or contaminated disks
4. Inform the client that temporary stinging is expected but to notify the physician if blurred vision or brow pain occurs
5. Instruct the client to check for the presence of the disk in the conjunctival sac daily at bedtime and upon arising
6. Since vision may change in the first few hours after the eye system is inserted, instruct the client to replace the disk at bedtime

IX. Beta-Adrenergic-Blocking Eye Medications (Box 64–8)

A. Description
1. Reduce intraocular pressure by decreasing sympathetic impulses and decreasing aqueous humor production without affecting **accommodation** or pupil size
2. Used to treat chronic open-angle **glaucoma**
3. Contraindicated in clients with asthma because systemic absorption can cause increased airway resistance
4. Use with caution in clients receiving oral beta blockers
B. Side Effects
1. Ocular irritation
2. Visual disturbances
3. Bradycardia
4. Hypotension
5. Bronchospasm
C. Implementation
1. Monitor vital signs, especially blood pressure and pulse before administering medication
2. If the pulse is 60 or below or if the systolic blood pressure is below 90 mmHg, hold the medication and contact the physician
3. Monitor for shortness of breath
4. Assess for risk of injury
5. Monitor I&O
6. Instruct the client to notify the physician if shortness of breath occurs
7. Instruct the client not to discontinue the medication abruptly

---

BOX 64–8. Beta-Adrenergic-Blocking Eye Medications

Betaxolol HCl (Betoptic)
Levobunolol HCl (Betagan Liquifilm)
Timolol maleate (Timoptic)

BOX 64–9. Carbonic Anhydrase Inhibitors: Eye Medications

Acetazolamide (Diamox)
Dichlorophenamide (Daranide)
Dorzolamide (Trusopt)
Methazolamide (Neptazane)

---

8. Instruct the client to change positions slowly to avoid orthostatic hypotension
9. Instruct the client to avoid hazardous activities
10. Instruct the client to avoid over-the-counter medications without the physician's approval

X. Carbonic Anhydrase Inhibitors (Box 64–9)

A. Description
1. Interfere with the production of carbonic acid, which leads to decreased aqueous humor formation and decreased intraocular pressure
2. Used for long-term treatment of open-angle **glaucoma**
3. Contraindicated in clients allergic to sulfonamides
B. Side Effects
1. Appetite loss
2. GI upset
3. Paresthesias in the fingers, toes, and face
4. Polyuria
5. Hypokalemia
6. Renal calculi
7. Photosensitivity
8. Lethargy
9. Drowsiness
10. Depression
C. Implementation
1. Monitor vital signs
2. Assess visual acuity
3. Assess for risk of injury
4. Monitor I&O
5. Monitor weight
6. Maintain oral hygiene
7. Monitor for side effects such as lethargy, anorexia, drowsiness, polyuria, nausea, and vomiting
8. Monitor electrolytes for hypokalemia
9. Increase fluid intake unless contraindicated
10. Advise the client to avoid prolonged exposure to sunlight
11. Encourage the use of artificial tears for dry eyes
12. Instruct the client not to discontinue the medication abruptly
13. Instruct the client to avoid hazardous activities while vision is impaired

---

BOX 64–10. Osmotic Medications for the Eye

Glycerin	Mannitol (Osmitrol)
Isosorbide (Ismotic)	Urea (Ureaphil)

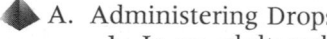

XI. Osmotic Medications (Box 64–10)

A. Description
  1. Lower intraocular pressure
  2. Used in emergency treatment of acute closed-angle **glaucoma**
  3. Used preoperatively and postoperatively to decrease vitreous humor volume
B. Side Effects
  1. Headache
  2. Nausea
  3. Vomiting
  4. Diarrhea
  5. Disorientation
  6. Electrolyte imbalances
C. Implementation
  1. Assess vital signs
  2. Assess visual acuity
  3. Assess for risk for injury
  4. Monitor I&O
  5. Monitor weight
  6. Monitor for electrolyte imbalances
  7. Increase fluid intake unless contraindicated
  8. Monitor for changes in level of orientation

XII. Otic Medication Administration (Box 64–11)

A. Administering Drops
  1. In an adult, pull the auricle up and back to straighten the external canal to instill ear drops
  2. Pull the auricle down and back for infants and children younger than 3 years of age
  3. Pull the auricle up and back for older children
B. Irrigation of the Ear
  1. Irrigation of the ear needs to be prescribed by the physician
  2. Ensure that there is direct visualization of the tympanic membrane
  3. Warm irrigating solution to 100°F because solutions that are not close to the client's body temperature will cause ear injury, nausea, and vertigo
  4. Irrigation must be done gently to avoid damage to the eardrum
  5. When irrigating, do not direct irrigation solution directly toward the eardrum
  6. If a perforation of the eardrum is suspected, irrigation is not done

XIII. Anti-Infective Ear Medications (Box 64–12)

A. Description
  1. Kill or inhibits growth of bacteria
  2. Used for otitis media or otitis externa
  3. Contraindicated if a prior hypersensitivity exists
B. Side Effects: Overgrowth of Nonsusceptible Organisms
C. Implementation
  1. Obtain vital signs
  2. Assess for allergies
  3. Assess pain
  4. Monitor for nephrotoxicity
  5. Instruct client to report dizziness, fatigue, fever, or sore throat, which may be indicative of a superimposed infection
  6. Instruct the client to complete the entire course of the medication
  7. Instruct the client to keep the ear canals dry

BOX 64–11. Medications That Affect Hearing Loss

ANTIBIOTICS

Amikacin (Amikin)
Chloramphenicol (Chloromycetin, Chloroptic, Ophthoclor)
Erythromycin (E-Mycin, ERYC, Ery-Tab, PCE Dispertabs, Ilotycin)
Gentamicin (Garamycin)
Streptomycin sulfate (Streptomycin)
Tobramycin sulfate (Nebcin)
Vancomycin (Vancocin)

DIURETICS

Acetazolamide (Diamox)
Furosemide (Lasix)
Ethacrynic acid (Edecrin)

OTHERS

Cisplatin (Platinol, Platinol-AQ)
Nitrogen mustard
Quinine (Quinamm)
Quinidine (Cardioquin, Quinaglute, Quinidex)

BOX 64–12. Anti-Infective Ear Medications

Amoxicillin (Amoxil)
Ampicillin trihydrate (Polycillin)
Cefaclor (Ceclor)
Clindamycin HCl (Cleocin)
Trimethoprim (TMP) and sulfamethoxazole (SMZ) (Bactrim, Cotrim, and Septra)
Erythromycin (Ilotycin, E-Mycin)
Penicillin V potassium (Pen-V)
Loracarbef (Lorabid)
Clarithromycin (Biaxin)
Chloramphenicol (Chloromycetin Otic)
Polymyxin B sulfate (Aerosporin)
Tetracycline HCl (Achromycin)
Acetic acid and aluminum acetate (Otic Domeboro)

XIV. Antihistamines and Decongestants
(Box 64–13)

A. Description
  1. Produce vasoconstriction
  2. Stimulate the receptors of the respiratory mucosa
  3. Reduce respiratory tissue hyperemia and edema to open obstructed eustachian tubes
  4. Used for acute otitis media
B. Side Effects
  1. Drowsiness
  2. Blurred vision
  3. Dry mucous membranes
C. Implementation
  1. Inform the client that drowsiness, blurred vision, and a dry mouth may occur
  2. Instruct the client to increase fluid intake unless contraindicated and to suck on hard candy to alleviate the dry mouth
  3. Instruct the client to avoid hazardous activities if drowsiness occurs

XV. Local Anesthetics

A. Description
  1. Block nerve conduction at or near the application site to control pain
  2. Used for pain associated with ear infections
B. Medication: Benzocaine (Americaine Otic; Tympagesic)
C. Side Effects
  1. Allergic reaction
  2. Irritation
D. Implementation
  1. Monitor for effectiveness if used for pain relief
  2. Assess for irritation or allergic reaction

XVI. Ceruminolytic Medications (Box 64–14)

A. Description
  1. Emulsify and loosen cerumen deposits
  2. Used to loosen and remove impacted wax from the ear canal
B. Side Effects
  1. Irritation
  2. Redness or swelling of the ear canal
C. Implementation

BOX 64–13. Antihistamines and Decongestants

Triprolidine and pseudoephedrine (Actifed)
Naphazoline HCl (Allerest, Albalon)
Chlorpheniramine (Chlor-Trimeton, Teldrin)
Brompheniramine (Bromphen, Dimetane)
Terfenadine (Seldane)
Clemastine (Tavist)
Cetirizine (Zyrtec)
Astemizole (Hismanal)

BOX 64–14. Ceruminolytic Medications

Carbamide peroxide (Debrox)
Boric acid (Ear-Dry)
Trolamine polypeptide oleate-condensate (Cerumenex)

---

  1. Instruct the client not to use drops more often than prescribed
  2. Moisten a cotton plug with medication before insertion
  3. Keep the container tightly closed and away from moisture
  4. Avoid touching the ear with the dropper
  5. Thirty minutes after instillation, irrigate the ear as prescribed gently with warm water using a soft rubber bulb ear syringe
  6. Irrigation may be done with hydrogen peroxide solution as prescribed, to flush cerumen deposits out of the ear canal
  7. For a chronic cerumen impaction, 1 to 2 drops of mineral oil will soften the wax
  8. Instruct the client to notify the physician if redness, pain, or swelling persists

PRACTICE QUESTIONS

1. In preparation for cataract surgery, the nurse is to administer cyclopentolate HCl (Cyclogyl) eye drops. The purpose of this medication is to:
   1 Provide lubrication to the operative eye
   2 Produce miosis of the operative eye
   3 Dilate the pupil of the operative eye
   4 Constrict the pupil of the operative eye

2. The home health nurse visits the client and instructs the client on the administration of the prescribed eye drops. Which of the following statements by the client indicates a need for further education?
   1 "I can tilt my head back, pull down on the lower lid, and place the drop in the lower lid."
   2 "I can lie down, pull down on the lower lid, and place the drop in the lower lid."
   3 "I can lie down, pull up on the upper lid, and place the drop in the lower lid."
   4 "I can lie on my side opposite to the eye I am going to place the drop. Put the drop in the corner of the lid nearest my nose, then slowly turn to my other side while blinking."

3. The most appropriate method to administer ear drops to the infant is to:
   1 Pull up and back on the auricle and direct the solution onto the eardrum
   2 Pull down and back on the auricle and direct the solution onto the eardrum
   3 Pull the ear down and back and direct the solution toward the wall of the canal
   4 Pull up and back on the earlobe and direct the solution toward the wall of the canal

4. To minimize the systemic effects that eye drops can produce, the nurse should instruct the client to:
   1 Eat before instilling the drops
   2 Swallow several times after instilling the drops
   3 Blink vigorously to encourage tearing after instilling the drops
   4 Occlude the nasolacrimal duct with a finger for several minutes after instilling the drops

5. The client is receiving both epinephrine HCl (Epifrin, Glaucon) and timolol maleate (Timoptic) eye drops. When instructing the client on the administration of the eye drops the nurse instructs the client to:
   1 Administer the epinephrine HCl first, followed by the timolol maleate
   2 Administer the timolol maleate first, followed by the epinephrine HCl
   3 Administer epinephrine HCl in the morning and the timolol maleate in the evening
   4 Wait 3 minutes between the instillation of each medication

6. The nurse is caring for a client with glaucoma. Which of the following medications, if prescribed for the client, does the nurse question?
   1 Carbachol (Miostat)
   2 Pilocarpine HCl (Isopto Carpine)
   3 Pilocarpine nitrate (Ocusert Pilo-20, Ocusert Pilo-40)
   4 Atropine sulfate (Isopto Atropine, Ocu-tropine)

7. A miotic medication has been prescribed for the client with glaucoma. The client asks the nurse about the purpose of the medication. Which of the following statements indicates accurate information regarding the medication?
   1 "The medication will lower the pressure in your eye and increase the blood flow to the retina."
   2 "The medication will help to dilate the eye to prevent pressure from occurring."
   3 "The medication will relax the muscles of the eyes and prevent blurred vision."
   4 "The medication will help to block the responses that are sent to the muscles in the eye."

8. Pilocarpine HCl (Isopto Carpine) is prescribed for the client with glaucoma. Which of the following medications does the nurse plan to have available in the event of systemic toxicity?
   1 Naloxone HCl (Narcan)
   2 Pindolol (Visken)
   3 Atropine sulfate
   4 Mesoridazine besylate (Serentil)

9. Betaxolol HCl (Betoptic) eye drops have been prescribed for the client with glaucoma. The home health nurse visits the client. Which of the following nursing actions is most appropriate related to monitoring for the side effects of this medication?
   1 Monitor temperature
   2 Monitor blood pressure
   3 Assess glucose level
   4 Assess peripheral pulses

10. The nurse prepares the client for an ear irrigation as prescribed by the physician. In performing the procedure, which of the following actions will the nurse take?
    1 Position the client to turn his or her head so that the ear to be irrigated is facing upward
    2 Warm the irrigating solution to 100°F
    3 Direct a slow steady stream of irrigation solution toward the eardrum
    4 Position the client with the affected side up following the irrigation

ANSWERS

1. **3**

Rationale: Cyclopentolate is a rapidly acting mydriatic and cycloplegic medication. It is effective in 25 to 75 minutes, and accommodation returns in 6 to 24 hours. Cyclopentolate is used for preoperative mydriasis.

Test-Taking Strategy: Use the process of elimination to answer the question. Options 2 and 4 present similar information. Miosis refers to a constricted pupil. Note that the question identifies a client being prepared for eye surgery. The pupil needs to be dilated for the surgical procedure. Review the action and purpose of this medication now if you had difficulty with this question!

Level of Cognitive Ability: Analysis
Phase of Nursing Process: Analysis
Client Needs: Physiological Integrity
Content Area: Pharmacology

Reference
Clark, J., Queener, S., & Karb, V. (1997). *Pharmacologic basis of nursing practice* (5th ed.). St. Louis: Mosby–Year Book. p. 833.

2. **3**

Rationale: The client can either lie down or sit with the head tilted back. The lower lid should be pulled downward with the thumb or fingers. The client holds the bottle like a pencil, with the tip downward, and squeezes the bottle gently allowing one drop to fall into the sac. The client gently closes the eye. An alternative method for clients who blink very easily is to place the client in the supine position with the head turned to one side. The eye to receive the eye drops should be uppermost. With the eye closed, drop the prescribed dose on the inner canthus of the eye. Have the client turn from side to midline and to the other side while blinking. The eye drops will move via gravity and surface tension into the conjunctival sac.

Test-Taking Strategy: Read the stem of the question carefully. The question asks for the option that indicates a need for further education. Use the process of elimination. Knowing that the client places drops into the eye by pulling down on the lower lid will direct you to the correct option for this question as stated. Review the procedure for the administration of eye medications now if you had difficulty with this question!

Level of Cognitive Ability: Analysis
Phase of Nursing Process: Evaluation
Client Needs: Health Promotion and Maintenance
Content Area: Pharmacology

Reference
Clark, J., Queener, S., & Karb, V. (1997). *Pharmacologic basis of nursing practice* (5th ed.). St. Louis: Mosby–Year Book. pp. 70–71.

3. 3

Rationale: In a child younger than 3 years, pull the ear down and straight back. The client should be turned on the side with the affected ear uppermost. With the nondominant hand pull down and back on the earlobe. Rest the wrist of the dominant hand on client's head. Administer the medication by aiming it at the wall of the canal rather than directly onto the eardrum. The client should remain with the affected ear uppermost for 10 to 15 minutes to retain the solution. In the adult or a child older than 3 years, pull up and back on the auricle to straighten the auditory canal.

Test-Taking Strategy: Eliminate options 1 and 2 because you would not direct ear solution directly onto the eardrum. Remembering that in a child younger than 3 years, pulling the ear down and straight back is the correct procedure for administering ear medications. Review the procedure for the administration of ear medications now if you had difficulty with this question!

Level of Cognitive Ability: Application
Phase of Nursing Process: Implementation
Client Needs: Physiological Integrity
Content Area: Pharmacology

Reference
Clark, J., Queener, S., & Karb, V. (1997). *Pharmacologic basis of nursing practice* (5th ed.). St. Louis: Mosby–Year Book. p. 71.

4. 4

Rationale: Applying pressure on the nasolacrimal duct prevents systemic absorption for the medication.

Test-Taking Strategy: Use the process of elimination to answer the question. Eating and swallowing are similar options and are not related to the systemic absorption of an eye medication. Blinking vigorously to produce tearing may result in the loss of the administered medication.

Level of Cognitive Ability: Application
Phase of Nursing Process: Implementation
Client Needs: Physiological Integrity
Content Area: Pharmacology

Reference
Clark, J., Queener, S., & Karb, V. (1997). *Pharmacologic basis of nursing practice* (5th ed.). St. Louis: Mosby–Year Book. p. 835.

5. 4

Rationale: When two or more drugs are to be administered, the client should wait 3 minutes between instillations.

Test-Taking Strategy: Knowledge regarding the administration of more than one eye medication is helpful to answer this question. Read all of the options carefully. Note that option 4, the correct option, is different from the other options and provides specific information related to the question.

Level of Cognitive Ability: Application
Phase of Nursing Process: Implementation
Client Needs: Health Promotion and Maintenance
Content Area: Pharmacology

Reference
Clark, J., Queener, S., & Karb, V. (1997). *Pharmacologic basis of nursing practice* (5th ed.). St. Louis: Mosby–Year Book. p. 835.

6. 4

Rationale: Options 1, 2, and 3 are miotic agents used in the treatment of glaucoma. Option 4, atropine sulfate, is a mydriatic and cycloplegic medication and its use is contraindicated in clients with glaucoma. Mydriatic medications dilate the pupil and can cause an increase in intraocular eye pressure.

Test-Taking Strategy: Knowledge regarding the classifications of the medications identified in the options will assist you in answering the question. Remember that my "d"riatics "d"ilate, and these medications are contraindicated in glaucoma.

Level of Cognitive Ability: Analysis
Phase of Nursing Process: Implementation
Client Needs: Safe, Effective Care Environment
Content Area: Pharmacology

Reference
Kee, J., & Hayes, E. (1997). *Pharmacology: A nursing process approach* (2nd ed.). Philadelphia: W. B. Saunders. pp. 299–300.

7. 1

Rationale: Miotics are used to lower the intraocular pressure, thereby increasing blood flow to the retina and decreasing retinal damage and loss of vision. Miotics cause a contraction of the ciliary muscle and a widening of trabecular meshwork.

Test-Taking Strategy: Knowledge regarding the action of miotics is required to answer this question. Read the question carefully and note that the question states that the client has glaucoma. This should provide you with the clue to direct you to the correct option. Prevention of increased intraocular pressure is the goal in clients with glaucoma. Options 2, 3, and 4 all describe actions related to mydriatic medications, which primarily dilate the pupils and relax the ciliary muscles.

Level of Cognitive Ability: Application
Phase of Nursing Process: Implementation
Client Needs: Health Promotion and Maintenance
Content Area: Pharmacology

Reference
Kee, J., & Hayes, E. (1997). *Pharmacology: A nursing process approach* (2nd ed.). Philadelphia: W. B. Saunders. p. 584.

8. 3

Rationale: Systemic absorption of pilocarpine HCl can produce toxicity and includes manifestations of vertigo, bradycardia, tremors, hypotension, syncope, cardiac dysrhythmias, and seizures. Atropine sulfate must be available in the event of systemic toxicity. Mesoridazine besylate is an antipsychotic medication. Pindolol is a beta-adrenergic blocker. Naloxone HCl is an opioid antagonist used to reverse narcotic-induced respiratory depression.

Test-Taking Strategy: Knowledge regarding antidotes related to various medications is required to answer this question. Knowledge related to the classifications of the medications presented in the options will assist in directing you to the correct option. Atropine sulfate is the antidote for systemic reactions that occur with pilocarpine. Take time now to review antidotes if you had difficulty with this question!

Level of Cognitive Ability: Analysis
Phase of Nursing Process: Planning
Client Needs: Physiological Integrity
Content Area: Pharmacology

Reference
Kee, J., & Hayes, E. (1997). *Pharmacology: A nursing process approach* (2nd ed.). Philadelphia: W. B. Saunders. p. 587.

9. **2**

Rationale: Hypotension manifested as dizziness, nausea, diaphoresis, headache, fatigue, constipation, and diarrhea are systemic effects of the medication. Nursing interventions include monitoring the blood pressure for hypotension and assessing the pulse for strength, weakness, irregular rate, and bradycardia. The nurse also monitors bowel activity and assesses for evidence of congestive heart failure (CHF) as manifested by dizziness, night cough, peripheral edema, and distended neck veins. Monitoring I&O and for an increase in weight and a decrease in urine output may also be indicative of CHF. This medication is an antiglaucoma medication and a beta-adrenergic blocker.

Test-Taking Strategy: Knowledge regarding the systemic effects related to this medication is required to answer the question. Read the question carefully and use the process of elimination in selecting the correct option. Remember the ABCs and this will direct you to option 2, circulation. Although option 4, peripheral pulses, is also related to circulation monitoring, the blood pressure is the more global

answer. Take time now to review the side effects of this medication if you had difficulty with this question!

Level of Cognitive Ability: Application
Phase of Nursing Process: Assessment
Client Needs: Physiological Integrity
Content Area: Pharmacology

Reference
Hodgson, B., & Kizior, R. (1999). *Saunders nursing drug handbook 1999.* Philadelphia: W. B. Saunders. pp. 109–111.

10. **2**

Rationale: Irrigation solutions that are not close to the client's body temperature can be uncomfortable and may cause injury, nausea, and vertigo. Position the client so that the ear to be irrigated is facing downward as this allows gravity to assist in the removal of the ear wax and solution. Following the irrigation, the client is to lie on the affected side for a period of time to finish the drainage of the irrigating solution. A slow, steady stream of solution should be directed toward the upper wall of the ear canal and not toward the tympanic membrane. Too much force could cause the tympanic membrane to rupture.

Test-Taking Strategy: Knowledge regarding the procedure for ear irrigation is necessary to answer the question. Use the process of elimination. Read each option carefully and remember that the nurse's concern is to prevent damage to the eardrum. Therefore, option 3 can be eliminated. Additionally, remember that the client should be positioned with the affected side downward to allow drainage of the irrigation solution.

Level of Cognitive Ability: Application
Phase of Nursing Process: Implementation
Client Needs: Safe, Effective Care Environment
Content Area: Pharmacology

Reference
Lammon, C., B., Foote, A. W., Leli, P. G., et al. (1995). *Clinical nursing skills.* Philadelphia: W. B. Saunders. pp. 313–314.

BIBLIOGRAPHY

Black, J. M., & Matassarin-Jacobs, E. (1997). *Medical-surgical nursing: Clinical management for continuity of care* (5th ed.). Philadelphia: W. B. Saunders.

Clark, J., Queener, S., & Karb, V. (1997). *Pharmacologic basis of nursing practice* (5th ed.). St. Louis: Mosby–Year Book.

Hodgson, B., & Kizior, R. (1999). *Saunders nursing drug handbook 1999.* Philadelphia: W. B. Saunders.

Kee, J., & Hayes, E. (1997). *Pharmacology: A nursing process approach* (2nd ed.). Philadelphia: W. B. Saunders.

Kuhn, M. (1998). *Pharmacotherapeutics: A nursing process approach* (4th ed.). Philadelphia: F. A. Davis.

Lammon, C., B., Foote, A. W., Leli, P. G., et al. (1995). *Clinical nursing skills.* Philadelphia: W. B. Saunders.

Lehne, R. (1998). *Pharmacology for nursing care* (3rd ed.). Philadelphia: W. B. Saunders.

UNIT XVII

The Adult Client with a Neurological Disorder

PYRAMID TERMS

Agnosia—The inability to use an object correctly.

Apraxia—The inability to carry out a purposeful activity.

Autonomic Dysreflexia—Also known as hyper-reflexia. Caused by visceral distention from a distended bladder or impacted rectum. A neurological emergency and must be treated immediately to prevent a hypertensive stroke. It occurs after the period of spinal shock is complete. Occurs with lesions above T6.

Babinski's Reflex—Indicates a disruption of the pyramidal tract. Dorsiflexion of the ankle and great toe with fanning of the other toes.

Brudzinski's Sign—Flexion of the head causes flexion of both thighs at the hips and knee flexion. Indicates meningeal irritation.

Decerebrate Posturing—Client stiffly extends one or both arms and possibly the legs. Indicates a brain stem lesion.

Decorticate Posturing—Client flexes one or both arms on the chest and may stiffly extend the legs. Indicates a nonfunctioning cortex.

Flaccid Posturing—Client displays no motor response in any extremity.

Glasgow Coma Scale—A method of assessing a client's neurological condition. A scoring system based on a scale of 1 to 15 points. A score below 8 indicates that coma is present. Eye-opening is the most important indicator.

Halo Traction—Pins or screws are inserted into the client's skull, and a circular fixation device and halo jacket or cast is applied.

Hemianopia—Blindness in half the visual field.

Homonymous Hemianopia—Blindness in the same visual field of both eyes.

Increased Intracranial Pressure—An increase in intracranial pressure caused by trauma, hemorrhage, growths or tumors, hydrocephalus, edema, or inflammation. Can impede circulation to the brain and absorption of cerebrospinal fluid (CSF), and can affect the functioning of nerve cells and lead to brain stem compression and death.

Kernig's Sign—Flex thigh and knee to right angles and, when they are extended, spasm of hamstring and pain occur. Indicates meningeal irritation.

Skull Tongs—Skull tongs are inserted into the outer aspect of the client's skull, just above the ears, and traction is applied.

Spinal Shock—Also known as neurogenic shock. A sudden depression of reflex activity in the spinal cord below the level of injury (areflexia). Occurs within the first hour of injury and can last days to months. The muscles become completely paralyzed and flaccid, and reflexes are absent.

Tensilon Test—Test is done to diagnose myasthenia gravis and to differentiate between myasthenic crisis and cholinergic crisis.

Unconscious Client—A state of depressed cerebral functioning with unresponsiveness to sensory and motor function. Some of the causes include head trauma, cerebral toxins, shock, hemorrhage, tumor, or infections.

PYRAMID TO SUCCESS

Pyramid points related to neurological disorders focus on monitoring for **increased intracranial pressure,** assessing level of consciousness, positioning clients, head injuries, spinal cord injuries, **spinal shock, autonomic dysreflexia,** implementation during a seizure, the cerebrovascular-accident (CVA) client, Parkinson's disease, myasthenia gravis, and the **Tensilon test.** Altered body image and psychosocial issues that occur as a result of the neurological disorder are also a focus of the Pyramid to Success.

NURSING PROCESS

ASSESSMENT

Airway
Level of consciousness
Vital signs
Respirations
Headache
Orientation to person, place, time
Pupils
Changes in personality
Numbness, weakness, dizziness, fainting, loss of consciousness
Speech and/or visual disturbance
Confusion

Alterations in memory, thinking, and judgment
Sensory and motor function
Pain
Reflexes
Posturing
Response to stimuli, both verbal and tactile
Response to painful stimuli: purposeful, nonpurposeful, posturing, or no response
Nutritional status
Bowel and bladder function
Psychosocial issues

ANALYSIS: Ineffective Airway Clearance

PLANNING	IMPLEMENTATION	EVALUATION
The client will maintain a respiratory rate of between 16 and 24 respirations per minute. The client performs coughing and deep breathing exercises and uses an incentive spirometry.	Assess respiratory status. Assess lung sounds. Encourage coughing and deep-breathing exercises. Instruct client on the use of an incentive spirometer.	Airway remains patent. Lungs remain clear and free of secretions. The client will not experience respiratory complications.

ANALYSIS: Altered Tissue Perfusion

PLANNING	IMPLEMENTATION	EVALUATION
The client remains oriented. The client will exhibit no further deterioration in neurological status.	Monitor vital signs. Monitor neurological status. Monitor level of consciousness. Assess sensory and motor abilities. Assess color, motion, and sensation in affected area. Monitor for adequate and palpable pulses. Monitor for signs of increased intracranial pressure. Monitor for signs of autonomic dysreflexia and spinal shock. Notify physician of changes in neurological status.	Vital signs and neurological status remain stable. Adequate tissue perfusion is maintained.

ANALYSIS: Alteration in Nutrition

PLANNING	IMPLEMENTATION	EVALUATION
The client drinks and eats adequate amounts of fluid and food.	Weigh client. Encourage foods and fluids. Monitor intake and output (I&O). Instruct client regarding the need for adequate fluids and fiber in the diet.	Nutritional status is adequate.

ANALYSIS: Potential for Infection

PLANNING	IMPLEMENTATION	EVALUATION
Temperature remains within normal limits. The client's surgical wound demonstrates signs of the healing process.	Monitor temperature. Monitor wound status. Change dressing as prescribed.	The client remains free of infection. Wound remains free of infection.

ANALYSIS: Alteration in Skin Integrity

PLANNING	IMPLEMENTATION	EVALUATION
Client remains free of skin breakdown as a result of immobility.	Turn and reposition client. Monitor skin integrity. Instruct client in the importance of turning and repositioning.	The client's skin remains intact.

ANALYSIS: Alteration in Comfort

PLANNING	IMPLEMENTATION	EVALUATION
The client reports reasonable comfort.	Assist client to identify comfort measures. Administer pain measures. Note and document effectiveness of pain measures. Instruct client regarding administration of prescribed medications and measures to reduce pain.	Client remains comfortable and reasonably free of pain.

ANALYSIS: Alteration in Mobility

PLANNING	IMPLEMENTATION	EVALUATION
The client learns to perform activities of daily living as independently as possible. The client verbalizes acceptance of mobility limitations.	Turn and reposition client. Assist client with mobility as necessary. Encourage out of bed activities as prescribed. Instruct client in the use of assistive devices.	The client complies with exercise programs and prescribed treatments. Client demonstrates correct use of assistive devices.

ANALYSIS: Self-Care Deficit

PLANNING	IMPLEMENTATION	EVALUATION
The client requests assistance with mobilization activities, as needed. The client participates in care.	Assess client's ability to perform self-care activities. Assist client in care, promoting independence as much as possible.	Client participates in self-care to optimal level. Client performs independent self-care activities to optimal level of functioning.

ANALYSIS: Alteration in Elimination Patterns

PLANNING	IMPLEMENTATION	EVALUATION
The client maintains controlled continence.	Assess bowel and bladder function. Assess bowel sounds. Monitor urinary output. Encourage optimal activity to stimulate bowel elimination. Initiate a bowel or bladder control program as appropriate.	Client remains free of elimination alterations.

ANALYSIS: Potential for Injury

PLANNING	IMPLEMENTATION	EVALUATION
The client avoids physical injury. The client achieves optimal level of independence without injury.	Assess client's motor and sensory deficit to determine safety needs. Provide appropriate assistive devices to prevent injury. Keep environment free of obstructions. Document client's safe performance of activities.	Client remains free of injury.

ANALYSIS: Ineffective Individual Coping

PLANNING	IMPLEMENTATION	EVALUATION
The client participates actively in the decision-making process.	Encourage client to make own decisions. Assist client to recognize own strengths and available support systems.	Client utilizes available support systems.

ANALYSIS: Body Image Disturbances

PLANNING	IMPLEMENTATION	EVALUATION
The client shares grief and loss with a significant person. The client verbalizes feelings about the physical disabilities.	Encourage client to express grief. Encourage client to verbalize grief with significant other. Mobilize support resources.	The client begins to cope with changes caused by the disability. Client verbalizes adjustment or adaptation to the disability.

CLIENT NEEDS

SAFE, EFFECTIVE CARE ENVIRONMENT

Advance directives
Advocacy
Client rights
Confidentiality
Informed consent for invasive procedures
Accident prevention related to neurological deficits
Asepsis with procedures and treatments
Standard precautions
Consultation and referrals

HEALTH PROMOTION AND MAINTENANCE

Expected body image changes resulting from neurological deficits
Prevention and early detection of health problems associated with neurological deficits
Neurological assessment
Home care instructions regarding care related to neurological disorder
Reinforcement regarding the importance of prescribed therapy

PSYCHOSOCIAL INTEGRITY

The ability to cope with feelings of isolation and loss of independence
Mobilizing coping mechanisms
Sensory and perceptual alterations

Grief and loss
Cultural, religious, and spiritual influences
Support systems and utilization of community resources
Body image changes

PHYSIOLOGICAL INTEGRITY

Use of assistive devices for mobility
Promoting normal elimination patterns
Measures to promote comfort
Promoting self-care measures
Pharmacological medications: actions, agents, side effects, and adverse effects
Complications related to procedures
Emergency care
Increased intracranial pressure
Assessing level of consciousness
Positioning clients
Head injuries
Spinal cord injuries
Spinal shock
Autonomic dysreflexia
Implementation during a seizure
The CVA client
Parkinson's disease
Myasthenia gravis
Tensilon test

REFERENCES

Black, J., & Matassarin-Jacobs, E. (1997). *Medical-surgical nursing: Clinical management for continuity of care* (5th ed.). Philadelphia: W. B. Saunders.

Luckmann, J. (1997). *Saunders manual of nursing care.* Philadelphia, W. B. Saunders.

National Council of State Boards of Nursing (eds.) (1997). *Test for the National Council Licensure Examination for Registered Nurses.* Chicago: Author.

CHAPTER 65

Neurological System

. . . .

I. Anatomy and Physiology of the Brain and Spinal Cord

A. Cerebrum
   1. Consists of the right and left hemispheres
   2. Each hemisphere receives sensory information from the opposite side of the body and controls the skeletal muscles of the opposite side
   3. Governs sensory and motor activity
   4. Governs thought and learning
B. Cerebral cortex (Box 65–1)
   1. Outer gray layer
   2. Divided into four lobes
   3. Responsible for the conscious activities of the cerebrum
C. Basal ganglia
   1. Cell bodies in white matter
   2. Assist cerebral cortex in producing smooth voluntary movements
D. Diencephalon
   1. Thalamus
      a. Relays sensory impulses to the cortex
      b. Provides a thalamic pain gate
      c. Part of the reticular activating system
   2. Hypothalamus

a. Regulates autonomic responses of the sympathetic and parasympathetic nervous systems
      b. Regulates stress response, sleep, appetite, body temperature, fluid balance, and emotions
      c. Responsible for the production of hormones secreted by the pituitary gland and hypothalamus
E. Brain stem
   1. Midbrain
      a. Responsible for motor coordination
      b. Visual reflex and auditory relay centers
   2. Pons
      a. Contains respiratory centers
      b. Regulates breathing
   3. Medulla oblongata
      a. Contains all afferent and efferent tracts
      b. Contains cardiac, respiratory, vomiting, and vasomotor centers
      c. Controls heart rate, respiration, blood vessel diameter, sneezing, swallowing, vomiting, and coughing
F. Cerebellum
   1. Coordinates smooth muscle movement
   2. Coordinates posture, equilibrium, and muscle tone
G. Spinal cord
   1. Provides neuron and synapse networks to produce involuntary responses to sensory stimulation
   2. Allows for control of the number of pain impulses that pass through on their way to the brain
   3. Carries sensory information to, and motor information from, the brain
   4. Extends from the first cervical to the second lumbar vertebra
   5. Protected by the meninges, cerebrospinal fluid, and adipose tissue
   6. Horns
      a. Inner column of gray matter contains two anterior and two posterior horns
      b. Posterior horns connect with afferent (sensory) nerve fibers

---

BOX 65–1. Cerebral Cortex

FRONTAL LOBE
Broca's area for speech
Prefontal lobe controls morals, emotions, and judgments

PARIETAL LOBE
Interprets pain, touch temperature, and pressure

TEMPORAL LOBE
Auditory center
Wernicke's area for sensory and speech

OCCIPITAL LOBE
Visual area

c. Anterior horns contain efferent (motor) nerve fibers
7. Nerve tracts
    a. White matter contains the nerve tract
    b. Ascending tract (sensory pathway)
    c. Descending tract (motor pathway)
H. Meninges
    1. Dura mater is the tough and fibrous membrane
    2. Arachnoid membrane is the delicate membrane and contains subarachnoid fluid
    3. Pia mater is the vascular membrane
    4. Subarachnoid space is formed by the arachnoid membrane and the pia mater
I. Cerebrospinal fluid
    1. Secreted in the ventricles and circulates through the ventricles to the subarachnoid layer of the meninges where it is reabsorbed
    2. Circulates in the subarachnoid space
    3. Normal pressure is 50 to 175 mm H_2O
    4. Normal volume is 125 to 150 mL
    5. Acts as a protective cushion
    6. Aids in the exchange of nutrients and wastes
J. Ventricles
    1. Four ventricles
    2. Communicate between the subarachnoid space
    3. Produce and circulate cerebrospinal fluid
K. Blood supply
    1. Right and left internal carotids
    2. Right and left vertebral arteries
    3. These arteries supply the brain via an anastomosis at the base of the brain called the circle of Willis
L. Neurotransmitters
    1. Acetylcholine
    2. Norepinephrine
    3. Dopamine
    4. Serotonin
    5. Amino acids
    6. Polypeptides
M. Neurons
    1. The cell body
    2. Contains the axons and dendrites
    3. Neurons carrying impulses to the central nervous system (CNS) are called sensory neurons
    4. Neurons carrying impulses away from the central nervous system (CNS) are called motor neurons
    5. Synapse is the chemical transmission of impulses from one neuron to another
N. Axons and dendrites
    1. The axon conducts impulses from the cell body
    2. The dendrites receive stimuli from the body and transmit them to the axons
    3. Protected and insulated by Schwann's cells
    4. The Schwann's cell sheath is called the neurolemma

5. Neurons do not reproduce after the neonatal period
6. If an axon or dendrite is damaged, it will die and be slowly replaced only if the neurolemma is intact and the cell body has not died
O. Spinal nerves
    1. Thirty-one pairs of spinal nerves
    2. Mixed nerve fibers are formed by the joining of the anterior motor and posterior sensory roots
    3. Posterior roots contain afferent (sensory) nerve fibers
    4. Anterior roots contain efferent (motor) nerve fibers
P. Autonomic nervous system
    1. Sympathetic (adrenergic) fibers dilate pupils, increase heart rate and rhythm, contract blood vessels, and relax smooth muscles of the bronchi
    2. Parasympathetic (cholinergic) fibers produce the opposite effect

II. Diagnostic Tests

A. Skull and spinal x-ray
    1. Description
        a. X-rays of the skull reveal the size and shape of the skull bones, suture separation in infants, fractures or bony defects, erosion, or calcification
        b. Spinal x-rays identify fractures, dislocation, compression, curvature, erosion, narrowed spinal cord, and degenerative processes
    2. Implementation preprocedure
        a. Provide nursing support for the confused, combative, or ventilator-dependent client
        b. Maintain immobilization of the neck if a spinal fracture is suspected
        c. Remove metal items from body parts
        d. If the client has thick and heavy hair, this should be documented, as it may affect interpretation of the x-ray film
    3. Implementation postprocedure: maintain immobilization until results are known
B. CT (computed tomography) scan
    1. Description
        a. A type of brain scanning that may or may not require an injection of a dye
        b. Used to detect intracranial bleeding, space-occupying lesions, cerebral edema, infarctions, hydrocephalus, cerebral atrophy, and shifts of brain structures
    2. Implementation preprocedure
        a. Obtain a consent if a dye is used
        b. Assess for allergies to iodine, contrast dyes, or shellfish if a dye is used
        c. Instruct the client in the need to lie still and flat during the test
        d. Instruct the client to hold the breath when requested

e. Initiate an IV if prescribed
f. Remove objects from the head such as wigs, barrettes, earrings, and hairpins
g. Assess for claustrophobia
h. Inform the client of possible mechanical noises as the scanning occurs
i. Inform the client that there may be a hot, flushed sensation and a metallic taste in the mouth when the dye is injected
j. Note that some clients may be given the dye even if they report an allergy, and are pretreated with an antihistamine and corticosteroids prior to the injection, to reduce the severity of a reaction
   3. Implementation postprocedure
      a. Provide replacement fluids because diuresis from the dye is expected
      b. Monitor for allergic reaction to the dye
      c. Assess the dye injection site for bleeding or hematoma, and monitor extremity for color, warmth, and the presence of distal pulses

C. Magnetic resonance imaging (MRI)
   1. Description
      a. A noninvasive procedure that identifies types of tissues, tumors, and vascular abnormalities
      b. Similar to the CT scan but provides more detailed pictures and does not expose the client to ionizing radiation
   2. Implementation preprocedure
      a. Remove all metal objects from the client
      b. Determine if the client has a pacemaker, implanted defibrillator, or metal implants such as a hip prosthesis or vascular clips because these clients cannot have this test performed
      c. Remove IV fluid pumps during the test
      d. Provide precautions for the client with pulse oximetry because it can cause a burn during testing if coiled around the body or a body part
      e. Provide an assessment of the client with claustrophobia
      f. Administer medication as prescribed for the client with claustrophobia
      g. Determine if the use of a contrast agent is to be used and follow the prescription related to the administration of food, fluids, and medications
      h. Instruct clients that they will need to remain still during the procedure
   3. Implementation postprocedure
      a. Client may resume normal activities
      b. Expect diuresis if a contrast agent was used

D. Lumbar puncture
   1. Description
      a. Insertion of a spinal needle through L3–L4 interspace into the lumbar subarachnoid space to obtain cerebrospinal fluid (CSF), measure CSF

fluid or pressure, or to instill air, dye, or medications
      b. Contraindicated in clients with **increased intracranial pressure,** because the procedure will cause a rapid decrease in pressure within the CSF around the spinal cord, leading to brain herniation
   2. Implementation preprocedure
      a. Obtain an informed consent
      b. Have clients empty their bladders
   3. Implementation during the procedure
      a. Position the client in a lateral recumbent position and have the client draw knees up to the abdomen and chin onto the chest
      b. Assist with the collection of specimens (label the specimens in sequence)
      c. Maintain strict asepsis
   4. Implementation postprocedure
      a. Monitor vital signs and neurological signs
      b. Position the client flat as prescribed
      c. Force fluids
      d. Monitor I&O

E. Myelogram
   1. Description: injection of dye or air into a subarachnoid space to detect abnormalities of the spinal cord and vertebrae
   2. Implementation preprocedure
      a. Obtain informed consent
      b. Provide hydration for at least 12 hours before the test
      c. Assess for allergies to iodine
      d. If the client is taking a phenothiazine, hold the medication because this medication lowers the seizure threshold
      e. Premedicate for sedation as prescribed
   3. Implementation postprocedure
      a. Vital signs and neurological assessment frequently as prescribed
      b. If a water-based dye is used, elevate the head 15 to 30 degrees for 8 hours as prescribed
      c. If an oil-based dye is used, keep the client flat 6 to 8 hours as prescribed
      d. If air is used, keep the head lower than the trunk
      e. Administer analgesics for headache or backache as prescribed
      f. Force fluids
      g. Monitor I&O
      h. Assess for bladder distention and voiding

F. Cerebral angiography
   1. Description: injection of a contrast through the femoral artery into the carotid arteries to visualize the cerebral arteries and assess for lesions
   2. Implementation preprocedure
      a. Obtain informed consent
      b. Assess client's allergies to iodine and shellfish
      c. Encourage hydration for 2 days before the test

    d. NPO 4 to 6 hours prior to the test as prescribed

    e. Obtain a baseline neurological assessment

    f. Mark the peripheral pulses

    g. Remove metal items from the hair

    h. Administer premedication as prescribed

  3. Implementation postprocedure

    a. Monitor neurological status and vital signs frequently until stable

    b. Monitor for swelling in the neck and for difficulty swallowing and notify the physician if these symptoms occur

    c. Maintain bed rest for 12 hours as prescribed

    d. Elevate the head of the bed 15 to 30 degrees only if prescribed

    e. Keep the bed flat if the femoral artery is used as prescribed

    f. Assess peripheral pulses

    g. Immobilize the puncture site for 12 hours as prescribed

    h. Apply sandbags and a pressure dressing to the injection site as prescribed

    i. Place ice on the puncture site as prescribed

    j. Force fluids

G. Electroencephalography (EEG)

  1. Description: a graphic recording of the electrical activity of the superficial layers of the cerebral cortex

  2. Implementation preprocedure

    a. Wash the client's hair

    b. Inform the client that electrodes are attached to the head and that electricity does not enter the head

    c. Withhold stimulants, antidepressants, tranquilizers, and anticonvulsants for 24 to 48 hours prior to the test as prescribed

    d. Allow the client to have breakfast if prescribed

    e. Premedicate for sedation as prescribed

  3. Implementation postprocedure

    a. Wash the client's hair

    b. Maintain side rails and safety precautions if the client was sedated

H. Caloric testing (oculovestibular testing)

  1. Description: provides information about the function of the vestibular portion of the eighth cranial nerve and aids in the diagnosis of cerebellum and brain stem lesions

  2. Procedure

    a. Patency of the external canal is confirmed

    b. Cold or warm water is introduced into the external auditory canal

    c. Stimulation of the auditory canal with warm water produces a horizontal nystagmus toward the side of the irrigated ear when the vestibular eighth cranial nerve is normal

    d. Stimulation of the auditory canal with cold water produces a horizontal nystagmus away from the side of the irrigated ear if the brain stem is intact

III. Neurological Assessment

A. Assessment of risk factors

  1. Trauma

  2. Hemorrhage

  3. Tumors

  4. Infection

  5. Toxicity

  6. Metabolic disorders

  7. Hypoxic conditions

  8. Deficiency conditions

  9. Hypertension

  10. Cigarette smoking

  11. Stress

B. Assessment of the cranial nerves

  1. Cranial nerve I (olfactory) sensory, smell

    a. Have the client close the eyes and occlude one nostril with a finger

    b. Ask the client to identify nonirritating odors such as coffee, tea, cloves, soap, chewing gum, and peppermint

    c. Repeat the test on the other nostril

  2. Cranial nerve II (optic) sensory, vision

    a. Assess visual acuity with a Snellen chart or newspaper or ask the client to count how many fingers the examiner is holding up

    b. Check visual fields by confrontation

    c. Have the client sit directly in front of examiner and stare at the examiner's nose

    d. The examiner slowly moves a finger from the periphery toward the center until the client says it can be seen

    e. Check color vision by asking the client to name the color of several nearby objects

  3. Cranial nerve III (oculomotor); cranial nerve IV (trochlear); cranial nerve VI (abducens)

    a. The motor functions of these nerves overlap; therefore, they need to be tested together

    b. First, inspect the eyelids for ptosis (drooping), then assess ocular movements and note any eye deviation

    c. Test accommodation and direct and consensual light reflexes

    d. Cranial nerve III (oculomotor) motor: assesses pupillary constriction, upper eyelid elevation, and most eye movement

    e. Cranial nerve IV (trochlear) motor: assesses downward and inward eye movement

    f. Cranial nerve VI (abducens): assesses lateral eye movement

  4. Cranial nerve V (trigeminal) sensory and motor

    a. Assesses sensation to the cornea, nasal and oral mucosa, facial skin, and mastication

b. To test motor function, ask the client to close the jaws tightly, then try to separate the clenched jaw

c. Test the corneal reflex by lightly touching the client's cornea with a cotton wisp

d. Check sensory function by asking the client to close the eyes, then lightly touch the forehead, cheeks, and chin, noting if the touch can be felt equally on both sides

5. Cranial nerve VII (facial) sensory and motor
   a. Test taste perception on the anterior two thirds of the tongue
   b. Have the client show the teeth
   c. Attempt to close the client's eyes against resistance and ask the client to puff out the cheeks
   d. Place sugar, salt, or vinegar on the front of the tongue and have the client identify these substances by their tastes

6. Cranial nerve VIII (acoustic) sensory
   a. The ability to hear tests the cochlear portion
   b. The sense of equilibrium tests the vestibular portion
   c. Check the client's ability to hear a watch ticking or a whisper
   d. Observe the client's balance and observe for swaying when walking or standing

7. Cranial nerve IX (glossopharyngeal) sensory and motor
   a. Assesses swallowing ability
   b. Assesses sensation to the pharyngeal soft palate and tonsillar mucosa, and taste perception on the posterior third of the tongue and salivation

8. Cranial nerve X (vagus) sensory and motor
   a. Assesses swallowing and phonation, sensation to the exterior ear's posterior wall, and sensation behind the ear
   b. Assesses sensation to the thoracic and abdominal viscera

9. Cranial nerve IX (glossopharyngeal); cranial nerve X (vagus)
   a. Have the client identify a taste at the back of the tongue
   b. Inspect the soft palate and observe for symmetrical elevation when the client says "aah"
   c. Touch the posterior pharyngeal wall with a tongue depressor to elicit a gag reflex

10. Cranial nerve XI (spinal accessory) motor
    a. Assesses uvula and soft palate movement, sternocleidomastoid and trapezius muscle
    b. Assesses upper portion of trapezius muscle, which governs shoulder movement and neck rotation
    c. Palpate and inspect the sternocleidomastoid muscle as the client pushes the chin against the examiner's hand
    d. Palpate and inspect the trapezius muscle

as the client shrugs shoulders against the examiner's resistance

11. Cranial nerve XII (hypoglossal) motor
    a. Assesses tongue movements involved in swallowing and speech
    b. Observe the tongue for asymmetry, atrophy, deviation to one side, and fasciculations
    c. Ask the client to push the tongue against a tongue depressor, then move the tongue rapidly in and out and from side to side

C. Assessment of level of consciousness
   1. Assesses cerebral function
   2. Assess client behavior to determine level of consciousness such as confusion, delirium, unconsciousness, stupor, and coma

D. Assessment of vital signs: monitor for blood pressure or pulse changes, which may indicate **increased intracranial pressure (ICP)**

E. Assessment of respirations (Box 65–2)

F. Assessment of temperature
   1. An elevated temperature increases the brain's metabolic rate
   2. An early rise in temperature indicates a dysfunction of the hypothalamus or brain stem
   3. A slow rise in temperature may indicate infection

G. Assessment of pupils
   1. Size
   2. Equality
   3. Reactions to light described as brisk, slow, or fixed
   4. Unusual eye movements
   5. Unilateral pupil dilation indicates compression of the third cranial nerve

---

BOX 65–2. Assessment of Respirations

CHEYNE-STOKES
Rhythmical with periods of apnea
Can indicate a metabolic dysfunction or dysfunction in the cerebral hemisphere or basal ganglia

NEUROGENIC HYPERVENTILATION
Regular rapid and deep sustained respirations
Indicates a dysfunction to the low midbrain and middle pons

APNEUSTIC
Irregular respirations with pauses at the end of inspiration and expiration
Indicates a dysfunction to the middle or caudal pons

ATAXIC
Totally irregular in rhythm and depth
Indicates a dysfunction in the medulla

CLUSTER
Clusters of breaths with irregularly spaced pauses
Indicates a dysfunction in the medulla and pons

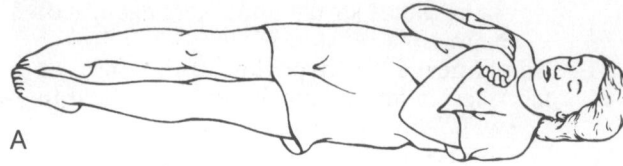

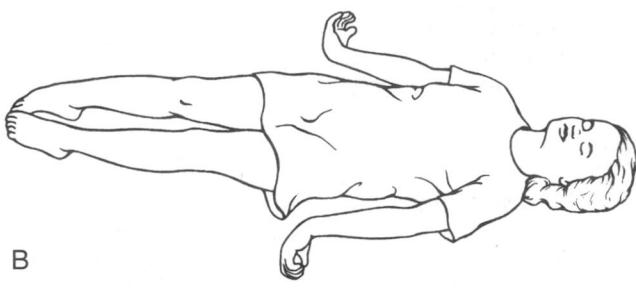

FIGURE 65–1. Posturing. *A,* Decorticate posturing. *B,* Decerebrate posturing. (From Ignatavicius, D., Workman, M., & Mishler, M. (1995). *Medical surgical nursing: A nursing process approach* (2nd ed.). Philadelphia: W.B. Saunders, p. 1111.)

6. Midposition; fixed pupil indicates midbrain injury
7. Pinpoint; fixed indicates pontine damage

H. Assessment of motor function
1. Muscle tone including strength and equality
2. Voluntary and involuntary movements
3. Purposeful and nonpurposeful movements

I. Assessment for posturing (Fig. 65–1)
1. Posturing indicates a deterioration of the condition
2. Flexor (**decorticate posturing**)
   a. Client flexes one or both arms on the chest and may stiffly extend the legs
   b. Indicates a nonfunctioning cortex
3. Extensor (**decerebrate posturing**)
   a. Client stiffly extends one or both arms and possibly the legs
   b. Indicates a brain stem lesion
4. **Flaccid posturing:** client displays no motor response in any extremity

---

BOX 65–3. Assessment of Reflexes

BABINSKI REFLEX

Dorsiflexion of the ankle and great toe with fanning of the other toes
Indicates a disruption of the pyramidal tract

CORNEAL REFLEX

Loss of the blink reflex
Indicates a dysfunction of cranial nerve V

GAG REFLEX

Loss of the gag reflex
Indicates a dysfunction of cranial nerves IX and X

BOX 65–4. Assessment of Meningeal Irritation

BRUDZINSKI'S SIGN

Flexion of the head causes flexion of both thighs at the hips and knee flexion

KERNIG'S SIGN

Flexion of the thigh and knee to right angles, and when extended, causes spasm of hamstring and pain

---

J. Assessment of reflexes (Box 65–3)
K. Assessment of meningeal irritation (Box 65–4)
1. Nuchal rigidity
2. Irritability
3. Fever
L. Assessment of the autonomic system
1. Sympathetic functions/adrenergic responses
   a. Increased pulse and blood pressure
   b. Dilated pupils
   c. Decreased peristalsis
   d. Increases perspiration
2. Parasympathetic function/cholinergic responses
   a. Decreased pulse and blood pressure
   b. Constricted pupils
   c. Increased salivation
   d. Increased peristalsis
   e. Dilated blood vessels
   f. Bladder contraction
M. Assessment of sensory function
1. Touch
2. Pressure
3. Pain
4. Bladder control
5. Bowel control

BOX 65–5. Glasgow Coma Scale

MOTOR RESPONSE POINTS

Obeys a simple response = 6
Localizes painful stimuli = 5
Normal flexion (withdrawal) = 4
Abnormal flexion (decorticate posturing) = 3
Extensor response (decerebrate posturing) = 2
No motor response to pain = 1

VERBAL RESPONSE POINTS

Oriented = 5
Confused conversation = 4
Inappropriate words = 3
Responds with incomprehensible sounds = 2
No verbal response = 1

EYE-OPENING POINTS

Spontaneous = 4
In response to sound = 3
In response to pain = 2
No response even to painful stimuli = 1

N. **Glasgow Coma Scale** (Box 65–5)
1. A method of assessing a client's neurological condition
2. A scoring system based on a scale of 1 to 15 points
3. A score below 8 indicates coma is present
4. Eye opening is the most important indicator

IV. The Unconscious Client

A. Description
1. A state of depressed cerebral functioning with unresponsiveness to sensory and motor function
2. Some of the causes include head trauma, cerebral toxins, shock, hemorrhage, tumor, or infections

B. Assessment
1. Unarousable
2. Primitive or no response to painful stimuli
3. Altered respirations
4. Decreased cranial nerve and reflex activity

C. Implementation (Box 65–6)

V. Increased Intracranial Pressure

A. Description
1. An **increase in intracranial pressure** caused by trauma, hemorrhage, growths or tumors, hydrocephalus, edema, or inflammation
2. Can impede circulation to the brain, impede the absorption of CSF, affect the functioning of nerve cells, and lead to brain stem compression and death

B. Assessment
1. Assess level of consciousness (LOC), which is the most sensitive and earliest indication of **increasing intracranial pressure**
2. Declining LOC from restlessness to confusion and coma
3. Headache
4. Abnormal respirations
5. Rise in blood pressure with widening pulse pressure
6. Slowing of pulse
7. Elevated temperature
8. Vomiting
9. Pupil changes
10. Changes in motor function from weakness to hemiplegia, a positive **Babinski reflex,** posturing as decorticate, decerebrate, and seizures
11. Late signs of **increased ICP** include increased systolic blood pressure, widened pulse pressure, and slowed heart rate

C. Implementation
1. Elevate the head of the bed 30 to 40 degrees as prescribed
2. Avoid Trendelenburg position
3. Prevent flexion of the neck and hips
4. Monitor respiratory status and prevent hypoxia

BOX 65–6. Care to the Unconscious Client

- Assess patency of airway and keep an airway and emergency equipment at the bedside
- Monitor blood pressure, pulse, and heart sounds
- Assess respiratory and circulatory status
- Maintain patent airway and ventilation because a high CO_2 level increases intracranial pressure
- Assess lung sounds for the accumulation of secretions
- Suction PRN
- Assess neurological status including LOC, pupillary reactions, motor and sensory function
- Position the client in semi-Fowler's position
- Change position of the client every 2 hours, avoiding injury when turning
- Avoid Trendelenburg position
- Use side rails at all times
- Assess for edema
- Monitor for dehydration
- Monitor I&O and daily weight
- Maintain NPO status until consciousness returns
- Maintain nutrition and fluid and electrolyte balance
- Check the gag and swallowing reflexes before resuming diet and begin with ice chips and fluids
- Provide intravenous or enteral feedings as prescribed
- Assess bowel sounds
- Monitor elimination patterns
- Monitor for constipation, impaction, and paralytic ileus
- Maintain urinary output to prevent stasis, infection, and calculus formation
- Monitor the status of skin integrity
- Initiate measures to prevent skin breakdown
- Provide frequent mouth care
- Remove dentures and contact lens
- Assess the eyes for corneal reflex and irritation and instill artificial tears or cover with eyepatches
- Monitor drainage from the ears or nose for the presence of cerebrospinal fluid
- Assume that the unconscious client can hear
- Avoid restraints
- Do not leave the client unattended if unstable
- Initiate seizure precautions if necessary
- Provide range-of-motion exercises to prevent contractures
- Use a footboard or high-top sneakers to prevent foot drop
- Use splints to prevent wrist deformities
- Initiate physical therapy as appropriate

5. Avoid the administration of morphine to prevent the occurrence of hypoxia
6. Maintain mechanical ventilation as prescribed, maintaining the $PaCO_2$ at 30 to 35 mmHg, which will result in vasoconstriction of the cerebral blood vessels, decreased blood flow, and therefore decreased **ICP**
7. Maintain body temperature
8. Prevent shivering, which can raise **intracranial pressure**
9. Decrease environmental stimuli

10. Monitor electrolyte levels and acid-base balance
11. Monitor I&O
12. Limit fluid intake to 1200 mL/day
13. Instruct client to avoid straining activities such as coughing and sneezing
14. Instruct client to avoid Valsalva maneuver

D. Medications (Box 65–7)
E. Surgical intervention (Box 65–8)

VI. Hyperthermia

A. Description
1. A temperature of 106° F, which increases the cerebral metabolism and increases the risk of hypoxia
2. The causes include infection, heat stroke, exposure to high environmental

---

BOX 65–7. Medications for ICP

MANNITOL (OSMITROL)

Hyperosmotic agent
Increases intravascular pressure by drawing fluid from the interstitial spaces and from the brain cells
Monitor renal function
Diuresis is expected

STEROIDS SUCH AS DEXAMETHASONE (DECADRON)

Stabilize the cell membrane and reduce the leakiness in the blood-brain barrier
Decrease cerebral edema
A histamine blocker may be administered to counteract the excess gastric secretion that occurs with the steroid
Clients must be withdrawn slowly from steroid therapy to reduce the risk of adrenal crisis

BLOOD PRESSURE MEDICATION

May be required to maintain cerebral perfusion at a normal level
Notify the physician if the blood pressure range is below 100 or above 150 mmHg systolic

ANTIPYRETICS AND MUSCLE RELAXANTS

Temperature reduction decreases metabolism, cerebral blood flow, and thus ICP
Muscle relaxants prevent shivering

ANTICONVULSANTS

May be given prophylactically to prevent seizures
Seizures increase metabolic requirements and cerebral blood flow and volume, thus increasing ICP

IV FLUIDS

Administered via infusion pump to minimize the amount of IV fluid administered
Hypertonic IVs are avoided because of the risk of promoting additional cerebral edema

---

BOX 65–8. Surgical Intervention for ICP

VENTRICULOPERITONEAL SHUNT

Description:
Shunts CSF from the ventricles into the peritoneum

Implementation postprocedure:
Position client supine and turn from back to unoperative side
Monitor for signs of increasing intracranial pressure due to shunt failure
Monitor for signs of infection

---

temperatures, and dysfunction of the thermoregulatory center

B. Assessment
1. Temperature of 106° F
2. Shivering
3. Nausea and vomiting

C. Implementation
1. Maintain a patent airway
2. Initiate seizure precautions
3. Monitor I&O and assess skin and mucous membranes for signs of dehydration
4. Monitor lung sounds
5. Monitor for dysrhythmias
6. Assess peripheral pulses for systemic blood flow
7. Induce normothermia with fluids, cool baths, fans, or hypothermia blanket

D. Inducing normothermia
1. Prevent shivering, which will increase cerebrospinal fluid pressure and oxygen consumption
2. Monitor neurological changes
3. Monitor for infection and respiratory complications such as hypothermia; may mask signs of infection
4. Monitor for cardiac dysrhythmias
5. Monitor I&O
6. Administer medications as prescribed to prevent shivering
7. Prevent trauma to the skin and tissues
8. Apply lotion to the skin frequently
9. Inspect for frostbite

E. Medications to prevent shivering (Box 65–9)

BOX 65–9. Medications to Prevent Shivering

CHLORPROMAZINE HYDROCHLORIDE (THORAZINE)

Depresses thermoregulation in the hypothalamus and reduces peripheral vasoconstriction, muscle tone, and shivering

MEPERIDINE HYDROCHLORIDE (DEMEROL)

Relaxes the smooth muscle and reduces shivering

◆ VII. Head Injury

A. Description
1. A trauma to the skull resulting in mild to extensive damage to the brain
2. Immediate complications include cerebral bleeding, hematomas, uncontrolled **increased ICP**, infections, and seizures
3. Changes in personality or behavior, cranial nerve deficits, and any other residual deficits depend on the area of the brain damage and the extent of the damage

B. Types of head injuries (Box 65–10)
1. Open
   a. Scalp lacerations
   b. Fractures in the skull
   c. Interruption of the dura mater
2. Closed
   a. Concussions
   b. Contusions
   c. Fractures

C. Hematoma
1. Description: can occur as a result of a subarachnoid hemorrhage or an intracerebral hemorrhage
2. Assessment
   a. Assessment findings will be dependent on the injury
   b. Clinical manifestations usually result from increased intracranial pressure
   c. Changing neurological signs in the client
   d. Level of consciousness
   e. Airway and breathing pattern
   f. Vital signs for signs of **increasing ICP**
   g. Headache, nausea, and vomiting
   h. Visual disturbances, pupillary changes, papilledema, and extraocular eye movements
   i. Nuchal rigidity
   j. CSF drainage from the ears or nose
   k. Weakness and paralysis
   l. Posturing
   m. Decreased sensation or absence of feeling
   n. Reflex activity
   o. Seizure activity
3. Implementation
   a. Monitor respiratory status and maintain a patent airway as increased CO_2 levels increase cerebral edema
   b. Monitor neurological status and vital signs, including temperature
   c. Monitor for **increased intracranial pressure (ICP)**
   d. Maintain head elevation to reduce venous pressure
   e. Prevent neck flexion
   f. Initiate normothermia measures for increased temperature
   g. Assess cranial nerve function, reflexes, and motor and sensory function
   h. Initiate seizure precautions
   i. Monitor for pain and restlessness

BOX 65–10. Types of Head Injuries

CONCUSSION

A jarring of the brain within the skull with temporary loss of consciousness

CONTUSION

A bruising type injury to brain
It may occur with subdural or extradural collection of blood

SKULL FRACTURES

Linear
Depressed
Compound
Comminuted

EPIDURAL HEMATOMA

The most serious type of hematoma, forms rapidly and results from an arterial bleed
Forms between the dura and the skull from a tear in the meningeal artery
A surgical emergency

SUBDURAL HEMATOMA

Forms slowly and results from a venous bleed
It occurs under the dura as a result of tears in the veins crossing the subdural space

SUBARACHNOID HEMORRHAGE

Bleeding directly into the brain, ventricles, or the subarachnoid space

INTRACEREBRAL HEMORRHAGE

Multiple hemorrhages around a contused area

j. Avoid morphine sulfate because it is a respiratory depressant and may **increase intracranial pressure (ICP)**
k. Monitor for drainage from the nose or ears because this fluid may be cerebrospinal fluid (CSF)
l. Do not attempt to clean the nose, suction, or allow the client to blow the nose if drainage occurs
m. Do not clean the ear if drainage is noted but apply a loose, dry, sterile dressing
n. Check drainage for presence of CSF
o. Notify the physician if drainage from the ears or nose is noted
p. Instruct the client to avoid coughing because this increases intracranial pressure
q. Monitor for signs of infection
r. Prevent complications of immobility

D. Craniotomy
1. Description
   a. A surgical procedure that involves an incision through the cranium to remove accumulated blood or a tumor
   b. Complications of the procedure include **increased intracranial pressure** from

BOX 65–11. Nursing Care Following Craniotomy

- Monitor vital signs and neurologic status every 30 minutes to 1 hour
- Monitor for increased intracranial pressure
- Monitor for decreased level of consciousness, motor weakness or paralysis, aphasia, visual changes, and personality changes
- Maintain mechanical ventilation and slight hyperventilation for the first 24 to 48 hours as prescribed to prevent increased intracranial pressure
- Assess the physician's orders regarding client positioning
- Avoid extreme hip or neck flexion and maintain the head in a midline neutral position
- Provide a quiet environment
- Monitor the head dressing frequently for signs of drainage
- Mark the area of drainage once each nursing shift for baseline comparison
- Monitor the Hemovac or Jackson-Pratt drain, which may be in place for 24 hours
- Maintain suction on the Hemovac or drain
- Measure drainage from the Hemovac or drain every 8 hours and record the amount and color
- Notify the physician if drainage is greater than the normal of 30 to 50 mL per shift
- Notify the physician immediately of excessive amounts of drainage or a saturated head dressing
- Record strict measurement of hourly I&O
- Maintain fluid restriction to 1500 mL/day as prescribed
- Monitor electrolyte values
- Monitor for dysrhythmias, which may occur as a result of fluid and electrolyte imbalance
- Apply ice packs or cool compresses as prescribed for periorbital edema and ecchymosis of one or both eyes, which is not an unusual occurrence
- Provide range-of-motion exercises every 8 hours
- Place antiembolism stockings on the client as prescribed
- Administer anticonvulsants, antacids, corticosteroids, and antibiotics as prescribed
- Administer analgesics such as codeine and acetaminophen as prescribed for pain

cerebral edema, hemorrhage, or obstruction of the normal flow of CSF
   c. Additional complications include hematomas, hypovolemic shock, hydrocephalus, respiratory and neurogenic complications, pulmonary edema, and wound infections
   d. Complications related to fluid and electrolyte imbalances include diabetes insipidus and inappropriate secretion of antidiuretic hormone
  2. Implementation preoperatively
   a. Explain procedure to the client and family
   b. Ensure that informed consent has been obtained
   c. Prepare to shave the client's head as

prescribed and cover it with appropriate covering
   d. Stabilize the client prior to surgery
  3. Implementation postoperatively (Box 65–11)
  4. Postoperative positioning (Box 65–12)

VIII. Spinal Cord Injury

A. Description
  1. Trauma to the spinal cord causing partial or complete disruption of the nerve tracts and neurons
  2. The injury can range from a contusion, laceration, or compression of the cord
  3. Spinal cord edema develops and necrosis of the spinal cord can develop as a result of compromised capillary circulation and venous return.
  4. Loss of motor function, sensation, reflex activity, and bowel and bladder control may result

BOX 65–12. Client Positioning Following Craniotomy

- Positions prescribed following craniotomy vary with the type of surgery and the specific postoperative physician's orders
- Always check the physician's orders regarding client positioning
- Incorrect positioning may cause serious and possibly fatal complications

REMOVAL OF A BONE FLAP FOR DECOMPRESSION

To facilitate brain expansion, the client should be turned from the back to the unoperative side, but not to the side operated on

POSTERIOR FOSSA SURGERY

To protect the operative site from pressure and minimize tension on the suture line, position the client on the side, with a pillow under the head for support, and not on the back

INFRATENTORIAL SURGERY

Involves surgery below the brain's tentorium
The physician may order a flat position without head elevation or may order the head of the bed to be elevated at 30 to 45 degrees
Do not elevate the head of the bed in the acute phase of care following surgery without a physician's order

SUPRATENTORIAL SURGERY

Involves surgery above the brain's tentorium
The physician may order the head of the bed to be elevated at 30 degrees to promote venous outflow through the jugular veins
Do not lower the head of the bed in the acute phase of care following surgery without a physician's order

5. The most common causes include motor vehicle accidents, falls, sporting and industrial accidents, and gunshot or stab wounds
6. Complications related to the injury include respiratory failure, **autonomic dysreflexia, spinal shock,** further cord damage, and death

B. Most frequently involved vertebrae
1. Cervical 5, 6, and 7
2. Thoracic 12
3. Lumbar 1

C. Transection of the cord
1. Complete transection of the cord
   a. The spinal cord is completely severed, with total loss of sensation, movement, and reflex activity below the level of injury
   b. If the cord has not suffered irreparable damage, early treatment is needed to prevent partial damage from developing into total and permanent damage
2. Partial transection of the cord
   a. The spinal cord is partially damaged or severed
   b. The symptoms depend on the extent and location of the damage

D. Types of injuries
1. Anterior cord syndrome
   a. Damage to the anterior portion of the gray and white matter of the spinal cord
   b. Motor function, pain, and temperature sensation are lost below the level of injury; however, the sensations of touch, position, and vibration remain intact
2. Posterior cord injury
   a. Damage to the posterior portion of the gray and white matter of the spinal cord
   b. Motor function remains intact but the client experiences a loss of vibratory sense, crude touch, and position sensation
3. Central cord syndrome
   a. Occurs from a lesion in the central portion of the spinal cord
   b. Loss of motor function is more pronounced in the upper extremities, and varying degrees and patterns of sensation remain intact
4. Brown-Séquard syndrome
   a. Results from penetrating injuries that cause hemisection of the spinal cord or injuries that affect half of the cord
   b. Motor function, proprioception, vibration, and deep touch sensations are lost on the same side of the body (ipsilateral) as the lesion
   c. On the opposite side of the body (contralateral) from the injury, the sensations of pain, temperature, and light touch are affected

E. Assessment of spinal cord injuries (Box 65–13)
1. Depends on the level of the cord injury

2. The level of spinal cord injury is the lowest spinal cord segment with intact motor and sensory function
3. Respiratory status
4. Motor and sensory changes below the level of injury
5. Total sensory loss and motor paralysis below the level of injury
6. Loss of reflexes below the level of injury
7. Loss of bladder and bowel control
8. Urinary retention and bladder distention
9. Presence of sweat, which does not occur on paralyzed areas

F. Cervical Injuries
1. C2 to C3 injury is usually fatal
2. C4 is the major innervation to the diaphragm by the phrenic nerve
3. Involvement above C4 causes respiratory difficulty and paralysis of all four extremities
4. Client may have movement in the shoulder if the injury is at C5 or below

G. Thoracic level injuries
1. Loss of movement of the chest, trunk, bowel, bladder, and legs, depending on the level of injury
2. Leg paralysis (paraplegia)
3. **Autonomic dysreflexia** with lesions above T6 and in cervical lesions
4. Visceral distention from a distended bladder or impacted rectum may cause reactions such as sweating, bradycardia, hypertension, nasal stuffiness, and gooseflesh

H. Lumbar and sacral level injuries
1. Loss of movement and sensation of the lower extremities
2. S2 and S3 center on micturation; therefore, below this level, the bladder will contract but not empty (neurogenic bladder)
3. Injury above S2 in males allows them to have an erection, but they are unable to ejaculate because of sympathetic nerve damage
4. Injury between S2 and S4 damages the sympathetic and parasympathetic response, preventing erection or ejaculation

I. Emergency implementation
1. Emergency management is critical because improper handling can cause further damage and loss of neurological function
2. Maintain a patent airway
3. Always suspect spinal cord injury until this injury is ruled out

---

BOX 65–13. Effects of the Spinal Cord Injury

QUADRIPLEGIA

Injury occurring from C1 through C8
Paralysis involving all four extremities

PARAPLEGIA

Injury occurring from T1 through L4
Paralysis involving only the lower extremities

4. Immobilize the client on a spinal backboard with the head in a neutral position to prevent an incomplete injury from becoming complete
5. Prevent head flexion, rotation, or extension
6. During immobilization, maintain traction and alignment on the head by placing the hands on either side of the head by the ears
7. Maintain an extended position
8. Log roll the client
9. No part of the body should be twisted or turned and the client should not be allowed to assume a sitting position
10. In the emergency room, a client who has sustained a severe cervical injury should be placed immediately in skeletal traction via skull tongs or halo vest to immobilize the cervical spine and reduce the fracture and dislocation

J. Implementation during hospitalization
1. Respiratory system
   a. Assess respiratory status because paralysis of the intercostal and abdominal muscles occurs with C4 injuries
   b. Monitor arterial blood gases and maintain mechanical ventilation if prescribed to prevent respiratory arrest, especially with cervical injuries
   c. Encourage deep breathing and the use of an incentive spirometer
   d. Monitor for signs of infection, particularly pneumonia
2. Cardiovascular system
   a. Monitor for cardiac dysrhythmias
   b. Assess for signs of hemorrhage or bleeding around the fracture site
   c. Assess for signs of shock such as hypotension, tachycardia, and a weak and thready pulse
   d. Assess lower extremities for deep vein thrombosis
   e. Measure circumference of the calf and thigh
   f. Apply thigh-high antiembolism stockings as prescribed
   g. Remove antiembolism stockings daily to assess the skin
   h. Monitor for orthostatic hypotension when repositioning the client
3. Neuromuscular system
   a. Assess neurological status
   b. Assess motor and sensory status to determine the level of injury
   c. Assess motor ability by testing client's ability to squeeze the hands, spread the fingers, move the toes, turn the feet
   d. Assess sensation by pinching skin or pricking with a pin, starting at the shoulders and working down the extremities
   e. Monitor for signs of **autonomic dysreflexia** and **spinal shock**

f. Immobilize the client to promote healing and prevent further injury
g. Assess pain
h. Initiate measures to reduce pain
i. Administer analgesics as prescribed
j. Monitor for complications of immobility
k. Prepare the client for decompression laminectomy, spinal fusion, or insertion of steel rods if prescribed
l. Collaborate with the physical therapist and occupational therapist to determine appropriate exercise techniques, to assess the need for hand and wrist splints, and to develop an appropriate plan to prevent footdrop
4. Gastrointestinal system
   a. Assess the abdomen for distention and hemorrhage
   b. Monitor bowel sounds and assess for paralytic ileus
   c. Prevent bowel retention
   d. Initiate a bowel control program as appropriate
   e. Maintain adequate nutrition and a high-fiber diet
5. Renal system
   a. Prevent bladder retention
   b. Initiate a bladder control program as appropriate
   c. Maintain fluid and electrolyte balance
   d. Maintain adequate fluid intake of 2000 mL daily
   e. Monitor for urinary tract infection and calculi
6. Integumentary system
   a. Assess skin integrity
   b. Turn the client every 2 hours
7. Psychosocial integrity
   a. Assess psychosocial status
   b. Encourage the client to express feelings of anger and depression
   c. Discuss sexual concerns of the client
   d. Promote self-care, setting realistic goals based on the client's potential functional level
   e. Encourage contact with appropriate community resources

K. **Spinal shock**
1. Description
   a. Also known as neurogenic shock
   b. A sudden depression of reflex activity in the spinal cord below the level of injury (areflexia)
   c. Occurs within the first hour of injury and can last days to months
   d. The muscles become completely paralyzed and flaccid and reflexes are absent
   e. **Spinal shock** ends when the reflexes are regained
2. Assessment
   a. Flaccid paralysis
   b. Hypotension

c. Bradycardia
d. Loss of reflex activity below the level of injury
e. Paralytic ileus

3. Implementation
   a. Monitor for signs of **spinal shock** following spinal cord injury
   b. Monitor for hypotension and bradycardia
   c. Monitor for reflex activity
   d. Assess bowel sounds
   e. Monitor for bowel and bladder retention
   f. Provide supportive measures as prescribed based on the presence of symptoms
   g. Monitor for the return of reflexes

L. **Autonomic dysreflexia**
1. Description
   a. Also known as hyperreflexia
   b. Commonly caused by visceral distention from a distended bladder or impacted rectum
   c. A neurologic emergency that must be treated immediately to prevent a hypertensive stroke
   d. It generally occurs after the period of **spinal shock** is resolved
   e. Occurs with lesions above T6 and in cervical lesions
2. Assessment
   a. Hypertension
   b. Bradycardia
   c. Flushing of the face and neck
   d. Severe, throbbing headache
   e. Nasal stuffiness
   f. Piloerection (gooseflesh)
   g. Sweating
   h. Nausea
   i. Restlessness
   j. Dilated pupils and blurred vision
3. Implementation
   a. Notify physician if signs of **autonomic dysreflexia** occur

b. Assess for potential cause and remove the stimulus
c. Monitor vital signs, particularly blood pressure, every 15 minutes
d. Raise the head of the bed to high Fowler's
e. Loosen tight clothing
f. Assess for bladder distention and prepare for urinary catheterization
g. If a urinary catheter is present, check for kinks in the tubing and for drainage
h. Assess for a fecal impaction and disimpact immediately
i. Administer antihypertensives as prescribed

M. Cervical traction for cervical injuries (Fig. 65–2)
1. Description
   a. Skeletal traction used to stabilize fractures or dislocations of the cervical or upper thoracic spine
   b. Two types of equipment used for cervical traction are **skull tongs** and **halo traction**
2. **Skull tongs**
   a. **Skull tongs** are inserted into the outer aspect of the client's skull and traction is applied
   b. Weights are attached to the tongs and the client is used as countertraction
   c. Monitor the neurological status of the client
   d. Determine the amount of weight prescribed to be added to the traction
   e. Ensure that weights hang securely and freely at all times
   f. Ensure the ropes for the traction remain within the pulley
   g. Maintain body alignment and maintain care of the client on Roto-Rest bed, Stryker, or Foster frame as prescribed
   h. Turn the client every 2 hours

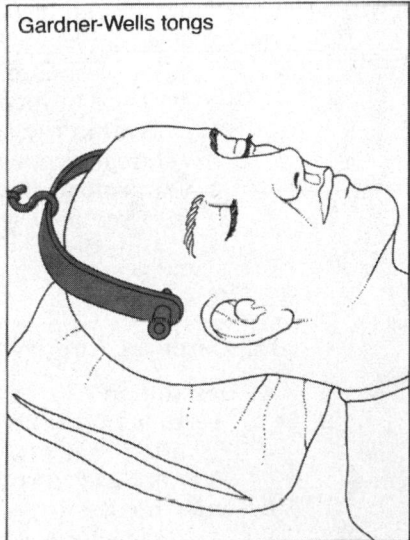

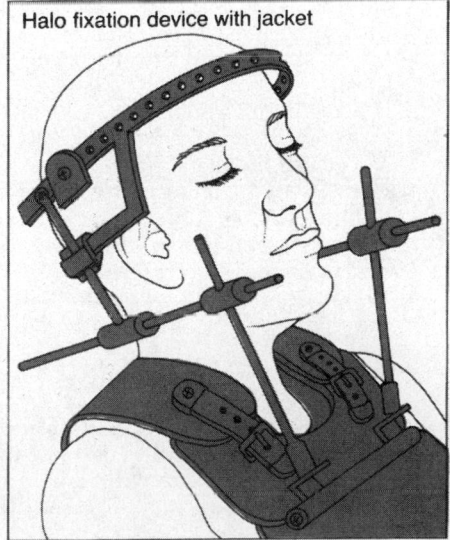

FIGURE 65–2. Types of cervical spine traction. (From Ignatavicius, D., Workman, M., & Mishler, M. (1995). *Medical-surgical nursing: A nursing process approach* (2nd ed.). Philadelphia, W.B. Saunders, p. 1188.)

i. Assess the insertion site of the tongs for infection

j. Provide a sterile pin site care as prescribed

3. **Halo traction**

a. Consists of a headpiece with four pins, two anterior and two posterior, inserted into the client's skull; then a halo jacket or cast is applied

b. Once the fracture is stable, the headpiece can be attached to a body jacket called a halo vest

c. Monitor the client's neurological status for changes in movement or decreased strength

d. Never move or turn the client by holding or pulling on the halo device

e. Assess for tightness of the jacket by ensuring that one finger can be placed under the jacket

f. Assess skin integrity to ensure that the jacket or cast is not causing pressure

g. Provide sterile pin site care as prescribed

4. Client education for a halo vest (Box 65–14)

N. Implementation for thoracic and lumbar/sacral injuries

1. Bed rest

BOX 65–14. Client Education for a Halo Device

- Notify the physician if the halo vest or ring bolts loosen
- Use fleece or foam inserts to relieve pressure points
- Keep the vest lining dry
- Clean the pin site daily
- Notify the physician if redness, swelling, drainage, open areas, pain, tenderness, or a clicking sound occurs from the pin site
- A sponge bath or tub bath is allowed; showers are prohibited
- Assess the skin under the vest daily for breakdown, using a flashlight
- Do not use any products other than shampoo on the hair
- When shampooing the hair, cover the vest with plastic
- When getting out of bed, roll onto the side and push on the mattress with the arms
- Never use the metal frame for turning or lifting
- Use a rolled towel or pillowcase between the back of the neck and the bed, or next to the cheek when lying on the side, and raise the head of the bed to increase sleep comfort
- Adapt clothing to fit over the halo
- Eat foods high in protein and calcium to promote bone healing
- Have the correct size wrench available at all times for an emergency
- If cardiopulmonary resuscitation is required, the anterior portion of the vest will be loosened and the posterior portion will remain in place to provide stability

---

2. Immobilization with a fiberglass or plastic body cast

3. Use of a brace or corset when the client is out of bed

O. Surgical implementation for thoracic and lumbar/sacral injuries

1. Decompressive laminectomy

a. Removal of one or more laminae

b. Allows for cord expansion from edema

c. Performed if conventional methods fail to prevent neurological deterioration

2. Spinal fusion and Harrington rod insertion

a. Used for thoracic spinal injuries

b. Insertion of a metal or steel rod to stabilize the thoracic spine

3. Implementation postoperatively

a. Monitor for respiratory impairment

b. Monitor vital signs, motor function, sensation, and circulatory status in lower extremities

c. Encourage breathing exercises

d. Assess for signs of fluid and electrolyte imbalance

e. Observe for complications of immobility

f. Keep the client flat

g. Provide cast care if the client is in a full body cast

h. Turn and reposition frequently by log rolling side to back to side using turning sheets and pillows between the legs to maintain alignment

i. Administer pain medication as prescribed

j. Maintain NPO status until the client is actively passing flatus

k. Monitor bowel sounds

l. Provide the use of a fracture bed pan

m. Monitor I&O

n. Provide diet high in protein, iron, and thiamine and low in calcium

P. Medications

1. Dexamethasone (Decadron)

a. Used for its anti-inflammatory and edema-reducing effects

b. May interfere with healing

2. Dextran

a. A plasma expander

b. Used to increase capillary blood flow within the spinal cord and to prevent or treat hypotension

3. Dantrolene (Dantrium)/Baclofen (Lioresal)

a. Used for clients with upper motor neuron injuries

b. Controls muscle spasticity

IX. Cerebral Aneurysm

A. Description

1. Dilation of the walls of a weakened cerebral artery

2. Can lead to rupture

B. Assessment

1. Headache

Table 65–1. **Types of Seizures**

Generalized Seizures	Partial Seizures
Tonic-Clonic (Grand Mal)	*Simple Partial*
May begin with an aura The tonic phase involves the stiffening or rigidity of the muscles of the arms and legs and usually lasts 10 to 20 seconds followed by loss of consciousness The clonic phase consists of hyperventilation and jerking of the extremities and usually lasts about 30 seconds Full recovery from the seizure may take several hours	Produces sensory symptoms accompanied by motor symptoms that are localized or confined to a specific area: the client remains conscious and may report an aura
Absence (Petit Mal)	*Complex Partial*
Brief seizure lasting seconds and the individual may or may not lose consciousness No loss or change in muscle tone occurs Seizures may occur several times during a day The victim appears to be daydreaming This type of seizure is more common in children	A psychomotor seizure The area of the brain most involved is the temporal lobe Characterized by periods of altered behavior that the client is not aware of The client loses consciousness for a few seconds
Myoclonic	
A seizure that presents as a brief generalized jerking or stiffening of extremities The victim may fall to the ground from the seizure	
Atonic or Akinetic (Drop Attacks)	
A sudden momentary loss of muscle tone The victim may fall to the ground as a result of the seizure	

2. Pain
3. Diplopia
4. Blurred vision
5. Tinnitus
6. Nausea
7. Hemiparesis
8. Nuchal rigidity
9. Irritability
10. Seizures

C. Implementation
 1. Maintain a patent airway (suction only with a physician's order)
 2. Administer oxygen as prescribed
 3. Monitor vital signs and for hypertension or dysrhythmias
 4. Avoid rectal temperatures
 5. Maintain bed rest in semi-Fowler's position or side-lying position
 6. Maintain a darkened room without stimulation
 7. Limit visitors
 8. Maintain fluid restrictions
 9. Monitor I&O
 10. Avoid stimulants in the diet

X. Seizures

A. Description
 1. An abnormal sudden excessive discharge of electrical activity within the brain
 2. Epilepsy is a disorder characterized by chronic seizure activity and indicates brain or CNS irritation
 3. Causes include genetic factors, trauma, tumors, circulatory or metabolic disorders, toxicity or infections

 4. Status epilepticus involves a rapid succession of epileptic spasms without intervals of consciousness; it is a potential complication that can occur with any type of seizure, and brain damage may result

B. Types of seizures (Table 65–1)
 1. Generalized seizures
  a. Tonic-clonic (grand mal)
  b. Absence (petit mal)
  c. Myoclonic
  d. Atonic or akinetic (drop attacks)
 2. Partial seizures
  a. Simple partial
  b. Complex partial

C. Assessment
 1. Seizure history
 2. Type of seizure
 3. Occurrences before, during, and after the seizure
 4. Prodromal signs as mood changes, irritability, and insomnia
 5. Aura, a sensation that warns the client of the impending seizure
 6. Loss of motor activity or bowel and bladder function or loss of consciousness during the seizure
 7. Occurrences during the postictal state such as headache, loss of consciousness, sleepiness, and impaired speech or thinking

D. Implementation
 1. Note the time and duration of the seizure
 2. Assess behavior at the onset of the seizure: if the client experienced an aura, if a change in facial expression occurred, or if a sound or cry occurred from the client

BOX 65–15. Neurological Assessment in CVA

Changes in level of consciousness (LOC)
Signs of increasing intracranial pressure (ICP)
Assessment of cranial nerves V, VII, IX, X, XII
Cranial nerve V—difficulty with chewing
Cranial nerve VII—facial paralysis or paresis
Cranial nerves IX and X—dysphagia
Cranial nerve IX—absent gag reflex
Cranial nerve XII—impaired tongue movement

3. If the client is standing, place the client on the floor and protect the head and body
4. Maintain a patent airway (do not force the jaws open)
5. Administer oxygen
6. Prepare to suction
7. Turn the client's head to the side
8. Prevent injury during the seizure
9. Remain with the client
10. Do not restrain the client
11. Loosen restrictive clothing
12. Note the type, character, and progression of the movements during the seizure
13. Monitor for incontinence
14. Administer medications IV diazepam (Valium), phenytoin (Dilantin), and phenobarbital sodium (Luminal) as prescribed to stop the seizure
15. Document the characteristics of the seizure
16. Monitor behavior following the seizure such as the state of consciousness, motor ability, and speech ability
17. Instruct the client on the importance of lifelong medication and the need for follow-up medication blood levels
18. Instruct the client to avoid alcohol, excessive stress, and fatigue
19. Encourage the client to contact available community resources such as the Epilepsy Foundation of America

◆ XI. Cerebrovascular Accident (CVA)

A. Description
   1. A sudden focal neurological deficit caused by cerebrovascular disease
   2. A syndrome in which the cerebral circulation is interrupted, causing neurological deficits
   3. Cerebral anoxia lasting longer than 10 minutes causes cerebral infarction with irreversible change
   4. Surrounding cerebral edema and congestion causes further dysfunction
   5. Diagnosis is determined by CT scan, EEG, and cerebral arteriography
   6. The permanent disability cannot be determined until the cerebral edema subsides
   7. The order in which function may return is facial, swallowing, lower limb, speech, and arms

Table 65–2. Left and Right Hemisphere Lesions

Assessment findings depend on area of brain affected
Lesions in the cerebral hemisphere result in manifestations on the contralateral side, which is the side of the body opposite the cerebral accident

Left Hemisphere Lesion	*Right Hemisphere Lesion*
Aphasia both expressive and receptive	Disoriented to time, place, and person
Agraphia—difficulty writing	Cannot recognize faces
Alexia—reading problems	Spatial—perceptual deficits
No memory deficit	Neglect of the left side
Deficits in the right visual field as reading problems and inability to discriminate words and letters	Client unaware of paralyzed side
	Loss of depth perception
No hearing deficit	Impulsive
Behavior slow, cautious, and disorganized	Unaware of neurologic deficits
	Confabulates
Anxious when attempting a new task	Euphoric, impaired sense of humor
	Constantly smiles
Depression	Denies illness
Sense of guilt	Poor judgment
Quick anger and frustration	Overestimates ability
Feelings of worthlessness	Loss of ability to hear tonal
Worries over the future	variations

B. Causes
   1. Thrombosis
   2. Embolism
   3. Hemorrhage from rupture of a vessel
   4. Transient ischemic attack (TIA)
C. Risk factors
   1. Atherosclerosis
   2. Hypertension
   3. Anticoagulation therapy
   4. Diabetes
   5. Stress
   6. Obesity
   7. Oral contraceptives
D. Assessment (Table 65–2; Box 65–15 and 65–16)
   1. Airway patency
   2. Slow bounding pulse
   3. Cheyne-Stokes respirations
   4. Hypertension
   5. Headache, nausea, and vomiting

BOX 65–16. Assessment Findings in a CVA

AGNOSIA

Inability to use an object correctly

APRAXIA

Inability to carry out a purposeful activity

HEMIANOPIA

Blindness in half of the visual field

HOMONYMOUS HEMIANOPIA

Blindness in the same side of both eyes
NOTE: With visual problems, client must turn the head to scan the complete range of vision

6. Dizziness and vertigo
7. Facial drooping
8. Nuchal rigidity
9. Diplopia and nystagmus
10. Papilledema
11. Blindness
12. Ataxia
13. Dysarthria
14. Dysphagia
15. Speech changes
16. Decreased sensation to pressure, heat, and cold
17. Bowel and bladder dysfunctions
18. Emotional changes
19. Paralysis

E. Aphasia
  1. Expressive
     a. Damage in Broca's area of the frontal brain
     b. The client understands what is said but is unable to communicate verbally
  2. Receptive
     a. Injury involving Wernicke's area in the temporoparietal area
     b. The client is unable to understand the spoken and often written word
  3. Global or mixed: language dysfunction in both the areas of expression and reception
  4. Implementation for aphasia
     a. Provide repetitive directions
     b. Break tasks down to one step at a time
     c. Repeat names of objects frequently used
     d. Use a picture board or communication board

F. Implementation during the acute phase of CVA
  1. Maintain a patent airway and administer oxygen as prescribed
  2. Monitor vital signs
  3. Maintain a blood pressure of 150/100 mmHg to maintain cerebral perfusion after a CVA
  4. Suction as prescribed but never suction nasally and for no longer than 10 seconds to prevent **increasing ICP**
  5. Monitor for **increasing ICP** because the client is at most risk during first 72 hours
  6. Position the client on the side with head of bed elevated 15 to 30 degrees as prescribed
  7. Monitor LOC, pupillary response, motor and sensory responses, cranial nerve function, and reflexes
  8. Maintain a quiet environment and provide minimal handling of the client to prevent further bleeding
  9. Administer IVs as prescribed
  10. Insert a Foley catheter as prescribed
  11. Maintain fluid and electrolyte balance
  12. Prepare to administer anticoagulants, antiplatelets, diuretics, antihypertensives, and anticonvulsants as prescribed
  13. Establish a form of communication

G. Implementation in the postacute phase of a CVA
  1. Continue with implementation from the acute phase
  2. Position the client 2 hours on the unaffected side, 20 minutes on the affected side
  3. Position the client in the prone position if necessary, for 30 minutes three times daily
  4. Provide skin, mouth, and eye care
  5. Perform passive range of motion exercises to prevent contractures
  6. Place antiembolism stockings on the client
  7. Measure thighs and calves for increase in size and assess for positive Homan's sign
  8. Monitor the gag reflex and ability to swallow
  9. Provide sips of fluids and slowly advance diet to foods that are easy to chew and swallow
  10. Provide soft and semisoft foods and fluids rather than liquids because clients are better able to tolerate these types of food
  11. When eating, position the client sitting in a chair, or sitting up in bed with the head and neck positioned slightly forward and flexed
  12. Place food in the back of the mouth on the unaffected side to prevent trapping of food in affected cheek

H. Implementation in the chronic phase of a CVA
  1. Provide eye care for visual deficits
  2. Approach the client from the nonaffected side
  3. Place the client's personal objects within the visual field
  4. Instruct the client with visual problems to turn head from side to side
  5. Place a patch over the affected eye if the client has diplopia
  6. Increase mobility as tolerated
  7. Encourage fluids and high-fiber diet
  8. Administer stool softeners as prescribed
  9. Encourage the client to express feelings
  10. Encourage independence in activities of daily living
  11. Assess the need for assistive devices such as a cane, walker, splints, or braces
  12. Teach transfer technique from bed to chair, and chair to bed
  13. Provide gait training
  14. Initiate physical and occupational therapy
  15. Refer to speech and language pathologist

XII. Multiple Sclerosis

A. Description
  1. A chronic, progressive, noncontagious, degenerative disease of the CNS characterized by demyelinization of the neurons
  2. It usually occurs between the ages of 20 and 40 and consists of periods of remission and exacerbation
  3. The causes are unknown but thought to be a result of autoimmune response or viral infection

4. Precipitating factors include pregnancy, fatigue, stress, infection, and trauma
5. EEG findings are abnormal
6. A lumbar puncture indicates increased gamma globulin but the serum globulin level is normal

B. Assessment
1. Fatigue and weakness
2. Ataxia and vertigo
3. Tremors and spasticity of the lower extremities
4. Parasthesias
5. Blurred vision and diplopia
6. Nystagmus
7. Dysphasia
8. Decreased perception to pain, touch, and temperature
9. Bladder and bowel disturbances including urgency, frequency, retention, and incontinence
10. Abnormal reflexes including hyperreflexia, absent reflexes, and positive **Babinski reflex**
11. Emotion changes such as apathy, euphoria, irritability, and depression
12. Memory changes and confusion

C. Implementation
1. Provide bed rest during exacerbation
2. Protect the client from injury by providing safety measures
3. Place an eyepatch on the eye for diplopia
4. Monitor for potential complications such as urinary tract infections, calculi, decubitus ulcers, respiratory tract infections, and contractures
5. Promote regular elimination by bladder and bowel training
6. Encourage independence
7. Assist the client to establish a regular exercise and rest program
8. Assess the need for and provide assistive devices
9. Initiate physical and speech therapy
10. Instruct the client to avoid fatigue, stress, infection, overheating, and chilling
11. Instruct clients to balance moderate activity with rest periods
12. Instruct clients to increase fluids and eat a balanced diet including low fat, high fiber, and foods high in potassium
13. Instruct the client in safety measures related to sensory loss, such as regulating the temperature of bathwater and avoiding heating pads
14. Instruct the client in safety measures related to motor loss, such as avoiding the use of scatter rugs and using assistive devices such as a walker or cane
15. Instruct the client in the self-administration of prescribed medications (Box 65–17)
16. Provide information about National Multiple Sclerosis Society

---

BOX 65–17. Medications Used with Multiple Sclerosis

STEROIDS

Used to reduce edema and the inflammatory response

Used to decrease the length of time the client's symptoms are exacerbated and improve the degree of recovery

IMMUNOSUPPRESSIVES

Used for the treatment of chronic progressive MS to stabilize the disease process

BACLOFEN (LIORESAL), DANTROLENE (DANTRIUM), or DIAZEPAM (VALIUM)

Used to lessen muscle spasticity

CARBAMAZEPINE (TEGRETOL)

Used to treated paresthesia

PROPRANOLOL (INDERAL) and CLONAZEPAM (CLONOPIN)

Used to treat cerebellar ataxia

BETHANECHOL (URECHOLINE)

Used to prevent urinary retention

OXYBUTYNIN CHLORIDE (DITROPAN)

Used to increase bladder capacity

XIII. Myasthenia Gravis

A. Description
1. A neuromuscular disease characterized by marked weakness and abnormal fatigue of the voluntary muscles
2. A defect in the transmission of nerve impulses at the myoneural junction occurs
3. Causes include insufficient secretion of acetylcholine, excessive secretion of cholinesterase, or unresponsiveness of the muscle fibers to acetylcholine

B. Assessment
1. Weakness and fatigue
2. Difficulty chewing
3. Dysphagia
4. Ptosis
5. Diplopia
6. Weak, hoarse voice
7. Difficulty breathing
8. Diminished breath sounds
9. Respiratory paralysis and failure

C. Implementation
1. Monitor respiratory status and ability to cough and deep breathe adequately
2. Monitor for respiratory failure
3. Maintain suctioning and emergency equipment at bedside
4. Monitor vital signs
5. Monitor speech and swallowing abilities to prevent aspiration

6. Encourage the client to sit up when eating
7. Assess muscle status
8. Instruct the client to conserve strength
9. Plan short activities that coincide with times of maximal muscle strength
10. Monitor for myasthenic and cholinergic crises
11. Administer anticholinesterase medications as prescribed
12. Instruct the client to avoid stress, infection, fatigue, and over-the-counter drugs
13. Instruct the client to wear a Medic-Alert bracelet
14. Inform clients about services from the Myasthenia Gravis Foundation

D. Anticholinesterase medications
  1. Action: increase levels of acetylcholine at myoneural junction
  2. Medications
     a. Neostigmine bromide (Prostigmin)
     b. Pyridostigmine bromide (Mestinon)
     c. Physostigmine (Antilirium)
     d. Edrophonium chloride (Tensilon)
  3. Side effects
     a. Sweating
     b. Salivation
     c. Nausea
     d. Diarrhea and abdominal cramps
     e. Bradycardia
     f. Hypotension
  4. Implementation
     a. Administer medications on time
     b. Administer medication 30 minutes before meals with milk and crackers to reduce GI upset
     c. Monitor and record muscle strength
     d. Note that excessive doses lead to cholinergic crisis
     e. Have the antidote (atropine) available

E. Myasthenic crisis
  1. Description
     a. Acute exacerbation of the disease
     b. Caused by a rapid, unrecognized progression of the disease, an inadequate amount of medication, infection, fatigue, or stress
  2. Assessment
     a. Weakness
     b. Dyspnea
     c. Dysphagia
     d. Restlessness
     e. Difficulty speaking
  3. Implementation
     a. Assess for signs of myasthenic crisis
     b. Increase anticholinesterase medication

F. Cholinergic crisis
  1. Description
     a. Depolarization of the motor end plates
     b. Caused by overmedication with anticholinesterase
  2. Assessment
     a. Restlessness

b. Weakness
c. Dysphagia
d. Dyspnea
e. Nausea, vomiting, and diarrhea
f. Fasciculations
g. Sweating
h. Salivation
i. Increased bronchial secretions
  3. Implementation
     a. Hold anticholinesterase medication
     b. Prepare to administer the antidote, atropine, if prescribed

G. Tensilon test
  1. Description: test done to diagnose myasthenia gravis and to differentiate between myasthenic crisis and cholinergic crisis
  2. To diagnose myasthenia gravis
     a. Tensilon injection is given to the client
     b. Positive for myasthenia: client shows improvement in muscle strength after the administration of Tensilon
     c. Negative for myasthenia: client shows no improvement in muscle strength, and strength may even deteriorate after injection of Tensilon
  3. To differentiate crisis
     a. Myasthenic crisis: Tensilon is administered and if strength improves, the client needs more medication
     b. Cholinergic crisis: Tensilon is administered and if weakness is more severe, an overdose of medication has occurred; administer atropine, the antidote, as prescribed

XIV. Parkinson's disease

A. Description (Box 65–18)
  1. A degenerative disease caused by the depletion of dopamine, which interferes with the inhibition of excitatory impulses
  2. It results in a dysfunction of the extrapyramidal system

BOX 65–18. Stages of Parkinson's Disease
STAGE 1 Unilateral involvement
STAGE 2 Bilateral involvement
STAGE 3 Impaired balance
STAGE 4 Fully developed severe disease
STAGE 5 Confinement to bed or a wheelchair

3. It is a slow, progressive disease that results in a crippling disability
4. The debilitation can result in falls, self-care deficits, depression, and failure of body systems
5. Mental deterioration occurs late in the disease

B. Assessment
1. Bradykinesia, abnormal slowness of movement, and sluggishness of physical and mental responses
2. Aching shoulders and arms
3. Monotonous speech
4. Handwriting that becomes progressively smaller
5. Tremors in the hands and fingers at rest (pill rolling)
6. Tremors increasing when fatigued and decreasing with purposeful activity or sleep
7. Rigidity with jerky interrupted movements
8. Restlessness and pacing
9. Blank facial expression
10. Drooling
11. Difficulty swallowing and speaking
12. Loss of coordination and balance
13. Shuffling steps, stooped position, and propulsive gait

C. Implementation
1. Assess neurological status
2. Assess ability to swallow and chew
3. Provide high-calorie, high-protein, high-fiber soft diet with small frequent feedings
4. Increase fluids to 2000 mL/day
5. Promote independence along with safety measures
6. Avoid rushing clients with activities
7. Assist with ambulation
8. Provide assistive devices
9. Instruct the client to wear low-heeled shoes
10. Encourage clients to lift feet when walking and to avoid prolonged sitting
11. Provide a firm mattress and position the client prone, without a pillow, to facilitate proper posture
12. Instruct proper posture by teaching the client to hold the hands behind the back to keep the spine and neck erect
13. Monitor for constipation
14. Promote physical therapy and rehabilitation
15. Administer anticholinergic medications as prescribed to treat tremors and rigidity and to inhibit the action of acetylcholine (Box 65–19)
16. Administer antiparkinsonian medications to increase the level of dopamine in the CNS (Box 65–19)
17. Instruct the client to avoid foods high in vitamin B_6 because they block the effects of antiparkinsonian medications
18. Instruct client to avoid monoamine oxidase (MAO) inhibitors because they will precipitate hypertensive crisis

---

BOX 65–19. Medications to Treat Parkinson's

Amantadine hydrochloride (Symadine, Symmetrel)
Ethopropazine hydrochloride (Parsidol)
Levodopa (Dopar, Larodopa)
Carbidopa and levodopa (Sinemet)
Trihexphenidyl hydrochloride (Artane)
Procyclidine hydrochloride (Kemadrin)
Benztropine mesylate (Cogentin)
Bromocriptine (Parlodel)

XV. Trigeminal Neuralgia

A. Description
1. A sensory disorder of the fifth cranial nerve
2. Results in severe, recurrent, sharp, facial pain along the trigeminal nerve

B. Assessment
1. Pain on the lips, gums, nose, or across the cheeks
2. Situations that stimulate symptoms such as cold, washing the face, chewing, or food or fluids of extreme temperatures

C. Implementation
1. Instruct clients to avoid hot or cold foods and fluids
2. Provide small feedings of liquid and soft foods
3. Instruct the client to chew food on the unaffected side
4. Administer medications as prescribed (Box 65–20)

D. Surgical implementation
1. An alcohol injection along affected portion of the nerve to produce anesthesia of the nerve may provide relief of pain for up to 16 months
2. Retrogasserian rhizotomy or total severance of the sensory root of the trigeminal nerve
3. Jannetta procedure, which surgically relocates the artery that is compressing the trigeminal nerve
4. Electrocoagulation or percutaneous radiofrequency rhizotomy to create a heat lesion

XVI. Bell's Palsy (Facial Paralysis)

A. Description
1. A lower motor neuron lesion of the seventh cranial nerve that may occur as a result of trauma, hemorrhage, meningitis, or a tumor

---

BOX 65–20. Medications to Treat Trigeminal Neuralgia

Carbamazepine (Tegretol)
Phenytoin (Dilantin)
Baclofen (Lioresal)

2. It results in paralysis of one side of the face
3. Recovery usually occurs in a few weeks without residual effects

B. Assessment
1. Flaccid facial muscles
2. Inability to raise the eyebrows, frown, smile, close the eyelids, or puff out the cheeks
3. Upward movement of the eye when attempting to close the eyelid
4. Loss of taste

C. Implementation
1. Encourage active facial exercise to prevent the loss of muscle tone
2. Provide a face sling to prevent stretching of weak muscles
3. Protect the eyes from dryness and to prevent injury
4. Promote good oral care
5. Instruct client to chew on the unaffected side
6. Administer analgesics and steroids as prescribed

XVII. Guillain-Barré Syndrome

A. Description
1. An acute infectious neuronitis of the cranial and peripheral nerves
2. The immune system overreacts to the infection and destroys the myelin sheath
3. It is usually preceded by a mild upper respiratory infection or gastroenteritis
4. The recovery is a slow process and can take years
5. The major concern is difficulty breathing

B. Assessment
1. Paresthesias
2. Weakness of lower extremities
3. Gradual progressive weakness of upper extremities and facial muscles
4. Can progress to respiratory failure
5. Cardiac dysrhythmias
6. Cerebrospinal fluid reveals an elevated protein level
7. EEG is abnormal

C. Implementation
1. Care is directed toward the treatment of symptoms
2. Monitor respiratory status
3. Provide respiratory treatments
4. Prepare to initiate respiratory support
5. Monitor cardiac status
6. Assess for complications of immobility
7. Provide client and family support

XVIII. Amyotrophic Lateral Sclerosis

A. Description
1. Also known as Lou Gehrig's disease
2. A progressive degenerative disease involving the motor system
3. The sensory and autonomic systems are not involved and mental status changes do not result from the disease
4. The cause of the disease may be related to an excess of glutamate, a chemical responsible for relaying messages between the motor neurons
5. As the disease progresses, muscle weakness and atrophy develop until a flaccid quadriplegia develops
6. Eventually the respiratory muscles become affected, leading to respiratory compromise, pneumonia, and death
7. There is no known cure and the treatment is symptomatic

B. Assessment
1. Fatigue
2. Fatigue while talking
3. Muscle weakness
4. Muscle atrophy
5. Tongue atrophy
6. Dysphagia
7. Weakness of the hands and arms
8. Fasciculations of the face
9. Nasal quality of speech
10. Dysarthria

C. Implementation
1. Care is directed toward the treatment of symptoms
2. Monitor respiratory status
3. Provide respiratory treatments
4. Prepare to initiate respiratory support
5. Assess for complications of immobility
6. Provide client and family support

XIX. Encephalitis

A. Description
1. An inflammation of the brain parenchyma and often the meninges
2. Affects the cerebrum, the brain stem, and/or the cerebellum
3. Most often caused by a viral agent, although bacteria, fungi, or parasites may also be involved
4. Viral encephalitis is almost always preceded by a viral infection

B. Transmission
1. Arboviruses can be transmitted to humans through the bite of an infected mosquito or tick
2. Echovirus, coxsackievirus, poliovirus, herpes zoster, and viruses that cause mumps and chickenpox are common enteroviruses associated with encephalitis
3. Herpes simplex type 1 virus can cause viral encephalitis
4. Amebic meningoencephalitis can enter the nasal mucosa of people swimming in warm fresh water, ponds, and lakes

C. Assessment
1. Presence of cold sores, lesions, or ulcerations of the oral cavity

2. History of insect bites and swimming in fresh water
3. Exposure to infectious diseases
4. Travel to areas where the disease is prevalent
5. Fever
6. Nausea and vomiting
7. Stiff neck
8. Changes in LOC and mental status
9. Symptoms of **increased ICP**
10. Motor dysfunction and focal neurological deficits

D. Implementation
1. Monitor vital and neurological signs
2. Assess LOC using the **Glasgow Coma Scale**
3. Assess mental status changes and personality and behavior changes
4. Assess for signs of **increased intracranial pressure**
5. Assess for presence of nuchal rigidity and a positive Kernig's or **Brudzinski's sign** indicating meningeal irritation
6. Assist the client to turn, cough, and deep breathe frequently
7. Elevate the head of the bed 30 to 45 degrees
8. Assess for muscle and neurological deficits
9. Administer acyclovir (Zovirax) as prescribed
10. Initiate rehabilitation as needed for motor dysfunction or neurological deficits

XX. Meningitis

A. Description
1. Inflammation of the arachnoid and pia mater of the brain and spinal cord
2. Caused by bacterial and viral organisms, although fungal and protozoal meningitis also occur
3. Predisposing factors include skull fractures, brain or spinal surgery, sinus or upper respiratory infections, the use of nasal sprays, and individuals with compromised immune systems
4. CSF fluid is analyzed to determine the diagnosis and the type of meningitis

B. Transmission
1. Direct contact, including droplet spread
2. Occurs in areas of high population density, crowded living areas, and prisons

C. Assessment
1. Mild lethargy
2. Memory changes
3. Short attention span
4. Bewilderment
5. Personality and behavior changes
6. Severe headache
7. Generalized muscle aches and pains
8. Nausea and vomiting
9. Fever and chills
10. Tachycardia
11. Deterioration in the level of consciousness
12. Red, macular rash with meningococcal meningitis

13. Abdominal and chest pain with viral meningitis
14. Photophobia
15. Signs of meningeal irritation such as nuchal rigidity and a positive Kernig's and **Brudzinski's sign**

D. Implementation
1. Monitor vital signs and neurological signs
2. Assess for signs of **increasing ICP**
3. Initiate seizure precautions
4. Monitor for seizure activity
5. Monitor for signs of meningeal irritation
6. Perform cranial nerve assessment
7. Assess vascular status
8. Maintain isolation precautions as necessary with bacterial meningitis
9. Maintain urine and stool precautions with viral meningitis
10. Maintain respiratory isolation for the client with pneumococcal meningitis
11. Elevate the head of the bed 30 degrees and avoid neck flexion and extreme hip flexion
12. Prevent stimulation and restrict visitors
13. Administer analgesics as prescribed
14. Administer antibiotics as prescribed

PRACTICE QUESTIONS

1. The client is experiencing chronic insomnia. The nurse interprets that which of the following areas of the nervous system is involved?
   1 Hippocampus and frontal lobe
   2 Temporal lobe and frontal lobe
   3 Reticular activating system and cerebral hemispheres
   4 Limbic system and cerebral hemispheres

2. The client has an impairment of cranial nerve II. Specific to this impairment, the nurse plans to do which of the following to ensure client safety?
   1 Provide a clear path for ambulation without obstacles
   2 Test the temperature of the shower water
   3 Speak loudly to the client
   4 Check the temperature of the food on the dietary tray

3. The client has a neurological deficit involving the limbic system. Specific to this type of deficit, the nurse documents which of the following information related to the client's behavior?
   1 Demonstrates inability to add and subtract; does not know who is president
   2 Cannot recall what was eaten for breakfast today
   3 Disoriented to person, place, and time
   4 Affect flat, with periods of emotional lability

4. The client has a cerebellar lesion. The nurse evaluates that the client is adapting successfully to this problem if the client demonstrates proper use of which of the following items?

1 Adaptive eating utensils
2 Walker
3 Raised toilet seat
4 Slider board

5. The nurse is planning to test the function of the trigeminal nerve (cranial nerve V). The nurse gathers which of the following items to perform the test?
   1 Flashlight, pupil size chart, or millimeter ruler
   2 Tuning fork and audiometer
   3 Safety pin, hot and cold water in test tubes, cotton wisp
   4 Snellen chart, ophthalmoscope

6. The nurse is testing the coordinated functioning of cranial nerves III, IV, and VI. To do this correctly, the nurse tests the
   1 Corneal reflex
   2 Six cardinal fields of gaze
   3 Pupil response to light
   4 Pupil response to light and accommodation

7. The client has dysfunction of the cochlear division of the vestibulcochlear nerve (cranial nerve VIII). The nurse evaluates that the client is adequately adapting to this problem if the client states a plan to obtain a
   1 Hearing aid
   2 Walker
   3 Pair of eyeglasses
   4 Bath thermometer

8. The nurse is assessing the muscle strength of the client. The nurse asks the client to hold the arms up and supinated, as if holding a tray, and then asks the client to close the eyes. The client's left hand turns and moves downward slightly. The nurse interprets that the client has
   1 Hyperreflexia
   2 Ataxia
   3 Pronator drift
   4 Nystagmus

9. The nurse is assessing the motor function of an unconscious client. The nurse plans to use which of the following to test the client's peripheral response to pain?
   1 Sternal rub
   2 Pressure on the orbital rim
   3 Squeezing of the sternocleidomastoid muscle
   4 Nailbed pressure

10. The nurse is testing the client for astereognosis. The nurse asks the client to close the eyes and to
    1 Think of a number and write it on a piece of paper
    2 Identify three objects placed in the hand, one at a time
    3 State whether one or two skin pricks are felt, after pricking the client's skin bilaterally in the same place
    4 Identify the smallest distance where two pricks can be felt, after pricking the client's skin with two pins at varying distances

11. The client has an impaired corneal reflex on one side. The client demonstrates the best understanding of how to protect the eye by stating intention to
    1 Wear an eyepatch
    2 Tape the eye shut during the day
    3 Use sterile saline drops every few hours to keep the eye moist
    4 Wipe inside the lower eyelid with a cotton-tipped applicator three times a day

12. The nurse is assessing the client's gait, which is characterized by unsteadiness and staggering steps. The nurse interprets this gait as being
    1 Spastic
    2 Ataxic
    3 Festinating
    4 Dystrophic or broad-based

13. The nurse is planning care for the client who displays confusion secondary to a neurological problem. Which of the following approaches by the nurse is least helpful in assisting this client?
    1 Giving simple, clear directions
    2 Providing a stable environment
    3 Providing sensory cues
    4 Encouraging multiple visitors at one time

14. The client with a neurological impairment experiences urinary incontinence. Which of the following nursing actions is most useful in helping the client adapt to this alteration?
    1 Establishing a toileting schedule
    2 Inserting a Foley catheter
    3 Using adult diapers
    4 Padding the bed with an absorbent cotton pad

15. The nurse is conducting a neurological assessment including a health history on a client with a neurological disorder. The client appears to have difficulty in answering the questions. The nurse should
    1 Defer the health history and proceed with the neurological examination
    2 Defer both the health history and neurological examination
    3 Ask a family member to stay during the interview
    4 Ask a second nurse to be present during the interview

16. The nurse has obtained a personal and family history for the client with a neurological disorder. Which of the following factors in the client's

history does not give the client added risk for neurological problems?
1 Previous back injury
2 Allergy to pollen
3 History of hypertension
4 History of headaches

17. The nurse has formulated a nursing diagnosis of Ineffective Breathing Pattern for a client with a neurological disorder. The nurse avoids including which of the following activities in the care plan for this client?
1 Keep the head and neck in good alignment
2 Elevate the head of the bed 30 degrees
3 Keep the client lying in a supine position
4 Keep suction equipment at the bedside

18. The client with a neurological problem has a nursing diagnosis of Hyperthermia. Which of the following measures does the nurse avoid while trying to lower the client's body temperature?
1 Giving tepid sponge baths
2 Administering acetaminophen (Tylenol) per protocol
3 Applying a hypothermia blanket
4 Placing ice packs in the axilla and groin areas

19. The client with right leg hemiplegia has a nursing diagnosis of Impaired Physical Mobility. The nurse evaluates that the family needs reinforcement of teaching if the nurse observes which of the following being done by the family?
1 Encouraging the client to stand unassisted on the leg
2 Active range of motion (ROM) to the affected leg
3 Passive ROM to the affected leg
4 Application of a premolded splint

20. The nurse is preparing a client who is scheduled to have a cerebral angiogram performed. The nurse assesses the client for
1 Allergy to salmon
2 Allergy to iodine or shellfish
3 Claustrophobia
4 Excessive weight

21. The client admitted with a neurological problem indicates to the nurse that magnetic resonance imaging (MRI) may be done. The nurse interprets that the client may be ineligible for this diagnostic procedure based on the client's history of
1 Hypertension
2 Chronic obstructive pulmonary disorder
3 Heart failure
4 Prosthetic valve replacement

22. The client is having a lumbar puncture (LP) performed. The nurse positions the client in which of the following positions for the procedure?
1 Side-lying, with legs pulled up and head bent down onto the chest
2 Side-lying, with a pillow under the hip
3 Prone, in slight Trendelenburg
4 Prone, with a pillow under the abdomen

23. The client is somewhat nervous about having an MRI. Which of the following statements by the nurse provides the most reassurance to the client about the procedure?
1 "It is necessary to remove any metal or metal-containing objects before having the MRI done to prevent the metal from being drawn into the magnetic field."
2 "The MRI machine is a long, hollow narrow tube and may make you feel somewhat claustrophobic."
3 "Even though you are alone in the scanner, you will be in voice communication with the technologist during the procedure."
4 "You will be able to eat before the procedure unless you get nauseated easily. If so, you should eat lightly."

24. The client has just undergone computed tomography (CT) scanning with a contrast medium. The nurse evaluates that the client understands postprocedure care if the client verbalizes to
1 Eat lightly for the remainder of the day
2 Rest quietly for the remainder of the day
3 Hold medications for at least 4 hours
4 Force fluids for the day

25. The nurse is assisting with caloric testing of the oculovestibular reflex of an unconscious client. Cold water is injected into the left auditory canal. The client exhibits horizontal nystagmus toward the right. The nurse understands that this indicates the client has
1 A cerebral lesion
2 A temporal lesion
3 An intact brain stem
4 Brain death

26. The nurse is admitting the client to the short stay unit following a myelogram. A water-based contrast agent was used. The nurse plans which of the following activity restrictions for the client?
1 Bed rest for 6 to 8 hours, with head of the bed elevated 15 to 30 degrees
2 Bed rest for 2 to 4 hours, with head of the bed elevated 15 to 30 degrees
3 Bed rest for 6 to 8 hours, with the head of the bed flat
4 Bed rest for 2 to 4 hours, with the head of the bed flat

27. The nurse is administering mouth care to an unconscious client. The nurse should avoid doing which of the following?
   1 Positioning the client on the side
   2 Using products with lemon or alcohol
   3 Cleansing the mucous membranes with Toothettes
   4 Brushing the teeth with a small toothbrush

28. The nurse has formulated a nursing diagnosis of Altered Nutrition: Less Than Body Requirements for the unconscious client. Which of the following outcomes indicates to the nurse that the goals have not yet been fully met?
   1 Stable weight
   2 Intake equaling output
   3 BUN 12 mg/dL
   4 Total protein 4.5 g/dL

29. The nurse assigned to an unconscious client is making initial daily rounds. Upon entering the room, the nurse notes that the client is lying supine in bed, with the head of bed elevated approximately 5 degrees. The nasogastric tube feeding is running at 70 mL/hour as ordered. The nurse auscultates adventitious breath sounds. Which of the following nursing diagnoses does the nurse formulate for that client?
   1 Risk for Altered Nutrition: Less Than Body Requirements
   2 Risk for Injury
   3 Risk for Aspiration
   4 Risk for Fluid Volume Deficit

30. The nurse is trying to help the family of an unconscious client cope with the situation. Which of the following interventions does the nurse plan to incorporate into the care routine for the client?
   1 Discouraging the family from touching the client
   2 Explaining equipment and procedures on an ongoing basis
   3 Ensuring adherence to visiting hours to ensure client's rest
   4 Encouraging family not to "give in" to their feelings of grief

31. The nurse is suctioning the unconscious client with a tracheostomy. The nurse should avoid which of the following actions?
   1 Keeping a supply of suction catheters at the bedside
   2 Auscultating breath sounds to determine the need for suctioning
   3 Hyperoxygenating the client before, during, and after suctioning
   4 Suctioning for longer than 10 seconds

32. The nurse has implemented a bowel training program for the unconscious client. The nurse evaluates the plan as successful if which of the following methods stimulates a bowel movement?
   1 Fleet enema
   2 Soap solution enema (SSE)
   3 Glycerin suppository
   4 Fecal disimpaction

33. The nurse checks the gastric residual of an unconscious client receiving nasogastric tube feedings continuously at 50 mL/hour. The nurse notes that every 4 hours or so, the residual is greater than 100 mL. The nurse interprets that the client is experiencing
   1 Too slow an infusion rate
   2 Delayed gastric emptying
   3 Early signs of peptic ulcer
   4 Air in the stomach

34. The nurse has formulated the nursing diagnosis Risk for Impaired Skin Integrity for an unconscious client. The nurse does not include which of the following interventions when writing the plan of care?
   1 Reposition every 2 hours and massage bony prominences
   2 Apply protective pads to heels and elbows
   3 Add a small amount of alcohol to the daily bathwater
   4 Provide perineal care every 8 hours and after incontinence

35. The nurse has applied a hypothermia blanket to a client with a fever. The nurse inspects the skin frequently to detect which complication of hypothermia blanket use?
   1 Skin breakdown
   2 Frostbite
   3 Arterial insufficiency
   4 Venous insufficiency

36. The home care nurse has placed a hyperthermic client in a bath of tepid water. The nurse evaluates that the client can safely come out of the tub when the client's temperature descends to at least
   1 98.6°F
   2 99°F
   3 102°F
   4 104°F

37. The nurse is caring for an unconscious client who is experiencing persistent hyperthermia with no signs and symptoms of infection. The nurse interprets that there may be damage to the client's thermoregulatory center in the
   1 Cerebrum
   2 Cerebellum
   3 Hippocampus
   4 Hypothalamus

38. The nurse has an order to administer medication to the client who is shivering because of hyper-

thermia. Which of the following medications does the nurse plan to administer?
1 Prochlorperazine (Compazine)
2 Chlorpromazine (Thorazine)
3 Thioridazine (Mellaril)
4 Fluphenazine (Prolixin)

39. The client seeking treatment for an episode of hyperthermia is being discharged to home. The nurse evaluates that the client needs clarification of discharge instructions if the client states to
1 Stay in a cool environment when possible
2 Increase fluid intake for the next 24 hours
3 Monitor voiding for adequacy of urine output
4 Resume full activity level immediately

40. The nurse is caring for the client with an increased intracranial pressure (ICP). The nurse assesses which of the following trends in vital signs if the intracranial pressure is rising?
1 Increasing temperature, increasing pulse, increasing respirations, decreasing BP
2 Increasing temperature, decreasing pulse, decreasing respirations, increasing BP
3 Decreasing temperature, decreasing pulse, increasing respirations, decreasing BP
4 Decreasing temperature, increasing pulse, decreasing respirations, increasing BP

41. The nurse is caring for a client with an ICP monitoring device. The nurse becomes most concerned if the ICP readings drifted to and stayed in the vicinity of
1 3 mmHg
2 8 mmHg
3 11 mmHg
4 15 mmHg

42. The nurse is planning care for the client with ICP monitoring. Which of the following interventions is contraindicated in the plan of care?
1 Using strict aseptic technique when touching the monitoring system
2 Assessing the insertion site for signs and symptoms of infection
3 Leveling the transducer at the lowest point of the ear
4 Checking all stopcocks and connections for leaks

43. The nurse is positioning the client with increased ICP. Which of the following positions does the nurse avoid?
1 Head turned to the side
2 Head midline
3 Neck in neutral position
4 Head of the bed elevated 30 to 45 degrees

44. The client recovering from head injury is arousable and participating in care. The nurse evalu-

ates that the client understands measures to prevent elevations in intracranial pressure if the nurse observes the client doing which of the following activities?
1 Exhaling during repositioning
2 Isometric exercises
3 Blowing the nose
4 Coughing vigorously

45. The family of an unconscious client with increased intracranial pressure is talking at the client's bedside. They are discussing the gravity of the client's condition and wondering if the client will ever recover. The nurse intervenes, based on the understanding that
1 The family needs immediate crisis intervention
2 The family could benefit from a conference with the physician
3 It is possible the client can hear the family
4 The client might have wanted a visit from the hospital chaplain

46. The client is being hyperventilated by a mechanical ventilator to decrease the ICP. The nurse plans to monitor arterial blood gas results and report values that are outside which of the following ranges?
1 PaO_2 60 to 100 mmHg, $PaCO_2$ 25 to 30 mmHg
2 PaO_2 60 to 100 mmHg, $PaCO_2$ 30 to 35 mmHg
3 PaO_2 80 to 100 mmHg, $PaCO_2$ 35 to 40 mmHg
4 PaO_2 80 to 100 mmHg, $PaCO_2$ 25 to 30 mmHg

47. The nurse is providing care to the client with ICP. Which of the following approaches may not be beneficial in controlling the client's ICP from an environmental viewpoint?
1 Maintaining a calm atmosphere
2 Reducing environmental noise
3 Clustering nursing activities to be done all at one time
4 Allowing the client uninterrupted time for sleep

48. The client is recovering from an injury that caused an ICP. The nurse evaluates that the client has the best return of neurological functioning if the client has which of the following sets of scores on the Glasgow Coma Scale?
1 Best eye-opening response 3, best motor response 8, best verbal response 6
2 Best eye-opening response 5, best motor response 4, best verbal response 8
3 Best eye-opening response 4, best motor response 6, best verbal response 5
4 Best eye-opening response 6, best motor response 5, best verbal response 4

49. The client has clear fluid leaking from the nose following basilar skull fracture. The nurse assesses that this is CSF if the fluid
    1 Clumps together on the dressing and has a pH of 7
    2 Separates into concentric rings and tests positive for glucose
    3 Is grossly bloody in appearance and has a pH of 6
    4 Is clear in appearance and tests negative for glucose

50. The home care nurse is making extended follow-up visits to a client discharged from the hospital after a moderately severe head injury. The family states that the client is behaving differently than before the accident. The client is more fatigued and irritable, and has some memory problems. The client, who was previously very even-tempered, is prone to outbursts of temper now. The nurse counsels the family based on an understanding that these behaviors
    1 Are short-term problems that will resolve in about a month
    2 Will probably be long-term sequelae of the injury
    3 Indicate a worsening of the original injury
    4 Will come and go as intracranial pressure changes

51. The client is admitted for observation after an auto accident with probable minor head injury. The nurse plans on leaving the cervical collar in place until
    1 The physician makes rounds
    2 The family comes to visit
    3 The results of spinal x-rays are known
    4 The nurse needs to do physical care

52. The client with a head injury has begun putting out copious amounts of urine through the Foley catheter. The client's urine output for the previous shift was 3000 mL. The nurse implements a new physician order to administer
    1 Desmopressin (DDAVP)
    2 Dexamethasone (Decadron)
    3 Ethacrynic acid (Edecrin)
    4 Mannitol (Osmitrol)

53. The client was seen and treated in the emergency department for treatment of a concussion. The nurse evaluates that the family need reinforcement of the discharge instructions if they verbalize to call the physician for which of the following client signs and symptoms?
    1 Difficulty speaking
    2 Difficulty awakening
    3 Vomiting
    4 Minor headache

54. The nurse is caring for the client in the emergency department after head injury. The client momentarily lost consciousness at the time of the injury, then regained it. The client has now lost consciousness again. The nurse takes quick action, knowing this is compatible with
    1 Skull fracture
    2 Concussion
    3 Subdural hematoma
    4 Epidural hematoma

55. The nurse is conducting home visits for a head-injured client with residual cognitive deficits. The client has problems with memory, shortened attention span, easy distractibility, and slow processing of information. The nurse plans to talk with the primary physician about a referral to a
    1 Psychologist
    2 Neuropsychologist
    3 Social worker
    4 Vocational rehabilitation specialist

56. The nurse is caring for a client who has undergone craniotomy with a supratentorial incision. The nurse uses which of the following postoperative positions?
    1 Head of the bed flat, head and neck midline
    2 Head of the bed flat, head turned to the nonoperative side
    3 Head of the bed elevated 30 to 45 degrees, head and neck midline
    4 Head of the bed elevated 30 to 45 degrees, head turned to the operative side

57. The nurse is evaluating the status of the client who had a craniotomy 3 days ago. The nurse suspects the client is developing meningitis as a complication of surgery if the client exhibits
    1 Positive Brudzinski's sign
    2 Negative Kernig's sign
    3 Absence of nuchal rigidity
    4 Glasgow Coma Scale score of 15

58. The nurse is assessing the fluid balance of a client after craniotomy. The nurse assesses for which of the following signs of overhydration, which would aggravate cerebral edema?
    1 Shift intake 950 mL, output 900 mL
    2 Unchanged weight
    3 BUN 10 mg/dL
    4 Serum osmolality 280 mOsm/kg H_2O

59. The nurse is preparing to give the postcraniotomy client medication for incisional pain. The family asks the nurse why the client is receiving codeine and not "something stronger." In formulating a response, the nurse incorporates the understanding that codeine
    1 Is one of the strongest narcotic analgesics available
    2 Cannot lead to physical or psychological dependence

3 Does not cause gastrointestinal upset or constipation as other narcotics do

4 Does not alter respirations or mask neurologic signs as other narcotics do

60. The nurse is developing a discharge teaching plan for the postcraniotomy client, including home care considerations. Which of the following items does the nurse not include in the teaching plan?

1 Tub bath or shower is permitted, but keep the scalp dry until sutures are removed

2 Use a check-off system for anticonvulsant medications to avoid missing doses

3 The client after craniotomy will not hear sounds clearly unless they are loud

4 If the client is prone to seizures or gets dizzy spells, someone should be with the client while walking

61. The nurse has an order to give "dexamethasone (Decadron) 4 mg IV now" to the postcraniotomy client. The nurse administers the medication

1 IV push over 1 minute

2 IV push over 4 minutes

3 IV piggyback over 10 minutes

4 IV piggyback over 30 minutes

62. The nurse has formulated a nursing diagnosis of Body Image Disturbance for the client after craniotomy. The nurse evaluates that the client has not met the outcome criteria by discharge if the client

1 Wears a turban to cover the incision

2 States an intention to purchase a hairpiece until the hair has grown back

3 Verbalizes that periorbital bruising will disappear over time

4 Indicates that facial puffiness will be a permanent problem

63. The client with a spinal cord injury at the level of C5 has a weakened respiratory effort, ineffective cough, and is using accessory neck muscles in breathing. The nurse carefully monitors the client and formulates which of the following nursing diagnoses?

1 Ineffective Breathing Pattern

2 Impaired Gas Exchange

3 Risk for Aspiration

4 Risk for Injury

64. The client with a cervical spine injury has Crutchfield tongs applied in the emergency department. The nurse avoids which of the following when planning care for this client?

1 Use of a Roto-Rest bed

2 Assessment of the integrity of the weights and pulleys

3 Comparing the amount of ordered traction with the amount in use

4 Removing the weights to reposition the client

65. The client with spinal cord injury becomes angry and belligerent whenever the nurse tries to administer care. The nurse should

1 Advise the client that rehabilitation progresses more quickly with cooperation

2 Acknowledge the client's anger and continue to encourage participation in care

3 Leave the client alone until ready to participate

4 Ask the family to deliver the care

66. The nurse has completed discharge instructions for the client with application of a Halo vest. The nurse evaluates that the client needs further clarification of the instructions if the client states to

1 Use caution because the vest alters balance

2 Wash the skin daily under the lamb's wool liner of the vest

3 Use a straw for drinking

4 Drive only during the daytime

67. The nurse is caring for the client who suffered a spinal cord injury 48 hours ago. The nurse detects gastrointestinal complications by assessing for

1 Flattened abdomen

2 Hematest-positive nasogastric tube (NGT) drainage

3 Hyperactive bowel sounds

4 History of diarrhea

68. The client with spinal cord injury expresses little interest in food and is very particular about the choice of meals that are actually eaten. The nurse interprets that

1 Meal choices represent an area of client control and should be encouraged as much as is nutritionally reasonable

2 Anorexia is a sign of clinical depression, and a referral to a psychologist is needed

3 The client has compulsive habits, which should be ignored as long as they are not harmful

4 The client probably has a naturally slow metabolism, and the decreased nutritional intake won't matter

69. The client with paraplegia has a Risk for Injury related to spasticity of leg muscles. Which of the following items does the nurse not include in a plan to minimize the risk of injury to the client?

1 Removing potentially harmful objects near the spastic limbs

2 Performing range of motion to the affected limbs

3 Use of padded restraints to immobilize the limb

4 Use of PRN orders for muscle relaxants such as baclofen (Lioresal)

70. The nurse is teaching the paraplegic client measures to promote skin integrity. Which of the following instructions will be least helpful to the client?
    1. Shifting weight every 2 hours while in a wheelchair
    2. Using a mirror to inspect for redness and breakdown twice a week
    3. Checking the bottom sheet for wetness and wrinkles
    4. Using a pressure relief pad while in a wheelchair

71. The client who is paraplegic after spinal cord injury has been taught muscle-strengthening exercises for the upper body. The nurse evaluates that the client will derive the least muscle-strengthening benefit from which of the following activities?
    1. Doing push-ups in a prone position
    2. Extending the arms while holding weights
    3. Doing active range of motion to the finger joints
    4. Squeezing rubber balls

72. The nurse is caring for the client who has suffered spinal cord injury. The nurse further assesses the client for other signs of autonomic dysreflexia if the client experiences
    1. Severe, throbbing headache
    2. Pallor of the face and neck
    3. Sudden tachycardia
    4. Severe and sudden hypotension

73. The family of a spinal cord–injured client rushes to the nursing station saying that the client needs immediate help. Upon entering the room, the nurse notes that the client is diaphoretic with a flushed face and neck, and complains of severe headache. The pulse is 40 and BP is 230/100 mmHg. The nurse acts quickly, knowing the client is experiencing:
    1. Spinal shock
    2. Malignant hypertension
    3. Pulmonary embolism
    4. Autonomic dysreflexia

74. The client with spinal cord injury is prone to experiencing autonomic dysreflexia. The nurse avoids which of the following measures to minimize the risk of recurrence?
    1. Strict adherence to a bowel retraining program
    2. Limiting bladder catheterization to once every 12 hours
    3. Keeping the linen wrinkle-free under the client
    4. Avoiding unnecessary pressure on the lower limbs

75. The client with spinal cord injury suddenly experiences an episode of autonomic dysreflexia. After checking vital signs, the nurse immediately
    1. Lowers the head of the bed and administers an antihypertensive agent
    2. Removes the noxious stimulus and administers an antihypertensive agent
    3. Lowers the head of the bed and removes the noxious stimulus
    4. Raises the head of the bed and removes the noxious stimulus

76. The nurse is planning care for the client in spinal shock. Which of the following actions are least helpful in minimizing the effects of vasodilatation below the level of the injury?
    1. Monitoring vital signs before and during position changes
    2. Using vasopressor medications as prescribed
    3. Moving the client quickly as one unit
    4. Applying thromboembolic disease stockings (TEDS) or compression stockings

77. The nurse is caring for a client admitted with spinal cord injury in spinal shock. The nurse minimizes the risk of compounding the injury most effectively by
    1. Keeping the client on a stretcher
    2. Log rolling the client on a firm mattress
    3. Log rolling the client on a soft mattress
    4. Placing the client on a Stryker frame

78. The nurse is evaluating the neurological signs of the male client in spinal shock following spinal cord injury. Which of the following observations by the nurse indicates that spinal shock persists?
    1. Presence of bulbospongiosis reflex
    2. Hyperreflexia
    3. Inability to elicit a Babinski response
    4. Reflex emptying of the bladder

79. The nurse is caring for a client with intracranial aneurysm who was previously alert. Which of the following assessments is not an early indication that the level of consciousness (LOC) is deteriorating?
    1. Slight slurring of speech
    2. Ptosis of the left eyelid
    3. Mild drowsiness
    4. Less frequent, spontaneous speech

80. The nurse is planning to put aneurysm precautions in place for the client with a cerebral aneurysm. Which of the following items is not included as part of the precautions?
    1. Avoidance of pushing or straining, such as with defecation
    2. Maintaining the head of the bed at 15 degrees
    3. Limiting cigarettes to three per day
    4. Provision of physical aspects of care by the nurse

81. The client with ruptured intracranial aneurysm has surgery delayed until the client becomes stable. The nurse administers which of the fol-

lowing medications as ordered to prevent clot lysis and breakdown?
1 Aminocaproic acid (Amicar)
2 Heparin sodium (Heparin)
3 Warfarin (Coumadin)
4 Alteplase (Activase)

82. The nurse has taught the client with subarachnoid hemorrhage about the effects of nimodipine (Nimotop), which has been prescribed for 3 weeks. The nurse evaluates that the client understands the purpose of this medication if the client states that it is a
1 Beta adrenergic blocker that will decrease blood pressure
2 Vasodilator that has an affinity for cerebral blood vessels
3 Calcium channel blocker, which will reduce the blood pressure
4 Calcium channel blocker, which will decrease spasm in cerebral blood vesssels

83. The nurse is assessing the client who is experiencing seizure activity. The nurse does not need to determine information about which of the following items as part of routine assessment of seizures?
1 Duration of the seizure
2 What the client ate in the 2 hours preceding the seizure activity
3 Seizure progression and type of movements
4 Changes in pupil size or eye deviation

84. The nurse is planning to institute seizure precautions for a client who is being admitted from the emergency department. Which of the following measures does the nurse avoid in planning for the client's safety?
1 Placing an airway and oxygen and suction equipment at the bedside
2 Padding the side rails of the bed
3 Putting a padded tongue blade at the head of the bed
4 Having IV equipment ready for insertion of IV access

85. The nurse is caring for the client who begins to experience seizure activity while in bed. Which of the following actions by the nurse is contraindicated?
1 Loosening restrictive clothing
2 Removing pillow and raising padded side rails
3 Restraining the client's limbs
4 Positioning the client to the side if possible, with head flexed forward

86. The nurse has given medication instructions to the client receiving phenytoin (Dilantin). The nurse evaluates that the client has adequate understanding if the client states

1 The medication dose may be self-adjusted, depending on side effects
2 Alcohol is not contraindicated while taking this medication
3 Good oral hygiene is needed, including brushing and flossing
4 The morning dose of the medication should be taken before a serum drug level is drawn

87. The nurse is planning care for the client with hemiparesis of the right arm and leg. The nurse incorporates in the care plan to place objects
1 Within the client's reach, on the right side
2 Within the client's reach, on the left side
3 Just out of the client's reach, on the right side
4 Just out of the client's reach, on the left side

88. The client with CVA has residual dysphagia. When a diet order is initiated, the nurse avoids doing which of the following?
1 Giving the client thin liquids
2 Thickening liquids to the consistency of oatmeal
3 Placing food on the unaffected side of the mouth
4 Allowing plenty of time for chewing and swallowing

89. The nurse has instructed the family of a CVA client who has homonymous hemianopsia about measures to help the client overcome the deficit. The nurse evaluates that the family understand the measures to use if they state to
1 Place objects in the client's impaired field of vision
2 Approach the client from the impaired field of vision
3 Remind the client to turn the head to scan the lost visual field
4 Discourage the client from wearing eyeglasses

90. The nurse is assessing the adaptation of the client to changes in functional status after CVA. The nurse assesses that the client is adapting most successfully if the client
1 Experiences bouts of depression and irritability
2 Consistently uses adaptive equipment in dressing self
3 Has difficulty with using modified feeding utensils
4 Gets angry with family if they interrupt a task

91. The nurse has formulated a nursing diagnosis of Unilateral Neglect for the client with CVA. Which of the following strategies is not used by the nurse in planning to help the client adapt to this deficit?
1 Move commode and chair to the affected side
2 Place bedside articles on the affected side
3 Approach the client from the unaffected side
4 Teach the client to scan the environment

92. The nurse is trying to communicate with a CVA client with aphasia. Which of the following actions by the nurse is least helpful to the client?
    1 Speaking to the client at a slower rate
    2 Completing the sentences that the client cannot finish
    3 Looking directly at the client during attempts at speech
    4 Allowing plenty of time for the client to respond

93. The client with diplopia has been taught to use an eyepatch to promote better vision and prevent injury. The nurse evaluates that the client has correct understanding of the use of the patch if the client states to
    1 Use the patch only when vision is especially troublesome
    2 Wear the patch for 1 hour at a time
    3 Wear the patch continuously, alternating eyes each day
    4 Wear the patch continuously, alternating eyes each week

94. A client receives a dose of edrophonium (Tensilon) intravenously. The client shows improvement in muscle strength for a period of time following the injection. The nurse interprets that this finding is compatible with
    1 Multiple sclerosis
    2 Amyotrophic lateral sclerosis
    3 Myasthenia gravis
    4 Muscular dystrophy

95. The client with myasthenia gravis is having difficulty speaking. The speech is dysarthritic and has a nasal tone. The nurse avoids using which of the following communication strategies when working with this client?
    1 Repeating what the client said to verify the message
    2 Encouraging the client to speak quickly
    3 Using a communication board when necessary
    4 Asking yes and no questions when able

96. The client with myasthenia gravis has a Risk for Ineffective Airway Clearance and Risk for Ineffective Breathing Pattern. The nurse keeps which of the following available at the client's bedside?
    1 Incentive spirometer and cough pillow
    2 Oxygen and metered dose inhaler
    3 Pulse oximeter and intermittent positive-pressure breathing (IPPB) machine
    4 Ambu bag and suction equipment

97. The client has experienced an episode of myasthenic crisis. The nurse assesses whether the client has precipitating factors such as

1 Too little exercise
2 Increased intake of fatty foods
3 Omitted doses of medication
4 Excess medication

98. The nurse is teaching the client with myasthenia gravis about prevention of myasthenic and cholinergic crises. The nurse tells the client that this is most effectively done by
    1 Doing all chores early in the day while less fatigued
    2 Taking medications on time to maintain therapeutic blood levels
    3 Doing muscle-strengthening exercises
    4 Eating large, well-balanced meals.

99. The home health nurse is visiting the client with myasthenia gravis, and is discussing methods to minimize the risk of aspiration during meals because of decreased muscle strength. Which of the following suggestions does the nurse avoid giving to the client?
    1 Sit straight up in the chair while eating
    2 Cut food into very small pieces, chewing thoroughly
    3 Swallow when the chin is tipped slightly downward to the chest
    4 Lift the head while swallowing liquids

100. The nurse has instructed the client with myasthenia gravis about ways to manage own health at home. The nurse evaluates that the client needs more information if the client makes which of the following statements?
    1 "I should take my medications an hour before mealtime."
    2 "I've made arrangements to get a portable resuscitation bag and home suction equipment."
    3 "Going to the beach will be a nice, relaxing form of activity."
    4 "Here's the Medic-Alert bracelet I obtained."

101. The client with Parkinson's disease has a Risk for Falls related to abnormal gait. The nurse assesses that the client's gait is
    1 Broad based and waddling
    2 Accelerating with walking on toes
    3 Unsteady and staggering
    4 Shuffling and propulsive

102. The client with Parkinson's disease is embarrassed about the symptoms of the disorder and is bored and lonely. The nurse plans which of the following approaches as most therapeutic in assisting the client to cope with the disease?
    1 Plan only a few activities for the client during the day
    2 Assist the client with activities of daily living (ADL) as much as possible
    3 Encourage and praise perseverance in exercising and performing ADLs

4 Cluster activities at the end of the day when the client is most bored

103. The client with Parkinson's disease is experiencing a parkinsonian crisis. The nurse immediately places the client
    1 In a quiet, dim room with respiratory and cardiac support available
    2 In a high Fowler's position, with a nasogastric tube at the bedside
    3 In a room near the nursing station, which is near the code cart
    4 In a bed with padded side rails, with limb restraints nearby

104. The nurse has given instructions to the client with Parkinson's disease about maintaining mobility. The nurse evaluates that the client understands the directions if the client states to
    1 Exercise in the evening to combat fatigue
    2 Rock back and forth to start movement with bradykinesia
    3 Sit in soft, deep chairs
    4 Buy clothes with many buttons to maintain finger dexterity

105. The client with trigeminal neuralgia asks the nurse what causes the painful episodes associated with the condition. The nurse's response is based on an understanding that the symptoms can be triggered by
    1 Stimulation of the affected nerve by pressure and temperature
    2 A hypoglycemic effect on the cranial nerve
    3 Release of catecholamines with infection or stress
    4 A local reaction to nasal stuffiness

106. The nurse is administering medications to the client with trigeminal neuralgia. The nurse brings which of the following prescribed medications to the client for pain relief?
    1 Meperidine (Demerol) and hydroxyzine (Vistaril)
    2 Carbemazepine (Tegretol) and phenytoin (Dilantin)
    3 Acetaminophen (Tylenol) and codeine
    4 Oxycodone and aspirin (Percodan)

107. The nurse has given suggestions to the client with trigeminal neuralgia about strategies to minimize episodes of pain. The nurse evaluates that the client needs reinforcement of information if the client makes which of the following statements?
    1 "I will wash my face with cotton pads."
    2 "I'll have to start chewing on the unaffected side."
    3 "I should rinse my mouth sometimes if toothbrushing is painful."

4 "I'll try to eat my food either very hot or very cold."

108. The client with Bell's palsy asks the nurse what caused this problem to occur. The nurse's response is based on an understanding that the etiology is
    1 Unknown, but possibly includes ischemia, viral infection, or an autoimmune problem
    2 Unknown, but possibly includes long-term tissue malnutrition and cellular hypoxia
    3 Primarily genetic in origin and triggered by exposure to neurotoxins
    4 Primarily genetic in origin but triggered by exposure to meningitis

109. The client with onset of Bell's palsy is very upset and crying about the change in facial appearance. The nurse plans to emotionally support the client by telling the client that
    1 This is similar to a CVA, but all symptoms will reverse without treatment
    2 This is not a CVA, and many clients recover in 3 to 5 weeks
    3 This is caused by a small tumor that is easily removed
    4 This is a temporary problem, with treatment similar to that for migraine headaches

110. The nurse is reinforcing information given to the client with Bell's palsy about medications used to decrease edema of nerve tissue. The nurse gives the client specific information about which of the following medications?
    1 Acetylsalicylic acid (aspirin)
    2 Ibuprofen (Motrin)
    3 Dexamethasone (Decadron)
    4 Prednisone (Deltasone)

111. The nurse has given the client with Bell's palsy instructions on preserving muscle tone in the face and preventing denervation. The nurse evaluates that the client needs additional information if the client states to
    1 Expose the face to cold and drafts
    2 Massage the face with a gentle upward motion
    3 Wrinkle the forehead, blow out the cheeks, and whistle
    4 Use a device for electrical stimulation of the face

112. The client is admitted to the hospital with a diagnosis of Guillain-Barré syndrome (polyradiculitis). The nurse inquires during the nursing admission interview if the client has a history of
    1 Back injury or trauma to the spinal cord
    2 Seizures or trauma to the brain
    3 Respiratory or gastrointestinal infection during the previous month
    4 Meningitis during the past 5 years

113. The client with Guillain-Barré syndrome has ascending paralysis and is intubated and receiving mechanical ventilation. Which of the following strategies does the nurse incorporate in the plan of care to help the client cope with this illness?
    1 Giving client full control over care decisions and restricting visitors
    2 Providing information, giving positive feedback, and using distraction
    3 Providing IV sedatives, reducing distractions, and limiting visitors
    4 Providing positive feedback and encouraging active range of motion (ROM)

114. The nurse is admitting a client with Guillain-Barré syndrome to the nursing unit. The client has an ascending paralysis to the level of the waist. Knowing the complications of the disorder, the nurse brings which of the following items into the client's room?
    1 Nebulizer and pulse oximeter
    2 Flashlight and incentive spirometer
    3 ECG monitoring electrodes and intubation tray
    4 Blood pressure cuff and flashlight

115. The nurse is evaluating respiratory outcomes for the client with Guillain-Barré syndrome. The nurse evaluates that which of the following is the least favorable outcome for the client?
    1 Adventitious breath sounds
    2 Spontaneous breathing
    3 Oxygen saturation 98%
    4 Vital capacity within normal range

116. The client is admitted with an exacerbation of multiple sclerosis (MS). The nurse is assessing the client for possible precipitating risk factors. Which of the following factors, if stated by the client, does the nurse assess as being unrelated to the exacerbation?
    1 A stressful week at work
    2 Ingestion of more fruits and vegetables
    3 A recent bout of the flu
    4 Inability to sleep well

117. The client with MS is experiencing muscle weakness, spasticity, and an ataxic gait. Based on this information, the nurse formulates which of the following nursing diagnoses for the client?
    1 Impaired Physical Mobility
    2 Activity Intolerance
    3 Impaired Tissue Integrity
    4 Self-Care Deficit

118. The nurse is planning care for the client with a neurogenic bladder due to MS. Which of the following plans for fluid administration of at least 2000 mL/day would be most helpful to this client?
    1 400 to 500 mL with each meal, additional fluids in the morning but not after midday
    2 400 to 500 mL with each meal, 500 to 600 mL in the evening prior to bedtime
    3 400 to 500 mL with each meal, 200 to 250 mL at midmorning, midafternoon, and late afternoon
    4 400 to 500 mL with each meal, with all extra fluid concentrated in the afternoon and evening

119. The nurse is caring for the client with an exacerbation of MS. Which of the following scheduled medications will the nurse administer to hasten recovery from the exacerbation?
    1 Baclofen (Lioresal) by mouth and diazepam (Valium) intravenously
    2 Carbamazepine (Tegretol) and phenytoin (Dilantin) by mouth
    3 Dexamethasone (Decadron) intravenously, then tapered to oral route
    4 Methylprednisolone (Solu-Medrol) and adrenocorticotropic hormone (ACTH) intravenously

120. The home health nurse has been discussing interventions to prevent constipation in the client with MS. The nurse evaluates that the client is using the information most effectively if the client reports
    1 Use of an enema every morning before breakfast
    2 Initiating a BM every other day, 45 minutes after the largest meal of the day
    3 Drinking a total of 1500 mL/day
    4 Taking stool softeners daily and using a glycerin suppository once a week

ANSWERS

1. **3**

Rationale: The reticular activating system in conjunction with the cerebral hemispheres is responsible for arousal. Insomnia, agitation, mania, and delirium are examples of elevations in this area of neurological functioning. The temporal lobe, hippocampus, and frontal lobe are responsible for memory. The limbic system is responsible for feelings and affect.

Test-Taking Strategy: It may be useful to you in questions of this nature to look at the word "activating" in reticular activating system. This may help you to recall that this area is responsible for wake and sleep patterns. Review the basic functions of the different areas of the brain briefly if you have difficulty with this question!

Level of Cognitive Ability: Analysis
Phase of Nursing Process: Analysis
Client Needs: Physiological Integrity
Content Area: Adult Health/Neurological

Reference

Black, J., & Matassarin-Jacobs, E. (1997). *Medical-surgical nursing: Clinical management for continuity of care* (5th ed.). Philadelphia: W. B. Saunders. p. 710.

2. **1**

Rationale: Cranial nerve II is the optic nerve, which governs vision. The nurse can provide safety for the visually impaired client by clearing the path of obstacles when ambulating. Testing the shower water temperature would be useful if there is impairment of peripheral nerves. Speaking loudly may help overcome deficit of cranial nerve VIII (vestibulocochlear). Cranial nerves VII (facial) and IX (glossopharyngeal) control taste from the anterior two thirds and posterior one third of the tongue, respectively.

Test-Taking Strategy: Knowledge of the cranial nerves is needed to answer this question accurately. Review them briefly if you had difficulty with this question!

Level of Cognitive Ability: Application
Phase of Nursing Process: Planning
Client Needs: Safe, Effective Care Environment
Content Area: Adult Health/Neurological

Reference

Black, J., & Matassarin-Jacobs, E. (1997). *Medical-surgical nursing: Clinical management for continuity of care* (5th ed.). Philadelphia: W. B. Saunders. pp. 712–713, 719.

3. **4**

Rationale: The limbic system is responsible for feelings (affect) and emotions. Calculation ability and knowledge of current events relate to function of the frontal lobe. The cerebral hemispheres with specific regional functions control orientation. Recall of recent events (for example, breakfast) is controlled by the hippocampus.

Test-Taking Strategy: A basic understanding of the functions of the different areas of the brain is necessary to answer this question. Review these functions now if you had difficulty with this question!

Level of Cognitive Ability: Application
Phase of Nursing Process: Implementation
Client Needs: Psychosocial Integrity
Content Area: Adult Health/Neurological

Reference

Black, J., & Matassarin-Jacobs, E. (1997). *Medical-surgical nursing: Clinical management for continuity of care* (5th ed.). Philadelphia: W. B. Saunders. p. 710.

4. **2**

Rationale: The cerebellum is responsible for balance and coordination. A walker provides stability for the client during ambulation. Adaptive eating utensils may be beneficial when the client has partial paralysis of the hand. A raised toilet seat is useful when the client does not have the mobility or ability to flex the hips. A slider board is used in transferring a client from a bed to a stretcher or wheelchair.

Test-Taking Strategy: To answer this question correctly, you must know that the cerebellum controls balance and coordination. This would immediately help you eliminate options 3 and 4. To help you choose between options 1 and 2, adaptive eating utensils are used when there is loss of fine motor coordination, such as with cerebrovascular accident. The walker helps the client maintain balance.

Level of Cognitive Ability: Analysis
Phase of Nursing Process: Evaluation
Client Needs: Health Promotion and Maintenance
Content Area: Adult Health/Neurological

Reference

Black, J., & Matassarin-Jacobs, E. (1997). *Medical-surgical nursing: Clinical management for continuity of care* (5th ed.). Philadelphia: W. B. Saunders. p. 712.

5. **3**

Rationale: The trigeminal nerve (cranial nerve V) has a motor and sensory division. The motor division innervates the muscles for chewing (mastication). The sensory division innervates the entire face, scalp, cornea, and nasal and oral cavities. The sensations of pain, temperature, and touch can be assessed using each of the respective items noted in option 3. The corneal reflex (motor division) can also be tested using the cotton wisp. The supplies noted in options 1, 2, and 4 are used for testing cranial nerves III, VIII, and II, respectively.

Test-Taking Strategy: Questions related to cranial nerves are difficult unless you know the differences between them. Review them now if you have the need!

Level of Cognitive Ability: Application
Phase of Nursing Process: Planning
Client Needs: Safe, Effective Care Environment
Content Area: Adult Health/Neurological

Reference

Black, J., & Matassarin-Jacobs, E. (1997). *Medical-surgical nursing: Clinical management for continuity of care* (5th ed.). Philadelphia: W. B. Saunders. p. 720.

6. **2**

Rationale: Cranial nerves III (oculomotor), IV (trochlear), and VI (abducens) have only motor components and control in a coordinated manner the six cardinal fields of gaze. This is tested by moving an object in six directions (involving horizontal and diagonal movements). Corneal reflex is the function of the trigeminal nerve (cranial nerve V). Pupillary response and accommodation are the functions of cranial nerve III alone.

Test-Taking Strategy: If you look at this question carefully, you will see that each of the incorrect responses has to do with pupillary reactions of some type. The correct answer in this case is the response that is different from the others. Being able to move the eyes through the six cardinal fields of gaze is a coordinated effort of three cranial nerves. Review cranial nerve testing if you had difficulty with this question!

Level of Cognitive Ability: Application
Phase of Nursing Process: Implementation
Client Needs: Physiological Integrity
Content Area: Adult Health/Neurological

Reference

Black, J., & Matassarin-Jacobs, E. (1997). *Medical-surgical nursing: Clinical management for continuity of care* (5th ed.). Philadelphia: W. B. Saunders. p. 720.

7. **1**

Rationale: The cochlear division of cranial nerve VIII is responsible for hearing. Clients with hearing difficulty may benefit from use of a hearing aid. The vestibular portion of this nerve controls equilibrium, so difficulty with this division may be controlled with the use of a walker. Eyeglasses would correct visual problems (cranial nerve II), whereas a bath thermometer would be of use to clients with sensory deficits of peripheral nerves, such as with diabetic neuropathy.

Test-Taking Strategy: Questions related to cranial nerves are difficult unless you know the differences between them. Knowing that the name of this nerve has two parts to it may be of use to you in remembering that it has to do with the two functions of the ear (hearing and balance). This helps you eliminate options 3 and 4. You need to be able to discriminate between the vestibular and cochlear portions of this nerve to select the correct option of the two remaining ones. Review cranial nerve testing if you had difficulty with this question!

Level of Cognitive Ability: Analysis
Phase of Nursing Process: Evaluation
Client Needs: Health Promotion and Maintenance
Content Area: Adult Health/Neurological

Reference
Black, J., & Matassarin-Jacobs, E. (1997). *Medical-surgical nursing: Clinical management for continuity of care* (5th ed.). Philadelphia: W. B. Saunders. pp. 720–721.

8. **3**

Rationale: Pronator drift occurs when a client cannot maintain the hands in a supinated position with the arms extended and eyes closed. This assessment may be done to detect small changes in muscle strength that might not otherwise be noted. Hyperreflexia is an excessive reflex action. Ataxia is a disturbance in gait. Nystagmus is characterized by fine, involuntary eye movements.

Test-Taking Strategy: Looking at everyday meanings of words may help you with this question. The word "drift" means to move slightly or without effort, which may give you a clue as to the correct response for this item.

Level of Cognitive Ability: Analysis
Phase of Nursing Process: Analysis
Client Needs: Physiological Integrity
Content Area: Adult Health/Neurological

Reference
Black, J., & Matassarin-Jacobs, E. (1997). *Medical-surgical nursing: Clinical management for continuity of care* (5th ed.). Philadelphia: W. B. Saunders. p. 722.

9. **4**

Rationale: Motor testing in the unconscious client can only be done by testing the response to painful stimuli. Nailbed pressure tests a basic peripheral response. Cerebral responses to pain are tested by using a sternal rub, placing upward pressure on the orbital rim, or squeezing the clavicle or sternocleidomastoid muscle.

Test-Taking Strategy: If you evaluate this question from the viewpoint of the location of each of the body parts described, you may easily determine the correct response. The nailbed is the most distal of all the choices, and is therefore the most peripheral. Each of the other responses may elicit a generalized response but not a localized one. Peripheral testing can be done on a limb that is unresponsive to the stimulus used to test the cerebral response. Review the process of peripheral testing if you had difficulty with this question!

Level of Cognitive Ability: Application
Phase of Nursing Process: Planning
Client Needs: Safe, Effective Care Environment
Content Area: Adult Health/Neurological

Reference
Black, J., & Matassarin-Jacobs, E. (1997). *Medical-surgical nursing: Clinical management for continuity of care* (5th ed.). Philadelphia: W. B. Saunders. p. 723.

10. **2**

Rationale: Astereognosis is the inability to discern the form or configuration of common objects using the sense of touch. Option 1 describes testing for agraphia, the inability to express thoughts in writing. Options 3 and 4 test for the extinction phenomenon and two-point stimulation, respectively.

Test-Taking Strategy: This question is difficult because you need to know common difficulties with proprioception to correctly identify the method used to test each. Take a few moments now to review these if they are unfamiliar!

Level of Cognitive Ability: Application
Phase of Nursing Process: Implementation
Client Needs: Physiological Integrity
Content Area: Adult Health/Neurological

Reference
Black, J., & Matassarin-Jacobs, E. (1997). *Medical-surgical nursing: Clinical management for continuity of care* (5th ed.). Philadelphia: W. B. Saunders. p. 724.

11. **3**

Rationale: With loss of the corneal (blink) reflex, the client is at risk of the eyes becoming dry, and also of suffering corneal abrasions if foreign matter comes in contact with the eye. Use of sterile saline drops is indicated to keep the eyes lubricated. An eyepatch would have to be used carefully because corneal abrasion could result if the cornea comes in contact with the patch. Introduction of a cotton-tipped applicator (foreign object) inside the lower eyelid also risks corneal abrasion. Taping the eye shut could impair the client's vision, putting the client at risk for other injury, such as falls.

Test-Taking Strategy: The best way to approach this question is from the viewpoint of potential trauma to the client. Notice that the stem includes the word "best." This indicates that other responses may be fully or partially correct. Each of the incorrect responses carries some degree of risk to the client. Additionally, options 1 and 2 are similar because they both address covering the eye. Therefore, both of these options can be eliminated when selecting the correct choice.

Level of Cognitive Ability: Analysis
Phase of Nursing Process: Evaluation
Client Needs: Health Promotion and Maintenance
Content Area: Adult Health/Neurological

Reference
Smeltzer, S., & Bare, B. (1996). *Brunner and Suddarth's textbook of medical-surgical nursing* (8th ed.). Philadelphia: Lippincott-Raven. p. 1722.

12. **2**

Rationale: An ataxic gait is characterized by unsteadiness and staggering. A spastic gait is characterized by stiff, short steps with legs held together, hip and knees flexed, and with toes that catch and drag. A festinating gait is best described as walking on toes with an accelerating pace. Dystrophic or broad-based gait is seen as waddling, with weight shifting from side to side and with legs far apart.

Test-Taking Strategy: Options 1 and 4 should be eliminated first because the names of these gaits do not seem to coincide with that in the stem. Of the two remaining, it may help you to remember that an ataxic gait is one of the more common gait alterations. Review the various types of gait now if you had difficulty with this question!

Level of Cognitive Ability: Analysis
Phase of Nursing Process: Analysis
Client Needs: Physiological Integrity
Content Area: Adult Health/Neurological

Reference
Black, J., & Matassarin-Jacobs, E. (1997). *Medical-surgical nursing: Clinical management for continuity of care* (5th ed.). Philadelphia: W. B. Saunders. p. 722.

13. **4**

Rationale: Clients with cognitive impairment from neurological dysfunction respond best to a stable environment, which is limited in the amounts and type of sensory input. The nurse can provide sensory cues and give clear, simple directions in a positive manner. Confusion and agitation can be minimized by reducing environmental stimuli (such as television or multiple visitors) and keeping familiar personal articles (such as family pictures) at the bedside.

Test-Taking Strategy: This question asks for the least helpful action, which makes you look for an incorrect response. The client who is confused can handle limited amounts of information at one time, which makes option 4 the correct answer to this question.

Level of Cognitive Ability: Application
Phase of Nursing Process: Planning
Client Needs: Psychosocial Integrity
Content Area: Adult Health/Neurological

Reference
Smeltzer, S., & Bare, B. (1996). *Brunner and Suddarth's textbook of medical-surgical nursing* (8th ed.). Philadelphia: Lippincott-Raven. p. 1708.

14. **1**

Rationale: A bladder retraining program, such as use of a toileting schedule, may be helpful to clients experiencing urinary incontinence. A Foley catheter should be used only when necessary because of risk of infection. Use of diapers or pads is the least acceptable alternative because the risk of skin breakdown is great.

Test-Taking Strategy: This question can be answered most easily by looking at it from a client safety viewpoint. Since Foley catheters carry risk of infection, and the use of diapers or pads carries the risk of skin breakdown, the only acceptable answer is the toileting schedule.

Level of Cognitive Ability: Application
Phase of Nursing Process: Implementation
Client Needs: Physiological Integrity
Content Area: Adult Health/Neurological

Reference
Smeltzer, S., & Bare, B. (1996). *Brunner and Suddarth's textbook of medical-surgical nursing* (8th ed.). Philadelphia: Lippincott-Raven. pp. 348, 1708.

15. **3**

Rationale: The health history and physical assessment conducted on a client with a neurological problem are very similar to those of any other client, with perhaps a more intense neurological exam. If the client is confused or agitated, or has difficulty hearing or speaking, the nurse should ask a significant other or family member to stay with the client during history taking to ensure accurate data.

Test-Taking Strategy: This question is asking which approach the nurse should take to get the health history information that is needed. Neither option 1 nor 2 accomplishes this, so they should be discarded first. A second nurse is of no added benefit to the client who is having difficulty answering. The logical response is to have a family member remain with the client.

Level of Cognitive Ability: Application
Phase of Nursing Process: Implementation
Client Needs: Psychosocial Integrity
Content Area: Adult Health/Neurological

Reference
Ignatavicius, D., Workman, M., & Mishler, M. (1995). *Medical-surgical nursing: A nursing process approach* (2nd ed.). Philadelphia: W. B. Saunders. p. 1100.

16. **2**

Rationale: Previous neurological problems such as headaches or back injuries place the client more at risk for development of a neurological disorder. Chronic diseases such as hypertension and diabetes mellitus also place the client at greater risk. Assessment of allergies is a routine part of the health history, regardless of the nature of the client's problem.

Test-Taking Strategy: This question is fairly straightforward. Each of the incorrect responses for the question has an actual or potential neurological association. Allergies indicate a disturbance of the immune system. Review the risks associated with neurological problems now if you had difficulty with this question!

Level of Cognitive Ability: Analysis
Phase of Nursing Process: Analysis
Client Needs: Physiological Integrity
Content Area: Adult Health/Neurological

Reference
Ignatavicius, D., Workman, M., & Mishler, M. (1995). *Medical-surgical nursing: A nursing process approach* (2nd ed.). Philadelphia: W. B. Saunders. p. 1100.

17. **3**

Rationale: The nurse maintains a patent airway for the client by keeping the head and neck in good alignment and elevating the head of bed 30 degrees unless contraindicated. Suction equipment is kept at the bedside if secretions need to be cleared. The client should be kept in a side-lying position whenever possible to minimize the risk of aspiration.

Test-Taking Strategy: This question tests a fundamental concept. Options 1 and 2 can be eliminated first because these are safe nursing actions. Option 4 addresses suctioning that refers to maintaining a patent airway. You would choose option 3 as the answer to the question, because it puts the client at greater risk of aspiration.

Level of Cognitive Ability: Application
Phase of Nursing Process: Planning
Client Needs: Safe, Effective Care Environment
Content Area: Adult Health/Neurological

Reference
Smeltzer, S., & Bare, B. (1996). *Brunner and Suddarth's textbook of medical-surgical nursing* (8th ed.). Philadelphia: Lippincott-Raven. pp. 1706–1707.

18. **4**

Rationale: Standard measures to lower body temperature include removing bed covers, providing cool sponge baths, using an electric fan in the room, administering acetaminophen, and placing a hypothermia blanket under the client. Ice packs are avoided because they could cause shivering, which increases cellular oxygen demands and could increase the intracranial pressure. If shivering occurs, it is managed with chlorpromazine (Thorazine).

Test-Taking Strategy: It may be helpful to look at this question from the body surface area that would be benefited by each of the measures above. Tepid sponge baths and a hyperthermia blanket would affect a good portion of the client's skin to reduce heat. Tylenol has an antipyretic effect. The ice packs are the incorrect option because they would affect the skin only in the area of the axilla and groin, giving less generalized cooling and increasing the risk of shivering. Review nursing care related to the client with hyperthermia now if you had difficulty with this question!

Level of Cognitive Ability: Application
Phase of Nursing Process: Implementation
Client Needs: Physiological Integrity
Content Area: Adult Health/Neurological

Reference
Smeltzer, S., & Bare, B. (1996). *Brunner and Suddarth's textbook of medical-surgical nursing* (8th ed.). Philadelphia: Lippincott-Raven. p. 1708.

19. **1**

Rationale: The question is worded to elicit an unsafe action on the part of the family. Depending on the client's functional ability, either passive or active ROM is indicated to keep the joint moving freely. Application of a premolded splint would also keep the limb aligned and in good position. The client should not attempt to stand unsupported on a weak or paralyzed limb. The inability to bear weight will cause the client to fall.

Test-Taking Strategy: This question tests fundamental concepts of impaired mobility and corrective actions. If you had any difficulty with this question, you may want to review these concepts now!

Level of Cognitive Ability: Analysis
Phase of Nursing Process: Evaluation
Client Needs: Health Promotion and Maintenance
Content Area: Adult Health/Neurological

Reference
Smeltzer, S., & Bare, B. (1996). *Brunner and Suddarth's textbook of medical-surgical nursing* (8th ed.). Philadelphia: Lippincott-Raven. p. 1707.

20. **2**

Rationale: The client undergoing cerebral angiography is assessed for possible allergy to the contrast dye, which can be determined by questioning the client about allergies to iodine or shellfish. Salmon is irrelevant to the question. Claustrophobia and excessive weight are areas of concern with magnetic resonance imaging.

Test-Taking Strategy: This concept is fundamental for angiography of any group of blood vessels. Memorize this now if you have not already. It is likely you could encounter this type of question in some form!

Level of Cognitive Ability: Application
Phase of Nursing Process: Assessment
Client Needs: Physiological Integrity
Content Area: Adult Health/Neurological

Reference
Ignatavicius, D., Workman, M., & Mishler, M. (1995). *Medical-surgical nursing: A nursing process approach* (2nd ed.). Philadelphia: W. B. Saunders. p. 1111.

21. **4**

Rationale: The client having an MRI has all metallic objects removed because of the magnetic field generated by the device. A careful history is done to determine if any metal objects are inside the client, such as orthopedic hardware, pacemakers, artificial heart valves, aneurysm clips, or intra-uterine devices. These may heat up, become dislodged, or malfunction during this procedure. The client may be ineligible if there is significant risk.

Test-Taking Strategy: You will note that each of the incorrect options is a medical disorder. The correct answer is the name of a surgical procedure in which an artificial valve (sometimes metal) is implanted. An important concept with regard to MRI is the avoidance of any metal objects in the vicinity of the machine. Review the contraindications related to this procedure now if you had difficulty with this question!

Level of Cognitive Ability: Analysis
Phase of Nursing Process: Analysis
Client Needs: Physiological Integrity
Content Area: Adult Health/Neurological

Reference
Smeltzer, S., & Bare, B. (1996). *Brunner and Suddarth's textbook of medical-surgical nursing* (8th ed.). Philadelphia: Lippincott-Raven. p. 1698.

22. **1**

Rationale: The client undergoing LP is positioned lying on the side, with the legs pulled up to the abdomen, and with the head bent down onto the chest. This position helps to open the spaces between the vertebrae.

Test-Taking Strategy: Knowing that an LP is the introduction of a needle into the subarachnoid space, it is reasonable that the position of the client must facilitate this. The correct answer is the only position that flexes the vertebrae for easier needle insertion. Review positioning procedures for an LP now if you had difficulty with this question!

Level of Cognitive Ability: Application
Phase of Nursing Process: Implementation
Client Needs: Safe, Effective Care Environment
Content Area: Adult Health/Neurological

Reference
Black, J., & Matassarin-Jacobs, E. (1997). *Medical-surgical nursing: Clinical management for continuity of care* (5th ed.). Philadelphia: W. B. Saunders. p. 733.

23. **3**

Rationale: The MRI scanner is a hollow tube that gives some clients a feeling of claustrophobia. Metal objects must be removed before the procedure so they are not drawn in to the magnetic field. The client may eat and take all prescribed medications before the procedure. If a contrast medium is used, the client may wish to eat lightly if the client has a tendency to get nauseated easily. The client lies supine on a padded table, which moves into the imager. The client must lie still during the procedure. The imager makes tapping noises while scanning. The client is alone in the imager, but the nurse can reassure the client that the technician is in voice communication with the client at all times during the procedure.

Test-Taking Strategy: The statement in each of the options is correct. However, the question asks which statement will give the most reassurance to the client. While all statements are factually true, the correct option is the only one that provides a measure of reassurance to the client. Review MRI now if you had difficulty with this question!

Level of Cognitive Ability: Application
Phase of Nursing Process: Implementation
Client Needs: Psychosocial Integrity
Content Area: Adult Health/Neurological

Reference
Black, J., & Matassarin-Jacobs, E. (1997). *Medical-surgical nursing: Clinical management for continuity of care* (5th ed.). Philadelphia: W. B. Saunders. p. 732.

24. **4**

Rationale: After CT scanning, the client may resume all usual activities. The client should be encouraged to take in extra fluids to replace those lost with diuresis from the contrast dye.

Test-Taking Strategy: Looking at the available choices, option 3 makes the least sense and should be eliminated first. Knowing that there is no special aftercare lets you eliminate options 1 and 2 next. Review the procedure related to CT scanning now if you had difficulty with this question!

Level of Cognitive Ability: Analysis
Phase of Nursing Process: Evaluation
Client Needs: Health Promotion and Maintenance
Content Area: Adult Health/Neurological

Reference
Black, J., & Matassarin-Jacobs, E. (1997). *Medical-surgical nursing: Clinical management for continuity of care* (5th ed.). Philadelphia: W. B. Saunders. p. 731.

25. **3**

Rationale: Caloric testing provides information about the vestibular portion of the eighth cranial nerve, which aids in differentiating between cerebellar and brain stem lesions. After determining patency of the ear canal, either warm or cold water is injected into the auditory canal. Normally, nystagmus occurs in the same direction as the irrigated ear if warm water is used, and away from the irrigated ear if cold water is used. Nystagmus indicates that the brain stem is intact. If death of the brain stem has occurred, nystagmus will not occur.

Test-Taking Strategy: In order to answer this question accurately, you must understand the purpose and nature of the test. It will be helpful to remember that this test is used as an adjunct to determine brain death. This would limit the realistic choices to option 3 or 4. Knowledge of the test is needed to differentiate between the two. Review the test now if you had difficulty with this question!

Level of Cognitive Ability: Analysis
Phase of Nursing Process: Analysis
Client Needs: Physiological Integrity
Content Area: Adult Health/Neurological

Reference
Black, J., & Matassarin-Jacobs, E. (1997). *Medical-surgical nursing: Clinical management for continuity of care* (5th ed.). Philadelphia: W. B. Saunders. p. 740.

26. **1**

Rationale: Following a myelogram, the client is placed on bed rest for 6 to 8 hours after the procedure. When a water-based contrast medium is used, the client is positioned with the head of bed elevated 15 to 30 degrees. With use of an oil-based medium, the head of bed is positioned flat (even though the contrast is aspirated out after the procedure).

Test-Taking Strategy: This question is asking for knowledge of two separate items: length of bed rest and head position. With a myelogram procedure, if you reason that the longer the bed rest, the less likelihood of complications, then you can narrow your choices to options 1 and 3. If you can remember that "oil rises, so keep the head low," you will be able to choose correctly. Review postprocedure care following a myelogram now if you had difficulty with this question!

Level of Cognitive Ability: Application
Phase of Nursing Process: Planning
Client Needs: Safe, Effective Care Environment
Content Area: Adult Health/Neurological

Reference
Black, J., & Matassarin-Jacobs, E. (1997). *Medical-surgical nursing: Clinical management for continuity of care* (5th ed.). Philadelphia: W. B. Saunders. pp. 735–736.

27. **2**

Rationale: The unconscious client is positioned on the side during mouth care to prevent aspiration. The teeth are brushed at least twice daily using a small toothbrush. The gums, tongue, roof of mouth, and oral mucous membranes are cleansed with Toothettes to avoid encrustation and infection. The lips are coated with water-soluble lubricant to prevent drying, cracking and encrustation. The use of products with lemon or alcohol should be avoided, because they have a drying effect.

Test-Taking Strategy: The question asks what the nurse should avoid. Standard mouth care procedures include use of toothbrush and Toothettes, so these may be eliminated first. Knowing that the unconscious client is at risk of aspiration tells you that option 1 is correct also. This leaves option 2 as incorrect because repeated use of these products could dry and crack the oral mucous membranes.

Level of Cognitive Ability: Application
Phase of Nursing Process: Implementation
Client Needs: Physiological Integrity
Content Area: Adult Health/Neurological

Reference
Black, J., & Matassarin-Jacobs, E. (1997). *Medical-surgical nursing: Clinical management for continuity of care* (5th ed.). Philadelphia: W. B. Saunders. p. 758.

28. **4**

Rationale: Expected outcomes for this nursing diagnosis in an unconscious client include stable weight, intake equaling output, evidence of wound healing, and normal BUN, total protein, and hemoglobin levels. Normal adult values are: BUN 5 to 20 mg/dL, total protein 6 to 8 g/dL, and hemoglobin 13.5 to 18.0 g/dL (male), 12 to 16 g/dL (female).

Test-Taking Strategy: The answer to this question is an item that is evidence of bad nutrition. Since stable weight and equal intake and output are satisfactory indicators, these can be eliminated. To discriminate between the last two, knowing that the BUN is normal allows you to select total protein as the answer to this question. Review these normal laboratory values now if you had difficulty with this question!

Level of Cognitive Ability: Analysis
Phase of Nursing Process: Evaluation
Client Needs: Health Promotion and Maintenance
Content Area: Adult Health/Neurological

References
Black, J., & Matassarin-Jacobs, E. (1997). *Medical-surgical nursing: Clinical management for continuity of care* (5th ed.). Philadelphia: W. B. Saunders. p. 758.
Jaffee, M., & McVan, B. (1997). *Davis's laboratory and diagnostic test handbook*. Philadelphia: F. A. Davis. pp. 1365, 1372, 1377.

29. **3**

Rationale: Risk for Aspiration is defined by NANDA as "the state in which an individual is at risk for entry of GI secretions, oropharyngeal secretions, or solids or fluids into tracheobronchial passages." Major defining characteristics specific for this client include reduced level of consciousness, depressed cough and gag reflexes, and gastrointestinal tube with tube feedings.

Test-Taking Strategy: Use the ABCs, Airway, Breathing, and Circulation, to answer the question. Given the description in the stem, it is easy to eliminate options 1 and 4 first. Of the two remaining, aspiration is one form of injury that the client could sustain. It is more specific, and therefore it is the better choice.

Level of Cognitive Ability: Analysis
Phase of Nursing Process: Analysis
Client Needs: Physiological Integrity
Content Area: Adult Health/Neurological

References
Cox, H., et al. (1997). *Clinical applications of nursing diagnosis: Adult, child, women's psychiatric, gerontic and home health considerations* (3rd ed.). Philadelphia: F. A. Davis. p. 100.
Smeltzer, S., & Bare, B. (1996). *Brunner and Suddarth's textbook of medical-surgical nursing* (8th ed.). Philadelphia: Lippincott-Raven. p. 1719.

30. **2**

Rationale: Families often need assistance to cope with the sudden, severe illness of a loved one. The nurse can help the family of an unconscious client by assisting them to work through their feelings of grief. The nurse should explain all equipment, treatments, and procedures, and supplement or reinforce information given by the physician. Family should be encouraged to touch and speak to the client, and to become involved in the client's care to the extent they are comfortable. The nurse should allow the family to stay with the client to the extent possible, and should encourage them to eat and sleep adequately to maintain their strength.

Test-Taking Strategy: The options seem to revolve around two themes: the adjustment of the family to the situation and the involvement or interaction with the client and care. Each of the incorrect options either inhibits the family's coping or distances the family from the client or the client's care. Avoid selecting these types of options.

Level of Cognitive Ability: Application
Phase of Nursing Process: Planning
Client Needs: Psychosocial Integrity
Content Area: Adult Health/Neurological

Reference
Black, J., & Matassarin-Jacobs, E. (1997). *Medical-surgical nursing: Clinical management for continuity of care* (5th ed.). Philadelphia: W. B. Saunders. p. 762.

31. **4**

Rationale: Suction equipment should be kept at the bedside of an unconscious client, regardless of whether an artificial airway is used. The nurse auscultates breath sounds every 2 to 4 hours, or more frequently if there is need. The client should be hyperoxygenated before, during, and after suctioning to minimize cerebral hypoxia. The client should not be suctioned for longer than 10 seconds at one time, to prevent cerebral hypoxia and a rise in intracranial pressure.

Test-Taking Strategy: The question is worded to make you seek an incorrect nursing action. Each of the first three options is standard suctioning procedure. The only option that is different, and dangerous, is option 4. If you had difficulty with this question, review suctioning procedures now!

Level of Cognitive Ability: Application
Phase of Nursing Process: Implementation
Client Needs: Physiological Integrity
Content Area: Adult Health/Neurological

Reference
Ignatavicius, D., Workman, M., & Mischler, M. (1995). *Medical-surgical nursing: a nursing process approach* (2nd ed.). Philadelphia: W. B. Saunders. pp. 663–665, 1276.

32. **3**

Rationale: The least amount of invasiveness needed to produce a bowel movement is best. Fecal disimpaction is done only when the client has become impacted from constipation as a result of inattention or failure of other measures. Enemas may be needed on an every other day basis, but they are used cautiously (even if not contraindicated) because the Valsalva maneuver can increase the intracranial pressure. Glycerin suppositories are the least invasive and usually stimulate bowel evacuation within a half hour. Stool softeners may be prescribed on a regular schedule to avoid hard, dry stools.

Test-Taking Strategy: The stem of the question includes the phrase "successful," which means that more than one (or all) of the options are correct. Working backward from most invasive to least invasive, you would eliminate the disimpaction first, followed by the SSE and Fleet enemas, leaving the glycerin suppository as the correct answer. Review the procedure for implementing an effective bowel training program now if you had difficulty with this question!

Level of Cognitive Ability: Analysis
Phase of Nursing Process: Evaluation
Client Needs: Health Promotion and Maintenance
Content Area: Adult Health/Neurological

References

Black, J., & Matassarin-Jacobs, E. (1997). *Medical-surgical nursing: Clinical management for continuity of care* (5th ed.). Philadelphia: W. B. Saunders. p. 761.
Smeltzer, S., & Bare, B. (1996). *Brunner and Suddarth's textbook of medical-surgical nursing* (8th ed.). Philadelphia: Lippincott-Raven. pp. 1722–1723.

33. **2**

Rationale: If the gastric residual is elevated on a persistent basis, the client may be experiencing delayed gastric emptying. The physician should be notified. First assess whether abdominal girth is enlarged, and auscultate bowel sounds to rule out intestinal obstruction. Some clients benefit from administration of metoclopramide (Reglan) to stimulate gastric emptying. The infusion rate cannot be too slow (option 1) if the client cannot tolerate that rate. Air in the stomach would be accompanied by abdominal distention and increased abdominal girth. Early peptic ulcer could be detected by Hematest-positive gastric aspirate.

Test-Taking Strategy: Increased gastric residual indicates the client is not tolerating the tube feedings. Possible causes of this include too rapid an infusion rate, bowel obstruction, or delayed gastric emptying. The only option that coincides with these possibilities is option 2.

Level of Cognitive Ability: Analysis
Phase of Nursing Process: Analysis
Client Needs: Physiological Integrity
Content Area: Adult Health/Neurological

Reference

Black, J., & Matassarin-Jacobs, E. (1997). *Medical-surgical nursing: Clinical management for continuity of care* (5th ed.). Philadelphia: W. B. Saunders. p. 760.

34. **3**

Rationale: Unconscious clients are completely immobile, having lost the protective reflexes to shift body weight (present even during normal sleep). It is up to the nurse to minimize the risk of prolonged pressure that could cause skin ischemia and breakdown. This is accomplished by repositioning the client every 2 hours and massaging bony prominences to stimulate circulation. Protective pads can be applied to the heels and elbows to reduce friction and shear. Appropriate perineal care is essential to keep waste products from excoriating the skin. The nurse can reduce skin dryness and irritation by adding a superfatty solution (such as baby oil or castile soap) to the daily bathwater. Drying agents, such as alcohol, are avoided because dry skin can crack and break down.

Test-Taking Strategy: This question can be analyzed by looking at the degree of skin risk with each of the options. It is apparent that each of the incorrect options poses no risk to the client. In fact, they are part of standard nursing care. The only option to avoid is the one that would dry the skin, that is, using alcohol in the bathwater. Remember, the question asks which intervention would not be included in the care plan.

Level of Cognitive Ability: Application
Phase of Nursing Process: Planning
Client Needs: Health Promotion and Maintenance
Content Area: Adult Health/Neurological

Reference

Black, J., & Matassarin-Jacobs, E. (1997). *Medical-surgical nursing: Clinical management for continuity of care* (5th ed.). Philadelphia: W. B. Saunders. p. 758.

35. **1**

Rationale: When a hypothermia blanket is used, the skin is inspected frequently for pressure points, which over time could lead to skin breakdown.

Test-Taking Strategy: Options 3 and 4 may be eliminated first because they are other health problems. The temperature of the blanket is not cold enough to produce frostbite. This leaves skin breakdown as the correct answer. Review the complications associated with the use of a hypothermia blanket now if you had difficulty with this question!

Level of Cognitive Ability: Application
Phase of Nursing Process: Assessment
Client Needs: Physiological Integrity
Content Area: Adult Health/Neurological

Reference

Black, J., & Matassarin-Jacobs, E. (1997). *Medical-surgical nursing: Clinical management for continuity of care* (5th ed.). Philadelphia: W. B. Saunders. p. 800.

36. **3**

Rationale: Clients should take tepid baths or receive cool sponge baths until the temperature has decreased to at least 102°F. The cool water helps dissipate body heat. The nurse should take care not to overchill the client, which could cause shivering. Maintaining the temperature at 102°F or less will prevent febrile seizures.

Test-Taking Strategy: This question has the word "safe" and the phrase "at least," which means the answer could also be a lower value. The question, however, is seeking the highest acceptable value. In this case, discard option 4 because this is much too high. A rebound temperature from that level could result in seizure activity. The other values are on the low side and should also be discarded.

Level of Cognitive Ability: Analysis
Phase of Nursing Process: Evaluation
Client Needs: Physiological Integrity
Content Area: Adult Health/Neurological

Reference

Cox, H., et al. (1997). *Clinical applications of nursing diagnosis: Adult, child, women's psychiatric, gerontic and home health considerations* (3rd ed.). Philadelphia: F. A. Davis. pp. 145–146.

37. **4**

Rationale: Hypothalamic damage causes hyperthermia, which may also be called "central fever." It is characterized by a persistent high fever with no diurnal variation. There is also an absence of sweating.

Test-Taking Strategy: Knowledge of the location of the brain's thermoregulatory center is needed to answer this question. Eliminate options 1 and 2 first because they are responsible for higher mental functions and balance, respectively. A quick trick may be to remember that hyper*thermia* is related to the hypo*thalamus*.

Level of Cognitive Ability: Analysis
Phase of Nursing Process: Analysis
Client Needs: Physiological Integrity
Content Area: Adult Health/Neurological

Reference
Ignatavicius, D., Workman, M., & Mishler, M. (1995). *Medical-surgical nursing: A nursing process approach* (2nd ed.). Philadelphia: W. B. Saunders. p. 1273.

38. **2**

Rationale: Chlorpromazine is used to control shivering in hyperthermic states. It is a phenothiazine and has antiemetic and antipsychotic uses, especially when psychosis is accompanied by increased psychomotor activity. Prochlorperazine is a phenothiazine that is an antiemetic and antipsychotic. Thioridazine and fluphenazine are phenothiazines that are used as antipsychotics.

Test-Taking Strategy: Knowledge of the different medications in this class is needed to help you differentiate among them. Eliminate options 3 and 4 first, because they are not used for other reasons in medical-surgical clients. Of the two remaining, remember that compazine is often used for nausea and thorazine is used for shivering. Review the action and purpose of this medication now if you had difficulty with this question!

Level of Cognitive Ability: Application
Phase of Nursing Process: Planning
Client Needs: Physiological Integrity
Content Area: Pharmacology

References
Deglin, J., & Vallerand, A. (1997). *Davis's drug guide for nurses* (5th ed.). Philadelphia: F. A. Davis. pp. 261, 509, 1010, 1151.
Smeltzer, S., & Bare, B. (1996). *Brunner and Suddarth's textbook of medical-surgical nursing* (8th ed.). Philadelphia: Lippincott-Raven. p. 1712.

39. **4**

Rationale: Discharge instructions for the client hospitalized for hyperthermia include prevention of heat related disorders, increased fluid intake for 24 hours, self-monitoring of voiding, and the importance of staying in a cool environment and resting.

Test-Taking Strategy: This question is worded to elicit the least appropriate activity upon discharge. Options 2 and 3 relate to maintaining and monitoring fluid balance, and are therefore eliminated. A cool environment is appropriate, so this is eliminated also. Resumption of full activity is not helpful; rather rest periods are indicated, so this is the correct option.

Level of Cognitive Ability: Analysis
Phase of Nursing Process: Evaluation
Client Needs: Health Promotion and Maintenance
Content Area: Adult Health/Neurological

Reference
Luckmann, J. (1997). *Saunders manual of nursing care*. Philadelphia: W. B. Saunders. p. 1735.

40. **2**

Rationale: A change in vital signs may be a late sign of increased ICP. Trends include increasing temperature and blood pressure, and decreasing pulse and respirations. Respiratory irregularities may also arise.

Test-Taking Strategy: This question looks complex but can be logically answered. If you remember that temperature rises, then you are able to eliminate options 3 and 4. If you know that the client becomes bradycardic, or know that the BP rises, you are able to make the correct choice. Review the signs of increased intracranial pressure now if you had difficulty with this question!

Level of Cognitive Ability: Application
Phase of Nursing Process: Assessment
Client Needs: Physiological Integrity
Content Area: Adult Health/Neurological

Reference
Smeltzer, S., & Bare, B. (1996). *Brunner and Suddarth's textbook of medical-surgical nursing* (8th ed.). Philadelphia: Lippincott-Raven. p. 1713.

41. **4**

Rationale: Normal ICP readings range from zero to 10 mmHg pressure. Sustained elevations above 15 mmHg are a cause for concern because they are considered abnormally high.

Test-Taking Strategy: Familiarity with the normal ICP pressures is needed to answer this question accurately. However, since elevated ICP is a clinical concern (no one ever speaks of low ICP), then you should be able to eliminate at least the two lowest numbers. Remembering that 15 mm is the "magic number" alerting you to be concerned helps you choose the correct option. Familiarity with the normal ICP pressures is needed to answer this question accurately.

Level of Cognitive Ability: Analysis
Phase of Nursing Process: Analysis
Client Needs: Physiological Integrity
Content Area: Adult Health/Neurological

Reference
Smeltzer, S., & Bare, B. (1996). *Brunner and Suddarth's textbook of medical-surgical nursing* (8th ed.). Philadelphia: Lippincott-Raven. p. 1717.

42. **3**

Rationale: To obtain accurate ICP pressure readings, the transducer is zeroed at the level of the foramen of Munro, which is approximated by placing the transducer 1 inch above the level of the ear. Serial ICP readings should be done with the client's head in the same position.

Test-Taking Strategy: Begin by eliminating options 1 and 2. Because there is a foreign body embedded in the client's brain, vigilant aseptic technique must be carried out. Of the two remaining options, it makes sense to ensure there are no leaks in the system, because bacteria could enter the system or incorrect pressure readings could be obtained. By elimination, the answer is the position of the transducer. Review the procedure related to ICP monitoring now if you had difficulty with this question!

Level of Cognitive Ability: Application
Phase of Nursing Process: Planning
Client Needs: Safe, Effective Care Environment
Content Area: Adult Health/Neurological

Reference
Smeltzer, S., & Bare, B. (1996). *Brunner and Suddarth's textbook of medical-surgical nursing* (8th ed.). Philadelphia: Lippincott-Raven. p. 1717.

43. 1

Rationale: The head of the client with increased ICP should be positioned so the head is in a neutral, midline position. The nurse should avoid flexing or extending the neck, or turning the neck side to side. The head of bed should be raised to 30 to 45 degrees. Use of proper positions promotes venous drainage from the cranium to keep intracranial pressure down.

Test-Taking Strategy: This question is asking which position will be detrimental to the client with increased ICP. This would be one that interferes either with arterial circulation to the brain or with venous drainage from the brain. The only position that meets one of these criteria is option 1. Review client positioning with ICP now if you had difficulty with this question!

Level of Cognitive Ability: Application
Phase of Nursing Process: Implementation
Client Needs: Physiological Integrity
Content Area: Adult Health/Neurological

Reference
Ignatavicius, D., Workman, M., & Mishler, M. (1995). *Medical-surgical nursing: A nursing process approach* (2nd ed.). Philadelphia: W. B. Saunders. p. 1273.

44. 1

Rationale: Activities that increase intrathoracic and intra-abdominal pressures cause indirect elevation of the ICP. Some of these activities include isometric exercises, Valsalva maneuver, coughing, sneezing, and blowing the nose. Exhaling during activities such as repositioning or pulling up in bed opens the glottis, which prevents intrathoracic pressure from rising.

Test-Taking Strategy: Evaluate each of the options in terms of the tension it puts on the body. Doing so will help you eliminate each of the incorrect options systematically. Review the measures that will reduce or prevent increased intracranial pressure if you had difficulty with this question!

Level of Cognitive Ability: Analysis
Phase of Nursing Process: Evaluation
Client Needs: Health Promotion and Maintenance
Content Area: Adult Health/Neurological

Reference
Smeltzer, S., & Bare, B. (1996). *Brunner and Suddarth's textbook of medical-surgical nursing* (8th ed.). Philadelphia: Lippincott-Raven. p. 1714.

45. 3

Rationale: Some clients who have awakened from an unconscious state have reported they remember hearing specific voices and conversations. Family and staff should assume the client's sense of hearing is still intact, and act accordingly. Research has also demonstrated that positive outcomes are associated with coma stimulation, that is, speaking to and touching the client.

Test-Taking Strategy: The nurse does not infer that the client wants a visit from the chaplain based on the family speaking over the client at the bedside, so that can be eliminated first. The family demonstrates no evidence of crisis, and they seem to be well informed. This eliminates options 1 and 2. Option 3 is the only correct choice.

Level of Cognitive Ability: Analysis
Phase of Nursing Process: Analysis
Client Needs: Psychosocial Integrity
Content Area: Adult Health/Neurological

Reference
Black, J., & Matassarin-Jacobs, E. (1997). *Medical-surgical nursing: Clinical management for continuity of care* (5th ed.). Philadelphia: W. B. Saunders. p. 762.

46. 4

Rationale: Hyperventilation with a $PaCO_2$ of 25 to 30 mmHg causes cerebral vasoconstriction, which decreases intracranial blood volume and intracranial pressure. The PaO_2 is not allowed to fall below 80 mmHg to prevent cerebral vasodilatation from hypoxemia.

Test-Taking Strategy: Since the bottom parameter of the arterial oxygen values in options 1 and 2 is too low, these options are eliminated first. Knowing that the normal $PaCO_2$ ranges from 35 to 45 mmHg, hyperventilation should cause these values to drop. Thus, option 4 is the correct answer, since the $PaCO_2$ value in option 3 is normal. Review hyperventilation and its relationship to intracranial pressure now if you had difficulty with this question!

Level of Cognitive Ability: Application
Phase of Nursing Process: Planning
Client Needs: Safe, Effective Care Environment
Content Area: Adult Health/Neurological

Reference
Ignatavicius, D., Workman, M., & Mishler, M. (1995). *Medical-surgical nursing: A nursing process approach* (2nd ed.). Philadelphia: W. B. Saunders. p. 1273.

47. 3

Rationale: Nursing interventions should be spaced out over the shift to minimize the risk of a sustained rise in ICP. If possible, activities known to raise the ICP should be avoided where possible. Other interventions to control the ICP include maintaining a calm, quiet environment and avoiding emotional stress and interruption of sleep.

Test-Taking Strategy: This question tests the concept that stimulation raises the ICP. If you know this, you will be able to discard each of the incorrect options as you read them. Review nursing care to the client with increased intracranial pressure now if you had difficulty with this question!

Level of Cognitive Ability: Application
Phase of Nursing Process: Implementation
Client Needs: Safe, Effective Care Environment
Content Area: Adult Health/Neurological

Reference
Smeltzer, S., & Bare, B. (1996). *Brunner and Suddarth's textbook of medical-surgical nursing* (8th ed.). Philadelphia: Lippincott-Raven. p. 1714.

48. 3

Rationale: The Glasgow Coma Scale is divided into three subsets as noted above. The client receives a numerical score for each subset. The highest possible score is 15; the lowest score is 3. Choices in the "best eye-opening response" category include spontaneously (4), to speech (3), to pain (2), no response (1). Choices in the "best motor response" category include obeys verbal commands (6), localizes pain (5), flexion, withdrawal (4), flexion, abnormal (3), extension, abnormal (2), no response (1). Choices in the "best verbal response" category include oriented × 3 (5), conversation, confused (4), speech, inappropriate (3), sounds, incomprehensible (2), no response (1). The higher the scores, the better the chance for recovery.

Test-Taking Strategy: A familiarity with this scale is needed to answer this question. If you know that the maximum score is 15, you would eliminate options 1 and 2 automatically. There are more motor response options than any other category, which may help you choose the correct option of the two remaining. Remember, the higher the better. Review the Glasgow Coma Scale now if you had difficulty with this question!

Level of Cognitive Ability: Analysis
Phase of Nursing Process: Evaluation
Client Needs: Physiological Integrity
Content Area: Adult Health/Neurological

Reference
Luckmann, J. (1997). *Saunders manual of nursing care.* Philadelphia: W. B. Saunders. p. 679.

49. **2**

Rationale: Leakage of CSF from the ears or nose may accompany basilar skull fracture. It can be distinguished from other body fluids because the drainage will separate into bloody and yellow concentric rings on dressing material, called Halo's sign. It also tests positive for glucose.

Test-Taking Strategy: The key to answering this question lies in knowing that CSF contains glucose, whereas other secretions, such as mucus, do not. Knowing that CSF separates into rings will also help you with this particular question. Review testing for CSF fluid now if you had difficulty with this question!

Level of Cognitive Ability: Analysis
Phase of Nursing Process: Assessment
Client Needs: Physiological Integrity
Content Area: Adult Health/Neurological

References
Ignatavicius, D., Workman, M., & Mishler, M. (1995). *Medical-surgical nursing: A nursing process approach* (2nd ed.). Philadelphia: W. B. Saunders. p. 1271.
Smeltzer, S., & Bare, B. (1996). *Brunner and Suddarth's textbook of medical-surgical nursing* (8th ed.). Philadelphia: Lippincott-Raven. p. 1789.

50. **2**

Rationale: Clients with moderate to severe head injury usually have residual physical and cognitive disabilities. These include personality changes, increased fatigue and irritability, mood alterations, and memory changes. The client may also require frequent to constant supervision. The nurse assesses the family's ability to cope and makes appropriate referrals to respite services, support groups, and state or local chapters of the National Head Injury Foundation.

Test-Taking Strategy: The stem states that the client had a moderately severe head injury. Knowing that deficits remain with the client helps you to eliminate options 3 and 4. Because the injury was more than minor, option 2 is more reasonable than option 1.

Level of Cognitive Ability: Analysis
Phase of Nursing Process: Analysis
Client Needs: Psychosocial Integrity
Content Area: Adult Health/Neurological

Reference
Ignatavicius, D., Workman, M., & Mishler, M. (1995). *Medical-surgical nursing: A nursing process approach* (2nd ed.). Philadelphia: W. B. Saunders. p. 1278.

51. **3**

Rationale: There is a significant association between cervical spine injury and head injury. For this reason, the nurse leaves any form of spinal immobilization in place until lateral cervical spinal x-rays rule out fracture or other damage.

Test-Taking Strategy: This question is rather straightforward. The reason for spinal immobilization is to protect the spine from movement, which could cause further damage if the cervical spine is injured. If x-ray results are negative, there is no reason to leave the collar in place. Take a few moments to review emergency care if this question was difficult. In this scenario, the results of the x-ray are the key to further intervention.

Level of Cognitive Ability: Application
Phase of Nursing Process: Planning
Client Needs: Safe, Effective Care Environment
Content Area: Adult Health/Neurological

Reference
Black, J., & Matassarin-Jacobs, E. (1997). *Medical-surgical nursing: Clinical management for continuity of care* (5th ed.). Philadelphia: W. B. Saunders. pp. 824–825.

52. **1**

Rationale: A complication of closed-head injury is diabetes insipidus (DI). This can occur with insult to the hypothalamus, the antidiuretic hormone storage vesicles, or the posterior pituitary gland. Urine output that exceeds 9 liters per day generally requires treatment with desmopressin. Dexamethasone, a glucocorticoid, is administered to treat cerebral edema. This medication may already be ordered for the client with a head injury. Ethacrynic acid and mannitol are both diuretics, which would be contraindicated.

Test-Taking Strategy: To answer this question, you need to know that a complication of head injury is DI. Knowing that DI results in excretion of very large amounts of dilute urine, options 3 and 4 can be eliminated immediately. You would choose option 1 over option 2 by knowing the actions of these two medications. Review the action and purpose of desmopressin now if you had difficulty with this question!

Level of Cognitive Ability: Application
Phase of Nursing Process: Implementation
Client Needs: Physiological Integrity
Content Area: Pharmacology

Reference
Black, J., & Matassarin-Jacobs, E. (1997). *Medical-surgical nursing: Clinical management for continuity of care* (5th ed.). Philadelphia: W. B. Saunders. p. 825.

53. **4**

Rationale: A concussion after head injury is a temporary loss of consciousness (from a few seconds to a few minutes) without evidence of structural damage. After concussion, the family is taught to monitor the client and to call the physician or return the client to the emergency department for several signs and symptoms, including confusion, difficulty awakening or speaking, one-sided weakness, vomiting, or severe headache. Minor headache is expected.

Test-Taking Strategy: To answer this question, you need to be familiar with neurologic signs and symptoms of ICP. Vomiting and neurologic deficits (in this case, speaking), indicate increased intracranial pressure. Decreasing LOC (difficulty arousing) is an early sign of increasing ICP. For these reasons, eliminate each of these responses and choose the minor headache, which is expected.

Level of Cognitive Ability: Analysis
Phase of Nursing Process: Evaluation
Client Needs: Health Promotion and Maintenance
Content Area: Adult Health/Neurological

Reference

Smeltzer, S., & Bare, B. (1996). *Brunner and Suddarth's textbook of medical-surgical nursing* (8th ed.). Philadelphia: Lippincott-Raven. p. 1790.

54. **4**

Rationale: The changes in neurologic signs from an epidural hematoma begin with loss of consciousness, as arterial blood collects in the epidural space and exerts pressure. The client regains consciousness as the CSF is rapidly reabsorbed to compensate for the rising ICP. As the compensatory mechanisms fail, even small amounts of additional blood cause the ICP to rise rapidly, and the client's neurologic status deteriorates quickly.

Test-Taking Strategy: Begin to answer this question by ruling out skull fracture and concussion as responsible for fluctuating neurological signs. Recall that a subdural hematoma is a collection of venous blood, which may accumulate more slowly and cause steadier deterioration of neurological signs. This may help you discriminate between epidural and subdural hematomas. Review the clinical manifestations associated with the various types of head injury now if you had difficulty with this question!

Level of Cognitive Ability: Analysis
Phase of Nursing Process: Analysis
Client Needs: Physiological Integrity
Content Area: Adult Health/Neurological

Reference

Smeltzer, S., & Bare, B. (1996). *Brunner and Suddarth's textbook of medical-surgical nursing* (8th ed.). Philadelphia: Lippincott-Raven. p. 1790.

55. **2**

Rationale: Clients with cognitive deficits after head injury may benefit from referral to a neuropsychologist, who specializes in evaluating and treating cognitive problems. The neuropsychologist plans an individual program of therapy and initiates counseling to help the client reach maximal potential. The neuropsychologist works in collaboration with other disciplines that are involved with the client's care and rehabilitation.

Test-Taking Strategy: Begin by eliminating the social worker referral as the least likely choice for this problem. A vocational rehabilitation specialist may not be indicated because the stem gives no information about employment. Of the two remaining, the neuropsychologist is a more specialized practitioner, who would be of more benefit in this situation. The question addresses a client with a neurological condition; therefore, the neuropsychologist is the best choice!

Level of Cognitive Ability: Application
Phase of Nursing Process: Planning
Client Needs: Psychosocial Integrity
Content Area: Adult Health/Neurological

Reference

Smeltzer, S., & Bare, B. (1996). *Brunner and Suddarth's textbook of medical-surgical nursing* (8th ed.). Philadelphia: Lippincott-Raven. p. 1796.

56. **3**

Rationale: Following supratentorial surgery, the head is kept at a 30- to 45-degree angle. The head and neck should not be angled either anteriorly or laterally, but rather should be kept in a neutral (midline) position. This will promote venous return through the jugular veins, which will help prevent a rise in intracranial pressure.

Test-Taking Strategy: This question tests knowledge of differences in positioning the craniotomy client with an infratentorial versus supratentorial incision. If you know that with supra- "keep the head up," and with infra- "keep the head down," you will eliminate options 1 and 2. Knowing how to position the head for optimal venous drainage helps you to select option 3 over option 4. Review client positioning following craniotomy now if you had difficulty with this question!

Level of Cognitive Ability: Application
Phase of Nursing Process: Implementation
Client Needs: Safe, Effective Care Environment
Content Area: Adult Health/Neurological

Reference

Black, J., & Matassarin-Jacobs, E. (1997). *Medical-surgical nursing: Clinical management for continuity of care* (5th ed.). Philadelphia: W. B. Saunders. p. 853.

57. **1**

Rationale: Signs of meningeal irritation compatible with meningitis include nuchal rigidity, positive Brudzinski's sign, and positive Kernig's sign. Nuchal rigidity is characterized by a stiff neck and soreness, which is especially noticeable when the neck is flexed. Kernig's sign is positive when the client feels pain and spasm of the hamstring muscles when the knee is straightened while the hip is flexed at a 90-degree angle. Brudzinski's sign is positive when the client flexes the hips and knees in response to the nurse gently flexing the head and neck onto the chest. A Glasgow Coma Scale score of 15 is a perfect score and indicates the client is awake and alert with no neurological deficits.

Test-Taking Strategy: This question tests classic signs and symptoms of meningeal irritation. If you are not familiar with them, you should take a few moments to review them now!

Level of Cognitive Ability: Analysis
Phase of Nursing Process: Analysis
Client Needs: Physiological Integrity
Content Area: Adult Health/Neurological

Reference

Ignatavicius, D., Workman, M., & Mishler, M. (1995). *Medical-surgical nursing: A nursing process approach* (2nd ed.). Philadelphia: W. B. Saunders. p. 1141.

58. **4**

Rationale: A 50-mL difference in intake and output for an 8-hour shift is insignificant. Stable weight indicates that there is neither fluid excess nor fluid deficit. The BUN of 10 mg/dL is within normal range (5 to 20 mg/dL) and does not indicate over- or underhydration. The normal serum osmolality is 285 to 295 mOsm/kg H_2O. A higher value indicates dehydration; a lower value indicates overhydration. After craniotomy the goal is to keep the serum osmolality on the high side of normal. This would minimize excess body water and control cerebral edema.

Test-Taking Strategy: To answer this question, you need to be familiar with common laboratory values, such as the BUN and serum "osmo." An easy way to remember serum osmo trends is to remember that "high is dry." By remembering this, you will know that the converse is also true; that is, a low value indicates excess body water (overhydration).

Level of Cognitive Ability: Analysis
Phase of Nursing Process: Assessment
Client Needs: Physiological Integrity
Content Area: Adult Health/Neurological

Reference

Ignatavicius, D., Workman, M., & Mishler, M. (1995). *Medical-surgical nursing: A nursing process approach* (2nd ed.). Philadelphia, W. B. Saunders. p. 1288.

59. **4**

Rationale: Codeine is the narcotic analgesic of choice for clients after craniotomy. It is often combined with a non-narcotic analgesic such as acetaminophen for added effect. It does not alter the respiratory rate or mask neurologic signs as other narcotics do. Side effects of codeine include gastrointestinal upset and constipation. The drug can lead to physical and psychological dependence with chronic use.

Test-Taking Strategy: This question tests your knowledge of codeine as a narcotic analgesic. General knowledge about narcotic analgesics as a class helps you to eliminate options 2 and 3. Because codeine is not the strongest narcotic available, you eliminate option 1 next. This leaves the correct answer, which is codeine's advantage of not masking neurologic signs.

Level of Cognitive Ability: Analysis
Phase of Nursing Process: Analysis
Client Needs: Physiological Integrity
Content Area: Pharmacology

References

Black, J., & Matassarin-Jacobs, E. (1997). *Medical-surgical nursing: Clinical management for continuity of care* (5th ed.). Philadelphia: W. B. Saunders. p. 855.
Deglin, J., & Vallerand, A. (1997). *Davis's drug guide for nurses* (5th ed.). Philadelphia: F. A. Davis. p. 292.

60. **3**

Rationale: Seizures are a potential complication that can occur for up to 1 year after surgery. For this reason, the client must diligently take anticonvulsant medications. The client and family are encouraged to keep track of doses administered. The family should learn seizure precautions and accompany the client while ambulating if dizziness or seizures tend to occur. The suture line is kept dry until sutures are removed to prevent infection. The postcraniotomy client is typically sensitive to loud noises, and can find them irritating (for example, loud television). Awareness control of environmental noise by others is helpful to this client.

Test-Taking Strategy: Begin to answer this question by eliminating option 1 first, since it is a general teaching point appropriate after many types of surgery. If you know that seizures are a potential postoperative risk up to a year after surgery, this eliminates options 2 and 4 as well. This leaves option 3 as the correct answer. Many clients after craniotomy have sensitivity to or are irritated by loud noises.

Level of Cognitive Ability: Application
Phase of Nursing Process: Planning
Client Needs: Health Promotion and Maintenance
Content Area: Adult Health/Neurological

Reference

Smeltzer, S., & Bare, B. (1996). *Brunner and Suddarth's textbook of medical-surgical nursing* (8th ed.). Philadelphia: Lippincott-Raven. p. 1741.

61. **1**

Rationale: Dexamethasone is an adrenocorticosteroid administered after craniotomy to control cerebral edema. It is given by IV push, and single doses are administered over 1 minute. Dexamethasone doses are changed to oral route after 24 to 72 hours and are tapered in dose until discontinued.

Test-Taking Strategy: Specific knowledge of this medication is needed to answer this question. This medication can be ordered for a variety of client problems, so it is worth reviewing if you had difficulty with this question!

Level of Cognitive Ability: Application
Phase of Nursing Process: Implementation
Client Needs: Physiological Integrity
Content Area: Pharmacology

References

Deglin, J., & Vallerand, A. (1997). *Davis's drug guide for nurses* (5th ed.). Philadelphia: F. A. Davis. p. 551.
Smeltzer, S., & Bare, B. (1996). *Brunner and Suddarth's textbook of medical-surgical nursing* (8th ed.). Philadelphia: Lippincott-Raven. p. 1737.

62. **4**

Rationale: After craniotomy, clients may experience difficulty with altered personal appearance. The nurse can help by listening to client concerns and by clarifying any misconceptions about facial edema, periorbital bruising, and hair loss (which are temporary). The nurse can encourage the client to participate in self-grooming and use personal articles of clothing. Finally, the nurse can suggest the use of a turban, followed by a hairpiece, to help the client adapt to the temporary change in appearance.

Test-Taking Strategy: The wording of this question makes you look for an incorrect statement or a maladaptive response. Options 1 and 2 both indicate adaptive responses and are therefore eliminated. Knowing that facial edema and bruising are temporary helps you to choose option 4 over option 3.

Level of Cognitive Ability: Analysis
Phase of Nursing Process: Evaluation
Client Needs: Psychosocial Integrity
Content Area: Adult Health/Neurological

Reference

Smeltzer, S., & Bare, B. (1996). *Brunner and Suddarth's textbook of medical-surgical nursing* (8th ed.). Philadelphia: Lippincott-Raven. p. 1741.

63. **1**

Rationale: Ineffective Breathing Pattern is diagnosed when the respiratory rate, depth, rhythm, timing, or chest wall movements are insufficient for optimal ventilation of the client. This is a risk for clients with spinal cord injury in the lower cervical area. Impaired Gas Exchange is used when oxygenation or carbon dioxide elimination is altered at the alveolar-capillary membrane. Risk for Aspiration and Risk for Injury are unrelated to the question as it is stated.

Test-Taking Strategy: This question discriminates among the various nursing diagnoses that relate to respiration. The client's clinical signs do not provide the best match for the defining characteristics of Risk for Aspiration and Risk for Injury. Knowing that the respiratory difficulty is a result of a motor problem helps you choose Ineffective Breathing Pattern over Impaired Gas Exchange. Additionally, the question states that the client has a weakened respiratory effort, ineffective cough, and is using accessory neck muscles in breathing. This indicates an ineffective breathing pattern.

Level of Cognitive Ability: Analysis
Phase of Nursing Process: Analysis
Client Needs: Physiological Integrity
Content Area: Adult Health/Neurological

References

Cox, H., et al. (1997). *Clinical applications of nursing diagnosis: Adult, child, women's, psychiatric, gerontic and home health considerations* (3rd ed.). Philadelphia: F. A. Davis. pp. 269, 327.
Ignatavicius, D. Workman, M., & Mishler, M. (1995). *Medical-surgical nursing: A nursing process approach* (2nd ed.). Philadelphia: W. B. Saunders. p. 1185.
Smeltzer, S., & Bare, B. (1996). *Brunner and Suddarth's textbook of medical-surgical nursing* (8th ed.). Philadelphia: Lippincott-Raven. p. 1801.

64. **4**

Rationale: Crutchfield tongs are applied after drilling holes in the client's skull under local anesthesia. Weights are attached to the tongs, which exert pulling pressure on the longitudinal axis of the cervical spine. Serial x-rays of the cervical spine are taken, with weights being gradually added until x-ray reveals that the vertebral column is realigned. After that, weights may be gradually reduced to a point that maintains alignment. The client with Crutchfield tongs is placed on a Stryker frame or Roto-Rest bed. The nurse ensures that weights hang freely and the amount of weight matches the current order. The nurse also inspects the integrity and position of the ropes and pulleys. The nurse does not remove the weights to administer care.

Test-Taking Strategy: The question asks for an action that is to be avoided, so the correct answer is an item that would be contraindicated. Knowing the basics of traction is sufficient to answer this question. Since options 2 and 3 are correct, and option 4 is not, then option 4 must be the answer to the question as stated. Review nursing care related to the client with cervical tongs now if you had difficulty with this question!

Level of Cognitive Ability: Application
Phase of Nursing Process: Planning
Client Needs: Safe, Effective Care Environment
Content Area: Adult Health/Neurological

References

Ignatavicius, D., Workman, M., & Mishler, M. (1995). *Medical-surgical nursing: A nursing process approach* (2nd ed.). Philadelphia: W. B. Saunders. pp. 1187–1188.
Smeltzer, S., & Bare, B. (1996). *Brunner and Suddarth's textbook of medical-surgical nursing* (8th ed.). Philadelphia: Lippincott-Raven. p. 1799–1800.

65. **2**

Rationale: Adjusting to paralysis is difficult both physically and psychosocially for the client and family. The nurse recognizes that the client goes through the grieving process in adjusting to the loss, and may move back and forth among the stages of grief. The nurse acknowledges the client's feelings while continuing to meet the client's physical needs and encouraging independence.

Test-Taking Strategy: This question can be answered easily by examining the impact or outcome of each of the options. The nurse cannot neglect the client until the client is ready (option 3), so this can be eliminated first. The family is also in crisis and needs the nurse's support (option 4), and should not be relied upon for care. Option 1 represents a factual but noncaring approach to the client, which is also not therapeutic. This leaves option 2 as the best choice of the available responses. Also, option 2 acknowledges the client's feelings.

Level of Cognitive Ability: Application
Phase of Nursing Process: Implementation
Client Needs: Psychosocial Integrity
Content Area: Adult Health/Neurological

Reference

Black, J., & Matassarin-Jacobs, E. (1997). *Medical-surgical nursing: Clinical management for continuity of care* (5th ed.). Philadelphia: W. B. Saunders. p. 910.

66. **4**

Rationale: The Halo device alters balance and can cause fatigue because of its weight. The client should cleanse the skin daily under the vest to protect the skin from ulceration, and should use powder or lotions sparingly or not at all. The wool liner should be changed if odor becomes a problem. The client should have food cut into small pieces to facilitate chewing and use straws for drinking. Pin care is done as instructed. The client may not drive because the device impairs the range of vision.

Test-Taking Strategy: To answer this question successfully, it is necessary to know that a Halo brace or vest is used to allow mobility for the client who needs continuous cervical traction. It maintains the head and spine in a neutral position. With this in mind, it may be fairly easy to choose option 4 as the correct answer to the question as stated. The inability to turn the head without turning the torso would make driving contraindicated. Review client education points related to a Halo vest now if you had difficulty with this question!

Level of Cognitive Ability: Analysis
Phase of Nursing Process: Evaluation
Client Needs: Health Promotion and Maintenance
Content Area: Adult Health/Neurological

Reference

Ignatavicius, D., Workman, M., & Mishler, M. (1995). *Medical-surgical nursing: A nursing process approach* (2nd ed.). Philadelphia: W. B. Saunders. p. 1193.

67. **2**

Rationale: After spinal cord injury, the client can develop paralytic ileus, which is characterized by absence of bowel sounds and abdominal distention. Development of a stress ulcer can be detected by Hematest-positive NGT aspirate or stool. A history of diarrhea is irrelevant.

Test-Taking Strategy: Knowing the basics of abdominal assessment and the physiologic stress response guarantees correct choice of an answer to this question. Review these concepts briefly if this question is problematic!

Level of Cognitive Ability: Application
Phase of Nursing Process: Assessment
Client Needs: Physiological Integrity
Content Area: Adult Health/Neurological

Reference

Ignatavicius, D., Workman, M., & Mishler, M. (1995). *Medical-surgical nursing: A nursing process approach* (2nd ed.). Philadelphia: W. B. Saunders. p. 1186.

68. **1**

Rationale: Depression is frequently seen in the client with spinal cord injury and may be exhibited as a loss of appetite. The client should be allowed to choose the types of food to eat and when they are eaten as much as is feasible, since it is one of the few areas of control that the client has left.

Test-Taking Strategy: The nurse does not make the diagnosis of clinical depression, which makes this an unreasonable choice. For the same reason, the option related to compulsive habits should be discarded. There is no evidence in the stem to demonstrate that the client has a slow metabolic rate, so this is eliminated next. The option that is left is the correct choice, that is, leaving the client as much control as possible.

Level of Cognitive Ability: Analysis
Phase of Nursing Process: Analysis
Client Needs: Psychosocial Integrity
Content Area: Adult Health/Neurological

Reference

Black, J., & Matassarin-Jacobs, E. (1997). *Medical-surgical nursing: Clinical management for continuity of care* (5th ed.). Philadelphia: W. B. Saunders. p. 898.

69. **3**

Rationale: Range-of-motion exercises are beneficial in stretching muscles, which may diminish spasticity. Removing potentially harmful objects is a good safety measure. Use of muscle relaxants is also indicated if the spasms cause discomfort to the client or pose a risk to the client's safety. Use of limb restraints will not alleviate spasticity and could harm the client.

Test-Taking Strategy: The wording of the question guides you to look for a response that is potentially harmful to the client. Each of the incorrect options can be eliminated systematically if you evaluate the options by looking for those interventions that would pose a risk to the client. Restraints should be avoided.

Level of Cognitive Ability: Application
Phase of Nursing Process: Planning
Client Needs: Safe, Effective Care Environment
Content Area: Adult Health/Neurological

Reference

Black, J., & Matassarin-Jacobs, E. (1997). *Medical-surgical nursing: Clinical management for continuity of care* (5th ed.). Philadelphia: W. B. Saunders. pp. 900–901.

70. **2**

Rationale: To prevent pressure ulcers from developing, the paraplegic client should shift weight in the wheelchair every 2 hours and should use a pressure relief pad. While in bed, the bottom sheet should be free of wrinkles and wetness. The client should use a mirror to inspect the skin twice a day (morning and evening) to assess for redness, edema, and breakdown. General additional measures include a nutritious diet and meticulous skin care.

Test-Taking Strategy: This question asks for a least helpful measure. Each of the responses appears reasonable on first inspection. With a closer look, however, you will notice that the time frame for inspecting the skin is much too infrequent, making this the correct response to the question as stated. Prioritization is required to answer this question!

Level of Cognitive Ability: Application
Phase of Nursing Process: Implementation
Client Needs: Health Promotion and Maintenance
Content Area: Adult Health/Neurological

Reference

Smeltzer, S., & Bare, B. (1996). *Brunner and Suddarth's textbook of medical-surgical nursing* (8th ed.). Philadelphia: Lippincott-Raven. p. 1806–1807.

71. **3**

Rationale: Range of motion to the finger joints prevents contractures but does not actively strengthen muscle groups needed for self-mobilization with paraplegia. Other activities that are more effective include push-ups from a prone position, sit-ups from a sitting position, extending the arms while holding weights, and squeezing rubber balls or crumpling newspaper.

Test-Taking Strategy: This question can be answered by thinking about the energy expenditure of the muscle groups involved in the activities listed in each option. The one that will involve the least energy expenditure (and therefore the least amount of muscle development) is the range-of-motion exercises, which makes it the correct answer to this question as stated.

Level of Cognitive Ability: Analysis
Phase of Nursing Process: Evaluation
Client Needs: Health Promotion and Maintenance
Content Area: Adult Health/Neurological

Reference

Smeltzer, S., & Bare, B. (1996). *Brunner and Suddarth's textbook of medical-surgical nursing* (8th ed.). Philadelphia: Lippincott-Raven. p. 1806.

72. **1**

Rationale: The client with spinal cord injury is at risk for autonomic dysreflexia with an injury above the level of T7. It is characterized by severe, throbbing headache, flushing of the face and neck, bradycardia, and sudden severe hypertension. Other signs include nasal stuffiness, blurred vision, nausea, and sweating. It is a life-threatening syndrome triggered by a noxious stimulus below the level of the injury.

Test-Taking Strategy: To answer this question correctly, it is necessary to know what causes autonomic dysreflexia. It results from the sudden exaggerated response of the sympathetic nervous system to a noxious stimulus. A massive sympathetic nervous system response causes severe hypertension. This would account for the throbbing headache (the correct answer), and cause flushing of the face and neck. Baroreceptors sense the sudden hypertension, causing a reflex bradycardia. The pulse and BP changes with autonomic dysreflexia are actually the opposite of what would occur with hypovolemic shock. Review the signs of autonomic dysreflexia now if you had difficulty with this question!

Level of Cognitive Ability: Application
Phase of Nursing Process: Assessment
Client Needs: Physiological Integrity
Content Area: Adult Health/Neurological

References

Black, J., & Matassarin-Jacobs, E. (1997). *Medical-surgical nursing: Clinical management for continuity of care* (5th ed.). Philadelphia: W. B. Saunders. pp. 894–895.

Ignatavicius, D., Workman, M., & Mishler, M. (1995). *Medical-surgical nursing: A nursing process approach* (2nd ed.). Philadelphia: W. B. Saunders. p. 1182.

73. **4**

Rationale: The client with spinal cord injury is at risk for autonomic dysreflexia with an injury above the level of T7. It is characterized by severe, throbbing headache, flushing of the face and neck, bradycardia, and sudden severe hypertension. Other signs include nasal stuffiness, blurred vision, nausea, and sweating. It is a life-threatening syndrome triggered by a noxious stimulus below the level of the injury.

Test-Taking Strategy: Begin to answer this question by eliminating options 1 and 3. The client in spinal shock would be hypotensive (not hypertensive), and the client's clinical picture does not match pulmonary embolism. (It may be useful to know also that autonomic dysreflexia does not occur until spinal shock resolves.) The word "hypertension" may have caught your eye in option 2, but knowing that this disorder, in option 2, occurs with anesthesia would cause you to discard this option as well.

Level of Cognitive Ability: Analysis
Phase of Nursing Process: Analysis
Client Needs: Physiological Integrity
Content Area: Adult Health/Neurological

References

Black, J., & Matassarin-Jacobs, E. (1997). *Medical-surgical nursing: Clinical management for continuity of care* (5th ed.). Philadelphia: W. B. Saunders. pp. 894–895.

Ignatavicius, D., Workman, M., & Mishler, M. (1995). *Medical-surgical nursing: A nursing process approach* (2nd ed.). Philadelphia: W. B. Saunders. p. 1182.

74. **2**

Rationale: The most frequent cause of autonomic dysreflexia is a distended bladder. Straight catheterization should be done every 4 to 6 hours, and Foley catheters should be checked frequently to prevent kinks in the tubing. Constipation and fecal impaction are other causes, so maintaining bowel regularity is important. Other causes include stimulation of the skin from tactile, thermal, or painful stimuli. The nurse administers care to minimize risk in these areas.

Test-Taking Strategy: The easiest way to answer questions of this nature is to remember that autonomic dysreflexia is caused by noxious stimuli to the bowel, bladder, or skin. With this in mind, you can easily eliminate each of the incorrect options for this question. Review the measures to minimize the risk of autonomic dysreflexia now if you had difficulty with this question!

Level of Cognitive Ability: Application
Phase of Nursing Process: Implementation
Client Needs: Safe, Effective Care Environment
Content Area: Adult Health/Neurological

Reference

Smeltzer, S., & Bare, B. (1996). *Brunner and Suddarth's textbook of medical-surgical nursing* (8th ed.). Philadelphia: Lippincott-Raven. p. 1804.

75. **4**

Rationale: Key nursing actions are to sit the client up in bed, remove the noxious stimulus, and bring the blood pressure under control with antihypertensive medication per protocol. The nurse can also clearly label the client's chart, identifying the risk for autonomic dysreflexia. Client and family should be taught to recognize, and later manage, the signs and symptoms of this syndrome.

Test-Taking Strategy: Note the word "immediately" in the stem. This is a clue that the first item in each option must be the first action. If you know to raise the head of the client's bed first (to try to minimize cerebral hypertension), then this eliminates each of the incorrect responses. Review immediate nursing interventions for the client experiencing autonomic dysreflexia if you had difficulty with this question!

Level of Cognitive Ability: Application
Phase of Nursing Process: Implementation
Client Needs: Physiological Integrity
Content Area: Adult Health/Neurological

Reference

Smeltzer, S., & Bare, B. (1996). *Brunner and Suddarth's textbook of medical-surgical nursing* (8th ed.). Philadelphia: Lippincott-Raven. p. 1804.

76. **3**

Rationale: Reflex vasodilatation below the level of spinal cord injury places the client at risk of orthostatic hypotension, which may be profound. Measures to minimize this include measuring vital signs before and during position changes, use of a tilt table in early mobilization, and changing the client's position slowly. Venous pooling can be reduced by using TEDs or pneumatic boots. Vasopressor medications are used per protocol.

Test-Taking Strategy: Reflex vasodilatation below the level of the injury causes hypotension. The question asks which is the least helpful in minimizing the hypotensive effect. Venous compression (option 4) is helpful and so is eliminated as the correct answer. Options 1 and 2 are helpful and are eliminated next. Knowing that quick position changes and movement would aggravate hypotension helps you be sure that you have selected the correct option.

Level of Cognitive Ability: Application
Phase of Nursing Process: Planning
Client Needs: Physiological Integrity
Content Area: Adult Health/Neurological

Reference

Smeltzer, S., & Bare, B. (1996). *Brunner and Suddarth's textbook of medical-surgical nursing* (8th ed.). Philadelphia: Lippincott-Raven. p. 1804.

77. **4**

Rationale: Spinal immobilization is necessary after spinal cord injury to prevent further damage and insult to the spinal cord. Whenever possible, the client is placed on a Stryker frame, which allows the nurse to turn the client to prevent complications of immobility while maintaining alignment of the spine. If a Stryker frame is not available, a firm mattress with a bedboard under it should be used.

Test-Taking Strategy: To answer this question quickly and accurately, you must be familiar with a Stryker frame and its use. Take a few moments now to review this if you had difficulty with this question!

Level of Cognitive Ability: Application
Phase of Nursing Process: Implementation
Client Needs: Safe, Effective Care Environment
Content Area: Adult Health/Neurological

Reference

Smeltzer, S., & Bare, B. (1996). *Brunner and Suddarth's textbook of medical-surgical nursing* (8th ed.). Philadelphia: Lippincott-Raven. p. 1797.

78. 3

Rationale: Resolution of spinal shock is occurring when there is return of reflexes (especially flexors to noxious cutaneous stimuli), a state of hyperreflexia rather than flaccidity, return of bulbospongiosis reflex in the male, and a positive Babinski reflex.

Test-Taking Strategy: Recall that spinal shock is characterized by loss of movement by skeletal muscles, bowel or bladder wall, or by reflex action. Return of any of these indicates that spinal shock is beginning to resolve. The inability to elicit any Babinski response indicates that spinal shock is ongoing. Thus, this is the correct answer to the question as stated. Review signs of spinal shock now if you had difficulty with this question!

Level of Cognitive Ability: Analysis
Phase of Nursing Process: Evaluation
Client Needs: Physiological Integrity
Content Area: Adult Health/Neurological

Reference

Black, J., & Matassarin-Jacobs, E. (1997). *Medical-surgical nursing: Clinical management for continuity of care* (5th ed.). Philadelphia: W. B. Saunders. p. 895.

79. 2

Rationale: Ptosis of the eyelid is caused by pressure on and dysfunction of cranial nerve III. Once this occurs, this is ongoing and does not relate to LOC. Early changes in LOC relate to alertness and verbal responsiveness. Less frequent speech, slight slurring of speech, and mild drowsiness are early signs of decreasing LOC.

Test-Taking Strategy: The question asks which assessment is not an early sign of LOC deterioration. Thus, the answer is either a later sign or one that is unrelated. If you know that LOC includes orientation, awareness, and verbal responsiveness, then you would eliminate each of the incorrect options systematically. Review the early signs of decreasing LOC now if you had difficulty with this question!

Level of Cognitive Ability: Application
Phase of Nursing Process: Assessment
Client Needs: Physiological Integrity
Content Area: Adult Health/Neurological

Reference

Smeltzer, S., & Bare, B. (1996). *Brunner and Suddarth's textbook of medical-surgical nursing* (8th ed.). Philadelphia: Lippincott-Raven. p. 1766.

80. 3

Rationale: Aneurysm precautions include placing the client on bed rest in a quiet setting. Lights are kept dim to minimize environmental stimulation. Any activity that increases BP or impedes venous return from the brain is prohibited, such as pushing, pulling, sneezing, coughing, or straining. The nurse provides all physical care to minimize increases in BP. For the same reason, visitors, radio, television, and reading materials are prohibited or limited. Stimulants such as caffeine and nicotine are prohibited; decaffeinated coffee or tea may be used.

Test-Taking Strategy: To answer this question you must understand that a global principle in aneurysm precautions is to limit the amount of stimulation (in any form) that the client receives and to prevent increased intracranial pressure (ICP). Options 1 and 2 are effective in promoting venous drainage from the brain (to keep ICP down) and are part of the precautions. Option 4 limits the amount of stimulation and exertion by the client and is also part of the precautions. Nicotine must be completely eliminated, which makes this the answer to the question. Review aneurysm precautions now if you had difficulty with this question!

Level of Cognitive Ability: Application
Phase of Nursing Process: Planning
Client Needs: Safe, Effective Care Environment
Content Area: Adult Health/Neurological

Reference

Smeltzer, S., & Bare, B. (1996). *Brunner and Suddarth's textbook of medical-surgical nursing* (8th ed.). Philadelphia: Lippincott-Raven. p. 1766.

81. 1

Rationale: Aminocaproic acid is an antifibrinolytic agent that prevents clot breakdown or dissolution. It is commonly ordered after subarachnoid hemorrhage if surgery is delayed or contraindicated. Heparin and coumadin are anticoagulants, which interfere with propagation or growth of a clot. Alteplase is a fibrinolytic, which actively breaks down clots.

Test-Taking Strategy: If you know that heparin and coumadin are anticoagulants, you eliminate options 2 and 3 immediately because they are contraindicated. Knowing that alteplase is a fibrinolytic causes you to eliminate this option also, since this drug would actively dissolve the clot (also contraindicated). This leaves you with aminocaproic acid as the correct response. Review the action and use of aminocaproic acid now if you had difficulty with this question!

Level of Cognitive Ability: Application
Phase of Nursing Process: Implementation
Client Needs: Physiological Integrity
Content Area: Pharmacology

References

Deglin, J., & Vallerand, A. (1997). *Davis's drug guide for nurses* (5th ed.). Philadelphia: F. A. Davis. pp. 46, 585, 1156, 1229.
Smeltzer, S., & Bare, B. (1996). *Brunner and Suddarth's textbook of medical-surgical nursing* (8th ed.). Philadelphia: Lippincott-Raven. p. 1765.

82. 4

Rationale: Nimodipine is a calcium channel blocking agent that has an affinity for cerebral blood vessels. It is used to prevent or control vasospasm in cerebral blood vessels, thereby reducing the chance for rebleeding. It is typically ordered for 3 weeks' duration.

Test-Taking Strategy: Knowledge of this medication and its use is needed to answer this question correctly. If you know that nimodipine is a calcium channel blocking agent, you limit your options to 3 and 4. Knowing that calcium channel blockers decrease vasospasm helps you choose option 4 over option 3. Review the purpose of nimodipine now if you had difficulty with this question!

Level of Cognitive Ability: Analysis
Phase of Nursing Process: Evaluation
Client Needs: Health Promotion and Maintenance
Content Area: Pharmacology

References

Deglin, J., & Vallerand, A. (1997). *Davis's drug guide for nurses* (5th ed.). Philadelphia: F. A. Davis. pp. 200, 205.
Smeltzer, S., & Bare, B. (1996). *Brunner and Suddarth's textbook of medical-surgical nursing* (8th ed.). Philadelphia: Lippincott-Raven. p. 1766.

83. 2

Rationale: Typically, seizure assessment includes the time the seizure began, part(s) of the body affected, the type of movements and progression of the seizure, changes in pupil size, eye deviation or nystagmus, client's condition during the seizure, and postictal status.

Test-Taking Strategy: The response about the client's intake prior to the seizure suggests worry about vomiting and subsequent aspiration. The nurse is concerned about aspiration, not from vomiting but from inhalation of the client's own saliva. Since all other options are standard assessments, this is the answer to the question. Review nursing assessment during a seizure if you had difficulty answering this question!

Level of Cognitive Ability: Application
Phase of Nursing Process: Assessment
Client Needs: Physiological Integrity
Content Area: Adult Health/Neurological

Reference

Ignatavicius, D., Workman, M., & Mishler, M. (1995). *Medical-surgical nursing: A nursing process approach* (2nd ed.). Philadelphia: W. B. Saunders. pp. 1135–1136.

84. 3

Rationale: Seizure precautions may vary somewhat from agency to agency, but they generally have some commonalities. Usually an airway and oxygen and suctioning equipment are kept available at the bedside. The side rails of the bed are padded, and the bed is kept in the lowest position. The client has an IV access in place to have a readily accessible route if IV anticonvulsant medications must be administered. The use of padded tongue blades is highly controversial, and they should not be kept at the bedside. Forcing a tongue blade into the mouth during a seizure will more likely harm the client who bites down during seizure activity. Risks include blocking the airway from improper placement, chipping the client's teeth, and subsequent risk of aspirating tooth fragments. If the client has an aura before the seizure, it may give the nurse enough time to place an oral airway before seizure activity begins.

Test-Taking Strategy: This question must be evaluated from the perspective of causing possible harm. No harm can come to the client from any of the options except for the tongue blade. Review seizure precautions now if you had difficulty with this question!

Level of Cognitive Ability: Application
Phase of Nursing Process: Planning
Client Needs: Safe, Effective Care Environment
Content Area: Adult Health/Neurological

Reference

Ignatavicius, D., Workman, M., & Mishler, M. (1995). *Medical-surgical nursing: A nursing process approach* (2nd ed.). Philadelphia: W. B. Saunders. p. 1134.

85. 3

Rationale: Nursing actions during a seizure include providing for privacy, loosening restrictive clothing, removing the pillow and raising the side rails in the bed, and placing the client on one side with the head flexed forward, if possible, to allow the tongue to fall forward and facilitate drainage. The limbs are never restrained because the strong muscle contractions could cause the client harm. If the client is not in bed when seizure activity begins, the nurse lowers the client to the floor if possible, protects the head with a pad against injury, and moves furniture that may injure the client. Other aspects of care are as described for the client who is in bed.

Test-Taking Strategy: This question must be evaluated from the perspective of causing possible harm. No harm can come to the client from any of the options except for restraining the limbs. Avoid restraints! Review care to a client during a seizure now if you had difficulty with this question!

Level of Cognitive Ability: Application
Phase of Nursing Process: Implementation
Client Needs: Physiological Integrity
Content Area: Adult Health/Neurological

Reference

Smeltzer, S., & Bare, B. (1996). *Brunner and Suddarth's textbook of medical-surgical nursing* (8th ed.). Philadelphia: Lippincott-Raven. p. 1783.

86. 3

Rationale: Typical anticonvulsant medication instructions include taking the dose daily to keep the blood level of the drug constant; having a serum drug level drawn before taking the morning dose; avoiding abruptly stopping the medication; avoiding alcohol; checking with the physician before taking OTC medications; avoiding activities where alertness and coordination are required until medication effects are known; providing good oral hygiene and getting regular dental care; and carrying a Medic-Alert bracelet or tag.

Test-Taking Strategy: Options 1 and 2 can be eliminated fairly easily because they are the least likely choices for being correct. Of the two remaining, medications are not generally taken just prior to drawing therapeutic serum levels, because the results would be artificially high. This leaves oral hygiene as the correct answer because of the risk of gingival hyperplasia. Review client education related to phenytoin now if you had difficulty with this question!

Level of Cognitive Ability: Analysis
Phase of Nursing Process: Evaluation
Client Needs: Health Promotion and Maintenance
Content Area: Adult Health/Neurological

Reference

Smeltzer, S., & Bare, B. (1996). *Brunner and Suddarth's textbook of medical-surgical nursing* (8th ed.). Philadelphia: Lippincott-Raven. p. 1786.

87. 2

Rationale: Hemiparesis is a weakness of the face, arm, and leg on one side. The client with one-sided hemiparesis benefits from having objects placed on the unaffected side and within reach. Other helpful activities with hemiparesis include ROM exercises to the affected side and muscle-strengthening exercises to the unaffected side.

Test-Taking Strategy: Begin to answer this question by eliminating options 3 and 4 as potentially hazardous to the client. This question tests your ability to distinguish between hemiparesis and unilateral neglect. The client with hemiparesis has weakness on one side, and therefore objects should be place on the stronger side. With unilateral neglect, objects are placed on the affected side to train the client to attend to that part of the environment. Knowing this, you would pick option 2 over option 1. Review care to the client with hemiparesis now if you had difficulty with this question!

Level of Cognitive Ability: Application
Phase of Nursing Process: Planning
Client Needs: Safe, Effective Care Environment
Content Area: Adult Health/Neurological

Reference
Smeltzer, S., & Bare, B. (1996). *Brunner and Suddarth's textbook of medical-surgical nursing* (8th ed.). Philadelphia: Lippincott-Raven. p. 1728.

88. **1**

Rationale: Before the client with dysphagia is started on a diet, the gag and swallow reflexes must have returned. The client is assisted with meals as needed and is given ample time to chew and swallow. Food is placed on the unaffected side of the mouth. Liquids are thickened to avoid aspiration.

Test-Taking Strategy: This question asks you to identify an incorrect item. Option 4 is generally a good action for all clients. Option 3 is correct because the client has better sensation and motion on the unaffected side of the mouth. This narrows your options to two opposing concepts: thin versus thick liquids. Thickened liquids are easier for the client with impaired facial motion and swallowing ability to manage. Knowing this enables you to choose option 1 as the action to avoid. Review care to the client with residual dysphagia now if you had difficulty with this question!

Level of Cognitive Ability: Application
Phase of Nursing Process: Implementation
Client Needs: Physiological Integrity
Content Area: Adult Health/Neurological

References
Black, J., & Matassarin-Jacobs, E. (1997). *Medical-surgical nursing: Clinical management for continuity of care* (5th ed.). Philadelphia: W. B. Saunders. p. 796.
Smeltzer, S., & Bare, B. (1996). *Brunner and Suddarth's textbook of medical-surgical nursing* (8th ed.). Philadelphia: Lippincott-Raven. p. 1728.

89. **3**

Rationale: Homonymous hemianopsia is loss of one half of the visual field. The client with homonymous hemianopsia should have objects placed in the intact field of vision, and the nurse should approach the client from the intact side. The nurse instructs the client to scan the environment to overcome the visual deficit, and does client teaching from within the intact field of vision. The nurse encourages the use of personal eyeglasses if they are available.

Test-Taking Strategy: To answer this question accurately, you must be able to distinguish between homonymous hemianopsia and unilateral neglect. Clients are approached differently with these two deficits. The similarity is that the client must be taught to scan the environment, which is also the answer to this question. Review the concept of homonymous hemianopsia if you are unfamiliar with it!

Level of Cognitive Ability: Analysis
Phase of Nursing Process: Evaluation
Client Needs: Health Promotion and Maintenance
Content Area: Adult Health/Neurological

Reference
Smeltzer, S., & Bare, B. (1996). *Brunner and Suddarth's textbook of medical-surgical nursing* (8th ed.). Philadelphia: Lippincott-Raven. p. 1728.

90. **2**

Rationale: Clients are evaluated as coping successfully with lifestyle changes after CVA if they make appropriate lifestyle alterations, use the assistance of others, and have appropriate social interactions.

Test-Taking Strategy: Options 1 and 4 are behaviors that may be expected in the client with CVA, but they are not adaptive responses. Rather, they are a result of the insult to the brain. Options 2 and 3 indicate that the client is trying to adapt, but option 2 has the better outcome.

Level of Cognitive Ability: Analysis
Phase of Nursing Process: Assessment
Client Needs: Psychosocial Integrity
Content Area: Adult Health/Neurological

Reference
Black, J., & Matassarin-Jacobs, E. (1997). *Medical-surgical nursing: Clinical management for continuity of care* (5th ed.). Philadelphia: W. B. Saunders. p. 806.

91. **3**

Rationale: Unilateral neglect is an unawareness of the paralyzed side of the body, which increases the client's risk for injury. The nurse's role is to refocus the client's attention to the affected side. The nurse moves personal care items and belongings to the affected side, as well as bedside chair and commode. The nurse teaches the client to scan the environment to become aware of that half of the body, and approaches the client from that side to further increase awareness. Review care to the client with unilateral neglect if you had difficulty with this question!

Test-Taking Strategy: With unilateral neglect, the client loses awareness of the half of the world that is on the affected side. If you know that the client needs to be trained to attend to that side, you can eliminate each of the incorrect options.

Level of Cognitive Ability: Application
Phase of Nursing Process: Planning
Client Needs: Safe, Effective Care Environment
Content Area: Adult Health/Neurological

Reference
Black, J., & Matassarin-Jacobs, E. (1997). *Medical-surgical nursing: Clinical management for continuity of care* (5th ed.). Philadelphia: W. B. Saunders. p. 806.

92. **2**

Rationale: Clients with aphasia after CVA often fatigue easily and have a short attention span. General guidelines when trying to communicate with the aphasic client include speaking more slowly and allowing adequate response time, listening to and watching attempts to communicate, and trying to put the client at ease with a caring and understanding manner. Avoid shouting (the client is not deaf), appearing rushed for a response, and letting family members give all the responses for the client.

Test-Taking Strategy: This question tests a fundamental concept in communicating with the aphasic client. If this question was difficult, take a few moments now to review these communication strategies!

Level of Cognitive Ability: Application
Phase of Nursing Process: Implementation
Client Needs: Psychosocial Integrity
Content Area: Adult Health/Neurological

Reference

Black, J., & Matassarin-Jacobs, E. (1997). *Medical-surgical nursing: Clinical management for continuity of care* (5th ed.). Philadelphia: W. B. Saunders. p. 805.

93. **3**

Rationale: Placing an eyepatch over one eye in the client with diplopia removes the second image and restores more normal vision. The patch is alternated on a daily basis to maintain the strength of the extraocular muscles of the eyes.

Test-Taking Strategy: Knowing that an eyepatch will help diplopia only while it is worn, you first eliminate options 1 and 2 as not helpful. If you know that the extraocular muscles weaken with eyepatch use, you may select option 3 over 4, because these are small muscles that would lose strength fairly rapidly.

Level of Cognitive Ability: Analysis
Phase of Nursing Process: Evaluation
Client Needs: Health Promotion and Maintenance
Content Area: Adult Health/Neurological

Reference

Black, J., & Matassarin-Jacobs, E. (1997). *Medical-surgical nursing: Clinical management for continuity of care* (5th ed.). Philadelphia: W. B. Saunders. p. 803.

94. **3**

Rationale: Myasthenia gravis can often be diagnosed based on clinical signs and symptoms. The diagnosis can be confirmed by injecting the client with a dose of Tensilon. This drug inhibits the breakdown of an enzyme in the neuro-muscular junction, so more acetylcholine binds onto receptors. If the muscle is strengthened for 3 to 5 minutes after this injection, it confirms a diagnosis of myasthenia gravis. Another medication, neostigmine (Prostigmin) may also be used because the effect lasts for 1 to 2 hours, giving a better analysis. For either medication, atropine should be available as the antidote.

Test-Taking Strategy: Knowledge of the purpose and expected findings of the Tensilon test is required to answer this question successfully. If this is unfamiliar, it is recommended that you review this test briefly. You are likely to see questions related to the Tensilon test!

Level of Cognitive Ability: Analysis
Phase of Nursing Process: Analysis
Client Needs: Physiological Integrity
Content Area: Pharmacology

Reference

Black, J., & Matassarin-Jacobs, E. (1997). *Medical-surgical nursing: Clinical management for continuity of care* (5th ed.). Philadelphia: W. B. Saunders. pp. 884–885.

95. **2**

Rationale: The client has speech that is nasal in tone and dysarthritic owing to cranial nerve involvement of the muscles governing speech. The nurse listens attentively and verbally, verifies what the client has said, asks questions requiring a yes or no response, and develops alternative communication methods (letter board, picture board, pen and paper, flash cards). Encouraging the client to speak quickly is unsuccessful and counterproductive.

Test-Taking Strategy: There are some techniques that are useful in communicating with clients with speech impairment, regardless of the specific cause of the difficulty. Options 3 and 4 are classic examples of alternative communication methods that are useful, so you would eliminate them as from the choices of items to avoid. Since option 1 is also helpful, this leaves option 2 as the correct answer to the question as stated. Speaking quickly is difficult for a client with a speech impairment.

Level of Cognitive Ability: Application
Phase of Nursing Process: Implementation
Client Needs: Psychosocial Integrity
Content Area: Adult Health/Neurological

References

Ignatavicius, D., Workman, M., & Mishler, M. (1995). *Medical-surgical nursing: A nursing process approach* (2nd ed.). Philadelphia: W. B. Saunders. p. 1227.
Smeltzer, S., & Bare, B. (1996). *Brunner and Suddarth's textbook of medical-surgical nursing* (8th ed.). Philadelphia: Lippincott-Raven. p. 1780.

96. **4**

Rationale: The client with myasthenia gravis may experience episodes of respiratory distress if excessively fatigued, or if the client develops myasthenic crisis or cholinergic crisis. For this reason, an Ambu bag, intubation tray, and suction equipment should be available at the bedside.

Test-Taking Strategy: Note that there are two items in each option. In order for the option to be correct, both parts of the answer must be correct. Knowing that the client with myasthenia gravis is at risk for aspiration and respiratory failure helps you to choose option 4 over each of the others. Additionally, option 4 addresses the maintenance of a patent airway!

Level of Cognitive Ability: Application
Phase of Nursing Process: Implementation
Client Needs: Safe, Effective Care Environment
Content Area: Adult Health/Neurological

Reference

Ignatavicius, D., Workman, M., & Mishler, M. (1995). *Medical-surgical nursing: A nursing process approach* (2nd ed.). Philadelphia: W. B. Saunders. p. 1224.

97. **3**

Rationale: Myasthenic crisis is often caused by undermedication and responds to administration of cholinergic medications such as neostigmine (Prostigmin) and pyridostigmine (Mestinon). Cholinergic crisis (the opposite problem) is caused by excess medication and responds to withholding of medications. Too little exercise and fatty food intake are incorrect. Overexertion and overeating could possibly trigger myasthenic crisis.

Test-Taking Strategy: To answer this question most easily, it is necessary to know that undermedication is a common cause of myasthenic crisis. Take a few moments to review the causes if you are unfamiliar with them!

Level of Cognitive Ability: Application
Phase of Nursing Process: Assessment
Client Needs: Physiological Integrity
Content Area: Adult Health/Neurological

References

Black, J., & Matassarin-Jacobs, E. (1997). *Medical-surgical nursing: Clinical management for continuity of care* (5th ed.). Philadelphia: W. B. Saunders. p. 885.

Ignatavicius, D., Workman, M., & Mishler, M. (1995). *Medical-surgical nursing: A nursing process approach* (2nd ed.). Philadelphia: W. B. Saunders. p. 1228.

---

98. 2

Rationale: Clients with myasthenia gravis are taught to space out activities over the day to conserve energy and restore muscle strength. It is very important to take medications correctly to maintain blood levels that are not too low or too high. Muscle-strengthening exercises are not helpful and can fatigue the client. Overeating is a cause of exacerbation of symptoms, as well as exposure to heat, crowds, erratic sleep habits, and emotional stress.

Test-Taking Strategy: If you know that common causes of myasthenic and cholinergic crises are undermedication and overmedication, respectively, you should be able to easily eliminate each of the incorrect options to this question. No other option would prevent both of those complications. It is extremely important that these clients take medications on time to maintain therapeutic blood levels. Review measures to prevent myasthenic and cholinergic crises now if you are unfamiliar with them!

Level of Cognitive Ability: Application
Phase of Nursing Process: Implementation
Client Needs: Health Promotion and Maintenance
Content Area: Adult Health/Neurological

Reference

Ignatavicius, D., Workman, M., & Mishler, M. (1995). *Medical-surgical nursing: A nursing process approach* (2nd ed.). Philadelphia: W. B. Saunders. p. 1234.

---

99. 4

Rationale: The client avoids swallowing any type of food or drink with the head lifted upward, which could actually cause aspiration by opening the glottis. The client should be advised to sit bolt upright while eating, cut food into very small pieces, chew thoroughly, tip the chin downward to swallow, and not talk with food in the mouth (glottis is open).

Test-Taking Strategy: If you look at the construct of this question, you will see that options 3 and 4 oppose each other. This makes it likely that one of the two is correct. In examining each of them, option 4 is the better choice. Lifting the head opens the airway, which will increase the risk of aspiration during drinking or eating.

Level of Cognitive Ability: Application
Phase of Nursing Process: Implementation
Client Needs: Physiological Integrity
Content Area: Adult Health/Neurological

Reference

Black, J., & Matassarin-Jacobs, E. (1997). *Medical-surgical nursing: Clinical management for continuity of care* (5th ed.). Philadelphia: W. B. Saunders. p. 885.

---

100. 3

Rationale: Most ongoing treatment for myasthenia gravis is done in outpatient settings, and the client needs to be aware of the lifestyle changes needed to maintain independence. Taking medications an hour before mealtime gives greater muscle strength for chewing, and is indicated. The client should have portable suction equipment and a portable resuscitation bag available in case of respiratory distress. The client should carry medical identification about the condition. The client should avoid activities that could worsen the symptoms, including stress, infection, heat, surgery, or alcohol.

Test-Taking Strategy: Options 2 and 4 are very reasonable courses of action, and so they are eliminated as possible answers to this question as stated. To discriminate between the remaining two options, you would need to know that medication an hour before meals gives strength to the muscles (for chewing and swallowing), and that heat and infection (crowds at the beach) trigger myasthenic crisis. Review client education points with myasthenia gravis!

Level of Cognitive Ability: Analysis
Phase of Nursing Process: Evaluation
Client Needs: Health Promotion and Maintenance
Content Area: Adult Health/Neurological

References

Ignatavicius, D., Workman, M., & Mishler, M. (1995). *Medical-surgical nursing: A nursing process approach* (2nd ed.). Philadelphia: W. B. Saunders. p. 1234.

Smeltzer, S., & Bare, B. (1996). *Brunner and Suddarth's textbook of medical-surgical nursing* (8th ed.). Philadelphia: Lippincott-Raven. p. 1780.

---

101. 4

Rationale: The Parkinsonian gait is characterized by short, accelerating, shuffling steps. The client leans forward with head, hips, and knees flexed, and has difficulty starting and stopping. A dystrophic gait is broad based and waddling. A festinating gait is accelerating with walking on toes. An ataxic gait is staggering and unsteady.

Test-Taking Strategy: Knowledge of the different types of gait disorders is helpful in answering this question. However, if you know the signs and symptoms of Parkinson's disease, you know that the client has bradykinesia and difficulty in initiating movement. The gait is difficult to start, but it accelerates once it has begun. This would help you eliminate options 1 and 3. To discriminate between options 2 and 4, the client with Parkinson's disease shuffles but does not walk on the toes.

Level of Cognitive Ability: Analysis
Phase of Nursing Process: Assessment
Client Needs: Physiological Integrity
Content Area: Adult Health/Neurological

References

Black, J., & Matassarin-Jacobs, E. (1997). *Medical-surgical nursing: Clinical management for continuity of care* (5th ed.). Philadelphia: W. B. Saunders. p. 722.

Smeltzer, S., & Bare, B. (1996). *Brunner and Suddarth's textbook of medical-surgical nursing* (8th ed.). Philadelphia: Lippincott-Raven. p. 1772.

---

102. 3

Rationale: The client with Parkinson's disease tends to become withdrawn and depressed, and should become an active participant in own care to prevent this. There should be planned activities throughout the day to inhibit daytime sleeping and boredom. The nurse gives the client encouragement and praises the client for perseverance. Exercise helps prevent progression of the disease and self-care improves self-esteem.

Test-Taking Strategy: Options 1 and 4 are the least plausible of all available answers, and so they may be eliminated first. Option 2 is well-intentioned but is not therapeutic in helping the client to cope with the disease. Option 3 is the best choice.

Level of Cognitive Ability: Application
Phase of Nursing Process: Planning
Client Needs: Psychosocial Integrity
Content Area: Adult Health/Neurological

Reference

Smeltzer, S., & Bare, B. (1996). *Brunner and Suddarth's textbook of medical-surgical nursing* (8th ed.). Philadelphia: Lippincott-Raven. p. 1774–1775.

---

103. **1**

Rationale: Parkinsonian crisis can occur with emotional trauma or sudden withdrawal of medications. The client exhibits severe tremors, rigidity, and bradykinesia. The client also displays anxiety, is diaphoretic, and has tachycardia and hyperpnea. The client should be placed in a quiet, dim room and respiratory and cardiac support should be available.

Test-Taking Strategy: Option 4 is not indicated and is eliminated first. Option 3 is not an immediate concern and is also discarded. Of the remaining two, there is nothing about parkinsonian crisis that warrants placement of an NG tube. This leaves the correct option, which is to put the client in a dim, quiet room and provide for support of cardiac and respiratory symptoms. Review nursing care for parkinsonian crisis now if you had difficulty with this question!

Level of Cognitive Ability: Application
Phase of Nursing Process: Implementation
Client Needs: Safe, Effective Care Environment
Content Area: Adult Health/Neurological

Reference

Black, J., & Matassarin-Jacobs, E. (1997). *Medical-surgical nursing: Clinical management for continuity of care* (5th ed.). Philadelphia: W. B. Saunders. p. 879.

---

104. **2**

Rationale: The client with Parkinson's disease should exercise in the morning when energy levels are highest. The client should avoid sitting in soft, deep chairs, because they are difficult to get up from. The client can rock back and forth to initiate movement. The client should buy clothes with Velcro fasteners and slide locking buckles to support the ability to dress self.

Test-Taking Strategy: Option 1 is not useful to clients with fatigue from any disorder, so this option may be eliminated first. Knowing that the client with Parkinson's has difficulty with movement and dexterity helps you eliminate options 3 and 4 next. Thus you are left with the correct answer, which is rocking back and forth to start movement. Review client teaching points with Parkinson's disease now if you had difficulty with this question!

Level of Cognitive Ability: Analysis
Phase of Nursing Process: Evaluation
Client Needs: Health Promotion and Maintenance
Content Area: Adult Health/Neurological

Reference

Black, J., & Matassarin-Jacobs, E. (1997). *Medical-surgical nursing: Clinical management for continuity of care* (5th ed.). Philadelphia: W. B. Saunders. p. 881.

---

105. **1**

Rationale: The paroxysms of pain that accompany this neuralgia are triggered by stimulation of the terminal branches of the trigeminal nerve. Symptoms can be triggered by pressure from washing the face, brushing the teeth, shaving, eating, and drinking. Symptoms can also be triggered by thermal stimuli such as a draft of cold air.

Test-Taking Strategy: Options 2 and 4 are the least plausible of the four choices and may be eliminated first. Of the remaining two, option 3 represents a chemical stimulus, while option 1 represents mechanical and thermal stimuli. Since trigeminal neuralgia is triggered by mechanical and thermal events, this is the correct choice.

Level of Cognitive Ability: Analysis
Phase of Nursing Process: Analysis
Client Needs: Physiological Integrity
Content Area: Adult Health/Neurological

Reference

Smeltzer, S., & Bare, B. (1996). *Brunner and Suddarth's textbook of medical-surgical nursing* (8th ed.). Philadelphia: Lippincott-Raven. p. 1816.

---

106. **2**

Rationale: The anticonvulsant medications carbemazepine and phenytoin help relieve the pain in many clients with trigeminal neuralgia. They act by inhibiting the reactivity of neurons in the trigeminal nerve. Narcotic analgesics (meperidine, codeine, oxycodone) are not very effective in controlling pain caused by trigeminal neuralgia.

Test-Taking Strategy: Note the similarities of all the incorrect options. They each have a narcotic analgesic as part of the option. In this case, looking for the option that is different will enable you to select the correct choice. The narcotic analgesics are not the best choice for these clients. The anticonvulsant medications have an unlabeled use to manage nerve pain, and they do this rather effectively. Review the actions and purposes of these medications now if you are unfamiliar with them!

Level of Cognitive Ability: Application
Phase of Nursing Process: Implementation
Client Needs: Physiological Integrity
Content Area: Pharmacology

Reference

Black, J., & Matassarin-Jacobs, E. (1997). *Medical-surgical nursing: Clinical management for continuity of care* (5th ed.). Philadelphia: W. B. Saunders. p. 930.

---

107. **4**

Rationale: Facial pain can be minimized by using cotton pads to wash the face and using room-temperature water. The client should chew on the unaffected side of the mouth, eat a soft diet, and take in foods and beverages at room temperature. If toothbrushing triggers pain, sometimes an oral rinse after meals is helpful instead.

Test-Taking Strategy: To answer this question most easily, you should know that the pain of trigeminal neuralgia is triggered by mechanical or thermal stimuli. This will help you eliminate each of the incorrect options systematically. Very hot or cold foods are likely to trigger the pain, not relieve it. Review client education points now if you had difficulty with this question!

Level of Cognitive Ability: Analysis
Phase of Nursing Process: Evaluation
Client Needs: Health Promotion and Maintenance
Content Area: Adult Health/Neurological

Reference
Smeltzer, S., & Bare, B. (1996). *Brunner and Suddarth's textbook of medical-surgical nursing* (8th ed.). Philadelphia: Lippincott-Raven. p. 1818.

108. **1**

Rationale: Bell's palsy is a one-sided facial paralysis from compression of the facial nerve (cranial nerve VII). The exact cause is unknown. Possible causes include vascular ischemia, exposure to viruses such as herpes zoster or simplex, autoimmune disease, or a combination of these items.

Test-Taking Strategy: If you know that the etiology of Bell's palsy is uncertain, you are able to eliminate options 3 and 4 automatically. Since option 2 looks more unrealistic than option 1, you might choose option 1. The role of viruses and the immune system is a popular item of investigation at this time.

Level of Cognitive Ability: Analysis
Phase of Nursing Process: Analysis
Client Needs: Physiological Integrity
Content Area: Adult Health/Neurological

Reference
Smeltzer, S., & Bare, B. (1996). *Brunner and Suddarth's textbook of medical-surgical nursing* (8th ed.). Philadelphia: Lippincott-Raven. p. 1818.

109. **2**

Rationale: Clients with Bell's palsy should be reassured that they have not experienced a stroke and that symptoms often disappear spontaneously in 3 to 5 weeks. The client is given supportive treatment for symptoms. It is not usually caused by a tumor, and the treatment is not similar to that for migraine headaches.

Test-Taking Strategy: Bell's palsy is not similar to CVA, which rules out option 1 first. It is not caused by an easily removed tumor nor is it treated like a migraine headache, which eliminates each of the other incorrect responses.

Level of Cognitive Ability: Application
Phase of Nursing Process: Planning
Client Needs: Psychosocial Integrity
Content Area: Adult Health/Neurological

Reference
Smeltzer, S., & Bare, B. (1996). *Brunner and Suddarth's textbook of medical-surgical nursing* (8th ed.). Philadelphia: Lippincott-Raven. pp. 1818–1819.

110. **4**

Rationale: Bell's palsy is typically treated with prednisone. The drug reduces inflammation and edema, allowing return of normal circulation to the nerve. If given early, the drug reduces the severity of the palsy, reduces pain, and preserves substantial, if not all, nerve function.

Test-Taking Strategy: It is useful to know that the corticosteroid medications are helpful in the treatment of nervous system disorders. This eliminates options 1 and 2. You would need to know how Bell's palsy is treated to differentiate between the last two. Review Bell's palsy and the action and purposes of these medications now if you had difficulty with this question!

Level of Cognitive Ability: Application
Phase of Nursing Process: Implementation
Client Needs: Physiological Integrity
Content Area: Pharmacology

Reference
Smeltzer, S., & Bare, B. (1996). *Brunner and Suddarth's textbook of medical-surgical nursing* (8th ed.). Philadelphia: Lippincott-Raven. p. 1819.

111. **1**

Rationale: Prevention of muscle atrophy with Bell's palsy is accomplished with the use of facial massage, facial exercises, and electrical stimulation of the nerves. Exposure to cold or drafts is avoided. Local application of heat to the face may improve blood flow and provide comfort.

Test-Taking Strategy: Evaluate each of the options with regard to their effect on preserving muscle tone in the face. Options 2, 3, and 4 are plausible choices. Option 1 is unrelated to muscle tone and is also contraindicated in clients with this condition. Because of this, option 1 is the answer to this question as stated.

Level of Cognitive Ability: Analysis
Phase of Nursing Process: Evaluation
Client Needs: Health Promotion and Maintenance
Content Area: Adult Health/Neurological

Reference
Smeltzer, S., & Bare, B. (1996). *Brunner and Suddarth's textbook of medical-surgical nursing* (8th ed.). Philadelphia: Lippincott-Raven. p. 1819.

112. **3**

Rationale: Guillain-Barré syndrome is a clinical syndrome of unknown origin that involves cranial and peripheral nerves. Many clients report a history of respiratory or GI infection in the 1 to 4 weeks before the onset of neurologic deficits. Occasionally it has been triggered by vaccination or surgery.

Test-Taking Strategy: If you examine the options for this question, each of the incorrect answers relates to trauma or infections of the nervous system. The time frames for these are also unstated or lengthy. In this case, the correct option is the one that is different from the others. That is, a history of respiratory or GI infection within a month is different from each of the other responses; it is the correct answer to this question.

Level of Cognitive Ability: Application
Phase of Nursing Process: Assessment
Client Needs: Physiological Integrity
Content Area: Adult Health/Neurological

Reference
Smeltzer, S., & Bare, B. (1996). *Brunner and Suddarth's textbook of medical-surgical nursing* (8th ed.). Philadelphia: Lippincott-Raven. p. 1820.

113. **2**

Rationale: The client with Guillain-Barré syndrome experiences fear and anxiety from the ascending paralysis and sudden onset of the disorder. The nurse can alleviate these by providing accurate information about the client's condition, giving expert care, giving positive feedback to the client, and encouraging relaxation and distraction. The family can become involved with selected care activities and provide diversion for the client as well.

Test-Taking Strategy: Option 1 should be eliminated first, because it is not practical to think that a client would be given full control over all care decisions. The client who is paralyzed cannot participate in active ROM, which eliminates option 4. Of the two remaining, it is obvious that option 2 is more beneficial in assisting the client to cope than option 3.

Level of Cognitive Ability: Application
Phase of Nursing Process: Planning
Client Needs: Psychosocial Integrity
Content Area: Adult Health/Neurological

Reference

Smeltzer, S., & Bare, B. (1996). *Brunner and Suddarth's textbook of medical-surgical nursing* (8th ed.). Philadelphia: Lippincott-Raven. p. 1821.

114. 3

Rationale: The client with Guillain-Barré syndrome is at risk for respiratory failure because of ascending paralysis. An intubation tray should be available for use. Another complication of this syndrome is cardiac dysrhythmias, which necessitates the use of ECG monitoring. Because the client is immobilized, the nurse should routinely assess for deep-vein thrombosis and pulmonary embolism.

Test-Taking Strategy: With an ascending paralysis, the client is at risk for involvement of respiratory muscles and subsequent respiratory failure. This knowledge makes you look for an option that coincides with this line of thought. Option 3 is the only option that includes an intubation tray, which would be needed if the client status deteriorated to needing intubation and mechanical ventilation. This option most directly addresses airway.

Level of Cognitive Ability: Application
Phase of Nursing Process: Implementation
Client Needs: Safe, Effective Care Environment
Content Area: Adult Health/Neurological

Reference

Smeltzer, S., & Bare, B. (1996). *Brunner and Suddarth's textbook of medical-surgical nursing* (8th ed.). Philadelphia: Lippincott-Raven. p. 1821.

115. 1

Rationale: Satisfactory respiratory outcomes include clear breath sounds on auscultation, spontaneous breathing, normal vital capacity, and normal arterial blood gases and pulse oximetry.

Test-Taking Strategy: There is only one option that does not represent full respiratory function. This should help you eliminate each of the incorrect items systematically. Note that this question asks for the least optimal outcome for the client.

Level of Cognitive Ability: Analysis
Phase of Nursing Process: Evaluation
Client Needs: Physiological Integrity
Content Area: Adult Health/Neurological

Reference

Smeltzer, S., & Bare, B. (1996). *Brunner and Suddarth's textbook of medical-surgical nursing* (8th ed.). Philadelphia: Lippincott-Raven. p. 1822.

116. 2

Rationale: The onset or exacerbation of MS is preceded by a number of different factors. These include emotional stress, fatigue, infection, physical injury, and pregnancy. There are no known methods of primary prevention. Intake of fruit and vegetables is an unrelated item.

Test-Taking Strategy: If you examine each of the options, all but the fruit and vegetables option involve physiological or psychological stress. Since this is the option that is different from the others, it is a likely choice for being the correct answer. Review the precipitating risk factors associated with MS now if you had difficulty with this question!

Level of Cognitive Ability: Analysis
Phase of Nursing Process: Assessment
Client Needs: Physiological Integrity
Content Area: Adult Health/Neurological

Reference

Black, J., & Matassarin-Jacobs, E. (1997). *Medical-surgical nursing: Clinical management for continuity of care* (5th ed.). Philadelphia: W. B. Saunders. p. 873.

117. 1

Rationale: Impaired Physical Mobility has been defined by the North American Nursing Diagnosis Association (NANDA) as "a state in which the individual experiences a limitation of ability for independent physical movement." The client's muscle weakness, muscle spasticity, and ataxic gait meet the defining characteristics for this nursing diagnosis. In addition, neuromuscular impairment is listed as a related factor.

Test-Taking Strategy: The stem gives you no information about skin condition or ADLs, so these nursing diagnoses are eliminated first. To discriminate between the last two, you must know that defining characteristics for Activity Intolerance include cardiopulmonary symptoms with exertion. Since the stem makes no mention of these, the correct answer is the Impaired Physical Mobility.

Level of Cognitive Ability: Analysis
Phase of Nursing Process: Analysis
Client Needs: Physiological Integrity
Content Area: Adult Health/Neurological

Reference

Cox, H., et al. (1997). *Clinical applications of nursing diagnosis: Adult, child, women's, psychiatric, gerontic and home health considerations* (3rd ed.). Philadelphia: F. A. Davis. p. 362.

118. 3

Rationale: Spacing fluid intake over the day helps the client with a neurogenic bladder to establish regular times for successful voiding. Omitting intake after the evening meal minimizes incontinence or the need to empty the bladder during the night.

Test-Taking Strategy: Options 2 and 4 should be eliminated first, because they could cause or aggravate nocturia. Of the two remaining, option 3 provides fluids at times that coincide with toileting schedules for bladder training. Option 1 would not accomplish this, which leaves option 3 as the correct answer.

Level of Cognitive Ability: Application
Phase of Nursing Process: Planning
Client Needs: Health Promotion and Maintenance
Content Area: Adult Health/Neurological

Reference

Black, J., & Matassarin-Jacobs, E. (1997). *Medical-surgical nursing: Clinical management for continuity of care* (5th ed.). Philadelphia: W. B. Saunders. p. 875.

119. 4

Rationale: Methylprednisolone and adrenocorticotropic hormone are administered intravenously to accelerate recovery from exacerbation of MS. Carbamazepine and phenytoin would be ordered for dysesthesias and trigeminal neuralgia. Baclofen and diazepam are used to treat muscle spasticity. Dexamethasone is another type of corticosteroid.

Test-Taking Strategy: Options 1 and 2 may be ordered for the client with MS to treat manifestations of the disorder, but not to treat an exacerbation. Of the two remaining, option 4 is the current treatment protocol, because methylprednisolone provides corticosteroids, while ACTH stimulates the adrenal gland to also produce more. Review these medications now if you had difficulty with this question!

Level of Cognitive Ability: Application
Phase of Nursing Process: Implementation
Client Needs: Physiological Integrity
Content Area: Pharmacology

Reference
Black, J., & Matassarin-Jacobs, E. (1997). *Medical-surgical nursing: Clinical management for continuity of care* (5th ed.). Philadelphia: W. B. Saunders. p. 874.

120. 2

Rationale: To effectively manage constipation, the client should take in a high-fiber diet, bulk formers, and stool softeners. A fluid intake of 2000 mL/day is recommended. The client should initiate the bowel program on an every other day basis. This should be done approximately 45 minutes after the largest meal of the day, to use the gastrocolic reflex. A glycerin suppository, bisacodyl suppository, or digital stimulation may be used to initiate the process. Laxatives and enemas should be avoided whenever possible because they lead to dependence.

Test-Taking Strategy: Option 1 is eliminated first as bad practice. Option 3 promotes constipation from insufficient fluid intake, and promotes dry, hard stools. Option 4 is insufficient in frequency. The client should not be allowed to go for one week without a bowel movement. Option 2 is then correct, promoting a BM every other day at a time when the GI motility is best.

Level of Cognitive Ability: Analysis
Phase of Nursing Process: Evaluation
Client Needs: Health Promotion and Maintenance
Content Area: Adult Health/Neurological

Reference
Black, J., & Matassarin-Jacobs, E. (1997). *Medical-surgical nursing: Clinical management for continuity of care* (5th ed.). Philadelphia: W. B. Saunders. p. 876.

BIBLIOGRAPHY

Black, J., & Matassarin-Jacobs, E. (1997). *Medical-surgical nursing: Clinical management for continuity of care* (5th ed.). Philadelphia: W. B. Saunders.

Chernecky, C, & Berger, B. (1997). *Laboratory tests and diagnostic procedures* (2nd ed.). Philadelphia: W. B. Saunders.

Cox, H., et al. (1997). *Clinical applications of nursing diagnosis: Adult, child, women's, psychiatric, gerontic and home health considerations* (3rd ed.). Philadelphia: F. A. Davis.

Deglin, J., & Vallerand, A. (1997). *Davis's drug guide for nurses* (5th ed.). Philadelphia: F. A. Davis.

Hodgson, B., & Kizior, R. (1999). *Saunders nursing drug handbook 1999.* Philadelphia: W. B. Saunders.

Ignatavicius, D., Workman, M., & Mishler, M. (1995). *Medical-surgical nursing: A nursing process approach* (2nd ed.). Philadelphia: W. B. Saunders.

Jaffee, M., & McVan, B. (1997). *Davis's laboratory and diagnostic test handbook.* Philadelphia: F. A. Davis.

Lammon, C., Foote, A., & Leli, P., et al. (1995). *Clinical nursing skills.* Philadelphia: W. B. Saunders.

Lehne, R. (1998). *Pharmacology for nursing care* (2nd ed.). Philadelphia: W. B. Saunders.

Luckmann, J. (1997). *Saunders manual of nursing care.* Philadelphia: W. B. Saunders.

Martini, F. (1995). *Fundamentals of anatomy and physiology* (3rd ed.). Upper Saddle River, NJ: Prentice-Hall.

O'Toole, M. (ed.). (1997). *Miller-Keane encyclopedia & dictionary of medicine, nursing, & allied health* (6th ed.). Philadelphia: W. B. Saunders.

Pinnell, N. (1996). *Nursing pharmacology.* Philadelphia: W. B. Saunders.

Smeltzer, S., & Bare, B. (1996). *Brunner and Suddarth's textbook of medical-surgical nursing* (8th ed.). Philadelphia: Lippincott-Raven.

CHAPTER 66

Neurological Medications

. . . .

I. Skeletal Muscle Relaxants

A. Description
1. Act directly on the neuromuscular junction or indirectly on the central nervous system (CNS)
2. Centrally acting muscle relaxants depress neuron activity in the spinal cord or brain
3. Peripherally acting muscle relaxants act directly on the skeletal muscles
4. Used to prevent or relieve muscle spasms, to treat spasticity associated with spinal cord disease or lesions, for painful musculoskeletal conditions, and for chronic debilitating disorders, such as multiple sclerosis, cerebrovascular accident (CVA), or cerebral palsy
5. Contraindicated in severe liver or renal disease and in severe heart disease
6. Should not be taken with CNS depressants, such as barbiturates, narcotics, and alcohol; sedatives; hypnotics; or tricylic antidepressants
7. Chronic high dose therapy can cause physical dependence; withdrawal should be done slowly
B. Medications (Box 66–1)
C. Side effects
1. Dizziness
2. Drowsiness
3. Dry mouth
4. Nausea
5. Gastrointestinal (GI) upset
6. Hypotension
7. Photosensitivity
8. Liver toxicity
D. Implementation
1. Obtain a medical and medication history
2. Monitor vital signs
3. Monitor for CNS side effects
4. Assess for risk of injury
5. Assess involved joints and muscles for pain and mobility
6. Monitor liver function tests as hepatotoxicity can occur
7. Monitor renal function studies
8. Instruct client to take medication with food to decrease GI upset
9. Instruct client to report side effects
10. Instruct client to avoid alcohol and CNS depressants
11. Instruct client to avoid activities requiring alertness

II. Antimyasthenic Medications

A. Description
1. Relieve muscle weakness associated with myasthenia gravis by blocking acetylcholine breakdown at the neuromuscular junction
2. Used to treat or diagnose myasthenia gravis or to distinguish cholinergic crisis from myasthenic crisis
3. Neostigmine bromide (Prostigmin), pyridostigmine bromide (Mestinon), and ambenonium (Mytelase) are used to control myasthenic symptoms

---

BOX 66–1. Skeletal Muscle Relaxants

Baclofen (Lioresal)
Carisoprodol (Soma)
Cyclobenzaprine HCl (Flexeril)
Dantrolene (Dantrium)
Diazepam (Valium)
Methocarbamol (Robaxin)
Orphenadrine (Norflex)
Chlorzoxazone (Paraflex, Parafon Forte)
Chlorphenesin carbamate (Maolate)
Meprobamate (Equanil, Miltown)

BOX 66–2. Antimyasthenic Medications

Edrophonium chloride (Tensilon)
Neostigmine bromide (Prostigmin)
Pyridostigmine bromide (Mestinon)
Ambenonium (Mytelase)

4. Edrophonium chloride (Tensilon) is used to diagnose myasthenia gravis and to distinguish cholinergic crisis from myasthenic crisis
B. Medications (Box 66–2)
C. Side effects: Cholinergic crisis (Box 66–3)
D. Implementation
1. Assess neuromuscular status, including reflexes, muscle strength, and gait
2. Monitor client for signs and symptoms of medication overdose (cholinergic crisis) and underdose (myasthenic crisis)
3. Instruct client to take medications on time to prevent weakness, as weakness can impair the client's ability to breathe and swallow
4. Instruct client to take medication before meals for best absorption
5. Instruct client to wear a MedicAlert bracelet
6. Note that antimyasthenic therapy is lifelong therapy
7. Evaluate for medication effectiveness, which is based on the improvement of neuromuscular symptoms or strength without cholinergic signs and symptoms
8. When administering edrophonium (Tensilon), have emergency resuscitation equipment on hand and atropine available for cholinergic crisis
E. **Tensilon test**
1. Tensilon is injected IV
2. The **tensilon test** can cause ventricular fibrillation and cardiac arrest
3. Atropine is the antidote for overdose
4. To diagnose:
a. If ptosis is immediately corrected after administration of the drug, the diagnosis is most likely myasthenia gravis
b. Most myasthenic clients will show a marked improvement in muscle tone within 30 to 60 seconds after injection,

and the muscle improvement lasts 4 to 5 minutes
5. To determine cholinergic crisis (overdose with anticholinesterase) or myasthenic crisis (undermedication):
a. In cholinergic crisis, muscle tone does not improve after the administration of Tensilon, and muscle twitching may be noted around the eyes and face
b. A tensilon injection makes the client in cholinergic crisis temporarily worse (negative tensilon test)
c. A tensilon injection temporarily improves the condition when the client is in myasthenic crisis (positive tensilon test)

III. Antiparkinsonian Medications

A. Description
1. Restore the balance of the neurotransmitters acetylcholine and dopamine in the CNS, decreasing the signs and symptoms of Parkinson's disease
2. These medications include the dopaminergics, which stimulate the dopamine receptors, and the anticholinergics, which block the cholinergic receptors
3. Used for drug-induced parkinsonism, in which neuroleptic agents block dopamine receptors in the CNS, leading to functional loss of dopamine activity
4. Used for Parkinson's disease, in which dopamine-containing neurons in the basal ganglia are destroyed or deficient, which causes loss of fine motor control
B. Dopaminergic medications
1. Description
a. Stimulate the dopamine receptors
b. Increase the amount of dopamine available in the CNS or enhance neurotransmission of dopamine
c. Contraindicated in cardiac, renal or psychiatric disorders
d. Levodopa taken with monoamine oxidase inhibitor (MAOI) antidepressant can cause a hypertensive crisis
2. Medications (Box 66–4)

BOX 66–3. Signs of Cholinergic Crisis

GI disturbances	Miosis
Nausea	Hypertension
Vomiting	Sweating
Diarrhea	Increased bronchial
Abdominal cramps	secretions
Increased salivation and tearing	

BOX 66–4. Dopaminergic Medications

Amantadine (Symmetrel)
Bromocriptine (Parlodel)
Carbidopa
Levodopa; carbidopa (Sinemet)
Pergolide (Permax)
Selegiline hydrochloride (Eldepryl)

3. Side effects
   a. Dyskinesia
   b. Involuntary body movements
   c. Tachycardia
   d. Nausea
   e. Vomiting
   f. Urinary retention
   g. Constipation
   h. Dizziness
   i. Orthostatic hypotension
   j. Confusion
   k. Mood changes
   l. Hallucinations
4. Implementation
   a. Assess vital signs
   b. Assess for risk for injury
   c. Instruct client to take medication with food if nausea and vomiting occur
   d. Assess for signs and symptoms of parkinsonism, such as rigidity, tremors, akinesia, and bradykinesia; a stooped forward posture; shuffling gait; and masked facies
   e. Monitor for signs of dyskinesia
   f. Instruct clients on carbidopa-levodopa (Sinemet) to eat low-protein foods, as high-protein diets interfere with medication transport to the CNS
   g. Instruct client to change positions slowly to minimize orthostatic hypotension
   h. Instruct clients not to discontinue the medication abruptly
   i. Instruct client to report side effects and symptoms of dyskinesia
   j. Instruct the client to avoid alcohol
   k. Monitor client for improvement in signs and symptoms of parkinsonism without the development of severe side effects from the medications
   l. Inform client that urine or perspiration may be discolored and that this is harmless, but it may stain clothing
   m. Advise the diabetic client that glucose testing should not be done through urine testing as the results will not be reliable
   n. When administering levodopa, instruct client to avoid excessive vitamin B$_6$ intake to prevent medication interactions

IV. Anticholinergic-Blocking Medications

A. Description
   1. Block the cholinergic receptors in the CNS, thereby suppressing acetylcholine activity
   2. Reduce the rigidity and some of the tremors but have a minimal effect on the bradykinesia
   3. Contraindicated in clients with glaucoma
   4. Clients with chronic obstructive lung diseases can develop dry, thick mucus secretions
B. Medications (Box 66–5)
C. Side effects
   1. Blurred vision
   2. Dry mouth

BOX 66–5. Anticholinergic Blocking Medications

Benztropine mesylate (Cogentin)
Trihexyphenidyl HCl (Artane)
Biperiden HCl (Akineton)
Ethopropazine HCl (Parsidol)
Orphenadrine HCl (Disipal)
Orphenadrine citrate (Banflex, Norflex)
Procyclidine HCl (Kemadrin)

   3. Dry secretions
   4. Increased pulse rate
   5. Constipation
   6. Urinary retention
   7. Restlessness and confusion
   8. Photophobia
D. Implementation
   1. Obtain a medication and medical history
   2. Monitor vital signs
   3. Assess for risk of injury
   4. Assess for signs and symptoms of parkinsonism, such as rigidity, tremors, akinesia, and bradykinesia; a stooped forward posture; shuffling gait; and masked facies
   5. Monitor client for improvement in signs and symptoms
   6. Assess client's bowel and urinary function and monitor for urinary retention and constipation
   7. Monitor for involuntary movements
   8. Encourage client to avoid alcohol, smoking, caffeine, and aspirin to decrease gastric acidity
   9. Instruct client to consult with physician before taking any nonprescription medications
   10. Instruct client to minimize dry mouth by increasing fluid intake and by using ice chips, hard candy, or gum
   11. Instruct client to reduce constipation by increasing fluid and fiber in the diet
   12. Instruct client to use sunglasses in direct sun because of possible photophobia
   13. Instruct client to have routine eye examinations to assess for intraocular pressure

V. Anticonvulsant Medications (Table 66–1)

A. Description
   1. Used to depress abnormal neuronal discharges and prevent the spread of seizures
   2. Use with caution in clients on anticoagulants, aspirin, sulfonamides, cimetidine (Tagamet), and antipsychotics
   3. Absorption is decreased with the use of antacids, calcium preparations, and antineoplastic medications
B. Implementation for clients on anticonvulsants
   1. Initiate seizure precautions

Table 66-1. Anticonvulsant Medications

Medication	Therapeutic Serum Range
Phenytoin (Dilantin)	10–20 μg/mL
Carbamazepine (Tegretol)	3–14 μg/mL
Mephenytoin (Mesantoin)	25–40 μg/mL
Ethotoin (Peganone)	10–50 μg/mL
Phenobarbital (Luminal)	15–40 μg/mL
Primidone (Mysoline)	5–10 μg/mL
Amobarbital (Amytal)	1–5 μg/mL
Mephobarbital (Mebaral)	15–40 μg/mL
Clonazepam (Klonopin)	20–80 ng/mL
Lorazepam (Ativan)	50–240 ng/mL
Ethosuximide (Zarontin)	40–100 μg/mL
Valproic acid (Depakene)	40–100 μg/mL

2. Monitor urinary output
3. Monitor liver and renal function tests
4. Monitor for signs of medication toxicity, which would include CNS depression, ataxia, nausea, vomiting, drowsiness, dizziness, restlessness, and visual disturbances
5. Instruct client to take anticonvulsants with food to decrease GI irritation but to avoid milk and antacids, which impair the absorption of anticonvulsants
6. Instruct client taking liquid medication to shake it well before ingesting
7. Instruct client not to discontinue medication
8. Instruct client not to consume alcohol
9. Instruct client to use caution when driving or performing activities that require alertness
10. Instruct client to wear a MedicAlert bracelet
11. Encourage client to follow up with periodic blood studies related to determining toxicity
12. Instruct client to avoid over-the-counter medications
13. Instruct diabetic client to monitor serum glucose levels closely
14. Inform client that urine may be a harmless pink-red or red-brown color
15. Instruct client to maintain good oral hygiene and to use a soft toothbrush
16. Instruct the client in the need for preventive dental check-ups
17. Instruct client to report symptoms of sore throat, bruising, and nosebleeds, which may indicate a blood dyscrasia
18. Instruct client to inform physician if adverse reactions occur, such as gingivitis, nystagmus, slurred speech, rash, or dizziness
19. If a seizure occurs, assess seizure activity, including location and duration
20. Protect client from hazards in the environment during a seizure
C. Hydantoins (Box 66-6)
   1. Used to treat seizures
   2. Phenytoin (Dilantin) is also used to treat dysrhythmias
   3. Side effects
      a. Gingival hyperplasia
      b. Reddened gums that bleed easily

BOX 66-6. Hydantoins

Phenytoin (Dilantin)
Mephenytoin (Mesantoin)
Ethotoin (Peganone)

   c. Slurred speech
   d. Confusion
   e. Depression
   f. Nausea
   g. Vomiting
   h. Constipation
   i. Headaches
   j. Blood dyscrasias
   k. Decreased platelet count
   l. Decreased white blood cell (WBC) count
   m. Elevated blood glucose
   n. Alopecia
   o. Hirsutism
   4. Implementation
      a. Oral tube feedings may interfere with the absorption of oral phenytoin and diminish the medication's effectiveness; therefore feedings should be scheduled as far as possible from the phenytoin administration
      b. Monitor therapeutic serum levels to assess for toxicity
      c. Monitor for signs of toxicity
      d. When administering IV phenytoin, dilute in normal saline, because dextrose causes the medication to precipitate
      e. When administering IV phenytoin, infuse no faster than 50 mg per minute; otherwise hypotension and cardiac dysrhythmias can occur
      f. Instruct client about the importance of good oral hygiene and regular dental examinations
      g. Instruct client to consult with physician before taking other medications to ensure compatibility with anticonvulsants
D. Barbiturates
   1. Used for grand mal seizures and acute episodes of seizures caused by status epilepticus
   2. May also be used as adjuncts to anesthesia
   3. Medications (Box 66-7)
   4. Side effects
      a. Drowsiness
      b. Dizziness

BOX 66-7. Barbiturates

Phenobarbital (Luminal)
Primidone (Mysoline)
Amobarbital (Amytal)
Mephobarbital (Mebaral)

BOX 66–8. Benzodiazepines

Clonazepam (Klonopin)
Clorazepate (Tranxene)
Diazepam (Valium)
Lorazepam (Ativan)

---

c. Hypotension
d. Respiratory depression
e. Tolerance to the medication
E. Benzodiazepines
1. To treat absence (petit mal) seizures
2. Diazepam (Valium) is used to treat status epilepticus, anxiety, and skeletal muscle spasms
3. Clorazepate (Tranxene) is used as adjunctive therapy for partial seizures
4. Medications (Box 66–8)
5. Side effects
a. Ataxia
b. Respiratory and cardiac depression
c. Medication tolerance
d. Drug dependency
F. Succinimides
1. Used to treat absence (petit mal) seizures
2. Medications (Box 66–9)
3. Side effects
a. Anorexia
b. Nausea
c. Vomiting
d. Blood dyscrasias
G. Oxazolidinediones
1. Used for absence (petit mal) seizures
2. Medications (Box 66–10)
3. Side effects
a. Sedation
b. Photophobia
H. Iminostilbenes
1. Used in treating seizure disorders that have not responded to other anticonvulsants
2. Used to treat trigeminal neuralgia
3. Medication: Carbamazepine (Tegretol)
4. Side effects
a. Drowsiness
b. Dizziness
c. Nausea
d. Vomiting
e. Constipation or diarrhea
f. Visual abnormalities
g. Dry mouth
h. Headache
i. Water retention

BOX 66–9. Succinimides

Ethosuximide (Zarontin)
Methsuximide (Celontin)
Phensuximide (Milontin)

BOX 66–10. Oxazolidinediones

Paramethadione (Paradione)
Trimethadione (Tridione)

---

j. increased sweating
I. Valproates
1. Used to treat grand mal, petit mal, myoclonic, and psychomotor seizures
2. Medications (Box 66–11)
3. Side effects
a. Nausea
b. Vomiting
c. Abdominal cramps
d. Diarrhea
e. Constipation
f. Hepatotoxicity

VI. Central Nervous System Stimulants

A. Description
1. Amphetamines and caffeine stimulate the cerebral cortex of the brain
2. Analeptics and caffeine act on the brain stem and medulla to stimulate respiration
3. Anorexiants act on the cerebral cortex and hypothalamus to suppress appetite
4. Used to treat narcolepsy and attention deficit disorders
5. Used to treat respiratory depression after anesthesia
6. Used as adjunctive therapy for exogenous obesity
B. Amphetamines
1. Medications (Box 66–12)
2. Side effects
a. Sleeplessness
b. Tremors
c. Irritability
d. Restlessness
e. Tachycardia
f. Heart palpitations
g. Hypertension
h. Dry mouth
i. Anorexia
j. Weight loss
k. Diarrhea or constipation
l. Impotence
m. Dependence and tolerance
C. Anorexiants
1. Medications (Box 66–13)
2. Side effects
a. Nervousness

BOX 66–11. Valproates

Valproic acid (Depakene)
Divalproex sodium (Depakote)

BOX 66–12. Amphetamines

Amphetamine sulfate
Dextroamphetamine sulfate (Dexedrine)
Methamphetamine hydrochloride (Desoxyn)
Methylphenidate hydrochloride (Ritalin)
Pemoline (Cylert)

---

    b. Restlessness
    c. Irritability
    d. Insomnia
    e. Heart palpitations
    f. Hypertension
D. Analeptics
    1. Medications
      a. Caffeine (Tirend, Vivarin)
      b. Theophylline, also a bronchodilator, may be used for newborn infants with apnea to stimulate respirations
    2. Side effects
      a. Nervousness
      b. Restlessness
      c. Tremors
      d. Twitching
      e. Palpitations
      f. Insomnia
      g. Diuresis
      h. GI irritation
      i. Tinnitus
E. CNS stimulant for migraines
    1. Sumatriptan succinate (Imitrex)
    2. Promotes vasoconstriction of the carotid arteries
F. Respiratory stimulant
    1. Doxapram hydrochloride (Dopram)
    2. Used to treat sedative hypnotic overdose to correct respiratory depression
G. Implementation for CNS stimulants
    1. Monitor vital signs
    2. Assess mental status
    3. Assess height, weight, and growth of children
    4. Monitor complete blood count (CBC), white

BOX 66–13. Anorexiants

Diethylpropion hydrochloride (Tenuate, Tepanil, Dospan)
Fenfluramine hydrochloride (Pondimin)
Mazindol (Sanorex, Mazanor)
Phendimetrazine tartrate (Adipost, Anorex, Trimcaps, Prelu-2)
Phenmetrazine hydrochloride (Preludin)
Phentermine hydrochloride (Fastin, Ionamin, Adipex-P)
Benzphetamine hydrochloride (Didrex)
Dextroamphetamine sulfate (Dexedrine)
Phenylpropanolamine hydrochloride (Acutrim, Control, Dexatrim, Prolamine)

---

blood cell (WBC), and platelet counts before and during therapy
    5. Monitor for side effects
    6. Monitor sleep patterns
    7. Monitor for such withdrawal symptoms as nausea, vomiting, weakness, and headache
    8. Instruct client to take the medication before meals
    9. Instruct client to avoid foods and beverages containing caffeine to prevent additional stimulation
    10. Instruct client to read labels on over-the-counter products because many contain caffeine
    11. Instruct client to avoid alcohol
    12. Instruct client not to discontinue the medication abruptly
    13. Instruct client to take the last daily dose of CNS stimulants at least 6 hours before bedtime to prevent insomnia
    14. Monitor for drug dependence and abuse with amphetamines
    15. If a child is taking a CNS stimulant, instruct the parents to notify the school nurse
    16. Monitor for calming effects of CNS stimulants within 3 to 4 weeks on children with attention deficit disorder
    17. Monitor growth in children on long-term therapy with methylphenidate HCl (Ritalin)

VII. Non-Narcotic Analgesics

A. Nonsteroidal anti-inflammatory drugs (NSAIDs)
    1. Description
      a. NSAIDs are aspirin and aspirin-like medications that inhibit the synthesis of prostaglandins
      b. They act as an analgesic to relieve pain, as an antipyretic to reduce body temperature, and as an anticoagulant to inhibit platelet aggregation
      c. Used to relieve inflammation and pain and in the treatment of rheumatoid arthritis, bursitis, tendinitis, osteoarthritis, and acute gout
      d. Contraindicated in hypersensitivity or liver or renal disease
      e. Aspirin should not be taken by children with flu symptoms because of the risk of Reye's syndrome
      f. Aspirin should not be taken if the client is on an anticoagulant
      g. Aspirin and an NSAID should not be taken together because aspirin decreases the blood level and the effectiveness of the NSAID
      h. NSAIDs can increase the effects of warfarin (Coumadin), sulfonamides, cephalosporins, and phenytoin (Dilantin)
      i. Hypoglycemia may result if ibuprofen (Motrin) is taken with insulin or an oral hypoglycemic medication

---

BOX 66–14. Nonsteroidal Anti-Inflammatory Drugs (NSAIDs)

Aspirin (ASA; Bayer, Ecotrin)
Diflunisal (Dolobid)
Indomethacin (Indocin)
Sulindac (Clinoril)
Tolmetin (Tolectin)
Phenylbutazone (Butazolidin)
Fenoprofen calcium (Nalfon)
Flurbiprofen sodium (Ansaid, Ocufen)
Ibuprofen (Motrin, Advil, Nuprin, Medipren)
Ketoprofen (Orudis)
Naproxen (Naprosyn)
Oxaprozin (Daypro)
Meclofenamate (Meclomen)
Mefenamic acid (Ponstel)
Piroxicam (Feldene)
Diclofenac sodium (Voltaren)
Etodolac (Lodine)
Ketorolac tromethamine (Toradol)

---

j. A high risk of toxicity exists if ibuprofen is taken concurrently with calcium blockers
2. Medications (Box 66–14)
3. Side effects (Table 66–2)
4. Implementation
   a. Assess client for allergies
   b. Obtain a medication history and medical history on the client
   c. Assess for history of gastric upset or bleeding or liver disease
   d. Assess the client for GI upset during medication administration
   e. Monitor for edema
   f. Monitor serum salicylate (aspirin) level when client is taking high doses
   g. Monitor for signs of bleeding, such as tarry stools, bleeding gums, petechiae, ecchymosis, and purpura
   h. Instruct client to take medication with water, milk, or food
   i. Enteric-coated form or buffered form of aspirin can be taken to decrease gastric distress
   j. Instruct client that enteric-coated tablets cannot be crushed or broken
   k. Advise clients to inform other health care professionals that they are taking high doses of aspirin
   l. Note that aspirin should be discontinued 3 to 7 days prior to surgery to reduce the risk of bleeding
   m. Instruct client to avoid alcoholic beverages
B. Acetaminophen (Tylenol)
   1. Description
      a. Inhibits prostaglandin synthesis
      b. Used to decrease pain and fever
      c. Contraindicated in hepatic or renal disease, alcoholism, and hypersensitivity
   2. Side effects
      a. Anorexia
      b. Nausea
      c. Vomiting
      d. Rash
      e. Hypoglycemia
      f. Oliguria
      g. Hepatotoxicity
   3. Implementation
      a. Monitor vital signs
      b. Assess client for history of liver dysfunction
      c. Monitor for hepatic damage, which includes nausea, vomiting, diarrhea, and abdominal pain
      d. Monitor liver function tests
      e. Instruct client that self-medication should not be used longer than 10 days for an adult and 5 days for a child
      f. Note that the antidote for Tylenol is acetylcysteine (Mucomyst)
      g. Evaluate for the effectiveness of the medication

VIII. Narcotic Analgesics

A. Description
   1. Suppress pain impulses but can suppress respiration and coughing by acting on the respiratory and cough center in the medulla of the brain stem
   2. Can produce euphoria or sedation
   3. Can cause physical dependence
   4. Used for relief of mild, moderate, or severe pain
B. Medications (Box 66–15)
   1. Codeine sulfate
      a. Effective cough suppressant at low doses
      b. Can cause constipation
   2. Hydromorphone hydrochloride (Dilaudid)
      a. Can decrease respiration
      b. Can cause constipation
   3. Meperidine (Demerol)
      a. Can decrease blood pressure and cause dizziness
      b. Can increase intracranial pressure in head injuries

Table 66–2. Side Effects of Aspirin and NSAIDs

Aspirin	NSAIDs
Drowsiness	Hypotension
Tinnitus	Sodium and water retention
Headaches	Gastric irritation
Flushing	Blood dyscrasias
Dizziness	Dizziness
GI symptoms	Tinnitus
Visual changes	Pruritus

BOX 66–15. Narcotic Analgesics

Codeine sulfate
Hydromorphone hydrochloride (Dilaudid)
Meperidine (Demerol)
Morphine sulfate
Oxycodone hydrochloride with acetaminophen (Percocet)
Oxycodone with aspirin (Percodan)
Propoxyphene napsylate (Darvon-N)
Propoxyphene hydrochloride (Darvon)
Buprenorphine hydrochloride (Buprenex)
Butorphanol tartrate (Stadol)
Dezocine (Dalgan)
Nalbuphine hydrochloride (Nubain)
Methadone hydrochloride (Dolophine)
Pentazocine (Talwin)
Pentazocine hydrochloride (Talwin Compound)
Hydrocodone (Hycodan)
Levorphanol tartrate (Levo-Dromoran)
Fentanyl (Duragesic, Sublimaze)
Sufentanil citrate (Sufenta)
Oxycodone hydrochloride (Roxicodone)
Oxymorphone hydrochloride (Numorphan)

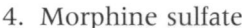

4. Morphine sulfate
   a. Can cause respiratory depression, orthostatic hypotension, and constipation
   b. May cause nausea and vomiting because of increased vestibular sensitivity
5. Oxycodone with aspirin (Percodan)
   a. Should not be taken by clients allergic to aspirin
   b. Can cause gastric irritation and should be taken with food or plenty of liquids
6. Propoxyphene napsylate (Darvon-N) and propoxyphene hydrochloride (Darvon)
   a. Darvon compound contains aspirin and should not be taken by clients allergic to aspirin
   b. Darvocet-N contains acetaminophen
7. Buprenorphine hydrochloride (Buprenex): Possesses agonist and antagonist properties
8. Butorphanol tartrate (Stadol): Possesses agonist and antagonist properties
9. Dezocine (Dalgan): Possesses agonist and antagonist properties
10. Nalbuphine hydrochloride (Nubain)
    a. Possesses agonist and antagonist properties
    b. Preferable for treating the pain of a myocardial infarction (MI) because it reduces the oxygen needs of the heart without reducing blood pressure
11. Methadone hydrochloride (Dolophine)
    a. Dilute doses of the oral concentrate with at least 90 mL of water
    b. Dilute dispersible tablets in at least 120 mL of water, orange juice, or acidic fruit beverage.
    c. Used as a replacement drug for opiate dependence or to facilitate withdrawal

12. Pentazocine (Talwin) and Pentazocine hydrochloride (Talwin Compound)
    a. Possesses agonist and antagonist properties
    b. Increases blood pressure and cardiac workload
    c. Causes dysphoria rather than euphoria
13. Hydrocodone (Hycodan): Frequently used for cough suppression
C. Implementation for narcotic analgesics
   1. Monitor vital signs
   2. Assess client thoroughly before administering pain medication
   3. Initiate nursing measures such as massage, distraction, deep breathing and relaxation exercises, the application of heat or cold as prescribed, and provide care and comfort prior to administering the narcotic analgesic
   4. Administer medications 30 to 60 minutes before painful activities
   5. Monitor the respiratory rate, and if the rate is less than 12 breaths per minute in an adult, withhold medication unless ventilatory support is being provided
   6. Monitor pulse, and if bradycardia develops, withhold the dose and notify the physician
   7. Monitor blood pressure for hypotension
   8. Auscultate breath sounds, because narcotic analgesics suppress the cough reflex
   9. Encourage activities such as turning, deep breathing, and incentive spirometry to prevent atelectasis and pneumonia
   10. Monitor level of consciousness (LOC)
   11. Initiate safety precautions such as side rails and a night light, and supervised ambulation and discourage smoking
   12. Monitor I&O
   13. Assess for urinary retention
   14. Instruct client to take oral doses with milk or a snack to reduce gastric irritation
   15. Instruct client to avoid alcohol
   16. Instruct client to avoid activities that require alertness
   17. Have narcotic antagonist, oxygen, and resuscitation equipment available
D. Morphine sulfate
   1. Description
      a. Used for acute pain due to MI or cancer, for dyspnea due to pulmonary edema, and as a preoperative medication
      b. Contraindicated in severe respiratory disorders, head injury or **increased intracranial pressure,** severe renal disease, or seizure activity
      c. Used with caution in clients with shock or blood loss
   2. Side effects
      a. Respiratory depression
      b. Orthostatic hypotension
      c. Urinary retention
      d. Nausea
      e. Vomiting

f. Constipation

g. Cough suppression

h. Reduction in pupillary size

i. Miosis

3. Implementation

   a. Note that the antidote for morphine overdose is naloxone (Narcan)

   b. Assess vital signs

   c. Note rate and depth of respirations

   d. Respirations of less that 10 per minute can indicate respiratory distress

   e. Monitor urinary output, which should be at least 600 mL/day

   f. Monitor bowel sounds for decreased peristalsis as constipation can occur

   g. Monitor for pupil changes as pinpoint pupils can indicate morphine overdose

   h. Avoid alcohol or CNS depressants as they can cause respiratory depression

   i. Instruct client to report dizziness or difficulty in breathing

   j. Assess risk for injury

   k. Assist client with activities and ambulation

   l. To administer morphine IV, dilute in at least 5 mL of sterile water or normal saline for injection and administer at a rate of 15 mg or less over 4 to 5 minutes

E. Meperidine (Demerol)

1. Description

   a. Used for acute pain and as a preoperative medication

   b. Contraindicated in head injuries and **increased intracranial pressure,** respiratory disorders, hypotension, shock, and severe hepatic and renal disease and in clients taking MAOI

   c. Should not be taken with alcohol or sedative hypnotics because it may increase the CNS depression

2. Side effects

   a. Hypotension

   b. Respiratory depression

   c. Tachycardia

   d. Drowsiness

   e. Mental clouding

   f. Constipation

   g. Urinary retention

   h. Nausea

   i. Vomiting

   j. Headache

   k. Dizziness

   l. Blurred vision

   m. Tinnitus

   n. Tremors

3. Implementation

   a. Monitor vital signs

   b. Monitor for respiratory dysfunction and hypotension

   c. Have naloxone (Narcan) available for overdose

   d. Monitor for urinary retention

e. Monitor bowel sounds and for constipation

f. Monitor mental status

g. Initiate safety precautions

h. Instruct client not to consume alcohol

i. Note effectiveness of medication

j. To administer IV, dilute in at least 5 mL of sterile water or normal saline for injection and administer the dose over 4 to 5 minutes

IX. Narcotic Antagonists

A. Used to treat respiratory depression from narcotic overdose

B. Medication: Naloxone (Narcan)

C. Implementation

1. Monitor blood pressure, pulse, and respiratory rate every 5 minutes initially, tapering to every 15 minutes, then every 30 minutes until stable

2. Place client on a cardiac monitor and monitor cardiac rhythm

3. Auscultate breath sounds

4. Monitor I&O

5. Auscultate bowel sounds

6. Have resuscitation equipment available

7. Do not leave client unattended

8. Monitor client closely for several hours because when the effects of the antagonist wear off, the client may again display signs of narcotic overdose

X. Osmotic Diuretics (Box 66–16)

A. Description

1. Increase osmotic pressure of the glomerular filtrate, inhibiting reabsorption of water and electrolytes

2. Used for oliguria and to prevent renal failure

3. Used to decrease intracranial pressure

4. Used to decrease intraocular pressure in narrow-angle glaucoma

5. Mannitol is used with chemotherapy to induce diuresis

B. Side effects

1. Fluid and electrolyte imbalances

2. Pulmonary edema from the rapid shifts of fluid

3. Nausea and vomiting

4. Tachycardia from the rapid fluid loss

5. Hyponatremia and dehydration

C. Implementation

1. Monitor vital signs

2. Monitor weight

3. Monitor urine output

BOX 66–16. Osmotic Diuretics

Mannitol (Osmitrol)

Urea (Ureaphil)

4. Monitor electrolyte levels
5. Monitor lungs and heart sounds for signs of pulmonary edema
6. Monitor for signs of dehydration
7. Monitor neurological status
8. Assess for signs of decreasing intracranial pressure if appropriate
9. Change client's position slowly to prevent orthostatic hypotension
10. Monitor for crystallization in the vial of mannitol prior to administering the medication; if crystallization is noted, do not administer the medication

XI. Corticosteroids (Box 66–17)

A. Description
  1. Inhibit accumulation of inflammatory cells at inflammation sites
  2. Prevent and suppress cell and tissue immune reactions
  3. Used to treat cerebral edema
  4. Side effects can occur primarily if the medication is prescribed long-term
B. Side effects
  1. Hyperglycemia
  2. Edema
  3. Sodium and water retention
  4. Hypokalemia
  5. Muscle wasting
  6. Osteoporosis
  7. Growth retardation in children
  8. Peptic ulcer
  9. Hypertension
  10. Convulsions
  11. Mood swings
  12. Cataracts and glaucoma
  13. Fragile skin
  14. Hirsutism
  15. Altered fat distribution
  16. Can mask the signs and symptoms of infection
C. Implementation
  1. Monitor vital signs
  2. Monitor serum electrolytes and blood glucose
  3. Monitor for hypokalemia and hyperglycemia
  4. Monitor weight
  5. Monitor for hypertension

BOX 66–17. Corticosteroids

Betamethasone (Celestone)
Cortisone acetate (Cortone)
Dexamethasone (Decadron)
Hydrocortisone (Cortef, Hydrocortone)
Methylprednisolone (Depo-Medrol, Medrol, Solu-Medrol)
Prednisolone (Delta-Cortef, Hydeltrasol)
Prednisone (Deltasone)

---

6. Monitor for edema
7. Monitor urine output
8. Assess medical history for glaucoma, cataracts, peptic ulcer, psychiatric problems, or diabetes
9. Monitor the older client for signs and symptoms of increased osteoporosis
10. Assess for changes in muscle strength
11. Prepare a schedule for the client on short-term tapered doses
12. Instruct client to take at mealtime or with food
13. Advise client to eat foods high in potassium
14. Instruct the client to avoid individuals with respiratory infections
15. Advise clients to inform all health care providers that they are taking the medication
16. Instruct client to report signs and symptoms of a drug overdose or Cushing's syndrome, including a moon face, puffy eyelids, edema in the feet, increased bruising, dizziness, bleeding, and menstrual irregularities
17. Note that the client may need additional doses during periods of stress, such as surgery
18. Instruct client not to stop medication abruptly as abrupt withdrawal can result in severe adrenal insufficiency
19. Advise client to consult with physician before receiving any vaccinations
20. Advise client to wear MedicAlert bracelet

PRACTICE QUESTIONS

1. The nurse is caring for a client in the emergency department who is diagnosed with Bell's palsy. The client has been taking acetaminophen (Tylenol), and a Tylenol overdose is suspected. The nurse anticipates that the antidote to be prepared is:
   1 Auranofin (Ridaura)
   2 Fludarabine (Fludara)
   3 Acetylcysteine (Mucomyst)
   4 Pentostatin (Nipent)

2. The client with trigeminal neuralgia tells the nurse that acetaminophen (Tylenol) is taken on a frequent daily basis for relief of generalized discomfort. Which of the following indicates toxicity associated with the medication?
   1 Platelet count of 400,000 cells/μL
   2 A direct bilirubin level of 2 mg/dL
   3 Prothrombin time of 12 seconds
   4 Sodium of 140 mEq/L

3. The nurse prepares to administer acetylcysteine (Mucomyst) to the client with an overdose of acetaminophen (Tylenol). Which of the following is an appropriate action when administering this antidote?
   1 Mixing the medication in a flavored ice drink and allowing the client to drink the medication through a straw

2 Administering the medication IV, mixed in 50 mL of normal saline and piggybacked through the main IV line

3 Administering the medication IM in the gluteal muscle

4 Administering the medication SC in the deltoid muscle

4. The client is receiving baclofen (Lioresal) for muscle spasms due to a spinal cord injury. Which of the following indicates a side effect related to this medication?
   1 Photosensitivity
   2 Slurred speech
   3 Hypertension
   4 Muscle pain

5. The client is suspected of having myasthenia gravis. Edrophonium (Tensilon), 2 mg IV, is administered to determine the diagnosis. Which of the following indicates the diagnosis of myasthenia gravis?
   1 An increase in muscle strength within 1 to 3 minutes following administration of the medication
   2 A decrease in muscle strength within 1 to 3 minutes following administration of the medication
   3 Joint pain following administration of the medication
   4 Feelings of faintness, dizziness, hypotension, and signs of flushing in the client

6. The client with myasthenia gravis is suspected of having cholinergic crisis. Which of the following symptoms indicates that this crisis exists?
   1 Hypotension
   2 Hypertension
   3 Mouth sores
   4 Ataxia

7. The client with myasthenia gravis is receiving pyridostigmine (Mestinon). The nurse monitors for signs and symptoms of cholinergic crisis caused by overdose of the medication. The nurse plans to have the antidote for cholinergic crisis available. Which of the following medications is the antidote for cholinergic crisis?
   1 Vitamin K
   2 Protamine sulfate
   3 Acetylcysteine (Mucomyst)
   4 Atropine sulfate

8. The client with myasthenia gravis becomes increasingly weaker. The physician prepares to identify whether the client is reacting to an overdose of the medication (cholinergic crisis) or an increasing severity of the disease (myasthenic crisis). An injection of edrophonium is administered. Which of the following indicates that the client is in cholinergic crisis?
   1 An improvement of the weakness
   2 A temporary worsening of the condition

3 No change in the condition
4 Complaints of muscle spasms

9. The client with myasthenia gravis verbalizes complaints of feeling much weaker than normal. The physician plans to implement a diagnostic test to determine whether the client is experiencing a myasthenic crisis. The physician administers edrophonium. Which of the following indicates that the client is experiencing a myasthenic crisis?
   1 Increasing weakness
   2 No change in the condition
   3 A temporary improvement in the condition
   4 An increase in muscle spasms

10. Levodopa (Carbidopa) is prescribed for the client with Parkinson's disease. The nurse monitors the client for adverse reactions to the medication. Which of the following indicates that the client is experiencing an adverse reaction?
    1 Pruritus
    2 Hypertension
    3 Tachycardia
    4 Impaired voluntary movements

11. Phenytoin (Dilantin), 100 mg PO three times daily, has been prescribed for the client for seizure control. The home health nurse visits the client and provides teaching regarding the medication. Which of the following statements, if made by the client, indicates effective teaching?
    1 "It's OK to break the capsules to make it easier for me to swallow them."
    2 "I will use a soft toothbrush to brush my teeth."
    3 "If I forget to take my medication, I can wait until the next dose and eliminate that dose."
    4 "If my throat becomes sore, it's a normal effect of the medication and it's nothing to be concerned about."

12. The client is taking phenytoin (Dilantin) for seizure control. Blood for a serum drug level is drawn. Which of the following indicates a therapeutic serum drug range?
    1 5 to 10 μg/mL
    2 10 to 20 μg/mL
    3 20 to 30 μg/mL
    4 30 to 40 μg/mL

13. The nurse is preparing an IV infusion of phenytoin (Dilantin) as prescribed by the physician for the client with seizures. Which of the following solutions will the nurse plan to use to dilute this medication?
    1 Lactated Ringer's
    2 5% Dextrose
    3 5% Dextrose and 1/2 normal saline
    4 Normal saline solution

14. The home health nurse visits a client who is taking phenytoin (Dilantin) for control of seizures. During the assessment, the nurse notes that the client is taking birth control pills. Which of the following should the nurse include in the teaching plan?
    1 The increased risk of thrombophlebitis while taking phenytoin and birth control pills together
    2 The potential decreased effectiveness of the birth control pills while taking Dilantin
    3 The client may stop the medication if it is causing severe gastrointestinal effects
    4 Pregnancy should be avoided while taking phenytoin

15. A client with trigeminal neuralgia is being treated with carbamazepine (Tegretol), 400 mg PO daily. Which of the following indicates that the client is experiencing an adverse reaction to the medication?
    1 WBC count of 3000/μL
    2 BUN, 15 mg/dL
    3 Sodium, 140 mEq/L
    4 Uric acid, 5.0 ng/dL

16. A client with multiple sclerosis is receiving diazepam (Valium), a centrally acting skeletal muscle relaxant. Which of the following, if noted during assessment of the client, indicates that the client is experiencing a side effect related to this medication?
    1 Headache
    2 Increased salivation
    3 Urinary retention
    4 Drowsiness

17. The nurse is caring for a client receiving morphine, 10 mg SC every 4 hours, for pain. Since morphine has been prescribed for this client, which of the following nursing actions would be included in the plan of care?
    1 Monitor the client's temperature
    2 Force fluids
    3 Maintain the client in a supine position
    4 Encourage the client to cough and deep breathe

18. Meperidine (Demerol) is prescribed for the client with pain. Which of the following would the nurse monitor as a side effect of this medication?
    1 Hypertension
    2 Bradycardia
    3 Diarrhea
    4 Urinary retention

19. The nurse is caring for a client with severe back pain. Codeine sulfate has been prescribed for the client. Which of the following does the nurse include in the plan of care while the client is taking this medication?
    1 Monitor for hypertension
    2 Monitor fluid balance

3 Monitor bowel activity
4 Monitor peripheral pulses

20. Dantrolene (Dantrium) is prescribed for a client with spinal cord injury for discomfort caused by spasticity. Which of the following laboratory values should the nurse monitor while the client is taking this medication?
    1 Sedimentation rate
    2 WBC count
    3 Liver function studies
    4 Creatinine

21. The client with epilepsy is taking the prescribed dose of phenytoin (Dilantin) to control seizures. Results of a Dilantin blood level study reveal a level of 35 μg/mL. Which of the following symptoms would be expected as a result of this laboratory result?
    1 No symptoms as this is a normal therapeutic Dilantin level
    2 Slurred speech
    3 Tachycardia
    4 Nystagmus

22. The physician initiates levodopa therapy for the client with Parkinson's disease. A few days after the client starts the medication, the client complains of nausea and vomiting. The nurse's best instruction to the client to alleviate the nausea is that:
    1 This is an expected side effect
    2 Eating a snack before taking the medication will help prevent the nausea
    3 Taking an antiemetic is the best measure to prevent the nausea
    4 The nausea and vomiting will decrease when the dose of levodopa is stabilized

23. Mannitol (Osmitrol) is prescribed for the client with increased intracranial pressure following a head injury. Which of the following indicates the therapeutic action of this medication?
    1 Induces diuresis by raising the osmotic pressure of the glomerular filtrate, thereby inhibiting tubular reabsorption of water and solutes
    2 Induces diuresis by promoting the reabsorption of sodium and water in the loop of Henle
    3 Prevents the filtration of sodium and water through the kidneys
    4 Prevents the filtration of sodium and potassium through the kidneys

24. Dexamethasone (Decadron) IV is prescribed for the client with cerebral edema. The nurse prepares the medication for administration. Which of the following indicates the appropriate preparation of this medication?
    1 Mixing the medication in 100 mL of lactated Ringer's solution
    2 Mixing the medication in 1000 mL of 5% dextrose

3 Preparing an undiluted direct injection of the medication

4 Diluting the medication in lactated Ringer's solution and preparing to administer as a direct injection

25. The client arrives at the emergency department complaining of back spasms. The client states, "I have been taking 2 to 3 aspirin every 4 hours for the last week and it hasn't helped my back." Aspirin intoxication is suspected. Which of the following symptoms indicates aspirin intoxication?

1 Diarrhea
2 Constipation
3 Tinnitus
4 Photosensitivity

ANSWERS

1. **3**

Rationale: The antidote for acetaminophen is acetylcysteine (Mucomyst). The normal therapeutic serum level is 5 to 20 μg/mL. A toxic level is greater than 50 μg/mL, and levels of greater than 200 μg/mL could indicate hepatotoxicity. Auranofin (Ridaura) is a gold preparation used in rheumatoid arthritis. Fludarabine (Fludara) and pentostatin (Nipent) are antineoplastic agents.

Test-Taking Strategy: Knowledge regarding the antidote for acetaminophen and the medications noted in the options will assist you in answering this question. It is important to know the antidote for various medications. If you had difficulty with this question, take time now to review antidotes!

Level of Cognitive Ability: Analysis
Phase of Nursing Process: Planning
Client Needs: Physiological Integrity
Content Area: Pharmacology

Reference
Kee, J., & Hayes, E. (1997). *Pharmacology: A nursing process approach* (2nd ed.). Philadelphia: W. B. Saunders. p. 232.

2. **2**

Rationale: In adults, overdose of acetaminophen causes liver damage. Option 2 is an indicator of liver function and is the only option that indicates an abnormal laboratory value. The normal direct bilirubin is 0 to 0.4 mg/dL. The normal platelet count is 150,000 to 400,000 cells/μL. The normal prothrombin time is 10 to 13 seconds. The normal sodium level is 135 to 145 mEq/L.

Test-Taking Strategy: Knowledge that acetaminophen causes liver damage and knowledge of the normal laboratory results will be helpful in answering this question. Utilize the process of elimination and your knowledge regarding normal laboratory values in the options will direct you to option 2, the abnormal value. Also, of all of the options, the bilirubin is the most directly related laboratory value to liver function.

Level of Cognitive Ability: Analysis
Phase of Nursing Process: Analysis
Client Needs: Physiological Integrity
Content Area: Pharmacology

Reference
Clark, J., Queener, S., & Karb, V. (1997). *Pharmacologic basis of nursing practice* (5th ed.). St. Louis: Mosby–Year Book. p. 367.

3. **1**

Rationale: Because acetylcysteine has a pervasive flavor of rotten eggs, it must be disguised in a flavored ice drink and is preferably drunk through a straw to minimize contact with the mouth. Acetylcysteine is the antidote for acetaminophen. It is a solution that is also used as a mucolytic agent; therefore, it is to be administered as an antidote by the oral route.

Test-Taking Strategy: Knowledge of the medication acetylcysteine will assist you in answering this question. Knowing that the medication is a solution that is also used for nebulization treatments will assist you in selecting the option that indicates an oral route. Note that options 2, 3, and 4 indicate parenteral administration and option 1, the correct option, indicates oral administration.

Level of Cognitive Ability: Application
Phase of Nursing Process: Implementation
Client Needs: Physiological Integrity
Content Area: Pharmacology

Reference
Clark, J., Queener, S., & Karb, V. (1997). *Pharmacologic basis of nursing practice* (5th ed.). St. Louis: Mosby–Year Book. pp. 361, 368.

4. **2**

Rationale: Side effects of baclofen include drowsiness, dizziness, weakness, and nausea. Occasional side effects include headache, paresthesia of the hands and feet, constipation or diarrhea, anorexia, hypotension, confusion, and nasal congestion. Paradoxical CNS excitement and restlessness can occur along with slurred speech, tremor, dry mouth, nocturia, and impotence.

Test-Taking Strategy: Knowledge regarding the medication is required to answer the question. Use the process of elimination. Option 2 is the option that is most closely associated with a neurological disorder. If you had difficulty with this question, take time now to review the side effects related to baclofen!

Level of Cognitive Ability: Analysis
Phase of Nursing Process: Assessment
Client Needs: Physiological Integrity
Content Area: Pharmacology

Reference
Hodgson, B., & Kizior, R. (1998). *Saunders nursing drug handbook 1998.* Philadelphia: W. B. Saunders. pp. 95–96.

5. **1**

Rationale: Edrophonium is a short-acting acetylcholinesterase inhibitor used as a diagnostic agent. When a new client with suspected myasthenia gravis is given 2 mg of the medication intravenously, an increase in muscle strength should be seen in 1 to 3 minutes. If no response occurs, another 4 to 10 mg of edrophonium is given over the next

2 minutes, and muscle strength is again tested. If no increase in muscle strength occurs with this higher dose, the muscle weakness is not caused by myasthenia gravis. Clients receiving injections of this medication commonly demonstrate a drop of blood pressure, feel faint and dizzy, and are flushed.

Test-Taking Strategy: Knowledge regarding this medication as a diagnostic tool for myasthenia gravis is required to answer this question. You are likely to see questions related to this medication and diagnostic test on NCLEX-RN. Take time now to review this medication as a diagnostic tool for suspected myasthenia gravis!

Level of Cognitive Ability: Analysis
Phase of Nursing Process: Assessment
Client Needs: Physiological Integrity
Content Area: Pharmacology

Reference
Clark, J., Queener, S., & Karb, V. (1997). *Pharmacologic basis of nursing practice* (5th ed.). St. Louis; Mosby–Year Book. pp. 448–449.

6. **2**

Rationale: Cholinergic crisis occurs with an overdose of medication. Indications of cholinergic crisis include GI disturbances, nausea, vomiting, diarrhea, abdominal cramps, increased salivation and tearing, miosis, hypertension, sweating, and increased bronchial secretions.

Test-Taking Strategy: Knowledge regarding both cholinergic crisis and myasthenic crisis is required to answer this question. You are likely to see questions on NCLEX-RN related to these conditions. Take time now to review both cholinergic and myasthenic crisis if you had difficulty with this question!

Level of Cognitive Ability: Analysis
Phase of Nursing Process: Assessment
Client Needs: Physiological Integrity
Content Area: Pharmacology

Reference
Clark, J., Queener, S., & Karb, V. (1997). *Pharmacologic basis of nursing practice* (5th ed.). St. Louis; Mosby–Year Book. p. 449.

7. **4**

Rationale: The antidote for cholinergic crisis is atropine sulfate. Vitamin K is the antidote for Coumadin. Protamine sulfate is the antidote for heparin, and acetylcysteine is the antidote for acetaminophen.

Test-Taking Strategy: Knowledge regarding antidotes for the various medications is required to answer this question. Review antidotes now, if you had difficulty with this question!

Level of Cognitive Ability: Application
Phase of Nursing Process: Planning
Client Needs: Physiological Integrity
Content Area: Pharmacology

Reference
Kee, J., & Hayes, E. (1997) *Pharmacology: A nursing process approach* (2nd ed.). Philadelphia: W. B. Saunders. p. 315.

8. **2**

Rationale: An edrophonium injection makes the client in cholinergic crisis temporarily worse. This is known as a negative Tensilon test.

Test-Taking Strategy: Knowledge regarding the use of this medication as a diagnostic tool to differentiate between cholinergic and myasthenic crisis is required to answer this question. You are likely to see questions related to this medication on NCLEX-RN. Take time now to review this diagnostic test and the differences between cholinergic and myasthenic crisis!

Level of Cognitive Ability: Analysis
Phase of Nursing Process: Assessment
Client Needs: Physiological Integrity
Content Area: Pharmacology

Reference
Clark, J., Queener, S., & Karb, V. (1997). *Pharmacologic basis of nursing practice* (5th ed.). St. Louis; Mosby–Year Book. p. 449.

9. **3**

Rationale: Edrophonium is administered to determine whether the client is reacting to an overdose of a medication (cholinergic crisis) or an increasing severity of the disease (myasthenic crisis). When the edrophonium injection is given and the condition improves temporarily, the client is in myasthenic crisis. This is known as a positive Tensilon test.

Test-Taking Strategy: Knowledge regarding the use of this medication as a diagnostic tool to differentiate between cholinergic and myasthenic crisis is required to answer this question. You are likely to see questions related to this medication on NCLEX-RN. Take time now to review this diagnostic test and the differences between cholinergic and myasthenic crisis!

Level of Cognitive Ability: Analysis
Phase of Nursing Process: Assessment
Client Needs: Physiological Integrity
Content Area: Pharmacology

Reference
Clark, J., Queener, S., & Karb, V. (1997). *Pharmacologic basis of nursing practice* (5th ed.). St. Louis; Mosby–Year Book. p. 449.

10. **4**

Rationale: Dyskinesia and impaired voluntary movement may occur with high levodopa dosages. Nausea, anorexia, dizziness, orthostatic hypotension, bradycardia, and akinesia (the temporary muscle weakness that lasts 1 minute to 1 hour, also known as "on-off" phenomenon) are frequent side effects of the medication.

Test-Taking Strategy: Knowledge regarding the adverse effects of levodopa is required to answer this question. Use the process of elimination. Options 2 and 3 are cardiac-related options, so these options can be eliminated first. Note that the question asks for an adverse reaction; therefore, select option 4 over option 1 as the correct answer. Review the adverse effects of carbidopa now, if you had difficulty with this question!

Level of Cognitive Ability: Analysis
Phase of Nursing Process: Assessment
Client Needs: Physiological Integrity
Content Area: Pharmacology

Reference
Kee, J., & Hayes, E. (1997) *Pharmacology: A nursing process approach* (2nd ed.). Philadelphia: W. B. Saunders. p. 311.

11. 2

Rationale: Phenytoin is an anticonvulsant. Gingival hyperplasia, bleeding, swelling, and tenderness of the gums can occur with the use of this medication. The client needs to be taught good oral hygiene, gum massage, and the need for regular dentist visits. The client should not skip medication doses as this could precipitate a seizure. Capsules should not be chewed or broken, and they must be swallowed. The client needs to be instructed to report a sore throat, fever, glandular swelling, or any skin reaction, as this indicates hematological toxicity.

Test-Taking Strategy: Utilize the process of elimination in selecting the correct option. Note that the question asks which of the statements if made by the client indicates that the teaching was effective. Eliminate option 3 as the client needs to be encouraged to take medications on time. Also, eliminate option 4 because the client needs to report these symptoms to the physician. Remember, Dilantin capsules should not be broken. Take time now to review the side effects related to phenytoin, if you had difficulty with this question!

Level of Cognitive Ability: Analysis
Phase of Nursing Process: Evaluation
Client Needs: Health Promotion and Maintenance
Content Area: Pharmacology

Reference
Kee, J., & Hayes, E. (1997) *Pharmacology: A nursing process approach* (2nd ed.). Philadelphia: W. B. Saunders. p. 244.

12. 2

Rationale: The therapeutic serum drug level range for phenytoin is 10 to 20 µg/mL.

Test-Taking Strategy: Knowledge regarding the therapeutic serum range of this medication is required to answer the question. A helpful hint may be to remember that the theophylline therapeutic range and the acetaminophen therapeutic range are the same as the Dilantin therapeutic range. Remembering this may assist you when answering questions related to these three medications.

Level of Cognitive Ability: Analysis
Phase of Nursing Process: Assessment
Client Needs: Physiological Integrity
Content Area: Pharmacology

Reference
Kee, J., & Hayes, E. (1997) *Pharmacology: A nursing process approach* (2nd ed.). Philadelphia: W. B. Saunders. p. 245.

13. 4

Rationale: Intravenous infusion of Dilantin should be administered by injection into a large vein. The medication may be diluted in saline solution; however, dextrose solution should be avoided because of drug precipitation. The medication is administered as intermittent doses. Continuous IV infusions should not be used. Infusion rates of more than 50 mg/min may cause hypotension or cardiac dysrhythmias, especially with elderly and debilitated clients.

Test-Taking Strategy: Knowledge regarding compatible IV solutions with phenytoin is required to answer this question. In most, but not all, situations, medications can be diluted in normal saline, so this would be your safe option to select if you were unfamiliar with the IV administration of this medication.

Level of Cognitive Ability: Application
Phase of Nursing Process: Planning
Client Needs: Physiological Integrity
Content Area: Pharmacology

Reference
Kee, J., & Hayes, E. (1997) *Pharmacology: A nursing process approach* (2nd ed.). Philadelphia: W. B. Saunders. p. 244.

14. 2

Rationale: Phenytoin enhances the rate of estrogen metabolism, which can decrease the effectiveness of some birth control pills.

Test-Taking Strategy: Knowledge regarding medication interactions while taking Dilantin is required to answer the question. Use the process of elimination to select the correct option. Option 1 would cause anxiety in the client. A client should not be instructed to stop anticonvulsant medication, as indicated in option 3. Pregnancy does not need to be "avoided." Review medication interactions related to phenytoin now, if you had difficulty with this question!

Level of Cognitive Ability: Analysis
Phase of Nursing Process: Implementation
Client Needs: Health Promotion and Maintenance
Content Area: Pharmacology

Reference
Clark, J., Queener, S., & Karb, V. (1997). *Pharmacologic basis of nursing practice* (5th ed.). St. Louis; Mosby–Year Book. p. 688.

15. 1

Rationale: Adverse effects of carbamazepine appear as blood dyscrasias, including aplastic anemia, agranulocytosis, thrombocytopenia, leukopenia, cardiovascular disturbances, thrombophlebitis, dysrhythmias, and dermatological effects.

Test-Taking Strategy: Knowledge regarding the adverse effects related to this medication is required to answer the question. Utilize the process of elimination. If you are familiar with normal laboratory values, you will note that the only option that indicates an abnormal value is option 1. Review the signs of adverse reactions related to this medication now, if you had difficulty with this question!

Level of Cognitive Ability: Analysis
Phase of Nursing Process: Assessment
Client Needs: Physiological Integrity
Content Area: Pharmacology

Reference
Hodgson, B., & Kizior, R. (1998). *Saunders nursing drug handbook 1998.* Philadelphia: W. B. Saunders. pp. 147–148.

16. 4

Rationale: Incoordination and drowsiness are common side effects resulting from this medication.

Test-Taking Strategy: Knowledge regarding multiple sclerosis and skeletal muscle relaxants is required to answer the question. Note that the question addresses a centrally acting skeletal muscle relaxant. This may assist you in the process of elimination and direct you to the correct option of drowsiness. If you had difficulty with this question, take time now to review the side effects associated with Valium!

Level of Cognitive Ability: Analysis
Phase of Nursing Process: Assessment
Client Needs: Physiological Integrity
Content Area: Pharmacology

Reference
Clark, J., Queener, S., & Karb, V. (1997). *Pharmacologic basis of nursing practice* (5th ed.). St. Louis; Mosby–Year Book. p. 706.

17. 4

Rationale: Morphine suppresses the cough reflex. Clients need to be encouraged to cough and deep breathe to prevent pneumonia.

Test-Taking Strategy: Utilize the process of elimination when answering this question. The question is specifically asking about nursing implementation related to this medication. Knowledge that morphine suppresses the cough reflex and the respiratory reflex would lead you to the correct option. Additionally, use your ABCs when selecting the correct option. Remember: Airway, Breathing, and Circulation!

Level of Cognitive Ability: Application
Phase of Nursing Process: Planning
Client Needs: Physiological Integrity
Content Area: Pharmacology

Reference
Hodgson, B., & Kizior, R. (1998). *Saunders nursing drug handbook 1998.* Philadelphia: W. B. Saunders. p. 706.

18. 4

Rationale: Side effects of this medication include respiratory depression, orthostatic hypotension, tachycardia, drowsiness and mental clouding, constipation, and urinary retention.

Test-Taking Strategy: Knowledge regarding side effects associated with narcotic analgesics will assist you in answering the question. From here, use the process of elimination. If you had difficulty with this question, take time now to review the medication!

Level of Cognitive Ability: Analysis
Phase of Nursing Process: Assessment
Client Needs: Physiological Integrity
Content Area: Pharmacology

Reference
Kee, J., & Hayes, E. (1997). *Pharmacology: A nursing process approach* (2nd ed.). Philadelphia: W. B. Saunders. p. 235.

19. 3

Rationale: While the client is taking codeine sulfate, the nurse would monitor vital signs and assess for hypotension. The nurse should also increase fluid intake, palpate the bladder for urinary retention, auscultate bowel sounds, and monitor the pattern of daily bowel activity and stool consistency. The nurse should monitor respiratory status and initiate breathing and coughing exercises. Additionally, the nurse monitors the effectiveness of the pain medication.

Test-Taking Strategy: Knowledge regarding side effects related to this medication will assist you in determining the most significant nursing intervention. Use the process of elimination in answering the question. Remember that codeine can cause constipation. If you had difficulty with this question, take time now to review nursing measures related to the administration of codeine sulfate!

Level of Cognitive Ability: Application
Phase of Nursing Process: Planning
Client Needs: Physiological Integrity
Content Area: Pharmacology

Reference
Hodgson, B., & Kizior, R. (1998). *Saunders nursing drug handbook 1998.* Philadelphia: W. B. Saunders. p. 251.

20. 3

Rationale: Dantrolene can cause liver damage, and the nurse should monitor the liver function studies. Baseline liver function studies are done before therapy starts, and regular liver function studies are performed throughout therapy. Dantrolene is discontinued if no relief of spasticity is achieved in 6 weeks.

Test-Taking Strategy: Knowledge regarding the effects of this medication is required to answer this question. Knowledge that this medication is hepatotoxic will direct you to the correct option. If you had difficulty with this question, take time now to review!

Level of Cognitive Ability: Analysis
Phase of Nursing Process: Assessment
Client Needs: Physiological Integrity
Content Area: Pharmacology

Reference
Clark, J., Queener, S., & Karb, V. (1997). *Pharmacologic basis of nursing practice* (5th ed.). St. Louis: Mosby–Year Book. p. 707.

21. 2

Rationale: The therapeutic Dilantin level is 10 to 20 μg/mL. At greater than 20 μg/mL, involuntary movements of the eyeballs (nystagmus) appear. At greater than 30 μ/mL, ataxia and slurred speech arise.

Test-Taking Strategy: Knowledge regarding the therapeutic Dilantin level is required to answer this question. Take time now to review therapeutic levels and associated signs, if you had difficulty with this question!

Level of Cognitive Ability: Analysis
Phase of Nursing Process: Analysis
Client Needs: Physiological Integrity
Content Area: Pharmacology

Reference
Clark, J., Queener, S., & Karb, V. (1997). *Pharmacologic basis of nursing practice* (5th ed.). St. Louis; Mosby–Year Book. p. 688.

22. 2

Rationale: The best instruction by the nurse is that snacks will prevent the nausea. Vomiting should not occur and needs to be alleviated if it occurs. Nonpharmacological approaches should be utilized first. Option 4 is inaccurate.

Test-Taking Strategy: Read the stem of the question carefully. The key word is "best." It is best to utilize nonpharmacological approaches first to alleviate the nausea. Focusing on the issue of the question will direct you to option 2.

Level of Cognitive Ability: Application
Phase of Nursing Process: Implementation
Client Needs: Physiological Integrity
Content Area: Pharmacology

Reference
Clark, J., Queener, S., & Karb, V. (1997). *Pharmacologic basis of nursing practice* (5th ed.). St. Louis: Mosby–Year Book. p. 700.

23. 1

Rationale: Mannitol is an osmotic diuretic that induces diuresis by raising the osmotic pressure of the glomerular filtrate, thereby inhibiting tubular reabsorption of water and solutes. It is used to reduce intracranial pressure in the client with head trauma.

Test-Taking Strategy: Read the question carefully, noting that it presents a client with increased intracranial pressure. Read the options carefully. The only option that suggests an action that will produce diuresis and thus reduce intracranial pressure is option 1. If you had difficulty with this question, take time now to review the action of mannitol!

Level of Cognitive Ability: Analysis
Phase of Nursing Process: Analysis
Client Needs: Physiological Integrity
Content Area: Pharmacology

Reference

Wilson, B., Shannon, M., & Stang, C. (1997). *Nurses drug guide.* Stamford, CT: Appleton & Lange. pp. 815–817.

24. **3**

Rationale: Dexamethasone may be given by direct IV injection or IV infusion. For IV infusion, it may be mixed with 0.9% sodium chloride or 5% dextrose.

Test-Taking Strategy: Utilize the process of elimination to answer the question. Eliminate option 2 because 1000 mL of solution is a very large amount to use to dilute this medication, particularly in a client with cerebral edema. Eliminate options 1 and 4 as they are similar in addressing the use of lactated Ringer's solution. This leaves option 3 as the correct option. If you had difficulty with this question, take time now to review the administration of Decadron!

Level of Cognitive Ability: Application
Phase of Nursing Process: Implementation
Client Needs: Physiological Integrity
Content Area: Pharmacology

Reference

Hodgson, B., & Kizior, R. (1998). *Saunders nursing drug handbook 1998.* Philadelphia: W. B. Saunders. pp. 296–297.

25. **3**

Rationale: Mild intoxication with acetylsalicylic acid (aspirin) is called salicylism and is commonly experienced when the daily dosage is more than 4 g. Tinnitus (ringing in the ears) is the most frequent effect noted with intoxication. Hyperventilation may occur because salicylate stimulates the respiratory center. Fever may result because salicylate interferes with the metabolic pathways coupling oxygen consumption and heat production.

Test-Taking Strategy: Knowledge regarding toxicity related to acetylsalicylic acid (aspirin) is required to answer this question. Note that the stem of the question refers to aspirin intoxication. Options 1 and 2 relate to GI symptoms. Option 3, the correct answer, is the indicator of toxicity. If you had difficulty with this question, take time now to review aspirin intoxication!

Level of Cognitive Ability: Analysis
Phase of Nursing Process: Assessment
Client Needs: Physiological Integrity
Content Area: Pharmacology

Reference

Clark, J., Queener, S., & Karb, V. (1997). *Pharmacologic basis of nursing practice* (5th ed.). St. Louis: Mosby–Year Book. p. 369

BIBLIOGRAPHY

Clark, J., Queener, S., & Karb, V. (1997). *Pharmacologic basis of nursing practice* (5th ed.). St. Louis: Mosby–Year Book.

Hodgson, B., & Kizior, R. (1998). *Saunders nursing drug handbook 1998.* Philadelphia: W. B. Saunders.

Kee, J., & Hayes, E. (1997). *Pharmacology: A nursing process approach* (2nd ed.). Philadelphia: W. B. Saunders.

Lehne, R. (1998). *Pharmacology for nursing care* (3rd ed.). Philadelphia: W. B. Saunders

Wilson, B., Shannon, M., & Stang, C. (1997). *Nurses drug guide.* Stamford, CT: Appleton & Lange.

UNIT XVIII

· ·

The Adult Client with a Musculoskeletal Disorder

PYRAMID TERMS

Casts—Made of plaster or fiber glass to provide immobilization of bone and joints after a fracture or injury.

Compartment Syndrome—Increased pressure within one or more compartments causing massive compromise of circulation to an area and causing irreversible neuromuscular damage within 4 to 6 hours of its onset if not treated.

External Fixation—Stabilization of a fracture by the use of an external frame, with multiple pins applied through the bone.

Fat Embolism—An embolism that can occur 24 to 48 hours following a fracture or within the first 72 hours.

Internal Fixation—Stabilization of a fracture that involves the application of screws, plates, pins, or nails to hold the fragments in alignment.

Reduction—The procedure that restores the bone to proper alignment.

Traction—Force applied in two directions to reduce and immobilize a fracture.

PYRAMID TO SUCCESS

The Pyramid to Success focuses on the emergency care to a client who sustains a fracture or other musculoskeletal injury, monitoring for complications related to fractures, and interventions if complications occur. Nursing care related to casts and traction is emphasized. Skill related to instructing the client in the use of an assistive device such as a cane, walker, or crutches is a pyramid point. Pyramid points also include postoperative care following hip surgery or amputation, and care to the client with rheumatoid arthritis, osteoporosis, or autoimmune disease. Focus on the points related to the psychosocial effects as a result of the musculoskeletal disorder, such as unexpected body image changes, and the mobilization of appropriate and available support services needed for the client.

NURSING PROCESS

ASSESSMENT

Fatigue and weakness
Fever
Weight loss
Inability to perform activities
Limited range of motion
Loss of movement
Asymmetry of limbs or deformed appearance
Tenderness, pain, stiffness, and swelling
Loss of sensory perception
Numbness or tingling of extremities
Muscle atrophy
Problems with balance or gait

ANALYSIS: Alteration in Comfort

PLANNING	IMPLEMENTATION	EVALUATION
Client reports the presence of pain. Client uses nonpharmacological measures to reduce pain.	Assess for pain. Assist client to identify comfort measures to reduce pain. Provide comfort measures. Instruct client in nonpharmacological measures to reduce pain. Administer pain medication as appropriate. Instruct client regarding administration of prescribed medications. Document the effectiveness of pain reduction techniques.	Client remains comfortable and free of pain.

ANALYSIS: Potential for Ineffective Airway Clearance

PLANNING	IMPLEMENTATION	EVALUATION
Client performs coughing and deep breathing exercises. Client tolerates ambulation activities as prescribed.	Monitor respiratory status for complications related to immobility. Encourage coughing and deep breathing. Turn and reposition client. Perform range-of-motion exercises as prescribed. Encourage out-of-bed activities as prescribed.	Lungs remain clear and free of secretions.

ANALYSIS: Potential for Alteration in Tissue Perfusion

PLANNING	IMPLEMENTATION	EVALUATION
Client reports adequate sensation in affected area.	Assess color, motion, and sensation in affected area. Monitor for adequate and palpable pulses.	Palpable pulses are noted. Adequate tissue perfusion in affected area is maintained.

ANALYSIS: Potential for Infection

PLANNING	IMPLEMENTATION	EVALUATION
Client remains free of infection.	Monitor temperature. Monitor wound status. Monitor for signs of infection.	Temperature remains within normal limits. Wound remains free of infection.

ANALYSIS: Potential for Injury

PLANNING	IMPLEMENTATION	EVALUATION
Client identifies factors that may cause injury. Client avoids situations that may cause physical injury.	Assess client's motor and sensory deficit to determine safety needs. Provide appropriate assistive devices to prevent injury. Instruct client in the use of assistive devices. Keep environment free of obstructions. Document client's safe performance of activities.	Client demonstrates correct use of assistive devices. Client achieves optimal level without injury. Client remains free of injury.

ANALYSIS: Alteration in Skin Integrity

PLANNING	IMPLEMENTATION	EVALUATION
Client remains free of skin breakdown as a result of immobility. Client's surgical wound demonstrates signs of the healing process.	Assess skin integrity. Turn and reposition client. Monitor surgical wound for signs of healing. Encourage ambulation and out-of-bed activity.	Surgical wound heals. Client's skin remains intact.

ANALYSIS: Alteration in Mobility

PLANNING	IMPLEMENTATION	EVALUATION
Client requests assistance with mobilization activities. Client identifies mobility limitations and restrictions.	Assess mobility limitations. Assist client with mobility. Provide assistive devices as appropriate for ambulation. Instruct client in the use of assistive devices. Encourage verbalization regarding mobility limitations and restrictions.	Client accepts mobility limitations. Client utilizes assistive devices appropriately.

ANALYSIS: Self-Care Deficit

PLANNING	IMPLEMENTATION	EVALUATION
Client verbalizes the need for assistance. Client participates in self-care to optimal level.	Assess the need for assistance with self-care. Assist client with self-care needs as necessary. Assist client in care promoting independence as much as possible.	Client performs independent self-care activities to optimal level of functioning.

ANALYSIS: Potential for Alteration in Elimination Patterns

PLANNING	IMPLEMENTATION	EVALUATION
Client verbalizes the presence of optimal elimination patterns.	Monitor intake and output. Assess bowel sounds. Assess dietary habits. Encourage optimal activity to stimulate bowel elimination. Instruct client regarding the need for adequate fluids and fiber in the diet.	Client remains free of elimination alterations related to immobility.

PLANNING	IMPLEMENTATION	EVALUATION
Client shares grief and loss with a significant person. Client actively participates in the decision-making process.	Encourage client to express grief and loss. Assist client to recognize own strengths and available support systems.	Client utilizes available support systems.

CLIENT NEEDS

SAFE, EFFECTIVE CARE ENVIRONMENT

Client rights

Confidentiality regarding disorder and plan of care

Informed consent for diagnostic treatments and surgical procedures

Physical therapy and occupational therapy referrals

Dietary consultation

Asepsis related to wounds

Standard precautions

Preventing injury from accidents

HEALTH PROMOTION AND MAINTENANCE

The aging process and disease prevention

Health promotion related to diet and activity

Physical assessment related to the musculoskeletal system

Home care instructions regarding care related to musculoskeletal disorder

Reinforcement regarding the importance of prescribed therapy

PSYCHOSOCIAL INTEGRITY

Grief and loss related to mobility limitations and restrictions

The ability to cope with feelings of isolation and loss of independence

Mobilizing coping mechanisms

Sensory and perceptual alterations

Cultural, religious, and spiritual influences

Situational role changes as a result of musculoskeletal disorder

Unexpected body image changes as a result of injury or disease

Available support systems and utilization of community resources

PHYSIOLOGICAL INTEGRITY

Use of assistive devices for mobility, such as canes, walkers, and crutches

Promoting normal elimination patterns

Measures to promote comfort

Promoting self-care measures

Pharmacological medications, actions, agents, side effects, and adverse effects

Complications related to procedures or injuries

Emergency care for a fracture or other injury

Complications of a fracture

Care related to casts and traction

Postoperative interventions

Rheumatoid arthritis

Osteoporosis

Autoimmune disorders

REFERENCES

Black, J., & Matassarin-Jacobs, E. (1997). *Medical-surgical nursing: Clinical management for continuity of care* (5th ed). Philadelphia: W. B. Saunders

Luckmann, J. (1997). *Saunders manual of nursing care.* Philadelphia: W. B. Saunders.

National Council of State Boards of Nursing (eds.) (1997). *Test for the National Council Licensure Examination for Registered Nurses.* Chicago: Author.

O'Toole, M. 9ed.). (1997). *Miller-Keane encyclopedia & dictionary of medicine, nursing & allied health* (6th ed.). Philadelphia: W. B. Saunders.

CHAPTER 67

The Musculoskeletal System

I. Anatomy and Physiology

A. Skeleton
1. Axial portion
   a. Cranium
   b. Vertebrae
   c. Ribs
2. Appendicular portion
   a. Limbs
   b. Shoulders
   c. Hips

B. Bones
1. Types of bones
   a. Long
   b. Short
   c. Flat
   d. Irregular
2. Spongy bone
   a. Located in the ends of long bones and the center of flat and irregular bones
   b. Can withstand forces applied in many directions
3. Dense (compact) bones
   a. Covers spongy bone
   b. Cylinder around a central marrow cavity
   c. Can withstand force predominantly in one direction
4. Characteristics of the bones
   a. Support and protect structures of the body
   b. Provide attachments for muscles, tendons, and ligaments
   c. Contain tissue in the central cavities, which aids in formation of blood cells
   d. Assist in regulating calcium and phosphate concentrations
5. Bone growth
   a. The length of bone growth is a result of the ossification of the epiphyseal cartilage at the ends of bones, and bone growth stops between the ages of 18 and 25 years
   b. The width of bone growth is a result of the activity of osteoblasts and occurs

throughout life but does slow down with the aging process
   c. Bone absorption around the bone marrow continues throughout life; therefore, bones become weaker with aging

C. Types of joints
1. Synarthrosis
   a. Fibrous or fixed joints
   b. No movement associated with these joints
2. Amphiarthrosis
   a. Cartilaginous joints
   b. Slightly movable joints
3. Diarthrosis
   a. Synovial joints
   b. Ball-and-socket joints
4. Condyloid
   a. Freely movable joints
   b. Synovial joints allow frictionless, painless movement
5. Characteristics of the joints
   a. Allow the movement between bones
   b. Formed where two bones join
   c. Surfaces are covered with cartilage
   d. Enclosed in a capsule
   e. Contain a cavity filled with synovial fluid
   f. Ligaments hold the bone and joint in the correct position
   g. Articulation is the meeting point of two or more joints
6. Synovial fluid
   a. Found in joint capsule
   b. Formed by synovial membrane, which lines joint capsule
   c. Lubricates the cartilage
   d. Cushion for shocks

D. Muscles
1. Characteristics of muscles
   a. Made up of bundles of muscle fibers
   b. Provide the force to move bones
   c. Assist in maintaining posture
   d. Assist with heat production

2. The process of contraction and relaxation
   a. Muscle contraction and relaxation require large amounts of adenosine triphosphate (ATP)
   b. Contraction also requires calcium, which functions as a catalyst
   c. Acetylcholine released by the motor end plate of the motor neuron initiates an action potential
   d. Acetylcholine is then destroyed by acetylcholinesterase
   e. Calcium is required to contract muscle fibers and acts as a catalyst for the enzyme needed for the sliding together action of actin and myosin
   f. Following contraction, ATP transports calcium out in order to allow actin and myosin to slide apart and allow the muscle to relax
3. Skeletal muscles
   a. Are attached to two bones and cross at least one joint
   b. The point of origin is the point of attachment on the bone closest to the trunk
   c. The point of insertion is the point of attachment on the bone farthest from the trunk
   d. Skeletal muscles act in groups
   e. Prime movers contract to produce movement
   f. Antagonists relax
   g. Synergists contract to stabilize
   h. Nerves activate and control the muscles

II. Diagnostic Tests

A. X-rays
   1. Description: a commonly used procedure to diagnose disorders of the musculoskeletal system
   2. Implementation
      a. Handle injured area carefully
      b. Administer analgesics as prescribed prior to the procedure particularly if the client is in pain
      c. Remove any radiopaque objects such as jewelry
      d. Shield client's testes, ovaries, or pregnant abdomen
      e. Client must lie still during the x-ray
      f. Inform client that exposure to radiation is minimal and not dangerous
      g. Health care provider is to wear a lead apron if staying in the room with the client
B. Magnetic resonance imaging (MRI)
   1. Description: a noninvasive procedure that identifies types of tissues and identifies tumors and vascular abnormalities
   2. Implementation preprocedure
      a. Remove metal objects from the client

b. Determine if the client has a pacemaker or metal implants such as a hip prosthesis or vascular clips because these clients cannot have this test performed
   c. Provide an assessment of the client with claustrophobia
   d. Administer medication as prescribed for the client with claustrophobia
C. Arthrogram
   1. Description
      a. A radiographic examination of the soft tissues of the joint structures
      b. Used to diagnose trauma to the joint capsule or ligaments
      c. A local anesthesia is used for the procedure
      d. A contrast medium or air is injected into the joint cavity and the joint is moved through range of motion as a series of x-rays is taken
   2. Implementation
      a. Inform the client to fast from food and fluids for 8 hours prior to the procedure
      b. Assess for client allergies to iodine or seafood prior to the procedure
      c. Obtain a consent form
      d. Have the client void before the procedure
      e. Inform the client of the need to remain as still as possible except when asked to reposition
      f. Minimize the use of the joint for 12 hours following the procedure
      g. Instruct the client that the joint may be edematous and tender for 1 to 2 days after the procedure and may be treated with ice packs and analgesics as prescribed
      h. Inform the client that if edema and tenderness last longer than 2 days to notify the physician
      i. If knee arthrography was performed, an Ace wrap over the knee may be prescribed for 3 to 4 days
      j. If air was used for injection, crepitus may be felt in the joint for up to 2 days
D. Bone scan
   1. Description
      a. Radioisotope is injected IV and is taken after migration to the bone
      b. The isotope will collect in areas, which indicates abnormal bone metabolism and some fractures if they exist
      c. The isotope is excreted in urine and feces within 48 hours and is not harmful to others
   2. Implementation
      a. Hold fluids for 4 hours prior to the procedure
      b. Obtain a consent form
      c. Remove all jewelry and metal objects
      d. Following the injection of the

radioisotope, the client must drink 32 ounces of water to promote renal filtering of excess isotope

e. From 1 to 3 hours after injection, have the client void, and then the scanning procedure is performed

f. Inform the client of the need to lie supine during the procedure

g. Inform the client that the procedure is not painful

h. No special precautions are required after the procedure because a minimal amount of radioactivity exists in the isotope

i. Assess the injection site for redness and swelling

j. Encourage oral fluid intake following the procedure

E. Gallium scan
 1. Description
   a. An isotope is used and is taken up or migrates to the bone slowly
   b. The isotope is given to client 2 to 3 hours before the scan
 2. Implementation
   a. Obtain a consent form preprocedure
   b. No special follow-up care is required

F. Tomography
 1. Description
   a. An x-ray film that views detailed structures otherwise hidden by bone
   b. Allows views of tissue at various planes as if slices have been made through the tissue
 2. Implementation: no special preparation is required

G. Bone or muscle biopsy
 1. Description: may be done during surgery or through aspiration or punch or needle biopsy
 2. Implementation
   a. Obtain a consent form preprocedure
   b. Monitor vital signs
   c. Monitor for bleeding, swelling, and hematoma or severe pain
   d. Elevate the site for 24 hours following the procedure to reduce edema
   e. Apply ice packs as prescribed to prevent the development of a hematoma
   f. Monitor for signs of infection following the procedure
   g. Inform the client that mild to moderate discomfort is normal following the procedure

H. Arthroscopy
 1. Description
   a. Provides an endoscopic examination of various joints
   b. Articular cartilage abnormalities can be assessed, loose bodies can be removed, and the cartilage trimmed
   c. A biopsy may be performed during the procedure

d. Complications of the procedure include infection, hemarthrosis, swelling, synovial rupture, joint injury, or thrombophlebitis

 2. Implementation
   a. Instruct the client to fast for 8 to 12 hours prior to the procedure
   b. Obtain a consent form
   c. Administer pain medication as prescribed postprocedure
   d. Resume a normal diet following the procedure
   e. An elastic wrap should be worn for 2 to 4 days as prescribed
   f. Instruct the client that walking without weight bearing is usually permitted after sensation returns but to limit activity for 1 to 4 days as prescribed
   g. Instruct the client to elevate the extremity as often as possible for 2 days and to place ice on the site to minimize swelling
   h. Instruct the client in the use of crutches, which may be used for 5 to 7 days postprocedure when walking
   i. Advise the client to notify the physician if fever, increased knee pain, or edema continues for more than 3 days

I. Arthrocentesis
 1. Description
   a. Involves aspirating synovial fluid, blood, or pus via a needle inserted into a joint cavity
   b. Medication may be instilled into the joint if necessary to alleviate inflammation
 2. Implementation
   a. Obtain a consent form preprocedure
   b. Apply a compress bandage as prescribed
   c. Instruct the client to rest the joint for 8 to 24 hours
   d. Instruct the client to notify the physician if a fever or swelling of the joint occurs

J. Electromyography (EMG)
 1. Description
   a. Assesses lower motor neuron lesions
   b. Measures electrical potential associated with skeletal muscle contractions
   c. Needles are inserted into the muscle and recordings of muscular electrical activity are traced on recording paper through an oscilloscope
 2. Implementation
   a. Obtain consent
   b. Instruct the client that the needle insertion is uncomfortable
   c. Instruct clients not to take any stimulants or sedatives 24 hours prior to the procedure
   d. Inform the client that slight bruising may occur at needle insertion sites

III. Laboratory Studies

A. Antinuclear antibody (ANA)
  1. A blood test used in the differential diagnosis of rheumatic diseases, and to detect antinucleoprotein factors and patterns associated with certain autoimmune diseases
  2. Positive at a titer of 1:20 or 1:40 depending on the laboratory
  3. A positive result does not necessarily confirm a disease
B. Anti-dsDNA antibody test
  1. A blood test done specifically to identify or differentiate DNA antibodies found in systemic lupus erythematosus (SLE) or other rheumatic diseases
  2. Supports a diagnosis, monitors disease activity and response to therapy, and establishes a prognosis for SLE
  3. Values
      a. Negative: less than 70 units by enzyme-linked immunosorbent assay (ELISA)
      b. Borderline: 70 to 200 units
      c. Positive: greater than 200 units
C. Rheumatoid (RA) factor
  1. A blood test used to diagnose rheumatoid arthritis
  2. Values
      a. Nonreactive: 0 to 39 IU/mL
      b. Weakly reactive: 40 to 79 IU/mL
      c. Reactive: greater than 80 IU/mL

IV. Fractures

A. Description: a break in the continuity of the bone caused by trauma, twisting as a result of muscle spasm or indirect loss of leverage, or bone decalcification and disease that result in osteopenia
B. Types
  1. Closed or simple: skin over the fractured area remains intact
  2. Greenstick: one side of the bone is broken and the other is bent; most commonly seen in children
  3. Transverse: the bone is fractured straight across
  4. Oblique: the break extends in an oblique direction
  5. Spiral: the break partially encircles the bone
  6. Comminuted: the bone is splintered or crushed, with three or more fragments
  7. Complete: the bone is completely separated by a break into two parts
  8. Incomplete: a partial break in the bone
  9. Open-compound: the bone is exposed to air through a break in the skin, and soft tissue injury and infection are common
  10. Impacted: a part of a fractured bone is driven into another bone
  11. Depressed: bone fragments are driven inward
  12. Compression: a fractured bone compressed by another bone

13. Pathological: a fracture caused by weakening of the bone structure by pathological processes such as neoplasia or osteomalacia; also called spontaneous fracture
C. Assessment of a fracture of an extremity
  1. Pain or tenderness over the involved area
  2. Loss of function
  3. Obvious deformity
  4. Crepitation
  5. Ecchymosis
  6. Erythema
  7. Edema
  8. Muscle spasm
  9. Impaired sensation
D. Initial care of a fracture of an extremity (Box 67–1)
  1. Immobilize affected extremity
  2. If a compound fracture exists, splint the extremity and cover the wound with a sterile dressing
E. **Reduction**: restoring the bone to proper alignment
  1. Closed **reduction**
      a. Performed by manual manipulation
      b. May be performed under local or general anesthesia
      c. A **cast** may be applied following **reduction**
  2. Open **reduction**
      a. Involves a surgical intervention
      b. May be treated with **internal fixation** devices
      c. The client may be placed in **traction** or a **cast** following the procedure
F. Fixation
  1. Internal **fixation**
      a. Follows open **reduction**
      b. Involves the application of screws, plates, pins, or nails to hold the fragments in alignment
      c. May involve the removal of damaged bone and replacement with a prosthesis
      d. Provides immediate bone strength
      e. Risk of infection is associated with the procedure
  2. External **fixation**
      a. An external frame is utilized with multiple pins applied through the bone
      b. Provides more freedom of movement than with **traction**
G. **Traction**
  1. Description
      a. The exertion of a pulling force applied in two directions to reduce and immobilize a fracture

BOX 67–1. Interventions for a Fracture	
Reduction	Traction
Fixation	Casts

b. Provides proper bone alignment and reduces muscle spasms
2. Implementation
   a. Maintain proper body alignment
   b. Ensure that the weights hang freely and do not touch the floor
   c. Do not remove or lift weights without a physician's order
   d. Ensure that pulleys are not obstructed
   e. Ensure that the ropes in the pulleys move freely
   f. Place knots in the ropes to prevent slipping
   g. Check the ropes for fraying
H. Skeletal **traction** (Fig. 67–1)
   1. Description: mechanically applied to bone using pins, wires, or tongs
   2. Implementation
      a. Monitor color, motion, and sensation (CMS) of the affected extremity
      b. Monitor the insertion sites for redness, swelling, or drainage
      c. Provide insertion site care as prescribed
   3. Cervical tongs
      a. Inserted into the outer aspect of the client's skull
      b. Traction and weight are applied as prescribed to reduce the fracture
      c. Weights should hang freely at all times because releasing the traction can cause further neurological damage
      d. Ensure that the ropes for the traction remain within the pulley
      e. Maintain body alignment
      f. Monitor for neurological changes
      g. Monitor for signs of infection at the pin insertion site
      h. Provide sterile pin site care as prescribed with solutions such as saline and hydrogen peroxide or ointments such as bacitracin and povidone-iodine (Betadine)
      i. The client is placed on a Roto-Rest bed or Stryker or Foster frame to maintain the spine in proper alignment and to allow the client to be turned
   4. Halo fixation device (Box 67–2)
      a. Four pins or screws are inserted into the client's skull
      b. The circular fixation device and halo jacket (vest) are then applied

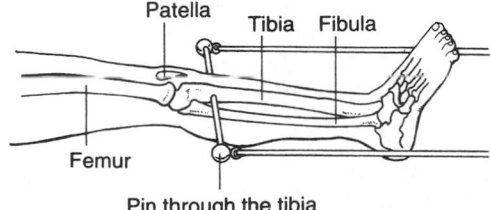

Patella   Tibia   Fibula

Femur

Pin through the tibia

FIGURE 67–1. Skeletal traction. (From Lammon, C., et al. [1995]. *Clinical nursing skills.* Philadelphia: W. B. Saunders. p. 281.)

BOX 67–2. Client Education: Use of a Halo Device

- The weight of the halo device alters balance
- Wear loose clothing with large openings for head and arms
- Obtain advice from the physician regarding bathing in a shower
- Wash under the lamb's wool liner of the vest to prevent rashes or sores
- Use powders or lotions sparingly under the vest
- Obtain assistance to change the liner if it becomes odorous
- Support the head with a small pillow when sleeping to prevent unnecessary pressure and discomfort
- Resume usual activities as much as possible
- The weight of the device may cause fatigue or weakness
- Do not drive, because vision is impaired with the device
- Use a straw for drinking fluids
- Cut meats and other foods in small pieces to facilitate chewing and swallowing
- In cold temperatures wrap the pins with cloth to prevent the metal from getting cold
- Assess the pin sites daily for reddening or drainage
- Have someone clean the pin sites as recommended by the physician
- Increase fluids and fiber in the diet to prevent constipation
- Use a position of comfort for sex
- If the bolts become loose notify the physician
- When getting out of bed, roll onto the side and push on the mattress with the arms
- Sitting straight up puts too much stress on the front pins
- Never use the metal frame for turning or lifting
- Eat foods high in protein and calcium to promote bone healing
- Have the correct size wrench with you in case of an emergency
- The anterior portion of the vest including the anterior bolts will need to be loosened
- The posterior portion of the vest should remain in place to provide stability for the spine during cardiopulmonary resuscitation

---

   c. Monitor neurological status for changes in movement or decreased strength after the halo device is applied
   d. Never move or turn the client by holding or pulling the halo device
   e. Assess the skin for pressure points from the jacket or cast
   f. The nurse should be able to insert one finger under the jacket or cast
I. Skin **traction** (Box 67–3; Table 67–1)
   1. Description: **traction** applied by the use of elastic bandages or adhesive
   2. Cervical skin **traction**
      a. Relieves muscle spasms and compression in upper extremities and neck

Table 67–1. **Common Methods of Applying Traction**

Type	Use	Nursing Care
Skin Traction		
Buck's	Straight traction to immobilize fractures of the hip or femur; may be unilateral or bilateral	Assess for proper body alignment, nerve and circulatory impairment, skin breakdown, and allergic reaction to adhesive tape; make sure the weights hang freely
Bryant's	An adaptation of Buck's traction; used to stabilize fractured femurs or correct congenital hip dislocations in children who weigh less than 40 pounds; traction is applied to both legs with a spreader bar attached to maintain leg alignment	Assess for pressure at the bony prominences; the client's buttocks should clear the mattress by 1 inch (see also nursing care for Buck's traction)
Russell's	Unilateral suspension traction used to immobilize fractures of the femur	Assess the sling for wrinkles and slippage (see also nursing care for Buck's traction)
Cervical head halter	Intermittent or continuous skin traction to relieve muscle spasm and nerve compression in the neck	Assess for pressure at the chin, occipital area, and ears; maintain the client's good body alignment; be sure the weights hang freely
Pelvic belt or girdle	Provides traction to the client's hips to relieve back, hip, and leg pain	Keep the body in proper alignment: assess for pressure and skin irritation under the device; be sure the weights hang freely
Dunlop's	Horizontal traction to align fractures of the humerus; vertical traction maintains the forearm in proper alignment	(See Buck's traction)

Table 67–1. **Common Methods of Applying Traction** *Continued*

Type	*Use*	*Nursing Care*
Skeletal Traction		
Thomas leg splint with Pearson attachment	Balanced suspension traction to stabilize fractures of the femur, acetabulum, hip, or lower leg	Assess for infection at the pin site: care for the pin site; maintain the person's body in good alignment to provide countertraction; the client may lift his or her buttocks for a bedpan or skin care without disturbing the traction; assess pressure areas for skin breakdown

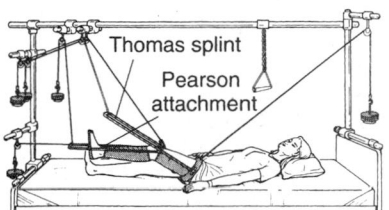

| Crutchfield tongs and other skull tongs | Provide immobilization of the cervical and upper thoracic vertebrae; halo traction is a variation that allows the client to move about freely while maintaining cervical traction | Maintain the client's body alignment; assess for infection at the pin site; care for the pin site |

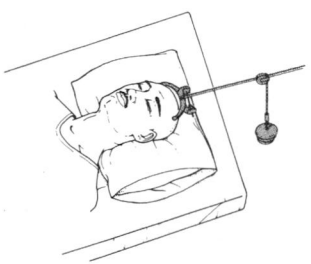

From Lammon, C., et al. (1995). *Clinical Nursing Skills.* Philadelphia: W.B. Saunders. pp. 282–283.

b. Uses a head halter and a chin pad to attach the **traction**
c. Use powder to protect the ears from friction rub
d. Position the client with the head of the bed elevated 30 to 40 degrees and attach the weights to a pulley system over the head of the bed
3. Buck's skin traction
   a. Used to alleviate muscle spasms; immobilizes a lower limb by maintaining a straight pull on the limb with the use of weights
   b. Apply a boot appliance to attach to the **traction**
   c. Attach weight to a pulley and allow the weights to hang freely over the edge of the bed
   d. Not more than 8 to 10 pounds of weight should be applied

BOX 67–3. Types: Skin Traction

Cervical traction	Russell's traction
Buck's traction	Pelvic traction
Bryant's traction	

e. Elevate the foot of the bed to provide the **traction**
4. Bryant's skin **traction**
   a. Used to stabilize a fractured femur
   b. Used to correct a congenital hip disorder in children
   c. Position the client flat with a 90-degree hip flexion
5. Russell's skin **traction**
   a. Used to stabilize a fractured femur prior to surgery
   b. Similar to Buck's **traction** but provides a double pull with the use of a knee sling
   c. **Traction** pulls at the knee and foot
   d. Position the client with the foot of the bed slightly elevated
6. **Pelvic skin traction**
   a. Used to relieve low back, hip, or leg pain and to reduce muscle spasm
   b. Apply the **traction** snugly over the pelvis and iliac crest and attach to weights
   c. Use measures as prescribed to prevent the client from slipping down in bed
J. Balanced suspension (Box 67–4)
   1. Description
      a. Used with skin or skeletal **traction**
      b. Used to approximate fractures of the femur, tibia, or fibula

BOX 67-4. Balanced Suspension

Thomas splint with Pearson attachment
Steinmann pin
Kirschner wires

c. Produced by a counterforce other than the client
2. Implementation
   a. Position the client in low-Fowler's, either on the side or back
   b. Maintain a 20-degree angle from the thigh to the bed
   c. Protect the skin from breakdown
   d. Provide pin care if pins are used with the skeletal **traction**
   e. Clean the pin site with sterile normal saline and hydrogen peroxide or Betadine as prescribed or per agency procedure
K. Dunlop's traction
   1. Description: horizontal traction to align fractures of the humerus; vertical traction maintains the forearm in proper alignment
   2. Implementation: nursing care is similar to Buck's traction
L. **Casts**
   1. Description: made of plaster or fiberglass to provide immobilization of bone and joints after a fracture or injury
   2. Implementation
      a. Keep the **cast** and extremity elevated
      b. Allow a wet **cast** 24 to 48 hours to dry (synthetic casts set in 20 minutes)
      c. Handle a wet **cast** with the palms of the hand until dry
      d. Turn the extremity unless contraindicated, so that all sides of the wet **cast** will dry
      e. Heat can be used to dry the **cast**
      f. The **cast** will change from a dull to a shiny substance when dry

g. Examine the skin and **cast** for pressure areas
h. Monitor the extremity for circulatory impairment such as pain, swelling, discoloration, tingling, numbness, coolness, or diminished pulse
i. Notify the physician immediately if circulatory compromise occurs
j. Prepare for bivalving or cutting the **cast** if circulatory impairment occurs
k. Petal the **cast;** maintain smooth edges around the **cast** to prevent crumbling of the **cast** material (Fig. 67-2)
l. Monitor the client's temperature
m. Monitor for the presence of a foul odor, which may indicate infection
n. Monitor drainage by circling the area of drainage on the **cast**
o. Monitor for warmth on the **cast**
p. Monitor for wet spots, which may indicate a need for drying, or the presence of drainage under the **cast**
q. If an open draining area exists on the affected extremity, a cut-out portion of the **cast** or a window will be made
r. Instruct the client not to stick objects inside the **cast**
s. Teach the client to keep the **cast** clean and dry
t. Instruct the client on isometric exercises to prevent muscle atrophy
M. Applying a sling
   1. Position the open sling with a binder center under the arm with the pointed end at the wrist and the base of the triangle at the elbow
   2. Pull the ends up, encasing the arm in the sling, bent at the elbow
   3. Position the arm across the chest
   4. Bring the top of the binder point over the neck on the unaffected side
   5. Bring the other binder point over the neck on the affected side

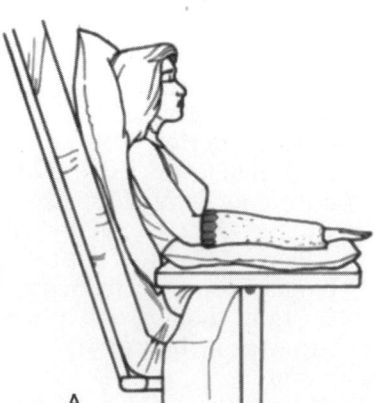

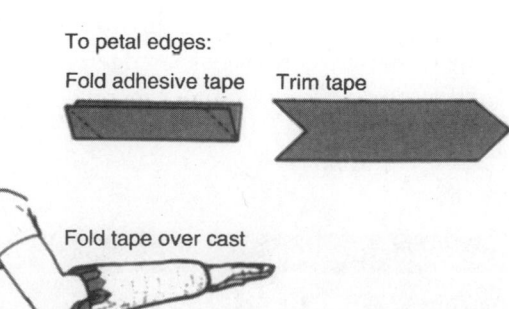

FIGURE 67-2. Petaling the edges of a cast. (From Lammon, C., et al. [1995]. *Clinical nursing skills.* Philadelphia: W. B. Saunders. p. 279.)

6. Position the arm with the wrist above the elbow
7. Tie the ends behind the neck in a square knot
8. Place gauze between the neck and sling knot to pad the area
9. Fold the remaining bandage around the elbow for support and fasten with a safety pin

◆ V. Crutch Walking

A. Description
   1. An accurate measurement of the client for crutches is important because an incorrect measurement could damage the brachial plexus
   2. The distance between the axilla and arm pieces on the crutches should be two finger-widths in the axilla space
   3. The elbows should be slightly flexed 20 to 30 degrees when walking
   4. When ambulating with the client, stand on the affected side
   5. Instruct the client never to rest the axillae on the axillary bars
   6. Instruct the client to look up and outward when ambulating
   7. Instruct the client to stop ambulation if numbness or tingling in the hands or arms occurs
B. Four-point gait (Fig. 67–3)
   1. Used when the client can bear weight on each leg
   2. Steps
     a. Move right crutch forward
     b. Move left foot forward
     c. Move left crutch forward
     d. Move right foot forward
C. Three-point gait (Fig. 67–4)

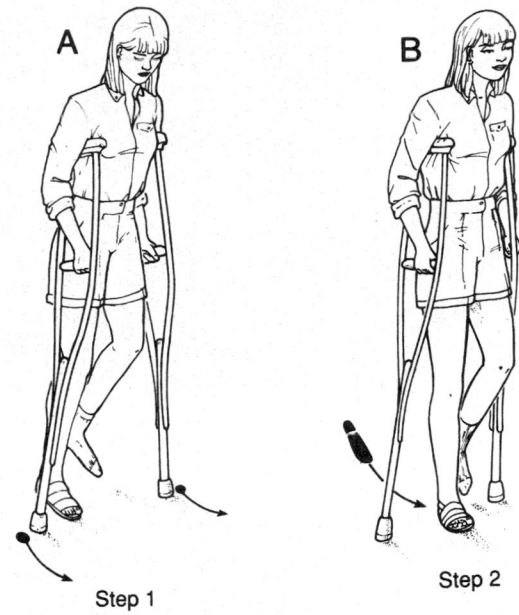

FIGURE 67–4. Three-point gait. (From Lammon, C., et al. [1995]. *Clinical nursing skills.* Philadelphia: W. B. Saunders. p. 242.)

   1. Used when the client can bear little or no weight on one leg
   2. Two crutches support the affected leg
   3. Steps
     a. Move both crutches and the affected leg forward
     b. Move the unaffected leg forward
D. Two-point gait (Fig. 67–5)
   1. Use when weight bearing is allowed on both feet and requires more balance
   2. Used when weight bearing is allowed on both feet
   3. Only two points are in contact with the floor
   4. Resembles normal walking

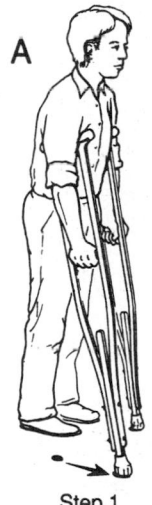 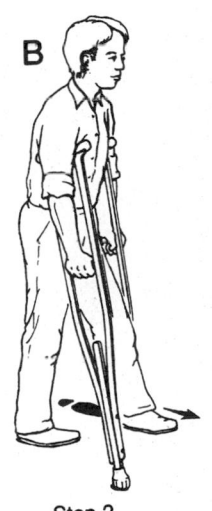 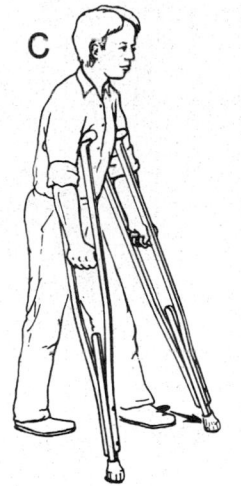 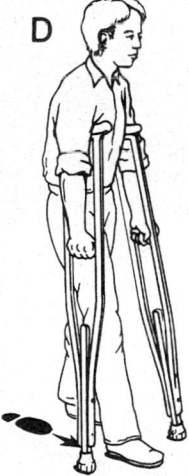

FIGURE 67–3. Four-point gait. (From Lammon, C., et al. [1995]. *Clinical nursing skills.* Philadelphia: W. B. Saunders. p. 241.)

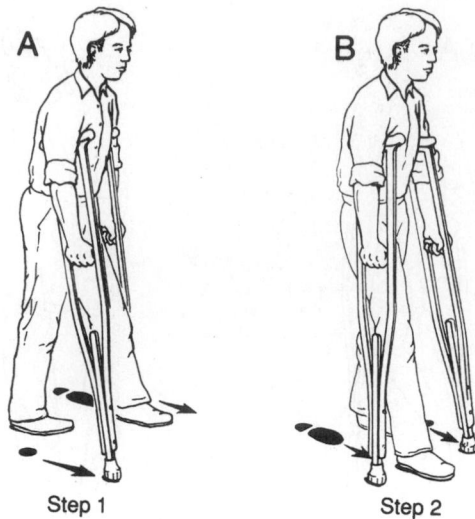

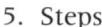

FIGURE 67–5. Two-point gait. (From Lammon, C., et al. [1995]. *Clinical nursing skills*. Philadelphia: W. B. Saunders. p. 241.)

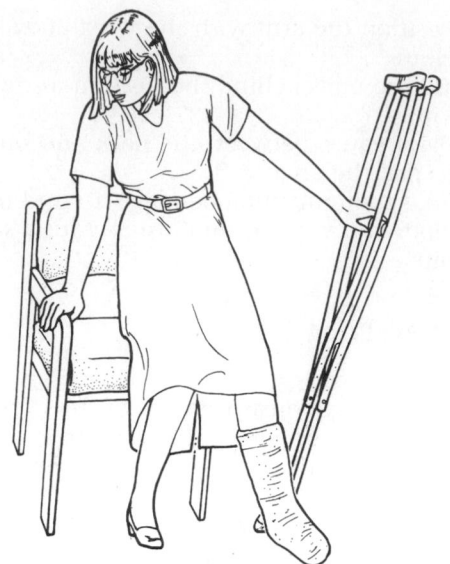

FIGURE 67–6. Standing from a sitting position. (From Lammon, C., et al. [1995]. *Clinical nursing skills*. Philadelphia: W. B. Saunders. p. 244.)

5. Steps
   a. Advance the right crutch and the left foot forward
   b. Advance the right foot and the left crutch forward
E. Assisting the client with crutches to sit and stand
   1. Place the unaffected leg against the front of the chair
   2. Move the crutches to the affected side and grasp the chair's arm with the hand on the unaffected side
   3. Flex the knee of the unaffected leg to lower self into the chair while placing the affected leg straight out in front
   4. Reverse steps to move from a sitting to a standing position (Fig. 67–6)
F. Going up and down stairs (Fig. 67–7)
   1. Up the stairs
      a. The client moves the unaffected leg up first

      b. The client moves the affected leg and the crutches up
   2. Down stairs
      a. The client moves the crutches and the affected leg down
      b. The client moves the unaffected leg down

VI. Canes and Walkers

A. Description: made of a lightweight material with a rubber suction tip at the bottom
B. Implementation
   1. Stand at the affected side of the client when ambulating
   2. The handle should be at the level of the client's greater trochanter

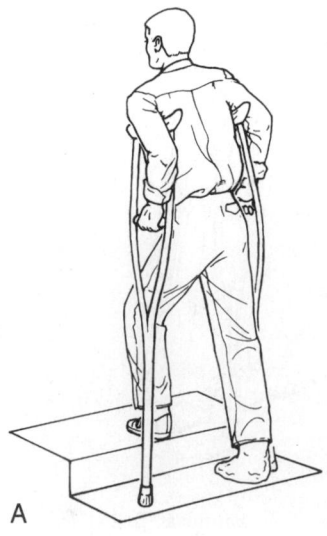

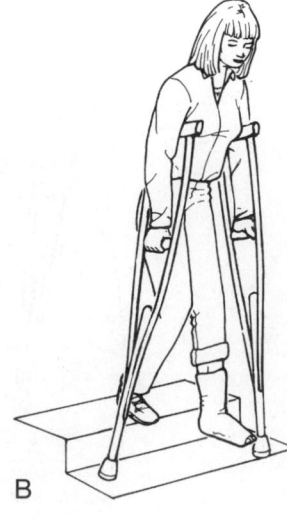

FIGURE 67–7. *A,* Going up stairs. *B,* Going down stairs. (From Lammon, C., et al. [1995]. *Clinical nursing skills*. Philadelphia: W. B. Saunders. p. 243.)

BOX 67–5. Risk Factors Associated with Musculoskeletal Disorders

Trauma and injury
Falls
Autoimmune disorders
Infection
Degenerative conditions such as rheumatoid arthritis
Obesity
Calcium deficiency
Postmenopausal states
Metabolic disorders such as diabetes
Neoplastic disorders
Hyperuricemia
Medications such as corticosteroids

---

3. The client's elbow should be flexed at a 25- to 30-degree angle
4. Instruct the client to hold the cane close to the body
5. Instruct the client to hold the cane in the hand on the unaffected side so that the cane and weaker leg can work together with each step
6. Instruct the client to move the cane at the same time as the affected leg
7. Instruct the client to inspect the rubber tips regularly for worn places

C. Hemicanes or quadripod canes
1. Used for clients who have the use of only one upper extremity
2. Hemicanes provide more security than a quadripod cane; however, both types provide more security than a single-tipped cane
3. Position the cane at the client's unaffected side with the straight nonangled side adjacent to the body
4. Position the cane 6 inches from the client's side with the hand grips level with the greater trochanter

D. Walker
1. Stand adjacent to the client on the affected side
2. Instruct the client to put all four points of the walker flat on the floor before putting weight on the hand pieces
3. Instruct the client to move the walker forward and to walk into it

◆ **VII. Complications of Fractures** (Box 67–6)

A. Fat embolism
1. Description
   a. An embolism originating in the bone marrow that occurs after a fracture
   b. Clients with long bone fractures are at the greatest risk for development of **fat embolism**
   c. Usually occurs within 48 hours following the injury

2. Assessment
   a. Restlessness
   b. Mental status changes
   c. Tachycardia
   d. Tachypnea
   e. Dyspnea
   f. Hypotension
   g. Petechial rash over the upper chest and neck
3. Implementation
   a. Notify the physician immediately
   b. Treat symptoms as prescribed to prevent respiratory failure and death

B. **Compartment syndrome**
1. Description
   a. Increased pressure within one or more compartments causing massive compromise of circulation to an area
   b. Leads to decreased perfusion and tissue anoxia
   c. Within 4 to 6 hours after the onset of **compartment syndrome**, neuromuscular damage is irreversible
2. Assessment
   a. Swelling
   b. Increased pain
   c. Pain with passive motion
   d. Inability to move joints
   e. Loss of sensation (paresthesia)
   f. Pulselessness
3. Implementation: notify the physician immediately

C. Infection
1. Description: can be caused by the interruption of the integrity of the integument
2. Assessment
   a. Local or systemic infection
   b. Fever
   c. Pain
   d. Erythema in the area surrounding the fracture
   e. Tachycardia
   f. Elevated WBC count
3. Implementation
   a. Notify the physician of signs of infection
   b. Prepare to initiate aggressive antibiotic therapy as prescribed

D. Avascular necrosis
1. Description: an interruption in the blood supply to the bony tissue, which results in the death of the bone
2. Assessment
   a. Pain
   b. Decreased sensation

BOX 67–6. Complications of Fractures

Compartment syndrome	Avascular necrosis
Fat emboli	Pulmonary emboli
Infection	

---

3. Implementation
   a. Notify the physician if pain or decreased sensation occurs
   b. Prepare the client for removal of necrotic tissue because it serves as a focus for infection
E. Pulmonary embolism
   1. Description: caused by immobility precipitated by a fracture
   2. Assessment
      a. Restlessness and apprehension
      b. Dyspnea
      c. Diaphoresis
      d. Blood gas changes
   3. Implementation
      a. Notify the physician if signs of emboli are present
      b. Prepare to administer anticoagulant therapy as prescribed

VIII. Fractured Hip

A. Types
   1. Intracapsular
      a. Bone is broken inside the joint
      b. Skin **traction** is applied preoperatively to immobilize and prevent pain
      c. Treatment includes a total hip replacement or **internal fixation** with replacement of the femoral head with an Austin Moore prosthesis
      d. Avoid hip flexion to prevent displacement
   2. Extracapsular
      a. Fracture can occur at the greater trochanter or can be an intertrochanteric fracture
      b. Trochanteric fracture is outside the joint
      c. Preoperative treatment includes balanced suspension **traction**
      d. Avoid hip flexion to prevent displacement
      e. Surgical treatment includes **internal fixation** with nail plate, screws, or wires
B. Implementation preoperatively
   1. Maintain skin **traction** to decrease pain and immobilize the leg
   2. Turn the client every 2 hours from back to unaffected side
C. Implementation of hip pinning and hip prosthesis
   1. Turn the client from the back to the unaffected side
   2. Maintain leg abduction to prevent internal or external rotation
   3. Trochanter roll to prevent external rotation
   4. Ensure that hip flexion angle does not exceed 60 to 80 degrees
   5. Elevate the head of the bed 30 to 45 degrees for meals only
   6. Ambulate as prescribed in 2 to 4 days with partial weight bearing
   7. Avoid hip flexion when getting the client out of bed
   8. Avoid the use of low chairs

D. Implementation of total hip replacement
   1. Maintain the leg and hip in proper alignment
   2. Prevent flexion or external or internal rotation
   3. Use an abduction pillow
   4. Position the client to the back and unaffected side
   5. Do not position to the affected side unless prescribed by the physician
   6. Elevate the head of the bed 30 to 45 degrees for meals only
   7. Monitor the wound for hemorrhage
   8. Monitor the wound for infection
   9. Monitor circulation and sensation of the affected side
   10. Maintain the Hemovac if in place
   11. Maintain compression on the Hemovac to facilitate drainage
   12. Monitor and record the Hemovac output
   13. Hemovac drainage should continuously decrease in amount, and by 48 hours postoperatively, drainage should be approximately 30 mL in an 8-hour period
   14. Maintain the use of antiembolism stockings and encourage the client to flex and extend the feet and ankles
   15. Provide continuous passive motion (CPM) the first day postoperatively with increasing degrees of flexion up to 90 degrees as prescribed
   16. Ambulate 1 to 2 days postoperatively as prescribed
   17. Keep the operative leg extended, supported, and elevated when getting the client out of bed
   18. Avoid weight bearing on the affected leg; instruct the client on the use of a walker to avoid weight bearing
   19. Avoid hip flexion greater than 90 degrees and avoid low chairs when out of bed
   20. Instruct the client to avoid crossing the legs and bending-over activities
   21. Begin physical therapy by day 6 postoperatively as prescribed

IX. Total Knee Replacement

A. Description: implantation of a device to substitute for the femoral condyles and the tibial joint surfaces
B. Implementation postoperative
   1. Monitor the incision for drainage and infection
   2. Maintain the Hemovac if in place
   3. Begin CPM 24 to 48 hours postoperatively as prescribed to exercise the knee and provide moderate flexion and extension
   4. Administer analgesics before CPM to decrease pain

5. The leg should not be dangled, to prevent dislocation
6. Maintain an Ace wrap or antiembolism stockings if prescribed
7. Out of bed 2 to 3 days postoperatively as prescribed
8. Avoid weight bearing and instruct the client in crutch walking

X. Herniation: Intervertebral Disk

A. Description: nucleus of disk protrudes into the annulus, causing nerve compression
B. Cervical disk
   1. Occurs at C5 to C6 and C6 to C7 interspaces
   2. Diagnosis is determined by cervical myelography
   3. Causes pain and stiffness in the neck, top of the shoulders, scapula, upper extremities, and head
   4. Produces paresthesia and numbness of the upper extremities
   5. Implementation
      a. Provide bed rest to relieve pressure and reduce inflammation and edema
      b. Provide immobilization as prescribed via a cervical collar, **traction,** or brace
      c. Apply hot, moist compresses as prescribed to increase the blood flow and relax spasms
      d. Instruct the client to avoid flexing, extending, or rotating the neck
      e. Instruct the client that while sleeping to avoid the prone position and keep the head in a neutral position using a feather pillow
      f. Instruct the client to avoid long automobile rides
      g. Instruct the client in the use of analgesics, sedatives, and anti-inflammatory agents as prescribed
      h. Instruct the client to take steroids if prescribed with food or antacids
      i. Monitor for blood dyscrasias if the client is taking steroids
      j. Instruct the client regarding the administration of pain medications as prescribed
      k. Prepare for corticosteroid injection into the epidural space if prescribed
   6. Cervical collar
      a. Used for cervical disk herniation
      b. Holds the head in a neutral or slightly flexed position
      c. The client may have to wear a cervical collar 24 hours a day
      d. Inspect skin under the collar for irritation
      e. When pain subsides, the client is taught cervical isometric exercises to strengthen the muscles
   7. Cervical **traction**
      a. Used for cervical disk herniation

   b. Consists of a head halter attached to a pulley and weight
   c. The head of the bed is elevated to provide countertraction
   d. Pad the halter to prevent skin irritation
C. Lumbar disk
   1. Occurs at L4 to L5 or L5 to S1 interspaces
   2. Diagnosis is determined by lumbar myelography
   3. Postural deformity occurs
   4. Produces muscle weakness and sensory loss
   5. Tendon reflexes are altered
   6. The client experiences low back pain and muscle spasms with radiation of the pain into one hip and down the leg (sciatica)
   7. The client experiences pain radiating into the leg on straight leg raises
   8. Pain is aggravated by bending, lifting, straining, sneezing, and coughing and is relieved by bed rest
   9. Implementation
      a. Bed rest on a firm mattress in a semi-Fowler's with moderate hip and knee flexion
      b. Apply moist heat and massage as prescribed
      c. Instruct the client to sleep on the side, with knees and hips in a position of flexion with a pillow between the legs
      d. Apply pelvic **traction** as prescribed to relieve muscle spasms
      e. Begin ambulation gradually as the inflammation and edema subside
      f. Instruct the client in the use of muscle relaxants, anti-inflammatory medications, and steroids as prescribed
      g. Instruct the client in the use of a corset or brace as prescribed
      h. Instruct the client regarding correct posture while sitting, standing, walking, and working
      i. Instruct the client to lift objects by bending the knees and keeping the back straight, avoiding lifting anything above the elbows
      j. Instruct the client regarding a weight control program as prescribed
      k. Instruct the client in an exercise program to strengthen abdominal and back muscles
D. Disk surgery (Box 67–7)
   1. Implementation preoperatively
      a. Reassure the client that surgery will not weaken the back
      b. Instruct the client regarding coughing and deep-breathing exercises
      c. Instruct the client about log-rolling and range-of-motion exercises
   2. Implementation postoperative: cervical disk
      a. Monitor vital signs
      b. Monitor for respiratory difficulty
      c. Encourage coughing and deep breathing

> **BOX 67–7. Types of Disk Surgery**
>
> Diskectomy: Removal of herniated disk tissue and related matter
> Laminectomy: Removal of the lamina
> Laminotomy: Division of the lamina of a vertebrae
> Diskectomy with fusion: Fusion of vertebrae with bone graft
> Chemolysis: Injections to dissolve affected disk

    d. Monitor for hoarseness and inability to cough effectively because this may indicate laryngeal nerve damage

    e. Use throat sprays or lozenges for a sore throat and do not use those that may numb the throat, to avoid choking

    f. Monitor the wound for drainage

    g. Provide a soft diet if the client complains of dysphagia

    h. Monitor for sudden return of radicular pain, which may indicate that the cervical spine has become unstable

  3. Implementation postoperative: lumbar disk

    a. Monitor vital signs

    b. Monitor for wound hemorrhage

    c. Monitor sensation and motor ability of lower extremities as well as color, temperature, and sensation of toes

    d. Monitor for urinary retention, paralytic ileus, and constipation

    e. Initiate measures to prevent constipation such as high-fiber diet, increased fluids, and stool softeners as prescribed

    f. When turning and repositioning the client, place bed in a flat position and a pillow between the legs; turn the client as a unit (log roll) without twisting the client's back

    g. When positioning the client, a pillow is placed under the head with the knees slightly flexed

    h. Avoid extreme knee flexion when the client is lying on the side

    i. To assist the client out of bed, raise the head of the bed while the client lies on the side; the client's head and shoulders are supported by the first nurse as the client pushes self to a sitting position, while the second nurse eases the legs over side of bed

    j. Instruct the client to avoid sitting because it places a strain on the surgical site

    k. Administer narcotics and sedatives as prescribed to relieve pain and anxiety

    l. Encourage early ambulation

    m. Assist the client with the use of a back brace or corset if prescribed

XI. Amputation

A. Description: the surgical removal of a limb or part of a limb

B. Implementation postoperatively

  1. Monitor vital signs

  2. Monitor for infection

  3. Monitor for hemorrhage

  4. Mark bleeding and drainage on the dressing if occur

  5. Keep a tourniquet at the bedside

  6. Monitor for pulmonary emboli

  7. Observe and prevent contractures

  8. Monitor for signs of necrosis and neuroma

  9. Evaluate for phantom limb pain; explain the sensation to the client; medicate client as prescribed

  10. During the first 24 hours, elevate the foot of the bed to reduce edema, then keep the bed flat to prevent hip flexion contractures as prescribed

  11. Do not elevate the stump itself because elevation can cause flexion contracture of the hip joint

  12. After 24 to 48 hours postoperatively, position the client prone as prescribed to stretch the muscles and prevent flexion contractures of the hip

  13. In the prone position, place a pillow under the abdomen and stump and keep the legs close together to prevent abduction

  14. Maintain application of an Ace wrap or elastic stump shrinker as prescribed to provide stump shrinkage

  15. Remove and rewrap the Ace bandage or elastic stump shrinker three to four times daily as prescribed

  16. Wash the stump with mild soap or water and apply lanolin to the skin if dry

  17. Massage the skin toward the suture line to increase circulation

  18. Prepare for a **cast** application if prescribed to prepare the stump for prosthesis

  19. Encourage the client to look at the stump

  20. Identify the client's reactions to the loss of a body part

  21. Encourage verbalization regarding the loss of a body part

  22. Assist the client to identify coping mechanisms to deal with the loss

C. Implementation of below the knee amputation

  1. Prevent edema

  2. Do not allow the stump to hang over the edge of the bed

  3. Do not allow the client to sit for long periods of time

D. Implementation of above the knee amputation

  1. Prevent internal or external rotation of the limb

  2. Place a sandbag or rolled towel along the outside of the thigh to prevent rotation

E. Rehabilitation

  1. Instruct the client in crutch walking

  2. Prepare the stump for prosthesis

  3. Prepare the client for the fitting of the stump for prosthesis

4. Instruct the client in exercises to maintain range of motion
5. Provide psychosocial support to the client

◆ XII. Rheumatoid Arthritis (RA)

A. Description
1. Chronic systemic inflammatory disease; the cause is unknown
2. Leads to destruction of connective tissue and synovial membrane within joints
3. Weakens and leads to dislocation of the joint and permanent deformity
4. Formation of pannus occurs at the junction of synovial tissue and articular cartilage projecting into the joint cavity and causing necrosis
5. Exacerbations are increased by physical or emotional stress
6. Risk factors include exposure to infectious agents; fatigue and emotional stress can exacerbate the condition
7. Vasculitis can cause malfunction and eventual failure of an organ or system

B. Assessment
1. Inflammation, tenderness, and stiffness of the joints
2. Moderate to severe pain and morning stiffness lasting longer than 30 minutes
3. Joint deformities
4. Spongy, soft feeling in joints
5. Muscle atrophy
6. Decreased range of motion
7. Low-grade temperature
8. Fatigue and weakness
9. Anorexia, weight loss, and anemia
10. Paresthesia
11. Pericarditis
12. Vasculitis
13. Fibrotic lung disease
14. Renal disease
15. Ocular involvement
16. Subcutaneous nodules
17. Sjögren's syndrome
18. Elevated sedimentation rate and positive rheumatoid factor
19. X-ray showing joint deterioration
20. Synovial tissue biopsy presents inflammation

C. Pain
1. Salicylates
   a. Administer salicylates as prescribed until a therapeutic serum level of 20 to 25 mg/ 100 mL is achieved
   b. When symptoms are relieved decrease dosage of salicylate as prescribed to achieve a maintenance level of 15 to 20 mg/100 mL
   c. Monitor for side effects including tinnitus, GI upset, or prolonged bleeding time
   d. Administer with meals or a snack
   e. Monitor for abnormal bleeding or bruising

2. Nonsteroidal anti-inflammatory drugs (NSAIDs)
   a. Administer in combination with salicylates as prescribed if pain and inflammation are not decreased within 6 to 12 weeks following salicylate therapy
   b. Monitor for side effects such as GI upset, CNS manifestations, skin rash, hypertension, fluid retention, and changes in renal function
3. Corticosteroids
   a. Administer as prescribed during exacerbations or severe involvement when commonly used agents are ineffective
   b. Monitor the client for Cushing-like symptoms such as moon face and acne
   c. Monitor for complications such as diabetes mellitus, infection, hypertension, osteoporosis, and glaucoma
4. Antineoplastic medications
   a. Administer as prescribed in clients with life-threatening RA
   b. Monitor for bone marrow depression, rashes, alopecia, hemorrhagic cystitis, and immune suppression
5. Gold salts
   a. Administer as prescribed in combination with salicylates and NSAIDs to induce remission and decrease pain and inflammation
   b. Monitor for side effects: dermatitis, rash, blood dyscrasia, nephropathy

D. Physical mobility
1. Preserve joint function
2. Provide range-of-motion (ROM) exercises to maintain joint motion and muscle strengthening
3. Balanced rest and activity
4. Splints during acute inflammation to prevent deformity
5. Prevent flexion contractures
6. Apply heat or cold therapy as prescribed to joints
7. Apply paraffin baths and massage as prescribed
8. Encourage consistency with exercise program
9. Instruct the client to stop exercise if pain increases
10. Exercise only to the point of pain
11. Avoid weight bearing on inflamed joints

E. Self-Care (Box 67–8)
1. Assess the need for assistive devices such as higher level toilet seats, chairs, and wheelchairs to facilitate mobility
2. Collaborate with occupational therapy to obtain assistive adaptive devices
3. Instruct the client in alternative strategies to providing activities of daily living (ADL)

BOX 67–8. Client Education for RA and DJD

- Assist the client to identify and correct hazards in the home
- Instruct the client in the correct use of assistive adaptive devices
- Instruct in energy conservation measures
- Review prescribed exercise program
- Instruct the client to sit in a chair with a high, straight back
- Instruct the client to use a small pillow only when lying down
- Instruct the client in measures to protect joints such as turning doorknobs counterclockwise and using two hands instead of one to hold objects
- Instruct the client regarding the prescribed medications
- Stress the importance of follow-up visits with the physician

---

F. Fatigue
　1. Identify factors that may contribute to fatigue
　2. Assess for anemia
　3. Administer iron, folic acid, and vitamin supplements as prescribed
　4. Assess for medication-related blood loss by testing the stool for occult blood
　5. Instruct the client in measures to conserve energy such as pacing activities and obtaining assistance when possible

G. Body image disturbance
　1. Assess the client's reaction to body change
　2. Encourage the client to verbalize feelings
　3. Assist the client with self-care activities and grooming
　4. Encourage the client to wear street clothes
　5. Provide patience and understanding and be aware that the client may be manipulative and demanding

H. Surgical implementation
　1. Synovectomy: surgical removal of the synovia to help maintain joint function
　2. Arthrodesis: procedure bony fusion of a joint to regain some mobility
　3. Joint replacement (arthroplasty): surgical replacement of diseased joints with artificial joints to restore motion to a joint and function to the muscles, ligaments, and other soft tissue structures that control a joint

◆ **XIII. Osteoporosis**

A. Description
　1. An age-related metabolic disease
　2. Bone demineralization results in the loss of bone mass, leading to fragile and porous bones and subsequent fractures
　3. Greater bone resorption than bone formation occurs
　4. Occurs most commonly in the wrist, hip, and vertebral column
　5. Can occur postmenopausal or as a result of a metabolic disorder or calcium deficiency

B. Assessment
　1. Back pain after lifting, bending, or stooping
　2. Back pain that increases with palpation
　3. Pelvic or hip pain, especially with weight bearing
　4. Problems with balance
　5. Decline in height from vertebrae compression
　6. Kyphosis of the dorsal spine
　7. Constipation, abdominal distention, and respiratory impairment as a result of movement restriction and spinal deformity
　8. Pathological fractures
　9. Appearance of thin, porous bone on x-ray

C. Implementation
　1. Assess risk for injury
　2. Provide a safe and hazard-free environment and assist the client to identify hazards in the home environment
　3. Use side rails to prevent falls
　4. Move the client gently when turning and repositioning
　5. Encourage ambulation
　6. Assist with ambulation if the client is unsteady
　7. Instruct in the use of assistive devices such as a cane or walker
　8. Provide ROM exercises
　9. Instruct in the use of good body mechanics
　10. Instruct the client in exercises to strengthen abdominal and back muscles in order to improve posture and provide support for the spine
　11. Instruct the client to avoid activities that can cause vertebral compression
　12. Apply a back brace as prescribed during an acute phase to immobilize the spine and provide spinal column support
　13. Encourage the use of a firm mattress
　14. Provide a diet high in protein, calcium, vitamins C and D, and iron
　15. Encourage adequate fluid intake to prevent renal calculi
　16. Instruct the client to avoid alcohol and coffee
　17. Administer estrogen or androgens to decrease the rate of bone resorption as prescribed
　18. Administer calcium and vitamin D as prescribed for bone metabolism
　19. Administer calcitonin as prescribed to inhibit bone loss
　20. Administer analgesics, muscle relaxants, and anti-inflammatory medications as prescribed

XIV. Osteoarthritis (Degenerative Joint Disease, DJD)

A. Description
　1. Progressive degeneration of the joints caused by wear and tear

2. Causes the formation of bony build-up and the loss of articular cartilage in peripheral and axial joints
3. Affects the weight-bearing joints and joints that receive the greatest stress such as the knees, toes, and lower spine
4. The cause is unknown but may be caused by trauma, fractures, infections, or obesity

B. Assessment
1. Joint pain that early in the disease process diminishes after rest and intensifies after activity
2. As the disease progresses, pain occurs with slight motion or even at rest
3. Symptoms are aggravated by temperature change and humidity
4. Crepitus
5. Joint enlargement
6. Presence of Heberden's nodes or Bouchard's nodes
7. Limited ROM
8. Difficulty getting up after prolonged sitting
9. Skeletal muscle atrophy
10. Inability to perform ADLs
11. Compression of the spine as manifested by radiating pain, stiffness, and muscle spasms in one or both extremities

C. Pain
1. Administer NSAIDs, salicylates, and muscle relaxants as prescribed
2. Prepare the client for corticosteroid injections into joints as prescribed
3. Place the affected joint in a functional position
4. Immobilize the affected joint with a splint or brace
5. Avoid large pillows under the head or knees
6. Provide a bed or foot cradle
7. Position the client prone twice a day
8. Instruct the client on the importance of moist heat, hot packs or compresses, and paraffin dips as prescribed
9. Apply cold applications when the joint is acutely inflamed
10. Encourage adequate rest, recommending 10 hours of sleep at night and a 1- to 2-hour nap in the afternoon

D. Nutrition
1. Encourage a well-balanced diet
2. Encourage weight loss if necessary

E. Physical mobility (Box 67–8)
1. Reinforce the exercise program and the importance of participating in the program
2. Instruct the client that exercises should be active rather than passive and to exercise only to the point of pain
3. Instruct the client to stop exercise if pain is increased with exercising
4. Instruct the client to decrease the number of repetitions in an exercise when the inflammation is severe

F. Surgical management
1. Osteotomy: the bone is cut to correct joint deformity and promote realignment
2. Total joint replacement (TJR)
   a. Performed when all measures of pain relief have failed
   b. Hips and knees are most commonly replaced
   c. Contraindicated in the presence of infection, advanced osteoporosis, and severe inflammation

XV. Gout

A. Description
1. A systemic disease in which urate crystals deposit in joints and other body tissues
2. Leads to abnormal amounts of uric acid in the body
3. Primary gout results from a disorder of purine metabolism
4. Secondary gout involves excessive uric acid in the blood that is caused by another disease

B. Phases
1. Asymptomatic
   a. No symptoms
   b. Serum uric acid is elevated
2. Acute: excruciating pain and inflammation of one or more small joints, especially the great toe
3. Intermittent: asymptomatic period between acute attacks
4. Chronic
   a. Results from repeated episodes of acute gout
   b. Results in deposits of urate crystals under the skin and within the major organs, especially the renal system

C. Assessment
1. Excruciating pain in the involved joints
2. Swelling and inflammation of the joints
3. Tophi (hard, fairly large and irregular shaped deposits in the skin) may break open and discharge a yellow gritty substance
4. Low-grade fever
5. Malaise
6. Headache
7. Pruritus
8. Presence of renal stones
9. Elevated uric acid levels

D. Implementation
1. Provide a low-purine diet as prescribed
2. Instruct the client to avoid foods such as organ meats, wines, aged cheese
3. Encourage a high fluid intake of 2000 mL to prevent stone formation
4. Encourage a weight-reduction diet if required
5. Instruct the client to avoid alcohol and fat-starvation diets because they may precipitate a gout attack
6. Maintain urine pH above 6

7. Increase urinary pH by eating alkaline ash foods such as citrus fruits and juices, milk, and other dairy products
8. Provide bed rest during acute attacks
9. Monitor joint ROM ability and appearance of joints
10. Position the joint in mild flexion position during an acute attack
11. Elevate the affected extremity
12. Protect the affected joint from excessive movement or direct contact with sheets
13. Provide heat or cold for local treatments to the affected joint as prescribed
14. Administer NSAIDs and anti-gout medications as prescribed

XVI. Autoimmune and Connective Tissue Disorders

A. Polyarteritis nodosa
  1. Description
    a. A collagen disease that causes inflammation of the arteries and thickening and impairment of the circulation
    b. Treatment is similar to treatment for systemic lupus erythematosus
    c. Affects middle-aged men and involves every body system
    d. The cause is unknown and the prognosis is poor
    e. Renal disorders and cardiac involvement are the most frequent causes of death
  2. Assessment
    a. Malaise and weakness
    b. Low-grade fever
    c. Severe abdominal pain
    d. Bloody diarrhea
    e. Weight loss
    f. Elevated erythrocyte sedimentation rate (ESR)
  3. Implementation
    a. Provide supportive care as required
    b. Provide a well-balanced diet
    c. Administer corticosteroids and analgesics to control pain and inflammation
    d. Provide emotional support and encourage the client to verbalize feelings
    e. Initiate support services for the client

B. Pemphigus
  1. Description
    a. A rare disease that occurs predominantly between middle and old age
    b. The cause is unknown and the disorder is potentially fatal
    c. Initial lesions occur on the oral mucosa and then progress to a generalized distribution
    d. Treatment is aimed at suppressing the immune response that causes blister formation
  2. Assessment
    a. Lesions appear as fragile flaccid bullae

    b. Partial-thickness wounds that bleed, weep, and form crusts when bullae are disrupted
    c. Debilitation, malaise, and pain
    d. Chewing and swallowing difficulties
    e. Nikolsky's sign—separation of the epidermis caused by rubbing the skin
    f. Leukocytosis, eosinophilia, foul-smelling discharge from skin
  3. Implementation
    a. Provide supportive care
    b. Provide oral hygiene and increase fluid intake
    c. Soothe oral lesions
    d. Assist with oatmeal or potassium permanganate baths as prescribed for relief of symptoms
    e. Administer topical or systemic antibiotics as prescribed for secondary infections
    f. Administer corticosteroids and cytotoxic agents as prescribed to bring about remission

C. Systemic lupus erythematosus (SLE)
  1. Description
    a. A chronic, progressive, systemic inflammatory disease that can cause major organs and systems to fail
    b. Connective tissue and fibrin deposits in blood vessels on collagen fibers and on organs
    c. Leads to necrosis and/or inflammation in blood vessels, lymph nodes, GI tract, and pleura
    d. There is no cure for the disease
  2. Causes
    a. The cause is unknown and it is thought to be a result of a defect in the immunologic mechanisms or of genetic origin
    b. Precipitating factors include drugs, stress, genetic factors, sunlight or ultraviolet light, and pregnancy
  3. Assessment
    a. Precipitating factors such as sunlight, stress, and medications
    b. Dry, scaly, raised rash on the face or upper body
    c. Fever
    d. Weakness, malaise, and fatigue
    e. Anorexia
    f. Weight loss
    g. Photosensitivity
    h. Joint pain
    i. Erythema of palms
    j. Butterfly erythema of face
    k. Anemia
    l. Positive antinuclear antibodies (ANA) and LE prep
    m. Elevated sedimentation rate
  4. Implementation
    a. Monitor skin integrity and provide frequent oral care

b. Instruct the client to clean the skin with a mild soap, avoiding harsh and perfumed substances
c. Assist with the use of ointments and creams for rash as prescribed
d. Identify factors contributing to fatigue
e. Administer iron, folic acid, or vitamin supplements as prescribed if anemia occurs
f. Provide a high-vitamin and high-iron diet
g. Provide a high-protein diet if there is no evidence of kidney disease
h. Instruct in measures to conserve energy such as pacing activities and balancing rest with exercise
i. Administer topical or systemic corticosteroids, salicylates, and NSAIDs as prescribed for pain and inflammation
j. Administer hydroxychloroquine (Plaquenil) as prescribed to decrease the inflammatory response
k. Instruct the client to avoid exposure to sunlight and ultraviolet light
l. Monitor for proteinuria and red cell casts in the urine
m. Monitor for bruising, bleeding, and injury
n. Assist with plasmapheresis as prescribed to remove autoantibodies and immune complexes from the blood before organ damage occurs
o. Monitor for signs of organ involvement such as pleuritis, nephritis, pericarditis, neuritis, anemia, and peritonitis
p. Note that lupus nephritis occurs early in the disease process
q. Provide supportive therapy as major organs become affected
r. Provide emotional support and encourage the client to verbalize feelings
s. Provide information regarding support groups and encourage use of community resources

D. Scleroderma (progressive systemic sclerosis)
  1. Description
    a. A chronic connective tissue disease, similar to SLE, characterized by inflammation, fibrosis, and sclerosis
    b. Affects the connective tissue throughout the body
    c. Causes fibrotic changes involving the skin, synovial membranes, esophagus, heart, lungs, kidneys, and GI tract
    d. Treatment is directed toward forcing the disease into remission and slowing its progress
  2. Assessment
    a. Pain
    b. Stiffness and muscle weakness
    c. Pitting edema of the hands and fingers that progresses to the rest of the body
    d. Taut and shiny skin that is free from wrinkles

e. Skin tissue is tight, hard and thick, and loses its elasticity
f. Mask-like hard skin that adheres to underlying structures
g. Dysphagia
h. Decreased range of motion
i. Joint contractures
j. Inability to perform ADLs

  3. Implementation
    a. Encourage activity as tolerated
    b. Maintain a constant room temperature
    c. Provide small frequent meals, eliminating foods that stimulate gastric secretions such as spicy foods, caffeine, and alcohol
    d. Advise the client to sit up for 1 to 2 hours after meals if esophageal involvement exists
    e. Provide supportive therapy as major organs become affected
    f. Administer corticosteroids as prescribed for inflammation
    g. Provide emotional support and encourage the use of resources as necessary

PRACTICE QUESTIONS

1. The client is complaining of knee pain. The knee is swollen, reddened, and warm to the touch. The nurse interprets that the client's signs and symptoms are not compatible with
   1 Inflammation
   2 Degenerative disease
   3 Infection
   4 Recent injury

2. The client is treated in the physician's office after a fall that sprained the ankle. X-ray has ruled out fracture. Before sending the client home, the nurse plans to teach the client about which of the following items that is to be avoided in the next 24 hours?
   1 Application of a heating pad
   2 Application of an Ace wrap
   3 Resting the foot
   4 Elevating the ankle on a pillow while sitting or lying down

3. The nurse is doing a physical assessment of the musculoskeletal system. The nurse documents the presence of which of the following as a normal finding?
   1 Presence of fasciculations
   2 Muscle strength graded 3/5
   3 Hypertrophy on the client's dominant side
   4 Atrophy on the client's nondominant side

4. The nurse has given dietary instructions to a client to minimize the risk of osteoporosis. The nurse evaluates that the client understands the recommended changes if the client verbalized to increase intake of which of these preferred foods?

1 Rice
2 Yogurt
3 Sardines
4 Chicken

5. The nurse is conducting health screening for osteoporosis. The nurse interprets that which of the following clients is at greatest risk of developing this disorder?
   1 A 36-year-old male who has asthma
   2 A 25-year-old female who jogs
   3 A sedentary 65-year-old female who smokes cigarettes
   4 A 70-year-old male who consumes excess alcohol

6. The home health nurse is planning to teach the client with osteoporosis about home modifications to reduce the risk of falls. Which of the following recommendations are unnecessary to include in the teaching plan?
   1 Use of staircase railings
   2 Use of nightlights
   3 Removing wall-to-wall carpeting
   4 Placing handrails in the bathroom

7. The nurse is providing care to the client after bone biopsy. Which of the following actions by the nurse is not needed in the care of this client?
   1 Monitoring the site for swelling, bleeding, and hematoma
   2 Administering intramuscular narcotic analgesics
   3 Elevating the limb for 24 hours
   4 Monitoring vital signs every 4 hours

8. The nurse has given instructions to the client returning home after arthroscopy of the knee. The nurse evaluates that the client understands the instructions if the client states to
   1 Stay off the leg entirely for the rest of the day
   2 Resume regular exercise the following day
   3 Refrain from eating food for the remainder of the day
   4 Report fever or site inflammation to the physician

9. The nurse is caring for the client who is going to have an arthrogram using a contrast medium. Which of the following assessments by the nurse are of highest priority?
   1 Allergy to iodine or shellfish
   2 Ability of the client to remain still during the procedure
   3 Whether the client has any remaining questions about the procedure
   4 Whether the client wishes to void before the procedure

10. The client with a bone infection is to have indium imaging done. The client asks the nurse to explain how the procedure is done. The nurse's response is based on the understanding that
    1 Indium is injected into the bloodstream and collects in normal bone, but not in infected areas
    2 Indium is injected into the bloodstream and highlights the vascular supply to the bone
    3 A sample of the client's leukocytes is tagged with indium, and will subsequently accumulate in infected bone
    4 A sample of the client's red blood cells (RBCs) is tagged with indium, and will highlight normal bone

11. The client with possible rib fracture has never had a chest x-ray. The nurse plans to tell the client which of the following items about the procedure?
    1 The x-rays stimulate a small amount of pain
    2 It is necessary to remove jewelry and any other metal objects
    3 The client will be asked to breathe in and out during the x-ray
    4 The x-ray technologist will stand next to the client during the x-ray

12. The nurse is teaching the client who is to have a gallium scan about the procedure. The nurse includes which of the following items as part of the instructions?
    1 The gallium will be injected intravenously 2 to 3 hours before the procedure
    2 The procedure takes about 15 minutes to perform
    3 The client must stand erect during the filming
    4 The client should remain on bed rest for the remainder of the day after the scan

13. The client has had a bone scan done. The nurse evaluates that the client understands the elements of follow-up care if the client states to
    1 Report any feelings of nausea or flushing
    2 Ambulate at least three times before the end of the day
    3 Eat only small meals for the remainder of the day
    4 Drink plenty of water for a day or two following the procedure

14. The client seeks treatment in the emergency department for a lower leg injury. There is visible deformity to the lower aspect of the leg, and the injured leg appears shorter than the other. The area is painful, swollen, and beginning to become ecchymotic. The nurse interprets that this client has experienced a
    1 Contusion
    2 Fracture
    3 Sprain
    4 Strain

15. The nurse is one of several people who witness a vehicle hit a pedestrian at fairly low speed on a small street. The individual is dazed and tries to get up. The leg appears fractured. The nurse plans to
    1 Stay with the person and coax the person to remain still
    2 Assist the person to get up and walk to the sidewalk
    3 Leave the person for a few moments to call an ambulance
    4 Try to manually reduce the fracture

16. The nurse witnesses a client sustain a fall, and suspects the leg may be broken. Which of the following actions is the highest priority of the nurse?
    1 Take a set of vital signs
    2 Call the radiology department
    3 Reassure the client that everything will be fine
    4 Immobilize the leg before moving the client

17. The nurse in the emergency department is caring for a client with a fractured arm. The nurse evaluates that which of the following items is not necessary before reduction of the fracture in the casting room?
    1 Explanation of the procedure to the client
    2 Administration of an analgesic
    3 Anesthesia consent
    4 Consent for the procedure

18. The nurse plans to reduce the anxiety of a client who is going to have a plaster cast applied by teaching the client about the procedure. The nurse does not include which of the following items in the discussion?
    1 A stockinette will be placed over the leg area to be casted
    2 The cast edges may be trimmed with a cast knife
    3 The cast will give off heat as it dries
    4 The client may bear weight on the cast in one-half hour

19. The nurse is planning to teach the client with a left arm cast about measures to keep the left shoulder from becoming stiff and "frozen." Which of the following suggestions does the nurse include in the teaching plan?
    1 Lift the left arm up over the head
    2 Lift the right arm up over the head
    3 Make a fist with the hand of the casted arm
    4 Use a sling on the left arm

20. The client has a fiberglass (nonplaster) cast applied to the lower leg. The client asks the nurse when the client will be able to walk on the cast. The nurse replies that the client will be able to bear weight on the cast
    1 Within 20 to 30 minutes of application

2 In approximately 8 hours
3 In 24 hours
4 In 48 hours

21. The nurse has given the client with a nonplaster (fiberglass) leg cast instructions on cast care at home. The nurse evaluates that the client needs further instruction if the client makes which of the following statements?
    1 "I should avoid walking on wet, slippery floors."
    2 "It's OK to wipe dirt off the top of the cast with a damp cloth."
    3 "I'm not supposed to scratch the skin underneath the cast."
    4 "If the cast gets wet, I can dry it with a hair dryer turned to the warmest setting."

22. The client with a hip fracture asks the nurse why Buck's extension traction is being applied before surgery. The nurse's response is based on the understanding that Buck's extension traction primarily
    1 Provides rigid immobilization of the fracture site
    2 Provides comfort by reducing muscle spasms, and provides fracture immobilization
    3 Lengthens the fractured leg to prevent severing of blood vessels
    4 Allows bony healing to begin before surgery

23. The client has just had skeletal traction pins inserted. The weights have been attached to the pins using a wire bow and a rope pulley system. Which of the following nursing interventions should the nurse plan once assessment of the traction set-up is complete?
    1 Cover the ends of the traction pins with cork or tape
    2 Perform pin site care
    3 Provide for distraction such as television
    4 Teach the client about pin care

24. The client in skeletal leg traction with an over-bed frame is not allowed to turn from side to side. Which of the following actions by the nurse is most useful in trying to provide good skin care to the client?
    1 Ask the client to lift up by digging into the mattress with the unaffected leg
    2 Push down on the mattress of the bed while administering care
    3 Have another nurse tilt the client anyway
    4 Ask the client to pull up on a trapeze to lift the hips off the bed

25. The nurse is evaluating the pin sites of a client in skeletal traction. The nurse is least concerned with which of the following findings?
    1 Purulent drainage
    2 Serous drainage
    3 Pain at a pin site
    4 Inflammation

26. The client immobilized in skeletal leg traction complains of being bored and restless. Based on these complaints, the nurse formulates which of the following nursing diagnoses for this client?
    1 Diversional Activity Deficit
    2 Powerlessness
    3 Self-Care Deficit
    4 Impaired Physical Mobility

27. The client has Buck's extension traction applied to the right leg. The nurse plans which of the following interventions to prevent complications of the device?
    1 Massage the skin of the right leg with lotion every 8 hours
    2 Give pin care once a shift
    3 Inspect the skin on the right leg at least once every 8 hours
    4 Release the weights on the right leg for range-of-motion exercises daily

28. The nurse is caring for the client who had skeletal traction applied to the left leg. The client is complaining of severe left leg pain. Which of the following actions should the nurse take first?
    1 Medicate the client with an analgesic
    2 Provide pin care
    3 Call the physician
    4 Check the client's alignment in bed

29. The nurse has suggested specific leg exercises for the client immobilized in right skeletal lower leg traction. The nurse evaluates that the client needs further instruction if the nurse observes the client
    1 Pulling up on the trapeze
    2 Flexing and extending the feet
    3 Performing active ROM to the right ankle and knee
    4 Doing quadriceps-setting and gluteal-setting exercises

30. The nurse is assessing the casted extremity of a client. The nurse assesses for which of the following signs and symptoms indicative of infection?
    1 Coolness and pallor of the extremity
    2 Presence of a "hot spot" on the cast
    3 Diminished distal pulse
    4 Dependent edema

31. The client has sustained a closed fracture and has just had a cast applied to the affected arm. The client is complaining of intense pain. The nurse has elevated the limb, applied an ice bag, and administered an analgesic with very little relief. The nurse interprets that this pain may be caused by
    1 Impaired tissue perfusion
    2 The newness of the fracture

3 The anxiety of the client
4 Infection under the cast

32. The nurse is admitting the client with multiple trauma to the nursing unit. The client has a leg fracture and had a plaster cast applied. In positioning the casted leg, the nurse should
    1 Keep the leg in a level position
    2 Keep the leg level for 3 hours, and elevate it for 1 hour
    3 Elevate the leg on pillows continuously for 24 to 48 hours
    4 Elevate the leg for 3 hours, and put it flat for 1 hour

33. The client is complaining of skin irritation from the edges of a cast applied the previous day. The nurse should take which of the following actions?
    1 Massage the skin at the rim of the cast
    2 Apply lotion to the skin at the rim of the cast
    3 Use a rough file to smooth the cast edges
    4 Petal the cast edges with adhesive tape

34. The client is being discharged to home after application of a plaster leg cast. The nurse evaluates that the client understands proper care of the cast if the client states to
    1 Avoid getting the cast wet
    2 Use the fingertips to lift and move the leg
    3 Cover the casted leg with warm blankets
    4 Use a padded coat hanger end to scratch under the cast

35. The client being measured for crutches asks the nurse why the crutches cannot rest up underneath the arm for extra support. The nurse's response is based on the understanding that this could result in
    1 Impaired range of motion while the client ambulates
    2 Skin breakdown in the area of the axilla
    3 Injury to the brachial plexus nerves
    4 A fall and further injury

36. The nurse is planning to teach the client how to stand on crutches. The nurse plans to incorporate into written instructions to tell the client to place the crutches
    1 8 inches to the front and side of the client's toes
    2 3 inches to the front and side of the client's toes
    3 20 inches to the front and side of the client's toes
    4 15 inches to the front and side of the client's toes

37. The nurse is giving the client with a left leg cast crutch-walking instructions using the three-point gait. The client is allowed touchdown of

the affected leg. The nurse tells the client to advance the
1 Left leg and right crutch, then right leg and left crutch
2 Crutches and then both legs simultaneously
3 Crutches and the right leg, then advance the left leg
4 Crutches and the left leg, then advance the right leg

38. The nurse has given the client instructions regarding crutch safety. The nurse evaluates that the client needs reinforcement of information if the client states
1 The need to have spare crutches and tips available
2 That crutch tips will not slip even when wet
3 Not to use someone else's crutches
4 That crutch tips should be inspected periodically for wear

39. The client has slight weakness in the right leg. Based on this assessment, the nurse determines that the client would benefit most from the use of a
1 Walker
2 Wooden crutch
3 Lofstrand crutch
4 Straight leg cane

40. A client who has experienced a CVA has partial hemiplegia of the left leg. The straight leg cane formerly used by the client is not quite sufficient now. The nurse interprets that the client could benefit from the somewhat greater support and stability provided by a
1 Quadripod cane
2 Wooden crutch
3 Lofstrand crutch
4 Wheelchair

41. The client with right-sided weakness needs to learn how to use a cane. The nurse plans to teach the client to position the cane by holding it with the
1 Left hand, and placing the cane in front of the left foot
2 Right hand, and placing the cane in front of the right foot
3 Left hand, and 6 inches lateral to the left foot
4 Right hand, and 6 inches lateral to the right foot

42. The client who is learning to use a cane is afraid it will slip with ambulation, causing a fall. The nurse provides the client with the greatest reassurance by telling the client that
1 Canes prevent falls, not cause them
2 The cane has a flared tip with concentric rings to give stability
3 The physical therapist will determine if the cane is inadequate

4 The cane would help to break a fall, even if the client does slip

43. The nurse is evaluating the client's use of a cane for left-sided weakness. The nurse intervenes and corrects the client if the nurse observes that the client
1 Holds the cane on the right side
2 Keeps the cane 6 inches out to the side of the right foot
3 Moves the cane when the right leg is moved
4 Leans on the cane when the right leg swings through

44. The client with a fractured femur experiences sudden dyspnea. A set of arterial blood gases reveal the following: pH 7.32, $PaCO_2$ 43, PaO_2 58, HCO_3^- 20. The nurse interprets that the client probably has experienced fat embolus because of the
1 $PaCO_2$
2 PaO_2
3 HCO_3^-
4 pH

45. The client with fat embolus is experiencing respiratory distress. The nurse plans to assist with which of the following therapies?
1 Administration of bronchodilators, intubation, mechanical ventilation
2 Administration of plasma expanders, oxygen mask, and suctioning
3 Administration of corticosteroids, intubation, mechanical ventilation with positive end-expiratory pressure (PEEP)
4 Administration of antihypertensives, high flow oxygen, continuous positive airway pressure (CPAP) mask

46. The client being mechanically ventilated after experiencing a fat embolus is visibly anxious. The nurse should
1 Encourage the client to sleep until arterial blood gas results improve
2 Ask the family members to stay with the client at all times
3 Ask the physician for an order for succinylcholine
4 Provide reassurance to the client and give small doses of morphine IV

47. The nurse is caring for a client being treated for fat embolus after multiple fractures. Which of the following data does the nurse evaluate as the most favorable indication of resolution of the fat embolus?
1 Arterial oxygen level 78 mmHg
2 Minimal dyspnea
3 Clear chest x-ray
4 Oxygen saturation 85%

48. The nurse is caring for the client who develops compartment syndrome from a severely fractured arm. The client asks the nurse how this can happen. The nurse's response is based on the understanding that
    1 An injured artery causes impaired arterial perfusion through the compartment
    2 The fascia expands with injury, causing pressure on underlying nerves and muscles
    3 A bone fragment has injured the nerve supply in the area
    4 Bleeding and swelling cause increased pressure in an area that cannot expand

49. The nurse is caring for a client with fresh application of a plaster leg cast. The nurse plans to prevent the development of compartment syndrome by instructing the licensed practical nurse to
    1 Elevate the limb and apply ice to the affected leg
    2 Elevate the limb and cover the limb with bath blankets
    3 Place the leg in a slightly dependent position and apply ice
    4 Keep the leg horizontal and apply ice to the affected leg

50. The client has undergone fasciotomy to treat compartment syndrome of the leg. The nurse provides which type of wound care to the fasciotomy site?
    1 Dry, sterile dressings
    2 Moist, sterile saline dressings
    3 Hydrocolloid dressings
    4 One-half strength Betadine dressings

51. The nurse has conducted teaching a client in an arm cast about signs and symptoms of compartment syndrome. The nurse evaluates that the client understands the information if the client states to report which of the following early symptoms of compartment syndrome?
    1 Pain that is relieved only by oxycodone (Percodan) and aspirin
    2 Pain that increases when the arm is dependent
    3 Cold, bluish fingers
    4 Numbness and tingling in the fingers

52. The nurse is assessing a confused elderly client admitted with a hip fracture. Which of the following data obtained by the nurse would not place the client at more risk for Altered Thought Processes?
    1 Stress induced by the fracture
    2 Hearing aid available and in working order
    3 Unfamiliar hospital setting
    4 Eyeglasses left at home

53. The elderly client is brought to the emergency department via ambulance after sustaining a fall. The client's left leg is shortened, adducted, and externally rotated. The nurse interprets these signs as consistent with
    1 Dislocated hip
    2 Dislocated knee
    3 Fracture of the femoral neck
    4 Fracture of the midshaft of the femur

54. The nurse is caring for an elderly client who had a hip pinned after being fractured. In planning nursing care, which of the following does the nurse avoid to minimize the chance for further injury?
    1 Siderails in the up position
    2 Use of a nightlight in the hospital room and bathroom
    3 Call bell placed within reach
    4 Delays in responding to call light

55. The nurse is repositioning the client who has returned to the nursing unit following internal fixation of a fractured right hip. The nurse uses a
    1 Pillow to keep the right leg abducted during turning
    2 Pillow to keep the right leg adducted during turning
    3 Trochanter roll to prevent external rotation while turning
    4 Trochanter roll to prevent abduction while turning

56. A client has been taught to use a walker to aid in mobility following internal fixation of a hip fracture. The nurse evaluates that the client is using the walker incorrectly if the client
    1 Holds the walker using the hand grips
    2 Leans forward slightly when advancing the walker
    3 Advances the walker with reciprocal motion
    4 Supports body weight on the hands while advancing the weaker leg

57. The client who has had a right total knee replacement asks the nurse how long the right leg must be kept in the continuous passive motion (CPM) machine. The nurse's response is based on the understanding that the device should be used
    1 For 30 minutes out of every hour
    2 Every other hour for 60 minutes
    3 For 3 hours at a time, followed by 1 hour of rest
    4 As much as the client can tolerate

58. The nurse has an order to get the client out of bed to a chair on the first postoperative day after total knee replacement. The nurse plans to do which of the following to protect the knee joint?
    1 Apply a knee immobilizer before getting the client up, and elevate the client's surgical leg while sitting

2 Apply an Ace wrap around the dressing, and put ice on the knee while sitting

3 Lift the client to the bedside chair leaving the CPM machine in place

4 Obtain a walker to minimize weight bearing by the client on the affected leg

59. The client who has had a total knee replacement tells the nurse that there is pain with extension of the knee. The nurse should
  1 Put the client's knee through full passive range of motion
  2 Immobilize the knee temporarily
  3 Administer an analgesic
  4 Notify the physician

60. The nurse has completed giving discharge instructions to the client after total knee replacement using a metal prosthesis. The nurse evaluates that the client does not fully understand the instructions if the client verbalizes to
  1 Report fever, redness, or increased pain
  2 Ignore changes in the shape of the knee
  3 Report bleeding gums or tarry stools
  4 Tell future caregivers about the metal implant

61. The client with diabetes mellitus has had a right below-knee amputation. The nurse is especially vigilant in assessing for which of the following signs and symptoms because of the history of diabetes?
  1 Edema of the stump
  2 Hemorrhage
  3 Separation of the wound edges
  4 Slight redness of the incision

62. A client is admitted to the nursing unit after a left below-the-knee amputation following a crush injury to the foot and lower leg. The client tells the nurse, "I think I'm going crazy. I can feel my left foot itching." The nurse interprets the client's statement to be
  1 A normal response, and indicates the presence of phantom limb sensation
  2 A normal response, and indicates the presence of phantom limb pain
  3 An abnormal response, and indicates the client needs more psychological support
  4 An abnormal response, and indicates the client is in denial about the limb loss

63. The nurse is planning to teach the client with below-knee amputation about skin care to prevent breakdown. Which of the following points does the nurse include while developing the teaching plan?
  1 A stump sock must be worn at all times and changed twice a week
  2 The residual limb is washed gently and dried every other day
  3 The socket of the prosthesis is washed with a harsh bactericidal agent daily

4 The socket of the prosthesis must be dried fully before using it

64. The nurse is caring for the client who had an above-knee amputation 2 days ago. The residual limb was wrapped with an elastic compression bandage, which has come off. The nurse immediately
  1 Calls the physician
  2 Rewraps the stump with an elastic compression bandage
  3 Applies ice to the site
  4 Applies a dry sterile dressing and elevates it on a pillow

65. The nurse has taught the client with a below-knee amputation about prosthesis and stump care. The nurse evaluates that the client has understood the instructions if the client states to
  1 Wear a clean nylon stump sock daily
  2 Toughen the skin of the stump by rubbing it with alcohol
  3 Prevent cracking of the skin of the stump by applying lotion daily
  4 Using a mirror to inspect all areas of the stump each day

66. The client is complaining of low back pain with radiation down the left posterior thigh. The nurse further assesses the client to see if the pain is worsened or aggravated by
  1 Bed rest
  2 Application of heat
  3 Bending or lifting
  4 Ibuprofen (Motrin)

67. The client with herniated intervertebral lumbar disk complains of knife-like, stabbing pain in the lower back, as well as pain radiating into the right buttock. The nurse interprets that the sharp stabbing pain is probably a result of
  1 Muscle spasm in the area of the herniated disk
  2 Pressure on the spinal cord
  3 Pressure on the spinal nerve root
  4 Excess cerebrospinal fluid production in the area

68. The nurse has an order to place the client with a herniated lumbar intervertebral disk on bedrest in Williams' position to minimize the pain. The nurse plans to put the bed
  1 In high-Fowler's position with the foot of bed flat
  2 In semi-Fowler's position with the knee gatch slightly raised
  3 In semi-Fowler's position with the foot of the bed flat
  4 Flat with the knee gatch raised

69. The client has just undergone spinal fusion after experiencing a herniated lumbar disk. The nurse

avoids which of the following to maintain client safety after this procedure?
1 Log-rolling technique for repositioning
2 Pillows under the length of the legs
3 Head of the bed flat
4 Overhead trapeze

70. The nurse has taught the client with a herniated lumbar disk about proper body mechanics and other items pertinent to low back care. The nurse evaluates that the client needs further instruction if the client verbalizes to
1 Get out of bed by sitting straight up and swinging the legs over the side of the bed
2 Increase fiber and fluids in the diet
3 Strengthen the back muscles by swimming or walking
4 Bend at the knees to pick up objects

71. The nurse is caring for the client who has had spinal fusion with insertion of hardware. The nurse is especially concerned with which of the following assessment findings?
1 Complaints of discomfort during repositioning
2 Temperature of 101°F oral
3 Old bloody drainage outlined on surgical dressing
4 Discomfort during coughing and deep-breathing exercises

72. The client who has had spinal fusion and insertion of hardware is extremely concerned with the perceived lengthy rehabilitation period. The client expresses concerns about finances and ability to return to prior employment. The nurse understands that the client's needs could best be addressed by referral to the
1 Surgeon
2 Clinical nurse specialist
3 Social worker
4 Physical therapist

73. The nurse is planning to teach the client proper use of a thoracic lumbar sacral orthosis (TLSO) after spinal fusion with instrumentation. The nurse plans to include which of the following teaching points in discussion with the client?
1 Areas of skin redness at the edges of the brace indicate a good, snug fit
2 The device is applied before getting out of bed in the morning
3 The brace should be applied directly next to the skin
4 The Velcro closures should be fairly loose to avoid constriction

74. The client is being transferred to the nursing unit from the postanesthesia care unit following spinal fusion with Harrington rod insertion. The nurse prepares to transfer the client from the stretcher to the bed by using

1 A bath blanket and the assistance of 3 people
2 A bath blanket and the assistance of 4 people
3 A slider board and the assistance of 2 people
4 A slider board and the assistance of 4 people

75. The client is being discharged to home following spinal fusion with insertion of Harrington rods. The nurse consults with the continuing care nurse regarding the need for follow-up modification of the home environment if the client states that
1 The bedroom and bath are on the second floor of the home
2 The bathroom has handrails in the shower
3 The family has rented a commode for use by the client
4 There are three steps to get up to the front door

76. The nurse in the emergency department is assessing a client with an open-leg fracture. The nurse inquires about the date of the client's last
1 Physical examination
2 Chest x-ray
3 Tetanus vaccine
4 Tuberculin test

77. The client who has experienced nonunion of a fracture is scheduled for bone grafting using cadaver bone. The client appears restless and anxious about the procedure. After determining that the client understands the surgical procedure, the nurse next explores
1 Concern about the level of postoperative pain
2 Potential worry about hepatitis or HIV infection
3 Whether the client needs a PRN order for an antianxiety agent
4 The availability of assistance for the client upon discharge

78. The client has just been admitted to the hospital with a fractured femur and pelvic fractures. The nurse plans to carefully monitor the client for which of the following signs and symptoms?
1 Tachycardia, hypotension
2 Bradycardia, hypertension
3 Fever, bradycardia
4 Fever, hypertension

79. The client with a left arm fracture exhibits loss of sensation in the left fingers, pallor, poor capillary refill, and diminished left radial pulse. The nurse should take which of the following actions?
1 Administer an analgesic
2 Check the circulation again in 30 minutes
3 Provide range of motion to the fingers of the left hand
4 Call the physician

80. The nurse is ambulating a client with a right leg fracture who has an order for partial weight-bearing status. The nurse evaluates that the client demonstrates compliance with this restriction if the client
    1 Does not bear weight on the right leg
    2 Allows the right leg to touch the floor only
    3 Puts 30% to 50% of the weight on the right leg
    4 Puts 60% to 80% of the weight on the right leg

81. The client is complaining of pain underneath a cast in the area of a bony prominence. The nurse interprets that this client may need
    1 To have the cast replaced with an air splint
    2 To have extra padding put over this area of the cast
    3 To have the cast bivalved
    4 To have a window cut in the cast

82. The nurse is planning to teach the client with a fractured leg in a long-leg cast about dietary measures to promote fracture healing. Which of the following suggestions are least helpful to the client?
    1 Take in a high-protein diet
    2 Take in a well-balanced diet
    3 Make sure to increase dietary fiber
    4 Drink extra amounts of fluids

83. The client is fearful about having an arm cast removed. Which of the following actions by the nurse is the most helpful?
    1 Telling the client that the saw makes a frightening noise
    2 Reassuring the client that no one has had an arm lacerated yet
    3 Stating that the hot cutting blades cause burns only very rarely
    4 Showing the client the cast cutter and explaining how it works

84. The client has just had a cast removed, and the underlying skin is yellow-brown and crusted. The nurse gives the client instructions for skin care. The nurse evaluates that the client has misunderstood the directions if the client states to
    1 Soak the skin and wash it gently
    2 Scrub the skin vigorously with soap and water
    3 Apply an emollient lotion to enhance softening
    4 Use a sunscreen on the skin if exposed for a period of time

85. The client has skeletal traction applied to the right leg, and has an overhead trapeze available for use. The nurse assesses which of the following as a high-risk area for pressure and breakdown?

    1 Scapulae
    2 Back of the head
    3 Right heel
    4 Left heel

86. The client has several fractures of the lower leg and has been placed in an external fixation device. The client is upset about the appearance of the leg, which is very edematous and misshapen. The nurse formulates which of the following nursing diagnoses for the client?
    1 Body Image Disturbance
    2 Activity Intolerance
    3 Risk for Impaired Physical Mobility
    4 Social Isolation

87. The nurse is planning measures to increase bed mobility for the client in skeletal leg traction. Which of the following items would the nurse consider to be most helpful for this client?
    1 Television
    2 Reading materials
    3 Overhead trapeze
    4 Fracture bedpan

88. The client has been placed in Buck's extension traction. The nurse can provide for countertraction to reduce shear and friction by
    1 Slightly elevating the head of the bed
    2 Slightly elevating the foot of the bed
    3 Providing an overhead trapeze
    4 Using a footboard

89. The nurse is evaluating goal achievement for the client in traction with Impaired Physical Mobility. The nurse evaluates that the client has not successfully met all of the goals formulated if which of the following outcomes is noted?
    1 Negative Homan's sign
    2 Active ROM of uninvolved joints
    3 Intact skin surfaces
    4 Bowel movement every 4 days

90. The client with Parkinson's disease has been prescribed benztropine (Cogentin). The nurse assesses for which of the following gastrointestinal side effects of this medication?
    1 Diarrhea
    2 Dry mouth
    3 Increased appetite
    4 Hyperactive bowel sounds

91. The client has been prescribed cyclobenzaprine (Flexeril) in the treatment of painful muscle spasms accompanying a herniated intervertebral disk. The nurse withholds the medication and questions the order if the client has concurrent orders to take
    1 Furosemide (Lasix)
    2 Valproic acid (Depakene)
    3 Ibuprofen (Motrin)
    4 Tranylcypromine (Parnate)

92. The nurse has administered diazepam (Valium) 5 mg IV to a client. The nurse plans to maintain the client on bed rest for at least
    1 30 minutes
    2 1 hour
    3 3 hours
    4 8 hours

93. The nurse is preparing to administer diazepam (Valium) 5 mg intravenously to a client. The nurse is careful to administer the medication over
    1 1 minute
    2 2 minutes
    3 30 seconds
    4 15 seconds

94. The nurse has given medication instructions to the client beginning therapy with carisoprodol (Soma). The nurse evaluates that the client understands the effects of the medication if the client states to
    1 Expect muscle spasticity as a side effect
    2 Take a missed dose when remembered, regardless of when the next dose is due
    3 Avoid alcohol while taking this medication
    4 Drive on city streets, but avoid highway driving

95. The client is receiving anticonvulsant therapy with phenytoin (Dilantin). The nurse assesses the results of which of the following laboratory tests with care?
    1 Complete blood count
    2 Serum sodium
    3 Serum potassium
    4 Blood urea nitrogen

96. The client who was started on anticonvulsant therapy with clonazepam (Klonopin) tells the nurse of increasing clumsiness and unsteadiness since starting the medication. The client is visibly upset by these manifestations and asks the nurse what to do. The nurse's response is based on the understanding that these symptoms
    1 Are most severe during initial therapy, and decrease or disappear with long-term use
    2 Indicate that the client is experiencing a severe untoward reaction to the drug
    3 Are probably the result of interaction with another medication
    4 Usually occur when the client takes the medication with food

97. The client is having the dosage of clonazepam (Klonopin) adjusted. The nurse plans to
    1 Monitor blood glucose levels
    2 Institute seizure precautions
    3 Weigh the client daily
    4 Observe for ecchymosis

98. The nurse has an order to administer phenytoin (Dilantin) 100 mg IV piggyback to a client. The nurse administers the medication after preparing it in
    1 5% dextrose in 0.45% normal saline
    2 Lactated Ringer's solution
    3 5% dextrose in water with an inline filter
    4 0.9% normal saline with an inline filter

99. The nurse in the physician's office is reviewing the results of a client's phenytoin (Dilantin) level drawn that morning. The nurse evaluates that the client had a therapeutic drug level if the client's result is
    1 3 μg/mL
    2 8 μg/mL
    3 15 μg/mL
    4 24 μg/mL

100. A client with a history of simple partial seizures is taking clorazepate (Tranxene). The client asks the nurse if there is a risk of addiction. The nurse's response is based on the understanding that clorazepate
    1 Is not physically or psychologically habit forming
    2 Leads to physical and psychological dependence with prolonged high-dose therapy
    3 Leads to physical tolerance, but only after 10 or more years of therapy
    4 Can result in psychological dependence only, due to the nature of the medication

101. The client has an order for valproic acid (Depakene) 250 mg once daily. To maximize the client's safety, the nurse should plan to schedule the medication
    1 At bedtime
    2 Before breakfast
    3 After breakfast
    4 With lunch

102. The client taking carbamazepine (Tegretol) asks the nurse what to do if the client misses a dose. The nurse responds that the carbamazepine should be
    1 Withheld until the next scheduled dose, which should then be doubled
    2 Withheld until the next scheduled dose
    3 Taken as long as it is not just prior to the next dose
    4 Taken when remembered

103. The nurse has given medication instructions to the client beginning anticonvulsant therapy with carbamazepine (Tegretol). The nurse evaluates that the client understands the use of the medication if the client states to
    1 Drive as long as it is not at night
    2 Use sunscreen when outdoors
    3 Keep tissues handy for excess salivation
    4 Discontinue the medication if fever or sore throat occurs

104. The client with vascular headaches is taking ergotamine (Ergostat). The home health nurse periodically assesses the client for
    1 Hypotension
    2 Dependent edema
    3 Constipation
    4 Cool, numb fingers and toes

105. The nurse is caring for a client with myasthenia gravis who has received edrophonium (Tensilon) intravenously. The client asks the nurse how long the improvement in muscle strength will last. The nurse's response is based on the understanding that the effects have a duration of approximately
    1 5 minutes
    2 15 minutes
    3 30 minutes
    4 60 minutes

106. The client with narcolepsy has been prescribed dextroamphetamine (Dexedrine). The client complains to the nurse that the client cannot sleep well anymore at night and does not want to take the medication any longer. Before making any specific comment, the nurse plans to investigate whether the client takes the medication at which of the following proper time schedules?
    1 At least 6 hours before bedtime
    2 2 hours before bedtime
    3 After supper each night
    4 Just prior to going to sleep

107. The client on the nursing unit has an order for dextroamphetamine (Dexedrine) 25 mg PO daily. The nurse collaborates with the dietitian to limit the amount of which of the following items on the client's dietary trays?
    1 Starch
    2 Caffeine
    3 Protein
    4 Fat

108. The client with Parkinson's disease has begun therapy with levodopa (L-dopa). The nurse evaluates that the client understands the action of the medication if the client verbalizes that results may not be apparent for
    1 24 hours
    2 2 to 3 days
    3 1 week
    4 2 to 3 weeks

109. The client is taking trihexyphenidyl (Artane) for the treatment of Parkinson's disease. The nurse assesses for which of the following untoward effects of this medication?
    1 Urinary incontinence
    2 Urinary retention
    3 Diarrhea
    4 Excessive perspiration

110. The client receiving therapy with carbidopa/levodopa (Sinemet) is upset and tells the home health nurse that the urine has turned a darker color since beginning this medication. The client wants to discontinue its use. In formulating a response to the client's concerns, the nurse interprets that this change is
    1 Indicative of developing toxicity
    2 A sign of interaction with another drug
    3 A harmless side effect of the medication
    4 A result of taking the medication with milk

111. The client with myasthenia gravis has difficulty chewing and has received a prescription for pyridostigmine (Mestinon). The nurse plans to check to see that the client takes the medication
    1 Just after meals
    2 Between meals
    3 With meals
    4 30 minutes before meals

112. A client with myasthenia gravis is taking neostigmine (Prostigmin). The client has frequent exacerbations of myasthenic crisis and cholinergic crisis. The nurse teaches the client that it is very important that this medication be
    1 Taken on time
    2 Double-dosed if one dose is missed
    3 Taken on an empty stomach
    4 Titrated for dosage depending on the symptoms

113. The client began taking amantadine (Symmetrel) approximately 2 weeks ago. The nurse evaluates that the medication is having a therapeutic effect if the client exhibits decreased
    1 White blood cell count
    2 Voiding
    3 Rigidity and akinesia
    4 Blood pressure

114. The nurse is obtaining a health history from a client and is assessing for risk factors associated with osteoporosis. Which of the following assessment findings is not an associated risk factor?
    1 High-calcium diet consumption
    2 Postmenopausal age
    3 Long-term use of corticosteroids
    4 Family history of osteoporosis

115. The nurse is discussing primary prevention measures to clients regarding osteoporosis. Which of the following is a primary prevention measure?
    1 Selecting shoes that have firm nonskid soles
    2 Installing telephones in most rooms of the house
    3 Applying nonskid strips on areas that get wet
    4 Maintaining body weight at or above minimum recommended levels

116. The nurse is providing instructions to a client with osteoporosis regarding appropriate food items to include in the diet. Which of the following food items provides the least amount of calcium?
    1 Plain yogurt
    2 Seafood
    3 Sardines
    4 Pork

117. The nurse is caring for a client with a diagnosis of gout. Which of the following laboratory values does the nurse expect to note in the client?
    1 Uric acid level of 8 mg/dL
    2 Calcium level of 9 mg/dL
    3 Phosphorus level of 3 mg/dL
    4 Uric acid level of 5 mg/dL

118. The home health nurse visits a client who is having an acute attack of gout. Which of the following is not a component of the plan of care for this client?
    1 Restricting fluids
    2 A low-purine diet
    3 Bed rest
    4 The administration of NSAIDs

119. The nurse is caring for a client with osteoarthritis. Which of the following are clinical manifestations associated with the disorder?
    1 Pain that is most severe later in the day
    2 An elevated platelet count
    3 Dull aching pain in the affected joints
    4 Elevated antinuclear antibody levels

120. The clinical nurse is performing an assessment on a client with a diagnosis of rheumatoid arthritis (RA). Which of the following does the nurse not expect to note during the assessment?
    1 Complaints of pain that is more severe following exercise
    2 Complaints of pain that is more severe upon arising in the morning
    3 Swollen, shiny joints
    4 Skin nodules near bony prominences

121. A client is suspected of having systemic lupus erythematous (SLE). Which of the following is a characteristic sign of SLE?
    1 Rash on the face across the bridge of the nose and on the cheeks
    2 Fatigue
    3 Fever
    4 Elevated red blood cell count

122. The home care nurse visits a client with SLE. Which of the following is not a component of the teaching plan for the client to manage fatigue?
    1 To avoid long periods of rest
    2 To sit whenever possible
    3 To take a hot bath in the evening
    4 To engage in moderate low-impact exercise when not fatigued

ANSWERS

1. **2**

Rationale: Redness and heat are associated with musculoskeletal inflammation, infection, or a recent injury. Degenerative disease is accompanied by pain, but there is no redness. Swelling may or may not occur.

Test-Taking Strategy: Swelling, redness, and warmth are signs of inflammation. The body's inflammatory response is triggered by inflammation, infection, and injury. This effectively rules out all of the incorrect options fairly easily.

Level of Cognitive Ability: Analysis
Phase of Nursing Process: Analysis
Client Needs: Physiological Integrity
Content Area: Adult Health/Musculoskeletal

Reference
Black, J., & Matassarin-Jacobs, E. (1997). *Medical-surgical nursing: Clinical management for continuity of care* (5th ed.). Philadelphia: W. B. Saunders. p. 2084.

2. **1**

Rationale: Soft-tissue injuries such as sprains are treated by RICE (Rest, Ice, Compression, Elevation) for the first 24 hours after the injury. Ice is applied intermittently for 20 to 30 minutes at a time. Heat is not used in the first 24 hours because it could increase venous congestion, which would increase edema and pain.

Test-Taking Strategy: It is likely that sprains should be rested and elevated, so these options are ruled out as the items to be avoided after a sprain. Use of an Ace wrap is also helpful in reducing the pain and swelling, so this cannot be the answer either. By the process of elimination, heat must be the item to avoid in the first 24 hours.

Level of Cognitive Ability: Application
Phase of Nursing Process: Planning
Client Needs: Physiological Integrity
Content Area: Adult Health/Musculoskeletal

Reference
Smeltzer, S., & Bare, B. (1996). *Brunner and Suddarth's textbook of medical-surgical nursing* (8th ed.). Philadelphia: Lippincott-Raven. p. 1909.

3. **3**

Rationale: Hypertrophy, or increased muscle size, on the client's dominant side of up to 1 cm is considered normal. Atrophy on either side is considered an abnormal finding. Muscle strength is graded from 0/5 (paralysis) to 5/5 (normal power). Fasciculations are fine muscle twitches that are not normally present.

Test-Taking Strategy: Options 2 and 4 should be ruled out first at face value. Atrophy is not a normal finding, and muscle strength of 3/5 is less than the maximum of 5/5, which is normal power. Knowing that fasciculations are not normal helps you to select option 3 over option 1.

Level of Cognitive Ability: Application
Phase of Nursing Process: Implementation
Client Needs: Health Promotion and Maintenance
Content Area: Adult Health/Musculoskeletal

Reference

Black, J., & Matassarin-Jacobs, E. (1997). *Medical-surgical nursing: Clinical management for continuity of care* (5th ed.). Philadelphia: W. B. Saunders. p. 2086.

4. 2

Rationale: The major dietary source of calcium is from dairy foods, including milk, yogurt, and a variety of cheeses. Calcium may also be added to certain products, such as orange juice, which are then advertised as being "fortified" with calcium. Calcium supplements are available and recommended for those with typically low-calcium intake.

Test-Taking Strategy: This question is reasonably straightforward. To answer this question, you need to know that dairy products are rich in calcium, and that yogurt is a dairy product. Each of the other options does not belong to that food group.

Level of Cognitive Ability: Analysis
Phase of Nursing Process: Evaluation
Client Needs: Health Promotion and Maintenance
Content Area: Adult Health/Musculoskeletal

Reference

Black, J. & Matassarin-Jacobs, E. (1997). *Medical-surgical nursing: Clinical management for continuity of care* (5th ed.). Philadelphia: W. B. Saunders. p. 2101.

5. 3

Rationale: Risk factors for osteoporosis include being female, postmenopausal, of advanced age, low-calcium diet, excessive alcohol intake, being sedentary, and smoking cigarettes. Long-term use of corticosteroids, anticonvulsants, and furosemide also increases risk.

Test-Taking Strategy: Option 2 is eliminated first. The 25-year-old female who jogs (exercise using the long bones) has negligible risk. The 36-year-old male with asthma is eliminated next because his only risk factor might be long-term corticosteroid use. Of the two remaining, the 65-year-old female has more risk (age, gender, postmenopausal, sedentary, smoking) than the 70-year-old male (age, alcohol consumption). By elimination option 3 is the correct choice.

Level of Cognitive Ability: Analysis
Phase of Nursing Process: Analysis
Client Needs: Health Promotion and Maintenance
Content Area: Adult Health/Musculoskeletal

Reference

Black, J., & Matassarin-Jacobs, E. (1997). *Medical-surgical nursing: Clinical management for continuity of care* (5th ed.). Philadelphia: W. B. Saunders. p. 2102.

6. 3

Rationale: Home modifications to reduce the risk for falls include use of railings on all staircases, ample lighting, removing scatter rugs, and placing handrails in the bathroom. Removal of wall-to-wall carpeting is not warranted.

Test-Taking Strategy: Begin to answer this question by eliminating options 1 and 4. Both of these items provide physical support to the client and are needed. Use of nightlights will enhance vision for the client getting up at night to use the bathroom, and is also warranted. The only remaining option, which is the correct answer, is the wall-to-wall carpeting. This does not pose a risk to the client and does not need to be removed.

Level of Cognitive Ability: Application
Phase of Nursing Process: Planning
Client Needs: Health Promotion and Maintenance
Content Area: Adult Health/Musculoskeletal

Reference

Black, J., & Matassarin-Jacobs, E. (1997). *Medical-surgical nursing: Clinical management for continuity of care* (5th ed.). Philadelphia: W. B. Saunders. p. 2103.

7. 2

Rationale: Nursing care after bone biopsy includes monitoring the site for swelling, bleeding, and hematoma formation. The biopsy site is elevated for 24 hours to reduce edema. The vital signs are monitored every 4 hours for 24 hours. The client usually requires mild analgesics; more severe pain usually indicates that complications are arising.

Test-Taking Strategy: One way to approach this question is to look at the method of anesthesia used for this procedure. If you know that this procedure is done under local anesthesia, it makes sense that monitoring vital signs every 4 hours is probably sufficient (option 4). The nurse routinely monitors for complications (option 1). This narrows the choices to site elevation or narcotic analgesics. Of these two, site elevation makes sense to reduce edema, whereas narcotic administration by the IM route seems excessive for a local procedure. Thus, option 2 is the answer to the question as stated.

Level of Cognitive Ability: Application
Phase of Nursing Process: Implementation
Client Needs: Safe, Effective Care Environment
Content Area: Adult Health/Musculoskeletal

Reference

Black, J., & Matassarin-Jacobs, E. (1997). *Medical-surgical nursing: Clinical management for continuity of care* (5th ed.). Philadelphia: W. B. Saunders. p. 2095.

8. 4

Rationale: After arthroscopy, the client can usually walk carefully on the leg once sensation has returned. The client is instructed to avoid strenuous exercise for at least a few days. The client may resume the usual diet. Signs and symptoms of infection should be reported to the physician.

Test-Taking Strategy: Options 2 and 3 are the least plausible, and may be eliminated first. To differentiate between the last two, you would need to know that the client can walk on the affected leg once sensation has returned. This would help you to eliminate that option. The client is always taught signs and symptoms of infection to report to the physician.

Level of Cognitive Ability: Analysis
Phase of Nursing Process: Evaluation
Client Needs: Health Promotion and Maintenance
Content Area: Adult Health/Musculoskeletal

Reference

Black, J., & Matassarin-Jacobs, E. (1997). *Medical-surgical nursing: Clinical management for continuity of care* (5th ed.). Philadelphia: W. B. Saunders. p. 256.

9. **1**

Rationale: Because of the risk of allergy to contrast dye, the nurse places highest priority on assessing whether the client has an allergy to iodine or shellfish. The nurse also reinforces information about the test, tells the client about the need to remain still during the procedure, and encourages the client to void before the procedure for comfort.

Test-Taking Strategy: Note that this question asks which option is of the "highest priority." This tells you that more than one or all of the options are correct (in fact, they all are). While options 2, 3, and 4 all compete for your priority, only option 1 (allergy to iodine or shellfish) takes obvious first preference. The consequence of possible anaphylactic shock (physiological risk) makes this the correct choice.

Level of Cognitive Ability: Application
Phase of Nursing Process: Assessment
Client Needs: Safe, Effective Care Environment
Content Area: Adult Health/Musculoskeletal

Reference

Black, J., & Matassarin-Jacobs, E. (1997). *Medical-surgical nursing: Clinical management for continuity of care* (5th ed.). Philadelphia: W. B. Saunders. p. 2094

10. **3**

Rationale: A sample of the client's blood is collected, and the leukocytes are tagged with indium. The leukocytes are then reinjected into the client. They accumulate in infected areas of bone, and can be detected with scanning. No special preparation or aftercare is necessary.

Test-Taking Strategy: This question is difficult if you are not familiar with the procedure. Look at the information. The client has a bone infection. With any type of infection, leukocytes migrate to the area (and bone is not a highly vascular area). This might suggest option 3 to you as the correct choice in answering this question.

Level of Cognitive Ability: Analysis
Phase of Nursing Process: Analysis
Client Needs: Safe, Effective Care Environment
Content Area: Adult Health/Musculoskeletal

Reference

Black, J., & Matassarin-Jacobs, E. (1997). *Medical-surgical nursing: Clinical management for continuity of care* (5th ed.). Philadelphia: W. B. Saunders. pp. 2094–2095.

11. **2**

Rationale: An x-ray is a photographic image of a part of the body on a special film, which is used to diagnose a wide variety of conditions. The x-ray itself is painless; any discomfort would arise from repositioning a painful part for filming. The nurse may want to premedicate a client who is at risk for pain. Any radiopaque objects such as jewelry or other metal must be removed. The client is asked to breathe in deeply, and then hold the breath while the chest x-ray is taken. To minimize risk of radiation exposure, the x-ray technologist stands in a separate area protected by a lead wall. The client also wears a lead shield over the gonads.

Test-Taking Strategy: Options 1 and 4 are obviously incorrect and are eliminated first. Of the two remaining, you would eliminate option 3 because the client needs to be still during the x-ray. Option 2 is the better choice, and is the correct answer to this question.

Level of Cognitive Ability: Application
Phase of Nursing Process: Planning
Client Needs: Safe, Effective Care Environment
Content Area: Adult Health/Musculoskeletal

Reference

Black, J., & Matassarin-Jacobs, E. (1997). *Medical-surgical nursing. Clinical management for continuity of care* (5th ed.). Philadelphia: W. B. Saunders. p. 250

12. **1**

Rationale: A gallium scan is similar to a bone scan, but with injection of gallium isotope instead of technetium Tc^{99m}. Gallium is injected 2 to 3 hours before the procedure. The procedure takes 30 to 60 minutes to perform. The client must lie still during the procedure. There is no special aftercare.

Test-Taking Strategy: If you know that a gallium scan is similar to a bone scan, then you can begin by eliminating options 3 and 4. The time frame in option 2 is rather brief, which allows you to choose option 1 as the correct answer.

Level of Cognitive Ability: Application
Phase of Nursing Process: Implementation
Client Needs: Safe, Effective Care Environment
Content Area: Adult Health/Musculoskeletal

Reference

Black, J., & Matassarin-Jacobs, E. (1997). *Medical-surgical nursing: Clinical management for continuity of care* (5th ed.). Philadelphia: W. B. Saunders. p. 2094.

13. **4**

Rationale: There are no special restrictions following a bone scan. The client is encouraged to drink large amounts of water for 24 to 48 hours to flush the radioisotope from the system. There are no hazards to the client or staff from the minimal amount of radioactivity of the isotope.

Test-Taking Strategy: There is no purpose for options 2 or 3, which allows you to eliminate them first. Nausea and flushing could accompany dye injection during a procedure, but this procedure uses radioisotopes and the question relates to care after the procedure. Thus, this option is eliminated also. The only option left is pushing fluids, which will hasten elimination of the isotope from the client's system.

Level of Cognitive Ability: Analysis
Phase of Nursing Process: Evaluation
Client Needs: Health Promotion and Maintenance
Content Area: Adult Health/Musculoskeletal

Reference

Black, J., & Matassarin-Jacobs, E. (1997). *Medical-surgical nursing: Clinical management for continuity of care* (5th ed.). Philadelphia: W. B. Saunders. p. 2094.

14. **2**

Rationale: Typical signs and symptoms of fracture include pain, loss of function in the area, deformity, shortening of the extremity, crepitus, swelling, and ecchymosis. Not all fractures lead to the development of every sign. A contusion results from a blow to soft tissue and causes pain, swelling, and ecchymosis. A sprain is an injury to a ligament caused by a wrenching or twisting motion. Symptoms include pain, swelling, and inability to use the joint or bear weight normally. A strain results from a pulling force on the muscle. Symptoms include soreness and pain with muscle use.

Test-Taking Strategy: Within the list of signs and symptoms in the stem, note the one that states one leg is shorter than another. Only a fractured bone (which shortens with displacement) could cause this sign. This makes it easy to eliminate each of the other incorrect options.

Level of Cognitive Ability: Analysis
Phase of Nursing Process: Analysis
Client Needs: Physiological Integrity
Content Area: Adult Health/Musculoskeletal

Reference
Smeltzer, S., & Bare, B. (1996). *Brunner and Suddarth's textbook of medical-surgical nursing* (8th ed.). Philadelphia: Lippincott-Raven. pp. 1908, 1910.

15. **1**

Rationale: With a suspected fracture, the client is not moved unless it is dangerous to remain in that spot. The nurse should remain with the client, and have someone else call for emergency help. A fracture is not reduced at the scene. Before moving the client, the site of fracture is immobilized to prevent further injury.

Test-Taking Strategy: Options 2 and 4 are the worst choices and should be eliminated first. Either of these options could result in further injury to the client. Of the two remaining choices, the more prudent action would be for the nurse to remain with the client and have someone else call for emergency assistance.

Level of Cognitive Ability: Application
Phase of Nursing Process: Planning
Client Needs: Physiological Integrity
Content Area: Adult Health/Musculoskeletal

Reference
Black, J., & Matassarin-Jacobs, E. (1997). *Medical-surgical nursing: Clinical management for continuity of care* (5th ed.). Philadelphia: W. B. Saunders. p. 2134.

16. **4**

Rationale: When a fracture is suspected, it is imperative that the area is splinted before the client is moved. Emergency help should be called for if the client is not hospitalized, and a physician is called for the hospitalized client. The nurse should remain with the client and provide realistic reassurance.

Test-Taking Strategy: This question asks for the highest priority of the nurse, which tells you that more than one option may be correct. In this instance, eliminate option 2 because the nurse does not order x-rays. Option 3 is eliminated next because the nurse never tells a client that "everything will be fine." Of the last two choices, immobilizing the limb is imperative for the client's safety, which makes it a better choice than taking vital signs.

Level of Cognitive Ability: Application
Phase of Nursing Process: Implementation
Client Needs: Physiological Integrity
Content Area: Adult Health/Musculoskeletal

Reference
Black, J., & Matassarin-Jacobs, E. (1997). *Medical-surgical nursing: Clinical management for continuity of care* (5th ed.). Philadelphia: W. B. Saunders. p. 2134.

17. **3**

Rationale: Before a fracture is reduced, the client is informed about the procedure, and consent is obtained. An analgesic is given as prescribed because the procedure is painful. Administration of anesthesia may or may not be done, depending on severity. Closed reductions may be done in the emergency department without anesthesia. If anesthesia is used, the procedure is done in the operating room.

Test-Taking Strategy: Options 1 and 4 are obviously needed, so these options are eliminated first. The stem specifically states that the procedure is going to be done in the cast room, which helps you to choose option 3 (anesthesia consent) as the unnecessary item.

Level of Cognitive Ability: Analysis
Phase of Nursing Process: Evaluation
Client Needs: Physiological Integrity
Content Area: Adult Health/Musculoskeletal

Reference
Smeltzer, S., & Bare, B. (1996). *Brunner and Suddarth's textbook of medical-surgical nursing* (8th ed.). Philadelphia: Lippincott-Raven. p. 1912.

18. **4**

Rationale: The procedure for casting involves washing and drying the skin and placing a stockinette material over the area to be casted. A roll of padding is then applied smoothly and evenly. The plaster is rolled onto the padding, and the edges are trimmed or smoothed as needed. A plaster cast gives off heat as it dries. A plaster cast can tolerate weight bearing once it is dry, which varies from 24 to 72 hours depending on the nature and thickness of the cast.

Test-Taking Strategy: Familiarity with the different types of casting materials and their differences helps you to answer this question with ease. Options 1, 2, and 3 are all true for plaster casts. Option 4 is true for nonplaster casts. Because of this, the nurse does not include option 4 in the discussion, and it is the answer to this question as stated.

Level of Cognitive Ability: Application
Phase of Nursing Process: Planning
Client Needs: Psychosocial Integrity
Content Area: Adult Health/Musculoskeletal

Reference
Smeltzer, S., & Bare, B. (1996). *Brunner and Suddarth's textbook of medical-surgical nursing* (8th ed.). Philadelphia: Lippincott-Raven. p. 1851.

19. **1**

Rationale: Immobility and the weight of a casted arm may cause the shoulder above an arm fracture to become stiff. The shoulder of a casted arm should be lifted over the head periodically as a preventive measure. The use of slings further immobilizes the shoulder and may be contraindicated. Making fists with the left hand provides good isometric exercise to maintain muscle strength. Range of motion of the affected fingers is also a useful measure. Lifting the right arm is of no particular value.

Test-Taking Strategy: Imagine each of the movements and think about the muscle groups that are moved with each. Options 2 and 4 provide for no movement of the left arm and are eliminated first. Making a fist with the hand on the casted arm provides good isometric exercise to the muscles surrounding the fracture, but again, does nothing for the shoulder. The only viable option is raising the arm over the head, which provides some range of motion for the shoulder joint.

Level of Cognitive Ability: Application
Phase of Nursing Process: Planning
Client Needs: Health Promotion and Maintenance
Content Area: Adult Health/Musculoskeletal

Reference
Black, J., & Matassarin-Jacobs, E. (1997). *Medical-surgical nursing: Clinical management for continuity of care* (5th ed.). Philadelphia: W. B. Saunders. p. 2151.

20. 1

Rationale: A fiberglass cast is made of water-activated polyurethane materials, which are dry to the touch within minutes, and reach full rigid strength in about 20 minutes. Because of this, the client can bear weight on the cast within 20 to 30 minutes.

Test-Taking Strategy: Familiarity with nonplaster casts is needed to answer this question precisely. Options 3 and 4 should be eliminated first, because these time frames are similar to the drying times for plaster casts. Knowing that the nonplaster type of cast is lighter and dries extremely quickly may help you to choose the 20- to 30-minute time frame as correct.

Level of Cognitive Ability: Application
Phase of Nursing Process: Implementation
Client Needs: Health Promotion and Maintenance
Content Area: Adult Health/Musculoskeletal

References
Black, J., & Matassarin-Jacobs, E. (1997). *Medical-surgical nursing: Clinical management for continuity of care* (5th ed.). Philadelphia: W. B. Saunders. p. 2147.
Smeltzer, S., & Bare, B. (1996). *Brunner and Suddarth's textbook of medical-surgical nursing* (8th ed.). Philadelphia: Lippincott-Raven. p. 1850.

21. 4

Rationale: Client instructions should include to avoid walking on wet, slippery floors to prevent falls. Surface soil on a cast may be removed with a damp cloth. If the cast gets wet, it can be dried with a hair dryer set to a cool setting to prevent skin breakdown. If the skin under the cast itches, cool air from a hair dryer may be used to relieve it. The client should never scratch under a cast because of the risk of skin breakdown and ulcer formation.

Test-Taking Strategy: Options 1 and 3 are certainly true, and are therefore eliminated as potential answers, given the wording of this question. Knowledge of nonplaster cast material is needed to discriminate between the last two. A fiberglass cast may be wiped with a damp cloth because it is water resistant. It may be helpful to remember never to use a hair dryer on a cast, or on the skin under any cast, with the dryer set at the warmest setting; only cool settings are used, to prevent burns.

Level of Cognitive Ability: Analysis
Phase of Nursing Process: Evaluation
Client Needs: Health Promotion and Maintenance
Content Area: Adult Health/Musculoskeletal

Reference
Smeltzer, S., & Bare, B. (1996). *Brunner and Suddarth's textbook of medical-surgical nursing* (8th ed.). Philadelphia: Lippincott-Raven. p. 1853.

22. 2

Rationale: Buck's extension traction is a type of skin traction often applied after hip fracture before the fracture is reduced in surgery. It reduces muscle spasms and helps to immobilize the fracture. It does not lengthen the leg for the purpose of preventing blood vessel severance. It also does not allow for bony healing to begin.

Test-Taking Strategy: Options 3 and 4 are the least plausible of all the choices, and should be eliminated first. To discriminate between the last two, look at the words "rigid immobilization" in option 1. Since skin traction uses lighter weights than skeletal traction, this type of traction cannot be said to provide rigid immobilization. At the same time, skin traction is very useful in reducing muscle spasms while immobilizing an area, which makes option 2 the answer to the question.

Level of Cognitive Ability: Analysis
Phase of Nursing Process: Analysis
Client Needs: Physiological Integrity
Content Area: Adult Health/Musculoskeletal

Reference
Black, J., & Matassarin-Jacobs, E. (1997). *Medical-surgical nursing: Clinical management for continuity of care* (5th ed.). Philadelphia: W. B. Saunders. p. 2138.

23. 1

Rationale: After insertion of skeletal traction pins, the ends are covered with tape or cork to prevent injury to the client or to health care personnel.

Test-Taking Strategy: Eliminate option 3 first because it is the least plausible. Option 4 is not timely, so that is eliminated also. Performing skin care (option 2) is not the priority at this time. This leaves option 1 as correct. Covering traction pins provides for the protection of clients and staff.

Level of Cognitive Ability: Application
Phase of Nursing Process: Planning
Client Needs: Safe, Effective Care Environment
Content Area: Adult Health/Musculoskeletal

Reference
Smeltzer, S., & Bare, B. (1996). *Brunner and Suddarth's textbook of medical-surgical nursing* (8th ed.). Philadelphia: Lippincott-Raven. p. 1862.

24. 4

Rationale: If the client in skeletal traction may not turn from side to side, the nurse should have the client pull up on a trapeze and try to lift the hips off the bed for skin care, bedpan use, and linen changes. If the client is unable to pull up on a trapeze, the nurse can push down on the mattress with one hand while administering care with the other.

Test-Taking Strategy: Option 3 is contraindicated because it ignores a medical order. Option 1 is not feasible as stated. The client cannot lift up from the bed using one foot only. Options 2 and 4 are both acceptable alternatives. Since the question asks which would be most useful, the answer is option 4. Providing care to the client who can lift the hips off the bed using a trapeze is easier and more efficient than providing care to one who cannot.

Level of Cognitive Ability: Application
Phase of Nursing Process: Implementation
Client Needs: Physiological Integrity
Content Area: Adulth Health/Musculoskeletal

Reference
Smeltzer, S., & Bare, B. (1996). *Brunner and Suddarth's textbook of medical-surgical nursing* (8th ed.). Philadelphia: Lippincott-Raven. p. 1862.

25. 2

Rationale: A small amount of serous oozing is expected at pin insertion sites. Signs of infection such as inflammation, purulent drainage, and pain at the pin site are not expected findings, and should be reported to the physician.

Test-Taking Strategy: Options 1 and 4 seem to indicate an infectious problem, and are eliminated as answers to be "least concerned with." To discriminate between options 2 and 3, look at them carefully. The complaint of pain is at "a pin site" only. It gives no indication that the pain is related to the fracture or muscle spasm. Since serous drainage is an expected finding, choose this over the complaint of pain as the answer to the question.

Level of Cognitive Ability: Analysis
Phase of Nursing Process: Evaluation
Client Needs: Physiological Integrity
Content Area: Adult Health/Musculoskeletal

Reference
Smeltzer, S., & Bare, B. (1996). *Brunner and Suddarth's textbook of medical-surgical nursing* (8th ed.). Philadelphia: Lippincott-Raven. p. 1863.

26. 1

Rationale: A major defining characteristic of Diversional Activity Deficit is expression of boredom by the client. The question does not identify difficulties with coordination, range of motion, or muscle strength, which would indicate Impaired Physical Mobility. The question also does not relate client feelings of inability to perform ADLs (Self-Care Deficit) or lack of control (Powerlessness).

Test-Taking Strategy: The key to answering this question lies in the complaints of boredom and restlessness. Compare these complaints to each of the listed nursing diagnoses, and you should be able to eliminate each of the incorrect options systematically.

Level of Cognitive Ability: Analysis
Phase of Nursing Process: Analysis
Client Needs: Psychosocial Integrity
Content Area: Adult Health/Musculoskeletal

Reference
Cox, H., Hinz, M., Lubno, M., et al. (1997). *Clinical applications of nursing diagnosis: Adult, child, women's, psychiatric, gerontic and home health considerations* (3rd ed.). Philadelphia: F. A. Davis. p. 301.

27. 3

Rationale: Buck's extension traction is a type of skin traction. The nurse inspects the skin of the limb in traction at least once every 8 hours for irritation or inflammation. Massaging the skin with lotion is not indicated. The nurse never releases the weights of traction unless specifically ordered by the physician. There are no pins to care for with skin traction.

Test-Taking Strategy: A baseline knowledge of Buck's extension traction allows you to eliminate options 2 and 4 easily. There are no pins, and the nurse never removes weights without a specific order to do so. Since the apparatus would have to be removed to apply lotion, which is unnecessary, the answer is to assess the skin integrity.

Level of Cognitive Ability: Application
Phase of Nursing Process: Planning
Client Needs: Safe, Effective Care Environment
Content Area: Adult Health/Musculoskeletal

Reference
Ignatavicius, D., Workman, M., & Mishler, M. (1995). *Medical-surgical nursing: A nursing process approach* (2nd ed.). Philadelphia: W. B. Saunders. pp. 1462–1463.

28. 4

Rationale: A client who complains of severe pain may need realignment or may have traction weights ordered that are too heavy. The nurse realigns the client, and if ineffective, calls the physician. Severe leg pain, once traction has been established, indicates a problem. Medicating the client should be done after trying to determine and treat the cause. Providing pin care is unrelated to the problem as described.

Test-Taking Strategy: On first reading, the only option that can be readily eliminated is option 2, providing pin care. The question asks you which should be done "first," which tells you that more than one answer is correct. Since it would be unwise to medicate a client without determining the true cause of the pain, this option is also eliminated. Of the remaining choices, checking the client's alignment is a prudent choice before calling the physician. At the very least, it provides one more piece of data for the physician to work with.

Level of Cognitive Ability: Application
Phase of Nursing Process: Implementation
Client Needs: Physiological Integrity
Content Area: Adult Health/Musculoskeletal

Reference
Ignatavicius, D., Workman, M., & Mishler, M. (1995). *Medical-surgical nursing: A nursing process approach* (2nd ed.). Philadelphia: W. B. Saunders. p. 1463.

29. 3

Rationale: Exercise is indicated within therapeutic limits for the client in skeletal traction to maintain muscle strength and range of motion. The client may pull up on the trapeze, perform active ROM with uninvolved joints, and do isometric muscle setting exercises (such as quadriceps- and gluteal-setting exercises). The client may also flex and extend the feet.

Test-Taking Strategy: Options 1 and 4 are most easily identified as correct actions, and are therefore eliminated as possible answers to this question. To discriminate between options 2 and 3, imagine the lines of pull on the fracture site with the movements described. While flexing and extending the feet do not disrupt the line of pull from the traction, performing active ROM to the affected knee and ankle does. Thus active ROM is the answer to the question, which is seeking an item that is an incorrect action.

Level of Cognitive Ability: Analysis
Phase of Nursing Process: Evaluation
Client Needs: Health Promotion and Maintenance
Content Area: Adult Health/Musculoskeletal

Reference
Smeltzer, S., & Bare, B. (1996). *Brunner and Suddarth's textbook of medical-surgical nursing* (8th ed.). Philadelphia: Lippincott-Raven. p. 1863.

30. 2

Rationale: Signs and symptoms of infection under a casted area include odor or purulent drainage from the cast, or the presence of "hot spots," which are areas of the cast that are warmer than others. The physician should be notified if any of these occur. Signs of impaired circulation in the distal limb include coolness and pallor of the skin, diminished arterial pulse, and edema.

Test-Taking Strategy: Begin to answer this question by thinking of what you would expect to find with infection: redness, swelling, heat, and purulent drainage. With these in mind, options 1 and 3 can be eliminated easily. To discriminate between options 2 and 4, "dependent edema" is not necessarily indicative of infection. Swelling is continuous. The "hot spot" on the cast could signify infection underneath that area, and is the correct answer to the question.

Level of Cognitive Ability: Application
Phase of Nursing Process: Assessment
Client Needs: Physiological Integrity
Content Area: Adult Health/Musculoskeletal

References
Black, J., & Matassarin-Jacobs, E. (1997). *Medical-surgical nursing: Clinical management for continuity of care* (5th ed.). Philadelphia: W. B. Saunders. p. 2150.
Smeltzer, S., & Bare, B. (1996). *Brunner and Suddarth's textbook of medical-surgical nursing* (8th ed.). Philadelphia: Lippincott-Raven. p. 1852.

31. **1**

Rationale: Most pain associated with fractures can be minimized with rest, elevation, application of cold, and administration of analgesics. Pain that is not relieved from these measures should be reported to the physician, because it may be a result of impaired tissue perfusion, tissue breakdown, or necrosis. Since this is a new closed fracture and cast, infection would not have had time to set in.

Test-Taking Strategy: Of the possible choices, options 2 and 3 are the least plausible given the description in the stem. These should be eliminated first. Since the fracture and cast are so new, it is extremely unlikely that infection could have possibly set in. The most likely alternative is impaired tissue perfusion because pain from ischemia is not relieved by comfort measures and analgesics.

Level of Cognitive Ability: Analysis
Phase of Nursing Process: Analysis
Client Needs: Physiological Integrity
Content Area: Adult Health/Musculoskeletal

Reference
Smeltzer, S., & Bare, B. (1996). *Brunner and Suddarth's textbook of medical surgical nursing* (8th ed.). Philadelphia: Lippincott-Raven. p. 1851.

32. **3**

Rationale: A casted extremity is elevated continuously for the first 24 to 48 hours to minimize swelling, and to promote venous drainage.

Test-Taking Strategy: To answer this question accurately, you should know that edema sets in after fracture, and can be augmented by casting. For this reason, options 1 and 2 are the least helpful, and can be eliminated first. There is no useful purpose for the timing in option 4. Thus option 3 is correct.

Level of Cognitive Ability: Application
Phase of Nursing Process: Implementation
Client Needs: Physiological Integrity
Content Area: Adult Health/Musculoskeletal

Reference
Black, J., & Matassarin-Jacobs, E. (1997). *Medical-surgical nursing: Clinical management for continuity of care* (5th ed.). Philadelphia: W. B. Saunders. p. 2150.

33. **4**

Rationale: The nurse petals the edges of the cast with tape to minimize skin irritation. If a client has a cast applied and returns home, the client can be taught to do the same.

Test-Taking Strategy: Options 1 and 2 are similar, and neither helps to get rid of the cause of the irritation, so they are eliminated first. Imagine the use of a "rough file"; it would create plaster chips and dust that could go underneath the cast, and is not practical. By the process of elimination, the nurse would petal the cast to cushion the skin from the irritating cast material.

Level of Cognitive Ability: Analysis
Phase of Nursing Process: Analysis
Client Needs: Physiological Integrity
Content Area: Adult Health/Musculoskeletal

Reference
Smeltzer, S., & Bare, B. (1996). *Brunner and Suddarth's textbook of medical-surgical nursing* (8th ed.). Philadelphia: Lippincott-Raven. pp. 1851, 1853.

34. **1**

Rationale: A plaster cast must remain dry to keep its strength. The cast should be handled using the palms of the hands, not the fingertips, until fully dry. Air should circulate freely around the cast to help it dry; the cast also gives off heat as it dries. The client should never scratch under the cast; a cool hair dryer may be used to eliminate an itch.

Test-Taking Strategy: Knowledge of cast care is needed to answer this question. Knowing that a wet cast can be dented with the fingertips, causing pressure underneath, helps you to discard option 2 first. Knowing that the cast needs to dry makes you eliminate option 3 next. Option 4 is dangerous to skin integrity and is immediately eliminated. This leaves option 1 as correct. Plaster casts, once they have dried after application, should not become wet.

Level of Cognitive Ability: Analysis
Phase of Nursing Process: Evaluation
Client Needs: Health Promotion and Maintenance
Content Area: Adult Health/Musculoskeletal

Reference
Smeltzer, S., & Bare, B. (1996). *Brunner and Suddarth's textbook of medical-surgical nursing* (8th ed.). Philadelphia: Lippincott-Raven. pp. 1849–1850, 1853.

35. **3**

Rationale: Crutches are measured so that the tops are 3 to 4 finger breadths or 1 to 2 inches from the axillae. This ensures that the client's axillae are not resting on the crutch, or bearing the weight of the crutch. This could result in injury to the nerves of the brachial plexus.

Test-Taking Strategy: Of the possible choices, options 1 and 4 should be eliminated first as the least likely of all available answers. To discriminate between the last two choices, knowledge of the complications of improper crutch measurement is needed. It is possible that skin breakdown could occur from friction. However, the more dangerous hazard is the risk of brachial nerve plexus injury, which is the answer to the question.

Level of Cognitive Ability: Analysis
Phase of Nursing Process: Analysis
Client Needs: Physiological Integrity
Content Area: Adult Health/Musculoskeletal

Reference

Smeltzer, S., & Bare, B. (1996). *Brunner and Suddarth's textbook of medical-surgical nursing* (8th ed.). Philadelphia: Lippincott-Raven. p. 338.

36. **1**

Rationale: The classic tripod position is taught to the client before giving instructions on gait. The crutches are placed anywhere from 6 to 10 inches in front and to the side of the client, depending on the client's body size. This provides a wide enough base of support to the client and improves balance.

Test-Taking Strategy: Three inches (option 2) and 20 inches (option 3) seem excessively short and long, respectively. These two options should be eliminated first. Of the two remaining, 8 inches seems more in keeping with the normal length of a stride than 15 inches for someone wearing a cast, and it is the answer to the question.

Level of Cognitive Ability: Application
Phase of Nursing Process: Planning
Client Needs: Health Promotion and Maintenance
Content Area: Adult Health/Musculoskeletal

Reference

Potter, P., & Perry, A. (1997). *Fundamentals of nursing: Concepts, process, and practice* (4th ed.). St. Louis: Mosby–Year Book. p. 936.

37. **4**

Rationale: A three-point gait requires good balance and arm strength. The crutches are advanced with the affected leg, and then the unaffected leg is moved forward. Option 1 describes a two-point gait. Option 2 describes a swing-to gait. Option 3 describes the three-point gait used for a right leg problem.

Test-Taking Strategy: Option 1 does not provide the support needed for the casted extremity described in the stem, and should be eliminated as a possible answer. Option 2 is not necessary if the client is allowed to let the extremity touch the floor, and is eliminated next. Of the two remaining, option 4 is the choice that provides support to the left leg, and is the correct answer.

Level of Cognitive Ability: Application
Phase of Nursing Process: Implementation
Client Needs: Health Promotion and Maintenance
Content Area: Adult Health/Musculoskeletal

Reference

Lammon, C., Foote, A., Leli, P., et al. (1995). *Clinical Nursing Skills.* Philadelphia: W. B. Saunders. p. 242.

38. **2**

Rationale: Crutch tips should remain dry. Water could cause slipping by decreasing the surface friction of the rubber tip on the floor. If crutch tips get wet, the client should dry them with a cloth or paper towel. The client should use only crutches measured for the client. The tips should be inspected for wear, and spare crutches and tips should be available if needed.

Test-Taking Strategy: The wording of the question directs you to look for a statement that is incorrect. Option 3 is certainly a correct statement, and is therefore eliminated as

a possible answer to this question. Options 1 and 4 are also true, and must be discarded also. This leaves option 2 as the correct answer. Crutch tips can slip when they get wet, posing a possible threat to the unsuspecting client.

Level of Cognitive Ability: Analysis
Phase of Nursing Process: Evaluation
Client Needs: Health Promotion and Maintenance
Content Area: Adult Health/Musculoskeletal

Reference

Potter, P., & Perry, A. (1997). *Fundamentals of nursing: Concepts, process, and practice* (4th ed.). St. Louis: Mosby–Year Book. p. 936.

39. **4**

Rationale: A straight-leg cane is useful for the client with slight weakness in one leg. A walker is beneficial to the client with greater or bilateral weakness, or is at risk for falls. Wooden crutches are often used by clients with a leg cast. Lofstrand crutches aid clients who need crutches, but have limited arm strength.

Test-Taking Strategy: Giving a walker to a client with a slight leg weakness is excessive, and is eliminated first. Since there is no evidence in the situation of the question that the client has weight-bearing difficulty, crutches are not indicated either. This leaves the straight-leg cane as the correct choice.

Level of Cognitive Ability: Analysis
Phase of Nursing Process: Analysis
Client Needs: Physiological Integrity
Content Area: Adult Health/Musculoskeletal

Reference

Potter, P., & Perry, A. (1997). *Fundamentals of nursing: Concepts, process, and practice* (4th ed.). St. Louis: Mosby–Year Book. p. 935.

40. **1**

Rationale: A quad cane may be used by the client requiring greater support and stability than is provided by a straight-leg cane. The quad cane provides a four-point base of support and is indicated for use by clients with partial or complete hemiplegia. Neither crutches nor a wheelchair is indicated for use with a client such as described in the stem.

Test-Taking Strategy: Giving a wheelchair to a client with partial hemiplegia is excessive, and is eliminated first. Wooden crutches are not indicated because there is no restriction in weight bearing. A Lofstrand crutch is useful for clients with bilateral weakness. This leaves the quad cane as the correct choice.

Level of Cognitive Ability: Analysis
Phase of Nursing Process: Analysis
Client Needs: Physiological Integrity
Content Area: Adult Health/Musculoskeletal

References

Potter, P., & Perry, A. (1997). *Fundamentals of nursing: Concepts, process, and practice* (4th ed.). St. Louis: Mosby–Year Book. p. 935.
Smeltzer, S., & Bare, B. (1996). *Brunner and Suddarth's textbook of medical-surgical nursing* (8th ed.). Philadelphia: Lippincott-Raven. p. 341.

41. **3**

Rationale: The client is taught to hold the cane on the opposite side of the weakness. This is because with normal walking, the opposite arm and leg move together (called reciprocal motion). The cane is placed 6 inches lateral to the fifth toe.

Test-Taking Strategy: Knowing that the cane is held at the client's side, not in front, helps you to eliminate options 1 and 2 first. Knowing that the preferred method is to have the cane positioned on the stronger side helps you to choose option 3 over option 4. Remember these important points!

Level of Cognitive Ability: Application
Phase of Nursing Process: Planning
Client Needs: Health Promotion and Maintenance
Content Area: Adult Health/Musculoskeletal

Reference

Potter, P., & Perry, A. (1997). *Fundamentals of nursing: Concepts, process, and practice* (4th ed.). St. Louis: Mosby–Year Book. p. 935.

42. 2

Rationale: A cane should have a slightly flared tip with flexible concentric rings. This tip acts as a shock absorber and provides optimal stability. Other advantages include greater speed with ambulation and less fatigue.

Test-Taking Strategy: Options 1 and 4 are the least plausible of all the choices and may be eliminated first. Neither of these statements provides any reassurance for the client. Option 3 also provides no information to relieve the client's anxiety. Option 2 is the best answer. It is a true statement, and addresses, in a factual way, the client's concerns about safety.

Level of Cognitive Ability: Application
Phase of Nursing Process: Implementation
Client Needs: Psychosocial Integrity
Content Area: Adult Health/Musculoskeletal

Reference

Smeltzer, S., & Bare, B. (1996). *Brunner and Suddarth's textbook of medical-surgical nursing* (8th ed.). Philadelphia: Lippincott-Raven. p. 341.

43. 3

Rationale: The cane is held on the stronger side to minimize stress on the affected extremity, and to provide a wide base of support. If necessary, the cane would be used on the affected side. The cane is held 6 inches lateral to the fifth great toe. The cane is moved forward with the affected leg. The client leans on the cane for added support while the stronger side swings through.

Test-Taking Strategy: The wording of this question guides you to look for an incorrect action. Knowing that the cane is held on the stronger side helps you eliminate options 1 and 2 first. These are both correct. To discriminate between the two remaining choices, recall that the client moves the cane with the weaker leg, and leans on it for support when the stronger leg swings through. This will help you to choose option 3 as the answer to this question.

Level of Cognitive Ability: Analysis
Phase of Nursing Process: Evaluation
Client Needs: Health Promotion and Maintenance
Content Area: Adult Health/Musculoskeletal

Reference

Smeltzer, S., & Bare, B. (1996). *Brunner and Suddarth's textbook of medical-surgical nursing* (8th ed.). Philadelphia: Lippincott-Raven. p. 341.

44. 2

Rationale: A key feature of fat embolism is a significant degree of hypoxemia, with a PaO_2 often less than 60 mmHg. Other features that distinguish fat embolism from pulmo-nary embolism are the higher fever and presence of fat in the blood with fat embolus, and the chest pain with respira-tion that characterizes pulmonary embolism.

Test-Taking Strategy: To answer this question correctly, you need to know that fat embolus causes significant hypox-emia, which can rapidly lead to respiratory failure. This knowledge will help you to choose the correct answer quickly and easily.

Level of Cognitive Ability: Analysis
Phase of Nursing Process: Analysis
Client Needs: Physiological Integrity
Content Area: Adult Health/Musculoskeletal

Reference

Black, J., & Matassarin-Jacobs, E. (1997). *Medical-surgical nursing: Clinical management for continuity of care* (5th ed.). Philadelphia: W. B. Saunders. p. 2141.

45. 3

Rationale: Respiratory failure is the most common cause of death after fat embolus. The client may be intubated and mechanically ventilated with positive end-expiratory pres-sure (PEEP) to treat the significant hypoxemia and pulmo-nary edema. Corticosteroids are given to treat inflammatory lung reactions and control cerebral edema.

Test-Taking Strategy: Fat embolus does not cause broncho-constriction or bronchospasm, which may help to eliminate option 1. The stem makes no mention of hypovolemia, so the plasma expanders in option 2 have no use. That option may be eliminated also. To discriminate between options 3 and 4, it is helpful to know that corticosteroids are used for the inflammatory lung reaction, and that hypertension may not be part of the clinical picture.

Level of Cognitive Ability: Application
Phase of Nursing Process: Planning
Client Needs: Physiological Integrity
Content Area: Adult Health/Musculoskeletal

Reference

Black, J., & Matassarin-Jacobs, E. (1997). *Medical-surgical nursing: Clinical management for continuity of care* (5th ed.). Philadelphia: W. B. Saunders. p. 2141.

46. 4

Rationale: The nurse always speaks to the client calmly and provides reassurance to the anxious client. Morphine is often prescribed for pain and anxiety for the client receiving mechanical ventilation.

Test-Taking Strategy: In option 1, the nurse does nothing to reassure or help the client, so it is incorrect. Family members are also stressed, not just because of the complica-tion, but because of the original injury. It is not beneficial to ask the family to take on the burden of remaining with the client at all times. Succinylcholine (option 3) is a para-lyzing agent, but has no antianxiety properties. Thus, this option is incorrect also. This leaves option 4 as the answer to the question. The nurse communicates with the client to relieve anxiety, and can provide the client with prescribed morphine, which alleviates anxiety while helping the client tolerate the ventilator.

Level of Cognitive Ability: Application
Phase of Nursing Process: Implementation
Client Needs: Psychosocial Integrity
Content Area: Adult Health/Musculoskeletal

Reference
Smeltzer, S., & Bare, B. (1996). *Brunner and Suddarth's textbook of medical-surgical nursing* (8th ed.). Philadelphia: Lippincott-Raven. p. 1917.

47. **3**

Rationale: A clear chest x-ray is a good indicator that fat embolus is resolving. When fat embolism occurs, there is a "snowstorm" appearance to chest x-ray. Eupnea, not minimal dyspnea, is a normal sign. Arterial oxygen levels should be 80 to 100 mmHg. Oxygen saturation should be greater than 95%.

Test-Taking Strategy: Knowledge of normal baseline respiratory values is helpful in answering this question. Knowing that the arterial oxygen and oxygen saturation levels are below normal helps you to eliminate these as possible correct answers. Dyspnea, even at a minimal level, is not normal and can be eliminated quickly. A clear chest x-ray is a normal finding, and is the answer to the question as stated.

Level of Cognitive Ability: Analysis
Phase of Nursing Process: Evaluation
Client Needs: Physiological Integrity
Content Area: Adult Health/Musculoskeletal

Reference
Smeltzer, S., & Bare, B. (1996). *Brunner and Suddarth's textbook of medical-surgical nursing* (8th ed.). Philadelphia: Lippincott-Raven. p. 1917.

48. **4**

Rationale: Compartment syndrome is caused by bleeding and swelling within a compartment, which is lined by fascia that does not expand. The bleeding and swelling put pressure on the nerves, muscles, and blood vessels in the compartment, triggering the symptoms.

Test-Taking Strategy: A basic understanding of the concept of a compartment is needed to answer this question. Option 1 should be eliminated first because it is not the result of an arterial injury. Knowing that the fascia itself cannot expand eliminates option 2. To discriminate between the last two, it is necessary to know that bleeding and swelling cause the symptoms, not a nerve injury.

Level of Cognitive Ability: Analysis
Phase of Nursing Process: Analysis
Client Needs: Physiological Integrity
Content Area: Adult Health/Musculoskeletal

Reference
Black, J., & Matassarin-Jacobs, E. (1997). *Medical-surgical nursing: Clinical management for continuity of care* (5th ed.). Philadelphia: W. B. Saunders. p. 2139.

49. **1**

Rationale: Compartment syndrome is prevented by controlling edema. This is achieved most optimally with the use of elevation and application of ice.

Test-Taking Strategy: Knowing that edema is controlled or prevented with limb elevation helps you to eliminate options 3 and 4 as possible choices. To discriminate between the last two choices, look at the effects of ice versus bath blankets. Ice will further control edema, whereas bath blankets will produce heat and prevent air circulation needed for the cast to dry. This comparison helps you to choose option 1 over option 2.

Level of Cognitive Ability: Application
Phase of Nursing Process: Planning
Client Needs: Safe, Effective Care Environment
Content Area: Adult Health/Musculoskeletal

Reference
Smeltzer, S., & Bare, B. (1996). *Brunner and Suddarth's textbook of medical-surgical nursing* (8th ed.). Philadelphia: Lippincott-Raven. p. 1917.

50. **2**

Rationale: The fasciotomy site is not sutured, but is left open to relieve pressure and edema. The site is covered with moist, sterile saline dressings. After 3 to 5 days, when perfusion is adequate and edema subsides, the wound is débrided and closed.

Test-Taking Strategy: This question can be answered by knowing what a fasciotomy involves and knowing the basics of wound care. With fasciotomy, the skin is not sutured closed but left open for pressure relief. Moist tissue needs to remain moist, which eliminates option 1. A hydrocolloid dressing is not indicated for use with clean, open incisions, which eliminates option 3. The incision is clean, not dirty, so there should be no reason to require Betadine. Knowing that Betadine can be irritating to normal tissues is an additional reason to choose option 2 over option 4.

Level of Cognitive Ability: Application
Phase of Nursing Process: Implementation
Client Needs: Physiological Integrity
Content Area: Adult Health/Musculoskeletal

Reference
Smeltzer, S., & Bare, B. (1996). *Brunner and Suddarth's textbook of medical-surgical nursing* (8th ed.). Philadelphia: Lippincott-Raven. p. 1917.

51. **4**

Rationale: The earliest symptom of compartment syndrome is paresthesias (numbness and tingling in the fingers). Other symptoms include pain unrelieved by narcotics, pain that increases with limb elevation, and pallor and coolness to the distal limb. Cyanosis is a late sign.

Test-Taking Strategy: This question asks for an early symptom of compartment syndrome. Since cyanosis is a late sign, option 3 is eliminated first. Knowing that compartment syndrome is characterized by insufficient circulation and ischemia secondary to pressure, look for symptoms that are consistent with this process. Pain is increased with elevation rather than dependency, so option 2 can be eliminated also. Because pain of ischemia is generally not relieved with analgesics, this cannot be an early symptom either. This leaves numbness and tingling as the answer.

Level of Cognitive Ability: Analysis
Phase of Nursing Process: Evaluation
Client Needs: Health Promotion and Maintenance
Content Area: Adult Health/Musculoskeletal

Reference
Black, J., & Matassarin-Jacobs, E. (1997). *Medical-surgical nursing: Clinical management for continuity of care* (5th ed.). Philadelphia: W. B. Saunders. p. 2139.

52. **2**

Rationale: Confusion in the elderly client with hip fracture could result from the unfamiliar hospital setting, stress caused by the fracture, concurrent systemic diseases, cerebral ischemia, or side effects of medications. Use of eyeglasses and hearing aids enhances the client's interaction with the environment, and can reduce disorientation.

Test-Taking Strategy: The wording of the question asks you to look for an option that will keep the client at the highest possible level of functioning from a cognitive perspective. Stress from the fracture (option 1) and unfamiliar setting (option 3) are not likely to help the client's functional level, and are eliminated as possible choices. Eyeglasses and hearing aids are both useful adjuncts in communicating with a client. Since the eyeglasses were left at home, they are of no use at the time. The working hearing aid is the answer to the question.

Level of Cognitive Ability: Analysis
Phase of Nursing Process: Assessment
Client Needs: Psychosocial Integrity
Content Area: Adult Health/Musculoskeletal

Reference
Smeltzer, S., & Bare, B. (1996). *Brunner and Suddarth's textbook of medical-surgical nursing* (8th ed.). Philadelphia: Lippincott-Raven. p. 1930.

53. **3**

Rationale: Typical signs and symptoms following femoral neck fracture include shortening of the affected leg, adduction, and external rotation. The client may report slight groin pain, or pain in the medial side of the knee. Moving the fractured extremity significantly increases the pain.

Test-Taking Strategy: Knowledge of basic signs and symptoms of hip fracture is necessary to answer this question. A dislocated knee and a fracture of the midshaft of the femur are the least likely choices of the four, and should be eliminated first. Of the two remaining, elderly clients are much more likely to fracture the hip after sustaining a fall than to dislocate it. On this basis alone you could choose option 3 as the correct answer.

Level of Cognitive Ability: Analysis
Phase of Nursing Process: Analysis
Client Needs: Physiological Integrity
Content Area: Adult Health/Musculoskeletal

Reference
Smeltzer, S., & Bare, B. (1996). *Brunner and Suddarth's textbook of medical-surgical nursing* (8th ed.). Philadelphia: Lippincott-Raven. p. 1926.

54. **4**

Rationale: Safe nursing actions intended to prevent injury to the client include keeping side rails up, setting the bed in a low position, and providing a call bell that is within the client's reach. Responding promptly to the client's use of the call light minimizes the chance that the client will try to get up alone, which could result in a fall.

Test-Taking Strategy: The wording of this question asks you to identify an incorrect or potentially harmful item. Since options 1 and 3 (side rails up and call bell in reach) are standard nursing actions, they are eliminated as possible choices. Use of a nightlight would help prevent falls, which is also helpful, and can be eliminated as a choice. This leaves the delay in answering the call light as the correct answer. Delays will give the client reason to try to get up unattended, and risk another fall and possible injury.

Level of Cognitive Ability: Application
Phase of Nursing Process: Planning
Client Needs: Safe, Effective Care Environment
Content Area: Adult Health/Musculoskeletal

Reference
Smeltzer, S., & Bare, B. (1996). *Brunner and Suddarth's textbook of medical-surgical nursing* (8th ed.). Philadelphia: Lippincott-Raven. p. 1930.

55. **1**

Rationale: Following internal fixation of a hip fracture, the client is turned to the affected side or the unaffected side as prescribed by the surgeon. Before moving the client, the nurse places a pillow between the client's legs to keep the affected leg in abduction. The client is then repositioned while proper alignment and abduction are maintained.

Test-Taking Strategy: A trochanter roll is useful in preventing external rotation, but it is used once the client has been repositioned. It is not used while turning the client. Thus, options 3 and 4 may be readily eliminated. To discriminate between options 1 and 2, use of a pillow keeps the legs abducted, not adducted. Thus, option 1 is the answer to the question.

Level of Cognitive Ability: Application
Phase of Nursing Process: Implementation
Client Needs: Physiological Integrity
Content Area: Adult Health/Musculoskeletal

Reference
Smeltzer, S., & Bare, B. (1996). *Brunner and Suddarth's textbook of medical-surgical nursing* (8th ed.). Philadelphia: Lippincott-Raven. p. 1928.

56. **3**

Rationale: The client should use the walker by placing the hands on the hand grips for stability. The client lifts the walker to advance it, and leans forward slightly while moving it. The client walks into the walker, supporting the body weight on the hands while moving the weaker leg. A disadvantage of the walker is that it does not allow for reciprocal walking motion. If the client were to try to use reciprocal motion with a walker, the walker would advance forward one side at a time as the client walks; thus the client would not be supporting the weaker leg with the walker during ambulation.

Test-Taking Strategy: The question asks for an incorrect movement on the part of the client. Holding the walker using the hand grips is an obvious correct action, and is eliminated first. The client must lean forward slightly in order to move the walker forward, so this option is eliminated as well. Reciprocal motion is moving one leg and the opposite arm at the same time. If the client were trying to do this with a walker, the client would be twisting the walker from side to side as it advances. This would be incorrect, and is therefore the answer to the question as it is stated.

Level of Cognitive Ability: Analysis
Phase of Nursing Process: Evaluation
Client Needs: Health Promotion and Maintenance
Content Area: Adult Health/Musculoskeletal

Reference
Smeltzer, S., & Bare, B. (1996). *Brunner and Suddarth's textbook of medical-surgical nursing* (8th ed.). Philadelphia: Lippincott-Raven. p. 341.

57. **4**

Rationale: The client who has received a total knee replacement often has the leg put into a CPM machine while in the postanesthesia care unit. The device increases circulation and movement of the knee joint. It should be used as much as possible.

Test-Taking Strategy: Knowledge of the purpose and effects of a CPM machine is needed to answer this question correctly. If this question was difficult for you, take a few moments now to review these concepts.

Level of Cognitive Ability: Analysis
Phase of Nursing Process: Analysis
Client Needs: Physiological Integrity
Content Area: Adult Health/Musculoskeletal

Reference
Smeltzer, S., & Bare, B. (1996). *Brunner and Suddarth's textbook of medical-surgical nursing* (8th ed.). Philadelphia: Lippincott-Raven. p. 1877.

58. **1**

Rationale: The nurse assists the client to get out of bed on the first postoperative day after putting a knee immobilizer on the affected joint for stability. The surgeon orders the weight-bearing limits on the affected leg. The leg is elevated while the client is sitting in the chair to minimize edema.

Test-Taking Strategy: A compression dressing should already be in place on the wound, so option 2 should be eliminated first. Since the CPM machine is used only while the client is in bed, option 3 is incorrect and is eliminated also. To discriminate between the last two options, knowing that ambulation is not started until the second postoperative day would help you choose correctly. The knee immobilizer should be a natural choice when answering a question about protecting a knee joint.

Level of Cognitive Ability: Application
Phase of Nursing Process: Planning
Client Needs: Safe, Effective Care Environment
Content Area: Adult Health/Musculoskeletal

Reference
Smeltzer, S., & Bare, B. (1996). *Brunner and Suddarth's textbook of medical-surgical nursing* (8th ed.). Philadelphia: Lippincott-Raven. p. 1877.

59. **3**

Rationale: Pain with knee extension is a common complaint of clients after knee replacement. This is because preoperatively the client placed the knee in flexion to reduce pain, and flexion contracture has resulted. The nurse should encourage the client to keep the knee extended, and administer analgesics as needed.

Test-Taking Strategy: The stem of the question states that there is pain with extension only. Immobilizing the knee will not help, so this option may be eliminated first. Putting the joint through full range of motion may be more than the client can tolerate; also, the client usually has a CPM machine, which controls the amount of flexion and extension of the joint. To discriminate between the last two options, you need to know that flexion contracture may occur, which leads you to choose medicating the client rather than notifying the physician.

Level of Cognitive Ability: Application
Phase of Nursing Process: Implementation
Client Needs: Physiological Integrity
Content Area: Adult Health/Musculoskeletal

Reference
Black, J., & Matassarin-Jacobs, E. (1997). *Medical-surgical nursing: Clinical management for continuity of care* (5th ed.). Philadelphia: W. B. Saunders. p. 2119.

60. **2**

Rationale: After total knee replacement, clients should report signs and symptoms of infection, and any changes in the shape of the knee. Any of these could indicate developing complications. With a metal implant, the client must be on anticoagulant therapy, and should report adverse effects of this therapy, including bleeding from a variety of sources. With a metal implant, the client must notify caregivers, because MRI will need to be avoided, and the client will need antibiotic prophylaxis for invasive procedures.

Test-Taking Strategy: The stem states that there is a metal prosthesis, which indicates that anticoagulant therapy is indicated. This would make options 3 and 4 correct. It is important to report signs and symptoms of infection (option 1), so that is eliminated as the answer to this question as well. By default, the correct answer is option 2. The client also needs to report changes in the shape of the knee, as this could indicate developing complications with the prosthesis.

Level of Cognitive Ability: Analysis
Phase of Nursing Process: Evaluation
Client Needs: Health Promotion and Maintenance
Content Area: Adult Health/Musculoskeletal

Reference
Luckmann, J. (1997). *Saunders manual of nursing care*. Philadelphia: W. B. Saunders. p. 1610.

61. **3**

Rationale: Clients with diabetes mellitus are more prone to wound infection and delayed wound healing as a result of the disease. Postoperative stump edema and hemorrhage are complications in the immediate postoperative period that apply to any client with an amputation. Slight redness of the incision is considered normal, as long it is dry and intact.

Test-Taking Strategy: The stem guides you to look for complications that are primarily from the coexisting condition of diabetes mellitus. Knowing that diabetes increases the client's chances of developing infection and delayed wound healing helps you to eliminate options 1 and 2 first. Choose option 3 over option 4 because separation of wound edges is a more serious problem than a slight redness to the incision line, which is considered normal.

Level of Cognitive Ability: Application
Phase of Nursing Process: Assessment
Client Needs: Physiological Integrity
Content Area: Adult Health/Musculoskeletal

Reference
Black, J., & Matassarin-Jacobs, E. (1997). *Medical-surgical nursing: Clinical management for continuity of care* (5th ed.). Philadelphia: W. B. Saunders. p. 1420.

62. **1**

Rationale: Phantom limb sensations are felt in the area of the amputated limb. These can include itching, warmth, and cold. The sensations are a result of intact peripheral nerves in the amputed area. Whenever possible, clients should be prepared for these sensations. The client may also feel painful sensations in the amputated limb, called phantom limb pain. The origin of the pain is less well understood, but the client should be prepared for this, too, whenever possible.

Test-Taking Strategy: Knowing that sensation and pain may be felt in the residual limb helps you to eliminate options 3 and 4 first, because the sensations are not abnormal responses. Select option 1 over option 2 because the client has described an itching sensation but has not complained of pain in the residual limb.

Level of Cognitive Ability: Analysis
Phase of Nursing Process: Analysis
Client Needs: Psychosocial Integrity
Content Area: Adult Health/Musculoskeletal

Reference

Black, J., & Matassarin-Jacobs, E. (1997). *Medical-surgical nursing: Clinical management for continuity of care* (5th ed.). Philadelphia: W. B. Saunders. p. 1421.

63. **4**

Rationale: A stump sock must be worn at all times to absorb perspiration and is changed daily. The residual limb is washed, dried, and inspected for breakdown twice each day. The socket of the prosthesis is cleansed with a mild detergent, and rinsed and dried fully each day. A harsh bactericidal agent would not be used.

Test-Taking Strategy: To answer this question accurately, you need the baseline knowledge that the prosthesis is cared for daily, and the stump is cared for twice a day. With this in mind, you can eliminate option 1 easily. Wearing a stump sock for 3 to 4 days is excessive and not conducive to maintaining intact, clean skin. Option 2 is eliminated for the same reason. The frequency of care is insufficient because it should be done twice daily. To discriminate between options 3 and 4, you should know that a mild cleanser is used. Even without this knowledge, you may be able to pick the correct option by knowing that the prosthesis should be fully dry before use.

Level of Cognitive Ability: Application
Phase of Nursing Process: Planning
Client Needs: Health Promotion and Maintenance
Content Area: Adult Health/Musculoskeletal

Reference

Smeltzer, S., & Bare, B. (1996). *Brunner and Suddarth's textbook of medical-surgical nursing* (8th ed.). Philadelphia: Lippincott-Raven. p. 1943.

64. **2**

Rationale: If the client with amputation has a cast or elastic compression bandage that slips off, the nurse must immediately wrap the stump with another elastic compression bandage. Otherwise excessive edema will rapidly form, which could cause a significant delay in rehabilitation. If the client had a cast that slipped off, the nurse would also have to call the physician so that a new one could be applied.

Test-Taking Strategy: Eliminate option 4 first as the least plausible of options. Elevation on one pillow is not going to greatly impede the development of edema once compression is released. For the same reason, option 3 is discarded. Ice is of limited value in controlling edema from this cause. Of the remaining two, the better option is to reapply the compression bandage. If the physician were called, the order would likely be to reapply the compression dressing anyway. If the question dealt with a cast that came off, the area should still be wrapped with a compression bandage, but then the physician needs to be called immediately also.

Level of Cognitive Ability: Application
Phase of Nursing Process: Implementation
Client Needs: Physiological Integrity
Content Area: Adult Health/Musculoskeletal

Reference

Smeltzer, S., & Bare, B. (1996). *Brunner and Suddarth's textbook of medical-surgical nursing* (8th ed.). Philadelphia: Lippincott-Raven. p. 1939.

65. **4**

Rationale: The client should wear a clean woolen stump sock each day. The stump is cleansed daily with a gentle soap and water, and is dried carefully. Alcohol is avoided because it could cause drying or cracking of the skin. Oils and creams are also avoided because they are too softening to the skin for safe prosthesis use. The client should inspect all surfaces of the stump daily for irritation, blisters, or breakdown.

Test-Taking Strategy: Nylon is a synthetic material that does not allow the best air circulation and holds in moisture. For this reason, a stump sock is not made of nylon, and option 1 is incorrect. Either alcohol or lotion can interfere with the natural condition of the skin, increasing the likelihood of breakdown either from drying or from excess moisture. For these reasons, options 2 and 3 are also incorrect. By elimination, the answer is option 4. It is very important that the client assess skin integrity of the stump at least daily.

Level of Cognitive Ability: Analysis
Phase of Nursing Process: Evaluation
Client Needs: Health Promotion and Maintenance
Content Area: Adult Health/Musculoskeletal

Reference

Black, J., & Matassarin-Jacobs, E. (1997). *Medical-surgical nursing: Clinical management for continuity of care* (5th ed.). Philadelphia: W. B. Saunders. p. 1423.

66. **3**

Rationale: Low back pain with radiation into one leg (sciatica) is consistent with a herniated lumbar disk. The nurse assesses the client to see if the pain is aggravated by events that increase intraspinal pressure such as bending, lifting, sneezing, coughing, or with lifting the leg straight up while supine (straight-leg raising test).

Test-Taking Strategy: To answer this question successfully, you need to know the basic causes of back pain and factors that alleviate or aggravate it. With this knowledge you know that bed rest, heat (or sometimes ice), and nonsteroidal anti-inflammatory agents usually relieve back pain, whereas bending, lifting, and straining aggravate it. If this question was difficult, review these concepts briefly now because they are fundamental.

Level of Cognitive Ability: Application
Phase of Nursing Process: Assessment
Client Needs: Physiological Integrity
Content Area: Adult Health/Musculoskeletal

Reference

Smeltzer, S., & Bare, B. (1996). *Brunner and Suddarth's textbook of medical-surgical nursing* (8th ed.). Philadelphia: Lippincott-Raven. p. 1813.

67. **1**

Rationale: Compression of a nerve results in inflammation, which then irritates adjacent muscles, putting them into spasm. The pain of muscle spasm is continuous, knife-like, and localized in the affected area. Knowledge of pain characteristics and causes is useful to the nurse in planning appropriate measures to relieve them.

Test-Taking Strategy: Eliminate option 4 first as the least plausible of all the choices. Pressure on a spinal nerve root causes the symptoms of sciatica, so option 3 can be eliminated next. Pressure on the spinal cord itself could result in a variety of manifestations, depending on the area involved. The pain of muscle spasm has the characteristics described in the question, which helps you choose option 1 over option 2. Additionally, a herniated disk is stated in the question and again in the answer, option 1.

Level of Cognitive Ability: Analysis
Phase of Nursing Process: Analysis
Client Needs: Physiological Integrity
Content Area: Adult Health/Musculoskeletal

Reference
Ignatavicius, D., Workman, M., & Mishler, M. (1995). *Medical-surgical nursing: A nursing process approach* (2nd ed.). Philadelphia: W. B. Saunders. p. 1171.

68. **2**

Rationale: Clients with low back pain are often more comfortable when placed in Williams' position. The bed is placed in semi-Fowler's position with the knee gatch raised sufficiently to flex the knees. This relaxes the muscles of the lower back and relieves pressure on the spinal nerve root.

Test-Taking Strategy: Knowledge of this specific position helps you to answer this question quickly and easily. If you are not familiar with it, however, look at the information in the stem. The client has back pain with a ruptured intervertebral disk. Positions that relieve this discomfort include those that provide slight flexion of low back muscles, which relieves pressure and avoids extension of the spine. Keeping the foot of the bed flat will enhance extension of the spine, so options 1 and 3 should be eliminated first. Option 4 would excessively stretch the lower back and put the client at risk for thrombophlebitis. By the process of elimination, the correct answer is option 2.

Level of Cognitive Ability: Application
Phase of Nursing Process: Planning
Client Needs: Safe, Effective Care Environment
Content Area: Adult Health/Musculoskeletal

Reference
Ignatavicius, D., Workman, M., & Mishler, M. (1995). *Medical-surgical nursing: A nursing process approach* (2nd ed.). Philadelphia: W. B. Saunders. p. 1172.

69. **4**

Rationale: Following spinal fusion, the head of the bed is generally kept in a flat position. The client is log-rolled from side to side as ordered. Pillows may be placed under the entire length of the legs by surgeon preference to relieve tension on the lower back. The use of an overhead trapeze is contraindicated because its use could promote twisting of the spine after surgery.

Test-Taking Strategy: After spinal surgery, the nurse uses positioning techniques and aids that will keep the spine in good alignment. Thus, options 1 and 3 are obviously indicated, and are therefore eliminated as items to avoid as this question asks. To discriminate between the last two items, using pillows under the length of the legs promotes slight flexion of the spine while avoiding pressure on the popliteal

space (which predisposes to thrombophlebitis). This may be a helpful item. Using an overbed trapeze could allow the client to twist the spine, which is directly contraindicated. Thus, option 4 is the item to avoid.

Level of Cognitive Ability: Application
Phase of Nursing Process: Implementation
Client Needs: Safe, Effective Care Environment
Content Area: Adult Health/Musculoskeletal

Reference
Black, J., & Matassarin-Jacobs, E. (1997). *Medical-surgical nursing: Clinical management for continuity of care* (5th ed.). Philadelphia: W. B. Saunders. pp. 923–924.

70. **1**

Rationale: Clients are taught to get out of bed by sliding near to the edge of the mattress. The client then rolls onto one side and pushes up from the bed using one or both arms. The back is kept straight and the legs are swung over the side. Increasing fluids and dietary fiber helps prevent straining at stool, thereby preventing increases in intraspinal pressure. Walking and swimming are excellent exercises for strengthening low back muscles. Proper body mechanics include bending at the knees, not the waist, to lift objects.

Test-Taking Strategy: The wording of this question guides you to look for an incorrect action. Options 3 and 4 are examples of classic interventions that are indicated, and so they are eliminated as answers to this question as stated. Clients with low back pain should avoid events that increase intraspinal pressure. Option 2 prevents increases in intraspinal pressure. Option 1 causes an increase in intraspinal pressure if you think of the body mechanics involved in getting out of bed this way. Therefore, choose option 1 as the answer to the question as it is phrased.

Level of Cognitive Ability: Analysis
Phase of Nursing Process: Evaluation
Client Needs: Health Promotion and Maintenance
Content Area: Adult Health/Musculoskeletal

Reference
Black, J., & Matassarin-Jacobs, E. (1997). *Medical-surgical nursing: Clinical management for continuity of care* (5th ed.). Philadelphia: W. B. Saunders. p. 918.

71. **2**

Rationale: The nursing assessment conducted following spinal surgery is similar to that done after other surgical procedures. For this specific type of surgery, the nurse assesses the neurovascular status of the lower extremities, watches for signs and symptoms of infection, and inspects the surgical site for evidence of CSF leakage (drainage is clear and tests positive for glucose). A mild temperature is expected after insertion of hardware, but a temperature over 101°F should be reported because it might possibly require that the hardware be removed.

Test-Taking Strategy: Each of the options contains at least a slight deviation from normal. The question asks which option would cause the nurse to be "especially concerned." Thus, you are looking for the option that has the greatest deviation from normal. Options 1 and 4 are expected after surgery, and although the nurse tries to minimize discomfort, the client is likely to have some discomfort even with proper analgesic use. The words "old" and "outlined" in option 3 indicate that this is not a new occurrence, and is not alarming either. This leaves the temperature of 101°F, which is excessive, and should be reported.

Level of Cognitive Ability: Application
Phase of Nursing Process: Assessment
Client Needs: Physiological Integrity
Content Area: Adult Health/Musculoskeletal

Reference

Black, J., & Matassarin-Jacobs, E. (1997). *Medical-surgical nursing: Clinical management for continuity of care* (5th ed.). Philadelphia: W. B. Saunders. p. 923.

72. 3

Rationale: Following spinal surgery, concerns about finances and employment are best handled by referral to a social worker, who has the best well-rounded information about resources available to the client.

Test-Taking Strategy: An understanding of the roles of the various members of the health care team helps you to answer this question quickly and without hesitation. The physical therapist has the best knowledge of techniques for increasing mobility and endurance. An occupational therapist would have knowledge of techniques for ADLs and items related to occupation, but this is not one of the options. The clinical nurse specialist and physician do not have information related to financial resources. In fact, it is the need for information related to finances that is the real key to answering this question, and points to the social worker as the optimal resource in this instance.

Level of Cognitive Ability: Analysis
Phase of Nursing Process: Analysis
Client Needs: Psychosocial Integrity
Content Area: Adult Health/Musculoskeletal

Reference

Black, J., & Matassarin-Jacobs, E. (1997). *Medical-surgical nursing: Clinical management for continuity of care* (5th ed.). Philadelphia: W. B. Saunders. p. 923.

73. 2

Rationale: A back brace or thoracolumbarsacral orthosis is individually fitted to the client. The brace should not irritate the skin with proper fitting. The brace is applied in the morning before getting out of bed. The closures should be secure, but not overly loose or tight. A layer of clothing is worn between the orthosis and the skin.

Test-Taking Strategy: Skin irritation (option 1) is not likely to be a good sign, and should be eliminated first. Loose connections are also not likely to indicate proper fit, so option 4 should be eliminated next. Of the two remaining, you would not choose option 3 because the orthosis is likely to become soiled with perspiration or cause skin irritation. Thus, you are left with option 2, the correct choice. The brace is applied in the morning before getting out of bed to maintain the spine in good alignment and give it proper support.

Level of Cognitive Ability: Application
Phase of Nursing Process: Planning
Client Needs: Physiological Integrity
Content Area: Adult Health/Musculoskeletal

Reference

Luckmann, J. (1997). *Saunders manual of nursing care.* Philadelphia: W. B. Saunders. pp. 1565, 1567, 1611.

74. 4

Rationale: Following spinal fusion, with or without instrumentation, the client is transferred from stretcher to bed using a slider board and the assistance of four people. This permits optimal stabilization and support of the spine while allowing the client to be moved smoothly and gently.

Test-Taking Strategy: This question can be answered by analyzing the level of comfort and stability provided to the client's spine with the amounts of assistance given in each option. Using this approach, you can systematically eliminate each of the incorrect options.

Level of Cognitive Ability: Application
Phase of Nursing Process: Implementation
Client Needs: Safe, Effective Care Environment
Content Area: Adult Health/Musculoskeletal

Reference

Black, J., & Matassarin-Jacobs, E. (1997). *Medical-surgical nursing: Clinical management for continuity of care* (5th ed.). Philadelphia: W. B. Saunders. p. 923.

75. 1

Rationale: Stair climbing may be restricted or limited for several weeks following spinal fusion with instrumentation. The nurse ensures that resources are in place prior to discharge so that the client may sleep and perform all ADLs on a single living level.

Test-Taking Strategy: Options 2 and 3 are obviously useful to the client, and can therefore be eliminated as answers to the question as stated. To discriminate between options 1 and 4 (both of which involve stairs), option 4 is the least problematic, while option 1 poses a significant problem to the client who is restricted from stair climbing. Thus, option 1 is the answer to the question as it is stated.

Level of Cognitive Ability: Application
Phase of Nursing Process: Implementation
Client Needs: Safe, Effective Care Environment
Content Area: Adult Health/Musculoskeletal

Reference

Ignatavicius, D., Workman, M., & Mishler, M. (1995). *Medical-surgical nursing: A nursing process approach* (2nd ed.). Philadelphia: W. B. Saunders. p. 1181.

76. 3

Rationale: With an open fracture, the client is at risk of developing osteomyelitis, gas gangrene, and tetanus. The nurse assesses for the date of the last tetanus immunization to ensure that the client has tetanus prophylaxis.

Test-Taking Strategy: With an open-leg fracture, the client is at risk for infection; therefore, you need to look for an answer that is somehow related to this complication. Physical examination and chest x-ray are ruled out because they are unrelated to this problem. Of the remaining two, the client would be at risk for developing tetanus with this injury, but not tuberculosis. Thus, the answer is to inquire about the date of the last tetanus vaccine.

Level of Cognitive Ability: Application
Phase of Nursing Process: Assessment
Client Needs: Health Promotion and Maintenance
Content Area: Adult Health/Musculoskeletal

Reference

Smeltzer, S., & Bare, B. (1996). *Brunner and Suddarth's textbook of medical-surgical nursing* (8th ed.). Philadelphia: Lippincott-Raven. p. 1914.

77. 2

Rationale: Clients who use cadaver bone can develop psychological problems because of worry about contracting the HIV virus or hepatitis from the cadaver bone. Clients need reassurance and information about the donor screening that is done to ensure that this does not occur.

Test-Taking Strategy: Options 3 and 4 are the least likely options of the four available, so these are eliminated first. Both options 1 and 2 are realistic possibilities. The level of pain that will be experienced in the postoperative period should be included as part of the basic preparation of the client for surgery. Knowing that a common concern is contracting disease from cadaver bone leads you to select this option over concern about postoperative pain. Additionally, option 2 is specific to the information contained in the question.

Level of Cognitive Ability: Analysis
Phase of Nursing Process: Analysis
Client Needs: Psychosocial Integrity
Content Area: Adult Health/Musculoskeletal

Reference

Black, J., & Matassarin-Jacobs, E. (1997). *Medical-surgical nursing: Clinical management for continuity of care* (5th ed.). Philadelphia: W. B. Saunders. pp. 2145–2146.

78. 1

Rationale: Clients who experience fractures of the femur, pelvis, thorax, and spine are at risk for hypovolemic shock. Bone fragments can damage blood vessels, leading to hemorrhage into the abdominal cavity and the thigh. This can occur with closed fractures as well as with open fractures. Signs of hypovolemic shock include tachycardia and hypotension.

Test-Taking Strategy: To answer this question successfully, two things are required: first, you must know that hypovolemic shock is a complication after these types of fractures; second, you must know the signs and symptoms of hypovolemic shock. This helps you eliminate options 2, 3, and 4 because fever, bradycardia, and hypertension are not part of the clinical picture with hypovolemic shock. If you were looking for fat embolism as the complication, you would not find any options that match because these signs would include fever, tachycardia, tachypnea, and hypoxia.

Level of Cognitive Ability: Application
Phase of Nursing Process: Planning
Client Needs: Physiological Integrity
Content Area: Adult Health/Musculoskeletal

Reference

Black, J., & Matassarin-Jacobs, E. (1997). *Medical-surgical nursing: Clinical management for continuity of care* (5th ed.). Philadelphia: W. B. Saunders. p. 2139.

79. 4

Rationale: The client with pallor, slow capillary refill, weakened or lost pulse, and absence of sensation or motion to the distal limb may have arterial damage from a lacerated, contused, thrombosed, or severed artery. These signs can occur with constriction from a tight cast as well. Regardless of the cause, the nurse notifies the physician immediately. Emergency intervention is needed, which could include removal of the constricting bandage, fracture reduction, or surgery to repair the area.

Test-Taking Strategy: Knowing that these signs indicate insufficient arterial circulation, you know that this can lead to irreversible ischemia and damage. Because of this, you eliminate options 1 and 3 first as not being helpful. Rechecking the circulation in 30 minutes loses valuable time for action to restore the impaired circulation, and is a poor choice. The physician should be notified immediately.

Level of Cognitive Ability: Application
Phase of Nursing Process: Implementation
Client Needs: Physiological Integrity
Content Area: Adult Health/Musculoskeletal

Reference

Black, J., & Matassarin-Jacobs, E. (1997). *Medical-surgical nursing: Clinical management for continuity of care* (5th ed.). Philadelphia: W. B. Saunders. p. 2139.

80. 3

Rationale: The client who has partial weight-bearing status places 30% to 50% of the body weight on the affected limb. Full weight-bearing status is placing full weight on the limb. Nonweight-bearing status does not allow the client to let the limb touch the floor. Touchdown weight bearing allows the client to let the limb touch the floor but not bear weight. There is no classification for 60% to 80% weight-bearing status.

Test-Taking Strategy: To answer this question with ease, you need to be familiar with the different categories of weight bearing. Begin by eliminating options 1 and 2 first, using general knowledge. The word "partial" to describe weight bearing does not seem to fit either of these. Option 3 is a better descriptor than option 4 for partial also, which may help you to select this one as the correct answer.

Level of Cognitive Ability: Analysis
Phase of Nursing Process: Evaluation
Client Needs: Health Promotion and Maintenance
Content Area: Adult Health/Musculoskeletal

Reference

Black, J., & Matassarin-Jacobs, E. (1997). *Medical-surgical nursing: Clinical management for continuity of care* (5th ed.). Philadelphia: W. B. Saunders. p. 2156.

81. 4

Rationale: A window may be cut in a dried cast to relieve pressure, assess pulses, relieve discomfort, or remove drains. Bivalving the cast involves splitting the cast along both sides to allow swelling, to facilitate taking x-rays, or to make a half-cast for use as an intermittent splint. Padding is not placed on top of a cast. The use of an air splint is not indicated.

Test-Taking Strategy: The key phrase in the stem of this question is "bony prominence." Wherever there is a bony prominence, there is a risk of pressure and skin breakdown. If the pressure area is under a cast, the cast must be removed in that area to relieve the pressure. Therefore, options 1 and 3 can be readily eliminated. Since extra padding *over* the area of the cast does no good either, that option can be eliminated next. This leaves putting a window in the cast as the correct answer. This will relieve the pressure in that one area without disrupting the cast.

Level of Cognitive Ability: Analysis
Phase of Nursing Process: Analysis
Client Needs: Physiological Integrity
Content Area: Adult Health/Musculoskeletal

Reference

Black, J., & Matassarin-Jacobs, E. (1997). *Medical-surgical nursing: Clinical management for continuity of care* (5th ed.). Philadelphia: W. B. Saunders. p. 2149.

82. **1**

Rationale: Clients who are casted have some degree of decreased mobility, and should optimize nutrition to aid in healing. This can be accomplished by increasing intake of dietary fiber, drinking extra fluids, and taking in a well-balanced diet.

Test-Taking Strategy: The concepts that are useful in answering this question relate to wound healing and decreased mobility. The wording of the question is such that you are looking for an incorrect item. Knowing that wound healing requires balanced nutrition helps you to eliminate option 2. With decreased mobility there is a risk of constipation, so one needs increased fluid and dietary fiber to prevent this. Therefore, the option that does not fit with these requirements is the high-protein diet, which is the answer to the question as stated. Remember, the question asks for the item that will be least helpful.

Level of Cognitive Ability: Application
Phase of Nursing Process: Planning
Client Needs: Health Promotion and Maintenance
Content Area: Adult Health/Musculoskeletal

Reference

Black, J., & Matassarin-Jacobs, E. (1997). *Medical-surgical nursing: Clinical management for continuity of care* (5th ed.). Philadelphia: W. B. Saunders. p. 2151.

83. **4**

Rationale: Clients may be fearful of having a cast removed due to misconceptions about the cast-cutting blade. The nurse should show the cast cutter to the client before it is used, and explain that the client may feel heat, vibration, and pressure. The cast cutter resembles a small electric saw with a circular blade. The nurse should reassure the client that the blade does not cut like a saw, but instead cuts the cast by vibrating side to side.

Test-Taking Strategy: Note the question asks for the "most helpful" action, which tells you that more than one option may be partially or totally correct. Option 2 gives no information although it may be well intentioned, and is eliminated first. Options 1 and 3 give accurate information, but are not reassuring. Option 4 gives the client the most reassurance because it best prepares the client for what will occur when the cast is removed.

Level of Cognitive Ability: Application
Phase of Nursing Process: Implementation
Client Needs: Psychosocial Integrity
Content Area: Adult Health/Musculoskeletal

Reference

Black, J., & Matassarin-Jacobs, E. (1997). *Medical-surgical nursing: Clinical management for continuity of care* (5th ed.). Philadelphia: W. B. Saunders. p. 2152.

84. **2**

Rationale: The skin under a casted area may be discolored and crusted with dead skin layers. The client should gently soak and wash the skin for the first few days. The skin should be patted dry, and a lubricating lotion should be applied. Clients often want to scrub the dead skin away, which irritates the skin. The client should avoid overexposing the skin to the sunlight.

Test-Taking Strategy: The question is worded to make you look for an incorrect item. Option 3 is obviously helpful, and therefore cannot be the answer to the question as stated. Option 4 is good advice if the skin has been covered, and is eliminated next. Options 1 and 2 seem to oppose each other, making it likely that one of them is correct. Because vigorous scrubbing is more likely to be irritating than providing gentle soaking, it is the most likely choice as the answer to the question.

Level of Cognitive Ability: Analysis
Phase of Nursing Process: Evaluation
Client Needs: Health Promotion and Maintenance
Content Area: Adult Health/Musculoskeletal

Reference

Black, J., & Matassarin-Jacobs, E. (1997). *Medical-surgical nursing: Clinical management for continuity of care* (5th ed.). Philadelphia: W. B. Saunders. pp. 2152–2153.

85. **4**

Rationale: Common areas that are under pressure and are at risk for breakdown include the elbows (if they are used for repositioning instead of a trapeze) and the heel of the good leg (which is used as a brace when pushing up in bed). Other pressure points caused by the traction include the ischial tuberosity, popliteal space, and Achilles tendon.

Test-Taking Strategy: The question asks for an area at high risk for breakdown. Thus, you would compare each of the options in terms of their relative risk, and choose the one that is greatest. The right heel is eliminated first because it is off the bed in the traction set-up. The overhead trapeze would diminish the likelihood that the scapulae and back of the head would be immobile. This leaves the left heel as the answer to the question. This makes sense, given that the client would use the unaffected heel to push into the mattress during repositioning. With repeated use, this could cause the left heel to become reddened and break down.

Level of Cognitive Ability: Application
Phase of Nursing Process: Assessment
Client Needs: Physiological Integrity
Content Area: Adult Health/Musculoskeletal

Reference

Smeltzer, S., & Bare, B. (1996). *Brunner and Suddarth's textbook of medical-surgical nursing* (8th ed.). Philadelphia: Lippincott-Raven, p. 1862.

86. **1**

Rationale: The client is at risk for Body Image Disturbance related to a change in the structure and function of the affected leg. There are no data in the stem to support a diagnosis of (actual) Activity Intolerance or Social Isolation. The client does have an actual Impaired Mobility because of the fixation device.

Test-Taking Strategy: The key words in the stem include "external fixation device," "edematous," and "misshapen." Given these descriptions, the defining characteristics for Body Image Disturbance match most readily. The only other option that is plausible given the information in the stem is the Impaired Physical Mobility. However, this is an actual problem for the client, whereas option 3 identifies this as a risk diagnosis, making option 3 incorrect.

Level of Cognitive Ability: Analysis
Phase of Nursing Process: Analysis
Client Needs: Psychosocial Integrity
Content Area: Adult Health/Musculoskeletal

References

Cox, H., Hinz, M., Lubno, M., et al. (1997). *Clinical applications of nursing diagnosis: Adult, child, women's, psychiatric, gerontic and home health considerations* (3rd ed.). Philadelphia: F. A. Davis. p. 506.

Ignatavicius, D., Workman, M., & Mishler, M. (1995). *Medical-surgical nursing: A nursing process approach* (2nd ed.). Philadelphia: W. B. Saunders. p. 1464.

87. 3

Rationale: The use of an overhead trapeze is extremely helpful in helping a client to move about in bed, and to get on and off the bedpan. This device has the greatest value in increasing overall bed mobility. A fracture bedpan is useful in reducing discomfort with elimination. Television and reading materials are helpful in reducing boredom and providing distraction.

Test-Taking Strategy: Note the phrase "most helpful" in the stem, which is seeking to identify options that will increase bed mobility. Although all options are useful to the client in skeletal traction, the only one that helps with overall bed mobility is the trapeze.

Level of Cognitive Ability: Application
Phase of Nursing Process: Planning
Client Needs: Health Promotion and Maintenance
Content Area: Adult Health/Musculoskeletal

Reference

Smeltzer, S., & Bare, B. (1996). *Brunner and Suddarth's textbook of medical-surgical nursing* (8th ed.). Philadelphia: Lippincott-Raven. p. 1862.

88. 2

Rationale: The part of the bed under an area in traction is usually elevated to aid in countertraction. For the client in Buck's extension traction (which is applied to a leg), the foot of the bed is elevated.

Test-Taking Strategy: To answer this question accurately, you need to understand the principles of traction and countertraction, and to be familiar with Buck's extension traction. Option 3 is not used for the purpose of countertraction, and is eliminated as a possible answer. Knowing that Buck's extension traction is applied to the leg helps to eliminate option 1. Of the two remaining choices, option 4 places undue pressure on the client's unaffected foot. Furthermore, a footboard is not used for the purpose of providing countertraction. Option 2 provides a force that opposes the traction force effectively without harming the client, and is the answer to the question.

Level of Cognitive Ability: Application
Phase of Nursing Process: Implementation
Client Needs: Safe, Effective Care Environment
Content Area: Adult Health/Musculoskeletal

Reference

Black, J., & Matassarin-Jacobs, E. (1997). *Medical-surgical nursing: Clinical management for continuity of care* (5th ed.). Philadelphia: W. B. Saunders. p. 2137.

89. 4

Rationale: Expected outcomes for Impaired Physical Mobility for the client in traction include absence of thrombophlebitis (measurable by negative Homan's sign), active baseline ROM to uninvolved joints, clear lung sounds, intact skin, and bowel movement every other day.

Test-Taking Strategy: This question can be answered systematically by evaluating the degree of normalcy of each of the options. The only abnormal option is option 4. A bowel movement every 4 days is insufficient. Constipation is a known complication of immobility.

Level of Cognitive Ability: Analysis
Phase of Nursing Process: Evaluation
Client Needs: Physiological Integrity
Content Area: Adult Health/Musculoskeletal

Reference

Black, J., & Matassarin-Jacobs, E. (1997). *Medical-surgical nursing: Clinical management for continuity of care* (5th ed.). Philadelphia: W. B. Saunders. p. 2143.

90. 2

Rationale: Common gastrointestinal side effects of benztropine therapy include constipation and dry mouth. Other GI side effects include nausea and ileus. These effects are the result of the anticholinergic properties of the drug.

Test-Taking Strategy: In examining the options, diarrhea and hyperactive bowel sounds are similar, so it is not likely that either of them is the correct answer. To discriminate between the last two, knowing that the medication is an anticholinergic helps you to choose dry mouth over increased appetite as the side effect to assess for.

Level of Cognitive Ability: Application
Phase of Nursing Process: Assessment
Client Needs: Physiological Integrity
Content Area: Pharmacology

Reference

Hodgson, B., & Kizior, R. (1998). *Saunders nursing drug handbook 1998.* Philadelphia: W. B. Saunders. pp. 102–104.

91. 4

Rationale: The client should not receive cyclobenzaprine if the client has taken monoamine oxidase (MAO) inhibitors such as tranylcypromine (Parnate) or phenelzine (Nardil) within the last 14 days. Otherwise, the client could experience hyperpyretic crisis, convulsions, or death.

Test-Taking Strategy: To answer this question correctly, it is necessary to know that cyclobenzaprine may not have been taken with MAO inhibitors within the last 14 days. If you had difficulty with this question, take a few moments now to review this medication.

Level of Cognitive Ability: Analysis
Phase of Nursing Process: Analysis
Client Needs: Safe, Effective Care Environment
Content Area: Pharmacology

Reference

Hodgson, B., & Kizior, R. (1999). *Saunders nursing drug handbook 1999.* Philadelphia: W. B. Saunders. pp. 269–270.

92. 3

Rationale: The client should remain in bed for at least 3 hours following a parenteral dose of diazepam. The drug is a centrally acting skeletal muscle relaxant and also has antianxiety, sedative-hypnotic, and anticonvulsant properties. Cardiopulmonary side effects of the drug include apnea, hypotension, bradycardia, or cardiac arrest. For this reason, resuscitative equipment is also kept nearby.

Test-Taking Strategy: Knowledge of the effects of diazepam administered intravenously would help to eliminate the 30- and 60-minute time frames as too brief. Eight hours, on the other hand, is excessive, which leaves the 3-hour time frame as the correct answer. This is a prudent choice.

Level of Cognitive Ability: Application
Phase of Nursing Process: Planning
Client Needs: Safe, Effective Care Environment
Content Area: Pharmacology

Reference

Hodgson, B., & Kizior, R. (1999). *Saunders nursing drug handbook 1999.* Philadelphia: W. B. Saunders. pp. 307–309.

93. 1

Rationale: The recommended rate of infusion of diazepam is to give each 5 mg of the drug over at least 1 minute. This will prevent adverse side effects including apnea, bradycardia, hypotension, or possibly cardiac arrest.

Test-Taking Strategy: A majority of medications administered intravenously to a client must be given over at least 1 minute. Because of this, you eliminate options 3 and 4 first as excessively brief. Of the two remaining, it is much more likely that it is given over 1 minute than 2. This is because the administration rate would be 5 mg/minute (option 1) rather than 2.5 mg/minute (option 2).

Level of Cognitive Ability: Application
Phase of Nursing Process: Implementation
Client Needs: Physiological Integrity
Content Area: Pharmacology

Reference

Hodgson, B., & Kizior, R. (1999). *Saunders nursing drug handbook 1999.* Philadelphia: W. B. Saunders. pp. 307–309.

94. 3

Rationale: Carisoprodol, a centrally acting skeletal muscle relaxant, may cause CNS side effects of drowsiness and dizziness. For this reason, the client avoids other CNS depressants, such as alcohol, while taking this medication. Driving or other activities requiring mental alertness are also avoided until the client's reaction to the medication is known. The drug is used to reduce muscle spasticity and pain. Missed doses should be taken if remembered within 1 hour.

Test-Taking Strategy: Begin to answer this question by eliminating option 4, because driving is either indicated or not indicated. Knowing that this medication is a skeletal muscle relaxant helps you to eliminate option 1 next because this medication relieves muscle spasms. To discriminate between the last two, knowing that alcohol should not be taken while on any medication that affects the CNS helps you to choose option 3 over option 2 as the correct answer.

Level of Cognitive Ability: Analysis
Phase of Nursing Process: Evaluation
Client Needs: Health Promotion and Maintenance
Content Area: Pharmacology

Reference

Hodgson, B., & Kizior, R. (1999). *Saunders nursing drug handbook 1999.* Philadelphia: W. B. Saunders. pp. 151, 1187.

95. 1

Rationale: The nurse carefully monitors the client's blood counts, since hematological side effects of this therapy include aplastic anemia, agranulocytosis, leukopenia, and thrombocytopenia. Other values that warrant monitoring include serum calcium levels, and the results of urinalysis, hepatic, and thyroid function tests.

Test-Taking Strategy: To answer this question accurately, you should understand that phenytoin has a number of hematological side effects. This would allow you to eliminate each of the other options systematically. If this question was difficult, review this medication again briefly now. It is commonly ordered, and has specific side effects to watch for and prevent.

Level of Cognitive Ability: Application
Phase of Nursing Process: Assessment
Client Needs: Physiological Integrity
Content Area: Pharmacology

Reference

Hodgson, B., & Kizior, R. (1999). *Saunders nursing drug handbook 1999.* Philadelphia: W. B. Saunders. pp. 823–825.

96. 1

Rationale: Drowsiness, unsteadiness, and clumsiness are expected effects of the drug during early therapy. They are dose related, and usually diminish or disappear altogether with continued use of the drug. They do not indicate that a severe side effect is occurring. They are also unrelated to interaction with another medication. The client is encouraged to take this medication with food to minimize GI upset.

Test-Taking Strategy: To answer this question successfully, you need to know that these effects occur early in the course of therapy. If needed, take a few moments now to review this medication.

Level of Cognitive Ability: Analysis
Phase of Nursing Process: Analysis
Client Needs: Physiological Integrity
Content Area: Pharmacology

Reference

Hodgson, B., & Kizior, R. (1999). *Saunders nursing drug handbook 1999.* Philadelphia: W. B. Saunders. pp. 238–240.

97. 2

Rationale: Clonazepam is a benzodiazepine that is used as an anticonvulsant. During initial therapy and during periods of dosage adjustment, the nurse should initiate seizure precautions for the client.

Test-Taking Strategy: Knowing that the medication is an anticonvulsant, the natural choice for the answer is the seizure precautions. The key information in the stem that leads you to this is the information about the dosage being adjusted. This could put the client at risk for return of seizure activity and makes it the only reasonable choice given the wording of the question.

Level of Cognitive Ability: Application
Phase of Nursing Process: Planning
Client Needs: Safe, Effective Care Environment
Content Area: Pharmacology

Reference

Hodgson, B., & Kizior, R. (1999). *Saunders nursing drug handbook 1999.* Philadelphia: W. B. Saunders. pp. 238–240.

98. 4

Rationale: Precipitation will occur if phenytoin is admixed with any solution other than 0.9% normal saline (NS). This is especially true of solutions containing dextrose. An inline filter reduces the chance of precipitants entering the blood stream. Phenytoin is very irritating to the vein wall or other tissues.

Test-Taking Strategy: A very important concept related to intravenous phenytoin (Dilantin) administration is that the medication can only be mixed in 0.9% NS. It cannot be mixed in a dextrose solution. This helps you to eliminate options 1 and 3 first. To choose between 2 and 4 without specifically knowing that 0.9% NS is the answer, knowing that phenytoin precipitates easily may help you to choose the correct answer, because option 4 also includes the use of an inline filter.

Level of Cognitive Ability: Application
Phase of Nursing Process: Implementation
Client Needs: Physiological Integrity
Content Area: Pharmacology

Reference

Hodgson, B., & Kizior, R. (1999). *Saunders nursing drug handbook 1999.* Philadelphia: W. B. Saunders. pp. 823–825.

99. **3**

Rationale: The therapeutic range for serum phenytoin levels is 10 to 20 µg/mL in clients with normal serum albumin levels and renal function. A level below this range indicates that the client is not receiving sufficient medication and is at risk for seizure activity. The medication dose should be adjusted upward. A level above this range indicates that the client is entering the toxic range and is at risk for toxic side effects of the medication. In this case, the dose should be adjusted downward.

Test-Taking Strategy: To answer this question accurately, you need to know the therapeutic drug level. This is a helpful value range to memorize now.

Level of Cognitive Ability: Analysis
Phase of Nursing Process: Evaluation
Client Needs: Health Promotion and Maintenance
Content Area: Pharmacology

Reference

Hodgson, B., & Kizior, R. (1999). *Saunders nursing drug handbook 1999.* Philadelphia: W. B. Saunders. pp. 823–825.

100. **2**

Rationale: Clorazepate is classified as an anticonvulsant, antianxiety agent, and sedative/hypnotic (benzodiazepine). One of the nursing implications of clorazepate therapy is that the medication can lead to physical or psychological dependence when there is prolonged therapy at high doses. For this reason, the amount of medication that is readily available to the client at any one time is restricted.

Test-Taking Strategy: Knowing that the medication is a benzodiazepine leads you to conclude that this medication can lead to physical as well as psychological dependence. This helps you eliminate each of the incorrect options in turn.

Level of Cognitive Ability: Analysis
Phase of Nursing Process: Analysis
Client Needs: Psychosocial Integrity
Content Area: Pharmacology

Reference

Hodgson, B., & Kizior, R. (1999). *Saunders nursing drug handbook 1999.* Philadelphia: W. B. Saunders. pp. 242–243.

101. **1**

Rationale: Valproic acid is an anticonvulsant that causes CNS depression. For this reason, the side effects of the medication include sedation, dizziness, ataxia, and confusion. When the client is taking this medication as a single daily dose,

administering it at bedtime negates the risk of injury from sedation and enhances client safety.

Test-Taking Strategy: Begin to answer this question by recalling that this medication is an anticonvulsant with CNS depressant properties. This train of thought leads you to think of sedation as a key side effect. Looking at the choices given for dosage times, the one that makes the most sense is the bedtime administration. This would allow the sedative effects of the medication to occur at a time when the client is sleeping, with less likelihood that the client will become injured because of the drug's effects.

Level of Cognitive Ability: Application
Phase of Nursing Process: Planning
Client Needs: Safe, Effective Care Environment
Content Area: Pharmacology

Reference

Lehne, R. (1998). *Pharmacology for nursing care* (3rd ed.). Philadelphia: W. B. Saunders. pp. 212–213, 274, 318.

102. **3**

Rationale: Carbamazepine is an anticonvulsant that should be taken around the clock, precisely as directed. If a dose is omitted, the client should take the dose as soon as it is remembered, as long as it is not immediately prior to the next dose. The medication should not be double-dosed. If more than once dose is omitted, the client should call the physician.

Test-Taking Strategy: A general rule of client teaching with medication is that medications are not double-dosed if one dose is missed. Therefore, eliminate option 1 first as an answer. To choose among the remaining options, knowing that the medication is an anticonvulsant may help you eliminate option 2 next. It is important for the client to receive the medication to suppress seizure activity. The same reasoning may also help you to choose option 3 over option 4.

Level of Cognitive Ability: Application
Phase of Nursing Process: Implementation
Client Needs: Physiological Integrity
Content Area: Pharmacology

Reference

Deglin, J., & Vallerand, A. (1997). *Davis's drug guide for nurses* (5th ed.). Philadelphia: F. A. Davis. p. 215.

103. **2**

Rationale: Carbamazepine acts by depressing synaptic transmission in the CNS. Because of this, the client should avoid driving or doing other activities that require mental alertness until the effect on the client is known. The client should use protective clothing and sunscreen to avoid photosensitivity reactions. The medication may cause dry mouth, and the client should be instructed to provide good oral hygiene and use sugarless candy or gum as needed. The medication should not be abruptly discontinued, because it could cause return of seizures or status epilepticus. Fever and sore throat (leukopenia) should be reported to the physician.

Test-Taking Strategy: Begin to answer this question by recalling that this is an anticonvulsant medication with CNS depressant properties. This leads you to discard option 1 first, because driving in general could be hazardous, but it has nothing to do with night vision. Option 4 is eliminated next because an anticonvulsant is not abruptly discontinued because side effects or infection occurs. Rather, the physician should be called. To choose between the remaining alternatives, remembering that carbamazepine causes dry mouth may help you to eliminate option 3, and choose option 2 as the answer. Photosensitivity can occur with this medication.

Level of Cognitive Ability: Analysis
Phase of Nursing Process: Evaluation
Client Needs: Health Promotion and Maintenance
Content Area: Pharmacology

Reference
Lehne, R. (1998). *Pharmacology for nursing care* (3rd ed.). Philadelphia: W. B. Saunders. pp. 207, 211–212, 318.

104. **4**

Rationale: Ergotamine produces vasoconstriction by stimulating alpha-adrenergic receptors and suppresses vascular headaches when given at therapeutic dose range. The nurse periodically assess for hypertension; cool, numb fingers and toes; muscle pain; and nausea and vomiting.

Test-Taking Strategy: To answer this question, first recall that vascular headaches are caused by vasodilation of the blood vessels in the head. Following this train of thought you then recall that this medication must cause vasoconstriction. This helps you to eliminate each of the incorrect options. The only side effect consistent with vasoconstriction is option 4, the cool, numb fingers and toes.

Level of Cognitive Ability: Application
Phase of Nursing Process: Assessment
Client Needs: Physiological Integrity
Content Area: Pharmacology

Reference
Deglin, J., & Vallerand, A. (1997). *Davis's drug guide for nurses* (5th ed.). Philadelphia: F. A. Davis. p. 438.

105. **3**

Rationale: Edrophonium is commonly given to test for myasthenic crisis. If the client is in myasthenic crisis, muscle strength improves after administration of the medication and lasts for about 30 minutes.

Test-Taking Strategy: This question is difficult to answer as stated without specific knowledge of the medication. You might eliminate options 1 and 2 as excessively brief, but you need to know that it lasts for 30 minutes to choose between options 3 and 4. This is a very important medication with which to be familiar. Take the time to review this medication now.

Level of Cognitive Ability: Analysis
Phase of Nursing Process: Analysis
Client Needs: Physiological Integrity
Content Area: Pharmacology

Reference
Hodgson, B., & Kizior, R. (1999). *Saunders nursing drug handbook 1999*. Philadelphia: W. B. Saunders. p. 1135.

106. **1**

Rationale: Dextroamphetamine is a CNS stimulant that acts by releasing norepinephrine from nerve endings. The client should take the medication at least 6 hours before going to bed at night to prevent disturbances with sleep.

Test-Taking Strategy: To answer this question successfully, you should remember that this medication causes CNS stimulation, which interferes with sleep. Knowing this, you

evaluate each of the options in terms of how far removed the scheduled dose is from the client's bedtime. Evaluating the question in this fashion helps you to eliminate each of the other incorrect options easily.

Level of Cognitive Ability: Application
Phase of Nursing Process: Planning
Client Needs: Psychosocial Integrity
Content Area: Pharmacology

Reference
Deglin, J., & Vallerand, A. (1997). *Davis's drug guide for nurses* (5th ed.). Philadelphia: F. A. Davis. pp. 339, 341.

107. **2**

Rationale: Dextroamphetamine is a CNS stimulant. Caffeine is a stimulant also and should be limited in the client taking this medication. The client should be taught to limit personal caffeine intake as well.

Test-Taking Strategy: To answer this question quickly and accurately, you should remember that this medication is a CNS stimulant. You then evaluate each of the options in terms of the additive stimulation provided by the items listed as options. Knowing that caffeine is also a stimulant helps you choose this as the item to be limited.

Level of Cognitive Ability: Application
Phase of Nursing Process: Implementation
Client Needs: Safe, Effective Care Environment
Content Area: Pharmacology

Reference
Deglin, J., & Vallerand, A. (1997). *Davis's drug guide for nurses* (5th ed.). Philadelphia: F. A. Davis. p. 341.

108. **4**

Rationale: Signs and symptoms of Parkinson's disease usually begin to resolve within 2 to 3 weeks of starting therapy, although in some clients marked improvement may not be seen for up to 6 months. Clients need to understand this concept to aid in compliance with medication therapy.

Test-Taking Strategy: To answer this question accurately, you need to know when the drug begins to produce the expected effects. If this question was difficult, you should take a few moments to briefly review this medication.

Level of Cognitive Ability: Analysis
Phase of Nursing Process: Evaluation
Client Needs: Health Promotion and Maintenance
Content Area: Pharmacology

Reference
Deglin, J., & Vallerand, A. (1997). *Davis's drug guide for nurses* (5th ed.). Philadelphia: F. A. Davis. p. 694.

109. **2**

Rationale: Trihexyphenidyl is an anticholinergic medication. Because of this, it can cause urinary hesitancy and retention, constipation, dry mouth, and decreased sweating as side effects.

Test-Taking Strategy: The key to answering this question lies in knowing that this medication has anticholinergic action. By evaluating each of the options in terms of their consistency with anticholinergic effects, you eliminate each of the incorrect options. Also, because options 1 and 2 directly oppose each other, you may automatically be drawn to choose between one of them as the correct answer.

Level of Cognitive Ability: Application
Phase of Nursing Process: Assessment
Client Needs: Physiological Integrity
Content Area: Pharmacology

Reference

Hodgson, B., & Kizior, R. (1999). *Saunders nursing drug handbook 1999.* Philadelphia: W. B. Saunders. pp. 1027–1029.

110. 3

Rationale: With carbidopa/levodopa therapy, a darkening of the urine or sweat may occur. The client should be reassured that this is a harmless effect of the medication, and its use should be continued.

Test-Taking Strategy: Knowledge of the side effects of this medication is needed to answer this question. If you are unfamiliar with it, you may want to take a few moments now to review this medication. It is always helpful to alert the client to side effects that could possibly be considered distasteful.

Level of Cognitive Ability: Analysis
Phase of Nursing Process: Analysis
Client Needs: Psychosocial Integrity
Content Area: Pharmacology

Reference

Deglin, J., & Vallerand, A. (1997). *Davis's drug guide for nurses* (5th ed.). Philadelphia: F. A. Davis. p. 692.

111. 4

Rationale: Pyridostigmine is a cholinergic medication used to increase muscle strength for the client with myasthenia gravis. For the client who has difficulty chewing, the medication may be administered 30 minutes before meals to enhance the client's ability to eat.

Test-Taking Strategy: The key to answering this question is the client's difficulty with chewing. Knowing that the medication increases muscle strength may lead you to choose to give the medication 30 minutes before meals, so the client has the ability to chew the food.

Level of Cognitive Ability: Application
Phase of Nursing Process: Planning
Client Needs: Health Promotion and Maintenance
Content Area: Pharmacology

Reference

Hodgson, B., & Kizior, R. (1999). *Saunders nursing drug handbook 1999.* Philadelphia: W. B. Saunders. pp. 888–890, 1135.

112. 1

Rationale: The client should take neostigmine exactly on time. Taking the medication early or late could result in myasthenic or cholinergic crisis. Taking the medication on time is especially important for the client with dysphagia because the client may not be able to swallow the medication if it is given late. These clients are taught to set a battery alarm clock to remind them of dosage times. The client should never skip or double up on missed doses. The medication should be administered with food or milk to minimize side effects.

Test-Taking Strategy: The stem tells you that the client has frequent myasthenic and cholinergic crises. If you know that these are triggered by insufficient and excessive medication, respectively, then you automatically eliminate options 2 and 4 first. The same reasoning will help you to choose option 1 over option 3.

Level of Cognitive Ability: Application
Phase of Nursing Process: Implementation
Client Needs: Physiological Integrity
Content Area: Pharmacology

Reference

Hodgson, B., & Kizior, R. (1999). *Saunders nursing drug handbook 1999.* Philadelphia: W. B. Saunders. pp. 732–735, 1135.

113. 3

Rationale: Amantadine is an antiparkinsonian agent that potentiates the action of dopamine in the CNS. The expected effect of therapy is a decrease in akinesia and rigidity. Leukopenia, urinary retention, and hypotension are all adverse effects of the medication.

Test-Taking Strategy: Begin to answer this question by recalling that this medication is used to treat Parkinson's disease. This leads you to choose option 3 as the expected effects of the medication. Thorough knowledge of the medication reinforces that the other options are incorrect, because they are all side effects of the drug.

Level of Cognitive Ability: Analysis
Phase of Nursing Process: Evaluation
Client Needs: Physiological Integrity
Content Area: Pharmacology

Reference

Hodgson, B., & Kizior, R. (1999). *Saunders nursing drug handbook 1999.* Philadelphia: W. B. Saunders. pp. 35–37, 1126.

114. 1

Rationale: Risk factors associated with osteoporosis include a diet that is deficient in calcium. Options 2, 3, and 4 include risk factors associated with osteoporosis. Additional risk factors include sedentariness, cigarette smoking, excessive alcohol consumption, chronic illness, and long-term use of anticonvulsants and furosemide.

Test Taking Strategy: Knowledge regarding the risk factors associated with osteoporosis is required to answer this question. Review these risk factors now if you are not familiar with them.

Level of Cognitive Ability: Analysis
Phase of Nursing Process: Assessment
Client Needs: Health Promotion and Maintenance
Content Area: Adult Health/Musculoskeletal

Reference

Black, J., & Matassarin-Jacobs, E. (1997). *Medical-surgical nursing: Clinical management for continuity of care* (5th ed.). Philadelphia: W. B. Saunders. p. 2102.

115. 4

Rationale: Maintaining body weight at or above minimum recommended levels is a primary prevention measure. Additional primary prevention measures include achieving optimal calcium intake, performing regular exercise, avoiding smoking and alcohol consumption, avoiding a high-sodium and high-protein diet, and adequate amounts of vitamin D. Options 1, 2, and 3 include secondary preventive measures.

Test-Taking Strategy: Use knowledge regarding the differences between primary and secondary prevention measures to answer the question. If you are unfamiliar with the differences, review now. This knowledge will easily guide you to option 4.

Level of Cognitive Ability: Analysis
Phase of Nursing Process: Assessment
Client Needs: Health Promotion and Maintenance
Content Area: Adult Health/Musculoskeletal

Reference

Black, J., & Matassarin-Jacobs, E. (1997). *Medical-surgical nursing: Clinical management for continuity of care* (5th ed.). Philadelphia: W. B. Saunders. p. 2102.

116. 4

Rationale: Foods high in calcium include plain yogurt, dairy products, seafood, sardines, green vegetables, calcium-fortified orange juice, and cereal. Of the items listed, option 4 contains the least amount of calcium.

Test-Taking Strategy: Note the key word "least" in the stem of the question. By the process of elimination, you should easily be directed to option 4. Review foods high in calcium now, if you had difficulty with this question!

Level of Cognitive Ability: Analysis
Phase of Nursing Process: Analysis
Client Needs: Health Promotion and Maintenance
Content Area: Adult Health/Musculoskeletal

Reference

Black, J., & Matassarin-Jacobs, E. (1997). *Medical-surgical nursing: Clinical management for continuity of care* (5th ed.). Philadelphia: W. B. Saunders. p. 2105.

117. 1

Rationale: In addition to the presence of clinical manifestations, gout is diagnosed by the presence of persistent hyperuricemia greater than 7 mg/dL. Options 2, 3, and 4 all indicate normal laboratory values. Additionally, the presence of uric acid in an aspirated sample of synovial fluid confirms the diagnosis.

Test-Taking Strategy: Knowledge of normal laboratory values will easily direct you to option 1. Options 2, 3, and 4 identify normal lab values, whereas option 1 indicates an elevated value. Review normal laboratory values now if you had difficulty with this question!

Level of Cognitive Ability: Analysis
Phase of Nursing Process: Assessment
Client Needs: Physiological Integrity
Content Area: Adult Health/Musculoskeletal

Reference

Black, J., & Matassarin-Jacobs, E. (1997). *Medical-surgical nursing: Clinical management for continuity of care* (5th ed.). Philadelphia: W. B. Saunders. p. 2107.

118. 1

Rationale: Ample fluid intake is encouraged to promote excretion of uric acid. The client is placed on bed rest until the pain subsides. A diet low in purine is normally prescribed, which includes a decrease in red and organ meats. NSAIDs are used to reduce pain and inflammation. Colchicine, which also may be prescribed, reduces the migration of leukocytes to the synovial fluid.

Test-Taking Strategy: Note the key word "not" in the stem of the question. Also note the key word "acute." This will assist in eliminating options 3 and 4. Knowledge that a low-purine diet may be recommended for the client with gout will easily direct you to option 1. Review care to the client with gout now if you had difficulty with this question!

Level of Cognitive Ability: Application
Phase of Nursing Process: Implementation
Client Needs: Health Promotion and Maintenance
Content Area: Adult Health/Musculoskeletal

Reference

Black, J., & Matassarin-Jacobs, E. (1997). *Medical-surgical nursing: Clinical management for continuity of care* (5th ed.). Philadelphia: W. B. Saunders. p. 2102.

119. 3

Rationale: The stiffness and joint pain that occur in osteoarthritis increase with lack of activity, are usually more severe in the morning, and may be aggravated by cold, damp weather. No specific laboratory findings are useful in diagnosing osteoarthritis. The client may have a normal or slightly elevated sedimentation rate. Dull, aching pain occurs in the affected joints and unlike rheumatoid arthritis, systemic manifestations are absent and joint involvement is not symmetric. Elevated white blood cell counts, platelet counts, and antinuclear antibodies occur in rheumatoid arthritis.

Test-Taking Strategy: Knowledge regarding the differences between osteoarthritis and rheumatoid arthritis is required to answer this question. Review the characteristics of rheumatoid arthritis and osteoarthritis now, if you had difficulty with this question.

Level of Cognitive Ability: Analysis
Phase of Nursing Process: Assessment
Client Needs: Physiological Integrity
Content Area: Adult Health/Musculoskeletal

Reference

Black, J., & Matassarin-Jacobs, E. (1997). *Medical-surgical nursing: Clinical management for continuity of care* (5th ed.). Philadelphia: W. B. Saunders. p. 2109.

120. 2

Rationale: Rheumatoid arthritis is characterized by chronic joint pain of varying intensity, which is more severe upon rising in the morning. The nurse notes that joint involvement is symmetrical and the joints are swollen, shiny, reddened, and painful. Rheumatoid nodules, which are painless subcutaneous movable skin nodules near bony prominences, may occur anywhere on the body.

Test-Taking Strategy: Note that options 1 and 2 are similar in that both address the component of pain and its occurrence. This should lead you to suspect that one of these options is correct. Review the characteristics associated with RA now, if you had difficulty with this question!

Level of Cognitive Ability: Analysis
Phase of Nursing Process: Assessment
Client Needs: Physiological Integrity
Content Area: Adult Health/Musculoskeletal

Reference

Monahan, F., & Neighbors, M. (1998). *Medical-surgical nursing: Foundations for clinical practice* (2nd ed.). Philadelphia: W. B. Saunders. p. 891.

121. 1

Rationale: Skin lesions or a rash on the face across the bridge of the nose and on the cheeks is a characteristic sign of SLE. Fever and fatigue may occur before and during exacerbation. Anemia is most likely to occur in SLE.

Test-Taking Strategy: Note the key words "characteristic sign." Knowledge regarding the manifestations associated with SLE will easily direct you to option 1. If you are unfamiliar with this important disorder, review now.

Level of Cognitive Ability: Analysis
Phase of Nursing Process: Assessment
Client Needs: Physiological Integrity
Content Area: Adult Health/Musculoskeletal

Reference

Monahan, F., & Neighbors, M. (1998). *Medical-surgical nursing: Foundations for clinical practice* (2nd ed.). Philadelphia: W. B. Saunders. p. 1491.

122. **3**

Rationale: To help reduce fatigue in the client with SLE, the nurse should instruct the client to sit whenever possible, to avoid hot baths, to schedule moderate low-impact exercises when not fatigued, and to maintain a balanced diet. The client is instructed not to rest for long periods because it promotes joint stiffness.

Test-Taking Strategy: Note the key words "not" and "manage fatigue." By the process of elimination, you should easily be directed to option 3 as being the action that exacerbates fatigue. If you had difficulty with this question, take time now to review measures to prevent fatigue!

Level of Cognitive Ability: Analysis
Phase of Nursing Process: Implementation
Client Needs: Health Promotion and Maintenance
Content Area: Adult Health/Musculoskeletal

Reference

Monahan, F., & Neighbors, M. (1998). *Medical-surgical nursing: Foundations for clinical practice* (2nd ed.). Philadelphia: W. B. Saunders. p. 1493.

BIBLIOGRAPHY

Cox, H., Hinz, M., Lubno, M., et al. (1997). *Clinical applications of nursing diagnosis: Adult, child, women's, psychiatric, gerontic and home health considerations* (3rd ed.). Philadelphia: F. A. Davis.

Black, J., & Matassarin-Jacobs, E. (1997). *Medical-surgical nursing: Clinical management for continuity of care* (5th ed.). Philadelphia: W. B. Saunders.

Chernecky, C., & Berger, B. (1997). *Laboratory tests and diagnostic procedures* (2nd ed.). Philadelphia: W. B. Saunders.

Deglin, J., & Vallerand, A. (1997). *Davis's drug guide for nurses* (5th ed.). Philadelphia: F. A. Davis.

Hodgson, B., & Kizior, R. (1999). *Saunders nursing drug handbook 1999.* Philadelphia: W. B. Saunders.

Ignatavicius, D., Workman, M., & Mishler, M. (1995). *Medical-surgical nursing: A nursing process approach* (2nd ed.). Philadelphia: W. B. Saunders.

Lammon, C., Foote, A., Leli, P., et al. *Clinical Nursing Skills.* Philadelphia: W. B. Saunders.

Leahy, J., & Kizilay, P. (1998). *Foundations of nursing practice: A nursing process approach.* Philadelphia: W. B. Saunders.

Lehne, R. (1998). *Pharmacology for nursing care* (3rd ed.). Philadelphia: W. B. Saunders.

Luckmann, J. (1997). *Saunders manual of nursing care.* Philadelphia: W. B. Saunders.

McKenry, L., & Salerno, E. (1995). *Mosby's pharmacology in nursing* (19th ed.). St. Louis: Mosby–Year Book.

Monahan, F., & Neighbors, M. (1998). *Medical-surgical nursing: Foundations for clinical practice* (2nd ed.). Philadelphia: W. B. Saunders.

Potter, P., & Perry, A. (1997). *Fundamentals of nursing: Concepts, process, and practice* (4th ed.). St. Louis: Mosby–Year Book.

Smeltzer, S., & Bare, B. (1996). *Brunner and Suddarth's textbook of medical-surgical nursing* (8th ed.). Philadelphia: Lippincott-Raven.

CHAPTER 68

Musculoskeletal Medications

I. Skeletal Muscle Relaxants (Box 68–1)

A. Description
1. Act directly on the neuromuscular junction or indirectly on the central nervous system (CNS)
2. Centrally acting muscle relaxants depress neuron activity in the spinal cord or brain
3. Peripherally acting muscle relaxants act directly on the skeletal muscles
4. Used to prevent or relieve muscle spasms, to treat spasticity associated with spinal cord disease or lesions, for painful musculoskeletal conditions, and for chronic debilitating disorders such as multiple sclerosis, cerebrovascular accident (CVA), or cerebral palsy
5. Contraindicated in severe liver, renal, or heart disease
6. Should not be taken with CNS depressants such as barbiturates, narcotics, and alcohol; sedatives; hypnotics; or tricyclic antidepressants
7. Avoid use if client has a history of breast cancer because mammary malignancy could recur

B. Side effects
1. Dizziness

BOX 68–1. Skeletal Muscle Relaxants

Baclofen (Lioresal)
Carisoprodol (Soma)
Cyclobenzaprine hydrochloride (Flexeril)
Dantrolene (Dantrium)
Diazepam (Valium)
Methocarbamol (Robaxin)
Orphenadrine (Norflex)
Chlorzoxazone (Paraflex, Parafon Forte)
Chlorphenesin carbamate (Maolate)
Meprobamate (Equanil, Miltown)

---

2. Drowsiness
3. Dry mouth
4. Nausea
5. Gastrointestinal (GI) upset
6. Hypotension
7. Photosensitivity
8. Liver toxicity

C. Implementation
1. Obtain a medical and medication history
2. Monitor vital signs
3. Monitor for CNS side effects
4. Assess for risk of injury
5. Assess involved joints and muscles for pain and mobility
6. Monitor liver function tests since hepatotoxicity can occur
7. Monitor renal function studies
8. Instruct client to take medication with food to decrease GI upset
9. Instruct client to report side effects
10. Instruct client to avoid alcohol and CNS depressants
11. Instruct client to avoid activities requiring alertness

D. Nursing considerations
1. Baclofen (Lioresal)
   a. Causes CNS effects such as drowsiness, dizziness, weakness, and fatigue
   b. Frequently causes nausea, constipation, and urinary retention
   c. Can be administered by intrathecal infusion using an implantable pump
2. Dantrolene (Dantrium)
   a. Acts directly on skeletal muscles to relieve spasticity
   b. Liver damage is the most serious adverse effect
   c. Liver function tests should be monitored prior to the initiation of treatment and during treatment
   d. Can cause GI bleeding, urinary frequency, impotence, photosensitivity, and rash

e. Instruct client to wear protective clothing when in the sun

f. Instruct client to notify physician if rash, bloody or tarry stool, or yellow discoloration of skin or eyes occurs

3. Cyclobenzaprine hydrochloride (Flexeril)

a. Contraindicated in clients who have received monoamine oxidase (MAO) inhibitors within 14 days of initiation of Flexeril therapy, and in clients with cardiac disorders

b. Used with caution in clients with a history of urinary retention, angle-closure glaucoma, and increased intraocular pressure

c. Should be used only for short term (2 to 3 weeks of therapy)

4. Methocarbamol (Robaxin)

a. Parenteral form (IV or IM) is contraindicated in clients with renal impairment

b. Parenteral (IV or IM) form can cause anaphylaxis and seizures

c. IV injection can cause hypotension and bradycardia

d. May cause urine to turn brown, black, or green

e. Inform client to notify physician if blurred vision, nasal congestion, urticaria, or rash occurs

5. Chlorzoxazone (Paraflex, Parafon Forte)

a. Monitor for hypersensitivity reactions, such as urticaria, redness or itching, and possibly angioedema

b. May cause malaise and urine discoloration

6. Carisoprodol (Soma)

a. Advise client to take medication with food to prevent GI upset

b. Instruct client to report rash or hypersensitivity to the physician

II. Antigout Medications (Box 68–2)

A. Description

1. Decrease inflammation
2. Reduce uric acid production
3. Increase uric acid excretion
4. To prevent or relieve gout
5. To manage hyperuricemia
6. Used cautiously in clients with GI, renal, cardiac, and hepatic disease

---

BOX 68–2. Antigout Medications

Allopurinol (Zyloprim)
Colchicine
Probenecid (Benemid)
Sulfinpyrazone (Anturane)

---

7. Allopurinol (Zyloprim) can increase the effect of Coumadin and oral hypoglycemic agents

B. Side effects

1. Headaches
2. Diarrhea
3. Nausea
4. Vomiting
5. Bone marrow depression
6. Skin rash
7. Uric acid kidney stones
8. Blood dyscrasias
9. Flushed skin
10. Sore gums
11. Metallic taste

C. Implementation

1. Assess serum uric acid levels
2. Monitor intake and output (I&O)
3. Maintain a fluid intake of at least 2000 to 3000 mL a day to prevent kidney stones
4. Monitor complete blood count (CBC), and renal and liver function studies
5. Instruct client to avoid alcohol and caffeine because these products can increase uric acid levels
6. Instruct client not to take large doses of vitamin C while taking allopurinol (Zyloprim) as kidney stones may occur
7. Encourage client to comply with therapy to prevent elevated uric acid levels and trigger a gout attack
8. Instruct client to avoid foods high in purine such as wine, alcohol, organ meats, sardines, salmon, gravy
9. Instruct client to take medication with food
10. Instruct client to report side effects to the physician
11. Advise client to have a yearly eye examination because visual changes can occur from prolonged use of allopurinol
12. Caution client not to take aspirin with these medications as this could trigger a gout attack
13. Concurrent use of aspirin causes elevated uric acid levels; clients should be instructed to take acetaminophen (Tylenol)

III. Antiarthritic Medications

A. Nonsteroidal anti-inflammatory drugs (NSAIDs) (Box 68–3)

1. Description

a. NSAIDs are aspirin and aspirin-like medications that inhibit the synthesis of prostaglandins

b. They act as an analgesic to relieve pain, as an antipyretic to reduce body temperature, and as an anticoagulant to inhibit platelet aggregation

c. Used to relieve inflammation and pain and in the treatment of rheumatoid

BOX 68–3. Nonsteroidal Anti-Inflammatory Drugs (NSAIDs)

Aspirin (ASA; Bayer, Ecotrin)
Diflunisal (Dolobid)
Indomethacin (Indocin)
Sulindac (Clinoril)
Tolmetin (Tolectin)
Phenylbutazone (Butazolidin)
Fenoprofen calcium (Nalfon)
Flurbiprofen sodium (Ansaid, Ocufen)
Ibuprofen (Motrin, Advil, Nuprin, Medipren)
Ketoprofen (Orudis)
Naproxen (Naprosyn)
Oxaprozin (Daypro)
Meclofenamate (Meclomen)
Mefenamic acid (Ponstel)
Piroxicam (Feldene)
Diclofenac sodium (Voltaren)
Etodolac (Lodine)
Ketorolac tromethamine (Toradol)

BOX 68–4. Gold Therapy Medications

Auranofin (Ridaura)
Aurothioglucose (Solganal)
Gold sodium thiomalate (Myochrysine)

arthritis, bursitis, tendinitis, osteoarthritis, and acute gout

d. Contraindicated in hypersensitivity or liver or renal disease

e. Aspirin should not be taken by children with flu symptoms because of the risk of Reye's syndrome

f. Aspirin should not be taken if the client is on an anticoagulant

g. Aspirin and an NSAID should not be taken together because aspirin decreases the blood level and the effectiveness of the NSAID

h. NSAID's can increase the effects of Coumadin, sulfonamides, cephalosporins, and phenytoin (Dilantin)

i. Hypoglycemia may result if ibuprofen (Motrin) is taken with insulin or an oral hypoglycemic medication

j. A high risk of toxicity exists if ibuprofen is taken concurrently with calcium blockers

2. Side effects (Table 68–1)
3. Implementation
   a. Assess client for allergies
   b. Obtain a medication history and medical history from the client

c. Assess for history of gastric upset or bleeding, or liver disease

d. Assess the client for GI upset during medication administration

e. Monitor for edema

f. Monitor serum salicylate (aspirin) level when client is taking high doses

g. Monitor for signs of bleeding such as tarry stools, bleeding gums, petechiae, ecchymosis, and purpura

h. Instruct client to take medication with water, milk, or food

i. Enteric-coated form or buffered form of aspirin can be taken to decrease gastric distress

j. Instruct client that enteric-coated tablets cannot be crushed or broken

k. Advise client to inform other health care professionals if they are taking high doses of aspirin

l. Note that aspirin should be discontinued 3 to 7 days prior to surgery to reduce the risk of bleeding

m. Instruct client to avoid alcoholic beverages

B. Gold therapy (Box 68–4)
  1. Description
     a. Referred to as chrysotherapy or heavy metal therapy
     b. Depresses migration of leukocytes and suppresses prostaglandin activity
     c. Reduces inflammation by decreasing enzyme release and altering the immune response
     d. Primarily used for palliative relief of symptoms in rheumatoid arthritis
     e. Contraindications are listed in Box 68–5
  2. Side effects
     a. Dizziness
     b. Rash
     c. Dermatitis

Table 68–1. Side Effects

Aspirin	NSAIDs
Drowsiness	Hypotension
Tinnitus	Sodium and water retention
Pruritus	Gastric irritation
Flushing	Blood dyscrasias
Dizziness	Dizziness
GI symptoms	Tinnitus
Visual changes	Pruritus

BOX 68–5. Contraindications to Gold Therapy

Eczema
Urticaria
Colitis
Hemorrhagic conditions
Systemic lupus erythematosus
Renal or hepatic dysfunction
Uncontrolled diabetes mellitus
Congestive heart failure
Recent radiation therapy

d. Urticaria
e. Erythema
f. Alopecia
g. Stomatitis
h. Diarrhea
i. Hepatitis
j. Abdominal pain
k. Metallic taste in the mouth
l. Bone marrow suppression
m. Blood dyscrasias
n. Photosensitivity reactions
o. Gold toxicity
3. Implementation
a. Obtain client's health history
b. Monitor for blood dyscrasias before and during therapy
c. Monitor for proteinuria and hematuria before and during therapy
d. When giving gold injection, monitor client for 30 minutes for possible allergic reaction
e. Monitor for side effects
f. Instruct client to maintain good oral hygiene
g. Instruct client to use sunscreen and protective clothing to prevent photosensitivity reactions
h. Teach client about the signs and symptoms of gold toxicity, which include pruritus, skin rash, metallic taste, stomatitis, and diarrhea
i. If toxicity occurs, dimercaprol (BAL [British antilecuisite] in oil) may be prescribed to enhance gold excretion

PRACTICE QUESTIONS

1. Allopurinol (Zyloprim) has been prescribed for the client. Which of the following information is accurate concerning this medication?
   1 It is used for the lysis of thrombi obstructing coronary arteries
   2 It prevents calcium ion entry across cell membranes of the cardiac smooth muscle
   3 It decreases sympathetic outflow from the CNS
   4 It decreases uric acid production and reduces uric acid concentrations in both the serum and urine

2. The nurse is caring for a client who is taking allopurinol. Which of the following medications, if prescribed for the client, would the nurse question?
   1 Mebendazole (Vermox)
   2 Ergonovine maleate (Ergotrate)
   3 Warfarin sodium (Coumadin)
   4 Pentazocine (Talwin)

3. The community health nurse visits a client at home. The client is taking Zyloprim, 400 mg PO daily. Which of the following would be included in the teaching plan regarding this medication?

   1 Inform client that the effect of the medication will occur immediately
   2 Instruct client to drink 3000 mL of fluid per day
   3 Instruct client to take medication on an empty stomach
   4 Inform client that if swelling of the lips occurs, this is a normal, expected response

4. The nurse is caring for a client with unstable angina. The client is taking acetylsalicylic acid (aspirin) on a daily basis to reduce the risk of myocardial infarction (MI). Which of the following medication doses would the nurse expect the client to be taking?
   1 3 g daily
   2 300 to 325 mg daily
   3 1.3 g daily
   4 650 to 700 mg daily

5. Colchicine is prescribed for a client with a diagnosis of gout. This medication would be contraindicated in which of the following disorders?
   1 Renal failure
   2 Hypothyroidism
   3 Diabetes
   4 Myxedema

6. The home health nurse is caring for a client who is taking probenecid (Benemid). The client has been instructed to restrict the diet to low-purine foods. Which of the following foods would the nurse instruct the client to avoid?
   1 Potatoes
   2 Ice cream
   3 Spinach
   4 Scallops

7. The physician prescribes auranofin (Ridaura) for the client with rheumatoid arthritis. Which of the following indicates to the nurse that the client is experiencing toxicity related to the medication?
   1 Constipation
   2 Complaints of a metallic taste in the mouth
   3 Ringing in the ears
   4 Joint pain

8. A transcutaneous electrical nerve stimulation (TENS) is prescribed for a client with pain. The client asks the nurse about the purpose of the TENS unit. Which of the following is not a component of the nurse's response to the client?
   1 "Electrodes are attached to the skin."
   2 "The unit relieves pain."
   3 "The unit will reduce the needs for analgesics."
   4 "Hospitalization is required because the unit is not portable."

9. Diclofenac (Voltaren) is prescribed for the client with osteoarthritis. Which of the following medications, if noted on the client's record, alerts the nurse to consult with the physician?

1 Warfarin (Coumadin)
2 Mesoridazine besylate (Serentil)
3 Primidone (Mysoline)
4 Trifluoperazine hydrochloride (Stelazine)

10. A film-coated form of diflunisal (Dolobid) has been prescribed for a client for the treatment of chronic rheumatoid arthritis. The client calls the clinic nurse because of difficulty swallowing the tablets. Which of the following instructions would the nurse provide to the client?
    1 Crush the tablets and mix them with food
    2 Open the tablets and mix the contents with food
    3 Swallow the tablets with large amounts of water or milk
    4 Notify the physician for a medication change

11. The physician instructs an elderly client with rheumatoid arthritis to take ibuprofen (Motrin). The normal adult dose for this client is which of the following?
    1 100 mg PO BID
    2 200 mg PO BID
    3 300 mg PO TID
    4 1000 mg PO QID

12. Baclofen (Lioresal) is prescribed for the client with multiple sclerosis. The primary therapeutic effect of this medication is which of the following?
    1 Increased muscle tone
    2 Decreased muscle spasms
    3 Decreased local pain and tenderness
    4 Increased range of motion

13. The nurse is monitoring a client receiving baclofen for side effects related to the medication. Which of the following indicates that the client is experiencing a side effect?
    1 Drowsiness
    2 Diarrhea
    3 Polyuria
    4 Muscular excitability

14. The nurse is providing discharge instructions to a client receiving baclofen. Which of the following would be included in the teaching plan?
    1 Restrict fluid intake
    2 Avoid the use of alcohol
    3 Stop the medication if diarrhea occurs
    4 Notify the physician if fatigue occurs

15. The adult client with muscle spasms is taking an oral maintenance dose of baclofen. Which of the following represents a safe maintenance dose for this medication?
    1 15 mg QID
    2 25 mg QID
    3 30 mg QID
    4 40 mg QID

16. A client with acute muscle spasms has been taking baclofen. The client calls the clinic nurse because of continuous feelings of weakness and fatigue and asks the nurse about discontinuing the medication. Which of the following responses to the client is most appropriate?
    1 "It is best that you taper the dose if you intend to stop the medication."
    2 "Weakness and fatigue commonly occur and will diminish with continued medication use."
    3 "It is all right to stop the medication if you think that you can tolerate the muscle spasms."
    4. "You should never stop the medication."

17. Dantrolene sodium (Dantrium) is prescribed for the client experiencing flexor spasms. Which of the following identifies the therapeutic action of this medication?
    1 Acts within the spinal cord to suppress hyperactive reflexes
    2 Acts on the CNS to suppress spasms
    3 Acts directly on skeletal muscle to relieve spasticity
    4 Depresses spinal reflexes

18. The nurse is analyzing the laboratory studies on a client receiving Dantrium. Which of the following laboratory tests identifies an adverse effect associated with the administration of this medication?
    1 BUN
    2 Creatinine
    3 Liver function tests
    4 Hematological function tests

19. The client is receiving oral dantrolene sodium for the treatment of spasticity. The usual maintenance adult dosage of this medication is which of the following?
    1 50 mg daily
    2 100 mg daily
    3 100 mg BID
    4 200 mg QID

20. The physician is planning to administer a skeletal muscle relaxant to a client with a spinal cord injury. The medication is going to be administered intrathecally (within the spinal column). Which of the following medications would the nurse expect to be prescribed and administered by this route?
    1 Cyclobenzaprine hydrochloride (Flexeril)
    2 Chlorzoxazone (Paraflex)
    3 Dantrolene sodium (Dantrium)
    4 Baclofen (Lioresal)

21. The nurse is reviewing the record of a client who has been prescribed baclofen. Which of the following disorders, if noted in the client's history, would alert the nurse to contact the physician?
    1 Coronary artery disease
    2 Diabetes mellitus
    3 Seizure disorders
    4 Hyperthyroidism

22. Cyclobenzaprine hydrochloride (Flexeril) is pre-scribed for the client for muscle spasms. The nurse is reviewing the client's record. Which of the following disorders, if noted in the client's record, would indicate a need to contact the phy-sician regarding the administration of this medi-cation?
    1 Glaucoma
    2 Hyperthyroidism
    3 Emphysema
    4 Diabetes mellitus

23. The client is to receive a prescription for metho-carbamol (Robaxin). The nurse provides instruc-tions to the client regarding the medication. Which of the following client statements indicates a need for further education?
    1 "My urine may turn brown or green."
    2 "If my vision becomes blurred, I don't need to be concerned about it."
    3 "I might get some nasal congestion from this medication."

    4 "This medication is prescribed to help relieve my muscle spasms."

24. The nurse is administering an IV dose of metho-carbamol (Robaxin) to a client with multiple scle-rosis. For which of the following adverse effects would the nurse monitor?
    1 Hypertension
    2 Tachycardia
    3 Rapid pulse
    4 Bradycardia

25. The nurse is reviewing the physician's orders for an adult client who has been admitted to the hospital following a back injury. Carisoprodol (Soma) is prescribed for the client to relieve the muscle spasms. The physician has prescribed 350 mg to be administered QID. The nurse determines that this dosage is:
    1 The normal adult dosage
    2 A lower than normal dosage
    3 A higher than normal dosage
    4 A dosage requiring further clarification

ANSWERS

1. **4**

Rationale: Allopurinol (Zyloprim) is an antigout medica-tion. It decreases uric acid production by inhibition of xan-thine oxidase, an enzyme, and reduces uric acid concentra-tions in both serum and urine.

Test-Taking Strategy: Knowledge regarding this medication is required to answer the question. Use the process of elimi-nation. Note that options 1 and 2 are similar in that they both address a cardiac situation. This leaves options 3 and 4. Knowledge that this medication is in the antigout classi-fication will assist in directing you to the correct option. If you had difficulty with this question, take time now to review the action of allopurinol!

Level of Cognitive Ability: Analysis
Phase of Nursing Process: Analysis
Client Needs: Physiological Integrity
Content Area: Pharmacology

Reference
Hodgson, B., & Kizior, R. (1999). *Saunders nursing drug handbook 1999.* Philadelphia: W. B. Saunders. p. 24.

2. **3**

Rationale: Allopurinol is an antigout medication that may increase the effect of oral anticoagulants. Warfarin sodium (Coumadin) is an anticoagulant, and if this medication were prescribed for the client, the nurse would verify the order. Ergonovine maleate (Ergotrate) is an antimigraine medica-tion. Pentazocine (Talwin) is an opioid analgesic Schedule IV medication. Mebendazole (Vermox) is an anthelmintic.

Test-Taking Strategy: Knowledge regarding the medication interactions related to Zyloprim is required to answer this question. If you had difficulty with this question, take time now to review the drug interactions associated with this medication!

Level of Cognitive Ability: Application
Phase of Nursing Process: Implementation
Client Needs: Safe, Effective Care Environment
Content Area: Pharmacology

Reference
Hodgson, B., & Kizior, R. (1999). *Saunders nursing drug handbook 1999.* Philadelphia: W. B. Saunders. p. 24.

3. **2**

Rationale: Clients taking Zyloprim are encouraged to drink 3000 mL of fluid a day. A full therapeutic effect may take 1 or more weeks. Zyloprim is to be given with or immediately following meals or milk. Clients who develop a rash, irrita-tion of the eyes, or swelling of the lips or mouth should contact the physician, as this may indicate hypersensitivity.

Test-Taking Strategy: Knowledge regarding client instruc-tions related to this medication will assist you in answering the question. Option 4 can be easily eliminated because it indicates a hypersensitivity, which is not a normal expected response. From this point, use the process of elimination and your nursing knowledge in selecting the correct option. If you had difficulty with this question, take time now to review client instructions related to Zyloprim.

Level of Cognitive Ability: Analysis
Phase of Nursing Process: Planning
Client Needs: Health Promotion and Maintenance
Content Area: Pharmacology

Reference

Hodgson, B., & Kizior, R. (1999). *Saunders nursing drug handbook 1999*. Philadelphia: W. B. Saunders. p. 24.

4. 2

Rationale: Acetylsalicylic acid (aspirin) may be used to reduce the risk of recurrent transient ischemic attacks (TIA) or stroke, or to reduce the risk of MI in clients with unstable angina or with a history of a previous MI. The normal dose for clients being treated with acetylsalicylic acid (aspirin) to decrease thrombosis and MI is 300 to 325 mg daily. Clients being treated to prevent TIAs are usually prescribed 1.3 g daily in two to four divided doses. Clients with rheumatoid arthritis are treated with 3.2 to 6 g daily in divided doses.

Test-Taking Strategy: Knowledge regarding the use of acetylsalicylic acid (aspirin) as prophylaxis is required to answer this question. Read the question carefully. Note the key phrase in the question: "reduce the risk of MI." This should indicate to you that the client is receiving the medication as a preventive measure, directing you to the lowest dose of medication in the options. If you had difficulty with this question, take time now to review aspirin dosages!

Level of Cognitive Ability: Analysis
Phase of Nursing Process: Analysis
Client Needs: Physiological Integrity
Content Area: Pharmacology

Reference

Hodgson, B., & Kizior, R. (1999). *Saunders nursing drug handbook 1999*. Philadelphia: W. B. Saunders. p. 75.

5. 1

Rationale: Colchicine is contraindicated in severe GI, renal, hepatic, or cardiac disorders and in clients with blood dyscrasias. Clients with impaired renal function may exhibit myopathy and neuropathy manifested as generalized weakness. This medication should be used with caution in clients with impaired hepatic function and in elderly and debilitated clients.

Test-Taking Strategy: Knowledge regarding the pharmacokinetics related to this medication is required to answer the question. This medication is rapidly absorbed from the GI tract, with highest concentrations appearing in the liver, spleen, and kidneys. Use the process of elimination to answer the question. Note that options 2, 3, and 4 are all endocrine-related disorders. Option 1, the correct option, is different from the others.

Level of Cognitive Ability: Analysis
Phase of Nursing Process: Analysis
Client Needs: Physiological Integrity
Content Area: Pharmacology

Reference

Clark, J., Queener, S., & Karb, V. (1997). *Pharmacologic basis of nursing practice* (5th ed.). St. Louis: Mosby–Year Book. p. 376.

6. 4

Rationale: Uric acid is produced when purine is catabolized. Probenecid (Benemid) is a medication used for clients with gout to inhibit the reabsorption of uric acid by the kidney and promote excretion of uric acid in the urine. Clients are instructed to modify their diets and limit excessive purine intake. High-purine foods to avoid or limit include organ meats, roe, sardines, scallops, anchovies, broth, mincemeat, herring, shrimp, mackerel, gravy, and yeast.

Test-Taking Strategy: Knowledge regarding foods that are low in purine is helpful to answer this question. Use the process of elimination. Options 1 and 3 are high-nutrient foods, so eliminate these options first. From this point, use your knowledge regarding the purpose of the medication, the treatment for gout, and food sources high in purine to select the correct option. If you had difficulty with this question, take time now to review foods that are high in purine!

Level of Cognitive Ability: Application
Phase of Nursing Process: Implementation
Client Needs: Health Promotion and Maintenance
Content Area: Pharmacology

Reference

Clark, J., Queener, S., & Karb, V. (1997). *Pharmacologic basis of nursing practice* (5th ed.). St. Louis: Mosby–Year Book. p. 377.

7. 2

Rationale: Auranofin (Ridaura) is the one gold preparation that is given orally rather than by injection. Gastrointestinal reactions, including diarrhea, abdominal pain, nausea, and loss of appetite, are common early in therapy but usually subside in the first 3 months. Early symptoms of toxic reactions include a rash, purple blotches, pruritus, mouth lesions, and a metallic taste in the mouth.

Test-Taking Strategy: Knowledge that Ridaura is a gold preparation will assist you in answering the question. Use the process of elimination. Option 4, joint pain, can be eliminated because the medication is administered to reduce joint pain. Note that the question is asking for a toxic effect; therefore, from the options remaining, you should be directed to the correct option, metallic taste. Remember, gold is a metal! If you had difficulty with this question, take time now to review toxicity related to gold compounds!

Level of Cognitive Ability: Analysis
Phase of Nursing Process: Assessment
Client Needs: Physiological Integrity
Content Area: Pharmacology

Reference

Clark, J., Queener, S., & Karb, V. (1997). *Pharmacologic basis of nursing practice* (5th ed.). St. Louis: Mosby–Year Book. p. 453.

8. 4

Rationale: The TENS unit is portable, and the client controls the system for relieving pain and reducing the need for analgesics. It is attached to the skin of the body by electrodes.

Test-Taking Strategy: Knowledge regarding the use of the TENS unit is helpful to answer this question. Read each option carefully. Note the word "not" in the stem of the question. You should be directed to option 4, because it would not be a very cost-effective pain management technique if the client required hospitalization.

Level of Cognitive Ability: Analysis
Phase of Nursing Process: Implementation
Client Needs: Health Promotion and Maintenance
Content Area: Pharmacology

Reference

Monahan, F., & Neighbors, M. (1998). *Medical-surgical nursing: Foundations for clinical practice* (2nd ed.). Philadelphia: W. B. Saunders. p. 892.

9. 1

Rationale: Voltaren is an NSAID. Interactions may occur with anticoagulants. The nurse should consult with the physician regarding a potential medication interaction. Serentil and stelazine are antipsychotic medications. Mysoline is an anticonvulsant. These medications are not contraindicated when administering Voltaren.

Test-Taking Strategy: Knowledge regarding the contraindications associated with the administration of this medication is required to answer this question. Review this medication now, if you had difficulty with this question!

Level of Cognitive Ability: Analysis
Phase of Nursing Process: Analysis
Client Needs: Physiological Integrity
Content Area: Pharmacology

References
Monahan, F., & Neighbors, M. (1998). *Medical-surgical nursing: Foundations for clinical practice* (2nd ed.). Philadelphia: W. B. Saunders. p. 893.
Hodgson, B., & Kizior, R. (1999). *Saunders nursing drug handbook 1999*. Philadelphia: W. B. Saunders. pp. 646, 857, 1024.

10. 3

Rationale: Dolobid may be given with water, milk, or meals. The tablets should not be crushed or broken open.

Test-Taking Strategy: Eliminate option 4 first as the least likely option. Next, noting the words "film-coated," eliminate options 1 and 2. Additionally, these options are similar in that they both suggest breaking the tablets. If you had difficulty with this question, review the procedure for administration now!

Level of Cognitive Ability: Application
Phase of Nursing Process: Implementation
Client Needs: Health Promotion and Maintenance
Content Area: Pharmacology

Reference
Hodgson, B., & Kizior, R. (1999). *Saunders nursing drug handbook 1999*. Philadelphia: W. B. Saunders. p. 322.

11. 3

Rationale: For acute or chronic rheumatoid arthritis or osteoarthritis, the normal PO adult dose of ibuprofen for an elderly client is 300 to 800 mg three to four times daily.

Test-Taking Strategy: This may be a difficult question. Note the word "elderly" in the question. This will assist in eliminating option 4. Review the normal dosage for this medication now, if you had difficulty with this question!

Level of Cognitive Ability: Analysis
Phase of Nursing Process: Analysis
Client Needs: Physiological Integrity
Content Area: Pharmacology

Reference
Hodgson, B., & Kizior, R. (1999). *Saunders nursing drug handbook 1999*. Philadelphia: W. B. Saunders. p. 511.

12. 2

Rationale: Baclofen is a skeletal muscle relaxant and acts at the spinal cord level to decrease the frequency and amplitude of muscle spasms in clients with spinal cord injuries or diseases and multiple sclerosis.

Test-Taking Strategy: Knowledge that this medication is a skeletal muscle relaxant is required to answer this question.

If you knew the action of this medication, you would easily be directed to option 2. Review this medication now, if you had difficulty with this question!

Level of Cognitive Ability: Analysis
Phase of Nursing Process: Evaluation
Client Needs: Physiological Integrity
Content Area: Pharmacology

Reference
Lehne, R. (1998). *Pharmacology for nursing care* (3rd ed.). Philadelphia: W. B. Saunders. pp. 222–223.

13. 1

Rationale: Baclofen is a CNS depressant and frequently causes drowsiness, dizziness, weakness, and fatigue. It can also cause nausea, constipation, and urinary retention. Clients should be warned about the possible reactions.

Test-Taking Strategy: Knowledge that baclofen is a CNS depressant used to treat muscle spasticity will easily direct you to option 1. If you had difficulty with this question, review the side effects of this medication now!

Level of Cognitive Ability: Analysis
Phase of Nursing Process: Assessment
Client Needs: Physiological Integrity
Content Area: Pharmacology

Reference
Lehne, R. (1998). *Pharmacology for nursing care* (3rd ed.). Philadelphia: W. B. Saunders. pp. 222–223.

14. 2

Rationale: Baclofen is a CNS depressant. The client should be cautioned against the use of alcohol and other CNS depressants since baclofen potentiates the depressant activity of these agents. Constipation rather than diarrhea is an adverse effect of baclofen. It is not necessary to restrict fluids, but the client should be warned that urinary retention can occur. Fatigue is related to a CNS effect that is most intense during the early phase of therapy and diminishes with continued medication use. It is not necessary that the client notify the physician.

Test-Taking Strategy: Knowledge that baclofen is a CNS depressant will easily direct you to option 2. If you were unsure of the correct answer, use general principles related to medication administration to select the correct option. Alcohol should be avoided with the use of many medications!

Level of Cognitive Ability: Application
Phase of Nursing Process: Assessment
Client Needs: Health Promotion and Maintenance
Content Area: Pharmacology

Reference
Lehne, R. (1998). *Pharmacology for nursing care* (3rd ed.). Philadelphia: W. B. Saunders. pp. 222–223.

15. 1

Rationale: Baclofen is dispensed in tablets of 10 and 20 mg for oral use. Dosages are low initially and then gradually increased. Maintenance doses range from 15 to 20 mg administered three to four times a day.

Test-Taking Strategy: Knowledge regarding the normal adult maintenance dosage is required to answer this question. This may be a difficult question, and if you are unfamiliar with this maintenance dosage, learn it now!

Level of Cognitive Ability: Analysis
Phase of Nursing Process: Analysis
Client Needs: Physiological Integrity
Content Area: Pharmacology

Reference
Lehne, R. (1998). *Pharmacology for nursing care* (3rd ed.). Philadelphia: W. B. Saunders. pp. 222–223.

16. **2**

Rationale: The client should be instructed that symptoms such as drowsiness, weakness, and fatigue are more intense in the early phase of therapy and diminish with continued medication use. The client should be instructed never to withdraw abruptly or stop the medication because abrupt withdrawal can cause visual hallucinations, paranoid ideation, and seizures. It is best for the nurse to inform the client that these symptoms will subside and to encourage the client to continue the use of the medication.

Test-Taking Strategy: Note the key words "most appropriate." Eliminate option 4 first because it is a rather extreme nursing response. Next, eliminate options 1 and 3 because these responses do not represent the scope of nursing practice.

Level of Cognitive Ability: Application
Phase of Nursing Process: Implementation
Client Needs: Health Promotion and Maintenance
Content Area: Pharmacology

Reference
Lehne, R. (1998). *Pharmacology for nursing care* (3rd ed.). Philadelphia: W. B. Saunders. p. 225.

17. **3**

Rationale: Dantrium acts directly on skeletal muscle to relieve muscle spasticity. The primary action is the suppression of calcium release from the sarcoplasmic reticulum. This is turn decreases the ability of the skeletal muscle to contract.

Test-Taking Strategy: Options 1, 2, and 4 are all similar in that they address the CNS (spinal cord, CNS, spinal reflexes) and the depression of reflexes. Therefore, eliminate these options. Review this medication now, if you had difficulty with this question!

Level of Cognitive Ability: Analysis
Phase of Nursing Process: Analysis
Client Needs: Physiological Integrity
Content Area: Pharmacology

Reference
Lehne, R. (1998). *Pharmacology for nursing care* (3rd ed.). Philadelphia: W. B. Saunders. p. 223.

18. **3**

Rationale: Dose-related liver damage is the most serious adverse effect of Dantrium. To reduce the risk of liver damage, tests of liver function should be performed prior to treatment and throughout the treatment interval. It is administered in the lowest effective dosage for the shortest time necessary.

Test-Taking Strategy: Eliminate options 1 and 2 because these tests both assess kidney function. From the remaining options, it is necessary to recall that this medication affects liver function. Review this medication now, if you had difficulty with this question!

Level of Cognitive Ability: Analysis
Phase of Nursing Process: Assessment
Client Needs: Physiological Integrity
Content Area: Pharmacology

Reference
Lehne, R. (1998). *Pharmacology for nursing care* (3rd ed.). Philadelphia: W. B. Saunders. p. 223.

19. **3**

Rationale: For treatment of spasticity, dantrolene is administered orally. The initial dosage for adults is 25 mg once daily. The usual maintenance dosage is 100 mg two to four times daily. If beneficial effects do not develop within 45 days, dantrolene therapy should cease.

Test-Taking Strategy: This may be a difficult question. Knowledge of the adult oral dosage is required to answer this question. If you are unfamiliar with the maintenance dosage of this medication, review now!

Level of Cognitive Ability: Analysis
Phase of Nursing Process: Analysis
Client Needs: Physiological Integrity
Content Area: Pharmacology

Reference
Lehne, R. (1998). *Pharmacology for nursing care* (3rd ed.). Philadelphia: W. B. Saunders. p. 223.

20. **4**

Rationale: Baclofen is the only skeletal muscle relaxant that can be administered intrathecally within the spinal column.

Test-Taking Strategy: Knowledge regarding intrathecal administration of muscle relaxants is required to answer this question. If you are unfamiliar with this form of therapy, take time now to review!

Level of Cognitive Ability: Analysis
Phase of Nursing Process: Planning
Client Needs: Physiological Integrity
Content Area: Pharmacology

Reference
Kuhn, M. (1998). *Pharmacotherapeutics: A nursing process approach* (4th ed.). Philadelphia: F. A. Davis. p. 317.

21. **3**

Rationale: Clients with seizure disorders may have a lowered seizure threshold when baclofen is administered. Concurrent therapy may require an increase in the anticonvulsive medication.

Test-Taking Strategy: Knowledge regarding the contraindications and the cautions associated with the administration of baclofen is required to answer this question. If you are unfamiliar with these contraindications and cautions, review them now!

Level of Cognitive Ability: Analysis
Phase of Nursing Process: Implementation
Client Needs: Physiological Integrity
Content Area: Pharmacology

Reference
Kuhn, M. (1998). *Pharmacotherapeutics: A nursing process approach* (4th ed.). Philadelphia: F. A. Davis. p. 317.

22. **1**

Rationale: Because this medication has anticholinergic effects, it should be used with caution for clients with a history of urinary retention, angle closure glaucoma, and increased intraocular pressure. Flexeril should be used only for short-term, 2- to 3-week therapy.

Test-Taking Strategy: Knowledge that this medication has anticholinergic effects will easily direct you to option 1. If you are unfamiliar with this medication and the contraindications associated with its administration, review now!

Level of Cognitive Ability: Analysis
Phase of Nursing Process: Implementation
Client Needs: Physiological Integrity
Content Area: Pharmacology

Reference
Kuhn, M. (1998). *Pharmacotherapeutics: A nursing process approach* (4th ed.). Philadelphia: F. A. Davis. p. 317.

23. **2**

Rationale: The client needs to be told that the urine may turn brown, black, or green. Other adverse effects include blurred vision, nasal congestion, urticaria, and rash. The client needs to be instructed that if these adverse effects occur, the physician needs to be notified.

Test-Taking Strategy: Note the key words "need for further education." This may assist you in the process of elimination and direct you to option 2. If you had difficulty with this question, take time now to review!

Level of Cognitive Ability: Analysis
Phase of Nursing Process: Evaluation
Client Needs: Health Promotion and Maintenance
Content Area: Pharmacology

Reference
Kuhn, M. (1998). *Pharmacotherapeutics: A nursing process approach* (4th ed.). Philadelphia: F. A. Davis. p. 317.

24. **4**

Rationale: Intravenous administration of methocarbamol (Robaxin) can cause hypotension and bradycardia. The nurse needs to monitor for these side effects.

Test-Taking Strategy: Eliminate options 2 and 3 first because they are similar. Knowledge regarding the specific side effects related to the IV use of this medication will direct you to option 4. Review this medication now, if you had difficulty with this question!

Level of Cognitive Ability: Analysis
Phase of Nursing Process: Assessment
Client Needs: Physiological Integrity
Content Area: Pharmacology

Reference
Kuhn, M. (1998). *Pharmacotherapeutics: A nursing process approach* (4th ed.). Philadelphia: F. A. Davis. p. 317.

25. **1**

Rationale: The normal adult dosage for Soma is 350 mg PO three to four times daily.

Test-Taking Strategy: This question may be difficult if you are not familiar with the normal medication dosage. Review this medication now, if you had difficulty with this question!

Level of Cognitive Ability: Analysis
Phase of Nursing Process: Analysis
Client Needs: Physiological Integrity
Content Area: Pharmacology

Reference
Kuhn, M. (1998). *Pharmacotherapeutics: A nursing process approach* (4th ed.). Philadelphia: F. A. Davis. p. 318.

BIBLIOGRAPHY

Black, J., & Matassarin-Jacobs, E. (1997). *Medical-surgical nursing: Clinical management for continuity of care* (5th ed.). Philadelphia: W. B. Saunders.

Chernecky, C., & Berger, B. (1997). *Laboratory tests and diagnostic procedures* (2nd ed.). Philadelphia: W. B. Saunders.

Clark, J., Queener, S., & Karb, V. (1997). *Pharmacologic basis of nursing practice* (5th ed.). St. Louis: Mosby–Year Book.

Hodgson, B., & Kizior, R. (1999). *Saunders nursing drug handbook 1999.* Philadelphia: W. B. Saunders.

Ignatavicius, D., Workman, M., & Mishler, M. (1995). *Medical-surgical nursing: A nursing process approach* (2nd ed.). Philadelphia: W. B. Saunders.

Kuhn, M. (1998). *Pharmacotherapeutics: A nursing process approach* (4th ed.). Philadelphia: F. A. Davis.

Lehne, R. (1998). *Pharmacology for nursing care* (3rd ed.). Philadelphia: W. B. Saunders.

Luckmann, J. (1997). *Saunders manual of nursing care.* Philadelphia: W. B. Saunders.

Monahan, F., & Neighbors, M. (1998). *Medical-surgical nursing: Foundations for clinical practice* (2nd ed.). Philadelphia: W. B. Saunders.

O'Toole, M. (ed.) (1997). *Miller-Keane encyclopedia & dictionary of medicine, nursing, & allied health* (6th ed.). Philadelphia: W. B. Saunders.

UNIT XIX

....

The Adult Client with a Mental Health Disorder

PYRAMID TERMS

Abuse—An act of misuse, deceit, or exploitation. The wrong or improper use or action toward another individual that results in injury, damage, maltreatment, or corruption.

Addiction—Also known as drug dependence. Incorporates the concepts of loss of control with respect to the use of a drug, taking the drug despite related problems and complications, and a tendency to relapse.

Coping Mechanisms—Methods of adjusting to environmental stress without altering one's own goals or purposes. Can include both conscious and unconscious mechanisms.

Crisis—A temporary state of disequilibrium in which an individual's usual coping mechanisms or problem-solving methods fail. It can result in personality growth or personality disorganization.

Defense Mechanisms—Unconscious intrapsychic processes used to fight off anxiety by preventing the conscious awareness of threatening feelings. These mechanisms can be used in a healthy or unhealthy manner.

Milieu—The physical and social environment in which an individual lives. Milieu therapy focuses on positive physical and social environmental manipulation in order to produce positive change.

Restraints—Physical restraints include any manual method or mechanical device, material, or equipment that inhibits free movement. Chemical restraints include the administration of medications for the purpose of inhibiting a specific behavior or movement.

Seclusion—Placing a client alone in a specially designed room for protection and close supervision. It is the last measure in a process to maximize safety to the client and others.

Suicide—The ultimate act of self-destruction in which an individual purposefully ends his or her own life.

Suicide Attempt—Any willful, self-inflicted, or life-threatening attempt by an individual that has not led to death.

PYRAMID TO SUCCESS

The Pyramid to Success focuses on the therapeutic nurse-client relationship, client rights, hospital admission procedures, and the ethical and legal issues related to the care of the client with a mental health disorder. Pyramid points focus on the use of restraints, seclusion, and electroconvulsive therapy (ECT). Focus on care to the client with an addiction, such as an eating disorder or drug or alcohol disorder. Additional focus areas include anxiety, depression, suicide, abuse and violence, rape crisis interventions, post-traumatic stress disorders, obsessive-compulsive disorders, schizophrenia, and bipolar disorders. Pyramid points address the use of medications prescribed for the client with a mental health disorder, particularly lithium and the benzodiazepines.

NURSING PROCESS

ASSESSMENT

Physical, social, emotional, intellectual, spiritual, and cultural aspects

Presenting problem, current lifestyle, and life experiences

Physical appearance, such as dress, posture, gait, motor activity level, attitude, behavioral mannerisms, and speech

Affect and emotional state

Sensorium, such as attention and alertness, orientation, and memory

Intelligence, insight, and awareness of illness

Cognitions and cognitive processes, such as speed, associative abilities, organization, content, abstract thinking, and judgment

Personal strengths

Coping mechanisms

Support systems

ANALYSIS: Altered Nutrition

PLANNING	IMPLEMENTATION	EVALUATION
Client verbalizes willingness to consume adequate nutritional intake.	Assess likes and dislikes of client. Select food items with client as appropriate to meet client's physical and psychosocial needs. Monitor weight. Monitor laboratory values. Monitor and document food intake.	Client eats prescribed foods. Client maintains weight.

ANALYSIS: Self-Care Deficit

PLANNING	IMPLEMENTATION	EVALUATION
Client initiates and follows through with personal hygiene measures.	Schedule time to perform personal hygiene and assist client as necessary. Monitor client for maintenance of personal hygiene. Monitor dress and appearance for appropriateness.	Client participates in personal hygiene measures.

ANALYSIS: Sleep Pattern Disturbance

PLANNING	IMPLEMENTATION	EVALUATION
Client identifies techniques to induce sleep.	Monitor sleep patterns. Monitor frequency and length of time client is awake at night. Teach relaxation skills and exercises. Decrease intake of caffeine and other stimulants. Discourage daytime napping. Adhere to relaxing bedtime ritual.	Client utilizes sleep and relaxation techniques. Client sleeps through the night.

ANALYSIS: Anxiety

PLANNING	IMPLEMENTATION	EVALUATION
Client identifies symptoms that are indicators of anxiety. Client utilizes anxiety-reducing techniques. Client demonstrates ability to continue with necessary activities.	Assess and document client's level of anxiety. Encourage client to verbalize thoughts and feelings to externalize anxiety. Assist client to identify events that have precipitated anxiety in the past. Explore techniques that have and have not reduced anxiety in the past. Assist client to focus on the present situation as a means of identifying coping mechanisms to reduce anxiety. Encourage client to express feelings. Reduce excessive stimulation by providing a quiet environment, limited contact with others, and limited use of caffeine and other stimulants. Provide appropriate diversion to reduce anxiety. Provide positive reinforcement when client is able to continue with activities of daily living and activities necessary to progress to optimal wellness.	Client verbalizes reduction in anxiety. Client demonstrates ability to focus appropriately.

ANALYSIS: High Risk for Violence (Self and Others)

PLANNING	IMPLEMENTATION	EVALUATION
The client verbalizes anger. The client demonstrates ability to control anger. The client identifies effective ways to express anger in a nondestructive manner.	Identify behaviors that are cues of impending violence against self or others. Identify situations that provoke violence. Encourage client to verbalize anger. Set limits on client's behavior. Explore with client alternative ways of expressing anger. Encourage the use of positive coping mechanisms. Assess and document client's potential for suicide. Initiate suicide precautions as necessary. Assess the need for the use of seclusion and restraints. Follow agency policies and procedures regarding the use of restraints or seclusion.	Client does not harm self or others

ANALYSIS: Altered Pattern of Communication

PLANNING	IMPLEMENTATION	EVALUATION
Client will state feelings in a given situation. Client will directly ask for what he or she wants or needs.	Define the nurse-client relationship. Develop a therapeutic relationship. Discuss behavioral expectations and consequences. Encourage discussion of feelings by role modeling. Acknowledge and reward open communication.	The client is direct in communicating feelings and needs.

ANALYSIS: Disturbance in Self-Concept

PLANNING	IMPLEMENTATION	EVALUATION
The client accepts positive feedback from others. The client identifies things that enhance self-concept. The client practices new behaviors.	Encourage and accept expression of thoughts and feelings. Provide opportunities to problem solve. Encourage client to practice new behaviors in role-playing situations. Provide praise and recognition.	The client will maintain a positive self-concept.

ANALYSIS: Ineffective Individual Coping

PLANNING	IMPLEMENTATION	EVALUATION
The client will distinguish verbal thoughts from the need to act out thoughts. The client will seek out nursing staff and request time away from others to de-escalate feelings.	Reduce environmental stimulation. Assist client to express thoughts and feelings. Assess for aggressive or potentially self-destructive behaviors. Encourage client to verbalize the need for an environment necessary to de-escalate feelings.	The client maintains safety of self and others.

ANALYSIS: Altered Thought Processes

PLANNING	IMPLEMENTATION	EVALUATION
The client will share perceptions of reality with others. The client will list pros and cons of actions before making decisions.	Use a calm, nonthreatening, directive approach. Present reality in a matter of fact tone and manner. Orient client to person, place, time, and situation. Encourage reality-oriented conversation and activities.	The client validates reality.

ANALYSIS: Social Isolation

PLANNING	IMPLEMENTATION	EVALUATION
The client will allow contact with others. The client will interact with others.	Promote trust and a therapeutic nurse-client relationship. Assist client to set daily goals. Be realistic about client's tolerance for activity with others.	The client maintains contact with others.

ANALYSIS: Altered Family Processes

PLANNING	IMPLEMENTATION	EVALUATION
Client/family identifies coping patterns. Client/family participates in decision-making processes.	Assess interaction between client and family. Assess for potentially disruptive behaviors. Promote a trusting relationship with client and family. Encourage client and family to verbalize feelings. Assist client and family to identify personal strengths. Encourage family to participate in client's care. Provide positive reinforcement for effective use of coping mechanisms. Initiate a multidisciplinary client care conference involving the client and family in problem solving and communication. Encourage family to express concerns related to home care. Explore available community resources with the family. Mobilize support services as appropriate.	Client/family utilizes appropriate coping mechanisms. Client and family acknowledge change in family roles.

ANALYSIS: Powerlessness

PLANNING	IMPLEMENTATION	EVALUATION
The client follows rules regarding acceptable behavior.	Teach client about personal boundaries. Discuss role expectations with the client. Provide choices whenever possible.	The client accepts limits and takes responsibility for own feelings.

ANALYSIS: Noncompliance

PLANNING	IMPLEMENTATION	EVALUATION
The client takes medications at prescribed times.	Instruct client regarding importance of medication regimen. Initiate referral to community resources and other support services as appropriate.	The client complies with therapeutic regimen.

CLIENT NEEDS

SAFE, EFFECTIVE CARE ENVIRONMENT

Client advocacy
Client rights
Confidentiality
Informed consent related to treatments, such as restraints, seclusion, and electroconvulsive therapy (ECT)
Legal responsibilities related to reporting incidences of violence and abuse
Psychiatric consultations and referrals
Providing safety to client and others
Use of restraints and seclusion

HEALTH PROMOTION AND MAINTENANCE

Psychosocial assessment techniques
Health promotion programs related to addictions
Individual lifestyle choices

PSYCHOSOCIAL INTEGRITY

Therapeutic nurse-client relationship
Coping mechanisms
Counseling techniques
Grief and loss
Religious and spiritual influences on health

Stress management
Support systems
Behavioral interventions
Chemical dependency
Abuse/neglect
Domestic violence
Sexual abuse/rape
Crisis intervention
Therapeutic milieu

PHYSIOLOGICAL INTEGRITY

Personal hygiene measures
Nutrition
Rest and sleep
Elimination
Medication administration
Expected and untoward effects of medications
Potential complications related to medications and electroconvulsive therapy (ECT)
Laboratory values related to medication therapy
Abusive and self-destructive behavior
Alterations in body systems related to addictions
Pathophysiology related to mental health disorders

REFERENCES

Carson, V., & Arnold, E. (1996). *Mental health nursing: The nurse-patient journey.* Philadelphia: W. B. Saunders
National Council of State Boards of Nursing. (eds.) (1997). *Test for the National Council Licensure Examination for Registered Nurses.* Chicago: Author.

O'Toole, M. (ed.) (1997). *Miller-Keane encyclopedia & dictionary of medicine, nursing & allied health* (6th ed.). Philadelphia: W. B. Saunders.

CHAPTER 69

Foundations of Psychiatric Mental Health Nursing

....

I. Mental Health

A. A lifelong process of successful adaptation to a changing internal and external environment
B. The individual is in contact with reality and the environment and possesses the ability to love, work, and resolve conflicts within a framework of reasonability

II. Psychiatric/Mental Health Illness

A. Description
   1. Loss of the ability to respond to the environment in ways that are in accord with oneself or society's expectations
   2. Characterized by thought or behavior patterns that cause the individual distress or impaired functioning
B. Personality characteristics
   1. Is unaccepting of self and dislikes self
   2. Has an unrealistic perception of strengths and weaknesses
   3. Thoughts and perceptions may not be reality based
   4. Is unable to find meaning and purpose in life
   5. Lacks direction and productivity in life
   6. Has difficulty in meeting own needs
   7. Depends on others for thought and actions
C. Adaptations to stress
   1. Feels out of control with self and with the environment
   2. Has a negative perception of the environment
   3. Has ineffective **coping mechanisms**
D. Interpersonal relationships
   1. Is unable to love and care for others
   2. Is unable to feel loved by others or accept feelings from others

III. Coping and Defense Mechanisms

A. **Coping mechanisms**
   1. Coping involves any effort to decrease the stress response
   2. **Coping mechanisms** can be either constructive or destructive in nature, task oriented related to direct problem solving, or can be a defense-oriented regulating response to protect oneself
   3. Destructive **coping mechanisms** often cause a mental health disorder because the problem that causes the disorder is avoided
   4. Neurotic or psychotic behaviors can typically result when **coping mechanisms** become destructive
B. **Defense mechanisms** (Box 69–1)
   1. A mechanism used to defend against anxiety and stress and to relieve emotional conflict caused by uncomfortable situations that threaten self-esteem
   2. The purpose of using a **defense mechanism** is to reduce anxiety and reestablish equilibrium
C. Implementation
   1. Assess the client's use of the **defense mechanism**
   2. Determine if the use of the **defense mechanism** characterizes unhealthy adjustment
   3. Facilitate appropriate use of **defense mechanisms**
   4. Avoid criticizing the behavior and the use of **defense mechanisms**
   5. Assist the client to identify the source of the anxiety
   6. Assist the client to explore methods to reduce the anxiety

BOX 69-1. Types of Defense Mechanisms

COMPENSATION

Putting forth extra effort to achieve in areas where one has a real or imagined deficiency

CONVERSION

The expression of emotional conflicts through physical symptoms

DENIAL

Disowning consciously intolerable thoughts and impulses

DISPLACEMENT

Feelings toward one person are directed to another who is less threatening, thereby satisfying an impulse with a substitute object

DISSOCIATION

The blocking off of an anxiety-provoking event or period of time from the conscious mind

FANTASY

Gratification by imaginary achievements and wishful thinking

FIXATION

Never advancing to the next level of emotional development and organization. The persistence in later life of interests and behavior patterns appropriate to an earlier age

IDENTIFICATION

The unconscious attempt to change oneself to resemble an admired person

INSULATION

Withdrawing into passivity and becoming inaccessible in order to avoid further threatening situations

INTELLECTUALIZATION

Excessive reasoning to avoid feeling; the thinking is disconnected from feelings, and situations are dealt with at a cognitive level

INTROJECTION

A type of identification in which the individual incorporates the traits or values of another into self

ISOLATION

Response in which a person blocks feelings associated with an unpleasant experience

PROJECTION

Transferring one's internal feelings, thoughts, and unacceptable ideas and traits to someone else

RATIONALIZATION

An attempt to make unacceptable feelings and behavior acceptable by justifying the behavior

REACTION FORMATION

Developing conscious attitudes and behaviors and acting out behaviors opposite to what one really feels

REGRESSION

Returning to an earlier developmental stage to express an impulse in order to deal with reality

REPRESSION

An unconscious process in which the client blocks undesirable and unacceptable thoughts from conscious expression

SUBLIMATION

Replacement of an unacceptable need, attitude, or emotion with one more socially acceptable

SUBSTITUTION

The replacement of a valued unacceptable object with an object that is more acceptable to the ego

SUPPRESSION

The conscious, deliberate forgetting of unacceptable or painful thoughts, ideas, and feelings

SYMBOLIZATION

The conscious use of an idea or object to represent another actual event or object; many times the meaning is not clear because the symbol may be representative of something unconscious

UNDOING

Engaging in behavior that is considered to be opposite of a previously unacceptable behavior, thought, or feeling

---

◆ **IV. The Nurse-Client Relationship**

A. Principles
1. Value the client as an individual
2. Be aware of the client in a holistic manner, including physical needs
3. Maintain appropriate limits
4. Remember that empathy is therapeutic and sympathy is nontherapeutic
5. Maintain honest and open communication
6. Encourage expression of the client's feelings
7. Assist the client to develop resources

◆ B. Phases of the therapeutic relationship
1. Orientation/initiation phase
   a. Establish boundaries and trust with the client
   b. Identify the expectations of the relationship
   c. Assess the anxiety in the client
   d. Define goals with the client
2. Working/continuation phase
   a. Promote an attitude of acceptance
   b. Continue to assess and evaluate problems
   c. Assist the client to express feelings
   d. Identify problems
   e. Promote insight and the use of constructive **coping mechanisms**
   f. Increase the client's independence

3. Termination/separation phase
   a. Prepare the client for termination and separation on initial contact
   b. Evaluate progress and achievement of goals
   c. Identify and deal with termination and separation issues
   d. Encourage the client to discuss feelings about termination
   e. Transfer the client to other support systems
   f. Do not promise the client that you will continue the relationship

V. Therapeutic Communication Process

A. Principles
   1. Communication includes both verbal and nonverbal expression
   2. Successful communication includes appropriateness, efficiency, flexibility, and feedback
   3. Anxiety in either the nurse or client impedes communication
   4. Communication needs to be goal directed within a professional framework
B. Therapeutic communication techniques and block to communication (Table 69–1)

VI. Diagnostic and Statistical Manual of Mental Disorders of the American Psychiatric Association

A. A taxonomy used to determine a medical diagnosis
B. A multiaxial system in which diagnostic criteria are inclusive for each diagnosis but allow for individualized differences within a pattern of behavior

Table 69–1. Therapeutic Communication Techniques and Blocks to Communication

Therapeutic Techniques	Blocks
Listening	Giving advice
Being silent	Changing the subject
Respecting the client	Giving approval or disapproval
Providing recognition and acknowledgment	Challenging the client
Providing feedback	Making stereotypical comments
Offering to assist	Making value judgments
Focusing and refocusing	Providing false reassurance
Clarifying and validating	Placing the client's feelings on hold
Reflecting	
Making observations	Asking the client "Why?"
Giving information	Being defensive
Presenting reality	
Summarizing	
Using open-ended questions	
Providing nonverbal encouragement	
Maintaining neutral responses	
Encouraging formulation of plan of action	

C. Knowledge of the criteria for a particular medical diagnosis will assist the nurse in making a clinical decision about a nursing diagnosis

VII. Types of Mental Health Admissions and Discharges (Box 69–2)

A. Voluntary admission
   1. Sought by the client or the client's guardian through a written application to the facility
   2. Voluntary clients have the right to demand an obtained release
   3. If the client is a minor, the release may be contingent on the consent of the parents or guardian
B. Informal admission
   1. A form of voluntary admission
   2. Informal admission permits a client to make a verbal application for the admission similar to that made for the hospital admission for medical treatment
C. Involuntary admission
   1. Involuntary admission is made without the client's consent
   2. Involuntary admission may be necessary when a person is a danger to self or others or is in need of psychiatric treatment or physical care
D. Commitment procedures
   1. Judicial determination, administrative determination, and agency determination
   2. A specified number of physicians must certify that the client's mental health justifies detention and treatment
   3. May be emergency, observational or temporary, or indeterminate or extended
E. Emergency involuntary admission
   1. Most states provide for emergency involuntary admission or civil commitment for a specified period (1 to 10 days on average) to prevent dangerous behavior that is likely to cause harm to self or others
   2. Police officers, physicians, and mental health professionals may be designated by statute to authorize the detention of mentally ill persons who are dangerous to themselves or others
F. Observational or temporary involuntary admission
   1. Civil commitment for observational or temporary, involuntary admission is of longer duration than emergency admission
   2. The primary purpose is observation, diagnosis, and treatment of people who suffer from mental illness or pose a danger to themselves or others
   3. The length of time is specified by statute and varies markedly from state to state
   4. Application for this type of admission can be made by a guardian, family member, physician, or other public health officer
   5. Some states permit any citizen to make application for aid to another

6. States vary as to their procedural requirements for this type of involuntary admission
7. Medical certification by two or more physicians that a person is mentally ill and in need of treatment, or a judicial or administrative review and order are often required for involuntary admission

G. Indeterminate, or extended, involuntary hospital admission
1. Provides extended care and treatment of the mentally ill
2. Those who undergo extended involuntary admission are committed solely through judicial or administrative action or medical certification
3. States that do not require a judicial hearing before commitment often provide the client with an opportunity for the judicial review after commitment procedures
4. This type of involuntary admission generally lasts 60 to 180 days, but it may be for an indeterminant length of time
5. Clients who are involuntarily committed do not lose their right of informed consent
6. Clients must be considered legally competent until they have been declared incompetent through a legal proceeding
7. If the nurse believes that a client lacks competency, action should be initiated to have a legal guardian appointed from the court

H. Release from the hospital
1. Description
   a. Depends on the client's admission status
   b. Clients who sought informal or voluntary admission have the right to demand and receive release
   c. Some states do provide for conditional release of voluntary clients, which enables the treating physician or administrator to order continued treatment on an outpatient basis if the clinical needs of the client warrant further care
2. Conditional release
   a. Usually requires outpatient treatment for a specified period to determine the client's compliance with medication protocol, ability to meet basic needs, and ability to reintegrate into the community
   b. A voluntary client who is conditionally released cannot be reinstitutionalized without consent unless the institution complies with the procedures for involuntary hospitalization
   c. An involuntary client who is conditionally released may be reinstitutionalized while the commitment is still in effect without recommencement of formal admission procedures

---

BOX 69–2. Client Rights

Right to accessible health care
Right to a coordination and continuity of health care
Right to courteous and individualized health care
Right to information about the qualifications, names, and titles of personnel delivering care
Right to refuse observation by those not directly involved in care
Right to privacy and confidentiality
Right to informed consent
Right to treatment
Right to refuse treatment
Right to treatment in the least restrictive setting
Right not to be subjected to unnecessary restraints
Right to habeas corpus; may request a hearing at any time to be released from the hospital
Right to information about diagnosis, prognosis, and treatment
Right to information on the charges of service
Right to communicate with people outside the hospital through written correspondence, telephone, and personal visits
Right to keep clothing and personal effects
Right to be employed
Right to religious freedom
Right to execute wills
Right to retain licenses, privileges, or permits established by law, such as a driver's or professional license

---

3. Discharge
   a. Discharge (unconditional release) is the termination of the client-institution relationship
   b. This release may be court ordered or administratively ordered
   c. The administration officer of an institution has the discretion to discharge clients
   d. In most states, clients can institute a court proceeding to seek a judicial discharge (writ of habeas corpus)
   e. Follow-up care is critical for these clients
   f. Discharge planning is important for the continued well-being of the psychiatric client
   g. After-care case managers are needed to facilitate the client's adaptation back into the community and to provide early referral if the treatment plan is not followed

PRACTICE QUESTIONS

1. Unresolved feelings related to loss may be weakened during which phase of the therapeutic nurse-client relationship?
   1 Orientation phase
   2 Working phase
   3 Termination phase
   4 Trusting phase

2. A client with major depression who attempted suicide says to the nurse, "I should have died. I've always been a failure. Nothing ever goes right for me." The most therapeutic response by the nurse is
   1 "I don't see you as a failure."
   2 "Feeling like this is all part of being ill."
   3 "You've been feeling like a failure for a while?"
   4 "You have everything to live for."

3. The community health nurse visits a client at home who says, "I haven't slept at all the last couple of nights." Which of the following responses by the nurse illustrates the most therapeutic communication technique for this client?
   1 "Go on . . . "
   2 "Sleeping?"
   3 "The last couple of nights?"
   4 "You're having difficulty sleeping?"

4. While the male nurse is conducting a sexual interview with a female client, the client states, "I don't want to discuss this—it's private and personal." Which of the following statements, if made by the male nurse, indicates that the nurse is therapeutic?
   1 "This often happens to me. Perhaps you would find it easier to speak to a nurse who is female?"
   2 "I am a professional nurse and as such I'll have you know that all information is kept confidential."
   3 "I know that some of these questions are difficult for you, but as a professional nurse, I must legally respect your confidentiality."
   4 "This is difficult for you to speak about, but I am trying to perform a complete assessment and I am no different from a female nurse, if that's your problem. We are both professionals."

5. The nurse is caring for a Native American client who says, "I don't want you to touch me. I'll take care of myself!" Which of the following responses is the most therapeutic communication by the nurse?
   1 "I will respect your feelings. I'll just leave this cup for you to collect your urine in. After breakfast, I will take more blood from you."
   2 "If you didn't want our care, why did you come here?"
   3 "Why are you being so difficult? I only want to help you."
   4 "Sounds like you're feeling pretty troubled by all of us. Let's work together so you can do everything for yourself."

6. A client admitted to the psychiatric hospital is experiencing Altered Thought Processes. The client believes that the food is being poisoned. Which type of communication technique does

the nurse plan to use to encourage the client to eat?
   1 Using open-ended questions and silence
   2 Offering opinions about the necessity of adequate nutrition
   3 Identifying the reasons that the client may not want to eat
   4 Focusing on self-disclosure regarding food preferences

7. The nurse is working with a client who has sought counseling after trying to save a neighbor involved in a house fire. In spite of the client's efforts, the neighbor died. Which of the following actions does the nurse engage in with the client during the working phase of the nurse-client relationship?
   1 Exploring the client's potential for self-harm
   2 Exploring the client's ability to function
   3 Inquiring about the client's perception or appraisal of the neighbor's death
   4 Inquiring about and examining the client's feelings that may block adaptive coping

8. A client who has just been sexually assaulted is very quiet and calm. The nurse analyzes this behavior as indicative of which defense mechanism?
   1 Denial
   2 Projection
   3 Rationalization
   4 Intellectualization

9. The nurse completes the initial assessment of a client admitted to the psychiatric unit. The nurse analyzes the data obtained on assessment and determines that which of the following presents a potential concern?
   1 The presence of bruises on the client's body
   2 The client's report of not eating or sleeping
   3 The client's report of suicidal thoughts
   4 The significant other's disapproval of the treatment

10. Laboratory work is prescribed on a client who has been experiencing delusions. When the nurse approaches the client to obtain a specimen of the client's blood, the client begins to shout "You're all vampires. Let me out of here!" The most appropriate nursing response is which of the following?
    1 "I am not going to hurt you, I am going to help you!"
    2 "What makes you think that I am a vampire?"
    3 "I'll leave and come back later for your blood."
    4 "It must be fearful to think others want to hurt you."

11. An inebriated client is brought to the emergency department by the local police. The client is told that the physician will be in to see the client in about 30 minutes. The client becomes very loud

and offensive and wants to be seen by the physician immediately. The most appropriate nursing intervention is which of the following?

1 Attempt to talk with the client to deescalate behavior
2 Watch the behavior escalate before intervening
3 Inform the client that he or she will be asked to leave if the behavior continues
4 Offer to take the client to an examination room until he or she can be treated

12. A client is admitted to a psychiatric unit for treatment of psychotic behavior. The client is at the locked exit door, and is shouting, "Let me out. There's nothing wrong with me. I don't belong here." The nurse analyzes this behavior as

1 Projection
2 Denial
3 Regression
4 Rationalization

13. A home health nurse is consulting with the psychiatric nurse and says, "Now that the client is responding to the antidepressant, the suicidal risk is over and I can stop my home visits." After analyzing this nurse's statement, which of the following is the most appropriate response by the psychiatric nurse?

1 "I agree. Clients who want to kill themselves are only suicidal for a limited time. No one can feel self-destructive forever."
2 "I disagree. Your comment reflects a lack of knowledge that this disease runs in families."
3 "I agree. The suicidal threats were really attention seeking. Continuing to visit would reinforce the client's use of manipulation."
4 "I disagree. Most suicides occur within about 3 months after improvement begins because the client now has the energy to carry out the suicidal intentions."

14. The supervisor reprimands the nurse in charge of the nursing unit because the charge nurse has not adhered to the unit budget. Later that afternoon, the charge nurse accuses the nursing staff of wasting supplies. This behavior is an example of

1 Denial
2 Repression
3 Suppression
4 Displacement

15. The client says to the nurse, "I'm going to die, and I wish my family would stop hoping for a cure! I get so angry when they carry on like this! After all, I'm the one who's dying." The most therapeutic response by the nurse is

1 "You're feeling angry that your family continues to hope for you to be cured?"

2 "I think we should talk more about your anger with your family."
3 "Well, it sounds like you're being pretty pessimistic. After all, years ago people died of pneumonia."
4 "Have you shared your feelings with your family?"

16. The nurse employed in a psychiatric unit is assigned to care for a client admitted to the unit 2 days ago. On review of the client's record, the nurse notes that the admission was an informal voluntary admission. Based on this type of admission, the nurse anticipates which of the following?

1 The client will be very resistant to treatment measures
2 The client's family will be very resistant to treatment measures
3 The client will be angry and will refuse care
4 The client will participate in the planning of the care and treatment plan

17. A nurse enters a client's room, and the client is demanding release from the hospital. The nurse reviews the client's record and notes that the client was admitted 2 days ago for treatment of anxiety disorder, and that the admission was a voluntary admission. Which of the following nursing actions will the nurse take?

1 Tell the client that discharge is not possible at this time
2 Call the client's family
3 Contact the physician
4 Persuade the client to stay a few more days

18. A client is admitted to the psychiatric nursing unit. On admission assessment, the nurse notes that the client is admitted by involuntary status. Based on this type of admission, the nurse most likely expects that the client

1 Presents a harm to self
2 Requested the admission
3 Consented to the admission
4 Provided written application to the facility for admission

19. The nurse is caring for a client who is scheduled for electroconvulsive therapy (ECT). The nurse notes that an informed consent has not been obtained for the procedure. On review of the record, the nurse notes that the admission was an involuntary hospitalization. Based on this information, the nurse determines

1 That an informed consent does not need to be obtained
2 That an informed consent should be obtained from the family
3 That an informed consent needs to be obtained from the client
4 That the physician will obtain the informed consent

20. Following a group therapy session, a client approaches a nurse and verbalizes a need for seclusion because of uncontrollable feelings. The most appropriate nursing action is to
    1 Inform the client that seclusion has not been prescribed
    2 Obtain an informed consent
    3 Call the client's family
    4 Place the client in seclusion immediately

21. The nurse is providing care to a client admitted to the hospital with a diagnosis of acute anxiety disorder. The nurse is conversing with the client. The client says to the nurse, "I have a secret that I want to tell you. You won't tell anyone about it, will you?" The most appropriate nursing response is which of the following?
    1 "No, I won't tell anyone."
    2 "I cannot promise to keep a secret."
    3 "If you tell me the secret, I will tell it to your doctor."
    4 "If you tell me the secret, I will need to document it in your record."

22. The nurse in a psychiatric clinic is greeted by a neighbor in a local grocery store. The neighbor says to the nurse, "How is Carol doing? She is my best friend and is seen at your clinic every week." The most appropriate nursing response is which of the following?
    1 "I'm not supposed to discuss this, but since you are my neighbor, I can tell you that she is doing great!"
    2 "I'm not supposed to discuss this, but since you are my neighbor, I can tell you that she really has some problems!"
    3 "If you want to know about Carol, you need to ask her yourself."

    4 "I cannot discuss any client situation with you."

23. The client was involuntarily admitted to the psychiatric unit because of episodes of extremely violent behavior. The client is demanding to be discharged from the hospital. The nurse does not allow the client to leave. Which of the following represents the legal ramifications associated with the nurse's behavior?
    1 The nurse will be charged with imprisonment
    2 The nurse will be charged with assault
    3 The nurse will be charged with slander
    4 No charge will be made against the nurse because the nurse's actions are reasonable

24. The nurse is preparing the client for the termination phase of the nurse-client relationship. Which of the following nursing tasks is most appropriate for this phase?
    1 Identifying expected outcomes
    2 Planning short-term goals
    3 Making appropriate referrals
    4 Developing a realistic solution

25. During the termination phase of the nurse-client relationship, the nurse observes that the client continuously demonstrates bursts of anger. The most appropriate interpretation of the behavior is that the client
    1 Requires further treatment and is not ready to be discharged
    2 Is displaying typical behaviors that can occur during termination
    3 Needs to be admitted to the hospital
    4 Needs to be referred to the psychiatrist as soon as possible

ANSWERS

1. **3**

Rationale: Termination often weakens strong feelings in the nurse and client. Since this represents a loss for both, unresolved issues that have a loss component may be reawakened during the termination process.

Test-Taking Strategy: Note the key words "unresolved" and "weakened" in the question. Considering the phases of the therapeutic nurse-client relationship will easily direct you to option 3. Review these phases now if you had difficulty with this question!

Level of Cognitive Ability: Analysis
Phase of Nursing Process: Analysis
Client Needs: Psychosocial Integrity
Content Area: Mental Health

Reference
Varcarolis, E. (1998). *Foundations of psychiatric mental health nursing* (3rd ed.). Philadelphia: W. B. Saunders. p. 162.

2. **3**

Rationale: Responding to the feelings expressed by a client is an effective therapeutic communication technique. The correct option is an example of the use of restating. Options 1, 2, and 4 block communication because they minimize the client's experience and do not facilitate exploration of the client's expressed feelings.

Test-Taking Strategy: Knowledge of the techniques that facilitate therapeutic communication will help you choose the correct option. Select an option that directly addresses client feelings and concerns. Option 3 is the only option that is stated in the form of a question and is open-ended, thus will encourage the verbalization of feelings.

Level of Cognitive Ability: Application
Phase of Nursing Process: Implementation
Client Needs: Psychosocial Integrity
Content Area: Mental Health

Reference
Haber, J., et al. (1997). *Comprehensive psychiatric nursing* (5th ed.). St. Louis: Mosby–Year Book. p. 131.

3. 4

Rationale: The most therapeutic nursing communication technique is restatement. Although it is a technique that has a prompting component to it, it repeats the client's major theme, which assists the nurse to obtain a more specific perception of the problem from the client.

Test-Taking Strategy: Option 1 is not the most therapeutic response because it is a general lead and allows the client to direct the discussion when it needs to be more focused at this point. Option 2 is not the most therapeutic because it uses reflection that simply repeats the client's last words to prompt further discussion (which, again, is too open-ended). Option 3 focuses on the number of nights rather than the specific problem of sleep. Option 4 will provide the perception of the problem from the client's perspective.

Level of Cognitive Ability: Application
Phase of Nursing Process: Implementation
Client Needs: Health Promotion and Maintenance
Content Area: Mental Health

Reference
Glod, C. A. (1998). *Contemporary psychiatric-mental health nursing.* Philadelphia: F. A. Davis. pp. 57–61.

4. 3

Rationale: On reading the stem of the question, you cannot tell whether the client is responding to the nurse's gender or is simply uncomfortable sharing personal information of an intimate nature. The most therapeutic response for the male nurse is not to bring what may be his own gender issues into the response at this time.

Test-Taking Strategy: This question seeks to examine your analysis of a potentially sensitive situation. In option 1, the male nurse seems to be projecting his experiences onto the client. In any case, it is not therapeutic because the response clearly ignores the fact that this is not about the nurse, but is about the client and the client's discomfort. In option 2, the nurse becomes pompous and just a tad angry and supercilious, which is not therapeutic. In option 4, the nurse begins correctly with an empathic stance but becomes involved in a gender defense and somewhat defensive about the nurse's professional demeanor.

Level of Cognitive Ability: Analysis
Phase of Nursing Process: Evaluation
Client Needs: Psychosocial Integrity
Content Area: Mental Health

Reference
Glod, C. A. (1998). *Contemporary psychiatric-mental health nursing.* Philadelphia: F. A. Davis. pp. 58–60, 445–459.

5. 4

Rationale: The most therapeutic response is the one that reflects the client's feelings and empowers the client by offering the control of the client's care. In this way, the nurse avoids engaging in a regressive struggle with the client. Native Americans view touch very differently from other Americans.

Test-Taking Strategy: This question tests your knowledge of culturally congruent communications for Native American clients. In option 1, the nurse uses avoidance and information giving. Option 2 is an aggressive and nontherapeutic communication technique. Option 3 is social and nontherapeutic because it labels the client's behavior and is likely to provoke anger from the client.

Level of Cognitive Ability: Analysis
Phase of Nursing Process: Analysis
Client Needs: Psychosocial Integrity
Content Area: Mental Health

Reference
Stuart, G. W., & Laraia, M. T. (1998). *Principles and practice of psychiatric nursing* (6th ed.). St. Louis: Mosby–Year Book. pp. 17–61.

6. 1

Rationale: Open-ended questions and silence are strategies used to encourage clients to discuss their problem. Options 2 and 3 are not helpful to the client because they do not encourage the client to express feelings. The nurse should not offer opinions and should encourage the client to identify the reasons for the behavior. Option 4 is not a client-centered intervention.

Test-Taking Strategy: Use the process of elimination. Eliminate options 2 and 3 first because they do not support the client's expression of feelings. Eliminate option 4 next because it is not a client-centered response. This leaves option 1 as the correct choice. Focusing on the client's feelings will easily direct you to option 1.

Level of Cognitive Ability: Application
Phase of Nursing Process: Planning
Client Needs: Psychosocial Integrity
Content Area: Mental Health

Reference
Haber, J., et al. (1997). *Comprehensive psychiatric nursing* (5th ed.). St. Louis: Mosby–Year Book. pp. 129, 592–593.

7. 4

Rationale: The client must first deal with feelings and negative responses before the client is able to work through the meaning of the crisis. Option 4 pertains directly to the client's feelings. Options 1, 2, and 3 do not directly address the client's feelings.

Test-Taking Strategy: It is necessary to know the tasks pertaining to each nursing process phase as well as crisis intervention content. Use the process of elimination in selecting the option that focuses on the feelings of the client. Review the phases of the nurse-client relationship now if you had difficulty with this question!

Level of Cognitive Ability: Application
Phase of Nursing Process: Implementation
Client Needs: Psychosocial Integrity
Content Area: Mental Health

Reference
Johnson, B. S. (1997). *Psychiatric mental health nursing: Adaptation and growth* (4th ed.). Philadelphia: Lippincott-Raven. p. 798.

8. 1

Rationale: Denial is a response by victims of sexual abuse. It is described as an adaptive and protective reaction. Projection is blaming or "scapegoating." Rationalization is justifying the unacceptable attributes about him- or herself. Intellectualization is the excessive use of abstract thinking or generalizations to decrease painful thinking.

Test-Taking Strategy: Knowledge regarding defense mechanisms is required to answer the question. The key words in the question are "calm" and "quiet." These behaviors are indicative of denial in a sexually abused victim. If you had difficulty with this question, take time now to review content related to the sexually abused victim and defense mechanisms!

Level of Cognitive Ability: Analysis
Phase of Nursing Process: Analysis
Client Needs: Psychosocial Integrity
Content Area: Mental Health

Reference
Fortinash, K. M., & Holoday-Worret, P. A. (1996). *Psychiatric-mental health nursing.* St. Louis: Mosby–Year Book. p. 18.

9. **3**

Rationale: The client's thoughts are extremely important when verbalized. Suicidal thoughts direct the nurse to incorporate this information into the plan of care. The nurse has the legal responsibility to protect the client from harm. Options 1, 2, and 4 will all affect the treatment of the client but are not of greatest importance at this time.

Test-Taking Strategy: The client is the focus of the question; therefore, eliminate option 4. Use priorities when selecting the correct option. Eliminate option 2 as of the least concern among the remaining options. Select option 3 because it is global and if the client verbalizes suicidal thoughts, it is a priority concern!

Level of Cognitive Ability: Analysis
Phase of Nursing Process: Analysis
Client Needs: Psychosocial Integrity
Content Area: Mental Health

Reference
Brent, N. (1997). *Nurses and the law.* Philadelphia: W. B. Saunders. p. 415.

10. **4**

Rationale: This response helps the client to focus on the emotion underlying the delusion, but does not argue with it. If the nurse attempts to change the client's mind, the delusion may in fact be even more strongly held.

Test-Taking Strategy: Knowledge regarding the dynamics of delusions and how delusions meet the client's underlying needs is helpful to answer the question. Option 4 is the only option that recognizes the client's need. Additionally, option 4 focuses on the client's feelings!

Level of Cognitive Ability: Analysis
Phase of Nursing Process: Analysis
Client Needs: Psychosocial Integrity
Content Area: Mental Health

Reference
Haber, J., et al. (1997). *Comprehensive psychiatric nursing* (5th ed.). St. Louis: Mosby–Year Book. p. 592.

11. **4**

Rationale: Safety of the client, other clients, and staff is of prime concern. When dealing with an impaired individual, trying to talk may be out of the question. Medication may be needed, and it may be necessary to restrain or seclude a client temporarily until he or she is no longer a danger to others. Option 1 may be out of the question, given the fact that the client is inebriated and may not be able to be reasoned with. Option 2 would be a mistake because waiting to intervene could cause the client to become even more agitated and a threat to others. Option 3 would only

further aggravate an already agitated individual. Option 4 is in effect an isolation technique that allows for separation from others and provides a less stimulating environment where the client can maintain dignity.

Test-Taking Strategy: Identifying that the client is inebriated makes a tremendous difference in the option that is selected. Use this information and the process of elimination to select the correct option. Option 4 most directly addresses the situation and the behavior and feelings of the client!

Level of Cognitive Ability: Analysis
Phase of Nursing Process: Analysis
Client Needs: Psychosocial Integrity
Content Area: Mental Health

Reference
Carson, V., & Arnold, E. (1996). *Mental health nursing: The nurse-patient journey.* Philadelphia: W. B. Saunders. p. 348.

12. **2**

Rationale: Denial is refusal to admit to a painful reality, which is treated as if it does not exist. In projection, a person unconsciously rejects emotionally unacceptable features and attributes them to other people, objects, or situations. In regression, the client returns to an earlier, more comforting, although less mature way of behaving. Rationalization is justifying illogical or unreasonable ideas, actions, or feelings by developing acceptable explanations that satisfy the teller as well as the listener.

Test-Taking Strategy: Remember that defense mechanisms are misused by clients who are dealing with threats to their esteem. The key phrase in the question that should direct you to the correct option is "There's nothing wrong with me." Select the response that recognizes clients' attempts to avoid looking at the reality of their situation. If you had difficulty with this question, take time now to review defense mechanisms!

Level of Cognitive Ability: Analysis
Phase of Nursing Process: Analysis
Client Needs: Psychosocial Integrity
Content Area: Mental Health

Reference
Carson, V., & Arnold, E. (1996). *Mental health nursing: The nurse-patient journey.* Philadelphia: W. B. Saunders. pp. 695–698.

13. **4**

Rationale: The statement made by the home health nurse is a classic example of one of the myths or fables about suicide. The facts presented by the psychiatric nurse in the correct option are accurate. Most suicides do occur within 3 months after the beginning of the improvement, when the client has the energy to carry out the suicidal intentions. At all visits, the nurse must assess for the continuation of suicidal ideation.

Test-Taking Strategy: Knowledge regarding the facts of suicide is required to answer the question. Use the process of elimination to answer the question. In option 1, while it is true that suicidal ideation is usually time-limited, this depends upon whether the feelings of self-destruction are eradicated. A small segment of the population with mental illness learns to live successfully in spite of the persistence of self-destructive ideas throughout their lives. In option 2, the information is incorrect, because suicide is not inherited. In addition, the communication is hypercritical and puts down the visiting nurse. Option 3 presents a myth about suicide.

Level of Cognitive Ability: Analysis
Phase of Nursing Process: Analysis
Client Needs: Psychosocial Integrity
Content Area: Mental Health

Reference

Carson, V., & Arnold, E. (1996). *Mental health nursing: The nurse-patient journey.* Philadelphia: W. B. Saunders. pp. 932–936.

14. **4**

Rationale: Ego defense mechanisms are operations outside of a person's awareness that the ego calls into play to protect against anxiety. Displacement is the discharging of pent-up feelings on people less dangerous than those who initially aroused the emotion. Denial is the blocking out of painful or anxiety-inducing events or feelings. Suppression is consciously keeping unacceptable feelings and thoughts out of awareness. Repression is unconsciously keeping unacceptable feelings out of awareness.

Test-Taking Strategy: Knowledge of ego defense mechanisms is necessary to answer the question. Read the behavior identified in the question to assist you in determining the type of ego defense mechanism. If you had difficulty with this question, take time now to review defense mechanisms!

Level of Cognitive Ability: Analysis
Phase of Nursing Process: Analysis
Client Needs: Psychosocial Integrity
Content Area: Mental Health

Reference

Carson, V., & Arnold, E. (1996). *Mental health nursing: The nurse-patient journey.* Philadelphia: W. B. Saunders. p. 697.

15. **1**

Rationale: Reflection is the therapeutic communication technique that redirects the client's feelings back in order to validate what the client is saying. In this case, the client may be able to "see" the dynamics involved in the client-family relationship. Questions that the client will be able to deal with more effectively include exploring the client's unwillingness to maintain hope and the client's anger regarding the family's hopefulness.

Test-Taking Strategy: Use therapeutic communication techniques to answer the question. Option 1 uses the therapeutic technique of reflection. In option 2, the nurse attempts to use focusing but the attempt to discuss central issues seems premature. In option 3, the nurse makes a judgment and is nontherapeutic in the one-on-one relationship. In option 4, the nurse is attempting to assess the client's ability to openly discuss feelings with family members. Although this is an appropriate communication and assessment for this client, the timing is somewhat premature and closes off facilitation of the client's feelings.

Level of Cognitive Ability: Application
Phase of Nursing Process: Implementation
Client Needs: Psychosocial Integrity
Content Area: Mental Health

Reference

Leahy, J, & Kizilay, P. (1998). *Foundations of nursing practice: A nursing process approach.* Philadelphia: W. B. Saunders. pp. 224–226.

16. **4**

Rationale: Generally, voluntary admission is sought by the client or client's guardian through a written application to

the facility. An informal voluntary admission permits a client to make a verbal application for admission, similar to that made for hospital admission for medical treatment. If the client seeks voluntary admission, the most likely expectation is that the client will participate in the treatment program.

Test-Taking Strategy: Note the key words "informal voluntary admission." This should provide you with the clue that will easily direct you to option 4. Additionally, note that options 1, 2, and 3 are similar. Review the various types of hospital admission processes now if you had difficulty with this question!

Level of Cognitive Ability: Analysis
Phase of Nursing Process: Analysis
Client Needs: Psychosocial Integrity
Content Area: Mental Health

Reference

Varcarolis, E. (1998). *Foundations of psychiatric mental health nursing* (3rd ed.). Philadelphia: W. B. Saunders. p. 99.

17. **3**

Rationale: Generally, voluntary admission is sought by the client or client's guardian through a written application to the facility. Voluntary clients have the right to demand and obtain release. If the client is a minor, the release may be contingent on the consent of the parents or guardian. The nurse needs to be familiar with state and facility policies and procedures. Many states require that the client submit a written release notice to the facility staff, who reevaluate the client's condition for possible conversion to involuntary status, according to criteria established by law. The best nursing action is to contact the physician.

Test-Taking Strategy: Noting the type of hospital admission will assist in eliminating option 1. It is inappropriate to "persuade" a client to stay in the hospital. Option 2 should be eliminated based simply on the issue of client rights and the issue of confidentiality. Review the various types of hospital admission and discharge processes now if you had difficulty with this question!

Level of Cognitive Ability: Application
Phase of Nursing Process: Implementation
Client Needs: Safe, Effective Care Environment
Content Area: Mental Health

Reference

Varcarolis, E. (1998). *Foundations of psychiatric mental health nursing* (3rd ed.). Philadelphia: W. B. Saunders. p. 99.

18. **1**

Rationale: Involuntary admission is made without the client's consent. Involuntary admission is necessary when a person is a danger to self or others or is in need of psychiatric treatment or physical care. A specified number of physicians must certify that a person's mental health justifies detention and treatment. Options 2, 3, and 4 describe the process of voluntary admission.

Test-Taking Strategy: Note the key words "involuntary status." This should easily direct you to option 1. Note that options 2, 3, and 4 are all similar. Review the process of involuntary admission now if you had difficulty with this question!

Level of Cognitive Ability: Analysis
Phase of Nursing Process: Analysis
Client Needs: Psychosocial Integrity
Content Area: Mental Health

Reference
Varcarolis, E. (1998). *Foundations of psychiatric mental health nursing* (3rd ed.). Philadelphia: W. B. Saunders. p. 99.

19. 3

Rationale: Clients who are involuntarily admitted do not lose their right to informed consent. Clients must be considered legally competent until they have been declared incompetent through a legal proceeding. The informed consent needs to be obtained from the client.

Test-Taking Strategy: Knowledge regarding the hospital admission process and the client's rights is necessary to answer this question. If you had difficulty with this question, focus on the issue of client rights to direct you to option 3. Review client rights now if you had difficulty with this question!

Level of Cognitive Ability: Analysis
Phase of Nursing Process: Implementation
Client Needs: Safe, Effective Care Environment
Content Area: Mental Health

Reference
Varcarolis, E. (1998). *Foundations of psychiatric mental health nursing* (3rd ed.). Philadelphia: W. B. Saunders. p. 100.

20. 2

Rationale: A client may request to be secluded or restrained. Federal laws require the consent of the client, unless an emergency situation exists in which an immediate risk to the client or others can be documented. The use of seclusion and restraint is permitted only on the written order of a physician, which must be reviewed and renewed every 24 hours, and which also must specify the type of restraint to be used.

Test-Taking Strategy: Knowledge regarding the legal issues surrounding the use of seclusion and restraints and knowledge regarding the issue of clients rights will easily direct you to option 2. There is no reason to call the family at this time; therefore, eliminate option 3. Knowing that a physician's written order is necessary will assist in eliminating option 4. Option 1 is not the best choice because this information, if given to a client experiencing uncontrollable feelings, may cause escalation of the feelings.

Level of Cognitive Ability: Application
Phase of Nursing Process: Implementation
Client Needs: Safe, Effective Care Environment
Content Area: Mental Health

Reference
Varcarolis, E. (1998). *Foundations of psychiatric mental health nursing* (3rd ed.). Philadelphia: W. B. Saunders. pp. 100, 321.

21. 2

Rationale: The nurse should never promise to keep a secret. Secrets are appropriate in a social relationship but not in a therapeutic one. The nurse needs to be honest with the client and tell the client that a promise cannot be made to keep the secret.

Test-Taking Strategy: Read each option carefully. Option 1 can be easily eliminated because it is inappropriate. Also, options 3 and 4 are not only inappropriate but are to an extent threatening and may even block further communication.

Level of Cognitive Ability: Application
Phase of Nursing Process: Implementation
Client Needs: Safe, Effective Care Environment
Content Area: Mental Health

Reference
Carson, V., & Arnold, E. (1996). *Mental health nursing: The nurse-patient journey.* Philadelphia: W. B. Saunders. p. 87.

22. 4

Rationale: A nurse is required to maintain confidentiality regarding clients and their care. Confidentiality is basic to the therapeutic relationship and is a client's right. The most appropriate response to the neighbor is option 4. Option 3 is correct in a sense; however, it is a rather blunt statement. Both options 1 and 2 identify statements that do not maintain client confidentiality. Option 4 is most direct and correct.

Test-Taking Strategy: Focus on the issue of the question: maintaining confidentiality. This should easily assist you in eliminating options 1 and 2. From the remaining options, select option 4 over option 3 because it is most direct and correct. Option 3 is a rather blunt and somewhat rude statement. Review confidentiality issues now if you had difficulty with this question!

Level of Cognitive Ability: Application
Phase of Nursing Process: Implementation
Client Needs: Safe, Effective Care Environment
Content Area: Mental Health

Reference
Carson, V., & Arnold, E. (1996). *Mental health nursing: The nurse-patient journey.* Philadelphia: W. B. Saunders. p. 87.

23. 4

Rationale: False imprisonment is an act with the intent to confine a person to a specific area. A nurse can be charged with false imprisonment if the nurse prohibits a client from leaving the hospital if the client was voluntarily admitted and if there are no agency or legal policies for detaining the client. On the other hand, if the client was involuntarily admitted or had agreed to an evaluation before discharge, the nurse's actions are reasonable.

Test-Taking Strategy: Noting the key words "involuntarily admitted" will easily direct you to eliminate option 1 and direct you to option 4. Options 2 and 3 are unrelated to the issue of the question and can be easily eliminated. Review the issues related to false imprisonment and hospital admissions now if you had difficulty with this question!

Level of Cognitive Ability: Analysis
Phase of Nursing Process: Analysis
Client Needs: Safe, Effective Care Environment
Content Area: Mental Health

Reference
Varcarolis, E. (1998). *Foundations of psychiatric mental health nursing* (3rd ed.). Philadelphia: W. B. Saunders. p. 106.

24. 3

Rationale: Tasks of the termination phase include evaluating client performance, evaluating achievement of expected outcomes, evaluating future needs, making appropriate referrals, and dealing with the common behaviors associated with termination. Options 1, 2, and 4 identify the tasks of the working phase of the relationship.

Test-Taking Strategy: Noting the key words "termination phase" should easily direct you to option 3. If you are unfamiliar with the appropriate tasks of the phases of the nurse-client relationship, take time now to review!

Level of Cognitive Ability: Analysis
Phase of Nursing Process: Evaluation
Client Needs: Psychosocial Integrity
Content Area: Mental Health

Reference

Carson, V., & Arnold, E. (1996). *Mental health nursing: The nurse-patient journey.* Philadelphia: W. B. Saunders. p. 87.

25. **2**

Rationale: In the termination phase of a relationship, it is normal for a client to demonstrate a number of regressive behaviors that can be disturbing to the nurse. Typical be-haviors include return of symptoms, anger, withdrawal, and minimizing the relationship. The anger that the client is experiencing is a normal behavior during the termination phase and does not necessarily indicate the need for hospi-talization or treatment.

Test-Taking Strategy: Note the key words "termination phase." This alone may assist in directing you to option 2. Additionally, note the similarity between options 1, 3, and 4. These options address the need for further supervised treatment. If you are unfamiliar with the client behaviors associated with the termination phase, take time now to re-view!

Level of Cognitive Ability: Analysis
Phase of Nursing Process: Evaluation
Client Needs: Psychosocial Integrity
Content Area: Mental Health

Reference

Carson, V., & Arnold, E. (1996). *Mental health nursing: The nurse-patient journey.* Philadelphia: W. B. Saunders. p. 258.

BIBLIOGRAPHY

Brent, N. (1997). *Nurses and the law.* Philadelphia: W. B. Saunders.

Carson, V., & Arnold, E. (1996). *Mental health nursing: The nurse-patient journey.* Philadelphia: W. B. Saunders.

Fortinash, K. M., & Holoday-Worret, P. A. (1996). *Psychiatric-mental health nursing.* St. Louis: Mosby–Year Book.

Glod, C. A. (1998). *Contemporary psychiatric-mental health nursing.* Philadelphia: F. A. Davis.

Haber, J., et al. (1997). *Comprehensive psychiatric nursing* (5th ed.). St. Louis: Mosby–Year Book.

Johnson, B. S. (1997). *Psychiatric mental health nursing: Adaptation and growth* (4th ed.). Philadelphia: Lippincott-Raven.

Leahy, J, & Kizilay, P. (1998). *Foundations of nursing practice: A nursing process approach.* Philadelphia: W. B. Saunders.

O'Toole, M. (1997). *Miller-Keane encyclopedia & dictionary of medicine, nursing, & allied health* (6th ed.). Philadelphia: W. B. Saunders.

Stuart, G. W., & Laraia, M. T. (1998). *Principles and practice of psychiatric nursing* (6th ed.). St. Louis: Mosby–Year Book.

Varcarolis, E. (1998). *Foundations of psychiatric mental health nursing* (3rd ed.). Philadelphia: W. B. Saunders.

CHAPTER 70

Models of Care

I. Milieu Therapy

A. Description
1. **Milieu** is the physical and social environment in which an individual lives
2. Provides an environment that is adapted to the individual client's needs and also provides greater comfort and freedom of expression than has been experienced in the past by the client
3. Staffed by people trained to provide support and understanding and individual attention
4. All members contribute to the planning and functioning of the setting
5. The power hierarchy is diminished because all members are viewed as significant and valuable members of the community

B. Focus
1. Positive environmental manipulation, both physical and social, in order to effect a positive change
2. Client's rights through involvement in setting goals, freedom of movement, and informal relationships with staff
3. Group and social interaction
4. Use of community meetings, activity groups, social skills groups, and physical exercise programs

II. Psychotherapy

A. Description
1. Use of a group of techniques to modify feelings, attitudes, and behaviors in clients
2. Therapist uses both verbal and nonverbal means of communication to build a relationship with the client

B. Focus
1. The basic concept involves understanding
2. The focus is on issues of importance to the client, purpose of the interaction, identification of the roles of the therapist and client, and the use of primarily verbal means of communication

3. Nonverbal techniques include silence, body language, facial expressions, and respect for personal space

C. Levels of psychotherapy
1. Supportive therapy
   a. Allows the client to express feelings, explore alternatives, and make decisions in a safe, caring environment
   b. It may be needed briefly or over a period of years
   c. There is no plan to introduce new methods of coping, instead the therapist reinforces the client's existing **coping mechanisms**
2. Reeducative therapy
   a. Involves learning new ways of perceiving and behaving
   b. The client explores alternatives in a planned systematic way, which requires a longer period than supportive therapy requires
   c. The client enters into a contract that specifies desired changes of behavior
   d. Reeducative therapy includes short-term psychotherapy, reality therapy, cognitive restructuring, and behavior modification
3. Reconstructive therapy
   a. Involves deep psychotherapy or psychoanalysis
   b. It may require 2 to 5 years of therapy or more and focuses on all aspects of the client's life
   c. Emotional and cognitive restructuring of self takes place
   d. Positive outcomes include greater understanding of self and others, more emotional freedom, and the development of potential abilities

III. Behavior and Behavior Modification

A. Behavior therapy
1. An approach to bring about behavioral change
2. It includes a group of diversified approaches for dealing with maladaptive behavior

1215

3. The belief is that most behaviors are learned
4. Maladaptive behavior is a way of dealing with stress, and the therapy is an approach to bring about a change in the behavior

B. Self-control therapy
1. Combination of cognitive and behavioral approaches
2. A basic theme is that talking to oneself can direct and control actions more effectively
3. Useful to deal with stress

C. Desensitization
1. The reduction of intense reactions to a stimulus by repeated exposure to the stimulus in a weaker and milder form
2. Gradually over a period of time, exposure is increased until the fear of the object or situation has ceased

D. Aversion therapy
1. Negative reinforcement is a technique to change behavior
2. A stimulus attractive to the client is paired with an unpleasant event in hopes of endowing it with negative properties

E. Modeling: the therapist provides a role model for specified identified behaviors and the client learns through imitation

F. Operant conditioning: entails rewarding a client for desired behaviors and is the basis for behavior modification

IV. Cognitive Therapy

1. An active, directive time-limited structured approach used to treat a variety of psychiatric disorders
2. Therapeutic techniques are designed to identify reality testing and correct distorted conceptualization and the dysfunctional belief underlying these cognitions
3. Clients learn to master problems in situations they previously considered insuperable by evaluating and correcting their thinking
4. The cognitive therapist helps clients to think and act more realistically and adaptively about their psychological problems so as to reduce symptoms
5. Various cognitive and behavioral strategies are used in cognitive therapy

V. Groups and Group Therapy

A. Stages of group development
1. Initial stage
   a. Involves superficial rather than open and trusting communication
   b. Members are becoming acquainted with each other and are searching for similarity between themselves and other group members
   c. Members may be unclear about the purpose or goals of the group
   d. A certain amount of structuring of group norms, roles, and responsibilities takes place
2. Working stage
   a. During this phase the real work of the group is accomplished
   b. Members are familiar with each other, the group leader, and the group roles, and they feel free to approach their problems and to attempt to solve their problems
   c. Conflict and cooperation surface during the group's work
3. Termination stage
   a. The group evaluates the experience and explores members' feelings about it and the impending separation
   b. Provides an opportunity for members who have difficulty with termination to learn to deal more realistically and comfortably with this normal part of human experience

B. Psychoanalytical group psychotherapy
1. Therapist holds a main position
2. Each client in the group has a relationship with the therapist
3. Communication is focused on three levels: unconscious, semiconscious, and conscious information

C. Transactional analysis (TA)
1. The three ego states of the individual, the parent, the child, and the adult are examined in TA groups
2. The goal is that individuals in the group will communicate from the proper ego states for the situation and the responses of others, thereby lessening conflict and promoting mature relationships

D. Rational emotive therapy: the therapist designs activities to eliminate the irrational ideas of the members of the group

E. Rogerian therapy
1. The therapist's goal is to help the members express their feelings toward one another during group sessions
2. The therapist's role is one of encouraging the expression of feelings, clarifying these feelings with clients, and accepting clients and their feelings nonjudgmentally

F. Gestalt therapy
1. Emphasis is on the "here and now"
2. Emphasizes self-expression, self-exploration, and self-awareness in the present
3. The client and therapist focus on everyday problems and try to solve them
4. The individual becomes aware of the total self and the surrounding environment
5. Awareness of the problem renders the client capable of change
6. The therapist's role is to help the members express their feelings and grow from their experiences

G. Interpersonal group therapy: to promote the

individual's comfort with others in the group, which then transfers to other relationships

H. Psychodrama groups
1. Explore truth through dramatic methods
2. The individual produces a topic to be explored
3. The therapist directs the individual through role playing
4. The audience experiences the feelings and identifies with the action on the stage
5. A catharsis occurs for the individual and the object

I. Community support groups
1. Promote identification, clarification, understanding, role modeling, feelings of togetherness, and group cohesion
2. Prevent the individual member from feeling lonely and isolated
3. Help members decrease levels of stress and increase levels of self-acceptance
4. Members are better able to deal with the problems that they brought to the group
5. The outcome is rewarding and the members develop new or more effective patterns of behavior
6. Some groups evolve into educational models that enhance communication, self-image, body image, problem solving, decision making, and growth processes

J. Family therapy
1. Specific intervention mode based on the premise that the members, with the presenting symptoms, signal the presence of pain in the whole family
2. The therapist works to assist the family to identify and express their thoughts and feelings, define family roles and rules, try new, more productive styles of relating, and restore strength to the family

PRACTICE QUESTIONS

1. An 18-year-old woman is admitted to an inpatient unit with the diagnosis of anorexia nervosa. A cognitive behavioral approach is used as part of her treatment plan. The purpose of this approach is to
   1 Help the client identify and examine dysfunctional thoughts and beliefs
   2 Emphasize social interaction with clients who withdraw
   3 Provide a supportive environment
   4 Examine intrapsychic conflicts and past issues

2. The nurse is providing reminiscence therapy for a group of clients. Which of the following clients would the nurse select for this group?
   1 A client who exhibits profound depression with moderate cognitive impairment
   2 A catatonic, immobile client with moderate cognitive impairment
   3 An undifferentiated schizophrenic client with moderate cognitive impairment

   4 A client with mild depression who demonstrates normal cognition

3. A client with major depression is considering cognitive therapy. The client says to the nurse, "How does this treatment work?" The nurse's response is
   1 "This type of treatment helps you examine how your thoughts and feelings contribute to your difficulties."
   2 "This type of treatment helps you examine how your past life has contributed to your problems."
   3 "This type of treatment helps you confront your fears by gradually exposing you to them."
   4 "This type of treatment will help you relax and develop new coping skills."

4. The nurse is speaking with a group of family members at a local support group regarding the importance of medication compliance. The nurse tells the group that of the following which is not known to increase medication compliance?
   1 Working with the psychiatrist to find the right medication at the right dose that provides the fewest side effects for the client
   2 Giving all medications just once per day
   3 Providing clients with the injectable, long-acting form of the medication
   4 Including the family in the medication planning process so that compliance can be reinforced at home

5. The nurse is assigned to care for a client who has an impaired sense of taste and touch. According to the nurse's theoretical framework, which of the following lobes of the brain is analyzed as impaired in processing this specialized information?
   1 Parietal
   2 Frontal
   3 Occipital
   4 Temporal

6. The primary locus of milieu therapy can best be described as which of the following?
   1 A form of behavior modification therapy
   2 A cognitive approach to changing behavior
   3 A living, learning, or working environment
   4 A behavioral approach to changing behavior

7. The use of disulfiram (Antabuse), a medication taken by individuals with alcohol problems works on the principle of which of the following therapies?
   1 Desensitization
   2 Self-control therapy
   3 Milieu therapy
   4 Aversion therapy

8. A client with a phobia is being treated for the condition. The client is introduced to short periods of exposure to the phobic object while in a relaxed state. This form of behavior modification can best be described as
   1 Systematic desensitization
   2 Self-control therapy
   3 Milieu therapy
   4 Aversion therapy

9. The client experiencing a great deal of stress and anxiety has been taught to use self-control therapy. Which of the following is not a component of this form of therapy?
   1 An advantage of this technique is that change is likely to last
   2 This form of therapy can be applied to new situations
   3 Talking to oneself is a basic component to this form of therapy
   4 It provides a negative reinforcement when stress is produced

10. The nurse is caring for a client with a chronic mental illness and is using a behavior modification approach (operant conditioning) in caring for the client. Which of the following is not a characteristic of this form of therapy?
    1 It uses negative reinforcement
    2 It increases the level of self-care in the client
    3 It increases social behaviors in the client
    4 It uses positive reinforcement

11. A client with an eating disorder is attending group meetings with Overeaters Anonymous. Which of the following is not a characteristic of this form of self-help group?
    1 People who have a similar problem are able to help others
    2 It is designed to serve people who have a common problem

3 The members provide support to each other
4 The leader is a nurse or psychiatrist

12. The client is attending a Gambler's Anonymous meeting for the first time. The prototype used by this group is the 12-step program developed by Alcoholics Anonymous. The first step in the 12-step program is which of the following?
    1 Stating that the gambling will be stopped
    2 Discontinuing relationships with friends who are gamblers
    3 Substituting gambling for other activities
    4 Admitting to having a problem

13. The nurse is conducting a group therapy session and a client with a manic disorder is monopolizing the group. The most appropriate nursing action is which of the following?
    1 Suggest that the client stop talking and try listening to others
    2 Ask the client to leave
    3 Tell the client to stop monopolizing the group
    4 Refer the client to another group

14. The nurse is planning to formulate a psychotherapy group. Several clients are interested in attending the session. The nurse plans the group knowing that the maximum number of group members is
    1 10
    2 12
    3 14
    4 16

15. The nurse is monitoring a group therapy session. During this session, the members are identifying tasks and boundaries. These activities are characteristic of which stage of group development?
    1 Forming
    2 Storming
    3 Norming
    4 Performing

ANSWERS

1. **1**

Rationale: Cognitive behavioral therapy is used to help clients identify and examine dysfunctional thoughts as well as identify and examine values and beliefs that maintain these thoughts. Options 2, 3, and 4 are incorrect.

Test-Taking Strategy: Note the key words "cognitive behavioral." Focusing on these key words should direct you to option 1. If you are unfamiliar with this type of therapy and its purpose, take time now to review!

Level of Cognitive Ability: Analysis
Phase of Nursing Process: Analysis
Client Needs: Psychosocial Integrity
Content Area: Mental Health

Reference
Varcarolis, E. (1998). *Foundations of psychiatric mental health nursing* (3rd ed.). Philadelphia: W. B. Saunders. p. 812.

2. **4**

Rationale: Reminiscence therapy is best for clients who meet the following criteria: normal to mild cognitive impairment; mild to moderate depression; withdrawn, socially isolated, understimulated behavior.

Test-Taking Strategy: This question tests your knowledge of the standards or criteria that are recommended for clients in the use of reminiscence therapy. Options 1, 2, and 3 describe inappropriate clients whose cognitive impairment would not be improved with this form of therapy. If you had difficulty with this question, take time now to review the characteristics of reminiscence therapy!

Level of Cognitive Ability: Application
Phase of Nursing Process: Implementation
Client Needs: Health Promotion and Maintenance
Content Area: Mental Health

Reference

Glod, C. A. (1998). *Contemporary psychiatric-mental health nursing.* Philadelphia: F. A. Davis. pp. 203–211.

3. 1

Rationale: Cognitive therapy is frequently used with clients who have depression. This type of therapy is based on exploring the client's subjective experience. It includes examining the client's thoughts and feelings about situations as well as how these thoughts and feelings contribute to and perpetuate the client's difficulties and mood.

Test-Taking Strategy: Focusing on the word "cognitive" will assist you in choosing the correct option. Look for a similar word or phrase used in the stem that is repeated in one of the options. Option 1 uses the word "thought" in describing the treatment.

Level of Cognitive Ability: Application
Phase of Nursing Process: Implementation
Client Needs: Health Promotion and Maintenance
Content Area: Mental Health

Reference

Carson, V., & Arnold, E. (1996). *Mental health nursing: The nurse-patient journey.* Philadelphia: W. B. Saunders. pp. 376–377.

4. 2

Rationale: Finding the right medication at the right dose that provides the fewest side effects for the client, providing clients with the injectable, long-acting form of the medication, and including the family in the medication planning process are measures that will promote compliance. Not all medications can be given on a once per day dosing regimen because of their short half-life. Lithium is an example of one such medication that must be dosed throughout the day to maintain steady serum drug levels.

Test-Taking Strategy: Be cautious of words such as "all," "none," "always," and "never." These imply that there are no exceptions and these words usually indicate an incorrect option. In the case of this question, not "all" medications may be dosed once a day because of their short half-life. Therefore, it is not appropriate to give all medications just once per day.

Level of Cognitive Ability: Analysis
Phase of Nursing Process: Analysis
Client Needs: Psychosocial Integrity
Content Area: Mental Health

Reference

Carson, V., & Arnold, E. (1996). *Mental health nursing: The nurse-patient journey.* Philadelphia: W. B. Saunders. pp. 518, 546, 562–564.

5. 1

Rationale: The brain is composed of four lobes. The parietal lobe, known as one of the association areas (because of its role in integrating sensory and motor information with the temporal and occipital lobes), along with the temporal lobe assists clients to focus on environmental events and receives specialized information (as well as higher-level information processing).

Test-Taking Strategy: This question tests your knowledge of the brain, its lobes, and its functions. Option 2 is incorrect because the frontal lobe, the most highly integrated brain area, assists clients to regulate arousal status, make decisions, and focus attention by processing input. Option 3 is incorrect because the occipital lobe is chiefly responsible for sight. Option 4 is incorrect because the temporal lobe integrates smell and hearing (as well as memory and emotional functioning).

Level of Cognitive Ability: Analysis
Phase of Nursing Process: Analysis
Client Needs: Physiological Integrity
Content Area: Mental Health

Reference

Glod, C. A. (1998). *Contemporary psychiatric-mental health nursing.* Philadelphia: F. A. Davis. pp. 75–81.

6. 3

Rationale: Milieu therapy, or "therapeutic community" has as its locus a living, learning, or working environment. Such therapy may be based on any number of therapeutic modalities, from structured behavioral therapy to spontaneous, humanistically oriented approaches. Although milieu may include behavioral approaches, its primary locus is described in option 3.

Test-Taking Strategy: Knowledge regarding the components of milieu therapy is required to answer this question. Note that options 1, 2, and 4 are similar and that option 3 identifies a global description.

Level of Cognitive Ability: Analysis
Phase of Nursing Process: Analysis
Client Needs: Psychosocial Integrity
Content Area: Mental Health

Reference

Varcarolis, E. (1998). *Foundations of psychiatric mental health nursing* (3rd ed.). Philadelphia: W. B. Saunders. p. 58.

7. 4

Rationale: Aversion therapy, also known as aversion conditioning or negative reinforcement, is a technique used to change behavior. In this therapy, a stimulus attractive to the client is paired with an unpleasant event in hopes of endowing it with negative properties.

Test-Taking Strategy: Knowledge that aversion therapy is a form of negative reinforcement will easily direct you to the correct option. If you had difficulty with this question, take time now to review this form of therapy!

Level of Cognitive Ability: Analysis
Phase of Nursing Process: Analysis
Client Needs: Psychosocial Integrity
Content Area: Mental Health

Reference

Varcarolis, E. (1998). *Foundations of psychiatric mental health nursing* (3rd ed.). Philadelphia: W. B. Saunders. p. 58.

8. 1

Rationale: Systematic desensitization is a form of therapy in which the client is introduced to short periods of exposure to the phobic object while in a relaxed state. Gradually exposure is increased until the anxiety about or fear of the object or situation has ceased.

Test-Taking Strategy: Read the description presented in the question carefully. This should assist in directing you to the correct option. If you had difficulty with this question, take time now to review systematic desensitization!

Level of Cognitive Ability: Analysis
Phase of Nursing Process: Analysis
Client Needs: Psychosocial Integrity
Content Area: Mental Health

Reference

Varcarolis, E. (1998). *Foundations of psychiatric mental health nursing* (3rd ed.). Philadelphia: W. B. Saunders. p. 58.

9. **4**

Rationale: Option 4 describes aversion therapy. Options 1, 2, and 3 are characteristics of self-control therapy.

Test-Taking Strategy: Note the key word "not" in the stem of the question. Think about the issue "self-control." This issue should easily direct you to option 4. If you are unfamiliar with self-control therapy, take time now to review!

Level of Cognitive Ability: Analysis
Phase of Nursing Process: Analysis
Client Needs: Psychosocial Integrity
Content Area: Mental Health

Reference

Varcarolis, E. (1998). *Foundations of psychiatric mental health nursing* (3rd ed.). Philadelphia: W. B. Saunders. p. 58.

10. **1**

Rationale: Operant conditioning entails rewarding a client for desired behaviors and is the basis for behavior modification. It uses a positive reinforcement approach. Options 2, 3, and 4 are accurate characteristics of this form of therapy.

Test-Taking Strategy: Note the key word "not" in the stem of the question. Note the similarity between options 2, 3, and 4. This should easily direct you to the correct option. If you had difficulty with this question, take time now to review the characteristics of operant conditioning!

Level of Cognitive Ability: Analysis
Phase of Nursing Process: Analysis
Client Needs: Psychosocial Integrity
Content Area: Mental Health

Reference

Varcarolis, E. (1998). *Foundations of psychiatric mental health nursing* (3rd ed.). Philadelphia: W. B. Saunders. p. 56.

11. **4**

Rationale: The sponsor of a self-help group is an experienced member of the group. A nurse or psychiatrist may be asked by the group to serve as a resource but would not be the leader of the group. Options 1, 2, and 3 are characteristics of a self-help group.

Test-Taking Strategy: Note the key word "not" in the stem of the question. Note that options 1, 2, and 3 are all similar. This should easily direct you to option 4 as the correct answer. Review the characteristics of a self-help group now, if you had difficulty with this question!

Level of Cognitive Ability: Analysis
Phase of Nursing Process: Analysis
Client Needs: Psychosocial Integrity
Content Area: Mental Health

Reference

Varcarolis, E. (1998). *Foundations of psychiatric mental health nursing* (3rd ed.). Philadelphia: W. B. Saunders. p. 258.

12. **4**

Rationale: The first step in the 12-step program is to admit that a problem exists. Options 1 and 2 are unrealistic as a first step in the process to recovery. Although option 3 may be a strategy, it is not the first step.

Test-Taking Strategy: Note the key words "first step" in the question. This will easily assist in directing you to option 4. If you are unfamiliar with the 12-step program, take time now to review!

Level of Cognitive Ability: Analysis
Phase of Nursing Process: Assessment
Client Needs: Psychosocial Integrity
Content Area: Mental Health

Reference

Varcarolis, E. (1998). *Foundations of psychiatric mental health nursing* (3rd ed.). Philadelphia: W. B. Saunders. p. 258.

13. **1**

Rationale: If a client is monopolizing the group it is important that the nurse be direct and decisive. The best action is to suggest that the client stop talking and try listening to others. Although option 3 may be a direct response, option 1 is the most therapeutic direct statement. Options 2 and 4 are inappropriate.

Test-Taking Strategy: Eliminate options 2 and 4 first because they are similar. Use therapeutic communication techniques to assist in directing you to option 1. If you had difficulty with this question, take time now to review therapeutic communication techniques!

Level of Cognitive Ability: Application
Phase of Nursing Process: Implementation
Client Needs: Psychosocial Integrity
Content Area: Mental Health

Reference

Varcarolis, E. (1998). *Foundations of psychiatric mental health nursing* (3rd ed.). Philadelphia: W. B. Saunders. p. 262.

14. **1**

Rationale: The ideal number of clients in a psychotherapy group ranges from 7 to 10. Having more than 10 members is not recommended because the group will subdivide, which is counterproductive. Too large a group can also create more opportunities for acting out, as opposed to working through issues.

Test-Taking Strategy: Knowledge regarding the general guidelines related to establishing a psychotherapy group is required to answer this question. If you are unfamiliar with these guidelines, take time now to review!

Level of Cognitive Ability: Analysis
Phase of Nursing Process: Planning
Client Needs: Psychosocial Integrity
Content Area: Mental Health

Reference

Varcarolis, E. (1998). *Foundations of psychiatric mental health nursing* (3rd ed.). Philadelphia: W. B. Saunders. p. 261.

15. **1**

Rationale: In the forming or initial stage, the members are identifying tasks and boundaries. Storming involves responding emotionally to tasks. In the norming stage members express intimate personal opinions and feelings around personal tasks. In the performing stage, members direct group energy toward the completion of tasks.

Test-Taking Strategy: Note the key word "identifying" in the question. This key word should assist in directing you to option 1. If you had difficulty with this question, take time now to review the stages of group development!

Level of Cognitive Ability: Analysis
Phase of Nursing Process: Evaluation
Client Needs: Psychosocial Integrity
Content Area: Mental Health

Reference
Varcarolis, E. (1998). *Foundations of psychiatric mental health nursing* (3rd ed.). Philadelphia: W. B. Saunders. p. 264.

BIBLIOGRAPHY

Carson, V., & Arnold, E. (1996). *Mental health nursing: The nurse-patient journey.* Philadelphia: W. B. Saunders.

Glod, C. A. (1998). *Contemporary psychiatric-mental health nursing.* Philadelphia: F. A. Davis.

Varcarolis, E. (1998). *Foundations of psychiatric mental health nursing* (3rd ed.). Philadelphia: W. B. Saunders.

CHAPTER 71

Mental Health Disorders

I. Anxiety

A. Description
   1. A subjective, individual experience
   2. A normal response to stress
   3. A feeling of apprehension, uneasiness, uncertainty, or dread
   4. Occurs as a result of threats that may be misperceived or misinterpreted
   5. Occurs as a result of a threat to identity or self-esteem
   6. May result when values are threatened
   7. May precede new experiences

B. Types of anxiety
   1. Normal: a healthy type of anxiety
   2. Acute: precipitated by imminent loss or change that threatens the sense of security
   3. Chronic: anxiety that the individual has lived with for a long time

C. Levels of anxiety
   1. Mild
      a. Associated with the tension of everyday life
      b. The individual is alert
      c. The perceptual field is increased
      d. Can be motivating, produce growth and creativity, and increase learning
   2. Moderate
      a. The focus is on immediate concerns
      b. Narrows the perceptual field
      c. Selective inattentiveness occurs
      d. Learning and problem solving still take place
   3. Severe
      a. Feeling that something bad is about to happen
      b. A significant reduction in perceptual field occurs
      c. Focus is on specific details or scattered details
      d. All behavior is directed at relieving the anxiety

   e. Learning and problem solving are not possible
   f. The individual needs direction to focus
   4. Panic
      a. Associated with dread and terror and a sense of impending doom
      b. The personality is disorganized
      c. The individual is unable to communicate or function effectively
      d. Increased motor activity occurs
      e. Loss of rational thoughts with distorted perception
      f. Inability to concentrate
      g. If prolonged, panic can lead to exhaustion and death

D. Implementation
   1. Recognize the anxiety
   2. Establish trust
   3. Protect the client
   4. Do not attack **coping mechanisms**
   5. Do not force the client into situations that provoke anxiety
   6. Decrease stimulation in the environment
   7. Modify the environment by setting limits or limiting the interaction with others
   8. Provide creative outlets
   9. Provide activities that limit the amount of time for destructive behavior
   10. Promote relaxation techniques
   11. Administer antianxiety medications as prescribed

E. Implementation: mild to moderate levels
   1. Help the client identify the anxiety
   2. Encourage the client to talk about feelings and concerns
   3. Help the client identify thoughts and feelings that occur prior to the onset of anxiety
   4. Encourage problem solving
   5. Encourage gross motor exercise

F. Implementation: severe to panic levels
   1. Reduce the anxiety quickly

2. Use a calm manner
3. Always remain with the client
4. Minimize environmental stimuli
5. Provide clear, simple statements
6. Use a low-pitched voice
7. Attend to the physical needs of the client
8. Provide gross motor activity
9. Administer antianxiety medications as prescribed

II. Generalized Anxiety Disorder

A. Description
   1. An unrealistic anxiety in which the cause can usually be identified
   2. Physical symptoms occur
B. Assessment
   1. Chronic muscular tension
   2. Restlessness
   3. Episodes of trembling and shakiness
   4. Chronic fatigue
   5. Dizziness
   6. Inability to relax
   7. Inability to concentrate
   8. Sleep problems
   9. Inability to recognize the connection between anxiety and physical symptoms
   10. The client is focused on the physical discomfort
C. Panic disorder
   1. Description
      a. The cause usually cannot be identified
      b. It produces a sudden onset with feelings of intense apprehension and dread
      c. Severe, recurrent, intermittent anxiety attacks, lasting 5 to 30 minutes, occur
   2. Assessment
      a. Choking sensation
      b. Labored breathing
      c. Pounding heart
      d. Chest pain
      e. Dizziness
      f. Nausea
      g. Blurred vision
      h. Numbness or tingling of extremities
      i. A sense of unreality and helplessness
      j. A fear of being trapped
      k. A fear of dying
   3. Implementation
      a. Attend to physical symptoms
      b. Assist the client to identify the thoughts that arouse the anxiety and identify the basis for these thoughts
      c. Assist the client to change unrealistic thoughts to more realistic thoughts
      d. Use cognitive restructuring
      e. Administer antianxiety medications as prescribed

III. Post-Traumatic Stress Disorder

A. Description: after experiencing a psychologically traumatic event, outside the range of usual experience, the individual reexperiences the event via recurrent and intrusive dreams or flashbacks
B. Stressors
   1. A natural disaster
   2. Combat
   3. Victim of rape
   4. Accidents
   5. Victim of crime or violence
   6. Victim of sexual, physical, or emotional **abuse**
   7. Reexperiencing the event as flashbacks
C. Assessment
   1. Emotional numbness
   2. Detachment
   3. Depression
   4. Anxiety
   5. Sleep disturbances and nightmares
   6. Hypervigilance
   7. Guilt about surviving
   8. Poor concentration and avoidance of activities that trigger the memory of the event
D. Implementation
   1. Desensitization through gradual exposure to the event or situations similar to the event
   2. Instructing the client in relaxation techniques
   3. Providing individual therapy that addresses loss of control issues or anger
   4. Using support groups
   5. Using hypnotherapy

IV. Phobias

A. Description
   1. An irrational fear of an object or situation that persists although the person may recognize it as unreasonable
   2. Is associated with panic level anxiety and the anxiety is severe if the object, situation, or activity cannot be avoided
   3. **Defense mechanisms** commonly used include repression and displacement
B. Types
   1. Agoraphobia
      a. Fear of being alone in open or public places where escape might be difficult
      b. The individual may not leave home
      c. The individual experiences fear or a sense of helplessness or embarrassment if the attack occurs
      d. The individual avoids situations that may trigger the attack
   2. Social phobia
      a. Fear of situations in which one might be embarrassed or criticized and the fear of making a fool of oneself
      b. Can include the fear of eating in public, public speaking, or performing
   3. Specific phobia: a fear of a single object,

activity, or situation such as snakes, closed spaces, and flying

◆ C. Implementation
1. Stay with the client when the anxiety is high to promote safety and security
2. Identify the basis of the anxiety
3. Allow the client to verbalize feelings about the anxiety-producing object or situation; frequently talking about the feared object is the first step in the desensitization process
4. Desensitization by gradually introducing the individual to the feared object or situation in small doses
5. Teach relaxation techniques such as breathing exercises, muscle relaxation exercises, and visualization of pleasant situations
6. Do not force contact with the phobic object or situation

V. Obsessive-Compulsive Disorder

◆ A. Obsessions: preoccupation with persistent intrusive thoughts and ideas
◆ B. Compulsions
1. Repeated performance of rituals or purposeless behaviors designed to prevent some event, divert unacceptable thoughts, and decrease anxiety
2. Obsessions and compulsions often occur together and can disrupt normal activities
3. Anxiety occurs if obsessions or compulsions are resisted, and from being powerless to resist the thoughts or rituals
4. Obsessive thoughts can involve issues of violence, aggression, sexual behavior, orderliness, or religion
5. Intrusive thoughts uncontrollably interrupt conscious thoughts and the ability to function

◆ C. Behavior patterns
1. Decrease the anxiety
2. Are associated with the obsessive thoughts
3. Neutralize the thought
4. During stressful times, the ritualistic behavior increases
5. **Defense mechanisms** include repression, displacement, and undoing

◆ D. Implementation
1. Identify the situations that precipitate the behavior
2. Do not interrupt the compulsive behaviors
3. Allow time for the client to perform rituals
4. Provide for client safety related to the behaviors
5. Implement a schedule for the client that distracts from the behaviors
6. Set limits on rituals that may interfere with the client's physical well-being to protect from physical harm
7. Encourage the client to verbalize concerns
8. Gradually assist the client to decrease the frequency of compulsive behaviors by establishing a written contract

VI. Somatoform Disorders

A. Description (Box 71-1)
1. Characterized by persistent worry or complaints regarding physical illness when there is no supporting physical findings
2. The client focuses on the physical signs and symptoms and is unable to control the signs and symptoms
3. The physical signs and symptoms increase with psychosocial stressors
4. The anxiety is redirected into a somatic concern
B. Somatization disorder
1. Description
a. Occurs over a period of years and usually presents before age 30
b. The client has multiple physical complaints involving multiple systems
c. The emotional stress can result from anxiety, fear, depression, worry, or repressed anger
d. The client may unconsciously use somatization for secondary gains such as increased attention and decreased responsibilities
2. Assessment
a. Physical complaints of abdominal pain, denial of emotional problems, signs of anxiety, fear, and low self-esteem
b. Psychosexual symptoms
c. Secondary gain
C. Hypochondriasis
1. Description
a. The preoccupation with fears of having a serious disease
b. No evidence of physical illness exists
c. Causes a significantly impaired social and occupational functioning
2. Assessment
a. Preoccupation with physical functioning
b. Frequent somatic complaints
c. Difficulty expressing feelings
d. Extensive use of home remedies or nonprescription medications
e. Repeatedly visiting the doctor
f. Secondary gain
g. Fatigue and insomnia
h. Anxiety
D. Conversion disorder
1. Description

BOX 71-1. Types of Somatoform Disorders
Somatization disorder Hypochondriasis Conversion disorder

a. A physical symptom or a deficit suggesting loss or altered body function related to psychological conflict or a neurological disorder
b. An expression of a psychological conflict or need
c. The most common conversion symptoms are blindness, deafness, paralysis, and the inability to talk
d. There is no organic cause
e. Symptoms are not intentionally produced by client
f. Symptoms are directly related to conflict and decrease anxiety

2. Assessment
a. "La belle indifference"—unconcerned with symptoms
b. Physical limitation or disability
c. Feelings of guilt, anxiety, or frustration
d. Low self-esteem and feelings of inadequacy
e. Unexpressed anger or conflict
f. Secondary gain

3. Implementation
a. Obtain a nursing history and assess for physical problems
b. Do not reinforce the sick role
c. Discourage verbalization about physical symptoms by not responding with positive reinforcement
d. Explore with the client the needs being met by symptoms
e. Assist the client to identify alternative ways of meeting needs
f. Assist the client to relate feelings and conflicts to physical symptoms
g. Allow a specific time period to discuss physical complaints because the client will feel less threatened if this behavior is limited rather than stopped completely
h. Assure the client that physical illness has been ruled out
i. Explore the source of anxiety and stimulate verbalization of anxiety
j. Encourage the use of relaxation techniques as the anxiety increases
k. Convey understanding that symptoms are real to the client
l. Implement pain-reduction measures as required
m. Report and assess any new physical complaint
n. Encourage diversional activities to decrease the client's focus on self
o. Provide positive feedback for accomplishments to increase self-esteem
p. Assist clients in recognizing their feelings and emotions
q. Contract with the client to engage in relationships with others to redirect interest
r. Administer antianxiety medications as prescribed

VII. Dissociative Disorder

A. Description
1. A disruption in integrative functions of memory, consciousness, or identity
2. Associated with exposure to a traumatic event

B. Dissociative identity disorder (multiple personality)
1. Description
a. Two or more fully developed distinct and unique personalities within the person
b. Personalities may take full control of the client one at a time
c. The personalities may or may not be aware of each other
2. Assessment
a. The inability to recall important information too extensive to be explained by ordinary forgetfulness
b. Transition from one personality to the other is related to stress and is sudden
c. Dissociation is used as a method of distancing and defending self from anxiety and traumatizing experiences

C. Dissociative amnesia
1. Description
a. Inability to recall important personal information because it is anxiety provoking
b. Memory impairment may be partial or almost complete
2. Assessment
a. Localized—the client blocks out all memories about a specified period
b. Selective—the client recalls some but not all memories about a specified period
c. Generalized—loss of all memory about past life

D. Dissociative fugue
1. Description
a. The assumption of a new identity in a new environment
b. The disorder may occur suddenly
2. Assessment
a. May drift from place to place
b. Develops few social relationships
c. When the fugue lifts the client returns home and is unable to recall the fugue state

E. Depersonalization disorder
1. Description: an altered self-perception in which one's own reality is temporarily lost or changed
2. Assessment
a. Feelings of detachment
b. Intact reality testing

F. Implementation
1. Develop a trusting relationship with the client
2. Encourage verbal expression of painful experiences, anxiety, and concerns
3. Explore methods of coping
4. Identify sources of conflict
5. Focus on client's strengths and skills
6. Orient client
7. Provide nondemanding simple routines
8. Allow clients to progress at their own pace
9. Use stress-reduction techniques
10. Individual, group, and/or family psychotherapy to integrate dissociated aspects of personality or memory and to expand self-awareness

VIII. Bipolar Disorder

A. Description (Box 71–2)
1. Characterized by episodes of mania and depression with periods of normal mood and activity in between
2. The treatment medication of choice is lithium carbonate, which can be toxic and therefore requires the regular monitoring of serum lithium levels

---

BOX 71–2. Assessment of Bipolar Disorder

MANIA
Inappropriate affect
Restlessness
Flight of ideas
Inability to eat or sleep because of involvement in more important things
Extroverted personality
Delusional self-confidence
Initiation of activity
High and unstable affect
Becomes angry quickly
Pressure of speech
Grandiose and persecutory delusions
Inappropriate dress
Urgent motor activity
Significant decrease in appetite
Inability to sleep yet still active
Sexually promiscuous
Distracted by environmental stimuli
Unlimited energy

DEPRESSION
Decreased emotion and physical activity
Inability to make quick decisions
Introverted personality
Lack of initiative
Lack of self-confidence
Internalizing hostility
Loss of interest in appearance
Lack of energy
Easily fatigued
Withdrawn from groups
Lack of sexual interest

B. Implementation for mania
1. Remove hazardous objects from the environment
2. Monitor the client's sleep patterns
3. Assess the client closely for fatigue
4. Provide frequent rest periods
5. Use comfort measures to promote sleep
6. Provide a private room if possible
7. Administer hypnotic or sedative medication as prescribed
8. Encourage the client to ventilate feelings
9. Use calm, slow interactions
10. Help the client focus on one topic during the conversation
11. Ignore or distract the client from grandiose thinking
12. Present reality to the client
13. Don't argue with the client
14. Limit group activities and assess the client's tolerance level
15. Provide high-calorie finger foods and fluids
16. Supervise the client's choice of clothing
17. Reduce environmental stimuli
18. Set limits on inappropriate behaviors
19. Provide physical activities and outlets for tension
20. Avoid competitive games
21. Provide gross motor activities such as walking
22. Provide simple and direct explanations for routine procedures
23. Provide structured activities or one-on-one activities with the nurse
24. Supervise administration of medication

IX. Schizophrenia

A. Description
1. A group of mental disorders characterized by psychotic features, inability to trust others, disordered thought processes, and disrupted interpersonal relationships
2. Disturbances in affect, mood, behavior, and thought processes
B. Assessment
1. Physical characteristics
   a. Disheveled appearance
   b. Body image distortions
   c. Preoccupied with somatic complaints
   d. Neglects eating, sleeping, and elimination
2. Motor activity (Box 71–3)
   a. Catatonic posturing—holding bizarre postures for long periods of time
   b. Catatonic excitement—moving excitedly with no environmental stimuli
   c. May be totally immobilized
   d. Unable to respond to commands or responds only to commands
   e. Waxy flexibility
   f. Movements may be repetitive or stereotyped

BOX 71–3. Abnormal Motor Behaviors

DESCRIPTION

Abnormal motor behavior or activity, displayed by the mentally ill client, occurring as a result of a psychiatric disorder

TYPES OF ABNORMAL MOTOR BEHAVIORS

Akathisia

Displaying motor restlessness and muscular quivering; the client is unable to sit or lie quietly

Echolalia

Repeating the speech of another person

Echopraxia

Repeating the movements of another person

Parkinson-like Symptoms

Making mask-like faces, drooling, and having shuffling gait, tremors, and muscular rigidity

Waxy Flexibility

Having one's arms or legs placed in a certain position and holding that same position for hours

Dyskinesia

Impairment of the power of voluntary movements

BOX 71–4. Abnormal Thought Processes

DESCRIPTION

Abnormal thought processes, displayed by the mentally ill client, occur as a result of a psychiatric disorder

NEOLOGISMS

Words that an individual makes up that have meaning only for the individual; often part of a delusional system

LOOSENESS OF ASSOCIATION

The individual's thinking is haphazard, illogical, and confused and connections in thought are interrupted; seen mostly in schizophrenic disorders

FLIGHT OF IDEAS

A constant flow of speech in which the individual jumps from one topic to another in rapid succession; there is a connection between topics although it is sometimes difficult to identify; seen in manic states

BLOCKING

A sudden cessation of a thought in the middle of a sentence; the client is unable to continue the train of thought; often sudden new thoughts come up unrelated to the topic

CIRCUMSTANTIALITY

Before getting to the point or answering a question, the individual gets caught up in countless details and explanations.

CONFABULATION

Filling a memory gap with detailed fantasy believed by the teller; the purpose of confabulation is to maintain self-esteem; seen in organic conditions such as Korsakoff's psychosis

WORD SALAD

A mixture of words and phrases that have no meaning

---

g. Motor activity may be increased as evidenced by agitation, pacing, inability to sleep, loss of appetite and weight, and impulsiveness

h. May be unable to initiate activity, known as volition or anergia

3. Emotional characteristics
   a. Mistrust
   b. Views the world as threatening and unsafe
   c. Feelings not easily interpreted
   d. Ambivalence manifested as compulsive rituals, negativism, and overcompliance
   e. May display feelings of helplessness, anxiety, anger, guilt and depression, and decreased self-esteem

4. Compulsive rituals: attempts to solve conflicting feelings by constant, repetitive activity, which may be stereotyped or seem meaningless

5. Overcompliance: attempts to deny responsibility for any action by doing only what another exactly instructs

6. Affective disturbances
   a. Flat affect or inappropriate affect
   b. Altered thought processes

7. Thought processes (Box 71–4)
   a. Impaired reality testing
   b. Fragmentation of thoughts
   c. Blocking
   d. Loose associations
   e. Autistic thinking
   f. Perceives environment in a totally self-centered way

g. Neologisms

h. Magical thinking

i. Unable to conceptualize meaning in words or thoughts

j. Unable to organize facts logically

k. Delusions

8. Types of delusions (Box 71–5)
   a. Loss of reference in which the client believes that certain events, situations, or interactions are directly related to self
   b. Delusions of persecution in which clients believe that they are being harassed, threatened, or persecuted by some powerful force
   c. Delusions of grandeur in which the client attaches special significance to self in relation to others or the universe and has an exaggerated sense of self that has no basis in reality

BOX 71-5. Delusions

DESCRIPTION

A false belief held to be true even when there is evidence to the contrary

TYPES

Persecution
The thought that one is being singled out for harm by others

Grandeur
The false belief that one is a very powerful and important person

Jealousy
The false belief that one's partner or mate is going out with other people

---

d. Somatic delusions in which the client believes that his or her body is changing or responding in an unusual way, which has no basis in reality
9. Perceptual distortions
   a. Illusions that may be brief experiences with a misinterpretation or exaggeration of reality
   b. Hallucinations such as perceiving objects, sensations, or images with no basis in reality (Box 71-6)
10. Language and communication disturbances (Box 71-7)
    a. Related to disorders in thought process
    b. Unable to organize language
    c. Difficulty communicating clearly
    d. Inappropriate responses to a situation
    e. A single word or phrase may represent the whole meaning of the conversation, and clients may feel they have communicated adequately

BOX 71-6. Preoccupation in Thought Content

HALLUCINATION

A sense perception for which no external stimuli exists; can have an organic or functional etiology

TYPES

Visual
Seeing things that are not there

Auditory
Hearing voices when none are present

Olfactory
Smelling smells that do not exist

Tactile
Feeling touch sensations in the absence of stimuli

Gustatory
Experiencing taste in the absence of stimuli

BOX 71-7. Language and Communication Disturbance

Neologism—a new word devised that has special meaning only to the client
Echolalia—repetition of words or phrases heard from another person
Verbigeration—purposeless repetition of words or phrases
Metonymic speech—mental confusion exhibited by the use of a word that is not the precise term intended but is of similar meaning
Clang association—repetition of words or phrases that are similar in sound only
Word salad—form of speech in which words or phrases are connected meaninglessly
Stilted language—an inappropriate and overly formal communication pattern, usually written, that seems artificial and intellectual
Pressured speech—speaks as if the words are being forced out quickly
Mutism—absence of verbal speech

---

   f. May develop private language
C. Types of schizophrenia (Box 71-8)
   1. Paranoid schizophrenia
      a. Suspiciousness
      b. Hostility
      c. Delusions
      d. Auditory hallucinations
      e. Anxiety and anger
      f. Aloofness
      g. Persecutory themes
      h. Violence
   2. Disorganized schizophrenia
      a. Extreme social withdrawal
      b. Disorganized speech or behavior
      c. Flat or inappropriate affect
      d. Silliness unrelated to speech
      e. Stereotyped behaviors
      f. Grimacing mannerisms
      g. Inability to perform activities of daily living (ADLs)
   3. Catatonic schizophrenia
      a. Marked psychomotor disturbances
      b. Immobility
      c. Stupor
      d. Waxy flexibility
      e. Excessive purposeless motor activity
      f. Echolalia
      g. Automatic obedience
      h. Stereotyped or repetitive behavior

BOX 71-8. Types of Schizophrenia

Paranoid	Undifferentiated
Disorganized	Residual
Catatonic	

4. Undifferentiated schizophrenia
   a. Does not meet criteria for paranoid, disorganized, or catatonic schizophrenia
   b. Delusions and hallucinations
   c. Disorganized speech
   d. Disorganized or catatonic behavior
   e. Flat affect
   f. Social withdrawal
5. Residual schizophrenia
   a. Diagnosed as schizophrenic in the past
   b. Time limited between attacks but may last for many years
   c. The client exhibits marked social isolation and withdrawal and impaired role functioning
D. Implementation: active hallucinations (Box 71–9)
   1. Monitor for hallucination cues
   2. Intervene with a one-on-one contact
   3. Decrease stimuli or move the client to another area
   4. Avoid conveying to the client that you are also experiencing the hallucination
   5. Respond verbally to anything real that the client talks about
   6. Avoid touching the client
   7. Encourage the client to express feelings
   8. During hallucination attempt to engage the client's attention through a concrete activity
   9. Accept and do not joke about or judge the client's behavior
   10. Provide easy activities and a structured environment with routine ADLs
   11. Monitor for signs of increasing fear, anxiety, or agitation
   12. Provide **seclusion** as necessary
   13. Administer medications as prescribed
E. Implementation: delusions
   1. Interact on the basis of reality
   2. Encourage the client to express feelings
   3. Do not dispute with the client or try to convince the client that delusions are false
   4. Initially initiate activities on a one-on-one basis
   5. Alter hospital routines as necessary, such as using canned or packaged food or food from home
   6. Recognize accomplishments and provide positive feedback for successes

X. Paranoid Disorders

A. Description
   1. The client demonstrates suspiciousness and mistrust of others
   2. The client is often viewed by others as hostile, stubborn, and defensive
   3. Concrete, pervasive delusional system characterized by persecutory and grandiose beliefs
B. Behaviors
   1. Suspicious and mistrustful
   2. Emotionally distant

BOX 71–9. Implementation for Schizophrenia

Assess the client's physical needs

Set limits on the client's behavior when it interferes with others and becomes disruptive

Maintain a safe environment

Initiate one-on-one interactions and progress to small groups as tolerated

Spend time with the client even if the client is unable to respond

Monitor for Altered Thought Processes

Maintain ego boundaries and avoid touching the client

Limit the time of interaction with the client

Avoid an overly warm approach; a neutral approach is less threatening

Do not make promises to the client that cannot be kept

Establish daily routines

Assist the client to improve grooming and accept responsibility for personal care

Sit with the client in silence if necessary

Provide brief and frequent contact with the client

Tell the client when you are leaving

Tell the client when you don't understand

Do not "go along" with the client's delusions or hallucinations

Provide simple concrete activities such as puzzles or word games

Reorient the client as necessary

Help the client establish what is real and unreal

Stay with the client if the client is frightened

Speak to the client in a simple, direct, and concise manner

Reassure the client that the environment is safe

Remove the client from group situations if client behavior is too bizarre, disturbing, or dangerous to others

Set realistic goals

Initially do not offer choices to the client, and gradually assist the client in making own decisions

Assess physical needs

Use containers for food, especially with the paranoid schizophrenic client

Provide a radio or tape player at night for insomnia

Explain in detail everything you are doing

Set limits on the client's behavior if the client is unable to do so

Decrease excessive stimuli in the environment

Monitor for suicide risk

Assist the client to use alternative means to express feelings through music or art therapy or writing

---

3. Distorts reality
4. Poor insight
5. Hypervigilance
6. Low self-esteem
7. Highly sensitive, difficulty in admitting own error, and takes pride in being correct
8. Hypercritical and intolerant of others
9. Hostile, aggressive, and quarrelsome
10. Evasive
11. Concrete thinking

◆ C. Delusions
1. Serves purpose in establishing identity and self-esteem
2. Grandiose and persecutory delusions
3. Process of delusion includes denial, projection, and rationalization
4. As trust in others increases, the need for delusions decreases
D. Types (Box 71–10)
1. Paranoid personality
a. Suspicious
b. Nonpsychotic
c. No hallucinations or delusions
d. No symptoms of schizophrenia
2. Paranoid state
a. Onset abrupt in response to stress and subsides when stress decreases
b. No hallucinations but experiences paranoid delusions
c. May be sensitive and suspicious before development of delusions
d. Psychotic state
e. No symptoms of schizophrenia
3. Paranoia
a. Client appears normal except for delusional system
b. Single, highly organized delusional system
c. Not bizarre
d. No hallucinations
e. Reserved and sensitive before onset
f. Psychotic state
g. No symptoms of schizophrenia
4. Paranoid schizophrenia
a. Prior to onset client becomes cold, withdrawn, distrustful, resentful, argumentative, sarcastic, and defiant
b. Bizarre, numerous, and changeable delusions
c. Delusions become less logical as client becomes more disorganized
d. Persecutory hallucinations
e. Psychotic state
f. All symptoms of schizophrenia are present
E. Implementation (Box 71–11)

XI. Personality Disorders

A. Description
1. Includes various inflexible maladaptive behavior patterns or traits that may impair functioning and relationships
2. Individuals usually remain in touch with reality and typically have a lack of insight into their behavior

BOX 71–10. Types of Paranoid Disorders

Paranoid personality	Paranoia
Paranoid state	Paranoid schizophrenia

BOX 71–11. Implementation: Paranoid Disorders

Assess for suicide risk
Diminish suspicious behavior
Establish a trusting relationship
Promote increased self-esteem
Remain calm, nonthreatening, and nonjudgmental
Provide continuity of care
Respond honestly to the client
Follow through on commitments made to the client
Acknowledge clients' feelings but tell clients that you do not share their interpretation of an event
Provide a daily schedule of activities
Assist clients to identify diversionary activities
Gradually introduce the client to groups
Refocus conversation to reality-based topics
Use role playing to help the client identify thoughts and feelings
Provide positive reinforcement for successes
Do not argue with delusions
Use concrete, specific words
Do not be secretive with the client
Do not whisper in the client's presence
Assure clients they will be safe
Involve the client in noncompetitive tasks
Provide the client an opportunity to complete small tasks
Monitor eating, drinking, sleeping, and elimination patterns
Limit physical contact
Monitor for agitation and decrease stimuli as needed

3. Stress exacerbates manifestations of personality disorder
4. In severe cases personality disorder may deteriorate to a psychotic state
B. Characteristics
1. Poor impulse control
a. Acting out to manage internal pain
b. Forms of acting out include physical and verbal attacks, manipulation, substance **abuse**, promiscuous sexual behaviors, and **suicide attempts**
2. Mood characteristics
a. Experience abandonment and depression
b. Moods include rage, guilt, fear, and emptiness
3. Impaired judgment
a. Has difficulty with problem solving
b. Unable to perceive consequences of behavior
4. Impaired reality testing: distorts reality and often projects own feelings onto others
5. Impaired object relations: rigid and inflexible and has difficulty in intimate relationships
6. Impaired self-perception: distorted self-perception and experiences self-hate or self-idealization
7. Impaired thought processes
a. Concrete or diffuse thinking
b. Difficulty concentrating

c. Impaired memory
8. Impaired stimulus barrier
   a. Unable to regulate incoming sensory stimuli
   b. Increased excitability
   c. Excessive response to noise and light
   d. Poor attention span
   e. Agitated
   f. Insomnia

C. Schizoid personality disorder
   1. Description: characterized by an inability to form warm, close social relationships
   2. Assessment
      a. Social detachment and lack of close relationships
      b. Interest in solitary activities
      c. Aloof and indifferent
      d. Restricted expression of emotions
      e. Lack of interest in others

D. Schizotypal personality disorder
   1. Description: exhibits abnormal or highly unusual thoughts, perceptions, speech, and behavior patterns
   2. Assessment
      a. Suspicious
      b. Paranoid
      c. Magical thinking
      d. Odd thinking and speech
      e. Relationship deficits

E. Paranoid personality disorder
   1. Description: characterized by suspiciousness and mistrust of others
   2. Assessment
      a. Suspicious and distrusting
      b. Argumentative
      c. Hostile aloofness
      d. Rigid, critical, and controlling of others
      e. Grandiosity

F. Histrionic personality disorder
   1. Description
      a. Characterized by overly dramatic and intensely expressive behavior
      b. The client is lively and dramatic and enjoys being the center of attention
      c. Interpersonal relations may be poor
   2. Assessment
      a. Attention seeking
      b. Needs to be the center of attention
      c. Sexually seductive or provocative
      d. Self-dramatizing and theatrical
      e. Overly concerned with appearance
      f. Has romantic fantasies and controls partners
      g. Bores easily
      h. Displays dependency

G. Narcissistic personality disorder
   1. Description
      a. Characterized by an increased sense of self-importance
      b. The client is preoccupied with fantasies and unlimited success and has a constant need for attention and admiration
   2. Assessment
      a. Grandiosity
      b. Requires admiration and inflated accomplishments
      c. Overestimates abilities and underestimates contributions of others
      d. Lacks empathy and sensitivity to needs of others

H. Avoidant personality disorder
   1. Description: characterized by social withdrawal and extreme sensitivity to potential rejection
   2. Assessment
      a. Feelings of inadequacy
      b. Hypersensitive to reactions of others and reacts poorly to criticism
      c. Social inhibition
      d. Lack of support system

I. Dependent personality disorder
   1. Description
      a. The individual lacks self-confidence and the ability to function independently
      b. Passively allow others to make decisions and assume responsibility for major areas in their life
   2. Assessment
      a. Difficulty making decisions
      b. Lacks autonomy
      c. Cannot tolerate being alone and must always have a close relationship
      d. Needs others to assume responsibility and make decisions

J. Obsessive-compulsive personality disorder
   1. Description: the client has difficulty expressing warm and tender emotions and reflects perfectionism, stubbornness, the need to control others, and a devotion to work
   2. Assessment
      a. Orderliness and perfectionism
      b. Overly conscientious
      c. Inflexible and preoccupied with details and rules
      d. Devoted to work and lacks leisure activities and friendships
      e. Miserly and stubborn
      f. Hoards worthless objects

K. Antisocial personality disorder
   1. Description
      a. A pattern of irresponsible and antisocial behavior
      b. Characterized by selfishness, inability to maintain lasting relationships, poor sexual adjustment, failure to accept social norms, irritability, and aggressiveness
   2. Assessment
      a. Perceives the world as hostile
      b. Superficial charm and hostility
      c. No shame or guilt
      d. Self-centered
      e. Unreliable
      f. Easily bored

g. Poor work history

h. Unable to tolerate frustration

i. Views others as objects to be manipulated

j. Poor judgment

k. Impulsive

◆ L. Borderline personality disorder

1. Description

a. Characterized by instability in interpersonal relationships, mood, and self-image

b. Behavior may be impulsive and unpredictable

2. Assessment

a. Unclear identity

b. Unstable and intense

c. Extreme shifts in mood

d. Easily angered

e. Easily bored

f. Argumentative

g. Depression

h. Self-destructive behavior

i. Manipulation

j. Unable to tolerate anxiety

k. Chronic feelings of emptiness and fear of being alone

l. Splitting

M. Passive-aggressive personality disorder

1. Description

a. Characterized by a passively expressing covert aggression rather than dealing with it directly

b. The behavior can interfere with both social and work activities

2. Assessment

a. Procrastination

b. Stubbornness

c. Intentional inefficiency

d. Forgetfulness

e. Dependency

◆ N. Implementation

1. Maintain safety against self-destructive behaviors

2. Allow the client to make choices and be as independent as possible

3. Encourage the client to discuss feelings rather than act them out

4. Provide consistency in response to the client's acting-out behaviors

5. Discuss expectations and responsibilities with the client

6. Discuss the consequences that will follow certain behaviors

7. Inform the client that harm to self, others, and property is unacceptable

8. Identify splitting behavior

9. Assist the client to deal directly with anger

10. Develop a written contract with the client

11. Encourage the client to keep a journal recording daily feelings

12. Encourage the client to participate in group activities, and praise nonmanipulative behavior

13. Set and maintain limits to decrease manipulative behavior

14. Remove the client from group situations in which attention-seeking behaviors occur

15. Provide realistic praise for positive behaviors in social situations

XII. Electroconvulsive Therapy (ECT)

A. Description

1. An effective treatment for depression that consists of inducing a grand mal seizure by passing an electrical current through electrodes that are attached to the temples

2. The administration of a muscle relaxant minimizes seizure activity, preventing damage to long bones and cervical vertebrae

3. The usual course is 6 to 12 treatments given two to three times per week

4. Maintenance ECT once a month may help to decrease relapse rate for clients with recurrent depression

5. ECT is not a permanent cure

6. Not necessarily effective in clients with dysthymic depression or those with depression and personality disorders, those with drug dependence, or those with depression secondary to situational or social difficulties

7. At risk clients include those with recent myocardial infarction, cerebral vascular accident, or cerebral vascular malformation, or clients with intracranial mass lesions

B. Uses

1. Clients with major depressive and bipolar depressive disorders especially when psychotic symptoms are present such as delusions of guilt, somatic delusions, and delusions of infidelity

2. Clients who have depression with marked psychomotor retardation and stupor

3. Manic clients whose conditions are resistant to lithium and antipsychotic medications and in clients who are rapid cyclers (a client with a bipolar disorder who has many episodes of mood swings close together)

4. Clients with schizophrenia (especially catatonia), those with schizoaffective syndromes, and psychotic clients

C. Indications for use

1. When antidepressant medications have no effect

2. When there is a need for rapid definitive response such as when a client is suicidal or homicidal

3. The client is in extreme agitation or stupor

4. The risks of other treatments outweigh the risk of ECT

5. The client has a history of poor medication response, a history of good ECT response, or both

6. The client prefers it

D. Preprocedure
1. Explain procedure to the client
2. Encourage the client to discuss feelings, including myths regarding ECT
3. Teach the client and family what to expect
4. Informed consent must be obtained when voluntary clients are being treated
5. For involuntary clients, when informed consent cannot be obtained, permission may be obtained from the next of kin, although in some states the permission for ECT must be obtained from the court
6. NPO after midnight or at least 4 hours prior to treatment
7. Baseline vital signs are taken
8. The client is requested to void
9. Hairpins, contact lenses, and dentures are removed
10. Administer preoperative medication if prescribed; glycopyrrolate (Robinul) or atropine may be prescribed to prevent the potential for aspiration and to minimize bradydysrhythmias in response to electrical stimulants

E. During the procedure
1. Place a blood pressure cuff on one of the client's arms
2. An IV line is inserted and EEG and ECG electrodes are attached
3. A pulse oximeter is placed onto the client's finger
4. Blood pressure is monitored throughout treatment
5. Medications administered may include a short-acting anesthetic such as methohexital sodium (Brevital Sodium), thiopental sodium (Pentothal), and a muscle relaxant such as succinylcholine (Anectine)
6. 100% oxygen by mask via positive pressure is administered throughout the procedure
7. An airway or bite block is placed to prevent biting the tongue
8. Electrical stimulus is given and the seizure should last 30 to 60 seconds

F. Postprocedure
1. The client will be transported to a recovery room with the blood pressure cuff and oximeter in place, where oxygen, suction, and other emergency equipment is available
2. Once the client is awake, talk to the client and take vital signs
3. The client may be confused; provide frequent orientation (brief, distinct, and simple) and reassurance
4. The client returns to the nursing unit when a 90% oxygen saturation level is maintained, vital signs are stable, and mental status is satisfactory
5. Assess the gag reflex prior to giving the client fluids, food, or medication

G. Potential side effects
1. Major side effects with bilateral treatment are confusion, disorientation, and short-term memory loss
2. The client may be confused and disoriented upon awakening
3. Memory deficits may occur, but memory usually recovers completely, although some clients have memory loss lasting up to 6 months

XIII. Cognitive Impairment Disorders

A. Dementia and Alzheimer's disease
1. Dementia
   a. Organic syndrome with progressive deterioration in intellectual functioning
   b. Long- and short-term memory loss occurs with impairment in judgment, abstract thinking, problem-solving ability, and behavior
   c. Results in a Self-Care Deficit
   d. The most common type of dementia is Alzheimer's disease
2. Alzheimer's disease (Box 71–12)
   a. An irreversible form of senile dementia from nerve cell deterioration
   b. Individuals with Alzheimer's disease experience cognitive deterioration and progressive loss of ability to carry out ADLs
   c. The client experiences a steady decline in physical and mental functioning and

---

BOX 71–12. Stages of Alzheimer's Disease

STAGE 1

Duration of the disease is 1 to 3 years
Mild memory impairment
Difficulty remembering names, appointments, and where things are
Indifferent and occasionally irritable

STAGE 2

Duration of the disease is 2 to 10 years
Moderate memory impairment of recent events
Decrease in orientation
Restless nights
Aphasia
Apraxia
Indifferent and occasionally irritable
Restlessness and pacing
Delusions

STAGE 3

Duration of this stage is 8 to 12 years
Severely impaired cognitive function
Severe disorientation
Severe agitation
Blunted emotions
Limb rigidity and flexion posture
Urinary and fecal incontinence

usually requires nursing home placement in the final stages of illness

3. Implementation
   a. Identify and reinforce retained skills
   b. Provide continuity of care
   c. Orient to the environment
   d. Furnish the environment with familiar possessions
   e. Acknowledge the client's feelings
   f. Assist the client and family members to manage memory deficits and behavior changes
   g. Encourage family members to express feelings about caregiving
   h. Provide caregiver support and identify the resources and support groups available
   i. Monitor ADLs
   j. Remind how to perform self-care activities
   k. Maintain independence
   l. Provide consistent routines
   m. Provide exercise such as walking with an escort
   n. Avoid activities that tax the memory
   o. Allow plenty of time to complete a task
   p. Use constant encouragement in a step-by-step approach
   q. Provide activities that distract and occupy time, such as listening to music, coloring, watching TV
   r. Provide mental stimulation with simple games or activities

4. Wandering
   a. Provide a safe environment
   b. Prevent unsafe wandering
   c. Provide close supervision
   d. Close and secure doors
   e. Use identification bracelets and electronic surveillance

5. Communication
   a. Adapt to the communication level of the client
   b. Use a firm volume and low pitched voice to communicate
   c. Stand directly in front of the client and maintain eye contact
   d. Call the client by name and identify self; wait for a response
   e. Use a calm and reassuring voice
   f. Use pantomine gestures if the client is unable to understand spoken words
   g. Use slow, clear, verbal communication techniques
   h. Use short words and simple sentences
   i. Ask only one question at a time and give one direction at a time
   j. Repeat questions if necessary but do not rephrase

6. Impaired judgment
   a. Remove throw rugs, toxic substances, and dangerous electrical appliances from the environment
   b. Reduce water heater temperature

7. Altered thought processes
   a. Call the client by name
   b. Orient the client frequently
   c. Use familiar objects in the room
   d. Place a calendar and clock in a visible place
   e. Maintain familiar routines
   f. Allow the client to reminisce
   g. Make tasks simple
   h. Allow time for the client to complete a task
   i. Provide positive reinforcement for positive behaviors

8. Altered sleep patterns
   a. Allow clients to wander in a safe place until they become tired
   b. Prevent shadows in the room
   c. Avoid the use of hypnotics because they cause confusion and aggravate the sundown effect

9. Agitation
   a. Assess the precipitant of the agitation
   b. Reassure the client
   c. Remove items that can be hazardous during the time of agitation
   d. Approach the client slowly and calmly from the front, then speak, gesture, and move slowly
   e. Remove the client to a less stressful environment
   f. Use touch gently
   g. Do not argue with or restrain the client
   h. Distract the client with questions about the problem and gradually turn the attention to something else

B. Autistic disorder
   1. A rare developmental disorder that includes characteristics such as lack of social response and interaction
   2. Withdrawal from social contact
   3. Impaired communication
   4. Bizarre mannerisms
   5. If the child can talk the child uses speech not for communication but to repeat words or phrases meaninglessly
   6. The child may develop an unusual attachment to a significant object and display frequent rocking, spinning, twirling, or other bizarre behaviors

C. Attention deficit hyperactivity disorder (ADHD)
   1. Known as hyperactivity
   2. The client cannot sustain concentration to complete a task
   3. The client has little impulse control and exhibits continual, frequently disruptive activity
   4. The client has a short attention span and difficulty with organizing and completing schoolwork

D. Tourette's disorder
   1. Description: appears between ages 2 and 15

and is characterized by recurrent involuntary and rapid movements affecting various parts of the body accompanied by vocal noises such as barks, grunts, or profanities

  2. Implementation
     a. Assess **suicide** potential
     b. Remove dangerous objects from the environment
     c. Establish a trusting one-on-one relationship
     d. Maintain eye contact
     e. Protect the client from harm by providing a helmet or protective padding
     f. If the client is a child, allow the child to have a favorite toy or other object
     g. Provide positive reinforcement for appropriate behaviors
     h. Set limits on socially inappropriate or manipulative behaviors
     i. Encourage the client to confront tension and frustration before they emerge as inappropriate behaviors
     j. Provide noncompetitive group situations

XIV. Psychosexual Alterations

A. Sexuality
   1. One's sense of being a sexual individual
   2. Includes how one looks, behaves, and relates to others
B. Alterations in sexual expression
   1. Heterosexuality—male/female sexual relationships
   2. Homosexuality—sexual attraction to a member of the same sex
   3. Bisexuality—sexual attraction to and activity with both sexes
   4. Transvestism—obsession with wearing clothing of the opposite sex
C. Alterations in sexual behavior
   1. Transsexualism: feeling that one's sex is inappropriate and desiring to acquire sexual characteristics of the opposite sex
   2. Exhibitionism: sexual urges and fantasies and exposing genitals to strangers
   3. Fetishism: using nonliving objects for sexual gratification
   4. Pedophilia: desiring sexual activity with a child under age 13
   5. Sexual masochism: sexual gratification that involves receiving pain
   6. Sexual sadism: sexual gratification that involves inflicting pain
   7. Voyeurism: sexual gratification through observing others disrobing or engaging in sexual activity
   8. Zoophilia: intense sexual arousal or desire for sexual contact with animal
   9. Frotteurism: intense sexual arousal when rubbing against a nonconsenting person

D. Implementation
   1. Assessment of sexual history and the precipitating event for sexual disorder
   2. Encourage the client to explore personal beliefs
   3. Provide a nonjudgmental attitude
   4. Provide supportive psychotherapy
   5. Initiate psychoanalysis as prescribed

PRACTICE QUESTIONS

1. The nurse is caring for a client who has bipolar disorder with aggressive social behavior. Which of the following activities are most appropriate for this client?
   1 Ping-Pong
   2 Writing
   3 Chess
   4 Basketball

2. A client is admitted to the hospital with a diagnosis of major depression—severe, single episode. The nurse assesses the client and identifies as a major concern the client's altered nutrition related to poor nutritional intake. The most appropriate nursing intervention related to this diagnosis is
   1 Explain to the client the importance of a good nutritional intake
   2 Weigh the client three times per week, before breakfast
   3 Report the nutritional concern to the psychiatrist and obtain a nutritional consult as soon as possible
   4 Consult with the nutritionist, offer the client several small frequent meals per day, and schedule brief nursing interactions with the client during these times

3. In planning activities for the depressed client, especially during the early stages of hospitalization, which of the following plans is best?
   1 Provide an activity that is quiet and solitary to avoid increased fatigue, such as working on a puzzle or reading a book
   2 Plan nothing until the client asks to participate in milieu
   3 Offer the client a menu of daily activities and insist the client participate in all of them
   4 Provide a structured daily program of activities and encourage the client to participate

4. The depressed client verbalizes feelings of low self-esteem and self-worth typified by statements such as "I'm such a failure . . . I can't do anything right!" The best nursing response is
   1 To tell the client that this is not true; we all have a purpose in life
   2 To remain with the client and sit in silence; this will encourage the client to verbalize feelings
   3 To reassure the client that you know how the client is feeling and that things will get better
   4 To identify recent behaviors or accomplishments that demonstrate skill ability

5. A depressed client who is on tranylcypromine sulfate (Parnate) has been instructed on diet. The nurse feels confident that the client understands the diet when, given a choice of foods at a restaurant, the client selects
   1 Pepperoni pizza, salad, and Coca-Cola
   2 Roasted chicken, roasted potatoes, and beer
   3 Pickled herring, french fries, and milk
   4 Fried haddock, baked potato, and milk

6. A client with a diagnosis of Major Depression, Recurrent with Psychotic Features, is admitted to the unit. In an attempt to create a safe environment for the client, the nurse must most importantly devise a plan of care that deals specifically with the client's
   1 Altered Thought Processes
   2 Altered Nutrition
   3 Self-Care Deficit
   4 Knowledge Deficit

7. A client is being treated for depression with amitriptyline hydrochloride (Elavil). During the initial phases of treatment, the most important nursing intervention is
   1 Ordering the client an MAO–tyramine-free diet
   2 Recognizing that frequent blood levels are in order because there is a narrow range between therapeutic and toxic blood levels of this drug
   3 Getting baseline postural blood pressures on the client before administering the drug and each time the drug is dispensed to the client, especially during the initial days of treatment
   4 Assessing the client for anticholinergic effects

8. A depressed client is ready for discharge. The nurse feels comfortable that the client has a good understanding of the disease process "Depression" when the client states
   1 "I'll never let this happen to me again. I won't let my boss or my job or my family get to me!"
   2 "It's important for me to eat well, exercise, and to take my medication. If I begin to lose my appetite or not sleep well, I've got to get in to see my doctor."
   3 "I've learned I am a good person and that I am worthy of giving and receiving love. I don't need anyone; I have myself to rely on!"
   4 "I don't know what happened to me. I've always been able to make decisions for myself and for my business. I don't ever want to feel so weak or vulnerable again!"

9. The nurse assesses a client with the admitting diagnosis of bipolar affective disorder (mania). The symptom presentation that requires the nurse's immediate intervention is
   1 The client's outlandish behaviors and inappropriate dress
   2 The client's grandiose delusions of being a royal descendent of King Arthur

3 The client's nonstop physical activity and poor nutritional intake
4 The client's incessant talking that includes sexual innuendos and teasing the staff

10. The client in a manic state emerges from her room. She is topless and is making sexual remarks and gestures toward staff and peers. The best initial nursing response is
    1 Quietly approach the client, escort her to her room, and assist her in getting dressed
    2 Approach the client in the hallway and insist that she go to her room
    3 Confront the client on the inappropriateness of her behaviors and offer her a time-out
    4 Ask the other clients to ignore her behavior; eventually she will return to her room

11. A client who is on lithium carbonate (lithium) will be discharged at the end of the week. In formulating a discharge teaching plan, the nurse instructs the client that it is most important
    1 To avoid soy sauce, wine, and aged cheese
    2 To take medication only as prescribed because it can become addicting
    3 To check with the psychiatrist before using any over-the-counter medications or prescription drugs
    4 To have the lithium level checked every 2 weeks

12. A client who is on lithium carbonate (lithium) offers complaints of polydipsia and gastric irritation. Later that day, the client complains of drowsiness, muscle weakness, and lack of coordination. It is time for the client's 4:00 P.M. dose. The best nursing action is
    1 Give the 4:00 P.M. dose as scheduled and reeducate the client that these are normal side effects for the medication
    2 Give the 4:00 P.M. dose and document the client's complaints
    3 Give the 4:00 P.M. dose and notify the charge nurse of the client's complaints
    4 Hold the 4:00 P.M. dose and notify the psychiatrist of the client's complaints

13. The nurse reviews the activity schedule for the day and believes the best activity that the manic client could participate in is
    1 Brown-bag luncheon and a book review
    2 Walking
    3 Paint by number activity
    4 Deep breathing and progressive relaxation group

14. A client who is delusional says to the nurse, "The federal guards were sent to kill me." The nurse's best response is
    1 "The guards are not out to kill you."
    2 "I don't believe this is true."
    3 "I don't know anything about the guards. Do

you feel afraid that people are trying to hurt you?"
4 "What makes you think the guards were sent to hurt you?"

15. A woman comes into the emergency department in a severe state of anxiety following a car accident. The most important nursing intervention is
    1 Remain with the client
    2 Put the client in a quiet room
    3 Teach the client deep breathing
    4 Encourage the client to talk about her feelings and concerns

16. A male client with delirium becomes agitated and confused in his room at night. The best initial intervention by the nurse is
    1 Use a nightlight and turn off the television
    2 Keep the television on during the night and turn on a soft light
    3 Move the client next to the nurse's station
    4 Play soft music during the night, and maintain a well-lit room

17. Which of the following assessment data indicates to the nurse that the client with critical care unit (CCU) psychosis is improving?
    1 The client tells his brother, "The nurses are trying to kill me!"
    2 The client's blood gases are stabilizing although he keeps watching the CCU nurses
    3 The client demonstrates increased sleep and absence of injuries
    4 The client appears to be delirious but the grimacing is reduced

18. The client is diagnosed with undifferentiated schizophrenia. The nurse prepares a nursing care plan for the client and in the planning, the nurse understands that
    1 The client must be allowed to set the goals for the plan of care
    2 Until the client's thinking is cleared, the nurse may need to assist the client with grooming and nutrition
    3 Refraining from pointing out the inconsistencies of the client's communication is essential to initial treatment
    4 Letting the client act out and using the quiet room and restraints when needed is essential

19. The nurse is performing an admission assessment on a client who is actively hallucinating. Which of the following nursing statements is most therapeutic at this time?
    1 "I talked to the voices you're hearing and they won't hurt you now."
    2 "I can hear your voice and she wants you to come to dinner."
    3 "Sometimes people hear things or voices others can't hear."

4 "I know you feel 'they are out to get you,' but it's not true."

20. The visiting nurse calls on an agoraphobic client who experiences panic attacks. Which of the following assessment data indicates that the client is responding to behavioral and pharmacological treatment?
    1 "I went to the movies with my family and stayed through the whole film by sitting on the aisle."
    2 "I took extra alprazolam (Xanax) and got through the funeral fairly well."
    3 "Taking my fluoxetine (Prozac) and a Xanax before I leave has helped me to cross the bridge and go to work every morning."
    4 "I have noticed that I'm becoming anxious and I worry if I don't take my Xanax just before it's due, I'll go crazy. So I get it ready to take to calm down."

21. The psychiatric clinical nurse specialist visits the client with panic attacks at home and teaches the client using paradoxical intention. Which of the following describes the intervention the nurse employs for the client?
    1 Having the client confront the anxiety-provoking stimulus and providing support during the episode
    2 Using progressive relaxation toward the client's individual anxiety hierarchy (and increasing the level of difficulty) and pairing relaxation with the gradual exposure to reduce the client's anxiety
    3 Presenting the anxiety-provoking stimulus without any preparation of the client and having the client remain exposed until the anxiety subsides
    4 Instructing the client to hyperventilate to create a panic attack

22. The nurse is teaching the family of a recently diagnosed pediatric client who has developed a strep-induced obsessive-compulsive disorder (OCD). Which of the following indicates an understanding by the family members of the biological basis for pediatric autoimmune neuropsychiatric disorders (PANDAS)?
    1 "Are you saying that our son's strep infection resulted in the development of an antibody that attacked the hypothalamus of his brain rather than fighting off his infection?"
    2 "Are you saying that our son's strep infection resulted in the development of an antibody that attacked the basal ganglia of his brain rather than fighting off his infection?"
    3 "Are you saying that our son's strep infection resulted in the development of an antibody that attacked the cerebrum of his brain rather than fighting off his infection?"
    4 "Are you saying that our son's strep infection resulted in the development of an antibody

that attacked the parietal lobe of his brain rather than fighting off his infection?"

23. The young client tentatively diagnosed with a borderline personality disorder says to his parents in family therapy, "I don't know why I got my tattoo; it was for me. OK? Sometimes I do these things to get you mad and sometimes I do them 'cause I'm bored. That's what happened the night I crashed the family car. I wasn't drunk or suicidal or anything like the police thought. It was just for kicks!" Which of the following is the most appropriate response by the nurse?
    1 "Next time pick less dangerous and expensive ways to explode."
    2 "It is scary when you feel out of control with such feelings of emptiness and anger that you can't stop yourself."
    3 "It's a good thing that you don't abuse substances or you might be dead due to your reckless disregard."
    4 "What can you do to stop your behavior when it gets to that point the next time?"

24. The nurse is caring for a client with a diagnosis of depression. The nurse monitors for signs of constipation and urinary retention knowing that these problems are most likely a result of
    1 Inadequate dietary intake and dehydration
    2 Lack of exercise and poor diet
    3 Poor dietary choices
    4 Psychomotor retardation and side effects of medication

25. The client is admitted to the inpatient unit and is being considered for electroconvulsive therapy (ECT). The client appears calm but the family is hypervigilant and anxious. The client's mother begins to cry and states, "My son's brain will be destroyed. How can the doctor do this to him?" The nurse's best response to this remark is
    1 "It sounds as though you need to speak to the psychiatrist."
    2 "Your son has decided to have this treatment. You should be supportive of him."
    3 "Perhaps you'd like to see the ECT room and speak to the staff."
    4 "It sounds as though you have some concerns about the ECT procedure. Why don't we all sit down together and discuss any concerns you may have."

26. The nurse is performing an assessment on a client who is diagnosed with post-traumatic stress disorder (PTSD). In caring for this client, the nurse understands which neurotransmitter system is affected?
    1 Serotonin
    2 Norepinephrine
    3 Acetylcholine
    4 Gamma-aminobutyric acid (GABA)

27. The nurse is caring for a client who has been treated with long-term antipsychotic medication. As part of the nursing care plan, the nurse monitors for tardive dyskinesia (TD). In the event that TD occurs, the nurse most likely observes
    1 Abnormal movements and involuntary movements of the mouth, tongue, and face
    2 Abnormal breathing through the nostrils accompanied by a shrill
    3 Severe headache, flushing, tremor, and ataxia
    4 Severe hypertension, migraine headache, and "marbles in the mouth" syndrome

28. The client who is diagnosed with pedophilia and was recently paroled as a sex offender, says, "I'm in treatment and I have served my time, now this group has posters all over the neighborhood telling about me with my picture on them." Which of the following is the most appropriate response by the nurse?
    1 "You understand that people fear for their children but you're feeling unfairly treated."
    2 "When children are hurt as you hurt them, people want you isolated."
    3 "You seem angry but you have committed serious crimes against several children, so your neighbors are frightened."
    4 "You're lucky it doesn't escalate into something pretty scary after your crime."

29. Which of the following assessment data indicates a potential complication associated with dementia?
    1 Presence of personal hygienic care
    2 Improvement in sleeping
    3 Absence of sundowner syndrome
    4 Confabulation

30. Which of the following assessment data causes the nurse to suspect retrograde amnesia in a client who has received ECT?
    1 Following the procedure, the client has difficulty recalling information that was learned prior to ECT for 2 days
    2 The client has a memory loss for 2 days following the procedure
    3 The client had difficulty remembering information learned prior to ECT for over 4 months
    4 The client has difficulty recalling newly learned information for 2 weeks following the procedure

31. The community health nurse visits a recently retired client at home. The client states, "Lately I'm getting forgetful about things. Do you think I'm getting Alzheimer's disease?" Which of the following responses by the nurse is the most therapeutic communication technique?
    1 "Tell me more about your forgetfulness. It isn't unusual for forgetfulness to occur if memory is not exercised. Are you staying socially active?"
    2 "Oh, I'm certain it's not Alzheimer's disease because there's no family history of it."

3 "Now, I'm not going to discuss this with you because I think you're just normal."

4 "Me, too. I have to make out lists now to go shopping. So, I don't want you to be saying or thinking this."

32. The nurse is discharging a client with a history of command hallucinations to harm self or others. The nurse instructs the client about interventions for hallucinations and anxiety. The nurse knows the client understands this teaching when the client says
   1 "My medications won't make me anxious."
   2 "I can call my therapist when I'm hallucinating so that I can talk about my feelings and plans and not hurt anyone."
   3 "I'll go to support group and talk so that I don't hurt anyone."
   4 "I won't get anxious or hear things if I get enough sleep and eat well."

33. The nurse develops a nursing diagnosis of Self-Care Deficit for an elderly client with dementia. Which of the following is the most appropriate goal for this client?
   1 The client will be admitted to a long-term care facility to have ADL needs met
   2 The client will function at the highest level of independence possible
   3 The client will complete all ADLs independently within 1 hour
   4 The nursing staff will attend to all the client's ADL needs during the hospital stay

34. The nurse observes that a client is psychotic, pacing, agitated, and presenting aggressive gestures. The client's speech pattern is rapid and affect is belligerent. Based on these observations, the nurse's immediate priority of care is to
   1 Provide safety for the client and other clients on the unit
   2 Offer the client a less stimulating area to calm down and gain control
   3 Provide the clients on the unit with a sense of comfort and safety
   4 Assist the staff in caring for the client in a controlled environment

35. The nurse is caring for a male client diagnosed with catatonic stupor. The client is lying on the bed with his body pulled into a fetal position. The most appropriate nursing intervention is which of the following?
   1 Leave the client alone and intermittently check on him
   2 Take the client into the dayroom with other clients so they can help watch him
   3 Sit beside him in silence with occasional open-ended questions
   4 Ask direct questions to encourage talking

36. The nurse is providing instructions to a client taking lithium carbonate (Eskalith). The nurse most appropriately instructs the client to
   1 Take lithium on an empty stomach
   2 Decrease sodium intake
   3 Increase fluid intake to 1500–3000 mL daily
   4 Diarrhea is expected with the medication

37. The mother of a teenage client with an anxiety disorder is concerned about her daughter's progress upon discharge. She states that her daughter "stashes food, eats all the wrong things that make her hyperactive, and hangs out with the wrong crowd." In helping the mother prepare for her daughter's discharge, the nurse instructs her to
   1 Restrict the daughter's socializing time with her friends
   2 Consider taking time from work to help her daughter readjust to the home environment
   3 Restrict the amount of chocolate and caffeine products in the home
   4 Keep her daughter out of school until she can adjust to the school environment

38. The client is admitted to the unit with a diagnosis of schizophrenia. A nursing diagnosis formulated for the client is Altered Thought Process, secondary to paranoia. In formulating a nursing care plan with the team, the nurse includes instruction to the staff to
   1 Avoid laughing or whispering in front of the client
   2 Increase socialization of the client with peers
   3 Have the client sign a release of information to appropriate parties so that adequate data can be obtained for assessment purposes
   4 Begin to educate the client about social supports in the community

39. A client is admitted with a diagnosis of depression. The nurse develops a plan of care for the client. Which of the following activities is most appropriate to include in the plan?
   1 Encourage the client to read
   2 Allow the client to select the activity
   3 Encourage the client to attend all unit activities
   4 Provide structure to the daily plan for the client

40. When planning the discharge of a client with chronic anxiety, the nurse directs the goals at promoting a safe environment at home. The most appropriate maintenance goal should focus on which of the following?
   1 Continued contact with a crisis counselor
   2 Identifying anxiety-producing situations
   3 Ignoring feelings of anxiety
   4 Eliminating all anxiety from daily situations

41. The client is unwilling to go out of the house for fear of "doing something crazy in public." Because of this fear, the client remains homebound except when accompanied outside by the spouse. The nurse analyzes these data and determines that the diagnosis is indicated as
    1 Social phobia
    2 Agoraphobia
    3 Claustrophobia
    4 Hypochondria

42. The nurse is developing a plan of care for a client who is scheduled to have electroconvulsive therapy (ECT). Which of the following nursing diagnoses is a priority for this client?
    1 Fear
    2 Anxiety
    3 Risk for Aspiration
    4 Body Image Disturbance

43. A depressed client is wandering the halls and the nurse notes that the client has long shreds of torn sheets wrapped around the throat. The most appropriate nursing diagnosis for this client is
    1 Risk for Injury
    2 Ineffective Individual Coping
    3 Hopelessness
    4 Risk for Loneliness

44. The client reports that crying spells have been a major problem over the past several weeks, and that the doctor said that depression is probably the reason. The nurse observes that the client is sitting slumped in the chair and the clothes that the client is wearing are not fitting well. The nurse interprets that further assessment should focus on
    1 Sleep patterns
    2 Onset of the crying spells
    3 Weight loss
    4 Medication compliance

45. The client with the diagnosis of major depression becomes more anxious on the unit, reports sleeping poorly, and seems be more irritable with staff and family. The nurse interprets the client's behavior as
    1 The client is at increased risk for suicide
    2 This is a normal response to hospitalization
    3 The client is dealing with pertinent issues
    4 The client may need some time off the unit

46. Which of the following assessment data does the nurse determine as indicating that the client is experiencing a major depressive episode?
    1 The client is a male
    2 The client states, "Since my wife died last week, I've been waking up hours before I should and I'm tired all day."
    3 The client uses marijuana
    4 The client states, "The last 3 weeks, I'm doing all the things I used to do but I'm not enjoying them."

47. A client was admitted to a medical unit with acute blindness. Many tests are performed and there seems to be no organic reason why this client cannot see. The nurse later learns that the client became blind after witnessing a hit-and-run car accident, in which a family of three was killed. The nurse suspects that the client may be experiencing a
    1 Psychosis
    2 Conversion disorder
    3 Dissociative disorder
    4 Repression

48. The manic client announces to everyone in the dayroom that a stripper is coming to perform this evening. When the psychiatric orderly firmly states that this will not happen, the manic client becomes verbally abusive and threatens physical violence to the orderly. Based on the analysis of this situation, the nurse determines that the most appropriate action is
    1 With assistance, escort the manic client to his or her room and administer PRN haloperidol (Haldol)
    2 Tell the client that smoking privileges are revoked for 24 hours
    3 Orient the client to time, person, and place
    4 Tell the client that the behavior is not appropriate

49. The nurse is reviewing the record of a client scheduled for ECT. Which of the following medical diagnoses, if noted on the client's record, indicates a need to contact the physician scheduled to perform the ECT?
    1 Recent myocardial infarction
    2 Diabetes mellitus
    3 Hyperthyroidism
    4 Peripheral vascular disease

50. The nurse is preparing a client for ECT, which is scheduled for the following morning. Which of the following is not a component of the plan of care?
    1 Withhold food and fluids for 6 hours prior to the treatment
    2 Have the client void before the procedure
    3 Remove dentures and contact lenses prior to the procedure
    4 Administer tap water enemas on the evening before the procedure

ANSWERS

1. **2**

Rationale: Solitary activities that require a short attention span with mild physical exertion are the most appropriate activities initially with a client who is aggressive. Writing (journaling), walks with the staff, and finger painting are activities that minimize stimuli and provide a constructive release for tension. Competitive games should be avoided because they can stimulate aggression and increase psychomotor activity.

Test-Taking Strategy: Knowledge of nursing interventions to meet the needs of the manic client is required to answer this question. Options 1, 3, and 4 are similar in that they are activities that the client cannot do alone. Option 2 is an activity that the client can do alone. It is the option that is different.

Level of Cognitive Ability: Application
Phase of Nursing Process: Implementation
Client Needs: Psychosocial Integrity
Content Area: Mental Health

Reference
Varcarolis, E. (1998). *Foundations of psychiatric mental health nursing* (3rd ed.). Philadelphia: W. B. Saunders. p. 606.

2. **4**

Rationale: Change in appetite is one of the major symptoms of depression, coupled with depressed mood, increased fatigue, feelings of worthlessness, diminished ability to think or indecisiveness, and psychomotor agitation or retardation. Offering the client several small frequent meals and the nurse's presence at that time to support, encourage, or perhaps even feed the client is an effective application of knowledge regarding the disease process and how it may affect the client.

Test-Taking Strategy: Option 4 is the only option that addresses the altered nutrition concretely and designs methods in which the client will feasibly increase the nutritional intake. Eliminate option 1 because the client is experiencing poor concentration; hence, even if the client does understand the rationale, the client still may not be able to complete tasks. Weighing the client does not address how to increase nutritional intake. Reporting to the psychiatrist and the nutritionist is to some degree correct, but lacks the method as to how one might increase food intake.

Level of Cognitive Ability: Application
Phase of Nursing Process: Implementation
Client Needs: Physiological Integrity
Content Area: Mental Health

Reference
Varcarolis, E. (1998). *Foundations of psychiatric mental health nursing* (3rd ed.). Philadelphia: W. B. Saunders. p. 566.

3. **4**

Rationale: A depressed person often suffers with depressed mood and is often withdrawn. Also, the person experiences difficulty concentrating, loss of interest or pleasure, low energy, fatigue, and feelings of worthlessness and poor self-esteem. The plan of care needs to provide successful experiences in a stimulating yet structured environment.

Test-Taking Strategy: The depressed client requires a structured/stimulating program. Options 1 and 2 are too "restrictive" and offer little or no structure and stimulation.

Option 3 is eliminated because the word "all" is in the selection. Option 4 is the only reasonable selection.

Level of Cognitive Ability: Application
Phase of Nursing Process: Planning
Client Needs: Safe, Effective Care Environment
Content Area: Mental Health

Reference
Varcarolis, E. (1998). *Foundations of psychiatric mental health nursing* (3rd ed.). Philadelphia: W. B. Saunders. p. 566.

4. **4**

Rationale: Feelings of low self-esteem and worthlessness are common symptoms of the depressed client. An effective plan of care is to provide successful experiences for the client that are challenging but will not be met with failure to enhance the client's personal self-esteem. Reminders of the client's past accomplishments or personal successes are ways to interrupt the client's negative self-talk and distorted cognitive self-view.

Test-Taking Strategy: Communication blocks are evident in options 1 and 3 because the nurse gives advice or devalues the client's feelings. Option 2, silence, may be interpreted as agreement. Option 4 provides the client with information based upon fact and promotes positive thoughts.

Level of Cognitive Ability: Application
Phase of Nursing Process: Implementation
Client Needs: Psychosocial Integrity
Content Area: Mental Health

Reference
Varcarolis, E. (1998). *Foundations of psychiatric mental health nursing* (3rd ed.). Philadelphia: W. B. Saunders. p. 566.

5. **4**

Rationale: Tranylcypromine sulfate (Parnate) is an MAO inhibitor used to treat depression. A tyramine-restricted diet is required while on this medication to avoid hypertensive crisis, a life-threatening side effect of the medication. Foods to be avoided are meats prepared with tenderizer, smoked or pickled fish, beef or chicken liver, and dry sausage (salami, pepperoni, bologna). In addition, figs, bananas, aged cheese, yogurt and sour cream, beer, red wine, and all other alcoholic beverages, soy sauce, yeast extract, chocolate, caffeine, and any aged, pickled, fermented, or smoked foods need to be avoided. Many over-the-counter medications also include tyramine and must be avoided as well.

Test-Taking Strategy: A knowledge of the MAO inhibitor medications and the foods and medications that are to be avoided is necessary to answer this question. Take time now to review these medications if you had difficulty with this question!

Level of Cognitive Ability: Analysis
Phase of Nursing Process: Evaluation
Client Needs: Health Promotion and Maintenance
Content Area: Mental Health

Reference
Varcarolis, E. (1998). *Foundations of psychiatric mental health nursing* (3rd ed.). Philadelphia: W. B. Saunders. p. 576.

6. **1**

Rationale: Major Depression, Recurrent, with Psychotic Features alerts the nurse that in addition to the criteria that designate the diagnosis of major depression, one must also deal with a client's psychosis. Psychosis is defined as a state in which a person's mental capacity to recognize reality, communicate, and relate to others is impaired, thus interfering with the person's capacity to deal with life's demands. Altered Thought Processes generally indicates a state of increased anxiety in which hallucinations and delusions prevail.

Test-Taking Strategy: All of the nursing diagnoses listed may be appropriate for a client diagnosed with major depression. The key to the answer lies with the specifier "psychotic features" in which the client often suffers with Altered Thought Processes such as hallucinations and delusions.

Level of Cognitive Ability: Application
Phase of Nursing Process: Planning
Client Needs: Safe, Effective Care Environment
Content Area: Mental Health

Reference
Antai-Otong, D. (1995). *Psychiatric nursing: Biological and behavioral concepts.* Philadelphia: W. B. Saunders. pp. 241, 249.

7. **3**

Rationale: Amitriptyline hydrochloride (Elavil) is a tricyclic antidepressant often used to treat depression. The client may experience some side effects such as sedation, dry mouth, constipation, or blurred vision (anticholinergic). These are annoying at best and can seem debilitating at worst. However, these are transient and will diminish as time goes on. More commonly, orthostatic changes can produce hypotension and tachycardia. This can be frightening to the client and dangerous (it may result in dizziness and the client falling). The client must be instructed to move slowly from a lying to a sitting to a standing position to avoid injury if these changes are experienced.

Test-Taking Strategy: Knowledge of tricyclic medications is required to answer this question. If you had difficulty with this question, take time now to review this medication!

Level of Cognitive Ability: Application
Phase of Nursing Process: Implementation
Client Needs: Physiological Integrity
Content Area: Mental Health

Reference
Hodgson, B., & Kizior, R. (1999). *Saunders nursing drug handbook 1999.* Philadelphia: W. B. Saunders. p. 51.

8. **2**

Rationale: The exact causes of depression are not known but are believed to be related to a biochemical disruption of neurotransmitters in the brain. Diet, exercise, and medication are recognized treatment of the disease process.

Test-Taking Strategy: Option 2 is the only answer that incorporates a holistic treatment approach, good nutrition, exercise, and medication as well as the client's knowledge of the signs of possible relapse. Options 1, 3, and 4 offer no insight into the disease process. In addition, option 1 reflects possible blaming or personal failure; option 3, an unwillingness to reach out to others.

Level of Cognitive Ability: Analysis
Phase of Nursing Process: Evaluation
Client Needs: Health Promotion and Maintenance:
Content Area: Mental Health

Reference
Varcarolis, E. (1998). *Foundations of psychiatric mental health nursing* (3rd ed.). Philadelphia: W. B. Saunders. pp. 563–566.

9. **3**

Rationale: Mania is a mood characterized by excitement, euphoria, hyperactivity, excessive energy, decreased need for sleep, and impaired ability to concentrate or complete a single train of thought. It is a period when the mood is predominantly elevated, expansive, or irritable. All selections reflect a client's possible symptomatology. Option 3, however, clearly presents a nursing problem, which compromises one's physiological integrity and needs to be addressed immediately (Maslow's hierarchy of needs).

Test-Taking Strategy: All four options reflect symptomatology related to a manic state. The stem of the question asks for an immediate intervention. Option 3 indicates a potential disruption in the client's physiological status. Use Maslow's hierarchy of needs theory to assist in answering the question.

Level of Cognitive Ability: Analysis
Phase of Nursing Process: Analysis
Client Needs: Physiological Integrity
Content Area: Mental Health

Reference
Antai-Otong, D. (1995). *Psychiatric nursing: Biological and behavioral concepts.* Philadelphia: W. B. Saunders. p. 130.

10. **1**

Rationale: A person who is experiencing mania lacks insight and judgment, has poor impulse control, and is highly excitable. The nurse must take control without creating increased stress or anxiety to the client. A quiet, firm approach while distracting the client (walking her to her room and assisting her to get dressed) achieves the goal of having her dressed appropriately and preserving her psychosocial integrity.

Test-Taking Strategy: The goal of the interaction is to have the client dress appropriately. Option 4 is immediately discarded as a selection. Although options 1, 2, and 3 are all similar, "insisting" the client go to her room may meet with a great deal of resistance; confronting the client and offering her a consequence of time-out may be meaningless to her. The nurse is using knowledge of the disease process to achieve the client's goals.

Level of Cognitive Ability: Application
Phase of Nursing Process: Implementation
Client Needs: Psychosocial Integrity
Content Area: Mental Health

Reference
Varcarolis, E. (1998). *Foundations of psychiatric mental health nursing* (3rd ed.). Philadelphia: W. B. Saunders. p. 606.

11. **3**

Rationale: Lithium is recognized as the medication of choice to treat manic-depressive illness. Its exact mechanism of action remains speculative; however, an equilibrium of Na and K must be maintained at the intracellular membrane to maintain therapeutic effects. Lithium competes with Na in the cell. Many over-the-counter medications contain Na, and often prescription medications (diuretics) change the Na:K ratios of the cell, thus affecting lithium concentrations and the therapeutic levels of the medication.

Test-Taking Strategy: A strong knowledge base relating to medication is required. Food restriction (tyramine-restricted diet) is associated with MAO inhibitors. Antianxiety agents (not lithium) are generally of an addictive nature. Lithium blood levels are recommended but are generally every 3 to 4 months. It is important that the nurse remembers that the Na:K ratio must be maintained for lithium to remain effective. A disruption at the cell membrane of these two electrolytes can yield to decrease lithium level or lithium toxicity.

Level of Cognitive Ability: Application
Phase of Nursing Process: Implementation
Client Needs: Health Promotion and Maintenance
Content Area: Mental Health

Reference
Hodgson, B., & Kizior, R. (1999). *Saunders nursing drug handbook 1999.* Philadelphia: W. B. Saunders. p. 600.

12. **4**

Rationale: The side effects of lithium include fine hand tremors, polyuria, mild thirst, and transient and mild nausea. Diarrhea, vomiting, nausea, drowsiness, muscle weakness, and lack of coordination may be early signs of toxicity. The medication is held and the psychiatrist notified so that the client may be further evaluated (lithium blood level) to determine toxicity.

Test-Taking Strategy: Options 1, 2, and 3 all require that the nurse give the medication. Option 4 requires the nurse to hold the medication, analyze and evaluate the data, and develop a plan of care to meet the client's needs. Review this important medication now if you had difficulty with this question!

Level of Cognitive Ability: Application
Phase of Nursing Process: Implementation
Client Needs: Physiological Integrity
Content Area: Mental Health

Reference
Antai-Otong, D. (1995). *Psychiatric nursing: Biological and behavioral concepts.* Philadelphia: W. B. Saunders. p. 557.

13. **2**

Rationale: A person who is experiencing mania is overactive, full of energy, lacks concentration, and has poor impulse control. The client needs an activity that will allow the client to use excess energy, yet not endanger others during the process.

Test-Taking Strategy: Options 1, 3, and 4 are relatively sedate activities that require concentration—a quality that is lacking in the manic state. Such activities may lead to increased frustration and anxiety for the client. Tetherball is an exercise that uses the large muscle groups of the body and is a great way to expend the increased energy this client is experiencing. Review the appropriate interventions for a manic client now if you had difficulty with this question!

Level of Cognitive Ability: Analysis
Phase of Nursing Process: Planning
Client Needs: Physiological Integrity
Content Area: Mental Health

Reference
Varcarolis, E. (1998). *Foundations of psychiatric mental health nursing* (3rd ed.). Philadelphia: W. B. Saunders. p. 606.

14. **3**

Rationale: Disagreeing with delusions may make the client more defensive and the client may cling to the delusions even more. It is most therapeutic for the nurse to empathize with the client's experience.

Test-Taking Strategy: Use therapeutic communication techniques with the client experiencing delusions. Eliminate options 1 and 2 because they are similar and are statements that disagree with the client. Option 4 is encouraging discussion regarding the delusion. Review communication techniques with the client experiencing delusions now if you had difficulty with this question!

Level of Cognitive Ability: Application
Phase of Nursing Process: Implementation
Client Needs: Psychosocial Integrity
Content Area: Mental Health

Reference
Varcarolis, E. (1998). *Foundations of psychiatric mental health nursing* (3rd ed.). Philadelphia: W. B. Saunders. pp. 191, 640.

15. **1**

Rationale: If a client is left alone with severe anxiety, the client may feel abandoned and become overwhelmed. Placing the client in a quiet room is also indicated but the nurse must stay with the client. It is not possible to teach clients deep breathing or relaxation until anxiety decreases. Encouraging the client to discuss concerns and feelings cannot take place until the anxiety has decreased.

Test-Taking Strategy: Note the key words "most important" and "severe." This question requires you to prioritize. Eliminate options 3 and 4 first, knowing that these actions are not possible when the client is in a severe state of anxiety. From the remaining options, the best action is to remain with the client!

Level of Cognitive Ability: Application
Phase of Nursing Process: Implementation
Client Needs: Psychosocial Integrity
Content Area: Mental Health

Reference
Varcarolis, E. (1998). *Foundations of psychiatric mental health nursing* (3rd ed.). Philadelphia: W. B. Saunders. p. 349.

16. **1**

Rationale: It is important to provide a consistent daily routine and a low-stimulating environment when the client is disoriented. Noise levels including radio and television may add to the confusion and disorientation. Moving the client next to the nurses' station is not the initial action.

Test-Taking Strategy: Note the key word "initial" in the stem of the question. Eliminate options 2 and 4 first because they are similar. Focusing on the key word will easily direct you to option 1. Review measures related to the client with delirium now if you had difficulty with this question!

Level of Cognitive Ability: Application
Phase of Nursing Process: Implementation
Client Needs: Psychosocial Integrity
Content Area: Mental Health

Reference
Haber, J., Krainovich-Miller, B., McMahon, A., & Price-Hoskins, P. (1997). *Comprehensive psychiatric nursing* (5th ed.). St. Louis: Mosby–Year Book. p. 676.

17. **3**

Rationale: Being bombarded with several lines, tubes, and even restraints such as confinement to a hospital bed on the CCU can cause feelings of powerlessness. In addition, clients who are on ventilators are aware of their immobilization and pose a risk for psychiatric symptoms and CCU psychosis. When the client leaves the unit the prognosis for CCU psychosis is one that is consistent with the medical condition. Improvement from CCU psychosis is evidenced by decreased hallucinations, anxiety, and aggressive behavior along with increased sleep and absence of injuries.

Test-Taking Strategy: This question tests your knowledge of CCU psychosis. Options 1, 2, and 4 do not indicate that the client is improving. Options 1 and 2 describe the client as actively hallucinating. CCU psychosis is often mistaken for delirium or dementia such as in option 4.

Level of Cognitive Ability: Analysis
Phase of Nursing Process: Evaluation
Client Needs: Physiological Integrity
Content Area: Mental Health

Reference
Glod, C. A. (1998). *Contemporary psychiatric-mental health nursing.* Philadelphia: F. A. Davis. pp. 273–274.

18. **2**

Rationale: As the nurse plans care for the schizophrenic client, it is important to understand the client's developmental stage and ability to accept the disease. Because of the severe decompensation in thinking, the client lacks insight and may not even acknowledge illness. In the acute phase, the nurse will take the lead in planning for the client's basic human needs such as nutrition, hygiene, sleep, and ADLs.

Test-Taking Strategy: Option 4 can easily be eliminated first. In clients with schizophrenia, it is important to provide a structured routine. It is important to expect the client to fulfill basic needs either by self-care or with the nurse's assistance. In option 3, while the nurse would let the client know that the nurse does not see or hear the voices the client speaks of, it is also important not to react to them as if they were real. Review care to the client with schizophrenia now if you had difficulty with this question!

Level of Cognitive Ability: Application
Phase of Nursing Process: Planning
Client Needs: Physiological Integrity
Content Area: Mental Health

Reference
Glod, C. A. (1998). *Contemporary psychiatric-mental health nursing.* Philadelphia: F. A. Davis. pp. 325–328.

19. **3**

Rationale: It is important for the nurse to let the client know that what the client is saying is not understood by the nurse. It is not appropriate to reinforce the client's altered reality. Allow the client to express concerns but reinforce the reality not the delusions. The nurse will want to avoid confronting the client but will want to say such supportive things as, "This must be very frightening to you" or "It's difficult to understand all that you are experiencing right now."

Test-Taking Strategy: Read each option carefully and note that options 1, 2, and 4 all indicate reinforcement to the client that the voices are real. Option 3 is the only statement that indicates reality. Review nursing interventions related to the client who is hallucinating now if you had difficulty with this question!

Level of Cognitive Ability: Application
Phase of Nursing Process: Implementation
Client Needs: Psychosocial Integrity
Content Area: Mental Health

Reference
Glod, C. A. (1998). *Contemporary psychiatric-mental health nursing.* Philadelphia: F. A. Davis. pp. 324–328.

20. **1**

Rationale: Clients generalizing their fears to any place or situation earmarks agoraphobia. Improvement is observed when the client is able to demonstrate appropriate coping behaviors for anxiety reduction.

Test-Taking Strategy: This question assesses your knowledge of client outcome criteria for agoraphobia with panic disorders. Options 2 and 3 do not indicate improvement because the client is learning to take extra medication to cope rather than internal empowerment. Option 4 is inappropriate because the client is demonstrating "clock watching" with regard to the medication schedule.

Level of Cognitive Ability: Analysis
Phase of Nursing Process: Evaluation
Client Needs: Psychosocial Integrity
Content Area: Mental Health

Reference
Glod, C. A. (1998). *Contemporary psychiatric-mental health nursing.* Philadelphia: F. A. Davis. pp. 382–387.

21. **4**

Rationale: In cognitive-behavioral therapy, the client with panic attacks will receive a mix of cognitive restructuring, exposure therapy, and paradoxical intention. In paradoxical intention, the client is instructed by the therapist to hyperventilate in order to cause a panic attack. When this occurs, the nurse teaches the client to stop struggling to prevent the anxiety by a variety of coping mechanisms. This assists the client to regain an internal locus of control or feeling of empowerment or mastery about the anxiety-provoking issue, situation, or person.

Test-Taking Strategy: This question tests your knowledge of the cognitive behavioral therapies that are used to treat clients in the community who suffer from panic attacks. Option 1 describes in vivo therapy, which is a type of exposure therapy. Option 2 describes systematic desensitization, another type of exposure therapy. Option 3 describes flooding, which is probably the most intensive therapy.

Level of Cognitive Ability: Analysis
Phase of Nursing Process: Analysis
Client Needs: Psychosocial Integrity
Content Area: Mental Health

Reference
Glod, C. A. (1998). *Contemporary psychiatric-mental health nursing.* Philadelphia: F. A. Davis. pp. 382–387.

22. **2**

Rationale: There are essentially six subsystems of the brain: cerebrum, diencephalon, basal ganglia, limbic system, brain stem, and the cerebrum. PANDAS is the acronym for the first identifiable biological marker, the antibody D8/17, which seems to attack the basal ganglia of the brain leading to hoarding, checking, and ritualistic behaviors observed in obsessive-compulsive children.

Test-Taking Strategy: Options 1, 3, and 4 provide incorrect regions of the brain regarding this condition. If you are unfamiliar with this condition and had difficulty with this question, take time now to review!

Level of Cognitive Ability: Analysis
Phase of Nursing Process: Evaluation
Client Needs: Psychosocial Integrity
Content Area: Mental Health

Reference
Glod, C. A. (1998). *Contemporary psychiatric-mental health nursing.* Philadelphia: F. A. Davis. pp. 75–90.

23. 2

Rationale: Reflection is a technique that prompts the client by repeating the major theme in the client's process in order to obtain a clearer view of the client's perception of the problem. Reflection allows the client time to review what the client is saying and is a therapeutic communication technique.

Test-Taking Strategy: This question assesses your knowledge of the most therapeutic response by the family therapist for a young client who is tentatively diagnosed with borderline personality disorder. In option 1, the family therapist inappropriately uses a sardonic response, which is nontherapeutic, because it gives advice. In option 3, the family therapist is nontherapeutic because the response starts by agreeing and ends up bordering on being slightly threatening. Option 4 is not the most therapeutic because it is premature in the therapy.

Level of Cognitive Ability: Application
Phase of Nursing Process: Implementation
Client Needs: Psychosocial Integrity
Content Area: Mental Health

Reference
Glod, C. A. (1998). *Contemporary psychiatric-mental health nursing.* Philadelphia: F. A. Davis. pp. 56–61.

24. 4

Rationale: Constipation can be related to inadequate food intake, lack of exercise, and poor diet; however, these factors would not account for urinary retention. Side effects of medications is the only choice that can satisfy complaints of both constipation and urinary retention.

Test-Taking Strategy: Options 1, 2, and 3 are all similar and address diet. Option 4 relates to both constipation and urinary retention. If you had difficulty with this question, take time now to review interventions for a client with depression and the effects of medications prescribed for this disorder!

Level of Cognitive Ability: Application
Phase of Nursing Process: Assessment
Client Needs: Physiological Integrity
Content Area: Mental Health

Reference
Varcarolis, E. (1998). *Foundations of psychiatric mental health nursing* (3rd ed.). Philadelphia: W. B. Saunders. p. 567.

25. 4

Rationale: Basic therapeutic communication techniques are what is being addressed in this question. Therapeutic communication fosters an active collaborative process that facilitates problem solving, change, learning, and growth.

Test-Taking Strategy: Basic understanding of therapeutic communication is being tested. Options 1, 2, and 3 avoid dealing with the client/family concerns. Furthermore, option 2 sounds punitive toward the family. In option 4, the nurse encourages the family and client to verbalize fears and concerns. Once the nurse has heard these, the nurse can then help to allay these fears and impart information.

Level of Cognitive Ability: Application
Phase of Nursing Process: Implementation
Client Needs: Psychosocial Integrity
Content Area: Mental Health

Reference
Varcarolis, E. (1998). *Foundations of psychiatric mental health nursing* (3rd ed.). Philadelphia: W. B. Saunders. p. 579.

26. 2

Rationale: There are four major neurotransmitters in the brain that can cause psychiatric disorders: biogenic amines, cholinergics, neuropeptides, and amino acids. PTSD involves the neurotransmitter norepinephrine.

Test-Taking Strategy: This question assesses your knowledge of the neurotransmitter system, which is involved in PTSD. Options 1, 3, and 4 are all incorrect. Serotonin is the neurotransmitter involved in depression; acetylcholine is the neurotransmitter involved in Alzheimer's disease; and GABA is the neurotransmitter involved in anxiety disorders and schizophrenia. Review PTSD now if you had difficulty with this question!

Level of Cognitive Ability: Analysis
Phase of Nursing Process: Analysis
Client Needs: Physiological Integrity
Content Area: Mental Health

Reference
Glod, C. A. (1998). *Contemporary psychiatric-mental health nursing.* Philadelphia: F. A. Davis. pp. 75–82.

27. 1

Rationale: Tardive dyskinesia is a severe reaction associated with long-term use of antipsychotic medication. The clinical manifestations of TD are abnormal movements (dyskinesia) and involuntary movements of the mouth, tongue ("fly catcher" tongue), and face. In its more severe form, TD involves fingers, arms, trunk, and respiratory muscles. When this occurs, the medication is discontinued.

Test-Taking Strategy: Knowledge regarding the clinical manifestations of TD is required to answer this question. Options 2, 3, and 4 do not identify the characteristics of TD. If you had difficulty with this question, take time now to review the characteristics associated with TD!

Level of Cognitive Ability: Analysis
Phase of Nursing Process: Assessment
Client Needs: Physiological Integrity
Content Area: Mental Health

Reference
Glod, C. A. (1998). *Contemporary psychiatric-mental health nursing.* Philadelphia: F. A. Davis. pp. 116–120.

28. 1

Rationale: The use of the therapeutic communication techniques of focusing and verbalizing the implied is the most therapeutic communication because it assists the client to clarify thinking and to look at what the client is really saying. Option 1 is the only option that reflects the use of therapeutic communication techniques.

Test-Taking Strategy: Use therapeutic communication techniques to answer the question. Eliminate option 2 first. This option is straightforward but somewhat insensitive and anxiety provoking. Eliminate option 3 because it is not therapeutic and does not help the client to express feelings. Option 4 is incorrect because it gives advice and does not help the client to express feelings.

Level of Cognitive Ability: Application
Phase of Nursing Process: Implementation
Client Needs: Psychosocial Integrity
Content Area: Mental Health

Reference
Glod, C. A. (1998). *Contemporary psychiatric-mental health nursing.* Philadelphia: F. A. Davis. pp. 58–60, 445–459.

29. **4**

Rationale: The clinical picture of dementia varies from the development of mild cognitive defects to severe, life-threatening alterations in neurological functioning. The client may employ confabulation or the fabrication of events or experiences to fill in memory gaps. Often, lack of inhibitions on the part of the client may constitute the first indication of anything being wrong to the client's significant others (the client may undress in front of people or demonstrate slovenly table manners). As the dementia progresses, the client will have episodes of wandering or sundowning.

Test-Taking Strategy: Knowledge regarding the manifestations associated with dementia is required to answer this question. If you had difficulty with this question, take time now to review!

Level of Cognitive Ability: Analysis
Phase of Nursing Process: Analysis
Client Needs: Physiological Integrity
Content Area: Mental Health

Reference
Glod, C. A. (1998). *Contemporary psychiatric-mental health nursing.* Philadelphia: F. A. Davis. pp. 233–258.

30. **3**

Rationale: When ECT is performed, the client may experience disorientation, attention difficulty, and transient neurological abnormalities, which usually resolve within a few hours or days. The most prominent adverse reaction is short-term anterograde and retrograde amnesia. Anterograde amnesia is defined as the loss of the client's ability to retain newly learned information. This kind of amnesia usually resolves within the first few weeks after ECT treatments. Retrograde amnesia is defined as difficulty recalling information learned prior to ECT. This kind of amnesia may last longer.

Test-Taking Strategy: This question assesses your understanding of anterograde and retrograde amnesia and its occurrence in clients after ECT treatments. Option 1 describes short-term anterograde amnesia, which is a self-remitting side effect. Option 2 describes short-term retrograde amnesia, which is a self-remitting side effect. Option 4 describes short-term retrograde amnesia, which is a self-remitting side effect. Review the side effects associated with ECT now if you had difficulty with this question!

Level of Cognitive Ability: Analysis
Phase of Nursing Process: Analysis
Client Needs: Physiological Integrity
Content Area: Mental Health

Reference
Haber, J., et al. (1997). *Comprehensive psychiatric nursing* (5th ed.). St. Louis: Mosby–Year Book. pp. 39–43, 641–643.

31. **1**

Rationale: The most effective communication technique is the one in which the nurse is giving information. With regard to memory functioning, the normal older adult who ages will find that the time required for memory scanning is longer for both recent and remote memory recall. Dementia of the Alzheimer's type involves a disorder characterized by a syndrome of symptomatology in which onset is slow and insidious with a generally progressive and deteriorating course.

Test-Taking Strategy: This question tests your knowledge of therapeutic communication techniques and the normal course of memory functioning in aging versus the clinical manifestations of Alzheimer's disease. In option 2, the nurse gives false reassurance, which devalues the client's feelings and discourages the client from expressing feelings for fear of ridicule. In option 3, the nurse is rejecting the client by refusing to consider the client's ideas or demonstrating ridicule or contempt for the client's ideas or behavior. In option 4, the nurse makes a social not a professional comment and belittles the client's concerns, which will discourage the expression of feelings.

Level of Cognitive Ability: Application
Phase of Nursing Process: Implementation
Client Needs: Psychosocial Integrity
Content Area: Mental Health

Reference
Stuart, G. W., & Laraia, M. T. (1998). *Principles and practice of psychiatric nursing* (6th ed.). St. Louis: Mosby–Year Book. pp. 17–61.

32. **2**

Rationale: There may be an increased risk for impulsive and/or aggressive behavior if a client is receiving command hallucinations to harm self or others. Clients should be asked if they have intentions to hurt themselves or others. Talking about auditory hallucinations can interfere with subvocal muscular activity associated with a hallucination.

Test-Taking Strategy: Use the process of elimination. Options 1, 3, and 4 are all interventions that a client can do to aid wellness. Option 2 is a specific agreement to seek help and evidences self-responsible commitment and control over own behavior.

Level of Cognitive Ability: Analysis
Phase of Nursing Process: Evaluation
Client Needs: Health Promotion and Maintenance
Content Area: Mental Health

Reference
Haber, J., et al. (1997). *Comprehensive psychiatric nursing* (5th ed.). St. Louis: Mosby–Year Book. pp. 580, 592–593.

33. **2**

Rationale: All clients, regardless of age, need to be encouraged to perform at the highest level of independence possible. This contributes to the client's sense of control and well-being.

Test-Taking Strategy: Options 3 and 4 are eliminated because the word "all" appears in the selections. Option 1 is eliminated because one does not know what the "self-care deficit" entails. To assume that the client requires long-term care on such little data would be erroneous!

Level of Cognitive Ability: Application
Phase of Nursing Process: Planning
Client Needs: Health Promotion and Maintenance
Content Area: Mental Health

Reference
Luckmann, J. (1997). *Saunders manual of nursing care.* Philadelphia: W. B. Saunders. p. 584.

34. 1

Rationale: Safety to the client and other clients is the priority. Option 1 is the only response that addresses the client and other clients' safety needs. Option 2 addresses the client's needs. Option 3 addresses other clients' needs. Option 4 is not client centered.

Test-Taking Strategy: Use Maslow's hierarchy of needs theory to prioritize. Note the words "belligerent," "agitated," and "aggressive." Safety is the key issue. Option 1 is the global response and addresses the safety of all.

Level of Cognitive Ability: Application
Phase of Nursing Process: Planning
Client Needs: Safe, Effective Care Environment
Content Area: Mental Health

Reference
Carson, V., & Arnold, E. (1996). *Mental health nursing: The nurse-patient journey.* Philadelphia: W. B. Saunders. p. 348.

35. 3

Rationale: Clients who are withdrawn may be immobile and mute, and require consistent, repeated approaches. Intervention includes establishment of interpersonal contact. Communication with withdrawn clients requires much patience from the nurse. The nurse facilitates communication with the client by sitting in silence, asking open-ended questions, and pausing to provide opportunities for the client to respond.

Test-Taking Strategy: Eliminate option 1 because you would not leave the client alone. Option 2 relies on other clients to care for this client and this is an inappropriate expectation. Asking direct questions to this client is not therapeutic. Option 3 is the best action because it provides for client supervision and communication as appropriate.

Level of Cognitive Ability: Application
Phase of Nursing Process: Implementation
Client Needs: Safe, Effective Care Environment
Content Area: Mental Health

Reference
Haber, J., et al. (1997). *Comprehensive psychiatric nursing* (5th ed.). St. Louis: Mosby–Year Book. pp. 582, 593.

36. 3

Rationale: Lithium is irritating to the gastric mucosa and is taken with meals. A low sodium intake causes an increase in lithium retention and can lead to toxicity. If diarrhea occurs, the physician needs to be notified. Option 3 is an appropriate instruction.

Test-Taking Strategy: Use the process of elimination to answer the question. Knowledge of the client teaching

points relating to lithium will easily direct you to option 3. Review these points if you had difficulty with this question.

Level of Cognitive Ability: Application
Phase of Nursing Process: Implementation
Client Needs: Health Promotion and Maintenance
Content Area: Mental Health

Reference
Varcarolis, E. (1998). *Foundations of psychiatric mental health nursing* (3rd ed.). Philadelphia: W. B. Saunders. p. 609.

37. 3

Rationale: It is strongly recommended that clients with anxiety disorder abstain from or limit their intake of caffeine, chocolate, and alcohol. These products have the potential of increasing anxiety. Options 1 and 4 are unreasonable and are an unhealthy approach. It may not be realistic for a family member to take time from work.

Test-Taking Strategy: Eliminate similar distractors. Options 1, 2, and 4 are concerned with monitoring or curtailing the client's physical activities, whereas option 3 addresses preparation of the environment. Option 3 also focuses on the concern or issue expressed in the question.

Level of Cognitive Ability: Application
Phase of Nursing Process: Implementation
Client Needs: Psychosocial Integrity
Content Area: Mental Health

Reference
Fontaine, K., & Fletcher, J. (1995). *Essentials of mental health nursing* (3rd ed.). Reading, MA: Addison-Wesley. pp. 177–178.

38. 1

Rationale: Altered Thought Processes secondary to paranoia is the client's problem and the plan of care must respond to this. The client is experiencing paranoia and is distrustful and suspicious of others. The treatment team needs to establish a rapport and trust with the client. Hence, laughing or whispering in front of the client is counterproductive.

Test-Taking Strategy: Use knowledge regarding this disorder to answer the question. Options 2, 3, and 4 ask the client to trust on a multitude of levels. These options are actions that are too intrusive for a client who is paranoid. Review this disorder now if you had difficulty with this question!

Level of Cognitive Ability: Application
Phase of Nursing Process: Implementation
Client Needs: Psychosocial Integrity
Content Area: Mental Health

Reference
Antai-Otong, D. (1995). *Psychiatric nursing: Biological and behavioral concepts.* Philadelphia: W. B. Saunders. p. 301.

39. 4

Rationale: A depressed person often suffers with depressed mood and is often withdrawn. Also, the person experiences difficulty concentrating, loss of interest or pleasure, low energy, fatigue, and feelings of worthlessness and poor self-esteem. The plan of care needs to provide a stimulating yet structured environment.

Test-Taking Strategy: The depressed client requires a structured and stimulating program. Options 1 and 2 are too restrictive and offer little or no structure and stimulation. Option 3 is eliminated because the word "all" is in the option. Option 4 is the only reasonable option that will provide a safe and effective environment!

Level of Cognitive Ability: Application
Phase of Nursing Process: Planning
Client Needs: Psychosocial Integrity
Content Area: Mental Health

Reference
Varcarolis, E. (1998). *Foundations of psychiatric mental health nursing* (3rd ed.). Philadelphia: W. B. Saunders. p. 566.

40. 2

Rationale: Recognizing situations that produce anxiety allows the client to prepare to cope with anxiety or avoid a specific stimulus. Counselors will not be available for all anxiety-producing situations. This option does not encourage the development of internal strengths. Ignoring feelings will not resolve anxiety. It is impossible to eliminate all anxiety from life.

Test-Taking Strategy: Eliminate option 4 first because of the word "all." Eliminate option 3 next because feelings should not be ignored. From the remaining two options, select option 2 over option 1 because this option is more client centered and provides the preparation for the client to deal with anxiety should it occur.

Level of Cognitive Ability: Application
Phase of Nursing Process: Planning
Client Needs: Health Promotion and Maintenance
Content Area: Mental Health

Reference
Fortinash, K., & Holoday-Worret, P. (1996). *Psychiatric-mental health nursing.* St. Louis: Mosby–Year Book. p. 238.

41. 2

Rationale: Agoraphobia is a fear of open spaces and the fear of being trapped in a situation from which there may not be an escape. Agoraphobia includes the possibility of experiencing a sense of helplessness or embarrassment if an attack occurs. Avoidance of such situations usually results in reduction of social and professional interactions. Social phobia focuses more on specific situations such as the fear of speaking, performing, or eating in public. Claustrophobia is a fear of closed-in places. Clients with hypochondriacal symptoms focus their anxiety on physical complaints and are preoccupied with their health.

Test-Taking Strategy: Knowledge regarding the specific types of phobias and associated client behaviors is required to answer this question. If you had difficulty with this question, take time now to review phobia types and associated client behaviors!

Level of Cognitive Ability: Analysis
Phase of Nursing Process: Analysis
Client Needs: Psychosocial Integrity
Content Area: Mental Health

Reference
O'Toole, M. (1997). *Miller-Keane encyclopedia & dictionary of medicine, nursing, & allied health* (6th ed.). Philadelphia: W. B. Saunders. p. 1242.

42. 3

Rationale: Aspiration is safeguarded against by keeping the client NPO for 6 to 8 hours before the treatment, removing dentures, and administering glycopyrrolate or atropine as prescribed. Although options 1 and 2 could also be contributory diagnoses, they are not the most important ones. There is no reason to imply that option 4 is even a consideration.

Test-Taking Strategy: Utilize Maslow's hierarchy of needs to correctly answer this question. Physiological needs must come first; select an answer that addresses these needs. Additionally, utilize the ABCs, Airway, Breathing, and Circulation. Airway is the concern with the risk of aspiration. If you had difficulty with this question, take time now to review procedures related to electroconvulsive therapy (ECT)!

Level of Cognitive Ability: Analysis
Phase of Nursing Process: Analysis
Client Needs: Physiological Integrity
Content Area: Mental Health

Reference
Varcarolis, E. (1998). *Foundations of psychiatric mental health nursing* (3rd ed.). Philadelphia: W. B. Saunders. p. 579.

43. 1

Rationale: Option 1 is clearly the correct answer. Knowledge of Maslow's hierarchy of needs dictates that the need for safety is foremost if a physiological need does not exist. Options 2 and 3 could be differential nursing diagnoses, but not the most appropriate ones. Option 4 may or may not be a consideration, and is not the best choice.

Test-Taking Strategy: This question uses the strategy of key words or phrases. In this case, "most appropriate" is the phrase to pay particular attention to. Also, use Maslow's hierarchy of needs. If a physiological need does not exist, safety is the priority!

Level of Cognitive Ability: Analysis
Phase of Nursing Process: Analysis
Client Needs: Physiological Integrity
Content Area: Mental Health

Reference
Iyer, P., Taptich, B., & Bernocchi-Losey, D. (1995). *Nursing process and nursing diagnosis.* Philadelphia: W. B. Saunders. p. 369.

44. 3

Rationale: All of the options are possible issues to address; however, the weight loss is the first item that needs assessment because an obvious ill fit of clothing could signify a substantial problem with physiological integrity. The client has told the nurse that the crying spells have been a problem, and medication has not been mentioned in the information given. Sleep is affected by depression and should be addressed; however, weight loss is the most important option with the data given.

Test-Taking Strategy: Use the process of elimination and Maslow's hierarchy of needs to answer the question. Since all of the information is important to assess at some point, the nurse must decide which has priority with the given situation. Significant weight loss is the most serious physiological concern!

Level of Cognitive Ability: Analysis
Phase of Nursing Process: Analysis
Client Needs: Physiological Integrity
Content Area: Mental Health

Reference

Johnson, B. S. (1997). *Psychiatric mental health nursing: Adaptation and growth* (4th ed.). Philadelphia: Lippincott-Raven. pp. 545–546.

45. **1**

Rationale: The behaviors mentioned may be manifested by the client who is contemplating suicide. Many of these are symptoms of the depressed client; however, with this client these behaviors have increased. Hospitalization may actually lessen these symptoms in the depressed client because a feeling of hope or relief may occur once treatment begins. Facing issues may be traumatic, but this is not the best answer for the question. Time off the unit for this client could put the client at risk for injury. Only when anxiety and irritability are controlled should the client safely leave the unit.

Test-Taking Strategy: Identify the client behaviors addressed in the question. Use the process of elimination in answering the question. Additionally, use Maslow's hierarchy of needs to assist in answering the question. Of the options presented, option 1 is the priority. If you had difficulty with this question, take time now to review the characteristics and client behaviors related to suicide!

Level of Cognitive Ability: Analysis
Phase of Nursing Process: Analysis
Client Needs: Physiological Integrity
Content Area: Mental Health

Reference

Carson, V., & Arnold, E. (1996). *Mental health nursing: The nurse-patient journey.* Philadelphia: W. B. Saunders. pp. 932–936.

46. **4**

Rationale: Major depression occurs twice as frequently in females as in males. Reacting to loss by experiencing altered sleep for 1 week is a normal grief response, whereas early morning awakening that extends over 2 weeks along with other symptomatology constitutes major depression. Although depression is often associated with substance abuse, it would, in and of itself, not constitute a major depression. Option 4 is the correct answer because it describes anhedonia (loss of pleasure in activities previously or usually enjoyed), which has extended over 3 weeks, a cardinal criterion for major depression according to DSM–IV.

Test-Taking Strategy: Knowledge of the epidemiology of and criteria for major depression will assist you to analyze the options accurately. Use the process of elimination in selecting the correct option. If you are unfamiliar with the content, you might be able to determine the correct option by considering the time frame noted in the option, which is one of the factors to be considered in the criteria for major depression according to DSM–IV. Take time now to review the assessment data related to depression if you had difficulty with this question!

Level of Cognitive Ability: Analysis
Phase of Nursing Process: Analysis
Client Needs: Psychosocial Integrity
Content Area: Mental Health

Reference

Varcarolis, E. (1998). *Foundations of psychiatric mental health nursing* (3rd ed.). Philadelphia: W. B. Saunders. p. 560.

47. **2**

Rationale: A conversion disorder is the alteration or loss of a physical function that cannot be explained by any known pathophysiological mechanism. It is thought to be an expression of a psychological need or conflict. In this scenario, the client witnessed an accident that was so psychologically painful, the client became blind. A dissociative disorder is a disturbance or alteration in the normally integrative functions of identity, memory, or consciousness. Psychosis is a state in which a person's mental capacity to recognize reality, communicate, and relate to others is impaired, thus interfering with the person's capacity to deal with life demands. Repression is a coping mechanism in which unacceptable feelings are kept out of awareness.

Test-Taking Strategy: Knowledge regarding defense mechanisms is required to answer the question. The key to the answer lies in the fact that the client evidences no organic reason to account for the blindness, hence a conversion disorder. If you had difficulty with this question, take time now to review defense mechanisms!

Level of Cognitive Ability: Analysis
Phase of Nursing Process: Analysis
Client Needs: Psychosocial Integrity
Content Area: Mental Health

Reference

Carson, V., & Arnold, E. (1996). *Mental health nursing: The nurse-patient journey.* Philadelphia: W. B. Saunders. pp. 697, 963–964.

48. **1**

Rationale: The client is at risk for injury to self and others and therefore should be escorted out of the dayroom. Hyperactive and agitated behavior usually responds to haloperidol (Haldol). Antipsychotic medications are useful to manage the manic client; lithium takes 1 to 3 weeks to become effective. Option 2 may increase the agitation that already exists in this client. Orientation will not halt the behavior. Telling the client that the behavior is not appropriate has already been attempted by the orderly.

Test-Taking Strategy: Use Maslow's hierarchy of needs and the process of elimination to answer the question. Look for the response that promotes safety of the client as well as other clients and staff. Knowledge of psychopharmacology is also helpful to answer this question correctly. If you had difficulty with this question, take time now to review the appropriate interventions in dealing with a manic client.

Level of Cognitive Ability: Analysis
Phase of Nursing Process: Analysis
Client Needs: Psychosocial Integrity
Content Area: Mental Health

Reference

Wilson, H. S., & Kneisl, C. R. (1996). *Psychiatric nursing* (5th ed.). Reading, MA: Addison-Wesley. pp. 347, 349.

49. **1**

Rationale: Several conditions present risks in the client scheduled for ECT. These include clients with recent myocardial infarction, cerebral vascular accident, and clients with cerebral vascular malformation or intracranial mass lesions.

Test-Taking Strategy: Knowledge regarding the risks associated with ECT is required to answer this question. Note the word "recent" in option 1. This key word should attract your attention as being the answer to this question. Review the risk factors associated with ECT now if you had difficulty with this question!

Level of Cognitive Ability: Analysis
Phase of Nursing Process: Analysis
Client Needs: Physiological Integrity
Content Area: Mental Health

Reference
Varcarolis, E. (1998). *Foundations of psychiatric mental health nursing* (3rd ed.). Philadelphia: W. B. Saunders. p. 578.

50. **4**

Rationale: Enemas are not a component of the pretreatment care for a client scheduled for ECT. Options 1, 2, and 3 are a part of the pretreatment plan. Additionally, an informed consent is required and the nurse should teach the client and family what to expect with ECT and allow the client to discuss feelings regarding the procedure.

Test-Taking Strategy: Knowledge regarding the pretreatment care for the client scheduled for ECT is required to answer this question. If you had difficulty with this question, take time now to review this procedure!

Level of Cognitive Ability: Application
Phase of Nursing Process: Planning
Client Needs: Physiological Integrity
Content Area: Mental Health

Reference
Varcarolis, E. (1998). *Foundations of psychiatric mental health nursing* (3rd ed.). Philadelphia: W. B. Saunders. p. 579.

BIBLIOGRAPHY

Antai-Otong, D. (1995). *Psychiatric nursing: Biological and behavioral concepts.* Philadelphia: W. B. Saunders.

Carson, V., & Arnold, E. (1996). *Mental health nursing: The nurse-patient journey.* Philadelphia: W. B. Saunders.

Fontaine, K., & Fletcher, J. (1995). *Essentials of mental health nursing* (3rd ed.). Reading, MA: Addison-Wesley.

Fortinash, K., & Holoday-Worret, P. (1996). *Psychiatric-mental health nursing.* St. Louis: Mosby–Year Book.

Glod, C. A. (1998). *Contemporary psychiatric-mental health nursing.* Philadelphia: F. A. Davis.

Haber, J, et al. (1997). *Comprehensive psychiatric nursing* (5th ed.). St. Louis: Mosby–Year Book.

Hodgson, B., & Kizior, R. (1999). *Saunders nursing drug handbook 1999.* Philadelphia: W. B. Saunders.

Iyer, P., Taptich, B., & Bernocchi-Losey, D. (1995). *Nursing process and nursing diagnosis.* Philadelphia: W. B. Saunders.

Johnson, B. S. (1997). *Psychiatric mental health nursing: Adaptation and growth* (4th ed.). Philadelphia: Lippincott-Raven.

Luckmann, J. (1997). *Saunders manual of nursing care.* Philadelphia: W. B. Saunders.

O'Toole, M. (1997). *Miller-Keane encyclopedia & dictionary of medicine, nursing, & allied health* (6th ed.). Philadelphia: W. B. Saunders.

Stuart, G. W., & Laraia, M. T. (1998). *Principles and practice of psychiatric nursing* (6th ed.). St. Louis: Mosby–Year Book.

Varcarolis, E. (1998). *Foundations of psychiatric mental health nursing* (3rd ed.). Philadelphia: W. B. Saunders.

Wilson, H. S., & Kneisl, C. R. (1996). *Psychiatric nursing* (5th ed.). Reading, MA: Addison-Wesley.

CHAPTER 72

Addictions

I. Eating Disorders

A. Description: Characterized by uncertain self-identification and grossly disturbed eating habits

B. Compulsive overeating
   1. Binge-like overeating without purging
   2. Food consumption is out of the individual's control and occurs in a stereotyped fashion
   3. Client may be repulsed by eating, and the eating relieves tension but does not produce pleasure
   4. Is aware that eating patterns are abnormal and feels depressed after eating
   5. Eats secretly during a binge and consumes high-calorie and easily digestible food
   6. Repeatedly tries to diet but without success
   7. Lacks interest in exercise programs and feels helpless and hopeless about weight
   8. When experiencing guilt, anger, depression, boredom, loneliness, inadequacy, or ambivalence, responds by eating

C. Anorexia nervosa
   1. Description
      a. The onset is often associated with a stressful life event
      b. The client intensely fears obesity
      c. Body image is distorted, and the client has a disturbed self-concept
      d. Preoccupied with foods that prevent weight gain and has a phobia against foods that produce weight gain
      e. The eating disorder can be life-threatening
      f. Death can occur from starvation, **suicide,** or electrolyte imbalance
   2. Assessment
      a. Refusal to eat and appetite loss
      b. Appetite denial
      c. Feelings of lack of control
      d. Self-induced vomiting and self-administered enemas
      e. Exercises compulsively
      f. Overachiever and perfectionist
      g. Decreased temperature, pulse, and blood pressure
      h. Weight loss
      i. Constipation
      j. Scaly, dry skin
      k. Gastrointestinal (GI) disturbances
      l. Sleep disturbances
      m. Electrolyte imbalances
      n. Hormone deficiencies
      o. Amenorrhea for at least three consecutive menstrual periods
      p. Teeth and gum deterioration
      q. Cyanosis and numbness of extremities
      r. Esophageal varices from vomiting
      s. Bone degeneration

D. Bulimia nervosa
   1. Description
      a. The client indulges in eating binges followed by purging behaviors
      b. Most clients remain within a normal weight range but feel that their lives are dominated by the eating-related conflict
   2. Assessment
      a. Consumes high-calorie and easily digested food in secret
      b. Binge, purge syndrome
      c. Attempts to lose weight through diets, vomiting, enemas, cathartics, and amphetamines or diuretics
      d. Preoccupied with body shape and weight
      e. Guilt about secretive eating
      f. Mood swings
      g. Low self-esteem
      h. Needs to control yet experiences feelings of powerlessness or loss of control
      i. Poor interpersonal relationships
      j. Overuse of laxatives and diuretics
      k. Loss of tooth enamel and dental decay
      l. Stomach ulcers and electrolyte imbalances
      m. Esophageal varies from vomiting
      n. Rectal bleeding
      o. Cardiac disease and hypertension
      p. Self-mutilating behavior
      q. Thoughts of and attempts at **suicide**

E. Implementation
   1. Assess the client's nutritional status

2. Establish a contract with the client concerning diet plan for the day
3. Assist the client in identifying precipitators of the eating disorder
4. Encourage the client to state feelings about the eating behavior
5. Be accepting and nonjudgmental, expressing neither approval nor disapproval of the behavior
6. Encourage behavior modification techniques
7. Provide praise and positive reinforcement for accomplishments
8. Supervise client during mealtimes and for a specified period after meals
9. Set a time limit for each meal
10. Provide a pleasant, relaxed environment for eating
11. Monitor for signs of physical complications related to the eating disorder
12. Record intake and output (I&O)
13. Weigh the client daily at the same time, using the same scale, after the client voids
14. When weighing the client, ensure that the client is wearing the same clothing as when the previous weight was taken
15. Monitor and restore fluid and electrolyte balance
16. Monitor elimination patterns
17. Assess and limit client's activity level
18. Encourage client to participate in diversional activities
19. Assess client's **suicide** potential
20. Administer antidepressant medication as prescribed
21. Encourage psychotherapy as prescribed
22. Refer client to support groups

II. Substance Abuse Disorders

A. Description: Behavioral changes associated with regular substance **abuse** that affects the central nervous system (CNS)
B. Substance dependence (Box 72–1)
   1. Pattern of repeated use of a substance, which usually results in tolerance, withdrawal, and compulsive drug-taking behavior
   2. Client takes substances in larger amounts

BOX 72–1. CAGE Screening Test for Substance Abuse

C—Have you ever felt the need to cut down on your drinking/drug use?
A—Have you ever been annoyed at criticism of your drinking/drug use?
G—Have you ever felt guilty about something you have done when you have been drinking or taking drugs?
E—Have you ever had an eye opener, taking drugs first thing in the morning to get going or to avoid withdrawal symptoms?

---

and over longer periods of time than was intended
3. Client has the desire to cut down but has unsuccessful efforts to decrease or discontinue use
4. Daily activities revolve around the use of a substance
C. Substance tolerance: The need for increased amounts of the substance to achieve the desired effect
D. Substance **abuse**
   1. Client recurrently uses substances
   2. Client experiences recurrent, significant harmful consequences related to the use of substances
   3. Client has legal problems related to substance **abuse**
E. Substance withdrawal
   1. Physiological and/or substance-specific cognitive symptoms
   2. Occurs when blood levels decrease in an individual with prolonged heavy use of a substance
F. Precipitating factors of substance **abuse**
   1. Rebellion and peer group pressure in adolescence
   2. Pleasure-seeking experience as the substance decreases physical and emotional pain
   3. Group influence and peer pressure
   4. Depression
   5. Loss and grieving
G. Dysfunctional behaviors of clients with substance **abuse**
   1. Insensitive to self and others
   2. Manipulative
   3. Impulsiveness
   4. Anger, including physical and verbal **abuse**
   5. Avoidance of relationships, with physical and emotional distancing
   6. Sense of self-importance and requiring special treatment
   7. Denial, blaming everything but the substance
   8. Codependence, modifying self behaviors and response to others
   9. Low self-esteem
   10. Depression

III. Alcohol Abuse

A. Description
   1. Alcohol is a CNS depressant affecting all body tissues
   2. Physical dependence is a biological need for alcohol to avoid physical withdrawal symptoms
   3. Psychological dependence is a craving for the subjective effect of alcohol
B. Risk factors
   1. Biological predisposition
   2. Depressed and highly anxious characteristics
   3. Low self-esteem
   4. Poor self-control

5. History of rebelliousness, poor school performance, delinquency
6. Poor parental relationships

C. Assessment
1. Slurred speech
2. Uncoordinated movements
3. Unsteady gait
4. Restlessness
5. Belligerence
6. Confusion
7. Sneaking drinks, drinking in the morning, and experiencing blackouts
8. Binge drinking
9. Arguments about drinking
10. Missing work
11. Increased tolerance to alcohol
12. Intoxication, with blood alcohol levels greater than or equal to 0.1%

D. Physical symptoms
1. Hepatitis
2. Cirrhosis of the liver
3. Esophagitis and gastritis
4. Pancreatitis
5. Anemias
6. Immune system dysfunctions
7. Brain damage
8. Peripheral neuropathy
9. Cardiac disorders
10. Telangiectasia
11. Acne rosacea

E. Psychological symptoms
1. Depression
2. Hostility
3. Suspiciousness
4. Rationalization
5. Irritability
6. Isolation
7. Decrease in inhibitions
8. Decrease in self-esteem
9. Denial that a problem exists

IV. Alcohol Withdrawal

A. Description
1. Occurs when an addicted person stops ingesting alcohol
2. Can occur 6 to 8 hours after drinking has ended or decreased, and symptoms can last 5 days or longer
3. Alcohol withdrawal is highly individual, and some clients experience mild withdrawal symptoms requiring minimal medical supervision; others experience severe symptoms that can be life-threatening

B. Stages of withdrawal
1. Stage 1
   a. May begin 6 to 8 hours after last ingestion or significant decrease in usual consumption of alcohol
   b. Anxiety
   c. Anorexia
   d. Insomnia
   e. Tremor
   f. Hyperalertness
   g. Internal shaking
   h. Nausea and vomiting
   i. Headache
   j. Increased pulse and blood pressure
   k. Depression
2. Stage 2
   a. May begin 8 to 12 hours after the last ingestion or a significant decrease in usual consumption of alcohol
   b. Profound confusion
   c. Gross tremor
   d. Nervousness
   e. Disorientation
   f. Illusions
   g. Nightmares
   h. Auditory and visual hallucinations
3. Stage 3
   a. May begin 12 to 48 hours after the last ingestion or significant decrease in usual consumption of alcohol
   b. Severe hallucinations
   c. Grand mal seizures
4. Stage 4
   a. May begin 3 to 5 days after the last ingestion or significant decrease in usual alcohol consumption
   b. Confusion, disorientation, clouding of consciousness, and delirium
   c. Hypertension, diaphoresis, tachycardia
   d. Visual and tactile hallucinations
   e. Fluctuating levels of consciousness
   f. Fever (103° to 104°F)
   g. Tremors
   h. Uncontrolled tachycardia
   i. Severe psychomotor activity
   j. Agitation
   k. Sleeplessness
   l. Hallucinations
   m. A medical emergency

C. Implementation
1. Initiate seizure precautions
2. Administer chlordiazepoxide (Librium) as prescribed for withdrawal and anticonvulsive effects
3. Administer diazepam (Valium) or pentobarbital (phenobarbital) as prescribed to produce sedation and control withdrawal
4. Administer phenytoin (Dilantin) as prescribed to prevent seizures
5. Administer vitamin B_1 (thiamine) as prescribed for malnutrition and to prevent Wernicke's encephalopathy
6. Administer magnesium sulfate as prescribed to increase the effectiveness of vitamin B_1 and help reduce postwithdrawal seizures
7. Hydrate the client
8. Monitor vital signs frequently
9. Monitor I&O
10. Orient client frequently
11. Maintain minimal stimuli

BOX 72–2. Hallucinogens	
Lysergic acid diethylamide (LSD)	Mescaline
Phencyclidine (PCP)	Peyote

BOX 72–3. Opiates	
Opium	Morphine
Heroin	Codeine
Meperidine hydrochloride (Demerol)	Methadone

12. Approach client in an accepting and nonjudgmental manner
13. Assist client to use assertive techniques rather than manipulation to meet needs
14. Set limits on manipulative behavior
15. Direct client to focus on the substance **abuse** problem
16. Limit the client's blame-placing or rationalizing to explain the substance **abuse** problem
17. Encourage client to participate in group therapy and support groups
18. Encourage client to attend weekly Alcoholics Anonymous (AA) meetings

D. Complications associated with chronic alcohol use
  1. Vitamin deficiencies
  2. Vitamin B deficiency causing peripheral neuropathies
  3. Thiamine deficiency causing Korsakoff's syndrome
  4. Alcohol-induced persistent amnesic disorder causing severe memory problems
  5. Wernicke's encephalopathy, causing confusion, ataxia, and abnormal eye movements

E. Disulfiram (Antabuse) therapy
  1. Description
    a. An alcohol deterrent used for alcoholic dependence
    b. The medication sensitizes the client to alcohol, so a disulfiram-alcohol reaction occurs if alcohol is ingested
    c. The client must abstain from alcohol for at least 12 hours before the initial dose is administered
    d. The client must avoid drinking for 14 days after Antabuse therapy has been discontinued, otherwise client is at risk for disulfiram-alcohol reaction
  2. Negative physiological responses
    a. Throbbing headache
    b. Flushing
    c. Nausea
    d. Copious vomiting
    e. Diaphoresis
    f. Dizziness
    g. Blurred vision and confusion
    h. Hypotension
    i. Dyspnea
    j. Palpitations
    k. Tachycardia
    l. Chest pain

3. Client education
    a. Educate as to the effects of the medication
    b. Instruct client that the effects of medication may occur for several days after discontinuance
    c. Ensure that client agrees to abstain from alcohol and any alcohol-containing substances
    d. Instruct client to avoid substances such as cough medicines, rubbing compounds, vinegar, mouthwashes, and aftershave lotions

V. Hallucinogens (Box 72–2)

A. Cause psychosis, with distorted perception, heightened sense of awareness, grandiosity, hallucinations, mystical experiences, and distortions of time and space
B. May harm self when under influence
C. No withdrawal syndrome when discontinued, but flashbacks may occur for several months after use stops
D. Bad trips may result in panic and unpredictable psychotic behaviors

VI. Marijuana

A. Causes altered state of awareness, relaxation, and mild euphoria
B. Decreases inhibitions
C. Decreased motivation from prolonged use
D. Can cause possible psychosis
E. Physiological effects include slowed reflexes
F. Causes drying of mucous membranes and reddening of eyes

VII. Opiates (Box 72–3)

A. Description
  1. Cause mental and physical deterioration
  2. High risk for infection with HIV virus or hepatitis virus if taken intravenously

BOX 72–4. Sedatives and Depressants	
Barbital	Chloral hydrate
Amytal	Glutethimide (Doriden)
Phenobarbital	Methaqualone
Nembutal	Benzodiazepines
Seconal	

---

3. Cause decreased response to pain, respiratory depression, constriction of pupils, euphoria, apathy, impaired judgment

B. Opiate withdrawal
   1. Methadone blocks the action of opiates and may be used to assist with withdrawal
   2. Signs of withdrawal include anxiety; yawning; diaphoresis; cramping; rhinorrhea; achiness and muscle twitching; anorexia; insomnia; increased temperature, respiration, and blood pressure; nausea and vomiting; diarrhea; and restlessness
   3. Overdose of opiates can lead to coma, respiratory depression, and death

VIII. Sedatives and Depressants (Box 72–4)

A. Description
   1. Act as a depressant, sedative, and hypnotic
   2. Cause physical and psychological dependence
   3. Cause euphoria
   4. Can cause depression and hostility
   5. Impaired judgment and lack of coordination can occur
   6. Slurring of speech and decreased inhibitions can occur
   7. Tolerance can develop

B. Withdrawal: causes increased temperature, tachycardia, postural hypotension, insomnia, tremors, agitation, apprehension, weakness, grand mal seizures, and psychosis

IX. Stimulants (Box 72–5)

A. Description
   1. Stimulants lead to alertness and extra energy and are used in obesity and narcolepsy; also used for hyperactive children
   2. Effects include euphoria, hyperactivity, insomnia, anorexia and weight loss, tachycardia and hypertension, psychotic behavior
   3. Psychological dependence and tolerance can occur
   4. Sudden death has been associated with cocaine **abuse**

B. Withdrawal
   1. Crash
   2. Depression
   3. Lack of energy

X. Antianxiety Medications (Box 72–6)

A. Description
   1. Cause physical and psychological addictiveness
   2. Cause relaxation, drowsiness, ataxia, and hypotension
   3. Withdrawal can produce seizures

B. Withdrawal
   1. Initiate seizure precautions
   2. Hydrate the client
   3. Monitor vital signs every hour
   4. Monitor I&O
   5. Orient client frequently
   6. Maintain minimal stimuli
   7. Approach client in an accepting and nonjudgmental manner
   8. Direct client's focus to the substance **abuse** problem
   9. Identify with client situations that precipitate angry feelings
   10. Limit the client's blame-placing or rationalizing to explain the substance **abuse** problem
   11. Assist client to use assertive techniques rather than manipulation to meet needs
   12. Set limits on manipulative behavior and verbal and physical **abuse**

13. Hold client firmly to reasonable limits, consistently reinforcing rules, with reasonable consequences for breaking rules
14. Hold client accountable for all behaviors
15. Assist client to explore strengths and weaknesses
16. Encourage time out if client is losing control
17. Encourage client to participate in unit activities
18. Encourage client to participate in group therapy and support groups
19. See Box 72–7 for a list of therapies
20. Box 72–8 delineates nursing care for clients

PRACTICE QUESTIONS

1. The nurse is caring for a client who was recently admitted for anorexia nervosa. When the nurse enters the room, the client is engaged in rigorous push-ups. Which of the following nursing actions would be most appropriate?
   1 Allow the client to complete the exercise program
   2 Tell the client that she is not allowed to exercise rigorously
   3 Interrupt the client and offer to take her for a walk
   4 Interrupt the client and weigh immediately

2. The nurse is caring for a client with anorexia nervosa. The nurse is monitoring the behavior of the client and understands that the client with anorexia nervosa manages anxiety by
   1 Always reinforcing self-approval
   2 Having the need always to make the right decision
   3 Engaging in immoral acts
   4 Observing rigid rules and regulations

3. The nurse is developing a plan of care for the hospitalized client with bulimia nervosa. Which of the following would not be a component of the plan of care?
   1 Monitoring intake and output (I&O)
   2 Monitoring electrolyte levels
   3 Observing for excessive exercise
   4 Assessing for the presence of laxatives and diuretics in the client's belongings

4. Alcohol withdrawal delirium is a medical emergency. Which of the following symptoms would alert the nurse to the potential for delirium tremens (DTs)?
   1 Fever, hypertension, changes in level of consciousness, hallucinations
   2 Hypertension, stupor, agitation, headache, auditory hallucinations
   3 Vomiting, ataxia, muscular rigidity, tactile hallucinations
   4 Coarse hand tremor, agitation, hallucinations, hypertension

5. The spouse of a client admitted for alcohol withdrawal says to the nurse, "I should get out of this bad situation." The best response by the nurse would be:
   1 "I agree with you. You should get out of this situation."
   2 "What do you find difficult about this situation?"
   3 "Why don't you tell your (spouse) about this."
   4 "This is not the best time to make that decision."

6. The nurse is assessing a client who has a history of opioid abuse. The nurse is monitoring the client for signs of withdrawal. Which of the following observations, if made by the nurse, is indicative of the clinical manifestations associated with withdrawal from opioids?
   1 Increased blood pressure (BP) and pulse, with low-grade fever, yawning, restlessness, anxiety, craving, diarrhea, and mydriasis
   2 Tachycardia, mild hypertension and fever, sweating, nausea, vomiting, and marked tremor
   3 Increased appetite, irritability, anxiety, restlessness, and altered concentration
   4 Depressed feelings, high drug craving, fatigue with a desire to sleep or altered sleep (insomnia or hypersomnia), agitation, and paranoia

7. The client who has experienced an uncomplicated postoperative course for 2 days and was to be discharged becomes diaphoretic, agitated, and confused as to time and place, and tries to leave the hospital in a hospital gown. The client's blood pressure is elevated and the pulse is 122. The client is known as a "heavy social drinker." If the client is treated for severe alcohol withdrawal delirium, what instrument will the nurse employ for the nursing care during this time?
   1 CAGE
   2 Short Michigan Alcoholism Screening Test (SMAST)
   3 Clinical Institute Withdrawal Assessment for Alcohol (CIWA)
   4 Blood alcohol level (BAL)

8. The community health nurse visits a client at home who is dependent on drugs. Which of the following assessment questions would assist the nurse to provide appropriate nursing care?
   1 "Why did you get started on these drugs?"
   2 "How long did you think you could take these drugs without someone finding out?"
   3 "How much do you use and what effect does it have on you?"
   4 The nurse does not ask any questions in fear that the client is in denial and will throw the nurse out of the home

9. Which of the following assessment data indicates a potential complication associated with a client taking benzodiazepines?
   1 "My doctor says I'm dependent on Valium but he gave it to me. Now he says it's not helpful and I don't need it anymore."
   2 "I'm on Prozac and doing well but I've had to increase my dose to 2 capsules a day. Do you think I'm addicted?"
   3 "My doctor says I'm addicted to my codeine. He gave it to me when I first fractured my ribs. Now he says I don't need it anymore, but I'm having pain without it."
   4 "I'm on Haldol and doing well, but I've had to increase my dose. Do you think I'm addicted?"

10. A client who has been drinking alcohol on a regular basis admits to having "a problem." The client is asking for assistance with the problem. The nurse would support the client to attend which of the following community groups?
   1 Al-Anon
   2 Alcoholics Anonymous
   3 Families Anonymous
   4 Fresh Start

11. A nurse is conducting group therapy for sexual addicts. At these meetings, sexual behaviors are discussed that would offend many people in the general public. The nurse knows that a guiding principle for effectively conducting this group is
   1 Accepting that sexual aberrations are always the result of inappropriate childhood experiences
   2 Knowledge that being nonjudgmental does not mean that one accepts the values and beliefs of others
   3 Conviction that sexual perverts must be identified publicly and forced to take hormone suppression drugs
   4 Knowledge that sexual behavior disorders always result from inadequate psychosocial response during sexual arousal

12. The client with a diagnosis of anorexia nervosa, who is in a state of starvation, is in a two-bed room. A newly admitted client will be assigned to this client's room. Which of the following would not be an appropriate choice for this client's roommate?
   1 A client with pneumonia
   2 A client with a fractured leg
   3 A client who could benefit from the client's assistance at mealtime
   4 A client who is not controlling

13. A female client with anorexia nervosa is a member of a predischarge group/support group. The client verbalizes that she would like to buy some new clothes, but her finances are limited. Group members brought some used clothes to the client to replace the client's old clothes. The client believed that these clothes were much too tight and reduced her calorie intake to 800 calories daily. The nurse analyzes this behavior as
   1 Normal behavior
   2 Indicative of the client's ambivalence about hospital discharge
   3 Evidence of the client's altered/distorted body image
   4 Regression as the client is moving toward the community

14. The nurse analyzes that the wife of an alcoholic client is benefiting from attending an Al-Anon group when the nurse hears the wife say
   1 "My attendance at the meetings has helped me see that I provoke my husband's violence."
   2 "I no longer feel that I deserve the beatings my husband inflicts on me."
   3 "I can tolerate my husband's destructive behaviors now that I know they are common with alcoholics."
   4 "I enjoy attending the meetings because they get me out of the house and away from my husband."

15. The client has been hospitalized and has participated in substance abuse therapy group sessions. Upon discharge, the client has consented to participate in Alcoholics Anonymous community groups. The nurse is monitoring the client's response to the substance abuse sessions. Which of the following statements by the client best indicates to the nurse that the client has assimilated session topics well, has coping response styles, and has processed information effectively for self-use?
   1 "I know I'm ready to be discharged; I feel like I can say no and leave a group of friends if they are drinking—no problem!"
   2 "This group has really helped a lot. I know it will be different when I go home. But I'm sure that my family and friends will all help me like the people in this group have . . . They'll all help me . . . I know they will . . . They won't let me go back to the old ways."
   3 "I'm looking forward to leaving here; I know that I will miss all of you. So, I'm happy and I'm sad, I'm excited and I'm scared. I know that I have to work hard to be strong and that everyone isn't going to be as helpful as you people."
   4 "I'll keep all my appointments, go to all my AA groups. I'll do everything I'm supposed to . . . Nothing will go wrong that way."

16. Which of the following assessment data indicates early signs of alcohol withdrawal?
   1 Anxiety, tremor, insomnia, tachycardia
   2 Disorientation, diaphoresis, insomnia
   3 Delusions, fever, vomiting, agitation
   4 Clouding of consciousness, tachycardia

17. A hospitalized client with a history of alcohol abuse tells the nurse, "I am leaving now. I have to go. I don't want any more treatment. I have things that I have to do right away." The client has not been discharged. In fact, the client is scheduled for an important diagnostic test to be performed in 1 hour. After the nurse discusses the client's concerns with the client, the client dresses and begins to walk out of the hospital room. The most appropriate nursing action is
   1 Restrain the client until the physician can be reached
   2 Call security to block all exit areas
   3 Tell the client that he or she cannot return to this hospital again if he or she leaves now
   4 Call the nursing supervisor

18. The psychiatric nurse is performing an admission assessment on a client with a diagnosis of bulimia nervosa. Which of the following is not a characteristic finding in this disorder?
   1 Enlarged parotid glands
   2 Dental erosion
   3 Electrolyte imbalances
   4 Body weight well below ideal range

ANSWERS

1. **3**

Rationale: Clients with anorexia nervosa are frequently preoccupied with rigorous exercise and push themselves beyond normal limits to work off caloric intake. The nurse must provide for appropriate exercise as well as place limits on rigorous activities.

Test-Taking Strategy: Focus on the key words "most appropriate" in the stem of the question. Knowledge of the seriousness of anorexia nervosa is essential in answering this question. Focus on the need for the nurse to set firm limits with clients who have this disorder. If you had difficulty with this question, take time now to review interventions for the client with anorexia nervosa!

Level of Cognitive Ability: Application
Phase of Nursing Process: Implementation
Client Needs: Physiological Integrity
Content Area: Mental Health

Reference
Varcarolis, E. (1998). *Foundations of psychiatric mental health nursing* (3rd ed.). Philadelphia: W. B. Saunders. p. 806.

2. **4**

Rationale: Clients with anorexia nervosa have the desire to please others. Their need to be correct or perfect interferes with rational decision-making processes. These clients are moralistic. Rules and rituals help the clients manage their anxiety.

Test-Taking Strategy: Avoid choices with absolutes, such as the word "always." They are usually incorrect. This would eliminate options 1 and 2. Option 3 is not characteristic of the information presented in the question, leaving only option 4 as the most feasible response.

Level of Cognitive Ability: Analysis
Phase of Nursing Process: Analysis
Client Needs: Psychosocial Integrity
Content Area: Mental Health

Reference
Thompson, J., McFarland, G., Hirsch, J., & Tucker, S. (1997)). *Mosby's clinical nursing* (4th ed.). St. Louis: Mosby–Year Book. p. 1348.

3. **3**

Rationale: Excessive exercise is a characteristic of anorexia nervosa, not a characteristic of clients with bulimia. Frequent vomiting, in addition to laxative and diuretic abuse, may lead to dehydration and electrolyte imbalance. Assessing for dehydration and electrolyte imbalance is an important nursing action, as these conditions can further complicate recovery.

Test-Taking Strategy: Note the key word "not" in the stem of the question. Options 1, 2, and 4 directly or indirectly imply concern about fluid and electrolyte balance. Option 3 is different from the others, and the correct response. Review the characteristics associated with bulimia nervosa now if you had difficulty with this question!

Level of Cognitive Ability: Analysis
Phase of Nursing Process: Planning
Client Needs: Physiological Integrity
Content Area: Mental Health

Reference
Townsend, M. (1996). *Psychiatric/mental health nursing: Concepts of care* (2nd ed.). Philadelphia: F. A. Davis. p. 611.

4. **1**

Rationale: The symptoms associated with DTs typically are anxiety, insomnia, anorexia, hypertension, disorientation, visual or tactile hallucinations, changes in level of consciousness, agitation, fever, and delusions.

Test-Taking Strategy: Knowledge regarding the clinical manifestations associated with DTs is required to answer this question. Review each option carefully to ensure that all the symptoms are contained in the correct option. Review these symptoms now if you had difficulty with this question!

Level of Cognitive Ability: Analysis
Phase of Nursing Process: Assessment
Client Needs: Physiological Integrity
Content Area: Mental Health

Reference
Varcarolis, E. (1998). *Foundations of psychiatric mental health nursing* (3rd ed.). Philadelphia: W. B. Saunders. p. 766.

5. **2**

Rationale: The most helpful response is one that encourages the client to problem solve. Giving advice implies that the nurse knows what is best and can also foster dependency. The nurse should not agree with the client nor should the nurse request that the client provide explanations.

Test-Taking Strategy: Use therapeutic communication techniques to answer this question. Eliminate option 3 because of the word "why," which should be avoided in communication. Eliminate option 1 because the nurse is agreeing with the client. Eliminate option 4 because this option places the client's feelings on hold. Option 2 is the only option that addresses the client's feelings!

Level of Cognitive Ability: Application
Phase of Nursing Process: Implementation
Client Needs: Psychosocial Integrity
Content Area: Mental Health

Reference
Varcarolis, E. (1998). *Foundations of psychiatric mental health nursing* (3rd ed.). Philadelphia: W. B. Saunders. p. 191.

6. **1**

Rationale: Opioids are central nervous system (CNS) depressants. They generally cause drowsiness and the feeling of being out of touch with the world. Option 1 identifies the manifestations associated with withdrawal. Recall that intoxication is exhibited by constricted pupils, euphoria, psychomotor retardation, "nodding out," insensitivity to pain, apathy, agitation, dysphoria, slurred speech, and/or drowsiness. Withdrawal occurs within 12 hours after the last dose and resembles influenza: dilated pupils, tearing, runny nose, and piloerection.

Test-Taking Strategy: This question tests your knowledge of the clinical manifestations of opioid abuse. Option 2 describes withdrawal from alcohol. Option 3 describes withdrawal from nicotine. Option 4 describes withdrawal from cocaine. If you had difficulty with this question, take time now to review the manifestations associated with withdrawal!

Level of Cognitive Ability: Analysis
Phase of Nursing Process: Assessment
Client Needs: Physiological Integrity
Content Area: Mental Health

Reference
Glod, C. A. (1998). *Contemporary psychiatric-mental health nursing.* Philadelphia: F. A. Davis. pp. 290–297.

7. **3**

Rationale: The Clinical Institute Withdrawal Assessment for Alcohol (CIWA) measures alcohol withdrawal symptoms by rating the following components: nausea and vomiting; tremor; paroxysmal sweats; anxiety; agitation; tactile, auditory, and visual disturbances; headache or fullness in the head; and orientation or clouding of the sensorium.

Test-Taking Strategy: This question assesses your knowledge of the appropriate tool to employ for the management of alcohol withdrawal. Option 1 is incorrect because the Short Michigan Alcoholism Screening Test (SMAST) is employed as a screening tool for alcohol dependence. Option 2 is incorrect because the CAGE Screening Test for Alcoholism and Substance Abuse asks four easy questions: 1. Have you ever felt you ought to Cut down on your drinking? 2. Have people Annoyed you by criticizing your drinking? 3. Have you ever felt Guilty about something you have done while inebriated? 4. Have you ever had a drink first thing in the morning to steady your nerves or get rid of a hangover (Eyeopener)? Option 4 is incorrect because the blood alco-

hol level (BAL) is a laboratory finding, not strictly a screening tool. Although it might be used periodically, it is not an assessment tool for caring for clients in alcohol withdrawal.

Level of Cognitive Ability: Application
Phase of Nursing Process: Planning
Client Needs: Physiological Integrity
Content Area: Mental Health

Reference
Glod, C. A. (1998). *Contemporary psychiatric-mental health nursing.* Philadelphia: F. A. Davis. pp. 289–293.

8. **3**

Rationale: Whenever the nurse employs an assessment for a client who is dependent on drugs, it is best for the nurse to attempt to elicit information by being nonjudgmental and direct. Asking the following questions assists the nurse who suspects that the client is dependent on drugs: "How much do you use and what effect does it have on you?"; "Do you have any withdrawal symptoms?"; "Have you ever tried to stop using this drug on your own?"; "How have you done it?"; "What happened?"; and "Do you spend too much time thinking about drugs or trying not to get caught?"

Test-Taking Strategy: This question tests your knowledge of the appropriate assessment questions for clients suspected of abusing drugs. Option 1 is incorrect because it is judgmental, off focus, and reflects the nurse's bias. Option 2 is incorrect because it is judgmental, insensitive, and aggressive, which is nontherapeutic. Option 4 is incorrect because it indicates passivity on the nurse's part and uses rationalization to avoid the therapeutic nursing intervention.

Level of Cognitive Ability: Application
Phase of Nursing Process: Assessment
Client Needs: Health Promotion and Maintenance
Content Area: Mental Health

Reference
Glod, C. A. (1998). *Contemporary psychiatric-mental health nursing.* Philadelphia: F. A. Davis. pp. 289–293.

9. **1**

Rationale: The only benzodiazepine presented in the options is diazepam (Valium). Benzodiazepines are effective only when used for short-term therapy. Short-acting benzodiazepines can produce withdrawal symptoms (insomnia, agitation, anxiety, irritability, nausea, and diaphoresis) within 1 to 2 days, and the long-acting benzodiazepines can produce withdrawal symptoms after 5 to 10 days following discontinuation.

Test-Taking Strategy: This question tests your knowledge of benzodiazepines and their management. Options 2, 3, and 4 are incorrect because they are not describing benzodiazepines. Take time now to review the benzodiazepines if you had difficulty with this question. You are likely to find questions related to these medications on NCLEX-RN!

Level of Cognitive Ability: Analysis
Phase of Nursing Process: Analysis
Client Needs: Physiological Integrity
Content Area: Mental Health

Reference
Glod, C. A. (1998). *Contemporary psychiatric-mental health nursing.* Philadelphia: F. A. Davis. pp. 92–127.

10. 2

Rationale: Alcoholics Anonymous is a major self-help organization for the treatment of alcoholism. Option 1 is a group for families of alcoholics. Option 3 is for parents of children who abuse substances. Option 4 is for nicotine addicts.

Test-Taking Strategy: If you are unfamiliar with these support groups, note the relationship between "drinking" in the question and "Alcoholics" in the correct option. Familiarize yourself with the purpose of specific support groups now, if you had difficulty with this question!

Level of Cognitive Ability: Application
Phase of Nursing Process: Implementation
Client Needs: Health Promotion and Maintenance
Content Area: Mental Health

Reference
Townsend, M. (1996). *Psychiatric/mental health nursing: Concepts of care* (2nd ed.). Philadelphia: F. A. Davis. p. 395.

11. 2

Rationale: A primary characteristic of an effective nurse is a nonjudgmental approach to clients. Nonjudgmental nurses allow clients to talk about feelings, and they respect clients as responsible people capable of making their own decisions. This allows the client to communicate openly and does not imply that the nurse accepts or condones the behavior of the client.

Test-Taking Strategy: Option 1 contains the word "always," thus a clue that it might not be the correct option. Option 3 is blatantly judgmental so obviously is not the correct option. Option 4 is rather narrow as compared with option 2. Option 2 is a basic tenet of psychiatric nursing and global in that it can be applied in all specialties.

Level of Cognitive Ability: Analysis
Phase of Nursing Process: Analysis
Client Needs: Psychosocial Integrity
Content Area: Mental Health

Reference
Fortinash, K., & Holoday-Worret, P. (1996). *Psychiatric mental health nursing.* St. Louis: Mosby–Year Book. pp. 149–150.

12. 1

Rationale: The client who has been starving has a compromised immune system. Having a roommate with pneumonia would put the client at risk for infection. The client with a fractured leg is an acceptable roommate. Clients should not be put in a position where they are able to focus on the nutritional needs of others or are being controlled by others, because this may contribute to sublimation and suppression of their own hunger.

Test-Taking Strategy: The key phrase is "in a state of starvation." Use the principle of prioritizing. The priority needs of the client with anorexia nervosa are physiological. The plan of care involves keeping the client free from opportunistic infections. This should direct you to option 1.

Level of Cognitive Ability: Application
Phase of Nursing Process: Planning
Client Needs: Safe, Effective Care Environment
Content Area: Mental Health

Reference
Wilson H., & Kneisl, C. (1996). *Psychiatric nursing* (5th ed.). Reading, MA: Addison-Wesley. pp. 427, 443.

13. 3

Rationale: Altered/distorted body image is a concern of clients with anorexia nervosa. Although the client may struggle with ambivalence and present with regressed behavior, the client's coping pattern relates to the basic issue of distorted body image. The nurse should address this need in the support group.

Test-Taking Strategy: Read the question carefully. Use the process of elimination to answer the question. The information provided in the question is directly related to an altered body image. This should direct you to the correct option.

Level of Cognitive Ability: Analysis
Phase of Nursing Process: Analysis
Client Needs: Psychosocial Integrity
Content Area: Mental Health

Reference
Varcarolis, E. (1998). *Foundations of psychiatric mental health nursing* (3rd ed.). Philadelphia: W. B. Saunders. p. 802.

14. 2

Rationale: Al-Anon support groups are a protected, supportive opportunity for spouses and significant others to learn what to expect and to obtain excellent pointers about successful behavioral changes. Option 2 is the most healthy response because it exemplifies an understanding that the alcoholic partner is responsible for his behavior and cannot be allowed to blame family members for loss of control. In option 1, the nonalcoholic partner should not feel responsible when the spouse loses control. Option 3 indicates that the wife remains codependent. Option 4 indicates that the group is being seen as an escape, not a place to work on issues.

Test-Taking Strategy: Use the process of elimination to answer the question. Identify the client of the question, and identify the option that most directly addresses the issue of the question, that is, benefiting from attending an Al-Anon group!

Level of Cognitive Ability: Analysis
Phase of Nursing Process: Evaluation
Client Needs: Psychosocial Integrity
Content Area: Mental Health

Reference
Carson, V., & Arnold, E. (1996). *Mental health nursing: The nurse-patient journey.* Philadelphia: W. B. Saunders. p. 1013.

15. 3

Rationale: In the defense mechanism of denial, the person denies reality. In option 3 the client is expressing real concern and ambivalence about discharge from the hospital. The client also demonstrates reality in the statement.

Test-Taking Strategy: Select the option that identifies the most realistic client verbalization. Knowing that in denial a person is unable to face reality, you can see that option 1 is blatant denial. In option 2, the client is relying heavily on others. The client's locus of control is external. In option 4, the client is concrete and procedure oriented; again the client denies that "nothing will go wrong that way" if the client follows all the directions. The client denies self and the value of self-input and choice within interactions.

Level of Cognitive Ability: Analysis
Phase of Nursing Process: Evaluation
Client Needs: Psychosocial Integrity
Content Area: Mental Health

Reference
Johnson, B. (1997). *Psychiatric–mental health nursing: Adaptation and growth* (4th ed.). Philadelphia: Lippincott-Raven. p. 8.

16. 1

Rationale: Early signs of alcohol withdrawal develop within a few hours after cessation or reduction of alcohol and peak after 24 to 48 hours. Early signs of withdrawal include anxiety, anorexia, insomnia, tremor, irritability, elevation in pulse and blood pressure, nausea, vomiting, and poorly formed hallucinations or illusions.

Test-Taking Strategy: Focus your attention on the use of the word "early" in this question. Knowledge of the early signs of withdrawal and alcohol withdrawal delirium will help you choose the correct option. If you are not familiar with the signs and symptoms of alcohol withdrawal and delirium, it would be helpful for you to review this now!

Level of Cognitive Ability: Analysis
Phase of Nursing Process: Assessment
Client Needs: Physiological Integrity
Content Area: Mental Health

Reference
Varcarolis, E. (1998). *Foundations of psychiatric mental health nursing* (3rd ed.). Philadelphia: W. B. Saunders. pp. 765–766.

17. 4

Rationale: A nurse can be charged with false imprisonment if a client is wrongfully made to believe that he or she cannot leave the hospital. Most health care facilities have documents that the client is asked to sign that relate to the client's responsibilities when he or she leaves against medical advice (AMA). The client should be asked to sign this document before leaving. The nurse should request that the client wait to speak to the physician before leaving, but if the client refuses to do so, the nurse cannot hold the client against her or his will. Restraining the client and calling security to block exits constitutes false imprisonment. Any client has a right to health care and cannot be told otherwise.

Test-Taking Strategy: Keeping the concept of false imprisonment in mind, eliminate options 1 and 2 as they are similar. Eliminate option 3 knowing that any client has a right to health care. From the options presented, the best action is option 4. Review the points related to false imprisonment now if you had difficulty with this question!

Level of Cognitive Ability: Application
Phase of Nursing Process: Implementation
Client Needs: Safe, Effective Care Environment
Content Area: Mental Health

Reference
Leahy, J., & Kizilay, P. (1998). *Foundations of nursing practice: A nursing process approach.* Philadelphia: W. B. Saunders. p. 68.

18. 4

Rationale: Clients with bulimia nervosa may not initially appear to be physically or emotionally ill. They are often at or slightly below ideal body weight. On further inspection, the client demonstrates enlargement of the parotid glands with dental erosion and caries if the client has been inducing vomiting. Electrolyte imbalances are present.

Test-Taking Strategy: Knowledge regarding the characteristics noted in bulimia nervosa and anorexia nervosa will assist in answering this question. Recall that in anorexia nervosa the body weight is normally below 85% of ideal body weight. Option 4 is a characteristic sign of anorexia nervosa. Review the characteristics of these disorders now if you had difficulty with this question!

Level of Cognitive Ability: Analysis
Phase of Nursing Process: Assessment
Client Needs: Physiological Integrity
Content Area: Mental Health

Reference
Varcarolis, E. (1998). *Foundations of psychiatric mental health nursing* (3rd ed.). Philadelphia: W. B. Saunders. p. 816.

BIBLIOGRAPHY

Carson, V., & Arnold, E. (1996). *Mental health nursing: The nurse-patient journey.* Philadelphia: W. B. Saunders.

Fortinash, K., & Holoday-Worret, P. (1996). *Psychiatric mental health nursing.* St. Louis: Mosby–Year Book.

Glod, C. A. (1998). *Contemporary psychiatric–mental health nursing.* Philadelphia: F. A. Davis.

Johnson, B. (1997). *Psychiatric–mental health nursing: Adaptation and growth* (4th ed.). Philadelphia: Lippincott-Raven.

Leahy, J., & Kizilay, P. (1998). *Foundations of nursing practice: A nursing process approach.* Philadelphia: W. B. Saunders.

Thompson, J., McFarland, G., Hirsch, J., & Tucker, S. (1997). *Mosby's clinical nursing* (4th ed.). St. Louis: Mosby–Year Book.

Townsend, M. (1996). *Psychiatric–mental health nursing* (2nd ed.). Philadelphia: F. A. Davis.

Varcarolis, E. (1998). *Foundations of psychiatric mental health nursing* (3rd ed.). Philadelphia: W. B. Saunders.

Wilson H., & Kneisl, C. (1996). *Psychiatric nursing* (5th ed.). Reading, MA: Addison-Wesley.

CHAPTER 73

Crisis Theory and Intervention

I. Crisis Intervention Therapy

A. Description
   1. **Crisis** is a temporary state of disequilibrium
   2. Decision making and problem solving are inadequate
   3. Treatment is immediate, supportive, and directly responsive to the immediate **crisis** to assist the client and/or the family through the stressful situation

B. Phases of a **crisis**
   1. Phase 1: External precipitating event
   2. Phase 2
      a. Perception of threat
      b. Increase in anxiety
      c. Client may cope or resolve **crisis**
   3. Phase 3
      a. Failure of coping
      b. Increasing disorganization
      c. Physical symptoms emerge
      d. Relationship problems
   4. Phase 4
      a. Mobilization of internal and external resources
      b. Resolutions related to pre**crisis** functioning include functioning at a higher level, at the same level, or at a lower level

C. **Crisis** intervention
   1. Treatment is immediate, supportive, and directly responsive to the immediate **crisis**
   2. Feelings of the client are acknowledged
   3. Goal-directed intervention
   4. Provides opportunities for expression and validation of feelings
   5. Connections are made between the meaning of the event and the **crisis**
   6. Explores alternative **coping mechanisms** and tries out new behaviors

II. Grieving

A. Description
   1. A normal human process that occurs in response to a loss
   2. Progresses through various stages, and the entire process may take up to 3 years

B. Assessment
   1. Crying
   2. Guilt and anger
   3. Depression
   4. Fatigue and lethargy
   5. Insomnia
   6. Agitation
   7. Anorexia
   8. Ambivalence
   9. Somatic complaints
   10. Sense of detachment and unreality
   11. Denial

C. Implementation
   1. Assess the client's progress through the grieving process
   2. Encourage the client to express feelings about the loss and its significance on life
   3. Encourage expression of angry feelings
   4. Explain the normal stages of the grieving process to the client
   5. Assist the client to make appropriate future plans related to changes caused by the loss
   6. Encourage the client to work through the feelings associated with the loss

III. Affective (Mood) Disorders

A. Description
   1. Illnesses that affect mood, ranging from elation or agitation to extreme sadness, emotional isolation
   2. Types of mood disorders may include depressive disorders, suicidal behavior, and bipolar (manic-depressive) disorders
   3. Can be maladaptive and incapacitating in nature

B. Precipitating factors
 1. Loss, which can be real or imagined and related to the person, status, self-esteem, a body part or function
 2. Major life events related to disruption of life patterns, conflict, or the entrance or exit of significant persons
 3. Role changes, such as marriage or divorce, parenting, or employment status
 4. Disruption in coping skills
 5. Physical changes due to medical illness or debilitating condition or drug-induced

IV. Depression

A. Description
 1. Affects feelings, thoughts, and behaviors
 2. Can occur after a loss, including loss of self-esteem, the end of a significant relationship, the death of a loved one, or a traumatic event
 3. The loss is followed by grief and mourning, and if this process does not resolve, depression results
 4. Depression may be mild, moderate, or severe
 5. Treatment includes antidepressant medication and electroconvulsive therapy (ECT)

B. Mild depression
 1. Triggered by an external event, and the experience follows the normal grief reaction
 2. Lasts less than 2 weeks
 3. Feeling sad
 4. Feeling let down or disappointed
 5. Mild alterations in sleep patterns
 6. Feeling less alert
 7. Irritability
 8. Disinterested in spending time with others
 9. Increased use of alcohol or drugs

C. Moderate depression
 1. Persists over time
 2. The person experiences a sense of change and often seeks help
 3. Despondent and gloomy
 4. Feels dejected
 5. Low self-esteem
 6. Helplessness and powerlessness
 7. May experience intense anxiety and anger
 8. Diurnal variation—may feel better at a certain time of the day, such as in the morning
 9. Slow thought processes and difficulty in concentrating
 10. Rumination—persistent thinking about and discussion of a particular subject
 11. Negative thinking and suicidal thoughts
 12. Sleep disturbances
 13. Social withdrawal
 14. Anorexia, weight loss, and fatigue
 15. Somatic complaints
 16. Menstrual changes
 17. Increased use of alcohol or drugs

D. Severe depression
 1. Intense and pervasive
 2. Despair and hopelessness
 3. Guilt and worthlessness
 4. Flat affect
 5. May show agitation and pace about
 6. Poor posture and unkempt appearance
 7. Decreased speech
 8. Self-destructive thoughts; however, client may lack energy to act on thought
 9. Social withdrawal
 10. Poor concentration and overwhelmed by simple tasks
 11. Severe psychomotor retardation
 12. Anorexia and marked weight loss
 13. Constipation and urinary retention
 14. Lack of sexual interest
 15. Terminal insomnia
 16. Diurnal variation—the person feels worse in the morning and better as the day goes on
 17. Delusions and hallucinations

E. Implementation
 1. Altered Thought Processes
 a. Encourage client to discuss losses or changes in life situation
 b. Encourage client to express sadness or anger and allow adequate time for verbal responses
 c. Assist in developing short-term goals
 d. Encourage the use of problem solving and positive thinking
 e. Limit decision making
 f. Spend short periods of time throughout the day with the client
 g. Be on time when a schedule is planned with the client
 h. Sit in silence with clients who are not verbalizing
 i. Use simple, concrete words when communicating
 j. Avoid a cheerful attitude
 2. Risk for self-harm
 a. Assess for **suicide** clues and intervene to provide safety precautions as necessary
 b. Ask client directly, "Have you thought of hurting yourself?"
 c. Assess lethality of plans
 d. Do not leave alone for extended periods
 e. If client has a suicidal plan, place on one-to-one supervision
 f. Form a suicide contract with client
 3. Activity intolerance
 a. Encourage daily exercise
 b. Assist with activities of daily living (ADLs) if client is unable to perform them
 c. Begin with one-to-one activities
 d. Provide activities for easy mastery to increase self-esteem and assist in alleviating guilt feelings
 e. Provide activities that require little orientation (card games, drawing)
 f. Engage in gross motor activities (walking)

g. Eventually bring client into small group activities, then large groups
4. Altered Nutrition
   a. Ensure adequate nutrition
   b. Offer small, high-calorie, high-protein snacks and fluids throughout the day
   c. Stay with the client during meals
   d. Weigh client weekly
   e. Assess bowel patterns for constipation
5. Sleep Pattern Disturbance
   a. Ensure adequate sleep
   b. Provide rest periods after activities
   c. Encourage client to dress and stay out of bed during the day
   d. Provide relaxation measures at bedtime
   e. Decrease environmental stimuli at bedtime
   f. Spend time with the client before bedtime

V. Suicidal Behavior

A. Description
   1. Suicidal clients characteristically have feelings of worthlessness, guilt, and hopelessness that are so overwhelming that they feel unable to go on with life and unfit to live
   2. The nurse caring for a depressed client always considers the possibility of suicide
B. High-risk groups
   1. Those with a history of previous **suicide attempts**
   2. Family history of **suicide attempts**
   3. Adolescents
   4. Disabled or terminally ill older adults
   5. Clients with personality disorders
   6. Clients with organic brain syndrome or dementia
   7. Depressed or psychotic clients
   8. Substance **abusers**
C. Clues
   1. Giving away personal, special, and prized possessions
   2. Canceling social engagements
   3. Making out or changing a will
   4. Taking out or changing insurance policies
   5. Positive or negative changes in behavior
   6. Poor appetite
   7. Sleeping difficulties
   8. Feelings of hopelessness
   9. Difficulty in concentrating
   10. Loss of interest in activities
   11. Client statements that indicate an intent to attempt suicide
   12. Sudden calmness or improvement in a depressed client
   13. Client questions about poisons, guns, or other lethal objects
D. Assessment
   1. The Plan
      a. Does the client have a plan?

b. What is the plan, how lethal is the plan, and how likely is death to occur?
      c. Does the client have the means to carry out the plan?
   2. Client history of attempts
      a. **Suicide attempts** in the past and the outcomes
      b. Was the client accidentally rescued?
      c. Have the past attempts and methods been the same, or have methods increased in lethality?
   3. Psychosocial
      a. Is the client alone or alienated from others?
      b. Is hostility or depression present?
      c. Do hallucinations exist?
      d. Is substance **abuse** present?
      e. Any recent losses or physical illness?
      f. Any environmental or lifestyle changes?
E. Implementation
   1. Initiate **suicide** precautions
   2. Remove harmful objects
   3. Do not leave client alone
   4. Provide one-to-one supervision at all times
   5. Provide a nonjudgmental, caring attitude
   6. Develop a contract, which is written, dated, and signed and indicates alternative behavior at times of suicidal thoughts
   7. Encourage the client to talk about feelings and to identify positive aspects about self
   8. Encourage active participation in own care
   9. Keep client active by assigning simple tasks
   10. Check that visitors do not leave harmful objects in the client's room
   11. Identify support systems
   12. Do not allow the client to leave the unit unless accompanied by a staff member
   13. Continue to assess the client's **suicide** potential

VI. Abusive Behaviors

A. Anger
   1. A feeling of annoyance that may be displaced onto an object or person
   2. Is used to avoid anxiety and gives a feeling of power in situations in which the person feels out of control
B. Violence: The physical force that is threatening to the safety of self and others
C. Aggression: Can be harmful and destructive when not controlled
D. Assessment
   1. History of violence or self-harm
   2. Poor impulse control and low tolerance of frustration
   3. Defiant and argumentative
   4. Verbal threats
   5. Increased pacing and agitation
   6. Muscle rigidity
   7. Flushed face
   8. Glaring

9. Loud voice
E. Implementation
   1. Acknowledge anger
   2. Set limits on behavior
   3. Listen actively and assist client to deal with consequences of anger
   4. Provide safety for expressing anger and safety to others
F. **Restraints** and **seclusion**
   1. Description
      a. Physical **restraints:** Any manual method or mechanical device, material, or equipment that inhibits free movement
      b. **Seclusion:** The last step in a process to maximize safety to a client and others, in which a client is placed alone in a specially designed room for protection and close supervision
      c. Chemical **restraints:** Medications given for a very specific purpose of inhibiting a specific behavior or movement; have an impact on the client's ability to relate to the environment
   2. Use of **restraints** and **seclusion**
      a. Should never be used as punishment or for the convenience of the staff
      b. The least restrictive means of **restraint** for the shortest duration should be used
      c. Used when behavior is physically harmful to the client or others
      d. Used when the disruptive behavior presents a danger to the facility
      e. Used when alternative or less restrictive measures are insufficient in protecting the client or others from harm
      f. Used when the client anticipates that a controlled environment would be helpful and requests **seclusion**
      g. Requires a written order by a physician, which must be reviewed and renewed every 24 hours and which also must specify the type of **restraint** to be used
      h. In an emergency, the charge nurse may place a client in **seclusion** or **restraint** and obtain a written or verbal order as soon as possible thereafter
      i. Laws require the consent of the client unless an emergency situation exists and can be documented
      j. The client must be removed from **restraints** when safer and quieter behavior is observed
      k. While in **restraints,** the client must be protected from all sources of harm
      l. The nurse must document the behavior leading to **restraint** or **seclusion** and the time the client is placed in and released from **restraint** or **seclusion**
      m. The client in **restraint** or **seclusion** must be assessed every 15 to 30 minutes for physical needs, safety, and comfort, and these observations are also documented

VII. Family Violence
A. Description
   1. The violence begins with threats or verbal or physical minor assaults, and the victim attempts to comply with the requests of the **abuser**
   2. The **abuser** loses control and becomes destructive and harmful while the victim attempts to protect him- or herself; the **abuser** then becomes loving and attempts to make peace
   3. The behavior may be an attempt for closeness and companionship
   4. The **abuser** believes that violence is normal and that the victim is responsible for the **abuse**
   5. Outsiders are not aware of what is happening in the family, and when outsiders try to enter the family, the family feels assaulted
   6. Family members are socially isolated and lack autonomy and trust among each other
   7. Caring and intimacy in the family are absent
   8. Family members expect other members in the family to meet their needs but none are able to do so
   9. The **abuser** threatens to abandon the family
B. Characteristics of **abusers**
   1. Impaired self-esteem
   2. Strong dependency needs
   3. Narcissistic and suspicious
   4. History of sexual **abuse** during childhood
   5. Perceive victims as their property and believe that they are entitled to **abuse** them
C. Characteristics of victims
   1. Feel trapped, dependent, helpless, and powerless
   2. Depressed
   3. Low self-esteem and blame themselves for the problems
D. Implementation
   1. Assess situations associated with family violence
   2. Assess for evidence of physical injuries
   3. Ensure privacy and confidentiality during assessment and provide a nonjudgmental and empathetic approach to foster trust
   4. Assist in resolving family dysfunction with prescribed therapies
   5. Encourage psychotherapy, counseling, group therapy, and support groups to assist family members in developing coping strategies
   6. Encourage individual therapy for victims that promotes coping with the trauma and prevents further psychological conflict
   7. Provide individual therapy for **abusers** that focuses on preventing violent behavior and repairing relationships
   8. Ensure that victim is not left alone with **abuser**
   9. Assist victim to understand his or her participation in the **abuse**

10. Assist victim to develop self-protective abilities and other problem-solving abilities
11. Provide support and assistance in coping with contacting the legal system
12. Assist family to identify an access to community and personal resources

VIII. Child Abuse

A. Description: Involves emotional or physical **abuse** or neglect, as well as sexual exploitation or molestation by caretakers or other individuals
B. Assessment
　1. Physical **abuse**
　　a. Unexplained bruises, burns, or fractures
　　b. Bald spots on scalp
　　c. Apprehensive child
　　d. Extreme aggressiveness or withdrawal
　　e. Fear of parents
　　f. Lack of crying when approached by a stranger
　2. Physical neglect
　　a. Inadequate weight gain
　　b. Poor hygiene
　　c. Consistent hunger
　　d. Inconsistent school attendance
　　e. Constant fatigue
　　f. Reports of lack of child supervision
　　g. Delinquency
　3. Emotional **abuse**
　　a. Speech disorders
　　b. Habit disorders, such as sucking, biting, rocking
　　c. Psychoneurotic reactions
　　d. Learning disorders
　　e. **Suicide attempts**
　4. Sexual **abuse**
　　a. Difficulty walking or sitting
　　b. Torn, stained, or bloody underclothing
　　c. Pain, swelling, or itching of the genitals
　　d. Bruises, bleeding, or lacerations in the genital or anal area
　　e. Unwillingness to change clothes or unwillingness to participate in gym activities
　　f. Poor peer relations
　　g. Delinquency
　　h. Changes in sleep performance
　　i. Self-disruptive behavior
C. Implementation
　1. Assess parents' strengths and weaknesses, normal **coping mechanisms,** and presence or absence of support systems
　2. Support child during a thorough physical assessment
　3. Assess injuries
　4. Report cases of suspected **abuse**
　5. Place child in an environment that is safe, thereby preventing further injury
　6. Move slowly around the child
　7. Avoid loud noises around the child

8. Communicate with the child at the child's eye level
9. Reassure the child that he or she is not a bad person, that the child is loved and not responsible for the **abuser's** behavior
10. Do not rescue the child from parents
11. Document in an objective manner information related to the suspected **abuse**
12. Assist the family in identifying stressors and alternative ways to express feelings
13. Provide education to the parents and refer parents to **crisis** hotlines and community support systems

IX. Elder Abuse

A. Description
　1. **Abuse** can be physical, sexual, psychological, or financial
　2. Neglect can include unintentional failure to care for the elder person's needs or an intentional neglect, such as abandonment
　3. Victims may attempt to dismiss injuries as accidental and **abusers** may prevent victims from receiving proper medical care to avoid discovery
　4. Victims are often socially isolated
　5. Victims may be care providers for the **abusers**
B. Assessment
　1. Physical **abuse**
　　a. Fractures
　　b. Lacerations
　　c. Punctures
　　d. Bruises
　　e. Burns
　2. Sexual **abuse**
　　a. Torn or stained underclothing
　　b. Discomfort or bleeding in the genital area
　　c. Difficulty in walking or sitting
　　d. Unexplained genital infections or disease
　3. Psychological **abuse**
　　a. Confusion
　　b. Fearful and agitated
　　c. Changes in appetite and weight
　　d. Withdrawn and loss of interest in self and social activities
　4. Financial **abuse**
　　a. Fearful when discussing finances
　　b. Confused, inaccurate, or no knowledge of finances
　　c. Inability to pay bills
　5. Neglect
　　a. Disheveled appearance
　　b. Dehydration and malnutrition
　　c. Dressed inadequately or inappropriately
　　d. Lacking physical needs, such as glasses, hearing aids, and dentures
　　e. Skin breaks
　　f. Signs of medication overdose
C. Implementation
　1. Assist with legal procedures, such as police

reports, order of protection, and court-ordered counseling
2. Explore alternative living arrangements that are least restrictive and disruptive to the victim
3. Assist with financial management protection
4. Encourage counseling and provide referrals to emergency community resources
5. Refer to protective services for adults
6. Arrange counseling and treatment for the **abuser**

◆ **X. Rape**

A. Description
1. Engaging another person in sexual intercourse through the use of force and without the consent of the sexual partner
2. The victim is not required by law to report the rape
3. The victim is often blamed by others and often receives no support from significant others
4. Acquaintance rapes involve someone known to the victim
5. Statutory rape is the act of sexual intercourse with someone under the age of legal consent even if there is consent from the minor

B. Assessment
1. Obtain the date of the last menstrual period
2. Determine form of birth control used and last act of intercourse before rape
3. Duration of intercourse, orifices violated, and penile penetration
4. Use of condom by perpetrator
5. Feelings of shame, embarrassment, humiliation, anger, and revenge
6. Fear of telling others for fear of not being believed

◆ C. Implementation
1. Encourage client not to shower, bathe, douche, or change clothing until examined
2. Assist with pelvic examination and obtaining specimens to detect semen
3. Preserve any evidence
4. Treat physical injuries
5. Provide client safety
6. Assist client in refraining from self-blame
7. Refer to **crisis** intervention and support groups

PRACTICE QUESTIONS

1. The nurse is reviewing the assessment data of a client admitted to the psychiatric unit. The nurse notes that the admission nurse has documented that the client is experiencing anxiety as a result of a situational crisis. The nurse determines that this type of crisis could be caused by
   1 A fire that destroyed the client's home
   2 A recent rape episode experienced by the client
   3 The death of a loved one
   4 Witnessing a murder

2. The nurse is conducting an initial assessment on a client in crisis. When assessing the client's perception of the precipitating event that led to the crisis, the most appropriate question to ask is
   1 "What leads you to seek help now?"
   2 "Who is available to help you?"
   3 "What do you usually do to feel better?"
   4 "With whom do you live?"

3. The nurse is developing a plan of care for the client experiencing anxiety following the loss of a job. The client is verbalizing concerns regarding the ability to meet role expectations and financial obligations. The most appropriate nursing diagnosis for this client is
   1 Altered Family Process
   2 Altered Thought Process
   3 Potential for Anxiety
   4 Ineffective Individual Coping

4. The nurse is developing a plan of care for the client in a crisis state. When developing the plan, the nurse will consider which of the following?
   1 Presenting symptoms in a crisis situation are similar for all individuals experiencing a crisis
   2 A crisis state indicates that the individual is suffering from an emotional illness
   3 A crisis state indicates that the individual is suffering from mental illness
   4 A client's response to a crisis is individualized, and what constitutes a crisis for one person may not constitute a crisis for another person

5. A client arrives in the emergency department in a crisis state. The client demonstrates signs of profound anxiety and is unable to focus on anything but the object of the crisis and the impact on self. The initial nursing assessment focuses on
   1 The object of the crisis
   2 The presence of support systems
   3 The physical condition of the client
   4 The client's coping mechanisms

6. The nurse is evaluating a client in crisis and is determining the potential for self-harm. Which of the following assessment data indicates that the client is a very high risk for suicide?
   1 The client is disorganized
   2 The client is impulsive
   3 The client has a history of suicide attempts
   4 The client has an immediate plan for a suicide attempt

7. The nurse observes that a client with a potential for violence is agitated, pacing up and down the hallway and making aggressive and belligerent gestures at other clients. Which of the following statements is most appropriate to make to this client?

1 "What is causing you to become agitated?"
2 "You need to stop that behavior now!"
3 "You will need to be restrained if you do not change your behavior."
4 "You will need to be placed in seclusion!"

8. The nurse in charge of a psychiatric unit is planning the staff/client assignment for the day. The most appropriate staff assignment to a male client who has a potential for violent behavior is which of the following?
1 A timid nurse
2 An inexperienced nurse
3 A male nurse
4 A mature, experienced female nurse

9. The clinic physician is planning to prescribe a medication for the client with major depression. Which of the following would be the first medication of choice for a client who has major depression?
1 Paroxetine hydrochloride (Paxil)
2 Amitriptyline (Elavil)
3 Tranylcypromine sulfate (Parnate)
4 Thioridazine hydrochloride (Mellaril)

10. The nurse is caring for a family with an 8-year-old female client who survived a mass murder of her teacher and classmates 1 week ago. The client's mother says, "She hasn't been eating well and keeps asking her father to start jogging with me. Is this normal?" The most appropriate therapeutic nursing response is
1 "It's common for school-aged children to respond to death by fearing separation and abandonment. If the loss of appetite continues overly long, we'll follow it more closely."
2 "It's common for school-aged children to respond to death by sadness and clinging to their parents, and having disrupted sleep. If the loss of appetite continues overly long, we'll follow it more closely."
3 "It's common for school-aged children to respond to death by acting out and withdrawing from their family. If the loss of appetite continues overly long, we'll follow it more closely."
4 "It's common for school-aged children to respond to death by being preoccupied with parents' health. If the loss of appetite continues overly long, we'll follow it more closely."

11. During a conversation with a depressed client on an inpatient unit, the client says to the nurse, "My family would be better off without me." The nurse's best response is
1 "Everyone feels this way when they are depressed."
2 "Have you talked to your family about this?"
3 "You sound very upset. Are you thinking of hurting yourself?"
4 "You will feel better once your medication begins to work."

12. Which of the following client statements alerts the nurse to the presence of low self-esteem associated with battered wife syndrome?
1 "I told him if he doesn't shape up, I'm leaving him."
2 "I stay because I like the money—he makes enough so I don't have to work."
3 "I love my husband very much. I need to do better. He's so stressed at work."
4 "I'm the luckiest woman in the world to be married to such a thoughtful man."

13. The community health nurse visits an older adult client who has recently lost her husband. The client says, "No one cares about me anymore. All the people I loved are dead." Which of the following responses by the nurse is the most therapeutic communication technique?
1 "That seems rather unlikely to me."
2 "You must be feeling all alone at this point."
3 "I don't believe that and neither do you."
4 "Right! Why not just pack it in?"

14. The nurse has been closely observing a client who has been displaying aggressive behaviors. The nurse observes that the behavior displayed by the client is escalating. Which of the following nursing interventions is least helpful to this client at this time?
1 Acknowledge the client's behavior
2 Maintain a safe distance from the client
3 Assist the client to an area that is quiet
4 Initiate confinement measures

15. The nurse is planning care for a client who is being hospitalized because the client has been displaying violent behavior and is at risk for potential harm to others. Which of the following is not a component of the plan of care?
1 Keep the door to the client's room open when providing care to the client
2 Assign the client to a room at the end of the hall to avoid disturbing the other clients
3 Face the client when providing care
4 Ensure that a security officer is within the immediate area

16. Which behaviors observed by the nurse might lead to the suspicion that the depressed female adolescent client may be suicidal?
1 The client becomes angry while speaking on the telephone and slams the receiver down on the hook
2 The client runs out of the therapy group, swearing at the group leader, and runs to her room
3 The client gets angry with her roommate when the roommate borrows the client's clothes without asking
4 The client gives away a prized CD and a cherished autographed picture of the performer

17. Which of these statements made by the nursing assistant to the nurse indicates to the nurse that the assistant understands suicide?
    1 "When a person talks about making suicide threats, the only thing the person wants is attention from family and friends."
    2 "Discussing suicide with a client is not harmful."
    3 "Depressed clients are the only persons who commit suicide."
    4 "Those clients who talk about suicide never do it."

18. A client is admitted to the psychiatric unit following a serious suicide attempt by hanging. The nurse's most important aspect of care is to maintain client safety. This is accomplished best by
    1 Assigning a staff member to the client who will remain with the client at all times
    2 Admitting the client to a seclusion room where all potentially dangerous articles are removed
    3 Removing the client's clothing and placing the client in a hospital gown
    4 Requesting that a peer remain with the client at all times

19. The nurse is caring for a suicidal client. The most appropriate nursing intervention in dealing with this client is to
    1 Demonstrate confidence in the client's ability to deal with stressors
    2 Provide hope and reassurance that the problems will resolve themselves
    3 Display an attitude of detachment, confrontation, and efficiency
    4 Provide authority, action, and participation

20. The police arrive at the emergency department with a client who has seriously lacerated both wrists. The initial nursing action is to
    1 Examine and treat the wound sites
    2 Secure and record a detailed history
    3 Encourage and assist client to ventilate feelings
    4 Administer an antianxiety agent

21. The nursing care plan indicates a nursing diagnosis of High Risk for Violence, self-directed, suicidal ideation with a plan. An expected outcome of this care plan is
    1 The client develops adequate coping and problem-solving skills
    2 The client displays less anxiety and agitation
    3 The client establishes a relationship with staff and peers
    4 The client denies suicidal ideation and identifies options to deal with stress

22. A depressed client is found unconscious on the floor in the day room. The nurse finds several empty bottles of a prescribed tricyclic antidepressant lying near the client. The immediate action of the nurse is to
    1 Call a "Code," as this incident presents a medical emergency
    2 Induce vomiting and notify the physician for further orders
    3 Call Poison Control
    4 Try to figure out the number of pills taken

23. The depressed client who appeared sullen, distraught, and hopeless a few days ago now suddenly appears calm, relaxed, and more energetic. The nurse's best response to the client's changes in behaviors is
    1 To feel comfortable that the client is adapting to the unit and is feeling safe
    2 To continue to assess the client's behaviors and document clearly in the chart
    3 To notify the team at staffing of these observations and alert them to the suspicion that the client is contemplating suicide
    4 To engage the client in one-to-one supervision, share with the client the observations that have been assessed, and ask whether the client is thinking about suicide

24. The nurse receives a telephone call from a male client who states that he wants to kill himself and has a bottle of sleeping pills in front of him. The best nursing action is to
    1 Insist that the client give you his name and address so that you can get the police there immediately
    2 Keep the client talking and allow the client to ventilate feelings
    3 Use therapeutic communications, especially the reflection of feelings
    4 Keep the client talking and signal to another staff member to trace the call so that appropriate help can be sent

25. Which of the following individuals is at the highest risk for committing suicide?
    1 A 24-year-old outpatient client who just had an argument with a coworker
    2 A 71-year-old client with severe cognitive deficits
    3 A 75-year-old male with cancer
    4 A 30-year-old newly divorced client who has custody of the children

26. A suicidal client is admitted to the hospital with a nursing diagnosis of Dysfunctional Grieving Related to the Loss of a Spouse. The client progresses well and is approaching discharge. Which of the following is an appropriate outcome for this nursing diagnosis?
    1 The client verbalizes stages of grief and plans to attend a community grief group
    2 The client verbalizes connections between significant losses and low self-esteem

3 The client verbalizes decreased desire for self-harm and discusses two alternatives to suicide
4 The client reports three additional coping strategies

27. A client comes to the emergency department following an assault and is extremely agitated, trembling, and hyperventilating. The most appropriate initial nursing action is to
    1 Encourage the client to discuss the assault
    2 Place the client in a quiet room alone to decrease stimulation
    3 Remain with the client until the anxiety decreases
    4 Begin to teach relaxation techniques

28. The nurse is caring for a client with severe depression. Which of the following activities is most appropriate for this client?
    1 Paint by number
    2 A puzzle
    3 Drawing
    4 Checkers

29. The client in a severe major depressive episode is unable to address activities of daily living. The most appropriate nursing intervention is to
    1 Feed, bathe, and dress the client as needed until the client can perform these activities independently
    2 Structure the client's day so that adequate time can be devoted to the client's assuming responsibility for the activities of daily living
    3 Offer the client choices and consequences to the failure to comply with the expectation of maintaining activities of daily living
    4 Have the client's peers confront the client about how the noncompliance in addressing activities of daily living affects the milieu

30. A woman comes into the emergency department following an assault. She presents with hyperventilation, pacing, rapid speech, and headache. The nurse correctly assesses the level of anxiety to be
    1 Panic
    2 Severe
    3 Moderate
    4 Psychotic

31. The visiting nurse is assessing an older, depressed client whose son was killed in an armed robbery after murdering two people. The client says, "I don't know what I did wrong. His dad died a hero in Vietnam when he was only 2 years old, but he's had everything. When he threw the cat up against the wall "to see if it landed on its feet" and stole money from me and denied it, his sister 'covered' for him." Which of the following is the most therapeutic response by the nurse?
    1 "It seems as if you and his sister feel regret."

    2 "Oh well, we can only love our children, do our very best, and hope they reflect our upbringing."
    3 "Do I hear you saying that you feel that your son's behavior was caused by the indulgence he received from his sister?"
    4 "Don't blame yourself. You seem to have been very caring. Some people just turn out evil despite all we do for them."

32. The nurse is preparing a hospitalized client for discharge. In evaluating the coping strategies learned during hospitalization, the nurse recognizes which of the following statements, if made by the client, as an indication that further teaching is needed?
    1 "I have learned ways to deal with the stresses in my life."
    2 "I know that I can't become depressed again."
    3 "I know that I can't be all things to all people."
    4 "I need to take my medications just as prescribed."

33. The nurse is monitoring a client who is in seclusion. The nurse determines that the client is safe to come out of seclusion when the client states
    1 "I am no longer a threat to myself or others."
    2 "I need to go to the bathroom."
    3 "I want to be alone for a while in my own room."
    4 "I can't breathe in here. The walls are closing in on me."

34. The nurse is preparing a discharge plan for the client who attempted suicide. The plan of care should focus on which of the following?
    1 Follow-up appointments
    2 Contracts and immediately available crisis resources
    3 Encouraging the family always to be with the client
    4 Providing the hospital phone number

35. The nursing instructor is teaching a group of nursing students about violence in the family. Which of the following statements is not a component of the teaching?
    1 Abusers usually have poor self-esteem
    2 Abusers use fear and intimidation
    3 Abusers are often jealous or self-centered
    4 Abuse occurs more in low-income families

36. A 2-year-old child is a suspected victim of child abuse. The nurse is interviewing the child's parent. Which statement, if made by the parent, indicates a characteristic associated with child abuse?
    1 "Once my child is potty trained, I can still expect her to have some 'accidents.'"
    2 "When I tell my child to do something once, I don't expect to have to tell her again."

3 "My child is expected to try to do things on her own, such as dress and feed."

4 "A 2-year-old's vocabulary is usually limited to about 200 words."

37. An elderly male client who is a victim of elder abuse and the family have been attending weekly counseling sessions. Which of the following statements, if made by the abusive family member, indicates that the family member has learned positive coping skills?
    1 "I will be more careful to make sure that my father's needs are met."
    2 "I am so sorry and embarrassed that the abusive event occurred. It won't happen again."
    3 "I feel better able to care for my father now that I know where to obtain assistance."
    4 "Now that my father is moving into my home, I will need to change my ways."

38. The moderately depressed client who was admitted 2 days ago suddenly begins smiling and reporting that the crisis is over. The client says to the nurse, "I'm finally cured." The nurse interprets this behavior as a cue to modify the treatment plan by
    1 Allowing the client off-unit privileges PRN
    2 Suggesting a reduction of medication
    3 Allowing increased "in-room" activities
    4 Increasing the level of suicide precautions

39. The nurse is planning care for the suicidal clients on the nursing unit. The nurse will prepare to provide additional precautions at which of the following times?
    1 Day shift
    2 Weekdays
    3 7 A.M. to 10 A.M.
    4 Weekends

40. The nurse is planning care for a client being admitted to the nursing unit who attempted suicide. Which of the following priority nursing interventions will the nurse include in the plan of care?
    1 Check whereabouts of client every 15 minutes
    2 Suicide precautions with 30-minute checks
    3 One-to-one suicide precautions
    4 Ask that the client report suicidal thoughts immediately

41. The emergency department nurse is caring for a client who has been identified as a victim of physical abuse. In planning care for the client, which of the following is the priority nursing action?
    1 Adhering to the mandatory abuse-reporting laws
    2 Obtaining treatment for the abusing family member
    3 Notifying the caseworker of the family situation

4 Removing the client from any immediate danger

42. An adolescent is returning home after an acute psychiatric hospitalization following a suicide attempt. Which of the following is least effective in preparing the client to return to a safe, effective care environment?
    1 Identify the family's strengths and weaknesses
    2 Suggest that the mother's boyfriend move out of the home
    3 Provide and offer the family options and resources
    4 Encourage sharing of feelings

43. A client tells the nurse that he/she is feeling out of control. The nurse observes that the client is pacing back and forth. Which approach by the nurse is most appropriate to maintain a safe environment?
    1 Administer the prescribed antianxiety medication immediately
    2 Move the client to a quiet room and talk about his/her feelings
    3 Isolate the client in a seclusion room
    4 Continue to monitor the client

44. The emergency department nurse is caring for an adult client who is a victim of family violence. Which of the following priority instructions is included in the discharge instructions?
    1 Explaining the importance of leaving the violent situation
    2 Information regarding the shelters
    3 Instructions regarding self-defense classes
    4 Instructions regarding calling the police

45. A female victim of a sexual assault is being seen in the crisis center. The client states that she still feels "as though the rape just happened yesterday" even though it has been a few months since the incident. The most appropriate nursing response is which of the following?
    1 "What do you think that you can do to alleviate some of your fears about being raped again?"
    2 "Tell me more about the incident that causes you to feel like the rape just occurred."
    3 "It will take some time to get over these feelings about your rape."
    4 "You need to try to be realistic. The rape did not just occur."

46. A client is admitted to the psychiatric unit following a serious suicidal attempt by a drug overdose. The priority nursing intervention is to
    1 Assign a staff member to the client for one to one supervision
    2 Admit the client to a seclusion room where all potentially dangerous articles are removed
    3 Remove the client's clothing from the client's room

4 Request that the client's roommate remain with the client at all times

47. The nurse in the emergency department is caring for a young female victim of sexual assault. The client's physical assessment is complete and physical evidence has been collected. The nurse notes that the client is withdrawn, confused, and at times physically immobile. These behaviors are interpreted by the nurse as:
    1 Evidence that the client is a high suicide risk
    2 Indicative of the need for hospital admission
    3 Signs of depression
    4 Normal reactions to a devastating event

48. The nurse has been working with a victim of rape in a clinic setting for the past 4 weeks. Which of the following short-term initial goals will not be a component of the plan of care?
    1 The client will resolve feelings of fear and anxiety related to the rape trauma
    2 Physical wounds will heal
    3 The client will verbalize feelings about the event

4 The client will participate in the treatment plan

49. The client who is experiencing suicidal thoughts states to the nurse, "It just doesn't seem worth it anymore. Why not just end it all?" The most appropriate initial nursing response is:
    1 "I'm sure your family loves you."
    2 "I know you don't feel good about yourself."
    3 "Did you sleep last night?"
    4 "What do you mean by that?"

50. A client comes to the clinic after losing all personal belongings in a hurricane. The nurse develops a nursing diagnosis of Ineffective Individual Coping. Which of the following is the least realistic goal for this client?
    1 The client will identify a realistic perception of stressors
    2 The client will develop adaptive coping patterns
    3 The client will express and share feelings regarding the present crisis
    4 The client will stop blaming self for the lack of insurance

ANSWERS

1. **3**

Rationale: A situational crisis arises from external rather than internal sources. External situations that could precipitate crisis include loss or change of a job, the death of a loved one, abortion, a change in financial status, divorce, the addition of new family members, pregnancy, and severe illness. Options 1, 2, and 4 identify adventitious crises. An adventitious crisis is not a part of everyday life; it is unplanned and accidental.

Test-Taking Strategy: Knowledge regarding the types of crisis situations is required to answer this question. You should be able to eliminate options 1, 2, and 4 because of the nature of their similarity. If you had difficulty with this question, review the types of crisis now!

Level of Cognitive Ability: Analysis
Phase of Nursing Process: Analysis
Client Needs: Psychosocial Integrity
Content Area: Mental Health

Reference
Varcarolis, E. (1998). *Foundations of psychiatric mental health nursing* (3rd ed.). Philadelphia: W. B. Saunders. pp. 368–369.

2. **1**

Rationale: A nurse's initial task when assessing a client in crisis is to assess the individual or family and the problem. The more clearly the problem can be defined, the better the chance a solution can be found. Option 1 will assist in determining data related to the precipitating event that led to the crisis. Options 2 and 4 assess situational supports. Option 3 assesses personal coping skills.

Test-Taking Strategy: Note the key words "precipitating event." Focus on these key words when selecting the correct option. Eliminate options 2 and 4 because these data will determine support systems. Eliminate option 3 because this question would be asked when determining coping skills.

Level of Cognitive Ability: Application
Phase of Nursing Process: Assessment
Client Needs: Psychosocial Integrity
Content Area: Mental Health

Reference
Varcarolis, E. (1998). *Foundations of psychiatric mental health nursing* (3rd ed.). Philadelphia: W. B. Saunders. pp. 370–371.

3. **4**

Rationale: Ineffective Individual Coping may be evidenced by inability to meet basic needs, inability to meet role expectations, alteration in social participation, use of inappropriate defense mechanisms, or impairment of usual patterns of communication. Altered Thought Processes is evidenced by altered attention span and distractibility or disorientation to time, place, person, and events. Altered Family Process may exist when the family has difficulty adapting or responding to the changes or traumatic experience of the member in crisis.

Test-Taking Strategy: Use the data presented in the question to direct you to the correct response. Option 3 can be easily eliminated because the client is presently experiencing anxiety. Eliminate option 1 because no data in the question addresses the family. Similarly, there are no data to suggest Altered Thought Processes, so this option is eliminated also, leaving option 4 as the correct option.

Level of Cognitive Ability: Analysis
Phase of Nursing Process: Planning
Client Needs: Psychosocial Integrity
Content Area: Mental Health

Reference
Varcarolis, E. (1998). *Foundations of psychiatric mental health nursing* (3rd ed.). Philadelphia: W. B. Saunders. p. 371.

4. 4

Rationale: Although each crisis response can be described in similar terms as far as presenting symptoms are concerned, what constitutes a crisis for one person may not constitute a crisis for another person because each is a unique individual. Being in the crisis state does not mean that the client is suffering from an emotional or mental illness.

Test-Taking Strategy: Eliminate option 1 because of the word "all." Next eliminate options 2 and 3 because a crisis does not indicate "illness." Review the characteristics of a crisis state now, if you had difficulty with this question.

Level of Cognitive Ability: Application
Phase of Nursing Process: Planning
Client Needs: Psychosocial Integrity
Content Area: Mental Health

Reference
Carson, V., & Arnold, E. (1996). *Mental health nursing: The nurse-patient journey.* Philadelphia: W. B. Saunders. p. 335.

5. 3

Rationale: The initial nursing assessment of a client in a crisis state is to evaluate the physical condition of the client, the potential for self-harm, and the potential for harm to others. Once this has been determined and appropriate interventions have been initiated, the nurse would then proceed with the psychiatric interview.

Test-Taking Strategy: Use Maslow's hierarchy of needs theory to answer the question. Physiological needs take priority over other needs. Option 3 is the only option that addresses a physiological need.

Level of Cognitive Ability: Analysis
Phase of Nursing Process: Assessment
Client Needs: Physiological Integrity
Content Area: Mental Health

Reference
Carson, V., & Arnold, E. (1996). *Mental health nursing: The nurse-patient journey.* Philadelphia: W. B. Saunders. p. 345.

6. 4

Rationale: The client presents a lethality potential if the client appears disorganized and impulsive. Clients at higher risk include those with a history of a dual diagnosis of mental illness and substance abuse or a personal or family history of suicide attempts, depression, alcoholism, or psychotic episodes. Having a plan, particularly if the method is immediate and available, makes the client a very high risk.

Test-Taking Strategy: Noting the key words "a very high risk" should easily direct you to option 4. Note the key words "immediate plan" in the correct option. If you are unfamiliar with the risk factors associated with suicide, review now. You are likely to see questions related to suicide on NCLEX-RN!

Level of Cognitive Ability: Analysis
Phase of Nursing Process: Analysis
Client Needs: Psychosocial Integrity
Content Area: Mental Health

Reference
Carson, V., & Arnold, E. (1996). *Mental health nursing: The nurse-patient journey.* Philadelphia: W. B. Saunders. p. 346.

7. 1

Rationale: The best statement is to ask the client what is causing the anger. This will assist the client to become aware of the behavior and may assist the nurse in planning appropriate interventions for the client. Option 2 is demanding behavior that could cause increased agitation in the client. Options 3 and 4 are threats to the client and are inappropriate.

Test-Taking Strategy: Eliminate option 2 because of the demand that it places on the client. Eliminate options 3 and 4 because they indicate threats to the client. Review appropriate nursing actions for the violent client now if you had difficulty with this question!

Level of Cognitive Ability: Application
Phase of Nursing Process: Implementation
Client Needs: Psychosocial Integrity
Content Area: Mental Health

Reference
Carson, V., & Arnold, E. (1996). *Mental health nursing: The nurse-patient journey.* Philadelphia: W. B. Saunders. p. 349.

8. 4

Rationale: A timid or inexperienced nurse should not be assigned to a potentially violent client. A mature, experienced nurse should be assigned to the client. Male clients may hesitate to strike or injure a female nurse. Additionally, female clients may be inclined to react negatively to another woman but positively to a male staff member.

Test-Taking Strategy: Options 1 and 2 can be easily eliminated. Gender can be a significant factor in determining a client assignment. Although you may be tempted to select option 3, note the key words "mature" and "experienced" in the correct option.

Level of Cognitive Ability: Application
Phase of Nursing Process: Implementation
Client Needs: Safe, Effective Care Environment
Content Area: Mental Health

Reference
Carson, V., & Arnold, E. (1996). *Mental health nursing: The nurse-patient journey.* Philadelphia: W. B. Saunders. p. 349.

9. 1

Rationale: Paxil is an antidepressant used in the treatment of major depression. Elavil is a tricyclic antidepressant (TCA) used to treat various forms of depression. Parnate is a monoamine oxidase (MAO) inhibitor used in the symptomatic treatment of severe depression in hospitalized or closely supervised clients, and Mellaril is an antipsychotic medication.

Test-Taking Strategy: Knowledge regarding the actions and the uses of the medications identified in the options is required to answer the question. If you are unfamiliar with these medications, take time now to review!

Level of Cognitive Ability: Analysis
Phase of Nursing Process: Analysis
Client Needs: Psychosocial Integrity
Content Area: Pharmacology

Reference

Hodgson, B., & Kizior, R. (1999). *Saunders nursing drug handbook 1999.* Philadelphia: W. B. Saunders. pp. 49, 787, 985, 1012.

10. **4**

Rationale: When school-aged children encounter death, it is perceived as associating death with punishment, mutilation, and violence. School-aged children may feel responsible for the death and usually do not perceive the finality of death until age 9 years. School-aged children have several common responses to death. They include school phobia, usually accompanied by reduced school performance, aggressive behavior, preoccupation with their parents' health, altered peer relationships, and/or reduction in appetite.

Test-Taking Strategy: This question assesses your knowledge of the ways in which children experience and understand death. Option 1 is incorrect because it describes behaviors that are common for infants/toddlers. Option 2 is incorrect because it describes the behaviors of 3- to 5-year-old children. Option 3 is incorrect because it describes the behaviors of adolescents.

Level of Cognitive Ability: Application
Phase of Nursing Process: Implementation
Client Needs: Psychosocial Integrity
Content Area: Mental Health

Reference

Glod, C. A. (1998). *Contemporary psychiatric-mental health nursing.* Philadelphia: F. A. Davis. pp. 634–639.

11. **3**

Rationale: Clients who are depressed may be at risk for suicide. It is critical for the nurse to assess suicidal ideation and plan. Ask the client directly if a plan for self-harm exists.

Test-Taking Strategy: Using therapeutic communication techniques will assist in directing you to the correct option. Option 3 is the only option that deals directly with the client's feelings. Additionally, clients at risk for suicide need to be directly assessed regarding the potential for self-harm.

Level of Cognitive Ability: Application
Phase of Nursing Process: Implementation
Client Needs: Psychosocial Integrity
Content Area: Mental Health

Reference

Varcarolis, E. (1998). *Foundations of psychiatric mental health nursing* (3rd ed.). Philadelphia: W. B. Saunders. p. 192.

12. **3**

Rationale: In the battering cycle, the client often vocalizes statements that reflect the low self-esteem and self-deprecation that combine to produce a victim of battering. The victim will assume the guilt for the abuse and persuade herself or himself that the punishment was deserved just as the perpetrator says.

Test-Taking Strategy: This question tests your knowledge of the dynamics of battered wife syndrome. In Phase I, the *tension-building phase,* which may last a few weeks to many months, the victim senses the perpetrator's growing frustration. In Phase II, the *acute battering incident,* which is the shortest and most violent phase, the batterer wants to "teach a lesson" to the victim. In Phase III, the *calm, loving respite* or *honeymoon phase,* the batterer believes the victim has been "taught a lesson" and won't act up again. The perpetrator is loving and charming to the victim. Options 1, 2, and 4 are all responses that are within the normal range for dyadic dialogue.

Level of Cognitive Ability: Analysis
Phase of Nursing Process: Assessment
Client Needs: Psychosocial Integrity
Content Area: Mental Health

Reference

Stuart, G. W., & Laraia, M. T. (1998). *Principles and practice of psychiatric nursing* (6th ed.). St. Louis: Mosby–Year Book. pp. 17–61.

13. **2**

Rationale: The client is experiencing loss and is feeling hopeless. The most therapeutic response by the nurse is the one that attempts to translate words into feelings.

Test-Taking Strategy: This question tests your knowledge of the therapeutic communication that will assist the client to express the loneliness that the client is feeling. In option 1, the nurse is voicing doubt, which is often used when a client verbalizes delusional ideas. In option 3, the nurse is disagreeing with the client, which implies that the nurse has passed judgment on the client's ideas or opinions. In option 4, the nurse uses sarcasm, which gives advice and is nontherapeutic as a nursing response.

Level of Cognitive Ability: Application
Phase of Nursing Process: Implementation
Client Needs: Psychosocial Integrity
Content Area: Mental Health

Reference

Stuart, G. W., & Laraia, M. T. (1998). *Principles and practice of psychiatric nursing* (6th ed.). St. Louis: Mosby–Year Book. pp. 17–61.

14. **4**

Rationale: During the escalation period, the client's behavior is moving toward loss of control. Nursing actions include taking control, maintaining safe distance, acknowledging behavior, moving the client to a quiet area, medicating the client if appropriate, and "showing force" if necessary. It is not appropriate during this period to initiate confinement measures. Initiating confinement measures is most appropriate during the crisis period.

Test-Taking Strategy: Note the key words "behavior" and "escalating." Nursing actions will vary depending on the level of aggressive behavior that the client is exhibiting. Knowledge of these levels and the appropriate nursing actions is required to answer this question. Review these levels and guidelines now if you had difficulty with this question!

Level of Cognitive Ability: Application
Phase of Nursing Process: Implementation
Client Needs: Psychosocial Integrity
Content Area: Mental Health

Reference

Carson, V., & Arnold, E. (1996). *Mental health nursing: The nurse-patient journey.* Philadelphia: W. B. Saunders. p. 350.

15. 2

Rationale: The client should be placed in a room near the nurses' station and not at the end of a long, relatively unprotected corridor. The nurse should not isolate self with a potentially violent client. The door to the client's room should be kept open, and the nurse should never turn away from the client. A security officer or male aide should be within immediate call should a suspicion of violence be imminent.

Test-Taking Strategy: Note the key word "not" in the stem of the question. Keeping in mind that safety is the issue, you should easily be able to select the correct option. If you had difficulty with this question, review guidelines on caring for the violent client!

Level of Cognitive Ability: Application
Phase of Nursing Process: Implementation
Client Needs: Safe, Effective Care Environment
Content Area: Mental Health

Reference
Carson, V., & Arnold, E. (1996). *Mental health nursing: The nurse-patient journey.* Philadelphia: W. B. Saunders. p. 349.

16. 4

Rationale: A depressed, suicidal client often gives away that which is of value as a way of saying "good-bye" and wanting to be remembered.

Test-Taking Strategy: Options 1, 2, and 3 are similar in that they deal with anger and "acting out behaviors" which are often typical of any adolescent. Option 4 is different in nature and an action that could indicate that the client may be "saying good-bye."

Level of Cognitive Ability: Analysis
Phase of Nursing Process: Analysis
Client Needs: Psychosocial Integrity
Content Area: Mental Health

Reference
Varcarolis, E. (1998). *Foundations of psychiatric mental health nursing* (3rd ed.). Philadelphia: W. B. Saunders. p. 730.

17. 2

Rationale: An open discussion of suicide will not encourage a client to make a decision to do so; it will, in fact, often help prevent it. Such a discussion offers the health care professional the opportunity to assess the reality of suicide for the client and take necessary precautions to keep the client safe.

Test-Taking Strategy: Note the key word "understands" in the question. Note the words "only" in options 1 and 3 and "never" in option 4. If you had difficulty with this question, take time now to review appropriate interventions for the suicidal client!

Level of Cognitive Ability: Analysis
Phase of Nursing Process: Evaluation
Client Needs: Psychosocial Integrity
Content Area: Mental Health

Reference
Varcarolis, E. (1998). *Foundations of psychiatric mental health nursing* (3rd ed.). Philadelphia: W. B. Saunders. p. 729.

18. 1

Rationale: Hanging is a serious suicide attempt. The plan of care must reflect action that will promote the client's safety.

Constant observation status (one-to-one) with a staff member who is never less than an arm's length away is the best selection.

Test-Taking Strategy: Eliminate option 2 because seclusion should not be the initial intervention. Eliminate option 4 next because the responsibility to safeguard a client is not the peer's responsibility. Eliminate option 3 because removing one's clothing will not maximize all possible safety strategies. Review nursing interventions for the client at risk for suicide now if you had difficulty with this question!

Level of Cognitive Ability: Analysis
Phase of Nursing Process: Planning
Client Needs: Safe, Effective Care Environment
Content Area: Mental Health

Reference
Varcarolis, E. (1998). *Foundations of psychiatric mental health nursing* (3rd ed.). Philadelphia: W. B. Saunders. p. 736.

19. 4

Rationale: A crisis is an acute, time-limited state of disequilibrium resulting from situational, developmental, or societal sources of stress. A person in this state is temporarily unable to cope with or adapt to the stressor by using previous problem solving. One who intervenes in this situation (the nurse) "takes over" for the client who is not in control and devises a plan (action) to secure and maintain the client's safety. Once this has occurred, the nurse works collaboratively with the client (participates) in developing new coping and problem-solving strategies.

Test-Taking Strategy: The client who experiences a "suicidal crisis" is in acute disequilibrium. Remember, in a "crisis," an authority figure must emerge to take action.

Level of Cognitive Ability: Application
Phase of Nursing Process: Implementation
Client Needs: Psychosocial Integrity
Content Area: Mental Health

Reference
Varcarolis, E. (1998). *Foundations of psychiatric mental health nursing* (3rd ed.). Philadelphia: W. B. Saunders. p. 369.

20. 1

Rationale: The initial nursing action is to assess and treat the self-inflicted injuries. Injuries from lacerated wrists can lead to a life-threatening situation. Other interventions may follow after the client has been treated medically.

Test-Taking Strategy: Use Maslow's hierarchy of needs theory to prioritize. Physiological needs come first. Option 1 addresses the physiological need!

Level of Cognitive Ability: Application
Phase of Nursing Process: Implementation
Client Needs: Physiological Integrity
Content Area: Mental Health

Reference
Carson, V., & Arnold, E. (1996). *Mental health nursing: The nurse-patient journey.* Philadelphia: W. B. Saunders. p. 346.

21. 4

Rationale: A suicidal client may have numerous diagnoses that encompass inadequate coping skills, anxiety, and strained interpersonal relationships. The question, however, directly and clearly designates that the problem that needs to be dealt with is the "High Risk for Violence, self-directed" and the client has both the "ideation and a plan." The answer is the option that the client no longer has suicidal ideations and has identified choices to deal with stress. Options 1, 2, and 3 are not directly related to the diagnosis as stated in the question.

Test-Taking Strategy: When presented with a question that identifies a nursing diagnosis, use the information in the question to assist in directing you to the correct option. Option 4 is the only option that offers a resolution to the nursing diagnosis of "suicidal ideation with a plan" in that the client denies the "suicidal ideation" and has identified other options.

Level of Cognitive Ability: Analysis
Phase of Nursing Progress: Planning
Client Needs: Psychosocial Integrity
Content Area: Mental Health

Reference
Antai-Otong, D. (1995). *Psychiatric nursing: Biological and behavioral concepts.* Philadelphia: W. B. Saunders. p. 351.

22. **1**

Rationale: Tricyclic antidepressants can be fatal when taken as an overdose regardless of the amount ingested. Serious, life-threatening symptoms can develop after an overdose. Immediate emergency medical attention and cardiac monitoring are necessary with an overdose of tricyclics.

Test-Taking Strategy: Note the key word "immediate" in the stem of the question. Options 3 and 4 would delay measures to provide immediate treatment. Eliminate option 2 because vomiting would not be induced in a client who is unconscious.

Level of Cognitive Ability: Application
Phase of Nursing Process: Implementation
Client Needs: Physiological Integrity
Content Area: Mental Health

Reference
Carson, V., & Arnold, E. (1996). *Mental health nursing: The nurse-patient journey.* Philadelphia: W. B. Saunders. p. 539.

23. **4**

Rationale: The sudden change in the depressed client's mood and affect may indicate that the client has come to a decision about suicide. The only way to be sure is to ask the client directly.

Test-Taking Strategy: The knowledge that all behavior has meaning is important. The only way to know what the behavior may mean is to ask the client. Safety of the client is the concern. Option 1 "assumes" meaning of the behavior. Option 2 offers no different strategy than would be used with any client. Option 3, "notifying" others of your concern, does nothing to address the problem directly.

Level of Cognitive Ability: Application
Phase of Nursing Process: Implementation
Client Needs: Physiological Integrity
Content Area: Mental Health

Reference
Carson, V., & Arnold, E. (1996). *Mental health nursing: The nurse-patient journey.* Philadelphia: W. B. Saunders. p. 937.

24. **4**

Rationale: In a crisis, the nurse must take an authoritative, active role to promote the client's safety. A bottle of sleeping pills in front of a client who verbalizes he wants to kill himself is a "crisis." The client's safety is of prime concern. Keeping the client on the phone and getting help to the client is the best intervention.

Test-Taking Strategy: Although each of the options may seem appropriate, the best option is option 4. It is the most global response and encompasses every necessary action. The word "insisting" may anger the client and he might hang up. Option 2 lacks the authoritative action stance of securing the client's safety. Using therapeutic communication is important, but overuse of "reflection" may sound uncaring or superficial and is lacking direction/solutions to the immediate problem of the client's safety.

Level of Cognitive Ability: Application
Phase of Nursing Process: Implementation
Client Needs: Safe, Effective Care Environment
Content Area: Mental Health

Reference
Varcarolis, E. (1998). *Foundations of psychiatric mental health nursing* (3rd ed.). Philadelphia: W. B. Saunders. p. 737.

25. **3**

Rationale: The individual at highest risk for suicide is the individual with a terminal illness. Other high-risk groups include adolescents; drug abusers; individuals with social problems, recent losses, and few or no social supports; and those with a history of suicide attempts and a suicide plan.

Test-Taking Strategy: Knowledge regarding the groups at high risk for suicide is required to answer this question. Use the process of elimination, and if you are unfamiliar with the risk factors and groups at risk for suicide, take time now to review!

Level of Cognitive Ability: Analysis
Phase of Nursing Process: Analysis
Client Needs: Psychosocial Integrity
Content Area: Mental Health

Reference
Carson, V., & Arnold, E. (1996). *Mental health nursing: The nurse-patient journey.* Philadelphia: W. B. Saunders. p. 934.

26. **1**

Rationale: The question is focused on the nursing diagnosis of Dysfunctional Grieving. The only option that deals with grief is option 1. Options 2, 3, and 4 are unrelated to this nursing diagnosis.

Test-Taking Strategy: When presented with a question that identifies a nursing diagnosis, use the information in the question to assist in directing you to the correct option. Option 1 is the only option focused on the nursing diagnosis of Dysfunctional Grieving. Additionally, note the word "grieving" in the question and the word "grief" in the correct option.

Level of Cognitive Ability: Analysis
Phase of Nursing Process: Planning
Client Needs: Health Maintenance and Promotion
Content Area: Mental Health

Reference
Varcarolis, E. (1998). *Foundations of psychiatric mental health nursing* (3rd ed.). Philadelphia: W. B. Saunders. p. 550.

27. **3**

Rationale: This client is in a severe state of anxiety. When a client is in a severe or panic state of anxiety, it is critical for the nurse to remain with the client. Processing the anxiety at this point will further increase the client's level of anxiety. The client in a severe state of anxiety would not be able to learn relaxation techniques.

Test-Taking Strategy: Knowledge of key nursing interventions with clients who present in a severe level of anxiety is necessary to assist you in answering this question. Remember to use therapeutic techniques. The best technique in this situation is to remain with the client. If you are unfamiliar with the symptoms of the different levels of anxiety and the interventions that are indicated, it would be important for you to review this information!

Level of Cognitive Ability: Application
Phase of Nursing Process: Implementation
Client Needs: Psychosocial Integrity
Content Area: Mental Health

Reference
Varcarolis, E. (1998). *Foundations of psychiatric mental health nursing* (3rd ed.). Philadelphia: W. B. Saunders. p. 349.

28. 3

Rationale: Concentration and memory are poor in severe depression. When a client has a diagnosis of severe depression, the nurse needs to provide activities that require little concentration. Activities that have no right or wrong choices or decisions minimize opportunities for clients to put themselves down.

Test-Taking Strategy: Knowledge of the nursing interventions that are indicated when working with clients who are depressed is required to assist you in answering this question. It is important to remember that clients with depression have difficulty concentrating and need activities that require little concentration. You must carefully select the option that meets this criterion.

Level of Cognitive Ability: Application
Phase of Nursing Process: Implementation
Client Needs: Psychosocial Integrity
Content Area: Mental Health

Reference
Varcarolis, E. (1998). *Foundations of psychiatric mental health nursing* (3rd ed.). Philadelphia: W. B. Saunders. p. 566.

29. 1

Rationale: The symptoms of major depression include depressed mood, loss of interest or pleasure, changes in appetite and sleep patterns, psychomotor agitation or retardation, fatigue, feelings of worthlessness/guilt, diminished ability to think or concentrate, and recurrent thoughts of death. Often the clients do not have the energy or interest to complete activities of daily living.

Test-Taking Strategy: Note the key words "severe major depressive episode." Often, severely depressed clients are unable to perform even the simplest of activities of daily living. The nurse assumes this role and completes these tasks with the client. In doing so, the nurse establishes a therapeutic relationship as the nurse demonstrates respect and acceptance of the client and contributes to fostering the client's self-esteem. Eliminate options 2 and 3 because the client lacks the energy and motivation to do these independently. In addition, option 3 may lead to increased feelings of worthlessness as the client fails to meet expectations. Option 4 will increase the client's feelings of poor self-esteem and unworthiness.

Level of Cognitive Ability: Application
Phase of Nursing Process: Implementation
Client Needs: Physiological Integrity
Content Area: Mental Health

Reference
Antai-Otong, D. (1995). *Psychiatric nursing: Biological and behavioral concepts.* Philadelphia: W. B. Saunders. pp. 170,183.

30. 2

Rationale: Clients who have severe anxiety have significant somatic complaints, ineffective functioning, loud or rapid speech, and purposeless activity. The client symptoms in the question do not relate to options 1, 3, and 4.

Test-Taking Strategy: Note the client symptoms carefully when trying to answer correctly a question similar to this one. Review the signs and symptoms associated with each level of anxiety now if you had difficulty with this question!

Level of Cognitive Ability: Analysis
Phase of Nursing Process: Assessment
Client Needs: Physiological Integrity
Content Area: Mental Health

Reference
Varcarolis, E. (1998). *Foundations of psychiatric mental health nursing* (3rd ed.). Philadelphia: W. B. Saunders. p. 346.

31. 1

Rationale: The most therapeutic communication by the nurse is one that seeks to help the client reframe a situation. By communicating with the client from the nurse's perception, the nurse reframes the client's limited thinking and problem solving (and recognizes the client's sense of guilt within the grieving, as well as rationalization of blame onto the sister).

Test-Taking Strategy: This question assesses your ability to identify the most therapeutic communication technique for the nurse to employ for clients who blame themselves for the behavior of others. In option 2, the nurse uses clichéd social, nontherapeutic communication. In option 3, the nurse uses an inappropriate and inaccurate dynamic interpretation, which is insensitive. In option 4, the nurse uses false reassurance, which is nontherapeutic.

Level of Cognitive Ability: Application
Phase of Nursing Process: Implementation
Client Needs: Psychosocial Integrity
Content Area: Mental Health

Reference
Glod, C. A. (1998). *Contemporary psychiatric–mental health nursing.* Philadelphia: F. A. Davis. pp. 56–61.

32. 2

Rationale: Depression may be a recurring illness for some people. The client needs to understand the symptoms and recognize when or if treatment needs to begin again. Options 1, 3, and 4 identify that the client has learned some coping skills, such as setting limits and taking medications.

Test-Taking Strategy: Option 2 is the correct option for this question as stated. Options 1, 3, and 4 are very positive and realistic. A client statement such as option 2 is the only unrealistic statement and thus indicates that further teaching is needed.

Level of Cognitive Ability: Analysis
Phase of Nursing Process: Evaluation
Client Needs: Health Promotion and Maintenance
Content Area: Mental Health

Reference
Johnson, B. S. (1997). *Psychiatric-mental health nursing: Adaptation and growth* (4th ed.). Philadelphia: Lippincott-Raven. pp. 558–561.

33. **1**

Rationale: Option 1 is clearly the best choice of the four options. The client in seclusion must be assessed at regular intervals (usually every 15 to 30 minutes) for physical needs, safety, and comfort. Option 2 indicates a physical need that could be met with a urinal or bedpan, if necessary. It does not indicate that the client has calmed down enough to leave the seclusion room. Option 3 could be an attempt to manipulate the nurse. It gives no indication that the client will control self when alone in the room. Option 4 indicates the need for supportive communication or possibly a PRN medication. It does not necessitate discontinuing seclusion.

Test-Taking Strategy: The issue of the question specifically relates to safety. Use the process of elimination to answer the question. You should easily be directed to option 1. Review seclusion procedure now if you had difficulty with this question!

Level of Cognitive Ability: Analysis
Phase of Nursing Process: Evaluation
Client Needs: Health Promotion and Maintenance
Content Area: Mental Health

Reference
Carson, V., & Arnold, E. (1996). *Mental health nursing: The nurse-patient journey.* Philadelphia: W. B. Saunders. pp. 348–349.

34. **2**

Rationale: Crisis times may occur between appointments. Contracts facilitate clients' feeling responsibility for keeping a promise. This gives the client control. Option 3 is unrealistic. Providing phone numbers will not assure available and immediate crisis intervention.

Test-Taking Strategy: The issue of the question relates to the availability of immediate resources for the client if needed. Eliminate option 3 first as this is unrealistic. Options 1 and 4 will not necessarily provide these immediate resources. Note the word "immediate" in the correct option. This key word will assist you in answering correctly!

Level of Cognitive Ability: Application
Phase of Nursing Process: Planning
Client Needs: Psychosocial Integrity
Content Area: Mental Health

Reference
Fortinash, K., & Holoday-Worret, P. (1996). *Psychiatric mental health nursing.* St. Louis: Mosby–Year Book. pp. 630, 634.

35. **4**

Rationale: Personal characteristics of abusers include low self-esteem, immaturity, dependence, insecurity, and jealousy. Abusers will often use fear and intimidation to the point where their victims will do anything just to avoid further abuse. The thought that abuse occurs more in lower socioeconomic groups is a myth.

Test-Taking Strategy: Note the key word "not" in the stem of the question. Options 1, 2, and 3 are all true statements. Only answer 4 is incorrect. If you had difficulty with this question, take time now to review the characteristics of an abuser and family violence!

Level of Cognitive Ability: Analysis
Phase of Nursing Process: Analysis
Client Needs: Psychosocial Integrity
Content Area: Mental Health

Reference
Carson, V., & Arnold, E. (1996). *Mental health nursing: The nurse-patient journey.* Philadelphia: W. B. Saunders. pp. 1044–1046.

36. **2**

Rationale: One characteristic of abusing parents is that they have expectations that are too high. As a result, the child cannot live up to the expectation. Unrealistic expectations result in the disappointment and frustration of the parent. The parent may even believe that the action of the child is intentional or done out of spite. The parent may react in an excessive manner, causing severe injury to the child.

Test-Taking Strategy: Options 1, 3, and 4 are true statements in that they are appropriate for the 2-year-old. Option 2 indicates an unrealistic expectation. Knowing normal growth and development activities for a 2-year-old will assist you to answer the question correctly. If you had difficulty with this question, take time now to review growth and development and the characteristics associated with child abuse!

Level of Cognitive Ability: Analysis
Phase of Nursing Process: Evaluation
Client Needs: Psychosocial Integrity
Content Area: Mental Health

Reference
Ashwill, J., & Droske, S. (1997). *Nursing care of children: Principles and practice.* Philadelphia: W. B. Saunders. pp. 1292–1293.

37. **3**

Rationale: Elder abuse is sometimes the result of family members who are being expected to care for their aging parents. This care can cause the family to become overextended, frustrated, or financially depleted. Knowing where to turn in the community for assistance in caring for aging family members can bring much-needed relief. Using these resources is a positive alternative coping strategy for many families.

Test-Taking Strategy: The stem of the question calls for a coping strategy. Only option 3 is a means of coping with the issues. The other responses are statements of good faith or promises that may or may not be kept in the future. Only option 3 outlines a definitive plan for how to handle the pressure associated with the father's care.

Level of Cognitive Ability: Analysis
Phase of Nursing Process: Evaluation
Client Needs: Health Promotion and Maintenance
Content Area: Mental Health

Reference
Carson, V., & Arnold, E. (1996). *Mental health nursing: The nurse-patient journey.* Philadelphia: W. B. Saunders. pp. 1070–1073.

38. **4**

Rationale: A client who is moderately depressed and has been in the hospital only 2 days is very unlikely to have such a dramatic cure. When a mood suddenly lifts, it is very likely that the client may have made the decision to harm self. Suicide precautions are necessary to keep the client safe.

Test-Taking Strategy: Options 1 and 2 support the client's notion that a cure has occurred, and the nurse must know that depression decreases over time. Option 3 allows the client to increase isolation and that would present a threat to the treatment plan. Safety is of the utmost importance now; therefore, option 4 is the choice.

Level of Cognitive Ability: Application
Phase of Nursing Process: Planning
Client Needs: Safe, Effective Care Environment
Content Area: Mental Health

Reference

Johnson, B. S. (1997). *Psychiatric-mental health nursing: Adaptation and growth* (4th ed.). Philadelphia: Lippincott-Raven. p. 862.

39. **4**

Rationale: There is less availability of nursing staff on the weekends, and the nurse should be alert to this high-risk time. Additionally, at shift change, many times there is less availability of staff. The psychiatric nurse and staff should increase precautions of identified clients at these times. The night shift is also more likely to have a suicide rather than the day shift.

Test-Taking Strategy: Options 1, 2, and 3 are similar and can be eliminated. The nurse could anticipate that times with less supervision of the client could be times of increased risks.

Level of Cognitive Ability: Application
Phase of Nursing Process: Planning
Client Needs: Safe, Effective Care Environment
Content Area: Mental Health

Reference

Johnson, B. S. (1997). *Psychiatric mental health nursing: Adaptation and growth* (4th ed.). Philadelphia: Lippincott-Raven. p. 862.

40. **3**

Rationale: One-to-one suicide precautions are required for the client who has attempted suicide. Options 1 and 2 may be appropriate but not at the present time, considering the situation. Option 4 may also be an appropriate nursing intervention, but the priority is stated in option 3. The best answer is constant supervision so that the nurse may intervene as needed if the client attempts to cause harm to self.

Test-Taking Strategy: Note the key word "priority" in the stem of the question. Options 1 and 2 can be easily eliminated. Focusing on the key word will easily direct you to option 3. Review interventions for the suicidal client now if you had difficulty with this question!

Level of Cognitive Ability: Application
Phase of Nursing Process: Implementation
Client Needs: Safe, Effective Care Environment
Content Area: Mental Health

Reference

Johnson, B. S. (1997). *Psychiatric-mental health nursing: Adaptation and growth* (4th ed.). Philadelphia: Lippincott-Raven. p. 871.

41. **4**

Rationale: Whenever the abused client remains in the abusive environment, priority must be placed on ascertaining whether the person is in any immediate danger. If so, emergency action must be taken to remove the client from the abusing situation. Options 1, 2, and 3 may be appropriate interventions but are not the priority.

Test-Taking Strategy: Use Maslow's hierarchy of needs, remembering that if a physiological need is not present, then safety is the priority. This guide should direct you to option 4, the only option that directly addresses client safety!

Level of Cognitive Ability: Application
Phase of Nursing Process: Planning
Client Needs: Safe, Effective Care Environment
Content Area: Mental Health

Reference

Carson, V., & Arnold, E. (1996). *Mental health nursing: The nurse-patient journey.* Philadelphia: W. B. Saunders. p. 1070.

42. **2**

Rationale: Option 2 is clearly the least effective response because there is no information in the stem which leads us to believe that the boyfriend's involvement has anything to do with the suicide attempt. Options 1, 3, and 4 are open-ended and offer helpful ways to enhance the family processes.

Test-Taking Strategy: The stem asks for the "least" effective option. Avoid reading into the question. There is no information in the stem that leads you to believe there is a problem with the boyfriend that led the adolescent to attempt suicide. It is important that a nurse remain nonjudgmental when dealing with clients. Additionally, options 1, 3, and 4 identify positive measures that will assure a safe environment for the client!

Level of Cognitive Ability: Application
Phase of Nursing Process: Implementation
Client Needs: Safe, Effective Care Environment
Content Area: Mental Health

Reference

Antai-Otong, D. (1995). *Psychiatric nursing: Biological and behavioral concepts.* Philadelphia: W. B. Saunders. p. 147.

43. **2**

Rationale: The anxiety symptoms demonstrated by this client require some form of intervention. Moving the client decreases environmental stimulus. Talking gives the nurse an opportunity to assess the cause of these feelings and to identify appropriate interventions. Seclusion is not appropriate. Medication is used only when other noninvasive approaches have been unsuccessful.

Test-Taking Strategy: Eliminate options 1 and 4 first. From the remaining two options, select option 2 over option 3 because it addresses the client's feelings. Remember, client's feelings are most important!

Level of Cognitive Ability: Application
Phase of Nursing Process: Implementation
Client Needs: Safe, Effective Care Environment
Content Area: Mental Health

Reference

Fortinash, K., & Holoday-Worret, P. (1996). *Psychiatric mental health nursing.* St. Louis: Mosby–Year Book. p. 231.

44. **2**

Rationale: Tertiary prevention of family violence includes assisting the victim once the abuse has already occurred. The nurse should provide the client with information about where to turn for help. This includes a specific plan for removing self from the abuser, information as to escaping, hot lines, and the location of shelters. An abused person is usually reluctant to call the police. Teaching the victim to fight back is not the appropriate action for the victim when dealing with a violent person.

Test-Taking Strategy: Focus on the issue of the question, which relates to providing the client with a safe environment. Use Maslow's hierarchy of needs theory to assist in directing you to option 2. If you had difficulty with this question, review the nursing measures for caring for a victim of family violence!

Level of Cognitive Ability: Application
Phase of Nursing Process: Implementation
Client Needs: Safe, Effective Care Environment
Content Area: Mental Health

Reference
Carson, V., & Arnold, E. (1996). *Mental health nursing: The nurse-patient journey.* Philadelphia: W. B. Saunders. pp. 1059–1061.

45. **2**

Rationale: Option 2 allows the client to express her ideas and feelings more fully and portrays a nonhurried, non-judgmental, supportive attitude. Clients need to be reassured that their feelings are normal and that they may freely express their concerns in a safe care environment.

Test-Taking Strategy: The client is seeking help. Option 1 places the problem solving totally on the client. Option 3 places the client's feelings on hold. Option 4 immediately blocks communication. Always address the client's feelings first!

Level of Cognitive Ability: Application
Phase of Nursing Process: Implementation
Client Needs: Psychosocial Integrity
Content Area: Mental Health

Reference
Carson, V., & Arnold, E. (1996). *Mental health nursing: The nurse-patient journey.* Philadelphia: W. B. Saunders. p. 1096.

46. **1**

Rationale: Drug overdose is a serious suicide attempt. The plan of care must reflect the action that will promote the client's safety. Constant observation status with a staff member who is never less than an arm's length away is the best selection.

Test-Taking Strategy: Eliminate option 4 first because it is not a roommate's responsibility to safeguard a client. Eliminate option 3 next because removing one's clothing does not maximize all possible safety strategies. From the remaining two options, select option 1 over option 2 because the correct option provides a constant supervision in this critical situation. You are likely to see questions similar to this on NCLEX-RN!

Level of Cognitive Ability: Application
Phase of Nursing Process: Implementation
Client Needs: Safe, Effective Care Environment
Content Area: Mental Health

Reference
Varcarolis, E. (1998). *Foundations of psychiatric mental health nursing* (3rd ed.). Philadelphia: W. B. Saunders. p. 736.

47. **4**

Rationale: The symptoms noted in the stem of the question indicate a normal reaction to a very intensely difficult crisis event. Although the client's initial reactions may be predictive of later problems, they do not indicate an abnormal initial response.

Test-Taking Strategy: During the acute phase of the rape crisis, the client can display a wide range of emotional and somatic responses. Use knowledge regarding client responses to devastating events and the process of elimination to answer the question. If you had difficulty with this question, take time now to review normal and abnormal client responses to dealing with devastating crisis events!

Level of Cognitive Ability: Analysis
Phase of Nursing Process: Analysis
Client Needs: Psychosocial Integrity
Content Area: Mental Health

Reference
Carson, V., & Arnold, E. (1996). *Mental health nursing: The nurse-patient journey.* Philadelphia: W. B. Saunders. pp. 1090–1092.

48. **1**

Rationale: Short-term goals will include the beginning stages of dealing with the rape trauma. Clients will be expected initially to keep appointments, participate in care, begin to explore feelings, and begin to heal physical wounds that were inflicted at the time of the rape.

Test-Taking Strategy: Note the key words "not" and "short-term initial goals." Use the process of elimination, considering each option and the reality of the option statement being achieved short-term. Note the word "resolved" in option 1. This word should provide you with the clue that this option is a long-term goal.

Level of Cognitive Ability: Application
Phase of Nursing Process: Planning
Client Needs: Psychosocial Integrity
Content Area: Mental Health

Reference
Carson, V., & Arnold, E. (1996). *Mental health nursing: The nurse-patient journey.* Philadelphia: W. B. Saunders. p. 1095.

49. **4**

Rationale: Option 4 allows the client to tell you more about what the current thoughts are. Option 1 is false reassurance and may close communication. While option 2 is offering empathy for the client, it does not further assess. Option 3 changes the subject and may close communication.

Test-Taking Strategy: Use the nursing process to select the correct option. Options 1 and 2 can be easily eliminated because they do not reflect assessment. Both options 3 and 4 relate to further assessment, but option 4 is directly related to the issue of the question.

Level of Cognitive Ability: Application
Phase of Nursing Process: Implementation
Client Needs: Psychosocial Integrity
Content Area: Mental Health

Reference
Johnson, B. S. (1997). *Psychiatric-mental health nursing: Adaptation and growth* (4th ed.). Philadelphia: Lippincott-Raven. pp. 866–871.

50. 4

Rationale: Options 1, 2, and 3 identify a positive movement toward increased self-esteem and problem solving. Option 4 places undue pressure on the client by implying that the client was negligent and contributed to the loss.

Test-Taking Strategy: Note the key phrase "least realistic." The words "realistic" and "adaptive," and the phrase "express and share feelings" in options 1, 2, and 3, respectively, identify positive goals. This should assist in directing you to option 4. Additionally, there is nothing in the question which indicates that the client lacked insurance, as option 4 reflects.

Level of Cognitive Ability: Analysis
Phase of Nursing Process: Planning
Client Needs: Psychosocial Integrity
Content Area: Mental Health

Reference
Antai-Otong, D. (1995). *Psychiatric nursing: Biological and behavioral concepts.* Philadelphia: W. B. Saunders. p. 147.

BIBLIOGRAPHY

Antai-Otong, D. (1995). *Psychiatric nursing: Biological and behavioral concepts.* Philadelphia: W. B. Saunders.

Ashwill, J., & Droske, S. (1997). *Nursing care of children: Principles and practice.* Philadelphia: W. B. Saunders.

Carson, V., & Arnold, E. (1996). *Mental health nursing: The nurse-patient journey.* Philadelphia: W. B. Saunders.

Fortinash, K., & Holoday-Worret, P. (1996). *Psychiatric mental health nursing.* St. Louis: Mosby–Year Book.

Glod, C. A. (1998). *Contemporary psychiatric-mental health nursing.* Philadelphia: F. A. Davis.

Hodgson, B., & Kizior, R. (1999). *Saunders nursing drug handbook 1999.* Philadelphia: W. B. Saunders.

Johnson, B. S. (1997). *Psychiatric-mental health nursing: Adaptation and growth* (4th ed.). Philadelphia: Lippincott-Raven.

Stuart, G. W., & Laraia, M. T. (1998). *Principles and practice of psychiatric nursing* (6th ed.). St. Louis: Mosby–Year Book.

Varcarolis, E. (1998). *Foundations of psychiatric mental health nursing* (3rd ed.). Philadelphia: W. B. Saunders.

CHAPTER 74

Psychiatric Medications

. . . .

I. Selective Serotonin Reuptake Inhibitors (SSRI) (Box 74–1)

A. Description
1. Inhibit serotonin uptake
2. Produce an antidepressant response

B. Side effects
1. Nausea
2. Diarrhea
3. Central nervous system (CNS) stimulation
4. Dry mouth
5. Photosensitivity
6. Insomnia
7. Headache
8. Nervousness
9. Dizziness
10. Weight loss

C. Implementation
1. Monitor vital signs
2. Monitor weight
3. Initiate safety precautions, particularly if dizziness occurs
4. Instruct client to take a single morning dose to prevent insomnia
5. Administer with a snack or with meals, which reduces the risk of dizziness and lightheadedness
6. Monitor suicidal client, especially during improved mood and increased energy levels
7. For clients on long-term therapy, monitor liver and renal function tests
8. Monitor white blood cell (WBC) and neutrophil counts and discontinue the medication, as prescribed, if levels fall below normal
9. If priapism (painful, prolonged penile erection) occurs, discontinue medication immediately and notify physician
10. Instruct client to change positions slowly to avoid hypotensive effect
11. Instruct client to avoid alcohol
12. Instruct client to report any visual changes to the physician

II. Tricyclic and Second-Generation Antidepressants (Box 74–2)

A. Description
1. Blocks the reuptake of norepinephrine and serotonin at the presynaptic neuron
2. Used to treat depression
3. May reduce seizure threshold
4. May reduce effectiveness of antihypertensive agents
5. Concurrent use with alcohol or antihistamines can cause CNS depression
6. Concurrent use with monoamine oxidase (MAO) inhibitors can cause hypertensive crisis

B. Side effects
1. Anticholinergic effects
2. Dry mouth
3. Decreased gastrointestinal (GI) motility and constipation
4. Difficulty in voiding
5. Dilated pupils and blurred vision
6. Photosensitivity
7. Cardiovascular disturbances
8. Tachycardia
9. Orthostatic hypotension
10. Dysrhythmias
11. Sedation
12. Weight gain
13. Anxiety, restlessness, and irritability
14. Decreased or increased libido with ejaculatory and erection disturbances

C. Implementation
1. Instruct client that the medication may take several weeks to produce the desired effect

---

BOX 74–1. Selective Serotonin Reuptake Inhibitors (SSRI)

Fluoxetine hydrochloride (Prozac)
Sertraline hydrochloride (Zoloft)
Paroxetine (Paxil)
Nefazodone (Serzone)
Trazodone (Desyrel)

> **BOX 74–2. Tricyclic and Second-Generation Antidepressants**
>
> Clomipramine hydrochloride (Anafranil)
> Amitriptyline hydrochloride (Elavil)
> Imipramine hydrochloride (Tofranil)
> Norpramine (Desipramine)
> Nortriptyline hydrochloride (Pamelor, Aventyl)
> Perphenazine and amitriptyline (Triavil)
> Doxepin hydrochloride (Sinequan)
> Chlordiazepoxide and amitriptyline (Limbitrol)
> Bupropion (Wellbutrin)
> Prozac (Fluoxetine)
> Trazodone (Desyrel)
> Amoxapine (Asendin)

2. Client response may not occur until 2 to 4 weeks after the first dose
3. Monitor for compliance of therapy
4. Monitor suicidal client, especially during improved mood and increased energy levels
5. Instruct client to change positions slowly to avoid hypotensive effect
6. Monitor pattern of daily bowel activity
7. Assess for urinary retention by bladder palpation
8. For clients on long-term therapy, monitor liver and renal function tests
9. Administer with food or milk if GI distress occurs
10. Administer the entire daily oral dose at one time, preferably at bedtime
11. Instruct client on fluoxetine (Prozac) to take medication early in the day to avoid interference with sleep
12. Instruct client to avoid alcohol and nonprescription medications to prevent adverse medication interactions
13. Instruct client to avoid driving and other activities requiring alertness
14. When the medication is discontinued, it should be tapered gradually

III. Monoamine Oxidase Inhibitors (MAOIs) (Box 74–3)

A. Description
   1. Inhibit MAO enzyme, which is present in the brain, blood platelets, liver, spleen, and kidneys
   2. Inhibition of the MAO enzyme metabolizes amines, norepinephrine, and serotonin, and the concentration of these amines increases

> **BOX 74–3. Monoamine Oxidase Inhibitors (MAOIs)**
>
> Isocarboxazid (Marplan)
> Phenelzine sulfate (Nardil)
> Tranylcypromine sulfate (Parnate)

3. Used for depression in clients who have not responded to other antidepressant therapy, including electroconvulsive therapy
4. Concurrent use with amphetamines, antidepressants, dopamine, epinephrine, guanethidine, levodopa, methyldopa, nasal decongestants, norepinephrine, reserpine, tyramine-containing foods, and vasoconstrictors may cause hypertensive crisis
5. Concurrent use with narcotic analgesics may cause hypertension or hypotension, coma, or seizures

B. Side effects
   1. Orthostatic hypotension
   2. Restlessness
   3. Insomnia
   4. Dizziness
   5. Lethargy
   6. Weakness
   7. GI upset
   8. Dry mouth
   9. Weight gain
   10. Peripheral edema
   11. Anticholinergic effects
   12. CNS stimulation, including anxiety, agitation, and mania
   13. Delay in ejaculation

C. Hypertensive crisis
   1. Hypertension
   2. Occipital headache radiating frontally
   3. Neck stiffness and soreness
   4. Nausea and vomiting
   5. Sweating
   6. Fever and chills
   7. Clammy skin
   8. Dilated pupils
   9. Palpitations
   10. Tachycardia or bradycardia
   11. Constricting chest pain
   12. Antidote for hypertensive crisis: 5 mg of phentolamine (Regitine) by IV injection

D. Implementation
   1. Monitor blood pressure frequently for hypertension
   2. Monitor for signs of hypertensive crisis
   3. If palpitations or frequent headaches occur, discontinue medication and notify physician
   4. Administer with food if GI distress occurs
   5. Instruct client that the medication effect may be noted during the first week of therapy, but maximum benefit may take up to 3 weeks
   6. Instruct client to report headache, neck stiffness, or neck soreness immediately
   7. Instruct client to change positions slowly to prevent orthostatic hypotension
   8. Instruct client to avoid caffeine or over-the-counter preparations such as weight-reducing pills or medications for hay fever and colds
   9. Monitor for client compliance with medication administration

---

BOX 74–4. Tyramine Foods to Avoid

Cheese, especially aged, except cottage cheese
Sour cream
Pickled herring
Avocados
Bananas
Papaya
Broad beans
Figs
Overripe fruit
Brewer's yeast
Meat extracts and tenderizers
Yogurt
Sausage, bologna, pepperoni, salami
Soy sauce
Raisins
Red wine, beer, sherry
Beef and chicken livers
Caffeine as coffee, tea, or chocolate

---

10. Instruct client to carry a Medic-Alert card indicating the taking of a MAOI medication
11. Avoid administering the medication in the evening because insomnia may result
12. MAO inhibitors should be tapered and discontinued 7 to 14 days before surgery
13. When the medication is discontinued, it should be discontinued gradually
14. Instruct client to avoid foods that require bacteria/molds for their preparation/preservation or those that contain tyramine (Box 74–4)

IV. Antimanic Medications (Box 74–5)

A. Description
   1. Affect cellular transport mechanism, alter both the presynaptic and postsynaptic events affecting serotonin, thus enhancing serotonin function
   2. Concurrent use with diuretics, fluoxetine, methyldopa, or nonsteroidal anti-inflammatory medications increases lithium reabsorption by the kidney, or inhibits lithium excretion, either of which increases the risk of lithium toxicity
   3. Acetazolamide, aminophylline, phenothiazines, and sodium bicarbonate may increase renal excretion of lithium, reducing its effectiveness
   4. The therapeutic dose is only slightly less than the amount producing toxicity

---

BOX 74–5. Antimanic Medications

Lithium carbonate (Eskalith, Lithane, Lithobid)
Lithium citrate (Cibalith-S)

---

5. The therapeutic drug serum level is 0.5 to 1.3 mEq/L
6. The causes of an increase in lithium level include decreased sodium intake, fluid and electrolyte loss associated with severe sweating, dehydration, diarrhea, diuretic therapy or illness, and overdose
7. Serum lithium levels should be checked every 1 to 2 months or whenever any behavioral change suggests an altered serum level
8. Blood samples to check serum lithium levels should be drawn in the morning, 12 hours after the last dose

B. Side effects
   1. Polyuria
   2. Polydipsia
   3. Anorexia
   4. Nausea
   5. Dry mouth
   6. Mild thirst
   7. Weight gain
   8. Abdominal bloating
   9. Soft stools or diarrhea
   10. Fine hand tremors
   11. Inability to concentrate
   12. Muscle weakness
   13. Lethargy
   14. Fatigue
   15. Headache
   16. Hair loss

C. Implementation
   1. Monitor suicidal client, especially during improved mood and increased energy levels
   2. Administer medication with food to minimize GI irritation
   3. Instruct client to maintain a fluid intake of 6 to 8 glasses of water a day
   4. Instruct client to avoid excessive amounts of coffee, tea, or cola, which have a diuretic effect
   5. Instruct client to maintain an adequate salt intake
   6. Do not administer diuretics while the client is taking lithium
   7. Instruct client to avoid alcohol
   8. Instruct the client to avoid over-the-counter medications
   9. Instruct clients that they may take a missed dose within 2 hours of the scheduled time; otherwise they should skip the missed dose and take the next dose at the scheduled time
   10. Instruct client not to adjust the dosage without consulting the physician as lithium should be tapered off and not discontinued abruptly
   11. Instruct client about the signs and symptoms of lithium toxicity
   12. Instruct client to notify the physician if polyuria, prolonged vomiting, diarrhea, or fever occurs
   13. Instruct client that the therapeutic response

to the medication will be noted in 1 to 3
weeks
14. Monitor electrocardiogram (ECG), renal
function tests, and thyroid tests
D. Lithium toxicity
1. Description
a. Occurs when ingested lithium cannot be
detoxified and excreted by the kidneys
b. Occurs when the serum lithium level
exceeds 2.0 mEq/L
2. Mild toxicity
a. Serum lithium level above 1.5 mEq/L
b. Apathy
c. Lethargy
d. Diminished concentration
e. Mild ataxia
f. Coarse hand tremors
g. Slight muscle weakness
3. Moderate toxicity
a. Serum lithium level of 1.5 to 2.5 mEq/L
b. Nausea
c. Vomiting
d. Severe diarrhea
e. Mild to moderate ataxia and
incoordination
f. Slurred speech
g. Tinnitus
h. Blurred vision
i. Muscle twitching
j. Irregular tremors
4. Severe toxicity
a. Serum lithium level above 2.5 mEq/L
b. Nystagmus
c. Muscle fasciculations
d. Deep tendon hyperreflexia
e. Visual or tactile hallucinations
f. Oliguria or anuria
g. Impaired level of consciousness (LOC)
h. Grand mal seizure or coma leading to
death
5. Implementation for lithium toxicity
a. Withhold lithium and notify physician
b. Monitor vital signs and LOC
c. Monitor cardiac status
d. Prepare to obtain lithium level;
electrolyte, blood urea nitrogen (BUN),
and creatinine counts; and CBC
e. Monitor for suicidal tendencies and
institute suicide precautions

V. Antianxiety or Anxiolytic Medications

A. Description
1. Depress the CNS, thereby increasing the
effects of gamma-aminobutyric acid (GABA),
which produces relaxation and may depress
the limbic system
2. Benzodiazepines have anxiety-reducing
(anxiolytic), sedative-hypnotic, muscle-
relaxing, and anticonvulsant actions (Box
74–6)

BOX 74–6. Benzodiazepines

Diazepam (Valium)	Estazolam (ProSom)
Alprazolam (Xanax)	Chlordiazepoxide
Clorazepate (Tranxene)	(Librium)
Oxazepam (Serax)	Clonazepam (Klonopin)
Flurazepam (Dalmane)	Halazepam (Paxipam)
Temazepam (Restoril)	Prazepam (Centrax)
Triazolam (Halcion)	Quazepam (Doral)
Lorazepam (Ativan)	

B. Side effects
1. Daytime sedation
2. Ataxia
3. Dizziness
4. Headaches
5. Blurred or double vision
6. Hypotension
7. Tremor
8. Amnesia
9. Slurred speech
10. Urinary incontinence
11. Constipation
12. Paradoxical CNS excitement
C. Acute toxicity
1. Somnolence
2. Confusion
3. Diminished reflexes and coma
4. Flumazenil (Romazicon), a benzodiazepine
antagonist, administered IV, will reverse
benzodiazepine intoxication in 5 minutes
5. Clients being treated for an overdose of
benzodiazepines may experience agitation,
restlessness, discomfort, and anxiety
D. Implementation
1. Monitor for motor responses, such as
agitation, trembling, and tension
2. Monitor for autonomic responses, such as
cold, clammy hands and sweating
3. Monitor for paradoxical CNS excitement
during early therapy, particularly in elderly
and debilitated people
4. Monitor for visual disturbances since the
medications can worsen glaucoma
5. Monitor liver and renal function tests and
blood counts
6. Reduce the medication dose as prescribed for
older adult clients and for clients with
impaired liver function
7. Initiate safety precautions because older
clients are at risk for falling when taking
these medications for sleep or anxiety
8. Assist with ambulation if drowsiness or
lightheadedness occurs
9. Instruct client that drowsiness usually
disappears during continued therapy
10. Instruct client to avoid tasks that require
alertness until the response to the
medication is established
11. Instruct client to avoid alcohol

12. Instruct client not to take other medications without consulting the physician
13. Instruct client not to withdraw the medication abruptly
E. Withdrawal
   1. To lessen withdrawal symptoms, the dosage of benzodiazepines should be tapered gradually over 2 to 6 weeks
   2. Abrupt or too rapid withdrawal results in:
      a. Restlessness
      b. Irritability
      c. Insomnia
      d. Hand tremors
      e. Abdominal or muscle cramps
      f. Sweating
      g. Vomiting
      h. Seizures

VI. Medications for Insomnia and Anxiety (Box 74–7)

A. Description
   1. Depress the reticular activating system by promoting the inhibitory synaptic action of the neurotransmitter GABA
   2. Used for short-term treatment of insomnia or for sedation to relieve anxiety, tension, and apprehension
B. Side effects
   1. Confusion
   2. Irritability
   3. Allergic reactions
   4. Agranulocytosis
   5. Thrombocytopenic purpura
   6. Megaloblastic anemia
C. Overdose
   1. Tachycardia
   2. Hypotension
   3. Cold and clammy skin
   4. Dilated pupils
   5. Weak and rapid pulse
   6. Signs of shock
   7. Depressed respirations
   8. Absent reflexes
   9. Coma and death may result from respiratory and cardiovascular collapse

---

BOX 74–7. Barbiturates

Amobarbital (Amytal)
Aprobarbital (Alurate)
Butabarbital (Butisol)
Pentobarbital (Nembutal)
Phenobarbital (Luminal)
Secobarbital (Seconal)
Buspirone (BuSpar)
Chloral hydrate
Ethchlorvynol (Placidyl)
Hydroxyzine hydrochloride (Atarax)
Meprobamate (Equanil)
Zolpidem tartrate (Ambien)

D. Withdrawal
   1. Severe withdrawal symptoms begin within 24 hours after the medication is discontinued in an individual with severe drug dependence
   2. Gradual withdrawal is used to detoxify a dependent person
   3. Anxiety
   4. Insomnia
   5. Nightmares
   6. Daytime agitation
   7. Tremors
   8. Delirium
   9. Seizures
E. Implementation
   1. Administer lower doses as prescribed for elderly clients
   2. Medications should be used with caution in clients who are suicidal or have a history of drug addiction
   3. Maintain safety by supervising ambulation and using side rails at night
   4. Instruct client to take medication as directed
   5. Instruct client to avoid driving or operating hazardous equipment if drowsiness, dizziness, or unsteadiness occurs
   6. Instruct client to avoid alcohol
   7. For insomnia, instruct client to take the medication 30 minutes before bedtime
   8. Instruct the client that a hangover effect may occur in the morning
   9. Instruct the client not to discontinue the medication abruptly
   10. Instruct the client taking chloral hydrate to take the medication with food or a full glass of water, fruit juice, or ginger ale to improve taste and to minimize gastric irritation

VII. Antipsychotic Medications (Box 74–8)

A. Description
   1. Improve the thought processes and behavior of clients with psychotic symptoms, especially those with schizophrenia
   2. Block dopamine receptors in the brain, thereby reducing the psychotic symptoms
   3. Block the chemoreceptor trigger zone and vomiting center in the brain, producing an antiemetic effect
   4. Phenothiazines lower the seizure threshold
   5. Antipsychotics should not be given with other antipsychotic or antidepressant medications
B. Side effects
   1. Anticholinergic effects
   2. Dry mouth
   3. Increased heart rate
   4. Urinary retention
   5. Constipation
   6. Hypotension
   7. Drowsiness
   8. Blood dyscrasias

BOX 74–8. Antipsychotic Medications

PHENOTHIAZINES

Chlorpromazine hydrochloride (Thorazine)
Promazine hydrochloride (Sparine)
Triflupromazine (Vesprin)
Fluphenazine hydrochloride (Prolixin)
Perphenazine (Trilafon)
Prochlorperazine maleate (Compazine)
Acetophenazine maleate (Tindal)
Trifluoperazine hydrochloride (Stelazine)
Mesoridazine besylate (Serentil)
Thioridazine hydrochloride (Mellaril)

NONPHENOTHIAZINES

Droperidol (Inapsine)
Haloperidol (Haldol)
Loxapine (Loxitane)
Chlorprothixene hydrochloride (Taractan)
Thiothixene hydrochloride (Navane)

OTHER ANTIPSYCHOTICS

Clozapine (Clozaril)
Molindone hydrochloride (Moban)
Risperidone (Risperdal)

9. Pruritus
10. Photosensitivity

C. Extrapyramidal syndrome
   1. Parkinsonism
      a. Tremors
      b. Mask-like facies
      c. Rigidity
      d. Shuffling gait
   2. Dystonia
      a. Facial grimacing
      b. Abnormal or involuntary eye movements
   3. Akathisia
      a. Restlessness
      b. Constant moving about
   4. Tardive dyskinesia
      a. Protrusion of the tongue
      b. Chewing motion
      c. Involuntary movement of the body and extremities

D. Implementation
   1. Monitor vital signs
   2. Monitor for extrapyramidal syndrome
   3. Monitor for symptoms of neuroleptic malignant syndrome
   4. Monitor urine output
   5. Monitor for blood dyscrasias
   6. Note that clients taking antipsychotic medications may require long-term medication for parkinsonian symptoms
   7. For oral use, the liquid form might be preferred because some clients hide tablets to avoid taking them
   8. Administer medication with food or milk to decrease gastric irritation
   9. Note that the absorption rate is faster with the liquid form
   10. Avoid skin contact with liquid concentrates to prevent contact dermatitis
   11. Protect liquid concentrates from light
   12. Dilute liquid concentrates with fruit juice
   13. Inform client that a full therapeutic effect of the medication may not be evident for 3 to 6 weeks following initiation of therapy; however, an observable therapeutic response may be apparent after 7 to 10 days
   14. Inform client that phenothiazines may cause a harmless pinkish to red-brown urine color
   15. Instruct client to use sunscreen, hats, and protective clothing when outdoors
   16. Instruct client to avoid alcohol or other CNS depressants
   17. Instruct client to change positions slowly to avoid orthostatic hypotension
   18. Instruct client to report signs of agranulocytosis, including sore throat, fever, and malaise
   19. Instruct client to report signs of liver dysfunction, including jaundice, malaise, fever, right upper abdominal pain
   20. When discontinuing antipsychotics, the medication dosage should be reduced gradually to avoid sudden recurrence of psychotic symptoms

VIII. Neuroleptic Malignant Syndrome

A. Description
   1. A potentially fatal syndrome that may occur at any time during therapy with neuroleptic medications (antipsychotic or antischizophrenic medications)
   2. Although it is rare, it is more commonly seen at the initiation of therapy, after clients are changed from one medication to another, after a dosage increase, or when a combination of medications is used

B. Assessment
   1. Dyspnea or tachypnea
   2. Tachycardia or irregular pulse rate
   3. Fever
   4. High or low blood pressure
   5. Increased sweating
   6. Loss of bladder control
   7. Skeletal muscle rigidity
   8. Pale skin
   9. Excessive weakness or fatigue
   10. Altered level of consciousness
   11. Seizures
   12. Severe extrapyramidal side effects
   13. Difficulty in swallowing
   14. Excessive salivation
   15. Oculogyric crisis
   16. Dyskinesia
   17. Elevated WBC count
   18. Elevated liver function tests
   19. Elevated creatine phosphokinase (CPK) level

C. Implementation
   1. Notify physician

2. Monitor vital signs
3. Initiate safety and seizure precautions
4. Discontinue neuroleptic medication
5. Monitor LOC
6. Administer antipyretics as prescribed
7. Use a cooling blanket to lower temperature
8. Monitor electrolytes and administer IV fluids as prescribed

PRACTICE QUESTIONS

1. A client receiving lithium carbonate complains of loose, watery stools and difficulty in walking. The nurse expects the serum lithium level to be which of the following?
   1 0.7 mEq/L
   2 1.0 mEq/L
   3 1.3 mEq/L
   4 1.7 mEq/L

2. When teaching a client who is being started on imipramine hydrochloride (Tofranil), the nurse would inform the client that the desired effects
   1 May start during the first week of administration
   2 May start during the second week of administration
   3 May not occur for 2 to 3 weeks after administration
   4 May not occur until after a month of administration

3. A client receiving thioridazine (Mellaril) complains that he feels very "faint" when trying to get out of bed in the morning. The nurse recognizes this complaint as a symptom of
   1 Psychosomatic problems
   2 Cardiac dysrhythmias
   3 Respiratory insufficiency
   4 Postural hypotension

4. A client who is on lithium carbonate therapy is scheduled for surgery. The nurse informs the client that
   1 The medication will be discontinued several days before surgery and resumed by injection in the immediate postoperative period
   2 The medication is to be taken until the day of surgery and resumed by injection immediately postoperatively
   3 The medication will be discontinued 1 to 2 days before the surgery and resumed as soon as full oral intake is allowed
   4 The medication will be discontinued a week before the surgery and resumed a week postoperatively

5. The client receiving tricyclic antidepressants arrives at the mental health clinic. Which observation indicates that the client is correctly following the medication plan?
   1 Reports sleeping 12 hours per night and 3 to 4 hours during the day
   2 Arrives at the clinic neat and appropriate in appearance
   3 Reports not going to work for this past week
   4 Complains of not being able to "do anything" anymore

6. The nurse is performing a follow-up teaching session with a client discharged 1 month ago. The client is taking fluoxetine (Prozac). What information is important for the nurse to gather, during this client visit, regarding the adverse effects related to the medication?
   1 Problems with excessive sweating
   2 Gastrointestinal (GI) dysfunctions
   3 Cardiovascular symptoms
   4 Problems with mouth dryness

7. The client taking buspirone hydrochloride (BuSpar) for 1 month returns for a postdischarge assessment. Which of the following manifestations indicates medication effectiveness?
   1 No report of alcohol withdrawal symptoms
   2 No paranoid thought process
   3 No rapid heartbeat or anxiety
   4 No thought broadcasting or delusions

8. A client taking lithium carbonate reports vomiting, abdominal pain, diarrhea, blurred vision, tinnitus, and tremors. The lithium level is assessed as a part of the routine follow-up. The level is 3.0 mEq/L. The nurse knows this level is
   1 Normal
   2 Slightly above normal
   3 Excessively below normal
   4 Toxic

9. A client is placed on chloral hydrate for short-term treatment. What nursing action indicates a clear understanding of the major side effect of this medication?
   1 Monitor neurological signs every 2 hours
   2 Monitor blood pressure every 4 hours
   3 Instruct client to call for ambulation assistance
   4 Lower bed and clear a path to the bathroom at bedtime

10. The home health nurse visits the client. The client gives the nurse a bottle of clomipramine (Anafranil). The nurse notes that the medication has not been taken by the client in 2 months. What behaviors observed in the client validate noncompliance with this medication?
    1 Frequent handwashing with hot, soapy water
    2 Complaints of weight gain
    3 Complaints of dry mouth
    4 Complaints of insomnia

11. An adult client is administered haloperidol (Haldol), 3 mg PO BID for a psychotic disorder. The nurse develops a plan of care and determines that the priority assessment is to

1 Check vital signs, compare the data, and record

2 Assess the physical safety of other unit clients

3 Monitor client's nutritional intake

4 Assess client's orientation and delusional status

12. Diphenhydramine hydrochloride (Benadryl) is used in the treatment of allergic rhinitis for a hospitalized client with a chronic psychotic disorder. This medication will not be continued at home because the nurse is aware that
   1 Allergic symptoms are short-term in duration
   2 Poor compliance causes this medication to fail to reach its therapeutic blood level
   3 Addictive properties are enhanced in the presence of psychotropic medications
   4 This medication promotes long-term extrapyramidal symptoms

13. The home health nurse visits the client at home. The client tells the nurse that she has been doubling the daily dosage of bupropion (Wellbutrin) to aid her in getting better faster. Which ongoing nursing assessment is required, based on this information?
   1 Monitor for orthostatic hypotension
   2 Monitor for seizure activity
   3 Monitor for weight gain
   4 Monitor for insomnia

14. Immediately after taking a routine evening dose of alprazolam (Xanax), a client says "I'm not sure I should have taken that stuff." The best response by the nurse is
   1 "You are afraid of the media claims about this medication."
   2 "Your depression will fade once the medication begins to work."
   3 "Anxiety is expected with any new experience."
   4 "Let's talk about how you feel about Xanax for a while."

15. Of the following actions by the nurse, which one demonstrates an understanding of safe administration of sertraline hydrochloride (Zoloft)?
   1 Administering the medication TID, as prescribed
   2 Administering the medication daily at 9:00 A.M.
   3 Administering the medication on an empty stomach
   4 Withholding the medication if tearfulness or melancholia is present

16. The physician orders phenobarbital sodium (Luminal), 10 mL by mouth daily. The medication bottle is labeled 20 mg/5 mL. What will the nurse administer?
   1 18.2 mg
   2 40 mg
   3 18.2 mL
   4 36.4 mL

17. A client is discharged on phenobarbital sodium, 100 mg by mouth BID. Which of the following statements, if made by the client, reflects an accurate understanding of safety precautions with this medication?
   1 "I must take my medication at the same time daily."
   2 "Using a daily dosing system container is helpful to the prevention of an overdose."
   3 "Drinking one beer may change the way my medication works."
   4 "I can take my medication with food if I need to."

18. A 20-year-old client takes thiothixene (Navane) at 9:00 A.M. daily. This is the first week of therapy with this medication. In planning a 10:00 A.M. bowling activity, which of the following is important?
   1 Noting the client's history of psychotic features
   2 Listening to the client's desire for 8 hours of sleep
   3 Planning nutritional snacks
   4 Developing a long-term relationship

19. Fluphenazine (Prolixin) is administered to a client daily. The nurse monitors for the common side effects of the medication. Which of the following does the nurse include in the plan of care?
   1 Monitor the blood pressure every 2 hours
   2 Review the WBC results daily
   3 Offer a nutritious snack between meals
   4 Offer hard candy or gum periodically

20. An 83-year-old client with dementia and dysphagia is frequently agitated and hyperactive due to insomnia. Secobarbital (Seconal), 100 mg by mouth, is prescribed and will be administered at home each evening by a family member. Seconal is supplied in 50-mg and 100-mg tablets. Which of the following instructions is most appropriate regarding the administration of the medication to this client?
   1 Administer one 100-mg tablet each evening
   2 Administer two 50-mg tablets each evening
   3 Administer the medication sprinkled evenly over the evening meal
   4 Administer the medication crushed in 1 tablespoon of applesauce

ANSWERS

1. 4

Rationale: The therapeutic serum level of lithium is 1.0 to 1.5 mEq/L for clients with acute mania and 0.6 to 0.8 mEq/L for maintenance levels. Serum lithium concentrations of 1.5 to 2.0 mEq/L may produce vomiting, diarrhea, drowsiness, incoordination, coarse hand tremors, muscle twitching, ECG T wave depression, and mental confusion.

Test-Taking Strategy: Knowledge regarding lithium carbonate and serum lithium levels is required to answer the question. Take time now to review this information. You will see questions related to this content on NCLEX-RN!

Level of Cognitive Ability: Analysis
Phase of Nursing Process: Analysis
Client Needs: Physiological Integrity
Content Area: Pharmacology

Reference
Hodgson, B., & Kizior, R. (1999). *Saunders nursing drug handbook 1999.* Philadelphia: W. B. Saunders. pp. 598–600.

2. 3

Rationale: The therapeutic effects of administration of imipramine hydrochloride may not occur for 2 to 3 weeks after the antidepressant therapy has been initiated.

Test-Taking Strategy: Knowledge regarding the therapeutic effect of imipramine hydrochloride is required to answer this question. Take time now to review this information. Client information regarding the medication needs to be thorough and accurate!

Level of Cognitive Ability: Application
Phase of Nursing Process: Implementation
Client Needs: Health Promotion and Maintenance
Content Area: Pharmacology

Reference
Hodgson, B., & Kizior, R. (1999). *Saunders nursing drug handbook 1999.* Philadelphia: W. B. Saunders. p. 522.

3. 4

Rationale: Neuroleptic medications can cause postural hypotension. The client needs to be taught to get out of bed slowly and to rise from a sitting position slowly because of this untoward effect related to the medication.

Test-Taking Strategy: The key phrase in the question is "feeling faint." This phrase will direct you to the correct option. Postural hypotension is a common complaint of clients taking neuroleptic medications.

Level of Cognitive Ability: Analysis
Phase of Nursing Process: Analysis
Client Needs: Physiological Integrity
Content Area: Pharmacology

Reference
Townsend, M. C. (1996). *Psychiatric-mental health nursing: Concepts of care* (2nd ed.). Philadelphia: F. A. Davis. p. 288.

4. 3

Rationale: The client who is on lithium carbonate must be off the medication from 1 to 2 days before the surgery and can resume the medication when full oral intake is ordered after the surgery.

Test-Taking Strategy: Use the process of elimination to answer the question. Lithium carbonate is an oral medication. It cannot be given as an injection. Therefore, eliminate options 1 and 2. Option 4 identifies a period of time that is unreasonable. Therefore, select option 3.

Level of Cognitive Ability: Application
Phase of Nursing Process: Implementation
Client Needs: Physiological Integrity
Content Area: Pharmacology

Reference
Hodgson, B., & Kizior, R. (1999). *Saunders nursing drug handbook 1999.* Philadelphia: W. B. Saunders. pp. 598–600.

5. 2

Rationale: Depressed individuals will sleep for long periods, are not able to go to work, and feel as if they cannot "do anything." Once they have had some therapeutic effect from their medication, they will report resolution of many of these complaints as well as demonstrate an improvement in their appearance.

Test-Taking Strategy: Use the process of elimination to answer the question. The symptoms stated in options 1, 3, and 4 are all symptoms of depression. The improvement in appearance indicates a therapeutic response to the medication, thus compliance with the medication regimen.

Level of Cognitive Ability: Analysis
Phase of Nursing Process: Evaluation
Client Needs: Physiological Integrity
Content Area: Pharmacology

Reference
Lehne, R. (1998). *Pharmacology for nursing care* (3rd ed.). Philadelphia: W. B. Saunders. p. 300.

6. 2

Rationale: Excessive sweating or dry mouth are not associated side effects of this medication. The most common adverse reactions related to this medication include central nervous system and GI dysfunction. Fluoxetine (Prozac) affects the GI system by causing nausea and vomiting, cramping, and diarrhea.

Test-Taking Strategy: Knowledge regarding the side effects and adverse reactions related to Prozac is required to answer this question. Take time now to review this information if you had difficulty with this question!

Level of Cognitive Ability: Application
Phase of Nursing Process: Assessment
Client Needs: Physiological Integrity
Content Area: Pharmacology

Reference
Kaplan, H., & Sadock, B. (1996). *Pocket handbook of psychiatric drug treatment* (2nd ed.). Baltimore: Williams & Wilkins. p. 146.

7. 3

Rationale: Buspirone hydrochloride is not recommended for the treatment of drug or alcohol withdrawal, thought disorders, or schizophrenia. BuSpar is most often indicated for the treatment of anxiety and aggression.

Test-Taking Strategy: Read all four options carefully. Use the process of elimination. Knowledge regarding the use of BuSpar will direct you to the correct option. Take time now to review this medication if you had difficulty with this question!

Level of Cognitive Ability: Analysis
Phase of Nursing Process: Evaluation
Client Needs: Physiological Integrity
Content Area: Pharmacology

References
Pinnell, N. (1996). *Nursing pharmacology.* Philadelphia: W. B. Saunders. p. 161.
Kaplan, H., & Sadock, B. (1996). *Pocket handbook of psychiatric drug treatment* (2nd ed.). Baltimore: Williams & Wilkins. p. 65.

8. **4**

Rationale: Routine maintenance serum levels of lithium are 0.6 to 0.8 mEq/L. Mild to moderate lithium intoxication occurs at 1.5 to 2.0 mEq/L. Levels of less than 0.4 mEq/L do not produce a therapeutic effect. Severe toxic levels are reached at levels greater than 2.5 mEq/L. Lithium toxicity requires immediate medical attention, with lavage and possible peritoneal dialysis or hemodialysis.

Test-Taking Strategy: Knowledge regarding lithium carbonate and serum lithium levels is required to answer the question. Take time now to review this information. You will see questions related to this content on NCLEX-RN!

Level of Cognitive Ability: Analysis
Phase of Nursing Process: Analysis
Client Needs: Physiological Integrity
Content Area: Pharmacology

References
Pinnell, N. (1996). *Nursing pharmacology.* Philadelphia: W. B. Saunders. p. 204.
Kaplan, H., & Sadock, B. (1996). *Pocket handbook of psychiatric drug treatment* (2nd ed.). Baltimore: Williams & Wilkins. p. 130.

9. **3**

Rationale: Monitoring neurological signs every 2 hours is not indicated. This medication does not cause serious neurological impairment. Blood pressure decreases to critical levels are rare in the absence of other BP problems. There may be residual daytime sedation and impairment of motor coordination; therefore, instruct the client to call for ambulation assistance.

Test-Taking Strategy: Read the options carefully. The time frames identified in options 1 and 2 are not necessary in this situation. Risk for injury is the issue of the question. The bedtime precautions in option 4 allow the client to ambulate independently, placing the client at risk. This leaves option 3 as the correct answer.

Level of Cognitive Ability: Analysis
Phase of Nursing Process: Analysis
Client Needs: Safe, Effective Care Environment
Content Area: Pharmacology

Reference
Kaplan, H., & Sadock, B. (1996). *Pocket handbook of psychiatric drug treatment* (2nd ed.). Baltimore: Williams & Wilkins. p. 79.

10. **1**

Rationale: Handwashing is a common obsessive-compulsive behavior. Clomipramine is commonly used in the treatment of this disorder. Weight gain is a common side effect of taking this medication. A dry mouth is an often-seen side effect. Sedation may be a side effect. Insomnia may occur as a seldom-seen side effect.

Test-Taking Strategy: Knowledge of the purpose of this medication is required to answer the question. From this point, use the process of elimination to select the correct option. Review the purpose of this medication now if you had difficulty with this question!

Level of Cognitive Ability: Application
Phase of Nursing Process: Assessment
Client Needs: Physiological Integrity
Content Area: Pharmacology

Reference
Kaplan, H., & Sadock, B. (1996). *Pocket handbook of psychiatric drug treatment* (2nd ed.). Baltimore: Williams & Wilkins. p. 174.

11. **4**

Rationale: Haloperidol is used to treat psychotic features in clients. Vital signs are routine and not specific to this situation. The physical safety of other clients is not a direct assessment of this client. Monitoring nutritional intake has no specific value as outlined in this situation. Hallucinations, delusions, and altered thought processes may cause clients to be a danger to themselves and others.

Test-Taking Strategy: Review the situation for data that give clues to acuity and urgency. Note that the question asks for the "first" action. Identify the client of the question and eliminate option 2. Vital signs and nutritional status are routine observations in this situation and may be delayed until potential crisis assessments are performed.

Level of Cognitive Ability: Analysis
Phase of Nursing Process: Assessment
Client Needs: Physiological Integrity
Content Area: Pharmacology

References
Pinnell, N. (1996). *Nursing pharmacology.* Philadelphia: W. B. Saunders. p. 190.
Kaplan, H., & Sadock, B. (1996). *Pocket handbook of psychiatric drug treatment* (2nd ed.). Baltimore: Williams & Wilkins. p. 107.

12. **3**

Rationale: Allergic symptoms may be constant as long as allergens are present. Poor compliance is a problem in psychotic clients. This variable is not a priority in this situation. Benadryl may become addictive when used with psychiatric medications. Benadryl may be used as a primary management tool for extrapyramidal symptoms and mild medication-induced movement disorders.

Test-Taking Strategy: Knowledge regarding the properties of diphenhydramine hydrochloride is required to answer this question. This knowledge will assist in directing you to the correct option. Take time now to review this medication if you had difficulty with this question!

Level of Cognitive Ability: Analysis
Phase of Nursing Process: Analysis
Client Needs: Physiological Integrity
Content Area: Pharmacology

Reference
Kaplan, H., & Sadock, B. (1996). *Pocket handbook of psychiatric drug treatment* (2nd ed.). Baltimore: Williams & Wilkins. p. 43

13. **2**

Rationale: Bupropion (Wellbutrin) does not cause significant orthostatic blood pressure changes. Seizure activity is common in dosages greater than 450 mg daily. Wellbutrin frequently causes a drop in body weight. Insomnia is a side effect, but seizure activity causes a greater client risk.

Test-Taking Strategy: Knowledge regarding the medication bupropion is required to answer the question. Note that the question asks for the assessment that is required. This information will assist in directing you to the correct option. Take time now to review this medication if you had difficulty with this question!

Level of Cognitive Ability: Analysis
Phase of Nursing Process: Assessment
Client Needs: Physiological Integrity
Content Area: Pharmacology

Reference
Fortinash, K., & Holoday-Worret, P. (1996). *Psychiatric mental health nursing.* St. Louis: Mosby–Year Book. p. 550.
Kaplan, H., & Sadock, B. (1996). *Pocket handbook of psychiatric drug treatment* (2nd ed.). Baltimore: Williams & Wilkins. p. 64.

14. **4**

Rationale: The nurse would add anxiety to the client by mentioning media concerns. Xanax is used to treat anxiety, not depression. Cliché responses do not express genuine concern. The nurse should focus on assessing the reason for the client's concern and provide teaching for this client.

Test-Taking Strategy: Identify the communication tools and communication blocks noted in the options. Use the process of elimination to assist you in selecting the correct option. Always address the client's feelings first, as noted in the correct option!

Level of Cognitive Ability: Application
Phase of Nursing Process: Implementation
Client Needs: Psychosocial Integrity
Content Area: Pharmacology

Reference
Fortinash, K., & Holoday-Worret, P. (1996). *Psychiatric mental health nursing.* St. Louis: Mosby–Year Book. p. 533.

15. **2**

Rationale: Sertraline hydrochloride (Zoloft) is generally administered once every 24 hours (QD). The medication may be administered without food or with food if GI distress occurs. Zoloft is classified as an antidepressant. The symptoms of tearfulness or melancholia would indicate a need for medication.

Test-Taking Strategy: Knowledge of the medication Zoloft is required to answer this question. The question asks about the "safe" administration. This key word should assist you in selecting the correct option. Review this medication now if you had difficulty with this question!

Level of Cognitive Ability: Analysis
Phase of Nursing Process: Analysis
Client Needs: Safe, Effective Care Environment
Content Area: Pharmacology

Reference
Kaplan, H., & Sadock, B. (1996). *Pocket handbook of psychiatric drug treatment* (2nd ed.). Baltimore: Williams & Wilkins. p. 155.

16. **2**

Rationale: 20 mg are administered in each 5 mL of the medication. 10 mL of medication is administered with each dose. $20 \times 2 = 40$.

Test-Taking Strategy: This is a simple math calculation. However, be careful in reading the dose prescribed and the label on the medication bottle when calculating the medication dosage!

Level of Cognitive Ability: Application
Phase of Nursing Process: Implementation
Client Needs: Physiological Integrity
Content Area: Pharmacology

Reference
Kaplan, H., & Sadock, B. (1996). *Pocket handbook of psychiatric drug treatment* (2nd ed.). Baltimore: Williams & Wilkins. p. 46.

17. **3**

Rationale: Taking the medication at the same time daily is a good medication administration policy. Dose containers are helpful to prevent dose omissions. Hypnotics should be used with caution to prevent additive effects with other central nervous system agents. The medication may be taken without regard to meals.

Test-Taking Strategy: Read the stem of the question carefully. Use the process of elimination in answering the question. Remember, alcohol should not be consumed when taking hypnotics.

Level of Cognitive Ability: Analysis
Phase of Nursing Process: Evaluation
Client Needs: Health Promotion and Maintenance
Content Area: Pharmacology

References
Hodgson, B., & Kizior, R. (1999). *Nursing drug handbook 1999.* Philadelphia: W. B. Saunders. pp. 815–816.
Kaplan, H., & Sadock, B. (1996). *Pocket handbook of psychiatric drug treatment* (2nd ed.). Baltimore: Williams & Wilkins. p. 46.

18. **1**

Rationale: Thiothixene reaches therapeutic levels in 5 to 10 days. Psychotic behaviors may not have disappeared in 1 week. A bowling activity, with its sounds and heavy ball, may increase symptoms. Sleep beyond 8 hours may be nontherapeutic. Snacks and a long-term relationship are not the priority in this situation.

Test-Taking Strategy: Use the process of elimination to answer this question. Also, remember that assessment is the first stem in the nursing process. Option 1 reflects assessment!

Level of Cognitive Ability: Application
Phase of Nursing Process: Planning
Client Needs: Physiological Integrity
Content Area: Pharmacology

References
Fortinash, K., & Holoday-Worret, P. (1996). *Psychiatric mental health nursing.* St. Louis: Mosby–Year Book. p. 535.
Kaplan, H., & Sadock, B. (1996). *Pocket handbook of psychiatric drug treatment* (2nd ed.). Baltimore: Williams & Wilkins. p. 94

19. **4**

Rationale: Dry mouth is a common side effect. Frequent mouth rinsing with water, sucking on hard candy, and chewing gum will alleviate this common side effect. Hypotension and hypertension are rare side effects of fluphenazine. Leukopenia is common but not viewed as a serious health threat, and the WBC would not be obtained on a daily basis. Weight gain is a common side effect, and frequent snacks will enhance this problem.

Test-Taking Strategy: The key phrase in the question is "common side effect." Knowledge regarding side effects related to this medication is required to answer the question. Eliminate options 1 and 2. It is unlikely that the client would need BP monitoring every 2 hours or that a WBC would be drawn daily. Offering a nutritious snack is not specific. Review the common side effects related to Prolixin now if you had difficulty with this question!

Level of Cognitive Ability: Application
Phase of Nursing Process: Implementation
Client Needs: Physiological Integrity
Content Area: Pharmacology

Reference
Kaplan, H., & Sadock, B. (1996). *Pocket handbook of psychiatric drug treatment* (2nd ed.). Baltimore: Williams & Wilkins. p. 107.

20. **4**

Rationale: If swallowing is difficult, avoid tablets and capsules when possible. Sprinkling the medication over the evening meal cannot ensure that all the dose will be consumed. Crushed medication placed in a small quantity of sweet food facilitates ease in swallowing and provides a pleasant taste. The potential for choking is a high priority in this situation.

Test-Taking Strategy: Read the question carefully. Note that the client is described as having dementia and dysphagia. Also note that the stem of the question asks for the "most appropriate" instructions. Read all four options and use the process of elimination. Dementia and dysphagia are key words. The risk of aspiration is a concern, therefore eliminate options 1 and 2 as these options are not the most appropriate instructions. Option 3 can be eliminated because this medication should be given at bedtime, not at the evening meal.

Level of Cognitive Ability: Application
Phase of Nursing Process: Implementation
Client Needs: Health Promotion and Maintenance
Content Area: Pharmacology

Reference
Fortinash, K., & Holoday-Worret, P. (1996). *Psychiatric–mental health nursing.* St. Louis: Mosby–Year Book. p. 387.

BIBLIOGRAPHY

Clark, J., Queener, S., & Karb, V. (1997). *Pharmacologic basis of nursing practice* (5th ed.). St. Louis: Mosby–Year Book.

Fortinash, K., & Holoday-Worret, P. (1996). *Psychiatric mental health nursing.* St. Louis: Mosby–Year Book.

Hodgson, B., & Kizior, R. (1999). *Saunders nursing drug handbook 1999.* Philadelphia: W. B. Saunders.

Kaplan, H., & Sadock, B. (1996). *Pocket handbook of psychiatric drug treatment* (2nd ed.). Baltimore: Williams & Wilkins.

Kee, J., Hayes, E. (1997). *Pharmacology: a nursing process approach* (2nd ed.). Philadelphia: W. B. Saunders.

Lehne, R. (1998). *Pharmacology for nursing care* (3rd ed.). Philadelphia: W. B. Saunders.

Pinnell, N. (1996). *Nursing pharmacology.* Philadelphia: W. B. Saunders.

Townsend, M. C. (1996). *Psychiatric-mental health nursing: Concepts of care* (2nd ed.). Philadelphia: F. A. Davis.

UNIT XX

··

The Gerontological Client

PYRAMID TERMS

Abuse—The willful infliction of pain, injury, or mental anguish. Unreasonable confinement or willful deprivation of services, including medical care. Abuse can include failure to prevent injury, verbal assaults, the demand to perform demeaning tasks, theft, or mismanagement of personal belongings.

Aging—The biopsychosocial process of change occurring between birth and death.

Alzheimer's Disease—An irreversible form of senile dementia. Individuals with Alzheimer's disease experience cognitive deterioration and progressive loss of ability to carry out the activities of daily living. The client experiences a steady decline in physical and mental functioning that frequently requires caregivers to seek outside resources for assistance.

Dementia—Organic syndrome identified by gradual and progressive deterioration in intellectual functioning. Long- and short-term memory loss occurs, with impairment in judgment, abstract thinking, problem-solving ability, and behavior.

Results in a self-care deficit. The most common type of dementia is Alzheimer's disease.

Depression—A functional disorder of mood that is not linked with aging. The depression may be precipitated by losses related to aging. Depression can be manifested by cognitive impairment or may be the cause of a decline in mental status. Depression can be identified by feelings of sadness, hopelessness, and worthlessness and a decreased interest in activities.

Exploitation—Illegal or improper use of the individual's resources.

Gerontology—The study of the process of aging.

Neglect—The lack of providing services necessary for physical or mental health.

Self-Neglect—The person chooses to avoid medical care or other services that could improve optimal function. Unless declared legally incompetent, an individual has the right to refuse care.

PYRAMID TO SUCCESS

The Pyramid to Success focuses on safety issues, the prevention of injury, restraints, **abuse** and **neglect**, **depression**, **dementia**, and **Alzheimer's disease**. Pyramid points also focus on methods of communication, particularly when deficits exist. When a question is presented on NCLEX-RN, if an age is identified in the case of the question, note the age. If the age represents an elderly client, use gerontological nursing concepts when answering the question.

NURSING PROCESS

ASSESSMENT

Vision
Hearing
Ability to communicate
Food and fluid intake
Arm and leg function
Basic activities of daily living
Skin integrity
Bowel and bladder function
Risk for infection
Risk for injury
Environmental hazards
Mental status
Social support systems

ANALYSIS: Sensory and Perceptual Alterations

PLANNING	IMPLEMENTATION	EVALUATION
The client utilizes measures that will assist with orientation.	Assess visual abilities and for the presence of cataracts. Assess for hearing loss. Utilize methods and devices that will assist with sensory deficits. Orient to environment.	The client remains oriented.

ANALYSIS: Altered Nutrition

PLANNING	IMPLEMENTATION	EVALUATION
The client consumes adequate food and fluids.	Assess nutritional status, including weight and hydration. Offer and provide frequent snacks, considering client's personal and cultural preferences.	The client maintains appropriate weight and hydration status. Nutritional and hydration status are within normal, expected limits.

ANALYSIS: Impaired Physical Mobility

PLANNING	IMPLEMENTATION	EVALUATION
The client uses adaptive devices safely for mobility.	Assess upper and lower extremities and the ability to ambulate. Instruct client in the safe use of assistive devices for mobilization.	The client achieves an optimal level of physical mobility.

ANALYSIS: Self-Care Deficit

PLANNING	IMPLEMENTATION	EVALUATION
The client communicates needs. The client performs some measures of care to self.	Maintain and enhance self-care abilities. Assist with activities of daily living. Supervise self-care. Support self-functioning to maintain independence.	The client maintains optimal level of independence.

ANALYSIS: Alteration in Skin Integrity

PLANNING	IMPLEMENTATION	EVALUATION
Client remains free of skin breakdown as a result of immobility.	Turn and reposition client. Monitor skin integrity. Instruct client in the importance of turning and repositioning.	The client's skin remains intact.

ANALYSIS: Altered Urinary and Bowel Elimination

PLANNING	IMPLEMENTATION	EVALUATION
The client establishes a toileting routine. The client determines causes of urinary and bowel dysfunction. The client identifies practices that may contribute to bowel dysfunction.	Assess urinary and bowel function. Identify bowel habits. Identify factors that affect normal bowel function. Provide measures to promote normal urinary and bowel function. Instruct client in measures to eliminate bowel dysfunction.	The client adheres to the prescribed bladder and bowel program. The client utilizes measures to eliminate bowel dysfunction. The client demonstrates normal urinary and bowel patterns.

ANALYSIS: Infection

PLANNING	IMPLEMENTATION	EVALUATION
Vital signs remain within baseline.	Assess for the risk of infection. Monitor vital signs and for signs of infection.	The client remains free from infection.

ANALYSIS: Risk for Injury

PLANNING	IMPLEMENTATION	EVALUATION
The client identifies behaviors that can cause injury. The client avoids injuries.	Determine client's ability related to safety and functional self-care. Maintain safety precautions. Institute measures to prevent falls. Position bed in low position. Provide handrails in bathrooms and halls. Assure that rooms are uncluttered. Provide adequate, nonglare lighting.	The client remains free of injury.

ANALYSIS: Altered Thought Processes

PLANNING	IMPLEMENTATION	EVALUATION
The client performs behaviors that are appropriate.	Monitor for disorientation. Assess mental status and for memory changes. Establish trust. Encourage psychosocial activity.	The client demonstrates optimal thought processes.

ANALYSIS: Ineffective Individual or Family Coping

PLANNING

The client and family participate in developing the plan of care. The client and family identify methods of coping.

IMPLEMENTATION

Involve the client and significant others in the assessment process and in planning care. Determine the degree of impact that the disability may have on independence. Assure that care options selected fit within the person's lifestyle. Utilize other health care professionals when planning care. Display nonjudgmental attitudes. Assist in selecting activities for the client that maintain self-identity and lifelong interests. Encourage attending activities to maintain social interaction. Encourage verbalization about the past. Assess available support systems. Provide resources to the family to obtain respite care.

EVALUATION

The client and/or family identify resources and support services available.

CLIENT NEEDS

SAFE, EFFECTIVE CARE ENVIRONMENT

Advance directives
Client rights and advocacy
Confidentiality
Continuity of care
Informed consent
The use of restraints
Appropriate procedures for safety
Accident prevention

HEALTH PROMOTION AND MAINTENANCE

Aging process
Expected body image changes
Family systems
Lifestyle choices
Client and family education
The prevention and early detection of disorders associated with **aging**
The importance of safety, exercise, and nutrition
The safe use of medications
The importance of follow-up visits to the physician

PSYCHOSOCIAL INTEGRITY

Coping mechanisms
Grief and loss

Religious and spiritual resources
Sensory/perceptual alterations
Changes and adjustment in role function
Situational role changes
Adjustment to potential deterioration in physical and mental health and well-being
Loss of the quantity and quality of relationships
The threat to independent functioning
Abuse and **neglect**
Crisis intervention
The use of resources for the client and family

PHYSIOLOGICAL INTEGRITY

Assistive devices
Elimination
Mobility and immobility
Nutrition and oral hydration
Personal hygiene
Rest and sleep
Safe medication administration
Alterations in body systems and the related risks due to the aging process

REFERENCES

Black, J., & Matassarin-Jacobs, E. (1997). *Medical-surgical nursing: Clinical management for continuity of care* (5th ed.). Philadelphia: W. B. Saunders.

Leahy, J., & Kizilay, P. (1998). *Foundations of nursing practice: A nursing process approach*. Philadelphia: W. B. Saunders.

National Council of State Boards of Nursing. (eds.) (1997). *Test for the National Council Licensure Examination for Registered Nurses.* Chicago: Author.

O'Toole, M. (ed.) (1997). *Miller-Keane encyclopedia & dictionary of medicine, nursing & allied health* (6th ed.). Philadelphia: W. B. Saunders.

CHAPTER 75

The Gerontological Client

I. Physiological Changes of Aging (Box 75–1)

A. Integumentary system
1. Loss of pigment in hair and skin
2. Increased nail thickness and decreased nail growth
3. Thinning of the epidermis
4. Easy bruising and tearing of the skin
5. Reduction in blood flow to the skin
6. Decreased skin turgor
7. Loss of elasticity and subcutaneous fat
8. Wrinkling of the skin
9. Dry, itchy, cracked skin
10. Inadequate sweating
11. Seborrheic dermatitis and keratosis formation

B. Neurological system
1. Changes in mental status
2. Slowed reflexes
3. Loss of balance
4. Dizziness and syncope
5. Slight tremors
6. Difficulty with fine motor movement
7. Changes in sleep patterns, such as decreased total sleep with earlier risings
8. Increased susceptibility to hypothermia and hyperthermia

C. Musculoskeletal system
1. Posture and stature changes causing a decrease in height
2. Kyphosis of the dorsal spine
3. Muscle mass decreases and muscles atrophy
4. Joint capsule components deteriorate
5. Decreased mobility, range of motion, flexibility, and stability
6. Increased stiffness
7. Decrease in physical strength
8. Decrease in muscular coordination
9. Change of gait, with shortened step and wider base
10. Increased brittleness of the bones
11. Decrease in deep tendon reflexes

D. Cardiopulmonary system
1. Energy and endurance diminish
2. Lowered tolerance to exercise
3. Decreased stretch and compliance of the chest wall
4. Decreased rib mobility and lung tone
5. Decreased strength and function of respiratory muscles
6. Decreased depth of respirations and oxygen intake
7. Decreased ability to cough
8. Decreased ability to expectorate
9. Decreased size and number of alveoli
10. Decreased compliance of the heart
11. Heart valves become thicker and more rigid
12. Decreased efficiency of blood return to the heart and decreased cardiac output
13. Decreased resting heart rate of 60 to 84 beats per minute
14. Average increase in blood pressure from 140/90 to 160/100
15. Susceptible to postural hypotension

E. Hematologic and immune systems
1. Hemoglobin and hematocrit levels remain within normal range but average toward the low end of normal
2. Lymphocyte counts tend to be lower
3. Decreased resistance to infection and disease
4. Prone to increased blood clotting

F. Gastrointestinal system
1. Decreased appetite, thirst, and intake
2. Decreased need for calories

BOX 75–1. Classification of Late Adulthood	
Young old	65–74 years old
Middle old	75–84 years old
Old old	85–99 years old
The elite old	100 years old or more

3. Decreased stomach-emptying time
4. Increased tendency toward constipation
5. Tooth loss
6. Difficulty in chewing and swallowing food
7. Digestive disturbances
8. Decreased glucose tolerance
9. Decreased absorption of carbohydrates, proteins, fats, and vitamins
10. Decreased lean body weight
11. Hiatal hernias common

G. Endocrine system
1. Decreased secretion of hormones, with specific changes related to each hormone function
2. Decreased metabolic rate
3. Decreased glucose tolerance
4. Resistance to insulin in peripheral tissues

H. Renal system
1. Decreased kidney size, function, and ability to concentrate urine
2. Decreased glomerular filtration rate
3. Decreased capacity of the bladder
4. Increased residual urine and increased incidence of infection and incontinence
5. Impaired drug excretion

I. Reproductive system
1. Decreased testosterone production and decreased size of testes
2. Changes in the prostate leading to urinary problems
3. Decreased secretion of hormones with the cessation of menses
4. Vaginal changes, including decreased muscle tone and lubrication

J. Special senses
1. Decreased visual acuity
2. Decreased accommodation in eyes
3. Decreased peripheral vision and increased sensitivity to glare
4. Increased adjustment time to changes in light
5. Presbyopia and cataract formation
6. Possible loss of hearing ability
7. Inability to discern taste of food
8. Decreased smell acuity
9. Changes in touch
10. Decreased pain awareness

II. Psychosocial Aspects of Aging (Box 75–2)

A. Changes in role function
B. Adjustments to retirement and loss of income
C. Changes in social life
D. Adjustment to potential deterioration in physical and mental health and well-being
E. Diminished quantity and quality of relationships
F. Threat to independent functioning
G. Loss of skills and competencies developed early in life
H. Coping with change and new life situations
I. Coping and stress of caring for dependent loved ones
J. Coping with loss

BOX 75–2. Concerns of the Older Population

Adequate income
Functional limitations from chronic illness and disability
Ability to maintain independence
Becoming a burden to loved ones
Isolation
Dependence on governmental and social systems
Access to social support systems

III. Elder Abuse and Neglect

A. Description
1. Involves physical, psychological, financial, and social **abuse**
2. Can involve a violation of client's rights
3. Individuals at most risk include those that are dependent, usually because of confusion, immobility, or the need for personal hygiene
4. Factors that contribute to **abuse** and **neglect** include long-standing family violence, caregiver stress, and the individual's increasing dependence.

B. Types
1. **Abuse**
   a. The willful infliction of pain, injury, or mental anguish
   b. Unreasonable confinement or willful deprivation of services, including medical care
   c. Can include failure to prevent injury, verbal assaults, the demand to perform demeaning tasks, theft, or mismanagement of personal belongings
2. **Neglect:** The lack of providing services necessary for physical or mental health
3. **Self-Neglect**
   a. The person chooses to avoid medical care or other services that would improve optimal functioning
   b. Unless declared legally incompetent, an individual has the right to refuse care
4. **Exploitation:** Illegal or improper use of the individual's resources
5. Assessment of **Abuse** and **Neglect**
   a. Abrasions, lacerations, and bruises
   b. Burns
   c. Sprains, fractures, or dislocations
   d. Pressure sores
   e. Injuries inconsistent with history
   f. Frequent falls
   g. Untreated medical problems
   h. Inappropriate dress and poor hygiene
   i. Excessive drowsiness
   j. Over- or undermedication
   k. Malnutrition
   l. Dehydration
   m. Expression of fear in response to touch
6. Implementation
   a. Assess for signs of **abuse** and **neglect**

b. Report cases of **abuse** and **neglect** as mandated by all states
c. Initiate protective services
d. Assess for dysfunctional family systems
e. Promote family functioning and self-care

IV. Use of Restraints

A. Physical restraints used to prevent injury are to be avoided, and alternative methods to provide safety must be assessed prior to the use of physical restraints
B. A physician's order must be obtained for the use of restraints
C. Discuss the use of restraints with the client and family
D. Obtain client/family consent for the use of restraints
E. Utilize the least restrictive device for restraint
F. Use only restraints that have been manufactured as a safety restraint
G. Observe the client frequently, and monitor for alterations in skin integrity and in circulation as a result of the restraints
H. Restraints need to be removed at frequent intervals to assess for complications and to allow for mobility and range of motion exercises
I. Always follow the institutional policy regarding the use of restraints

V. Medications

A. Major problems with prescription medications include adverse effects, medication interactions, medication errors, noncompliance, and the cost
B. Determine the use of over-the-counter medications
C. Keep the use of medications to a minimum
D. Begin with doses at one third to one half of normal adult doses
E. Closely monitor for adverse effects and response to therapy because of the increased risk for drug toxicity
F. Note that a common sign of an adverse reaction in the elderly is an acute change in mental status
G. Assess for medication interactions in client taking multiple medications
H. Advise the client to use one pharmacy and notify the consulting physicians of medications taken
I. Administration of medications
 1. Check for mouth dryness as medication may stick and dissolve in mouth
 2. Place client in sitting position when administering medication
 3. Crush tablets if necessary and give with textured food (nectar, applesauce) if not contraindicated
 4. Do not crush enteric-coated tablets and do not open capsules
 5. Administer liquid preparations if the client has difficulty in swallowing tablets
 6. If administering a suppository, do not insert suppository immediately after removing from the refrigerator
 7. A suppository may take longer to dissolve due to decreased body core temperature
 8. When administering parenteral medication, monitor the site as it may ooze medication or bleed due to decreased tissue elasticity
 9. Do not use an immobile limb for administering parenteral medication
 10. Monitor client compliance with taking prescribed medications
 11. Monitor for safety in correctly taking medications
 12. Use a medication cassette to facilitate proper administration of medication

VI. Decubiti

A. Description
 1. An impairment of skin integrity
 2. Localized areas of necrosis of the skin and subcutaneous tissue due to pressure
 3. Prevention of skin breakdown is a major role of the nurse, particularly in caring for the bedridden or immobile client
B. Assessment
 1. Stage 1
  a. A reddened area that returns to normal skin color after 15 to 20 minutes of pressure relief, such as turning the client to another position
  b. The skin is intact; the area is red and does not blanch with external pressure
 2. Stage 2
  a. Area in which the top layer of skin is missing
  b. The ulcer usually is shallow with a pinkish-red base, and a white or yellow eschar may be present
 3. Stage 3
  a. Deep ulcers that extend into the dermis and subcutaneous tissues
  b. White, gray, or yellow eschar is usually present at the bottom of the ulcer, and the ulcer crater may have a lip or edge
  c. Purulent drainage is common
 4. Stage 4
  a. Deep ulcers that extend into muscle and bone
  b. Stage 4 ulcers have a foul smell, and the eschar is brown or black
  c. Purulent drainage is common
C. Implementation
 1. Institute measures to prevent decubiti
 2. Monitor for an alteration in skin integrity
 3. Relieve or remove pressure on the skin
 4. Turn and reposition the immobile client every 2 hours or more frequently if necessary
 5. Ambulate the client
 6. Provide active and passive range of motion exercises every 8 hours

7. Keep the skin clean and dry and the sheets wrinkle-free
8. Apply moisture barrier as prescribed to protect the skin
9. Use assistive devices to prevent pressure, such as an alternating air pressure mattress or sheepskin padding
10. Assess the nutritional status of the client
11. Provide adequate nutritional intake to promote tissue integrity

VII. Dementia

A. Description
   1. Organic syndrome with progressive deterioration in intellectual functioning
   2. Long- and short-term memory loss occurs, with impairments in judgment, abstract thinking, problem-solving ability, and behavior
   3. Results in a self-care deficit
   4. The most common type of **dementia** is **Alzheimer's disease**
B. **Alzheimer's disease**
   1. An irreversible form of senile **dementia**
   2. Individuals with **Alzheimer's disease** experience cognitive deterioration and progressive loss of ability to carry out the activities of daily living
   3. The client experiences a steady decline in physical and mental functioning that frequently requires caregivers to seek outside resources for assistance
C. Assessment
   1. Stage I
      a. Duration of this stage is 1 to 3 years
      b. Mild memory impairment
      c. Difficulty in remembering names, appointments, and where things are
      d. Client is indifferent and occasionally irritable
   2. Stage II
      a. Duration of this stage is 2 to 10 years
      b. Moderate memory impairment of recent events
      c. Decrease in orientation
      d. Restless nights
      e. Aphasia
      f. Apraxia
      g. Client is indifferent and occasionally irritable
      h. Restlessness and pacing
      i. Delusions
   3. Stage III
      a. Duration of this stage is 8 to 12 years
      b. Severely impaired cognitive function
      c. Severe disorientation
      d. Severe agitation
      e. Blunted emotions
      f. Limb rigidity and flexion posture
      g. Urinary and fecal incontinence

D. Implementation
   1. Identify and reinforce retained skills
   2. Assist client and family members to manage memory deficits and behavior changes
   3. Encourage family members to express feelings about caregiving
   4. Provide caregiver support and identify the resources and support groups available
   5. Provide continuity of care
   6. Orient client to the environment
   7. Furnish environment with familiar possessions
   8. Acknowledge the client's feelings
   9. Monitor activities of daily living
   10. Remind client how to perform self-care activities
   11. Maintain independence
   12. Provide consistent routines
   13. Provide exercise with supervision, such as walking
   14. Avoid activities that tax the memory
   15. Allow plenty of time to complete a task
   16. Use constant encouragement in a step-by-step approach
   17. Provide activities that distract and occupy time, such as listening to music, drawing, and watching TV
   18. Provide mental stimulation with simple games or activities
E. Implementation for specific behaviors
   1. Wandering
      a. Provide a safe environment
      b. Prevent unsafe wandering
      c. Provide close supervision
      d. Close and secure doors
      e. Use identification bracelets and electronic surveillance devices
   2. Communication
      a. Adapt to the communication level of the client
      b. Use a firm volume and low pitch of voice to communicate
      c. Use a calm and reassuring voice
      d. Use pantomine gestures if the client is unable to understand spoken words
      e. Use slow, clear, verbal communication techniques
      f. Use short words and simple sentences
      g. Call the client by name, identify yourself, and wait for a response
      h. Ask only one question at a time, and give one direction at a time
      i. Repeat questions if necessary but do not rephrase
      j. Stand directly in front of the client and maintain eye contact
      k. Listen for feeling and emotion expressed by the client
   3. Impaired judgment
      a. Eliminate from the environment throw rugs, toxic substances, dangerous

electrical appliances, or any other objects that can present a risk of injury
  b. Reduce hot water heater temperature
4. Altered thought processes
  a. Orient client frequently
  b. Place a calendar and clock in a visible place
  c. Call the client by name
  d. Use familiar objects in the room
  e. Maintain familiar routines
  f. Make tasks simple
  g. Allow time for client to complete a task
  h. Allow client to reminisce
5. Altered sleep patterns
  a. Allow clients to wander in a safe place until they become tired
  b. Prevent shadows in the room
  c. Avoid the use of hypnotics as they cause confusion and aggravate the sundown effect
6. Agitation
  a. Assess the precipitant of the agitation
  b. Reassure the client
  c. Remove items that can be hazardous during the time of agitation
  d. Approach the client slowly and calmly from the front, then speak, gesture and move slowly
  e. Remove the client to a less stressful environment
  f. Use touch gently
  g. Do not argue with the client or restrain the client
  h. Distract the client with questions about the problem and gradually turn the attention to something else

VIII. Depression

A. Description
  1. A functional disorder of mood that is not linked with **aging**

2. The **depression** may be manifested by cognitive impairment or may be the cause of a decline in mental status
3. **Depression** can be identified by feelings of sadness, hopelessness, worthlessness, and a decreased interest in activities
B. Assessment
  1. Difficulty in concentrating
  2. Feelings of inadequacy and sadness
  3. Difficulty in sleeping or excessive sleeping
  4. Weight gain or loss
  5. Vegetative symptoms
  6. Constipation
  7. Loss of interest in activities
  8. Decreased endurance and energy
  9. Preoccupation with physical health
  10. Thoughts of death or suicide
C. Implementation
  1. Assess for signs associated with **depression**
  2. Monitor for the risk of suicide and notify physician
  3. Implement safety precautions for suicide risk
  4. Provide and reinforce positive experiences
  5. Motivate the client by positive reinforcements
  6. Provide a variation in daily schedule but limit changes, as change is anxiety-producing for the older client
  7. Allow client to talk and reminisce
  8. Maintain reality
  9. Initiate counseling as appropriate
  10. Table 75–1 lists some of the prescribed medications for depression

IX. Pain

A. Description
  1. Pain can occur from numerous causes and most often occurs from degenerative changes in the musculoskeletal system
  2. The failure to alleviate pain in the older

Table 75–1. Antidepressant Medications

Medications	Actions	Nursing Implications
Imipramine (Tofranil) Amitriptyline (Elavil) Nortriptyline (Pamelor) Desipramine (Norpramin)	Tricyclic antidepressants that increase synaptic concentrations of norepinephrine and/or serotonin	Monitor liver and renal function tests Monitor for bowel and urinary retention Monitor for hypotension and dysrhythmias Instruct client to change positions slowly Be alert to photosensitivity, which can occur Instruct client to use sunscreens Assess for visual disturbances Monitor for suicide potential Do not abruptly discontinue medication
Trazodone (Desyrel) Fluoxetine (Prozac)	Antidepressants that selectively inhibit serotonin reuptake in the brain	Monitor liver and renal function tests Monitor WBC and neutrophil counts Monitor for dizziness and lightheadedness Be alert to photosensitivity, which can occur Instruct client to use sunscreens Assess for visual disturbances Monitor for suicide potential Do not abruptly discontinue medication

client can lead to functional limitations affecting the ability to function independently

B. Assessment
1. Agitation
2. Moaning
3. Crying
4. Restlessness
5. Verbal reporting of pain

C. Implementation
1. Monitor the client for signs of pain
2. Identify the pattern of pain
3. Identify precipitating factor(s) for the pain
4. Monitor the impact of pain on activities of daily living
5. Provide pain relief through measures such as distraction, relaxation, massage, biofeedback
6. Administer pain medication as prescribed and instruct client in its use
7. Evaluate the effects of pain-reducing measures

X. Impaired Mobility

A. Description
1. Usually occurs secondary to multiple types of problems and diseases
2. Impaired mobility can occur due to decreased physical function related to cardiovascular, pulmonary, musculoskeletal, and neurological disease, or accidents

B. Assessment
1. Existing disease processes
2. Ambulation
3. Ability to care for self

C. Implementation
1. Assess risk of injury
2. Determine cause of mobility restriction
3. Assess mobility restrictions related to disease processes
4. Monitor limitations related to all self-care activities
5. Provide rest periods between activities and in the afternoon
6. Break up activities to last no longer than 20 minutes
7. Perform activities that require a high level of energy in the morning
8. Maintain mobility through exercise and guided activities
9. Determine the best assistive aid or adaptive device for the client
10. Demonstrate and monitor the safe use of the assistive device
11. Monitor skin for integrity
12. Provide range of motion exercises to prevent deformities and contractures
13. Monitor respiratory status and encourage deep breathing to promote lung expansion

D. Assistive devices
1. Canes
   a. Made of a lightweight material with a rubber suction tip at the bottom
   b. Stand at the affected side of the client when the client is ambulating
   c. The handle should be at the level of the greater trochanter
   d. The client's elbow should be flexed at a 25 to 30° angle
   e. Instruct client to hold cane close to the body
   f. Instruct client to hold cane in the hand on the unaffected side so that cane and weaker leg can work together with each step
   g. Instruct the client to move the cane at the same time as the affected leg
2. Hemi or quadripod canes
   a. Used for clients who have the use of only one upper extremity
   b. Hemi canes provide more security than a quad cane; however, both types provide more security than a single-tipped cane
   c. Position cane at client's unaffected side, with the straight, nonangled side adjacent to the body
   d. Position the cane 6 inches from client's side, with the hand grips level with the greater trochanter
3. Walkers
   a. Stand adjacent to the client on the affected side
   b. Instruct the client to put all four points of the walker flat on the floor before putting weight on the hand pieces
   c. Instruct the client to move the walker forward and to walk into it

XI. Fractured Hip

A. Description
1. Bone is broken inside the joint (intracapsular), or the fracture can occur at the greater trochanter (extracapsular) outside the joint
2. Fractured hips occurring in the elderly are most likely due to a fall

B. Assessment
1. Safety
2. Pain
3. Swelling
4. Asymmetry of hip
5. X-ray film to confirm fracture

C. Preoperative implementation
1. Maintain skin traction as prescribed to immobilize the leg and decrease pain
2. Turn client every 2 hours from back to unaffected side
3. Instruct in coughing and deep-breathing exercises and the use of incentive spirometry

D. Postoperative implementation
1. Hip pinning and hip prosthesis
   a. Turn from back to unaffected side
   b. Maintain leg abduction to prevent internal or external rotation

    c. Place a trochanter roll to prevent external rotation

    d. Assure that hip flexion angle does not exceed 60 to 80°

    e. Avoid hip flexion when getting client out of bed

    f. Avoid the use of low chairs

    g. Elevate head of the bed 30 to 45° for meals only

    h. Ambulate as prescribed in 2 to 4 days, with partial weight bearing

2. Total hip replacement

    a. Prevent hip flexion or external or internal rotation

    b. Use an abduction pillow

    c. Position to back and unaffected side

    d. Do not position to affected side unless prescribed by the physician

    e. Maintain leg and hip in proper alignment

    f. Elevate head of the bed 30 to 45° for meals only

    g. Maintain Hemovac (suction device) if in place

    h. Maintain compression on Hemovac to facilitate drainage

    i. Monitor and record Hemovac output

    j. Hemovac drainage should continuously decrease in amount and by 48 hours postoperatively should be approximately 30 mL in an 8-hour period

    k. Maintain the use of antiembolism stockings and encourage client to flex and extend feet and ankles

    l. Provide continuous passive motion (CPM) first day postoperatively, with increasing degrees of flexion up to 90° as prescribed

    m. Ambulate 1 to 2 days postoperatively as prescribed

    n. To avoid hip strain and bending, do not position bed too low when getting client out of bed

    o. Keep operative leg extended, supported, and elevated when getting client out of bed

    p. Avoid weight bearing on the affected leg and instruct client on the use of a walker to prevent weight bearing

    q. Avoid hip flexion greater than 80° and avoid low chairs when out of bed

    r. Instruct client to avoid crossing legs and bending-over activities

    s. Monitor wound for hemorrhage and infection

    t. Monitor circulation and sensation of the affected side

    u. Begin physical therapy postoperatively as prescribed

XII. Pneumonia

A. Description: The causes of pneumonia in the older client include the effects of the **aging** process on the respiratory system, weakness and the inability to cough, malnutrition, and the use of medications

B. Assessment

1. Acute change in mental status
2. Confusion
3. Cough
4. Fever
5. Rapid respiratory rate
6. Chest pain
7. Dyspnea
8. Chest radiograph confirmation

C. Implementation

1. Monitor vital signs
2. Assess lung sounds
3. Administer oxygen as prescribed
4. Administer respiratory therapy as prescribed
5. Administer antibiotics as prescribed
6. Provide adequate rest with some progressive activity
7. Mobilize the bed rest client as soon as possible
8. Provide adequate nutrition and hydration
9. Encourage client to receive immunization against influenza and pneumococcal pneumonia to prevent infection

XIII. Nutritional Intake

A. Description

1. Physiological requirements decrease with age
2. The older client is at risk for inadequate nutritional and fluid intake due to inability to prepare food, loss of dentition, loss of appetite, lack of exercise, loss of taste and smell sensation, loss of interest in eating, **depression,** or lack of financial resources

B. Assessment

1. Appetite
2. Hydration status
3. Body weight
4. Ability to feed self
5. Ability to chew and swallow
6. Fluid and calorie intake
7. Ability to prepare food and mobilize the resources to shop

C. Implementation

1. Assess appetite
2. Monitor for signs of dehydration and malnutrition
3. Monitor body weight
4. Assess ability to chew and swallow
5. Monitor intake of food and fluids
6. Assess food likes and dislikes
7. Provide small, frequent, nutritious meals
8. Offer nutritious drinks
9. Assess ability to prepare food and to shop for food
10. Provide resources necessary to supply client with adequate food

XIV. Constipation

A. Description
1. Normal elimination does not occur due to a structural problem or disease state
2. Constipation is the most frequent complaint regarding bowel function of older people

B. Assessment
1. Frequency of defecation
2. Usual time for defecation
3. Dietary habits
4. Use of laxatives or enemas

C. Implementation
1. Determine the cause of constipation
2. Re-establish typical bowel habits
3. Maintain regular defecation
4. Promote comfort and privacy during defecation
5. Increase fluid intake
6. Add fiber to the diet
7. Provide anal lubricant
8. Administer stool softeners as prescribed
9. Use suppositories sparingly, limiting type to glycerin or Dulcolax as prescribed
10. Use enemas sparingly, limiting the use to small, cleansing enemas such as Fleet, as prescribed
11. Avoid the use of mineral oil because of problems associated with the absorption of fat-soluble vitamins and the risk of aspiration

XV. Diarrhea

A. Description
1. Frequent defecation of loose or liquid stools
2. Infections may cause diarrhea
3. Fecal impaction may cause overflow diarrhea, with stool oozing around the impaction
4. Antibiotic-associated diarrhea, such as that caused by *Clostridium difficile*, is a problem for older individuals, particularly if they are hospitalized

B. Assessment
1. Frequency of defecation
2. Usual time for defecation
3. Dietary habits
4. Use of laxatives or enemas
5. Stool oozing
6. Signs of dehydration
7. Electrolyte values

C. Implementation
1. Assess causative factor
2. Initiate interventions as prescribed based on causative factor
3. Assess for fluid deficit and dehydration
4. Monitor intake and output (I&O) and electrolyte levels
5. Increase dietary bulk and fiber
6. Monitor skin around anal area

XVI. Urinary Incontinence

A. Description
1. The involuntary release or leakage of urine
2. The physiological changes that occur in the kidney and bladder as a result of the **aging** process may lead to the urinary incontinence problems experienced by some older clients

B. Assessment
1. Contributing factors
2. I&O
3. Urinary incontinence patterns
4. Urinary retention
5. Signs of urinary infection, such as burning, frequency, foul odor, or confusion
6. Urinalysis results

C. Implementation
1. Monitor I&O
2. Monitor urinary patterns
3. Assess contributing factors such as a bladder infection, distance to the bathroom, difficulty ambulating or removing clothing, or coughing, sneezing, or laughing
4. Establish toileting schedule such as every 2 hours, or before and after activities, meals, sleep, and rest periods
5. Provide easy access to bathroom
6. Ensure adequate fluid intake
7. Provide protection plan for accidents to avoid embarrassment
8. Instruct the client about the use of such incontinence aids as pads or briefs
9. Provide skin care and monitor for skin breakdown
10. Teach Kegel exercises to control stress and urge incontinence
11. Kegel exercises
   a. Contract pubococcygeus muscle
   b. Hold contraction for 10 seconds
   c. Relax for 10 seconds
   d. Work up to 25 repetitions three times a day

XVII. Impaired Vision and Hearing

A. Description
1. Due to the physiological changes that occur with the **aging** process, clients develop decreased visual and hearing acuity
2. Such conditions as loss of sight and hearing, cataracts, glaucoma, and presbyopia can develop

B. Assessment
1. Risk for injury
2. Ability to see and hear adequately
3. Cataract development
4. The need for assistive devices
5. Frequently asking people to repeat statements
6. Better understanding of speech when in small groups
7. Avoiding large groups

8. Withdrawing from social interactions
9. Straining to hear
10. Turning head to favor one ear or leaning forward
11. Shouting in conversation
12. Ringing in the ears
13. Failing to respond when not looking in the direction of the sound
14. Irritability
15. Answering questions incorrectly
16. Raising the volume of the television or radio

C. Implementation
   1. Impaired vision
     a. Alert the client when approaching
     b. When speaking to the client who has limited sight, use a normal tone of voice
     c. Orient the client to the environment
     d. Use a focal point and provide further orientation to the environment from that focal point
     e. Allow the client to touch objects in the room
     f. Utilize the clock placement of foods on the meal tray to orient the client
     g. When ambulating, allow the client to grasp the nurse's arm at the elbow, and keep the arm close to the nurse's body so the client can detect the direction of movement
     h. Instruct the client to remain one step behind the nurse when ambulating
     i. Provide radios, TVs, and clocks that give the time orally
     j. Promote independence as much as possible
   2. Impaired hearing
     a. Use written words if the client is able to see, read, and write
     b. Talk in a room without distracting noises
     c. Talk in lower tones, as shouting is not helpful
     d. Move close to the client and speak slowly and clearly
     e. Use telephone amplifiers
     f. Use flashing lights that are activated by the ringing of telephone or doorbell
     g. Use of specially trained dogs that help the client to be aware of sound and to alert the client to potential dangers
     h. Use lip reading and sign language, which combines speech with hand movements that signify letters, words, or phrases
     i. Encourage the client to wear glasses when talking to someone to improve vision for lip reading
     j. Face the client when speaking
     k. Provide plenty of light in the room
     l. Get the attention of the client before you begin to speak
     m. Keep hands and other objects away from the mouth when talking to the client
     n. Validate with the client the understanding of statements made, by asking the client to repeat what was said
     o. Rephrase sentences and repeat information
     p. Move closer to the better-hearing ear
   3. Hearing aids (Box 75–3)
     a. Encourage client to start using the hearing aid slowly to develop appreciation of hearing via the hearing aid device
     b. Teach client to concentrate on the sounds that are to be heard and to filter out background noise

---

BOX 75–3. Client Education in the Use of a Hearing Aid

- Clean the ear mold with mild soap and water
- Avoid excessive wetting, and keep the hearing aid dry
- Clean the ear cannula of the hearing aid with a toothpick or pipe cleaner
- Turn off the hearing aid and remove the battery when it is not in use
- Keep extra batteries on hand
- Keep in a safe place
- Avoid dropping and avoid exposure of hearing aid to extremes of heat and cold
- Adjust the volume to the minimal hearing level to prevent feedback squeaking
- Prevent hair sprays, oils, or other hair and face products to come in contact with the receiver

---

PRACTICE QUESTIONS

1. Which of the following statements, if made by the nurse, indicates an understanding of hearing loss that can occur in the elderly?
   1 "The elderly are often distracted."
   2 "The elderly respond to low-pitched tones."
   3 "The elderly have middle ear changes."
   4 "The elderly develop moist cerumen production."

2. An elderly male client is admitted with malnutrition. Which one of the following laboratory data indicates a protein deficiency?
   1 Creatinine, 0.6 mg/dL
   2 Transferrin, 90 mg/dL
   3 Calcium, 4.5 mEq/L
   4 Sodium, 138 mEq/L

3. To reduce the risk of aspiration during meals, an elderly client should be positioned:
   1 Upright in a chair
   2 On the left side in bed
   3 In low Fowler's position with legs elevated
   4 On the right side in bed

4. Prior to feeding an elderly client via a nasogastric tube, the nurse should:
   1 Check the placement of the tube
   2 Check the last time medications were given

3 Rinse the Asepto syringe with warm water

4 Warm the feeding to 103°F

5. An elderly hypertensive client is taking lisinopril (Prinivil, Zestril), 10 mg PO QD. Which statement, if made by the client, indicates to the visiting nurse that further teaching is necessary?
   1 "I take the pill after breakfast each day."
   2 "I need to change my position slowly."
   3 "If I get a bad headache, I should call my doctor immediately."
   4 "I can skip a dose once a week."

6. Which of the following clients may be a victim of elder abuse?
   1 A 90-year-old woman with advanced Parkinson's disease
   2 A 68-year-old man with newly diagnosed cataracts
   3 A 70-year-old woman with early-diagnosed Lyme disease
   4 A 75-year-old man with moderate hypertension

7. An elderly female client confides to the visiting nurse that she is afraid she will fall while going to the bathroom at night. Which suggestion, if made by the nurse, indicates that the nurse understands the visual changes affecting the elderly?
   1 "Use a bell to call your daughter if you need to get up."
   2 "Keep a red light on in the bathroom at night."
   3 "Use a commode in your bedroom at night."
   4 "Limit your fluid intake during the day."

8. Which nursing intervention, if performed by the nurse, may calm an agitated elderly client with Alzheimer's disease?
   1 Playing a radio
   2 Turning the lights out
   3 Putting an arm around the client's waist
   4 Encouraging group participation

9. Which of the following activities would best promote health and maintenance among older adults?
   1 Gardening every day for an hour
   2 Cycling three times a week for 20 minutes
   3 Sculpting once a week for 40 minutes
   4 Walking three to five times a week for 30 minutes

10. Which statement, if made by an elderly client with myasthenia gravis, indicates to the nurse that further teaching is necessary?
    1 "I can change the time of my medication on the mornings that I feel strong."
    2 "I rest each afternoon after my walk."
    3 "If I get abdominal cramps and diarrhea, I should call my doctor."

4 "I cough and deep breathe many times during the day."

11. Which of the following activities performed by the nurse fosters reminiscence among the elderly?
    1 Displaying calendars and clocks
    2 Encouraging client participation in pottery class
    3 Setting up pet therapy sessions
    4 Having story-telling hours

12. Which nursing diagnosis would have the highest priority for an elderly client?
    1 Altered Oral Mucous Membrane
    2 Ineffective Airway Clearance
    3 Impaired Memory
    4 Risk for Loneliness

13. Which situation in the home of an elderly client, if found by a visiting nurse, requires immediate attention?
    1 An operable smoke detector
    2 A prefilled medication tray
    3 Unsecured scatter rugs
    4 Clear exit passageways

14. To encourage an elderly female client's participation in recreational therapy, what nursing intervention should the nurse perform first?
    1 Change the client's soiled disposable brief
    2 Introduce the client to group members
    3 Have the client's hair washed and cut
    4 Encourage the client to wear supportive shoes

15. Which statement, if made by an elderly client, indicates to the nurse that further teaching about bowel elimination is necessary?
    1 "I drink 6 to 8 glasses of water per day."
    2 "I walk 1 to 2 miles per day."
    3 "I need to decrease fiber in my diet."
    4 "I have a bowel movement every other day."

16. Which of the following situations, if practiced by a nurse, portrays ageism?
    1 Accepting differences among older adults
    2 Allowing older adults to make decisions
    3 Informing the elderly of their rights
    4 Advising older adults to forego aggressive treatment

17. Which of the following age-related body changes may cause digitalis toxicity in the frail elderly?
    1 Decreased cough efficiency and decreased vital capacity
    2 Decreased lean body mass and decreased glomerular filtration rate
    3 Decreased salivation and decreased gastrointestinal motility
    4 Decreased muscle strength and loss of bone density

18. Which of the following nursing actions would contribute to encouraging autonomy in an elderly male client in a nursing home?
    1 Scheduling his barber appointments
    2 Allowing him to choose social activities
    3 Decorating his room
    4 Planning his meals

19. Which of the following clinical signs, if exhibited by a terminally ill elderly client, indicates to the nurse that death may be imminent?
    1 Cold, clammy skin and irregular, noisy breathing
    2 Eupnea and normal body temperature
    3 Presence of swallowing reflex and active bowel sounds
    4 Rubor and paresthesias

20. The elderly client is less able to regulate hot and cold bodily changes, due to alterations in the activity of the:
    1 Parotid glands
    2 Thymus gland
    3 Pineal gland
    4 Sweat glands

21. Which behavior, if engaged in by an elderly widow, indicates ineffective coping?
    1 Visiting her husband's grave once a month
    2 Participating in a senior citizens program
    3 Looking at old snapshots of her family
    4 Neglecting her personal grooming

22. When communicating with an elderly client who is hearing impaired, the nurse initially:
    1 Stands in front of the client
    2 Exaggerates lip movements
    3 Obtains a sign language interpreter
    4 Pantomimes and writes the client notes

23. Which statement, if made by an elderly client, indicates that further teaching concerning improving sleep is necessary?
    1 "I drink hot chocolate before bedtime."
    2 "I have stopped smoking cigars."
    3 "I swim three times a week."
    4 "I read for 40 minutes before bedtime."

24. The visiting nurse observes that the elderly male client is confined by his daughter-in-law to his room. When the nurse suggests he walk to the den and join the family, he says, "I'm in everyone's way, my son needs for me to stay here." The most important action for the nurse to take is to:
    1 Suggest to the client and daughter-in-law that they consider a nursing home for the client
    2 Suggest appropriate resources to the client and daughter-in-law, such as respite care and senior citizens groups

    3 Say nothing, as it is best for the nurse to remain neutral and wait to be asked for help
    4 Say to the son, "Confining your father to his room is inhumane."

25. The community health nurse visits a frail, 80-year-old male client at home. The client has several bruises on his back, hips, and chest. The medication count and the client's mental status indicate that he is receiving too much sedation. The client says, "My son gets tired having to tend to me at night. I'm always wet and it's all my fault. My son can't help being a little rough." Which of the following responses by the nurse is appropriate?
    1 "You're saying that when you're incontinent at night, you feel at fault and that you feel your son can't help being rough?"
    2 "Oh, he can't, can he? I intend to report this abusive behavior to the police."
    3 "Well, I know you feel that you're a bother, but you pay your way and then some. I'll talk with your son and clear this right up."
    4 "Let's not dwell on this. After all, you are doing quite well and maybe we can arrange for you to go to a nursing home on weekends."

26. Which of the following assessment data indicates a potential complication associated with the skin of an aging client?
    1 Wrinkling, baldness, and gray hair
    2 Thinning and loss of elasticity in the skin
    3 Deepening of expression lines, and wrinkling
    4 Crusting and thinning of skin

27. Which of the following assessment data indicates a potential complication associated with age-related changes in the musculoskeletal system?
    1 Decrease in height
    2 Decrease in lean body mass
    3 Overall sclerotic lesions
    4 Changes in structural bone tissue

28. Which of the following assessment data indicates a potential complication associated with the eyes of older adult clients?
    1 Vision is 20/20
    2 Irregular lens or cornea
    3 Vision is 20/30
    4 Lens opacification

29. Which of the following assessment data indicates that the elder client with Alzheimer's disease has entered Stage III?
    1 Loss of speech
    2 Loss of locomotion
    3 Forgets own phone number
    4 Urinary and fecal incontinence

30. Which nursing intervention, if performed by the nurse for an elderly immobilized client, may prevent respiratory complications?
    1 Monitoring vital signs every shift
    2 Decreasing oral fluid intake
    3 Changing the client's position every 2 hours
    4 Instructing the client to bear down every hour and hold the breath

ANSWERS

1. **2**

Rationale: Presbycusis refers to the age-related irreversible degenerative changes of the inner ear leading to decreased hearing acuity. As a result of these changes, the elderly have a decreased response to high-frequency sounds. Low-pitched tones of voice are more easily heard and interpreted by the elderly.

Test-Taking Strategy: Knowledge regarding the physiological changes that occur with hearing among the elderly is required to answer this question. There is only one correct response. Options 1, 3, and 4 are not accurate statements. If you had difficulty with this question, take time now to review the characteristics of presbycusis.

Level of Cognitive Ability: Application
Phase of Nursing Process: Assessment
Client Needs: Physiological Integrity
Content Area: Fundamental Skills

Reference
Ignatavicius, D., Workman, M., & Mishler, M. (1995). *Medical-surgical nursing: A nursing process approach* (2nd ed.). Philadelphia: W. B. Saunders. pp. 152, 1352.

2. **2**

Rationale: Serum transferrin is an iron-transport protein that can be measured directly or calculated as an indirect measurement of total iron-binding capacity. It is a more sensitive indicator of protein status than is albumin. When serum transferrin is less than 100 mg/dL, the level of visceral protein depletion is severe. The normal creatinine level is 0.6 to 1.3 mg/dL. The normal calcium level is 9 to 11 mg/dL, or 4.5 to 5.5 mEq/L. The normal sodium level is 135 to 145 mEq/L.

Test-Taking Strategy: Use the process of elimination in answering the question. The key word in the question is "protein." The only option that refers to the analysis of protein is option 2. Additionally, if you were familiar with the normal laboratory values, you would eliminate options 1, 3, and 4. Take time now to review these laboratory values if you had difficulty with this question!

Level of Cognitive Ability: Analysis
Phase of Nursing Process: Analysis
Client Needs: Physiological Integrity
Content Area: Fundamental Skills

Reference
Ignatavicius, D., Workman, M., & Mishler, M. (1995). *Medical-surgical nursing: A nursing process approach* (2nd ed.). Philadelphia: W. B. Saunders. pp. 1768, 1776.

3. **1**

Rationale: It is preferable to get clients out of bed and sitting in a chair for meals. This position facilitates chewing and swallowing and prevents reflux of stomach contents.

Test-Taking Strategy: To protect the client from aspiration, the nurse must know proper positioning for feeding. Use the process of elimination to select the correct option. Option 1 is the only correct response.

Level of Cognitive Ability: Application
Phase of Nursing Process: Planning
Client Needs: Safe, Effective Care Environment
Content Area: Fundamental Skills

Reference
Craven, R., & Hirnle, C. (1996). *Fundamentals of nursing: Human health and function* (2nd ed.). Philadelphia: J. B. Lippincott. p. 1048.

4. **1**

Rationale: To prevent aspiration while administering a tube feeding, the nurse should position the client in an upright sitting position or elevate the head of the bed at least 30°. Before the feeding, the nurse checks the placement of the tube by aspirating gastric contents and measuring the pH. Formulas are given at room temperature as a bolus feeding, as intermittent feedings, or by continuous infusion.

Test-Taking Strategy: To prevent the complication of aspiration when feeding a client with a nasogastric tube, the nurse's first priority would be to assess accurate placement of the tube. Take time now to review the principles related to nasogastric tube feedings if you had difficulty with this question!

Level of Cognitive Ability: Application
Phase of Nursing Process: Implementation
Client Needs: Safe, Effective Care Environment
Content Area: Fundamental Skills

Reference
Black, J., & Matassarin-Jacobs, E. (1997). *Medical-surgical nursing: Clinical management for continuity of care* (5th ed.). Philadelphia: W. B. Saunders. pp. 1752–1753.

5. **4**

Rationale: Lisinopril is an antihypertensive, angiotensin-converting enzyme inhibitor (ACE inhibitor). The usual dosage range is 10 to 20 mg daily. Adverse effects include headache, dizziness, fatigue, orthostatic hypotension, tachycardia, and angioedema. Specific client education points include taking one pill a day, not stopping the medication without consulting the physician, and monitoring for side effects and adverse reactions that include gastrointestinal (GI) upset, skin rash, dizziness, lightheadedness, headache, and fatigue. The client should notify the physician if side effects occur.

Test-Taking Strategy: Knowledge regarding the indications and the side effects of lisinopril will assist in answering the question. Use the process of elimination to answer the question, noting that the question asks for the inaccurate client statement. Options 1, 2, and 3 are accurate statements. Option 4 is the inaccurate statement. If you had difficulty with this question, take time now to review this medication!

Level of Cognitive Ability: Analysis
Phase of Nursing Process: Evaluation
Client Needs: Health Promotion and Maintenance
Content Area: Pharmacology

Reference

Hodgson, B., & Kizior, R. (1999). *Saunders nursing drug handbook 1999.* Philadelphia: W. B. Saunders. pp. 596–597.

6. **1**

Rationale: Elder abuse is widespread and occurs among all subgroups of the population. It includes physical and psychological abuse, misuse of property, and violation of rights. The typical abuse victim is a woman of advanced age with few social contacts and at least one physical or mental impairment that limits the ability to perform activities of daily living (ADL). In addition, this client lives alone or with the abuser and depends on the abuser for care.

Test-Taking Strategy: To answer this question, the nurse needs to identify which of the clients, as presented in the options, is most defenseless as the result of the disease process. Identifying that point will assist in directing you to the correct option. If you had difficulty with this question, take time now to review content related to elder abuse!

Level of Cognitive Ability: Analysis
Phase of Nursing Process: Assessment
Client Needs: Psychosocial Integrity
Content Area: Fundamental Skills

Reference

Black, J., & Matassarin-Jacobs, E. (1997). *Medical-surgical nursing: Clinical management for continuity of care* (5th ed.). Philadelphia: W. B. Saunders. pp. 89–90.

7. **2**

Rationale: Because it takes older people longer for their eyes to adapt to changes from dark to light and vice versa, they are at a greater risk of falls and injuries. Any place where there is a sudden change from dark to light or from light to dark can be dangerous. Entering theaters and getting up at night are two hazardous situations that may be risky for older adults. Eyes adapt to the dark by using the rod receptors, which are sensitive to short blue-green wavelengths. Red wavelengths are longer and are perceived by the cones. Thus, a red light in the bathroom at night will allow for adequate vision to function in the dark without the need for adaptation.

Test-Taking Strategy: To answer this question, the nurse needs to know the physiological eye changes that occur in the elderly. Although options 1 and 3 are not incorrect, they do not meet the client's need for independence. Option 4 is incorrect because the elderly need to be encouraged to drink at least 2 liters of fluid a day to prevent dehydration. Option 2 reflects the nurse's understanding of the visual changes affecting the elderly and how to best help this client's aging eyes and maintain independence.

Level of Cognitive Ability: Analysis
Phase of Nursing Process: Analysis
Client Needs: Physiological Integrity
Content Area: Fundamental Skills

Reference

Black, J., & Matassarin-Jacobs, E. (1997). *Medical-surgical nursing: Clinical management for continuity of care* (5th ed.). Philadelphia: W. B. Saunders. p. 940.

8. **3**

Rationale: Nursing interventions for the Alzheimer client who is angry, frustrated, or hostile include decreasing environmental stimuli, approaching the client calmly and with assurance, not demanding anything from the client, and distracting the client. It is important that the nurse reach out, touch, hold a hand, put an arm around the waist or in some way maintain physical contact.

Test-Taking Strategy: There is only one correct option. Playing a radio may increase stimuli and turning the lights out may produce more agitation. The client with Alzheimer's would not be a candidate for group work if he or she is agitated. Calmly touching the client or putting an arm around the waist tends to distract the client and decrease the fear, frustration, or anger being experienced by the client.

Level of Cognitive Ability: Application
Phase of Nursing Process: Planning
Client Needs: Psychosocial Integrity
Content Area: Fundamental Skills

Reference

Polaski, A. L., & Tatro, S. E. (1996). *Luckmann's core principles and practice of medical-surgical nursing.* Philadelphia: W. B. Saunders. p. 371.

9. **4**

Rationale: Exercise and activity are essential for health promotion and maintenance in the older adult and to achieve an optimal level of functioning. Approximately half the physical deterioration of the elderly is caused by disuse rather than by the aging process or disease. One of the best exercises for an older adult is walking, progressing to 30-minute sessions three to five times each week. Swimming and dancing are also beneficial.

Test-Taking Strategy: This question is asking for the best activity the elderly should engage in. Options 1, 2, and 3, although possible, are not the best activities. Option 4 is the best exercise for an older adult.

Level of Cognitive Ability: Analysis
Phase of Nursing Process: Analysis
Client Needs: Health Promotion and Maintenance
Content Area: Fundamental Skills

Reference

Black, J., & Matassarin-Jacobs, E. (1997). *Medical-surgical nursing: Clinical management for continuity of care* (5th ed.). Philadelphia: W. B. Saunders. p. 85.

10. **1**

Rationale: The client with myasthenia gravis and the family should be taught information about myasthenia gravis and its treatment. They should be aware of adverse reactions of anticholinesterase medications and steroids and should be taught that timing of anticholinesterase medication is critical. It is important to instruct the client to administer the medication on time to maintain a chemical balance at the neuromuscular junction. If not given on time, the client may become too weak to swallow.

Test-Taking Strategy: There is only one correct option. Use the process of elimination to answer the question. A client who does not understand the importance of the anticholinesterase medication regimen needs further teaching. Options 2, 3, and 4 include all the necessary information that the client requires to understand how to maintain health with this neurological degenerative disease.

Level of Cognitive Ability: Analysis
Phase of Nursing Process: Evaluation
Client Needs: Health Promotion and Maintenance
Content Area: Fundamental Skills

Reference

Polaski, A. L., & Tatro, S. E. (1996). *Luckmann's core principles and practice of medical-surgical nursing.* Philadelphia: W. B. Saunders. p. 382.

11. **4**

Rationale: The older adult searches for emotional integration and acceptance of the past and present, as well as acceptance of physiological decline without fear of death. Older adults who like to retell stories or past events need to be provided the opportunity to do so. This phenomenon is called life review, or reminiscence. In a sense, it is a way for an older adult to relive and restructure life experiences and is a part of achieving ego identity.

Test-Taking Strategy: Use the process of elimination to answer the question. Option 1 indicates reality orientation techniques. Options 2 and 3 indicate socialization and physical activity. Story-telling hours would allow older adults to engage in memories that provided them satisfaction or a resolution of experiences.

Level of Cognitive Ability: Analysis
Phase of Nursing Process: Analysis
Client Needs: Psychosocial Integrity
Content Area: Fundamental Skills

Reference

Taylor, C., Lillis, C., & LeMone, P. (1997). *Fundamentals of nursing: The art and science of nursing care* (3rd ed.). Philadelphia: J. B. Lippincott. p. 161.

12. **2**

Rationale: High-priority diagnoses pose the greatest threat to the client's well-being. Maslow's Hierarchy of Needs Theory, client preference, and anticipation of future problems are guides for prioritizing client problems. Although options 1, 3, and 4 may be appropriate nursing diagnoses, option 2 identifies airway, the highest priority.

Test-Taking Strategy: Physiological needs of the client must be addressed first. Use the ABCs to answer the question. The order of priority is Airway, Breathing, and Circulation. The nursing diagnosis of Ineffective Airway Clearance should be identified by the nurse as a priority nursing diagnosis!

Level of Cognitive Ability: Analysis
Phase of Nursing Process: Analysis
Client Needs: Physiological Integrity
Content Area: Fundamental Skills

Reference

Taylor, C., Lillis, C., & LeMone, P. (1997). *Fundamentals of nursing: The art and science of nursing care* (3rd ed.). Philadelphia: J. B. Lippincott. p. 278.

13. **3**

Rationale: Trauma for the elderly in the home may come about because of an unsteady gait, the presence of unsecured scatter rugs, cluttered passageways, smoking in bed, inoperable smoke detectors, a history of previous falls, a history of substance abuse, or the presence of an unsecured, loaded gun in the house.

Test-Taking Strategy: Use the process of elimination to answer the question. Read the options carefully. There is one

unsafe situation among the options, the presence of unsecured scatter rugs. To prevent falls, these rugs need to be secured. The other options presented all ensure safety for the client.

Level of Cognitive Ability: Analysis
Phase of Nursing Process: Assessment
Client Needs: Safe, Effective Care Environment
Content Area: Fundamental Skills

Reference

Taylor, C., Lillis, C., & LeMone, P. (1997). *Fundamentals of nursing: The art and science of nursing care* (3rd ed.). Philadelphia: J. B. Lippincott. p. 534.

14. **1**

Rationale: According to Maslow's hierarchy of needs theory, lower needs must be met before a person can focus on higher ones. Client needs may be prioritized according to the following: physiological needs, safety needs, love and belonging needs, self-esteem needs, and self-actualization needs. Option 1 addresses a physiological need.

Test-Taking Strategy: Use the process of elimination and do not read into the question. Basic physiological needs are a priority in administering nursing care. Although options 2, 3, and 4 address the client's needs, the priority would be to keep the client clean and dry and to avoid embarrassment.

Level of Cognitive Ability: Application
Phase of Nursing Process: Implementation
Client Needs: Physiological Integrity
Content Area: Fundamental Skills

Reference

Taylor, C., Lillis, C., & LeMone, P. (1997). *Fundamentals of nursing: The art and science of nursing care* (3rd ed.). Philadelphia: J. B. Lippincott. p. 278.

15. **3**

Rationale: Adequate dietary fiber is one of the most important factors in aiding bowel function. Dietary fiber increases fecal weight and water content and accelerates the transit of fecal mass through the GI tract. The retention of water by the fiber has the ability to soften stools and promote regularity.

Test-Taking Strategy: Read the stem carefully. The question asks for an inaccurate statement concerning bowel elimination. Options 1, 2, and 4 are correct statements. Fluids and exercise facilitate bowel elimination. Also remember that the client's elimination pattern is individual.

Level of Cognitive Ability: Analysis
Phase of Nursing Process: Evaluation
Client Needs: Health Promotion and Maintenance
Content Area: Fundamental Skills

Reference

Leahy, J., & Kizilay, P. (1998). *Foundations of nursing practice: A nursing process approach.* Philadelphia: W. B. Saunders. p. 928.

16. **4**

Rationale: Ageism is a form of prejudice in which older adults are stereotyped by characteristics found in only a few members of their group. Fundamental to ageism is the view that older people are different from "me" and will remain different from "me"; therefore, they do not experience the same desires, needs, and concerns. Industrialism and technological advances have placed a high priority on productivity, so that retired people may be said to have "outlived their usefulness."

Test-Taking Strategy: Understanding the definition of ageism is necessary to answer this question. From this point, use the process of elimination. Options 1, 2, and 3 are supportive roles that the nurse engages in when dealing with the elderly. Option 4 suggests that the nurse does not think the elderly are worthy of aggressive treatment and demonstrates ageism.

Level of Cognitive Ability: Analysis
Phase of Nursing Process: Analysis
Client Needs: Psychosocial Integrity
Content Area: Fundamental Skills

Reference
Taylor, C., Lillis, C., & LeMone, P. (1997). *Fundamentals of nursing: The art and science of nursing care* (3rd ed.). Philadelphia: J. B. Lippincott. p. 165.

17. **2**

Rationale: The frail elderly are at risk of developing digitalis toxicity because of decreased lean body mass and age-associated decreased glomerular filtration rate. Serum potassium is closely monitored. The combination of hypokalemia and digitalis therapy can lead to lethal dysrhythmias.

Test-Taking Strategy: Use the process of elimination and knowledge regarding the physiological changes associated with aging. This should direct you to option 2, the correct option. Also, note that option 2 is the only option that addresses renal excretion. The other options are age-related body changes, but they would not cause digitalis toxicity in the frail elderly. If you had difficulty with this question, take time now to review the physiological changes associated with aging.

Level of Cognitive Ability: Analysis
Phase of Nursing Process: Analysis
Client Needs: Physiological Integrity
Content Area: Fundamental Skills

Reference
Black, J., & Matassarin-Jacobs, E. (1997). *Medical-surgical nursing: Clinical management for continuity of care* (5th ed.). Philadelphia: W. B. Saunders. p. 93.

18. **2**

Rationale: Autonomy is the personal freedom to direct one's own life as long as it does not impinge on the rights of others. An autonomous person is capable of rational thought. This individual can identify problems, search for alternatives, and select solutions that allow continued personal freedom as long as the rights and property of others are not harmed. Loss of autonomy, and therefore of independence, is a very real fear among elderly people.

Test-Taking Strategy: Use the process of elimination to answer the question. Understanding the definition of autonomy will direct you to the correct option. To promote independence in clients, it is essential to give them choices. Option 2 is the only option that allows the client to be a decision maker.

Level of Cognitive Ability: Application
Phase of Nursing Process: Planning
Client Needs: Psychosocial Integrity
Content Area: Fundamental Skills

Reference
Black, J., & Matassarin-Jacobs, E. (1997). *Medical-surgical nursing: Clinical management for continuity of care* (5th ed.). Philadelphia: W. B. Saunders. p. 102.

19. **1**

Rationale: The clinical signs of impending or approaching death include inability to swallow, pitting edema, decreased gastrointestinal and urinary tract activity, bowel and bladder incontinence, loss of motion sensation and reflexes, elevated temperature but cold or clammy skin, cyanosis, lowered blood pressure, noisy or irregular respiration, and Cheyne-Stokes respirations.

Test-Taking Strategy: Use the process of elimination and eliminate options 2 and 3 as these identify normal findings. Option 4 does not imply approaching death. Option 1, the correct option, identifies two main clinical signs of approaching death. If you had difficulty with this question, take time now to review the signs associated with impending or approaching death.

Level of Cognitive Ability: Analysis
Phase of Nursing Process: Assessment
Client Needs: Physiological Integrity
Content Area: Fundamental Skills

Reference
Taylor, C., Lillis, C., & LeMone, P. (1997). *Fundamentals of nursing: The art and science of nursing care* (3rd ed.). Philadelphia: J. B. Lippincott. p. 784.

20. **4**

Rationale: Functions of the skin include protection, sensory reception, homeostasis, and temperature regulation. The skin helps regulate the body temperature in two ways, by dilation and constriction of blood vessels and by activity of the sweat glands. As aging progresses, alterations in sweat gland activity make the glands less effective in temperature regulation, so the aging person is less able to regulate hot and cold bodily changes.

Test-Taking Strategy: Use the process of elimination to answer the question. The parotid glands are responsible for the drainage of saliva, which plays an important role in digestion. The pineal gland is a major site of melatonin biosynthesis. The thymus gland plays an immunological role throughout life. Sweat glands control temperature regulation. If you had difficulty with this question, take time now to review the functions of the glands identified in each option.

Level of Cognitive Ability: Analysis
Phase of Nursing Process: Analysis
Client Needs: Physiological Integrity
Content Area: Fundamental Skills

Reference
Polaski, A. L., & Tatro, S. E. (1996). *Luckmann's core principles and practice of medical-surgical nursing.* Philadelphia: W. B. Saunders. pp. 1326–1327.

21. **4**

Rationale: Coping mechanisms are behaviors used to decrease stress and anxiety. Typical behaviors include physical activity and exercise, smoking and drinking, lack of eye contact, and withdrawal. In response to a death, ineffective coping is manifested by an extreme behavior that in some instances may be harmful to the individual either physically or psychologically.

Test-Taking Strategy: Use the process of elimination and note that the question asks for the ineffective coping behavior. Options 1, 2, and 3 are positive activities that the individual is engaging in to get on with her life. Option 4 is indicative of a behavior that identifies an ineffective coping behavior in the grieving process.

Level of Cognitive Ability: Analysis
Phase of Nursing Process: Analysis
Client Needs: Psychosocial Integrity
Content Area: Fundamental Skills

Reference

Taylor, C., Lillis, C., & LeMone, P. (1997). *Fundamentals of nursing: The art and science of nursing care* (3rd ed.). Philadelphia: J. B. Lippincott. pp. 760, 796.

22. **1**

Rationale: The nurse would ensure that the hearing-impaired client can see the nurse when speaking by providing adequate lighting and by standing in front of the client. The nurse should enunciate words clearly but not exaggerate lip movements. If the client is profoundly hearing impaired and uses signing, a sign language interpreter should be obtained. If a client cannot understand by reading lips, the nurse would try using gestures, pantomiming or writing notes.

Test-Taking Strategy: The word "initially" is a key word and should direct you toward the correct option. The nurse may at some time utilize options 3 and 4, but to communicate effectively with a hearing-impaired client, the nurse first makes sure that the client can see her or him. If you had difficulty with this question, take time now to review the nursing interventions for the hearing impaired.

Level of Cognitive Ability: Application
Phase of Nursing Process: Implementation
Client Needs: Psychosocial Integrity
Content Area: Fundamental Skills

Reference

Black, J., & Matassarin-Jacobs, E. (1997). *Medical-surgical nursing: Clinical management for continuity of care* (5th ed.). Philadelphia: W. B. Saunders. p. 1000.

23. **1**

Rationale: Many nonpharmacologic sleep aids can be used to influence sleep. The client should avoid caffeinated beverages and stimulants such as tea, cola, and chocolate and foods containing tyrosine, such as cheddar cheese. The client should exercise regularly, as exercise enhances sleep by burning off tension that accumulates during the day. A 20- to 30-minute walk, swim, or bicycle ride three times a week is helpful. The client should sleep on a good bed with a firm mattress. Smoking and alcohol should be avoided. The client should avoid large meals, peanuts, beans, fruit and raw vegetables that produce gas, and snacks high in fat that are difficult to digest.

Test-Taking Strategy: Read the question carefully. Note that the question asks for a response that indicates the need for further teaching. Options 2, 3, and 4 are positive responses indicating that the client has learned about ways of improving sleep. Option 1 indicates that the client does not know that chocolate is a stimulant and will interfere with a good night's rest.

Level of Cognitive Ability: Analysis
Phase of Nursing Process: Evaluation
Client Needs: Physiological Integrity
Content Area: Fundamental Skills

Reference

Black, J., & Matassarin-Jacobs, .E. (1997). *Medical-surgical nursing: Clinical management for continuity of care* (5th ed.). Philadelphia: W. B. Saunders. p. 408.

24. **2**

Rationale: It is thought that between 1 and 2 million elders may suffer from neglect, abuse, or exploitation, but few incidents are actually reported. Assisting clients and families to become knowledgeable about community support systems that are available, and making the public aware of the problems involved, are only two of the many roles and responsibilities of the nurse. Stress management techniques will also be invaluable to the nurse in helping the caregivers develop patience and high levels of interpersonal giving.

Test-Taking Strategy: Use the process of elimination to answer the question. In option 1, the suggestion to commit the client to a nursing home is premature. While the data provided tells you this elder requires nursing care, you don't know the extent of nursing care. Observing that the client has begun to be confined to his room makes it necessary for the nurse to intervene legally and ethically, so option 3 is not appropriate and is passive in terms of advocacy. Option 4 is incorrect and judgmental. Caregiver stress and burn-out is thought to account for much elder abuse.

Level of Cognitive Ability: Application
Phase of Nursing Process: Implementation
Client Needs: Psychosocial Integrity
Content Area: Fundamental Skills

References

Haber, J. (1997). *Comprehensive psychiatric nursing* (5th ed.). St. Louis: Mosby–Year Book. pp. 777–802.
Johnson, B. S. (1997). *Psychiatric–mental health nursing: Adaptation and growth* (4th ed.). Philadelphia: Lippincott-Raven. pp. 817–858.

25. **1**

Rationale: The correct answer summarizes and focuses upon the content of the client's message. In addition, it restates so the client can hear himself making excuses about his son's physical abuse. The abused elder classically excuses the abuser.

Test-Taking Strategy: This question assesses your ability to intervene in elder abuse. Use the process of elimination. In option 2, the nurse is sarcastic and without further investigation moves to report the incident. In option 3, the nurse confirms the client's fear that he is a "bother," begins to insinuate that his son is using his money, and that this situation will be cleared up just by the nurse's talking with the client's son. Option 4 is incorrect because it advocates avoiding the issue and then, incongruously, states "things are proceeding well" but that the client can go to a "nursing home on the weekends."

Level of Cognitive Ability: Application
Phase of Nursing Process: Implementation
Client Needs: Safe, Effective Care Environment
Content Area: Fundamental Skills

References

Haber, J. (1997). *Comprehensive psychiatric nursing* (5th ed.). St. Louis: Mosby–Year Book. pp. 777–802.
Johnson, B. S. (1997). *Psychiatric–mental health nursing: Adaptation and growth* (4th ed.). Philadelphia: Lippincott-Raven. pp. 817–858.

26. **4**

Rationale: The integument of older adults consists of three layers: the epidermis, the dermis, and subcutaneous tissue that lies beneath the dermis. The normal physiological changes that occur in the skin of older adults include thinning and loss of elasticity and deepening of expression lines. Other normal age-related changes in the skin of older adults include wrinkles, gray hair, sagging skin, and baldness. Crusting of the skin and thinning of skin would indicate a potential complication.

Test-Taking Strategy: Read the question carefully and note the key phrase "potential complication." This question requires you to clarify the normal changes that occur in the skin and those that are common disorders seen in the integumentary system of aging clients. The first three options describe normal physiological changes in the skin. The fourth option adds crusting of the skin, which is a common disorder that can occur. More than 90% of older adults have some kind of skin disorder. Such disorders can be caused by external sources, such as sunlight, climate, and allergic reactions to medications. The internal causes of skin disorders include diabetes, stress, malignancy, and obesity. Option 4 is the only option that identifies a potential complication.

Level of Cognitive Ability: Analysis
Phase of Nursing Process: Analysis
Client Needs: Physiological Integrity
Content Area: Fundamental Skills

References

Black, J. M., & Matassarin-Jacobs, E. (1997). *Medical-surgical nursing: Clinical management for continuity of care* (5th ed.). Philadelphia: W. B. Saunders. pp. 1943–1953.
Luckmann, J. (1997). *Saunders manual of nursing care.* Philadelphia: W. B. Saunders. pp. 1617–1636.
Matteson, M. A., McConnell, E. S., & Linton, A. D. (1997). *Gerontological nursing concepts and practice* (2nd ed.). Philadelphia: W. B. Saunders. pp. 176–179.

27. **3**

Rationale: Sclerotic or osteoblastic lesions occur as bone resorption increases and results in replacement of original bone with fibrous material. This condition occurs in Paget's disease, an age-related disorder. The normal age-related changes in bone structure include an increase in the ratio of cortical bone to trabecular bone loss, a decrease in stature, and a loss of 1.2 cm over 20 years, leading to a decrease in height. In addition, the amount of lean body mass decreases, and the amount of subcutaneous fat distribution increases.

Test-Taking Strategy: Note the key phrase "potential complication." This question assesses your knowledge of age-related changes in the musculoskeletal system as well as abnormal changes. Options 1, 2, and 4 are incorrect options and correct for normal, age-related changes in the musculoskeletal system. Option 3 is the correct answer because it describes the excessive resorption and deposit of bone that earmarks Paget's disease.

Level of Cognitive Ability: Analysis
Phase of Nursing Process: Analysis
Client Needs: Physiological Integrity
Content Area: Fundamental Skills

References

Black, J. M., & Matassarin-Jacobs, E. (1997). *Medical-surgical nursing: Clinical management for continuity of care* (5th ed.). Philadelphia: W. B. Saunders. pp. 1905–1908.
Luckmann, J. (1997). *Saunders manual of nursing care.* Philadelphia: W. B. Saunders. pp. 1523–1524; 1587–1588.
Matteson, M. A., McConnell, E. S., & Linton, A. D. (1997). *Gerontological nursing: Concepts and practice* (2nd ed.). Philadelphia: W. B. Saunders. pp. 197–200.

28. **4**

Rationale: One of the eye complications for older adults is cataracts. Cataracts, caused by the progressive, degenerative changes occurring after 50 years of age, are an abnormal eye condition that result in a loss of opacity of the crystalline lens, causing visual disturbances. Ninety-five percent of persons over 65 years of age suffer from some degree of lens opacity, and almost 1.5 million cataract extractions are performed annually. The lens (and ciliary body) is located behind the iris at the pupillary opening. The lens of the eye acts like a camera lens, refracting and focusing light onto the retina. Composed of transparent fibers in an elastic membrane, the lens capsule contains no blood vessels, nerves, or connective tissue. Lens thickness is controlled by the ciliary body (which contains the thickened part of the vascular coat of the eye that joins the iris and choroid).

Test-Taking Strategy: Note the key phrase "potential complication." This question is assessing your knowledge of the abnormal eye findings across the life span. Although this question specifically tests your knowledge of the changes that occur in the eyes of older adults, it uses life span differences that may have cued you regarding the correct option. Option 1 describes normal vision. Option 2 describes an astigmatism, which is a common visual problem in children. Option 3 describes the normal visual acuity for an infant. If you had difficulty answering this question, review the physical assessment findings for normal and abnormal eyes of clients across the life span. Understanding the anatomy and physiology of the eyes will enhance your ability to understand the pathophysiology and its treatment as well as the nursing care.

Level of Cognitive Ability: Analysis
Phase of Nursing Process: Analysis
Client Needs: Physiological Integrity
Content Area: Fundamental Skills

References

Black, J. M., & Matassarin-Jacobs, E. (1997). *Medical-surgical nursing: Clinical management for continuity of care* (5th ed.). Philadelphia: W. B. Saunders. pp. 833–834; 848–851.
Luckmann, J. (1997). *Saunders manual of nursing care.* Philadelphia: W. B. Saunders. pp. 760–768.
Matteson, M. A., McConnell, E. S., & Linton, A. D. (1997). *Gerontological nursing: Concepts and practice* (2nd ed.). Philadelphia: W. B. Saunders. p. 360.

29. **3**

Rationale: Stage I reflects mild memory impairment. In Stage II, moderate memory impairment exists. In Stage III, severe disorientation occurs, and the client can't recall the home phone number, has trouble choosing proper clothing, and requires coaxing to bathe.

Test-Taking Strategy: This question requires knowledge of the progression of Alzheimer's disease. If you had difficulty with this question, take time now to review this important content and the assessment findings associated with the disease!

Level of Cognitive Ability: Analysis
Phase of Nursing Process: Analysis
Client Needs: Physiological Integrity
Content Area: Fundamental Skills

References

Black, J. M., & Matassarin-Jacobs, E. (1997). *Medical-surgical nursing: Clinical management for continuity of care* (5th ed.). Philadelphia: W. B. Saunders. pp. 691–694; 773–780.

Luckmann, J. (1997). *Saunders manual of nursing care.* Philadelphia: W. B. Saunders. pp. 578; 713–717.

Matteson, M. A., McConnell, E. S., & Linton, A. D. (1997). *Gerontological nursing: Concepts and practice* (2nd ed.). Philadelphia: W. B. Saunders. pp. 295–298.

30. **3**

Rationale: The nurse should assess the client's vital signs every 4 hours to identify an elevated temperature that suggests infection. The nurse would encourage fluid intake to loosen secretions and thus enable the client to expectorate more easily. Frequent position change helps mobilize lung secretions and prevent pooling. It is important to encourage coughing and deep breathing to mobilize lung secretions. Clients should be instructed to avoid the Valsalva maneuver or any activity involving holding the breath.

Test-Taking Strategy: Read the question carefully, noting the key phrase "prevent respiratory complications." Use the process of elimination to answer the question. Changing the position of the immobilized client every 2 hours will help prevent pooling of lung secretions. The other options do not assist the client to improve ventilatory efforts.

Level of Cognitive Ability: Application
Phase of Nursing Process: Implementation
Client Needs: Physiological Integrity
Content Area: Fundamental Skills

Reference

Black, J. M., & Matassarin-Jacobs, E. (1997). *Medical-surgical nursing: Clinical management for continuity of care* (5th ed.). Philadelphia: W. B. Saunders. p. 1134.

BIBLIOGRAPHY

Black, J. M., & Matassarin-Jacobs, E. (1997). *Medical-surgical nursing: Clinical management for continuity of care* (5th ed.). Philadelphia: W. B. Saunders.

Craven, R., & Hirnle, C. (1996). *Fundamentals of nursing: human health and function* (2nd ed.). Philadelphia: J. B. Lippincott.

Eliopoulos, C. (1997). *Gerontological nursing* (4th ed.). Philadelphia: Lippincott-Raven.

Haber, J. (1997). *Comprehensive psychiatric nursing* (5th ed.). St. Louis: Mosby–Year Book.

Hodgson, B., & Kizior, R. (1999). *Saunders nursing drug handbook 1999.* Philadelphia: W. B. Saunders.

Ignatavicius, D., Workman, M., & Mishler, M. (1995). *Medical-surgical nursing: A nursing process approach* (2nd ed.). Philadelphia: W. B. Saunders.

Johnson, B. S. (1997). *Psychiatric-mental health nursing: Adaptation and growth* (4th ed.). Philadelphia: Lippincott-Raven.

Leahy, J., & Kizilay, P. (1998). *Foundations of nursing practice: A nursing process approach.* Philadelphia: W. B. Saunders.

Luckmann, J. (1997). *Saunders manual of nursing care.* Philadelphia: W. B. Saunders.

Matteson, M. A., McConnell, E. S. & Linton, A. D. (1997). *Gerontological nursing: Concepts and practice.* (2nd ed.). Philadelphia: W. B. Saunders.

Polaski, A. L., & Tatro, S. E. (1996). *Luckmann's core principles and practice of medical-surgical nursing.* Philadelphia: W. B. Saunders.

Taylor, C., Lillis, C., & LeMone, P. (1997). *Fundamentals of nursing: the art and science of nursing care* (3rd ed.). Philadelphia: J. B. Lippincott.

Comprehensive Test Questions

1. The client is beginning to take a solid oral diet following subtotal gastrectomy. The nurse would do which of the following to minimize the risk of dumping syndrome?
   1 Have the client avoid taking fluids with the meal
   2 Ask the client to sit up for an hour after eating
   3 Provide concentrated, high-carbohydrate foods
   4 Give the client two large meals per day

2. The nurse is caring for a newborn infant after surgical intervention for imperforate anus. Which of the following positions is most appropriate for the newborn in the postoperative period?
   1 Supine with no head elevation
   2 Supine with the head elevated 30°
   3 Side-lying with the legs extended
   4 Side-lying with the legs flexed

3. The mother of a child with hepatitis A tells the home care nurse that she is very concerned because the jaundice in the child seems to be worse. Which of the following responses is most appropriate?
   1 "You need to call the physician."
   2 "The child is probably infectious again."
   3 "You need to change the child's diet."
   4 "In many situations, the jaundice worsens before it resolves."

4. A client recently admitted to the hospital in the manic phase of bipolar disorder is dehydrated, unkempt, taking antipsychotic medications, and complaining of abdominal "fullness" and discomfort. The nurse determines that an appropriate intervention for these complaints is to
   1 Teach self-grooming skills
   2 Force fluids and reward cleanliness with unit privileges
   3 Encourage frequent fluid intake and a high-fiber diet
   4 Monitor the adequacy of the antipsychotic dosage

5. The nurse is caring for a poorly controlled Type I (insulin-dependent) diabetic client. As part of the nursing care plan, the nurse monitors for diabetic ketoacidosis (DKA). In the event that DKA does occur, the nurse anticipates that the most likely medication to be prescribed is
   1 Regular insulin
   2 NPH insulin
   3 Glucagon
   4 Glyburide (DiaBeta)

6. The client with severe psoriasis has a nursing diagnosis of Self-Esteem Disturbance. The nurse plans to incorporate which of the following behaviors when working with this client?

   1 Keep communications brief
   2 Approach client in a formal manner
   3 Listen attentively
   4 Avoid looking at affected skin areas

7. The nurse is caring for a client with a wound infection. The culture report reveals the presence of *Pseudomonas aeruginosa*. Which of the following does the nurse anticipate to be prescribed to treat the wound?
   1 A glycerin emollient
   2 Aspercreme
   3 Myoflex
   4 Acetic acid solution

8. The client has an order for an injection to be administered by the intradermal route. The nurse avoids which of the following actions when administering this medication?
   1 Insert the needle at a 10 to 15° angle
   2 Inject the medication slowly
   3 Massage the area after removing the needle
   4 Make a circular mark around the injection site

9. The client is admitted to the emergency department following burn injury in a house fire. The skin on the client's trunk is tan-colored, dry, and hard. It is edematous but not painful. The nurse interprets that this client's burn should be classified as:
   1 Superficial partial thickness (first-degree)
   2 Moderate partial thickness (second-degree)
   3 Deep partial thickness (second-degree)
   4 Full thickness (third-degree)

10. The client who is being evaluated for thermal burn injuries to the arms and legs complains of thirst and asks the nurse for a drink. Which of the following actions by the nurse is most appropriate?
    1 Give the client small glasses of clear liquids
    2 Keep the client NPO
    3 Allow the client to have full liquids
    4 Order the client a full meal tray with extra liquids

11. The elderly client has sustained a superficial skin tear to the arm. The nurse applies which of the following types of dressings?
    1 Dry, sterile dressing
    2 Wet to dry dressing
    3 Gelfoam sponge dressing
    4 Semipermeable film dressing

12. The client is NPO and has a nasogastric tube in place after suffering bilateral burns to the legs. The nurse evaluates that the client's gastrointestinal (GI) status is least satisfactory if which of the following is noted on reassessment?
    1 Gastric pH of 3
    2 Presence of hypoactive bowel sounds

3 GI drainage that is guaiac negative
4 Absence of abdominal discomfort

13. The client with a large abdominal wound is starting to develop a skin irritation in the area where dressing tape is applied to the skin. The nurse interprets that the client would benefit most from
   1 Obtaining a wound culture
   2 Cleansing the irritated area with povidine-iodine
   3 Use of Montgomery straps
   4 Use of nonallergenic tape

14. The client has a nursing diagnosis of Sleep Pattern Disturbance. The nurse plans to encourage which of the following nutritional behaviors on the part of the client to best enhance nighttime sleep?
   1 Eat a large bedtime snack
   2 Drink a glass of milk at bedtime
   3 Eat a bedtime snack with spicy ingredients
   4 Avoid caffeine products 1 hour prior to sleep

15. The nurse is providing mouth care to the unconscious client. The nurse should avoid which of the following actions during this procedure?
   1 Turning the head to one side
   2 Using a bite stick or padded tongue blade
   3 Using oral suction equipment
   4 Rinsing with a large volume of fluid

16. The nurse is administering eye care to the client with an artificial eye. The nurse first separates the upper and lower eyelids with the dominant hand and cups the nondominant hand under the eye. The nurse then removes the eye by applying pressure with the index finger below the
   1 Eye
   2 Brow
   3 Inner canthus
   4 Outer canthus

17. The nurse has given the client with a continuous passive motion (CPM) device instructions about the device and its use. The nurse evaluates that the client has misunderstood one of the points if the client states
   1 How to use the "stop-go" button
   2 To report any discomfort in the knee to the nurse
   3 To reset the degrees of flexion or extension according to comfort
   4 That the knee should stay aligned with the hinged joint on the machine

18. The client has been instructed in crutch-walking techniques and has been fitted for crutches. Before beginning ambulation, the nurse checks the fit of the crutches to ensure that there is a space between the axilla and the top crutch pad of

1 1 inch
2 2 inches
3 3 inches
4 4 inches

19. The nurse is setting up a transcutaneous electrical nerve stimulation (TENS) unit for a client with chronic pain. As the nurse turns up the level of stimulation, the client complains of discomfort. The nurse interprets this to mean that
   1 The maximal stimulation has been reached and that it should be decreased slightly
   2 The maximal stimulation has been far exceeded and should be decreased by half
   3 This is a temporary effect, and the stimulation should continue to be increased
   4 This is a complication of the device's use, and it should be discontinued immediately

20. The hospitalized client who has been placed on "contact precautions" has been ordered to have a chest x-ray film in the radiology department. The nurse should plan to do which of the following upon receipt of this order?
   1 Place a mask on the client in preparation for transport
   2 Place a sterile gown on the client
   3 Transport through empty corridors only
   4 Question the physician about whether a portable chest film may be obtained

21. The client who had surgery for treatment of glaucoma has a nursing diagnosis of Risk for Injury. The home care nurse evaluates that the nursing diagnosis is not resolved if the client does which of the following?
   1 Scans environment, turning head side to side
   2 Uses grab bars in bathroom or holds wall for added stability
   3 Takes in sufficient fluid and fiber to avoid constipation
   4 Takes off eye shield applied to use during sleep

22. A group of postmenopausal women are learning to do breast self-examination. The nurse teaches the group which of the following points about this procedure?
   1 Use the tips of the fingers to increase the likelihood of feeling lumps
   2 Examine the left breast with the left hand, and vice versa
   3 Do the examination on the same day of every month
   4 Do the examination 7 days after the start of the menstrual cycle

23. The nurse is monitoring the fluid balance of the client with a burn injury. The nurse assesses that the client is less than adequately hydrated if which of the following data is noted during assessment?

1 Urine output of 40 mL/hr
2 Urine color that is pale yellow
3 Urine specific gravity of 1.032
4 Urine pH of 6

24. The client is recovering well 24 hours after cranial surgery but is fatigued. The neurosurgeon advances the client from NPO status to clear liquids. The nurse interprets that which of the following data is the least reliable in determining the client's readiness to take in fluids?
    1 Bowel sounds
    2 Appetite
    3 Absence of nausea
    4 Presence of swallow reflex

25. The home care nurse is making a visit to a client who is wheelchair-bound after a spinal cord injury sustained 4 months ago. Just prior to leaving the home, the nurse ensures that which of the following has been done to prevent an episode of autonomic dysreflexia?
    1 Recording the amount of urine obtained with catheterization
    2 Leaving the client in an unchilled area of the room
    3 Noting a bowel movement (BM) on the client progress note
    4 Updating the home safety sheet

26. The client who had cranial surgery for cancer of the brain 5 days ago has a few cognitive deficits and does not seem to be progressing as quickly as the client or family hoped. Which of the following approaches by the nurse is most helpful to the client and family at this time?
    1 Emphasize progress in a realistic manner
    2 Inform client and family of standardized goals of care
    3 Set high goals to give the client something to "aim for"
    4 Tell the family to be extremely optimistic with the client

27. The client is being treated on the medical nursing unit for a cerebrovascular accident (CVA). The client at 8 A.M. was awake and alert, with vital signs of T 98.8°F oral, P 80, RR 18, BP 138/80. At 12 noon, the client is confused and arousable only to tactile stimuli, and vital signs are T 99°F oral, P 62, RR 20, BP 166/72. The nurse should take which of the following most important actions?
    1 Retake the vital signs
    2 Reorient the client
    3 Administer a PRN antihypertensive
    4 Call the physician

28. The nurse is teaching the client with a seizure disorder and the spouse about safety precautions after discharge. The nurse evaluates that

the client needs more information if the client states to
    1 Take all prescribed medications on time
    2 Have the spouse nearby when showering
    3 Drink alcohol in small amounts only on weekends
    4 Refrain from smoking alone

29. An outbreak of head lice has occurred at the local school. The school nurse is providing instructions to the mothers of the children attending the school regarding the application of malathion (Ovide). Which of the following instructions does the nurse provide?
    1 Leave lotion on for 8 to 12 hours and then wash hair with nonmedicated shampoo
    2 Apply immediately after washing the hair
    3 Pour onto the hair and then rinse immediately
    4 Allow to remain on hair 10 minutes and then rinse with water

30. The client has had a transsphenoidal resection of the pituitary gland. The nurse notes drainage on the nasal dressing. Suspecting cerebrospinal fluid (CSF) leakage, the nurse would look for drainage that is
    1 Bloody with very small clots
    2 Sanguineous, surrounded by clear to straw-colored fluid
    3 Serosanguineous only
    4 Sanguineous only with no clot formation

31. The client arrives in the emergency department with closed head injury to the right side of the head from assault with a baseball bat. The nurse assesses the client neurologically, looking primarily for motor response deficits that involve
    1 The left side of the body
    2 The right side of the body
    3 Both sides of the body equally
    4 Cranial nerves only, such as speech and pupillary response

32. The nurse has an order to begin aneurysm (subarachnoid) precautions on a client with a subarachnoid hemorrhage secondary to aneurysm rupture. The nurse plans to incorporate which of the following items in controlling the environment for this client?
    1 Keep the window blinds open
    2 Turn on a small spotlight above the client's head
    3 Make sure the door to the room is open at all times
    4 Prohibit or limit radio, television, and newspapers

33. The nurse is caring for the client on bed rest as part of subarachnoid (aneurysm) precautions. The nurse would avoid doing which of the fol-

lowing when giving respiratory care to this client to prevent atelectasis?
1 Reposition gently side to side every 2 hours
2 Assist with incentive spirometer
3 Encourage hourly coughing
4 Encourage hourly deep breathing

34. At the end of the work shift, the nurse is reviewing the respiratory status of a client admitted with acute cerebrovascular accident (CVA) earlier in the day. The nurse evaluates that the client's airway is patent if which of the following data is identified?
1 Respiratory rate 24, oxygen saturation 94%, breath sounds clear
2 Respiratory rate 18, oxygen saturation 98%, breath sounds clear
3 Respiratory rate 16, oxygen saturation 85%, wheezes bilaterally
4 Respiratory rate 20, oxygen saturation 92%, diminished breath sounds in bases

35. The nurse is assessing for changes in skin color in a dark-skinned client. The nurse finds which of the following areas least helpful in assessing for pallor or cyanosis?
1 Sclera
2 Tongue
3 Mucous membranes
4 Nailbeds

36. The nurse has an order to get a paraplegic client out of bed into a chair. The nurse interprets that which of the following items would be best to put in the chair under the client?
1 Plastic-lined absorbent pad
2 Pillow
3 Air ring
4 Gel pad

37. A client is seen in the clinic for complaints of pubic itching that has been persistent over the past several weeks. Following an assessment, it has been determined that the client has pubic lice. Lindane (Kwell) shampoo is prescribed, and the nurse provides instruction to the client regarding the use of the medication. Which of the following instructions would the nurse provide to the client?
1 Leave shampoo on for 8 to 12 hours and then remove by washing
2 Work into dry hair and leave in place for 4 minutes
3 Apply the shampoo as prescribed for 2 days in a row
4 Apply to the entire pubic area, lower abdomen, and upper thighs

38. The client is experiencing chronic pruritus. Which of the following items should the nurse teach the client to promote hydration of the skin?

1 Maintain humidity less than 40%
2 Use very hot or very cold water for bathing
3 Avoid bathing in the shower or tub daily
4 Apply emollients once skin is thoroughly dry

39. The client has undergone laser surgery to remove two nevi. The nurse evaluates that the client has understood discharge instructions if the client verbalizes to
1 Protect the areas from direct sunlight for at least 3 months
2 Report any signs of swelling or redness immediately to the physician
3 Cleanse the areas daily, using scrubbing motions
4 Expect significant discomfort after the procedure

40. The physician has prescribed BenGay topical cream for a client with a muscular sprain. The nurse provides instructions to the client regarding the medication. Which of the following statements, if made by the client, indicates an understanding of this prescribed treatment?
1 "I will apply a heating pad to the area after applying the medication."
2 "The medication may make me sleepy but will stop the muscle spasms."
3 "The medication will act as a local anesthetic."
4 "The medication is addicting."

41. The ambulatory care nurse is working with a 22-year-old female client who has been diagnosed with pelvic inflammatory disease (PID). The nurse incorporates which of the following items in a teaching plan for this individual?
1 Avoid frequent douching
2 Intrauterine devices are a good birth control method
3 Undergarments made of nylon are best
4 It is necessary to change sanitary pads only every 8 hours

42. The mother of an 18-month-old child tells the clinic nurse that her child has been having some mild diarrhea and describes the child's stools as "mushy." The mother tells the nurse that the child is tolerating fluids and solid foods. The most appropriate suggestion regarding the child's diet is to
1 Give the child applesauce, strained bananas, and strained carrots
2 Give the child rice and mashed potatoes diluted with skim milk
3 Give the child gelatin, strained cabbage, and custard
4 Give the child fluids only until the "mushy" stools stop

43. The nurse provides home care instructions to the mother of a child who had a cleft palate repair. Which of the following statements, if made by the mother, indicates the need for further instructions?
    1 "I will use a short nipple on the bottle."
    2 "I will give my child baby foods or baby food mixed with water."
    3 "I need to buy some straws for drinking."
    4 "I can give my child the pacifier in 2 weeks."

44. The client with bipolar disorder is receiving lithium carbonate (Eskalith). The nurse knows that lithium is used primarily to treat
    1 The depressive phase of bipolar disease
    2 Manic episodes of bipolar disease
    3 Both depressive and manic episodes
    4 Hypertensive emergencies

45. The nurse has been caring for a client who recently went through divorce proceedings and attempted suicide. The individual crisis intervention sessions centered on the divorce and the suicide attempt. Which of the following is the best indicator that the client has resolved the perception and meaning of this crisis event?
    1 Motivation to seek additional therapy centered on old conflicts re-emerging from the divorce and suicide attempt
    2 The client identifies support systems
    3 The client reviews the cultural view to therapy
    4 The client identifies self-capabilities

46. A couple is seen in the fertility clinic. Following several tests, it has been determined that the husband is not sterile and that the wife has nonpatent fallopian tubes. The nurse is preparing the woman and her husband for an in vitro fertilization. Which of the following statements, if made by the woman or her husband, indicates a need for further education?
    1 "Ova and sperm are collected and allowed to incubate."
    2 "A fertilized ovum is transferred into the woman's uterus."
    3 "The procedure is a method of medically assisted reproduction."
    4 "The procedure is performed by artificial insemination of sperm through the vagina."

47. The nurse in the gynecological clinic is reviewing the record of a pregnant woman after the first prenatal visit. The nurse notes that the physician has documented that the woman has a platypelloid pelvis. Based on this documentation, the nurse determines that this type of pelvis
    1 Is a normal female pelvis
    2 Has a flat shape
    3 Has an oval shape
    4 Is heart shaped

48. The nurse is caring for an infant with esophageal atresia with tracheocsophageal fistula (TEF). Surgery is scheduled to be performed in 1 hour. IV fluids have been initiated, and a nasogastric (NG) tube has been inserted by the physician. The nursing intervention of highest priority during this preoperative period is to:
    1 Monitor temperature
    2 Irrigate the NG tube every 5 to 10 minutes
    3 Aspirate the NG tube every 5 to 10 minutes
    4 Monitor the blood pressure

49. A mother brings her child to the well-child clinic and expresses concern to the nurse because the child was exposed to hepatitis in school. Based on this information, which of the following is not a component of the nursing assessment?
    1 The presence of left upper quadrant abdominal pain
    2 Hepatomegaly
    3 The presence of jaundice
    4 The character and color of the stools and urine

50. The pediatric nurse educator provides a teaching session to parents regarding the substances that cause lead poisoning. Which of the following is not a known environmental substance that can lead to this problem?
    1 Vinyl blinds
    2 Paint chips
    3 Solder used in plumbing
    4 Properly glazed pottery

51. The client asks the nurse to re-explain what is involved in an intravenous fluorescein angiography study. The nurse incorporates which of the following statements in the reply?
    1 "No contrast dye is used."
    2 "Food is restricted for 4 hours prior to the procedure."
    3 "Dilating drops will be instilled prior to the procedure."
    4 "The study predicts the success of radial keratotomy."

52. The nurse is planning to teach a group of adolescents about the use of condoms as part of a risk reduction program for sexually transmitted diseases (STDs). The nurse plans to include which of the following items in the teaching plan?
    1 Use condoms whenever the partner seems risky
    2 Condoms should not be lubricated
    3 Natural membrane condoms are as effective as latex
    4 Always apply the condom before inserting the penis into the vagina

53. The ambulatory care nurse is seeing a client for a follow-up visit after being treated for toxic

shock syndrome (TSS). The nurse asks the client if which of the following signs and symptoms have disappeared?
1 Low-grade fever, nausea, and vaginal bleeding
2 Low-grade fever, vomiting, and greenish vaginal discharge
3 High fever, abdominal pain, vomiting, and diarrhea
4 High fever, purulent vaginal discharge, and abdominal pain

54. At the beginning of the work shift, the nurse is assessing the client who has returned from the postanesthesia care unit following transurethral resection of the prostate (TURP). The client has a bladder irrigation running via a three-way Foley catheter. The nurse assesses which of the following colors in the urinary drainage tubing as most favorable?
1 Pale pink
2 Dark pink with clots
3 Bright red
4 Tea-colored

55. A child is diagnosed with Hirschsprung's disease. The mother asks the nurse about the cause of the disease. The most appropriate response is which of the following?
1 "It is the inability to digest fully the protein part of wheat, barley, rye, and oats."
2 "It is the inability to tolerate sugar found in dairy products."
3 "It results from the absence of special cells in the rectum."
4 "It results from increased bowel motility that leads to spasm and pain."

56. Lindane (Kwell) is prescribed for the treatment of scabies. This medication therapy is contraindicated in which of the following clients?
1 A 42-year-old woman with coronary artery disease
2 A 17-year-old with seizure disorders
3 An elderly diabetic client
4 A 52-year-old man with hypertension

57. The nurse caring for a client immediately following transurethral resection of the prostate (TURP) notices that the client has suddenly become confused and disoriented. Which of the following actions by the nurse is most important?
1 Ensure that a clock and calendar are in the room
2 Notify the physician
3 Reorient the client
4 Speed up the flow rate of the IV

58. The nurse is caring for the 25-year-old client who will undergo bilateral orchidectomy for testicular cancer. Which of the following ap-

proaches by the nurse is most helpful in exploring client concerns about loss of reproductive ability?
1 "Has the doctor told you that you will not be able to have children?"
2 "You must be sad that you won't be able to have children after surgery."
3 "Do you feel that the doctor has told you all you need to know about the upcoming surgery?"
4 "Can you share with me any concerns about how this surgery will affect you in the future?"

59. The nurse is participating in a prostate screening clinic for men. Which of the following items is not assessed by the nurse as a sign of prostatism?
1 Unusual force in urinary stream
2 Hesitancy when initiating urinary stream
3 Inability to stop voiding quickly
4 Postvoid dribbling of urine

60. The female client being seen in the ambulatory care clinic has a history of syphilis infection. The nurse assessing the client for reinfection would expect to observe a lesion on the labia that
1 Has a cauliflower-like appearance
2 Is painless and indurated
3 Appears as one or more vesicles that then rupture
4 Is erythematous and papular in appearance

61. The home care nurse visits a child recently discharged from the hospital with a diagnosis of hepatitis A virus (HAV). The mother asks the nurse when the child can return to school. The most appropriate nursing response is
1 "When the jaundice disappears."
2 "In about 1 month."
3 "Within 1 week after the onset of jaundice."
4 "At the beginning of the next academic year."

62. The parents of a child with a cleft palate are concerned and ask the nurse when the palate will be repaired. The nurse bases the response on the knowledge that
1 Cleft palate repair is usually performed between 6 months and 2 years of age
2 Cleft palate repair is usually performed by 2 months of age
3 Cleft palate repair is usually performed by age 4 weeks
4 Cleft palate cannot be repaired

63. A child with a diagnosis of tetralogy of Fallot exhibits an increased depth and rate of respirations. On further assessment, the nurse notes increased hypoxemia. The nurse interprets these findings as indicating
1 Immediate physician notification
2 A hypercyanotic episode

3 Anxiety
4 A temper tantrum

64. The nurse is applying a topical glucocorticoid to a client with psoriasis. The nurse would be least concerned about the potential for systemic absorption of the medication if the medication was being applied to which of the following body areas?
   1 Back
   2 Axilla
   3 Scalp
   4 Neck

65. The mother of a child being discharged following heart surgery asks the nurse when the child will be able to return to school. The most appropriate response is
   1 "The child may return to school in 1 week."
   2 "The child may return to school in 1 week but needs to go half days for the first 2 weeks."
   3 "The child may return to school in 3 weeks but needs to go half days for the first few days."
   4 "The child will not be able to return to school during this academic year."

66. During a home visit, the nurse speaks with the client and establishes mutual goals to help the client become more independent. In this role, the nurse is functioning as
   1 A researcher
   2 A resource linker
   3 An advocate
   4 A collaborator

67. As a home health case manager, the nurse functions as a coordinator of client care. This means that the nurse
   1 Reports to all members of the client's care team daily to advise of plans
   2 Teaches client and significant others daily about the case management process
   3 Plans weekly meetings with all individuals involved in the care to assess status
   4 Organizes, manages, and balances health care services needed for the client

68. The client who was diagnosed with toxic shock syndrome (TSS) has developed petechiae, oozing from puncture sites, and coolness of the digits of the hands and feet. The results of the client's clotting studies are prolonged. The nurse interprets that the client's symptoms are most compatible with
   1 Vitamin K deficiency
   2 Factor VIII deficiency
   3 Heparin overdose
   4 Disseminated intravascular coagulopathy (DIC)

69. The hospitalized client has a diagnosis of pelvic inflammatory disease (PID). In which of the following positions in bed would it be most therapeutic for the nurse to place the client?
   1 Prone with head flat
   2 Supine in semi-Fowler's position
   3 Left side-lying
   4 Right side-lying

70. The school nurse has conducted a class on testicular self-examination at the local high school. The nurse evaluates that the information was correctly interpreted if one of the students states to
   1 Perform the examination after a cold shower
   2 Expect the examination to be slightly painful
   3 Roll the testicle between thumb and forefinger
   4 Perform the self-examination every other month

71. The client is admitted to the same-day surgery unit for postoperative monitoring following cataract removal surgery. The nurse assesses the normal postoperative cornea with a flashlight, noting it to be
   1 Clear
   2 Cloudy
   3 Spotted
   4 Sanguineous

72. A topical glucocorticoid is prescribed for an infant with dermatitis in the gluteal area. The nurse provides instructions to the mother regarding the use of the medication. Which of the following, if stated by the mother, indicates an understanding of the use of the medication?
   1 "The medication will help relieve the inflammation."
   2 "I should place a diaper and plastic pants on my child after I apply the medication, to protect the area."
   3 "I should massage the medication into the skin."
   4 "I need to apply the medication in a thick layer to protect the skin."

73. A child with severe seborrheic dermatitis is receiving treatments of topical glucocorticoid applications over an extensive area of the body, followed by the application of an occlusive dressing. Which systemic effect can occur as a result of this treatment?
   1 Local infection
   2 Thinning of the skin
   3 Growth retardation
   4 Adrenal hyperactivity

74. A client with acute seborrheic dermatitis of the back, chest, and legs is receiving treatments with salicylic acid. Which of the following indicates

the presence of a systemic toxicity from this medication?

1 Dizziness
2 Lower leg pain
3 Nausea
4 Decreased respirations

75. Immediately following cataract repair, the client's affected conjunctiva and eyelids are edematous. The nurse interprets that

1 This is grossly abnormal and should be reported at once
2 This is normal and should subside within 3 days
3 This is abnormal, because the conjunctiva should not be affected
4 This is abnormal, because only the eyelids should be affected

76. A homebound client confidentially discusses suicidal plans with the nurse. Based on the professional duty to observe confidentiality, the nurse

1 Cannot tell anyone what that client said
2 Must have the client go to the local mental health center daily for counseling
3 Asks the client not to talk about suicidal plans if a nurse cannot share it with anyone
4 Must override the duty to observe confidentiality and notify the client's physician about the suicidal ideation

77. The nurse is planning a presentation on noise prevention for a display booth at a local health fair. The nurse plans to incorporate which of the following concepts in the display that is designed to minimize individual risk of hearing loss?

1 Sitting near loud music is not harmful
2 Ear plugs or other protectors are necessary only with power tools
3 Don't worry about prolonged ringing in the ears after loud noises
4 Cup hands over the ears if loud noise is expected suddenly

78. The nurse is instructing the nursing assistant in the care of the client with a hearing aid. Which of the following items does the nurse include in the discussion?

1 Check the battery to ensure that it is working before use
2 Leave the hearing aid in place while showering
3 Hearing aids do not require any care
4 A water-soluble lubricant is used on the aid before insertion

79. The nurse has given the client at risk for motion sickness suggestions about medications that can prevent an occurrence. The nurse evaluates that the client has correctly learned the information

if the client states to take medication at what time before the triggering event?

1 At least one half day before
2 At least 1 hour before
3 At least the day before
4 At least 2 days before

80. At the beginning of the shift, the nurse is assessing the status of the client wearing a halo brace. The nurse determines that which of the following items noted needs correction?

1 Exposed metal edges of screws
2 Tightened screws
3 Fingerwidth space between jacket and skin
4 Clean, dry lamb's wool jacket lining

81. The community health nurse is providing an educational session to the members of a local community. Which of the following, if provided during the session, best describes health promotion and primary disease prevention activities?

1 Personal health care services directed toward the pathological process of disease
2 Activities that focus on case finding and screening surveys
3 Activities focusing on retraining individuals to maximize use of remaining capacities
4 Activities that focus on health education, good standards of nutrition that have been adjusted to the developmental phases of life, and attention to personality development

82. The nurse is teaching the mother of a newborn infant measures to maintain health in the infant. Which of the following is an example of primary prevention activities for the infant?

1 Selective placement of the infant
2 PKU (phenylketonuria) testing at birth
3 Administration of an antibiotic for an umbilical cord staphylococcal infection
4 Periodic well-baby examinations

83. The psychiatric nurse is reviewing the discharge plan of a hospitalized client. The nurse reviews the plan bearing in mind that the prominent problem in the management of mentally ill clients in the community is

1 Client's noncompliance with medication therapy, resulting in unstable blood levels
2 Family reaction to keeping the client in the community
3 Community opposition
4 Increased incidence of social problems

84. The client is admitted to the visiting nurse services for observation after being discharged from the hospital for new-onset congestive heart failure (CHF). The nurse teaches the client about the dietary restrictions that must be followed. Which of the following statements, if made by the client, indicates that further teaching is needed?

1 "I'm going to have a ham and cheese sandwich with potato chips for lunch."
2 "I'm going to weigh myself daily to be sure I don't gain too much fluid."
3 "I can have most fresh fruits and fresh vegetables."
4 "I'm not supposed to eat cold-cuts."

85. The prenatal clinic nurse is performing a nutritional assessment on a pregnant adolescent. The primary reason why pregnant teenagers are at greater risk for nutritional deficiencies is
   1 Their parents may be upset about the pregnancy
   2 They are still going through a growth stage
   3 They don't go to school
   4 They have missed classes on good nutrition

86. During a home visit, the nurse suspects that a young daughter of the client is bulimic. The nurse bases the suspicion on which of the primary characteristics of bulimia?
   1 Eating binges and purging
   2 Eating only vegetables and fruits
   3 Refusal to eat
   4 Hoarding of food

87. The nurse is employed in a fertility clinic. A woman and her husband are seen by the physician, and an in vitro fertilization has been discussed with the couple. The couple asks the nurse about this procedure. The nurse plans the response based on which of the following accurate descriptions of the procedure?
   1 Ova and sperm are collected and immediately transferred into the woman's uterus
   2 A fertilized ovum is transferred into the woman's uterus
   3 Ova and sperm must be obtained from a donor other than the potential parents, and it may take some time to locate the donor
   4 Artificial insemination of sperm through the vagina with a syringe is commonly employed

88. The nurse in the gynecological clinic is reviewing the record of a pregnant woman after the first prenatal visit. The nurse notes that the physician has documented that the woman has a gynecoid pelvis. Based on this documentation, the nurse determines that this type of pelvis
   1 Is a normal female pelvis
   2 Has a flat shape
   3 Has an oval shape
   4 Is heart shaped

89. Topical azelaic acid (Azelex) is prescribed for a client. The clinic nurse is providing instructions regarding the use of this medication. Which of the following statements, if made by the client, indicates a need for further instruction?

1 "The medication is to treat my eczema."
2 "I need to wash and dry my skin before I apply the medication."
3 "I need to apply the medication twice daily."
4 "I need to gently massage a thin film onto the affected area."

90. The client with spinal cord injury resulting in paraplegia suddenly complains of severe headache and nausea. The client is diaphoretic, with piloerection and flushing of skin. The client's blood pressure is 210 mmHg systolic. The nurse immediately suspects
   1 Return of spinal shock
   2 Malignant hypertension
   3 Impending cerebrovascular accident
   4 Autonomic dysreflexia

91. The client with stroke has right-sided hemianopsia. The nurse plans to do which of the following to help the client adapt to this visual deficit?
   1 Place all objects within the left visual field
   2 Place all objects within the right visual field
   3 Ensure that the family brings client's eyeglasses to hospital
   4 Teach the client to scan the environment

92. The client has just had a Foley catheter removed and is to be started on a bladder retraining program. Which of the following prescribed interventions gives the caregivers the most useful information about the client's ability to empty the bladder?
   1 Calculating fluid intake total for the shift
   2 Measuring postvoid residual
   3 Assisting client to the bathroom every 2 hours
   4 Recording the amount of the client's voidings

93. The nurse is performing a full physical examination of the client. The nurse selects which of the following items to test the function of cranial nerve II (optic)?
   1 Flashlight
   2 Ophthalmoscope
   3 Reflex hammer
   4 Snellen chart

94. Minoxidil solution (Rogaine) is prescribed for the client to treat hair loss. The nurse provides instructions to the client regarding the application of the medication. Which of the following statements if made by the client would indicate that the teaching is effective?
   1 "I will apply the prescribed amount of solution two times a day."
   2 "I will apply the prescribed amount of solution at bedtime."
   3 "I will apply the prescribed amount of solution three times a day."
   4 "I will apply the prescribed amount of solution four times a day."

95. A client receiving total parenteral nutrition (TPN) suddenly develops chest pain, dyspnea, tachycardia, cyanosis, and a decreased level of consciousness. Which complication of TPN should the nurse suspect?
    1 Hyperglycemia
    2 Catheter-related sepsis
    3 Allergic reaction to the TPN catheter
    4 Air embolism

96. The nurse is caring for the client who has undergone intravenous fluorescein angiography. The nurse tells the client to avoid which of the following activities immediately after the procedure?
    1 Watching large-screen TV
    2 Reading newsprint
    3 Lying down
    4 Listening to music

97. The nurse is caring for a client who had surgery for glaucoma. The nurse teaches the client to avoid activities that increase intraocular pressure (IOP). Which action would the nurse instruct the client to avoid?
    1 Bending at the waist
    2 Watching television
    3 Reading books with small type
    4 Reading books with large type

98. The client is seen in the ambulatory care clinic for a first-degree burn to the arm. The nurse assesses the skin for which of the following characteristics?
    1 Weeping blister
    2 Waxy white color
    3 Insensitivity to pain and cold
    4 Bright pink or red color

99. The home health nurse has instructed the parents about home safety measures with children. The nurse evaluates that the parents have misunderstood instructions if one of them states to
    1 Store medications in childproof containers
    2 Refer to medication as "candy for when you are sick"
    3 Label all toxic substances and place in a locked area
    4 Keep syrup of ipecac in the house at all times

100. The home health nurse is visiting a client who has been started on therapy with clotrimazole (Lotrimin). The nurse plans to monitor the effectiveness of this medication by documenting which of the following with each visit?
    1 Sore throat
    2 Rash
    3 Fever
    4 Pain relief

101. The nurse is preparing to bathe a 1-day-old newborn infant. Which of the following indicates an inaccurate intervention regarding the procedure?
    1 Immersing the infant in water
    2 Ensuring that the water temperature does not exceed 100°F
    3 Supporting the infant's body during the bath
    4 Ensuring that the water temperature is warm

102. Following the delivery of a baby, the nurse performs an initial assessment of the newborn infant. The nurse plans to perform the Apgar score
    1 Immediately at birth, 1 minute after birth, and 5 minutes after birth
    2 Immediately at birth, 3 minutes after birth, and 10 minutes after birth
    3 One minute after birth, 5 minutes after birth, and 10 minutes after birth
    4 One minute after birth, after the cord is cut, and after the mother delivers the placenta

103. The nurse is performing an Apgar scoring on a neonate immediately following birth. The nurse notes that the heart rate is greater than 100, the respiratory effort is good, muscle tone is active, the newborn sneezes when suctioned by the bulb syringe, and the skin color is pink. The nurse would most appropriately document which of the following Apgar scores for the newborn infant?
    1 3
    2 5
    3 7
    4 10

104. The nurse is preparing a client for electroconvulsive therapy (ECT). The family of the client asks the nurse about the treatments. Which of the following is not accurate regarding the procedure?
    1 Memory loss will occur but will disappear with time
    2 Some confusion may be noted following the procedure
    3 This treatment is tried prior to the use of medications
    4 The average series involves 8 to 12 treatments

105. The nurse is caring for a pregnant woman with a diagnosis of severe pre-eclampsia. Which of the following is not a component of the plan of care?
    1 Out of bed activity as tolerated
    2 Seizure precautions
    3 Keeping the room semidark
    4 Padding the side rails of the bed

106. The nurse is performing a health screening with a 54-year-old client. The client has a blood pressure of 128/82, total cholesterol of 190 mg/dL, and fasting blood glucose level of 184. The nurse

interprets that the client has which of the following modifiable risk factors for coronary artery disease (CAD)?
1 Hypertension
2 Glucose intolerance
3 Age
4 Hyperlipidemia

107. The nurse is planning a stress management seminar for clients in an ambulatory care setting. Which of the following concepts should the nurse plan to include in the content of the seminar?
1 Guided imagery is a wonderful technique but requires video equipment for its use
2 Confrontation is a useful method for solving potentially stressful conflicts with others
3 Biofeedback has the advantage of using no equipment at all
4 Progressive muscle relaxation techniques are useful for easing tension from many causes

108. The nurse is trying to determine the ability of the client with myocardial infarction to manage independently at home after discharge. Which of the following statements made by the client indicates that the client may have the most difficulty after discharge?
1 "I don't have anyone to help me with doing heavy housework at home."
2 "I think I have a good understanding of what all my medications are for."
3 "I will be sure to keep my appointment with the cardiologist."
4 "I need to start exercising more to improve my health."

109. The home care nurse has taught the client with a nursing diagnosis of Decreased Cardiac Output about helpful lifestyle adaptations to promote health. The nurse evaluates that the client best understood the information if the client stated to
1 Eat enough daily fiber to prevent straining at stool
2 Drink 2 to 3 ounces of liquor each night to promote vasodilatation
3 Drink 3000 mL/day to promote renal perfusion
4 Try to exercise vigorously to strengthen cardiac reserve

110. The client is started on tolbutamide (Orinase) once daily. The client should be advised by the nurse to take this medication
1 Before going to bed at night
2 At suppertime
3 Between breakfast and lunch
4 At breakfast

111. The client has begun oral medication therapy with cisapride (Propulsid). The nurse evaluates

that the client is experiencing anticipated effects of the medication if the client reports relief of
1 Heartburn
2 Diarrhea
3 Abdominal pain
4 Constipation

112. The nurse is planning a teaching session with the client with chronic renal failure (CRF) about managing the condition between dialysis treatments. The nurse plans to include that weight gain between dialysis treatments is ideally no more than
1 0.5 to 1.0 kg
2 1 to 1.5 kg
3 2 to 4 kg
4 5 to 6 kg

113. The client has a nursing diagnosis of "Activity Intolerance, related to underlying cardiovascular disease as evidenced by exertional fatigue and increased blood pressure." Which of the following observations made by the nurse best indicates client progress in meeting goals for this nursing diagnosis?
1 Chooses a healthy diet that meets caloric needs
2 Sleeps without awakening throughout the night
3 Verbalizes the benefits of increasing activity
4 Ambulates 10 feet farther each day

114. The physician has written an order for a client to have an echocardiogram. The nurse takes which of the following actions to prepare the client for the procedure?
1 Questions the client about allergies to iodine or shellfish
2 Keeps the client NPO for 2 hours prior to the procedure
3 Tells the client that the procedure is painless and takes 30 to 60 minutes
4 Has the client sign a consent for invasive procedures

115. The nurse in the newborn nursery is performing admission vital signs on the newborn infant. Which of the following findings indicates a normal heart rate?
1 110 beats per minute
2 130 beats per minute
3 160 beats per minute
4 180 beats per minute

116. The nurse is performing an assessment on a newborn infant admitted to the nursery following birth. On assessment of the neonate's head, which of the following would the nurse most likely expect to note?
1 A depressed anterior fontanel
2 A soft and flat anterior fontanel
3 An anterior fontanel measuring 1 cm
4 An anterior fontanel measuring 6 cm

117. The client with coronary artery disease is scheduled to have diagnostic exercise stress testing. Which of the following items should the nurse plan to include in client teaching about this procedure?
    1 Avoid cigarettes for 30 minutes before the procedure
    2 Wear loose clothing with a shirt that buttons in front
    3 Eat a light snack just prior to the procedure
    4 Wear firm, rigid shoes such as work boots

118. A client is going to have cardiac catheterization to diagnose the extent of coronary artery disease. The nurse places highest priority on teaching the client to report which of the following sensations during the procedure?
    1 Pressure at the insertion site
    2 Urge to cough
    3 Warm, flushed feeling
    4 Chest pain

119. The client recovering from pulmonary edema is preparing for discharge. The nurse plans to teach the client to do which of the following to manage or prevent recurrent symptoms after discharge?
    1 Take a double dose of diuretic if peripheral edema is noted
    2 Withhold digoxin (Lanoxin) if slight respiratory distress occurs
    3 Weigh self on a daily basis
    4 Sleep with the head of the bed flat

120. A client is scheduled to undergo cardiac catheterization for the first time. Which of the following client statements made to the nurse indicates a clear understanding of the procedure?
    1 "I will have to go to the operating room for this procedure."
    2 "I will probably feel tired after the test from lying on a hard x-ray table for a few hours."
    3 "It will really hurt when the catheter is first put in."
    4 "I will receive general anesthesia for the procedure."

121. The labor room nurse assists with the administration of an epidural regional block. The nurse monitors for the major side effect associated with this type of regional anesthesia by
    1 Taking the mother's temperature
    2 Taking the mother's apical pulse
    3 Assessing the mother's reflexes
    4 Monitoring the mother's blood pressure

122. The client admitted with coronary artery disease complains of dyspnea at rest. The nurse uses which of the following items as the best means to monitor respiratory status on an ongoing basis?

    1 Oxygen flowmeter
    2 Oxygen saturation monitor
    3 Telemetry cardiac monitor
    4 Apnea monitor

123. The nurse has a standing order to remove the nasogastric (NG) tube from a postcardiac surgery client on the first postoperative day. The nurse would most certainly question the order if which of the following assessments was made by the nurse?
    1 Bowel sounds are absent
    2 Abdomen is slightly distended
    3 NG tube drainage is Hematest negative
    4 The client is drowsy

124. The client recovering from cardiac surgery has a left pleural effusion and is having a thoracentesis. The nurse places the client in which of the following positions for the procedure?
    1 Upright and leaning forward with arms on an over-the-bed table
    2 Right side-lying, with legs curled up into a fetal position
    3 Left lateral, with right arm supported by a pillow
    4 Dorsal recumbent

125. The nurse is caring for a child with increased intracranial pressure. On review of the chart, the nurse notes that a transtentorial herniation has occurred. The nurse notes that this type of herniation does not include which of the following?
    1 The brain herniates downward and around the tentorium cerebelli
    2 The herniation can be unilateral or bilateral
    3 It involves only anterior portions of the brain
    4 It can cause death if large amounts of tissue are involved

126. A client with total parenteral nutrition (TPN) via a central intravenous (IV) line is scheduled to receive an antibiotic by the IV route. Which action by the nurse is appropriate before hanging the antibiotic solution?
    1 Ensure a separate IV access for the antibiotic
    2 Turn off the TPN for 30 minutes before administering the antibiotic
    3 Check with the pharmacy to be sure the antibiotic can be hung through the TPN line
    4 Flush the central line with 60 mL of normal saline before hanging the antibiotic

127. A client receiving total parenteral nutrition has a history of congestive heart failure. The physician has ordered furosemide (Lasix), 40 mg daily, to prevent fluid overload. Which laboratory value should be closely monitored by the nurse to prevent adverse effects from this medication treatment?

1 Glucose
2 Sodium
3 Potassium
4 Magnesium

128. The nurse notes on rounds that a client's total parenteral nutrition solution is 4 hours behind. What is the appropriate nursing action?
   1 Hang the TPN using gravity flow because the infusion pump is malfunctioning
   2 Replace the TPN solution with 10% dextrose and restart TPN the following day
   3 Assess the equipment to be sure it is functioning properly and at the correct rate, re-time the TPN solution bag, and notify the physician
   4 Increase the infusion rate to a rate that allows the infusion volume to correct itself within a 2-hour period

129. The nurse is reviewing the chart of a child with a head injury. The nurse notes that the level of consciousness has been documented as obtunded. Which of the following would the nurse expect on assessment of the child?
   1 Awake, alert, interacting with the environment
   2 The ability to think clearly and rapidly is lost
   3 The ability to recognize place or person is lost
   4 Sleeps unless aroused and once aroused has limited interaction with the environment

130. The nurse is performing an assessment on a child with a head injury. The nurse notes an abnormal flexion of the upper extremities and an extension of the lower extremities. The nurse documents this type of positioning as which of the following?
   1 Decorticate posturing
   2 Decerebrate posturing
   3 Flexion of the arms and legs
   4 A normal expected positioning following head injury

131. During a home care visit, the elderly client complains of chronic constipation. A dietary recommendation that the nurse could include in the plan of care is
   1 Increasing rice and bananas in the diet
   2 Increasing intake of sugar-free products
   3 Increasing fluids to at least 8 glasses a day and increasing dietary fiber
   4 Increasing potassium in the diet

132. The client has undergone cataract removal but has not had an intraocular implant. The client is visibly upset because vision is blurry. Which of the following approaches should the nurse plan to take when giving emotional support to this client?
   1 Explore the meaning of the new permanent vision loss

2 Determine whether any relatives have lost vision permanently
3 Explain that vision will improve with adjustment to aphakic lenses
4 Reassure the client that disability benefits will definitely apply

133. The client with a history of ear problems is going on vacation by aircraft. The nurse advises the client to avoid which of the following to prevent barotrauma during ascent and descent of the airplane?
   1 Sucking hard candy
   2 Swallowing
   3 Yawning
   4 Keeping mouth motionless

134. The client has had same-day surgery to insert a ventilating tube in the tympanic membrane. The nurse evaluates that the client understands discharge instructions if the client states to
   1 Use a shower cap if taking a shower
   2 Swim only with head above water
   3 Wash the hair in 2 minutes or less
   4 Avoid taking any medication for pain

135. The adult client seeks treatment in an ambulatory care clinic for complaints of left earache, nausea, and a full feeling in the left ear. The client has an elevated temperature. The nurse first questions the client about
   1 History of recent brain abscess
   2 History of recent upper respiratory infection (URI)
   3 Whether acetaminophen relieves the pain
   4 Whether hearing is magnified in that ear

136. The nurse is caring for a child with a head injury. On review of the records the nurse notes that the physician has documented decorticate posturing. This type of posturing indicates which of the following?
   1 Damage to the midbrain
   2 Damage to the pons
   3 Damage to the diencephalon
   4 A lesion in the cerebral hemisphere

137. The nurse is reviewing the record of a newborn infant in the nursery and notes that the physician has documented the presence of a cephalhematoma. Based on this documentation, the nurse expects to note which of the following?
   1 Swelling of the soft tissues of the head and scalp
   2 Edema resulting from bleeding below the periosteum of the cranium
   3 A suture split greater than 1 cm
   4 A hard, rigid, immobile suture line

138. The clinic nurse of a well-baby clinic is assessing the language and communication developmental milestones of a 4-month-old infant.

Which of the following does the nurse expect to note based on the age of the infant?
1 Use of gestures
2 Babbling sounds
3 Cooing sounds
4 Increased interest in sounds

139. The mother of a 4-month-old infant brings the infant to the well-baby clinic for immunization. Knowing that the infant has received all the recommended immunizations to date, which of the following immunizations does the nurse prepare to administer?
1 DTP#1, OPV#1, HBV#1, Hib#1
2 DTP#2, OPV#2, HBV#2, Hib#2
3 DTP#3, OPV#3, HBV#3, Hib#3
4 DPT#4, TB skin test, MMR#1, varicella

140. The nurse in a well-baby clinic is providing nutrition instructions to the mother of a 1-month-old infant. Which of the following instructions is most appropriate?
1 Offer rice cereal mixed with breast milk or formula
2 Introduce strained vegetables one at a time
3 Introduce strained fruits one at a time
4 Breast milk or formula is the main food

141. The clinic nurse of a well-baby clinic is assessing the motor development of a 24-month-old child. Which of the following does the nurse expect to note in the child at this age?
1 The child builds a tower of two blocks
2 The child opens a door knob
3 The child snaps large snaps
4 The child puts on simple clothes independently

142. The pediatric nurse is caring for a hospitalized toddler. The nurse determines that the most appropriate play activity for the child is which of the following?
1 Playing with a push-pull toy
2 Playing peek-a-boo
3 Hand-sewing a picture
4 Listening to music

143. The nurse is admitting to the hospital a child with a diagnosis of lactose intolerance. Which of the following data does the nurse expect to obtain on assessment?
1 Reports of frothy diarrhea
2 Reports of profuse, watery diarrhea and vomiting
3 Reports of foul-smelling ribbon stools
4 Reports of diffuse abdominal pain unrelated to meals or activity

144. The nurse is providing dietary instructions to the mother of a child with celiac disease. Which of the following food items does the nurse instruct the mother not to include in the child's nutritional plan?
1 Rice
2 Oatmeal
3 Corn
4 Vitamin supplements

145. The nurse is admitting a newborn infant to the nursery and notes that the physician has documented that the baby has an omphalocele. Which of the following best describes this condition?
1 Viscera are inside the abdominal cavity and under the dermis
2 Viscera are inside the abdominal cavity and under the skin
3 Viscera are outside the abdominal cavity but inside a translucent sac covered with peritoneum and amniotic membrane
4 Viscera are outside the abdominal cavity and not covered with a sac

146. A child is diagnosed with intussusception. Which of the following most appropriately describes a characteristic of this disorder?
1 Incomplete development of the anus
2 Invagination of a section of the intestine into the distal bowel
3 The infrequent and difficult passage of dry stools
4 The presence of fecal incontinence

147. The administration of mineral oil has been prescribed for the child with constipation. The nurse provides instructions to the mother regarding the administration of the mineral oil. Which of the following statements, if made by the mother, indicates effective teaching?
1 "I will administer the mineral oil followed by a glass of warm water."
2 "I will mix the mineral oil with 8 ounces of warm juice prior to administration."
3 "I will mix the mineral oil with chilled chocolate milk prior to administration."
4 "I will administer the mineral oil prior to each meal."

148. The home care nurse visits the mother of a 1-month-old infant to provide bottle-feeding instructions. The nurse provides instructions regarding the amount of formula to be given, knowing that the stomach capacity for a 1-month-old is
1 10 to 20 mL
2 30 to 90 mL
3 75 to 100 mL
4 90 to 150 mL

149. The nurse is caring for a 1-year-old child following cleft palate repair. Following feeding, which

of the following is the most appropriate action?
1 Rinse the mouth with water
2 Clean the mouth with diluted hydrogen peroxide
3 Use cotton swabs saturated with half-strength Betadine solution to clean the mouth
4 Use a soft lemon-and-glycerine swab to clean the mouth

150. The newborn infant is diagnosed with gastro-esophageal reflux (GER). The mother of the baby asks the nurse to explain the diagnosis. The nurse bases the response on which of the following descriptions of this disorder?
1 A portion of the stomach protrudes through the esophageal hiatus of the diaphragm
2 Abdominal contents herniate through an opening of the diaphragm
3 Gastric contents regurgitate back into the esophagus
4 The esophagus terminates before it reaches the stomach

151. The nurse is assessing a newborn infant with a diagnosis of hiatal hernia. Which of the following assessment findings does the nurse most specifically expect to note in the newborn infant?
1 Excessive oral secretions
2 Coughing, wheezing, and short periods of apnea
3 Bowel sounds heard over the chest
4 Hiccuping and spitting up after a meal

152. The nurse is reviewing the laboratory results of an infant suspected of having hypertrophic pyloric stenosis. Which of the following does the nurse most likely expect to note in this infant?
1 Respiratory acidosis
2 Respiratory alkalosis
3 Metabolic acidosis
4 Metabolic alkalosis

153. A client with a history of recent upper respiratory infection presents to the urgent care center with chest pain. The nurse interprets that the pain is most likely of respiratory origin if the client states which of the following about the pain?
1 "It hurts on the left side of my chest."
2 "I have never had this pain before."
3 "The pain is about a 6 on a scale of 1 to 10."
4 "It hurts more when I breathe in."

154. A client with a history of angina pectoris tells the nurse that chest pain usually occurs after going up 2 flights of stairs or after walking 4 blocks. The nurse interprets that the client is experiencing which of the following forms of angina?
1 Stable
2 Unstable
3 Variant
4 Intractable

155. A client with a first-degree heart block has an ECG taken during an episode of chest pain. The nurse interprets that which of the following ECG changes is due to the first-degree heart block?
1 Prolonged PR interval
2 Widened QRS complex
3 Tall, peaked T waves
4 Presence of Q waves

156. The nurse is teaching the client with angina pectoris about disease management and lifestyle changes that are necessary to control disease progression. Which of the following items is not included by the nurse when developing the teaching plan?
1 Take nitroglycerin whenever chest discomfort begins
2 Use muscle relaxation to cope with stressful situations
3 It is best to exercise once a week for an hour
4 Avoid using table salt with meals

157. A home health nurse is visiting an elderly client whose family has gone out for the day. The client experiences chest pain that is unrelieved by three sublingual nitroglycerin tablets given by the nurse. Which of the following actions by the nurse would be most appropriate at this time?
1 Notify a family member who is next of kin
2 Inform the home care agency supervisor that the visit may be prolonged
3 Call for an ambulance to transport the client to the emergency department
4 Drive the client to the physician's office

158. The ambulatory care nurse is working with a client who has been diagnosed with Prinzmetal's (variant) angina. The nurse plans to reinforce to the client that this form of angina
1 Is most effectively managed by beta-blocking agents
2 Is generally treated with calcium channel–blocking agents
3 Has the same risk factors as stable and unstable angina
4 Improves with a low-sodium, high-potassium diet

159. The nurse working in a long-term-care facility is assessing a client experiencing chest pain. The nurse would interpret that the pain is most likely due to myocardial infarction (MI) if which

of the following observations is made by the nurse?

1 The client is not experiencing nausea or vomiting

2 The client says the pain began while trying to open a stuck dresser drawer

3 The pain has not been relieved by rest and 3 nitroglycerin tablets

4 The pain is described as substernal and radiating to the left arm

160. The client is admitted with a diagnosis of myocardial infarction and is going to have a nitroglycerin drip started by IV. Noting that the client does not have an intra-arterial monitoring line in place, the nurse obtains which of the following pieces of equipment for use at the bedside?

1 Central venous pressure (CVP) insertion tray

2 Noninvasive blood pressure monitor

3 Defibrillator

4 Pulse oximeter

161. The client with myocardial infarction has been transferred from the coronary care unit (CCU) to the general medical unit. The nurse encourages the client to do which of the following activities immediately after transfer?

1 Ad lib activities since the client will be discharged soon

2 Unsupervised hallway ambulation with distances up to 200 feet

3 Bathroom privileges and self-care activities

4 Strict bed rest for 24 hours after transfer

162. A client with no history of heart disease has experienced acute myocardial infarction and has been given thrombolytic therapy with t-PA (tissue plasminogen activator). The nurse interprets that the client is most likely experiencing complications of this therapy if which of the following assessments is made?

1 Tarry stools

2 Nausea and vomiting

3 Decreased urine output

4 Orange-colored urine

163. The 15-year-old client who is pregnant and unwed says, "My life was unbearable before I met Johnny. My mother beats me up every day and my Dad has been sleeping with me since I was 10 years old!" Which of the following responses is the most therapeutic communication technique by the nurse?

1 "Why didn't you just report your parents for abuse?"

2 "What are you saying? Your parents abused you so you got pregnant?"

3 "Sounds like you decided to have a baby so you'd have someone for yourself."

4 "It seems that you needed help to separate from your family. Do you feel you are ready to have a baby with Johnny before separating?"

164. The client who lost his home and family to a tornado says to the nurse, "I have found great sustenance in helping others who were hit like me." In preparing a plan for the client, the nurse will need to understand that this client

1 Will probably experience anger and other emotions about his plight before rebuilding his life

2 Is reorganizing his life

3 Has poor judgment and could panic and require lethality assessment

4 Is in a state of shock

165. The client undergoing hemodialysis begins to experience muscle cramping. The hemodialysis nurse should take which one of the following corrective actions?

1 Administer magnesium sulfate

2 Administer hypotonic saline

3 Increase the ultrafiltration rate

4 Decrease the ultrafiltration rate

166. The client has had surgery to repair a fractured left hip. The nurse plans to use which of the following most important items when repositioning the client from side to side in the bed?

1 Bed pillow

2 Overhead trapeze

3 Abductor splint

4 Adductor splint

167. The client with a stable 4-day-old lumbar vertebral fracture is experiencing muscle spasms. The nurse avoids using which of the following in efforts to relieve the spasm?

1 Prescribed intermittent traction

2 Analgesics

3 Heat

4 Cold

168. The nurse has reviewed activity restrictions with a client who is being discharged following insertion of a femoral head prosthesis. The nurse evaluates that the client understands the material presented if the client states to

1 Use a raised toilet seat

2 Exercise the leg past the point of 90° flexion

3 Bend carefully to put on socks and shoes

4 Sit in chairs without arms for better mobility

169. The nurse is talking to the client who underwent a below-knee amputation 2 days earlier. The client says to the nurse, "I hate looking at this; I feel that I'm not even myself anymore." The nurse formulates which of the following nursing diagnoses based on the statement by this client?

1 Altered Health Maintenance

2 Self-Care Deficit

3 Body Image Disturbance
4 Ineffective Individual Coping

170. The client receiving heparin sodium by continuous IV infusion removes the tubing from the pump to change the hospital gown. The nurse is concerned that the client received a bolus of medication. After requesting an order for a stat PTT (partial thromboplastin time) level, the nurse checks to see whether which medication is available in the medication cart?
    1 Aminocaproic acid (Amicar)
    2 Vitamin K (AquaMEPHYTON)
    3 Enoxaparin (Lovenox)
    4 Protamine sulfate

171. The client returning to the medical nursing unit following cardiac catheterization has a stat order to receive a dose of procainamide. The nurse uses which of the following pieces of equipment to determine most adequately the client's response to this medication?
    1 Cardiac monitor
    2 Noninvasive blood pressure cuff
    3 Pulse oximeter
    4 Glucometer

172. The 10-year-old female client who has been reported for drawing sexually explicit scenes in her textbooks says to the psychiatric nurse, "I just felt like it." Which of the following responses would be the most therapeutic communication for the nurse to employ to assess abuse-related symptoms?
    1 "I am concerned about you. Are you now or have you ever been abused?"
    2 "Well, a picture paints a thousand words."
    3 "You just felt like destroying your textbooks?"
    4 "Your parents and teachers are very concerned about your drawings."

173. In the nursing assessment, the client says, "My daughter was murdered in her New York apartment, and her estranged husband called to tell me. I can't stop myself from wondering if he killed her, but the police have ruled him out as a suspect." Which of the following responses would be the most therapeutic communication technique?
    1 "It feels terrible to lose a daughter. I'd have suspicions about him too."
    2 "Have you shared your concerns with the police?"
    3 "I don't think you should blame yourself one little bit."
    4 "I agree. What do you want to bet he did it?"

174. The nurse is assessing a coronary care unit client who seems to fluctuate in the ability to focus during the day. Which of the following diagnoses would be selected by the nurse?

1 Delirium related to "CCU psychosis"
2 Alcohol withdrawal delirium
3 Dementia related to "CCU psychosis"
4 Substance intoxication dementia

175. The nurse is discussing smoking cessation with a client diagnosed with coronary artery disease. Which of the following statements is correct for the nurse to make to the client to try to motivate the client to quit smoking?
    1 "If you quit now, your risk of cardiovascular disease will decrease to that of a nonsmoker in 3 to 4 years."
    2 "Since most of the damage has already been done, it will be all right to cut down a little at a time."
    3 "If you totally quit smoking right now, you can cut your cardiovascular risk to zero within a year."
    4 "None of the cardiovascular effects is reversible, but quitting might prevent lung cancer."

176. The client with heart failure is scheduled to be discharged to home with digoxin (Lanoxin) and furosemide (Lasix) as ongoing medications. The nurse teaches the client to report which of the following items that indicates that the medications are not having the intended effect?
    1 Cough accompanied by other signs of respiratory infection
    2 Sudden increase in appetite
    3 Weight gain of 2 to 3 pounds in a few days
    4 High urine output during the day

177. The client has experienced an episode of pulmonary edema. The nurse determines that the client's respiratory status is improving after this event if which of the following breath sounds is noted?
    1 Rales to the apices
    2 Crackles in bases
    3 Wheezes
    4 Rhonchi

178. The client with pulmonary edema has morphine sulfate ordered to be given intravenously. The nurse evaluates that the client experienced an intended effect of the medication if which of the following assessment data is noted?
    1 Relief of apprehension
    2 Decreased urine output
    3 Increased pulse rate
    4 Increased blood pressure

179. The client with myocardial infarction is recovering from cardiogenic shock. The nurse would interpret that which of the following observations of the client's clinical condition is most favorable?

1 Central venous pressure (CVP) of 15 mmHg
2 Frequent premature ventricular contractions (PVCs)
3 Urine output of 40 mL/hr
4 Heart rate, 110 beats per minute

180. A client receiving total parenteral nutrition is demonstrating signs and symptoms of an air embolism. What is the first action by the nurse?
1 Notify the physician
2 Stop the TPN
3 Place the client in high Fowler's position
4 Lay the client on the left side in Trendelenburg's position

181. The client has been started on medication therapy with amrinone (Inocor). The nurse evaluates that the client is not experiencing anticipated therapeutic benefit if the client has a noticeable decrease in
1 Weight
2 Lung crackles
3 Peripheral edema
4 Blood pressure

182. The elderly client takes cascara sagrada for ongoing management of chronic constipation. The nurse assesses the client's laboratory results for which of the following electrolyte imbalances related to long-term use of this medication?
1 Hypokalemia
2 Hyperkalemia
3 Hyponatremia
4 Hypernatremia

183. The client has been started on cyclobenzaprine (Flexeril) for the management of muscle spasms in the cervical spine. The client is experiencing drowsiness, dizziness, and dry mouth. The nurse interprets that
1 These represent an allergic reaction to the medication
2 These are the most common side effects of this medication
3 These effects are dose related; the client should cut the medication dose in half
4 These effects are related to the problem with the cervical spine

184. The client has been given a prescription for diphenhydramine (Benadryl). The nurse plans to teach the client to avoid which of the following until the client's response to the medication is known?
1 Drinking alcohol
2 Using nighttime sedative medication
3 Driving
4 Using mouth lozenges

185. The nurse is monitoring a child with a brain tumor for complications associated with increased intracranial pressure (ICP). Which of the following if noted by the nurse indicates the presence of diabetes insipidus (DI)?

1 Urine specific gravity above 1.020
2 Weight gain
3 Hypertension
4 A high urine output

186. Enoxacin (Penetrex) is prescribed for the client with cervical gonorrhea. Which of the following instructions does the nurse provide to the client regarding the administration of this medication?
1 Take the medication with milk
2 Take the medication with meals
3 Take the medication 1 hour before meals
4 Take the medication with an antacid

187. A child is receiving edetate calcium disodium (calcium EDTA) by intravenous infusion for the treatment of lead poisoning. The physician prescribes a blood level concentration measurement. Which of the following is the most appropriate nursing intervention?
1 Irrigate the IV with normal saline prior to drawing blood for the lead concentration level
2 Stop the IV infusion for 1 hour prior to obtaining blood for the lead concentration level
3 Obtain blood for the lead concentration level from the extremity that is not receiving the intervention infusion
4 Maintain NPO status 12 hours prior to obtaining blood for the serum lead concentration

188. The nurse is providing instructions to a client receiving enalapril maleate (Vasotec). Which of the following is not a component of the instructions?
1 Rise slowly from a lying to sitting position
2 Notify the physician if nausea occurs
3 Notify the physician if a sore throat occurs
4 Several weeks of therapy may be required for the full therapeutic effect

189. Enoxaparin sodium (Lovenox) is prescribed for the client following hip replacement surgery. The nurse prepares to have which of the following available in the event that an overdose of the medication occurs?
1 Vitamin K
2 Protamine sulfate
3 Epinephrine
4 Adrenaline

190. The nurse is teaching the client how to perform the four-point gait for crutch-walking. Which of the following indicates the correct procedure for instructing the client?
1 Move the right crutch forward, move the left foot forward, move the left crutch forward, move the right foot forward
2 Move the left foot forward, move the right crutch forward, move the right foot forward, move the left crutch forward

3 Move both crutches forward and then move the left foot forward followed by the right foot forward

4 Move the left foot forward, move the right foot forward, followed by both crutches forward

191. During the physical examination, the young African American client complains of fatigue, weakness, fever, hematuria without pain, severe joint pain in multiple sites, and recurrent infections. A diagnosis of sickle cell anemia is made. Which of the following statements, if made by the client, indicates a need for further instruction?
   1 "When I'm feeling better, I'm returning to the football team."
   2 "I'm using a schedule to maintain my increased fluid intake."
   3 "I'm joining a group of students interested in antiques."
   4 "I've learned to knit and sew my own clothes."

192. The nurse is performing an initial physical examination on a young female client who complains of fatigue, weakness, malaise, muscle pain, joint pain at multiple sites, anorexia with slight weight loss, and photosensitivity. Systemic lupus erythematosus (SLE) is suspected. Which of the following additional symptomatology indicates a diagnosis of SLE?
   1 Presence of two hemoglobin S genes
   2 Ascites
   3 Emboli
   4 Butterfly rash on cheeks and bridge of nose

193. The nurse is assessing the arterial blood gases on the child being monitored for increased intracranial pressure (ICP). Which of the following values indicates a normal ICP?
   1 PaO_2 greater than 80 mmHg and $PaCO_2$ less than 45 mmHg
   2 PaO_2 greater than 70 mmHg and $PaCO_2$ less than 50 mmHg
   3 PaO_2 greater than 60 mmHg and $PaCO_2$ less than 35 mmHg
   4 PaO_2 greater than 50 mmHg and $PaCO_2$ less than 30 mmHg

194. The nurse is trying to speak to a client who is hard of hearing. The nurse incorporates which of the following strategies into communication with this client?
   1 Shout as loudly as possible
   2 Approach the client from behind
   3 Stand in front of the client while speaking
   4 Overenunciate words

195. The nurse is caring for a client with terminal cancer who is close to death. In reviewing the care plan, the nurse determines that a priority for nursing care is
   1 Keeping the client well sedated so the client is totally unaware of what is actually happening
   2 Making sure the family has privacy and is kept informed of what is happening
   3 Carrying out the physician's orders so all the prescribed treatments are given
   4 Management of symptoms to maintain client self-esteem and to make the client comfortable

196. The community health nurse is visiting a client who has been diagnosed with obstructive sleep apnea (OSA). Which of the following statements by the client indicates the most therapeutic response to treatment?
   1 "Since I have been using the device to keep my airway open, I sleep much better."
   2 "My wife says my snoring is as loud as ever."
   3 "I just don't feel like I've slept much when I wake up, even now."
   4 "My wife is happy because I don't snore as loudly or as frequently as I used to."

197. On assessment, the client tells the nurse, "I wake up in the morning and I'm exhausted before I get up." The most therapeutic response by the nurse is
   1 "For us to obtain an accurate picture of your patterns of sleep, would you fill out a sleep diary every day for at least 2 weeks?"
   2 "You poor dear. This must be very distressing to you."
   3 "How long have you been experiencing sleeplessness?"
   4 "I'm going to have the physician order a sleeping medication for you."

198. The forensic nurse is caring for an incarcerated client who constantly compliments the nurse. Which of the following responses is the most therapeutic communication technique by the nurse?
   1 "Thank you for the compliment, but please keep your comments to yourself from now on. Your remarks are irrelevant to the reason I am working with you."
   2 "Thank you."
   3 "Keep your compliments to yourself, if you please."
   4 "I'm very complimented, but let's return to you."

199. The nurse is teaching the client with gastroesophageal reflux disease (GERD) about dietary management of the disorder. The nurse incorporates which of the following statements in the discussion?
   1 Avoid eating or drinking for 3 hours prior to sleep

2 Eat large meals to stimulate digestion
3 Drink beverages that are very warm or cold
4 Limit fluid intake with meals

200. The client with esophageal cancer, being fed by a gastrostomy tube, has a nursing diagnosis of Ineffective Individual Coping, related to body image changes and potentially terminal diagnosis. Which of the following behaviors exhibited by the client indicates that the nursing diagnosis has not been resolved?
1 Participates in self-care activities
2 Asks questions about nursing care
3 Interacts with family during visiting hours
4 Avoids looking at feeding gastrostomy tube

201. The nurse has given the client with hepatitis instructions about postdischarge management during convalescence. The nurse evaluates that the client needs further teaching if the client states to
1 Eat a high-carbohydrate, low-fat diet
2 Avoid alcohol and aspirin
3 Resume full activity level within 1 week
4 Take prescribed amounts of vitamin K

202. The nurse has given discharge instructions to the client who has had ocular surgery of the right eye. The nurse evaluates that the client needs further instruction if the client states to
1 Report a temperature of 99°F or greater
2 Wear sunglasses during the day
3 Wear an eyeshield at night
4 Sleep on the back or left side

203. The client with glaucoma has suffered significant eye damage prior to diagnosis and now has impaired vision. The nurse evaluates that the client needs further assistance in adapting to this situation if the client states that
1 The family will drive the client when eye examinations are needed
2 There is no difficulty driving at dusk
3 Nightlights have been placed in the hallways for night use
4 It is important to have periodic eye examinations

204. A client in the emergency department is diagnosed with Bell's palsy. The nurse assessing this client should expect to find which of the following?
1 Narrowing of the palpebral fissure
2 A lag in closing the bottom eyelid
3 A symmetrical smile
4 Paroxysms of excruciating pain in the lips and cheek

205. A nurse is assessing a client with Guillain-Barré syndrome. Which of the following is of greatest concern?

1 A blood pressure decrease from 106/60 to 98/58
2 Respiratory vital capacity of 10 mL/kg
3 Difficulty in articulating words
4 Paralysis progressing from the toes to the waist

206. The nurse is mixing the morning dose of 10 units (U) of Regular and 35 units of NPH insulin SC for a client with insulin-dependent diabetes mellitus (IDDM). The nurse prepares an insulin syringe, gently agitates the insulin solutions, cleans the tops of the correct vials of insulin, and injects an amount of air equal to the dose ordered into each vial. Which of the following actions indicates that the nurse understands the principles of mixing insulins correctly?
1 Draws up 35 U of NPH insulin and checks syringe contents with another nurse before drawing up the Regular insulin
2 Draws up 10 U of Regular insulin and checks syringe contents with another nurse before drawing up the NPH insulin
3 Draws up 10 U of Regular insulin, draws up 35 U of NPH insulin, and checks syringe contents with another nurse
4 Draws up 35 U of NPH insulin, draws up 10 U of Regular insulin, and checks syringe contents with another nurse

207. During a routine visit to the physician's office for monitoring of diabetic control, the elderly client complains to the nurse of vision changes. The client describes blurring of the vision, with difficulty in reading and with driving at night. Given the client's history, the nurse interprets that the client is probably developing
1 Detached retina
2 Papilledema
3 Glaucoma
4 Cataracts

208. The client with primary open angle glaucoma has been prescribed timolol (Timoptic) ophthalmic drops. The client asks the nurse how this medication works. The nurse tells the client that the medication lowers intraocular pressure by
1 Reducing intracranial pressure
2 Increasing contractions of the ciliary muscle
3 Constricting the pupil
4 Reducing production of aqueous humor

209. The client is scheduled to begin therapy with acetazolamide (Diamox) for the management of glaucoma. The nurse assesses the client for history of allergy or sensitivity to
1 Corticosteroids
2 Nonsteroidal anti-inflammatory agents
3 Penicillin
4 Sulfa drugs

210. During the physical examination, a 10-year-old child complains of mild to severe ear pain that is aggravated by palpation of the auricle. A foul-smelling, yellow, tenacious discharge is evident in the ear canal, and a diagnosis of acute otitis externa is made. Which of the following statements, if made by the child, indicates that the nurse's instruction is effective?
    1 "I know that I'll have to live with slight dizziness, but I'll report any increase in dizziness that lasts over 5 minutes."
    2 "I will go with my mother to have special ear testing annually."
    3 "I won't put anything smaller than my elbow into my ear from now on."
    4 "I will use cotton swabs instead of a face cloth to clean my ears."

211. The nurse is planning to instruct the client with chronic vertigo about safety measures to prevent exacerbation of symptoms or injury. The nurse plans to teach the client that it is important to
    1 Drive at times when the client does not feel dizzy
    2 Go to the bedroom and lie down when vertigo is experienced
    3 Remove throw rugs and clutter in the home
    4 Turn the head slowly when spoken to

212. The nurse is assessing the client to determine adjustment to presbycusis. Which of the following factors assessed by the nurse indicates successful adaptation to this problem?
    1 Denial of hearing impairment
    2 Proper use of hearing aid
    3 Withdrawal from social activities
    4 Reluctance to answer the telephone

213. The client has a decubitus ulcer on the sacrum. The ulcer has partial thickness skin loss and formation of a blister. The nurse categorizes the ulcer as
    1 Stage I
    2 Stage II
    3 Stage III
    4 Stage IV

214. The client is receiving topical corticosteroid therapy in the treatment of psoriasis. The nurse maximizes the effectiveness of this therapy by
    1 Carefully rubbing the application into the skin
    2 Applying a dry, sterile dressing over the affected area
    3 Covering the application with a warm, moist dressing and an occlusive outer wrap
    4 Placing the area under a heat lamp for 20 minutes

215. The nurse is counseling the client about decreasing the risk for cervical cancer. The nurse would not include which of the following statements in the discussion?
    1 Keep appointments for Pap smears at the frequency advised by physician
    2 Seek prompt treatment for vaginitis
    3 Condoms are needed only if the client doesn't trust new partners
    4 A partner who is uncircumcised may provide increased risk

216. The nurse has given instructions to the client with a cystocele about Kegel exercises. The nurse evaluates that the client has not fully understood the directions if the client states to
    1 Begin voiding and then stop the stream, holding residual urine for an hour
    2 Stop and start the stream of urine several times during a voiding
    3 Tighten perineal muscles for up to 10 seconds several times a day
    4 Tighten perineal muscles for up to 5 minutes three or four times a day

217. The client has been given a prescription for gemfibrozil (Lopid). The nurse plans to instruct the client to limit which of the following foods while taking this medication?
    1 Fish
    2 Beef
    3 Spicy foods
    4 Citrus products

218. The client recovering from an exacerbation of left-sided heart failure has a nursing diagnosis of Activity Intolerance. The nurse evaluates that the client is best tolerating mild exercise if the client exhibits which of the following changes in vital signs during activity?
    1 Pulse rate increased from 80 to 104 beats per minute
    2 Respiratory rate increased from 16 to 19 breaths per minute
    3 Oxygen saturation decreased to 91% from 96%
    4 Blood pressure decreased from 140/86 mmHg to 112/72 mgHg

219. The client has just been told by the physician of the diagnosis of breast cancer. The client responds, "Oh, no, does this mean I'm going to die?" The nurse interprets that the client's initial reaction is one of
    1 Anxiety
    2 Fear
    3 Denial
    4 Rage

220. The client who had a body cast applied 2 days earlier begins to complain of anorexia, nausea, and abdominal discomfort. Which of the follow-

ing is the most important action for the nurse to take?
1 Test the client's stool for guaiac
2 Administer a dose of antacid ordered PRN
3 Administer an antiemetic ordered PRN
4 Notify the physician

221. The nurse is giving the client instructions over the telephone about preparation for mammography. The nurse plans to include which of the following items in the directions?
1 Use only lanolin-based skin lotions on the day of the test
2 Avoid using underarm deodorant before the test
3 The client may wear metal jewelry
4 The client should have clear liquids only on the day of the test

222. The nurse notes blanching, coolness, and edema at the peripheral intravenous (IV) site. Which of the following should the nurse do first?
1 Check for a blood return
2 Discontinue the IV
3 Apply a warm compress
4 Measure the area of infiltration

223. The goal for the client with partial premature separation of the placenta is "no signs of fetal distress during the episode." Which of the following outcomes written by the nurse indicates this goal has been achieved?
1 Fetal heart rate (FHR) of 160 to 180 bpm
2 No accelerations of fetal heart rate
3 Variable decelerations present
4 Short-term variability present

224. The client who is noted to handle stress by family violence, is now engaged in group therapy sessions. The client is yelling at another client in the therapy session and screams, "I can't listen to this . . . You people are no different from the ones at home." The client stands up and tips the chair over backwards. The nurse's immediate action is to
1 Call security immediately to the group therapy session
2 Explore other client's responses to the client's yelling behavior
3 Firmly reinforce group rules to the client, stating that aggressive yelling is not acceptable in the group
4 Inform the yelling client that he or she must leave the group immediately

225. The client is preparing to be discharged to an outpatient status. The nurse is discussing termination and follow-up plans with the client. Which of the following client statements most concerns the nurse about the client's discharge and indicates the need for follow-up treatment?

1 "I want to say thank you. I think I've worked hard . . . and you too. I know I'm not finished yet . . . I need to come back for appointments. I'm glad . . . I don't think I could leave totally on my own."
2 "I think I really couldn't have worked that job even if the man had given me the time he should have during the interview. It's just as well. I really didn't want a job where I had to work such long hours. But I had good reason to get depressed and end up here. But it all worked out . . . I really didn't want that job anyway."
3 "This has been the hardest trip here for me, but I have made progress in learning how to communicate . . . especially with my family. I'm ready to go. I feel I'm ready this time . . . more than the last!"
4 "I really tried to listen to what people said in the groups this time. Sometimes it was hard, but I tried to listen. I think we really helped each other. I think I've learned to listen better rather than my jumping too quickly into something."

226. A child has been tentatively diagnosed with rheumatic fever. The nurse interprets that this diagnosis is consistent with which of the following laboratory results obtained for this client?
1 Negative C-reactive protein (CRP) level
2 Unchanged erythrocyte sedimentation rate (ESR)
3 Elevated antistreptolysin O (ASO) titer
4 Negative antinuclear antibody (ANA) level

227. The client is being discharged after being treated for infective endocarditis. The nurse should plan to give the client which of the following discharge instructions?
1 Take acetaminophen (Tylenol) if chest pain worsens
2 Use a firm-bristled toothbrush and floss vigorously to prevent cavities
3 Take antibiotics until chest pain is fully resolved
4 Notify all health care providers of medical history before any invasive procedures

228. The nurse has given the client with atrial fibrillation instructions to take one aspirin daily. The client says to the nurse, "Why do I need to take this? I don't get any pain with my heart rhythm." Which of the following responses by the nurse is most correct?
1 "This will help prevent clot formation in your heart as a result of your heart's rhythm."
2 "This will prevent any inflammation from occurring on the walls of your heart."
3 "This will most likely keep you from ever having a heart attack."
4 "This will keep you from experiencing chest pain."

229. The client has been treated for pleural effusion with thoracentesis. The nurse evaluates that this therapy has been most effective if the client has
1 Decreased severity of cough
2 Absence of dyspnea
3 Decreased tactile fremitus
4 Dull percussion notes

230. The client did not seek medical treatment for a previous respiratory infection and subsequently developed empyema. The nurse assesses the client for which of the following signs and symptoms associated with this problem?
1 Pleural pain and fever
2 Hyperresonant breath sounds
3 Decreased respiratory rate
4 Diaphoresis during the day

231. The client with long-standing empyema undergoes decortication of the affected lung area. Postoperatively, the nurse uses which of the following as the most effective position for the client?
1 Supine
2 Sims'
3 Side-lying
4 Semi-Fowler's

232. The nurse is caring for a client who has a subtotal gastrectomy. The nurse assesses the client for which of the following signs and symptoms of dumping syndrome?
1 Abdominal pain, elevated temperature, and weakness
2 Fever, constipation, and rectal bleeding
3 Diarrhea, chills, and hiccups
4 Weakness, diaphoresis, and diarrhea

233. The nurse is concerned about the adequacy of peripheral tissue perfusion in the post–cardiac surgery client. Which of the following actions does the nurse plan to avoid when giving care to this client?
1 Use of knee gatch
2 Covering legs lightly when sitting in chair
3 Range of motion exercises to the ankles
4 Application of pneumatic boots

234. The nurse is instructing the post–cardiac surgery client about activity limitations for the first 6 weeks after hospital discharge. The nurse includes which of the following items in the instruction?
1 Resume activities that involve straining as long as they do not cause pain
2 Driving is permitted as long as lap and shoulder seatbelts are worn
3 Lift any object that does not weigh more than 25 pounds
4 Use the arms for balance, not weight support, when getting out of bed or a chair

235. The nurse is assessing an ECG rhythm strip of a client. The P waves and QRS complexes are regular. The PR interval is 0.14 second, and QRS complexes measure 0.08 second. The overall heart rate is 82. The nurse interprets the cardiac rhythm to be
1 Sinus bradycardia
2 Sick sinus syndrome
3 Normal sinus rhythm
4 First-degree heart block

236. The client's ECG strip shows atrial and ventricular rates of 70 complexes per minute. The PR interval is 0.16 second, the QRS complex measures 0.06 second, and the PP interval is slightly irregular. The nurse interprets this rhythm to be
1 Sinus bradycardia
2 Normal sinus rhythm
3 Sinus tachycardia
4 Sinus arrhythmia

237. The nurse is watching the cardiac monitor and notices that the rhythm suddenly changes. There are no P waves or QRS complexes. Instead there are wavy lines on the monitor screen. The nurse interprets that the client is experiencing
1 Premature ventricular contractions (PVCs)
2 Sinus tachycardia
3 Ventricular tachycardia
4 Ventricular fibrillation

238. The client with myocardial infarction is experiencing new, multiform premature ventricular contractions (PVCs). Knowing that the client is allergic to lidocaine hydrochloride, the nurse plans to have which one of the following medications available for immediate use?
1 Digoxin (Lanoxin)
2 Metoprolol (Lopressor)
3 Verapamil (Isoptin)
4 Procainamide (Pronestyl)

239. The client has received antidysrhythmic therapy for treatment of premature ventricular contractions (PVCs). The nurse evaluates this therapy as most effective if the client's PVCs continue to
1 Be multifocal in appearance
2 Occur in pairs
3 Decrease to a frequency of less than 6 per minute
4 Fall on the second half of the T wave

240. The client with chronic atrial fibrillation is being started on quinidine sulfate (Quinidex Extentabs) as maintenance therapy for dysrhythmia suppression. Which of the following would not be included by the nurse in a teaching plan about this medication?
1 Stop taking the prescribed anticoagulant after starting this new medication
2 Take the medication with food if GI upset occurs

3 Avoid chewing the sustained-release tablets

4 Take the dose at the same time each day

241. The adult client has been defibrillated three times unsuccessfully for ventricular fibrillation, and cardiopulmonary resuscitation (CPR) is resumed. The nurse concludes that CPR is being administered most effectively by noting that
   1 The ratio of compressions to ventilations is 5:1
   2 Respirations are given at a rate of 12 breaths per minute
   3 The chest compressions are given at a depth of 1.5 to 2 inches
   4 The carotid pulse is palpable with each compression

242. The nurse is assessing the client's condition after cardioversion. Which of the following observations is of highest priority to the nurse?
   1 Status of airway
   2 Oxygen flow rate
   3 Level of consciousness
   4 Blood pressure

243. The nurse is assigned to care for a child with a brain injury. On review of the records the nurse notes that the child has a temporal lobe herniation. Which of the following is not characteristic of this type of herniation?
   1 A shifting of the temporal lobe laterally across the tentorial notch occurs
   2 It produces compression of the 6th cranial nerve
   3 It can cause ipsilateral pupil dilation
   4 Flaccid paralysis, pupil fixation, and death can occur if the intracranial pressure continues to rise

244. The nurse notes redness, warmth, and a yellowish drainage at the insertion site of a central venous catheter in a client receiving total parenteral nutrition. What is the rationale for immediate notification of the physician?
   1 Infections of a central catheter site can lead to septicemia
   2 The client is experiencing an allergy to the TPN solution
   3 The TPN solution has infiltrated and must be stopped
   4 The client is allergic to the dressing material covering the site

245. A client with cancer is placed on permanent total parenteral nutrition. For what reason must the nurse consider psychosocial support when planning care for this client?
   1 Death is imminent
   2 TPN requires disfiguring surgery for permanent port implantation
   3 The client will need to adjust to the idea of living without eating by the usual route

4 Nausea and vomiting occur regularly with this type of treatment and will prevent the client from social activity

246. In the female Offenders Group, the offender client says, "I was abused by my father and then my husband, so I finally stabbed him when he came after me, but no one on the jury believed me 'cause my husband, the 'big shot,' can lie to anyone and be believed." If no one in the group responds, which of the following is the most therapeutic response by the nurse?
   1 "Seems as if you went from one abusing man to another. Do you really think you're here because your husband is a good liar and a 'big shot'?"
   2 "Your story is very much like every woman's here. I think you had other options besides violence, don't you?"
   3 "Yes. Everyone here was ill used and abused, but what makes you think that this is a reason to stab someone?"
   4 "A pretty horrible experience for you to undergo. Does anyone in the group want to respond?"

247. The family nurse practitioner is assessing the incarcerated client's mental status. Based upon knowledge of the forensic client, which of the following findings is most likely to be discovered in the offender client's history?
   1 Cirrhosis of the liver
   2 Severe or chronic mental illness
   3 Substance abuse
   4 Cardiac disease

248. Which of the following is the most needed by a homeless female, elderly client who has tuberculosis?
   1 Commitment to a sanatorium
   2 Food, clothing, and basic hygiene
   3 Safe shelter, food, and medication
   4 Money to buy groceries and obtain an apartment

249. Which one of the following data is associated with functionally impaired behavior in dementia?
   1 Incontinence and poor personal hygiene
   2 Hitting and kicking behaviors
   3 Screaming and complaining
   4 Wandering and pacing

250. The nurse is caring for a client with Alzheimer's disease who is having difficulty recognizing objects that are well known, including people. Which of the following would the nurse report?
   1 Aphasia
   2 Agnosia
   3 Apraxia
   4 Ataxia

251. The nurse is providing instructions to the client regarding the use of a walker. Which of the following is not a component of the teaching plan?
    1 The rubber tips should be inspected daily
    2 Pick up the walker and move it forward and then walk into the walker one step at a time
    3 Be certain that there is 35° to 40° of flexion at the client's elbow to ensure correct length of the walker
    4 The client should wear shoes when ambulating with the walker

252. The nurse is caring for a newborn infant. The laboratory report shows the total calcium level to be 8.0 mg/dL. The nurse interprets this laboratory value to be
    1 Lower than normal
    2 Higher than normal
    3 A normal value
    4 Requiring physician notification

253. The nurse is caring for an infant with a tracheostomy and prepares to suction the infant. Which of the following identifies an inaccurate nursing intervention?
    1 Insert the catheter the length of the tracheostomy tube with the suction off
    2 Apply intermittent suction and withdraw the catheter with a twisting motion
    3 Limit insertion and suctioning time to 10 seconds to prevent hypoxia
    4 Reoxygenate between suction catheter passage and allow sufficient recovery time with each pass

254. The nurse is preparing to suction a neonate through a tracheostomy. Which of the following suction settings is appropriate for this procedure?
    1 60 to 80 mmHg
    2 80 to 90 mmHg
    3 80 to 100 mmHg
    4 100 to 120 mmHg

255. The nurse is preparing to administer an intramuscular injection to a 4-year-old child. The nurse prepares to administer the injection in the ventral gluteal muscle. Which of the following indicates the maximum amount of medication volume that can be safely injected?
    1 0.5 mL
    2 1 mL
    3 1.5 mL
    4 2.0 mL

256. The nurse is administering an acetaminophen (Tylenol) suppository to a child with a fever. The nurse prepares to insert the suppository into the rectum a distance of
    1 No more than 0.5 cm
    2 No more than 1 cm
    3 No more than 2 cm
    4 No more than 2.5 cm

257. The nurse is administering ear drops to a 2-year-old child. Which of the following indicates the appropriate method of administration?
    1 Pull the pinna of the ear back and down
    2 Pull the pinna of the ear back and up
    3 Place the child in a prone position with the ear to receive the drop facing downward
    4 Place the child in a side-lying position with the ear to receive the drop downward

258. The schizophrenic client says to the nurse, "Will you protect me from the Grand Duchess?" and points to an older adult client who is sitting reading a book. Which of the following is the most therapeutic communication technique by the nurse?
    1 "Where is she? I'll talk to her."
    2 "The Grand Duchess, huh? Well, I'm the Queen and I will order her to stay away from you."
    3 "You will be safe here. Your thinking will be clearer after your medication starts to work."
    4 "I can see no Grand Duchess. You will need to trust me on that."

259. The client interrupts the nurse manager on rounds and says, "I need to get out of here so I can work on my computer project to save the world!" The night nurse reported that the client was admitted after attacking his father with an iron for interrupting him at the computer. Which of the following is the most therapeutic response by the nurse manager?
    1 "I will be able to talk with you in 15 minutes after you take your medication."
    2 "You have a project to save the world? I'd really like to hear about that after I finish rounds."
    3 "Well, sit right down and eat your breakfast. You're not going to save the world on an empty stomach."
    4 "You hurt your father because of these thoughts and you won't leave here until you can control yourself better."

260. A multiple sclerosis client who has received home health care due to progressive neurological deterioration states increasing difficulty in transferring from the bed to a chair but wants to remain at home. The home health care nurse would
    1 Observe the client demonstrating the transfer technique
    2 Itemize the number of falls that the client has had in recent weeks
    3 Seize the opportunity to discuss potential nursing home placement
    4 Start a restorative nursing program before more deterioration occurs

261. The community health nurse is making a home visit to a client who has an implantable cardioverter/defibrillator (ICD). The nurse reviews the postoperative teaching concerning pacemakers and dysrhythmias with the client. Which of the following statements indicates that further teaching is necessary?
    1 "If I feel an internal defibrillator shock, I should sit down."
    2 "I can stop taking my antidysrhythmic medicine now since I have a pacemaker."
    3 "My wife knows how to call the emergency medical services if I need it."
    4 "I have to avoid airport metal detectors and magnetic resonance imaging equipment."

262. The home health nurse discusses the home regimen with the postoperative cardiac surgery client. The client states, "I get dizzy in the shower." Based on the client's statement, which of the following does the nurse assess first?
    1 The temperature of the water of the client's shower
    2 The bathroom environment in the home
    3 Client's insurance plan for reimbursement of medical equipment
    4 The client's insurance plan regarding coverage of home health aides

263. The nurse is preparing to care for a client with a cervical-uterine radiation implant. The plan of care for the client will include all the following except
    1 The client will be in a private room
    2 Visitors are restricted
    3 A lead shield is kept at the bedside
    4 A radiation sign will be posted outside the client's room

264. A client seen in the health care clinic is diagnosed with syphilis, and the physician orders an intramuscular injection of penicillin G benzathine (Bicillin). After administering the intramuscular injection of medication, the nurse should
    1 Administer subcutaneous epinephrine
    2 Monitor the client for 30 minutes
    3 Encourage the client to ambulate
    4 Apply a topical anesthetic spray to the injection site

265. The nurse visits a schizophrenic client and finds the walls and windows of the client's home covered with aluminum foil. The client says, "It filters out the radio waves they've been sending to infect me!" If the nurse were assessing the client's hallucinations completely, which of the following questions would the nurse ask?
    1 "Are the auditory hallucinations loud or soft?"
    2 "How effective do you feel the foil has been

and how long have you been feeling that this is happening?"
    3 "Does the foil ever wear out?"
    4 "Where did you obtain the aluminum foil?"

266. The nurse is performing a mental status examination with a client who answers, "Glass breaks if you throw stones or shoot at it with a gun. My cousin shoots guns at the police all the time at target practice. People who live in glass houses shouldn't throw stones." Which of the following interpretations by the nurse is the most appropriate?
    1 Speech is distractable and contains flight of ideas
    2 Speech is incoherent and tangential
    3 Speech is pressured and contains clang associations
    4 Speech is illogical and loosely associated

267. The nurse is caring for a schizophrenic client who states, "I decided not to take my medication because I realize that it really can't help me. Only I can help me." Which of the following responses would be the most therapeutic communication technique by the nurse?
    1 "Only you can help?"
    2 "You decided not to take your medication?"
    3 "Your doctor wants you to continue with this medication because it is helping you. Do you recall needing to be hospitalized because you stopped your medication?"
    4 "If you can make this wise an observation, you probably don't need your medication any longer."

268. The forensic nurse must have excellent mental health skills. Which of the following skills is the most critical for the forensic nurse?
    1 The ability to evaluate the risk for violence in incarcerated clients
    2 The ability to work in a setting with blurred boundaries
    3 The ability to perform a follow-up physical assessment
    4 The ability to teach social skills to incarcerated clients

269. The nurse is instructing the client to perform a two-point gait for crutch-walking. Which of the following indicates appropriate instructions for this type of crutch-walking?
    1 Move the left foot forward and the left crutch forward, followed by the right crutch and the right foot
    2 Advance the right crutch and the left foot forward, followed by advancing the right foot and the left crutch forward
    3 Advance both crutches forward, followed by the left foot and then the right foot
    4 Advance the right foot, then the left foot, followed by both crutches

270. The nurse is caring for a client who has just returned from the operating room following the creation of a colostomy. The nurse is assessing the drainage in the pouch attached to the site where the colostomy was formed and notes serosanguineous drainage. Which of the following is the most appropriate nursing action based on this assessment?
 1 Notify the physician
 2 Document the amount and characteristics of the drainage
 3 Apply ice to the stoma site
 4 Apply pressure to the stoma site

271. The client with complete heart block has had a permanent-demand ventricular pacemaker inserted. The nurse assesses for proper pacemaker function by examining the ECG strip for the presence of pacemaker spikes
 1 Just after each T wave
 2 Before each QRS complex
 3 Just after each P wave
 4 Before each P wave

272. The nurse is monitoring a client with leukemia who is receiving doxorubicin (Adriamycin) by IV infusion. Which of the following assessment signs indicates toxicity of the medication?
 1 Elevated blood urea nitrogen (BUN)
 2 Elevated creatinine
 3 ECG changes
 4 A red coloration of the urine

273. A client who was hospitalized 5 days ago has developed left calf tenderness and has a positive Homans' sign. The nurse assigned to this client next assesses the client for
 1 Coolness and pallor of the affected limb
 2 Diminished distal peripheral pulses
 3 Increased calf circumference
 4 Bilateral edema

274. The nurse is implementing a plan of care for the client with deep vein thrombosis of the right leg. Which of the following interventions does the nurse avoid when delivering care to this client?
 1 Elevation of the right leg
 2 Ambulation in the hall twice per shift
 3 Application of moist heat to the right leg
 4 Administration of acetaminophen (Tylenol)

275. A client has been diagnosed with thromboangiitis obliterans (Buerger's disease). The nurse is considering measures to help the client cope with lifestyle changes needed to control the disease process. The nurse plans to refer the client to a
 1 Medical social worker
 2 Dietitian
 3 Smoking cessation program
 4 Pain management clinic

276. A child is diagnosed with impetigo. The physician prescribes a topical medication for treatment. The nurse anticipates that which of the following medications will be prescribed?
 1 Triple antibiotic
 2 Acyclovir (Zovirax)
 3 Mupirocin (Bactroban)
 4 Masoprocol (Actinex)

277. Coal tar has been prescribed for the client with psoriasis. The nurse provides instruction to the client regarding this treatment. Which of the following statements if made by the client indicates a need for further education?
 1 "The medication can cause diarrhea."
 2 "The medication can cause phototoxicity."
 3 "The medication has an unpleasant odor."
 4 "The medication can stain the skin and hair."

278. The community health nurse is conducting an education session for community members regarding measures to prevent skin cancer. The nurse is instructing the members regarding the use of sunscreen protection. The nurse evaluates that teaching was effective if a community member states that chemical sunscreens are most effective when applied
 1 Immediately after swimming
 2 15 minutes before exposure to the sun
 3 Immediately before exposure to the sun
 4 One hour before exposure to the sun

279. PolySkin is prescribed to cover a peripheral IV site. The home health nurse is preparing a plan of care for the client regarding the IV site dressing changes. Which of the following is most appropriate to include in the plan?
 1 Change PolySkin daily
 2 Apply PolySkin over a dry, sterile dressing
 3 Change PolySkin weekly
 4 Change PolySkin at least every 2 to 3 days

280. The nurse is caring for a client with a burn injury to the chest. Nitrofurazone (Furacin) is prescribed to be applied to the site of injury. Which of the following is not a component of the plan of care regarding the use of this treatment measure?
 1 Apply saline-soaked dressings over the medication
 2 Wash burn site daily
 3 Apply 1/16-inch film directly to the burn sites
 4 Apply medication with a sterile gloved hand

281. Mafenide (Sulfamylon) is prescribed for the client with a burn injury to the hand. Which of the following does the nurse include in the instructions to the client regarding the use of this medication?
 1 It is normal to experience local discomfort and burning after applying the medication

2 If local pain occurs after applying the medication, notify the physician

3 Apply a thinner film to the burn site than prescribed if burning develops

4 If burning occurs, discontinue the medication

282. The burn client is receiving treatments of topical mafenide (Sulfamylon) to the site of injury. Which of the following systemic effects can occur from the use of this medication?
1 Alkalosis
2 Acidosis
3 Hypotension
4 Hypertension

283. A Vigilon nonocclusive burn dressing is prescribed for the client with a partial thickness burn to the hand. Which of the following will be included in the plan of care regarding this treatment?
1 Change dressing every 3 days
2 Secure dressing over wound with gauze
3 Change dressing weekly
4 Apply over a sterile, dry dressing

284. Sodium hypochlorite (Dakin's) solution is prescribed for a client with a wound on the left foot. The wound is draining purulent material. Which of the following treatments does the nurse expect to be prescribed?
1 Irrigation of the wound
2 Place solution in wound and cover with an occlusive dressing
3 Soak sterile dressing with solution and pack into the wound
4 Foot soaks for 20 minutes daily

285. Tretinoin (Retin-A) is prescribed for a client with acne. The nurse provides instructions to the client regarding the medication. Which of the following is not a component of the teaching plan?
1 "Avoid exposure to the sun."
2 "You should start to see results in 2 to 3 weeks."
3 "If your skin begins to peel, notify the physician."
4 "Cleanse the skin thoroughly before applying the medication."

286. The nurse provides instructions to a client regarding the use of tretinoin (Retin-A). Which of the following statements if made by the client would indicate a need for further education?
1 "I will wash my hands thoroughly after applying medication."
2 "I should begin to see results in about 3 weeks."
3 "I will apply the medication liberally to the skin."
4 "I cannot use any cosmetics while I am using this medication."

287. Isotretinoin (Accutane) is prescribed for a client to treat severe cystic acne. The nurse provides instructions to the client regarding the medication. Which of the following indicates a need for further instruction?
1 "I need to take the medication with food."
2 "I can crush the tablets if I have difficulty in swallowing them."
3 "I will need to take the medication for 15 to 20 weeks."
4 "I will be taking the medication two times a day."

288. Isotretinoin (Accutane) is prescribed for a client with severe acne. The nurse instructs the client regarding the importance of follow-up to evaluate which of the following?
1 Triglyceride level
2 Sedimentation rate
3 Complete blood count
4 Cholesterol level

289. The physician prescribes isotretinoin (Accutane) for a client with severe acne. The nurse reviews the client's record. Which of the following medications, if noted on the client's record, requires physician notification?
1 Phenytoin (Dilantin)
2 Tetracycline (Achromycin)
3 Digoxin (Lanoxin)
4 Furosemide (Lasix)

290. The registered nurse is observing a newly hired nurse perform a dressing change on a client with a leg ulcer. Fibrinolysin and desoxyribonuclease (Elase) dry powder is prescribed. Which of the following observations indicates an inaccurate procedure regarding this treatment?
1 The nurse cleans the wound with a sterile solution prior to applying Elase
2 The nurse covers the Elase application with a dry, sterile dressing
3 The nurse covers the Elase application with a petrolatum gauze
4 The nurse prepares the solution just prior to use

291. Sutilains (Travase) is prescribed to treat a skin ulcer. Which of the following nursing interventions is not a component of the plan of care regarding this treatment?
1 Cleaning the wound with a sterile solution
2 Covering the Travase application with a dry, sterile dressing
3 Moistening the wound with sterile normal saline and then applying the Travase
4 Placing the Travase in the refrigerator following use

292. The nurse is preparing to change a dressing on a client with a decubitus ulcer. Dextranomer (Debrisan) is prescribed. Which of the following

is not a component of the plan of care regarding this treatment?

1 The wound is moistened prior to application of the Debrisan

2 The Debrisan is lightly packed into the wound

3 The Debrisan is applied carefully into the wound, avoiding the surrounding tissues

4 The wound bed is thoroughly dried prior to applying the medication

293. The home health nurse is visiting the client who has had a prosthetic valve replacement for severe mitral valve stenosis. Which statement by the client reflects an understanding of specific postoperative care for this surgery?

1 "I threw away my straight razor and bought an electric razor."

2 "I have to go to the bathroom several times a night."

3 "I count my pulse every day."

4 "I still do my deep-breathing exercises."

294. The nurse is planning to teach the client with peripheral arterial disease about measures to limit disease progression. The nurse does not include which of the following items in a list of suggestions to be given to the client?

1 Cut down on the amount of fats consumed in the diet

2 Use a heating pad on the legs to aid vasodilatation

3 Walk each day to increase circulation to the legs

4 Be careful not to injure the legs or feet

295. The home health nurse visits a client recovering from cardiogenic shock secondary to an anterior myocardial infarction. The nurse reviews the importance of planned rest periods and instructs the client to seek medical attention with symptoms of angina immediately. Which statement by the client indicates an understanding of the importance of these topics in rehabilitation?

1 "I wear a Medic-alert bracelet."

2 "I have planned periods of rest at 10 A.M. and 3 P.M. daily."

3 "I've lost 4 pounds since discharge."

4 "My daily pulse has remained between 65 and 80 beats/minute."

296. The home health nurse is reviewing medications with the client receiving colchicine for the treatment of gout. The nurse evaluates that the medication is effective if the client reports a decrease in

1 Blood glucose

2 Blood pressure

3 Joint inflammation

4 Headaches

297. The client has an order to receive enoxaparin (Lovenox). The nurse administers this medication by which of the following routes?

1 Oral

2 Subcutaneous

3 Intramuscular

4 Intravenous

298. The client states to the home health nurse, "I get so frustrated. I can't even do my gardening." The nurse questions the client regarding the activity level since coronary artery bypass surgery. Which response indicates a need for further teaching?

1 "I plan regular rest periods during the day."

2 "I pace my activities throughout the day."

3 "I avoid outdoor physical activity during the heat of the day."

4 "I try to walk immediately after lunch, after I've finished my morning house cleaning."

299. The home health nurse is observing the caregiver change the sternotomy dressing of the postoperative client. Which action identifies correct principles of infection control?

1 The caregiver selects a previously opened gauze to cover the sternal wound

2 The caregiver washes hands prior to removal of the soiled dressing and again before applying the clean dressing

3 The caregiver covers the mouth with the hand when sneezing, then continues with the dressing change

4 The caregiver dons gloves prior to removal of the old dressing and then applies the new dressing

300. The nurse is reviewing the laboratory results of an infant suspected of having hypertrophic pyloric stenosis. Which of the following does the nurse most likely expect to note in this infant?

1 A blood pH of 7.50

2 A blood pH of 7.30

3 A blood bicarbonate of 22 mEq/L

4 A blood bicarbonate of 19 mEq/L

ANSWERS

1. **1**

Rationale: Factors to minimize dumping syndrome after gastric surgery include having the client maintain a low Fowler's position while eating and lie down for at least 30 minutes after eating; giving small, frequent meals; avoiding liquids with meals; and avoiding high-carbohydrate food sources. Antispasmodic medications are also prescribed as needed to delay gastric emptying.

Test-Taking Strategy: Note the key words "minimize the risk" in the question. Use your knowledge of dumping syndrome and its causes to eliminate each of the incorrect options. The name of the condition, "dumping syndrome," should assist in directing you to the correct option.

Level of Cognitive Ability: Application
Phase of Nursing Process: Implementation
Client Needs: Health Promotion and Maintenance
Content Area: Adult Health/Gastrointestinal

Reference

Monahan, F., & Neighbors, M. (1998). *Medical-surgical nursing: Foundations for clinical practice* (2nd ed.). Philadelphia: W. B. Saunders. p. 1040.

2. **4**

Rationale: Following surgical intervention for imperforate anus, a side-lying position with the legs flexed or a prone position to keep the hips elevated can reduce edema and pressure on the surgical site.

Test-Taking Strategy: Consider the anatomical location of this surgical procedure. Eliminate options 1 and 2 first because these positions will cause pressure on the surgical site. For this same reason, option 3 can be eliminated. Review postoperative care following this surgical procedure now if you had difficulty with this question!

Level of Cognitive Ability: Application
Phase of Nursing Process: Implementation
Client Needs: Physiological Integrity
Content Area: Child Health

Reference

Ashwill, J., & Droske, S. (1997). *Nursing care of children: Principles and practice*. Philadelphia: W. B. Saunders. p. 748.

3. **4**

Rationale: The parents should be told that the jaundice may appear to get worse before it resolves. Options 1, 2, and 3 are incorrect.

Test-Taking Strategy: Use knowledge regarding the pathophysiology associated with hepatitis and therapeutic communication skills to answer the question. Options 1 and 2 place the mother's concerns on hold and add to the existing concern. Specific dietary measures assist in providing rest to the liver and are unrelated to the development of jaundice. If you had difficulty with this question, take time now to review the physiology associated with jaundice in a child with hepatitis!

Level of Cognitive Ability: Application
Phase of Nursing Process: Implementation
Client Needs: Psychosocial Integrity
Content Area: Child Health

Reference

Ashwill, J., & Droske, S. (1997). *Nursing care of children: Principles and practice*. Philadelphia: W. B. Saunders. p. 765.

4. **3**

Rationale: Constipation is a common elimination problem of clients in a manic phase of bipolar disorder. Constipation may occur as the result of a combination of factors, including taking antipsychotic medications, suppressing the urge to defecate, and decreasing fluid intake as the result of the manic activity level. The symptoms listed in the question—"dehydration," "unkempt," "abdominal fullness and discomfort," and "antipsychotic medications"—in combination are indicators of constipation. A high-fiber diet and increased fluids can reduce constipation.

Test-Taking Strategy: Focus on the complaints identified in the question. Use Maslow's hierarchy of needs theory. Option 3 is the only option that addresses physiological integrity!

Level of Cognitive Ability: Analysis
Phase of Nursing Process: Analysis
Client Needs: Physiological Integrity
Content Area: Mental Health

Reference

Wilson, H., & Kneisl, C. (1996). *Psychiatric nursing* (5th ed.). Reading, MA: Addison-Wesley. p. 350.

5. **1**

Rationale: Regular insulin intravenously is the treatment choice for DKA. This short-acting insulin is the only insulin that can be given IV and monitored/titrated carefully to the client's high blood sugar levels. NPH insulin is an intermediate-acting insulin and thus not appropriate for treatment in emergency DKA. Glucagon is used to treat hypoglycemia because it increases blood glucose levels, and glyburide is an oral hypoglycemic agent used to treat Type II diabetes. Both these agents are also inappropriate.

Test-Taking Strategy: Knowledge of medications used in treatment of diabetes and DKA is necessary to answer this question. Knowledge that DKA is characterized by extremely high blood sugar levels will assist in eliminating options 3 and 4. Recalling that Regular insulin is the only type of insulin that can be administered IV will direct you to option 1. Review the treatment for DKA now if you had difficulty with this question!

Level of Cognitive Ability: Analysis
Phase of Nursing Process: Analysis
Client Needs: Physiological Integrity
Content Area: Adult Health/Endocrine

Reference

Black, J., & Matassarin-Jacobs, E. (1997). *Medical-surgical nursing: Management for continuity of care* (5th ed.). Philadelphia: W. B. Saunders. p. 1985.

6. **3**

Rationale: Clients with chronic skin disorders may have Self-Esteem Disturbance because of the disorder itself and possible rejection by others. The nurse demonstrates acceptance of the client by using a quiet, unhurried manner, and by using appropriate visual contact, facial expression, and therapeutic touch. Communications that seem brief and formal may reinforce the feelings of rejection, as does avoidance of looking at the affected skin areas.

Test-Taking Strategy: Use basic concepts related to therapeutic communication to answer this question. The wording of the question tells you that there is only one correct response. Review therapeutic communication techniques now if you had difficulty with this question!

Level of Cognitive Ability: Application
Phase of Nursing Process: Planning
Client Needs: Psychosocial Integrity
Content Area: Adult Health/Integumentary

Reference
Burrell, P., Gerlach, M., & Pless, B. (1997). *Adult nursing: Acute and community care* (2nd ed.). Stamford, CT: Appleton & Lange. p. 1983.

7. 4

Rationale: Acetic acid solution is used for irrigating, cleansing, and packing wounds infected by *Pseudomonas aeruginosa*. Glycerin is an emollient that is used for dry, cracked, and irritated skin. Aspercreme and Myoflex are used to treat muscular aches.

Test-Taking Strategy: Note the key words *"Pseudomonas aeruginosa."* These key words and knowledge of the products indicated in the options will assist in directing you to option 4. Review these products now if you had difficulty with this question!

Level of Cognitive Ability: Analysis
Phase of Nursing Process: Analysis
Client Needs: Physiological Integrity
Content Area: Pharmacology

Reference
Kuhn, M. (1998). *Pharmacotherapeutics: A nursing process approach* (4th ed.). Philadelphia: F. A. Davis. p. 988.

8. 3

Rationale: An intradermal injection is administered with the needle bevel facing upward at a 10 to 15° angle. The medication is injected slowly, and a bleb should form under the skin with injection. After withdrawing the needle, the area may be patted dry with a 2×2 sterile gauze pad. The area should not be rubbed, to prevent spread of the medication beyond the area of injection. All equipment is then disposed of, and the area of injection is outlined for later reference.

Test-Taking Strategy: Note the key word in the question, "avoid." This tells you that the correct answer is the option that represents incorrect nursing practice. Use knowledge of basic administration techniques to answer this question. Review the procedure for intradermal injections now if you had difficulty with this question!

Level of Cognitive Ability: Application
Phase of Nursing Process: Implementation
Client Needs: Physiological Integrity
Content Area: Fundamental Skills

Reference
Leahy, J., & Kizilay, P. (1998). *Foundations of nursing practice: A nursing process approach.* Philadelphia: W. B. Saunders. p. 485.

9. 4

Rationale: Third-degree (full-thickness) burns involve the epidermis, the full dermis, and some of the subcutaneous fat layer. The burn appears to be a tan or fawn color, with skin that is hard, dry, and inelastic. The area may be edematous and compresses tissue underneath from eschar formation. The nerve endings have been damaged, so the area is insensitive to touch or to pain.

Test-Taking Strategy: Specific knowledge of the characteristics of various thickness burns is needed to answer this question correctly. If needed, review the characteristics of the various burn depths at this time!

Level of Cognitive Ability: Analysis
Phase of Nursing Process: Analysis
Client Needs: Physiological Integrity
Content Area: Adult Health/Integumentary

Reference
Burrell, P., Gerlach, M., & Pless, B. (1997). *Adult nursing: Acute and community care* (2nd ed.). Stamford, CT: Appleton & Lange. p. 2030.

10. 2

Rationale: The client should be maintained on NPO (nothing by mouth) status because burns frequently cause paralytic ileus. The client should also be told that fluids could cause vomiting because of the effect of burn injury on gastrointestinal (GI) tract functioning. Mouth care should be given as appropriate to alleviate the sensation of thirst.

Test-Taking Strategy: To answer this question correctly, it is necessary to understand the effects of a major physiological stressor, such as burns, on the client's system. Apply nursing knowledge and knowledge of the "fight or flight" response in answering this question!

Level of Cognitive Ability: Application
Phase of Nursing Process: Implementation
Client Needs: Physiological Integrity
Content Area: Adult Health/Integumentary

Reference
Burrell, P., Gerlach, M., & Pless, B. (1997). *Adult nursing: Acute and community care* (2nd ed.). Stamford, CT: Appleton & Lange. p. 2038.

11. 4

Rationale: Semipermeable film dressings, such as Op-Site or Duoderm, are used on superficial ulcers and occasionally on some deep, draining, or necrotic ulcers. These dressings have the advantage of staying in place for several days, allowing tissues to heal underneath. Dry, sterile dressings would stick to the wound and are inappropriate. Wet to dry dressings are not necessary, since the tissue does not need debridement. Gelfoam sponge dressings are a type of enzyme dressing used in the treatment of necrotic tissue.

Test-Taking Strategy: Specific knowledge of the various types of dressing materials and their uses is needed to answer this question. If needed, take a few moments to review this important content area at this time!

Level of Cognitive Ability: Application
Phase of Nursing Process: Implementation
Client Needs: Physiological Integrity
Content Area: Adult Health/Integumentary

Reference
Burrell, P., Gerlach, M., & Pless, B. (1997). *Adult nursing: Acute and community care* (2nd ed.). Stamford, CT: Appleton & Lange. p. 1997.

12. 1

Rationale: The gastric pH should be maintained at 7 or greater with the use of prescribed antacids and histamine H_2 receptor–blocking agents. Lowered pH in the absence of food or tube feedings can lead to erosion of the gastric lining and ulcer development. The client's bowel sounds may be expected to be hypoactive in the absence of oral or nasogastric tube (NGT) intake. Absence of discomfort and bleeding are normal findings.

Test-Taking Strategy: Use knowledge of the effects of physiological stressors on the GI tract to eliminate each of the incorrect options. The key words in the question, "least satisfactory," tell you that the correct answer is an abnormal or unexpected piece of data.

Level of Cognitive Ability: Analysis
Phase of Nursing Process: Evaluation
Client Needs: Physiological Integrity
Content Area: Adult Health/Integumentary

Reference

Burrell, P., Gerlach, M., & Pless, B. (1997). *Adult nursing: Acute and community care* (2nd ed.). Stamford, CT: Appleton & Lange. p. 2040.

13. **3**

Rationale: The use of Montgomery straps is recommended to prevent skin breakdown with frequent dressing changes. This limits the friction and shear that could irritate skin with frequent removal and reapplication of tape. Hypoallergenic tape is used on clients with either thin and fragile skin or on those clients whose skin is sensitive to standard tape, and who require less frequent dressing changes. Cleansing with povidone-iodine and obtaining a wound culture are not indicated.

Test-Taking Strategy: Use knowledge of basic concepts related to skin integrity and wound care materials to answer this question. Note that the question has the key words "benefit most from." This implies that more than one option may be partially correct. Review basic measures related to maintaining skin integrity now if you had difficulty with this question!

Level of Cognitive Ability: Analysis
Phase of Nursing Process: Analysis
Client Needs: Physiological Integrity
Content Area: Fundamental Skills

Reference

Leahy, J., & Kizilay, P. (1998). *Foundations of nursing practice: A nursing process approach.* Philadelphia: W. B. Saunders. p. 603.

14. **2**

Rationale: Milk contains the essential amino acid tryptophan, which enhances sleep by promoting production of the neurotransmitter serotonin in the brain. In this instance, research has supported what has been known as an "old wives' tale." The client should avoid spicy foods and a large intake just prior to bedtime. The client should also avoid caffeine after 12 noon.

Test-Taking Strategy: Note that the question contains the key word "best." This tells you that more than one option may be partially or totally correct. Use prioritizing skills to select the best option. Options 1 and 3 can be easily eliminated. From the remaining options, note the time frame "1 hour" in option 4. This should assist in eliminating this option!

Level of Cognitive Ability: Application
Phase of Nursing Process: Planning
Client Needs: Health Promotion and Maintenance
Content Area: Fundamental Skills

References

Leahy, J., & Kizilay, P. (1998). *Foundations of nursing practice: A nursing process approach.* Philadelphia: W. B. Saunders. p. 711.
Lutz, C., & Przytulski, K. (1997). *Nutrition and diet therapy* (2nd ed.). Philadelphia: F. A. Davis. p. 92.

15. **4**

Rationale: The client who is unconscious is at great risk of aspiration. The nurse assesses the client for the presence of a gag reflex. The nurse turns the client's head to the side and places an emesis basin underneath the mouth. A bite stick or padded tongue blade is used to open the mouth; use of the nurse's gloved fingers is avoided to prevent injury to the caregiver. Small volumes of fluid are used in rinsing the mouth, and oral suctioning is used to prevent aspiration.

Test-Taking Strategy: The key word in the question is "avoid." This tells you that the correct response is an incorrect nursing action. Use basic nursing knowledge related to hygiene measures to choose correctly. Keep in mind the issue related to the risk for aspiration. Noting the word "large" in option 4 will assist in directing you to that option!

Level of Cognitive Ability: Application
Phase of Nursing Process: Implementation
Client Needs: Safe, Effective Care Environment
Content Area: Fundamental Skills

Reference

Leahy, J., & Kizilay, P. (1998). *Foundations of nursing practice: A nursing process approach.* Philadelphia: W. B. Saunders. p. 547.

16. **1**

Rationale: The nurse removes the eye prosthesis by retracting the lower eyelid and applying gentle pressure just below the eye.

Test-Taking Strategy: Use basic nursing knowledge related to care of the client with an eye prosthesis to answer this question. If you are unfamiliar with this procedure, take a few moments to review it at this time!

Level of Cognitive Ability: Application
Phase of Nursing Process: Implementation
Client Needs: Physiological Integrity
Content Area: Fundamental Skills

Reference

Leahy, J., & Kizilay, P. (1998). *Foundations of nursing practice: A nursing process approach.* Philadelphia: W. B. Saunders. p. 554.

17. **3**

Rationale: The client is instructed about how to stop and start the machine, and to notify the nurse about knee discomfort. The client should also be aware of proper positioning, so that the nurse can be notified if the leg slips. The client should not try to adjust the flexion and extension settings. These are decided on by the orthopedic surgeon and are maintained as ordered. Other key actions by the nurse with the use of this device are to assess the neurovascular status of the extremity, and to ensure that the device is padded with manufactured disposable padding before the client's leg is placed in the device.

Test-Taking Strategy: Familiarity with the concepts and operation of this device is needed to answer this question correctly. If needed, take a few moments to review the key points of this apparatus!

Level of Cognitive Ability: Analysis
Phase of Nursing Process: Evaluation
Client Needs: Safe, Effective Care Environment
Content Area: Fundamental Skills

Reference

Monahan, F., & Neighbors, M. (1998). *Medical-surgical nursing: Foundations for clinical practice* (2nd ed.). Philadelphia: W. B. Saunders. p. 868.

18. **2**

Rationale: To prevent injury to the brachial nerve plexus and still provide sufficient support, there should be a distance of 2 inches between the client's axilla and the top of the crutch pad. This measurement is determined with the client holding the crutches with the elbows bent at a 30° angle.

Test-Taking Strategy: Use concepts related to basic client mobility to answer this question. Since crutches are commonly used in the treatment of selected orthopedic problems, take the time to review this material if you are not familiar with it!

Level of Cognitive Ability: Application
Phase of Nursing Process: Assessment
Client Needs: Physiological Integrity
Content Area: Adult Health/Musculoskeletal

Reference
Lammon, C., Foote, A., & Leli, P., et al. (1995). *Clinical nursing skills*. Philadelphia: W. B. Saunders. p. 240

19. **1**

Rationale: Using a TENS unit involves application of electrodes to the skin and adjusting the level of stimulation to the electrodes. The amount of stimulation is increased until the client feels discomfort, which indicates that the maximal stimulation necessary to block pain stimuli has been reached. The volume is then reduced by a small amount until no further muscle contractions occur. The other responses are incorrect.

Test-Taking Strategy: Familiarity with this device and its application is needed to answer this question accurately. If needed, take a few moments at this time to review the highlights of this increasingly popular method of pain control!

Level of Cognitive Ability: Analysis
Phase of Nursing Process: Analysis
Client Needs: Physiological Integrity
Content Area: Fundamental Skills

Reference
Monahan, F., & Neighbors, M. (1998). *Medical-surgical nursing: Foundations for clinical practice* (2nd ed.). Philadelphia: W. B. Saunders. p. 892.

20. **4**

Rationale: The client who is placed on contact precautions has a high microorganism count in some type of body secretion (such as feces or wound drainage). This client is placed in a private room whenever possible and is removed from the room only when absolutely necessary. Clients should be transported only for essential purposes, and precautions are maintained to minimize the risk of transmission of microorganisms.

Test-Taking Strategy: Use knowledge related to transmission of infection and isolation procedures to answer this question. Eliminate options 2 and 3 first as being the least plausible of all the options. Choose option 4 over option 1 because the source of infection has not been identified in the stem, and because it is the most comprehensive solution.

Level of Cognitive Ability: Application
Phase of Nursing Process: Planning
Client Needs: Safe, Effective Care Environment
Content Area: Fundamental Skills

Reference
Leahy, J., & Kizilay, P. (1998). *Foundations of nursing practice: A nursing process approach*. Philadelphia: W. B. Saunders. p. 1237.

21. **4**

Rationale: The client could sustain injury postoperatively from increased intraocular pressure, from trauma, or from impaired vision resulting in falls or other injury. The client should take action to avoid activities that could precipitate any of these. Scanning the environment and using grab bars are good for prevention of falls. Increasing fiber and fluids helps avoid constipation; straining from constipation could increase intraocular pressure. Taking off an eye patch prescribed during sleep could result in injury to the eye and should be avoided.

Test-Taking Strategy: Note that the key words in the question are "not resolved." This tells you that the correct answer is an incorrect action on the part of the client. Use knowledge of principles related to postoperative care following eye surgery to answer this question.

Level of Cognitive Ability: Analysis
Phase of Nursing Process: Evaluation
Client Needs: Health Promotion and Maintenance
Content Area: Adult Health/Eye

Reference
Beare, P., & Myers, J. (1998). *Adult health nursing* (3rd ed.). St. Louis: Mosby–Year Book. p. 1120.

22. **3**

Rationale: Women who are postmenopausal are taught to do breast self-examination on the same day of every month. Before menopause, women should do the procedure 7 days after the start of the menstrual cycle, when the breasts are least tender. Each breast is examined with the opposite hand. The pads of the fingers should be used for palpation, not the fingertips. The client may use a circular, up and down, or wedge method of assessment. Consistency of use of the same method is more important than the actual method used.

Test-Taking Strategy: Note that the key word in the question is "postmenopausal." This tells you that the correct answer is the assessment technique that is appropriate for this population. With this in mind, eliminate option 4 first. Use knowledge of physical assessment techniques to correctly choose among the three remaining options.

Level of Cognitive Ability: Application
Phase of Nursing Process: Implementation
Client Needs: Health Promotion and Maintenance
Content Area: Adult Health/Oncology

Reference
Beare, P., & Myers, J. (1998). *Adult health nursing* (3rd ed.). St. Louis: Mosby–Year Book. p. 1639.

23. **3**

Rationale: The client who is underhydrated will have a urine specific gravity of greater than 1.030. Normal values for urine specific gravity are 1.010 to 1.030. Pale yellow urine is a normal finding, as is a urine output of 40 mL per hour (minimum is 30 mL/hour). A urine pH of 6 is adequate (4.5 to 8.0 is normal), but this value is not used in monitoring hydration status.

Test-Taking Strategy: Use knowledge of signs of dehydration and normal fluid balance to answer this question. Note that the wording of the question guides you to look for data that are out of the normal range. Knowledge of the normal values will easily direct you to the correct option!

Level of Cognitive Ability: Analysis
Phase of Nursing Process: Assessment
Client Needs: Physiological Integrity
Content Area: Adult Health/Integumentary

Reference

Burrell, P., Gerlach, M., & Pless, B. (1997). *Adult nursing: Acute and community care* (2nd ed.). Stamford, CT: Appleton & Lange. p. 2040.

24. 2

Rationale: To begin and tolerate oral intake after cranial or any other type of surgery, the client must have bowel sounds. The client must also have intact swallow and gag reflexes and should be free of nausea and vomiting. The client is likely to be easily fatigued, which may decrease appetite. Thus, appetite is the least reliable indicator regarding when intake should be started.

Test-Taking Strategy: Use basic principles of postoperative care to answer this question. Note that the wording of the question states "least reliable." This tells you that the correct answer is an option that is of little use in directing nursing actions related to diet.

Level of Cognitive Ability: Analysis
Phase of Nursing Process: Analysis
Client Needs: Physiological Integrity
Content Area: Adult Health/Neurological

Reference

Burrell, P., Gerlach, M., & Pless, B. (1997). *Adult nursing: Acute and community care* (2nd ed.). Stamford, CT: Appleton & Lange. p. 932.

25. 2

Rationale: The most common cause of autonomic dysreflexia is visceral stimuli, such as with blockage of urinary drainage or with constipation. Barring these, other causes include noxious mechanical and thermal stimuli, particularly pressure and overchilling. For this reason, the nurse ensures that the client is positioned with no pinching or pressure on paralyzed body parts and ensures that the client will be sufficiently warm.

Test-Taking Strategy: Note that the key word in the stem of the question is "prevent." This implies an action orientation on the part of the nurse. Each of the incorrect options contains an item related to documentation, rather than an action to be taken just prior to leaving.

Level of Cognitive Ability: Application
Phase of Nursing Process: Implementation
Client Needs: Health Promotion and Maintenance
Content Area: Adult Health/Neurological

Reference

Burrell, P., Gerlach, M., & Pless, B. (1997). *Adult nursing: Acute and community care* (2nd ed.). Stamford, CT: Appleton & Lange. p. 959.

26. 1

Rationale: The most helpful approach by the nurse is to emphasize progress that is being made in a realistic manner. The nurse does not offer false hope but does provide factual information in a clear test positive manner. The nurse encourages the family to be realistic in their expectations and attitudes as well. The plan of care should be individualized for each client.

Test-Taking Strategy: Use knowledge of basic communication strategies to answer this question. Note that the question contains the key words "most helpful." This tells you that more than one option may be partially correct.

Level of Cognitive Ability: Application
Phase of Nursing Process: Implementation
Client Needs: Psychosocial Integrity
Content Area: Adult Health/Neurological

Reference

Burrell, P., Gerlach, M., & Pless, B. (1997). *Adult nursing: Acute and community care* (2nd ed.). Stamford, CT: Appleton & Lange. p. 933.

27. 4

Rationale: The most important nursing action is to call the physician. The deterioration in neurological status, increasing pulse, and increasing BP with a widening pulse pressure all indicate that the client is experiencing increased intracranial pressure. This requires immediate treatment to prevent further complications and possible death. The nurse should recheck the vital signs to assure accuracy and should reorient the client to surroundings. If the client's blood pressure falls within parameters for PRN antihypertensive medication, this should also be administered. All of the distracters are secondary nursing actions.

Test-Taking Strategy: Note that the key words in this question are "most important." This tells you that some or all of the options may be partially or totally correct. Use your nursing knowledge and priority-setting ability to choose the correct option.

Level of Cognitive Ability: Application
Phase of Nursing Process: Implementation
Client Needs: Physiological Integrity
Content Area: Adult Health/Neurological

Reference

Burrell, P., Gerlach, M., & Pless, B. (1997). *Adult nursing: Acute and community care* (2nd ed.). Stamford, CT: Appleton & Lange. p. 907.

28. 3

Rationale: The client should avoid intake of alcohol. Alcohol could interact with the client's seizure medications, or the alcohol itself could precipitate seizure activity. The other options are all correct. The client should take all medications on time to avoid drops in therapeutic medication levels that could precipitate seizures. The client should not bathe in the shower or tub alone and should not smoke alone, to minimize risk of injury should a seizure occur.

Test-Taking Strategy: The key words in the question are "safety precautions" and "needs more information." The first phrase guides you to think about appropriate safety measures that should be used in the home. The phrase "needs more information" guides you to look for an option that is an incorrect statement. Use your nursing knowledge to determine the correct option!

Level of Cognitive Ability: Analysis
Phase of Nursing Process: Evaluation
Client Needs: Health Promotion and Maintenance
Content Area: Adult Health/Neurological

Reference

Burrell, P., Gerlach, M., & Pless, B. (1997). *Adult nursing: Acute and community care* (2nd ed.). Stamford, CT: Appleton & Lange. p. 911.

29. 1

Rationale: The instructions for the use of Ovide include sprinkle lotion on dry hair and rub gently until the scalp is moistened; allow to dry naturally; after 8 to 12 hours wash hair with nonmedicated shampoo; rinse, and use a fine-toothed comb to remove lice; repeat in 7 to 9 days if needed.

Test-Taking Strategy: Knowledge regarding the use of this lotion is required to answer this question. If you are unfamiliar with the use of this treatment, review the important client teaching points now!

Level of Cognitive Ability: Application
Phase of Nursing Process: Implementation
Client Needs: Health Promotion and Maintenance
Content Area: Pharmacology

Reference

Kuhn, M. (1998). *Pharmacotherapeutics: A nursing process approach* (4th ed.). Philadelphia: F. A. Davis. p. 991.

30. 2

Rationale: CSF leakage following cranial surgery may be detected by noting drainage that is serosanguineous (due to surgery) and surrounded by an area of straw-colored or pale drainage. The typical appearance of CSF drainage is that of a "halo." The other options are incorrect. The nurse would also further verify actual CSF drainage by testing the drainage for glucose, which would be positive.

Test-Taking Strategy: To answer this question accurately, it is necessary to be familiar with the appearance and assessment of CSF drainage. Since this is an important concept, take the time to review this material if the question was difficult!

Level of Cognitive Ability: Application
Phase of Nursing Process: Assessment
Client Needs: Physiological Integrity
Content Area: Adult Health/Neurological

Reference

Burrell, P., Gerlach, M., & Pless, B. (1997). *Adult nursing: Acute and community care* (2nd ed.). Stamford, CT: Appleton & Lange. p. 933.

31. 1

Rationale: Motor responses such as weakness and decreased movement will be seen on the side of the body that is opposite an area of head injury. Contralateral deficits result from compression of the cortex of the brain or the pyramidal tracts. Depending on the severity of injury, the client may have a variety of neurological deficits.

Test-Taking Strategy: Begin to answer this question by eliminating option 4. Absolute words such as "only" in an option make it unlikely to be the correct choice. Use knowledge of anatomy and physiology and nursing assessment to choose correctly among the three remaining options.

Level of Cognitive Ability: Application
Phase of Nursing Process: Assessment
Client Needs: Physiological Integrity
Content Area: Adult Health/Neurological

Reference

Burrell, P., Gerlach, M., & Pless, B. (1997). *Adult nursing: Acute and community care* (2nd ed.). Stamford, CT: Appleton & Lange. p. 907.

32. 4

Rationale: Environmental stimuli are kept to a minimum with subarachnoid precautions in order to prevent and/or minimize increases in intracranial pressure. For this reason, lighting is reduced by closing window blinds and the door to the client's room. Overhead lighting is also avoided for the same reasons. The nurse prohibits television, radio, or newspapers, unless this is so stressful for the client that it would be counterproductive. In that instance, minimal amounts of stimuli by these means are allowed with approval of the physician.

Test-Taking Strategy: To answer this question correctly, it is necessary to understand the rationale behind aneurysm precautions. Analyze each of the options, then, in terms of how the item could affect the intracranial pressure. Review aneurysm precautions now if you had difficulty with this question!

Level of Cognitive Ability: Application
Phase of Nursing Process: Planning
Client Needs: Safe, Effective Care Environment
Content Area: Adult Health/Neurological

Reference

Burrell, P., Gerlach, M., & Pless, B. (1997). *Adult nursing: Acute and community care* (2nd ed.). Stamford, CT: Appleton & Lange. p. 1000.

33. 3

Rationale: With subarachnoid precautions, any activity that could raise the client's intracranial pressure (ICP) is avoided. For this reason, activities such as straining, coughing, blowing the nose, and even sneezing are avoided whenever possible. The other interventions (repositioning, deep breathing, and incentive spirometry) do not provide an added risk of increasing ICP and are beneficial in reducing respiratory complications of bed rest.

Test-Taking Strategy: Note that the key word in this question is "avoid." This tells you that the correct answer to the question will be an item that is an incorrect nursing action. Use principles related to increased intracranial pressure to make your selection.

Level of Cognitive Ability: Application
Phase of Nursing Process: Implementation
Client Needs: Physiological Integrity
Content Area: Adult Health/Neurological

Reference

Burrell, P., Gerlach, M., & Pless, B. (1997). *Adult nursing: Acute and community care* (2nd ed.). Stamford, CT: Appleton & Lange. p. 1000.

34. 2

Rationale: The client's airway is patent if all the respiratory parameters measured fall within normal limits. Therefore, the respiratory rate ideally should be 16 to 20, oxygen saturation greater than 95%, and breath sounds clear. The only option that meets all three criteria is option 2.

Test-Taking Strategy: Use knowledge of physical assessment data to answer this question. Remember that when there are multiple parts to an option, all the parts of that option must be correct in order for that option to be correct.

Level of Cognitive Ability: Analysis
Phase of Nursing Process: Evaluation
Client Needs: Physiological Integrity
Content Area: Adult Health/Neurological

Reference

Burrell, P., Gerlach, M., & Pless, B. (1997). *Adult nursing: Acute and community care* (2nd ed.). Stamford, CT: Appleton & Lange. p. 989.

35. **1**

Rationale: Skin color may be more difficult to assess in the client with dark skin. The best areas to use to detect pallor and cyanosis include the tongue, mucous membranes, and nailbeds. The sclera are most useful in evaluating jaundice.

Test-Taking Strategy: Note that the key words in this question are "least helpful." This tells you that the answer to the question is the area that will not give reliable assessment data. Visualize each of the responses in terms of the vascularity of that area in making your selection.

Level of Cognitive Ability: Application
Phase of Nursing Process: Assessment
Client Needs: Physiological Integrity
Content Area: Adult Health/Integumentary

Reference

Burrell, P., Gerlach, M., & Pless, B. (1997). *Adult nursing: Acute and community care* (2nd ed.). Stamford, CT: Appleton & Lange. p. 1978.

36. **4**

Rationale: The client who cannot shift weight unaided should have a pressure relief pad in place under the buttocks to prevent skin breakdown. The best products to accomplish this are devices that have a tendency to equalize the client's weight on the pad. These include foam, water, gel, or alternating-air products. A plastic-lined pad provides no pressure relief. A pillow provides cushion but does not redistribute weight equally. An air ring relieves pressure in some spots, but causes pressure in others by virtue of design.

Test-Taking Strategy: The key words in the question are "best" and "paraplegic." Use nursing knowledge about skin breakdown and preventive measures to answer this question.

Level of Cognitive Ability: Analysis
Phase of Nursing Process: Analysis
Client Needs: Physiological Integrity
Content Area: Adult Health/Integumentary

Reference

Burrell, P., Gerlach, M., & Pless, B. (1997). *Adult nursing: Acute and community care* (2nd ed.). Stamford, CT: Appleton & Lange. p. 1995.

37. **2**

Rationale: Kwell is worked into dry hair and left in place for 4 minutes. After this, the shampoo is rinsed off with warm water. Dead nits can be removed with a comb or tweezers. Although one treatment is usually sufficient, a second application in 7 days may be required. Sexual partners should be treated concurrently.

Test-Taking Strategy: Knowledge regarding the use of Kwell in the treatment of pubic lice is required to answer this question. If you are unfamiliar with the use of this medication, take time now to review!

Level of Cognitive Ability: Application
Phase of Nursing Process: Implementation
Client Needs: Health Promotion and Maintenance
Content Area: Pharmacology

Reference

Lehne, R. (1998). *Pharmacology for nursing care* (3rd ed.). Philadelphia: W. B. Saunders. p. 1003.

38. **3**

Rationale: Several things may be done to promote hydration of the skin. Room temperature should be maintained at greater than 40%. The client should take tub baths or showers only every 2 to 3 days and should sponge bath between times. Bath water should be between 95° and 100°F (tepid) and not very hot or very cold. Harsh soaps should be avoided, and emollients should be applied generously to the skin while it is still damp.

Test-Taking Strategy: Use principles of basic hygiene and skin care to answer this question. The wording of the question tells you that only one of the responses will be correct.

Level of Cognitive Ability: Application
Phase of Nursing Process: Implementation
Client Needs: Health Promotion and Maintenance
Content Area: Adult Health/Integumentary

Reference

Burrell, P., Gerlach, M., & Pless, B. (1997). *Adult nursing: Acute and community care* (2nd ed.). Stamford, CT: Appleton & Lange. p. 1985.

39. **1**

Rationale: After laser surgery to remove any type of skin lesion, the skin should be protected from direct sunlight for a minimum of 3 months. There should be minimal or no discomfort following the procedure, and if present, it should be easily relieved with acetaminophen. The area should be cleansed gently with half strength hydrogen peroxide twice a day after the Telfa dressing is removed (24 hours postprocedure). Redness and swelling are expected after this procedure.

Test-Taking Strategy: The wording of the question tells you that the correct response will be worded as a correct statement. Familiarity with aftercare following laser surgery is needed to answer this question. If needed, take a few moments now to review this content area.

Level of Cognitive Ability: Analysis
Phase of Nursing Process: Evaluation
Client Needs: Health Promotion and Maintenance
Content Area: Adult Health/Integumentary

Reference

Burrell, P., Gerlach, M., & Pless, B. (1997). *Adult nursing: Acute and community care* (2nd ed.). Stamford, CT: Appleton & Lange. pp. 1992–1993.

40. **3**

Rationale: BenGay is one of the many products used for the temporary relief of muscular aches, rheumatism, arthritis, sprains, and neuralgia. These types of products contain combinations of antiseptics, local anesthetics, analgesics, and counterirritants. A heating pad should not be applied because irritation or burning of the skin may occur. The medication is not addicting, does not act in a systemic manner, nor cause sleepiness.

Test-Taking Strategy: Noting the key words "topical cream" may assist in eliminating options 2 and 4. Recalling the principles related to heat application will assist in eliminating option 1. Review the client teaching points related to the use of this medication now if you had difficulty with this question!

Level of Cognitive Ability: Analysis
Phase of Nursing Process: Evaluation
Client Needs: Health Promotion and Maintenance
Content Area: Pharmacology

Reference
Kuhn, M. (1998). *Pharmacotherapeutics: A nursing process approach* (4th ed.). Philadelphia: F. A. Davis. p. 988.

41. **1**

Rationale: The client who has been diagnosed with PID should avoid frequent douching, because this decreases the natural flora that control growth of infectious organisms. The client should also avoid strong soaps, sprays, powders, and so on, which irritate the perineum. The client should wear cotton undergarments that "breathe," and clothes should not fit tightly. Sanitary pads are changed optimally every 4 hours, or at least every 6 hours. Tampons should be changed with the same frequency after recovery and should not be used during the acute infection. Some health care providers may recommend avoiding them indefinitely. Intrauterine devices increase the client's susceptibility to PID.

Test-Taking Strategy: Familiarity with PID and its risk factors is needed to answer this question correctly. If needed, take a few moments to review this important content area for women's health now!

Level of Cognitive Ability: Application
Phase of Nursing Process: Planning
Client Needs: Health Promotion and Maintenance
Content Area: Adult Health/Reproductive

Reference
Beare, P., & Myers, J. (1998). *Adult health nursing* (3rd ed.). St. Louis: Mosby–Year Book. p. 1657.

42. **1**

Rationale: If mild diarrhea occurs in a child younger than 2 years of age, a soft diet is advised as long as the child is tolerating solids. The ABCs (applesauce, strained bananas, and strained carrots), rice, potatoes, and other bland foods without dairy products are advised. Extra fluids may also be needed and may be given by adding 1 to 2 extra ounces of water to each bottle of formula or juice.

Test-Taking Strategy: Note the key word "mild" and the child's age in the question. This should assist in eliminating option 4. Recalling that dairy products and foods that irritate the GI tract should be avoided will assist in eliminating options 2 and 3.

Level of Cognitive Ability: Application
Phase of Nursing Process: Implementation
Client Needs: Physiological Integrity
Content Area: Child Health

Reference
Ashwill, J., & Droske, S. (1997). *Nursing care of children: Principles and practice.* Philadelphia: W. B. Saunders. p. 688.

43. **3**

Rationale: The mother needs to be instructed that straws, pacifiers, spoons, or fingers must be kept away from the child's mouth for 7 to 10 days. Additionally, the mother should be advised to avoid taking an oral temperature. Options 1, 2, and 4 are accurate measures following cleft palate repair.

Test-Taking Strategy: Consider the anatomical location of the surgical procedure in answering the question. Also, note the key phrase "indicate the need for further instructions" in the stem of the question. These clues will assist in directing you to the correct option. Review postoperative care following cleft palate repair now if you had difficulty with this question!

Level of Cognitive Ability: Application
Phase of Nursing Process: Implementation
Client Needs: Health Promotion and Maintenance
Content Area: Child Health

Reference
Ashwill, J., & Droske, S. (1997). *Nursing care of children: Principles and practice.* Philadelphia: W. B. Saunders. p. 705.

44. **2**

Rationale: Lithium is an antimanic medication and is used to treat the manic phase of a manic-depressive disorder.

Test-Taking Strategy: Knowledge regarding the use of lithium is required to answer this question. If you had difficulty with this question, take time now to review this important medication. You are likely to see a question regarding this medication on NCLEX-RN!

Level of Cognitive Ability: Analysis
Phase of Nursing Process: Analysis
Client Needs: Physiological Integrity
Content Area: Pharmacology

Reference
Hodgson, B., & Kizior, R. (1999). *Saunders nursing drug handbook 1999.* Philadelphia: W. B. Saunders. p. 598.

45. **1**

Rationale: Option 1 addresses tasks of the evaluative process of crisis intervention. Options 2, 3, and 4 identify important issues and client expectations that reflect the movement toward resolution of the conflict but do not specifically indicate resolution.

Test-Taking Strategy: Note the key words "best indicator that the client has resolved." Reading each option carefully, focusing on these key words, should easily direct you toward option 1. Review crisis intervention now if you had difficulty with this question!

Level of Cognitive Ability: Analysis
Phase of Nursing Process: Evaluation
Client Needs: Psychosocial Integrity
Content Area: Mental Health

Reference
Johnson, B. S. (1997). *Psychiatric–mental health nursing: Adaptation and growth.* Philadelphia: Lippincott-Raven. p. 802.

46. **4**

Rationale: In vitro fertilization is a method of medically assisted reproduction for women with nonpatent, diseased, or missing fallopian tubes, or with infertility of unknown etiology. Ova and sperm are obtained from potential parents or donors, placed in a nutrient medium, and allowed to incubate; then the fertilized ovum is transferred into the woman's uterus. The woman houses the pregnancy throughout gestation and gives birth. Option 4 describes the procedure for artificial insemination. Options 1, 2, and 3 are correct statements regarding this procedure.

Test-Taking Strategy: Note the key words "need for further education" in the stem of the question. Option 3 can be easily eliminated. Knowledge regarding the procedure associated with in vitro fertilization will assist in eliminating options 2 and 3. Option 4 describes the procedure of artificial insemination. Review this procedure now if you had difficulty with this question!

Level of Cognitive Ability: Analysis
Phase of Nursing Process: Evaluation
Client Needs: Health Promotion and Maintenance
Content Area: Maternity

Reference
Nichols, F., & Zwelling, E. (1997). *Maternal-newborn nursing: Theory and practice.* Philadelphia: W. B. Saunders. p. 161.

47. **2**

Rationale: A platypelloid pelvis has a flat shape. A gynecoid pelvis is a normal female pelvis. An anthropoid pelvis has an oval shape, and an android pelvis is heart shaped.

Test-Taking Strategy: Knowledge regarding the four classic types of pelvis is required to answer this question. However, if you are unfamiliar with these types of pelvis, take time now to review!

Level of Cognitive Ability: Analysis
Phase of Nursing Process: Analysis
Client Needs: Physiological Integrity
Content Area: Maternity

Reference
Nichols, F., & Zwelling, E. (1997). *Maternal-newborn nursing: Theory and practice.* Philadelphia: W. B. Saunders. p. 177.

48. **3**

Rationale: Esophageal atresia with tracheoesophageal fistula (TEF) represents a critical neonatal surgical emergency. While the infant is awaiting transfer to surgery, management centers on prevention of aspiration. The infant is kept supine or prone, with the head of the bed elevated, to decrease the chance of gastric secretions from entering the lungs. IV fluids are essential. An NG tube must be in place and aspirated every 5 to 10 minutes to keep the proximal pouch clear of secretions.

Test-Taking Strategy: Note the key phrase "highest priority" in the stem of the question. You can easily eliminate options 1 and 4, as these are normal, standard procedures. From the remaining options, select option 3 over option 2 by recalling that the risk of aspiration is of highest concern. Additionally, you would not want to instill fluid into the stomach of a preoperative infant. Review nursing care of this disorder now if you had difficulty with this question!

Level of Cognitive Ability: Application
Phase of Nursing Process: Implementation
Client Needs: Physiological Integrity
Content Area: Child Health

Reference
Ashwill, J., & Droske, S. (1997). *Nursing care of children: Principles and practice.* Philadelphia: W. B. Saunders. p. 708.

49. **1**

Rationale: Assessment findings in a child with hepatitis include right upper quadrant tenderness and hepatomegaly. The stools will be pale and clay-colored, and urine will be dark and "frothy." Jaundice may be present and will be best assessed in the sclera, nailbeds, and mucous membranes.

Test-Taking Strategy: Note the key word "not" in the stem of the question. Knowledge regarding the anatomical location will easily direct you to option 1. If you had difficulty with this question, take time now to review the assessment findings in a child with hepatitis!

Level of Cognitive Ability: Application
Phase of Nursing Process: Assessment
Client Needs: Physiological Integrity
Content Area: Child Health

Reference
Ashwill, J., & Droske, S. (1997). *Nursing care of children: Principles and practice.* Philadelphia: W. B. Saunders. p. 765.

50. **4**

Rationale: Paint chips, soil contaminated with lead, lead solder used in plumbing, vinyl blinds, and improperly glazed pottery can cause lead poisoning.

Test-Taking Strategy: Note the key word "not" in the stem of the question. Reading each option carefully will easily direct you to option 4 because of the word "properly" in this option. Take time to review these poisonous substances now if you had difficulty with this question!

Level of Cognitive Ability: Application
Phase of Nursing Process: Assessment
Client Needs: Health Promotion and Maintenance
Content Area: Child Health

Reference
Ashwill, J., & Droske, S. (1997). *Nursing care of children: Principles and practice.* Philadelphia: W. B. Saunders. pp. 337–340.

51. **3**

Rationale: This study is used to evaluate intraocular conditions, including retinopathy and tumors. An injection of IV contrast dye is performed after ocular dilating medications are administered. There are no food or fluid restrictions prior to the procedure. Other related concepts are similar to those concerning injection of any contrast dye.

Test-Taking Strategy: Familiarity with this procedure is needed to answer this question correctly. If needed, take a few moments to review this material. The key word "angiography" in the stem should give you a framework to use when selecting your response.

Level of Cognitive Ability: Application
Phase of Nursing Process: Implementation
Client Needs: Physiological Integrity
Content Area: Adult Health/Eye

Reference
Beare, P., & Myers, J. (1998). *Adult health nursing* (3rd ed.). St. Louis: Mosby–Year Book. p. 1111.

52. **4**

Rationale: Condoms must be applied before any vaginal penetration occurs to be effective. A condom must be used with every sexual encounter to be safe. A lubricated condom may be used to increase sensitivity of the glans. Natural membrane condoms are less effective in preventing the spread of some STDs.

Test-Taking Strategy: The wording of the question tells you that the correct option will also be a true statement. Use knowledge of STDs and contraceptive methods to eliminate each of the incorrect options. Review prevention of STDs now if you had difficulty with this question!

Level of Cognitive Ability: Application
Phase of Nursing Process: Planning
Client Needs: Health Promotion and Maintenance
Content Area: Fundamental Skills

Reference
Burrell, P., Gerlach, M., & Pless, B. (1997). *Adult nursing: Acute and community care* (2nd ed.). Stamford, CT: Appleton & Lange. p. 1717.

53. **3**

Rationale: The classic symptoms of TSS are high fever (101°F or higher), vomiting, and severe diarrhea. Other typical symptoms include headache, myalgia, chills, abdominal pain, dizziness, lethargy, possible confusion, and agitation. Vaginal bleeding or discharge is not part of the clinical picture. TSS typically is caused by *Staphylococcus aureus* infection associated with tampon use during menses.

Test-Taking Strategy: Remember that for an option to be correct, all parts of that option must be correct. With this in mind, eliminate options 1 and 2 first, since the client presents with a high-grade fever. Knowing the etiology of TSS will help you eliminate option 4. The syndrome is caused by tampon use during menses and is not associated with purulent discharge.

Level of Cognitive Ability: Analysis
Phase of Nursing Process: Assessment
Client Needs: Physiological Integrity
Content Area: Fundamental Skills

Reference
Burrell, P., Gerlach, M., & Pless, B. (1997). *Adult nursing: Acute and community care* (2nd ed.). Stamford, CT: Appleton & Lange. p. 1724.

54. **1**

Rationale: If the bladder irrigation is infusing at a sufficient rate, the drainage through the Foley tubing will be pale pink. A dark pink color (sometimes referred to as punch-colored) indicates that the speed of the irrigation should be increased. Bright red bleeding should be reported to the surgeon, as it could indicate complications. Tea-colored urine is not seen after TURP but may be described in the client with renal failure.

Test-Taking Strategy: To answer this question correctly, recall that hemorrhage is a complication following any surgical procedure. Remember also that the purpose of bladder irrigation is to flush out blood and clots that could otherwise accumulate in the bladder following surgery. With this in mind, it is relatively easy to conclude that pale pink drainage would indicate sufficient irrigation flow.

Level of Cognitive Ability: Application
Phase of Nursing Process: Assessment
Client Needs: Physiological Integrity
Content Area: Adult Health/Renal

Reference
Burrell, P., Gerlach, M., & Pless, B. (1997). *Adult nursing: Acute and community care* (2nd ed.). Stamford, CT: Appleton & Lange. p. 1784.

55. **3**

Rationale: Hirschsprung's disease is also known as congenital aganglionosis or megacolon. It results from the absence of ganglion cells in the rectum and to varying degrees up into the colon. Option 1 describes celiac disease. Option 2 describes lactose intolerance. Option 4 describes irritable bowel syndrome.

Test-Taking Strategy: Knowledge regarding the description and cause of Hirschsprung's disease is required to answer this question. If you are unfamiliar with this disorder, take time now to review!

Level of Cognitive Ability: Application
Phase of Nursing Process: Implementation
Client Needs: Physiological Integrity
Content Area: Child Health

Reference
Ashwill, J., & Droske, S. (1997). *Nursing care of children: Principles and practice.* Philadelphia: W. B. Saunders. p. 735.

56. **2**

Rationale: Lindane can penetrate the intact skin and can cause convulsions if absorbed in sufficient quantities. Clients at highest risk for convulsions are premature infants, children, and clients with pre-existing seizure disorders. Lindane should not be used on pediatric clients unless safer medications have failed to control infection.

Test-Taking Strategy: Knowledge regarding the contraindications associated with the use of Lindane is required to answer this question. If you are unfamiliar with these contraindications, learn them now!

Level of Cognitive Ability: Analysis
Phase of Nursing Process: Analysis
Client Needs: Physiological Integrity
Content Area: Pharmacology

Reference
Lehne, R. (1998). *Pharmacology for nursing care* (3rd ed.). Philadelphia: W. B. Saunders. p. 1003.

57. **2**

Rationale: The client who suddenly becomes disoriented and confused following TURP could be experiencing early signs of hyponatremia. This may occur because the flushing solution used during the operative procedure is hypotonic. If enough solution is absorbed through the prostate veins during surgery, the client experiences increased circulating volume and dilutional hyponatremia. The nurse should notify the physician of these symptoms. Reorienting the client and ensuring that clock and calendar are visible may be helpful but do not correct the problem. The nurse does not increase the flow rate of an IV without an order. In addition, speeding up the flow rate could potentially worsen the problem, depending on the solution that is hanging.

Test-Taking Strategy: Note that the key words in the question are "most important." This tells you that more than one or all of the options may be partially or totally correct. In this case, option 4 is wrong and should be eliminated first. You would choose correctly among the three remaining options by knowing the reason for the symptoms, and that it requires medical intervention to adequately treat it.

Level of Cognitive Ability: Analysis
Phase of Nursing Process: Analysis
Client Needs: Physiological Integrity
Content Area: Adult Health/Renal

Reference

Burrell, P., Gerlach, M., & Pless, B. (1997). *Adult nursing: Acute and community care* (2nd ed.). Stamford, CT: Appleton & Lange. p. 1784.

58. **4**

Rationale: One of the most helpful approaches in exploring client concerns is to use open-ended questions. These tend to elicit more descriptive responses on the part of the client. This is the reason that option 4 is correct. Options 1 and 3 are closed-ended questions that may be answered with a "yes" or "no" response. Option 2 imposes the nurse's opinion on the client and does not value the client's perspective.

Test-Taking Strategy: Use basic principles related to therapeutic communication and interviewing skills to answer this question. Knowledge of blocks to communication will help you eliminate each of the incorrect responses systematically.

Level of Cognitive Ability: Application
Phase of Nursing Process: Implementation
Client Needs: Psychosocial Integrity
Content Area: Fundamental Skills

Reference

Taylor, C., Lillis, C., & LeMone, P. (1997). *Fundamentals of nursing: The art and science of nursing care* (3rd ed.). Philadelphia: Lippincott-Raven. p. 370.

59. **1**

Rationale: Signs of prostatism that may be reported to the nurse are reduced force and size of urinary stream, intermittent stream, hesitancy in beginning the flow of urine, inability to stop urinating quickly, a sensation of incomplete bladder emptying after voiding, and an increase in episodes of nocturia. These symptoms are the result of pressure of the enlarging prostate on the client's urethra.

Test-Taking Strategy: Remember that options that are similar are not likely to be correct. In this case, each of the incorrect options represents a difficulty with properly emptying the bladder. Using the process of elimination, this leads to option 1 as the correct choice.

Level of Cognitive Ability: Application
Phase of Nursing Process: Assessment
Client Needs: Health Promotion and Maintenance
Content Area: Adult Health/Renal

Reference

Burrell, P., Gerlach, M., & Pless, B. (1997). *Adult nursing: Acute and community care* (2nd ed.). Stamford, CT: Appleton & Lange. pp. 1778–1779.

60. **2**

Rationale: The characteristic lesion of syphilis is painless and indurated. The lesion is referred to as a chancre. Genital warts are characterized by cauliflower-like growths, or growths that are soft and fleshy. Genital herpes is accompanied by the presence of one or more vesicles that then rupture and heal. Scabies is characterized by erythematous, papular eruptions.

Test-Taking Strategy: To answer this question accurately, it is necessary to be familiar with the clinical signs of various sexually transmitted diseases. This knowledge would allow you to eliminate each of the incorrect options systematically.

Level of Cognitive Ability: Analysis
Phase of Nursing Process: Assessment
Client Needs: Physiological Integrity
Content Area: Fundamental Skills

Reference

Burrell, P., Gerlach, M., & Pless, B. (1997). *Adult nursing: Acute and community care* (2nd ed.). Stamford, CT: Appleton & Lange. p. 1719.

61. **3**

Rationale: Because hepatitis A is not infectious within 1 week after the onset of jaundice, the child may return to school at that time if the child feels well enough.

Test-Taking Strategy: Knowledge regarding the infectious period of hepatitis A is required to answer this question. Take time now to review the infectious period of HAV if you had difficulty with this question!

Level of Cognitive Ability: Application
Phase of Nursing Process: Implementation
Client Needs: Health Promotion and Maintenance
Content Area: Child Health

Reference

Ashwill, J., & Droske, S. (1997). *Nursing care of children: Principles and practice.* Philadelphia: W. B. Saunders. p. 765.

62. **1**

Rationale: Cleft palate repair is individualized and based on the degree of deformity and size of the child. Cleft palate repair is usually performed between the ages of 6 months and 2 years. Early closure facilitates speech development.

Test-Taking Strategy: Knowledge regarding the repair of cleft palate is required to answer the question. Option 4 can be easily eliminated first. Eliminate options 2 and 3 next, because the time frames are very close. Review the management of cleft palate repair now if you had difficulty with this question!

Level of Cognitive Ability: Analysis
Phase of Nursing Process: Analysis
Client Needs: Psychosocial Integrity
Content Area: Child Health

Reference

Ashwill, J., & Droske, S. (1997). *Nursing care of children: Principles and practice.* Philadelphia: W. B. Saunders. p. 703.

63. **2**

Rationale: Children with tetralogy of Fallot or with physiology similar to that seen with this disorder may experience hypercyanotic episodes, or "tet spells." These episodes are characterized by increased respiratory rate and depth and increased hypoxia.

Test-Taking Strategy: Knowledge regarding the manifestations associated with this condition will assist in selecting the correct option. Options 3 and 4 can be easily eliminated. From the remaining options, select option 2 over option 1. "Immediate" physician notification is not necessary, except in a life-threatening situation. Additionally, the nurse should appropriately position the child prior to calling the physician.

Level of Cognitive Ability: Analysis
Phase of Nursing Process: Analysis
Client Needs: Physiological Integrity
Content Area: Child Health

Reference
Ashwill, J., & Droske, S. (1997). *Nursing care of children: Principles and practice.* Philadelphia: W. B. Saunders. p. 923.

64. **1**

Rationale: Topical glucocorticoids can be absorbed into the systemic circulation. Absorption is higher from regions where the skin is especially permeable (scalp, axilla, face, eyelids, neck, perineum, genitalia), and lower from regions where penetrability is poor (back, palms, soles).

Test-Taking Strategy: Note the key words "least concerned." Focus on the issue of the question, "permeability and the potential for systemic absorption." Think about the permeability of the skin area presented in the options. This should direct you to option 1.

Level of Cognitive Ability: Analysis
Phase of Nursing Process: Analysis
Client Needs: Physiological Integrity
Content Area: Pharmacology

Reference
Lehne, R. (1998). *Pharmacology for nursing care* (3rd ed.). Philadelphia: W. B. Saunders. p. 1055.

65. **3**

Rationale: Following heart surgery, the child may return to school in 3 weeks but needs to go half days for the first few days. The mother should also be told that the child cannot participate in physical education for 2 months.

Test-Taking Strategy: Option 4 can be easily eliminated because this is not realistic or reasonable. Next, eliminate options 1 and 2 because they are similar. If you had difficulty with this question, take time now to review guidelines related to the child returning to school after heart surgery!

Level of Cognitive Ability: Application
Phase of Nursing Process: Implementation
Client Needs: Health Promotion and Maintenance
Content Area: Child Health

Reference
Ashwill, J., & Droske, S. (1997). *Nursing care of children: Principles and practice.* Philadelphia: W. B. Saunders. p. 922.

66. **3**

Rationale: A client's advocate is a person who speaks out for or supports the best interests of the client. This includes encouraging independence as well as speaking for the client. Option 1 is incorrect because the researcher's goal is to identify factors that alter health care outcomes. Option 2 is incorrect because a resource linker is a person who helps the client make contact with the appropriate community agency. Option 4 is incorrect because in the role of collaborator the nurse works with the client, family, community, and other health care providers to organize the plan of care.

Test-Taking Strategy: Note the key words "become more independent." These key words and knowledge of the functions of a researcher, resource linker, and collaborator will easily direct you to the correct option.

Level of Cognitive Ability: Application
Phase of Nursing Process: Implementation
Client Needs: Safe, Effective Care Environment
Content Area: Fundamental Skills

Reference
Stanhope, M., & Lancaster, J. (1996). *Community health nursing: Promoting health of aggregates, families and individuals* (4th ed.). St. Louis: Mosby–Year Book. p. 98.

67. **4**

Rationale: The role of the case manager is to organize, manage, and balance health care services needed for the client. Although options 1, 2, and 3 may be functions of the case manager, it is highly unlikely that these can be done in accordance with the time frames given when in a home health situation.

Test-Taking Strategy: The key words "case manager" will assist in directing you to the correct option. If you are unsure of the functions of the case manager, take time now to review!

Level of Cognitive Ability: Analysis
Phase of Nursing Process: Analysis
Client Needs: Safe, Effective Care Environment
Content Area: Fundamental Skills

Reference
Clark, M. J. (1996). *Nursing in the community* (2nd ed.). Stamford, CT: Appleton & Lange. pp. 65–67.

68. **4**

Rationale: Toxic shock syndrome is caused by infection and is often associated with tampon use. The client's symptoms in this question are compatible with disseminated intravascular coagulopathy, which is a complication of TSS. The nurse assesses the client at risk and notifies the physician promptly when a pattern of signs and symptoms is noted. Although signs of bleeding may be seen with each of the conditions listed in the distracters, the initial diagnosis of TSS makes DIC the logical choice.

Test-Taking Strategy: Note that the stem contains the key word "most." Familiarity with TSS and DIC is necessary to answer this question. If needed, take a few moments to review each of these disorders and their correlation at this time.

Level of Cognitive Ability: Analysis
Phase of Nursing Process: Analysis
Client Needs: Physiological Integrity
Content Area: Fundamental Skills

Reference
Beare, P., & Myers, J. (1998). *Adult health nursing* (3rd ed.). St Louis: Mosby–Year Book. p. 1659.

69. **2**

Rationale: Placing the client supine in semi-Fowler's position allows gravity to aid in drainage of the abdominal cavity. This helps prevent the formation of abscesses high in the abdomen. Abscesses in this location could rupture and cause peritonitis. The color, odor, and amount of vaginal secretions are also noted and recorded.

Test-Taking Strategy: Note that the stem of the question contains the key words "most therapeutic." This implies that more than one answer may be partially correct. Use knowledge of this disorder and basic nursing measures to assist in directing you to option 2.

Level of Cognitive Ability: Application
Phase of Nursing Process: Implementation
Client Needs: Physiological Integrity
Content Area: Fundamental Skills

Reference
Beare, P., & Myers, J. (1998). *Adult health nursing* (3rd ed.). St. Louis: Mosby–Year Book. p. 1657.

70. **3**

Rationale: Testicular self-examination is an excellent self-screening program for testicular cancer, which predominantly affects men in their late teens and twenties. The examination is performed once a month, as is breast self-examination. As an aid to remember to do it, the examination should be done on the same day each month. The scrotum is held in one hand, and the testicle is rolled between the thumb and forefinger of the other hand. The examination should not be painful. It is easiest to do either during or after a warm shower (or bath) when the scrotum is relaxed.

Test-Taking Strategy: The wording of the question tells you that one option is correct, while the other three are incorrect statements. Use knowledge of physical assessment techniques and the process of elimination to choose correctly. Review this procedure now if you had difficulty with this question!

Level of Cognitive Ability: Analysis
Phase of Nursing Process: Evaluation
Client Needs: Health Promotion and Maintenance
Content Area: Fundamental Skills

Reference

Beare, P., & Myers, J. (1998). *Adult health nursing* (3rd ed.). St. Louis: Mosby–Year Book. p. 1640.

71. **1**

Rationale: The cornea following cataract surgery should be clear, round, and smooth. Either a cloudy or spotty appearance or a scattering of the light could indicate that there is infection or increased intraocular pressure. The term sanguineous denotes blood; there should be no bleeding in the corneal area postoperatively.

Test-Taking Strategy: Note the key words "following cataract removal." Specific knowledge of expected postoperative findings is needed to answer this question accurately. If needed, take a few moments to review the principles of care following cataract removal surgery.

Level of Cognitive Ability: Application
Phase of Nursing Process: Assessment
Client Needs: Physiological Integrity
Content Area: Adult Health/Eye

Reference

Beare, P., & Myers, J. (1998). *Adult health nursing* (3rd ed.). St. Louis: Mosby–Year Book. p. 1126.

72. **1**

Rationale: The mother should be advised not to apply a tight-fitting diaper or plastic pants because these items will act as an occlusive dressing. Avoid the use of occlusive dressings (bandages or plastic wraps) to cover the affected site following the application of the topical glucocorticoid, unless the physician specifically prescribes wound coverage. The medication is gently rubbed into the skin after a thin layer is applied.

Test-Taking Strategy: Note the key words "indicates an understanding." The words "thick" in option 4 and "should massage" in option 3 should assist you in eliminating these options. Knowledge that occlusive dressings are avoided or knowledge of the action of the glucocorticoid will direct you to the correct option. If you had difficulty with this question, take time now to review this medication!

Level of Cognitive Ability: Analysis
Phase of Nursing Process: Evaluation
Client Needs: Health Promotion and Maintenance
Content Area: Pharmacology

Reference

Lehne, R. (1998). *Pharmacology for nursing care* (3rd ed.). Philadelphia: W. B. Saunders. p. 1055.

73. **3**

Rationale: Topical glucocorticoids can be absorbed in sufficient amounts to produce systemic toxicity. Principal concerns are growth retardation (in children) and adrenal suppression in all age groups. Systemic toxicity is more likely under extreme conditions of use, such as with prolonged therapy in which extensive surfaces are treated with high doses of high-potency agents in conjunction with occlusive dressings.

Test-Taking Strategy: Options 1 and 2 can be eliminated first because they are local reactions. From the remaining two options, knowledge regarding the concerns related to systemic toxicity is required to answer the question. Review these systemic effects now if you had difficulty with this question!

Level of Cognitive Ability: Analysis
Phase of Nursing Process: Analysis
Client Needs: Physiological Integrity
Content Area: Pharmacology

Reference

Lehne, R. (1998). *Pharmacology for nursing care* (3rd ed.). Philadelphia: W. B. Saunders. p. 1055.

74. **1**

Rationale: Salicylic acid is readily absorbed through the skin, and systemic toxicity (salicylism) can result. Symptoms include tinnitus, hyperpnea, dizziness, and psychological disturbances. Constipation and diarrhea are not associated with salicylism.

Test-Taking Strategy: Noting the name of the medication will assist in directing you to the correct option if you can recall the toxic effects that occur with acetyl"salicylic" acid (aspirin). If you are unfamiliar with the toxic effects of salicylic acid, take time now to review!

Level of Cognitive Ability: Analysis
Phase of Nursing Process: Assessment
Client Needs: Physiological Integrity
Content Area: Pharmacology

Reference

Lehne, R. (1998). *Pharmacology for nursing care* (3rd ed.). Philadelphia: W. B. Saunders. p. 1056.

75. **2**

Rationale: Edema of the conjunctiva, sclera, and eyelids is normal following cataract removal surgery. This results from the trauma of surgery and should be gone in 3 days or less following surgery.

Test-Taking Strategy: To answer this question accurately, it is necessary to be familiar with the postoperative course of the client following this procedure. If needed, take a few moments to review the highlights of postoperative eye care at this time.

Level of Cognitive Ability: Analysis
Phase of Nursing Process: Analysis
Client Needs: Physiological Integrity
Content Area: Adult Health/Eye

Reference
Beare, P., & Myers, J. (1998). *Adult health nursing* (3rd ed.). St. Louis: Mosby–Year Book. p. 1126.

76. 4

Rationale: Option 1 is incorrect because the nurse has a moral obligation to protect the client. Option 2 is incorrect because the client is homebound; the client must be seen in the home. Option 3 is incorrect because the nurse has a moral obligation to intervene when clients tell the nurse of their ideas or plans to harm themselves or others. Option 4 is the only correct response. The nurse must override the duty to observe confidentiality and notify the client's physician about the client's suicidal ideation.

Test-Taking Strategy: Remember that the nurse must override confidentiality when it will conflict with other duties toward the client, conflict with duties toward identified others, and conflict with the duties toward unidentified others or the rights and interests of society. Review the issues surrounding confidentiality now if you had difficulty with this question!

Level of Cognitive Ability: Application
Phase of Nursing Process: Implementation
Client Needs: Safe, Effective Care Environment
Content Area: Mental Health

Reference
Stanhope, M., & Lancaster, J. (1996). *Community health nursing: Promoting health of aggregates, families and individuals* (4th ed.). St. Louis: Mosby–Year Book. p. 98.

77. 4

Rationale: A variety of ear protective devices are available commercially. These include a variety of disposable and reusable ear plugs, headbands, and foam-filled muffs. They should be used around any type of loud noise, such as power tools, machinery, lawnmowers, chainsaws, and such. Sitting near loud music should be avoided whenever possible. If a loud, sudden noise is anticipated, the ears should be covered for protection. The client should see a physician for tinnitus or hearing loss after exposure to a loud noise.

Test-Taking Strategy: The wording of the question guides you to select an option that is a correct action. This question tests basic concepts related to noise control and ear protection. If this question was difficult, be sure to review this content area now!

Level of Cognitive Ability: Application
Phase of Nursing Process: Planning
Client Needs: Health Promotion and Maintenance
Content Area: Adult Health/Ear

Reference
Beare, P., & Myers, J. (1998). *Adult health nursing* (3rd ed.). St. Louis: Mosby–Year Book. p. 1161.

78. 1

Rationale: The battery of the hearing aid should be checked before use. In addition, once it is positioned the client should be asked whether the device is working properly. The hearing aid should be removed for showering, since it should not get wet. It should also be put away in its case at night. It should be cleaned according to manufacturer's directions, which usually consist of washing with warm, soapy water followed by thorough drying. Care is taken not to discard the device in the unit linen bags, and a sign or notation about the device is made on the unit Kardex or client worksheet. Lubricants or other solvents are not used on the devices.

Test-Taking Strategy: Specific knowledge of these commonly used devices is needed to answer this question accurately. By the process of elimination, you should be easily directed to the correct option. If needed, take a few minutes now to review these concepts.

Level of Cognitive Ability: Application
Phase of Nursing Process: Implementation
Client Needs: Safe, Effective Care Environment
Content Area: Adult Health/Ear

Reference
Beare, P., & Myers, J. (1998). *Adult health nursing* (3rd ed.). St. Louis: Mosby–Year Book. p. 1165.

79. 2

Rationale: To be maximally effective, medications to prevent motion sickness should be taken at least an hour before the triggering event. Medications that are commonly used for this purpose include dimenhydrinate (Dramamine), scopolamine (Transderm Scop), meclizine (Bonine), promethazine (Phenergan), and prochlorperazine (Compazine).

Test-Taking Strategy: Specific knowledge about the optimal time frames for this type of medication is needed to answer this question correctly. If needed, take a few moments to review this area now!

Level of Cognitive Ability: Analysis
Phase of Nursing Process: Evaluation
Client Needs: Physiological Integrity
Content Area: Adult Health/Ear

Reference
Beare, P., & Myers, J. (1998). *Adult health nursing* (3rd ed.). St. Louis: Mosby–Year Book. p. 1179.

80. 1

Rationale: The metal edges of the halo brace screws should be covered with rubber tips or corks to diminish the sound if the brace is bumped. The screws should all be properly tightened. A clean, dry lamb's wool lining should be in place underneath the jacket, and there should be a fingerwidth space between the jacket and the skin. In addition, the client should wear a clean, white cotton tee-shirt next to the skin to help prevent itching.

Test-Taking Strategy: The key words in the question are "needs correction." This tells you that the correct answer is an option that represents a problem with the assessment data. If this device is not familiar to you, take a few minutes to review the key principles involved in the care of this device.

Level of Cognitive Ability: Application
Phase of Nursing Process: Assessment
Client Needs: Safe, Effective Care Environment
Content Area: Adult Health/Neurological

Reference
Burrell, P., Gerlach, M., & Pless, B. (1997). *Adult nursing: Acute and community care* (2nd ed.). Stamford, CT: Appleton & Lange. p. 958.

81. 4

Rationale: Personal health care services that provide the first contact with the health care system and are directed toward the pathological process constitute primary care. Activities that focus on case finding, screening surveys, and the prevention of the complications of sequelae are secondary prevention. Activities that focus on retraining and re-education of individuals for the maximum use of remaining capacities are tertiary prevention. Activities that focus on health education, good standards of nutrition that have been adjusted to the developmental phases of life, and attention to personality development are all part of health promotion.

Test-Taking Strategy: Knowledge of the activities that constitute health promotion and primary prevention will easily direct you to the correct option. If you had difficulty with this question, take time now to review primary, secondary, and tertiary levels of prevention!

Level of Cognitive Ability: Analysis
Phase of Nursing Process: Analysis
Client Needs: Health Promotion and Maintenance
Content Area: Fundamental Skills

Reference

Stanhope, M., & Lancaster, J. (1996). *Community health nursing: Promoting health of aggregates, families and individuals* (4th ed.). St. Louis: Mosby–Year Book. pp. 36, 270.

82. 4

Rationale: Primary prevention activities are actions designed to prevent a disease from occurring and reduce the probability of the occurrence of a specific illnesses. Periodic selective well-baby examinations focus on health education and good standards of nutrition adjusted for the developmental level of the client, and address issues of adequate housing, recreation, and genetics. This also includes active protection against any unnecessary stressors or threats.

Test-Taking Strategy: Selective placement of the infant is vague and does not give any specific information, therefore eliminate option 1. Option 2 is eliminated because PKU testing at birth is an example of secondary prevention because it is early diagnosis and treatment. Option 3 is eliminated because it is actual treatment with an antibiotic for an umbilical cord staphylococcal infection. The purpose of periodic well-baby examinations is early diagnosis and treatment, which represents a primary prevention activity.

Level of Cognitive Ability: Analysis
Phase of Nursing Process: Analysis
Client Needs: Health Promotion and Maintenance
Content Area: Maternity

Reference

Stanhope, M., & Lancaster, J. (1996). *Community health nursing: Promoting health of aggregates, families and individuals* (4th ed.). St. Louis: Mosby–Year Book. pp. 36, 270, 612.

83. 1

Rationale: Option 1 is correct because clients often forgetting to take medications as scheduled is the prominent problem. Options 2, 3, and 4 may occur, but they are not the prominent problem and can be addressed and often controlled.

Test-Taking Strategy: Options 2, 3, and 4 can be easily eliminated because of their similarity. Knowledge about the lifestyles and problems of the mentally ill in the community

makes option 1 the correct answer. Additionally, option 1 is specifically client focused.

Level of Cognitive Ability: Analysis
Phase of Nursing Process: Analysis
Client Needs: Psychosocial Integrity
Content Area: Mental Health

Reference

Spradley, B. W., & Allender, J. A. (1996). *Community health nursing: Concepts and practice* (4th ed.). Philadelphia: Lippincott-Raven. pp. 559–561.

84. 1

Rationale: Ham, cheese (and most cold-cuts), as well as potato chips, are high in sodium. When a client has CHF, the goal is to reduce fluid accumulation. One way that this is done is sodium reduction. Daily weight is a good intervention to help the client monitor fluid overload. Most fresh fruits and vegetables are low in sodium.

Test-Taking Strategy: Note the key words "further teaching is needed." Knowledge of the pathophysiology of CHF and the implementations needed to achieve desired outcomes will easily direct you to the correct option. If you had difficulty with this question, take time now to review the pathophysiology associated with CHF!

Level of Cognitive Ability: Analysis
Phase of Nursing Process: Evaluation
Client Needs: Physiological Integrity
Content Area: Adult Health/Cardiovascular

Reference

Ignatavicius, D., Workman, M., & Mishler, M. *Medical surgical nursing: A nursing process approach* (2nd ed.). Philadelphia: W. B. Saunders. pp. 890, 894–895.

85. 2

Rationale: Teens are experiencing a major growth spurt. Normally, adolescent girls need more protein and iron and fewer calories. The pregnancy adds to these normal needs. Although all choices may have an impact on nutritional deficiencies, the primary reason is the growth spurt.

Test-Taking Strategy: Noting the issue of the question will easily direct you to option 2. Additionally, option 2 is the only option that directly addresses a physiological need. Review the stages of growth and development and the nutritional needs of the adolescent during pregnancy now if you had difficulty with this question!

Level of Cognitive Ability: Analysis
Phase of Nursing Process: Analysis
Client Needs: Physiological Integrity
Content Area: Maternity

Reference

Stanhope, M., & Lancaster, J. (1996). *Community health nursing: Promoting health of aggregates, families and individuals* (4th ed.). St. Louis: Mosby–Year Book. pp. 531–532.

86. 1

Rationale: Eating binges and purging are the characteristics seen in bulimia. Eating only certain types of foods may reflect a preference but does not indicate bulimia. Bulimic individuals usually do not refuse to eat, they binge and purge. Hoarding of food may indicate another problem.

Test-Taking Strategy: Knowledge of the major characteristics of bulimia will easily direct you to option 1. If you are unfamiliar with the characteristics of bulimia, take time now to review!

Level of Cognitive Ability: Analysis
Phase of Nursing Process: Assessment
Client Needs: Physiological Integrity
Content Area: Mental Health

Reference
Spradley, B. W., & Allender, J. A. (1996). *Community health nursing: Concepts and practice* (4th ed.). Philadelphia: Lippincott-Raven. p. 419.

87. **2**

Rationale: In vitro fertilization is a method of medically assisted reproduction for women with nonpatent, diseased, or missing fallopian tubes, or with infertility of unknown etiology. Ova and sperm are obtained from potential parents or donors, placed in a nutrient medium, and allowed to incubate; then the fertilized ovum is transferred into the woman's uterus. The woman houses the pregnancy throughout gestation and gives birth. Option 4 describes the procedure for artificial insemination. Options 1 and 3 are incorrect statements regarding this procedure.

Test-Taking Strategy: Knowledge regarding the procedure associated with in vitro fertilization will assist in eliminating options 1 and 3. Option 4 can be eliminated first because this describes the procedure of artificial insemination. Review this procedure now if you had difficulty with this question!

Level of Cognitive Ability: Analysis
Phase of Nursing Process: Planning
Client Needs: Physiological Integrity
Content Area: Maternity

Reference
Nichols, F., & Zwelling, E. (1997). *Maternal-newborn nursing: Theory and practice.* Philadelphia: W. B. Saunders. p. 161.

88. **1**

Rationale: A gynecoid pelvis is a normal female pelvis. A platypelloid pelvis has a flat shape. An anthropoid pelvis has an oval shape, and an android pelvis is heart shaped.

Test-Taking Strategy: Knowledge regarding the four classic types of pelvis is required to answer this question. Recalling that the gynecoid pelvis is a normal female pelvis will easily assist in directing you to the correct option. However, if you are unfamiliar with these types of pelvis, take time now to review!

Level of Cognitive Ability: Analysis
Phase of Nursing Process: Analysis
Client Needs: Physiological Integrity
Content Area: Maternity

Reference
Nichols, F., & Zwelling, E. (1997). *Maternal-newborn nursing: Theory and practice.* Philadelphia: W. B. Saunders. p. 177.

89. **1**

Rationale: Azelex is a topical medication used to treat mild to moderate acne. It appears to work by suppressing growth of *Propionibacterium acnes* and by decreasing proliferation of keratinocytes. Options 2, 3, and 4 are accurate statements regarding the use of this medication.

Test-Taking Strategy: Knowledge regarding the use of Azelex is required to answer this question. It is a relatively new medication used to treat mild to moderate acne. If you are unfamiliar with this medication, take time now to review!

Level of Cognitive Ability: Analysis
Phase of Nursing Process: Evaluation
Client Needs: Health Promotion and Maintenance
Content Area: Pharmacology

Reference
Lehne, R. (1998). *Pharmacology for nursing care* (3rd ed.). Philadelphia: W. B. Saunders. p. 1058.

90. **4**

Rationale: Autonomic dysreflexia (or hyperreflexia) results from sudden strong discharge of the sympathetic nervous system in response to a noxious stimulus. Signs and symptoms include pounding headache, nausea, nasal stuffiness, flushed skin, piloerection, and diaphoresis. Severe hypertension can occur, with systolic BP rising potentially as high as 300 mmHg. It often is triggered by thermal or mechanical events, such as kinked catheter tubing, constipation, urinary tract infection (UTI), or a variety of cutaneous stimuli. The nurse must recognize this situation immediately and take corrective action to remove the stimulus. If untreated, this medical emergency could result in stroke, status epilepticus, or possibly death.

Test-Taking Strategy: To answer this question accurately, it is necessary to be familiar with this potentially recurrent complication of spinal cord injury. Since this topic is important, take a few moments to review it now if needed.

Level of Cognitive Ability: Analysis
Phase of Nursing Process: Analysis
Client Needs: Physiological Integrity
Content Area: Adult Health/Neurological

Reference
Burrell, P., Gerlach, M., & Pless, B. (1997). *Adult nursing: Acute and community care* (2nd ed.). Stamford, CT: Appleton & Lange. p. 959.

91. **4**

Rationale: The client with hemianopsia is taught to scan the environment. This allows the client to take in the entirety of the visual field, which is necessary for proper functioning within the environment and helps prevent injury to the client. Eyeglasses are useful if the client already wears them, but they will not correct this visual field deficit. Neither option 1 nor 2 helps the client adapt to this visual impairment.

Test-Taking Strategy: Note that the key words in this question are "hemianopsia" and "adapt." This tells you that the correct response is the option that teaches the client a response to overcome the visual deficit. An understanding of the term hemianopsia is needed to choose correctly. Review interventions related to this disorder now if you had difficulty with this question!

Level of Cognitive Ability: Application
Phase of Nursing Process: Planning
Client Needs: Health Promotion and Maintenance
Content Area: Adult Health/Neurological

Reference
Burrell, P., Gerlach, M., & Pless, B. (1997). *Adult nursing: Acute and community care* (2nd ed.). Stamford, CT: Appleton & Lange. p. 991.

92. **2**

Rationale: Catheterization to measure postvoid residual gives specific information about the ability of the bladder to empty completely. Assisting the client to the bathroom will aid in the success of the bladder retraining program but does not specifically address the question presented. Recording intake and output are, again, useful general interventions but do not indicate how completely the client is emptying the bladder with each voiding.

Test-Taking Strategy: Note that the key phrases in this question are "most useful" and "ability to empty the bladder." Eliminate options 1 and 4 first as being the least specific interventions to address this question. Choose option 2 over option 3 because it is the most concrete measurement of the degree of bladder emptying.

Level of Cognitive Ability: Analysis
Phase of Nursing Process: Analysis
Client Needs: Health Promotion and Maintenance
Content Area: Adult Health/Renal

Reference
Burrell, P., Gerlach, M., & Pless, B. (1997). *Adult nursing: Acute and community care* (2nd ed.). Stamford, CT: Appleton & Lange. p. 991.

93. **4**

Rationale: Cranial nerve II (the optic nerve) is responsible for visual acuity. This may be tested by using a Snellen chart to assess distant vision. Another item that may be used to evaluate optic nerve II function is a Rosenbaum card to evaluate near-vision. This card is a handheld card for visual acuity; the nurse records the smallest line seen as well as the distance of the card from the client. A flashlight is used to test the pupillary reaction. An ophthalmoscope is used to examine the retina. A reflex hammer is used to test reflexes.

Test-Taking Strategy: Use knowledge of basic physical examination procedures to answer this question. If needed, do a brief review of cranial nerve assessment at this time!

Level of Cognitive Ability: Application
Phase of Nursing Process: Assessment
Client Needs: Physiological Integrity
Content Area: Adult Health/Eye

Reference
Beare, P., & Myers, J. (1998). *Adult health nursing* (3rd ed.). St. Louis: Mosby–Year Book. p. 1107.

94. **1**

Rationale: A 2% minoxidil solution is used for topical treatment of baldness. The usual dosage is 1 mL applied two times a day.

Test-Taking Strategy: Knowledge regarding the usual dosage for minoxidil solution is required to answer this question. If you are unfamiliar with this medication, take time now to review!

Level of Cognitive Ability: Analysis
Phase of Nursing Process: Evaluation
Client Needs: Health Promotion and Maintenance
Content Area: Pharmacology

Reference
Lehne, R. (1998). *Pharmacology for nursing care* (3rd ed.). Philadelphia: W. B. Saunders. p. 1061.

95. **4**

Rationale: Symptoms of air embolism include decreased level of consciousness, tachycardia, dyspnea, anxiety, feelings of impending doom, chest pain, cyanosis, and hypotension. The signs and symptoms in the question do not indicate an infection, allergic reaction, or hyperglycemia.

Test-Taking Strategy: Focus on the signs and symptoms identified in the question to assist in directing you to the correct option. Noting that the signs are cardiopulmonary and neurological should easily assist you to option 4. Review the signs of air embolism now if you had difficulty with this question!

Level of Cognitive Ability: Analysis
Phase of Nursing Process: Analysis
Client Needs: Physiological Integrity
Content Area: Fundamental Skills

Reference
Craven, R. F., & Hirnle, C. J. (1996). *Fundamentals of nursing: Human health and function* (2nd ed.). Philadelphia: Lippincott-Raven. p. 572.

96. **2**

Rationale: IV fluorescein angiography is used to evaluate the internal structures of the eye. After the procedure, the client should avoid activities that require near vision for up to 2 hours. This is because vision may be blurred due to the effect of dilating eye drops.

Test-Taking Strategy: Note that the question contains the key word "avoid." This tells you that the correct answer will be one that is not consistent with usual practice. Use knowledge of this procedure and aftercare to make your selection. Review this procedure now if you had difficulty with this question!

Level of Cognitive Ability: Application
Phase of Nursing Process: Implementation
Client Needs: Safe, Effective Care Environment
Content Area: Adult Health/Eye

Reference
Beare, P., & Myers, J. (1998). *Adult health nursing* (3rd ed.). St. Louis: Mosby–Year Book. p. 1111.

97. **1**

Rationale: Bending at the waist to do any number of activities can cause a rise in IOP. For this reason, any activity that involves bending should be avoided or modified. The client may read and watch television without specific risk of increasing IOP.

Test-Taking Strategy: Remember that options that are similar are not likely to be correct. For this reason, eliminate options 3 and 4 first. Use knowledge of effects of increased IOP to choose correctly between the two remaining options. Review the activities that increase IOP now, if you had difficulty with this question!

Level of Cognitive Ability: Application
Phase of Nursing Process: Implementation
Client Needs: Health Promotion and Maintenance
Content Area: Adult Health/Eye

Reference
Beare, P., & Myers, J. (1998). *Adult health nursing* (3rd ed.). St. Louis: Mosby–Year Book. p. 1122.

98. 4

Rationale: First-degree burns are bright pink or red in color without any blistering. The skin blanches to touch, may be edematous and painful, and heals on its own, usually within a week. Weeping blisters characterize moderate partial thickness (second-degree) burns. A waxy white color characterizes deep partial thickness (second-degree) burns. Third-degree burns are associated with insensitivity to pain and cold.

Test-Taking Strategy: Specific knowledge of the characteristics of various thickness burns is needed to answer this question correctly. Noting the key words "first-degree burn" may assist in directing you to option 4. If needed, review the differences between the various burn depths at this time!

Level of Cognitive Ability: Application
Phase of Nursing Process: Assessment
Client Needs: Physiological Integrity
Content Area: Adult Health/Integumentary

Reference
Burrell, P., Gerlach, M., & Pless, B. (1997). *Adult nursing: Acute and community care* (2nd ed.). Stamford, CT: Appleton & Lange. p. 2030.

99. 2

Rationale: Home safety measures are simple but important. Medications should be stored in childproof containers. The number of tablets in a container should be limited. Medicine should not be referred to as candy. Toxic substances should be labeled with green poison stickers on them and should be placed in a locked area out of reach of children. Syrup of ipecac should be readily available, and poison control numbers should be visible near all telephones.

Test-Taking Strategy: Use knowledge of basic safety measures to answer this question. The wording of the question guides you to look for a statement that is an incorrect response on the part of the parents. By the process of elimination, you should easily be directed to option 2!

Level of Cognitive Ability: Analysis
Phase of Nursing Process: Evaluation
Client Needs: Health Promotion and Maintenance
Content Area: Child Health

Reference
Ashwill, J., & Droske, S. (1997). *Nursing care of children: Principles and practice.* Philadelphia: W. B. Saunders. p. 491.

100. 2

Rationale: Clotrimazole is a topical antifungal used in the treatment of cutaneous fungal infections. The nurse monitors the effectiveness of this medication by noting the presence or absence of skin rash.

Test-Taking Strategy: Note the key words "monitor the effectiveness." Familiarity with this group of medications is needed to answer this question accurately. If needed, take a few moments to review this group of anti-infectives at this time!

Level of Cognitive Ability: Application
Phase of Nursing Process: Planning
Client Needs: Physiological Integrity
Content Area: Pharmacology

Reference
Hodgson, B., & Kizior, R. (1999). *Saunders nursing drug handbook 1999.* Philadelphia: W. B. Saunders. pp. 243–245.

101. 1

Rationale: Newborn infants may be immersed in water after the umbilical stump has healed. Water should be warm, not hot. A bath thermometer may be used to check the temperature of the water, which should not exceed 100°F. If a thermometer is not available, a temperature that is comfortable when tested on the inside of the wrist or elbow is appropriate. The infant's body must be supported at all times during the bath.

Test-Taking Strategy: Note the key word "inaccurate." Eliminate options 2 and 4 first as they are similar. Noting the age of the infant will assist in eliminating option 4. If you had difficulty with this question, take time now to review the appropriate procedure for bathing a neonate!

Level of Cognitive Ability: Analysis
Phase of Nursing Process: Analysis
Client Needs: Safe, Effective Care Environment
Content Area: Maternity

Reference
Ashwill, J., & Droske, S. (1997). *Nursing care of children: Principles and practice.* Philadelphia: W. B. Saunders. p. 435.

102. 1

Rationale: One of the earliest indicators of successful adaptation of the neonate is the Apgar score. This test is performed immediately at birth, 1 minute after birth, and 5 minutes after birth.

Test-Taking Strategy: Knowledge that the Apgar score is the earliest indicator of successful adaptation of the neonate will easily direct you to option 1. If you had difficulty with this question, take time now to review this test!

Level of Cognitive Ability: Application
Phase of Nursing Process: Planning
Client Needs: Physiological Integrity
Content Area: Maternity

Reference
Ashwill, J., & Droske, S. (1997). *Nursing care of children: Principles and practice.* Philadelphia: W. B. Saunders. p. 52.

103. 4

Rationale: One of the earliest indicators of successful adaptation of the newborn infant is the Apgar score. Scoring ranges from 0 to 10. Five criteria are used to measure the infant's adaptation. *Heart rate:* absent = 0; less than 100 = 1; greater than 100 = 2. *Respiratory effort:* absent = 0; slow or irregular weak cry = 1; good, crying lustily = 2. *Muscle tone:* limp or hypotonic = 0; some extremity flexion = 1; active, moving and well flexed = 2. *Irritability or reflexes* (measured by bulb suctioning): no response = 0; grimace = 1; cough, sneeze, or vigorous cry = 2. *Color:* cyanotic or pale = 0; acrocyanotic, cyanosis of extremities = 1; pink = 2.

Test-Taking Strategy: Knowledge that the Apgar scoring ranges from 0 to 10 and knowledge of the measures used in determining the score will assist in answering this question. Focus on the assessment signs noted in the question to assist in directing you to the correct option. If you had difficulty with this question, take time now to review this test!

Level of Cognitive Ability: Application
Phase of Nursing Process: Assessment
Client Needs: Physiological Integrity
Content Area: Maternity

Reference
Ashwill, J., & Droske, S. (1997). *Nursing care of children: Principles and practice.* Philadelphia: W. B. Saunders. p. 52.

104. **3**

Rationale: ECT as a form of treatment is considered when medication therapy has failed, when the client is at high risk for suicide or starvation, or when depression is judged to be overwhelmingly severe. Treatments are given three times a week, with an average series involving 8 to 12 treatments and a duration of 2 to 4 weeks. The most common side effects are amnesia of events occurring near the period of the treatment. Memory deficits may occur and tend to disappear with time.

Test-Taking Strategy: Eliminate options 1 and 2 first because they are similar. Knowledge that ECT is a form of treatment that is considered when medication therapy has failed will easily direct you to option 3. Review the procedure for ECT now if you had difficulty with this question!

Level of Cognitive Ability: Analysis
Phase of Nursing Process: Analysis
Client Needs: Physiological Integrity
Content Area: Mental Health

Reference
Carson, V., & Arnold, E. (1997). *Mental health nursing: The nurse-patient journey.* Philadelphia: W. B. Saunders. p. 785.

105. **1**

Rationale: Women with severe pre-eclampsia are maintained on strict bed rest in the lateral position but may have bathroom privileges. Options 2, 3, and 4 are correct interventions. Additionally, environmental stimuli such as visitors and a ringing phone are kept at a minimum to avoid stimulating the CNS and causing an eclamptic seizure.

Test-Taking Strategy: Note the key word "not" in the stem of the question. Eliminate options 2 and 4 first because they are similar. Padding side rails is a component of seizure precautions. Keep in mind the goal of care with this client: to prevent a seizure. This will assist in eliminating option 3 because this action would prevent CNS stimulation.

Level of Cognitive Ability: Application
Phase of Nursing Process: Implementation
Client Needs: Physiological Integrity
Content Area: Maternity

Reference
Nichols, F., & Zwelling, E. (1997). *Maternal-newborn nursing: Theory and practice.* Philadelphia: W. B. Saunders. p. 651.

106. **2**

Rationale: Hypertension, cigarette smoking, and hyperlipidemia are major modifiable risk factors that have been shown through research to be objective predictors of CAD. Glucose intolerance, obesity, and response to stress are contributing modifiable risk factors to CAD. Age greater than 40 years is a nonmodifiable risk factor. The nurse places priority on risk factors that can be modified.

Test-Taking Strategy: To answer this question correctly, it is necessary to know that risk for CAD is higher with age over 40 years, total cholesterol greater than 200 mg/dL, and in clients with diabetes mellitus (random blood glucose exceeding 120). Options 1 and 4 can be eliminated because these findings are within normal range. Being able to discriminate between modifiable and nonmodifiable risk factors enables you to choose option 2 over option 3.

Level of Cognitive Ability: Analysis
Phase of Nursing Process: Assessment
Client Needs: Health Promotion and Maintenance
Content Area: Adult Health/Cardiovascular

Reference
Black, J., & Matassarin-Jacobs, E. (1997). *Medical-surgical nursing: Clinical management for continuity of care* (5th ed.). Philadelphia: W. B. Saunders. pp. 1239, 1962.

107. **4**

Rationale: Biofeedback, progressive muscle relaxation, meditation, and guided imagery are techniques that the nurse can teach the client to reduce the physical impact of stress on the body and promote a feeling of self-control for the client. Biofeedback utilizes electronic equipment, whereas the others require no equipment after the technique is learned. Confrontation is not a stress management technique; it is a communication technique. Use of confrontation in communication is more likely to increase stress than relieve it.

Test-Taking Strategy: The wording of the question guides you to look for a true statement. Familiarity with the differences among stress management techniques guides you to eliminate each of the incorrect options. Take a few moments to review these now if you have the need.

Level of Cognitive Ability: Application
Phase of Nursing Process: Planning
Client Needs: Psychosocial Integrity
Content Area: Mental Health

Reference
Ignatavicius, D., Workman, M., & Mishler, M. (1995). *Medical-surgical nursing: A nursing process approach* (2nd ed.). Philadelphia: W. B. Saunders. p. 114.

108. **1**

Rationale: To ensure the best outcome, clients should be able to comply with instructions related to activity, diet, medications, and follow-up health care upon discharge from the hospital following myocardial infarction. All the options except option 1 indicate that the client will be successful in these key areas.

Test-Taking Strategy: To answer this question correctly, it is necessary to understand the key areas of information and resources needed by the client with myocardial infarction. This will help you eliminate each of the incorrect options systematically. Since these concepts related to disease self-management are so universal, you should review the elements of client teaching prior to discharge if you found this question difficult.

Level of Cognitive Ability: Analysis
Phase of Nursing Process: Evaluation
Client Needs: Health Promotion and Maintenance
Content Area: Adult Health/Cardiovascular

Reference
Luckmann, J. (1997). *Saunders manual of nursing care.* Philadelphia: W. B. Saunders. p. 1053.

109. **1**

Rationale: Standard home care instructions for a client with this nursing diagnosis include, among others, lifestyle changes such as decreased alcohol, avoiding activities that increase the demands on the heart, instituting a bowel regimen to prevent straining and constipation, and maintenance of fluid and electrolyte balance.

Test-Taking Strategy: The wording of the question tells you that there is only one option that is worded correctly, and that the other three responses are totally incorrect. Use your knowledge of events that increase cardiac workload to systematically eliminate options 2, 3, and 4.

Level of Cognitive Ability: Analysis
Phase of Nursing Process: Evaluation
Client Needs: Physiological Integrity
Content Area: Adult Health/Cardiovascular

Reference
Cox, H., Hinz, M., Lubno, M., et al. (1997). *Clinical applications of nursing diagnosis* (3rd ed.). Philadelphia: F. A. Davis. p. 284.

110. **4**

Rationale: Tolbutamide is an oral hypoglycemic agent that should be taken in the morning. It should be taken with breakfast to minimize gastric irritation and to enhance diabetic control.

Test-Taking Strategy: To answer this question accurately, it is necessary to know that this medication is an oral hypoglycemic. This would allow you to reason that it should be taken in the morning, so that it can stimulate the pancreas to produce the insulin that is needed during the day.

Level of Cognitive Ability: Application
Phase of Nursing Process: Implementation
Client Needs: Health Promotion and Maintenance
Content Area: Pharmacology

Reference
Deglin, J., & Vallerand, A. (1997). *Davis's drug guide for nurses* (5th ed.). Philadelphia: F. A. Davis. p. 619.

111. **1**

Rationale: Cisapride is classified as a gastrointestinal prokinetic agent. It is used in the management of nighttime gastric reflux that is associated with gastroesophageal reflux disease. Relief of heartburn is the intended effect. Constipation, diarrhea, and abdominal pain are all side effects of therapy with this medication.

Test-Taking Strategy: To answer this question accurately, it is necessary to know that this medication is a gastric stimulant. This would allow you to eliminate options 2 and 4. Specific knowledge related to medication action is needed to discriminate between the two remaining options.

Level of Cognitive Ability: Analysis
Phase of Nursing Process: Evaluation
Client Needs: Physiological Integrity
Content Area: Pharmacology

Reference
Deglin, J., & Vallerand, A. (1997). *Davis's drug guide for nurses* (5th ed.). Philadelphia: F. A. Davis. p. 264.

112. **2**

Rationale: A limit of 1 to 1.5 kg of weight gain between dialysis treatments helps prevent hypotension that occurs with removal of larger volumes of fluid. The nurse instructs the client about how to manage the daily fluid allotment to assist the client in staying within this low fluid intake range to prevent excess weight gain.

Test-Taking Strategy: It may be helpful in answering this question to recall that 1 liter of fluid weighs approximately 1 kg. Knowing that there are approximately 6 liters of blood

circulating, this would help you eliminate options 3 and 4 as being too large. Correspondingly, option 1 is eliminated because it is too small, representing only 500 to 1000 mL of fluid.

Level of Cognitive Ability: Application
Phase of Nursing Process: Planning
Client Needs: Health Promotion and Maintenance
Content Area: Adult Health/Renal

Reference
Lewis, S., Collier, I., & Heitkemper, M. (1996). *Medical-surgical nursing: Assessment and management of clinical problems* (4th ed.). St. Louis: Mosby–Year Book. p. 1400.

113. **4**

Rationale: The question asks you to select a response that gives the best indication that the nursing diagnosis is resolving. Each of the options indicates a positive outcome on the part of the client. However, option 1 would most likely indicate progress with a nursing diagnosis of Altered Nutrition. Option 2 would be a satisfactory outcome for Sleep Pattern Disturbance. Both options 3 and 4 relate to the nursing diagnosis of Activity Intolerance. However, since the question asks about progress in resolving the diagnosis, option 4 is more action oriented and is therefore the better choice.

Test-Taking Strategy: Knowledge of various nursing diagnoses is needed to answer this question. This would help you eliminate options 1 and 2. You would discriminate correctly between options 3 and 4 by choosing the option that indicates actual progress, rather than just a good intention.

Level of Cognitive Ability: Analysis
Phase of Nursing Process: Evaluation
Client Needs: Health Promotion and Maintenance
Content Area: Adult Health/Cardiovascular

Reference
Cox, H., Hinz, M., Lubno, M., et al. (1997). *Clinical applications of nursing diagnosis* (3rd ed.). Philadelphia: F. A. Davis. p. 252.

114. **3**

Rationale: Echocardiography is a noninvasive, risk-free, pain-free test that involves no special preparation. It is commonly done at the bedside or on an outpatient basis. The client must lie quietly for 30 to 60 minutes while the procedure is being performed. It is important to provide adequate information to eliminate unnecessary worry on the part of the client.

Test-Taking Strategy: To answer this question accurately, it is necessary to understand that echocardiography involves ultrasound, which is noninvasive and painless. This basic knowledge will help you eliminate each of the incorrect responses easily. If this question was difficult, review the basics of this procedure at this time.

Level of Cognitive Ability: Application
Phase of Nursing Process: Implementation
Client Needs: Safe, Effective Care Environment
Content Area: Adult Health/Cardiovascular

Reference
Ignatavicius, D., Workman, M., & Mishler, M. (1995). *Medical-surgical nursing: A nursing process approach* (2nd ed.). Philadelphia: W. B. Saunders. pp. 806–807.

115. **2**

Rationale: The normal heart rate for a neonate is 120 to 150 beats per minute.

Test-Taking Strategy: Knowledge regarding the normal heart rate of a newborn infant is required to answer this question. If you are unfamiliar with the normal ranges for neonatal vital signs, take time now to review!

Level of Cognitive Ability: Analysis
Phase of Nursing Process: Assessment
Client Needs: Physiological Integrity
Content Area: Maternity

Reference
Ashwill, J., & Droske, S. (1997). *Nursing care of children: Principles and practice*. Philadelphia: W. B. Saunders. p. 55.

116. **2**

Rationale: The anterior fontanel is diamond shaped and located on the top of the head. It should be flat and soft and may range in size from almost nonexistent to 4 to 5 cm across. It normally closes by 18 to 24 months of age. A depressed fontanel may indicate dehydration.

Test-Taking Strategy: Option 1 can be easily eliminated. Eliminate option 4 next knowing that 6 cm is rather large. From the remaining options, knowledge that the fontanel should be soft and flat will easily direct you toward that option. Review normal neonatal assessment now if you had difficulty with this question!

Level of Cognitive Ability: Analysis
Phase of Nursing Process: Assessment
Client Needs: Physiological Integrity
Content Area: Maternity

Reference
Ashwill, J., & Droske, S. (1997). *Nursing care of children: Principles and practice*. Philadelphia: W. B. Saunders. p. 55.

117. **2**

Rationale: The client should wear loose, comfortable clothing for the procedure. Easy ECG lead placement is enhanced if the client wears a shirt that buttons in front. The client should wear rubber-soled, supportive shoes such as sneakers. The client is NPO after bedtime, or for a minimum of 2 hours before the test. The client should avoid smoking, alcohol, and caffeine altogether on the day of the test. Inadequate or incorrect preparation can interfere with the test and possibly yield false-positive findings.

Test-Taking Strategy: The wording of the question tells you that there is only one correct response, and that each of the other choices is an incorrect statement. Read each option carefully. Noting the words "30 minutes," "just prior," and "work boots" in each of the incorrect options will assist in answering the question. Review this procedure now if you had difficulty with this question!

Level of Cognitive Ability: Application
Phase of Nursing Process: Planning
Client Needs: Safe, Effective Care Environment
Content Area: Adult Health/Cardiovascular

Reference
Ignatavicius, D., Workman, M., & Mishler, M. (1995). *Medical-surgical nursing: A nursing process approach* (2nd ed.). Philadelphia: W. B. Saunders. p. 806.

118. **4**

Rationale: The client is taught before cardiac catheterization to report chest pain or any unusual sensations immediately. The client is taught that a warm, flushed feeling may accompany dye injection and is normal. The client may be asked to cough or breathe deeply from time to time during the procedure. Because local anesthetic is used, the client is expected to feel pressure but not pain at the insertion site.

Test-Taking Strategy: The key words in the stem of the question are "highest priority." This tells you that more than one or all of the options may be partially or totally correct. An option such as chest pain is often a good choice in questions such as these, when the other options do not necessarily have a negative connotation or indicate an adverse effect.

Level of Cognitive Ability: Application
Phase of Nursing Process: Planning
Client Needs: Safe, Effective Care Environment
Content Area: Adult Health/Cardiovascular

Reference
Ignatavicius, D., Workman, M., & Mishler, M. (1995). *Medical-surgical nursing: A nursing process approach* (2nd ed.). Philadelphia: W. B. Saunders. p. 802.

119. **3**

Rationale: The client can best determine fluid status at home by weighing self on a daily basis. Increases of 2 to 3 pounds in a short time are reported to the physician. The client should sleep with the head of the bed elevated on a 6- to 10-inch foam wedge. During recumbent sleep, fluid (which has seeped into the interstitium by day with the assistance of the effects of gravity) is rapidly reabsorbed into the systemic circulation. Sleeping with the head of the bed flat is therefore avoided. The client does not modify drug dosages without consulting the physician.

Test-Taking Strategy: Eliminate options 1 and 2 first because it is unsafe for clients to regulate their own medication dosages based on symptoms. Knowing that weight is an excellent indicator of fluid volume status allows you to choose correctly between the remaining options.

Level of Cognitive Ability: Application
Phase of Nursing Process: Planning
Client Needs: Health Promotion and Maintenance
Content Area: Adult Health/Cardiovascular

Reference
Smeltzer, S., & Bare, B. (1996). *Brunner and Suddarth's textbook of medical-surgical nursing* (8th ed.). Philadelphia: Lippincott-Raven. p. 663.

120. **2**

Rationale: It is common for the client to be fatigued following the cardiac catheterization procedure. Other preprocedure teaching points include that the procedure is done in a darkened cardiac catheterization room. A local anesthetic is used so there is little to no pain with catheter insertion. General anesthesia is not used. The x-ray table is hard and may be tilted periodically, and the procedure may take up to 2 hours. The client may feel various sensations with catheter passage and dye injection.

Test-Taking Strategy: The wording of the question makes you look for a correct statement on the part of the client. Since this is not a surgical procedure, you would first eliminate options 1 and 4. The words "really hurt" in options 3 should cause you to eliminate that option next.

Level of Cognitive Ability: Analysis
Phase of Nursing Process: Evaluation
Client Needs: Safe, Effective Care Environment
Content Area: Adult Health/Cardiovascular

Reference
Black, J., & Matassarin-Jacobs, E. (1997). *Medical-surgical nursing: Clinical management for continuity of care* (5th ed.). Philadelphia: W. B. Saunders. p. 1231.

121. **4**

Rationale: The main effect of regional anesthesia is hypotension, which results from vasodilatation in the lower body and a reduction of venous return. After regional anesthesia, the blood pressure is taken every 1 to 2 minutes for 15 minutes, then every 10 to 15 minutes.

Test-Taking Strategy: Knowledge regarding the effects produced by regional anesthesia is required to answer this question. If you are unfamiliar with this type of anesthesia, take time now to review!

Level of Cognitive Ability: Application
Phase of Nursing Process: Implementation
Client Needs: Physiological Integrity
Content Area: Maternity

Reference
Nichols, F., & Zwelling, E. (1997). *Maternal-newborn nursing: Theory and practice.* Philadelphia: W. B. Saunders. p. 804.

122. **2**

Rationale: Dyspnea in the cardiac client is often accompanied by hypoxemia. This would be detected by an oxygen saturation monitor, especially if used continuously. An apnea monitor detects episodes when the client has stopped breathing briefly. Cardiac monitors detect dysrhythmias. An oxygen flowmeter is part of the set-up that is needed to deliver oxygen therapy.

Test-Taking Strategy: The key words in the stem of the question are "monitor," "respiratory," and "ongoing basis." This tells you that the correct option will be the piece of equipment that is best suited to help the nurse assess the client's respiratory status. Knowledge of basic items used in assessment of client status helps you to eliminate each of the incorrect options.

Level of Cognitive Ability: Application
Phase of Nursing Process: Implementation
Client Needs: Physiological Integrity
Content Area: Adult Health/Cardiovascular

Reference
Ignatavicius, D., Workman, M., & Mishler, M. (1995). *Medical-surgical nursing: A nursing process approach* (2nd ed.). Philadelphia: W. B. Saunders. p. 789.

123. **1**

Rationale: The NGT should remain in place until the client has bowel sounds. If not, the client could have paralytic ileus, which could result in distention and vomiting if the NGT is discontinued. It is normal for NGT drainage to be Hematest negative. The abdomen is likely to be slightly distended after surgery, and it is also likely that the client may be drowsy after experiencing a stressor such as cardiac surgery.

Test-Taking Strategy: The question guides you to look for an item that would make you leave the NGT in place. Note that the question contains the key words "most certainly question the order." This tells you that more than one or all of the options may be partially or totally correct. You must prioritize your answer based on which item is most critical to the client's well-being.

Level of Cognitive Ability: Application
Phase of Nursing Process: Implementation
Client Needs: Safe, Effective Care Environment
Content Area: Adult Health/Cardiovascular

Reference
Black, J., & Matassarin-Jacobs, E. (1997). *Medical-surgical nursing: Clinical management for continuity of care* (5th ed.). Philadelphia: W. B. Saunders. p. 1361.

124. **1**

Rationale: The client undergoing thoracentesis usually sits in an upright position, with the anterior thorax supported by pillows, or leaning over an over-the-bed table. The client must be positioned to enlist the aid of gravity in accessing and draining the effusion.

Test-Taking Strategy: Use the principles of gravity to answer this type of question. The correct option is the only one that allows the fluid to accumulate in an area that could easily be aspirated. Any form of side-lying position will cause fluid to accumulate under that side, which is inaccessible to the physician. The dorsal recumbent position will also be eliminated using similar thought processes.

Level of Cognitive Ability: Application
Phase of Nursing Process: Implementation
Client Needs: Physiological Integrity
Content Area: Adult Health/Cardiovascular

Reference
Potter, P., & Perry, A. (1997). *Fundamentals of nursing: Concepts, process, and practice* (4th ed.). St. Louis: Mosby–Year Book. p. 1215.

125. **3**

Rationale: Transtentorial herniation occurs when part of the brain herniates downward and around the tentorium cerebelli. It can be unilateral or bilateral and may involve anterior or posterior portions of the brain. If a large amount of tissue is involved, it can cause death because vital brain structures are compressed and become unable to perform their function.

Test-Taking Strategy: Note the key word "not" in the stem of the question. This key word and knowledge of this type of brain disorder will assist in directing you to the correct option. This question may be very difficult if you are unfamiliar with this disorder. Review this disorder now if you had difficulty with this question!

Level of Cognitive Ability: Analysis
Phase of Nursing Process: Analysis
Client Needs: Physiological Integrity
Content Area: Child Health

Reference
Ashwill, J., & Droske, S. (1997). *Nursing care of children: Principles and practice.* Philadelphia: W. B. Saunders. p. 1229.

126. **1**

Rationale: The TPN line is used only for administration of the TPN solution. Any other intravenous medication must be run though a separate IV access site.

Test-Taking Strategy: Some knowledge of TPN administration is needed to answer this question. Note the similarity between options 2, 3, and 4. These options all involve using the TPN line for administration of the antibiotic. Option 1 is the only option that identifies a separate access for the antibiotic. Review nursing care related to TPN now if you had difficulty with this question!

Level of Cognitive Ability: Application
Phase of Nursing Process: Implementation
Client Needs: Physiological Integrity
Content Area: Fundamental Skills

Reference

Craven, R. F., & Hirnle, C. J. (1996). *Fundamentals of nursing: Human health and function* (2nd ed.). Philadelphia: Lippincott-Raven. p. 572.

127. **3**

Rationale: Furosemide is a non–potassium-sparing diuretic, and insufficient replacement may lead to hypokalemia. Although the glucose, sodium, and magnesium levels will be monitored, these laboratory values are not specific to administering Lasix.

Test-Taking Strategy: Some knowledge of the action of furosemide is needed. As a non–potassium-sparing diuretic, the most critical laboratory value to watch with its use is the potassium level. Review this medication now if you had difficulty with this question!

Level of Cognitive Ability: Analysis
Phase of Nursing Process: Analysis
Client Needs: Physiological Integrity
Content Area: Pharmacology

Reference

Craven, R.F., & Hirnle, C.J. (1996). *Fundamentals of nursing: Human health and function* (2nd ed.). Philadelphia: Lippincott-Raven. p. 575.

128. **3**

Rationale: If an infusion falls behind schedule, the nurse should not increase the rate in an attempt to catch up because a hyperosmotic reaction could result. The solution should not be replaced by another and restarted the next day. An infusion pump should always be used to administer TPN.

Test-Taking Strategy: Knowledge regarding the administration of TPN is required to answer this question. Use the nursing process to assist in answering the question. Assess the system before taking any action. Review the principles related to the administration of TPN now if you had difficulty with this question!

Level of Cognitive Ability: Application
Phase of Nursing Process: Implementation
Client Needs: Physiological Integrity
Content Area: Fundamental Skills

Reference

Potter, P., & Perry, A. (1997). *Fundamentals of nursing: Concepts, process, and practice* (4th ed.). St. Louis: Mosby–Year Book. p. 1123.

129. **4**

Rationale: Obtunded indicates that the child sleeps unless aroused and once aroused has limited interaction with the environment. Full consciousness indicates that the child is alert, awake, and oriented and interacts with the environment. Confusion indicates that the ability to think clearly and rapidly is lost, and disorientation indicates that the ability to recognize place or person is lost.

Test-Taking Strategy: Knowledge regarding the descriptions associated with level of consciousness and neurological assessment is required to answer this question. If you are unfamiliar with these assessments, take time now to review!

Level of Cognitive Ability: Analysis
Phase of Nursing Process: Assessment
Client Needs: Physiological Integrity
Content Area: Child Health

Reference

Ashwill, J., & Droske, S. (1997). *Nursing care of children: Principles and practice.* Philadelphia: W. B. Saunders. p. 1231.

130. **1**

Rationale: Decorticate posturing is an abnormal flexion of the upper extremities and an extension of the lower extremities, with possible plantar flexion of the feet. Decerebrate posturing is an abnormal extension of the upper extremities with internal rotation of the upper arms and wrists and an extension of the lower extremities with some internal rotation.

Test-Taking Strategy: Options 3 and 4 can be easily eliminated first. From the remaining options, it is necessary to know the assessment finding that occurs with either decorticate or decerebrate posturing. If you had difficulty with this question, take time now to review.

Level of Cognitive Ability: Analysis
Phase of Nursing Process: Assessment
Client Needs: Physiological Integrity
Content Area: Child Health

Reference

Ashwill, J., & Droske, S. (1997). *Nursing care of children: Principles and practice.* Philadelphia: W. B. Saunders. p. 1230.

131. **3**

Rationale: Increase of fluid intake and dietary fiber will help change the consistency of the stool and make it easier for the client to pass. Increasing intake of rice and bananas will increase constipation; increasing sugar-free products and potassium will not be beneficial to the client.

Test-Taking Strategy: To answer this question correctly you must understand the physiological causes of constipation and factors that will alter consistency of stool. If you had difficulty with this question, take time now to review the interventions for constipation!

Level of Cognitive Ability: Analysis
Phase of Nursing Process: Planning
Client Needs: Physiological Integrity
Content Area: Fundamental Skills

Reference

Clark, M. J. (1996). *Nursing in the community.* (2nd ed.) Stamford, CT: Appleton & Lange. p. 539.

132. **3**

Rationale: The client with cataract removal without intraocular implant will have blurry vision. This improves with the wearing of aphakic lenses. Depending on the degree of visual impairment preoperatively, this may or may not be a worsening of the client's sight.

Test-Taking Strategy: Eliminate options 1 and 4 first because they contain absolute words such as "new permanent" and "definitely," respectively. Choose option 3 over option 2 by applying knowledge of intended effects of this surgery.

Level of Cognitive Ability: Application
Phase of Nursing Process: Planning
Client Needs: Psychosocial Integrity
Content Area: Adult Health/Eye

Reference
Beare, P., & Myers, J. (1998). *Adult health nursing* (3rd ed.). St. Louis: Mosby–Year Book. p. 1126.

133. **4**

Rationale: Clients who are prone to barotrauma should do any of a variety of mouth movements to equalize pressure in the ear, particularly during ascent and descent of an aircraft. These can include yawning, swallowing, drinking, chewing, or sucking on hard candy. The Valsalva maneuver may also be helpful. The client should avoid sitting with the mouth motionless during this time, as this aggravates pressure build-up behind the tympanic membrane.

Test-Taking Strategy: Note the word "avoid" in the stem of the question. Evaluate each of the options in terms of its movement. All the options but the correct one involve movement of the mouth. Remember that options that are similar are not likely to be correct.

Level of Cognitive Ability: Application
Phase of Nursing Process: Implementation
Client Needs: Health Promotion and Maintenance
Content Area: Adult Health/Ear

Reference
Beare, P., & Myers, J. (1998). *Adult health nursing* (3rd ed.). St. Louis: Mosby–Year Book. p. 1176.

134. **1**

Rationale: Following insertion of tubes in the ears, it is important to avoid getting water in the ears. For this reason, swimming, showering, or washing the hair is avoided after surgery until the time frame designated for each activity by the surgeon. A shower cap or ear plug may be used to shower if allowed by the physician. The client should take medication as advised for postoperative discomfort.

Test-Taking Strategy: The wording of the question guides you to look for an option that is a correct statement. Use knowledge of principles related to postoperative care and ear surgery to answer this question. Remember that options that are similar are not likely to be correct. This may help you eliminate options 2 and 3. Use general nursing knowledge to choose the correct option of the remaining two.

Level of Cognitive Ability: Analysis
Phase of Nursing Process: Evaluation
Client Needs: Health Promotion and Maintenance
Content Area: Adult Health/Ear

Reference
Beare, P., & Myers, J. (1998). *Adult health nursing* (3rd ed.). St. Louis: Mosby–Year Book. p. 1177.

135. **2**

Rationale: Otitis media in the adult is typically one-sided and presents as an acute process with earache, nausea, and possible vomiting, fever, and fullness in the ear. The client may complain of diminished hearing in that ear. The nurse takes a client history first, assessing whether the client has had a recent URI. It is unnecessary to question the client about brain abscess. The nurse may ask the client if anything relieves the pain, but ear infection pain is not usually relieved until antibiotic therapy is initiated.

Test-Taking Strategy: Note that the key word in the question is "first." This tells you that more than one or all of the options may be partially or totally correct. Use nursing knowledge related to history taking and ear disorders to answer this question. Review otitis media now if you had difficulty with this question!

Level of Cognitive Ability: Application
Phase of Nursing Process: Assessment
Client Needs: Physiological Integrity
Content Area: Adult Health/Ear

Reference
Beare, P., & Myers, J. (1998). *Adult health nursing* (3rd ed.). St. Louis: Mosby–Year Book. pp. 1172–1173.

136. **4**

Rationale: Decorticate posturing indicates a lesion in the cerebral hemisphere or disruption of the corticospinal tracts. Decerebrate posturing indicates damages in the diencephalon, midbrain, or pons.

Test-Taking Strategy: Knowledge regarding assessment findings related to head injuries is required to answer this question. If you are unfamiliar with decorticate and decerebrate posturing, take time now to review. You are likely to find questions related to this content on NCLEX-RN!

Level of Cognitive Ability: Analysis
Phase of Nursing Process: Analysis
Client Needs: Physiological Integrity
Content Area: Child Health

Reference
Ashwill, J., & Droske, S. (1997). *Nursing care of children: Principles and practice.* Philadelphia: W. B. Saunders. p. 1230.

137. **2**

Rationale: A cephalhematoma indicates edema resulting from bleeding below the periosteum of the cranium. It does not cross the suture line. It is most likely due to ruptured blood vessels from head trauma during birth. It develops within 24 to 48 hours after birth and may take 2 to 3 weeks to resolve. Option 1 identifies a caput succedaneum. Option 3 may indicate increased intracranial pressure. Option 4 may be associated with premature closure or craniosynostosis and should be investigated further.

Test-Taking Strategy: Knowledge regarding the normal and abnormal neonatal assessment findings is required to answer this question. If you had difficulty with this question, take time now to review!

Level of Cognitive Ability: Analysis
Phase of Nursing Process: Assessment
Client Needs: Physiological Integrity
Content Area: Maternity

Reference
Ashwill, J., & Droske, S. (1997). *Nursing care of children: Principles and practice.* Philadelphia: W. B. Saunders. p. 59.

138. **2**

Rationale: Babbling sounds are common between the ages of 3 and 4 months. Additionally, at this age crying becomes more differentiated. Between the ages of 1 and 3 months, the infant will produce cooing sounds. An increased interest in sounds occurs between 6 and 8 months, and the use of gestures occurs between 9 and 12 months.

Test-Taking Strategy: Noting the age of the infant will assist in eliminating options 1 and 4. From the remaining options, focus on the age to direct you to option 2, because cooing occurs very early in infancy. Review these developmental milestones now if you had difficulty with this question!

Level of Cognitive Ability: Analysis
Phase of Nursing Process: Assessment
Client Needs: Physiological Integrity
Content Area: Maternity

Reference
Ashwill, J., & Droske, S. (1997). *Nursing care of children: Principles and practice.* Philadelphia: W. B. Saunders. p. 85.

139. **2**

Rationale: DTP#1, OPV#1, HBV#1, and Hib#1 are the scheduled immunizations for an infant 1 to 2 months of age. DTP#2, OPV#2, HBV#2, and Hib#2 are administered at 4 months of age. DTP#3, OPV#3, HBV#3, and Hib#3 are administered at 6 months of age. DPT#4, TB skin test, MMR#1, and varicella are administered between 12 and 15 months of age.

Test-Taking Strategy: Noting the age of the infant will assist in easily eliminating options 3 and 4. Recalling the schedule for the administration of HBV may assist in directing you to option 2. If you had difficulty with this question, take time now to learn the immunization schedules. You are likely to see a question related to this content on NCLEX-RN!

Level of Cognitive Ability: Application
Phase of Nursing Process: Planning
Client Needs: Health Promotion and Maintenance
Content Area: Child Health

Reference
Ashwill, J., & Droske, S. (1997). *Nursing care of children: Principles and practice.* Philadelphia: W. B. Saunders. p. 92.

140. **4**

Rationale: Breast milk or formula is the main food throughout infancy. Rice cereal mixed with breast milk or formula is introduced at 4 months of age. Strained vegetables, fruits, and meats, introduced one at a time, can begin at 6 months of age.

Test-Taking Strategy: Focus on the age of the infant to direct you to the correct option. Noting the similarity in options 1, 2, and 3 will assist in directing you to option 4. These three options address food items. Review age-appropriate nutrition measures now if you had difficulty with this question!

Level of Cognitive Ability: Application
Phase of Nursing Process: Implementation
Client Needs: Health Promotion and Maintenance
Content Area: Child Health

Reference
Ashwill, J., & Droske, S. (1997). *Nursing care of children: Principles and practice.* Philadelphia: W. B. Saunders. p. 92.

141. **2**

Rationale: At age 15 months, the nurse would expect that the child could build a tower of two blocks. A 24-month-old would be able to open a door knob. At age 30 months, the child would be able to snap large snaps and put on simple clothes independently.

Test-Taking Strategy: Note the age of the child to assist in directing you to the correct option. Visualize each of the fine motor skills presented in the options to assist in selecting the correct one. Review these developmental milestones now if you had difficulty with this question!

Level of Cognitive Ability: Analysis
Phase of Nursing Process: Assessment
Client Needs: Physiological Integrity
Content Area: Child Health

Reference
Ashwill, J., & Droske, S. (1997). *Nursing care of children: Principles and practice.* Philadelphia: W. B. Saunders. p. 96.

142. **1**

Rationale: The toddler has increased use of motor skills and enjoys manipulating small objects such as toy people, cars, and animals. Push-pull toys are appropriate for this age. Option 2 is most appropriate for an infant. Option 3 is most appropriate for a school-aged child. Option 4 is most appropriate for an adolescent.

Test-Taking Strategy: Note the age group of the child and the related developmental stage to assist in answering the question. Option 2 can be eliminated because this activity is most appropriate for an infant. Next, eliminate option 4 knowing that this activity is most appropriate for an adolescent. From the remaining options, recalling that for the toddler play activities should meet the need for activity will assist in directing you to option 1. Review age-related activities and toys now if you had difficulty with this question!

Level of Cognitive Ability: Analysis
Phase of Nursing Process: Analysis
Client Needs: Psychosocial Integrity
Content Area: Child Health

Reference
Ashwill, J., & Droske, S. (1997). *Nursing care of children: Principles and practice.* Philadelphia: W. B. Saunders. p. 179.

143. **1**

Rationale: Lactose intolerance causes frothy, not fatty, stools. Abdominal distention, crampy abdominal pain, and excessive flatus may also occur. Option 2 is a clinical manifestation of celiac disease. Option 3 is a clinical manifestation of Hirschsprung's disease. Option 4 is a clinical manifestation of irritable bowel syndrome.

Test-Taking Strategy: Knowledge regarding the clinical manifestations associated with lactose intolerance is required to answer this question. Noting the word "intolerance" may assist in directing you to option 1. Review the clinical manifestations associated with this disorder now if you had difficulty with this question!

Level of Cognitive Ability: Analysis
Phase of Nursing Process: Assessment
Client Needs: Physiological Integrity
Content Area: Child Health

Reference
Ashwill, J., & Droske, S. (1997). *Nursing care of children: Principles and practice.* Philadelphia: W. B. Saunders. p. 731.

144. **2**

Rationale: Dietary management is the mainstay of treatment for the child with celiac disease. All wheat, rye, barley, and oats should be eliminated from the diet and replaced with corn and rice. Vitamin supplements, especially fat-soluble vitamins and folate, may be needed in the early period of treatment to correct deficiencies.

Test-Taking Strategy: Note the key word "not" in the stem of the question. Knowledge that wheat, rye, barley, and oats need to be eliminated from the diet will easily direct you to option 2. Review the diet for the child with celiac disease now if you had difficulty with this question!

Level of Cognitive Ability: Application
Phase of Nursing Process: Implementation
Client Needs: Health Promotion and Maintenance
Content Area: Child Health

Reference
Ashwill, J., & Droske, S. (1997). *Nursing care of children: Principles and practice.* Philadelphia: W. B. Saunders. p. 733.

145. **3**

Rationale: Omphalocele is an abdominal wall defect. It involves a large herniation of the gut into the umbilical cord. The viscera are outside the abdominal cavity but inside a translucent sac covered with peritoneum and amniotic membrane. Option 4 describes a gastroschisis. Options 1 and 2 describe an umbilical hernia.

Test-Taking Strategy: Eliminate options 1 and 2 first because they are similar. Knowledge that an omphalocele is an abdominal wall defect in which viscera are outside the abdominal cavity but inside a translucent sac covered with peritoneum and amniotic membrane will direct you to option 3. Review this disorder now if you are unfamiliar with it!

Level of Cognitive Ability: Analysis
Phase of Nursing Process: Analysis
Client Needs: Physiological Integrity
Content Area: Maternity

Reference
Ashwill, J., & Droske, S. (1997). *Nursing care of children: Principles and practice.* Philadelphia: W. B. Saunders. p. 742.

146. **2**

Rationale: Intussusception is an invagination of a section of the intestine into the distal bowel. It is the most common cause of bowel obstruction in children aged 3 months to 6 years. Option 1 describes imperforate anus, and this disorder is diagnosed in the neonatal period. Option 3 describes constipation. Option 4 describes encopresis. Constipation can affect any child at any time though it peaks at ages 2 to 3 years. Encopresis generally affects preschool and school-aged children.

Test-Taking Strategy: Options 3 and 4 can be eliminated first. Focusing on the word "child" in the question should assist in eliminating option 1 as this disorder is diagnosed in the neonatal period. Review this disorder now if you had difficulty with this question!

Level of Cognitive Ability: Analysis
Phase of Nursing Process: Analysis
Client Needs: Physiological Integrity
Content Area: Child Health

Reference
Ashwill, J., & Droske, S. (1997). *Nursing care of children: Principles and practice.* Philadelphia: W. B. Saunders. p. 749.

147. **3**

Rationale: Mineral oil is best tolerated when it is given chilled or mixed with cold drinks. Mixing the oil with chocolate milk, blending it with ice cubes and fruit juice, or chilling it helps disguise the taste.

Test-Taking Strategy: Eliminate options 1 and 2 because they are similar. From the remaining options, eliminate option 4 next because administering the mineral oil to a child prior to a meal will certainly affect the child's appetite and desire to eat.

Level of Cognitive Ability: Analysis
Phase of Nursing Process: Evaluation
Client Needs: Health Promotion and Maintenance
Content Area: Child Health

Reference
Ashwill, J., & Droske, S. (1997). *Nursing care of children: Principles and practice.* Philadelphia: W. B. Saunders. p. 744.

148. **4**

Rationale: The stomach capacity of a newborn infant is 10 to 20 mL, is 30 to 90 mL for a 1-week-old infant, is 75 to 100 mL for a 2- to 3-week-old infant, and is 90 to 150 mL for a 1-month-old.

Test-Taking Strategy: Knowledge regarding the pediatric differences in the upper gastrointestinal system is required to answer this question. Note the key words "1-month-old." This should assist in eliminating options 1 and 2. Attempt to visualize the amounts in options 3 and 4 to assist in selecting the correct answer. Review these pediatric differences now if you had difficulty with this question!

Level of Cognitive Ability: Analysis
Phase of Nursing Process: Implementation
Client Needs: Health Promotion and Maintenance
Content Area: Child Health

Reference
Ashwill, J., & Droske, S. (1997). *Nursing care of children: Principles and practice.* Philadelphia: W. B. Saunders. p. 699.

149. **1**

Rationale: Following cleft palate repair, the mouth is rinsed with water after feedings to clean the palate repair. Rinsing food and residual sugars from suture lines reduces the risk of infection. Options 2, 3, and 4 are incorrect procedures, and the solutions identified in these options should not be used.

Test-Taking Strategy: Consider the anatomical location of the surgical site to assist in answering this question. Note that the types of solutions identified in options 2, 3, and 4 can cause damage to the suture site. This focus should easily direct you to option 1. Review care for a child following cleft palate repair now if you had difficulty with this question!

Level of Cognitive Ability: Application
Phase of Nursing Process: Implementation
Client Needs: Physiological Integrity
Content Area: Child Health

Reference
Ashwill, J., & Droske, S. (1997). *Nursing care of children: Principles and practice.* Philadelphia: W. B. Saunders. p. 706.

150. 3

Rationale: GER is regurgitation of gastric contents back into the esophagus. Option 1 describes a hiatal hernia. Option 2 describes a congenital diaphragmatic hernia. Option 4 describes esophageal atresia.

Test-Taking Strategy: Careful reading of each option and noting the word "reflux" will identify a relationship in option 3 and assist in directing you to the correct choice. If you had difficulty with this question, take time now to review this disorder!

Level of Cognitive Ability: Analysis
Phase of Nursing Process: Analysis
Client Needs: Physiological Integrity
Content Area: Maternity

Reference

Ashwill, J., & Droske, S. (1997). *Nursing care of children: Principles and practice.* Philadelphia: W. B. Saunders. pp. 708, 712–713.

151. 2

Rationale: Clinical manifestations associated with hiatal hernia are similar to gastroesophageal reflux and specifically include vomiting, coughing, wheezing, short periods of apnea, and failure to thrive. Option 1 is a clinical manifestation of esophageal atresia and tracheoesophageal fistula. Option 3 is a clinical manifestation associated with congenital diaphragmatic hernia. Option 4 is a clinical manifestation of gastroesophageal reflux.

Test-Taking Strategy: Knowledge that a protrusion of a portion of the stomach through the esophageal hiatus of the diaphragm occurs in a hiatal hernia will assist in directing you to option 2. If you had difficulty with this question, take time now to review this important disorder!

Level of Cognitive Ability: Analysis
Phase of Nursing Process: Assessment
Client Needs: Physiological Integrity
Content Area: Maternity

Reference

Ashwill, J., & Droske, S. (1997). *Nursing care of children: Principles and practice.* Philadelphia: W. B. Saunders. pp. 708, 712–713.

152. 4

Rationale: Laboratory findings in an infant with hypertrophic pyloric stenosis include metabolic alkalosis caused by vomiting, including decreased serum potassium and sodium levels, increased pH and bicarbonate, and a decreased chloride level.

Test-Taking Strategy: Recalling the concepts related to acid-base balance and the clinical manifestation, the progressive projectile nonbilious vomiting that occurs in hypertrophic pyloric stenosis will easily direct you to option 4. Remember that metabolic alkalosis occurs from vomiting!

Level of Cognitive Ability: Analysis
Phase of Nursing Process: Assessment
Client Needs: Physiological Integrity
Content Area: Child Health

Reference

Ashwill, J., & Droske, S. (1997). *Nursing care of children: Principles and practice.* Philadelphia: W. B. Saunders. p. 718.

153. 4

Rationale: Chest pain is assessed using the standard pain assessment parameters, (e.g., characteristics, location, inten-

sity, duration, precipitating and alleviating factors, and associated symptoms). However, the answers to these questions may or may not help to discriminate the origin of pain accurately. Pain of pleuropulmonary origin usually becomes worse on inspiration.

Test-Taking Strategy: Key words in the stem of this question are "respiratory origin." This tells you that you are looking for an item that will discriminate respiratory from nonrespiratory conditions. Note also that the question has "most likely" as other key words. This tells you that more than one or all of the options may be partially or totally correct. You must use your knowledge of cardiac and respiratory assessment data to choose correctly among the options presented.

Level of Cognitive Ability: Analysis
Phase of Nursing Process: Assessment
Client Needs: Physiological Integrity
Content Area: Adult Health/Cardiovascular

Reference

Ignatavicius, D., Workman, M., & Mishler, M. (1995). *Medical-surgical nursing: A nursing process approach* (2nd ed.). Philadelphia: W. B. Saunders. pp. 788–789.

154. 1

Rationale: Stable angina is triggered by a predictable amount of effort or emotion. Unstable angina is triggered by an unpredictable amount of exertion or emotion, and it may occur at night; the attacks increase in number, duration, and severity over time. Variant angina is triggered by coronary artery spasm; the attacks are of longer duration than in classic angina and tend to occur early in the day and at rest. Intractable angina is chronic and incapacitating, and it is refractory to medical therapy.

Test-Taking Strategy: To answer this question accurately, you must be familiar with the different forms of angina pectoris. If needed, take a few moments to review them at this time. It may be helpful to think about the common definition of the word in each option to help guide you in selecting the correct answer.

Level of Cognitive Ability: Analysis
Phase of Nursing Process: Analysis
Client Needs: Physiological Integrity
Content Area: Adult Health/Cardiovascular

Reference

Black, J., & Matassarin-Jacobs, E. (1997). *Medical-surgical nursing: Clinical management for continuity of care* (5th ed.). Philadelphia: W. B. Saunders. p. 1254.

155. 1

Rationale: A prolonged PR interval indicates first-degree heart block. A widened QRS complex indicates delay in intraventricular conduction, such as bundle branch block. Tall, peaked T waves may indicate hyperkalemia. The development of Q waves indicates myocardial necrosis in the area covered by that lead. An ECG taken with pain is intended to capture ischemic changes, which include ST segment elevation or depression.

Test-Taking Strategy: To answer this question accurately, recall knowledge of how normal cardiac events are captured on ECG, and use your knowledge of the normal cardiac complex to determine which part of the ECG complex changes. Begin to answer this question by eliminating options 3 and 4 as least plausible, and use knowledge of the normal ECG complex to choose option 1 over option 2.

Level of Cognitive Ability: Analysis
Phase of Nursing Process: Analysis
Client Needs: Physiological Integrity
Content Area: Adult Health/Cardiovascular

Reference
Black, J., & Matassarin-Jacobs, E. (1997). *Medical-surgical nursing: Clinical management for continuity of care* (5th ed.). Philadelphia: W. B. Saunders. p. 1254.

156. **3**

Rationale: Exercise is most effective when done at least three times a week for 20 to 30 minutes to reach a target heart rate. Other good habits include limiting salt and fat in the diet and using stress management techniques. The client should also be taught to take nitroglycerin before any activity that causes pain, and to take the medication at the first sign of chest discomfort.

Test-Taking Strategy: The question asks you for an item that the nurse would not include. Therefore, you need to look for an item that is completely or partially incorrect. Options 1, 2, and 4 are correct items of information and are therefore eliminated. Exercise should be done at least three times a week for optimal benefit.

Level of Cognitive Ability: Application
Phase of Nursing Process: Planning
Client Needs: Health Promotion and Maintenance
Content Area: Adult Health/Cardiovascular

Reference
Smeltzer, S., & Bare, B. (1996). *Brunner and Suddarth's textbook of medical-surgical nursing* (8th ed.). Philadelphia: Lippincott-Raven. p. 644.

157. **3**

Rationale: Chest pain that is unrelieved by rest and 3 doses of nitroglycerin given 5 minutes apart may not be typical anginal pain but may signal myocardial infarction (MI). Since the risk of sudden cardiac death is greatest in the first 24 hours after MI, it is imperative that the client receive emergency cardiac care. A physician's office is not equipped to treat myocardial infarction. Communication with family or agency delays client treatment, which is needed immediately.

Test-Taking Strategy: The question asks for the "most appropriate" nursing action, which makes you prioritize among plausible nursing actions. Eliminate options 1 and 2 first as being the least plausible of your choices. Since myocardial infarction is a medical emergency, option 3 becomes the better choice of the two remaining.

Level of Cognitive Ability: Application
Phase of Nursing Process: Implementation
Client Needs: Physiological Integrity
Content Area: Adult Health/Cardiovascular

Reference
Smeltzer, S., & Bare, B. (1996). *Brunner and Suddarth's textbook of medical-surgical nursing* (8th ed.). Philadelphia: Lippincott-Raven. p. 642.

158. **2**

Rationale: Prinzmetal's angina results from spasm of the coronary vessels. The risk factors are unknown, and this form of angina is relatively unresponsive to nitrates. Beta-blockers are contraindicated because they may actually worsen the spasm. Diet therapy is not indicated.

Test-Taking Strategy: To answer this question most easily, recall that variant angina is a functional disorder that results from coronary spasm and is not due to atherosclerosis. The correct option, then, is one that is effective against spasm, which is option 2.

Level of Cognitive Ability: Application
Phase of Nursing Process: Planning
Client Needs: Health Promotion and Maintenance
Content Area: Adult Health/Cardiovascular

Reference
Luckmann, J. (1997). *Saunders manual of nursing care*. Philadelphia: W. B. Saunders. p. 1038.

159. **3**

Rationale: The pain of angina may radiate to the left shoulder, arm, neck, or jaw. It is often precipitated by exertion or stress, has few associated symptoms, and is relieved by rest and nitroglycerin. The pain of MI may also radiate to the left arm, shoulder, jaw, and neck. It typically begins spontaneously, lasts longer than 30 minutes, and is frequently accompanied by associated symptoms (such as nausea, vomiting, dyspnea, diaphoresis, anxiety). The pain of MI requires opioid analgesics such as morphine sulfate for relief.

Test-Taking Strategy: The question is seeking an item that differentiates anginal pain from that of MI, which may be similar at the onset. A classic hallmark of the pain from MI is that it is unrelieved by rest and nitroglycerin. Use knowledge of this concept to eliminate each of the incorrect options systematically.

Level of Cognitive Ability: Analysis
Phase of Nursing Process: Assessment
Client Needs: Physiological Integrity
Content Area: Adult Health/Cardiovascular

Reference
Ignatavicius, D., Workman, M., & Mishler, M. (1995). *Medical-surgical nursing: A nursing process approach* (2nd ed.). Philadelphia: W. B. Saunders. p. 990.

160. **2**

Rationale: Nitroglycerin dilates both arteries and veins, causing peripheral blood pooling and thus reducing preload, afterload, and myocardial work. This also accounts for the primary side effect of nitroglycerin, which is hypotension. In the absence of continuous direct arterial pressure monitoring, the nurse should use an automatic noninvasive pressure monitor.

Test-Taking Strategy: To answer this question accurately, you need to know the effects of nitroglycerin on the cardiovascular system. This will help you to eliminate systematically each of the other incorrect options.

Level of Cognitive Ability: Application
Phase of Nursing Process: Implementation
Client Needs: Safe, Effective Care Environment
Content Area: Adult Health/Cardiovascular

Reference
Smeltzer, S., & Bare, B. (1996). *Brunner and Suddarth's textbook of medical-surgical nursing* (8th ed.). Philadelphia: Lippincott-Raven. p. 650.

161. **3**

Rationale: Upon transfer from the CCU to an intermediate care or general medical unit, the client is allowed self-care activities and bathroom privileges. It is unnecessary and possibly harmful to limit the client to bed rest. The client should ambulate with supervision in the hall for brief distances, with the distances being gradually increased to 50, 100, and 200 feet.

Test-Taking Strategy: Eliminate options 1 and 2 first since they are excessive for the client who has just been transferred out of the CCU. Option 4 is not viable since the client would be doing less than in the CCU prior to transfer. CCU activities allow for bed rest with commode privileges.

Level of Cognitive Ability: Application
Phase of Nursing Process: Implementation
Client Needs: Physiological Integrity
Content Area: Adult Health/Cardiovascular

Reference
Black, J., & Matassarin-Jacobs, E. (1997). *Medical-surgical nursing: Clinical management for continuity of care* (5th ed.). Philadelphia: W. B. Saunders. p. 1264.

162. **1**

Rationale: Thrombolytic agents are used to dissolve existing thrombi, and the nurse must monitor the client for obvious or occult signs of bleeding. This includes assessment for obvious bleeding within the GI tract, urinary system, and skin. It also includes Hematesting secretions for occult blood.

Test-Taking Strategy: The word "thrombolytic," meaning to dissolve clots, focuses your attention on blood coagulation. Look for an item that has a hematological connection—in this case, option 1, which indicates bleeding from the GI tract.

Level of Cognitive Ability: Analysis
Phase of Nursing Process: Analysis
Client Needs: Physiological Integrity
Content Area: Adult Health/Cardiovascular

Reference
Smeltzer, S., & Bare, B. (1996). *Brunner and Suddarth's textbook of medical-surgical nursing* (8th ed.). Philadelphia: Lippincott-Raven. p. 996.

163. **4**

Rationale: Adolescent pregnancy outside of marriage (a complex subject issue) can arise from female low self-esteem, fears of inadequacy, and desperation to escape from an abusive and dysfunctional family. The most therapeutic communication technique is the one that uses restatement and repeats the main thought the client expressed. This assures the client that the nurse is listening and is attempting to validate what the client has said. The second therapeutic communication technique that the nurse employs is focusing. In this case, the nurse asks questions that help the client respond to the subject being asked about.

Test-Taking Strategy: This question assesses your ability to use the most therapeutic communication technique for a client from a complex, dysfunctional family. Options 1, 2, and 3 are all nontherapeutic. Option 1 reflects knowledge deficit on the nurse's part. Option 2 is insensitive and makes assumptions. Option 3 makes connections that are assumed and imply judgmental bias.

Level of Cognitive Ability: Application
Phase of Nursing Process: Implementation
Client Needs: Psychosocial Integrity
Content Area: Mental Health

Reference
Varcarolis, E. (1998). *Foundations of psychiatric mental health nursing* (3rd ed.). Philadelphia: W. B. Saunders. pp. 181–205.

164. **1**

Rationale: Crisis is the alteration caused in a client by a stressful event or perceived threat in which the client's ordinary problem-solving skills are no longer effective, so the client's resulting powerlessness increases stress, which may be adaptive or maladaptive. The crisis described here is adventitious in that it doesn't happen to everyone, and multiple losses can result from major environmental changes. The phases or stages are described as the *precrisis* or level of coping prior to the impact of the actual crisis. This first phase is characterized by shock, disbelief, panic, or intense fearfulness. The *second phase* involves the client's attempts to solve the problem constructively, usually by joining in team efforts to care for others or engage in "search and rescue." During the *honeymoon phase* (1 week to several months), the client continues to help others and to engage in life restructuring, which may be earmarked by psychological and behavioral problems. Finally, during the phase of *restructuring and reorganizing*, the client begins to cope with problems and to rebuild his or her own life, including business, home, and personal components.

Test-Taking Strategy: This question tests your knowledge of the phases or stages of crisis or a human disaster. Note the information provided in the question to direct you to the correct option. Option 2 describes the period of reconstruction and reorganization. Option 3 describes the impact phase of a human disaster. Option 4 describes the period of impact.

Level of Cognitive Ability: Analysis
Phase of Nursing Process: Planning
Client Needs: Psychosocial Integrity
Content Area: Mental Health

Reference
Varcarolis, E. (1998). *Foundations of psychiatric mental health nursing* (3rd ed.). Philadelphia: W. B. Saunders. pp. 365–425.

165. **4**

Rationale: Muscle cramps during hemodialysis are a common problem. They result either from too rapid removal of water and sodium, or from neuromuscular hypersensitivity. The nurse corrects this situation either by slowing down the ultrafiltration rate on the hemodialyzer, or by administering hypertonic or isotonic normal saline. Magnesium sulfate is not prescribed to correct this occurrence.

Test-Taking Strategy: Familiarity with this complication of hemodialysis and its treatment is needed to answer this question correctly. It would make sense that the ultrafiltration rate should be slowed if the client develops symptoms. Use knowledge of fluid and electrolytes and principles of hemodialysis to choose correctly.

Level of Cognitive Ability: Application
Phase of Nursing Process: Implementation
Client Needs: Physiological Integrity
Content Area: Adult Health/Renal

Reference
Lewis, S., Collier, I., & Heitkemper, M. (1996). *Medical-surgical nursing: Assessment and management of clinical problems* (4th ed.). St. Louis: Mosby–Year Book. p. 1401.

166. **3**

Rationale: Following surgery to repair a fractured hip, an abductor splint is used to maintain the affected extremity in good alignment. An overhead trapeze and bed pillow are also used, but they are not the priority item to be used in repositioning.

Test-Taking Strategy: Note that the key words in the stem of the question are "most important." This tells you that more than one or all of the options may be partially or totally correct. Use nursing knowledge to prioritize your answer. Remember that an abductor splint is used to maintain correct alignment in a client following repair of a fractured hip. This concept will assist in answering questions similar to this one.

Level of Cognitive Ability: Application
Phase of Nursing Process: Planning
Client Needs: Physiological Integrity
Content Area: Adult Health/Musculoskeletal

Reference
Lewis, S., Collier, I., & Heitkemper, M. (1996). *Medical-surgical nursing: Assessment and management of clinical problems* (4th ed.). St. Louis: Mosby–Year Book. p. 1864.

167. **4**

Rationale: Traction, analgesics, and heat may all be used to relieve the pain of muscle spasm in the client with a vertebral fracture. The use of ice is incorrect, because ice is applied to a site only for the first 24 hours after an injury. Application of ice to the spine of a client could result in feelings of being chilled and uncomfortable.

Test-Taking Strategy: Note the word "avoids" in the stem of the question. Option 2 can be easily eliminated. Next, eliminate option 1 because of the word "prescribed." Use concepts related to the principles of heat and cold to select from the remaining options. If this question was difficult, take a few moments to review this area at this time!

Level of Cognitive Ability: Application
Phase of Nursing Process: Implementation
Client Needs: Physiological Integrity
Content Area: Adult Health/Musculoskeletal

Reference
Lewis, S., Collier, I., & Heitkemper, M. (1996). *Medical-surgical nursing: Assessment and management of clinical problems* (4th ed.). St. Louis: Mosby–Year Book. p. 1869.

168. **1**

Rationale: The client who has had insertion of a femoral head prosthesis should use a raised toilet seat. The client should also maintain the leg in a neutral, straight position when lying, sitting, or walking. The leg should not be adducted, internally rotated, or flexed more than 90°. The client should sit in chairs that have arms so there will be assistance when the client is ready to rise from the sitting position. The client should avoid putting on own socks and shoes for 8 weeks after surgery, because doing so would force the leg into acute flexion.

Test-Taking Strategy: To answer this question correctly, it is necessary to be familiar with the limitations in motion needed following implantation of a hip prosthesis. Answer this question by evaluating each of the options in terms of the risk for prosthesis displacement that it carries. This concept will assist in eliminating options 2, 3, and 4.

Level of Cognitive Ability: Analysis
Phase of Nursing Process: Evaluation
Client Needs: Health Promotion and Maintenance
Content Area: Adult Health/Musculoskeletal

Reference
Lewis, S., Collier, I., & Heitkemper, M. (1996). *Medical-surgical nursing: Assessment and management of clinical problems* (4th ed.). St. Louis: Mosby–Year Book. p. 1867.

169. **3**

Rationale: Body Image Disturbance is characterized by negative verbalizations or feelings about a body part. This is a common response after amputation. The nurse supports the client and assists the client to work through these feelings. The client may also have the other nursing diagnoses listed in the distracters, but Body Image Disturbance is the nursing diagnosis that correlates best with the client's statement.

Test-Taking Strategy: Use knowledge of defining characteristics for the various nursing diagnoses to help you choose correctly. Focus on the client's statement in the question. The client's statement guides you to the correct response.

Level of Cognitive Ability: Analysis
Phase of Nursing Process: Analysis
Client Needs: Psychosocial Integrity
Content Area: Adult Health/Musculoskeletal

Reference
Lewis, S., Collier, I., & Heitkemper, M. (1996). *Medical-surgical nursing: Assessment and management of clinical problems* (4th ed.). St. Louis: Mosby–Year Book. p. 1876.

170. **4**

Rationale: If the tubing is removed from an IV pump and the tubing is not clamped, the client will receive a bolus of the solution and medication contained in the solution. The client who receives a bolus dose of heparin is at risk for bleeding. If the results of the next PTT are too high, the nurse may be required to give a dose of protamine sulfate, which is the antidote for heparin. Lovenox is an anticoagulant. Amicar is an antithrombinolytic (inhibits clot breakdown). Vitamin K is the antidote for warfarin.

Test-Taking Strategy: Knowledge regarding the complication that can occur in this situation and the antidote for heparin will easily direct you to the correct option. If this question was difficult, take a few moments to memorize this important information!

Level of Cognitive Ability: Application
Phase of Nursing Process: Implementation
Client Needs: Physiological Integrity
Content Area: Pharmacology

Reference
Deglin, J., & Vallerand, A. (1997). *Davis's drug guide for nurses* (5th ed.). Philadelphia: F. A. Davis. p. 1032.

171. **1**

Rationale: Procainamide is an antidysrhythmic medication, used often to treat ventricular dysrhythmias that do not adequately respond to lidocaine. The effectiveness of this medication is best determined by evaluating the client's cardiac rhythm. Thus, a cardiac monitor is of greatest value, although the blood pressure cuff and pulse oximeter will give general information about the client's cardiovascular status. A glucometer is not needed for this client with the information presented.

Test-Taking Strategy: Note that the key words in the stem are "determine most adequately." This tells you that more than one response may be partially or totally correct. To answer this question correctly, it is necessary to know that this medication is an antidysrhythmic medication. With this in mind, you can use prioritizing skills to deduce the correct answer.

Level of Cognitive Ability: Application
Phase of Nursing Process: Implementation
Client Needs: Physiological Integrity
Content Area: Pharmacology

Reference
Deglin, J., & Vallerand, A. (1997). *Davis's drug guide for nurses* (5th ed.). Philadelphia: F. A. Davis. pp. 1004–1006.

172. **1**

Rationale: The behaviors which this child engaged in are a warning signal of distress. All nurses need to incorporate questions that deal with the issue of current or past abuse into their nursing assessment. Although some adult clients may have repressed memories of abuse and other clients may not be able to open up during the assessment phase of the one-to-one relationship, the nurse who asks questions with sensitivity and in a straightforward manner opens the door to the painful disclosure that clients may need to make. The questions include, "Are you now or have you ever been sexually, and/or physically, and/or psychologically abused?" and "Are you presently safe now?"

Test-Taking Strategy: This question tests your knowledge of how to evaluate abuse-related symptoms during a nursing assessment. Symptoms include aggression and oppositional behaviors, age-inappropriate sexual behaviors, onset of school problems, and/or regressed behaviors. In Option 2, the nurse is insensitive, sarcastic, and intrusive. In option 3, the nurse is assessing the client's destructive behaviors, not the specific concerns of possible sexual abuse history. In option 4, although the nurse is trying to assess the client's abuse-related symptoms, the nurse uses indirect means rather than straightforward expressions of the nurse's concern.

Level of Cognitive Ability: Analysis
Phase of Nursing Process: Analysis
Client Needs: Psychosocial Integrity
Content Area: Mental Health

Reference
Varcarolis, E. (1998). *Foundations of psychiatric mental health nursing* (3rd ed.). Philadelphia: W. B. Saunders. pp. 387–440.

173. **2**

Rationale: Option 2 addresses the issue of the client's statement. Options 1 and 4 are statements that identify the process of agreeing with the client. Option 3 is not directly related to the issue of the client's statement.

Test-Taking Strategy: This question tests your knowledge of victimology and domestic violence. Use the process of elimination. Options 1 and 4 are nontherapeutic in that they use agreeing, which is a premature action that negates a full evaluation of the facts. Option 3 is not directly related to the issue of the question. This leaves option 2 as the correct answer to this question.

Level of Cognitive Ability: Analysis
Phase of Nursing Process: Analysis
Client Needs: Psychosocial Integrity
Content Area: Mental Health

Reference
Varcarolis, E. (1998). *Foundations of psychiatric mental health nursing* (3rd ed.). Philadelphia: W. B. Saunders. pp. 387–415.

174. **1**

Rationale: CCU psychosis occurs in some clients in critical care milieus. It fluctuates over the course of a day and usually is directly caused by sensory deprivation and/or medication-related or underlying medical conditions. There are no data in the question to indicate that alcohol is a concern. Options 3 and 4 both address dementia, and there are no data in the question to indicate that dementia exists.

Test-Taking Strategy: This question tests your knowledge of delirium and dementia and how to read the question correctly. Use the data presented in the question and the process of elimination to answer the question. Options 2, 3, and 4 are incorrect and reflect your knowledge deficit regarding these cognitive disorders. Eliminate options 3 and 4 as they are similar and both address dementia. Eliminate option 2 next because there are no data to indicate that alcohol is a concern.

Level of Cognitive Ability: Analysis
Phase of Nursing Process: Analysis
Client Needs: Psychosocial Integrity
Content Area: Mental Health

Reference
Varcarolis, E. (1998). *Foundations of psychiatric mental health nursing* (3rd ed.). Philadelphia: W. B. Saunders. pp. 681–723.

175. **1**

Rationale: The risks to the cardiovascular system from smoking are noncumulative and are not permanent. Three to four years after cessation, a client's cardiovascular risk is similar to that of a person who never smoked.

Test-Taking Strategy: Words that are absolute, such as "totally" in option 3 and "none" in option 4, would cause you to eliminate these options first. Knowledge about the cumulative risk of smoking on cardiovascular status is needed to discriminate accurately between options 1 and 2.

Level of Cognitive Ability: Application
Phase of Nursing Process: Implementation
Client Needs: Health Promotion and Maintenance
Content Area: Adult Health/Cardiovascular

Reference
Ignatavicius, D., Workman, M., & Mishler, M. (1995). *Medical-surgical nursing: A nursing process approach* (2nd ed.). Philadelphia: W. B. Saunders. p. 787.

176. **3**

Rationale: Clients with heart failure should immediately report weight gain, loss of appetite, shortness of breath with activity, edema, persistent cough, and nocturia. An increase in daytime voiding is expected while on diuretic therapy (Lasix). A cough due to respiratory infection does not necessarily indicate that heart failure is exacerbating.

Test-Taking Strategy: Eliminate option 1 first because the client's cough is accompanied by other signs of respiratory infection and does not indicate impending heart failure. Option 2 is eliminated next, because it is a positive sign. Option 4 is expected with diuretic therapy administered in the morning. This leaves option 3 as the correct option. Sudden weight gain would accompany fluid retention and should be reported.

Level of Cognitive Ability: Application
Phase of Nursing Process: Implementation
Client Needs: Health Promotion and Maintenance
Content Area: Adult Health/Cardiovascular

Reference

Smeltzer, S., & Bare, B. (1996). *Brunner and Suddarth's textbook of medical-surgical nursing* (8th ed.). Philadelphia: Lippincott-Raven. p. 671.

177. **2**

Rationale: Pulmonary edema is characterized by extreme breathlessness, dyspnea, air hunger, and production of frothy, pink-tinged sputum. Auscultation of the lungs reveals rales to the apices. As the client's condition improves, the amount of fluid in the alveoli decreases and may be detected by crackles in the bases. (Clear lung sounds indicate full resolution of the episode.) Wheezes and rhonchi are not associated with pulmonary edema.

Test-Taking Strategy: Fluid in the lungs from pulmonary edema produces sounds that are called rales or crackles, which eliminates options 3 and 4. Option 1 is less plausible than option 2 because rales throughout lung fields cannot possibly indicate an improvement in client condition.

Level of Cognitive Ability: Analysis
Phase of Nursing Process: Evaluation
Client Needs: Physiological Integrity
Content Area: Adult Health/Cardiovascular

Reference

Luckmann, J. (1997). *Saunders manual of nursing care.* Philadelphia: W. B. Saunders. p. 1072.

178. **1**

Rationale: Morphine reduces anxiety and dyspnea in the client with pulmonary edema. It also causes blood to pool in the periphery from decreased peripheral resistance. It decreases pulmonary capillary pressures, which reduces fluid migration into the alveoli. The client receiving morphine is monitored for signs and symptoms of respiratory depression and extreme drops in blood pressure, especially when administered intravenously.

Test-Taking Strategy: The question contains the key words "intended effect." To answer this question accurately, it is necessary to know the various effects of morphine as a narcotic agent. Knowing that it causes a drop in blood pressure and respiratory rate and provides some degree of euphoria allows you to eliminate systematically each of the incorrect responses.

Level of Cognitive Ability: Analysis
Phase of Nursing Process: Evaluation
Client Needs: Physiological Integrity
Content Area: Adult Health/Cardiovascular

Reference

Smeltzer, S., & Bare, B. (1996). *Brunner and Suddarth's textbook of medical-surgical nursing* (8th ed.). Philadelphia: Lippincott-Raven. p. 660.

179. **3**

Rationale: Urine output of greater than 30 mL/hour indicates that there is adequate perfusion to the kidneys, and therefore most likely other organs are equally perfused. Classic cardiovascular signs of cardiogenic shock include low blood pressure and tachycardia. The CVP rises as the backward effects of the left ventricular failure become ap-

parent. The normal value for the CVP is 0 to 5 when measuring in mmHg. Dysrhythmias commonly occur as a result of decreased oxygenation to the myocardium, but they are not a good sign.

Test-Taking Strategy: Note that the stem of the question contains the key words "most favorable." This tells you that you must prioritize the answer. Knowing the normal values for CVP helps you eliminate option 1 first. Next eliminate option 4 because it is higher than the normal range for heart rate. To discriminate between the last two options, recall that ventricular dysrhythmias are abnormal, whereas a urine output of 40 mL/hr is not.

Level of Cognitive Ability: Analysis
Phase of Nursing Process: Evaluation
Client Needs: Physiological Integrity
Content Area: Adult Health/Cardiovascular

Reference

Smeltzer, S., & Bare, B. (1996). *Brunner and Suddarth's textbook of medical-surgical nursing* (8th ed.). Philadelphia: Lippincott-Raven. p. 672.

180. **4**

Rationale: Lying on the left side may prevent air from flowing into the pulmonary veins. Trendelenburg's position increases intrathoracic pressure, which decreases the amount of blood pulled into the vena cava during inspiration.

Test-Taking Strategy: Knowledge regarding the complications associated with TPN, specifically air embolism, is required to answer this question. Note the key word "first" in the stem of the question. This will assist in eliminating option 1. Eliminate option 2 next because this action will not treat the problem. From the remaining options, think about the principles of gravity and the anatomy of the cardiopulmonary system to assist in directing you to option 4. Option 4 is the longest and most specific answer.

Level of Cognitive Ability: Application
Phase of Nursing Process: Implementation
Client Needs: Physiological Integrity
Content Area: Fundamental Skills

Reference

Craven, R.F., & Hirnle, C.J. (1996). *Fundamentals of nursing: Human health and function* (2nd ed.). Philadelphia: Lippincott-Raven. p. 572.

181. **4**

Rationale: Amrinone is an inotropic agent used to relieve the manifestations of heart failure. Therapeutic effects include decrease in edema, weight (fluid), dyspnea, and lung crackles. Blood pressure should remain stable or increase (if hypotensive). Hypotension is listed as a common cardiovascular adverse reaction.

Test-Taking Strategy: To answer this question correctly, it is necessary to know the intended actions and effects of this medication. This will allow you to use critical thinking skills to eliminate each of the incorrect options. If you are unfamiliar with this medication, take time now to review!

Level of Cognitive Ability: Analysis
Phase of Nursing Process: Evaluation
Client Needs: Physiological Integrity
Content Area: Pharmacology

Reference

Deglin, J., & Vallerand, A. (1997). *Davis's drug guide for nurses* (5th ed.). Philadelphia: F. A. Davis. p. 130.

182. **1**

Rationale: Hypokalemia can result from long-term use of cascara sagrada, which is a laxative medication. The medication stimulates peristalsis and alters fluid and electrolyte transport, thus helping fluid to accumulate in the colon. Long-term use of laxatives is generally discouraged, but their use among the elderly continues to be high.

Test-Taking Strategy: Specific knowledge related to the side effects of this medication is needed to answer this question accurately. Take a few moments now to review this medication if this question was difficult.

Level of Cognitive Ability: Application
Phase of Nursing Process: Assessment
Client Needs: Physiological Integrity
Content Area: Pharmacology

Reference

Deglin, J., & Vallerand, A. (1997). *Davis's drug guide for nurses* (5th ed.). Philadelphia: F. A. Davis. p. 228.

183. **2**

Rationale: Drowsiness, dizziness, and dry mouth are the most common side effects of cyclobenzaprine. This medication is a centrally acting skeletal muscle relaxant used in the management of muscle spasm that accompanies a variety of conditions.

Test-Taking Strategy: Specific knowledge related to the side effects of this medication is needed to answer this question accurately. Take a few moments now to review this medication if this question was difficult.

Level of Cognitive Ability: Analysis
Phase of Nursing Process: Analysis
Client Needs: Physiological Integrity
Content Area: Pharmacology

Reference

Deglin, J., & Vallerand, A. (1997). *Davis's drug guide for nurses* (5th ed.). Philadelphia: F. A. Davis. p. 304.

184. **3**

Rationale: Diphenhydramine is an antihistamine medication that causes drowsiness, anorexia, and dry mouth as the most common side effects. The nurse should plan to teach the client to avoid driving or doing any other activities that require mental acuity until the client's response to the medication is determined. Alcohol and CNS depressant medications should be avoided altogether while taking this medication. Lozenges may help relieve the side effect of dry mouth.

Test-Taking Strategy: Use knowledge of the common side effects of this frequently used medication to answer this question. Read the stem of the question carefully. The key words in the stem of this question are "avoid" and "until the client's response...is known." This tells you that the correct answer is one that is not totally contraindicated, thus eliminating options 1 and 2.

Level of Cognitive Ability: Application
Phase of Nursing Process: Planning
Client Needs: Health Promotion and Maintenance
Content Area: Pharmacology

Reference

Deglin, J., & Vallerand, A. (1997). *Davis's drug guide for nurses* (5th ed.). Philadelphia: F. A. Davis. p. 381.

185. **4**

Rationale: Diabetes insipidus can occur in a child with increased ICP. A specific gravity above 1.020, weight gain, and hypertension are indications of the syndrome of inappropriate antidiuretic hormone (SIADH). A high urine output would be indicative of DI.

Test-Taking Strategy: Knowledge regarding the signs and symptoms associated with the complications of increased ICP is required to answer this question. If you are unfamiliar with the clinical manifestations associated with DI and SIADH, take time now to review!

Level of Cognitive Ability: Analysis
Phase of Nursing Process: Assessment
Client Needs: Physiological Integrity
Content Area: Child Health

Reference

Ashwill, J., & Droske, S. (1997). *Nursing care of children: Principles and practice.* Philadelphia: W. B. Saunders. p. 1233.

186. **3**

Rationale: Enoxacin is administered 1 hour before or 2 hours after meals. Antacids may decrease absorption and should be given at least 4 hours before or 2 hours after the medication.

Test-Taking Strategy: Knowledge regarding the administration of this medication is required to answer this question. Note that options 1, 2, and 4 are similar in that they indicate administration of the medication with another substance (milk, meals, antacid). Therefore the best selection is option 3.

Level of Cognitive Ability: Application
Phase of Nursing Process: Implementation
Client Needs: Health Promotion and Maintenance
Content Area: Pharmacology

Reference

Hodgson, B., & Kizior, R. (1999). *Saunders nursing drug handbook 1999.* Philadelphia: W. B. Saunders. pp. 363–364.

187. **2**

Rationale: If the child is receiving an IV infusion of calcium EDTA, the infusion should be stopped for 1 hour prior to obtaining blood for a lead concentration level. Otherwise, the blood lead concentration will indicate a falsely elevated reading.

Test-Taking Strategy: This is a difficult question and one that requires knowledge regarding the procedure for obtaining blood for lead concentration level. Take time now to review the procedure related to this laboratory test if you had difficulty with this question!

Level of Cognitive Ability: Application
Phase of Nursing Process: Implementation
Client Needs: Physiological Integrity
Content Area: Child Health

Reference

Hodgson, B., & Kizior, R. (1999). *Saunders nursing drug handbook 1999.* Philadelphia: W. B. Saunders. p. 360.

188. **2**

Rationale: To reduce the hypotensive effect of this medication, the client is instructed to rise slowly from a lying to a sitting position and to permit legs to dangle from the bed momentarily before standing. If nausea occurs, it is not necessary to notify the physician. The client should be instructed to consume noncaffeinated carbonated beverages, unsalted crackers, or dry toast to alleviate the nausea. The client should report signs of a sore throat or fever as these may indicate infection. The client should be notified that several weeks may be needed for the full therapeutic effect of blood pressure reduction. The client should also be instructed not to skip doses or discontinue the medication, as severe rebound hypertension can occur.

Test-Taking Strategy: Note the key word "not" in the stem of the question. Knowing that this medication is an antihypertensive will assist in eliminating options 1 and 4. From the remaining options, use the skill of prioritizing. Option 3 indicates the possibility of infection and is the best indication of the need for physician notification, therefore select option 2 based on the wording of the stem of the question.

Level of Cognitive Ability: Application
Phase of Nursing Process: Implementation
Client Needs: Health Promotion and Maintenance
Content Area: Pharmacology

Reference
Hodgson, B., & Kizior, R. (1999). *Saunders nursing drug handbook 1999.* Philadelphia: W. B. Saunders. p. 361.

189. **2**

Rationale: Lovenox is an anticoagulant. Accidental overdose of this medication may lead to bleeding complications. The antidote is protamine sulfate. Vitamin K is the antidote for Coumadin. Epinephrine and adrenaline are the same medications and are normally used to treat hypersensitivity reactions or acute bronchial asthma attacks and bronchospasms.

Test-Taking Strategy: Eliminate options 3 and 4 first because they are the same medications. Knowledge that this medication is an anticoagulant and that the antidote is the same as for heparin will assist in directing you to option 2. Review this medication now if you had difficulty with this question!

Level of Cognitive Ability: Application
Phase of Nursing Process: Implementation
Client Needs: Physiological Integrity
Content Area: Pharmacology

Reference
Hodgson, B., & Kizior, R. (1999). *Saunders nursing drug handbook 1999.* Philadelphia: W. B. Saunders. pp. 365–366.

190. **1**

Rationale: The four-point gait is used for clients with muscle weakness or poor balance who can bear weight on both legs. The gait is safe but slow. The client always has three points in contact with the floor. Option 1 describes the appropriate procedure for performing the four-point gait.

Test-Taking Strategy: The key words "four-point gait" will assist in eliminating options 3 and 4. Recall that in this gait, the client always has three points in contact with the floor. Additionally, remember that in this gait, the crutch is moved forward first. These concepts will assist in correctly answering questions related to this type of crutch-walking.

Level of Cognitive Ability: Application
Phase of Nursing Process: Implementation
Client Needs: Safe, Effective Care Environment
Content Area: Fundamental Skills

Reference
Lammon, C., Foote, A., Leli, P., et al. (1995). *Clinical nursing skills.* Philadelphia: W. B. Saunders. p. 241.

191. **1**

Rationale: Clients with sickle cell anemia are advised to avoid strenuous activities (to conserve energy) and to avoid crowds (to prevent infection). Quiet activities as tolerated are recommended when the client is feeling well. Increasing fluid intake is encouraged to assist in preventing sickle cell crisis.

Test-Taking Strategy: This question tests your knowledge of sickle cell anemia and its nursing management. Note the key words "need for further instruction." Option 1 is the statement which indicates that the client does not understand the measures related to treatment. If you are unfamiliar with this disease, review the nursing measures required for care now!

Level of Cognitive Ability: Analysis
Phase of Nursing Process: Evaluation
Client Needs: Health Promotion and Maintenance
Content Area: Child Health

Reference
Jarvis, C. (1996). *Physical examination and health assessment* (2nd ed.). Philadelphia: W. B. Saunders. pp. 569–598.

192. **4**

Rationale: SLE, chiefly occurring in females 10 to 35 years of age, is a chronic inflammatory disease that affects multiple body systems. A butterfly rash on the cheeks and bridge of the nose is a key symptom of SLE. Other symptoms observed in SLE include alopecia, Raynaud's phenomenon, pericarditis, pleural effusion, myocarditis, nephritis, hepatomegaly, splenomegaly, mental status alterations, and convulsive disorders. Option 1 is found in sickle cell anemia. Options 2 and 3 are found in many conditions but not usually in SLE.

Test-Taking Strategy: Knowledge regarding the clinical manifestations associated with SLE is required to answer this question. Remember that the key symptom is a butterfly rash. This will assist in answering questions similar to this one. If you are unfamiliar with this disease, you will want to review the manifestations of SLE now!

Level of Cognitive Ability: Analysis
Phase of Nursing Process: Assessment
Client Needs: Physiological Integrity
Content Area: Adult Health/Musculoskeletal

Reference
Jarvis, C. (1996). *Physical examination and health assessment* (2nd ed.). Philadelphia: W. B. Saunders. pp. 569–598.

193. **1**

Rationale: Normal blood gas levels are PaO_2 of greater than 80 mmHg and $PaCO_2$ of less than 45 mmHg in a child with normal ICP. Options 2, 3, and 4 are incorrect.

Test-Taking Strategy: Note the key word "normal" in the question. Knowing that the normal PaO_2 is 80 to 100 mmHg will assist in eliminating options 2, 3, and 4. If you had difficulty with this question, take time now to review normal blood gas values!

Level of Cognitive Ability: Analysis
Phase of Nursing Process: Assessment
Client Needs: Physiological Integrity
Content Area: Child Health

Reference
Ashwill, J., & Droske, S. (1997). *Nursing care of children: Principles and practice.* Philadelphia: W. B. Saunders. p. 1230.

194. 3

Rationale: The nurse should stand in front of the client while speaking. The nurse should also approach the client from the front, or should raise the hand or touch the client's arm to get attention if necessary. Raising the voice is helpful, but it is not necessary to shout as loudly as one can. Overenunciation of words does not help the client who may be able partially to read lips as a compensatory mechanism for hearing loss.

Test-Taking Strategy: Use knowledge of basic communication strategies as well as knowledge of ear disorders to answer this question. If this question was difficult, take a few moments now to review these items!

Level of Cognitive Ability: Application
Phase of Nursing Process: Implementation
Client Needs: Psychosocial Integrity
Content Area: Adult Health/Ear

Reference
Beare, P., & Myers, J. (1998). *Adult health nursing* (3rd ed.). St. Louis: Mosby–Year Book. p. 1167.

195. 4

Rationale: The nurse needs to focus on the needs of the client, keep the client comfortable, and maintain dignity and self-esteem. Although the nurse needs to control the pain, it is not necessary to keep the client too sedated. The client should be able to interact with family members and make care decisions. The family needs are important, but the client needs are most important. As the client's needs change, the nurse needs to make decisions about the care needed and consult with the physician to update any orders.

Test-Taking Strategy: Focus on the key word "priority." Also note the client of the question. This will assist in eliminating option 2. Eliminate option 1 because of the word "sedated." Eliminate option 3 because of the word "all." The nurse has the responsibility to provide safe, effective care to clients. Options 1, 2, and 3 may be incorporated into the care but option 4 provides a framework for comprehensive, quality care and is the priority!

Level of Cognitive Ability: Analysis
Phase of Nursing Process: Analysis
Client Needs: Physiological Integrity
Content Area: Fundamental Skills

Reference
Leahy, J., & Kizilay, P. (1998). *Foundations of nursing practice: A nursing process approach.* Philadelphia: W. B. Saunders. p. 1154.

196. 1

Rationale: OSA is caused by a collapsed airway during sleep that blocks the client's breathing. OSA may result from obesity or from structural abnormalities (jaw, uvula, other tissues in the throat). Periods of apnea (lack of breathing for over 10 seconds) or hypopnea (periods of reduced airflow) that cause sleep alterations occur.

Test-Taking Strategy: This question tests your knowledge of OSA. Note the key phrase "most therapeutic." Options 2 and 4 are similar and should be eliminated first. In option 2, the client continues to report OSA. Option 3 is not

a response that the condition has improved. Review the treatment for OSA and the expected therapeutic response now if you had difficulty with this question!

Level of Cognitive Ability: Analysis
Phase of Nursing Process: Evaluation
Client Needs: Psychosocial Integrity
Content Area: Mental Health

Reference
Black, J., & Matassarin-Jacobs, E. (1997). *Medical-surgical nursing: Clinical management for continuity of care* (5th ed.). Philadelphia: W. B. Saunders. p. 401.

197. 1

Rationale: The question describes the client's complaint of tiredness on arising. A sleep diary is a method for documenting the exact sleep-wake patterns and/or disruptions the client is experiencing. The sleep diary assists the client to assess the frequency and severity of sleep disturbances. Simple and cost effective, sleep diaries can be employed to evaluate the effectiveness of intervention if used both before and after treatment.

Test-Taking Strategy: This question tests your knowledge of nursing interventions that can be used to increase understanding about sleep-wake patterns, sleep disorders and their causation, and factors affecting sleep. In option 2, the nurse expresses sympathy and provides a nontherapeutic and social response. In option 3, the nurse makes an assumption that the client's stated exhaustion is produced through sleeplessness. In option 4, the nurse is premature in suggesting that a sleeping medication would assist the client to sleep.

Level of Cognitive Ability: Application
Phase of Nursing Process: Implementation
Client Needs: Psychosocial Integrity
Content Area: Mental Health

Reference
Black, J., & Matassarin-Jacobs, E. (1997). *Medical-surgical nursing: Clinical management for continuity of care* (5th ed.). Philadelphia: W. B. Saunders. pp. 397–401.

198. 1

Rationale: Forensic nurses must continually be on guard to avoid any blurring or violations of boundaries in the professional one-to-one relationship. Many beginning nurses may find themselves uncertain as to how to acknowledge explicit remarks or compliments. It is important to remember that a simple "thank you" can easily be seen by the offender as a sign that the nurse wants the client to continue extending compliments. In addition, silence can cause the same reaction in the client. Any familiarity of any kind is out-of-line, and offenders are well aware of this. That is why a structured and specific response is crucial to the maintenance of a professional nurse-client relationship in this situation.

Test-Taking Strategy: This question tests your knowledge of how to maintain the boundaries of the nurse-client relationship. Options 2, 3, and 4 are all incorrect, and the rationale will assist you to determine the reasons for the response being inappropriate. Review appropriate and inappropriate responses now if you had difficulty with this question!

Level of Cognitive Ability: Application
Phase of Nursing Process: Implementation
Client Needs: Psychosocial Integrity
Content Area: Mental Health

Reference
Varcarolis, E. (1998). *Foundations of psychiatric mental health nursing* (3rd ed.). Philadelphia: W. B. Saunders. pp. 301–325, 507–535.

199. **1**

Rationale: The client with GERD should avoid eating or drinking within 3 hours of sleep to prevent episodes of nocturnal reflux. The client should eat small, frequent meals ranging from four to six per day. The client should drink fluids with meals to aid food passage in the GI tract. The client should avoid drinking very warm or cold beverages. The client should also avoid spices, citrus juices, fats, alcohol, coffee, and chocolate.

Test-Taking Strategy: Use knowledge of basic concepts related to digestion to help you answer this question. This will help you eliminate options 2 and 4. Knowledge of pathophysiology of GERD will help you choose option 1 over option 3. Review GERD now if you had difficulty with this question!

Level of Cognitive Ability: Application
Phase of Nursing Process: Implementation
Client Needs: Health Promotion and Maintenance
Content Area: Adult Health/Gastrointestinal

Reference
Black, J., & Matassarin-Jacobs, E. (1997). *Medical-surgical nursing: Clinical management for continuity of care* (5th ed.). Philadelphia: W. B. Saunders. pp. 1738–1739.

200. **4**

Rationale: Expected outcomes for a nursing diagnosis of Ineffective Individual Coping can include such behaviors as maintaining social interactions and activities, as well as involvement in the plan of care. The client who will not look at the feeding gastrostomy tube is either in denial or has not yet effectively coped with the altered route for supplying nutrition.

Test-Taking Strategy: Note that the key phrases in the question are "Ineffective Individual Coping" and "has not been resolved." Use basic nursing knowledge of coping skills and terminal illness to eliminate each of the incorrect options. This will assist in directing you to option 4 as the correct answer to this question!

Level of Cognitive Ability: Analysis
Phase of Nursing Process: Evaluation
Client Needs: Psychosocial Integrity
Content Area: Adult Health/Oncology

Reference
Black, J., & Matassarin-Jacobs, E. (1997). *Medical-surgical nursing: Clinical management for continuity of care* (5th ed.). Philadelphia: W. B. Saunders. p. 1745.

201. **3**

Rationale: The client with hepatitis is easily fatigued and may require several weeks to resume full activity level. It is important for the client to get adequate rest so that the liver may heal. The client should take in a high-carbohydrate and low-fat diet. The client should avoid hepatotoxic substances such as aspirin and alcohol. If prescribed for prolonged clotting times, the client should take vitamin K.

Test-Taking Strategy: The wording of the question guides you to look for an incorrect statement on the part of the client. Use your knowledge of liver disorders in general, and hepatitis in particular, to eliminate each of the incorrect options. Remember that fatigue is a troublesome problem in hepatitis and a lengthy period of convalescence is usually necessary!

Level of Cognitive Ability: Analysis
Phase of Nursing Process: Evaluation
Client Needs: Health Promotion and Maintenance
Content Area: Adult Health/Gastrointestinal

Reference
Black, J., & Matassarin-Jacobs, E. (1997). *Medical-surgical nursing: Clinical management for continuity of care* (5th ed.). Philadelphia: W. B. Saunders. pp. 1867, 1870–1871.

202. **1**

Rationale: The client is generally taught to report a temperature of 101°F or greater. The client should also report chills, pain unrelieved by medication, bleeding, foul-smelling drainage, or redness at the surgical site. The client should wear eyeglasses during the day and an eyeshield at night to protect the eye. The client should lie on the back or the nonoperative side unless otherwise instructed by the surgeon.

Test-Taking Strategy: Begin to answer this question by eliminating options 2 and 3 first. Remember that options that are similar (in this case related to eye protection) are not likely to be correct. Use knowledge of basic postoperative instructions to choose option 1 over option 4, according to the wording of this question.

Level of Cognitive Ability: Analysis
Phase of Nursing Process: Evaluation
Client Needs: Health Promotion and Maintenance
Content Area: Adult Health/Eye

Reference
Burrell, P., Gerlach, M., & Pless, B. (1997). *Adult nursing: Acute and community care* (2nd ed.). Stamford, CT: Appleton & Lange. p. 1877.

203. **2**

Rationale: The client who has adjusted to the impaired vision that may accompany glaucoma will take action to maintain safety in dim lighting. This includes moving carefully in dim lighting, using nightlights along paths traveled in the home at night, and avoidance of driving at dusk or dawn. Satisfactory adjustment is also indicated by recognition of the need for ongoing eye examinations and the presence of a supportive family.

Test-Taking Strategy: Remember that options that are similar are not likely to be correct. With this in mind, eliminate options 1 and 4 first. To discriminate between options 2 and 3, recall that vision is further impaired in dim lighting. This will guide you to choose option 2 over option 3, according to the wording of the question.

Level of Cognitive Ability: Analysis
Phase of Nursing Process: Evaluation
Client Needs: Psychosocial Integrity
Content Area: Adult Health/Eye

Reference
Burrell, P., Gerlach, M., & Pless, B. (1997). *Adult nursing: Acute and community care* (2nd ed.). Stamford, CT: Appleton & Lange. p. 1883.

204. **2**

Rationale: The facial drooping associated with Bell's palsy makes it difficult for the client to close the eyelid on the affected side. A widening of the palpebral fissure (the opening between the eyelids) and an asymmetrical smile are seen with Bell's palsy. Paroxysms of excruciating pain are seen with trigeminal neuralgia.

Test-Taking Strategy: Options 1 and 3 reflect findings opposite to those that would be expected with Bell's palsy. Option 4 relates to another disorder. Review the manifestations associated with Bell's palsy now if you had difficulty with this question!

Level of Cognitive Ability: Analysis
Phase of Nursing Process: Assessment
Client Needs: Physiological Integrity
Content Area: Adult Health/Neurological

Reference
Polaski, A., & Tatro, S. (1996). *Luckmann's core principles and practice of medical-surgical nursing.* Philadelphia: W. B. Saunders. p. 416.

205. **2**

Rationale: Respiratory compromise is a major concern in clients with Guillain-Barré syndrome. Clients are often intubated and mechanically ventilated when the vital capacity is less than 15 mL/kg. Although orthostatic hypotension is a problem with these clients, the BP drop is less than 10 mmHg and is not significant. Options 3 and 4 are expected, depending on the degree of paralysis that occurs.

Test-Taking Strategy: Remember the ABCs to answer the question. A vital capacity as identified in option 2 presents the greatest concern. Airway and breathing take priority!

Level of Cognitive Ability: Analysis
Phase of Nursing Process: Analysis
Client Needs: Physiological Integrity
Content Area: Adult Health/Neurological

Reference
Black, J., & Matassarin-Jacobs, E. (1997). *Medical-surgical nursing: Clinical management for continuity of care* (5th ed.). Philadelphia: W. B. Saunders. p. 877.

206. **2**

Rationale: Insulin dosages are verified by another nurse before administration. When two types of insulins are mixed, the doses must be verified after each is drawn up in order to verify the dosage for each one. The Regular (unmodified) insulin is drawn first. This prevents adding the acting modified insulin to the unmodified vial.

Test-Taking Strategy: Knowledge of technique for mixing insulins will assist you in answering this question. Remember that each insulin must be checked separately in order to verify the correct dosage. Remember RN, Regular before NPH! This will assist in directing you to the correct option!

Level of Cognitive Ability: Application
Phase of Nursing Process: Implementation
Client Needs: Safe, Effective Care Environment
Content Area: Pharmacology

Reference
Kozier, B., Erb, G., & Blais, K. (1998). *Fundamentals of nursing: Concepts, process, and practice* (5th ed.). Reading, MA: Addison-Wesley. pp. 1322–1323.

207. **4**

Rationale: Although the incidence of cataracts increases with age, the elderly client with diabetes is at greater risk for developing cataracts. The most frequent complaint is of blurred vision that is not accompanied by pain. The client may also experience difficulty with reading, night driving, and glare.

Test-Taking Strategy: Specific knowledge related to the risks for and signs and symptoms of common eye disorders is needed to answer this question. If this question was difficult, take a few moments to review the signs and symptoms of the eye disorders described in the options!

Level of Cognitive Ability: Analysis
Phase of Nursing Process: Analysis
Client Needs: Physiological Integrity
Content Area: Adult Health/Eye

Reference
Burrell, P., Gerlach, M., & Pless, B. (1997). *Adult nursing: Acute and community care* (2nd ed.). Stamford, CT: Appleton & Lange. p. 1878.

208. **4**

Rationale: Beta-adrenergic blocking agents such as timolol reduce intraocular pressure by decreasing the production of aqueous humor. Miotic agents (such as pilocarpine) increase contractions of the ciliary muscle and constrict the pupil, thereby increasing the outflow of aqueous humor.

Test-Taking Strategy: Specific knowledge about the action of this medication is needed to answer this question. Knowing that this medication is a beta-adrenergic blocking agent will assist in directing you to option 4. Additionally, knowing the pathophysiology associated with glaucoma will assist in directing you to the correct option. If needed, take a few moments to review the action of this medication now!

Level of Cognitive Ability: Application
Phase of Nursing Process: Implementation
Client Needs: Physiological Integrity
Content Area: Adult Health/Eye

Reference
Burrell, P., Gerlach, M., & Pless, B. (1997). *Adult nursing: Acute and community care* (2nd ed.). Stamford, CT: Appleton & Lange. p. 1882.

209. **4**

Rationale: Acetazolamide is the prototype of the proximal tubule diuretics that are sulfonamides. Prior to administration of this medication, clients should be assessed for allergy and should also be monitored during therapy for allergic reaction and photosensitivity.

Test-Taking Strategy: Visually, the options are divided into two groups: options 1 and 2 as anti-inflammatory agents, and options 3 and 4 as antibiotics. Knowing that Diamox belongs to neither of these groups, it makes sense that the chemical makeup of the medication must be similar to that of one of the options. Eliminate options 1 and 2 first as being least likely. It may help you to narrow your choice to know that a variety of medications have sulfa in them, which makes it the more likely option!

Level of Cognitive Ability: Application
Phase of Nursing Process: Assessment
Client Needs: Physiological Integrity
Content Area: Adult Health/Cardiovascular

Reference
Hodgson, B., & Kizior, R. (1999). *Saunders nursing drug handbook 1999.* Philadelphia: W. B. Saunders. pp. 8–10.

210. 3

Rationale: Children are constantly exploring their environments, and this includes their own bodies. It is not uncommon for children to put sharp or small objects such as cotton swabs into their ears, and these behaviors can cause injury. Acute otitis externa may cause a low-pitched tinnitus but not usually dizziness unless the condition has progressed to an otitis media. Audiography is performed in school screening every year, and this diagnosis may require more than the usual screening for children. Cotton-tipped applicators should not be used by children. A face cloth is an age-appropriate method for ear cleaning.

Test-Taking Strategy: Note the key words "instruction is effective." Options 1 and 4 can be easily eliminated. From the remaining options, basic principles related to care of the ears will easily direct you to option 3. If you had difficulty with this question, take time now to review teaching points related to this disorder!

Level of Cognitive Ability: Analysis
Phase of Nursing Process: Evaluation
Client Needs: Health Promotion and Maintenance
Content Area: Child Health

Reference
Jarvis, C. (1996). *Physical examination and health assessment* (2nd ed.). Philadelphia: W. B. Saunders. pp. 352–384.

211. 3

Rationale: The client with chronic vertigo should avoid driving and using public transportation. The sudden movements involved in each could precipitate an attack. To further prevent vertigo attacks, the client should change position slowly and should turn the entire body, not just the head, when spoken to. If vertigo does occur, the client should immediately sit down or grasp the nearest piece of furniture. The client should maintain the home in a state that is free of clutter and has throw rugs removed, since the effort of trying to regain balance after slipping could trigger the onset of vertigo.

Test-Taking Strategy: Begin to answer this question by eliminating options 1 and 2 first, since they put the client at greatest risk of injury secondary to vertigo. Choose option 3 over option 4 since it is the safer intervention of the two remaining ones.

Level of Cognitive Ability: Application
Phase of Nursing Process: Planning
Client Needs: Health Promotion and Maintenance
Content Area: Adult Health/Ear

Reference
Burrell, P., Gerlach, M., & Pless, B. (1997). *Adult nursing: Acute and community care* (2nd ed.). Stamford, CT: Appleton & Lange. p. 1933.

212. 2

Rationale: Presbycusis occurs as part of the aging process and is a progressive sensorineural hearing loss. Some clients may not adapt well to the impairment, denying its presence. Others withdraw from social interactions and contact with others, embarrassed by the problem and the need to wear a hearing aid. Clients show adequate adaptation by obtaining and regularly using a hearing aid.

Test-Taking Strategy: The key words in the question are "successful adaptation." A review of each of the options shows that the only option with positive wording is option 2. The incorrect options indicate a need for further adaptation.

Level of Cognitive Ability: Analysis
Phase of Nursing Process: Evaluation
Client Needs: Psychosocial Integrity
Content Area: Adult Health/Ear

Reference
Monahan, F., & Neighbors, M. (1998). *Medical-surgical nursing: Foundations for clinical practice* (2nd ed.). Philadelphia: W. B. Saunders. p. 2019.

213. 2

Rationale: A stage II ulcer is characterized by nonintact skin. There is partial thickness skin loss, and the wound may appear as an abrasion, shallow crater, or blister. A stage I ulcer is a reddened area that doesn't blanch but has intact skin. Stage III ulcer is full thickness, and Stage IV is full thickness with necrosis or damage to muscle, bone, or supportive tissue.

Test-Taking Strategy: An understanding of the different stages of pressure ulcer classification is needed to answer this question accurately. If needed, take a few moments to review this important content area now!

Level of Cognitive Ability: Analysis
Phase of Nursing Process: Analysis
Client Needs: Physiological Integrity
Content Area: Adult Health/Integumentary

Reference
Ignatavicius, D., Workman, M., & Mishler, M. (1995). *Medical-surgical nursing: A nursing process approach* (2nd ed.). Philadelphia: W. B. Saunders. p. 1936.

214. 3

Rationale: The nurse can enhance penetration of topical corticosteroid therapy to the client with psoriasis by applying warm, moist heat and an occlusive outer wrap. The wrap may consist of a plastic film, glove, bootie, or similar item. If large surface areas of skin are involved, the occlusive therapy may be limited to 12 hours per day to minimize local and systemic side effects.

Test-Taking Strategy: Note the key word in the stem, which is "maximizes." This implies that one option is better than the others for enhancing the effect of this therapy. Use principles related to heat therapy to eliminate each of the other incorrect options. Review treatment measures for psoriasis now if you had difficulty with this question!

Level of Cognitive Ability: Application
Phase of Nursing Process: Implementation
Client Needs: Physiological Integrity
Content Area: Adult Health/Integumentary

Reference
Ignatavicius, D., Workman, M., & Mishler, M. (1995). *Medical-surgical nursing: A nursing process approach* (2nd ed.). Philadelphia: W. B. Saunders. p. 1958.

215. 3

Rationale: Condoms should be used for adequate protection, especially with new partners. Sexually transmitted diseases (that could be acquired without condom use) do increase the client's risk of cervical cancer. It is true that uncircumcised partners may provide increased risk. The client should adhere to guidelines for early detection of cervical cancer (Pap smear) and should seek prompt treatment of vaginitis and cervicitis if they occur.

Test-Taking Strategy: The key words in the question are "not" and "cervical cancer." The wording of the question guides you to look for an incorrect statement. Knowledge of general measures to promote health guide you to eliminate options 1 and 2 first. Knowledge of STDs as a risk factor for cervical cancer helps you select option 3 over option 4.

Level of Cognitive Ability: Application
Phase of Nursing Process: Implementation
Client Needs: Health Promotion and Maintenance
Content Area: Adult Health/Oncology

Reference

Burrell, P., Gerlach, M., & Pless, B. (1997). *Adult nursing: Acute and community care* (2nd ed.). Stamford, CT: Appleton & Lange. p. 1734.

216. **1**

Rationale: Kegel muscles strengthen the perineal floor and are useful in prevention and management of cystocele, rectocele, and enterocele. There are several acceptable ways to perform Kegel exercises. These involve starting and stopping the flow of urine either once for up to 5 minutes, or several times during a single voiding for about 5 seconds. Since the muscles that control urination also are involved in defecation, these exercises can also be done once during defecation. Otherwise, they may be done by holding perineal muscles taut for up to 10 seconds several times a day, or for 5 minutes three to four times a day. Option 1 is not a correct method for performing Kegel exercises. Residual urine should not be held in the bladder for lengthy periods because it could promote urinary tract infection.

Test-Taking Strategy: A basic understanding of the purpose and procedure for these commonly prescribed exercises is necessary to answer this question. Note the key phrase "has not fully understood." General principles related to the prevention of urinary tract infections will direct you to option 1. If needed, take a few moments now to review the procedure for Kegel exercises!

Level of Cognitive Ability: Analysis
Phase of Nursing Process: Evaluation
Client Needs: Health Promotion and Maintenance
Content Area: Fundamental Skills

Reference

Burrell, P., Gerlach, M., & Pless, B. (1997). *Adult nursing: Acute and community care* (2nd ed.). Stamford, CT: Appleton & Lange. p. 1740.

217. **2**

Rationale: Gemfibrozil is a lipid-lowering agent. It is given as part of a therapeutic regimen that also includes dietary counseling—specifically, the limitation of saturated and other fats in the diet.

Test-Taking Strategy: To answer this question correctly, it is necessary to know the nature of the medication and the corresponding elements of the diet that should be altered. If this question was difficult, take a few moments to review this medication and these key concepts at this time!

Level of Cognitive Ability: Application
Phase of Nursing Process: Planning
Client Needs: Health Promotion and Maintenance
Content Area: Pharmacology

Reference

Hodgson, B., & Kizior, R. (1999). *Saunders nursing drug handbook 1999.* Philadelphia: W. B. Saunders. p. 461.

218. **2**

Rationale: Vital signs that remain near baseline indicate good cardiac reserve with exercise. The options with the pulse rate and oxygen saturation level changes are incorrect because they represent changes from normal values to abnormal ones. Blood pressure drops of more than 10 mmHg are not a good sign. Only the respiratory rate remains in the normal range, and it reflects a minimal increase.

Test-Taking Strategy: The key words in this question are "best tolerating." Use analytical skills and fundamental knowledge of vital signs to eliminate each of the incorrect options. The only option that identifies values that remain within the normal range is option 2.

Level of Cognitive Ability: Analysis
Phase of Nursing Process: Evaluation
Client Needs: Physiological Integrity
Content Area: Adult Health/Cardiovascular

Reference

Black, J., & Matassarin-Jacobs, E. (1997). *Medical-surgical nursing: Clinical management for continuity of care* (5th ed.). Philadelphia: W. B. Saunders. p. 1288.

219. **2**

Rationale: The client's response is one of fear. The client has verbalized the object of fear (dying), which makes anxiety incorrect. There is no evidence of denial or rage in the client's statement.

Test-Taking Strategy: Use knowledge of psychological responses and coping strategies to choose correctly. The wording of the question tells you that there is only one correct choice. The client's statement clearly identifies fear.

Level of Cognitive Ability: Analysis
Phase of Nursing Process: Analysis
Client Needs: Psychosocial Integrity
Content Area: Adult Health/Oncology

Reference

Burrell, P., Gerlach, M., & Pless, B. (1997). *Adult nursing: Acute and community care* (2nd ed.). Stamford, CT: Appleton & Lange. p. 1816.

220. **4**

Rationale: The client who has been placed in a body cast is at risk for developing cast syndrome. This results from pressure on the mesenteric artery and can lead to intestinal obstruction. The most important action of the nurse is to interpret the client's symptoms correctly and report them to the physician. Cast syndrome is usually treated with nasogastric decompression, intravenous therapy for hydration, and possibly application of a new cast.

Test-Taking Strategy: To answer this question correctly, it is necessary to interpret the client's symptoms correctly and to understand the severity of the problem. Note the key phrase "most important action" in the stem of the question. This should provide you with the clue that physician notification is required. If this question was difficult, take a few moments to review the complications of a body cast and the associated signs and symptoms!

Level of Cognitive Ability: Application
Phase of Nursing Process: Implementation
Client Needs: Physiological Integrity
Content Area: Adult Health/Musculoskeletal

Reference
Monahan, F., & Neighbors, M. (1998). *Medical-surgical nursing: Foundations for clinical practice* (2nd ed.). Philadelphia: W. B. Saunders. p. 856.

221. **2**

Rationale: Mammography is a type of radiographic procedure. Therefore, the client is advised not to wear jewelry or metal objects on the day of the examination. There is no special dietary preparation. The client should avoid use of lotions or underarm deodorant prior to the test.

Test-Taking Strategy: The wording of the question guides you to look for an option that is a correct statement. Use knowledge of procedures related to radiography and skin care to answer this question. Review this diagnostic procedure now if you had difficulty with this question!

Level of Cognitive Ability: Application
Phase of Nursing Process: Planning
Client Needs: Safe, Effective Care Environment
Content Area: Adult Health/Oncology

Reference
Burrell, P., Gerlach, M., & Pless, B. (1997). *Adult nursing: Acute and community care* (2nd ed.). Stamford, CT: Appleton & Lange. p. 1804.

222. **2**

Rationale: Blanching, coolness, and edema of the IV site are all classic signs of infiltration. As infiltration can be damaging to the surrounding tissue, the first action of the nurse is to discontinue the IV to prevent any further damage. The nurse should not depend solely on the blood return for assurance that the cannula is in the vein, as a blood return may be present even if the cannula is only partially in the vein. Warm compresses may be applied to the infiltrated area only after the IV is discontinued and only if the infiltrated solution is not damaging to the surrounding tissues. Measuring the area of infiltration should be done only after the IV has been discontinued so that further tissue damage is prevented.

Test-Taking Strategy: The stem of the question contains the key word "first." Although all the options may be appropriate, remember to prioritize. The signs presented in the question identify infiltration. Infiltration indicates that the IV needs to be discontinued. Review the signs of infiltration and the appropriate interventions now if you had difficulty with this question!

Level of Cognitive Ability: Application
Phase of Nursing Process: Implementation
Client Needs: Physiological Integrity
Content Area: Fundamental Skills

Reference
Ignatavicius, D., Workman, M., & Mishler, M. (1995). *Medical-surgical nursing: A nursing process approach* (2nd ed.). Philadelphia: W. B. Saunders. p. 287.

223. **4**

Rationale: Reassuring signs in the fetal heart tracing include a FHR of 120 to 160, accelerations of FHR, no variable decelerations, and the presence of short-term variability. Variable decelerations indicate cord compression. The short-term variability indicates that the infant is able to make the necessary adjustments to the stresses of labor.

Test-Taking Strategy: Knowledge of the normal fetal heart response to the labor process would help eliminate each of the incorrect options systematically. Review the normal and abnormal responses now if you had difficulty with this question!

Level of Cognitive Ability: Analysis
Phase of Nursing Process: Evaluation
Client Needs: Physiological Integrity
Content Area: Maternity

Reference
Lowdermilk, D., Perry, S., & Bobak, I. (1997). *Maternity & women's health care* (6th ed.). St. Louis: Mosby–Year Book. pp. 328–350.

224. **3**

Rationale: Knowledge of defense mechanisms is inherent in choosing the correct response. The client is displacing anger by yelling and throwing down the chair. The nurse first role-models setting limits on the client's behavior. The nurse reinforces group rules, physical safety, and a sense of control. Options 1 and 2 are premature at this point. This exploration may occur later in the group process. Option 4 may be the second action but only if the client presents with escalating behavior.

Test-Taking Strategy: Choosing the initial response requires organization of care with physiological safety as a primary concern. The nurse must deal with the "here and now" situation. The nurse sets limits on unacceptable behavior yet balances respect with safety. The nurse does not jump ahead to premature demands or call upon security until escalation occurs.

Level of Cognitive Ability: Application
Phase of Nursing Process: Implementation
Client Needs: Physiological Integrity
Content Area: Mental Health

Reference
Johnson, B. S. (1997). *Psychiatric-mental health nursing: Adaptation and growth.* Philadelphia: Lippincott-Raven. p. 9.

225. **2**

Rationale: Knowledge of the defense mechanisms is essential in choosing the correct response. Rationalization is substitution of acceptable reasons for actual reasons for behavior. In option 2, the client is rationalizing and is minimizing the response to loss. Options 1, 3, and 4 all indicate that the client is reviewing and evaluating certain valued perceptions of the treatment process prior to discharge.

Test-Taking Strategy: Note the key words "most concerns." Use the process of elimination and knowledge of defense mechanisms to answer the question. This should direct you to option 2 as the concern. If you had difficulty with this question, take time now to review defense mechanisms!

Level of Cognitive Ability: Analysis
Phase of Nursing Process: Evaluation
Client Needs: Physiological Integrity
Content Area: Mental Health

Reference
Johnson, B. S. (1997). *Psychiatric-mental health nursing: Adaptation and growth.* Philadelphia: Lippincott-Raven. p. 10.

226. **3**

Rationale: In the presence of rheumatic fever, the child will exhibit leukocytosis, positive CRP level, elevated ASO titer, and elevated ESR. A positive ANA test is used to diagnose a wide variety of collagen, vascular, and immune complex disorders and will be positive with rheumatic fever also.

Test-Taking Strategy: Specific knowledge of diagnostic tests used for inflammatory conditions is needed to answer this question. If this question was difficult, review either rheumatic fever or the various diagnostic tests identified in the options!

Level of Cognitive Ability: Analysis
Phase of Nursing Process: Analysis
Client Needs: Physiological Integrity
Content Area: Child Health

Reference

Monahan, F., & Neighbors, M. (1998). *Medical-surgical nursing: Foundations for clinical practice* (2nd ed.). Philadelphia: W. B. Saunders. p. 237.

227. **4**

Rationale: The client should alert any health care provider of a history of infective endocarditis prior to any procedure that involves instrumentation. The provider should place the client on prophylactic antibiotics. Antibiotics should be taken for the full course of therapy. The client should notify the physician if chest pain worsens or if dyspnea or other symptoms occur. The client should use a soft toothbrush and floss carefully to avoid any bleeding of the gums, which could provide a portal of entry for bacterial infection.

Test-Taking Strategy: Begin to answer this question by eliminating options 1 and 3, which are most obviously incorrect. Discriminate between the last two options by understanding the risks associated with infection for this client. Review the complications and risks associated with endocarditis now if you had difficulty with this question!

Level of Cognitive Ability: Application
Phase of Nursing Process: Planning
Client Needs: Health Promotion and Maintenance
Content Area: Adult Health/Cardiovascular

Reference

Monahan, F., & Neighbors, M. (1998). *Medical-surgical nursing: Foundations for clinical practice* (2nd ed.). Philadelphia: W. B. Saunders. p. 236.

228. **1**

Rationale: A daily aspirin is recommended to prevent embolus secondary to clot formation along the walls of the atria, which are fibrillating. Atrial fibrillation puts the client at risk for mural thrombi because of sluggish blood flow through the atria due to loss of the atrial kick. Although aspirin does have anti-inflammatory properties, it cannot prevent "any inflammation" from occurring, as stated in option 2. Options 3 and 4 are completely incorrect.

Test-Taking Strategy: An understanding of the altered dynamics of blood flow and the action of aspirin is needed to answer this question accurately. Options 3 and 4 can be eliminated first. Knowing that aspirin inhibits platelet aggregation will assist in directing you to option 1. If this question was difficult, take a few moments to review the action and purpose of aspirin!

Level of Cognitive Ability: Application
Phase of Nursing Process: Implementation
Client Needs: Health Promotion and Maintenance
Content Area: Pharmacology

Reference

Monahan, F., & Neighbors, M. (1998). *Medical-surgical nursing: Foundations for clinical practice* (2nd ed.). Philadelphia: W. B. Saunders. p. 247.

229. **2**

Rationale: The client who has undergone thoracentesis successfully should find relief of signs and symptoms experienced before the procedure. Typical signs and symptoms include dry, nonproductive cough, dyspnea (usually on exertion), decreased or absent tactile fremitus, and dull or flat percussion notes.

Test-Taking Strategy: A dull percussion note over lung tissue is abnormal and is eliminated first as a possible answer. Since options 1 and 3 specify "decreases" of a symptom, they are not totally effective and are also discarded. This leaves option 2, absence of dyspnea, as the answer. The client should be free of dyspnea after this procedure, with re-expansion of lung tissue.

Level of Cognitive Ability: Analysis
Phase of Nursing Process: Evaluation
Client Needs: Physiological Integrity
Content Area: Adult Health/Respiratory

Reference

Black, J., & Matassarin-Jacobs, E. (1997). *Medical-surgical nursing: Clinical management for continuity of care* (5th ed.). Philadelphia: W. B. Saunders. p. 1167.

230. **1**

Rationale: The client with empyema usually experiences dyspnea, pleural pain, night sweats, fever, anorexia, and weight loss. There is a decrease in breath sounds over the affected area, a flat sound to percussion, and decreased tactile fremitus.

Test-Taking Strategy: This question should be fairly easy to decipher, even without thorough knowledge of the signs and symptoms of empyema. Knowing that it can result from an infectious process, you would automatically choose the option that contains fever and pleural pain. If you are unfamiliar with the assessment signs associated with this condition, review them now!

Level of Cognitive Ability: Application
Phase of Nursing Process: Assessment
Client Needs: Physiological Integrity
Content Area: Adult Health/Respiratory

Reference

Smeltzer, S., & Bare, B. (1996). *Brunner and Suddarth's textbook of medical-surgical nursing* (8th ed.). Philadelphia: Lippincott-Raven. p. 503.

231. **4**

Rationale: Following any procedure involving thoracotomy, the nurse places the client in semi-Fowler's position. This position allows for maximal lung expansion and promotes drainage through chest tubes that were placed during surgery.

Test-Taking Strategy: Begin to answer this question by eliminating the supine and Sim's positions first. After thoracic surgery, the client needs to be more upright for ease of breathing. The same line of reasoning helps you choose semi-Fowler's position over side-lying. Review postoperative care following this procedure now if you had difficulty with this question!

Level of Cognitive Ability: Application
Phase of Nursing Process: Implementation
Client Needs: Physiological Integrity
Content Area: Adult Health/Respiratory

Reference
Smeltzer, S., & Bare, B. (1996). *Brunner and Suddarth's textbook of medical-surgical nursing* (8th ed.) Philadelphia: Lippincott-Raven. pp. 503, 577.

232. 4

Rationale: Dumping syndrome occurs after gastric surgery because food is not held as long in the stomach and is "dumped" into the small intestine as a hypertonic mass. This causes fluid to shift into the intestines, causing cardiovascular as well as GI symptoms. Symptoms typically include weakness, dizziness, diaphoresis, flushing, hypotension, abdominal pain and distention, hyperactive bowel sounds, and diarrhea.

Test-Taking Strategy: To answer this question correctly, it is necessary to have an understanding of the nature and causes of dumping syndrome following gastrectomy. If needed, take a few moments to review this material now!

Level of Cognitive Ability: Application
Phase of Nursing Process: Assessment
Client Needs: Physiological Integrity
Content Area: Adult Health/Gastrointestinal

Reference
Monahan, F., & Neighbors, M. (1998). *Medical-surgical nursing: Foundations for clinical practice* (2nd ed.). Philadelphia: W. B. Saunders. p. 1040.

233. 1

Rationale: The nurse plans postoperative measures to prevent venous stasis. They include applying elastic stockings or leg wraps, use of pneumatic compression boots, discouraging leg crossing, avoiding knee gatch, performing passive and active ROM, and omitting placement of pillows in the popliteal space. Covering the legs with a light blanket while sitting promotes warmth and vasodilatation of the leg vessels.

Test-Taking Strategy: The use of the word "avoid" in the stem guides you to look for an incorrect choice. Options 2, 3, and 4 are systematically eliminated because they are helpful actions. The use of knee gatch is contraindicated because it puts pressure on blood vessels in the popliteal area, impeding venous return. Thus it is the answer to the question as stated. Knowledge of standard nursing care procedures helps you answer this question quickly and successfully.

Level of Cognitive Ability: Application
Phase of Nursing Process: Planning
Client Needs: Physiological Integrity
Content Area: Adult Health/Cardiovascular

Reference
Smeltzer, S., & Bare, B. (1996). *Brunner and Suddarth's Textbook of medical-surgical nursing* (8th ed.). Philadelphia: Lippincott-Raven. p. 708.

234. 4

Rationale: Typical discharge activity instructions for the first 6 weeks include lift nothing heavier than 5 pounds, do not drive, and avoid any activities that cause straining. The client is taught to use the arms for balance, but not weight support, to avoid the effects of straining. These limitations are to allow for sternal healing, which takes approximately 6 weeks.

Test-Taking Strategy: This question is worded in the affirmative, so you are looking for a correct statement. Option

1 is eliminated first because it is contraindicated in several cardiac conditions. Option 3 is excessive, so that can be eliminated next. Of the remaining options, it is common practice after many surgical procedures to prohibit driving temporarily, which leaves you with the correct answer, which is option 4 (this option, incidentally, helps the client avoid straining).

Level of Cognitive Ability: Application
Phase of Nursing Process: Implementation
Client Needs: Health Promotion and Maintenance
Content Area: Adult Health/Cardiovascular

Reference
Black, J., & Matassarin-Jacobs, E. (1997). *Medical-surgical nursing: Clinical management for continuity of care* (5th ed.). Philadelphia: W. B. Saunders. p. 1363.

235. 3

Rationale: Normal sinus rhythm is defined as a regular rhythm with an overall rate of 60 to 100 beats/minute. The PR and QRS measurements are normal, measuring 0.12 to 0.20 second and 0.04 to 0.10 second, respectively.

Test-Taking Strategy: A baseline knowledge of normal ECG measurements can help you decipher questions such as these fairly readily. Take the time to review basic ECG rhythm interpretations now if needed. This area of knowledge has been added to the NCLEX-RN test plan!

Level of Cognitive Ability: Analysis
Phase of Nursing Process: Analysis
Client Needs: Physiological Integrity
Content Area: Adult Health/Cardiovascular

Reference
Black, J., & Matassarin-Jacobs, E. (1997). *Medical-surgical nursing: Clinical management for continuity of care* (5th ed.). Philadelphia: W. B. Saunders. p. 1296.

236. 4

Rationale: Sinus arrhythmia has all the characteristics of normal sinus rhythm, except there is an irregular PP interval. This occurs because of phasic changes in the rate of firing of the SA node, which may occur with vagal tone and with respiration. It does not affect the cardiac output.

Test-Taking Strategy: Eliminate option 2 because the rate in the rhythm described in the stem is irregular. Sinus tachycardia and sinus bradycardia are both rate-related dysrhythmias, but they are regular rhythms. This leaves sinus arrhythmia as the only possible choice.

Level of Cognitive Ability: Analysis
Phase of Nursing Process: Analysis
Client Needs: Physiological Integrity
Content Area: Adult Health/Cardiovascular

Reference
Black, J., & Matassarin-Jacobs, E. (1997). *Medical-surgical nursing: Clinical management for continuity of care* (5th ed.). Philadelphia: W. B. Saunders. p. 1299.

237. 4

Rationale: Ventricular fibrillation is characterized by absence of P waves and QRS complexes. The rhythm is instantly recognized by the presence of coarse or fine fibrillatory waves on the cardiac monitoring screen. Each of the incorrect options has a recognizable complex that appears on the monitoring screen.

Test-Taking Strategy: Eliminate options 2 and 3 first, since there are no complexes by which to count cardiac rate (tachycardia by definition is a rate greater than 100). PVCs are isolated ectopic beats superimposed on an underlying rhythm, so option 1 is eliminated next. There are no true complexes with ventricular fibrillation, which then becomes your choice as the correct option.

Level of Cognitive Ability: Analysis
Phase of Nursing Process: Analysis
Client Needs: Physiological Integrity
Content Area: Adult Health/Cardiovascular

Reference

Ignatavicius, D., Workman, M., & Mishler, M. (1995). *Medical-surgical nursing: A nursing process approach* (2nd ed.). Philadelphia: W. B. Saunders. p. 851.

238. **4**

Rationale: Procainamide is a Class 1 antidysrhythmic that is the medication of choice used to treat ventricular dysrhythmias in clients who are allergic to lidocaine. Other frequently ordered medications for ventricular dysrhythmias include bretylium tosylate (Bretylol) and magnesium sulfate. Digoxin is a cardiac glycoside; metoprolol is a beta-adrenergic blocking agent; verapamil is a calcium channel blocking agent. Whereas all these medications may be used in the treatment of a variety of cardiac conditions, none of them is indicated as a first-line antidysrhythmic.

Test-Taking Strategy: Medication knowledge is needed to answer this question accurately. If you are not familiar with first-line antidysrhythmic agents, take a few moments to review this medication classification now!

Level of Cognitive Ability: Application
Phase of Nursing Process: Planning
Client Needs: Physiological Integrity
Content Area: Adult Health/Cardiovascular

Reference

Ignatavicius, D., Workman, M., & Mishler, M. (1995). *Medical-surgical nursing: A nursing process approach* (2nd ed.). Philadelphia: W. B. Saunders. p. 850.

239. **3**

Rationale: PVCs are considered dangerous when they are frequent (over 6/minute), occur in pairs or couplets, are multifocal (multiform), or fall on the T wave. In each of these instances, the client's cardiac rhythm is likely to degenerate into ventricular tachycardia or ventricular fibrillation, both of which are potentially deadly dysrhythmias.

Test-Taking Strategy: Any questions you may see regarding PVCs would probably deal with recognition of when they become dangerous. Review these now, if needed, to increase the likelihood of successfully answering any questions in this area!

Level of Cognitive Ability: Analysis
Phase of Nursing Process: Evaluation
Client Needs: Physiological Integrity
Content Area: Adult Health/Cardiovascular

Reference

Black, J., & Matassarin-Jacobs, E. (1997). *Medical-surgical nursing: Clinical management for continuity of care* (5th ed.). Philadelphia: W. B. Saunders. p. 1305.

240. **1**

Rationale: Medication-specific teaching points for quinidine include to take the medication exactly as prescribed; do not chew the sustained-release tablets; take with food if GI upset occurs; wear a Medic-Alert bracelet or tag; and have periodic checks of heart rhythm and blood counts. The client should not stop taking a prescribed medication unless specifically ordered by the physician.

Test-Taking Strategy: This question is phrased to make you look for an incorrect statement. Options 3 and 4 are good general instructions for medication use and are therefore eliminated first. If you have difficulty choosing between options 1 and 2, look again at the wording of the options. It is not usual practice to "stop taking" a "prescribed" medication. This would lead you to choose option 1 as the correct answer.

Level of Cognitive Ability: Application
Phase of Nursing Process: Planning
Client Needs: Health Promotion and Maintenance
Content Area: Adult Health/Cardiovascular

Reference

Karch, A. (1997). *1997 Lippincott's nursing drug guide.* Philadelphia: Lippincott-Raven. p. 943.

241. **4**

Rationale: Correct procedure for basic life support with two rescuers includes a compression-to-ventilation ratio of 5 to 1. With adults, compressions are performed at a depth of 1.5 to 2 inches. The 5:1 ratio yields an effective rate of 12 respirations per minute. With effective compressions, carotid pulsations should be present. At its best, CPR produces only 30% of the normal cardiac output, so correct technique is vital.

Test-Taking Strategy: The question asks for the "best" indicator, implying more than one correct answer. In this case, all options are correct. However, options 1, 2, and 3 are procedural and do not reflect an outcome. The key words "most effectively" guide you to look for an end-result of the procedure, which is option 4.

Level of Cognitive Ability: Analysis
Phase of Nursing Process: Evaluation
Client Needs: Physiological Integrity
Content Area: Adult Health/Cardiovascular

Reference

Ignatavicius, D., Workman, M., & Mishler, M. (1995). *Medical-surgical nursing: A nursing process approach* (2nd ed.). Philadelphia: W. B. Saunders. pp. 876–878.

242. **1**

Rationale: Nursing responsibilities after cardioversion include maintenance of a patent airway, oxygen administration, assessment of vital signs and level of consciousness, and dysrhythmia detection. Use the basics of ABCs to answer this question—Airway, Breathing, and Circulation. Airway takes priority over other concerns that compete for the nurse's attention.

Test-Taking Strategy: Note that the stem of the question contains the key words "highest priority." This tells you that more than one or all of the options may be partially or totally correct. This question is relatively easy, though, since it follows the ABCs of life support. Airway comes first.

Level of Cognitive Ability: Analysis
Phase of Nursing Process: Assessment
Client Needs: Physiological Integrity
Content Area: Adult Health/Cardiovascular

Reference
Smeltzer, S., & Bare, B. (1996). *Brunner and Suddarth's textbook of medical-surgical nursing* (8th ed.). Philadelphia: Lippincott-Raven. p. 874.

243. **2**

Rationale: Temporal lobe herniation or uncal herniation refers to a shifting of the temporal lobe laterally across the tentorial notch. This produces compression of the third cranial nerve and ipsilateral pupil dilatation. If pressure continues to rise, flaccid paralysis, pupil dilatation, pupil fixation, and death will result.

Test-Taking Strategy: Note the key word "not" in the stem of the question. Knowledge regarding the pathophysiology associated with temporal lobe herniation is required to answer this question. Recalling the functions of the various cranial nerves may assist in directing you to the correct option. If you had difficulty with this question, take time now to review!

Level of Cognitive Ability: Analysis
Phase of Nursing Process: Analysis
Client Needs: Physiological Integrity
Content Area: Child Health

Reference
Ashwill, J., & Droske, S. (1997). *Nursing care of children: Principles and practice.* Philadelphia: W. B. Saunders. p. 1229.

244. **1**

Rationale: Redness, warmth, and purulent drainage are signs of an infection, not an allergic reaction. Infiltration causes the surrounding tissue to become cool and pale. An infection of a central catheter site can lead to septicemia.

Test-Taking Strategy: The issue of this question is to identify signs of infection. Key words in the question are "redness," "warmth," and "drainage." These key words and the skill of prioritizing will assist you to answer correctly. Infection and septicemia are serious complications of TPN!

Level of Cognitive Ability: Analysis
Phase of Nursing Process: Analysis
Client Needs: Physiological Integrity
Content Area: Fundamental Skills

Reference
Ignatavicius, D., Workman, M., & Mishler, M. (1995). *Medical-surgical nursing: A nursing process approach* (2nd ed.). Philadelphia: W. B. Saunders. pp. 284–285.

245. **3**

Rationale: Permanent TPN is indicated for clients who can no longer absorb nutrients via the enteral route. These clients may no longer be able to take nutrition orally. Options 1, 2, and 4 are incorrect statements.

Test-Taking Strategy: Note the key word "permanent" in the question. Knowledge regarding the purpose and considerations related to TPN is required to answer this question. Option 1 can be easily eliminated. Options 2 and 4 are inaccurate statements. Review TPN now if you had difficulty with this question!

Level of Cognitive Ability: Analysis
Phase of Nursing Process: Analysis
Client Needs: Psychosocial Integrity
Content Area: Adult Health/Oncology

Reference
Burrell, P., Gerlach, M., & Pless, B. (1997). *Adult nursing: Acute and community care* (2nd ed.). Stamford, CT: Appleton & Lange. p. 1354.

246. **4**

Rationale: The most therapeutic communication technique is one that uses reflection and facilitates the client's feelings. In addition, a supportive communication that encourages and supports other clients in the group to "connect" or relate to the client by responding to the client's statements is the most therapeutic group communication technique.

Test-Taking Strategy: This question tests your knowledge of the most therapeutic communication technique for the facilitation of clients' feelings in a group of women offenders. Option 1 makes an insensitive observation that might embarrass the client in the group. Option 2 is not therapeutic because it is judgmental and demonstrates bias. Option 3 minimizes the client's history of abuse.

Level of Cognitive Ability: Application
Phase of Nursing Process: Implementation
Client Needs: Psychosocial Integrity
Content Area: Mental Health

Reference
Varcarolis, E. (1998). *Foundations of psychiatric mental health nursing* (3rd ed.). Philadelphia: W. B. Saunders. pp. 181–205.

247. **3**

Rationale: Characteristics of the forensic client include the following: severe or chronic mental illness, drug abusers, poor judgment, limited reasoning abilities, and inability to learn from mistakes.

Test-Taking Strategy: This question tests your knowledge of the characteristics of the forensic client. Options 1 and 4 are incorrect. Option 2 cites a characteristic of the forensic client but one with a lower incidence than drug abuse. If you had difficulty with this question, take time now to review the characteristics of forensic clients!

Level of Cognitive Ability: Analysis
Phase of Nursing Process: Assessment
Client Needs: Psychosocial Integrity
Content Area: Mental Health

Reference
Varcarolis, E. (1998). *Foundations of psychiatric mental health nursing* (3rd ed.). Philadelphia: W. B. Saunders. pp. 301–352, 507–537.

248. **3**

Rationale: This question tests your knowledge of basic human needs and the treatment for tuberculosis. Option 1 cites an old-fashioned medical treatment of rest for healing. Option 2 cites fine measures but not necessarily priority ones. Option 4 is inappropriate because the client might just use the money inappropriately.

Test-Taking Strategy: The question asks you to think critically and to prioritize, using Maslow's hierarchy of needs and knowledge of the disease. Note the key word "medication" in the correct option. In this case, the nurse knows that safe shelter, medication, and food are priorities even over basic personal hygiene.

Level of Cognitive Ability: Analysis
Phase of Nursing Process: Assessment
Client Needs: Physiological Integrity
Content Area: Mental Health

Reference
Varcarolis, E. (1998). *Foundations of psychiatric mental health nursing* (3rd ed.). Philadelphia: W. B. Saunders. p. 450.

249. **1**

Rationale: In dementia, functionally impaired behaviors are those in which the ability to perform self-care is lost, and its expression may be aversive and burdensome. Vegetative behaviors are also examples of functionally impaired behaviors. In option 2, the data described consist of aggressive psychomotor behaviors illustrated by increases in gross motor movement, such as scratching, pushing, and assaultiveness, which can cause harm or repel another. In option 3, the data described consist of verbally aggressive behavior described as vocalizations, such as manipulation, negativism, and disruptiveness, which have the effect of repelling others. In option 4, the data described consist of nonaggressive psychomotor behavior that consists of an increase in gross motor movement without an apparent negative effect on others, but draws attention because of its repetitive nature, such as restlessness.

Test-Taking Strategy: This question tests your knowledge of what disturbing behaviors characterize dementia. Recalling that, in dementia, functionally impaired behaviors are those in which the ability to perform self-care is lost, will easily direct you to option 1. Review the behaviors associated with dementia now if you had difficulty with this question!

Level of Cognitive Ability: Analysis
Phase of Nursing Process: Assessment
Client Needs: Psychosocial Integrity
Content Area: Mental Health

Reference
Varcarolis, E. (1998). *Foundations of psychiatric mental health nursing* (3rd ed.). Philadelphia: W. B. Saunders. pp. 681–722.

250. **2**

Rationale: When the illness (Alzheimer's disease) affects the temporal-parietal-occipital association cortex, the client may experience inability to identify well-known objects and people. This is called agnosia.

Test-Taking Strategy: This question assesses your knowledge of the effects of illnesses on the temporal-parietal-occipital association cortex. Read the description of the client behavior to assist in answering the question. In option 1, difficulty in finding the right word to use is called aphasia. In option 3, an inability to perform familiar skilled activities is called apraxia. In Option 4, ataxia is altered motor functioning.

Level of Cognitive Ability: Application
Phase of Nursing Process: Implementation
Client Needs: Psychosocial Integrity
Content Area: Mental Health

Reference
Varcarolis, E. (1998). *Foundations of psychiatric mental health nursing* (3rd ed.). Philadelphia: W. B. Saunders. pp. 625–679.

251. **3**

Rationale: In a standing position, there should be 25° to 30° of flexion at the client's elbow. A walker of incorrect height will not allow the client's line of gravity to go through his or her base of support. The other options are correct regarding the use of a walker.

Test-Taking Strategy: Note the key word "not" in the stem of the question. Knowledge regarding the safe use of a walker will assist in answering the question. Options 1 and 4 can be easily eliminated first. Visualize the use of a walker to assist in eliminating option 2. Review the principles related to the safe use of a walker now if you had difficulty with this question!

Level of Cognitive Ability: Application
Phase of Nursing Process: Planning
Client Needs: Health Promotion and Maintenance
Content Area: Fundamental Skills

Reference
Lammon, C., Foote, A., Leli, P., et al. (1995). *Clinical nursing skills.* Philadelphia: W. B. Saunders. pp. 245–247.

252. **3**

Rationale: Total calcium levels are 7.0 to 12.0 mg/dL in a term infant younger than 1 week old and 8.0 to 10.5 mg/dL in a child. Neonatal hypocalcemia is defined as a total serum calcium concentration of less than 7.0 mg/dL.

Test-Taking Strategy: Knowledge regarding the normal calcium level in a newborn infant is required to answer this question. If you had difficulty with this question or are unfamiliar with these normal values, take time now to review!

Level of Cognitive Ability: Analysis
Phase of Nursing Process: Analysis
Client Needs: Physiological Integrity
Content Area: Maternity

Reference
Ashwill, J., & Droske, S. (1997). *Nursing care of children: Principles and practice.* Philadelphia: W. B. Saunders. p. 565.

253. **3**

Rationale: When suctioning a tracheostomy in an infant, it is necessary to limit insertion and suctioning time to 5 seconds to prevent hypoxia. Options 1, 2, and 4 indicate correct suctioning procedures for the infant.

Test-Taking Strategy: Note the key word "inaccurate" in the stem of the question. Knowledge regarding the procedure for suctioning an infant through a tracheostomy is required to answer this question. These principles will assist in eliminating options 1, 2, and 4. Noting the time frame of 10 seconds in option 3 will guide you to this option as the answer to the question as stated. This is a rather lengthy suctioning time for an infant!

Level of Cognitive Ability: Analysis
Phase of Nursing Process: Analysis
Client Needs: Physiological Integrity
Content Area: Child Health

Reference
Ashwill, J., and Droske, S. (1997). *Nursing care of children: Principles and practice.* Philadelphia: W. B. Saunders. p. 479.

254. **1**

Rationale: The suction setting for a tracheostomy for a neonate should be 60 to 80 mmHg. An infant setting is 80 to 100 mmHg, and for larger children 100 to 120 mmHg is appropriate.

Test-Taking Strategy: Knowledge regarding the appropriate amount of suction to use when suctioning a neonate is required to answer this question. Noting that the question addresses a neonate will assist you in selecting the option with the least amount of suction, option 1.

Level of Cognitive Ability: Analysis
Phase of Nursing Process: Analysis
Client Needs: Physiological Integrity
Content Area: Maternity

Reference
Ashwill, J., & Droske, S. (1997). *Nursing care of children: Principles and practice.* Philadelphia: W. B. Saunders. p. 479.

255. **3**

Rationale: In a young child aged 3 to 6 years old, the maximum volume of IM medication that can be safely injected into the ventral gluteal muscle is 1.5 mL.

Test-Taking Strategy: Knowledge regarding the safe administration of IM medications in a child is required to answer this question. Noting the age of the child and attempting to visualize the size of a child at this age may assist in selecting the correct option. If you had difficulty with this question, take time now to review!

Level of Cognitive Ability: Analysis
Phase of Nursing Process: Planning
Client Needs: Physiological Integrity
Content Area: Child Health

Reference
Ashwill, J., & Droske, S. (1997). *Nursing care of children: Principles and practice.* Philadelphia: W. B. Saunders. p. 495.

256. **3**

Rationale: The child's rectal vault is not as long as that of an adult, and the distance required to place medications is approximately 1 to 2 cm. After insertion, the buttocks should be held together until the urge to expel the suppository has passed.

Test-Taking Strategy: Knowledge regarding the anatomy of a child and the principles related to the administration of rectal medications is required to answer this question. If you did not know the answer to this question, take time now to review this procedure!

Level of Cognitive Ability: Application
Phase of Nursing Process: Planning
Client Needs: Physiological Integrity
Content Area: Child Health

Reference
Ashwill, J., & Droske, S. (1997). *Nursing care of children: Principles and practice.* Philadelphia: W. B. Saunders. p. 497.

257. **1**

Rationale: Because of the internal anatomy of the ear, the nurse should remember to pull the pinna of the ear back and down if the child is 3 years old or younger. If the child is older than 3 years, pull the pinna of the ear back and up. The child should lie on the unaffected side with the ear to receive the drops upward.

Test-Taking Strategy: Knowledge regarding the anatomy of a child and the principles related to the administration of ear medications is required to answer this question. If you did not know the answer to this question, take time now to review this procedure!

Level of Cognitive Ability: Analysis
Phase of Nursing Process: Analysis
Client Needs: Physiological Integrity
Content Area: Child Health

Reference
Ashwill, J., & Droske, S. (1997). *Nursing care of children: Principles and practice.* Philadelphia: W. B. Saunders. p. 499.

258. **3**

Rationale: The schizophrenic client is making paranoid statements. However, this is an example not of a hallucination but of a delusion that is focused on one other person. It is important that the nurse provide the client with supportive intervention but also be protective of the other client. The most therapeutic response to such clients is the one that assures the client of safety and states that the client's thinking will be less frightening and overwhelming. It is useless to argue with the clients as that will only place a strain on the trust issue of your relationship with the paranoid client and earn you a regressive struggle.

Test-Taking Strategy: This question tests your knowledge of how to respond to clients who are psychotic and, in this case, paranoid. Option 1 is not therapeutic because the nurse feeds into the client's psychosis by asking where the fantasy person is. Option 2 is not therapeutic because the nurse is sarcastic and belittling to the client. Option 4 is not therapeutic because while the nurse begins by presenting reality, the nurse then is demeaning to the client in the second statement.

Level of Cognitive Ability: Application
Phase of Nursing Process: Implementation
Client Needs: Psychosocial Integrity
Content Area: Mental Health

Reference
Glod, C. A. (1998). *Contemporary psychiatric–mental health nursing.* Philadelphia: F. A. Davis. pp. 305–340.

259. **1**

Rationale: The most therapeutic response is one that sets limits on the client's interruptive behavior and assesses the client's ability to control his behavior. It is not confrontational nor challenging but rather provides in neutral language a time for the client to see the nurse. If the client is unable to wait, then the nurse will assign one of the nursing staff to assist the client. In addition, the nurse manager has offered the client a therapeutic activity to engage in and use up energy. If the client refuses medication and cannot control his behavior, an intervention to assist the client to take medication will be instituted but only after attempting to elicit his compliance. Nevertheless, the nursing staff will use the least restrictive means possible.

Test-Taking Strategy: This question tests your knowledge of the most therapeutic nursing intervention to apply for a client who is delusional and presents with a recent history of violence. In option 2, the nurse uses restating and feeds into the client's delusional system, which is not therapeutic and belittles the client's mental status. In option 3, the nurse uses a "playful and mothering" type of social response that may escalate the client's behavior. Remember the concreteness of the client's thinking. In option 4, the nurse chastises the client for behavior that is not in his control, especially if the client has just had a first episode of psychosis and/or is schizophrenic and has been noncompliant with medication. (If this is the case, the client will be carefully and patiently retaught the importance of taking his medication.) If the client remains noncompliant, the psychiatrist may also consider using intramuscular medications to support the client's maintenance of health.

Level of Cognitive Ability: Application
Phase of Nursing Process: Implementation
Client Needs: Psychosocial Integrity
Content Area: Mental Health

Reference
Glod, C. A. (1998). *Contemporary psychiatric–mental health nursing.* Philadelphia: F. A. Davis. pp. 305–340.

260. **1**

Rationale: Starting a restorative program is a good choice but not unless an assessment has first been completed. Observation of the transfer techniques is recommended. Itemizing the number of falls is another important indicator but not as strong as actual observation. Discussing nursing home placement would be premature in light of the client's desire to stay at home.

Test-Taking Strategy: The focus in this question is an evaluation of needs, thereby eliminating the option of starting a restorative program. The client is in need of restorative care to effect continued independence in the home setting. There is one negative response that is automatically eliminated: nursing home placement. The number of falls may be an important indicator of level of function, but direct client observation is the best answer. Remember, assessment is the first step of the nursing process!

Level of Cognitive Ability: Application
Phase of Nursing Process: Implementation
Client Needs: Health Promotion and Maintenance
Content Area: Adult Health/Neurological

Reference
Rice, R. (1995). *Home health nursing procedures: Concepts & application.* St. Louis: Mosby–Year Book. p. 298.

261. **2**

Rationale: Clients with an ICD usually continue to receive antidysrhythmic medications after discharge from the hospital. The nurse should stress the importance of continuing to take these medications as prescribed. The nurse should provide clear instructions about the purposes of the medications, dosage schedule, and side effects to report. Options 1, 3, and 4 are correct.

Test-Taking Strategy: Note the key words "further teaching is necessary." Use the process of elimination. Basic principles related to the administration of prescribed medication will easily assist in directing you to the correct option. Review teaching points related to ICDs now if you had difficulty with this question!

Level of Cognitive Ability: Analysis
Phase of Nursing Process: Evaluation
Client Needs: Health Promotion and Maintenance
Content Area: Adult Health/Cardiovascular

Reference
Ignatavicius, D., Workman, M., & Mishler, M. (1995) *Medical-surgical nursing: A nursing process approach* (2nd ed.) Philadelphia: W. B. Saunders. p. 884.

262. **1**

Rationale: The client may be taking hot showers, which lead to vasodilatation and a decrease in venous return to the heart. Decreased venous return would decrease cerebral blood flow, thus causing symptoms of dizziness. By assessing the temperature of the shower first, the nurse may identify the problem and instruct the client to defer hot showers/baths until healing has occurred.

Test-Taking Strategy: Note the key word "first" in the stem of the question. Focus on the description of the client's complaint and safety in determining the first assessment. Options 3 and 4 can be eliminated first because they do not directly relate to client safety. From the remaining options, select option 1 as the item to be assessed first because it directly relates to the client's complaint.

Level of Cognitive Ability: Analysis
Phase of Nursing Process: Analysis
Client Needs: Safe, Effective Care Environment
Content Area: Adult Health/Cardiovascular

References
Lewis, S., Collier, I., & Heitkemper, M. (1996). *Medical-surgical nursing: Assessment & management of clinical problems* (4th ed.) St Louis: Mosby–Year Book. p. 922.

263. **2**

Rationale: The external radiation level associated with these implants necessitates that exposure to staff, other clients, and visitors be minimal. Therefore, clients undergoing internal radiation usually have private rooms. Visitors are limited, and women who are pregnant or who potentially may be pregnant should not enter the room. Visitation is allowed for individuals older than 16 years of age. Clients with radiation implants must have warning signs posted on their closed doors and charts to alert staff and visitors that radiation therapy is in process. A lead shield is kept at the bedside for use in preventing exposure to radiation when direct care is provided.

Test-Taking Strategy: Focus on the issue: to prevent exposure to radiation. This focus should assist in directing you to the correct option. Note the absolute word "restricted" in option 2. This should assist in directing you to this option. Review the nursing precautions for caring for clients with radiation implants now if you had difficulty with this question!

Level of Cognitive Ability: Application
Phase of Nursing Process: Planning
Client Needs: Safe, Effective Care Environment
Content Area: Adult Health/Oncology

Reference
Monahan, F., & Neighbors, M. (1998). *Medical-surgical nursing: Foundations for clinical practice* (2nd ed.). Philadelphia: W. B. Saunders. p. 1519.

264. **2**

Rationale: Anaphylactic shock is a possible reaction to penicillin therapy, and the onset of anaphylaxis is nearly always within 10 minutes of administration. The client should be observed for 30 minutes after intramuscular injection so that if anaphylaxis develops, help is immediately available.

Test-Taking Strategy: Eliminate options 1 and 4 first, knowing that these actions are not normal practice with the administration of penicillin G. From the remaining options, knowledge that anaphylaxis can occur following the administration of penicillin G will easily direct you to option 2.

Level of Cognitive Ability: Application
Phase of Nursing Process: Implementation
Client Needs: Physiological Integrity
Content Area: Pharmacology

Reference
Clark, J., Queener, S., & Karb, V. (1997). *Pharmacologic basis of nursing practice* (5th ed.). St Louis: Mosby–Year Book. p. 473.

265. **2**

Rationale: Schizophrenic clients experience auditory hallucinations in which they hear voices that aren't present, but this experience seems to be more somatic as it is related to the client's perception of infection. When the nurse needs to assess the client's hallucinations completely, appropriate questions include: Are the hallucinations solely auditory or do they include other senses? How long has the client experienced the hallucinations and have they changed in any way? What is the content of the hallucinations? How strongly does the client believe in the hallucinations?

Test-Taking Strategy: This question tests your knowledge of how to perform a comprehensive, individualized assessment for hallucinations. Options 3 and 4 can be easily eliminated first. Option 1 is inappropriate and additionally would not provide comprehensive assessment data.

Level of Cognitive Ability: Analysis
Phase of Nursing Process: Assessment
Client Needs: Psychosocial Integrity
Content Area: Mental Health

Reference
Varcarolis, E. (1998). *Foundations of psychiatric mental health nursing* (3rd ed.). Philadelphia: W. B. Saunders. pp. 625–679.

266. **4**

Rationale: Loose associations are speech patterns in which there is lack of a logical relationship between thoughts and ideas that causes speech and thought to seem inexact, vague, unfocused, and diffuse.

Test-Taking Strategy: This question tests your knowledge of terminology used to describe speech. Option 1 is an incorrect interpretation. Flight of ideas is overproductive speech characterized by the client's quickly switching from one subject to another with only a sense of fragmented ideas. Option 2 is an incorrect interpretation. Incoherence is characterized by speech that cannot be understood. Tangential speech is an inappropriate response to a statement in which the content of the statement is disregarded. The client's reply is directed toward an incidental aspect of the initial statement, the type of language used, the emotions of the sender, or another facet of the same subject. Option 3 is an incorrect interpretation. Clanging is a form of rhyming that is not comprehensible, but the client seems to be caught up in the sound of the words.

Level of Cognitive Ability: Analysis
Phase of Nursing Process: Analysis
Client Needs: Psychosocial Integrity
Content Area: Mental Health

Reference
Varcarolis, E. (1998). *Foundations of psychiatric mental health nursing* (3rd ed.). Philadelphia: W. B. Saunders. pp. 625–679.

267. **3**

Rationale: Noncompliance with antipsychotic medication is one of the chief reasons that clients with schizophrenia have relapses. The psychiatric nurse teaches schizophrenic clients to recognize the onset of symptoms that are associated with relapse.

Test-Taking Strategy: This question tests your knowledge of the appropriate therapeutic communication technique for the schizophrenic client who has decided not to take medication any longer. In options 1 and 2, the nurse is employing restating which, while therapeutic, is not useful to this client and to this client's situation. In option 4, the nurse is using an illogical, judgmental, and biased response that is not therapeutic.

Level of Cognitive Ability: Analysis
Phase of Nursing Process: Analysis
Client Needs: Psychosocial Integrity
Content Area: Mental Health

Reference
Varcarolis, E. (1998). *Foundations of psychiatric mental health nursing* (3rd ed.). Philadelphia: W. B. Saunders. pp. 301–326.

268. **1**

Rationale: The most critical skill for the forensic psychiatric nurse is the ability to evaluate the risk of violence in a client. Setting boundaries, performing a follow-up health history and examination, and teaching appropriate social skills, such as assertive communications, are also necessary. However, estimation of the risk for violence is crucial for the forensic nurse because the risk for violence is six times higher for incarcerated clients than for the general population.

Test-Taking Strategy: This question tests your knowledge of the competencies specific to the forensic nurse. In option 2, blurred boundaries would be very incorrect for clients in correctional facilities. In fact, the forensic nurse will be careful to maintain boundaries and to set limits for offenders, because less structure is viewed as nontherapeutic and confuses offenders. In options 3 and 4, the nurse's skills in this area, while needed, are not vital.

Level of Cognitive Ability: Analysis
Phase of Nursing Process: Analysis
Client Needs: Psychosocial Integrity
Content Area: Mental Health

Reference
Varcarolis, E. (1998). *Foundations of psychiatric mental health nursing* (3rd ed.). Philadelphia: W. B. Saunders. pp. 301–326.

269. **2**

Rationale: The two-point gait is faster than the four-point gait and requires more balance. It is used when weight-bearing is allowed on both feet. Only two points are in contact with the floor. The two-point gait closely resembles normal walking. Option 2 identifies the correct procedure for the two-point gait.

Test-Taking Strategy: Noting the name of this type of gait will assist in directing you to the correct option. Read the options carefully, and identify the option that describes the gait in which two points are in contact with the floor. This will easily assist you to option 2 and assist with answering questions similar to this one. Review this gait now if you had difficulty with this question!

Level of Cognitive Ability: Analysis
Phase of Nursing Process: Analysis
Client Needs: Safe, Effective Care Environment
Content Area: Fundamental Skills

Reference

Lammon, C., Foote, A., Leli, P., et al. (1995). *Clinical nursing skills.* Philadelphia: W. B. Saunders. p. 241.

270. 2

Rationale: During the first 24 to 72 hours following surgery, mucus and serosanguineous drainage are expected from the stoma. Options 2 and 3 are inappropriate actions. There is no need to notify the physician since this is an expected finding.

Test-Taking Strategy: Note the key words "just returned from the operating room" and "serosanguineous." This will assist in recalling that this type of drainage is expected at this time period. Review the expected findings following this type of surgery now if you had difficulty with this question!

Level of Cognitive Ability: Application
Phase of Nursing Process: Implementation
Client Needs: Physiological Integrity
Content Area: Adult Health/Gastrointestinal

Reference

Monahan, F., & Neighbors, M. (1998). *Medical-surgical nursing: Foundations for clinical practice* (2nd ed.). Philadelphia: W. B. Saunders. p. 1007.

271. 2

Rationale: If a ventricular pacemaker is functioning properly, there will be a pacer spike followed by a QRS complex. An atrial pacemaker spike precedes a P wave if an atrial pacemaker is implanted. A demand pacemaker fires only when needed and should therefore discharge only when there is no electrical activity occurring in the client's own heart.

Test-Taking Strategy: Knowledge of the normal cardiac conduction pathway as represented on the ECG complex can help you successfully navigate this question. Knowing that the QRS signals ventricular depolarization will lead you to the correct response. Review pacemakers now if you had difficulty with this question!

Level of Cognitive Ability: Application
Phase of Nursing Process: Assessment
Client Needs: Physiological Integrity
Content Area: Adult Health/Cardiovascular

Reference

Black, J., & Matassarin-Jacobs, E. (1997). *Medical-surgical nursing: Clinical management for continuity of care* (5th ed.). Philadelphia: W. B. Saunders. p. 1321.

272. 3

Rationale: Cardiotoxicity can occur with the use of Adriamycin. The medication can produce irreversible toxicity to the heart, including ECG changes and congestive heart failure. Elevated renal function tests (options 1 and 2) are not associated with the use of this medication. A harmless red discoloration of the urine may occur with the use of this medication.

Test-Taking Strategy: Options 1, 2, and 4 are similar in that they all address the renal system. In this situation, select the option that is different, option 3. If you are unfamiliar with this medication and the toxic effects that can occur with its use, take time now to review!

Level of Cognitive Ability: Analysis
Phase of Nursing Process: Assessment
Client Needs: Physiological Integrity
Content Area: Pharmacology

Reference

Clark, J., Queener, S., & Karb, V. (1997) *Pharmacologic basis of nursing practice* (5th ed.). St Louis: Mosby–Year Book. p. 595.

273. 3

Rationale: The client with thrombophlebitis, also known as deep vein thrombosis, exhibits redness and/or warmth of the affected leg, tenderness at the site, possible dilated veins (if superficial), low-grade fever, edema distal to the obstruction, positive Homans' sign, and increased calf circumference in the affected extremity. Pedal pulses are unchanged from baseline because this is a venous, not arterial, problem. Often clients silently develop thrombophlebitis, that is, they do not present with any signs and symptoms unless they experience pulmonary embolism as a complication.

Test-Taking Strategy: This question is worded in the affirmative, and looks for additional signs and symptoms of thrombophlebitis. Begin by eliminating options 1 and 2, which are symptoms of arterial, not venous, problems. Thrombophlebitis is usually a unilateral problem, which helps you eliminate option 4.

Level of Cognitive Ability: Application
Phase of Nursing Process: Assessment
Client Needs: Physiological Integrity
Content Area: Adult Health/Cardiovascular

Reference

Black, J., & Matassarin-Jacobs, E. (1997). *Medical-surgical nursing: Clinical management for continuity of care* (5th ed.). Philadelphia: W. B. Saunders. p. 1434.

274. 2

Rationale: Standard management of the client with deep vein thrombosis includes bed rest for 5 to 7 days, limb elevation, relief of discomfort with warm moist heat and analgesics as needed, anticoagulant therapy, and monitoring for signs of pulmonary embolism. Ambulation is contraindicated, as it increases the likelihood of dislodgment of the tail of the thrombus, which would travel to the lungs as a pulmonary embolism.

Test-Taking Strategy: This question is worded to make you look for an incorrect action, as noted by the word "avoid" in the stem. Application of heat and limb elevation are indicated to reduce inflammation and edema, so these options are not the correct answer. Tylenol relieves discomfort and is also incorrect. This leaves ambulation, which could lead to pulmonary embolism. This is the dangerous action and is the correct answer for this question as stated.

Level of Cognitive Ability: Application
Phase of Nursing Process: Implementation
Client Needs: Physiological Integrity
Content Area: Adult Health/Cardiovascular

Reference

Black, J., & Matassarin-Jacobs, E. (1997). *Medical-surgical nursing: Clinical management for continuity of care* (5th ed.). Philadelphia: W. B. Saunders. p. 1435.

275. 3

Rationale: Smoking is highly detrimental to the client with Buerger's disease, and it is recommended that clients stop completely. Since smoking is a form of chemical dependency, referral to a smoking cessation program may be helpful for many clients. For many clients, symptoms are relieved or alleviated once smoking stops.

Test-Taking Strategy: To answer this question quickly and accurately, it is necessary to understand the importance of smoking as an etiological agent. Since general treatment goals for this disorder are the same as for other peripheral vascular diseases, this option may be easily selected over the other unrelated choices.

Level of Cognitive Ability: Application
Phase of Nursing Process: Planning
Client Needs: Psychosocial Integrity
Content Area: Adult Health/Cardiovascular

Reference
Smeltzer, S., & Bare, B. (1996). *Brunner and Suddarth's textbook of medical-surgical nursing* (8th ed.). Philadelphia: Lippincott-Raven. p. 738.

276. **3**

Rationale: Bactroban is a topical antibacterial active against impetigo caused by staphylococcus or streptococcus. Acyclovir is a topical antiviral agent that inhibits DNA replication in the virus. It has activity against herpes simplex types 1 and 2, varicella-zoster, Epstein-Barr virus, and cytomegalovirus. Triple antibiotic would not be effective in treating herpes virus. Actinex is a keratolytic.

Test-Taking Strategy: Knowledge of the treatment for impetigo is required to answer this question. If you are not familiar with these medications, take time now to review!

Level of Cognitive Ability: Analysis
Phase of Nursing Process: Analysis
Client Needs: Physiological Integrity
Content Area: Pharmacology

Reference
Kuhn, M. (1998). *Pharmacotherapeutics: A nursing process approach* (4th ed.). Philadelphia: F. A. Davis. p. 989.

277. **1**

Rationale: Coal tar is used to treat psoriasis and other chronic disorders of the skin. It suppresses DNA synthesis, mitotic activity, and cell proliferation. It has an unpleasant odor, can frequently stain the skin and hair, and can cause phototoxicity. Systemic toxicity does not occur.

Test-Taking Strategy: Note the key words "a need for further education" in the stem of the question. The name of the medication will assist in eliminating options 3 and 4. It is necessary to know that the medication does not cause systemic effects to answer this question correctly. If you had difficulty with this question, review this treatment now!

Level of Cognitive Ability: Analysis
Phase of Nursing Process: Evaluation
Client Needs: Physiological Integrity
Content Area: Pharmacology

References
Lehne, R. (1998). *Pharmacology for nursing care* (3rd ed.). Philadelphia: W. B. Saunders. p. 1059.
Kuhn, M. (1998). *Pharmacotherapeutics: A nursing process approach* (4th ed.). Philadelphia: F. A. Davis. p. 989.

278. **4**

Rationale: Sunscreens are most effective when applied about 30 minutes to 1 hour before exposure to the sun so

that they can penetrate the skin. All sunscreens should be reapplied after swimming or sweating.

Test-Taking Strategy: Knowledge that sunscreens need to penetrate the skin will assist in eliminating options 2 and 3. Noting the key words "most effective" will assist in directing you to option 4. Review protective skin measures now if you had difficulty with this question!

Level of Cognitive Ability: Analysis
Phase of Nursing Process: Evaluation
Client Needs: Health Promotion and Maintenance
Content Area: Pharmacology

Reference
Kuhn, M. (1998). *Pharmacotherapeutics: A nursing process approach* (4th ed.). Philadelphia: F. A. Davis. p. 993.

279. **4**

Rationale: PolySkin is a self-adhering, transparent polyurethane dressing that is gas and oxygen permeable and is used to cover central and peripheral IV sites. It should be changed at least every 2 to 3 days.

Test-Taking Strategy: Note that the issue of this question relates to an IV site. Eliminate option 3 first. Knowledge regarding this type of dressing will assist in eliminating options 1 and 2. If you are unfamiliar with this type of protective dressing, take time now to review!

Level of Cognitive Ability: Application
Phase of Nursing Process: Planning
Client Needs: Physiological Integrity
Content Area: Pharmacology

Reference
Kuhn, M. (1998). *Pharmacotherapeutics: A nursing process approach* (4th ed.). Philadelphia: F. A. Davis. p. 993.

280. **1**

Rationale: Furacin is applied topically to the burn and has a broad spectrum of antibiotic activity. It is used in second- or third-degree burns in which bacterial resistance to other agents is a real or potential problem. A film of $1/16$ inch is applied directly to the burn using a sterile gloved hand. The burn site is washed daily. Saline-soaked dressings are not used.

Test-Taking Strategy: Knowledge regarding the use of this medication is required to answer this question. Note the key word "not" in the stem of the question. This should easily direct you to option 1 because infection is a major concern with the burn client, and a wet dressing can more easily harbor bacteria. Review the use of this medication for burn therapy now if you had difficulty with this question!

Level of Cognitive Ability: Analysis
Phase of Nursing Process: Analysis
Client Needs: Physiological Integrity
Content Area: Pharmacology

Reference
Kuhn, M. (1998). *Pharmacotherapeutics: A nursing process approach* (4th ed.). Philadelphia: F. A. Davis. p. 998.

281. **1**

Rationale: Mafenide is bacteriostatic for both gram-negative and gram-positive organisms and is used to treat second- and third-degree burns to reduce bacteria present in avascular tissues. The client should be informed that the medication will cause local discomfort and burning.

Test-Taking Strategy: Eliminate options 3 and 4 because it is not within the scope of nursing practice to advise a client to alter or discontinue a medication therapy. Knowledge that this is a normal expected occurrence will easily direct you to option 1. If you had difficulty with this question, take time now to review!

Level of Cognitive Ability: Application
Phase of Nursing Process: Implementation
Client Needs: Health Promotion and Maintenance
Content Area: Pharmacology

Reference
Kuhn, M. (1998). *Pharmacotherapeutics: A nursing process approach* (4th ed.). Philadelphia: F. A. Davis. p. 998.

282. 2

Rationale: Sulfamylon is a strong carbonic anhydrase inhibitor and can suppress renal excretion of acid, thereby causing acidosis. Clients receiving this treatment should be monitored for acid-base status, and if the acidosis becomes severe the medication should be discontinued for 1 to 2 days. An elevated blood pressure may be expected in the client with pain. Hypotension is not associated with the use of this medication.

Test-Taking Strategy: Knowledge regarding the systemic effects associated with the use of this medication is required to answer this question. Review the systemic effects of this medication now if you had difficulty with this question!

Level of Cognitive Ability: Analysis
Phase of Nursing Process: Analysis
Client Needs: Physiological Integrity
Content Area: Pharmacology

Reference
Kuhn, M. (1998). *Pharmacotherapeutics: A nursing process approach* (4th ed.). Philadelphia: F. A. Davis. p. 998.

283. 2

Rationale: A Vigilon dressing is used to clean small, partial thickness burns. It is a colloidal suspension on a polyethylene mesh support, is permeable to gases and water vapor, and provides a moist environment. It is changed daily. For nonocclusive use it is secured over the wound with gauze or tape. Option 4 is incorrect.

Test-Taking Strategy: Knowledge that the dressing is changed daily will assist in eliminating options 1 and 3. Knowledge regarding the use of this type of burn covering will assist in directing you to option 2. If you are unfamiliar with this type of burn covering, take time now to review!

Level of Cognitive Ability: Application
Phase of Nursing Process: Planning
Client Needs: Physiological Integrity
Content Area: Pharmacology

Reference
Kuhn, M. (1998). *Pharmacotherapeutics: A nursing process approach* (4th ed.). Philadelphia: F. A. Davis. p. 999.

284. 1

Rationale: Dakin's is a chloride solution that is used for irrigating and cleaning necrotic or purulent wounds. It can be used for packing necrotic wounds. It cannot be used to pack purulent wounds since the solution is inactivated by copious pus. It should not come in contact with healing or normal tissue, and it should be rinsed off immediately if used for irrigation. Solutions are unstable and must be prepared fresh for each use.

Test-Taking Strategy: Eliminate options 2, 3, and 4 because they are similar and indicate continuous contact of the solution with the wound. If you are unfamiliar with the use of this solution, take time now to review!

Level of Cognitive Ability: Analysis
Phase of Nursing Process: Analysis
Client Needs: Physiological Integrity
Content Area: Pharmacology

Reference
Kuhn, M. (1998). *Pharmacotherapeutics: A nursing process approach* (4th ed.). Philadelphia: F. A. Davis. p. 988.

285. 3

Rationale: Tretinoin decreases cohesiveness of the epithelial cells, increasing cell mitosis and turnover. It is potentially irritating, particularly when used correctly. Within 48 hours of use, the skin generally becomes red and begins to peel. It is not necessary to notify the physician if this occurs. Options 1, 2, and 4 are correct.

Test-Taking Strategy: Note the key word "not" in the stem of the question. Knowledge that within 48 hours of medication use the skin normally becomes red and begins to peel will easily direct you to option 3. If you are unfamiliar with the use of this medication, take time now to review!

Level of Cognitive Ability: Application
Phase of Nursing Process: Implementation
Client Needs: Health Promotion and Maintenance
Content Area: Pharmacology

Reference
Kuhn, M. (1998). *Pharmacotherapeutics: A nursing process approach* (4th ed.). Philadelphia: F. A. Davis. p. 997.

286. 4

Rationale: Tretinoin is applied liberally to the skin. The hands are washed thoroughly immediately after applying. Therapeutic results should be seen after 2 to 3 weeks but may not be optimal until after 6 weeks. The client may use cosmetics, but the skin needs to be cleansed thoroughly before applying the medication.

Test-Taking Strategy: Note the key words "need for further education" in the stem of the question. Knowledge regarding the use of the medication will assist in directing you to option 4. Review this medication now if you had difficulty with this question!

Level of Cognitive Ability: Analysis
Phase of Nursing Process: Evaluation
Client Needs: Health Promotion and Maintenance
Content Area: Pharmacology

Reference
Kuhn, M. (1998). *Pharmacotherapeutics: A nursing process approach* (4th ed.). Philadelphia: F. A. Davis. p. 997.

287. 2

Rationale: Isotretinoin is administered two times daily for 15 to 20 weeks. The usual adult dosage is 0.5 to 2 mg/kg/day. If needed, a second course may be given, but not until 2 months have elapsed after completing the first course. The medication needs to be taken with food to facilitate absorption. The tablets should be administered whole and not crushed.

Test-Taking Strategy: Knowledge regarding the use of this medication is required to answer this question. If you are unfamiliar with this treatment, take time now to review!

Level of Cognitive Ability: Analysis
Phase of Nursing Process: Evaluation
Client Needs: Health Promotion and Maintenance
Content Area: Pharmacology

Reference
Hodgson, B., & Kizior, R. (1999). *Saunders nursing drug handbook 1999.* Philadelphia: W. B. Saunders. p. 558.

288. **1**

Rationale: Accutane can elevate triglyceride levels. Blood triglyceride content should be measured prior to treatment and periodically thereafter until effects of triglycerides have been evaluated. The client needs to be instructed about the importance of follow-up to evaluate the triglyceride level.

Test-Taking Strategy: It is necessary to know that this medication can affect the triglyceride level in the client. Review the effects of this medication now if you had difficulty with this question!

Level of Cognitive Ability: Application
Phase of Nursing Process: Implementation
Client Needs: Physiological Integrity
Content Area: Pharmacology

Reference
Lehne, R. (1998). *Pharmacology for nursing care* (3rd ed.). Philadelphia: W. B. Saunders. p. 1059.

289. **2**

Rationale: Adverse effects of isotretinoin can be increased by the use of tetracyclines. Tetracyclines increase the risk of pseudotumor cerebri and papilledema. Because of the potential for increased toxicity, tetracyclines should be discontinued prior to isotretinoin therapy.

Test-Taking Strategy: Knowledge of the contraindications associated with the use of this medication is required to answer this question. If you are unfamiliar with this medication, take time now to review the contraindications associated with its use!

Level of Cognitive Ability: Analysis
Phase of Nursing Process: Implementation
Client Needs: Physiological Integrity
Content Area: Pharmacology

Reference
Lehne, R. (1998). *Pharmacology for nursing care* (3rd ed.). Philadelphia: W. B. Saunders. p. 1059.

290. **2**

Rationale: The wound should be cleansed with a sterile solution and gently patted dry. A thin layer of Elase is applied and covered with a petrolatum gauze. If a dry powder is used, for best effects the solution should be prepared just prior to use.

Test-Taking Strategy: Note the word "inaccurate" in the stem of the question. Noting this key word should assist in directing you to option 2. Review the method of application of Elase now if you had difficulty with this question!

Level of Cognitive Ability: Analysis
Phase of Nursing Process: Analysis
Client Needs: Safe, Effective Care Environment
Content Area: Pharmacology

Reference
Kuhn, M. (1998). *Pharmacotherapeutics: A nursing process approach* (4th ed.). Philadelphia: F. A. Davis. p. 1010.

291. **2**

Rationale: The wound should be cleansed with a sterile solution prior to treatment. The nurse then should thoroughly moisten the wound with normal saline or sterile water and apply a loose, thin dressing after applying a thin film of Travase extending ¼ to ½ inch beyond the area to be debrided. The ointment should be refrigerated.

Test-Taking Strategy: Note the word "not" in the stem of the question. Knowledge regarding the use of this medication is required to answer the question. Review the method of application of Travase now if you had difficulty with this question!

Level of Cognitive Ability: Application
Phase of Nursing Process: Planning
Client Needs: Physiological Integrity
Content Area: Pharmacology

Reference
Kuhn, M. (1998). *Pharmacotherapeutics: A nursing process approach* (4th ed.). Philadelphia: F. A. Davis. p. 1010.

292. **4**

Rationale: Debrisan is a cleansing rather than a debriding agent. It is effective in wet wounds only. It should not be packed into wounds tightly because maceration of surrounding tissue may result.

Test-Taking Strategy: Knowledge regarding the use of this medication is required to answer this question. If you are unfamiliar with the use of Debrisan, take time now to review!

Level of Cognitive Ability: Application
Phase of Nursing Process: Planning
Client Needs: Physiological Integrity
Content Area: Pharmacology

Reference
Kuhn, M. (1998). *Pharmacotherapeutics: A nursing process approach* (4th ed.). Philadelphia: F. A. Davis. p. 1012.

293. **1**

Rationale: Prosthetic valves require long-term anticoagulation to prevent clots from forming on the "foreign" tissue implanted in the client's body. Anticoagulation therapy requires clients to avoid any trauma or potential means of bleeding, such as straight razors. Options 2, 3, and 4 are not specifically related to postoperative care following prosthetic valve replacement.

Test-Taking Strategy: Key words in the question include "prosthetic" and "specific." Recalling that anticoagulant therapy is required following prosthetic valve replacement will easily direct you to option 1. Options 2, 3, and 4 are unrelated to specific postoperative care following prosthetic heart valve replacement. Prosthetic valves will require anticoagulation therapy for life, and the client must be instructed in safety measures. Review postoperative care now if you had difficulty with this question!

Level of Cognitive Ability: Analysis
Phase of Nursing Process: Evaluation
Client Needs: Physiological Integrity
Content Area: Adult Health/Cardiovascular

Reference
Lewis, S., Collier, I., & Heitkemper, M. (1996). *Medical-surgical nursing: Assessment and management of clinical problems* (4th ed.). St. Louis: Mosby–Year Book. p. 1030.

294. 2

Rationale: Long-term management of peripheral arterial disease consists of measures that increase peripheral circulation (exercise), promote vasodilatation (warmth), relieve pain, and maintain tissue integrity (foot care and nutrition). Application of heat directly to the extremity is contraindicated. The affected extremity may have decreased sensitivity and is at risk for burns. Also, the affected tissue does not get adequate circulation at rest. Direct application of heat raises oxygen and nutritional requirements of the tissue even further.

Test-Taking Strategy: To answer this question accurately, it is necessary to incorporate principles that help the client decrease the risk for tissue injury and progression of atherosclerosis. If this question was difficult, be sure to review this important content area now!

Level of Cognitive Ability: Application
Phase of Nursing Process: Planning
Client Needs: Health Promotion and Maintenance
Content Area: Adult Health/Cardiovascular

Reference
Ignatavicius, D., Workman, M., and Mishler, M. (1995). *Medical-surgical nursing: A nursing process approach* (2nd ed.). Philadelphia: W. B. Saunders. p. 941.

295. 2

Rationale: The client recovering from cardiogenic shock secondary to a myocardial infarction will require a progressive rehabilitation related to physical activity. The heart requires several months to heal from an uncomplicated myocardial infarction. The complication of cardiogenic shock will increase the recovery period for healing. Paced activities with planned rest periods will decrease the chance of experiencing angina or delayed healing. Options 1, 3, and 4 are not related to the instructions provided by the nurse.

Test-Taking Strategy: Focus on the issue in the question regarding the instructions that the nurse provides to the client. Use the process of elimination. Option 1 addresses the need to identify the client as a cardiac client but does not discuss the physical activity rehabilitation topic. Option 3 does not address the importance of pacing activity or reporting of chest pain. Option 4 does describe pulse rates but does not address the need for rest periods or the need to seek medical attention for chest pain.

Level of Cognitive Ability: Analysis
Phase of Nursing Process: Evaluation
Client Needs: Health Promotion and Maintenance
Content Area: Adult Health/Cardiovascular

Reference
Lewis, S., Collier, I., & Heitkemper, M. (1996). *Medical-surgical nursing: Assessment and management of clinical problems* (4th ed.). St. Louis: Mosby–Year Book. p. 135.

296. 3

Rationale: Colchicine is classified as an antigout agent. It interferes with the ability of the white blood cells to initiate and maintain an inflammatory response to monosodium urate crystals. The client should report a decrease in pain and inflammation in affected joints, as well as a decrease in the number of gout attacks.

Test-Taking Strategy: To answer this question accurately, it is necessary to be able to recall the classification of this medication. Referring to the diagnosis of the client in the question will assist in directing you to the correct option. If needed, take a few moments to review this medication now!

Level of Cognitive Ability: Analysis
Phase of Nursing Process: Evaluation
Client Needs: Health Promotion and Maintenance
Content Area: Pharmacology

Reference
Deglin, J., & Vallerand, A. (1997). *Davis's drug guide for nurses* (5th ed.). Philadelphia: F. A. Davis. p. 294.

297. 2

Rationale: Enoxaparin is an anticoagulant that is administered by the subcutaneous route. It is used in preventing thromboembolism in selected clients at risk. It may also be given in the home after discharge, with follow-up by a home health nurse.

Test-Taking Strategy: To answer this question accurately, it is necessary to be familiar with this medication and administration. If you are unfamiliar with this medication, take a few moments to review this medication now!

Level of Cognitive Ability: Application
Phase of Nursing Process: Implementation
Client Needs: Physiological Integrity
Content Area: Pharmacology

Reference
Deglin, J., & Vallerand, A. (1997). *Davis's drug guide for nurses* (5th ed.). Philadelphia: F. A. Davis. p. 586.

298. 4

Rationale: Exercise is an integral part of the rehabilitation program. It is necessary for optimal physiological functioning and psychological well-being. Postoperative physical rehabilitation must be progressive, with planned periods of rest. Exercise tolerance is judged by the client's response, such as heart rate and endurance. Options 1, 2, and 3 are all correct teaching included in cardiac rehabilitation. Option 4 lacks planned periods of rest and the client has grouped too many activities in a brief period of time, which would decrease endurance.

Test-Taking Strategy: Note the key words "need for further education." Use the process of elimination. Rehabilitative exercise post cardiovascular surgery is individually prescribed for the client. The client's exercise regimen is planned with scheduled rest periods, avoiding peak environmental heat times and prior to meals. Exercise after meals can decrease the client's tolerance due to shunting of blood to the gastrointestinal tract for digestion. Options 1 and 2 are similar and can be eliminated. Option 3 identifies a correct client action and thus can also be eliminated. Knowing that extreme heat increases the workload of the heart, thereby decreasing client endurance, will easily direct you to option 4.

Level of Cognitive Ability: Analysis
Phase of Nursing Process: Evaluation
Client Needs: Health Promotion and Maintenance
Content Area: Adult Health/Cardiovascular

Reference
Lewis, S., Collier, I., & Heitkemper, M. (1996). *Medical-surgical nursing: Assessment and management of clinical problems* (4th ed.). St. Louis: Mosby–Year Book. p. 924.

299. 2

Rationale: The single most effective technique to prevent the spread of germs/bacteria is good handwashing. The postoperative cardiovascular surgical client will perform clean dressing changes once discharged home. Options 1, 3, and 4 all increase the risk of wound contamination due to poor aseptic technique.

Test-Taking Strategy: The initial step for all aseptic procedures begins with handwashing. Handwashing prevents the spread of infection. Use the process of elimination to answer the question. Gauze that has been opened has been exposed to potential pathogens (option 1). In option 3, the nurse sneezed into the gloved hand and did not change the glove, thereby contaminating the dressing. In option 4, the nurse contaminates gloves by removing the old dressing, then contaminates the clean dressing with the contaminated glove.

Level of Cognitive Ability: Analysis
Phase of Nursing Process: Evaluation
Client Needs: Health Promotion and Maintenance
Content Area: Fundamental Skills

Reference
Smith, S., & Duell, D. (1996). *Clinical nursing skills* (4th ed.). Stamford, CT: Appleton and Lange. p. 338.

300. 1

Rationale: Laboratory findings in an infant with hypertrophic pyloric stenosis include metabolic alkalosis due to vomiting, including decreased serum potassium, sodium, and chloride levels and increased pH and bicarbonate level.

Test-Taking Strategy: Recalling the concepts related to acid-base balance and the clinical manifestation, the progressive, projectile, nonbilious vomiting that occurs in hypertrophic pyloric stenosis will easily direct you to option 1. Options 3 and 4 can be easily eliminated because these values are normal. In metabolic alkalosis, the pH is elevated, as is the bicarbonate level. Option 2 reflects an elevation in pH. Remember that metabolic alkalosis occurs from vomiting!

Level of Cognitive Ability: Analysis
Phase of Nursing Process: Assessment
Client Needs: Physiological Integrity
Content Area: Child Health

Reference
Ashwill, J., & Droske, S. (1997). *Nursing care of children: Principles and practice.* Philadelphia: W. B. Saunders. p. 718.

REFERENCES

Ashwill, J., & Droske, S. (1997). *Nursing care of children: Principles and practice.* Philadelphia: W. B. Saunders.

Bandman, E., & Bandman, B. (1995). *Nursing ethics through the life span.* Stamford, CT: Appleton & Lange.

Beare, P., & Myers, J. (1998). *Adult health nursing* (3rd ed.). St. Louis: Mosby–Year Book.

Black, J., & Matassarin-Jacobs, E. (1997). *Medical-surgical nursing: Management for continuity of care* (5th ed.). Philadelphia: W. B. Saunders.

Burrell, P., Gerlach, M., & Pless, B. (1997). *Adult nursing: Acute and community care* (2nd ed.). Stamford, CT: Appleton & Lange.

Carson, V., & Arnold, E. (1997). *Mental health nursing: The nurse-patient journey.* Philadelphia: W. B. Saunders.

Clark, J., Queener, S., & Karb, V. (1997). *Pharmacologic basis of nursing practice* (5th ed.). St Louis: Mosby–Year Book.

Clark, M. J. (1996). *Nursing in the community* (2nd ed.). Stamford, CT: Appleton & Lange.

Cox, H., Hinz, M., Lubno, M., et al. (1997). *Clinical applications of nursing diagnosis* (3rd ed.). Philadelphia: F. A. Davis.

Craven, R. F., & Hirnle, C. J. (1996). *Fundamentals of nursing: Human health and function* (2nd ed.). Philadelphia: Lippincott-Raven.

Deglin, J., & Vallerand, A. (1997). *Davis's drug guide for nurses* (5th ed.). Philadelphia: F. A. Davis.

Glod, C. A. (1998). *Contemporary psychiatric–mental health nursing.* Philadelphia: F. A. Davis.

Hodgson, B., & Kizior, R. (1999). *Saunders nursing drug handbook 1999.* Philadelphia: W. B. Saunders.

Ignatavicius, D., Workman, M., & Mishler, M. *Medical-surgical nursing: A nursing process approach* (2nd ed.). Philadelphia: W. B. Saunders.

Jarvis, C. (1996). *Physical examination and health assessment* (2nd ed.). Philadelphia: W. B. Saunders.

Johnson, B. S. (1997). *Psychiatric–mental health nursing: Adaptation and growth.* Philadelphia: Lippincott-Raven.

Karch, A. (1997). *1997 Lippincott's nursing drug guide.* Philadelphia: Lippincott-Raven.

Kozier, B., Erb, G., & Blais, K. (1998). *Fundamentals of nursing: Concepts, process, and practice* (5th ed.). Reading, MA: Addison-Wesley.

Kuhn, M. (1998). *Pharmacotherapeutics: A nursing process approach* (4th ed.). Philadelphia: F. A. Davis.

Lammon, C., Foote, A., Leli, P., et al. (1995). *Clinical nursing skills.* Philadelphia: W. B. Saunders.

Lehne, R. (1998). *Pharmacology for nursing care* (3rd ed.). Philadelphia: W. B. Saunders.

Lewis, S., Collier, I., & Heitkemper, M. (1996). *Medical-surgical nursing: Assessment and management of clinical problems* (4th ed.). St. Louis: Mosby–Year Book.

Lowdermilk, D., Perry, S., & Bobak, I. (1997). *Maternity & women's health care* (6th ed.). St. Louis: Mosby–Year Book.

Luckmann, J. (1997). *Saunders manual of nursing care.* Philadelphia: W. B. Saunders.

Monahan, F., & Neighbors, M. (1998). *Medical surgical nursing: Foundations for clinical practice* (2nd ed.). Philadelphia: W. B. Saunders.

Nichols, F., & Zwelling, E. (1997). *Maternal-newborn nursing: Theory and practice.* Philadelphia: W. B. Saunders.

Polaski, A., & Tatro, S. (1996). *Luckmann's core principles and practice of medical-surgical nursing.* Philadelphia: W. B. Saunders.

Potter, P., & Perry, A. (1995). *Basic nursing theory and practice* (3rd ed.). St. Louis: Mosby–Year Book.

Potter, P., & Perry, A. (1997). *Fundamentals of nursing: Concepts, process, and practice* (4th ed.). St. Louis: Mosby–Year Book.

Rice, R. (1995). *Home health nursing procedures: Concepts & application.* St. Louis: Mosby–Year Book.

Smeltzer, S., & Bare, B. (1996). *Brunner and Suddarth's textbook of medical-surgical nursing* (8th ed.). Philadelphia: Lippincott-Raven.

Smith, S., & Duell, D. (1996). *Clinical nursing skills* (4th ed.). Stamford, CT: Appleton & Lange.

Spradley, B. W., & Allender, J. A. (1996). *Community health nursing: Concepts and practice* (4th ed.). Philadelphia: Lippincott-Raven.

Stanhope, M., & Lancaster, J. (1996). *Community health nursing: Promoting health of aggregates, families, and individuals* (4th ed.). St. Louis: Mosby–Year Book.

Taylor, C., Lillis, C., & LeMone, P. (1997). *Fundamentals of nursing: The art and science of nursing care* (3rd ed.). Philadelphia: Lippincott-Raven.

Varcarolis, E. (1998). *Foundations of psychiatric mental health nursing* (3rd ed.). Philadelphia: W. B. Saunders.

Wilson, H., & Kneisl, C. (1996). *Psychiatric nursing* (5th ed.). Reading, MA: Addison-Wesley.

General Bibliography

Ashwill, J., & Droske, S. (1997). *Nursing care of children: Principles and practice.* Philadelphia: W. B. Saunders.

Antai-Otong, D., & Kongale, G. (1995). *Psychiatric nursing: Biological and behavioral concepts.* Philadelphia: W. B. Saunders.

Ball, J., & Bindler, R. (1995). *Pediatric nursing: Caring for children.* Stamford, CT: Appleton & Lange.

Beare, P., & Myers, J. (1998). *Adult health nursing* (3rd ed.). St Louis: Mosby–Year Book.

Black J., & Matassarin-Jacobs, E. (1997). *Medical-surgical nursing: Clinical management for continuity of care* (5th ed.). Philadelphia: W. B. Saunders.

Brent, N. (1997). *Nurses and the law.* Philadelphia: W. B. Saunders.

Burrell, L., Gerlach, M., & Pless, B. (1997). *Adult nursing: Acute and community care* (2nd ed.). Stamford, CT: Appleton & Lange.

Carpenito, L. (1997). *Nursing diagnosis: Application to clinical practice* (7th ed.). Philadelphia: Lippincott-Raven.

Carson, V., & Arnold, E. (1996). *Mental health nursing: The nurse-patient journey.* Philadelphia: W. B. Saunders.

Chernecky, C., & Berger, B. (1997). *Laboratory tests and diagnostic procedures* (2nd ed.). Philadelphia: W. B. Saunders.

Deglin, J., & Vallerand, A. (1997). *Davis's drug guide for nurses* (5th ed.). Philadelphia: F. A. Davis.

Glod, C. A. (1998). *Contemporary psychiatric–mental health nursing.* Philadelphia: F. A. Davis.

Gorrie, T., McKinney, E., & Murray, E. (1998). *Foundations of maternal-newborn nursing* (2nd ed.). Philadelphia: W. B. Saunders.

Hartshorn, J., Sole, M., & Lamborn, M. (1997). *Introduction to critical care nursing* (2nd ed.). Philadelphia: W. B. Saunders.

Hodgson, B., & Kizior, R. (1998). *Saunders nursing drug handbook 1998.* Philadelphia: W. B. Saunders.

Ignatavicius, D., Workman, M., & Mishler, M. (1995). *Medical surgical nursing: A nursing process approach* (2nd ed.). Philadelphia: W. B. Saunders.

Iyer, P., Taptich, B., & Bernocchi-Losey, D. (1995). *Nursing process and nursing diagnosis.* Philadelphia: W. B. Saunders.

Jaffee, M., & McVan, B. (1997). *Davis's laboratory and diagnostic test handbook.* Philadelphia: F. A. Davis.

Jarvis, C. (1996). *Physical examination and health assessment* (2nd ed.). Philadelphia: W. B. Saunders.

Johnson, B. S. (1997). *Psychiatric–mental health nursing: Adaptation and growth* (4th ed.). Philadelphia: J. B. Lippincott.

Kee, J., & Hayes, E. (1997). *Pharmacology: A nursing process approach* (2nd ed.). Philadelphia: W. B. Saunders.

Kee, J., & Marshall, S. (1996). *Clinical calculations* (3rd ed.). Philadelphia: W. B. Saunders.

Ladewig, P., London, M. & Olds, S. (1997). *Maternal-newborn nursing care: The nurse, the family, and the community* (4th ed.). Reading, MA: Addison-Wesley.

Lammon, C., Foote, A., & Leli, P., et al. (1995). *Clinical nursing skills.* Philadelphia: W. B. Saunders.

Leahy, J., & Kizilay, P. (1998). *Foundations of nursing practice: A nursing process approach.* Philadelphia: W. B. Saunders.

Lehne, R. (1998). *Pharmacology for nursing care* (3rd ed.). Philadelphia: W. B. Saunders.

Lewis, S., Collier, I., & Heitkemper, M. (1996). *Medical-surgical nursing: Assessment and management of clinical problems* (4th ed.). St. Louis: Mosby–Year Book.

Lipsey, S., & Ignatavicius, D. (1994). *Math for nurses: A problem solving approach.* Philadelphia: W. B. Saunders.

Lowdermilk, D., Perry, S., & Bobak, I. (1997). *Maternity & women's health care* (6th ed.). St. Louis: Mosby–Year Book.

Luckmann, J. (1997). *Saunders manual of nursing care.* Philadelphia: W. B. Saunders.

Lutz, C., & Przytulski, K. (1997). *Nutrition and diet therapy* (2nd ed.). Philadelphia: F. A. Davis.

Mahan, L., & Escott-Stump, S. (1996). *Krause's food, nutrition, & diet therapy* (9th ed.). Philadelphia: W. B. Saunders.

Matteson, M., McConnell, E., & Linton, A. (1996). *Gerontological nursing: Concepts and practice* (2nd ed.). Philadelphia: W. B. Saunders.

McKenry, L., & Salerno, E. (1998). *Mosby's pharmacology in nursing* (20th ed.). St. Louis: Mosby–Year Book.

Monahan, F., & Neighbors, M. (1998). *Medical-surgical nursing: Foundations for clinical practice* (2nd ed.). Philadelphia: W. B. Saunders.

Nichols, F., & Zwelling, E. (1997). *Maternal-newborn nursing: Theory and practice.* Philadelphia: W. B. Saunders.

O'Toole, M. (ed.). (1997). *Miller-Keane encyclopedia & dictionary of medicine, nursing, & allied health* (6th ed.). Philadelphia: W. B. Saunders.

Paul, S., & Hebra, J. (1997). *The nurse's guide to cardiac rhythm interpretation: Implications for patient care.* Philadelphia: W. B. Saunders.

Pillitteri, A. (1995). *Maternal & child health nursing: Care of the childbearing and childrearing family* (2nd ed.). Philadelphia: Lippincott-Raven.

Pinnell, N. (1996). *Nursing pharmacology.* Philadelphia, W. B. Saunders.

Polaski, A., & Tatro, S. (1996). *Luckmann's core principles and practices of medical-surgical nursing.* Philadelphia: W. B. Saunders.

Potter, P., & Perry, A. (1997). *Fundamentals of nursing: Concepts, process, and practice* (4th ed.). St. Louis: Mosby–Year Book.

Rice, R. (1996). *Home health nursing: Practices, concepts and application* (2nd ed.). St. Louis: Mosby–Year Book.

Rocchiccioli, J., & Tilbury, M. (1998). *Clinical leadership in nursing.* Philadelphia: W. B. Saunders.

Smeltzer, S., & Bare, B. (1996). *Brunner and Suddarth's textbook of medical-surgical nursing* (8th ed.). Philadelphia: Lippincott-Raven.

Swanson, J., & Nies, M. (1997). *Community health nursing: promoting the health of aggregates* (2nd ed.). Philadelphia: W. B. Saunders.

Taylor, C., Lillis, C., & LeMone, P. (1997). *Fundamentals of nursing: The art and science of nursing care* (3rd ed.). Philadelphia: Lippincott-Raven.

Thompson J., McFarland, G., Hirsch, J., & Tucker, S. (1997). *Mosby's clinical nursing.* St. Louis: Mosby–Year Book.

VanRiper, S., & VanRiper, J. (1997). *Cardiac diagnostic tests: A guide for nurses.* Philadelphia: W. B. Saunders.

Varcarolis, E. (1998). *Foundations of psychiatric mental health nursing* (3rd ed.). Philadelphia: W. B. Saunders.

Wong, D. (1997). *Essentials of pediatric nursing* (5th ed.). St. Louis: Mosby–Year Book.

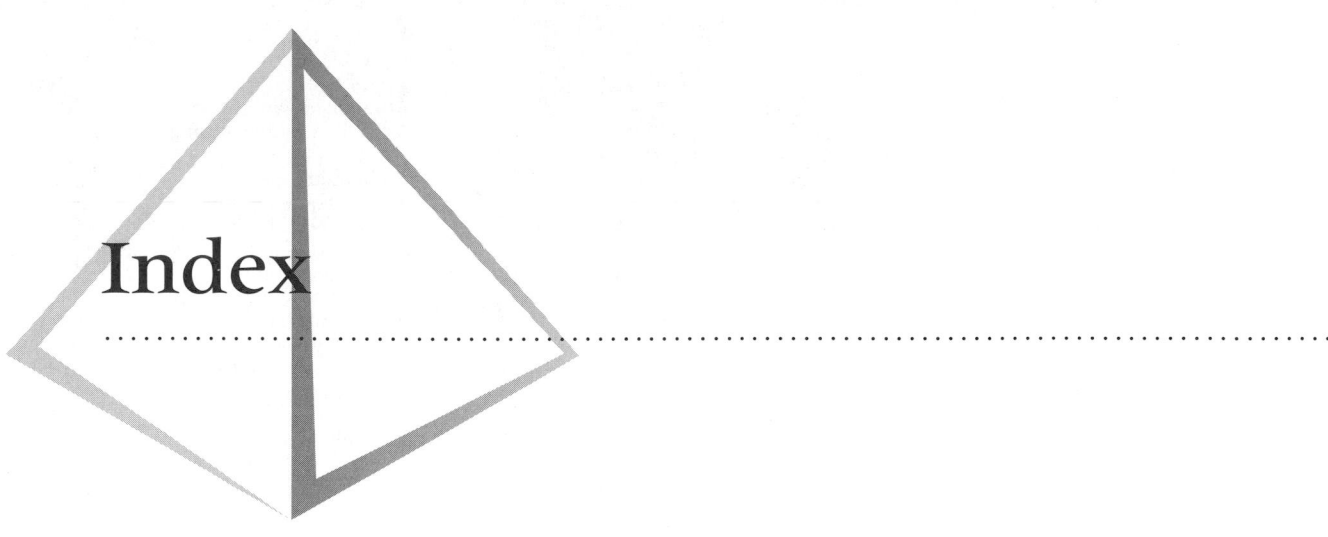

Index

Note: Page numbers in *italics* refer to figures; page numbers followed by t refer to tables; page numbers followed by b refer to text in boxes.

Bring home:

1) Reading book that you are doing your book report on.

2)